Benumof and Hagberg's

Airway
Management

Benumof and Hagberg's

THIRD EDITION

Airway Management

EDITED BY

Carin A. Hagberg, MD

Joseph C. Gabel Professor and Chair
Department of Anesthesiology
The University of Texas Medical School at Houston
Chief of Anesthesia and Director of Neuroanesthesia and Advanced
  Airway Management
Memorial Hermann Hospital
Houston, Texas

ELSEVIER
SAUNDERS

ELSEVIER
SAUNDERS

1600 John F. Kennedy Blvd.
Ste 1800
Philadelphia, PA 19103-2899

Notices

Knowledge and best practice in this field are constantly changing. As new research and experience
broaden our understanding, changes in research methods, professional practices, or medical
treatment may become necessary.

Practitioners and researchers must always rely on their own experience and knowledge in
evaluating and using any information, methods, compounds, or experiments described herein. In
using such information or methods they should be mindful of their own safety and the safety of
others, including parties for whom they have a professional responsibility.

With respect to any drug or pharmaceutical products identified, readers are advised to check
the most current information provided (i) on procedures featured or (ii) by the manufacturer of
each product to be administered, to verify the recommended dose or formula, the method and
duration of administration, and contraindications. It is the responsibility of practitioners, relying on
their own experience and knowledge of their patients, to make diagnoses, to determine dosages
and the best treatment for each individual patient, and to take all appropriate safety precautions.

To the fullest extent of the law, neither the Publisher nor the authors, contributors, or editors,
assume any liability for any injury and/or damage to persons or property as a matter of products
liability, negligence or otherwise, or from any use or operation of any methods, products,
instructions, or ideas contained in the material herein.

International Standard Book Number
978-1-4377-2764-7

Content Strategist: William Schmitt
Content Development Specialists: Julie Mirra, Julia Bartz
Publishing Services Manager: Patricia Tannian
Project Manager: Sarah Wunderly
Design Direction: Steven Stave

Printed in China

Last digit is the print number: 9 8 7 6 5 4 3 2 1

Dedicated in loving memory of two friends who positively influenced both my life and career

Dawn Iannucci for her devotion and tireless efforts on my behalf

and

Adranik Ovassapian, MD, for his inspiration and encouragement.

Both will be fondly remembered and greatly missed.

Contributors

Ronda E. Alexander, MD
Assistant Professor
Department of Otorhinolaryngology—Head and Neck
  Surgery
The University of Texas Medical School at Houston
Director
Texas Voice Performance Institute
Houston, Texas

Carlos A. Artime, MD
Assistant Professor
Department of Anesthesiology
The University of Texas Medical School at Houston
Houston, Texas

Paul A. Baker, MB, ChB, FANZCA
Senior Lecturer
Department of Anaesthesiology
University of Auckland School of Medicine
Consultant Anaesthetist
Paediatric Anaesthesia
Starship Children's Health
Auckland, New Zealand

David R. Ball, MBBS
Consultant Anaesthetist
Dumfries and Galloway Royal Infirmary
Dumfries, United Kingdom

Anis S. Baraka, MD, FRCA(Hon)
Emeritus Professor of Anesthesiology
American University of Beirut
Member of WFSA Advisory Group
Beirut, Lebanon

Irving Z. Basañez, MD
Resident Physician
Department of Otolaryngology
Vanderbilt University Medical Center
Nashville, Tennessee

Elizabeth C. Behringer, MD
Professor of Anesthesiology
Director of Critical Care Education
Cardiac Surgical Intensivist, Department of
  Anesthesiology
Cedars-Sinai Medical Center
Los Angeles, California

Jacqueline A. Bello, MD, FACR
Professor of Clinical Radiology and Neurosurgery
Director of Neuroradiology
Montefiore Medical Center
Albert Einstein College of Medicine
New York, New York

Jonathan L. Benumof, MD
Professor
Department of Anesthesiology
University of California San Diego School of Medicine
San Diego, California

Lauren C. Berkow, MD
Associate Professor of Anesthesia and Critical Care
  Medicine
Johns Hopkins School of Medicine
Baltimore, Maryland

James M. Berry, MD
Professor and Division Head (Adult Anesthesia)
Department of Anesthesiology
Vanderbilt University School of Medicine
Nashville, Tennessee

Nasir I. Bhatti, MD
Associate Professor
Departments of Otolaryngology—Head and Neck
  Surgery and Anesthesiology Critical Care Medicine
Director, Johns Hopkins Adult Tracheostomy and
  Airway Service
Johns Hopkins School of Medicine
Baltimore, Maryland

Archie I.J. Brain, MA, LMSSA, FFARCSI, FRCA(Hon), FANZCA(Hon)
Honorary Research Fellow
Institute of Laryngology
University of London
London, United Kingdom

Ansgar M. Brambrink, MD, PhD
Professor of Anesthesiology and Perioperative Medicine
Oregon Health and Science University
Portland, Oregon

Calvin A. Brown III, MD
Assistant Professor of Medicine
Harvard Medical School
Vice Chair
Department of Emergency Medicine
Faulkner Hospital
Attending Physician
Emergency Medicine
Brigham and Women's and Faulkner Hospitals
Boston, Massachusetts

Robert A. Caplan, MD
Staff Anesthesiologist
Virginia Mason Medical Center
Clinical Professor of Anesthesiology
University of Washington
Seattle, Washington

Davide Cattano, MD, PhD
Associate Professor and Director
Otolaryngology—Head and Neck Anesthesia
Medical Director
Preoperative Anesthesia Clinic
Department of Anesthesiology
The University of Texas Medical School at Houston
Houston, Texas

Laura F. Cavallone, MD
Assistant Professor
Department of Anesthesiology
Washington University in St. Louis
Saint Louis, Missouri

Erol Cavus, MD
Assistant Professor of Anesthesiology
Department of Anesthesiology and Intensive Care Medicine
University Hospital Schleswig-Holstein Campus Kiel
Kiel, Germany

Jacques E. Chelly, MD, PhD, MBA
Professor and Vice Chairman of Clinical Research
Director of the Division of Acute Perioperative Interventional Pain
Department of Anesthesiology
University of Pittsburgh School of Medicine
Director of Acute Perioperative Interventional Pain Service
UPMC Shadyside Hospital
Pittsburgh, Pennsylvania

T. Linda Chi, MD
Associate Professor of Neuroradiology
Division of Diagnostic Imaging
MD Anderson Cancer Center
Houston, Texas

Chris C. Christodoulou, MBChB Cum Laude, DA(UK), LMCC, FRCPC
Assistant Professor in Anesthesia
Department of Anesthesia and Perioperative Medicine
University of Manitoba
Winnipeg, Manitoba, Canada

Rebecca E. Claure, MD
Clinical Assistant Professor of Anesthesia
Department of Anesthesia
Stanford University Medical Center
Stanford
Pediatric Anesthesiologist
Lucile Packard Children's Hospital
Palo Alto, California

Edmond Cohen, MD
Professor of Anesthesiology
Director of Thoracic Anesthesia
Department of Anesthesiology
Mount Sinai School of Medicine
New York, New York

Neal H. Cohen, MD, MPH, MS
Professor of Anesthesia and Perioperative Care and Medicine
Vice Dean
University of California San Francisco School of Medicine
San Francisco, California

Lee Coleman, MD
Assistant Professor
Department of Anesthesiology
Cedars-Sinai Medical Center
Los Angeles, California

Tim M. Cook, BA, MBBS, FRCA
Consultant in Anaesthesia and Intensive Care Medicine
Royal United Hospital
Bath, United Kingdom

Richard M. Cooper, BSc, MSc, MD, FRCPC
Professor
Department of Anesthesia
University of Toronto
Anesthesiologist
Department of Anesthesia and Pain Management
University Health Network
Toronto General Hospital
Toronto, Ontario, Canada

Steven A. Deem, MD
Adjunct Professor of Anesthesiology and Medicine
University of Washington
Seattle, Washington

David A. Diaz Voss Varela, MD
Postdoctoral Fellow
Department of Otolaryngology Head and Neck Surgery
Johns Hopkins University School of Medicine
Baltimore, Maryland

Pierre Auguste Diemunsch, MD, PhD
Chairman
Department of Anesthesiology and Intensive Care
University Hospital of Hautepierre
Strasbourg, France

Stephen F. Dierdorf, MD
Professor and Vice Chair
Department of Anesthesia
Indiana University School of Medicine
Indianapolis, Indiana

Volker Dörges, MD
Professor of Anesthesiology
Department of Anesthesiology and Intensive Care
    Medicine
University Hospital Schleswig-Holstein Campus Kiel
Kiel, Germany

D. John Doyle, MD, PhD
Professor of Anesthesiology
Department of General Anesthesiology
Cleveland Clinic
Cleveland, Ohio

Lara Ferrario, MD
Assistant Professor
Director of Neuroanesthesia and Director of
    Neuroanesthesia Fellowships
Department of Anesthesiology
The University of Texas Medical School at Houston
Houston, Texas

David Z. Ferson, MD
Professor
Department of Anesthesiology and Perioperative
    Medicine
MD Anderson Cancer Center
Houston, Texas

Lorraine J. Foley, MD
Clinical Assistant Professor of Anesthesia
Department of Anesthesia
Tufts School of Medicine
Boston, Massachusetts
Winchester Anesthesia Associates
Winchester Hospital
Winchester, Massachusetts

Michael Frass, MD
Professor of Medicine
Medical University Vienna
Department of Medicine I
Vienna, Austria

Michael A. Gibbs, MD, FACEP
Professor and Chair
Department of Emergency Medicine
Carolinas Medical Center
University of North Carolina
Charlotte School of Medicine—Charlotte Campus
Charlotte, North Carolina

Katherine S.L. Gil, MD, BSc
Assistant Professor of Anesthesiology and Neurological
    Surgery
Department of Anesthesiology
Northwestern University Feinberg School of Medicine
Chicago, Illinois

Julian A. Gold, MD
Co-Chairman
Department of Anesthesiology
Cedars-Sinai Medical Center
Associate Professor of Clinical Anesthesiology
Department of Anesthesiology
Keck School of Medicine of University of Southern
    California
Los Angeles, California

Steven B. Greenberg, MD
Director of Critical Care Services
Evanston Hospital
NorthShore University HealthSystem
Evanston, Illinois
Clinical Assistant Professor
Department of Anesthesiology/Critical Care
University of Chicago
Chicago, Illinois

John A. Griswold, MD, FACS
Professor and Chairman
Department of Surgery
Texas Tech University Health Science Center
Medical Director
Timothy J. Harnar Regional Burn Center
Medical Director
University Medical Center Level 1 Trauma Center
Lubbock, Texas

Carin A. Hagberg, MD
Joseph C. Gabel Professor and Chair
Department of Anesthesiology
The University of Texas Medical School at Houston
Chief of Anesthesia and Director of Neuroanesthesia
    and Advanced Airway Management
Memorial Hermann Hospital
Houston, Texas

Gregory B. Hammer, MD
Professor
Anesthesia and Pediatrics
Stanford University School of Medicine
Stanford
Director of Anesthesia Research
Lucile Packard Children's Hospital
Palo Alto, California

Stephen Harvey, MD
Assistant Professor
Department of Anesthesiology
Vanderbilt University
Nashville, Tennessee

Alexander T. Hillel, MD
Assistant Professor
Department of Otolaryngology—Head and Neck
  Surgery
The Johns Hopkins University School of Medicine
Baltimore, Maryland

Orlando R. Hung, BSc (Pharmacy), MD, FRCPC
Professor
Anesthesia, Surgery, and Pharmacology
Dalhousie University
Halifax, Canada

Ranu R. Jain, MD
Assistant Professor
Department of Anesthesiology
The University of Texas Medical School at Houston
Houston, Texas

Aaron M. Joffe, DO
Assistant Professor
Department of Anesthesiology and Pain Medicine
University of Washington
Harborview Medical Center
Seattle, Washington

Girish P. Joshi, MBBS, MD, FFARCSI
Professor of Anesthesiology and Pain Management
Director of Perioperative Medicine and Ambulatory
  Anesthesia
University of Texas Southwestern Medical Center
Dallas, Texas

Jeffrey P. Keck Jr., MD
Assistant Clinical Professor
Virginia Commonwealth University
Richmond, Virginia
Director of Anesthesia Education
Subspecialty Chief, Trauma Anesthesia
Departments of Anesthesia and Critical Care
Pikeville Medical Center
Pikeville, Kentucky

Sofia Khan, MBChB, FRCA
Anaesthetic Consultant
Manchester Royal Infirmary
Manchester, United Kingdom

P. Allan Klock Jr., MD
Professor and Vice Chair for Clinical Affairs
Department of Anesthesia and Critical Care
University of Chicago
Chicago, Illinois

Prof. Peter Krafft, MBA, MD
Head
Department of Anesthesia and Intensive Care Medicine
Hospital Rudolfsstiftung
Vienna, Austria

Prof. Dr. Claude Krier, MBA
Professor and Medical Director
Klinikum Stuttgart
Stuttgart, Germany

Michael Seltz Kristensen, MD
Head of Section for Anesthesia for ENT-, Head-,
  Neck- and Maxillofacial Surgery
Department of Anaesthesia
Center of Head and Orthopaedics
Rigshospitalet
University Hospital of Copenhagen
Copenhagen, Denmark

Olivier Langeron, MD, PhD
Professor of Anesthesiology and Critical Care
Department of Anesthesiology and Critical Care
Université Pierre et Marie-Curie—Paris VI
CHU Pitié-Salpêtrière
Assistance Publique-Hôpitaux de Paris
Paris, France

Richard M. Levitan, MD
Professor
Department of Emergency Medicine
Jefferson Medical College
Attending Physician
Emergency Medicine
Thomas Jefferson University Hospital
Philadelphia, Pennsylvania

Brian L. Marasigan, MD
Assistant Professor of Cardiovascular Anesthesiology
Director of Core Residency Program
Department of Anesthesiology
The University of Texas Medical School at Houston
Houston, Texas

Lynette J. Mark, MD
Associate Professor of Anesthesiology and Critical Care
  Medicine
Associate Professor of Otolaryngology—Head and Neck
  Surgery
Department of Anesthesiology
Johns Hopkins University
Baltimore, Maryland

Eric C. Matten, MD
Clinical Assistant Professor
Department of Anesthesia and Critical Care
University of Chicago Pritzker School of Medicine,
  Chicago
Department of Anesthesia
NorthShore University HealthSystem
Evanston, Illinois

Barry E. McGuire, MBChB, FRCA, MRCGP
Consultant Anaesthetist
Department of Anaesthesia
Ninewells Hospital and Medical School
Dundee, United Kingdom

Joseph H. McIsaac III, MD, MS
Chief of Trauma Anesthesia
Department of Anesthesiology
Hartford Hospital
Hartford, Connecticut
Associate Clinical Professor of Anesthesiology
Department of Anesthesiology
University of Connecticut School of Medicine
Farmington, Connecticut
Associate Adjunct Professor of Biomedical Engineering
University of Connecticut Graduate School
Storrs, Connecticut

Leah Meisterling, DO, MBA
Neuroanesthesia Subspecialty Chair
Department of Anesthesiology
Intensivist
Surgical Intensive Care Unit
Hartford Hospital
Hartford, Connecticut
Associate Clinical Professor of Anesthesiology
Department of Anesthesiology
University of Connecticut
Farmington, Connecticut

Gabriel Mena, MD
Cardiovascular Fellow
DeBakey Methodist Hospital
Assistant Professor of Anesthesiology
Department of Anesthesiology and Perioperative
  Medicine
MD Anderson Cancer Center
Houston, Texas
Professor Ad Honorem
Department of Anesthesiology
Universidad de Antioquia
Medellin, Colombia

Nathan W. Mick, MD
Assistant Professor
Tufts University School of Medicine
Boston, Massachusetts
Director of Pediatric Emergency Medicine
Department of Emergency Medicine
Maine Medical Center
Portland, Maine

David M. Mirsky, MD
Pediatric Neuroradiology Fellow
The Children's Hospital of Philadelphia
University of Pennsylvania
Philadelphia, Pennsylvania

Thomas C. Mort, MD
Critical Care Medicine Subspecialty Chair
Senior Anesthesiologist and Associate Director
Surgical Intensive Care Unit
Hartford Hospital
Hartford, Connecticut
Associate Professor of Anesthesiology and Surgery
University of Connecticut School of Medicine
Storrs, Connecticut

Jessen Mukalel, MD
Assistant Professor
Department of Anesthesiology
The University of Texas Medical School at Houston
Houston, Texas

Uma Munnur, MD
Associate Professor of Anesthesiology
Department of Anesthesiology
Baylor College of Medicine
Houston, Texas

Michael F. Murphy, MD
Professor and Chair
Department of Anesthesiology and Pain Medicine
University of Alberta
Zone Chief of Anesthesiology
Department of Anesthesiology
Alberta Health
Edmonton, Alberta, Canada

Robert T. Naruse, MD
Assistant Clinical Professor
Department of Anesthesiology
Keck School of Medicine of The University of Southern
  California
Director of Neuroanesthesia
Department of Anesthesiology
Cedars-Sinai Medical Center
Los Angeles, California

Vladimir Nekhendzy, MD
Clinical Associate Professor of Anesthesia and
  Otolaryngology
Chief of Ear, Nose, and Throat Anesthesia Division
Director, Stanford Anesthesia Advanced Airway
  Management Program
Stanford University School of Medicine
Stanford, California

Kevin F. O'Grady, BASc, MHSc, MD, FRCSC
Plastic, Reconstructive, and Aesthetic Surgery
Private Practice
Richmond Hill, Ontario, Canada

Babatunde Ogunnaike, MD
Professor
Department of Anesthesiology and Pain Management
University of Texas Southwestern Medical Center
Vice Chairman and Chief of Anesthesia Services
Parkland Health and Hospital System
Dallas, Texas

Irene P. Osborn, MD
Associate Professor of Anesthesiology and Neurosurgery
Department of Anesthesiology
Mount Sinai School of Medicine
New York, New York

Anil Patel, MBBS, FRCA
Chairman
Department of Anaesthesia
Royal National Throat Nose and Ear Hospital and
    University College Hospital
London, United Kingdom

Bela Patel, MD
Associate Professor of Medicine
Director, Division of Critical Care Medicine
Department of Internal Medicine
Program Director of Pulmonary and Critical Medicine
    Fellow Program
Divisions of Critical Care, Pulmonary and Sleep
    Medicine
The University of Texas Medical School at Houston
Houston, Texas

Karen L. Posner, PhD
Research Professor
Department of Anesthesiology and Pain Medicine
University of Washington
Seattle, Washington

Mary F. Rabb, MD
Professor
Department of Anesthesiology
The University of Texas Medical School at Houston
Houston, Texas

Ali S. Raja, MD, MBA, MPH
Associate Director for Trauma
Department of Emergency Medicine
Brigham and Women's Hospital
Tactical Physician/Medical Director
Boston SWAT Team
Federal Bureau of Investigation
Boston, Massachusetts

Satya K. Ramachandran, MD, FRCA
Assistant Professor of Anesthesiology
University of Michigan Medical School
Director of Quality Assurance (Anesthesiology) and
    Post-Anesthesia Care
University Hospital
Ann Arbor, Michigan

Sivam Ramanathan, MD†
Professor Emeritus
University of Pittsburgh
Director of OB Anesthesia Research
Associate Director OB Anesthesia Fellowship
Department of Anesthesiology
Cedars-Sinai Medical Center
Los Angeles, California

Allan P. Reed, MD
Professor of the Practice of Anesthesiology
Department of Anesthesiology
Mount Sinai School of Medicine
New York, New York

William H. Rosenblatt, BA, MD
Professor of Anesthesia and Surgery
Department of Anesthesiology
Yale University School of Medicine
New Haven, Connecticut

Soham Roy, MD, FACS, FAAP
Associate Professor of Pediatric Otolaryngology
Department of Otorhinolaryngology
University of Texas Health Science Center
Houston, Texas

Kurt Rützler, MD
Department for Cardiothoracic and Vascular Anesthesia
    and Intensive Care Medicine
Medical University of Vienna
Vienna, Austria
Institute of Anaesthesiology
University Hospital Zürich
Zürich, Switzerland

Sebastian G. Russo, MD, PhD, DEAA
Department of Anaesthesiology, Emergency and
    Intensive Care Medicine
University of Göttingen
Göttingen, Germany

M. Ramez Salem, MD
Chair Emeritus
Department of Anesthesiology
Advocate Illinois Masonic Medical Center
Clinical Professor
Department of Anesthesiology
University of Illinois College of Medicine
Chicago, Illinois

Antonio Sanchez, MD
Senior Partner
Kaiser Permanente
Baldwin Park Medical Center
Baldwin Park, California

Jan-Henrik Schiff, MPH
Associate Professor
James Cook University School of Medicine and
    Dentistry
Queensland, Australia
Consultant Anaesthetist
Department of Anesthesiology and Operative Intensive
    Care Medicine
Katherinenhospital
Stuttgart, Germany

Bettina U. Schmitz, MD, PhD, DEAA
Associate Professor of Anesthesiology
Department of Anesthesiology
Texas Tech University Health Science Center
Lubbock, Texas

† Deceased

David E. Schwartz, MD, FCCP
Associate Dean for Clinical Affairs
Professor and Head
Department of Anesthesiology
University of Illinois College of Medicine at Chicago
Chicago, Illinois

Jeanette Scott, MB, ChB, FANZCA
Consultant Anaesthetist
Middlemore Hospital
Auckland, New Zealand

Torin Shear, MD
Clinical Assistant Professor
Department of Anesthesia
NorthShore University HealthSystem
Evanston, Illinois
Clinical Assistant Professor
University of Chicago Pritzker School of Medicine
Chicago, Illinois

Roy Sheinbaum, MD
Professor
Department of Anesthesiology
Director of Cardiothoracic and Vascular Anesthesiology
The University of Texas Medical School at Houston
Houston, Texas

Edward R. Stapleton, EMT-P
Associate Professor of Emergency Medicine
Department of Emergency Medicine
Stony Brook School of Medicine
Stony Brook, New York

Maya S. Suresh, MD
Professor and Chairman
Division Chief
Obstetric and Gynecology Anesthesiology
Baylor College of Medicine
Houston, Texas

Mark D. Tasch, MD
Associate Professor of Clinical Anesthesia
Department of Anesthesia
Indiana University School of Medicine
Indianapolis, Indiana

Arnd Timmermann, MD, DEAA, MME
Division Head
Department of Anesthesiology, Pain Therapy, Intensive
   Care and Emergency Medicine
DRK Kliniken Berlin Westend and Berlin Mitte
Berlin, Germany
Professor of Anesthesiology
University of Göttingen
Göttingen, Germany

Arthur J. Tokarczyk, MD
Clinical Assistant Professor
Department of Anesthesiology
University of Chicago Pritzker School of Medicine,
   Chicago
Anesthesiologist, Department of Anesthesiology
NorthShore University HealthSystem
Evanston, Illinois

Sonia Vaida, MD
Professor of Anesthesiology, Obstetrics and Gynecology
Director of Obstetric Anesthesia
Vice Chair of Research
Department of Anesthesiology
Penn State College of Medicine
Hershey, Pennsylvania

Jeffery S. Vender, MD, FCCP, FCCM, MBA
Professor and Chairman
Department of Anesthesiology
Director of Critical Care Services
Northwestern University Feinburg School of Medicine
Evanston Northwestern Healthcare
Evanston, Illinois

Chandy Verghese, MBBS, FRCA, DA
Consultant in Anaesthesia and Intensive Care
Royal Berkshire NHS Trust, Royal Berkshire Hospital
Reading, United Kingdom

Ashutosh Wali, MBBS, MD, FFARCSI
Associate Professor of Anesthesiology
Associate Professor of Obstetrics and Gynecology
Director of Advanced Airway Management
Baylor College of Medicine
Houston, Texas

Andreas Walther, PD
Professor and Chairman
Department of Anesthesiology and Intensive Care
Klinikum Stuttgart
Stuttgart, Germany

Mark A. Warner, MD
Dean
Mayo School of Graduate Medical Education
Professor of Anesthesiology
Mayo Clinic College of Medicine
Rochester, Minnesota

William C. Wilson, MD, MA
Clinical Professor and Vice Chairman
Chief of Division of Critical Care Medicine
Program Director of ACCM Fellowship
Department of Anesthesiology
University of California, San Diego
San Diego, California

Robert Wong, BS, MD
Anesthesia Resident
Department of Anesthesia
Cedars-Sinai Medical Center
Los Angeles, California

Mark Zakowski, MD
Adjunct Associate Professor of Anesthesiology
Charles R. Drew University of Medicine and Science
Chief of Obstetric Anesthesia and Obstetric
    Anesthesiology Fellowship Director
Department of Anesthesiology
Cedars-Sinai Medical Center
Los Angeles, California

Foreword

The development of airway management as a subspecialty was spurred by the findings from the American Society of Anesthesiologists (ASA) closed claims project in the early 1980s that adverse outcomes resulting from airway management were the single largest cause of malpractice lawsuits against anesthesiologists. When the first edition of *Airway Management* appeared in 1996, airway management was beginning to become a recognizable subspecialty, and the book gave the new subspecialty an intellectual spine. At the same time, the Society for Airway Management had just come into being and gave the subspecialty an administrative and educational spine. Also, the second iteration of the ASA Difficult Airway algorithm became known throughout the world at about this time, and was either practiced as published or in a slightly modified version. Research in airway management has since accelerated tremendously. Today, the large majority of training centers in the United States have a formalized teaching program (required resident rotation) in airway management. In addition, today, one just needs to walk up and down the aisles of the exhibit hall at any annual ASA meeting to find that airway management is an extremely robust and growing subspecialty, in all dimensions, throughout the world.

However, the bedrock of safe airway management, in my opinion, has not changed over the past 20 years. Safe airway management consists of the following: proper preairway management evaluation; securing the airway with the patient awake and spontaneously ventilating when difficulty with the airway is recognized (awake intubation); having plan B (and C, etc.) immediately available in case plan A does not work; allowing the patient to awaken and resume spontaneous ventilation in a timely fashion when various airway management plans are not successful; insisting on unequivocal confirmation of tracheal intubation; and finally, in this day and age of increasing incidence of morbid obesity and obstructive sleep apnea, placing the patient in the proper monitoring environment postextubation.

On top of this bedrock of safe airway management practice, new management techniques and insights make the successful application of the bedrock ever easier to apply to ever more challenging cases. The purpose and rationale of continuing a book like *Airway Management* are to keep pace with these new developments and bring the airway management community as close as possible to the advancing frontier.

The editor of the third edition of *Airway Management*, Dr. Carin Hagberg, is perfectly positioned to lead the anesthesia community as close as is realistically possible to the frontier of airway management. She is an experienced and mature practitioner of airway management and knows the bedrock. She has been a very significant person in the development of the Society of Airway Management, having held virtually every important position in the organization, and as such has great perspective on the educational and administrative needs of the airway community. She has performed research and knows what the questions are. In short, a "triple threat" leads the charge. Given the history of this subspecialty, this book, and the editor, if you want to be good at airway management today, then read and consult this book.

Jonathan L. Benumof, MD

Preface

There have been many advances in airway management over the past two decades and since the publication of the second edition of *Airway Management*. It is essential that clinicians become familiar with the most recent developments in equipment and scientific knowledge to allow the safe practice of airway management. In the third edition of this book, three new chapters (Ultrasonography of the Airway; Video Laryngoscopes; and Disaster Preparedness, Cardiopulmonary Resuscitation, and Airway Management) have been added. The remaining chapters have been substantially updated to address current thinking and practice, and the book is in full color for the first time. Also, at the end of each chapter, there are a summary, up to a dozen bulleted, concise Clinical Pearls, and selected references.

The basic structure and philosophy of the book have not changed. It is divided into seven parts. Part 1 provides basic clinical science considerations of airway management. Part 2 presents difficult airway terminology and recognition, as well as a thorough analysis of the American Society of Anesthesiologists Difficult Airway Algorithm. Part 3 emphasizes patient preparation and preintubation ventilation procedures. Part 4 covers specific methods and problems in securing an airway. Many new airway devices and techniques are reviewed, and the indications for and confirmation of tracheal intubation are provided. Part 5 covers management of difficult airway situations, such as in pediatric patients and the intensive care unit. Part 6 emphasizes postintubation procedures and discusses such issues as monitoring the airway and extubation. Part 7 presents societal considerations of airway management, including instruction and learning of airway management skills both in and out of the operating room, as well as effective dissemination of critical airway information and medical-legal considerations.

Competent and safe airway management is an essential component of anesthetic practice worldwide. The consequences of failure to adequately oxygenate and ventilate a patient's lungs can be catastrophic to both the patient and the practitioner. It is generally known that management improvements have led to a documented decline in the incidence of airway-related perioperative morbidity. Both the dissemination of information and the development of new techniques and devices have contributed to this. The modern-day anesthesia practitioner needs to learn not only the techniques of using a variety of airway devices, but also when use of each would be most appropriate in a given situation.

We are most fortunate to live in today's world of anesthesia practice. I look forward to future advances and what research will unfold in our specialty. This book will not provide competence in airway management but does offer a firm foundation upon which further training and education can be based. Effective airway management requires commitment to a process of ongoing learning, skill maintenance, and self-assessment that should last throughout the practitioner's professional career. This book should serve this commitment well.

Carin A. Hagberg, MD

Acknowledgments

The preparation of the third edition of *Airway Management* has required the help and cooperation of many. To each individual, I acknowledge my debt of gratitude. It has been both an honor and a privilege to have worked with all of the authors, including expert anesthesiologists, emergency room specialists, surgeons, radiologists, and basic scientists from across the world.

The staff at Elsevier has contributed in countless ways, with competence, patience, and hard work, particularly Julie Mirra and Sarah Wunderly, who kept me on task and played a vital role in the quality of the final written text. I would also like to thank Anne Starr for her fantastic organizational and secretarial assistance.

I especially wish to express my deep appreciation to Jon Benumof, MD, without whose mentorship I would not have become the editor of this book, and my heartfelt thanks to my family, especially my husband, Steven Roberts, without whose understanding, forbearance, and support this textbook would not have been possible.

Contents

Video Contents

PART 1

Basic Clinical Science Considerations

Chapter 1

Functional Anatomy of the Airway

LEE COLEMAN | MARK ZAKOWSKI | JULIAN A. GOLD | SIVAM RAMANATHAN

I. INTRODUCTION

The air passages starting from the nose and ending at the bronchioles are necessary for the delivery of respiratory gas to and from the alveoli. During clinical anesthesia, the anesthesiologist uses these air passages to deliver the anesthetic gases to the alveoli while, at the same time, maintaining vital respiratory gas transport. To accomplish proper airway management, anesthesiologists often gain access to the airways by means of an endotracheal tube (ETT) or other devices that are directly introduced into the patient's upper or lower air passages. In addition, anesthesiologists are called upon to establish access to the airways in certain dire emergencies. A general understanding of the airway structures is critical for establishing and maintaining the airway. For the purpose of description, the airway is divided into the *upper airway*, which extends from the nose to the glottis or thoracic inlet, and the *lower airway*, which includes the trachea, the bronchi, and the subdivisions of the bronchi. The airways also serve other important functions, such as olfaction, deglutition, and phonation. A detailed anatomic description of these structures is beyond the scope of this chapter. Structural details as they relate to function in health and disease and some important anesthetic implications are explained here. In addition, some advances in imaging techniques that give insight to functional anatomy are described.

II. UPPER AIRWAY

A. Nose

The airway functionally begins at the nares and the mouth, where air first enters the body. Phylogenetically, breathing was intended to occur through the nose. This arrangement not only enables the animal to smell danger but also permits uninterrupted conditioning of the inspired air while feeding. Resistance to airflow through the nasal passages is twice the resistance that occurs through the mouth. Therefore, during exercise or respiratory distress, mouth breathing occurs to facilitate a reduction in airway resistance and increased airflow.

The nose serves a number of functions: respiration, olfaction, humidification, filtration, and phonation. In the adult human, the two nasal fossae extend 10 to 14 cm from the nostrils to the nasopharynx. The two fossae are divided mainly by a midline quadrilateral cartilaginous septum together with the two extreme medial portions of the lateral cartilages. The nasal septum is composed mainly of the perpendicular plate of the ethmoid bone descending from the cribriform plate, the septal cartilage, and the vomer (Fig. 1-1). It is normally a midline structure but can be deviated to one side.[1] Disruption of the cribriform plate secondary to facial trauma or head injury may allow direct communication with the anterior cranial fossa. The use of positive-pressure mask ventilation in this scenario may lead to the entry of bacteria or foreign material, resulting in meningitis or sepsis. In addition, nasal airways, nasotracheal tubes, and nasogastric tubes may be inadvertently introduced into the subarachnoid space. The posterior portion of the septum is usually midline, but trauma-associated septal deviations and congenital choanal atresia can cause posterior obstruction (Fig. 1-2).

Each nasal fossa is convoluted and provides approximately 60 cm² surface area per side for warming and humidifying the inspired air.[2] The nose is also able to prewarm inspired air to a temperature of 32° C to 34° C, over a wide range of ambient temperatures from 8° C to

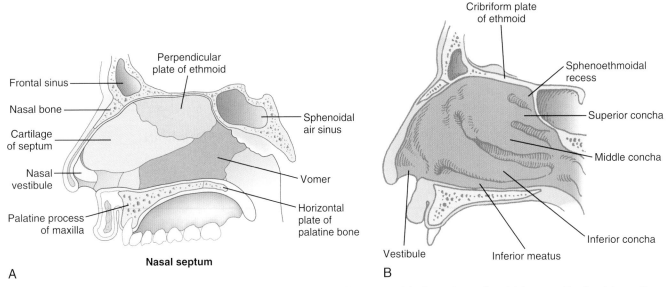

Nasal septum

A

B

Figure 1-1 A, Medial wall (septum) of the nasal cavity. The sphenoid sinus opens into the sphenoethmoidal recess. The frontal, maxillary, and ethmoidal sinuses open into meatuses of the nose. Notice that the nasal septum contains cartilage in front and bone in the back. **B,** Lateral wall of the nasal cavity. Conchae are also known as turbinate bones. (Modified from Ellis H, Feldman S: *Anatomy for anaesthetists*, ed 6, Oxford, 1993, Blackwell Scientific.)

Normal

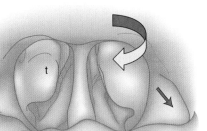

Choanal Atresia

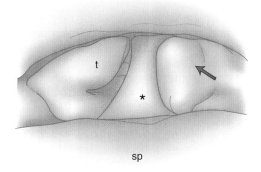

Figure 1-2 Posterior choanal atresia as seen by computed tomographic virtual endoscopy. Normal posterior nasopharynx is on the *top* and posterior choanal atresia is on the *bottom*. The curved arrow points to choanae, and the straight arrow in both figures points to the eustachian tube opening. ***, Characteristically thickened vomer; *sp*, soft palate; *t*, turbinates. (From Thomas BP: CT virtual endoscopy in the evaluation of large airway disease: review. *AJR Integrative Imaging*, 2008.)

40° C.[3] The nasal fossa is bounded laterally by inferior, middle, and superior turbinate bones (conchae),[4] which divide the fossa into scroll-like spaces called the inferior, middle, and superior meatuses (see Fig. 1-1).[2,5,6] The inferior turbinate usually limits the size of the nasotracheal tube that can be passed through the nose, and damage to the lateral wall may occur as a result of vigorous attempts during nasotracheal intubation. The arterial supply to the nasal cavity is mainly from the ethmoid branches of the ophthalmic artery, the sphenopalatine and greater palatine branches of the maxillary artery, and the superior labial and lateral nasal branches of the facial artery. Kiesselbach's plexus, where these vessels anastomose, is situated in Little's area on the anterior-inferior portion of the nasal septum. This is a common source of clinically significant epistaxis. The turbinates have a rich vascular supply that affords the nasal airway the ability to expand or contract according to the degree of vascular engorgement. The vascular mucous membrane overlying the turbinates can be damaged easily, leading to profuse hemorrhage. The paired paranasal sinuses—sphenoid, ethmoid, maxillary, and frontal—drain through apertures into the lateral wall of the nose. Prolonged nasotracheal intubation may lead to infection of the maxillary sinus due to obstruction of the ostia.[7]

The olfactory area is located in the upper third of the nasal fossa and consists of the middle and upper septum and the superior turbinate bone. The respiratory portion is located in the lower third of the nasal fossa.[6] The respiratory mucous membrane consists of ciliated columnar cells containing goblet cells and nonciliated columnar cells with microvilli and basal cells. The olfactory cells have specialized hairlike processes, called the olfactory hair, which are innervated by the olfactory nerve.[6]

The nonolfactory sensory nerve supply to the nasal mucosa is derived from the first two divisions of the trigeminal nerve, the anterior ethmoidal and maxillary nerves. Airborne chemical irritants cause firing of the trigeminal nerves, which presumably are responsible for reflexes such as sneezing and apnea.[8] The afferent pathway for the sneezing reflex originates at the histamine-activated type C neurons of the trigeminal nerve, and the efferent pathway consists of several somatic motor nerves. The act of sneezing is associated with an increased intrathoracic air pressure of up to 100 mm Hg and may produce airflow up to 100 mph.[8]

The parasympathetic autonomic nerves reach the mucosa from the facial nerve after relay through the sphenopalatine ganglion, and sympathetic fibers are derived from the plexus surrounding the internal carotid artery through the vidian nerve.[9] Approximately 10,000 L of ambient air passes through the nasal airway per day, and 1 L of moisture is added to this air in the process.[10] The moisture is derived partly from transudation of fluid through the mucosal epithelium and partly from secretions produced by glands and goblet cells. These secretions have significant bactericidal properties. Foreign body invasion is further minimized by the stiff hairs (vibrissae), the ciliated epithelium, and the extensive lymphatic drainage of the area.

A series of complex autonomic reflexes controls the blood supply to the nasal mucosa and allows it to shrink and swell quickly. Reflex arcs also connect this area with other parts of the body. For example, the Kratschmer reflex leads to bronchiolar constriction on stimulation of the anterior nasal septum in animals. A demonstration of this reflex may be seen in the postoperative period as a patient becomes agitated when the nasal passage is packed.[9]

B. Pharynx

The pharynx, 12 to 15 cm long, extends from the base of the skull to the level of the cricoid cartilage anteriorly and the inferior border of the sixth cervical vertebra posteriorly.[11] It is widest at the level of the hyoid bone (5 cm) and narrowest at the level of the esophagus (1.5 cm), which is the most common site for obstruction after foreign body aspiration. It is further subdivided into the nasopharynx, oropharynx, and laryngopharynx. The nasopharynx, which primarily has a respiratory function, lies posterior to the termination of the turbinates and nasal septum and extends to the soft palate. The oropharynx has primarily a digestive function, starts below the soft palate, and extends to the superior edge of the epiglottis. The laryngopharynx (hypopharynx) lies between the fourth and sixth cervical vertebrae, starts at the superior border of the epiglottis, and extends to the inferior border of the cricoid cartilage, where it narrows and becomes continuous with the esophagus (Fig. 1-3). The eustachian tubes open into the lateral walls of the nasopharynx.

In the lateral walls of the oropharynx are situated the tonsillar pillars of the fauces. The anterior pillar contains the glossopharyngeus muscle, and the posterior pillar contains the palatoglossus muscle.[12] The wall of the pharynx consists of two layers of muscles, an external

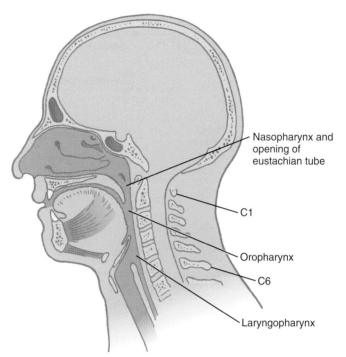

Figure 1-3 Diagrammatic representation of a sagittal section through head and neck to show divisions of the pharynx. Laryngopharynx is also known as the hypopharynx. (Modified from Ellis H, Feldman S: *Anatomy for anaesthetists*, ed 6, Oxford, 1993, Blackwell Scientific.)

Labels in figure: Nasopharynx and opening of eustachian tube; C1; Oropharynx; C6; Laryngopharynx

circular layer and an internal longitudinal layer. Each layer is composed of three paired muscles. The stylopharyngeus, salpingopharyngeus, and palatopharyngeus muscles form the internal layer. They elevate the pharynx and shorten the larynx during deglutition. The superior, middle, and inferior constrictors form the external layer; they advance the food in a coordinated fashion from the oropharynx into the esophagus.

The constrictors are innervated by filaments arising out of the pharyngeal plexus (formed by motor and sensory branches from the vagus, the glossopharyngeal, and the external branch of the superior laryngeal nerve). The inferior constrictor is additionally innervated by branches from the recurrent laryngeal and external laryngeal nerves. The internal layer is innervated by the glossopharyngeal nerve.

1. Defense Against Pathogens

Inhaled particles of size greater than 10 μm are removed by inertial impaction on the posterior nasopharynx. In addition, the inhaled airstream changes direction sharply (90 degrees) at the nasopharynx, resulting in some loss of momentum of the suspended particles. Being unable to remain suspended, the particles are trapped by the pharyngeal walls. The impacted particles are trapped by the circularly arrayed lymphoid tissue located at the entrance to the respiratory and alimentary tracts, known as the ring of Waldeyer (Fig. 1-4). The ring includes masses of lymphoid tissue or tonsils, including the two large palatine, lingual, eustachian tubal, and nasopharyngeal tonsils.

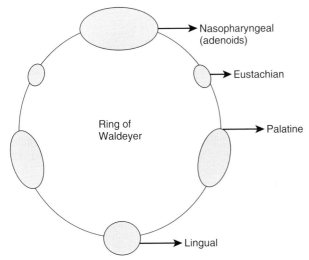

Figure 1-4 The ring of Waldeyer, a collection of lymphoid (tonsillar) tissue that guards against pathogen invasion. (Modified from Hodder Headline PLC, London.)

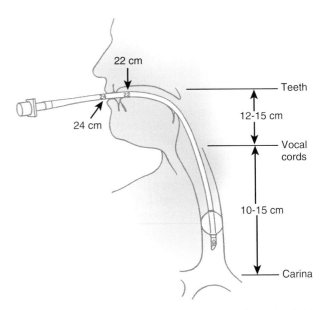

Figure 1-5 Important distances for proper endotracheal tube placement. (From Stone DJ, Bogdonoff DL: Airway considerations in the management of patients requiring long-term endotracheal intubation. *Anesth Analg* 74:276, 1992.)

The nasopharyngeal tonsils are also called adenoids.[13,14] These structures occasionally impede the passage of ETTs, especially if they are infected and enlarged. Specifically, enlarged adenoid tissue may impede passage of a nasotracheal tube or nasal airway or may simply obstruct the nasal airway passages. The lingual tonsils are located between the base of the tongue and the epiglottis. During routine anesthetic evaluation of the oropharynx, the lingual tonsils are typically not visible. Lingual tonsillar hypertrophy, which is usually asymptomatic, has been reported as a cause of unanticipated difficult intubation and fatal upper airway obstruction.[15] In addition, sepsis originating from one of the numerous lymphoid aggregates may lead to a retropharyngeal or peritonsillar abscess, which poses anesthetic challenges.[7]

Ciliary activity also works to clear trapped nonsoluble particles that are held in an outer mucus layer within the nares. This function is influenced by temperature, viscosity of the mucus, and the osmotic properties of the discharge. The ciliary movement can be negatively affected by many factors, such as viral infections or environmental agents, including air pollution and cigarette smoke. The loss of ciliary function leads to chronic and recurrent infections and can gradually severely injure the respiratory tract, leading to conditions such as chronic bronchitis, sinusitis, and otitis.[3]

2. Upper Airway Obstruction

a. SEDATION AND ANESTHESIA

The pharynx is the common pathway for food and the respiratory gases. Patency of the pharynx is vital to the patency of the airway and proper gas exchange in unintubated patients. Proper placement of an ETT requires an understanding of the distance relationships from the oropharynx to the vocal cords and carina. Complications such as a cuff leak at the level of the vocal cords and endobronchial intubation may thus be avoided (Fig. 1-5). Traditionally, it has been taught that upper airway obstruction in patients who are sedated or anesthetized

(without an ETT), or who have altered levels of consciousness for other reasons, occurs as a result of the tongue's falling back onto the posterior pharyngeal wall. Specifically, it is thought that a reduction in genioglossus muscle activity leads to posterior displacement of the tongue with subsequent obstruction.[16] However, a number of publications offer a different explanation. The velopharyngeal segment of the upper airway adjacent to the soft palate has recently become the primary focus. This area is particularly prone to collapse and has been found to be the predominant flow-limiting site during sedation and anesthesia,[17] speech disorders, and obstructive sleep apnea (OSA) (Fig. 1-6).

Nandi and colleagues, using lateral radiographs in patients under general inhalational anesthesia, showed that obstructive changes in the airway occurred at the level of the soft palate and epiglottis.[18] Shorten and coworkers, using magnetic resonance imaging (MRI), found that patients receiving intravenous sedation for anxiolysis with midazolam had anterior-posterior dimensional changes in the upper airway also at the level of the soft palate and epiglottis while sparing the tongue (see Fig. 1-6).[19] In addition, Mathru and coauthors, using MRI to evaluate volunteers receiving propofol anesthesia, found that obstruction occurs at the level of the soft palate and not the tongue.[20] Therefore, it appears that the soft palate and epiglottis may play a more significant role than the tongue in pharyngeal upper airway obstruction.

b. OBSTRUCTIVE SLEEP APNEA

Reduction in the size of the pharynx is also a factor in the development of respiratory obstruction in patients with OSA.[21] This problem has been studied with the use of imaging techniques including computed tomography (CT) and MRI, nasopharyngoscopy, fluoroscopy, and

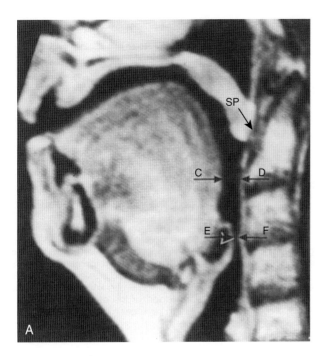

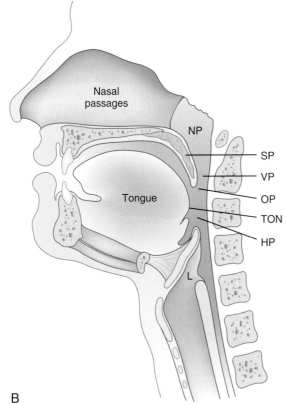

Figure 1-6 A, Medial sagittal view of upper airway showing site of airway obstruction in sedated patients. In the obstructed state, the soft palate is in contact with the posterior pharyngeal wall. CD, Minimum anteroposterior diameter at level of tongue; EF, minimum anteroposterior diameter at level of epiglottis. **B,** The velopharynx *(VP)* and its relation to the soft palate *(SP)*, nasopharynx *(NP)*, oropharynx *(OP)*, tonsil *(TON)*, hypopharynx *(HP)*, and larynx *(L)*. (From Shorten GD, Opie NJ, Graziotti P, et al: Assessment of upper airway anatomy in awake, sedated and anaesthetized patients using magnetic resonance imaging. *Anaesth Intensive Care* 22:165, 1994.)

acoustic reflection.[22] Structural changes that include tonsillar hypertrophy, retrognathia, and variations in craniofacial structures have been linked to sleep apnea risk, presumably by increasing upper airway collapsibility. CT and MRI studies in awake subjects have shown increased fatty tissue deposition and submucosal edema in the lateral walls of the pharynx, both of which can narrow the pharyngeal lumen and predispose to obstruction during sleep, when protective neuromuscular mechanisms wane.[23] Obesity, the major risk factor for OSA, has been shown to increase pharyngeal collapsibility through reductions in lung volumes, especially decreases in functional residual capacity (FRC), which are accentuated with the onset of sleep. This decrease in FRC may increase pharyngeal collapsibility through reductions in tracheal traction on the pharyngeal segment.[23,24] In awake male patients with OSA, CT has revealed a reduced airway caliber at all levels of the pharynx when compared with normal patients, with the narrowest portion posterior to the soft palate.[25]

The subatmospheric intra-airway pressure created by contraction of the diaphragm against the resistance of the nose can lead to a reduction in size of the pharyngeal airway. The collapsible segments of the pharynx are divided into three areas: retropalatal, retroglossal, and retroepiglottic. Patency depends on the contractile function of pharyngeal dilator muscles in these segments. The muscles involved are the tensor palatini, which retracts the soft palate away from the posterior pharyngeal wall; the genioglossus, which moves the tongue anteriorly; and the muscles that move the hyoid bone forward, including the geniohyoid, sternohyoid, and thyrohyoid muscles.[23,26] In patients with OSA, elevated genioglossal and tensor palatini muscle activity has been observed in the awake state. In contrast, normal subjects have lower activity in these muscles. Observations like these suggest that increased upper airway dilator muscle activity compensates for a more anatomically narrow upper airway in OSA. The reduction in upper airway muscle activity during sleep has been implicated in leading to increased likelihood of upper airway obstruction in patients with OSA compared with healthy subjects.[23,24] Studies also show that the configuration of the airway may differ in patients with OSA. Normally, the longer axis of the pharyngeal airway is transverse; however, in OSA patients the anterior-posterior axis is predominant. It is believed that this orientation is less efficient and may affect upper airway muscle function. Continuous positive airway pressure (CPAP) has been found to be effective in treating airway obstruction in these patients. The application of CPAP appears to increase the volume and cross-sectional area of the oropharynx, especially in the lateral axis.[27]

Clinical problems can arise from both the exaggeration and the depression of upper airway reflexes. A heightened reflex response can lead to laryngospasm and prolonged paroxysm of cough, whereas depressed reflexes can increase the risk of aspiration and compromised airway.[28]

The velopharynx, an area of the pharynx adjacent to the soft palate, is assuming increased importance in the understanding of OSA, speech disorders, and airway obstruction under anesthesia (see Fig. 1-6 B).[29] Fiberoptic nasendoscopy and MRI are recommended for studying velopharyngeal dysfunction.[29-31] Six skeletal muscles—the tensor veli palatini, levator veli palatini, musculus uvulae, palatoglossus, palatopharyngeus, and superior constrictor—help form the so-called velopharyngeal sphincter. The proper function of the sphincter is vital to opening and closing of the nasal passages to airflow during deglutition and normal breathing.

C. Larynx

The larynx, which lies in the adult neck opposite the third through sixth cervical vertebrae,[12] is situated at the crossroads between the food and air passages (or conduits). It is made up of cartilages forming the skeletal framework, ligaments, membranes, and muscles. Its primary function is to serve as the "watchdog" of the respiratory tract, allowing passage only to air and preventing secretions, food, and foreign bodies from entering the trachea. In addition, it functions as the organ of phonation. The larynx may be located somewhat higher in females and children. Until puberty, no differences in laryngeal size exist between males and females. At puberty, the larynx develops more rapidly in males than in females, almost doubling in the anteroposterior diameter. The female larynx is smaller and more cephalad.[12] The measurements of the length, transverse diameter, and sagittal diameter of the adult larynx are 44, 36, and 43 mm, respectively, in the male and 41, 36, and 26 mm, respectively, in the female.[32] Most larynxes develop somewhat asymmetrically.[33] The inlet to the larynx is bounded anteriorly by the upper edge of the epiglottis, posteriorly by a fold of mucous membrane stretched between the two arytenoid cartilages, and laterally by the aryepiglottic folds.[9]

1. Bones of the Larynx

The hyoid bone (Fig. 1-7) suspends and anchors the larynx during respiratory and phonatory movement. It is U shaped, and its name is derived from the Greek word *hyoeides*, meaning shaped like the letter upsilon. It has a body, which is 2.5 cm wide by 1 cm thick, and greater and lesser horns (cornu). The hyoid does not articulate with any other bone. It is attached to the styloid processes of the temporal bones by the stylohyoid ligament and to the thyroid cartilage by the thyrohyoid membrane and muscle. Intrinsic tongue muscles originate on the hyoid, and the pharyngeal constrictors are also attached there.[4,12,34]

2. Cartilages of the Larynx

Nine cartilages provide the framework of the larynx (Fig. 1-8; see also Fig. 1-7). These are the unpaired thyroid, cricoid, and epiglottis and the paired arytenoids, corniculates, and cuneiforms. They are connected and supported by membranes, synovial joints, and ligaments. The ligaments, when covered by mucous membranes, are called folds. The thyroid, cricoid, and arytenoid cartilages consist of hyaline cartilage, whereas the other cartilages are elastic cartilage. Hyaline cartilage tends to ossify in the adult, and this occurs earlier in men than in women.[3]

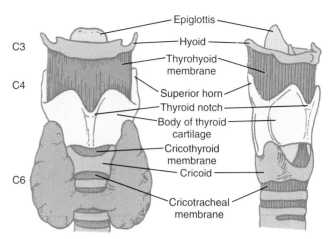

Figure 1-7 External frontal *(left)* and anterolateral *(right)* views of the larynx. Notice the location of cricothyroid membrane and thyroid gland in relation to thyroid and cricoid cartilage in the frontal view. The horn of the thyroid cartilage is also known as the cornu. In the anterolateral view, the shape of the cricoid cartilage and its relation to thyroid cartilage are shown. (Modified from Ellis H, Feldman S: *Anatomy for anaesthetists,* ed 6, Oxford, 1993, Blackwell Scientific.)

a. THYROID CARTILAGE

The thyroid cartilage, the longest laryngeal cartilage and the largest structure in the larynx, acquires its shieldlike shape from the embryologic midline fusion of the two distinct quadrilateral laminae.[35] In females, the sides join at an angle of approximately 120 degrees; in males, the angle is closer to 90 degrees. This smaller thyroid angle explains the greater laryngeal prominence ("Adam's apple"), longer vocal cords, and lower-pitched voice in

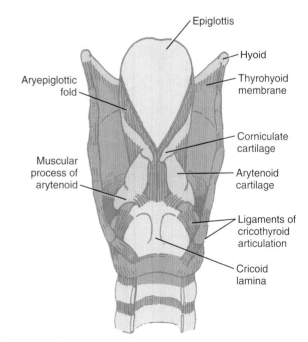

Figure 1-8 Cartilages and ligaments of the larynx seen posteriorly. Notice the location of the corniculate cartilage within the aryepiglottic fold. (Modified from Ellis H, Feldman S: *Anatomy for anaesthetists,* ed 6, Oxford, 1993, Blackwell Scientific.)

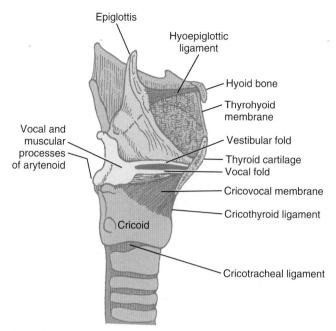

Epiglottis

Hyoepiglottic ligament

Hyoid bone

Thyrohyoid membrane

Vestibular fold

Vocal and muscular processes of arytenoid

Thyroid cartilage

Vocal fold

Cricovocal membrane

Cricothyroid ligament

Cricoid

Cricotracheal ligament

Figure 1-9 Sagittal (lateral) view of the larynx. The vocal and vestibular folds and the thyroepiglottic ligament attach to the midline of the inner surface of the thyroid cartilage. Also notice the relationship between the cricovocal membrane and the vocal folds. (Modified from Ellis H, Feldman S: *Anatomy for anaesthetists*, ed 6, Oxford, 1993, Blackwell Scientific.)

males.[36] The thyroid notch lies in the midline at the top of the fusion site of the two laminae.[37] On the inner side of this fusion line are attached the vestibular ligaments and, below them, the vocal ligaments (Fig. 1-9). The superior (greater) and inferior (lesser) cornua of the thyroid are slender, posteriorly directed extensions of the edges of the lamina. The lateral thyrohyoid ligament attaches the superior cornu to the hyoid bone, and the cricoid cartilage articulates with the inferior cornu at the cricothyroid joint. The movements of this joint are rotatory and gliding and result in changes in the length of the vocal folds.

b. CRICOID CARTILAGE

The cricoid cartilage (see Fig. 1-9) represents the anatomic lower limit of the larynx and helps support it.[35] The name *cricoid* is derived from the Greek words *krikos* and *eidos*, meaning shaped like a ring, and it is frequently said to have a signet-ring shape. It is thicker and stronger than the thyroid cartilage and represents the only complete cartilaginous ring in the airway. For this reason, cautious downward pressure on the cricoid cartilage to prevent passive regurgitation is possible without subsequent airway obstruction. Traditionally, it was thought that the pediatric airway was narrowest at the level of the cricoid, and recommendations for ETT size were made based on the size of the cricoid ring. However, studies done with video bronchoscopes on anesthetized and paralyzed children have shown that the glottic opening may be narrower than the cricoid region.[38] Therefore, an ETT tube may cause more damage to the vocal cords than to the subglottic area.

The bulky portion or lamina is located posteriorly. The tracheal rings are connected to the cricoid by ligaments and muscles. The cricoid lamina forms ball-and-socket synovial articulations with the arytenoids posterosuperiorly and with the thyroid cartilage inferolaterally and anteriorly.[35] It also attaches to the thyroid cartilage by means of the cricothyroid membrane (CTM), a relatively avascular and easily palpated landmark in most adults (see Figs. 1-8 and 1-9).

The inner diameters of the cricoid cartilage have been measured in cadavers, with great variability noted. Randestad and colleagues reported that the smallest diameter is in the frontal plane, which in females ranged from 8.9 to 17.0 mm (mean, 11.6 mm) and in males from 11.0 to 21.5 mm (mean, 15.0 mm).[39] They pointed out that placement of a standard size ETT (7 mm inner diameter for females, 8 mm for males) through the cricoid cartilage while preventing mucosal necrosis may be difficult in certain individuals.[39] The CTM represents an important identifiable landmark, providing access to the airway by percutaneous or surgical cricothyroidotomy.

The dimensions of the CTM have been identified in cadaveric specimens.[40-42] However, the actual methods of obtaining the anatomic measurements varied, making comparisons difficult to interpret. Caparosa and Zavatsky described the CTM as a trapezoid with a width ranging from 27 to 32 mm, representing the actual anatomic limit of the membrane, and a height of 5 to 12 mm.[41] Bennett and coauthors[40] reported the width as 9 to 19 mm and the height as 8 to 19 mm, whereas Dover and coworkers[42] reported a width of 6.0 to 11.0 mm and a height of 7.5 to 13.0 mm, using the distance between the cricothyroid muscles as their horizontal limit. The width and height of the membrane are reported to be smaller in females than in males.[10,42]

Anteriorly, vascular structures overlie the membrane and pose a risk of hemorrhage.[40,42-44] Cadaveric studies have reported the presence of a transverse cricothyroid artery, a branch of the superior thyroid artery, traversing the upper half of the membrane. Therefore, a transverse incision in the lower third of the membrane is recommended. The superior thyroid artery courses along the lateral edge of the membrane, and various branches of the superior and inferior thyroid veins and the jugular veins are also reported to traverse the membrane.

c. ARYTENOIDS

The two light arytenoid cartilages (see Fig. 1-8) are shaped like three-sided pyramids, and they lie in the posterior aspect of the larynx.[45] The arytenoid's medial surface is flat and is covered with only a firm, tight layer of mucoperichondrium.[45,46] The base of the arytenoid is concave and articulates by a true diarthrodial joint with the superior lateral aspect of the posterior lamina of the cricoid cartilage. It is described as a ball and socket with three movements—rocking or rotating, gliding, and pivoting—that control adduction and abduction of the vocal cords. All such synovial joints can be affected by rheumatoid arthritis. Cricoarytenoid arthritis is present in a majority of patients with rheumatoid arthritis and has been identified as a cause of life-threatening upper airway obstruction.[47] Cricoarytenoid arthropathy has also been reported as a rare but potentially fatal cause of acute upper airway obstruction in patients with systemic lupus erythematosus.[48]

The lateral extension of the arytenoid base is called the muscular process. Important intrinsic laryngeal muscles, the lateral and posterior cricoarytenoids, originate here. The medial extension of the arytenoid base is called the vocal process. Vocal ligaments, the bases of the true vocal folds, extend from the vocal process to the midline of the inner surface of the thyroid lamina (see Fig. 1-9). The fibrous membrane that connects the vocal ligament to the thyroid cartilage actually penetrates the body of the thyroid. This membrane is called Broyles' ligament. This ligament contains lymphatics and blood vessels and therefore can act as an avenue for extension of laryngeal cancer outside the larynx.[35,49] The relationship between the anterior commissure of the larynx and the inner aspect of the thyroid cartilage is important to otolaryngologists, who perform thyroplasties and supraglottic laryngectomies on the basis of its location. A study of cadavers reported that the anterior commissure of the larynx can usually be found above the midpoint of the vertical midline fusion of the thyroid cartilage ala.[46,50]

d. EPIGLOTTIS

The epiglottis is considered to be vestigial by many authorities.[51] Composed primarily of fibroelastic cartilage, the epiglottis does not ossify and maintains some flexibility throughout life.[35,45,52] It is shaped like a leaf and is found between the larynx and the base of the tongue (see Figs. 1-8 and 1-9).[34,46] The anterior surface of the epiglottis is concave, and this, in combination with laryngeal elevation, aids in airway protection during deglutition.[1] In approximately 1% of the population, the tip and posterior aspect of the epiglottis are visible during a pharyngoscopic view with the mouth opened and tongue protruded. Contrary to reports, this does not always predict ease of intubation.[53] The upper border of the epiglottis is attached by its narrow tip or petiole to the midline of the thyroid cartilage by the thyroepiglottic ligament (see Fig. 1-9). The hyoepiglottic ligament connects the epiglottis to the back of the body of the hyoid bone.[34,54] The mucous membrane that covers the anterior aspect of the epiglottis sweeps forward to the tongue as

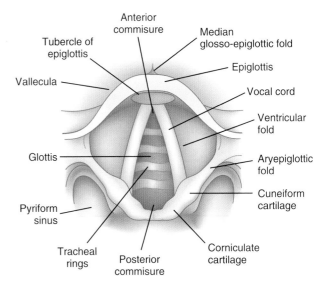

Figure 1-10 Larynx viewed from above with a laryngeal mirror. Notice the location of the anterior and posterior commissures of the larynx and the aryepiglottic fold. Elevations in the aryepiglottic folds are the cuneiform cartilages. (Modified from Tucker HM: Anatomy of the larynx. In Tucker HM, editor: *The larynx*, ed 2, New York, 1993, Thieme Medical, p 9.)

the median glossoepiglottic fold and to the pharynx as the paired lateral pharyngoepiglottic folds.[35] The pouch-like areas found between the median and lateral folds are the valleculae (Fig. 1-10). The tip of a properly placed Macintosh laryngoscope blade rests in this area. The vallecula is a common site of impaction of foreign bodies, such as fish bones, in the upper airway.

The introduction of advanced scanning techniques using contrast-enhanced multidetector computed tomography (MDCT) has enabled three-dimensional (3-D) and four-dimensional visualization of larger airways. Images of normal and diseased structures can be generated by using special postprocedure CT virtual endoscopy computer software. The presence of air-filled lumens of the upper airways makes it possible for the technical staff to build high-quality endoscopy-like images. Similar techniques have been applied to lower airways also. A virtual endoscopic picture of acute epiglottitis can be seen in Fig. 1-11.[55]

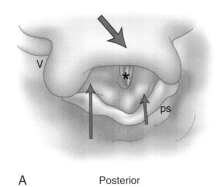
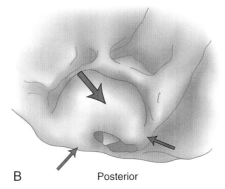

Figure 1-11 Acute epiglottitis. **A,** Virtual endoscopy showing normal appearance of the epiglottis *(large arrow)*, aryepiglottic fold *(long thin arrow)*, arytenoid prominence *(short thin arrow)*, and glottis *(astersisk)*. **B,** The appearance in acute epiglottitis. Notice the enlarged edematous epiglottis, indicated by the *large arrow*, and arytenoids *(thin arrows)*. *ps,* Pyriform sinus; *V,* vallecula. (From Thomas BP: CT virtual endoscopy in the evaluation of large airway disease: review. *AJR Integrative Imaging*, 2008.)

e. CUNEIFORM AND CORNICULATE CARTILAGES

The epiglottis is connected to the arytenoid cartilages by the laterally placed aryepiglottic ligaments and folds (see Figs. 1-8 and 1-10)). Two sets of paired fibroelastic cartilages are embedded in each aryepiglottic fold.[45] The sesamoid cuneiform cartilage is roughly cylindrical and lies anterosuperior to the corniculate in the fold. The cuneiform may be seen laryngoscopically as a whitish elevation through the mucosa (see Fig. 1-10). The corniculate is a small, triangular object visible directly over the arytenoid cartilage. The cuneiform and corniculate cartilages reinforce and support the aryepiglottic folds[35,46] and may help the arytenoids move.[12,52]

f. FALSE AND TRUE VOCAL CORDS

The thyrohyoid membrane (see Figs. 1-7 through 1-9), attaching the superior edge of the thyroid cartilage to the hyoid bone, provides cranial support and suspension.[12] It is separated from the hyoid body by a bursa that facilitates movement of the larynx during deglutition.[46] The thicker median section of the thyrohyoid membrane is the thyrohyoid ligament, and its thinner lateral edges are pierced by the internal branches of the superior laryngeal nerves.

Beneath the laryngeal mucosa is a fibrous sheet containing many elastic fibers, known as the fibroelastic membrane of the larynx. Its upper area, the quadrangular membrane, extends in the aryepiglottic fold between the arytenoids and the epiglottis. The lower free border of the membrane is called the vestibular ligament; it forms the vestibular folds, or false cords (see Figs. 1-9 and 1-10).[34,36,47]

The CTM joins the cricoid and thyroid cartilages. The thickened median area of this fibrous tissue, the "conus elasticus," extends up inside the thyroid lamina to the anterior commissure and continues and blends with the vocal ligament. The cricothyroid ligament thus connects the cricoid, thyroid, and arytenoid cartilages.[36,47] The thickened inner edges of the cricothyroid ligament, called the vocal ligament, form the base of the vocal folds (see Fig. 1-10).[12,46]

g. LARYNGEAL CAVITY

The laryngeal cavity (Fig. 1-12) extends from the laryngeal inlet to the lower border of the cricoid cartilage. When it is viewed laryngoscopically from above, two paired inward projections of tissue are visible in the laryngeal cavity: the superiorly placed vestibular folds, or false cords, and the more inferiorly placed vocal folds, or true vocal cords (see Fig. 1-10). The space between the true cords is called the rima glottidis, or the glottis (see Fig. 1-12). The glottis is divided into two parts. The anterior intermembranous section is situated between the two vocal folds. The two vocal folds meet at the anterior commissure of the larynx (see Fig. 1-10). The posterior intercartilaginous part passes between the two arytenoid cartilages and the mucosa, stretching between them in the midline posteriorly, forming the posterior commissure of the larynx (see Fig. 1-10).[36] At rest, the vocal processes are approximately 8 mm apart. The area extending from the laryngeal inlet to the vestibular folds

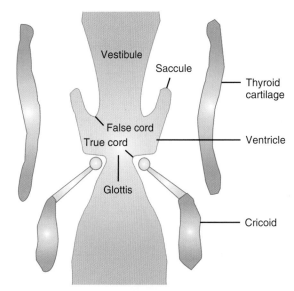

Figure 1-12 Diagrammatic representation of the laryngeal cavity. Notice the location of the false and true cords and laryngeal saccule. (Modified from Pectu LP, Sasaki CT: Laryngeal anatomy and physiology. *Clin Chest Med* 12:415, 1991.)

is known as the vestibule or supraglottic larynx (see Fig. 1-12). The laryngeal space from the free border of the cords to the cricoid cartilage is called the subglottic or infraglottic larynx.

On the basis of cadaver studies, the measurements of the subglottis have been identified.[41,56,57] Understanding the anatomic relationships between the cricothyroid space and the vocal folds is important to minimize complications after cricothyrotomy (Fig. 1-13).[58] Bennett and colleagues[40] reported this distance to be 9.78 mm. The region between the vestibular folds and the glottis is termed the ventricle or the sinus (see Fig. 1-12). The ventricle may expand anterolaterally to a pouchlike area with many lubricating mucous glands, called the laryngeal saccule (see Fig. 1-12).[35] The saccule is believed to help in voice resonance in apes.[46,51] The pyriform sinus lies laterally to the aryepiglottic fold within the inner surface of the thyroid cartilage (see Fig. 1-10).[46]

The epithelium of the vestibular folds is of the ciliated pseudostratified variety (respiratory), whereas the epithelium of the vocal folds is of the nonkeratinized squamous type.[37] Therefore, the entire interior of the larynx is covered with respiratory epithelium except for the vocal folds.[9]

Airway protection is enhanced by the orientation of the cords. The false cords are directed inferiorly at their free border. This position can help to stop egress of air during a Valsalva maneuver. The true cords are oriented slightly superiorly. This prevents air or matter from entering the lungs. Great pressure is required to separate adducted true cords.[52] Air trapped in the ventricle during closure pushes the false cords and the true cords more tightly together.[15,37,52]

3. Muscles, Innervation, and Blood Supply of the Larynx

The complex and delicate functions of the larynx are made possible by an intricate group of small muscles.

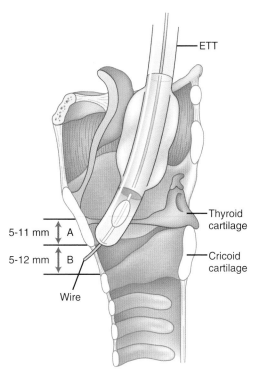

ETT

5-11 mm ↕ A

5-12 mm ↕ B

Wire

Thyroid cartilage

Cricoid cartilage

Figure 1-13 Schematic illustration showing the relationships of the larynx, thyroid, and cricoid cartilages, including the distance (range) from the vocal cords to the anteroinferior edge of the thyroid cartilage *(A)* and the distance (range) from the anteroinferior edge of the thyroid cartilage to the anterosuperior edge of the cricoid cartilage *(B)*. Also shown is the wire penetrating the cricothyroid membrane for retrograde intubation. *ETT,* Endotracheal tube. (From Kuriloff DB, Setzen M, Portnoy W: Laryngotracheal injury following cricothyroidotomy. *Laryngoscope* 99:125, 1989.)

These muscles can be divided into extrinsic and intrinsic groups.[51,54] The extrinsic group connects the larynx with its anatomic neighbors, such as the hyoid bone, and modifies the position and movement of the larynx. The intrinsic group facilitates the movements of the laryngeal cartilages against one another and directly affects glottic movement.

a. EXTRINSIC MUSCLES OF THE LARYNX

The suprahyoid muscles attach the larynx to the hyoid bone and elevate the larynx. These muscles are the stylohyoid, geniohyoid, mylohyoid, thyrohyoid, digastric, and stylopharyngeus muscles. In the infrahyoid muscle group are the omohyoid, sternothyroid, thyrohyoid, and sternohyoid muscles. These "strap" muscles, in addition to lowering the larynx, can modify the internal relationship of laryngeal cartilages and folds to one another. The inferior constrictor of the pharynx primarily assists in deglutition (Table 1-1).[12,35-37]

b. INTRINSIC MUSCLES OF THE LARYNX

The function of the intrinsic musculature is threefold: (1) to open the vocal cords during inspiration, (2) to close the cords and the laryngeal inlet during deglutition, and (3) to alter the tension of the cords during phonation.[12,35,59] The larynx can close at three levels: the aryepiglottic folds close by contraction of the aryepiglottic and oblique arytenoid muscles, the false vocal cords close by action of the lateral thyroarytenoids, and the true vocal cords by contraction of the interarytenoids, the lateral cricoarytenoids, and the cricothyroid.[12] The intrinsic muscles include the aryepiglottic and thyroepiglottic, thyroarytenoid and vocalis, oblique and transverse arytenoids, lateral and posterior cricoarytenoids, and cricothyroids (Fig. 1-14). All but the transverse arytenoid are paired.

Some authors consider the cricothyroid muscle to be both an extrinsic and an intrinsic muscle of the larynx because its actions affect both laryngeal movement and the glottic structures. It is the only intrinsic muscle found external to the larynx itself. The paired cricothyroid muscles join the cricoid cartilage and the thyroid cartilage (Fig. 1-15). The muscle has two parts. A larger, ventral section runs vertically between the cricoid and the inferior thyroid border. The smaller, oblique segment attaches to the posterior inner thyroid border and the lesser cornu of the thyroid. During swallowing, the muscle contracts and the ventral head draws the anterior part of the cricoid cartilage toward the relatively fixed lower border of the thyroid cartilage. The oblique head of the muscle rocks the cricoid lamina posteriorly. Because the arytenoids do not move, the vocal ligaments are tensed and the glottic length is increased 30%.[46,60]

The thick, posterior cricoarytenoid muscle originates near the entire posterior midline of the cricoid cartilage. Muscle fibers run superiorly and laterally to the posterior area of the muscular process of the arytenoid cartilage.[20]

TABLE 1-1

Extrinsic Muscles of the Larynx

Muscle	Function	Innervation
Sternohyoid	Indirect depressor of the larynx	Cervical plexus Ansa hypoglossi C1, C2, C3
Sternothyroid	Depresses the larynx Modifies the thyrohyoid and aryepiglottic folds	Same as above
Thyrohyoid	Same as above	Cervical plexus Hypoglossal nerve C1, C2
Thyroepiglottic	Mucosal inversion of aryepiglottic fold	Recurrent laryngeal nerve
Stylopharyngeus	Assists folding of thyroid cartilage	Glossopharyngeal
Inferior pharyngeal constrictor	Assists in swallowing	Vagus (pharyngeal plexus)

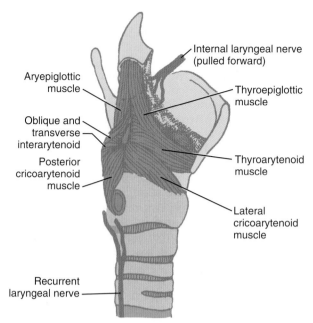

Figure 1-14 Intrinsic muscles of the larynx and their nerve supply. (Modified from Ellis H, Feldman S: *Anatomy for anaesthetists*, ed 6, Oxford, 1993, Blackwell Scientific.)

On contraction, the posterior cricoarytenoid rotates the arytenoids and moves the vocal folds laterally. The posterior cricoarytenoid is the only true abductor of the vocal folds.[36,45,46,52]

The lateral cricoarytenoid muscle joins the superior border of the lateral cricoid cartilage and the muscular process of the arytenoid. This muscle rotates the arytenoids medially, adducting the true vocal folds.[35] The unpaired transverse arytenoid muscle joins the posterolateral aspects of the arytenoids. This muscle, which is covered anteriorly by a mucous membrane, forms the posterior commissure of the larynx. Its contraction brings

the arytenoids together and ensures posterior adduction of the glottis.[35,36,45]

The oblique arytenoids (see Fig. 1-14) ascend diagonally from the muscular processes posteriorly across the cartilage to the opposite superior arytenoid and help close the glottis. Fibers of the oblique arytenoid may continue from the apex through the aryepiglottic fold as the aryepiglottic muscle, which attaches itself to the lateral aspect of the epiglottis. The aryepiglottic muscle and the oblique arytenoid act as a purse-string sphincter during deglutition.[46]

The thyroarytenoid muscle (see Fig. 1-14) is broad and sometimes is divided into three parts. It is among the fastest-contracting striated muscles.[52] The muscle arises along the entire lower border of the thyroid cartilage. It passes posteriorly, superiorly, and laterally to attach to the anterolateral surface and the vocal process of the arytenoid.

The segment of thyroarytenoid muscle that lies adjacent to the vocal ligament (and frequently surrounds it) is called the vocalis muscle. The vocalis is the major tensor of vocal fold and can "thin" the fold to achieve a high pitch. Beneath the mucosa of the fold, extending from the anterior commissure back to the vocal process, is a potential space called Reinke's space. This area can become edematous if traumatized. The more laterally attached fibers of the thyroarytenoid function as the prime adductor of the vocal folds.[46]

The most lateral section of the muscle, sometimes called the thyroepiglottic muscle, attaches to the lateral aspects of arytenoids, the aryepiglottic fold, and even the epiglottis. When it contracts, the arytenoids are pulled medially, down, and forward.[35,46] This shortens and relaxes the vocal ligament. The function and innervation of the extrinsic muscles are summarized in Table 1-1. Table 1-2 describes the intrinsic musculature of the larynx.

c. INNERVATION OF THE LARYNX

The main nerves of the larynx are the recurrent laryngeal nerves and the internal and external branches of the

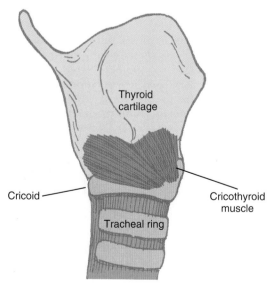

Figure 1-15 The cricothyroid muscle and its attachments. (Modified from Ellis H, Feldman S: *Anatomy for anaesthetists*, ed 6, Oxford, 1993, Blackwell Scientific.)

TABLE 1-2		
Intrinsic Muscles of the Larynx		
Muscle	**Function**	**Innervation**
Posterior cricoarytenoid	Abductor of vocal cords	Recurrent laryngeal
Lateral cricoarytenoid	Adducts arytenoids, closing glottis	Recurrent laryngeal
Transverse arytenoid	Adducts arytenoids	Recurrent laryngeal
Oblique arytenoid	Closes glottis	Recurrent laryngeal
Aryepiglottic	Closes glottis	Recurrent laryngeal
Vocalis	Relaxes the cords	Recurrent laryngeal
Thyroarytenoid	Relaxes tension cords	Recurrent laryngeal
Cricothyroid	Tensor of the cords	Superior laryngeal (external branch)

superior laryngeal nerves. The external branch of the superior laryngeal nerve supplies motor innervation to the cricothyroid muscle. All other motor supply to the laryngeal musculature is provided by the recurrent laryngeal nerve (see Fig. 1-14). The superior laryngeal and recurrent laryngeal nerves are derivatives of the vagus nerve.

The superior laryngeal nerve usually separates from the main trunk, off the inferior vagal ganglion, just outside the jugular foramen. At approximately the level of the hyoid bone, it divides into the smaller external and larger internal branches. The external branch travels below the superior thyroid artery to the cricothyroid muscle, giving off a branch to the inferior constrictor of the pharynx along the way. The internal branch travels along with the superior laryngeal artery and passes through the thyrohyoid membrane laterally between the greater cornu of the thyroid and the hyoid. The nerve and artery together pass through the pyriform recess, where the nerve may be anesthetized intraorally. The nerve divides almost immediately into a series of sensory branches and provides sensory innervation from the posterior aspect of the tongue base to as far down as the vocal cords. Sensory innervation of the epiglottis is dense, and the true vocal folds are more heavily innervated posteriorly than anteriorly.[52]

The left recurrent laryngeal nerve branches from the vagus in the thorax and courses cephalad after hooking around the arch of the aorta in close relation to the ligamentum arteriosum, at approximately the level of the fourth and fifth thoracic vertebrae. On the right, the nerve loops posteriorly beneath the subclavian artery, at approximately the first and second thoracic vertebrae, before following a cephalad course to the larynx. Both nerves ascend the neck in the tracheoesophageal groove before they reach the larynx. The nerves enter the larynx just posterior to, or sometimes anterior to, the cricothyroid articulation. The recurrent laryngeal nerve supplies all the intrinsic muscles of the larynx except the cricothyroid. The recurrent laryngeal nerve also provides sensory innervation to the larynx below the vocal cords. Parasympathetic fibers to the larynx travel along the laryngeal nerves, and the sympathetics from the superior cervical ganglion travel to the larynx with blood vessels. Tables 1-1 and 1-2 summarize the innervation of the laryngeal musculature.

GLOTTIC CLOSURE AND LARYNGEAL SPASM. Stimulation of the superior laryngeal nerve endings in the supraglottic region can induce protective closure of the glottis. This short-lived phenomenon is a polysynaptic involuntary reflex.[52] Triggering of other nerves, notably cranial nerves such as the trigeminal and glossopharyngeal, can produce a lesser degree of reflex glottic closure.[61,62] The nerve endings in the mammalian supraglottic area are highly sensitive to touch, heat, and chemical stimuli.[63] This sensitivity is especially intense in the posterior commissure of the larynx, close to where the pyriform recesses blend with the hypopharynx.[63,64] Complex sensory receptors, similar in structure to lingual taste buds, have been demonstrated here.[65] Instillation of water, saline, bases, or acids has been demonstrated to cause glottic closure in

vitro and in vivo.[66] Infants also respond to stimulation with prolonged apnea, although this response disappears later in life.[4]

The term *episodic paroxysmal laryngospasm* has been coined to describe laryngeal dysfunction that may or may not arise as a true episode of respiratory distress.[66,67] Postoperative superior laryngeal nerve injury has been reported to cause paroxysmal laryngospasm arising with stridor and acute airway obstruction. Superior laryngeal nerve blockade may be temporarily effective in some patients.[68]

Laryngospasm occurs when glottic closure persists long after removal of the stimulus.[62,64] This has led to speculation that laryngospasm represents a focal seizure of the adductors innervated by the recurrent laryngeal nerve.[69] This state is initiated by repeated superior laryngeal nerve stimulation.[62] It has been reported that the recurrent laryngeal nerve may also be responsible for laryngospasm.[70] Symptoms abate, perhaps through a central mechanism, as hypoxia and hypercarbia worsen.[71]

VOCAL CORD PALSIES. The recurrent laryngeal nerve may be traumatized during surgery on the thyroid and parathyroid glands.[14,72] Malignancy or benign processes of the neck, trauma, pressure from an ETT or a laryngeal mask airway, and stretching of the neck may also affect the nerve.[9,54,58,73] The left recurrent laryngeal nerve may be compressed by neoplasms in the thorax, aneurysm of the aortic arch, or an enlarged left atrium (mitral stenosis).[34] It may occasionally be injured during ligation of a patent ductus arteriosus. The left nerve is likely to be paralyzed twice as frequently as the right one because of its close relationship to many intrathoracic structures. Damage to the superior laryngeal nerve (external branch) during thyroidectomy is the most common cause of voice change.[74]

Under normal circumstances, the vocal cords meet in the midline during phonation (Fig. 1-16). On inspiration, they move away from each other. They return toward the midline on expiration, leaving a small opening between them. When laryngeal spasm occurs, both true and false vocal cords lie tightly in the midline opposite each other. To arrive at a clinical diagnosis, the position of the cords must be examined laryngoscopically during phonation and inspiration (Fig. 1-17; see Fig. 1-16).

The recurrent laryngeal nerve carries both abductor and adductor fibers to the vocal cords. The abductor fibers are more vulnerable, and moderate trauma causes

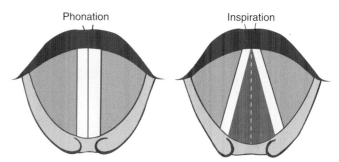

Figure 1-16 Position of vocal cords during phonation and inspiration. (From Hodder Headline PLC, London.)

Phonation   Inspiration

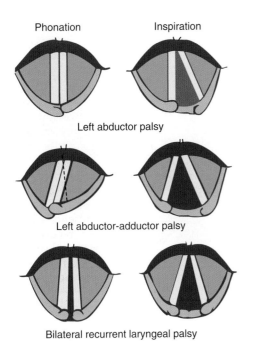

Left abductor palsy

Left abductor-adductor palsy

Bilateral recurrent laryngeal palsy

Figure 1-17 Diagrammatic representation of different types of vocal cord palsies. Notice that in complete bilateral recurrent laryngeal palsy (*bottom*), the vocal cords remain in the abducted position and the glottic opening is preserved. For details see text. (From Hodder Headline PLC, London.)

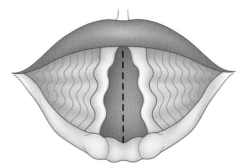

Figure 1-18 Cadaveric position of vocal cords. Notice the wavy appearance of the vocal cords. For details see text. (From Hodder Headline PLC, London.)

a pure abductor paralysis (Selmon's law).[75] Severe trauma causes both abductor and adductor fibers to be affected.[9] Pure adductor paralysis does not occur as a clinical entity. In the case of pure unilateral abductor palsy, both cords meet in the midline on phonation (because adduction is still possible on the affected side). However, only the normal cord abducts during inspiration (see Fig. 1-17). In the case of complete unilateral palsy of the recurrent laryngeal nerve, both abductors and adductors are affected. On phonation, the unaffected cord crosses the midline to meet its paralyzed counterpart, appearing to lie in front of the affected cord (see Fig. 1-17).[9] On inspiration, the unaffected cord moves to full abduction. When abductor fibers are damaged bilaterally (incomplete bilateral damage to the recurrent laryngeal nerve), the adductor fibers draw the cords toward each other, and the glottic opening is reduced to a slit, resulting in severe respiratory distress (see Fig. 1-17).[51,54] However, with a complete palsy, each vocal cord lies midway between abduction and adduction, and a reasonable glottic opening exists. Thus, bilateral incomplete palsy is more dangerous than the complete variety.

Damage to the external branch of the superior laryngeal nerve or to the superior laryngeal nerve trunk causes paralysis of the cricothyroid muscle (the tuning fork of the larynx), resulting in hoarseness that improves with time because of increased compensatory action of the opposite muscle. The glottic chink appears oblique during phonation. The aryepiglottic fold on the affected side appears shortened, and the one on the normal side is lengthened. The cords may appear wavy. The symptoms include frequent throat clearing and difficulty in raising the vocal pitch.[60] A total bilateral paralysis of vagus

nerves affects the recurrent laryngeal nerves and the superior laryngeal nerves. In this condition, the cords assume the abducted, cadaveric position.[5,9] The vocal cords are relaxed and appear wavy (Fig. 1-18).[9,60] A similar picture may be seen after the use of muscle relaxants.

Topical anesthesia of the larynx may affect the fibers of the external branch of the superior laryngeal nerve and paralyze the cricothyroid muscle, signified by a "gruff" voice. Similarly, a superior laryngeal nerve block may affect the cricothyroid muscle in the same manner as surgical trauma does. These factors must be taken into consideration when evaluating post-thyroidectomy vocal cord dysfunction after surgery.

d. BLOOD SUPPLY OF THE LARYNX

Blood supply to the larynx is derived from the external carotid and subclavian arteries. The external carotid gives rise to the superior thyroid artery, which bifurcates, forming the superior laryngeal artery. This artery courses with the superior laryngeal nerve through the thyrohyoid membrane to supply the supraglottic region. The inferior thyroid artery, derived from the thyrocervical trunk, terminates as the inferior laryngeal artery. This vessel travels in the tracheoesophageal groove with the recurrent laryngeal nerve and supplies the infraglottic larynx. There are extensive connections with the ipsilateral superior laryngeal artery and across the midline. A small cricothyroid artery may branch from the superior thyroid and cross the CTM. It most commonly travels near the inferior border of the thyroid cartilage.[46]

III. LOWER AIRWAY

A. Gross Structure of the Trachea and Bronchi

The adult trachea begins at the cricoid cartilage, opposite the sixth cervical vertebra (see Figs. 1-7 and 1-8). It is 10 to 20 cm long and 12 mm in diameter. It is flattened posteriorly and contains 16 to 20 horseshoe-shaped cartilaginous rings. At the sixth ring, the trachea becomes intrathoracic. The first and last rings are broader than the rest. The lower borders of the last ring split and curve interiorly between the two bronchi to form the carina at the level of the fifth thoracic vertebra (angle of Louis, second intercostal space). The posterior part of the trachea, void of cartilage, consists of a membrane of smooth muscle and fibroelastic tissue joining the ends of the cartilages. The muscle of the trachea is stratified with an inner circular and an outer longitudinal layer. The longitudinal bundles predominate in children but are virtually absent in adults.[45,51] Both the trachea and the proximal airways have extensive submucosal glands beneath the epithelium.[76]

It has been determined that the lengthening of the trachea during neck extension occurs mainly between the vocal cords and the sternal notch. This explains why ETTs fixed at the mouth ascend on average 2 cm in the trachea with neck extension.[77]

The tip of the tracheal tube moves toward the vocal cords, increasing the chance of accidental extubation. During flexion, the tube moves toward the carina or even the bronchus, depending on the original tube position and the extent of flexion. This is true in both adults and children.[77-79] It is therefore necessary to exercise constant vigil when the neck is moved in any direction to rule out displacement of the tube tip.

In the adult, the right main stem bronchus is wider and shorter and takes off at a steeper angle than the left main stem bronchus. Therefore, ETTs, suction catheters, and foreign bodies more readily enter the right bronchial lumen. However, the angulations of the two bronchi are almost equal in children younger than 3 years of age. The right main stem bronchus gives rise to three lobar bronchi, and the left to two. Both the main bronchi and the lower lobe bronchi are situated outside the lung substance. The large main bronchi are 7 to 12 mm in diameter; they divide into 20 bronchopulmonary divisions supplying each respective lobule's medium bronchi (4 to 7 mm) and small bronchi (0.8 to 4 mm). Bronchioles are bronchi that are smaller than 0.8 mm in diameter. Bronchioles do not have any cartilage in their walls.[46] The tracheobronchial airways occupy 1% of the lung volume, with the remaining 99% composed of large vessels and lung parenchyma.[76]

Bronchioles are of two types, terminal and respiratory. The terminal bronchioles do not bear any alveoli; they lead into the alveoli-bearing respiratory bronchioles. Each terminal bronchiole leads to three respiratory bronchioles, and each respiratory bronchiole leads to four generations of alveolar ducts (Fig. 1-19).[46] Although the diameter of each new generation of airway decreases progressively, the aggregate cross-sectional area increases. This is especially true for airways 2 mm or less in diameter, because further branching is not accompanied by concomitant decreases in caliber. The failure of the airway diameter to decrease with subsequent divisions produces the "inverted thumbtack" appearance on a graph depicting increasing surface area as a function of distance from the mouth (Fig. 1-20).[7]

The bronchi are surrounded by irregular cartilaginous rings that are similar in structure to the trachea except that the attachment of the posterior membrane is more anterior (Fig. 1-21).[47] The rings give way to discrete, cartilaginous plates as the bronchi become intrapulmonary at the lung roots (Fig. 1-22). Eventually, even these plates disappear, usually at airway diameters of approximately 0.6 mm.[47]

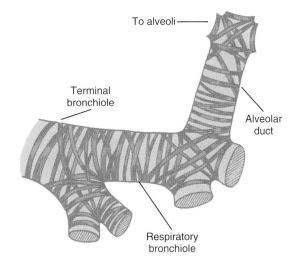

Figure 1-19 Bronchiolar division and geodesic network of muscle layer surrounding the airway. Two smooth muscle spirals run in opposite directions. This arrangement enables the muscles to constrict and shorten the airways at the same time. (Modified from Hodder Headline PLC, London.)

The rings or plates of the bronchi are interconnected by a strong fibroelastic sheath within which a myoelastic layer consisting of smooth muscle and elastic tissue is arrayed.[7] The myoelastic band is arranged in a special pattern called a geodesic network, representing the shortest distance between two points on a curved surface (see Fig. 1-19). This architectural design serves as the strongest and most effective mechanism for withstanding or generating pressures within a tube without fiber slippage along the length of the outer surface of the tube. The

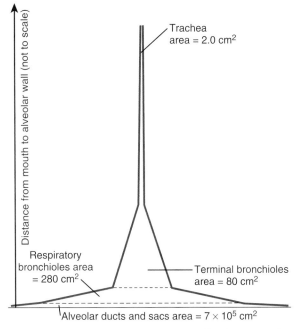

Figure 1-20 Relationship between cross-sectional area and generation of the airway. Notice the abrupt increase in cross section when the respiratory bronchiole is reached (inverted thumbtack arrangement). For details see text. (From Hodder Headline PLC, London.)

TRACHEA

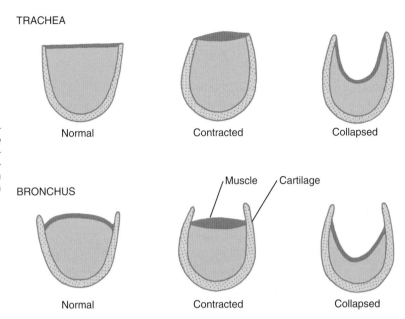

BRONCHUS

Figure 1-21 Cross-sectional view of trachea and bronchus. Notice the different sites of attachment of the posterior membrane in the tracheal and bronchial sections. Also notice the invagination of posterior membrane into the lumen in the collapsed state. (From Horsfield K: The relation between structure and function of the airways of the lung. *Br J Dis Chest* 68:145, 1974.)

network of smooth muscle runs around the airway in two opposing spirals. This arrangement helps in not only constricting the airway but shortening it.[80] The primary function of the muscular component is to change the size of the airway according to the respiratory phase. The smooth muscle tone (bronchomotor tone) is predominantly under the influence of the vagus nerve. The elastic layer runs longitudinally but encircles the bronchus at the points of division.[7]

The muscular layer becomes progressively thinner distally, but its thickness relative to the bronchial wall increases. Therefore, the terminal bronchiole with the narrowest lumen has perhaps the thickest muscle, almost 20% of the total thickness of the wall that lacks cartilaginous support.[46,47] For this reason, smaller bronchioles may be readily closed off by action of the musculature during prolonged bronchial spasm. Such an arrangement may facilitate closure of unperfused portions of the lung when a ventilation-perfusion mismatch occurs (e.g., pulmonary embolism). The smooth muscles and the glands of the cartilaginous airways are innervated by the autonomic nervous system. They are stimulated by the vagus and inhibited by sympathetic impulses derived from the upper thoracic ganglia. This smooth muscle mass can increase twofold to threefold in patients with severe asthma.[80]

B. Airway Epithelium and Airway Defense Mechanisms

The cartilaginous airways are lined by a tall, columnar, pseudostratified epithelium containing at least 13 cell types.[32] An important function of this lining is the production of mucus, a part of the respiratory defense mechanism. The mucus is steadily propelled to the outside by a conveyer belt mechanism. The large airways have a mucous secretory apparatus that consists of serous and goblet cells and submucous glands. The submucous glands empty into secretory tubules, which in turn connect with the larger connecting ducts. Several connecting ducts unite and form the ciliated duct that opens into the airway lumen. No mucous glands are present in the bronchioles.

The most numerous cells of the large airways are the ciliated epithelial cells, which bear 250 cilia per cell.[9,32] The length of the cilia decreases progressively in the smaller airways. On the surface of the cell are found small claws and microvilli. The microvilli probably regulate the volume of secretions through reabsorption, a function that may be shared with the brush cells scattered along the airways. The basal cell, more numerous in the large airways, imparts to the epithelium the pseudostratified appearance. The other cell types, except for the K cell,

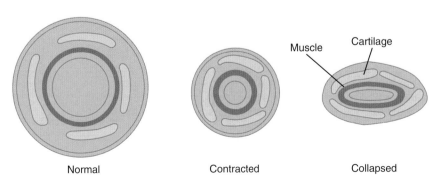

Figure 1-22 Cross-sectional views of medium bronchi (4 to 8 mm diameter) with peribronchial space. (From Horsfield K: The relation between structure and function of the airways of the lung. *Br J Dis Chest* 68:145, 1974.)

TABLE 1-3

Types of Tracheobronchial Cell

Cell	Probable Function
Epithelial	
Goblet	Mucous secretion
Serous	Mucous secretion
Ciliated	Mucous propulsion-resorption, supportive
Brush	Mucous resorption
Basal	Supportive, parent
Intermediate	Parent
Clara	Supportive, parent
Kulchitsky	Neuroendocrine; possible mechanoreceptor, chemoreceptor
Mesenchymal	
"Globule" leukocyte	Immunologic defense
Lymphocyte	Defense

Modified from Jeffrey PK, Reid L: New features of the rat airway epithelium: A quantitative and electron microscopic study. *J Anat* 120:295, 1975.

develop from the basal cell through the intermediate cell. This cell lies in the layer above the basal cell and differentiates into cells with secretory or ciliary function.[9,32,48] The K cell, or Kulchitsky-like cell, resembles the Kulchitsky cells of the gastrointestinal tract. These cells take up, decarboxylate, and store amine precursors, such as levodopa (L-dopa) and therefore are known as amine precursor uptake and decarboxylation (APUD) cells. The functions of the K cells are not definitely known, but proposed roles include mechanoreception (stretch) or chemoreception (carbon dioxide). Globule leukocytes are derived from subepithelial mast cells and interact with them to transfer immunoglobulin E to the secretions and to alter membrane permeability to locally produced or circulating antibodies. The ubiquitous lymphocytes and plasma cells defend against pathogens. Table 1-3 lists important cell types that constitute the airway epithelium.

The nonciliated bronchiolar epithelial cell, or Clara cell, largely makes up the cuboidal epithelium of the bronchioles. The Clara cells assume the role of basal cells as a stem cell in the bronchiole. Only six cell types have been recorded in the human bronchiole: the ciliated, brush, basal, K, and Clara cells and the globular leukocyte. These cells form a single-layered simple cuboidal epithelium.

C. Blood Supply

Bronchial arteries supply the bronchi and the bronchioles. Arterial supply extends into the respiratory bronchiole. Arterial anastomoses occur in the adventitia of the bronchiole. The branches enter the submucosa after piercing the muscle layer to form the submucosal capillary plexus. The venous radices arising from the capillary plexus reach the venous plexus in the adventitia by penetrating the muscle layer. When the muscle layer contracts, the arteries can maintain forward flow to the

capillary plexus. However, the capillaries cannot force the blood back into the venous plexus. Therefore, prolonged bronchial spasm can lead to mucous membrane swelling in the small airways.[7] The venous drainage of the bronchi occurs through the bronchial, azygous, hemiazygos, and intercostal veins. There is some communication between the pulmonary artery and the bronchiolar capillary plexus leading to normally occurring "anatomic shunting."

D. Function of the Lower Airway

1. Forces Acting on the Airway

Different forces act on the airway to alter its morphology continuously. These forces are modified by (1) the location of a given airway segment (intrathoracic or extrathoracic), (2) the phases of respiration, (3) lung volume, (4) gravity, (5) age, and (6) disease.[47,48]

Intrathoracic, intrapulmonary airways such as the distal bronchi and bronchioles are surrounded by a potential space, the peribronchial space (Fig. 1-23). The bronchi are untethered and therefore move longitudinally within this sheath. However, the bronchiolar adventitia is attached by an elastic tissue matrix to the adjoining elastic framework of the surrounding alveoli and parenchyma. Consequently, the bronchioles are subject to transmitted tissue forces.[9,43]

Many forces act in concert to modify the airway lumen (Fig. 1-24). The forces that tend to expand the lumen include the pressure of the gas in the bronchi bronchioles and the elastic tissue forces of the alveoli. Forces that tend to close the airway include the elasticity of the bronchial wall, which increases as the lumen expands; the forces related to bronchial muscle contraction; and the pressure of the gas in the surrounding alveoli. The

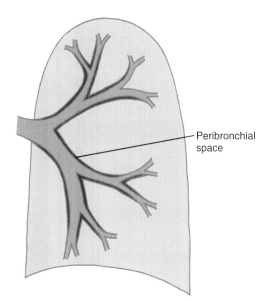

Figure 1-23 Diagram showing formation of peribronchial space by invagination of the visceral pleura. (From Horsfield K: The relation between structure and function of the airways of the lung. *Br J Dis Chest* 68:145, 1974.)

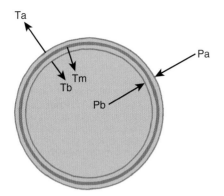

Figure 1-24 Vector diagram showing transmural forces influencing airway caliber: *Pa,* Alveolar gas pressure; *Pb,* barometric pressure; *Ta,* alveolar elastic forces; *Tb,* bronchial elastic forces; *Tm,* bronchial muscular forces. Arrow direction indicates the direction of the force. The algebraic sum of these forces determines the size of the airway lumen at any given time. (From Horsfield K: The relation between structure and function of the airways of the lung. *Br J Dis Chest* 68:145, 1974.)

algebraic sum of these forces at any given time determines the diameter of the airway.[46,47]

The lower part of the trachea and proximal bronchi are intrathoracic but extrapulmonary. Consequently, they are subject to the regular intrathoracic pressures (intrapleural pressure) but not to the tissue elastic recoil forces. The upper trachea is both extrathoracic and extrapulmonary. Although it is unaffected by the elastic recoil of the lung, it is subject to the effects of ambient pressure and cervical tissue forces.[43,47]

During spontaneous inspiration, the lung expands, which lowers the alveolar pressure more than it does the bronchial pressure, creating a pressure gradient that induces airflow. This increases the elastic retractive forces of the connective tissue and opens the intrathoracic airways. However, extrathoracic intraluminal pressure decreases relative to atmospheric pressure, with the result that the diameter of the upper trachea decreases. During expiration, alveolar pressure rises and exceeds the tissue retractive forces, thus decreasing the intrathoracic airway diameter. In this case, the extrathoracic intraluminal pressure rises above the atmospheric pressure, and the upper trachea expands. On forced expiration, alveolar pressure is greatly elevated, further reducing the diameter of the smaller airways.

The dynamic forces are altered by gravity such that the forces tending to expand the lung are greater at the top than at the bottom of the lung regardless of whether the patient is prone, supine, or erect.[49] The diameter and length of the airways of all sizes vary directly as the cube root of the lung volume varies when the lung expands.[50] On expiration below FRC, the retractive forces gradually decrease the airway size toward the point of closing volume. Because of the effect of gravity, the basal airways close first. The retractive forces of the elastic tissues decrease with aging, which explains why closing volume increases with age. This effect is exaggerated in diseases involving elastic tissue damage (e.g., pulmonary emphysema).

2. Relationship Between Structure and Function

The extent to which the retractive forces affect the airway morphology is related to the specific structure of the airway segment in question. When the fibromuscular membrane of the trachea contracts, the ends of the cartilages are approximated, and the lumen narrows in both the intrathoracic and the extrathoracic trachea. When the radial forces decrease airway diameter, the posterior membrane invaginates into the lumen (see Fig. 1-21). However, the rigid cartilaginous hoops prevent luminal occlusion. Extrapulmonary bronchi behave in a similar fashion.

The medium intrapulmonary bronchi within the peribronchial sheath are surrounded by cartilaginous plates. Although these plates add some rigidity to the wall, they do not prevent collapse, so these airways are dependent on the elastic retractive forces of the surrounding tissue (see Fig. 1-24).[47] Therefore, forced expiration can collapse many bronchioles in emphysema.

The miniature carinas at small airway bifurcations maintain airway lumens. Intrinsic bronchial muscles reduce the lumen and increase the mean velocity of the airflow during forced expiratory maneuvers, particularly in the peripheral airways with small flow rates. Here, two additional anatomic adaptations contribute to increasing flow rates. First, as the muscular ring contracts, the mucous lining is thrown into accordion-type folds that project into the lumen, further narrowing it (Fig. 1-25).[47] Second, the venous plexus situated between the muscle and the cartilage fills and invaginates into the lumen during muscle contraction. These mechanisms permit bronchoconstriction without distorting the surrounding tissues and minimize the muscular effort required to reduce the airway lumen. The drawback of such an arrangement is that even a small amount of fluid or sputum can result in complete occlusion of the small airways.[47] Therefore, it is not surprising that airway resistance is increased tremendously during an asthmatic attack that is characterized by both bronchospasm and increased secretions.[51,52,81] The small airways can also be affected by interstitial pulmonary edema, a condition in which the peribronchial space can accumulate fluid and isolate the bronchus from the surrounding retractive forces (see Fig. 1-25).

In severe asthma, thickening of the airway walls occurs due to increases in smooth muscle mass, infiltration with inflammatory cells, deposition of connective tissue, vascular changes, and mucous gland hyperplasia. Such a thickening is called *airway remodeling.* Airway remodeling occurs in milder and even asymptomatic cases of asthma. In the past, airway thickening was confirmed with the use of invasive techniques such as biopsy. More recently, scanning techniques have been used to study airway remodeling.[82] MDCT has been used to objectively assess airway remodeling in patients with severe asthma. MDCT used in conjunction with special software can yield reproducible results concerning airway remodeling, and the 3-D airway images allow for correlation of airway function with structural changes.[82] The indices of airway wall thickness measured by MDCT are inversely correlated

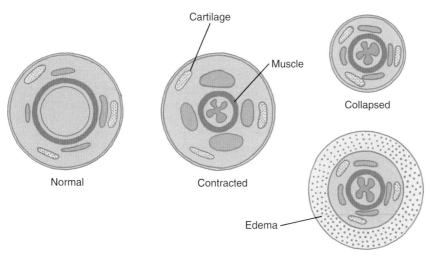

Cartilage

Muscle

Collapsed

Normal

Contracted

Edema

Interstitial pulmonary edema

Figure 1-25 Structure of small bronchi (0.8 to 4 mm in diameter). Notice that the mucous membrane is thrown into folds in contracted and collapsed states, reducing the airway lumen. Also shown is the accumulation of interstitial edema in the peribronchial space. (From Horsfield K: The relation between structure and function of the airways of the lung. *Br J Dis Chest* 68:145, 1974.)

with changes in the 1-second forced expiratory volume (FEV_1). Noninvasive measurements of airway thickness over a period of time has the ability to show responses to treatment with corticosteroids and bronchodilators.[82,83]

IV. CONCLUSIONS

This chapter describes certain salient features of the human respiratory passages as they relate to their functional anatomy in health and disease from the anesthesiologist's point of view. It also pointed out some recent advances in scanning technology that can shed light on changes in functional anatomy of the lower airway in disease states such as asthma. It is necessary for students of anesthesia to possess some knowledge of the structures that they will most frequently use as a passageway to care of patients in their professional career.

V. CLINICAL PEARLS

- Cricoarytenoid arthritis can lead to airway difficulties in patients with rheumatoid arthritis or systemic lupus erythematosus.

- To diagnose vocal cord dysfunction, it is necessary to examine the position of the vocal cords during inspiration and phonation.

- The recurrent laryngeal and superior laryngeal nerves may be injured during thyroid surgery, leading to severe vocal cord dysfunction.

- A bilateral partial recurrent nerve palsy is more dangerous than complete palsy.

- Neck movement during anesthesia can result in movement of the tip of the endotracheal tube (ETT).

- New imaging techniques such as virtual endoscopy and multidetector computed tomography (MDCT) are providing added insight into the structure and function of the airways in health and disease.

- Upper airway obstruction in sedated patients occurs at the level of soft palate and not at the level of the tongue.

SELECTED REFERENCES

All references can be found online at expertconsult.com.

3. Pohunek P: Development, structure and function of the upper airways. *Paediatr Respir Rev* 5:2–8, 2004.
23. Patil SP, Schneider H, Schwartz AR, Smith PL: Adult obstructive sleep apnea: Pathophysiology and diagnosis. *Chest* 132:325–337, 2007.
24. Isono S: Obstructive sleep apnea of obese adults: Pathophysiology and perioperative airway management. *Anesthesiology* 110:908–921, 2009.
28. Nishino T: Physiological and pathophysiological implications of upper airway reflexes in humans. *Jpn J Physiol* 50:3–14, 2000.
29. Rowe MR, D'Antonio LL: Velopharyngeal dysfunction: Evolving developments in evaluation. *Curr Opin Otolaryngol Head Neck Surg* 13:366–370, 2005.
47. Kolman J, Morris I: Cricoarytenoid arthritis: A cause of acute upper airway obstruction in rheumatoid arthritis. *Can J Anaesth* 49:729–732, 2002.
55. Thomas BP, Strother MK, Donnelly EF, Worrell JA: CT virtual endoscopy in the evaluation of large airway disease: Review. *AJR Am J Roentgenol* 192:S20–S30, 2009.
72. Fewins J, Simpson CB, Miller FR: Complications of thyroid and parathyroid surgery. *Otolaryngol Clin North Am* 36:189–206, 2003.
76. Hyde DM, Hamid Q, Irvin CG: Anatomy, pathology, and physiology of the tracheobronchial tree: Emphasis on the distal airways. *J Allergy Clin Immunol* 124:S72–S77, 2009.
77. Wong DT, Weng H, Lam E, et al: Lengthening of the trachea during neck extension: Which part of the trachea is stretched? *Anesth Analg* 107:989–993, 2008.

Chapter 2

Airway Imaging: Principles and Practical Guide

T. LINDA CHI | DAVID M. MIRSKY | JACQUELINE A. BELLO | DAVID Z. FERSON

I. INTRODUCTION

Interpretation of radiologic studies is not usually in the domain of anesthesiologists. However, imaging studies can provide a wealth of information regarding the airway. This information can be aptly used for formulating an anesthetic plan. Currently, radiology is not part of the curriculum of any anesthesia residency training program; for this reason, most anesthesiologists have only rudimentary skills in the interpretation of radiologic studies. The main goal of this chapter is to introduce anesthesiologists to normal airway anatomy as visualized on conventional radiography (plain x-ray films) and on cross-sectional imaging such as computed tomography (CT) and magnetic resonance imaging (MRI) and to illustrate the anatomic variants and pathologic processes that can compromise the airway. The technical aspects of each

imaging modality are reviewed briefly. Emphasis is placed on evaluation of the airway using available radiologic studies, which are most often performed for non-airway issues. Relevant information regarding the airway is readily available and ranges from conventional chest radiographs to high-resolution cross-sectional imaging of the neck or chest by CT or MRI. The clinical examples in this chapter focus on the pathologic processes involving the airway that are most relevant to anesthesiologists and include short discussions of some of the more common abnormalities.

Simplistically, the airway can be regarded as a tubular conduit for air inhaled from the nares to the tracheobronchial tree. The soft tissue structures bordering the airway have warranted more of the radiologist's attention. The integrity of the airway with its natural contrast is usually referenced with respect to extrinsic impression, compression, encroachment, or displacement. Segmentation of the airway into compartments (i.e., head and neck, chest) is artificial and is usually done only for the ease of discussion. However, imaging of this airspace as a unique entity is gaining popularity. Knowledge of the technical differences among imaging modalities can aid in ordering and interpreting the imaging study. This is especially important when selecting a study that will best depict the anatomic structures and pathologic processes of the airway.

II. IMAGING MODALITIES

A. Conventional Radiography (Plain Film)

Wilhelm Conrad Roentgen, a German physicist, discovered x-rays on November 8, 1895, while studying the behavior of cathode rays (electrons) in high-energy cathode ray tubes. By serendipity, he noticed that a mysterious ray that escaped the cathode tube penetrated objects differently, and he named this the *x-ray*. For his work, he was awarded the first Nobel Prize for Physics in 1901.[1]

X-rays are a type of electromagnetic radiation; as the name implies, they transport energy through space as a combination of electric and magnetic fields. Other types of electromagnetic radiation include radio waves, radiant heat, and visible light. In diagnostic radiology, the predominant energy source used for imaging is ionizing radiation (i.e., alpha, beta, gamma, and x-rays). The science of electromagnetic waves and x-ray generation is very complex and exceeds the scope of this text. In principle, x-rays are produced by energy conversion as a fast stream of electrons is suddenly decelerated in an x-ray tube.[2] The localized x-ray beam that is produced passes through the part of the body being studied. The final image is dependent on the degree of attenuation of the beam by matter.

Attenuation is the reduction in the intensity of the beam as it traverses matter of different constituents. It is caused by absorption or deflection of photons from the beam. The transmitted beam determines the final image, which is represented in shades of gray.[3–5] The lightest or brightest area on the film or image represents the greatest attenuation of the beam by tissue and the least amount of beam transmitted to film. For example, bone is a high-density material that attenuates much of the x-ray beam; images of bone on x-ray films are very bright or white. A plain film image is a one-dimensional collapsed or compressed view of the body part being imaged. This information can also be presented in a digital format without the use of traditional x-ray films.

Compared with other, more sophisticated imaging modalities, conventional radiography has limited range in the display of tissues of different density and spatial resolution. Its advantages are lower cost of the examination, overall lower radiation exposure compared with a more comprehensive CT examination, and presentation of anatomy with a larger field of view. The head, chest, abdomen, or extremity can be visualized on a single film or digitized image, and therefore the image appears more familiar to nonradiologists. Also, the plain x-ray film can be obtained quickly at the patient's bedside in any location in the hospital. The combination of x-radiography with cine mode allows radiologists to obtain dynamic images, which are used to evaluate organ function (e.g., barium swallow to evaluate deglutition, intravenous pyelogram to assess renal function, vascular studies).

B. Computed Tomography

After the discovery of x-rays, it became apparent that images of the internal structures of the human body could yield important diagnostic information. However, the usefulness of x-ray studies is limited because they project a three-dimensional (3-D) object onto a two-dimensional display. With x-rays, the details of internal objects are masked by the shadows of overlying and underlying structures. The goal of diagnostic imaging is to bring forth the organ or area of interest in detail while eliminating unwanted information. Various film-based traditional tomographic techniques were developed, culminating in the creation of computerized axial tomography or computed tomography (CT).[6] The first clinically viable CT scanner was developed by Hounsfield and commercially marketed by EMI Limited (Middlesex, England) for brain imaging in the early 1970s.[7] Since then, several generations of CT scanners have been developed.

As with conventional plain film radiography, CT technology requires x-rays as the energy source. Whereas conventional radiography employs a single beam of x-rays from a single direction and yields a static image, CT images are obtained with the use of multiple collimated x-ray beams from multiple angles, and the transmitted radiation is counted by a row or rows of detectors. The patient is enclosed in a gantry, and a fan-shaped x-ray source rotates around the patient. The radiation counted by the detectors is analyzed with the use of mathematical equations to localize and characterize tissues by density and attenuation measurements. A single cross-sectional image is produced with one rotation of the gantry.[6] The gantry must then "unwind" to prepare for the next slice while the table carrying the patient moves forward or backward by a distance that is predetermined by slice thickness. An intrinsic limitation of this technique is the time required for moving the mechanical parts.

The introduction of slip-ring technology in the 1990s and the development of faster computers, high-energy x-ray tubes, and multidetectors enabled continuous activation of the x-ray source without having to unwind the gantry and also allowed continuous movement of the tabletop. This process, known as *helical CT*, is used in the latest generation of CT scanners. Because the information acquired using helical CT is volumetric, in contrast to the single slice obtained with conventional CT, the entire thorax or abdomen can be scanned in a single breath-hold. Volumetric information makes it possible to identify small lesions more accurately and allows better 3-D reformation. Because of the higher speed of data acquisition, misregistration and image degradation caused by patient motion are no longer significant concerns. This is especially important when scanning uncooperative patients and trauma victims. The absorbed radiation dose used in multidetector helical CT (as compared with conventional single-detector row CT) is dependent on the scanning protocol and varies with the desired high-speed or high-quality study.[8]

Practically speaking, CT examinations have become routine. The spatial resolution of CT is the best of all the imaging modalities currently available. The advantage of CT technology is that it can depict accurately any pathology involving bones. Data acquisition is very quick. CT can be used to produce images in all three planes and to provide information for surface rendering and 3-D reformation, which allows the display of organs in an anatomic format that can be easily recognized by clinicians.

C. Magnetic Resonance Imaging

MRI has become one of the most widely used imaging modalities in diagnostic radiology. In contrast to conventional radiography and CT, MRI uses no ionizing radiation. Instead, imaging is based on the resonance of the atomic nuclei of certain elements such as sodium, phosphorus, and hydrogen in response to radio waves of the same frequency produced in a static magnetic field environment. Current clinical MRI units use protons from the nuclei of hydrogen atoms to generate images because hydrogen is the most abundant element in the body. Every water molecule contains two hydrogen atoms, and larger molecules, such as lipids and proteins, contain many hydrogen atoms. Powerful electromagnets are used to create a magnetic field, which influences the alignment of protons in hydrogen atoms in the body. When radio waves are applied, protons are knocked out of natural alignment, and when the radio wave is stopped, the protons return to their original state of equilibrium, realigning to the steady magnetic field and emitting energy, which is translated into weak radio signals. The time it takes for the protons to realign, referred to as a *relaxation time*, is dependent on the tissue composition and cellular environment.[9] The different relaxation times and signal strengths of the protons are processed by a computer, generating diagnostic images. With MRI, the chemical and physical properties of matter are examined at the molecular level. The relaxation times for each tissue type, designated T1 and T2, are expressed as constants at a given magnetic field strength. Imaging that optimizes T1 or T2 characteristics is referred to as T1-weighted or T2-weighted imaging, respectively. Tissue response to pathologic processes usually includes an increase in bound water (edema), which lengthens the T2 relaxation time and appears as a bright focus on T2-weighted images.[9]

MRI is more sensitive, but not necessarily more specific, in detecting pathology than CT, which depicts anatomy with unparalleled clarity. Imaging with MRI provides metabolic information at the cellular level, allowing one to link organ function and physiology to anatomic information. MRI and CT technologies also have other differences: (1) MRI shows poor bony detail, whereas CT provides excellent images of bony structures; (2) hemorrhage, especially if acute, is clearly visible on CT scans but may be difficult to diagnose with MRI because the appearance of blood varies temporally to the evolution of the breakdown products of hemoglobin; and (3) MRI is very susceptible to all types of motion artifacts, ranging from a patient's movement, breathing, swallowing, and phonation to vascular and cerebral spinal fluid pulsation and flow.

MRI scanners operate in a strong magnetic field environment, and strict precautions must be observed. Any item containing ferromagnetic substances that is introduced into the magnetic field environment can become a projectile and result in deleterious consequences for patients, personnel, and the MRI scanner itself. Therefore, no metal objects should be brought into the MRI suite if one is not absolutely certain about their composition. Only specially designed nonferromagnetic equipment is used in the MRI suite, including anesthesia machines, monitoring equipment, oxygen tanks, poles for intravenous equipment, infusion pumps, and stretchers. Pagers, telephones, handheld organizers and computers, credit cards, and analog watches must also be removed, because the strong magnetic field can cause malfunction or permanent damage to them. Patients must be carefully screened for implantable pacemakers, intracranial aneurysm clips, cochlear implants, and other metallic foreign objects before entering the MRI environment.

III. BASICS OF PLAIN FILM INTERPRETATION

To illustrate the usefulness of conventional radiography in evaluating the airway, this discussion focuses on the interpretation of plain films of the cervical spine, chest, and neck. Before the CT era, these were probably the most frequently ordered x-ray studies in the hospital setting, and they are ubiquitous in patients' film jackets and on picture archiving communication systems (PACS). As a composite, these studies provide a picture of the entire airway. Although these radiologic studies are usually obtained for reasons other than airway evaluation, it is actually in the group of patients who are "normal" or "cleared for surgery" that one may glean important observations about the airway. The anatomy and pathology displayed by plain film radiographs may alert the anesthesiologist to potential difficulties in securing the patient's airway and help him or her to develop an alternative anesthetic plan. In this sense, the information about the airway that is inherent to these x-ray examinations is gratuitous. The following sections address the basics of plain film interpretation with respect to imaging of the airway anatomy and pathology.

A. Cervical Spine Radiography

1. General Technique, Anatomy, and Basic Interpretation

The cervical spine connects the skull to the trunk; it articulates with the occiput above and the thoracic vertebrae below. The bony elements, muscles, ligaments, and intervertebral discs support and provide protection to the spinal cord. On plain films, one can appreciate the bony morphology of the vertebrae and the disc spaces and assess the alignment of the vertebral column very quickly. This indirectly provides information regarding the integrity of the ligaments, which are crucial in maintaining alignment of the cervical spine. However, individual ligaments and muscle groups all have the same or similar attenuation and cannot be differentiated from one another on plain film. A systematic approach is recommended to evaluate the spine for bony integrity, alignment, cartilage, joint space, and soft tissue abnormalities. The disadvantages of cervical spine radiography are the limited range of tissue attenuation and the loss of spatial resolution caused by overlapping bone structures.

The most common indications for obtaining cervical spine radiographs in today's medical practice are for the evaluation of trauma, spinal stability, and cervical spondylosis and in the search for radiopaque foreign bodies. Different views of the cervical spine are tailored to each clinical need. The most common views are the lateral, anteroposterior (AP), open-mouth odontoid, oblique, and pillar views (Fig. 2-1). In acute cervical spine injury, cross-table lateral, AP, and open-mouth odontoid views are recommended. A lateral view reveals the majority of injuries (Fig. 2-2); however, patients who are rendered quadriplegic by severe ligamentous injuries may demonstrate a normal lateral cervical spine radiograph. When the AP and then the open-mouth odontoid views are added to the cross-table lateral view of the cervical spine, the sensitivity of detecting significant injury is increased from 74% to 82% and then to 93%.[10] In today's practice, cross-sectional imaging (i.e., CT of the spine) has become a mainstay in the evaluation of the cervical spine, especially in the setting of acute trauma. MRI is particularly useful in evaluating the spinal cord.

In brief, a normal lateral cervical radiograph should demonstrate seven intact vertebrae and normal alignment of the anterior and posterior aspects of the vertebral bodies. This is especially important for trauma victims, because 7% to 14% of fractures are known to occur at the C7 or C7-T1 level.[11] The posterior vertebral body line is more reliable and must be intact. The anterior vertebral line is often encumbered by the presence of anterior osteophytes. Normal facet joints overlap in an orderly fashion, similar to shingles on a rooftop. The spinolaminar line, which is the dense cortical line representing the junction of the posterior laminae and the posterior spinous process, is uninterrupted. Relative uniformity of the interlaminar (interspinous) distances should be observed. The posterior spinal line (i.e., posterior cervical line), an imaginary line extending from the spinolaminar line of the atlas to C3 (Fig. 2-3), should demonstrate a continuous curve in parallel to the posterior vertebral body line; the distance between the two correlates with the spinal canal diameter.[12]

The anatomy and integrity of the craniocervical junction are crucial to the anesthesiologist. To achieve successful and safe endotracheal intubation, the anterior atlantodental interval (AADI), the vertical and anterior-posterior position of the dens, and the degree of extension of the head on the neck must be considered. The anterior arch of C1 bears a constant relationship to the dens; this is the AADI or predental space. It is defined as the space between the posterior surface of the anterior arch of C1 and the anterior surface of the dens. In flexion, because of the physiologic laxity of the cervicocranial ligaments, the anterior tubercle of the atlas assumes a more normal-appearing relationship to the dens, and the AADI increases in width, greater rostrally than caudally. In children and with flexion in adults, the AADI is normally about 5 mm. In adults, it is generally accepted that the AADI is 3 mm or less (Fig. 2-4).[12]

The bony structures of the atlantoaxial joint provide mobility (e.g., rotational movement) rather than stability. Therefore, the ligaments play a significant role in stability. The most important ligaments in the upper cervical spine are the transverse ligament, the alar ligaments, and the tectorial membrane. If the transverse ligament is disrupted and the alar and apical ligaments remain intact, up to 5 mm of movement at the atlantoaxial joint can be seen.[13] If all the ligaments have been disrupted, the AADI can measure 10 mm or larger. In atlantoaxial subluxation, the dens is invariably displaced posteriorly, which causes narrowing of the spinal canal and potential impingement of the spinal cord. The space available for the spinal cord is defined as the diameter of the spinal canal as measured in the AP plane, at the C1 level, that is not occupied by the odontoid process. In the normal spine, this space is approximately 20 mm.[13]

2. Pertinent Findings and Pathology

a. PSEUDOSUBLUXATION AND PSEUDODISLOCATION

Pseudosubluxation and *pseudodislocation* are terms applied to the physiologic anterior displacement of C2 on C3 that is frequently seen in infants and young children (Fig. 2-5). Physiologic anterior displacement of C2 on C3 and of C3 on C4 occurs in 24% and 14%, respectively, of children up to 8 years of age.[14]

In pediatric trauma cases, if C2 is anteriorly displaced and there are no other signs of trauma such as posterior arch fracture or prevertebral soft tissue hematoma, the spinolaminar lines of C1 through C3 should have a normal anatomic relationship. In a neutral position, the spinolaminar line of C2 lies on or up to 1 mm anterior or posterior to the imaginary posterior spinal line. If the C2 vertebra is intact, as the C2 body glides forward with respect to C3 during flexion, the spinolaminar line of C2 moves 1 to 2 mm anterior to the posterior spinal line. Similarly, with extension, the posterior translation of the C2 body is mirrored by similar posterior displacement of the spinolaminar line of C2 with respect to the posterior spinal line.

In traumatic spondylolisthesis, which is rare in children but more common in adults, the C2 body would translate anteriorly in flexion and posteriorly in extension, and the posterior spinal line would be maintained because of intact ligaments. However, flexion and extension films are not advisable if traumatic spondylolisthesis is suspected.

b. CONGENITAL AND DEVELOPMENTAL ANOMALIES

OCCIPITAL FUSION OF C1. Important to rigid laryngoscopy and endotracheal intubation is the distance between the

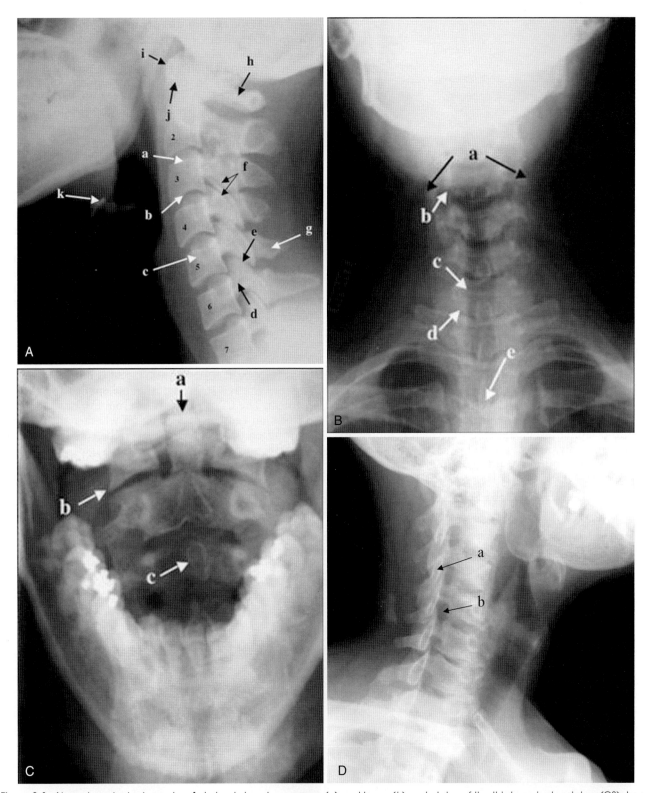

Figure 2-1 Normal cervical spine series. **A,** Lateral view shows upper (*a*) and lower (*b*) end plates of the third cervical vertebra (C3), transverse process (*c*), pedicle (*d*), facet joint (*e*), articulating facets (*f*), posterior spinous process (*g*), posterior arch of C1 (*h*), anterior arch of C1 (*i*), atlantoaxial distance (*j*), and hyoid bone (*k*). **B,** Anteroposterior view shows smoothly undulating cortical margins of the lateral masses (*a*), joint of Luschka (*b*), superior (*c*) and inferior (*d*) end plates, and a midline posterior spinous process (*e*). **C,** Open-mouth odontoid view shows the odontoid tip (*a*), centered between the lateral masses of the axis; symmetrical lateral margins of the lateral atlantoaxial joints (*b*); and a spinous process (*c*). **D,** Oblique view shows laminae of the articular masses (*a*), reflecting the shingling effect, and an intervertebral (neural) foramen (*b*).

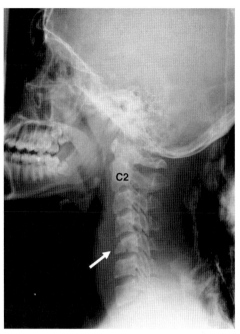

Figure 2-2 Cervical spine fracture. Lateral radiograph of the cervical spine demonstrates a compression fracture of the C5 vertebra (*arrow*). A retropulsed fragment impinges on the spinal canal.

head extension and contributes to difficult intubation.[13,15] Occipitalization of C1 with the occiput (atlanto-occipital fusion) not only limits head extension but also adds stress to the atlantoaxial joint. Although the majority of head extension occurs at the atlanto-occipital joint, some extension can also occur at C1-C2.[15] Nichol and Zuck observed that in patients with limited or no extension possible at the atlanto-occipital joint, general extension of the head actually brings the larynx "anterior," thus limiting the visibility of the larynx on laryngoscopy.[15]

NONFUSION OF ANTERIOR AND POSTERIOR ARCHES OF C1. Ossification of the atlas begins with the lateral masses during intrauterine life. At birth, neither the anterior nor the posterior arches are fused. Fusion of the anterior arch is complete between 7 and 10 years of age. During the second year, the center of the posterior tubercle appears, and by the end of the fourth year, the posterior arch becomes complete.[12] Nonfusion of the anterior or the posterior arch, or both, exists as a normal variant in adults and should not be mistaken for fracture (Fig. 2-7).

occiput and the posterior tubercle of C1, known as the atlanto-occipital distance (Fig. 2-6), which is quite variable from individual to individual. Head extension is limited by the abutment of the occiput to the posterior tubercle of C1. It has been proposed that a shorter atlanto-occipital distance decreases the effectiveness of

PSEUDOFRACTURES OF C2 AND DENS. The second cervical vertebra, the axis (C2), is the largest and heaviest cervical segment. The C2 vertebra arises from five or six separate ossification centers, depending on whether the centrum has one or two centers. The vertebral body is ossified at birth, and the posterior arch is partially ossified. They fuse posteriorly by the second or third year of life and unite with the body of the vertebra by the seventh year.

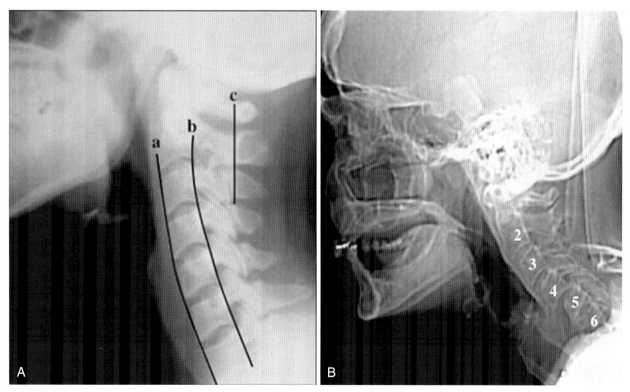

Figure 2-3 Normal lateral cervical spine radiograph **(A)** demonstrates normal alignment. *a,* Anterior spinal line; *b,* posterior vertebral line; *c,* posterior spinal line. **B,** Lateral scout view of a computed tomography scan demonstrates anterior subluxation of C4 on C5.

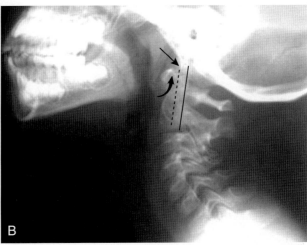

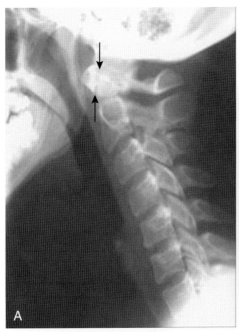

Figure 2-4   Anterior atlantodental interval (AADI). **A,** Lateral radiograph of the cervical spine in an adult patient. The AADI or predental space *(arrows)* is normally less than 3 mm. **B,** Lateral radiograph of the cervical spine in a pediatric patient. An AADI of up to 5 mm *(curved arrow)* can be normal in a child. The basion, the midpoint of the anterior border of the foramen magnum, is indicated by the *straight* arrow. The *dotted line* is an imaginary line indicating the inferior extension from the basion, and the posterior axial line is indicated by the *solid line.* The distance between the dotted line and the solid line is the basion-axial interval (BAI); it should be 12 mm or less for a normal occipitovertebral relationship in a child.

The odontoid process (dens) serves as the conceptual body of C1, around which the atlas rotates and bends laterally. In contrast to the other cervical vertebrae, C2 does not have a discrete pedicle. The dens is situated between the lateral masses of the atlas and is maintained in its normal sagittal relationship to the anterior arch of

Figure 2-5   Pseudosubluxation at C2-C3. T2-weighted sagittal magnetic resonance cervical spine study demonstrates physiologic anterior displacement of C2 on C3 in a child. Also seen are normal soft tissue masses encroaching on the airway from adenoids *(a),* palatine tonsils *(b),* and lingual tonsils at the base of the tongue *(c).*

C1 by several ligaments, the most important of which is the transverse atlantal ligament. Superiorly, the dentate (apical) ligament extends from the clivus to the tip of the dens. Alar ligaments secure the tip of the dens to the occipital condyles and to the lateral masses of the atlas. They are the second line of defense in maintaining the proper position of the dens. The tectorial membrane is a continuum of the posterior longitudinal ligament from the body of C2 to the upper surface of the occipital bone anterior to the foramen magnum.

The dens ossifies from two vertically oriented centers that fuse by the seventh fetal month. Cranially, a central cleft separates the tips of these ossification centers (Fig. 2-8), and it can mimic a fracture if ossification is incomplete. The ossiculum terminale, the ossification center for the tip of the dens, may be visible on plain films, conventional tomograms, or CT scans and unites with the body by age 11 or 12 years. Failure of the ossiculum terminale to develop or failure to unite with the dens may result in a bulbous cleft dens tip. A nonunited terminal dental ossification center, called the *os terminale,* may be mistaken for a fracture of the odontoid tip.

HYPOPLASIA OF C2. The position and anatomy of the dens with respect to the anterior arch of C1 and the foramen magnum are worthy of attention. Congenital anomalies of the odontoid process, such as hypoplasia, can result in a loss of the buttressing action of the dens during extension and subsequent compression of neural elements. Examples of conditions that are associated with odontoid hypoplasia are the Morquio, Klippel-Feil, and Down syndromes; neurofibromatosis; dwarfism; spondyloepiphyseal dysplasia; osteogenesis imperfecta; and congenital scoliosis.[13,16] Patients with these conditions are

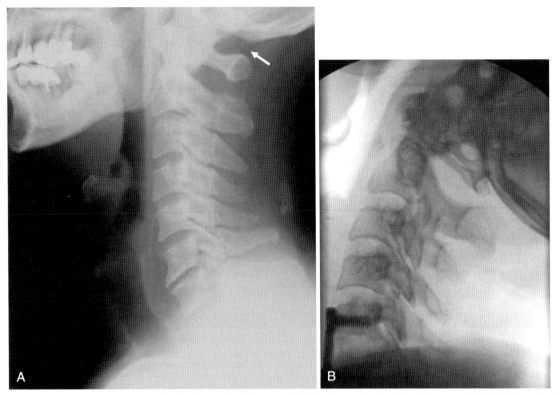

Figure 2-6 Atlanto-occipital distance. **A,** Lateral radiograph of the cervical spine in neutral position; the *arrow* indicates the atlanto-occipital distance. **B,** Lateral radiograph of the cervical spine in hyperextension. Head extension is limited by the abutment of the occiput to the posterior tubercle of C1.

predisposed to atlantoaxial subluxation and craniocervical instability, and hyperextension of the head for intubation should be avoided. In addition, congenital fusion of C2 and C3 (Fig. 2-9), whether occurring as an isolated anomaly or as part of Klippel-Feil syndrome, places added stress at the C1-C2 junction.

c. ACQUIRED PATHOLOGY

CERVICAL SPONDYLOSIS. Cervical spine radiographs are obtained for the evaluation of cervical spondylosis

(Fig. 2-10). The hypertrophic bone changes associated with this condition are well depicted on radiographic studies. Large anterior osteophytes that project forward may cause dysphagia and difficult intubation. The bone canal and neural foramina are assessed for stenosis; if stenosis is present, precautions can be taken when hyperextending

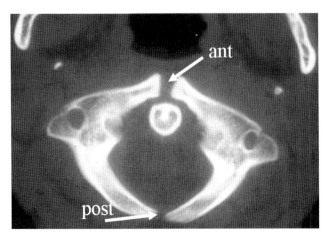

Figure 2-7 Nonfused anterior (*ant*) and posterior (*post*) arches of C1, normal variant (axial computed tomogram with bone algorithm).

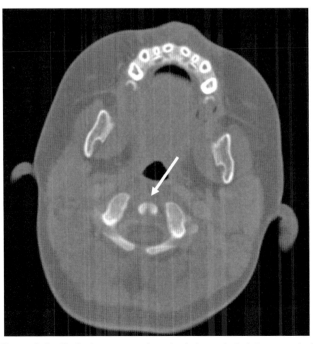

Figure 2-8 Cleft dens, normal variant (*arrow*) (axial computed tomogram with bone algorithm).

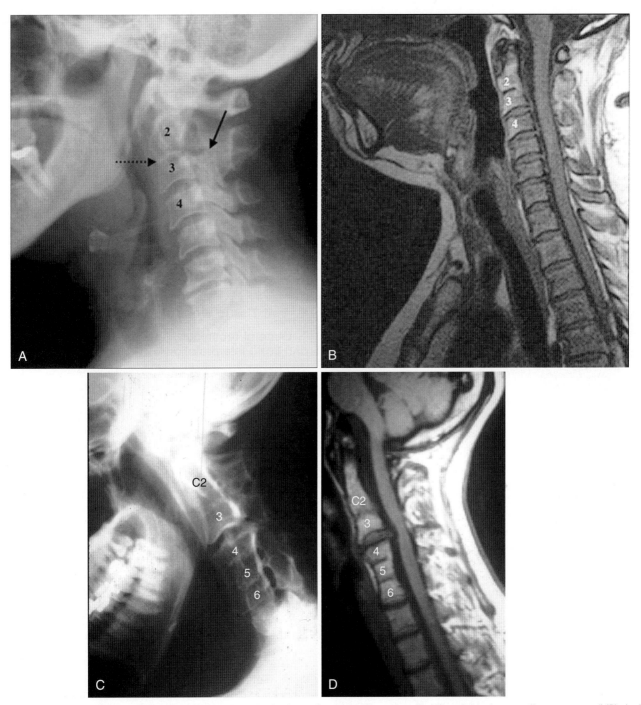

Figure 2-9   Congenital fusion of C2 and C3. Lateral cervical spine radiograph **(A)** and sagittal T1-weighted magnetic resonance (MR) study **(B)** demonstrate fusion of the C2 and C3 vertebral bodies *(dotted arrow)* and their lateral and posterior elements *(solid arrow)*. Lateral radiograph **(C)** and T1-weighted MR cervical spine study **(D)** of a patient with Klippel-Feil syndrome demonstrate fusion of C2 to C3 and fusion of C4 to C6. Not surprisingly, a disc herniation is present at the point of greatest mobility at C3-C4.

the neck and positioning the patient to avoid exacerbation of baseline neurologic symptomatology. Calcification and ossification are well depicted on radiographic studies.

Ossification of the anterior longitudinal ligament and diffuse idiopathic skeletal hyperostosis have been reported as causes of difficult intubation.[17] This can be readily appreciated on plain films. Another condition that may signal difficult intubation is calcification of the stylohyoid ligament (Fig. 2-11).[18]

INFLAMMATORY ARTHROPATHIES. Inflammatory arthropathies involving the atlantoaxial joint with subluxation are classically seen in patients with rheumatoid arthritis or ankylosing spondylitis. However, the underlying causes of atlantoaxial subluxation are quite different in these two entities. Ankylosing spondylitis is characterized by progressive fibrosis and ossification of ligaments and joint capsules. In rheumatoid arthritis, bone erosion, synovial overgrowth, and destruction of the ligaments occur.

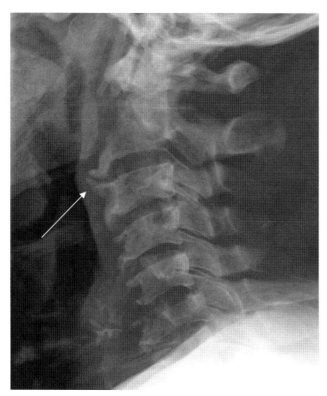

Figure 2-10 Cervical spondylosis. Lateral cervical spine radiograph demonstrates large anterior osteophytes *(arrow)* that indent the airway and oropharynx.

Patients with rheumatoid arthritis are not only susceptible to AP subluxation at the C1-C2 junction but also at risk for vertical subluxation of the dens. Whether this condition is referred to as "cranial settling," superior migration of the odontoid process, or basilar invagination, the end result is the same.[12] The odontoid process protrudes above the foramen magnum, narrowing the available space for the spinal cord and potentially leading to cord compression with the slightest head extension (Fig. 2-12).[13]

In response to the effective foreshortening of the spine that occurs secondary to the superior migration of the odontoid process from inflammatory or degenerative disease, there is acquired rotational malalignment between the spine and larynx.[19] The larynx and the trachea, because they are semirigid structures and as a result of the tethering effect of the arch of the aorta as it passes posteriorly over the left main bronchus, are predictably displaced caudally, deviated laterally to the left, rotated to the right, and anteriorly angulated. The effective neck length can be affected by superior migration of the dens, severe spondylosis with loss of disc space, or iatrogenic causes secondary to surgery. The soft tissues of the pharynx become more redundant owing to the relative shortening of the neck, which further obscures the view of the larynx. On laryngoscopy, the vocal cords are rotated clockwise. A rotated airway is suspected when the frontal view of the cervical spine demonstrates a deviated tracheal air column.

d. ANTHROPOLOGIC MEASUREMENTS

Historically, bony landmarks other than the spine that can be appreciated on a lateral cervical spine radiograph have been used in the anesthesia arena to preoperatively predict difficult laryngoscopy and endotracheal intubation on the basis of anatomic factors. Mandibular size, the ratios of the various measurements, and their relationship to the hyoid bone have been proposed as predictors of difficult laryngoscopy (Fig. 2-13).[20] These measurements are meant to reflect the oral capacity, the degree of mouth opening, and the level of larynx.[21,22] It is apparent that the causes of difficult laryngoscopy and endotracheal intubation are multifactorial. Combined with the clinical examination, anatomic measurements and findings assessed by x-ray studies can help alert the anesthesiologist to a potentially difficult airway. In this way, difficult laryngoscopy and endotracheal intubation can be anticipated and not unexpected.

B. Soft Tissue Neck Radiography

1. General Technique, Anatomy, and Basic Interpretation

The lateral cervical spine study with bone and soft tissue technique allows an incidental view of the aerodigestive tract and a gross assessment of the overall patency of the airway. Useful ossified cartilage or bony landmarks of the pharynx and larynx that can be appreciated on the lateral neck radiograph are the hard palate, hyoid bone, thyroid, and cricoid cartilages (Fig. 2-14). The hard palate is a bony landmark used to separate the nasopharynx from the oropharynx. The larynx can be thought of as being suspended from the hyoid bone. Muscles acting on the hyoid bone elevate the larynx and provide the primary protection from aspiration. The largest cartilage in the neck is the thyroid cartilage, which along with the cricoid cartilage acts as a protective shield for the inner larynx. The cricoid cartilage is the only complete cartilaginous ring in the respiratory system. It is located at the level where the larynx ends and the trachea begins.

Normal air-filled structures seen on lateral plain films are the nasopharynx, oropharynx, and hypopharynx. Air in the pharynx outlines the soft palate, uvula, base of the tongue, and nasopharyngeal airway (Fig. 2-15). Any sizable soft tissue pathology results in deviation or effacement of the airway. The tongue constitutes the bulk of the soft tissues at the level of the oropharynx. In children, and sometimes in adults, prominent lymphatic tissues such as adenoids and palatine tonsils may encroach on the nasopharyngeal and oral airways. Lingual tonsils are located at the base of the tongue above the valleculae, which are air-filled pouches between the tongue base and the free margin of the epiglottis.

The epiglottis is an elastic fibrocartilage shaped like a flattened teardrop or leaf that tapers inferiorly and attaches to the thyroid cartilage. The epiglottis tends to be more angular in infants than in adults. During the first several years of life, the larynx changes its position in the neck.[23,24] The free edge of the epiglottis in neonates is found at or near the C1 level, and the cricoid cartilage, representing the most caudal portion of the larynx, is at

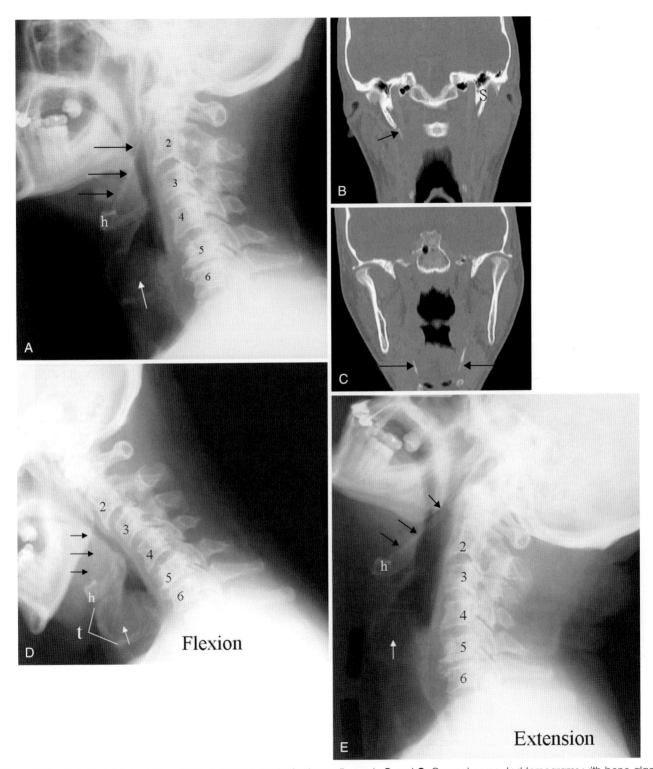

Figure 2-11 Calcified stylohyoid ligament. **A,** Lateral cervical spine radiograph. **B** and **C,** Coronal computed tomograms with bone algorithm. Lateral cervical spine flexion **(D)** and extension **(E)** views are also shown. *Black arrows* indicate calcified stylohyoid ligaments, and *white arrows* indicate the laryngeal ventricle (at the level of the vocal cords). Notice the change in the level of the hyoid bone and vocal cords with flexion and extension of the neck. *h,* Hyoid bone; *s,* styloid process; *t,* calcified thyroid cartilage.

the C4-C5 level. By adolescence, the epiglottis is found at the C2-C3 level and the cricoid is at the C6 level. The adult epiglottis is usually seen at the C3 level, with the cricoid at C6-C7. However, the position of these structures in the normal population varies by at least one vertebral body level.

Sometimes visualized by a cervical spine radiographic study with soft tissue neck technique or on the CT scout view or the MR sagittal view of the neck is a transversely oriented, air-containing lucent stripe, located just below the base of the aryepiglottic folds, which indicates the position of the air-filled laryngeal ventricle

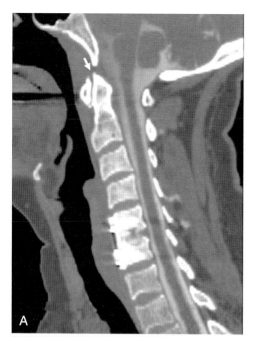

Figure 2-12 Position of the dens in a normal patient **(A)**, in a rheumatoid patient **(B)**, and in a nonrheumatoid patient with basilar invagination and platybasia **(C)**. **A,** Postmyelography computed tomogram with sagittal reformation demonstrates normal relationship of the dens with respect to the foramen magnum, brainstem, and anterior arch of C1. A normal atlantoaxial distance (AADI) is seen (*arrow*). **B,** T1-weighted sagittal magnetic resonance (MR) study of the cervical spine in a rheumatoid patient with erosion and pannus formation at the atlantoaxial joint resulting in increased AADI (*arrow*), posterior subluxation of the dens, and brainstem compression. **C,** Sagittal MR study of the brain in a nonrheumatoid patient shows normal AADI, but basilar invagination and platybasia have resulted in vertical subluxation of the dens and brainstem compression. The line drawn from the hard palate to the posterior lip of the foramen magnum is Chamberlain's line (*dotted line*); basilar invagination is defined as extension of the odontoid tip 5 mm or more above this line. Also notice the fusion of the C2 and C3 vertebrae. The small, linear, dark line at the mid-C2 level is the subdental synchondrosis (*white arrow*).

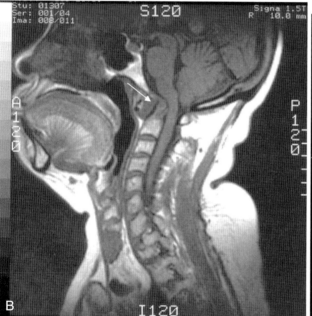

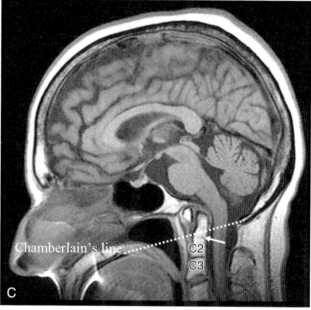

(Fig. 2-16). This marks the position of the true vocal cords, which are just below this lucent stripe. Lateral to the aryepiglottic fold is the pyriform sinus of the pharynx. This anterior mucosal recess lies between the posterior third of the thyroid cartilage and the aryepiglottic fold. The extreme lower aspect of the pyriform sinus is situated between the mucosa-covered arytenoids and the mucosa-covered thyroid cartilage, at the level of the true vocal cords. The air column caudally represents the cervical trachea. On the AP view, the false and true vocal cords above and below the laryngeal ventricles may be identified, as well as the subglottic region and the trachea.

The landmarks dorsal to the airway are shadows representing the normal soft tissue structures of the posterior wall of the nasopharynx, which is closely adherent to the anterior surface of the atlas and the axis and extends superiorly to the clivus and inferiorly to become continuous with the soft tissues of the posterior wall of the hypopharynx. The ligaments of the cervicocranium are critical to maintaining stability throughout this region; they are directly involved in the range of motion of the cervicocranium and anteriorly contribute to the prevertebral soft tissue shadow. Superimposed on these deep structures are the constrictor muscles and the mucosa of the posterior pharyngeal wall. The cervicocranial prevertebral soft tissue contour should normally be slightly posteriorly concave rostral to the anterior tubercle of C1, anteriorly convex in front of the anterior tubercle, and

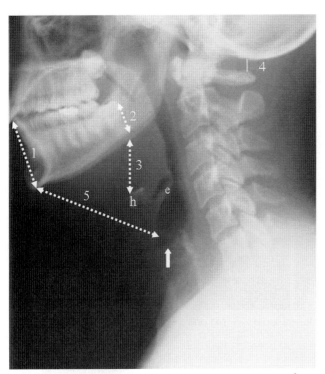

Figure 2-13   Mandibular and hyoid measurements proposed as predictors of difficult laryngoscopy: *1,* Anterior depth of mandible; *2,* posterior depth of mandible; *3,* mandibulohyoid distance; *4,* atlanto-occipital distance; *5,* thyromental distance. Laryngeal ventricle *(solid arrow)* demarcates the level of the larynx. The true vocal cords are just below the level of the laryngeal ventricle. *e,* Epiglottis; *h,* hyoid bone.

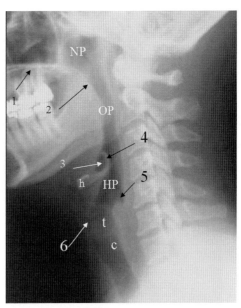

Figure 2-15   Normal airway structures seen on a lateral cervical spine radiograph: *1,* Hard palate; *2,* soft palate and uvula; *3,* air-filled vallecula; *4,* epiglottis; *5,* air-filled pyriform sinus; *6,* air-filled stripe of laryngeal ventricle; *C,* noncalcified cricoid cartilage; *h,* hyoid bone; *HP,* hypopharynx; *NP,* nasopharynx; *OP,* oropharynx; *t,* thyroid cartilage.

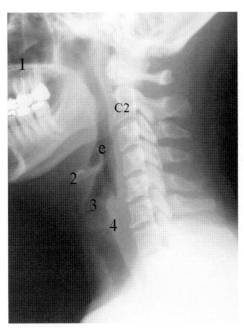

Figure 2-14   Normal bony landmarks on a lateral cervical spine radiograph: *1,* Hard palate; *2,* hyoid bone; *3,* calcified thyroid cartilage; *4,* calcified cricoid cartilage; *e,* epiglottis.

posteriorly concave caudal to the anterior tubercle, depending on the amount of adenoidal tissue and on the amount of air in the pharynx.

Adenoidal tissue appears as a homogeneous, smoothly lobulated mass of varying size and configuration. The anterior surface of the adenoid is demarcated by air anteriorly and inferiorly. The air inferior to the adenoids allows differentiation between adenoids and the presence of a nasopharyngeal hematoma, which is commonly associated with major midface fractures. In infants and young children, the soft tissues of the cervicocranium are lax and redundant. Depending on the phase of respiration and position, the thickness of the prevertebral soft tissues may appear to increase and may simulate a retropharyngeal hematoma. This finding may extend to the lower cervical spine. This anomaly becomes normal if imaging is repeated with the neck extended and during inspiration. By 8 years of age, the contour of the soft tissues should resemble that seen in adults. Of note, in pediatric patients, sedation may result in a decrease in AP diameter of the pharynx at the level of the palatine tonsils, in the soft palate, and at the level of the epiglottis.

In the lower neck (C3 to C7), the prevertebral soft tissue shadow differs from that in the cervicocranium because of the presence of the beginning of the esophagus and the prevertebral fascial space, which are recognized on the lateral radiograph as a fat stripe. By standard anatomic description, the esophagus begins at the level of C4; however, in vivo, the esophageal ostium may normally be found as high as C3 or as low as C6 and varies with the phase of swallowing and the flexion and extension of the cervical spine.[25] The prevertebral soft tissue thickness, the distance between the posterior pharyngeal

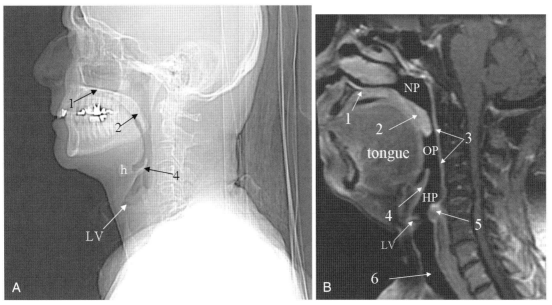

Figure 2-16 Normal airway structures seen on a computed tomographic lateral scout view **(A)** and on a T1-weighted, fat-suppressed post-contrast sagittal magnetic resonance cervical spine study **(B)**: *1*, Hard palate; *2*, soft palate and uvula; *3*, retropharyngeal or prevertebral soft tissue; *4*, epiglottis; *5*, arytenoid prominence; *6*, trachea air column; *h*, hyoid bone; *HP*, hypopharynx; *LV*, laryngeal ventricle; *NP*, nasopharynx; *OP*, oropharynx.

air column and the anterior portion of the third or fourth vertebra, should not exceed one half to three quarters of the diameter of the vertebral body. In the opinion of Harris and Mirvis, only the measurement at C3 is valid, and it should not exceed 4 mm (Fig. 2-17).[12]

More caudally, at the cervicothoracic junction, assessment of the prevertebral soft tissues is based on contour rather than actual measurement. This contour should parallel the arch formed by the anterior cortices of the lower cervical and upper thoracic vertebral bodies.

In truth, plain film diagnosis of upper airway diseases has been supplanted by cross-sectional imaging, except in a few situations in which plain radiographic findings are pathognomonic of the disease. Two classic examples of plain film radiologic diagnosis are acute epiglottitis and croup.

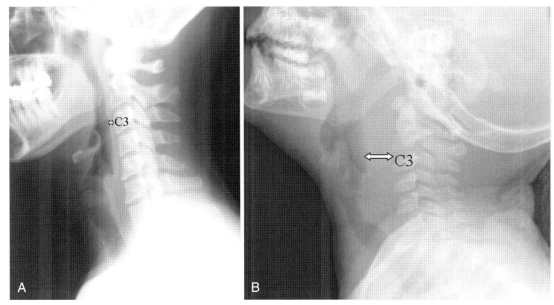

Figure 2-17 Prevertebral soft tissues seen on lateral cervical spine radiographic studies. **A,** Normal adult. **B,** Retropharyngeal abscess in a child. The arrow points to the anteriorly displace airway and increase in the prevertebral space between the vertebral column and the airway. (Courtesy of Dr. Alan Schlesinger, Texas Children's Hospital, Houston, TX.)

2. Classic Plain Film Diagnosis

a. ACUTE EPIGLOTTITIS

In acute epiglottitis (or supraglottitis, a more encompassing term), there is edema and swelling of the epiglottis with or without involvement of the aryepiglottic folds and arytenoids. The offending organism is usually *Haemophilus influenzae*. Airway compromise with a rapidly progressive course requiring emergency tracheostomy is a possibility if the entity goes unrecognized and untreated. In general, the infection is milder in adults than in children. This entity, usually a more indolent form, is making a comeback among patients with acquired immunodeficiency syndrome (AIDS).

The findings on plain film are swelling or enlargement of the epiglottis. On the conventional lateral radiograph of the neck, thickening of the free edge of the epiglottis can be appreciated and is referred to as the "thumb sign" (Fig. 2-18). The width of the adult epiglottis should be less than one third of the AP width of the C4 body. Cross-sectional imaging is superfluous. However, the degree of airway compromise can theoretically be quantified by 3-D reformation.

b. LARYNGOTRACHEOBRONCHITIS OR CROUP

In laryngotracheobronchitis or croup, the subglottic larynx is involved. This condition affects younger children and has a less fulminant course than acute epiglottitis. The swelling of the soft tissues in the subglottic neck can be appreciated on an AP view of the neck (Fig. 2-19). There is usually a long segment narrowing of the glottis and subglottic airway with loss of the normal angle

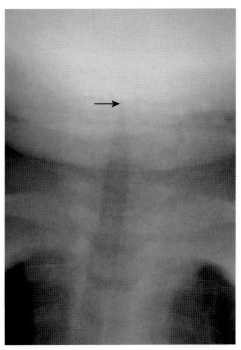

Figure 2-19 Croup. Anteroposterior soft tissue neck radiograph in an infant. Long segment narrowing of the subglottic airway is present *(arrow)* with loss of the normal angle between the vocal cords and the subglottic airway ("steeple sign"). (Courtesy of Dr. Alan Schlesinger, Texas Children Hospital, Houston.)

between the vocal cords and the subglottic airway. This has been referred to as the "steeple sign." The hypopharynx is usually dilated because of the airway obstruction distally.

c. FOREIGN BODY

Plain films are usually obtained in the initial assessment of suspected foreign body ingestion. In children, up to 50% of witnessed foreign body ingestions are asymptomatic.[26] Most foreign bodies are radiopaque, but wood and plastic usually are not visible on plain films. The radiopacity of ingested fishbone varies with the type of fish.[27] In the neck, ingested foreign bodies most often lodge at the level of the pyriform sinus (Fig. 2-20).

C. Chest Radiography

1. General Technique

Before the advent of CT, chest radiography was routinely ordered to assess pulmonary and cardiovascular status, and it is still a cost-efficient examination that yields a great deal of general information. The most common views of the chest are the posteroanterior (PA), anteroposterior (AP), and lateral projections (Fig. 2-21). The PA chest view is obtained with the patient's anterior chest closest to the film cassette and the x-ray beam directed from a posterior to an anterior direction. Alternatively, the AP chest view is done with the patient's back closest to the film cassette and the x-ray beam directed in the anterior to posterior direction. The part of the chest closest to the film cassette is the least magnified; therefore, the cardiac silhouette is larger on the AP projection.

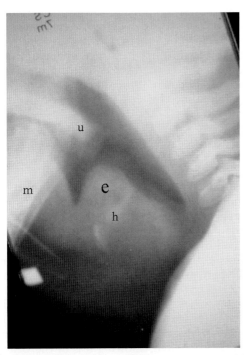

Figure 2-18 Epiglottitis. Lateral soft tissue examination of the neck during flexion in a child demonstrates an enlarged and swollen epiglottis ("thumb sign"). *e,* Epiglottis; *h,* hyoid; *m,* mandible; *u,* uvula. (Courtesy of Dr. Alan Schlesinger, Texas Children's Hospital, Houston.)

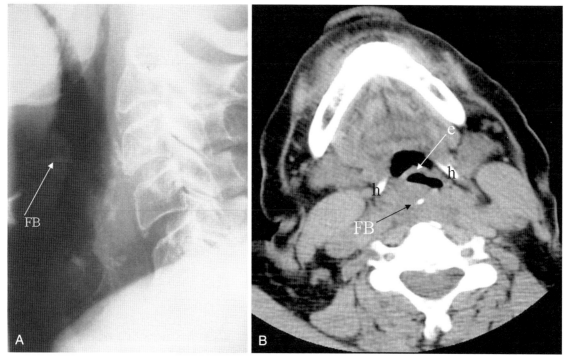

Figure 2-20 Foreign body, fishbone. **A,** Lateral radiograph of the cervical spine. **B,** Axial computed tomogram of the neck in a different patient. *e,* Tip of the epiglottis; *FB,* fishbone; *h,* hyoid.

The lateral projection is most often performed with the patient's left chest closest to the film cassette for better delineation of the structures in the left hemithorax, which is more obscured by the heart on a PA projection.

Other common projections include the oblique, decubitus, and lordotic views. The oblique view is useful for assessing a lesion with respect to other structures in the chest. The decubitus view is helpful to assess whether an apparent elevated hemidiaphragm is being caused by a large subpulmonic pleural effusion. The lordotic view is helpful to look for a suspected small apical pneumothorax, which can also be accentuated on an expiratory-phase examination.

It is useful to train one's eyes to analyze the chest radiograph systematically to cover the details of the chest wall, including the ribs, lungs (field and expansion), and mediastinal structures such as the heart and the outline of the tracheal-bronchial tree. On an adequate inspiratory film, the hemidiaphragms are below the anterior end of the sixth rib, or at least below the 10th posterior rib, and the lung expansion should be symmetrical. The right hemidiaphragm is usually half an interspace higher than the left, which is depressed by the heart (see Fig. 2-21A). Without doubt, the art of chest radiograph interpretation has diminished since the advent of CT, which demonstrates chest pathology with unparalleled clarity. However, chest radiography can still provide a composite survey of the chest at one quick glance. One can easily compare the lung volumes, identify the position of the mediastinum, determine the presence or absence of major airspace disease, and make a gross assessment of the cardiac status.

2. Interpretation of Pertinent Findings

a. LEVEL OF DIAPHRAGM

A high hemidiaphragm implies reduced lung volume, which can result from phrenic nerve paralysis, thoracic conditions causing chest pain that leads to splinting, or extrapulmonic processes such as an enlarged spleen or liver, pancreatitis, or subphrenic abscess. The presumed level of the hemidiaphragm is seen as an edge or transition between the aerated lungs and the opacity of the organs in the abdomen. If the thin leaves of the hemidiaphragm are outlined by air, a pneumoperitoneum should be considered (Fig. 2-22).

b. LUNG AERATION

A well-expanded lung should appear radiographically lucent but be traversed by "lung markings," thin threads of interstitium consisting of septa and arterial, venous, and lymphatic vessels. In most normal individuals, the lungs appear more lucent at the top owing to the distribution of the pulmonary vasculature, the effect of gravity, and overlying soft tissues such as breast tissues. In patients with congestive heart failure or pulmonary venous hypertension, this pattern is reversed, with "cephalization" and engorgement of the pulmonary veins in the upper lung zones (Fig. 2-23; also see Fig. 2-21D). In general, any process such as fluid, pus, or cells that replaces the airspaces of the lungs causes the x-ray beam to be more attenuated, allowing less of the beam to be transmitted through the patient to the film. This causes the affected areas to appear less dark or more opaque (white) on the film. A whole host of diseases could be responsible, depending on the clinical picture, including

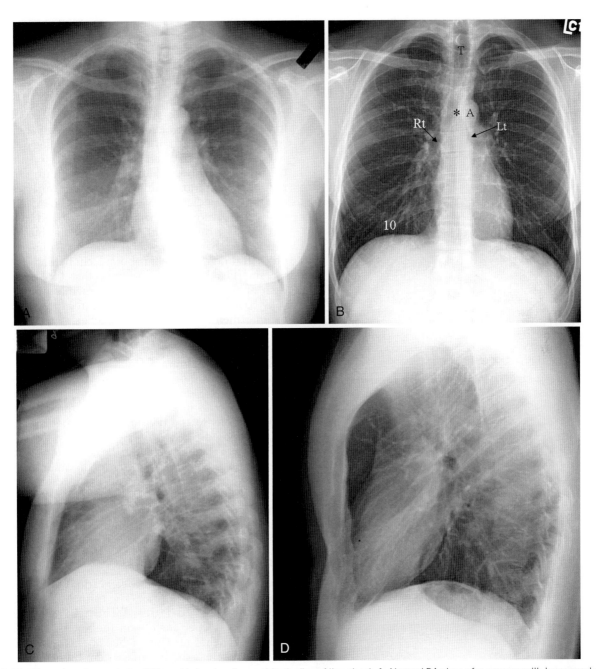

Figure 2-21   Normal posteroanterior (PA) and lateral radiographic studies of the chest. **A,** Normal PA view of a woman with increased density at the lung bases related to overlying breast tissues. **B,** PA view of a man with lucent lungs. **C,** Normal lateral chest view. **D,** Lateral view of a patient with chronic obstructive pulmonary disease showing barrel-shaped chest with increased retrosternal air; notice that the lung base appears progressively more lucent overlying the dorsal spine. The carina is indicated by an *asterisk. 10,* 10th posterior rib; *A,* aorta; *Lt,* left bronchus; *Rt,* right bronchus; *T,* trachea.

pleural effusion, pulmonary edema, pneumonia, lung mass, lung collapse or atelectasis, lung infarct or contusion, and metastatic disease (Fig. 2-24). The key from an anesthesiologist's point of view is not to make the correct pathologic diagnosis but to note the abnormality, which may affect ventilation, and adjust the anesthetic practice accordingly.

In contrast to the increased opacity of the lung caused by the preceding conditions is a hemithorax, which appears too lucent and devoid of the expected lung markings. Two entities should be considered. Foremost is a

pneumothorax (Fig. 2-25); if the pneumothorax is large, the collapsed lung will be medially applied against the mediastinum. If the mediastinum is shifted away from the midline, a *tension pneumothorax* may be present, and emergent management is required. More often than not, the cause is the presence in patients with chronic obstructive pulmonary disease of large emphysematous blebs, which are sometimes difficult to differentiate from a moderate to large pneumothorax.

More rare causes of a unilateral lucent lung are pulmonary oligemia with decreased pulmonary flow from a

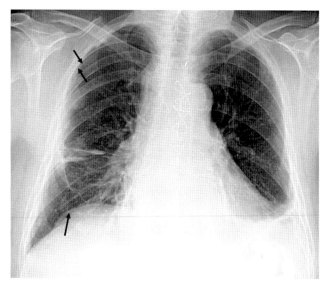

Figure 2-22 Pneumoperitoneum. Postoperative anteroposterior chest radiograph after thoracotomy. *Arrows* in right upper chest demarcate the thin pleural line defining a tiny pneumothorax. *Arrow* in right lower chest indicates the right hemidiaphragm outlined by a small pneumoperitoneum. This patient also has cardiomegaly and right midlung and left basilar atelectasis.

thromboembolism of the right or left pulmonary artery, pulmonary neoplasm, and obstructive hyperinflation. Bilateral lucent lungs are harder to appreciate. These are usually seen in patients with pulmonary stenosis secondary to cyanotic heart disease and right-to-left shunts. A discussion of the pediatric chest and congenital heart and lung diseases is beyond the scope of this chapter.

c. MEDIASTINUM AND HEART

The mediastinum lies centrally in the chest and contains the hila, tracheobronchial tree, heart and great vessels, lymph nodes, esophagus, and thymus. The mediastinum

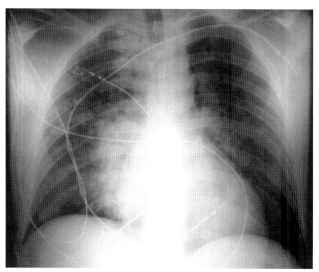

Figure 2-23 Congestive heart failure. Anteroposterior chest radiograph demonstrates engorgement of the perihilar vasculature. An endotracheal tube and a nasogastric tube are in place.

is extrapleural and is outlined by air in the adjacent lungs. Except for the air within the trachea and the main stem bronchi, the remainder of the mediastinal structures are soft tissues or of water density (including the fat) on conventional chest radiographs. Therefore, it is extremely difficult to localize a mediastinal lesion. Traditional pleural reflections or vertical lines have been described for a frontal chest radiograph that, if deviated, would suggest the presence of mediastinal pathology.

Felson proposed a radiologic approach to subdividing the mediastinum on a lateral radiograph into three compartments: anterior, middle, and posterior.[28] The anterior and middle mediastinum are divided by an imaginary line that extends along the back of the heart and front of the trachea. The middle and posterior mediastinal compartments are separated by a similar line that connects a point on each thoracic vertebra about 1 cm behind its anterior margin (Fig. 2-26).[28] Conditions that can be found in each of the compartments of the mediastinum are logically based on the anatomic structures found within the compartment. For example, tracheal, esophageal, and thyroid lesions would lie in the middle mediastinum. Neurogenic tumors and spinal problems would be in the posterior mediastinum. Cardiac and thymic lesions would occupy the anterior mediastinum. Certain diseases such as lymph node disorders, lymphoma, and aortic aneurysms may arise in any or all three compartments. Many modifications to the divisions of the mediastinum have been proposed.[29]

The great vessels and the heart should be centrally located on the AP view of the mediastinum. The aortic knob is usually on the left, and the cardiothoracic ratio on the AP view is roughly less than 50%. The hila are composed of the pulmonary arteries and their main branches, the upper lobe pulmonary veins, the major bronchi, and the lymph glands (Fig. 2-27).

d. TRACHEOBRONCHIAL TREE

The positions of the trachea, carina, and main stem bronchi are outlined by air. The carinal bifurcation angle is typically 60 to 75 degrees.[29] The right main stem bronchus has a steeper angle than the left (see Fig. 2-21); it usually branches off the trachea at an angle of 25 to 30 degrees, whereas the left main stem bronchus leaves the trachea at a 45- to 50-degree angle. The trachea is a tubular structure that extends from the cricoid cartilage to the carina, which is located approximately at the T5 level. C-shaped hyaline cartilage rings, which can calcify with age, outline the trachea anteriorly. The posterior trachea is membranous. The mean transverse diameter of the trachea is approximately 15 mm for women and 18 mm for men.[29] The trachea in the cervical region is midline, but it is deviated to the right in the thorax.

ENDOTRACHEAL TUBE POSITIONING. Adequate positioning of an endotracheal tube (ETT) in an intubated patient is usually documented by obtaining a chest radiograph. The tip should be intrathoracic and at a distance above the carina that ensures equal ventilation to both lungs. One should evaluate the position of the ETT with the patient's head and neck in a neutral position; however, this may not be possible in an intensive care unit setting. The tip

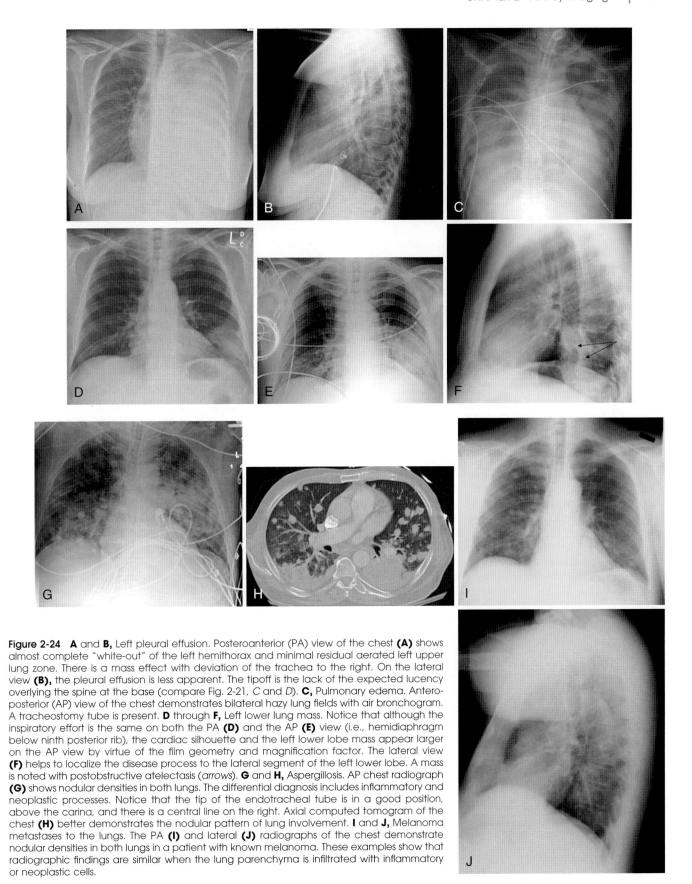

Figure 2-24 **A** and **B,** Left pleural effusion. Posteroanterior (PA) view of the chest **(A)** shows almost complete "white-out" of the left hemithorax and minimal residual aerated left upper lung zone. There is a mass effect with deviation of the trachea to the right. On the lateral view **(B),** the pleural effusion is less apparent. The tipoff is the lack of the expected lucency overlying the spine at the base (compare Fig. 2-21, *C* and *D*). **C,** Pulmonary edema. Antero-posterior (AP) view of the chest demonstrates bilateral hazy lung fields with air bronchogram. A tracheostomy tube is present. **D** through **F,** Left lower lung mass. Notice that although the inspiratory effort is the same on both the PA **(D)** and the AP **(E)** view (i.e., hemidiaphragm below ninth posterior rib), the cardiac silhouette and the left lower lobe mass appear larger on the AP view by virtue of the film geometry and magnification factor. The lateral view **(F)** helps to localize the disease process to the lateral segment of the left lower lobe. A mass is noted with postobstructive atelectasis (*arrows*). **G** and **H,** Aspergillosis. AP chest radiograph **(G)** shows nodular densities in both lungs. The differential diagnosis includes inflammatory and neoplastic processes. Notice that the tip of the endotracheal tube is in a good position, above the carina, and there is a central line on the right. Axial computed tomogram of the chest **(H)** better demonstrates the nodular pattern of lung involvement. **I** and **J,** Melanoma metastases to the lungs. The PA **(I)** and lateral **(J)** radiographs of the chest demonstrate nodular densities in both lungs in a patient with known melanoma. These examples show that radiographic findings are similar when the lung parenchyma is infiltrated with inflammatory or neoplastic cells.

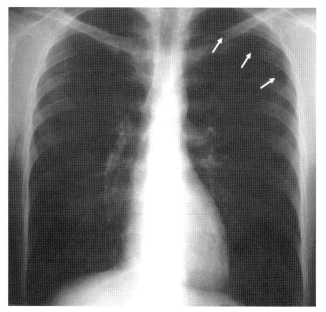

Figure 2-25 Pneumothorax. Posteroanterior chest radiograph in a young man with spontaneous pneumothorax *(arrows)*. (Courtesy of Dr. John Pagani, IRPA, Houston.)

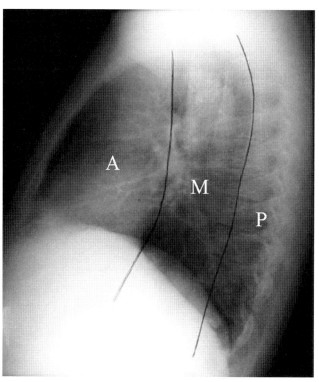

Figure 2-26 Mediastinal compartments. Lateral chest radiograph with imaginary lines drawn on the film to demonstrate the three mediastinal compartments. The anterior *(A)* and middle *(M)* mediastinal compartments are divided by a line extending along the back of the heart and front of the trachea. A line connecting each thoracic vertebra about 1 cm behind its anterior margin separates the middle from the posterior *(P)* mediastinal compartment.

of the ETT may move up or down by 1 to 2 cm with flexion or extension of the head. Rotation of the head and neck usually results in ascent of the tip.[29] The optimal position of the tip of the ETT is 3 to 5 cm above the carina, to allow enough latitude in movement of the tube with turning of the patient's head, and the inflated cuff should be below the vocal cords (Fig. 2-28).[30] Malpositioning of the cuff at the level of the vocal cords or pharynx increases the risk of aspiration. Overinflation of the cuff at the level of the vocal cords may lead to necrosis.[31] The inflated cuff of the ETT should fill the tracheal air column without changing its contour. Overall, the ETT size should be about two thirds of the diameter of

the tracheal lumen. At times, the tip of the ETT extends beyond the carina, resulting in intubation of the right main bronchus, which can be detected by asymmetrical breath sounds or on chest radiographs. If this condition goes unrecognized, atelectasis in the underaerated lung may result (Fig. 2-29).

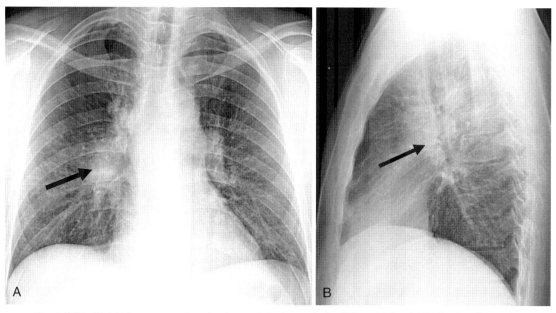

Figure 2-27 Right hilar mass and nodes *(arrows)*. Posteroanterior **(A)** and lateral **(B)** chest radiographs.

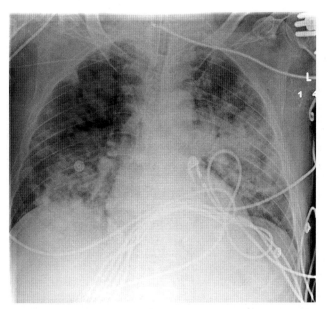

Figure 2-28 Anteroposterior (AP) portable chest radiograph. Most chest examinations in the intensive care unit are obtained with a portable x-ray machine in the AP projection. Notice the acceptable position of the ETT above the carina. A right subclavian central venous line is present with the tip in the superior vena cava. Multiple cables attached to monitors are crossing the chest.

NASOGASTRIC TUBE POSITIONING. If a nasogastric or orogastric tube is in place, it should more or less course inferiorly and to the left, toward the fundus of the stomach in the left upper quadrant, except for the unusual case of situs inversus. If the gastric tube has inadvertently intubated the bronchus, the errant course of the tube will be evident on the plain film.

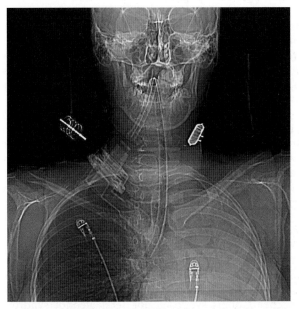

Figure 2-29 Endotracheal tube (ETT) in right main bronchus. Anteroposterior (AP) computed tomographic (CT) scout view obtained for CT soft tissue neck study reveals errant ETT in right main bronchus resulting in nonaeration of the left lung (white lung).

IV. CROSS-SECTIONAL ANATOMY AND PATHOLOGY: COMPUTED TOMOGRAPHY AND MAGNETIC RESONANCE IMAGING

The anatomy of the airway from the nasal cavity to the lungs is exceptionally well depicted by CT, and MRI can be a useful complement in the evaluation of these regions. MRI is superior to CT in the evaluation of tumor infiltration of soft tissues but lacks the ability to depict bone erosions secondary to tumor because cortical bone gives no MRI signal. Infiltration of the bone marrow and gross destruction of bone are appreciable on MRI. MRI takes longer to perform and therefore is susceptible to motion artifacts, including breathing and vascular pulsation artifacts, whereas spiral CT technology allows the entire neck or thorax to be scanned in a single breath-hold. Both techniques allow either direct scanning or 3-D volume acquisition with multiplanar postprocessing and reformation capabilities.

A. Midface

The development of the face, nose, and sinuses is complex but systematic. Therefore, the occurrence of congenital lesions and malformations in these areas is quite logical and predictable, depending on the time of prenatal insult. Face, nose, and sinus development is temporally and spatially related to the development of the optic nerve, globe, and corpus callosum, and this accounts for the frequency of concurrent anomalies in these regions.

The major features of the face develop during the fourth to eighth week of gestation as a result of the growth, migration, and merging of a number of processes bordering on the stomodeum, which is a slitlike invagination of the ectoderm that marks the location of the mouth. At the fourth gestational week, one unpaired and two paired prominences, derivatives of the first branchial arch, can be identified bordering the stomodeum. The unpaired median frontonasal prominence is located superiorly, the paired maxillary processes are lateral, and the paired mandibular processes are inferior.[32] The various cleft lip and palate and cleft face syndromes can be explained by the failure of these different processes to grow, migrate, and merge properly.[32]

Relevant to anesthetic practice is an awareness that midline craniofacial dysraphism can be categorized into two groups: an inferior group, in which the clefting primarily affects the upper lip, with or without the nose, and a superior group, in which the clefting primarily affects the nose, with or without involvement of the forehead and the upper lip. It is the inferior group that is associated with basal encephalocele (i.e., sphenoidal, sphenoethmoid, and ethmoid encephaloceles), callosal agenesis, and optic nerve dysplasias. The superior group is characterized by hypertelorism, a broad nasal root, and a median cleft nose, with or without a median cleft upper lip. The superior group is also associated with an increased incidence of frontonasal and intraorbital encephaloceles (Fig. 2-30).[32] The presence of these phenotypic features should alert the anesthesiologist to the possibility of an encephalocele intruding into the nasal cavity, and caution

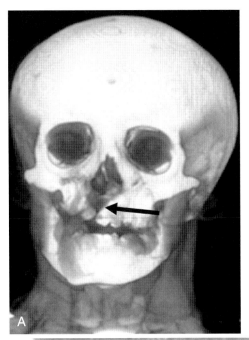

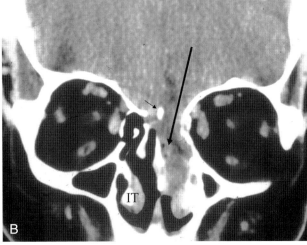

Figure 2-30 **A,** Cleft lip. Three-dimensional computed tomographic (CT) reconstruction demonstrates a bone cleft of the maxilla (*arrow*) resulting in communication between the nasal and oral cavities. **B,** Frontonasal encephalocele. Coronal CT demonstrates dehiscent left cribriform plate with soft tissue extending into the nasal cavity. The *long arrow* indicates the frontonasal encephalocele, and the *short arrow* indicates the crista galli. *IT,* Inferior turbinate.

can then be exercised when inserting a nasogastric tube (NGT) or nasal airway.

B. Nose and Nasal Cavity

The nose is pyramidal in shape and includes both the external apparatus and the nasal cavity. It is one of the two gateways to the aerodigestive tract. Most of the airflow to the lungs occurs through the nasal cavity. Mouth breathing is not physiologic; it is a learned action. The three physiologic functions of the nose are respiration, defense, and olfaction.[33] In respiration, airflow is modified by nasal resistance at the level of the nares and the nasal valves to allow efficient pulmonary ventilation.

A major portion of the nasal airflow passes through the middle meatus. The passage of inspired air through the nasal cavity allows humidification and warming.[33]

1. Imaging Anatomy Overview

Cross-sectional imaging of the nose and paranasal sinuses allows one to examine the air passage from the nares to the nasopharynx. A dedicated examination of the nose and sinuses yields detailed information about this region (Fig. 2-31). Incidental imaging of the sinuses and airway on a routine brain or spine study often allows general assessment of the airway that might be useful in the overall preoperative assessment of a patient (Fig. 2-32).

The bony housing of the nose and the nasal cavities is well depicted by CT. By changing the viewing windows and level, one can delineate the soft tissue component to better advantage. The nasal cavity is divided into two cavities separated by the nasal septum. The roof of the nasal cavity is formed by the cribriform plate of the ethmoid. The hard palate serves as the floor. Protruding into the nasal cavities along the lateral walls are mucosa-covered, scroll-like projections of bone called the inferior, middle, superior, and supreme turbinates or conchae. The supreme turbinates are seen in only 60% of people.[33] The air space beneath and lateral to each turbinate, into which the paranasal sinuses drain, is referred to as the meatus.

In addition to clearly defining the anatomy, cross-sectional imaging can also be a window to viewing physiologic function, in particular the nasal cycle (the cyclic variation in the thickness of the mucosa of the nasal cavity), which repeats every 20 minutes to 6 hours.[33,34] This physiologic change is manifested as alternating side-to-side swelling of the turbinates.

2. Pertinent Imaging Pathology

a. CONGENITAL AND DEVELOPMENTAL ABNORMALITIES

CONGENITAL CHOANAL STENOSIS AND ATRESIA. The development of the nasal cavity is complete by the second month of fetal life. From the second to the sixth month of prenatal life, the nostrils are closed by epithelial plugs that later recanalize to establish a patent nasal cavity. Failure of this process could account for the congenital stenoses and atresias that cause nasal airway obstruction and are often seen in conjunction with craniofacial anomalies.[32]

Congenital nasal airway obstruction most commonly occurs in the posterior nasal cavity secondary to choanal atresia (Fig. 2-33). The atresias may be bony, membranous, or both. At birth, severe respiratory difficulty and inability to insert an NGT more than 3 to 4 cm into the nose despite the presence of air in the trachea and lungs suggests the diagnosis of atresia. However, most atresias are unilateral, and may remain undetected until late in life.

Stenosis of the posterior nasal cavity (choanae) is probably more common than true atresia. About 75% of children with bilateral choanal stenosis or atresia have other congenital abnormalities such as Apert's syndrome, Treacher Collins syndrome, or fetal alcohol syndrome. Because the pathology is usually manifested as bony overgrowth, CT is the imaging modality of choice. The major feature of atresia is an abnormal widening of the vomer

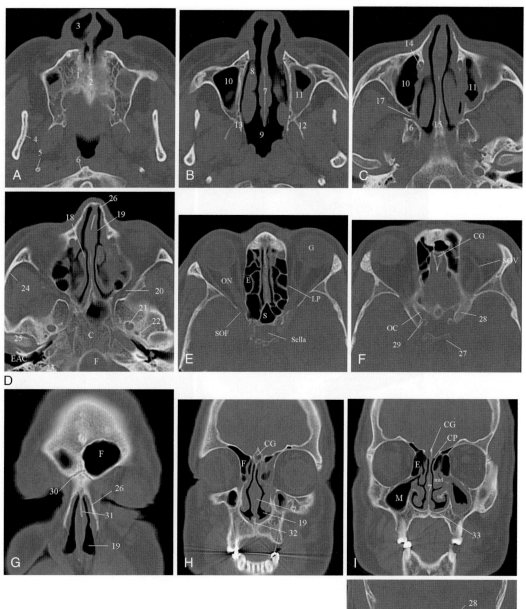

Figure 2-31 Axial (**A** through **F**) and coronal (**G** through **J**) computed tomographic studies showing the anatomy of the sinonasal cavity: *1,* Hard palate; *2,* base of nasal septum; *3,* nostril; *4,* ramus mandible; *5,* styloid process; *6,* anterior arch of C1; *7,* nasal septum; *8,* inferior turbinate; *9,* nasopharynx; *10,* right maxillary sinus; *11,* left maxillary sinus with inflammatory mucosal disease; *12,* lateral pterygoid plate; *13,* medial pterygoid plate; *14,* nasolacrimal duct; *15,* rostrum sphenoid; *16,* pterygoid process; *17,* pterygopalatine fossa; *18,* middle turbinate; *19,* nasal cavity; *20,* inferior orbital fissure; *21,* foramen ovale; *22,* foramen spinosum; *23,* carotid canal; *24,* zygomatic arch; *25,* mandibular head; *26,* nasal bone; *27,* dorsum sella; *28,* anterior clinoid; *29,* calcified carotid artery; *30,* nasofrontal suture; *31,* perpendicular plate of ethmoid; *32,* vomer; *33,* hard palate; *C,* clivus; *CG,* crista galli; *E,* ethmoid sinus; *EAC,* external auditory canal; *F,* foramen magnum; *G,* globe; *inf,* inferior turbinate; *mid,* middle turbinate; *OC,* optic canal; *ON,* optic nerve; *S,* sphenoid sinus; *SOF,* superior orbital fissure; *SOV,* superior ophthalmic vein.

(Fig. 2-34). Nasal airway obstruction may also result from rhinitis or turbinate hypertrophy.

DEVIATED SEPTUM. The cartilage of the nasal capsule, which is the foundation of the upper part of the face, eventually becomes ossified or atrophied with age. All that remains of the cartilage of the nasal capsule in adults is the anterior part of the nasal septum and the alar cartilages that surround the nostrils. The midline septal cartilage is continuous with the cartilaginous skull base. At birth, the lateral masses of the ethmoid are ossified, but the septal cartilage and the cribriform plates are still cartilaginous. Another ossification center appears in the septal cartilage anterior to the cranial base and becomes the perpendicular plate of the ethmoid. In about the third to sixth year of life, the lateral masses of the ethmoid

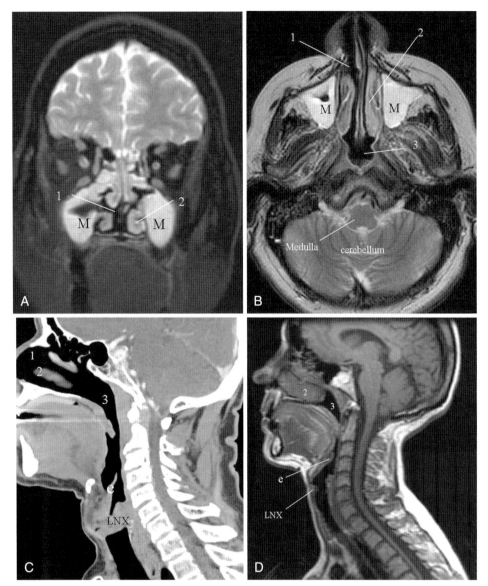

Figure 2-32 Airway as seen on routine studies. **A,** T2-weighted coronal magnetic resonance (MR) image of the brain demonstrates hyperintense, inflamed, thickened mucosa of the maxillary sinuses. **B,** T2-weighted axial MR image of the brain demonstrates sinus disease with a clear nasal cavity and nasopharynx. **C,** Sagittal reformation from computed tomographic neck examination demonstrates a clear airway from nose to trachea. **D,** T1-weighted sagittal MR cervical spine examination demonstrates signal void (black) of the air column of the airway. *1,* Nasal cavity; *2,* inferior turbinate; *3,* nasopharynx; *e,* epiglottis; *LNX,* larynx; *M,* maxillary sinus with thickened mucosa.

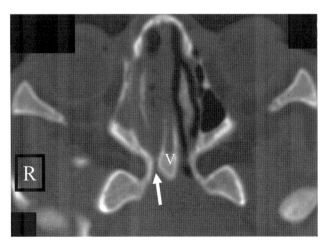

Figure 2-33 Choanal atresia. Axial computed tomographic scan demonstrates posterior aperture stenosis on the right (*arrow*). The vomer (*V*) is enlarged.

and the perpendicular plate become united across the roof of the nasal cavity by ossification of the cribriform plate, which unites with the vomer below somewhat later. Growth of the septal cartilage continues for a short time after craniofacial union is complete, and this probably accounts for what is commonly seen as deviated nasal septum.[32]

Acquired bases of deviated septum also exist (e.g., trauma), and there is a varying degree of septal deviation, which can be associated with a prominent bony beak. In most cases, septal deviation is not problematic for NGT or nasal airway insertion, but having prior knowledge of the anatomy of the nasal cavity allows one to choose the path of least resistance.

CONCHA BULLOSA. The term *concha bullosa* refers to an aerated turbinate, most often the middle turbinate, either unilateral or bilateral. In most cases it an incidental

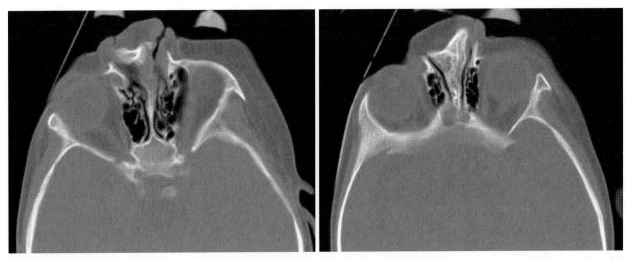

Figure 2-34 Congenital nasal deformity. Axial computed tomographic scans demonstrate abnormal nasal bone architecture with soft tissue cleft and the impact on nasal airways.

finding. However, it can be quite large and narrows the nasal air passage. Knowing which nasal cavity is narrowed by the presence of a concha bullosa helps guide the selection of which nasal cavity to cannulate (Fig. 2-35).

b. INFLAMMATORY CONDITIONS

RHINOSINUSITIS. In general, no imaging is required for work-up of uncomplicated rhinosinusitis. Views of the sinus are included in a routine CT brain study. The air within the sinuses abuts the bony sinus wall and appears black on both CT and MRI. To assess the bony structures, CT is preferred. However, MRI is extremely useful to differentiate inflammatory disease from tumor. Inflammatory sinus disease is characterized by increased water content; therefore, an increased T2 signal (i.e., bright signal) is produced on T2-weighted imaging. Common inflammatory sinus disease is most often seen as T2-hyperintense lining of the walls of the sinus, representing thickened mucosa. In contrast, with increased cellularity, tumor masses typically exhibit an isointense signal on T2-weighted imaging. The most common local complications of inflammatory sinusitis are swollen turbinates, polyps, and retention cysts.

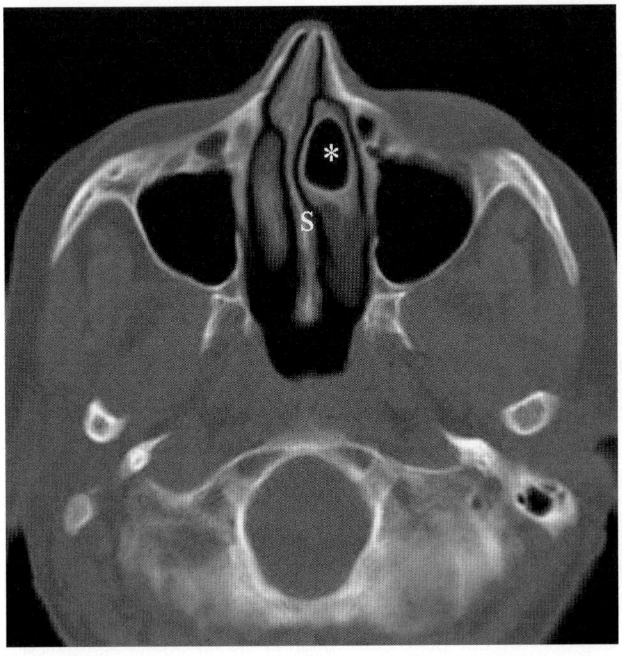

POLYPOSIS. Nasal airway obstruction may result from rhinitis, polyposis, or turbinate hypertrophy. These entities affecting the airway are easily recognizable on cross-sectional imaging. Sensibly, the presence of polyposis may discourage an anesthesiologist from attempting nasal intubation (Figs. 2-36 and 2-37).

c. TRAUMA

Facial fractures are often classified using the Le Fort system and its variants. This system is based on experiments predicting the course of fractures on the basis of lines of weakness in the facial skeleton. Nasal fractures are the most common facial fractures and may involve the nasal bones or the cartilaginous structures. If the nasal septum is fractured and a hematoma results, the vascular supply to the cartilage may be compromised, leading to cartilage necrosis. If the septal hematoma is not recognized and treated, it becomes an organized hematoma, which causes thickening of the septum and can result in impaired breathing (Fig. 2-38). Without doubt, CT is the modality of choice for evaluating trauma to the facial structures. Three-dimensional reconstruction and surface rendering can also be performed to better highlight fracture deformities. Even if all the details of a complex facial fracture are not known, an oral airway is preferable to a nasal airway, except in the case of mandibular fracture (Fig. 2-39), for which the nasal approach to intubation is preferred.

Figure 2-35 Concha bullosa. Axial computed tomographic scan demonstrates pneumatization (*asterisk*) of the left middle turbinate and deviated septum (*S*).

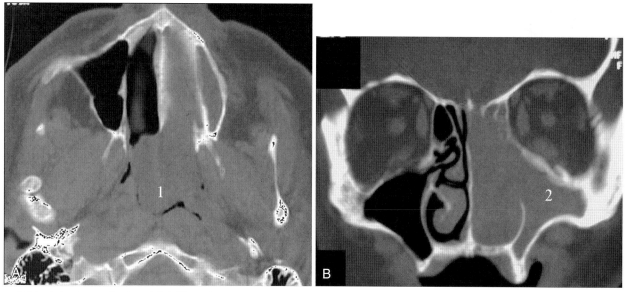

Figure 2-36 Antrochoanal polyp. Axial **(A)** and coronal **(B)** computed tomography scans demonstrate soft tissue obliterating the left nasal cavity and extending posteriorly into the nasopharynx (*1*) and laterally into the left maxillary sinus (*2*).

d. TUMORS AND OTHER CONDITIONS

MALIGNANT TUMORS. Malignant tumors of the nasal cavity and the paranasal sinuses are rare and have a poor prognosis because they are frequently diagnosed in an advanced stage. They are often accompanied by inflammatory disease. MRI is superior to CT in differentiating tumor from inflammatory disease and therefore is useful in delineating the tumor boundary from the often-associated inflammatory component. Inflammatory diseases involve a high water content; therefore, they have high T2-weighted intensity and appear bright on MRI. Nasal and paranasal tumors are usually cellular and have an intermediate-intensity signal on T2-weighted imaging (Fig. 2-40).[35,36] CT is useful for assessing bone involvement. The histology of the tumor can sometimes be suggested by the way in which the bone is affected: aggressive bone destruction is usually seen in squamous cell carcinomas (SCCs), metastatic lung and breast cancers, a few sarcomas, and rare fibrous histiocytomas (Fig. 2-41).

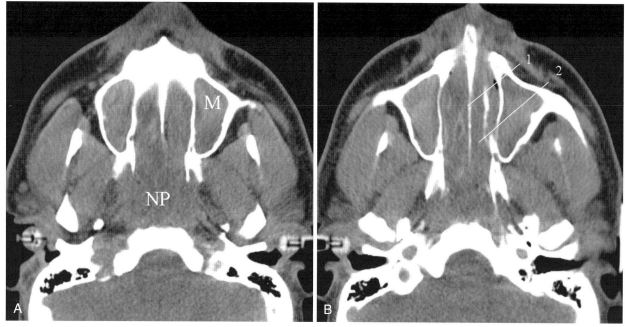

Figure 2-37 Nasal polyps. Axial computed tomography scans (**A** and **B**) demonstrate complete obliteration of the nasal passageways and pharynx by soft tissue polyps, resulting in chronic maxillary sinus inflammatory changes. *1,* Nasal septum; *2,* nasal cavity; *NP,* nasopharynx; *M,* maxillary sinus.

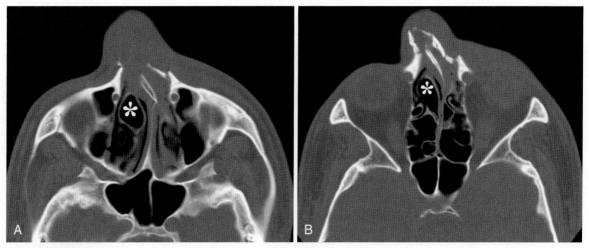

Figure 2-38 Nasal and septal fracture. Axial computed tomography scans (**A** and **B**) demonstrate comminuted fractures of the nasal bones bilaterally as well as a septal fracture. The nasal passages are further compromised by the incidental right concha bullosa (*asterisk*).

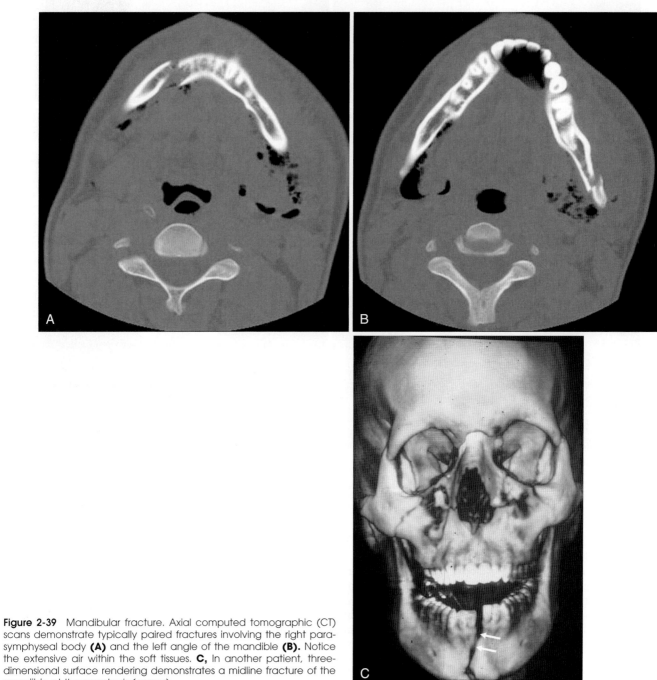

Figure 2-39 Mandibular fracture. Axial computed tomographic (CT) scans demonstrate typically paired fractures involving the right parasymphyseal body **(A)** and the left angle of the mandible **(B).** Notice the extensive air within the soft tissues. **C,** In another patient, three-dimensional surface rendering demonstrates a midline fracture of the mandible at the symphysis (*arrows*).

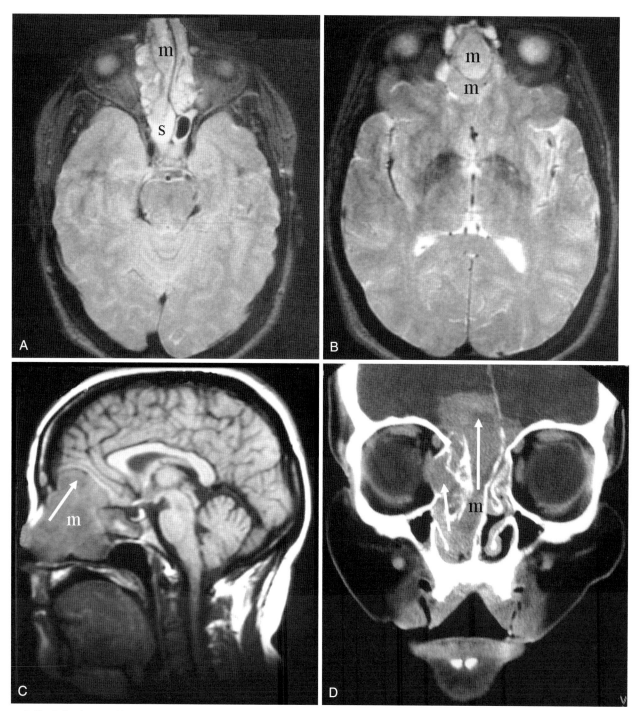

Figure 2-40 Esthesioneuroblastoma. **A** and **B,** T2-weighted axial magnetic resonance (MR) studies of the brain. Notice the large isointense soft tissue mass *(m)* in the nasal cavity, which is accompanied by obstructive inflammatory sinus disease of high T2 signal *(s)*. The extension of the mass intracranially, indicated by the *arrows,* is better appreciated on the sagittal T1-weighted MR image of the brain **(C)** and on the coronal computed tomogram (CT) with contrast **(D).** Coronal CT better demonstrates bone destruction and also extension of the tumor to the right orbit.

NONMALIGNANT DESTRUCTIVE TUMORS

Juvenile Nasopharyngeal Angiofibroma. Juvenile nasopharyngeal angiofibroma is a benign hypervascular tumor found almost exclusively in young adolescent men. It is a nonmalignant, locally destructive tumor of the sinonasal cavity. The most common presenting signs are unilateral nasal obstruction and spontaneous epistaxis. The tumor usually arises at the sphenopalatine foramen at the lateral nasopharyngeal wall and is locally destructive over time.[35]

The imaging characteristics consist of a nasal cavity and nasopharyngeal mass, a widened pterygopalatine fossa, anterior displacement of the posterior wall of the maxillary sinus, and erosion of the medial pterygoid plate (Fig. 2-42). Treatment is surgical resection, often with preoperative embolization to decrease the blood supply.

Wegener's Granulomatosis. Wegener's granulomatosis, a necrotizing vasculitis, usually affects the upper and lower

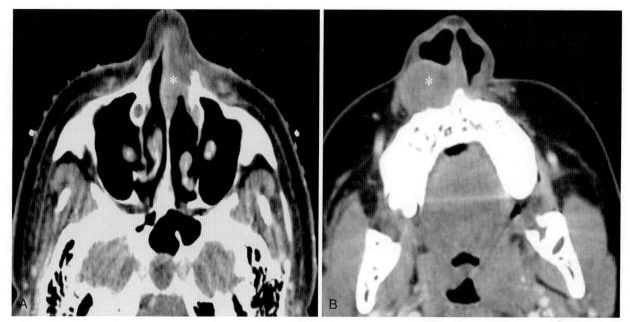

Figure 2-41 A, Lymphoma of the nasal septum. Axial computed tomographic (CT) scan shows an infiltrating lesion of the anterior nasal septum (*asterisk*) that extends into the left maxillary soft tissues. **B,** Rhabdomyosarcoma of the right nasal cavity and nasal ala. Axial CT scan demonstrates a soft tissue mass (*asterisk*) effacing the right nostril.

respiratory tracts and causes a renal glomerulonephritis. It is probably autoimmune in origin. It most often involves the nasal septum first and may arise as a chronic nonspecific inflammatory process. This process becomes diffuse, and septal ulcerations and perforations occur. Secondary bacterial infection often complicates the clinical and imaging picture (Fig. 2-43).[35]

Fibrous Dysplasia. Fibrous dysplasia, an idiopathic bone disorder, is not a tumor but can encroach on the airway and sinuses. Most patients are young at the time of diagnosis. There are monostotic and polyostotic forms. Craniofacial bones are more often involved in the polyostotic form (Fig. 2-44).[35]

C. Oral Cavity

The oral cavity, contiguous with the oropharynx, is the primary conduit to the gastrointestinal tract. The development of the mouth and that of the face are centered on a surface depression, the stomodeum, just below the developing brain. The ectoderm covering the forebrain extends into the stomodeum, where it lies adjacent to the foregut. The junctional zone between the ectoderm and the endoderm is the oropharyngeal membrane, which corresponds to Waldeyer's ring. Dissolution of the oropharyngeal membrane in the fourth gestational week results in establishing patency between the mouth and the foregut.[37]

The oral cavity is separated from the oropharynx by the circumvallate papillae, anterior tonsillar pillars, and soft palate. The anterior two thirds of the tongue (oral tongue), floor of the mouth, gingivobuccal and buccomasseteric regions, maxilla, and mandible are considered oral cavity structures. The anatomic distinction between the oral cavity and the oropharynx has clinical importance. Malignancies, especially SCCs, in

these two regions are different in their presentation and prognosis.

1. Imaging Anatomy Overview

CT and MRI are used extensively for evaluation of the oral cavity. The advantages of CT are the speed of data acquisition and the ability to detect calcifications pertinent in the evaluation of inflammatory diseases affecting the salivary glands. For evaluating the extent of tumor infiltration of the soft tissues, MRI is superior to CT; however, it is easily degraded by motion artifacts (Fig. 2-45).

The tongue consists of two symmetrical halves separated by a midline lingual septum. Each half of the tongue is composed of muscular fibers, which are divided into extrinsic and intrinsic muscles. There are four intrinsic tongue muscles: the superior longitudinal muscle, inferior longitudinal muscle, transverse muscles, and vertical muscles. The intrinsic muscles receive motor innervation from the hypoglossal nerve (cranial nerve [CN] XII) and participate in the enunciation of various consonants. The intrinsic muscles are difficult to distinguish on CT, but they are well visualized on MRI, because each muscle bundle is surrounded by high-intensity fibrofatty tissues.

The muscles that originate externally to the tongue but have distal muscle fibers that interdigitate within the substance of the tongue are considered to be extrinsic muscles of the tongue. The main extrinsic muscles are the genioglossus, hyoglossus, and styloglossus muscles. Sometimes the superior constrictors and the palatoglossus muscles are discussed with the extrinsic muscles of the tongue. The extrinsic muscles attach the tongue to the hyoid, mandible, and styloid process.

Motor innervation comes from the hypoglossal nerve, which courses between the mylohyoid and hyoglossus muscles. The sensory input from the anterior tongue is from the lingual nerve, which is a branch of the trigeminal nerve (CN V). Special sensory taste fibers from the

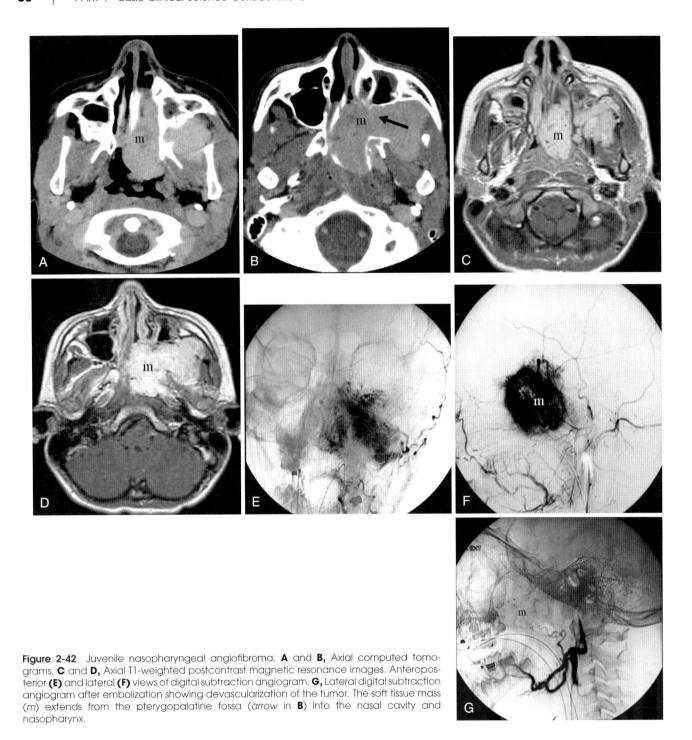

Figure 2-42 Juvenile nasopharyngeal angiofibroma. **A** and **B,** Axial computed tomograms. **C** and **D,** Axial T1-weighted postcontrast magnetic resonance images. Anteroposterior **(E)** and lateral **(F)** views of digital subtraction angiogram. **G,** Lateral digital subtraction angiogram after embolization showing devascularization of the tumor. The soft tissue mass (*m*) extends from the pterygopalatine fossa (*arrow* in **B**) into the nasal cavity and nasopharynx.

anterior two thirds of the tongue course with the lingual nerve before forming the chorda tympani nerve, which subsequently joins the facial nerve (CN VII). The special sensory fibers from the posterior one third of the tongue (tongue base) are supplied by the glossopharyngeal nerve (CN IX). The arterial blood supply to the tongue is from branches of the lingual artery, which itself is a branch of the external carotid artery. Venous drainage is to the internal jugular vein.[25,38]

The floor of the mouth is mainly composed of the mylohyoid muscles, the paired anterior bellies of the digastrics muscles, and the geniohyoid muscles. The space caudal to the mylohyoid muscle and above the hyoid bone is considered to be the suprahyoid neck. Through a gap between the free posterior border of the mylohyoid muscle and the hyoglossus muscle, the submandibular gland wraps around the dorsal aspect of the mylohyoid muscle.

Several named spaces and regions in the oral cavity are mentioned in brief because of their anatomic importance with respect to the structures contained within them. The *sublingual region* is below the mucosa of the floor of

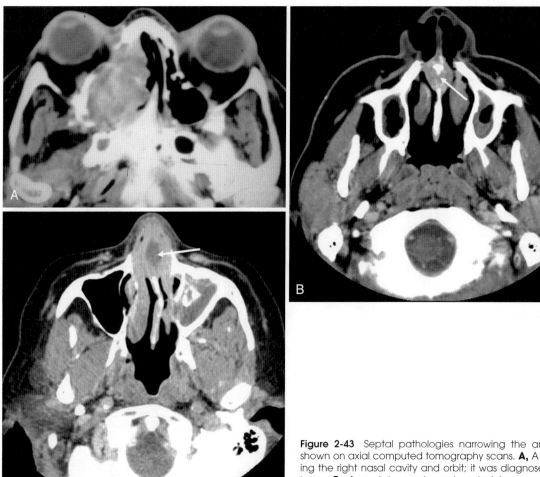

Figure 2-43 Septal pathologies narrowing the anterior nasal cavity are shown on axial computed tomography scans. **A,** A soft tissue mass is invading the right nasal cavity and orbit; it was diagnosed as Wegener's granuloma. **B,** A septal granuloma is noted in association with focal bone destruction. **C,** A ring-enhancing lesion of the anterior septum is seen, consistent with a septal abscess.

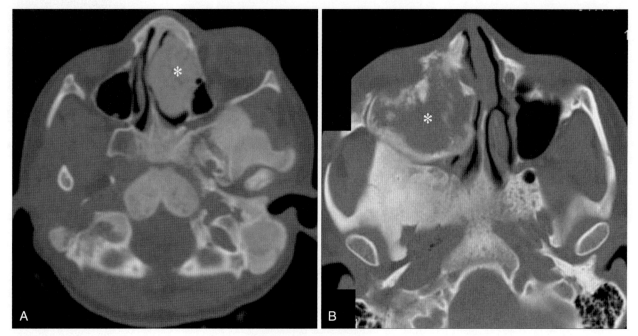

Figure 2-44 Fibrous dysplasia. **A,** Axial computed tomogram (CT) demonstrates a mass obliterating the left nasal cavity (*asterisk*) with the typical "ground glass" appearance of fibrous dysplasia involving the left skull base. **B,** Axial CT scan from a different patient demonstrates fibrous dysplasia with malignant degeneration to osteosarcoma invading the right nasal cavity and orbit (*asterisk*).

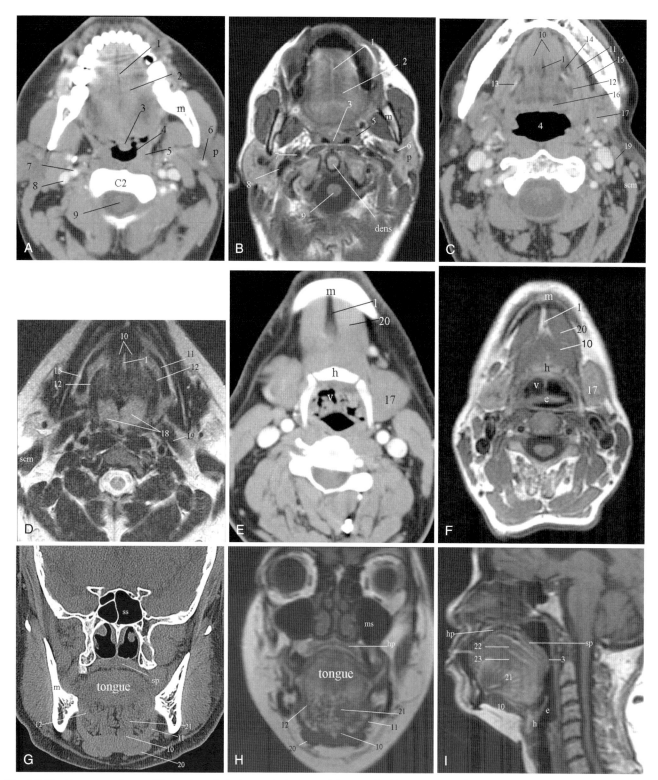

Figure 2-45 Normal anatomy of the oral cavity is demonstrated on axial computed tomographic (CT) images (**A, C,** and **E**) with corresponding axial magnetic resonance (MR) scans (**B, D,** and **F**), on coronal CT **(G)** and coronal T1-weighted MR **(H)** scans, and on a sagittal T1-weighted MR image **(I)**: *1,* Median raphe of tongue (fat is low density on CT and bright on T1-weighted MR images); *2,* tongue (transverse fibers are seen better on MR imaging); *3,* uvula; *4,* oropharynx; *5,* pharyngeal constrictor muscle; *6,* retromandibular vein; *7,* internal carotid artery; *8,* internal jugular vein; *9,* cervical cord; *10,* paired geniohyoid muscles; *11,* mylohyoid muscle; *12,* hyoglossus muscle; *13,* lingual artery and vein medial to hyoglossus muscle; *14,* Wharton's duct, hypoglossal nerve, and lingual nerve lateral to hyoglossus muscle; *15,* fat in sublingual space; *16,* tongue base; *17,* submandibular gland; *18,* palatine tonsils narrowing oropharynx; *19,* posterior belly of digastric muscle; *20,* paired anterior belly of digastric muscle; *21,* genioglossus muscle; *22,* superior longitudinal muscle; *23,* transverse muscle; *e,* epiglottis; *h,* body of hyoid bone; *hp,* hard palate; *m,* mandible; *ms,* maxillary sinus; *p,* parotid gland; *scm,* sternocleidomastoid muscle; *sp,* soft palate; *ss,* sphenoid sinus; *v,* vallecula.

the mouth, superomedial to the mylohyoid muscle and lateral to the genioglossus-geniohyoid muscles. It is primarily fat filled and is continuous with the submandibular region at the posterior margin of the mylohyoid muscle. The contents of this space include the sublingual gland and ducts, the submandibular gland duct (Wharton's duct) and sometimes a portion of the hilum of the submandibular gland, anterior fibers of the hyoglossus muscle, and the lingual artery and vein. The hyoglossus muscle is an important surgical landmark (see Fig. 2-45C). Lateral to this muscle, one can identify Wharton's duct, the hypoglossal nerve, and the lingual nerve; the lingual artery and vein lie medially. Wharton's duct runs anteriorly from the gland, traveling with the hypoglossal nerve and the lingual nerve (mandibular branch of the trigeminal nerve). Initially, it lies between the hyoglossus muscle and the mylohyoid muscle. More anteriorly, it lies between the genioglossus and mylohyoid muscles. The duct drains into the floor of the mouth, just lateral to the frenulum of the tongue.[39]

The *submandibular space* or fossa is defined as the space inferior to the mylohyoid muscle, between the mandible and the hyoid bone. At the posterior margin of the mylohyoid muscle, the submandibular space is continuous with the sublingual space and the anterior aspect of the parapharyngeal space. This communication allows the spread of pathology. The submandibular space is primarily fat filled and contains the superficial portion of the submandibular gland and lymph nodes, lymphatic vessels, and blood vessels. The anterior bellies of the digastric muscle lie in the paramedian location in this space. Branches of the facial artery and vein course lateral to the anterior digastric muscle in the fat surrounding the submandibular gland. The artery lies deep to the gland, and the anterior facial vein is superficial.[38] One important anatomic point is that pathology intrinsic to the submandibular gland displaces the facial vein laterally. Other masses lateral to

the gland, including nodes, can be identified with the vein interposed between the gland and the mass.[40]

The lips are composed of orbicularis muscle, which comprises muscle fibers from multiple facial muscles that insert into the lips and additional fibers proper to the lips. The innervation to the lips is from branches of the facial nerve (CN VII). The vestibule of the mouth, or the *gingivobuccal region*, is the potential space separating the lips and cheeks from the gums and teeth. The parotid gland ducts and mucous gland ducts of the lips and cheek drain into this space, which is contiguous posteriorly with the oral cavity through the space between the last molar tooth and the ramus of the mandible.[38]

2. Pertinent Imaging Pathology

a. MACROGLOSSIA

The tongue makes up the bulk of soft tissues in the oral cavity. Enlargement of the tongue, which is defined clinically as protrusion of the tongue beyond the teeth or alveolar ridge in the resting position, compromises the oral airway and makes the insertion of airway devices challenging. Larsson and colleagues defined the appearance of macroglossia on CT imaging as (1) base of the tongue more than 50 mm in the transverse dimension, (2) genioglossus muscle more than 11 mm in the transverse dimension, (3) midline cleft on the tongue surface, and (4) submandibular glands normal in size but bulging out of the platysma muscle owing to tongue enlargement.[41]

There are congenital and noncongenital causes of macroglossia. The congenital syndromes in which macroglossia can be seen are trisomy 21, Beckwith-Wiedemann syndrome, hypothyroidism, and mucopolysaccharidoses. The more common noncongenital causes are tumor of the tongue, lymphangioma, hemangioma, acromegaly, and amyloid (Figs. 2-46 and 2-47). Rarely, infection

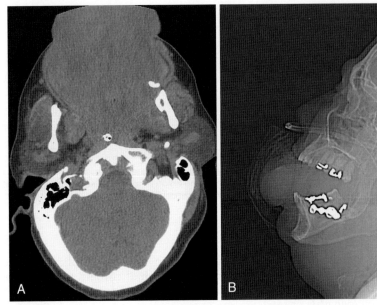

Figure 2-46 Macroglossia in a patient with a diagnosis of multiple myeloma and amyloid who developed an allergic reaction to amoxicillin clavulanate potassium (Augmentin). **A,** Axial computed tomographic (CT) image demonstrates the enlarged tongue occupying and extending beyond the oral cavity. There is no apparent oropharyngeal airway. A nasogastric tube is in place. **B,** Lateral CT scout view demonstrates the protrusion of the tongue beyond the confines of the oral cavity and diffuse soft tissue swelling on the neck.

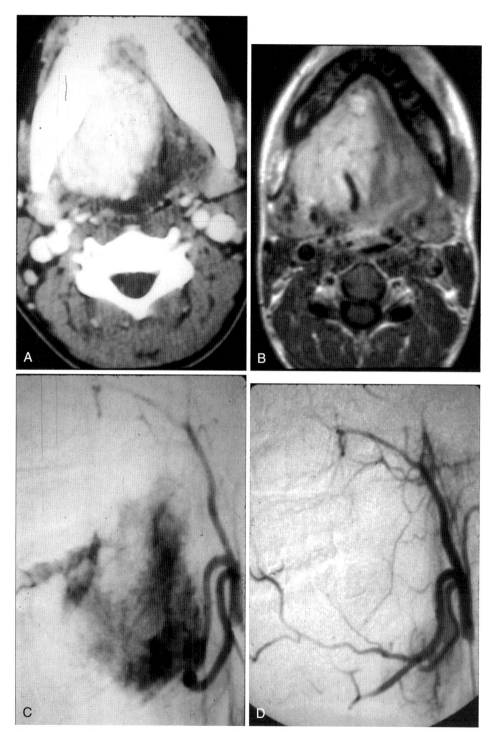

Figure 2-47 Tongue hemangioma. Contrast-enhanced computed tomography **(A)** and magnetic resonance imaging **(B)** demonstrate an enhancing right tongue lesion that almost fills the oral cavity. **C,** The vascularity of the lesion is further demonstrated in the lateral view of the right external carotid angiogram. **D,** Angiogram after embolization shows devascularization of the tumor.

can result in macroglossia, especially in an immune-compromised host (Fig. 2-48).

Posterior displacement of the tongue, or glossoptosis, may be observed with macroglossia, micrognathia or retrognathia, and neuromuscular disorders, including unilateral tongue paralysis secondary to hypoglossal nerve (CN XII) denervation. It can also occur in normal patients in

some cases. The obvious complication is relative airway obstruction, which, if chronic, results in a myriad of systemic complications.

b. MICROGNATHIA AND RETROGNATHIA

Micrognathia is a term used to describe an abnormally small mandible. *Retrognathia* is defined as abnormal

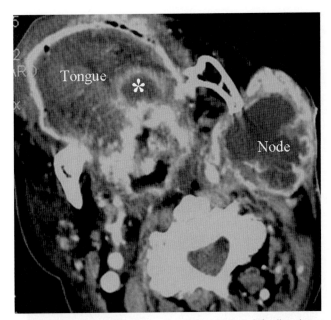

Figure 2-48 *Mycobacterium avium-intracellulare* infection in an immune-compromised patient. Axial computed tomogram with contrast demonstrates an irregular enhancement of lymph nodes and lymphoid tissue at the tongue base. The fungating tongue lesion (*asterisk*) compromises the oropharyngeal airway.

posterior placement of the mandible. These two findings often coexist. Abnormal growth or placement of the mandible can be caused by malformation, deformation, or connective tissue dysplasia.[42] The most familiar syndromic form featuring an abnormal mandible is in the Pierre Robin sequence. Other clinical entities include the Treacher Collins, Stickler, and DiGeorge syndromes. Thin-section CT with 2-D or 3-D reformation provides information regarding the size and proportions of the maxilla, nose, mandible, and airway. Micrognathia and retrognathia not only contribute to airway obstruction but also are possible indicators of difficult direct laryngoscopy and endotracheal intubation that can lead to life-threatening complications (Figs. 2-49 and 2-50).[42]

c. EXOSTOSIS

Hyperostosis of the hard palate or mandible is a benign disease that is usually of no clinical significance. Most often these are small exostoses. They may arise from the oral surface of the hard palate (torus palatinus), from the alveolar portion of the maxilla in the molar region along the lingual surface of the dental arch (torus maxillaris), or along the lingual surface of the mandible (torus mandibularis) (Fig. 2-51). Large lesions may restrict tongue motion and distort the airway, leading to speech disturbance.

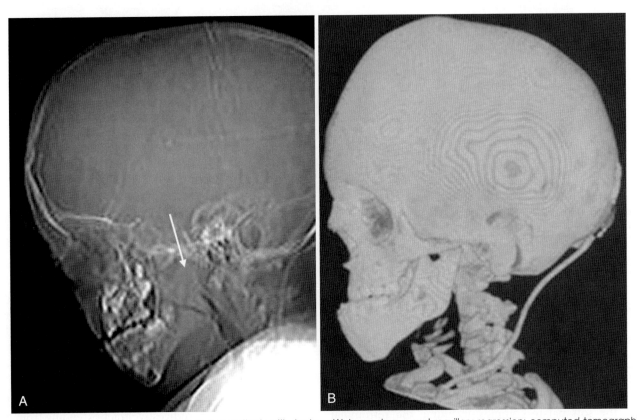

Figure 2-49 Midface regression syndrome in two patients with Jackson-Weiss syndrome and maxillary regression: computed tomographic scout view **(A)** and three-dimensional surface rendering **(B).** Notice the presence of a ventriculoperitoneal shunt; hydrocephalus may result from the craniosynostosis associated with this syndrome. The mandible is hypoplastic, and there is soft tissue obscuring the nasopharynx (*arrow*).

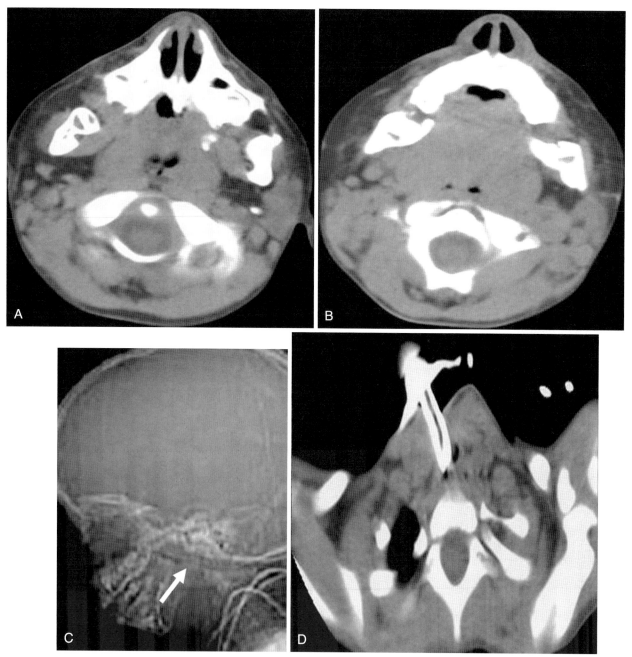

Figure 2-50 Treacher Collins syndrome. Axial computed tomographic (CT) scans at the level of the nasopharynx **(A)** and oropharynx **(B)** demonstrate almost complete obliteration of the airway by soft tissue, secondary to the facial microsomia. **C,** Lateral CT scout view demonstrates marked narrowing of the airway (*arrow*). **D,** Axial CT scan at the thoracic inlet demonstrates the tracheostomy necessitated by this condition.

d. TUMORS

Only 7% of oral cavity lesions are malignant; however, most of these malignant tumors are SCCs. Other neoplasms include minor salivary gland tumors, lymphomas, and sarcomas. Risk factors for SCC of the oral cavity include a long history of tobacco and alcohol use. SCC can arise anywhere in the oral cavity, but it has a predilection for the floor of the mouth, the ventrolateral tongue, and the soft palate complex including the retromolar trigone area and the anterior tonsillar pillar. Most lesions are moderately advanced at the time of presentation; 30% to 65% of patients with SCC of the oral cavity have nodal involvement at the time of diagnosis. The tumors of the oral cavity are usually less aggressive than SCCs arising from the oropharynx. Both CT and MRI are useful for assessing tumor extent and nodal involvement.[39]

D. Pharynx

The pharynx is a mucosa-lined tubular structure and is the portion of the aerodigestive tract extending from the skull base to the cervical esophagus. By convention and for ease of discussion, it is divided into three parts: nasopharynx, oropharynx, and hypopharynx. Anatomically,

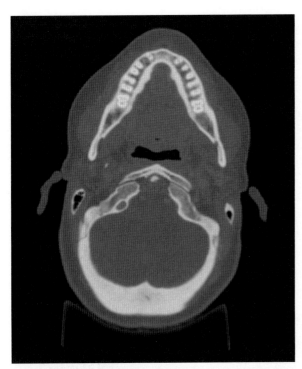

Figure 2-51 Torus mandibularis. Axial computed tomogram at the level of the mandible demonstrates cortical widening of the lingual surface of the mandible.

the nasopharynx is defined as extending from the skull base to the hard palate, the oropharynx from the hard palate to the hyoid bone, and the hypopharynx from the hyoid bone to the caudal margin of the cricoid cartilage. Below the level of the cricoid cartilage, the cervical esophagus begins. The hypopharynx can be further subdivided into the pyriform sinus region, the posterior wall, the postcricoid region, and the lateral surface of the aryepiglottic folds.[25,38]

The pharyngeal musculature includes the three overlapping constrictor muscles (the superior, middle, and inferior pharyngeal constrictors) and the cricopharyngeus, salpingopharyngeus, stylopharyngeus, palatopharyngeus, tensor veli palatini, and levator veli palatini muscles. Innervation is primarily from the pharyngeal plexus of nerves, to which the vagus (CN X) and glossopharyngeal nerve contribute. The vagus nerve primarily supplies motor innervation to the constrictors. The mandibular branch of the trigeminal nerve innervates the tensor veli palatini muscle. Sensory information travels along the glossopharyngeal nerve and the internal laryngeal branch of the superior laryngeal nerve, which arises from the vagus nerve.

The arterial supply to the pharynx is from branches of the external carotid artery, including the ascending pharyngeal artery, tonsillar branches of the facial artery, and the palatine branches of the maxillary artery. Superior and inferior thyroid arteries supply most of the lower pharynx. The primary venous drainage is through the superior and inferior thyroid veins and the pharyngeal veins into the internal jugular veins. The lymphatic drainage is complex and extensive to the jugular, retropharyngeal, posterior cervical, and paratracheal nodes.[25,43,44]

Imaging studies of the pharynx most commonly include plain radiographic films, barium studies, CT, and MRI. In contrast to CT and MRI, a barium study is a dynamic imaging technique that can demonstrate the sequential contractions of the pharyngeal musculature during deglutition. It can show whether the pharyngeal wall is fixed or pliable and may detect mucosal lesions not apparent on CT or MRI. CT and MRI are most commonly done with the patient in the supine position and the neck in the neutral position. Intravenous contrast is recommended with CT for evaluation of lymphadenopathy. The inherent differences in signal intensity between tumor, fat, and muscle on MRI often allow accurate delineation of the tumor extent without gadolinium, which is the contrast agent commonly used in clinical practice.[44] Because of the clinical concern for perineural spread of tumor in the head and neck region, MRI is usually performed with contrast.

1. Nasopharynx

a. IMAGING ANATOMY OVERVIEW

The nasopharynx is an air-containing cavity that occupies the uppermost extent of the aerodigestive tract. The roof and posterior wall of the nasopharynx are formed by the sphenoid sinus, the clivus, and anterior aspect of the first two cervical vertebrae. The inferior aspect of the nasopharynx is formed by the hard palate, the soft palate, and the ridge of pharyngeal musculature that opposes the soft palate when it is elevated (Passavant's ridge). The lateral nasopharyngeal walls are formed by the margins of the superior constrictor muscle. Anteriorly, the nasopharynx is in direct continuity with the nasal cavity through the posterior choanae. The nasopharynx is in direct communication with the middle ear cavity through the eustachian tubes (Fig. 2-52).[44]

b. PERTINENT IMAGING PATHOLOGY

ADENOIDAL HYPERTROPHY. The adenoids are lymphatic tissues that are located in the upper posterior aspect of the nasopharynx. Prominent adenoids are typical in children; by the age of 2 to 3 years, the adenoids can fill the entire nasopharynx and extend posteriorly into the posterior choanae. Regression of the lymphoid tissue starts during adolescence and continues into later life. By the age of 30 to 40 years, adenoidal tissue is minimal, although normal adenoidal tissue may occasionally be seen in adults in the fourth and fifth decades of life. Adenoid tissues appear isodense to muscle on CT imaging (see Fig. 2-52D). On MRI, the adenoids are isointense to muscle on T1-weighted imaging and hyperintense on T2-weighted imaging. If prominent adenoidal tissue is seen in an adult, human immunodeficiency virus (HIV) infection should be suspected.[44] Differentiation between lymphomatous involvement and hypertrophy of the adenoids is not possible on imaging, because both entities are hyperintense on T2-weighted imaging. Enlargement of the adenoids can cause partial obstruction of the nasopharyngeal airway and make insertion of an NGT difficult. They may also contribute to the symptom complex of obstructive sleep apnea.

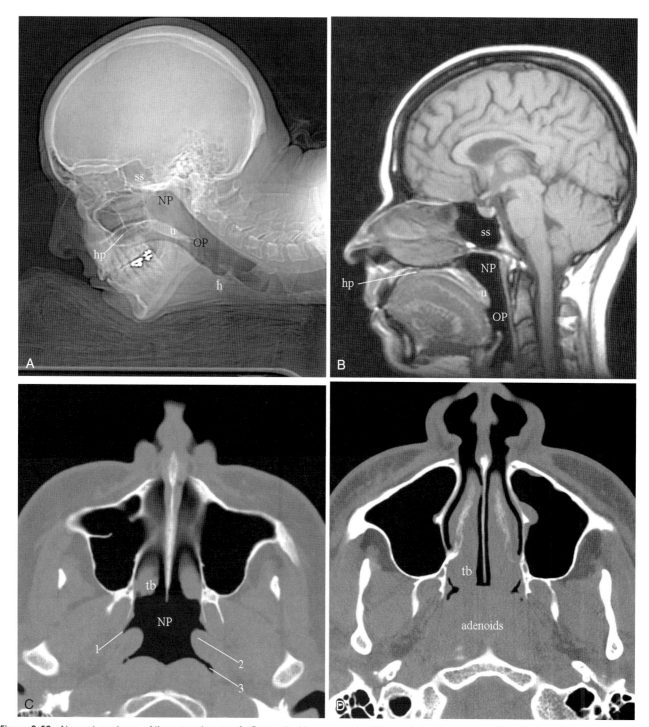

Figure 2-52 Normal anatomy of the nasopharynx. **A,** Computed tomographic (CT) scout view in prone position. **B,** T1-weighted sagittal brain magnetic resonance image. **C,** Normal nasopharynx on axial CT scan. **D,** Prominent adenoids effacing the nasopharyngeal airway. *1,* Opening of the eustachian tube; *2,* torus tubarius; *3,* fossa of Rosenmüller; *h,* hyoid; *hp,* hard palate; *NP,* nasopharynx; *OP,* oropharynx; *ss,* sphenoid sinus; *tb,* turbinate, *u,* uvula.

TORNWALDT'S CYST. Tornwaldt's cyst is a not uncommon incidental finding on MRI. It is usually midline and located between the longus capitis muscles in the posterior nasopharynx. It is a developmental anomaly in which the ascension of the notochord back into the skull base pulls a small tag of the developing nasopharyngeal mucosa with it, creating a midline pit or tract that closes over and results in a midline cyst, usually after pharyngitis. These lesions usually have a high signal intensity on T1- and T2-weighted imaging, probably because of the high protein content of the cyst fluid. Tornwaldt's cyst is usually infected by anaerobic bacteria, which may empty

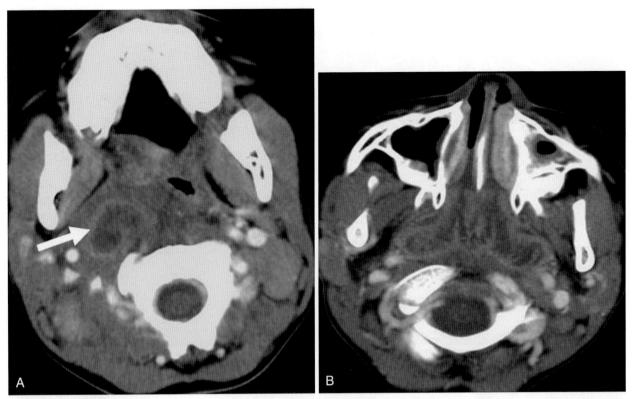

Figure 2-53 Suppurative adenitis seen on axial computed tomography scans. **A,** A ring-enhancing mass (*arrow*) in the right parapharyngeal space is deviating the oropharynx. **B,** Bilateral bulky adenopathy is present with abscess formation obliterating the nasopharynx.

into the nasopharynx and cause intermittent halitosis. The CT density of the cyst is similar to that of surrounding muscle and lymphoid tissue.

INFECTION AND ABSCESS. Abscess in the parapharyngeal space may result from tonsillar infection or from iatrogenic or traumatic perforation of the pharynx. The infection may extend from the skull base to the submandibular region and can be difficult to differentiate from a neoplastic process. If large enough, it may compromise the airway. Infection spreading to retropharyngeal nodes (suppurative adenitis) can also obliterate the nasopharynx airway (Fig. 2-53).

TUMORS AND OTHER CONDITIONS. SCC of the nasopharynx is a relatively rare cancer that accounts for only 0.25% of all malignancies in North America. It has a high rate of incidence in Asia, however, where it is the most common tumor in men, accounting for 18% of cancers in China.[43] SCC accounts for 70% or more of the malignancies arising in the nasopharynx, and lymphomas account for about 20%. The remaining 10% are a variety of lesions, including adenocarcinoma, adenoid cystic carcinoma, rhabdomyosarcoma, melanoma, extramedullary plasmacytoma, fibrosarcoma, and carcinosarcoma. Risk factors for SCC in the nasopharynx include the presence of immunoglobulin A antibodies against Epstein-Barr virus, human leukocyte antigens HLA-A2 and HLA-B-Sin histocompatibility loci, nitrosamines, polycyclic hydrocarbons, poor living conditions, and chronic sinonasal infections.[44] The most common presentation is nodal

disease. There is no correlation between primary tumor size and the presence of nodal disease. Imaging with CT and MRI is performed to map accurately the extent of the disease, not for histologic diagnosis (Fig. 2-54).

2. Oropharynx

a. IMAGING ANATOMY OVERVIEW

The oropharynx is the region posterior to the oral cavity that includes the posterior one third of the tongue (tongue base), the palatine tonsils, the soft palate, and the oropharyngeal mucosa and constrictor muscles. The posterior pharyngeal wall is at the level of the second and third cervical vertebrae. Laterally, there are two mucosa-lined faucial arches; the anterior arch is formed by the mucosa of the palatoglossus muscle, and the posterior arch is formed by the palatopharyngeus muscle. The palatine tonsils are located between the two faucial arches, and the lingual tonsils reside at the base of the tongue. Both sets of tonsils vary in size and can encroach on the airway.

The arterial supply to the oropharynx is mainly from branches of the external carotid artery: the tonsillar branch of the facial artery, the ascending pharyngeal artery, the dorsal lingual arteries, and the internal maxillary and facial arteries. The venous drainage is primarily through the peritonsillar veins, which pierce the constrictor musculature and drain into the common facial vein and the pharyngeal plexus. Lymphatic drainage is mainly to the jugulodigastric chain from the skull base to the cricoid cartilage, the retropharyngeal nodes, the posterior

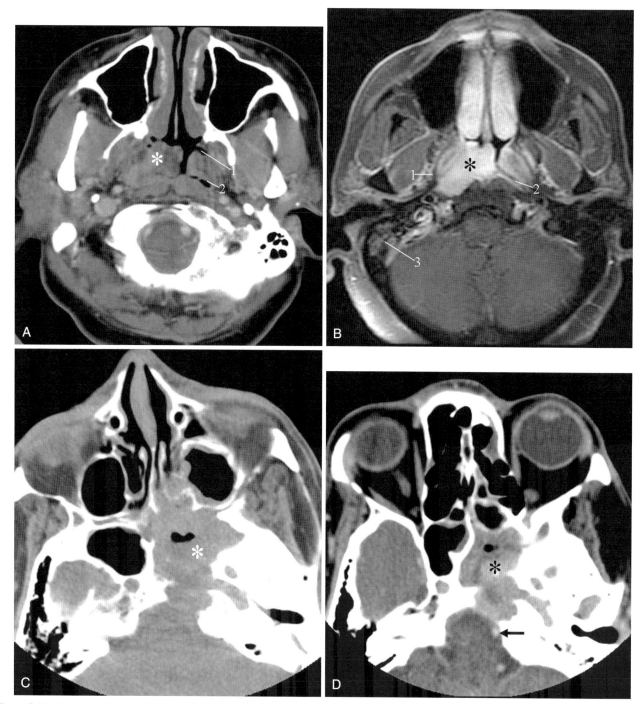

Figure 2-54 Squamous cell carcinoma (SCC) of the right nasopharynx. **A,** Axial computed tomogram (CT) with contrast demonstrates bulky soft tissue asymmetry in the nasopharynx with abnormal enhancement on the right. **B,** T1-weighted magnetic resonance image with gadolinium contrast confirms a right nasopharyngeal mass obstructing the eustachian canal and consequent opacification of the right mastoid air cells. **C,** Axial CT demonstrates SCC extending from the soft tissues of the left nasopharynx to the posterior fossa of the brain with bone destruction of the skull base. **D,** Axial CT after contrast enhancement. Notice the proximity of this invasive lesion to the vertebral artery (*arrow*) at the foramen magnum. If these findings are not appreciated at the time of surgery, an errant nasogastric tube can easily enter the cranium, damage the brainstem, and injure the vertebral artery. In each image, the mass is indicated by an *asterisk*. *1*, Eustachian tube; *2*, fossa of Rosenmüller; *3*, opacified mastoid air cells.

triangle nodes from the level of the skull base to the cricoid cartilage, and sometimes the parotid nodes.[44]

b. PERTINENT IMAGING PATHOLOGY

TONSILLAR HYPERTROPHY. During the third and fourth fetal months, lymphoid tissues invade the pharyngeal region of the adenoid tonsils, the palatine region (palatine tonsils), and the root of the tongue (lingual tonsils).[37] The adenoids are located in the roof of the nasopharynx. As mentioned previously, enlargement of the palatine and lingual tonsils may compromise the airway (Fig. 2-55).

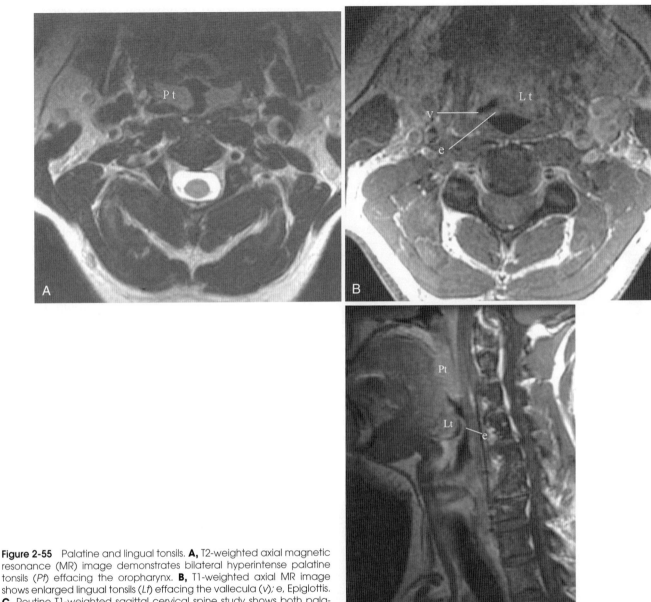

Figure 2-55 Palatine and lingual tonsils. **A,** T2-weighted axial magnetic resonance (MR) image demonstrates bilateral hyperintense palatine tonsils (*Pt*) effacing the oropharynx. **B,** T1-weighted axial MR image shows enlarged lingual tonsils (*Lt*) effacing the vallecula (*v*); e, Epiglottis. **C,** Routine T1-weighted sagittal cervical spine study shows both palatine tonsils (*Pt*) and lingual tonsils (*Lt*) effacing the airway. The lingual tonsils push the epiglottis (*e*) dorsally.

TONSILLITIS AND PERITONSILLAR ABSCESS. Acute bacterial tonsillitis is most commonly caused by β-hemolytic streptococcus, staphylococcus, pneumococcus, or *Haemophilus* species. It is usually a self-limited disease; however, uncontrolled infection of the tonsils may result in a peritonsillar abscess or, rarely, a tonsillar abscess. On CT imaging, the findings of acute or chronic tonsillitis are nonspecific. Focal homogeneous swelling of the palatine tonsils can be present and is difficult to differentiate from tumor. The imaging features of abscess formation are a low-density center and an enhancing rim of soft tissue (Fig. 2-56). Peritonsillar abscess is the accumulation of pus around the tonsils. The infection may extend to the retropharyngeal, parapharyngeal, or submandibular spaces.

RETROPHARYNGEAL PROCESS. Infection of the retropharyngeal space usually results from an infection at a site whose primary drainage is to the retropharyngeal lymph nodes, such as the nose, sinuses, throat, tonsils, oral cavity, or middle ear. The lymph nodes enlarge and undergo suppuration and eventually rupture into the retropharyngeal space, creating an abscess. It can be caused by a penetrating injury or by cervical spine osteomyelitis or diskitis. Before the advent of antibiotics, retropharyngeal infection was potentially life-threatening. A retropharyngeal space infection can extend from the skull base to the carina. On imaging, a retropharyngeal abscess expands the prevertebral space, with enhancement along its margins.

Included in the differential diagnosis of a retropharyngeal abscess is tendinitis of the longus colli, which is characterized by inflammation of the tendinous insertion of the longus colli muscle with deposition of calcium hydroxyapatite crystals. An effusion may extend from the

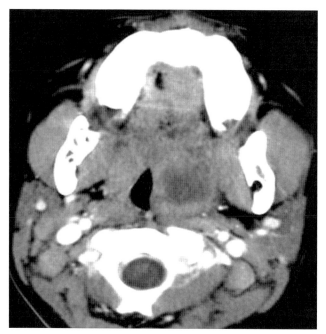

Figure 2-56 Tonsillar abscess. Axial computed tomogram with contrast demonstrates a left tonsillar fluid collection compressing the oropharynx.

prevertebral space into the retropharyngeal space and mimic a retropharyngeal abscess. Post-traumatic hematoma may also increase the width of the prevertebral space. In addition, cervical spine pathology can extend and enlarge the prevertebral space and cause the airway to deviate anteriorly.

TORTUOUS INTERNAL OR COMMON CAROTID ARTERY. If the course of either the common carotid artery or the internal carotid artery is directed medially, bulging of the submucosa of the oropharynx or hypopharynx may result. In this less protected location, the artery is more vulnerable to trauma. Imaging is useful to prevent unnecessary biopsy of this pseudosubmucosal mass (Fig. 2-57).

TUMORS AND OTHER CONDITIONS. SCC is the most common neoplasm of the oropharynx, and its predisposing factors include alcohol and tobacco use. Most recently, epidemiologic and molecular data have shown a strong association between human papillomavirus (HPV) infection—in particular, exposure to or infection with high-risk HPV-16—and the development of oropharyngeal cancer, especially tonsillar cancer. This subset of patients with oropharyngeal cancers present at a younger age and have distinct molecular and pathologic differences, with an as yet unexplained improved prognosis.[45] There is also a proven causal relationship between HPV-16 and the development of cervical cancer, and for this reason HPV infection is considered a sexually transmitted disease.

The site of origin determines the spread of the tumor; the most common locations are the anterior and posterior tonsillar pillars, tonsillar fossa, soft palate, and base of the tongue (Fig. 2-58). Staging of tumor in the oropharynx depends on the size of the tumor and whether it has invaded adjacent structures. Other neoplasms include lymphoma, minor salivary gland tumors, and mesenchymal tumors.

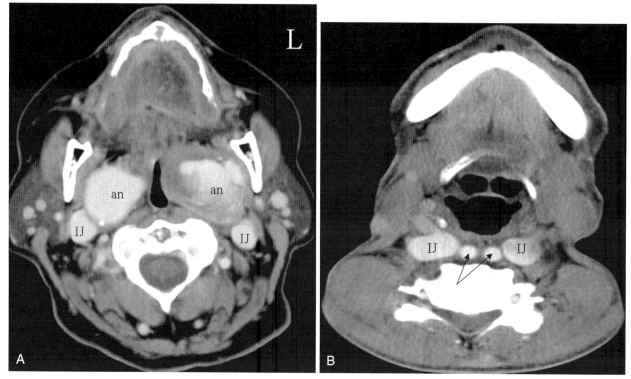

Figure 2-57 Anomalous course of carotids. **A,** Axial computed tomogram (CT) with contrast shows bilateral carotid aneurysms (*an*) effacing the oropharynx. Notice the presence of thrombus in the lumen of the aneurysm on the left. **B,** Axial CT with contrast demonstrates medially deviated carotids assuming a retropharyngeal location (*arrows*). *IJ,* Internal jugular vein.

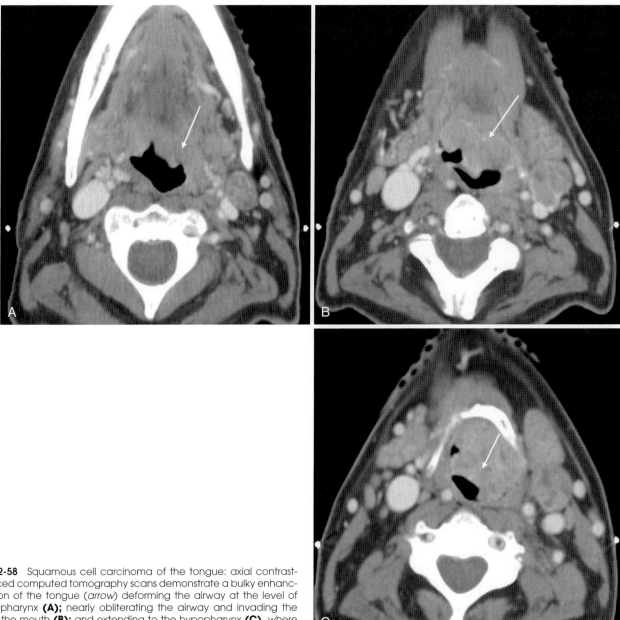

Figure 2-58 Squamous cell carcinoma of the tongue: axial contrast-enhanced computed tomography scans demonstrate a bulky enhancing lesion of the tongue (*arrow*) deforming the airway at the level of the oropharynx **(A)**; nearly obliterating the airway and invading the floor of the mouth **(B)**; and extending to the hypopharynx **(C)**, where it fills the pre-epiglottic space.

3. Hypopharynx

The boundary of the hypopharynx is classically defined as the segment of the pharynx that extends from the level of the hyoid bone and the valleculae to the cricopharyngeus or the lower level of the cricoid cartilage. By definition, the cervical esophagus starts at the caudal end of the cricoid cartilage. The cricopharyngeus muscle acts as the superior esophageal sphincter. It arises from the lower aspect of the inferior constrictor muscle attached to the cricoid. The upper esophageal sphincter is normally closed until a specific volume and pressure in the hypopharynx trigger relaxation of the cricopharyngeus muscle to allow a bolus of food to pass into the cervical esophagus. The cricopharyngeus muscle then closes to prevent reflux.[43]

a. IMAGING ANATOMY OVERVIEW

The hypopharynx can be divided into four regions: the pyriform sinuses, the posterior wall of the hypopharynx, the postcricoid region, and the lateral surface of the aryepiglottic folds. The pyriform sinus is the anterolateral recess of the hypopharynx. The anterior pyriform sinus mucosa abuts on the posterior paraglottic space. The most caudal portion of the pyriform sinus lies at the level of the true vocal cords. The lateral aspect of the aryepiglottic folds forms the medial wall of the pyriform sinus (Fig. 2-59). This is considered a marginal zone because the aryepiglottic folds are part of both the hypopharynx and the supraglottic larynx. Tumors involving the medial surface of the aryepiglottic folds behave like laryngeal tumors. The biologic behavior of tumors arising from the

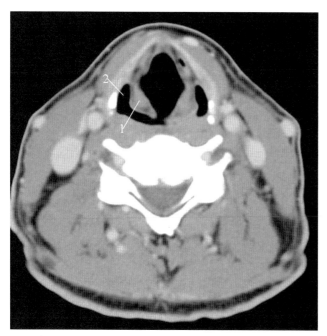

Figure 2-59 Aryepiglottic fold and pyriform sinus. Axial computed tomogram at the level of hypopharynx. *1*, Aryepiglottic fold; *2*, air-containing pyriform sinus.

lateral surface of the aryepiglottic folds is similar to that of the more aggressive pharyngeal tumors. The lateral wall of the pyriform sinus is formed by the thyroid membrane and cartilage.[44]

The posterior hypopharyngeal wall is continuous with the posterior wall of the oropharynx and begins at the level of the valleculae. It continues caudally as the posterior wall of the cricopharyngeus and the cervical esophagus. The retropharyngeal space lies behind the posterior pharyngeal wall. The anterior wall of the lower hypopharynx is referred to as the *postcricoid hypopharynx*: the larynx is anterior and the hypopharynx is posterior to this soft tissue boundary. It extends from the level of the arytenoid cartilages to the lower cricoid cartilage. On imaging, the transition from the hypopharynx to the cervical esophagus is denoted by a change in the shape of the aerodigestive tract, from crescentic or ovoid to round.

The arterial supply to the lower pharynx is mainly from the superior and inferior thyroid arteries. Venous drainage is through the superior and inferior thyroid veins and individual pharyngeal veins to the internal jugular vein.

b. PERTINENT IMAGING PATHOLOGY

PHARYNGITIS. In immunocompetent patients, imaging is usually not required for the diagnosis or management of pharyngitis. In AIDS patients, imaging may be helpful to evaluate the extent of disease. Bacterial etiology is not the only concern; opportunistic infection with *Candida* or cytomegalovirus may involve the hypopharynx. These entities do not compromise the airway, but the mucosa is friable and is susceptible to injuries from instrumentation.

PHARYNGOCELE. A pharyngocele is a broad-based outpouching of the pharyngeal mucosa of the upper pyriform sinus, which distends with phonation or during the Valsalva maneuver. These lesions are visible as air-filled structures on CT or as barium-filled areas on a barium swallow test.

ZENKER'S DIVERTICULUM. It is postulated that dyssynergy of the cricopharyngeus muscle plays a role in the formation of this pulsion diverticulum of the hypopharynx. The diverticulum typically extends posteriorly and laterally, usually to the left, and may appear as an incidental, air-filled structure in the hypopharynx on CT and MRI. If alerted to the presence of a diverticulum, one should take more caution during blind advancement of an NGT, which may take an errant course (Fig. 2-60).

TRAUMA

Hematomas. Direct trauma or iatrogenic trauma caused by instrumentation, surgery, or a foreign body may result in retropharyngeal hematoma. Hemophiliacs may be more susceptible to hematomas with minor trauma. The imaging finding is retropharyngeal or prevertebral soft tissue swelling.

Postradiation Changes. The edema that occurs after radiation therapy may persist for many months or years and reflects a radiation-induced obliterative endarteritis. In cases of edema, the pharyngeal and supraglottic mucosa appears swollen, bulging, and hypodense on CT, and the submucosa fat is thickened and streaky. The platysma muscle and skin are also thickened. The end result is fibrosis and loss of elasticity of the soft tissues. This increased rigidity of the soft tissues should be taken into account during laryngoscopy for endotracheal intubation and in selecting the correct size of a laryngeal mask airway (LMA). Specifically, the LMA needs to be one or even two sizes smaller than predicted by the patient's weight.

TUMORS AND OTHER CONDITIONS

Squamous Cell Carcinoma. The hypopharynx is lined by stratified squamous epithelium, and most tumors of the hypopharynx are SCCs (Fig. 2-61). The risk factors for SCC of the hypopharynx include alcohol abuse, smoking, and previous radiation therapy. Patients with Plummer-Vinson syndrome have a higher incidence of postcricoid carcinoma. Extensive submucosal growth is common and can be appreciated only on imaging. The airway may be effaced and displaced. Most patients have metastases to the cervical nodes at presentation. Between 4% and 15% of patients with SCC of the hypopharynx have a synchronous or metachronous second primary tumor.[44,46]

Lymphomas. Hodgkin's lymphoma predominantly affects adolescents and young adults, whereas non-Hodgkin's lymphoma is a disease of older patients. In contrast to patients with Hodgkin's disease, patients with non-Hodgkin's lymphoma present with disease in extranodal sites, such as Waldeyer's ring. The imaging features of extranodal head and neck lymphoma can be difficult to differentiate from those of SCC. Lymphadenopathy in Hodgkin's disease can be quite large without affecting the airways.

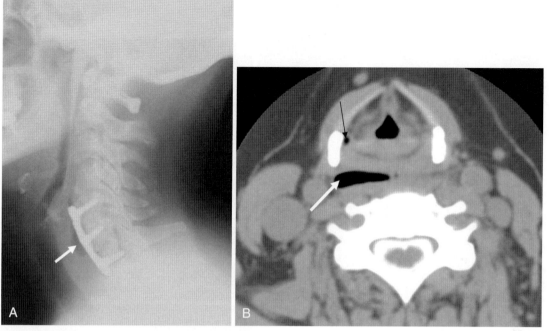

Figure 2-60 Zenker's diverticulum. **A,** Lateral cervical spine computed tomogram (CT) with soft tissue technique demonstrates an air-filled structure in the hypopharynx (*white arrow*) after anterior fusion. **B,** Axial CT at the level of the larynx shows the air-filled Zenker diverticulum to the right of midline (*white arrow*) and the tip of the right pyriform sinus (*black arrow*).

Other Malignancies. Less common primary cancers in the pharynx include minor salivary gland tumors (most often involving the soft palate), rhabdomyosarcomas, granular cell tumors, schwannomas and neurofibromas, hemangiomas, lipomas, amyloids, and metastases.[43,44]

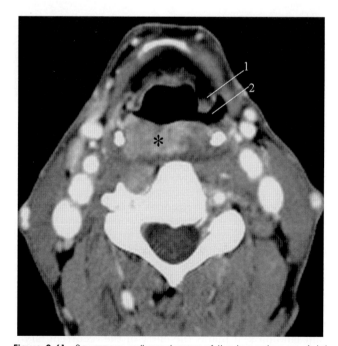

Figure 2-61 Squamous cell carcinoma of the hypopharynx. Axial computed tomogram with contrast demonstrates an enhancing mass (*asterisk*) involving the posterior wall of the hypopharynx with deformity of the airway. Notice the effacement of the right pyriform sinus. *1,* Aryepiglottic fold; *2,* pyriform sinus.

E. Larynx

1. Imaging Anatomy Overview

Before the advent of CT and MRI, examination of the larynx consisted of plain radiographic films, multidirectional tomography, barium swallow, and laryngography. On a sagittal view, one can easily identify the hyoid bone, epiglottis, aryepiglottic folds, and vestibule, which is the space extending from the epiglottis to the level of the false vocal cords. At the level of the thyroid cartilage, a tiny slit of air is seen directed in the anterior-posterior direction. This is the laryngeal ventricle, which separates the false vocal cords from the true vocal cords (see Fig. 2-15).

Barium swallow, which is still used today, provides dynamic information about the swallowing mechanism and any dysfunction or incoordination of the muscles of swallowing and respiration. CT and MRI allow visualization of structures deep to the mucosa (Fig. 2-62); however, breathing and swallowing movements make imaging of the larynx difficult. The faster CT scanning technology available today allows the entire neck to be scanned in a single breath-hold. Helical technology allows reformation of the airway in multiple planes with one acquisition. MRI examination of the larynx continues to be problematic because of motion artifacts intrinsic and extrinsic to the larynx and longer acquisition time compared with CT. The advantage of MRI over CT is its ability to distinguish greater soft tissue contrast. The multiplanar capability of both CT and MRI is helpful in the evaluation of the mucosal folds and spaces in the neck.

In brief, the larynx can be considered as a conduit to the lungs. It also provides airway protection against aspiration and allows vocalization. It has an outer supporting

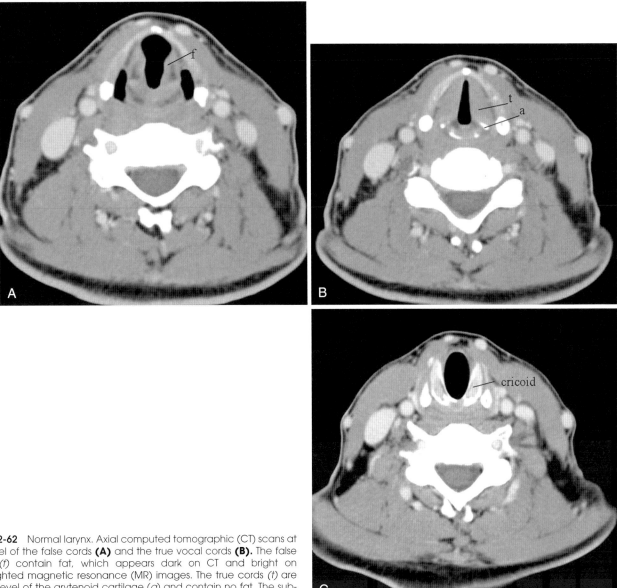

Figure 2-62 Normal larynx. Axial computed tomographic (CT) scans at the level of the false cords **(A)** and the true vocal cords **(B).** The false cords *(f)* contain fat, which appears dark on CT and bright on T1-weighted magnetic resonance (MR) images. The true cords *(t)* are at the level of the arytenoid cartilage *(a)* and contain no fat. The subglottic airway is ovoid in shape, as shown in an axial CT scan **(C).**

skeleton comprising a series of cartilages, fibrous sheets, muscles, and ligaments that provides structure and protection for the inner mucosal tube, the endolarynx. Between the cartilages and the mucosal surface lie the paraglottic and pre-epiglottic spaces, which contain loose areolar tissues, lymphatics, and muscles. Superiorly, the larynx is suspended from the hyoid bone, which is attached to the styloid process at the base of the skull by the stylohyoid ligament. Calcification of the stylohyoid ligament (see Fig. 2-11) has been proposed as a cause of difficult intubation.[18] Contraction of the muscles attached to the hyoid bone move it anterior and superior with consequent similar movements of the larynx. This sequence of movements also pulls the epiglottis to the horizontal plane, eventually inverting and closing the glottis and contributing to protection from aspiration.[47,48]

The parts of the exoskeleton of the larynx that are visible on plain radiography include the arytenoid cartilage, the cricoid cartilage, and the thyroid cartilage, which is the largest cartilage of the larynx. The thyroid cartilage is made up of two shieldlike laminae that fuse anteriorly to form the laryngeal prominence (Adam's apple). The angle of the fusion is usually more acute and more prominent in men. Paired superior and inferior cornua project from the posterior margin of the thyroid cartilage. The superior thyroid cornu is connected with the dorsal tip of the greater cornu of the hyoid bone by the thyrohyoid membrane. The inferior cornu articulates medially with the lateral wall of the cricoid cartilage to form the cricothyroid joint, where the thyroid cartilage rocks back and forth. Radiographically, this is an important landmark; it marks the entry of the recurrent laryngeal nerve to the larynx.[38] Muscles that attach to the external surface of the thyroid cartilage include the sternothyroid and thyrohyoid muscles and the inferior pharyngeal constrictors. The thyrohyoid membrane bridges

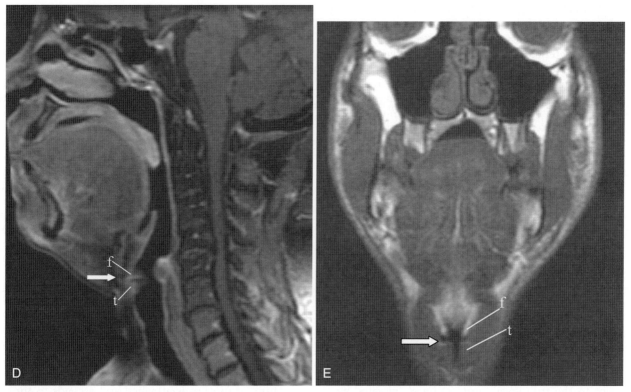

Figure 2-62, cont'd T-1 weighted sagittal **(D)** and coronal **(E)** MR images demonstrate the false cords *(f)* separated from the true cords *(f)* by the laryngeal ventricle *(arrow)*.

the gap between the upper surface of the thyroid cartilage and the hyoid bone. Likewise, the cricothyroid membrane spans the distance between the lower margin of the thyroid cartilage and the cricoid cartilage.[47]

The cricoid cartilage, which is shaped like a signet ring with the larger part facing posteriorly, is the base of the larynx. On the upper surface of the cricoid lamina are two paired articular facets, on which are situated the arytenoid cartilages. The arytenoid cartilages are important surgical and imaging landmarks.[25] Each cartilage is pyramidal in shape. The base is formed by two projections: the muscular process situated on the posterolateral margin and the vocal process located anteriorly. The muscular and vocal processes are at the level of the true vocal cords.

The corniculate cartilage sits at the apex of the pyramid and is located above the level of the laryngeal ventricle, at the level of the false vocal cords. The arytenoid cartilages are important in maintaining airway patency and participate in vocalization by altering the opening of the glottis and the tension of the vocal cords. This is achieved by movements between the arytenoid and cricoid cartilages: adduction, abduction, anterior-posterior sliding, and medial-lateral sliding.[25]

For surgical planning purposes, the endolarynx can be divided into three compartments: the supraglottic larynx, the glottic larynx (glottis), and the subglottic larynx. The supraglottic airway can be defined as extending from the tip of the epiglottis to the laryngeal ventricles; it includes the false vocal cords, epiglottis, aryepiglottic folds, and arytenoids. The glottis is defined

by the mucosal coverings of the true vocal cords and the anterior and posterior commissures. The subglottic larynx includes the undersurface of the true vocal cords and extends to the lower border of the cricoid cartilage.[38,47] The laryngeal ventricle demarcates two embryologically distinct laryngeal components: the supraglottic larynx and the subglottic larynx. The supraglottic larynx forms from primitive anlage and has richer lymphatics compared with the tracheobronchial buds. This embryologic and histologic difference accounts for the higher incidence of nodal metastasis at presentation of squamous cell cancer of the supraglottic larynx as compared to that of the glottic or subglottic primary.[47]

Several structures in the endoskeleton of the larynx are worth describing. The *epiglottis* is a yellow elastic fibrocartilage; its tip defines the cephalad margin of the supraglottic larynx. It has a flattened teardrop or leaf shape that tapers to an inferior point called the petiole of the epiglottis, where it attaches to the thyroid cartilage through the thyroepiglottic ligament. The superior and lateral edges are free. Most of the epiglottis extends behind the thyroid cartilage; the tip may be above the hyoid bone and sometimes can be seen through the oral cavity. It is held in place and stabilized by the hyoepiglottic and thyroepiglottic ligaments. The hyoepiglottic ligament is a tough, fibrous, fanlike ligament that extends from the ventral midline of the epiglottis to the dorsal margin of the hyoid cartilage. Immediately above the ligament are the pharyngeal recesses, the valleculae, which are situated just caudal to the tongue base. The epiglottis helps to guard against aspiration; during swallowing, the aryepiglottic folds pull the sides of the epiglottis down, thereby narrowing the entrance to the larynx.[25,48]

The *quadrangular membrane* stretches anteriorly from the upper arytenoid and corniculate cartilages to the lateral margin of the epiglottis and contributes to the support of the epiglottis.[47] The superior free margin of this membrane forms the support for the aryepiglottic fold, which stretches from the upper margin of the arytenoids to the lateral margin of the epiglottis. The corniculate and cuneiform cartilages within the aryepiglottic fold help support the edge of each fold. These small, mucosa-covered cartilages are visualized on laryngoscopy as two small protuberances at the posterolateral border of the rima glottidis.[25] The aryepiglottic folds form the lateral margin of the vestibule of the supraglottic airway. The upper part of the aryepiglottic fold is the aryepiglottic muscle, which functions like a purse string to close the opening of the larynx during swallowing. Lateral to the aryepiglottic folds are the pyriform sinuses. The apex, the most inferior aspect of the pyriform sinus, is at the level of the true vocal cords.

The inferior free margin of the quadrangular membrane forms the *ventricular ligament*, which extends anteriorly from the superior arytenoid cartilage to the inner lamina of the thyroid cartilage and supports the free edge of the false vocal cords. The false vocal cords are superior to the true vocal cords and are separated by a lateral pouching of the airway, the laryngeal ventricle.[47] A second set of ligaments, the vocal ligaments, lies parallel and inferior to the ventricular ligament. It also extends from the vocal process of the arytenoid cartilage to the inner lamina of the thyroid just above the anterior commissure. The vocal ligament provides medial support for the true vocal cords. The space between the left and right vocal cords is referred to as the rima glottis, through which air passes to allow breathing and vocalization. Extending from the vocal ligament is another fibrous membrane, the conus elasticus, which attaches inferiorly to the upper inner margin of the cricoid cartilage. The conus spans part of the gap between the thyroid and cricoid cartilages.[25,47]

The muscles of the larynx are categorized as intrinsic and extrinsic muscles. The intrinsic muscles regulate the aperture of the rima glottis: (1) the thyroarytenoid makes up the bulk of the true vocal cord and has a lateral and a medial belly; (2) the lateral cricoarytenoids extend from the muscular process of the arytenoid cartilage to the upper lateral cricoid cartilage and function to adduct the cords; (3) the posterior cricoarytenoids extend from the muscular process of the arytenoid cartilage to the posterior surface of the cricoid cartilage and abduct the cords laterally; and (4) the intra-arytenoid muscle stretches from one arytenoid to the other and functions to adduct the vocal cords.[25,47] The extrinsic muscle is the cricothyroid muscle, which extends from the lower thyroid cartilage anteriorly to the upper cricoid cartilage. The contraction of this muscle pivots the thyroid cartilage forward around an axis through the cricothyroid joint, which stretches and tenses the vocal cords, thus affecting pitch in vocalization.[25,47]

Because the vocal cords are not static structures, they are difficult to image. During normal respiration, the vocal cords are slightly abducted. During deep inspiration, the true vocal cords fully abduct against the lateral wall of the glottic airway. The airway opening becomes narrowed with medialization of the true cords during breath-holding with or without a Valsalva maneuver, expiration, and phonation. Extending below the true vocal cords to the cricoid cartilage is the infraglottic cavity. The trachea begins below the level of the cricoid cartilage.[47]

The larynx is innervated primarily by branches of the vagus nerve.[25] The recurrent laryngeal nerve innervates all the intrinsic muscles of the larynx. If vocal cord paralysis is present and nerve damage is suspected, imaging should be tailored to follow the course of the recurrent laryngeal nerve in the neck and upper chest. The vagus nerve, after exiting the jugular foramen, passes vertically down the neck within the carotid sheath, between the internal jugular vein and the internal carotid artery (which becomes the common carotid artery) to the root of the neck. In front of the right subclavian artery, the recurrent laryngeal nerve branches from the vagus nerve, loops around the right subclavian artery, and ascends to the side of the trachea behind the common carotid artery, in the tracheoesophageal groove. On the left side, the recurrent laryngeal nerve arises at the level of the aortic arch. It loops around the arch at the point where ligamentum arteriosum is attached and ascends to the side of the trachea in the tracheoesophageal groove. The recurrent laryngeal nerve enters the larynx behind the cricothyroid joint and innervates all the muscles of the larynx except the cricothyroid muscle, which is an extrinsic muscle of the anterior larynx that is innervated by the external laryngeal branch of the superior laryngeal nerve, a branch of the vagus nerve in the neck. Sensory input from the laryngeal mucosa is by the internal laryngeal branch of the superior laryngeal nerve, which perforates the posterior lateral portion of the thyrohyoid membrane.[25]

The blood supply to the larynx is from two branches of the external carotid artery: the superior and inferior laryngeal arteries. The superior laryngeal artery, a branch of the superior thyroid artery, travels with the internal branch of the superior laryngeal nerve. The inferior laryngeal artery, a branch of the inferior thyroid artery, which is a branch of the thyrocervical trunk, accompanies the recurrent laryngeal nerve into the larynx.[25]

2. Pertinent Imaging Pathology

a. TRAUMA

Fracture of the larynx, which usually occurs as a result of a vehicular accident, can involve the thyroid cartilage, the cricoid cartilage, or both. Laryngotracheal separation is usually fatal. Dislocation of the arytenoids relative to the cricoid cartilage may be encountered. Malalignment of the thyroid and cricoid cartilages results in dislocation of the cricothyroid joint. On imaging, the presence of air in the paraglottic soft tissues is an indication of laryngeal trauma (Fig. 2-63).

Foreign bodies may be present due to trauma but are more commonly the result of ingestion or aspiration. The pyriform sinus is a common location for a foreign body.

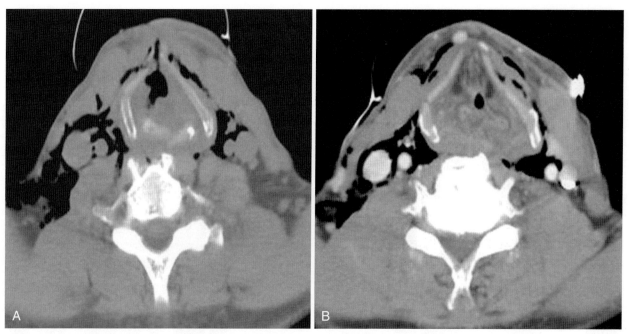

Figure 2-63 Laryngeal fracture. Precontrast **(A)** and postcontrast **(B)** axial computed tomography scans show extensive deep fascial emphysema as well as multiple fractures of the thyroid and cricoid cartilages.

If the foreign body enters the larynx, it usually passes through to the trachea or a bronchus. Burn injury to the larynx can be caused by inhalation or ingestion of hot material. The supraglottic larynx is most likely to be involved, and generalized edema can occur.

b. VOCAL CORD PARALYSIS

Vocal cord paralysis may be characterized as either a superior laryngeal nerve deficit, a recurrent laryngeal nerve deficit, or a total vagus nerve deficit. The entire course of the vagus nerve and the recurrent laryngeal nerve should be imaged when assessing vocal cord paralysis (Fig. 2-64).

The superior laryngeal nerve, through the external laryngeal branch, innervates only one muscle of the larynx—an extrinsic muscle, the cricothyroid muscle. This muscle extends between the thyroid and cricoid cartilages. As the muscle contracts, the anterior cricoid ring is pulled up toward the lower margin of the thyroid cartilage. This action rotates the upper cricoid lamina (and thus the arytenoids) posteriorly and puts tension on the true vocal cords. If one side is paralyzed, contraction of one muscle rotates the posterior cricoid to the contralateral paralyzed side.

More commonly, vocal cord paralysis is caused by recurrent laryngeal nerve pathology. All of the laryngeal muscles, except for the cricothyroid muscle, are innervated by this nerve. Most findings are secondary to atrophy of the thyroarytenoid muscle, the muscle that contributes to the bulk of the true vocal cords. The vocal cords become thinner and more pointed. Compensatory enlargement of the ventricle and the pyriform sinus is seen.[47] In the more acute phase, the paralyzed cord appears flaccid, prolapses medially because of the lack of muscular tone in the thyroarytenoid muscle, and

demonstrates a lack of movement during breathing maneuvers and phonation.

c. CONGENITAL LESIONS

The respiratory system is formed from an outpouching of the primitive pharynx.[42,47] A tracheoesophageal septum is formed and separates the trachea from the primitive foregut. The laryngeal lumen is initially occluded and later recanalizes. Congenital lesions are related to delays in the development and maturation of the respiratory system.[42,47]

LARYNGOMALACIA. Laryngomalacia represents a delay in the development of the laryngeal support system. The structures of the larynx are present but are not mature enough to keep the larynx open. Primarily, the supraglottic larynx is affected to a varying degree. The presentation in the infant may vary from a floppy epiglottis only to collapse of the entire supraglottic larynx on inspiration. This abnormality is self-limited, and the problem resolves with maturation.[42,47]

WEBS AND ATRESIAS. Webs can be seen at any level of the larynx, but they are usually at the level of the true vocal cords. Subglottic webs are sometimes associated with cricoid abnormalities. Atresia of the larynx results from incomplete recanalization. Although the trachea is formed, there is no air passage to it.[42,47]

STENOSIS. Stenosis of the larynx or the upper trachea may be caused by a congenital anomaly or by iatrogenic or therapeutic trauma. Congenital subglottic stenosis is secondary to soft tissue stenosis from the true cord down to the cricoid. The infant usually outgrows this problem.

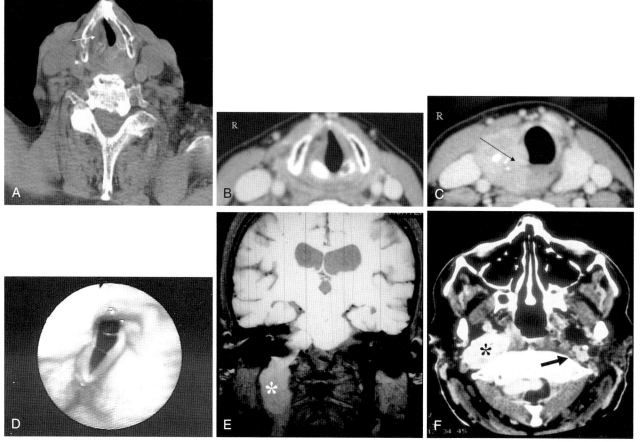

Figure 2-64 Causes of vocal cord paralysis in three different patients. In patient 1, there is right vocal cord paralysis secondary to tumor invasion. An axial computed tomographic (CT) scan **(A)** demonstrates squamous cell carcinoma invading the right vocal cord, which is medially deviated. In patient 2, there is right vocal cord paralysis secondary to tumor in the tracheoesophageal groove involving the recurrent laryngeal nerve. An axial contrast-enhanced CT scan **(B)** demonstrates a paralyzed right true vocal cord. In this case, denervation results from neural compromise in the tracheoesophageal groove due to papillary carcinoma of the right thyroid tumor **(C)**. The paralyzed right cord is visualized endoscopically in **D.** In patient 3, a contrast-enhanced coronal T1-weighted magnetic resonance image **(E)** and an axial CT scan **(F)** demonstrate an enhancing vagus nerve schwannoma (*asterisk*) in a patient with known neurofibromatosis. Notice the normal vagus nerve (*arrow*), which is located within the contralateral carotid sheath, together with the carotid artery and jugular vein. This patient presented with right vocal cord paralysis.

The most common cause of stenosis is prolonged tracheal intubation or tracheostomy. Typically, the pattern of involvement starts anteriorly and laterally before eventually circumferentially involving the membranous portion. Trauma-related stenosis has a more variable pattern. Ingestion of caustic material usually results in strictures along the posterior supraglottic airway and larynx.[42,47] Both plain radiographic studies and CT are good at assessing the extent and length of the stenotic segment.

d. TUMORS AND OTHER CONDITIONS

BENIGN TUMORS. Benign masses encountered in the larynx include vocal cord nodules, juvenile papillomatosis, and other nonepithelial tumors such as hemangiomas, lipomas, leiomyomas, rhabdomyomas, chondromas, neural tumors, paragangliomas, schwannomas, and granular cell tumors.[42]

CYSTS AND LARYNGOCELES. Mucus-retention cysts can occur along any mucosal surface, but they are most common in the supraglottic larynx. Laryngoceles may be internal, external, or both. The common finding in a supraglottic mass is its connection with the laryngeal ventricle (Fig. 2-65).[42,47]

MALIGNANT NEOPLASMS. Most laryngeal tumors are malignant, and SCC is the most common type. These cancers arise on the mucosal surface and can be readily visualized by direct endoscopy. Imaging with CT and MRI is used to define the extent of the disease. Cross-sectional imaging is useful to assess the degree and direction of airway compromise (Fig. 2-66). Other cell types found are adenocarcinoma, verrucous carcinoma, and anaplastic carcinoma. More rare tumors are sarcoma, melanoma, lymphoma, leukemia, plasmacytoma, fibrous histiocytoma, and metastatic disease.[47]

F. Trachea

The trachea is a tubular structure that extends from the cricoid cartilage, at approximately the C6 level, to the carina, usually at the T5 or T6 level. It is a conduit between the larynx and the lungs and is composed of 16 to 20 incomplete hyaline cartilaginous rings bound in a

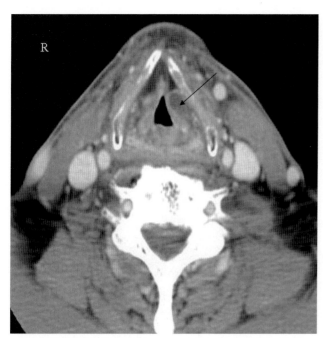

Figure 2-65 Laryngocele. Axial contrast-enhanced computed tomographic scan demonstrates a fluid-filled internal laryngocele on the left (*arrow*).

tight elastic connective tissue that is oriented longitudinally. The cartilage forms about two thirds of the circumference of the trachea; the posterior border is formed by a fibromuscular membrane. The trachea is approximately 10 to 13 cm long (average length, 11 cm). The diameter of the tracheal lumen depends on the height, age, and gender of the subject. In men, the tracheal diameter ranges from 13 to 25 mm in the coronal imaging plane and from 13 to 27 mm in the sagittal imaging plane. In women, the dimensions are 10 to 21 mm in the coronal plane and 10 to 23 mm in the sagittal plane.[49,50] Cross-sectional area correlates best with height in children.

The axial sections of the tracheal lumen assume the following successive shapes: round, lunate, flattened, and elliptical. The luminal shape is also affected by the respiratory cycle, maneuvers, and body position. During rapid and deep inspiration, the thoracic portion of the trachea widens and the cervical portion narrows; the opposite occurs with expiration. The innervation of the trachea is from the parasympathetic tracheal branches of the vagus nerve, the recurrent laryngeal nerve, and the sympathetic nerves. The trachea has a segmental blood supply from multiple branches of the inferior thyroidal arteries and bronchial arteries.[25]

1. Imaging Anatomy Overview

Radiologic evaluation of the trachea includes plain films of the neck and chest, CT, and MRI. A lateral view of the neck provides a good screening examination for the cervical trachea. Chest radiography allows an initial assessment of the thoracic trachea and mediastinal structures. CT, and especially helical CT, is superior for evaluation of the tracheal anatomy and pathology because it allows direct visualization of the cross-sectional trachea. With multiplanar reconstruction, the degree and length of

stenosis can be fully assessed. Virtual bronchoscopy, which is a 3-D reconstruction of helical CT data, allows simulated navigation through the tracheobronchial tree. MRI so far has limited use owing to its longer scanning time, intrinsic artifacts from breathing motion, and limited resolution.

2. Pertinent Imaging Pathology

Early detection of tracheal pathology is unusual because significant compromise of the airway can be present before symptoms manifest. More than 75% occlusion of the luminal diameter at rest, and more than 50% occlusion during exertion, must be present before symptoms of airway obstruction are manifested.[50] If symptoms are present, a superior mediastinal mass is often found on PA chest radiography. Also, the tracheal air column may be deviated or narrowed. Rarely, tracheal enlargement occurs as a result of tracheomalacia in patients with cystic fibrosis or Ehlers-Danlos complex. Pathology affecting the trachea can largely be classified as extrinsic or intrinsic diseases.

a. EXTRINSIC TRACHEAL PATHOLOGY

THYROID GOITER. One of the more common extrinsic pathologies affecting the cervical and substernal trachea is a goiter of the thyroid gland. The trachea is usually displaced laterally, and luminal compression is evident. Vocal cord paralysis, hoarseness, dyspnea, and dysphagia may be the presenting symptoms. These symptoms are all predictable and are predicated on the location of the goiter with respect to the trachea, the esophagus, and the recurrent laryngeal nerve. The lateral and posterior extension of abnormal soft tissue with respect to the larynx displaces the airway anteriorly and laterally and may be a cause of difficult intubation (Fig. 2-67).

THYROID CARCINOMA AND NODES. As in the case of thyroid goiter, any mass involving or enlarging the thyroid gland can result in airway displacement and compression (Fig. 2-68). Enlarged lymph nodes secondary to lymphoma or metastatic disease can also cause extrinsic compression of the trachea.

VASCULAR RINGS AND SLINGS. Vascular rings encircle both the trachea and the esophagus with airway compression. The most common example is the double aortic arch. Vascular slings are noncircumferential vascular anomalies that may cause airway compromise. The trachea may be compressed posteriorly from a pulmonary artery sling, in which the left pulmonary artery arises from the right pulmonary artery. It can also be compressed from the front by the innominate artery or an aberrant left subclavian artery.

b. INTRINSIC TRACHEAL PATHOLOGY

TRAUMA. External injury to the trachea more frequently results from blunt trauma than from penetrating trauma, and it is often associated with other significant injuries to the chest, cervical spine, and great vessels. Pneumothorax, pneumomediastinum, and subcutaneous emphysema may be the presenting signs, in addition to endotracheal bleeding and airway compromise. Internal injuries such

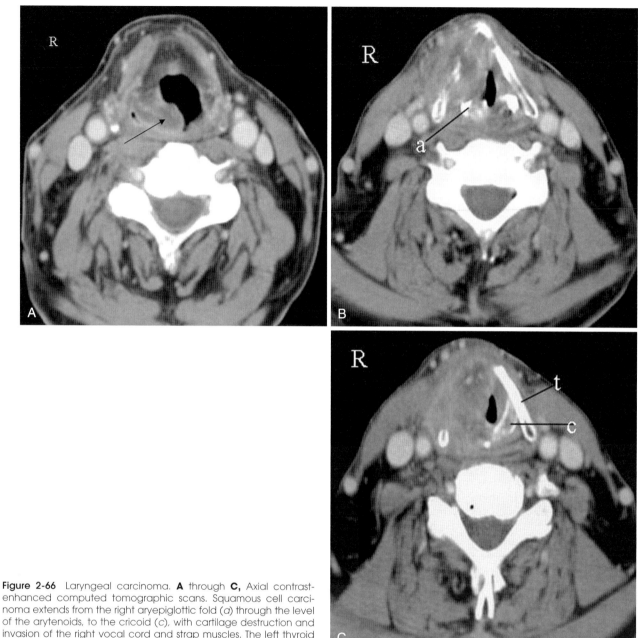

Figure 2-66 Laryngeal carcinoma. **A** through **C,** Axial contrast-enhanced computed tomographic scans. Squamous cell carcinoma extends from the right aryepiglottic fold (*a*) through the level of the arytenoids, to the cricoid (*c*), with cartilage destruction and invasion of the right vocal cord and strap muscles. The left thyroid cartilage (*f*) is intact, and the right is destroyed by tumor.

as chemical and thermal injury to the airway result in mucosal edema and subsequent airway compromise.

IATROGENIC INJURY. A late complication of translaryngeal intubation is stenosis at the cuff site, tip, or stoma site of the tracheostomy. Cuff trauma is related to pressure necrosis, in which the cuff pressure exceeds the capillary pressure. The incidence of this complication has decreased significantly since the introduction of the high-volume, low-pressure cuff, which is more pliable and can mold to the contours of the trachea. The blood supply to the anterior cartilages is susceptible to pressure effects, and anterior tracheal scarring may occur. With increased pressure, the posterior membranous part of the trachea can become affected, and the scarring becomes more circumferential. This type of injury is related to the position of the cuff and is seen radiographically as smooth tapering over one or two cartilage segments. Symptoms may arise from 2 weeks to months after extubation. Less common long-term complications of endotracheal intubation include tracheomalacia and tracheoesophageal fistula (TEF).[13,51]

Early tracheostomy complications are usually related to an abnormal angulation of the tube. In contrast to endotracheal intubation, tracheostomy is not affected by changes in head and neck position because it is not anchored at the nose or mouth. Angulation of the tracheostomy tube may result in increased airway resistance, difficulty in clearing secretions, erosion, or perforation of the trachea.

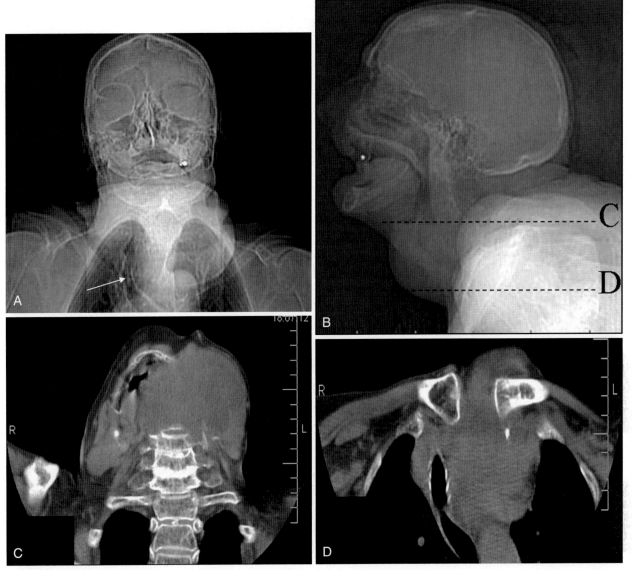

Figure 2-67   Goiter. Anteroposterior computed tomogram **(A)** and lateral scout film **(B)** demonstrate a clinically obvious thyroid mass. Notice the tracheal deviation in image **A** (*arrow*) and the anterior displacement of the airway in image **B. C** and **D,** Axial images (referenced on the lateral scout view) further demonstrate the mass effect on the airway from the level of the hyoid to the thoracic inlet.

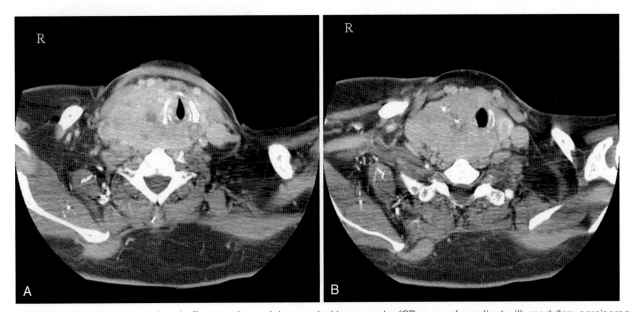

Figure 2-68   Tracheal displacement and effacement on axial computed tomography (CT) scans of a patient with medullary carcinoma of the thyroid. **A,** CT scan demonstrates the right thyroid mass displacing the airway anteriorly and to the contralateral side. **B,** The tumor has destroyed the cricoid cartilage on the right and abuts the subglottic airway.

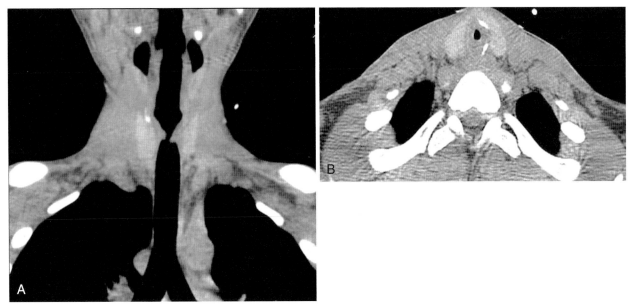

Figure 2-69 Tracheal stenosis. **A,** Coronal reformatted computed tomographic (CT) image in a child demonstrates marked subglottic narrowing of the trachea. **B,** Axial CT in the same patient further defines the severity of narrowing.

c. NON-NEOPLASTIC TRACHEAL NARROWING

The intrinsic pathology of diffuse tracheal narrowing results from trauma due to aspiration of heat or of caustic or acid chemicals, radiation therapy, or intubation injury; additional unusual causes include sarcoidosis, Wegener's granulomatosis, fungal infection, croup, and congenital conditions (Fig. 2-69).

TRACHEOMALACIA. Tracheomalacia is characterized by abnormal flaccidity of the trachea resulting in collapse of the thoracic tracheal segment during expiration. There is softening of the supporting cartilage and widening of the posterior membranous wall, which may balloon anteriorly into the airway. Tracheomalacia can be divided into primary intrinsic and secondary extrinsic forms. Patients may have minimal or severe symptoms depending on the degree of airway obstruction.

CONGENITAL STENOSIS (SUBGLOTTIC OR TRACHEAL). Congenital stenosis is uncommon and is usually associated with other congenital anomalies. The affected segment has rigid walls with a narrowed lumen, and the cartilages can be complete rings. The stenotic segment can be focal, or the entire trachea may be affected. Symptoms usually arise within the first few weeks or months of age. Most patients are treated conservatively.

TRACHEOESOPHAGEAL FISTULA. TEF is a common congenital anomaly, with an incidence of 1 in 3000 to 4000 births. TEF is often associated with esophageal atresia.[50] There are several forms of TEF. The most common is a proximal esophageal atresia with a distal TEF. This anomaly may be associated with severe neonatal respiratory distress and may necessitate emergent tracheostomy. It is not uncommon for more than one fistula to be present, and there may be other associated anomalies affecting the cardiovascular, gastrointestinal, renal, or central nervous system (Fig. 2-70).

d. TUMORS AND OTHER CONDITIONS

Most benign tracheal neoplasms are found in pediatric patients. Squamous cell papilloma, fibroma, and hemangioma are the most common types. In adults, the most common benign tumors are chondroma, papilloma, fibroma, hemangioma, and granular cell myoblastoma.

Primary malignant neoplasms of the trachea are uncommon; laryngeal and bronchial primary tumors are

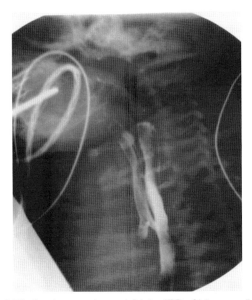

Figure 2-70 Tracheoesophageal fistula (TEF). Oblique radiograph from a swallow study with contrast outlines a classic H-type TEF. (Courtesy of Dr. Netta Marlyn Blitman, Montefiore Medical Center, Bronx, NY.)

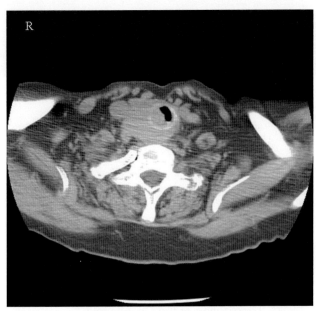

Figure 2-71 Tracheal invasion from follicular carcinoma of the thyroid. Axial computed tomography scan demonstrates a mass on the right that is deviating and invading the trachea.

much more common. In adults, however, primary neoplasms of the trachea are more common than benign tumors. The most common malignant tumor is SCC.[50]

The trachea may be secondarily involved by metastatic disease, either from a remote primary tumor or by direct invasion, such as from a thyroid primary (Fig. 2-71).

V. CONCLUSIONS

Rapid technological advances in the field of radiology now allow excellent visualization of airway structures and provide anesthesiologists with essential information to formulate a safe and effective anesthetic plan. However, radiology is not a part of the curriculum of any anesthesia residency training program, and therefore most anesthesiologists do not know how to analyze the radiologic studies, such as MRI and CT, that are usually a part of the preoperative surgical evaluation. We hope that this chapter, by updating anesthesiologists on the principles of MRI and CT and illustrating how airway structures are displayed by these new imaging modalities, can provide clinicians with good basic skills in gathering clinically useful information from these imaging studies. In addition, we hope that clinicians will not only incorporate the information from radiologic studies to provide better care to their patients but also consider using new imaging modalities as powerful research tools to study the airway.

VI. CLINICAL PEARLS

- In children and in adults during flexion, the anterior atlantodental interval (AADI) is normally about 5 mm.

In adults, it is generally accepted that the AADI is 3 mm or less.

- Although the majority of head extension occurs at the atlanto-occipital joint, some extension can also occur at C1-C2. In patients with limited or no extension possible at the atlanto-occipital joint, general extension of the head actually brings the larynx "anterior," thereby limiting the visibility of the larynx on laryngoscopy.

- A nonunited terminal dental ossification center (os terminale) may be mistaken for a fracture of the odontoid tip.

- Conditions that are associated with odontoid hypoplasia are the Morquio, Klippel-Feil, and Down syndromes; neurofibromatosis; dwarfism; spondyloepiphyseal dysplasia; osteogenesis imperfecta; and congenital scoliosis. Patients with these conditions are predisposed to atlantoaxial subluxation and craniocervical instability, and hyperextension of the head for intubation should be avoided.

- Counterclockwise rotation of the larynx should be suspected if the frontal view of the cervical spine demonstrates a deviated tracheal air column.

- In addition to partial or total choanal atresia, nasal airway obstruction may result from rhinitis or from turbinate hypertrophy.

- In a patient with radiation-induced changes to the neck, the increased rigidity of the soft tissues should be taken into account during laryngoscopy for endotracheal intubation and in selecting the correct size of a laryngeal mask airway (LMA). Specifically, the LMA needs to be one or even two sizes smaller than predicted by the patient's weight.

SELECTED REFERENCES

All references can be found online at expertconsult.com.

10. Streitwieser DR, Knopp R, Wales LR, et al: Accuracy of standard radiographic views in detecting cervical spine fractures. *Ann Emerg Med* 12:538–542, 1983.
12. Harris JH, Mirvis SE: *The radiology of acute cervical spine trauma*, ed 3, Baltimore, 1996, Williams & Wilkins.
13. Crosby ET, Lui A: The adult cervical spine: Implications for airway management. *Can J Anaesth* 37:77–93, 1990.
15. Nichol HC, Zuck D: Difficult laryngoscopy: The "anterior" larynx and the atlanto-occipital gap. *Br J Anaesth* 55:141–144, 1983.
19. Keenan MA, Stiles CM, Kaufman RL: Acquired laryngeal deviation associated with cervical spine disease in erosive polyarticular arthritis: Use of the fiberoptic bronchoscope in rheumatoid disease. *Anesthesiology* 58:441–449, 1983.
20. White A, Kander PL: Anatomical factors in difficult direct laryngoscopy. *Br J Anaesth* 47:468–474, 1975.
21. Chou HC, Wu TL: Mandibulohyoid distance in difficult laryngoscopy. *Br J Anaesth* 71:335–339, 1993.
22. Frerk CM, Till CB, Bradley AJ: Difficult intubation: Thyromental distance and the atlanto-occipital gap. *Anaesthesia* 51:738–740, 1996.
30. Goodman LR, Putman CE: *Intensive care radiology: Imaging of the critically ill*, Philadelphia, 1983, WB Saunders, p 19.
31. Bishop MJ, Weymuller EA, Jr, Fink BR: Laryngeal effects of prolonged intubation. *Anesth Analg* 63:335–342, 1984.

Chapter 3

Ultrasonography in Airway Management

MICHAEL SELTZ KRISTENSEN

I. INTRODUCTION

Ultrasonography (USG) has many potential advantages: It is safe, quick, repeatable, portable, and widely available and gives real-time dynamic images. USG must be used *dynamically* in direct conjunction with the airway procedures for maximum benefit in airway management. For example, if the transducer is placed on the neck, the endotracheal tube (ETT) can be visualized passing into the trachea or the esophagus *while* it is being placed, whereas the location of the ETT is difficult to visualize if the transducer is placed on the neck of a patient who already has an ETT in place.

II. THE ULTRASOUND IMAGE AND HOW TO OBTAIN IT

Ultrasound refers to sound frequencies beyond 20,000 Hz; frequencies from 2 to 15 MHz are typically used for medical imaging. Ultrasound transducers act as both transmitters and receivers of reflected sound. Tissues exhibit differing acoustic impedance values, and sound reflection occurs at the interfaces between different types of tissues. The impedance difference is greatest at interfaces of soft tissue with bone or air. Some tissues give a strong echo (e.g., fat, bone); these are called *hyperechoic* structures, and they appear *white*. Other tissues let the ultrasound beam pass easily (e.g., fluid collections, blood in vessels) and therefore create only a weak echo; these are *hypoechoic* structures and appear *black* on the screen. When the ultrasound beam reaches the surface of a bone, a strong echo (i.e., a strong white line) appears, and there is a strong absorption of ultrasound, resulting in depiction of only a limited depth of the bony tissue. Nothing is seen beyond the bone because of acoustic shadowing. Cartilaginous structures such as the thyroid cartilage, the cricoid cartilage, and the tracheal rings, appear homogeneously hypoechoic (black), but the cartilages tend to calcify with age.[1]

Muscles and connective tissue membranes are hypo-echoic but have a more heterogeneous, striated appearance than cartilage does. Glandular structures such as the submandibular and thyroid glands are homogeneous and mildly to strongly hyperechoic in comparison with adjacent soft tissues. Air is a very weak conductor of ultrasound, so when the ultrasound beam reaches the border between a tissue and air, a strong reflection (strong white line) appears, and everything on the screen beyond that point represents only artifacts, especially reverberation artifacts, which create multiple parallel white lines on the screen. However, the artifacts that arise from the pleura/lung border often reveal useful information. Visualization of structures such as the posterior pharynx, posterior commissure, and posterior wall of the trachea is prevented by intraluminal air.[1] In B-mode USG, an array of transducers simultaneously scans a plane through the body that can be viewed as a two-dimensional image on the screen, depicting a "slice" of tissue.

In M-mode USG (M = motion), a rapid sequence of B-mode scans representing one single line through the tissue is obtained. The images follow each other in sequence on the screen, enabling the sonographer to see and measure range of motion as the organ boundaries that produce reflections move relative to the probe. In color Doppler USG, velocity information is presented as a color-coded overlay on top of a B-mode image.

The higher the frequency of the ultrasound wave, the higher the image resolution and the less penetration in depth. All modern ultrasound transducers used in airway management have a range of frequencies that can be adjusted during scanning to optimize the image. The linear high-frequency transducer (Fig. 3-1) is the most suitable for imaging superficial airway structures (within 2 to 3 cm from the skin). The curved low-frequency transducer is most suitable for obtaining sagittal and parasagittal views of structures in the submandibular and supraglottic regions, mainly because of its wider field of view.[1] The micro convex transducer gives a wide view of the pleura between two ribs. If only one transducer must be chosen, then a linear high-frequency transducer will enable performance of most ultrasound examinations that are relevant for airway management.

Because air does not conduct ultrasound, the probe must be in full contact with the skin or mucosa without any interfacing air.[2] This is achieved by applying judicious amounts of conductive gel between the probe and the skin. Because of the prominent thyroid cartilage, it is sometimes a challenge to avoid air under the probe when performing a sagittal midline scan from the hyoid bone to the suprasternal notch in a male patient. Portable machines can provide accurate answers to basic questions and are sufficient for airway USG.[3]

III. VISUALIZING THE AIRWAY AND THE ADJACENT STRUCTURES

With conventional transcutaneous USG, the airway can be visualized from the tip of the chin to the midtrachea, along with the pleural aspect of the most peripheral alveoli and the diaphragm. Additional parts of the airway can be seen with special techniques: Trachea can be seen

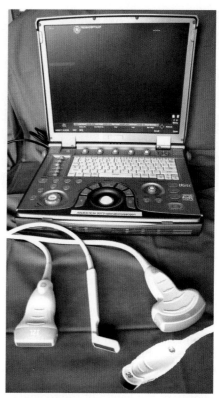

Figure 3-1 Laptop-sized ultrasound machine with transducers *(left to right):* linear 7- to 12-MHz high-frequency transducer; small linear 6- to 10-MHz high-frequency "hockey-stick" transducer; curved, convex 2- to 6-MHz low-frequency transducer; micro convex 4- to 10-MHz transducer *(foreground).* (From Kristensen MS: Ultrasonography in the management of the airway. *Acta Anaesthesiol Scand* 55:1155–1173, 2011.)

from the esophagus when performing transesophageal USG, and the tissue surrounding the more distal airway from the midtrachea to the bronchi can be visualized with endoscopic USG via a bronchoscope. These special techniques are not covered in detail in this chapter.

A. Mouth and Tongue

USG is a simple method for examination of the mouth and its contents. The tongue is composed of an anterior mobile part situated in the oral cavity and a fixed pharyngeal portion. The lingual musculature is divided into the extrinsic muscles (which have a bony insertion and alter the position of the tongue) and intrinsic muscles, whose fibers alter the shape of the tongue.[4] The tongue can be visualized from within the mouth, but the image may be difficult to interpret.[5,6]

The floor of the mouth and the tongue are easily visualized by placing the transducer submentally. If the transducer is placed in the coronal plane just posterior to the mentum and from there moved posteriorly until the hyoid bone is reached, one can perform a thorough evaluation of all the layers of the floor of the mouth, the muscles of the tongue, and any possible pathologic processes (Fig. 3-2). The scanning image will be flanked by the acoustic shadow of the mandible on each side. The dorsal lingual surface is clearly identified.[7] The width of

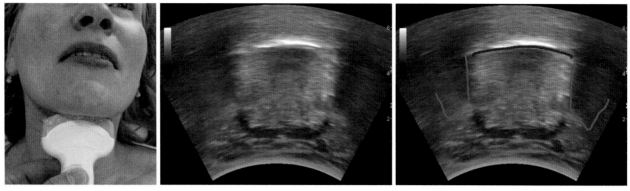

Figure 3-2 Transverse scan of the floor of the mouth and the tongue. *Left,* Placement of the transducer. *Middle,* The resulting ultrasound image. *Right,* The dorsal surface of the tongue is indicated by a red line, and shadows arising from the mandible are outlined in green. (From Kristensen MS: Ultrasonography in the management of the airway. *Acta Anaesthesiol Scand* 55:1155–1173, 2011.)

the tongue base can be measured in a standardized way by locating the two lingual arteries with Doppler ultrasound and measuring the distance between these arteries where they enter the tongue base at its lower lateral borders.[8] A longitudinal scan of the floor of the mouth and the tongue is obtained if the transducer is placed submentally in the sagittal plane. If a large convex transducer is used, the whole length of the floor of the mouth and the majority of the length of the tongue can be seen in one image (Fig. 3-3). The acoustic shadows from the symphysis of the mandible and from the hyoid bone form the anterior and posterior limits of this image. Detailed imaging of the function of the tongue, including bolus holding, lingual propulsion, lingual-palatal contact, tongue tip and dorsum motion, bolus clearance, and hyoid excursion, can be evaluated in this plane.[7]

When the tongue is in contact with the palate, the palate can be visualized; if there is no contact with the palate, the air at the dorsum of the tongue will make visualization of the palate impossible. An improved image is achievable if water is ingested and retained in the oral cavity. The water eliminates the air-tissue border and

allows visualization of most of the oral cavity including the palate (Fig. 3-4), as well as a better differentiation of the hard palate from the soft palate.[4]

The tongue can be visualized in detail with the use of three-dimensional USG.[9] In a child, the major anatomic components of the tongue and mouth are covered by four scanning positions: the midline sagittal, the parasagittal, the anterior coronal, and the posterior coronal planes.[10] In the transverse midline plane just cranial to the hyoid bone, the tongue base and the floor of the mouth are seen. In the transverse (axial) plane in the midline, the lingual tonsils and the valleculae can be imaged. The vallecula is seen just below the hyoid bone, and when the probe is angled caudally, the preglottic and paraglottic spaces and the infrahyoid part of the epiglottis are seen.[11]

B. Oropharynx

Imaging of a part of the lateral border of the mid-oropharynx can be obtained by placing the transducer vertically with its upper edge approximately 1 cm below

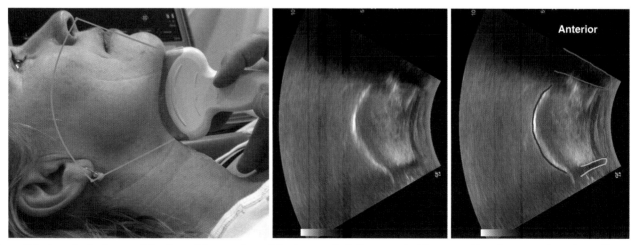

Figure 3-3 Longitudinal scan of the floor of the mouth and the tongue. *Left,* Placement of the curved low-frequency transducer. The area covered by the scan is outlined in light blue. *Middle,* The resulting ultrasound image. *Right,* The shadow from the mentum of the mandible is outlined in green, the muscles in the floor of the mouth in purple, the shadow from the hyoid bone in light orange, and the dorsal surface of the tongue in red. (From Kristensen MS: Ultrasonography in the management of the airway. *Acta Anaesthesiol Scand* 55:1155–1173, 2011.)

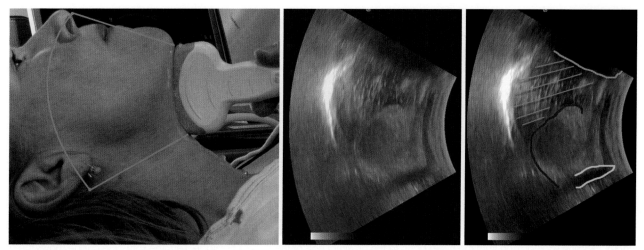

Figure 3-4 The tongue and the mouth are filled with water. Placement of the transducer is the same as in Figure 3-3. The shadow from the mentum of the mandible is outlined in green, the shadow from the hyoid bone in light orange, and the dorsal surface of the tongue in red. The blue lines indicate the water in the mouth. The large white line represents the strong echo from the hard palate. (From Kristensen MS: Ultrasonography in the management of the airway. *Acta Anaesthesiol Scand* 55:1155–1173, 2011.)

the external auditory canal.[7] The lateral pharyngeal border and the thickness of the lateral parapharyngeal wall can be determined.[12] The parapharyngeal space can also be visualized via the mouth by placing the probe directly over the mucosal lining of the lateral pharyngeal wall, but this approach is difficult for the patient to tolerate.[13]

C. Hypopharynx

By performing USG through the thyrohyoid membrane, cricothyroid space, cricothyroid membrane (CTM), and thyroidal cartilage lamina and along the posterior edge of the thyroid lamina, it is possible to locate and classify hypopharyngeal tumors with a success rate as high as that achieved with computed tomography (CT) scanning.[14]

D. Hyoid Bone

The hyoid bone is a key landmark that separates the upper airway into two scanning areas: the suprahyoid and infrahyoid regions. The hyoid bone is visible on the transverse view as a superficial, hyperechoic, inverted U–shaped, linear structure with posterior acoustic shadowing. On the sagittal and parasagittal views, the hyoid bone is visible in cross section (see Fig. 3-4) as a narrow, hyperechoic, curved structure that casts an acoustic shadow.[1]

E. Larynx

Because of the superficial location of the larynx, USG offers images of higher resolution than CT or magnetic resonance imaging (MRI) when a linear high-frequency transducer is used.[11] The different parts of the laryngeal skeleton have different sonographic characteristics.[15] The hyoid bone is calcified early in life, and its bony shadow is an important landmark. The thyroid and cricoid cartilages show variable but progressive calcification throughout life, whereas the epiglottis stays hypoechoic. The true

vocal cords overlie muscle that is hypoechoic, whereas the false cords contain echoic fat.

The thyrohyoid membrane runs between the caudal border of the hyoid bone and the cephalad border of the thyroid cartilage and provides a sonographic window through which the epiglottis can be visualized in all subjects when the linear transducer is oriented in the transverse plane (with varying degrees of cephalad or caudad angulation).[1] The midline sagittal scan through the upper larynx from the hyoid bone cranially to the thyroid cartilage distally (Fig. 3-5) reveals the thyrohyoid ligament, the pre-epiglottic space containing echogenic fat, and, posterior to that, a white line representing the laryngeal surface of the epiglottis.[15] On parasagittal view, the epiglottis appears as a hypoechoic structure with a curvilinear shape; on transverse view, it is shaped like an inverted C. It is bordered anteriorly by the hyperechoic, triangular pre-epiglottic space and lined posteriorly by a hyperechoic air-mucosa interface.[16] In a convenience sample of 100 subjects, the transverse midline scan cranially to the thyroid cartilage depicted the epiglottis in all subjects and revealed an average epiglottis thickness of 2.39 mm.[17]

In the cricothyroid region, the probe can be angled cranially to assess the vocal cords and the arytenoid cartilages and thereafter moved distally to access the cricoid cartilages and the subglottis.[11] With transverse scanning in the paramedian position, the following structures can be visualized (starting cranially and moving distally): faucial tonsils, lateral tongue base, lateral vallecula, strap muscles, laminae of the thyroid cartilage, the lateral cricoid cartilage, and, posteriorly, the piriform sinuses and the cervical esophagus.[11]

The laryngeal cartilage is noncalcified in the child, but calcification starts in some individuals before 20 years of age, and it increases with age. In subjects with non-calcified cartilage, the thyroid cartilage is visible on sagittal and parasagittal views as a linear, hypoechoic structure with a bright air-mucosa interface at its posterior surface. On the transverse view, it has an inverted V

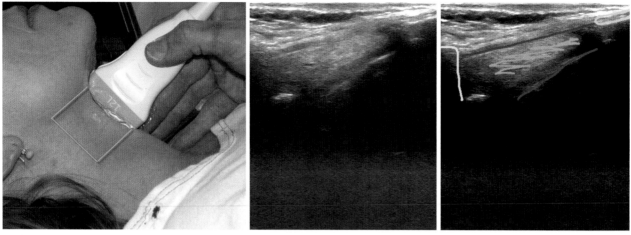

Figure 3-5 Midline sagittal scan from the hyoid bone to the proximal part of the thyroid cartilage. *Left,* The light blue outline shows the area covered by the scan. *Middle,* The scanning image. *Right,* The shadow from the hyoid bone is marked in yellow, the thyrohyoid membrane in red, the posterior surface of part of the epiglottis in blue, the pre-epiglottic fat in orange, and the thyroid cartilage in green. (From Kristensen MS: Ultrasonography in the management of the airway. *Acta Anaesthesiol Scand* 55:1155–1173, 2011.)

shape (Fig. 3-6), within which the true and false vocal cords are visible.[1] By 60 years of age, all individuals show signs of partial calcification, and approximately 40% of the cartilage at the level of the vocal cords is calcified.[18] The calcification is seen as a strong echo with posterior acoustic shadowing. Often the anatomic structures can be visualized despite the calcifications by angling the transducer. In a population of patients who were examined due to suspicion of laryngeal pathology, a sufficient depiction of the false cords was obtained in 60% of cases, of the vocal cords in 75%, of the anterior commissure in 64%, and of the arytenoid region in 71%; in 16% of cases, no endolaryngeal structures could be depicted.[18]

F. Vocal Cords

In individuals with noncalcified thyroid cartilages, the false and the true vocal cords can be visualized through the thyroid cartilage.[15] In individuals with calcified thyroid cartilage, the vocal cords and the arytenoid cartilages can still be seen by combining the scan obtained by placing the transducer just cranially to the superior thyroid notch angling it caudally with the scans obtained from the CTM in the midline and on each side with the transducer angled 30 degrees cranially.[11] In a study group of 24 volunteers with a mean age of 30 years, the thyroid cartilage provided the best window for imaging the vocal cords. In all participants, it was possible to visualize and distinguish the true and false vocal cords by moving the transducer in a cephalocaudad direction over the thyroid cartilage.[1]

The true vocal cords appear as two triangular, hypoechoic structures (the vocalis muscles) outlined medially by the hyperechoic vocal ligaments (see Fig. 3-6). They are observed to oscillate and move toward the midline during phonation.[1] In a study of 229 participants ranging in age from 2 months to 81 years, the true and false cords were visible in all female participants. In males, the visibility was 100% for those younger than 18 years and gradually decreased to less than 40% in males 60 years of age and older.[19] The false vocal cords lie parallel and cephalad to the true cords, are more hyperechoic in appearance, and remain relatively immobile during phonation.

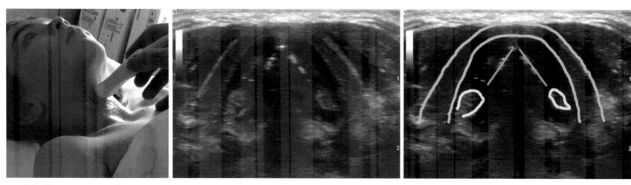

Figure 3-6 Transverse midline scan over the thyroid cartilage in an 8-year-old boy. *Left,* Placement of the transducer. *Middle,* The scanning image. *Right,* The thyroid cartilage is marked in green, the vocal cords in orange, the anterior commissure in red, and the arytenoid cartilages in yellow. (From Kristensen MS: Ultrasonography in the management of the airway *Acta Anaesthesiol Scand* 55:1155–1173, 2011.)

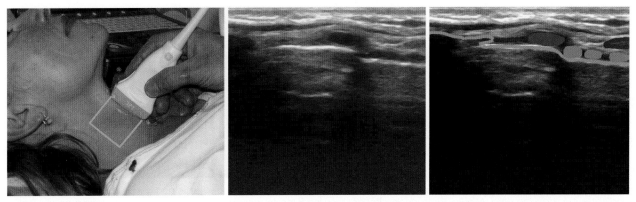

Figure 3-7 Cricothyroid membrane (CTM). *Left,* The linear high-frequency transducer is placed in the midsagittal plane. The scanning area is marked with light blue. *Middle,* The scanning image. *Right,* The thyroid cartilage is marked in green, the cricoid cartilage in dark blue, the tracheal rings in light blue, the CTM in red, the tissue-air border in orange, and the isthmus of the thyroid gland in brown. Below the orange line, only artifacts are seen. (From Kristensen MS: Ultrasonography in the management of the airway *Acta Anaesthesiol Scand* 55:1155–1173, 2011.)

G. Cricothyroid Membrane and Cricoid Cartilage

The CTM runs between the caudal border of the thyroid cartilage and the cephalad border of the cricoid cartilage. It is clearly seen on sagittal (Fig. 3-7) and parasagittal views as a hyperechoic band linking the hypoechoic thyroid and cricoid cartilages.[1] The cricoid cartilage has a round, hypoechoic appearance on the parasagittal view and an arch-like appearance on the transverse view.

H. Trachea

The location of the trachea in the midline of the neck makes it a useful reference point for transverse ultrasound imaging. The cricoid cartilage marks the superior limit of the trachea; it is thicker than the tracheal rings below and is seen as a hypoechoic, rounded structure. It serves as a reference point during performance of the sagittal midline scan (see Fig. 3-7). Often the first six tracheal rings can be imaged when the neck is in mild extension.[13] The trachea is covered by skin, subcutaneous fat, the strap muscles, and, at the level of the second or third tracheal ring, the isthmus of the thyroid gland (see Fig. 3-7). The strap muscles appear hypoechoic and are encased by thin hyperechoic lines from the cervical fascia.[13] A high-riding innominate artery may be identified above the sternal notch as a transverse anechoic structure crossing the trachea.[13] The tracheal rings are hypoechoic, and they resemble a "string of beads" in the parasagittal and sagittal plane (see Fig. 3-7). In the transverse view, they resemble an inverted U highlighted by a hyperechoic air-mucosa interface (Fig. 3-8) and by reverberation artifact posteriorly.[1]

I. Esophagus

The cervical esophagus is most often visible posterolateral to the trachea on the left side at the level of the suprasternal notch (see Fig. 3-8). The concentric layers of esophagus result in a characteristic "bull's-eye" appearance on USG. The esophagus can be seen to compress

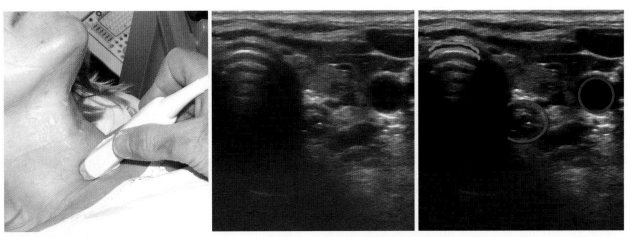

Figure 3-8 Trachea and esophagus. *Left,* A transverse scan is performed just cranial to the suprasternal notch and to the patient's left side of the trachea. *Middle,* The scanning image. *Right,* The anterior part of the tracheal cartilage is outlined in light blue, the esophagus in purple, and the carotid artery in red. (From Kristensen MS: Ultrasonography in the management of the airway. *Acta Anaesthesiol Scand* 55:1155–1173, 2011.)

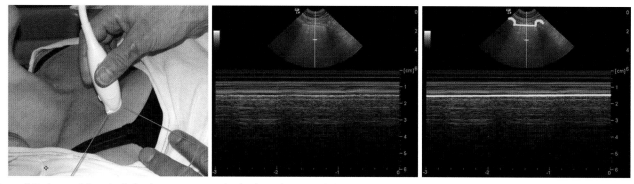

Figure 3-9 Lung sliding. *Left,* A micro convex probe is placed over an interspace between two ribs during normal ventilation. The light blue line indicates the scanning area. *Middle,* The scanning image, showing B-mode scanning above and M-mode scanning below. *Right,* The pleural line is marked in yellow and the ribs in orange (the curved lines at each end of the straight line). Notice that the outline of the ribs and the pleural line forms the image of a flying bat, the "bat sign." In the M-mode image, it is easy to distinguish the nonmoving tissue above the pleural line from the artifact caused by respiratory movement of the visceral pleura relative to the parietal pleura. This is called the "seashore sign" or the "sandy beach sign" because the nonmoving part resembles waves and the artifact pattern below resembles a sandy beach. (From Kristensen MS: Ultrasonography in the management of the airway. *Acta Anaesthesiol Scand* 55:1155–1173, 2011.)

and expand with swallowing, and this feature can be used for accurate identification.[13] The patient may be placed in a modified position for examining the esophagus by slightly flexing the neck with a pillow under the head and turning the head 45 degrees to the opposite side while the neck is scanned on either side; this technique makes the esophagus visible also on the right side in 98% of cases.[20]

J. Lower Trachea and Bronchi

Transesophageal USG displays a part of the lower trachea. When a saline-filled balloon is introduced in the trachea during cardiopulmonary bypass, it is possible to perform USG through the trachea, thus displaying the proximal aortic arch and the innominate artery.[21] The bronchial wall and its layers can be visualized from within the airway by passing a flexible ultrasound probe through the working channel of a flexible bronchoscope. This technique, called *end bronchial ultrasound*, reliably distinguishes between airway infiltration and compression by tumor.[22]

K. Peripheral Lung and Pleura

The ribs are identifiable by their acoustic shadow, and between two ribs a hyperechoic line is visible. This line, called the *pleural line*, represents the interface between the soft tissue of the chest wall and air (Fig. 3-9). In the normal breathing or ventilated subject, one can identify a kind of to-and-fro movement synchronous with ventilation; this is called "pleural sliding" or "lung sliding."[23] The movement is striking because the surrounding tissue is motionless.[24] Lung sliding is best seen dynamically, in real time or on video.[25]

The investigation should always start by placing the probe perpendicular to the ribs and in such a way that two rib shadows are identified. The succession of the upper rib, pleural line, and lower rib outlines a characteristic pattern, the "bat sign" (see Fig. 3-9) and must be recognized to correctly identify the pleural line and avoid interpretation errors due to a parietal emphysema. Lung

ultrasound examination should therefore be considered not feasible if the bat sign is not identified.[26] Lung sliding can be objectified using the time-motion mode, which highlights a clear distinction between a wave-like pattern located above the pleural line and a sand-like pattern below, called the "seashore sign" (see Fig. 3-9).[26]

In breath-holding or apnea, there is no lung sliding, but a "lung pulse"—small movements synchronous with the heartbeat—is seen instead (Fig. 3-10). The lung pulse can be explained as the vibrations of the heart are transmitted through a motionless lung. The lung pulse can also be demonstrated in the time-motion M-mode scanning. There is a strong echo from the pleural line, and dominant reverberation artifacts of varying strength are seen. They appear as lines parallel to the pleural line and spaced with the same distance as the distance from the skin surface to the pleural line. These "A-lines" are seen in both the normal and the pathologic lung.[26]

The "B-line" is an artifact with seven features: It is (1) a hydrometric comet-tail artifact that (2) arises from the pleural line, (3) is hyperechoic, (4) is well defined, (5) spreads up indefinitely (i.e., spreads to the edge of the screen without fading—up to 17 cm with a probe reaching 17 cm[26]), (6) erases A-lines, and (7) moves with lung sliding when lung sliding is present.[27] Sparse B-lines occur in normal lungs but three or more B-lines indicates pathology (e.g., interstitial syndrome).[27] B-lines are also called "ring-down" artifacts.[28]

L. Diaphragm

The diaphragm and its motion can be imaged by placing a convex transducer in the subxiphoid window in the middle upper abdominal region, just beneath the xiphoid process and the lower margin of the liver. The transducer is tilted 45 degrees cephalad, and bilateral diaphragm motion is noticed.[29] The bilateral diaphragm moves toward the abdomen when the lungs are ventilated and toward the chest during the relaxation phase. The liver and spleen movements represent the whole movement of the right and left diaphragm during respiration and can be visualized by placing the probe in the longitudinal

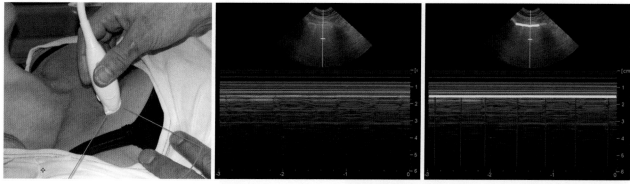

Figure 3-10 Lung pulse. *Left,* Placement of the transducer. *Middle,* The scanning image, showing B-mode scanning above and M-mode scanning below. In this nonventilated lung, the only movement is that caused by the heartbeat, which creates a subtle movement of the lungs and the pleura. This movement is visualized in the M-mode image synchronous with the heartbeat and is called the "lung pulse." *Right,* The pleural line is marked in yellow and the superficial outline of the ribs in orange. The red lines indicate the lung pulse. (From Kristensen MS: Ultrasonography in the management of the airway. *Acta Anaesthesiol Scand* 55:1155–1173, 2011.)

plane along the right anterior axillary line and the left posterior axillary line, respectively. The movement of the most caudal margin of the liver and spleen with respiration is measured.[30]

IV. CLINICAL APPLICATIONS

A. Prediction of Difficult Laryngoscopy in Surgical Patients

In a pilot study of 27 elective surgical patients, it was found that failure to identify the epiglottis and trachea with sublingual USG was a more accurate predictor of a Cormack-Lehane grade 3 or greater laryngoscopy score than the Mallampati classification was.[31] However, the interpretation of the sublingual USG approach was later reevaluated, and it remains to be determined whether this approach is useful in predicting airway difficulties.[6]

In 50 morbidly obese patients, the distance from the skin to the anterior aspect of the trachea, measured at the level of the vocal cords and the suprasternal notch, was significantly greater in those patients in whom laryngoscopy was difficult, even after optimization of laryngoscopy by laryngeal manipulation. However, these findings could not be reproduced when the end point was laryngoscopy grade without the use of laryngeal manipulation for optimization of the laryngoscopic view.[32,33]

B. Evaluation of Pathology That May Influence the Choice of Airway Management Technique

Subglottic hemangiomas, laryngeal stenosis, laryngeal cysts, and respiratory papillomatosis (Fig. 3-11) can be visualized with USG. A pharyngeal pouch (Zenker's diverticulum), representing a source of regurgitation and

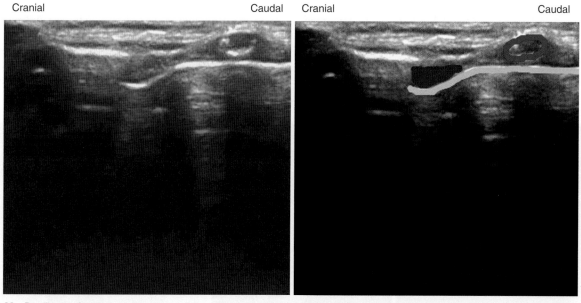

Cranial   Caudal   Cranial   Caudal

Figure 3-11 Papilloma. Sagittal midline scan of the anterior neck in a patient with a papilloma on the anterior tracheal wall immediately caudal to the anterior commissure. *Left,* The scanning image. *Right,* The tissue-air border is marked in yellow, the cricoid cartilage in blue, and the papilloma in reddish-brown. (From Kristensen MS: Ultrasonography in the management of the airway *Acta Anaesthesiol Scand* 55:1155–1173, 2011.)

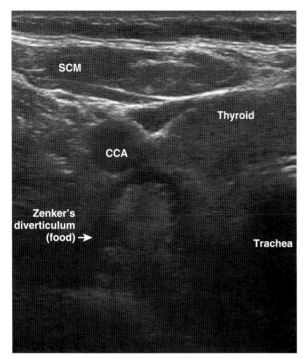

Figure 3-12 Zenker's diverticulum is seen laterally to the trachea on a transverse scan on the anterior neck above the suprasternal notch. *CCA,* Common carotid artery; *SCM,* sternocleidomastoid muscle. (Courtesy of Peter Cheng, Kaiser Permanente Riverside Medical Center, Riverside, CA.)

aspiration, is seen on a transverse linear high-frequency scan of the neck and is located at the posterolateral aspect of the left thyroid lobe (Fig. 3-12).[11,34-36] Malignancies and their relationship with the airway can be seen and quantified.

Fetal airway abnormalities, such as extrinsic obstruction caused by adjacent tumors (e.g., lymphatic malformation, cervical teratoma), can be visualized by prenatal USG (Fig. 3-13).[37] With this information, airway management can be planned, either at birth or as an ex utero intrapartum treatment (EXIT) procedure. The EXIT maneuver can consist of performing a cesarean section and endotracheal intubation or tracheostomy while the newborn is still attached to the umbilical cord and thus maintains fetal circulation.

C. Diagnosis of Obstructive Sleep Apnea

The width of the tongue base, measured by USG, was found to correlate with the severity of sleep-related breathing disorders, including a patient's sensation of choking during the night. The width was measured as the distance between the lingual arteries where they enter the tongue base at its lower lateral borders.[8] The thickness of the lateral pharyngeal wall, as measured with USG, is significantly higher in patients with obstructive sleep apnea than in patients without this condition.[12]

D. Evaluation of Prandial Status

Twenty subjects were randomized to either fasting or nonfasting status and had their stomach examined with USG. The technique was found to be specific in identifying a full stomach but only moderately reliable in identifying an empty stomach. After the subjects drank water, the stomach was identified 100% of the time by all observers in both conditions. Recent publications have suggested clinical usefulness of USG in determining prandial status.[38-40]

E. Prediction of the Appropriate Diameter of an Endotracheal, Endobronchial, or Tracheostomy Tube

In children and young adults, USG is a reliable tool for measuring the diameter of the subglottic upper airway and correlates well with MRI, which is the gold standard.[41,42]

The diameter of the left main stem bronchus, and therefore the proper size of a left-sided double-lumen tube, can be estimated with USG. Immediately before anesthesia in a series of patients, the outer diameter of the trachea was measured by USG just above the sternoclavicular joint in the transverse section. The ratio between the diameter of the trachea and that of the left main stem bronchus was obtained from CT images. The ratio between left main stem bronchus diameter on CT imaging and outer tracheal diameter measured with USG was 0.68. The results were comparable to those obtained with chest radiography as a guide for selecting left double-lumen tube size.[43]

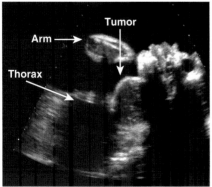
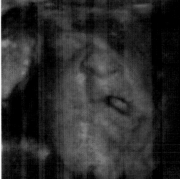
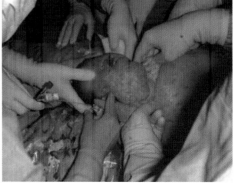

Figure 3-13 *Left,* A large tumor is seen on the neck of a fetus. *Middle,* Three-dimensional ultrasonographic image. *Right,* The head is delivered, and the airway is managed while the fetal circulation is still intact. (Courtesy of Connie Jørgensen, Rigshospitalet, Copenhagen, Denmark.)

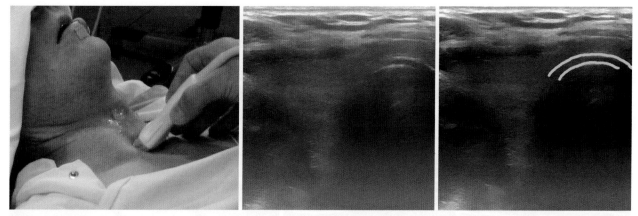

Figure 3-14 Tracheal deviation. *Left,* The transducer is placed transversely in the midline over the suprasternal notch. *Middle,* The scanning image reveals lateral deviation of the middle part of the trachea. *Right,* The cartilage of the tracheal ring (light blue) is deviated to the patient's left side. (From Kristensen MS: Ultrasonography in the management of the airway. *Acta Anaesthesiol Scand* 55:1155–1173, 2011.)

In children with tracheostomy, USG measurement of the tracheal width and of the distance from the skin to the trachea can be used to predict the size and shape of a potential replacement tracheostomy tube, and adequate images can be obtained by placing the ultrasound probe just superior to the stomach.[44]

F. Localization of the Trachea

Obesity, a short thick neck, neck mass, previous surgery or radiotherapy to the neck, and thoracic pathology resulting in tracheal deviation can make accurate localization of the trachea challenging and cumbersome. Even the addition of chest radiography and techniques of needle aspiration to locate the trachea may be futile.[45] This situation is even more challenging in emergency cases and in cases where awake tracheostomy is chosen because of a predicted difficult mask ventilation or difficult endotracheal intubation. Under such circumstances, preoperative USG for localization of the trachea (Fig. 3-14) is very useful.[45]

G. Localization of the Cricothyroid Membrane

The CTM plays a crucial role in airway management, but it was correctly identified by anesthesiologists in only 30% of cases when identification was based on surface landmarks and palpation alone.[46] USG allows reliable, quick, and easily learned identification of the CTM.[46-48] USG is a useful technique to identify the trachea before elective transtracheal cannulation or emergency cricothyrotomy. This was demonstrated by a case concerning an obese patient with Ludwig's angina in whom it was not possible to identify the trachea by palpation. A portable ultrasound machine was used to locate the trachea 2 cm lateral to the midline.[49] Accurate localization of the trachea allows the clinician to approach the difficult airway by placing a transtracheal catheter or performing a tracheostomy before anesthesia. In cases of awake intubation, it provides the added safety of having localized the CTM in advance in case the intubation should fail and an emergency transcricoid access should become necessary.

One method for localizing the CTM is described as follows: A transverse, midline scan is performed from the clavicles to the mandible with a 10-MHz linear array probe, and the CTM is identified by its characteristic echogenic artifact, the cricothyroid muscles lateral to it, and the thyroid cartilage cephalad.[48] In a study of 50 emergency department patients, the craniocaudal level of the CTM was located by performing a longitudinal sagittal midline scan and then sliding the probe bilaterally to localize the lateral borders of the CTM. The mean time to visualization of the CTM was 24.3 seconds.[47] A simple and systematic approach to localizing the CTM is shown in Figure 3-15.

H. Airway-Related Nerve Blocks

USG has casuistically been used to identify and block the superior laryngeal nerve as part of the preparation for awake fiberoptic intubation. The greater horn of the hyoid bone and the superior laryngeal artery were identified, and the local analgesic was injected between them.[50] In 100 ultrasound examinations for the superior laryngeal nerve space (i.e., the space delimited by the hyoid bone, the thyroid cartilage, the pre-epiglottic space, the thyrohyoid muscle, and the membrane between the hyoid bone and the thyroid cartilage), all components of the space were seen in 81% of cases, and there was a suboptimal, but still useful, depiction of the space in the remaining 19% of cases. The superior laryngeal nerve itself was not seen.[51]

I. Confirmation of Endotracheal Tube Placement

Confirmation of whether the ETT has entered the trachea or the esophagus can be made directly, in real time, by scanning the anterior neck during the intubation or indirectly by looking for ventilation at the pleural or the diaphragmatic level, or by a combination of these techniques. Direct confirmation has the advantage that an accidental esophageal intubation is recognized immediately, before ventilation is initiated and therefore before air is forced into the stomach resulting in an increased

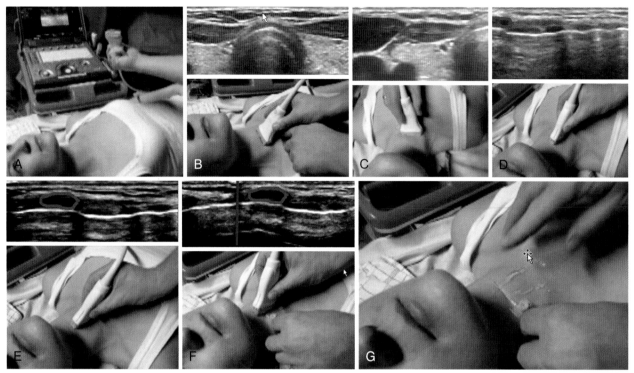

Figure 3-15 Localization of the cricothyroid membrane (CTM). **A,** The patient is lying supine, and the operator stands on the patient's right side, facing the patient. **B,** The linear high-frequency transducer is placed transversely over the neck just above the suprasternal notch (*below*), and the trachea is seen in the midline on the scan (*above*). **C,** The transducer is moved to the patient's right side so that the right border of the transducer is superficial to the midline of the trachea. **D,** The right end of the transducer is kept in the midline of the trachea while the left end is rotated into the sagittal plane, resulting in a longitudinal scan of the midline of the trachea. The caudal part of the cricoid cartilage is seen on the scan and is outlined in blue. **E,** The transducer is moved cranially, and the cricoid cartilage (blue) is seen as a slightly elongated structure that is significantly larger and located more anteriorly than the tracheal rings. **F,** A needle is moved under the transducer from the cranial end; it is used only as a marker. Its shadow (red line) is just cephalad to the cranial border of the cricoid cartilage (blue). **G,** The transducer is moved, and the needle indicates the distal part of the CTM. (From Kristensen MS: Ultrasonography in the management of the airway. *Acta Anaesthesiol Scand* 55:1155–1173, 2011.)

risk of emesis and aspiration. Confirmation at the pleural level has the advantage of distinguishing, at least to some extent, between tracheal and endobronchial intubation.

Both the direct and the indirect confirmation techniques have the advantage over capnography because they can be applied in very-low-cardiac-output situations. USG has the advantage over stethoscopy in that it can be performed in noisy environments, such as in helicopters. In a cadaver model in which a 7.5-MHz curved probe was placed longitudinally over the CTM, it was possible for residents given only 5 minutes of training in the technique to correctly identify esophageal intubation (97% sensitivity) with dynamic examination at the time of intubation. When the examination was performed after the intubation, statically, the sensitivity was very poor.[52]

In 40 elective patients, a 3- to 5-MHz curved transducer placed at the level of the CTM and held at a 45-degree angle facing cranially allowed detection of all five accidental esophageal intubations. Tracheal passage of the ETT was seen as a brief flutter deep to the thyroid cartilage, whereas esophageal intubation created a clearly visible bright (hyperechoic) curved line with a distal dark area (shadowing) appearing on one side of, and deep to, the trachea.[53]

In another study, 33 patients with normal airways were intubated electively in both trachea and esophagus in random order and had a linear 5- to 10-MHz probe placed transversely on the anterior neck just superior to the suprasternal notch. USG allowed detection of both tracheal and esophageal intubation in all 33 patients. It was concluded that skilled ultrasonographers, in a controlled operating room setting, can consistently detect the passage of an ETT into either the trachea or the esophagus in normal airways.[54]

In children, direct confirmation of ETT placement by scanning via the CTM required multiple views; the USG examination was apparently performed after the intubation, making comparison to other studies difficult, and the feasibility of that approach has been challenged.[55,56]

Indirect confirmation of ETT placement in 15 patients was performed with the use of a portable, handheld ultrasound machine and routine scanning in the third and fourth intercostal spaces on both sides during the phases of preoxygenation, apnea, bag-mask ventilation, intubation, and positive-pressure ventilation after intubation. ETT placement was determined in all cases.[57]

The color power Doppler function has been used as a supplement during observation of lung sliding to detect that a lung was ventilated.[57] The distinction between tracheal and endobronchial intubation can be made by scanning the lung bilaterally. If there is pleural sliding on one side and lung pulse on the other side, the tip of the tube is in the main stem bronchus on the side on which lung sliding is observed. The ETT is then withdrawn until lung sliding is observed bilaterally, indicating that the tip of the tube is again placed in the trachea.[58] Indirect confirmation of intubation by detection of a "sliding lung" was studied in fresh ventilated cadavers; the tip of the ETT was placed in either the esophagus, the trachea, or the right main stem bronchus. A high sensitivity (95% to 100%) was found for detection of esophageal versus airway (trachea or bronchus) intubation. The sensitivity for distinguishing a right main stem bronchus intubation from an endotracheal intubation was lower (69% to 78%), most likely because of transmitted movement of the left lung due to expansion of the right lung.[59]

Indirect confirmation of intubation by depiction of the movement of the diaphragm bilaterally was shown to be useful for distinguishing between esophageal and endotracheal intubation in a pediatric population.[29] However, when the technique was used to distinguish between main stem bronchus and endotracheal intubation, diaphragmatic ultrasound was not equivalent to chest radiography for determining ETT placement within the airway.[60]

The *combination* of the direct transverse scan on the neck at the level of the CTM and lung ultrasound detecting lung sliding in 30 emergency department patients who needed endotracheal intubation correctly detected the three cases of esophageal intubation, even in the presence of four cases of pneumohemothorax.[61] The combination of the direct transverse scan on the neck at the level of the thyroid lobes, combined with lung ultrasound, has casuistically demonstrated its value by enabling detection of esophageal intubation in a patient in whom laryngoscopy was difficult in the clinical emergency setting.[62]

Filling the cuff with fluid helps in seeing the cuff position on USG.[63] Use of a metal stylet does not augment visualization of the ETT.[64] In children, when the transducer was placed at the level of the glottis, the vocal cords were always visible; the passing of the ETT was visible in all children and was characterized by widening of the vocal cords.[65] USG is also useful in confirming the correct position of a double-lumen tube.[43]

The following procedure is recommended for USG confirmation of ETT placement: Perform a transverse scan over the trachea, just above the sternal notch. Note the location and appearance of the esophagus. Let the intubation be performed. If the ETT is visualized passing into the esophagus, remove it without starting to ventilate the patient and make another intubation attempt, possibly using another technique. If the ETT is not seen, or if it is seen in the trachea, have the patient ventilated via the tube. Move the transducer to the midaxillary lines and look for lung sliding bilaterally. If there is bilateral lung sliding, it is a confirmation that the ETT is in the airway, but a main stem bronchus intubation cannot be ruled out. If there is lung sliding on one side and lung pulse on the other side, then a main stem bronchus intubation is likely, and the tube can be removed gradually until bilateral sliding is present. If there is no lung sliding on either side but lung pulse is present, there is a small risk that the tube has entered the esophagus. If there is neither lung pulse nor lung sliding, then a pneumothorax should be expected.

J. Tracheostomy

Accurate localization of the trachea in the absence of surface landmarks can be very challenging and cumbersome. Preoperative USG for localization of the trachea (see Fig. 3-14) is very suitable for both surgical tracheostomy and percutaneous dilatational tracheostomy (PDT).[45] In children, preoperative USG is of value in verifying the precise tracheostomy position and thereby preventing subglottic damage to the cricoid cartilage and the first tracheal ring, hemorrhage due to abnormally placed or abnormally large blood vessels, and pneumothorax.[66]

K. Percutaneous Dilatational Tracheostomy

USG allows localization of the trachea, visualization of the anterior tracheal wall and pretracheal tissue including blood vessels, and selection of the optimal intercartilaginous space for placement of the tracheostomy tube.[67,68] The distance from the skin surface to the tracheal lumen can be measured to predetermine the length of the puncture cannula that is needed to reach the tracheal lumen without perforating the posterior wall.[69] The same distance can be used to determine the optimal length of the tracheostomy cannula.[70]

Ultrasound-guided PDT was applied in a case in which bronchoscope-guided technique had been abandoned.[69] Autopsy in cases of fatal bleeding after PDT revealed that the tracheostomy level was much more caudal than intended and that the innominate vein and the arch of the aorta had been eroded. It is likely that the addition of a USG examination to determine the level for the PDT and to avoid blood vessels could diminish this risk.[71] PDT results in a significantly lower rate of cranial misplacement of the tracheostomy tube compared with "blind" placement.[68] Bronchoscope-guided PDT often results in considerable hypercapnia, whereas Doppler ultrasound–guided PDT does not.[72]

In a prospective series of 72 PDTs, the combination of USG and bronchoscopy was applied. Before the procedures, all subjects had their pretracheal space examined with USG; the findings led to a change in the planned puncture site in 24% of cases and to a change of procedure to surgical tracheostomy in one case in which the ultrasound examination revealed a goiter with extensive subcutaneous vessels.[73] A different approach, namely trying to follow the needle during its course through the tissue overlying the trachea, was tried in a cadaver model. A small curved transducer was used in the transverse plane to localize the tracheal midline and was then turned to the longitudinal plane to allow needle puncture in the inline plane and to follow the needle's course from skin surface to trachea. After guidewire insertion a CT scan was performed that demonstrated that although all punctures had successfully entered the trachea on the first (89%) or second (11%) attempt, the guidewire was placed laterally to the ideal midline position in five of nine cadavers.[74] Another approach using real-time ultrasound guidance with visualization of the needle path by means of a linear high-frequency transducer placed transversely over the trachea was more successful and resulted in visualization of the needle path und satisfactory guide-wire placement in all of 13 patients.[75]

L. Confirmation of Gastric Tube Placement

Abdominal USG performed in the intensive care unit (ICU) had a 97% sensitivity for detecting correct gastric placement of a weighted-tip nasogastric (NG) tube. Immediately after insertion of the NG tube, the metal stylet was removed and a 2- to 5-MHz convex transducer was used to examine the duodenum in the middle gastric area. If the NG tube was not visualized, the probe was oriented toward the left upper abdominal quadrant to visualize the gastric area. If the NG tube tip was still not visible, 5 mL normal saline mixed with 5 mL air was injected into the tube to visualize the hyperechoic "fog" exiting the tip. The tip of the NG tube was considered to be correctly located when it was seen to be surrounded by fluid and echogenic moving formations (related to peristalsis). The tip of the NG tube was visualized by sonography in 34 of 35 cases. Radiography correctly identified all 35 catheters, but the radiographic confirmation lasted on average 180 minutes (range, 113 to 240 minutes); in contrast, the sonographic examinations lasted 24 minutes on average (range, 11 to 53 minutes). The authors concluded that bedside USG performed by nonradiologists is a sensitive method for confirming the position of weighted-tip NG feeding tubes, that it is easily taught to ICU physicians, and that conventional radiography can be reserved for cases in which USG is inconclusive.[76]

A Sengstaken-Blakemore tube may be applied for severe esophageal variceal bleeding, but there are considerable complications, including death, from esophageal rupture after inadvertent inflation of the gastric balloon in the esophagus.[77] USG of the stomach can aid in the rapid confirmation of correct placement. If the Sengstaken tube is not directly visible, inflation of 50 mL air via the gastric lumen (not the gastric balloon!) of the tube should lead to a characteristic jet of echogenic bubbles within the stomach. The gastric balloon is slowly inflated under direct USG control and usually appears as a growing echogenic circle within the stomach.[77]

M. Diagnosis of Pneumothorax

USG is as effective as chest radiography in detecting or excluding pneumothorax.[28] It is even more sensitive in the ICU setting: USG was able to establish the diagnosis in the majority of patients in whom a pneumothorax was invisible on plain radiographs but diagnosed by CT scan.[26] In patients with multiple injuries, USG was faster and had a higher sensitivity and accuracy compared to chest radiography.[78]

The presence of lung sliding or lung pulse on USG examination indicates that two pleural layers are in close proximity to each other at that specific point under the transducer (i.e., there is no pneumothorax there). If there is free air (pneumothorax) in the part of the pleural cavity underlying the transducer, no lung sliding or lung pulse will be seen, and A-lines (Fig. 3-16) will be more dominant.[26] In the M-mode, the "stratosphere sign" will

be seen: only parallel lines through all of the depth of the image (see Fig. 3-16). If the transducer is placed right at the border of the pneumothorax, where the visceral pleura intermittently is in contact with the parietal pleura, the lung point will be seen. This is a sliding lung alternating with A-lines, synchronous with ventilation. The lung point is pathognomonic for pneumothorax (see Fig. 3-16). If a pneumothorax is suspected, the rib interspaces of the thoracic cavity can be systematically "mapped" to confirm or rule out a pneumothorax. An online video is available to view the lung point (http://www.airwaymanagement.dk/index.php?option=com_content&view=article&id=3&Itemid=2 [accessed January 2011]).[25]

The detection of lung sliding has a negative predictive value of 100%, meaning that when lung sliding is seen, a pneumothorax of the part of the lung beneath the ultrasound probe is ruled out.[24] For diagnosis of occult pneumothorax, the abolition of lung sliding alone had a sensitivity of 100% and a specificity of 78%. Absent lung sliding plus the A-line sign had a sensitivity of 95% and a specificity of 94%. The lung point had a sensitivity of 79% and a specificity of 100%.[26]

A systematic approach is recommended when examining the supine patient. The anterior chest wall can be divided into quadrants and the probe first placed at the most superior aspect of the thorax with respect to gravity (i.e., the lower part of the anterior chest wall in supine patients). The probe is then positioned on each of the four quadrants of the anterior area, followed by the lateral chest wall between the anterior and posterior axillary lines and the rest of the accessible part of the thorax.[26]

If the suspicion of a pneumothorax arises intraoperatively, USG is the fastest way to confirm or rule it out, especially considering that an anterior pneumothorax is often undiagnosed in a supine patient subjected to plain anteroposterior radiography and that CT, the gold standard, is very difficult to apply in this situation. USG is an obvious first choice in diagnostics if a pneumothorax is suspected during or after central venous cannulation or nerve blockade, especially if USG is already in use for the procedure itself and thus immediately available.

N. Differentiation Among Different Types of Lung and Pleura Pathology

Seventy percent of the pleural surface is accessible to ultrasound examination.[28] In a study of 260 dyspneic medical-ICU patients with acute respiratory failure, the results of lung USG (performed by a dedicated specialist in lung USG) on initial presentation in the ICU were compared with the final diagnosis by the ICU team. Three items were assessed: artifacts (horizontal A-lines or vertical B-lines indicating interstitial syndrome), lung sliding, and alveolar consolidation or pleural effusion or both. Predominant A-lines plus lung sliding indicated asthma or chronic obstructive pulmonary disease with 89% sensitivity and 97% specificity. Multiple anterior diffuse B-lines with lung sliding indicated pulmonary edema with 97% sensitivity and 95% specificity. The use of these profiles would have provided correct diagnoses

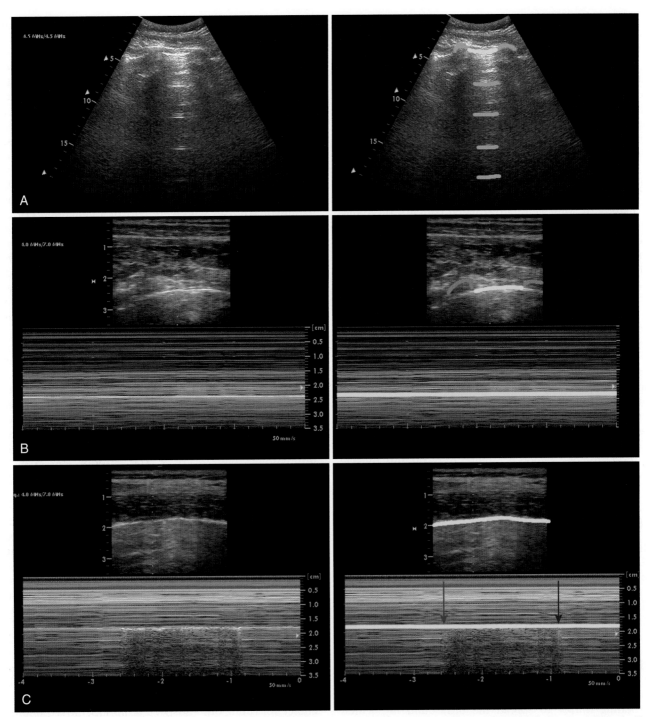

Figure 3-16 Pneumothorax. The scanning images are shown on the *left* and the marked-up images on the *right*. **A,** Image obtained with a convex transducer in a rib interspace. The pleural line *(yellow)* represents the surface of the parietal pleura. The ribs *(orange)* create underlying shadows. The "A-lines" *(light blue)* are reverberation artifacts from the pleural line; notice that they are dispersed with the same distance between the A-lines as between the skin surface and the pleural line. **B,** Again, the pleural line is marked in *yellow* and the ribs in *orange*. Everything posterior to the pleural line is artifact. There is absence of pleural sliding and absence of lung pulse. The M-mode image consists only of parallel lines, called the "stratosphere sign." **C,** The *green arrow* represents the "lung point," the moment in which the visceral pleura just comes in contact with the parietal pleura at the exact location of the transducer. For the time interval from the green to the *blue arrow*, the two pleural layers are in contact with each other and form the "lung sliding" pattern. After the time represented by the blue arrow, the two pleural layers are no longer in contact, and the "stratosphere sign" is seen. The lung point can be difficult to see on the static B-mode image, whereas it is easy to recognize with dynamic, real time, B-mode scanning. (**C,** Courtesy of Erik Sloth, Aarhus University Hospital, Skejby, Denmark.) (From Kristensen MS: Ultrasonography in the management of the airway. *Acta Anaesthesiol Scand* 55:1155–1173, 2011.)

in 90.5% of cases. It was concluded that lung ultrasound can help the clinician make a rapid diagnosis in patients with acute respiratory failure.[27]

USG can detect pleural effusion and differentiate between pleural fluid and pleural thickening, and it is more accurate and preferable to radiographic measurement in the quantification of pleural effusion.[28] Routine use of lung USG in the ICU setting can lead to a reduction of the number of chest radiographs and CT scans performed.[79]

O. Prediction of Successful Extubation

In a study of adult ventilator-treated patients, the transducer was placed on the CTM with a transverse view of the larynx. The width of the air column was significantly smaller in the group of patients who developed postextubation stridor.[80] However, the number of patients in the stridor group was small ($n = 4$), and these results need to be evaluated in larger studies.

Intubated patients receiving mechanical ventilation in a medical ICU had their breathing force evaluated by USG. The probe was placed along the right anterior axillary line and the left posterior axillary line for measurement of liver and spleen displacement in craniocaudal aspects, respectively. The cutoff value of diaphragmatic displacement for predicting successful extubation was determined to be 1.1 cm. The liver and spleen displacements measured in the study were thought to reflect the "global" functions of the respiratory muscles, and this method provided a good parameter of respiratory muscle endurance and predictor of extubation success.[30]

V. SPECIAL TECHNIQUES AND FUTURE ASPECTS

The lateral position of a laryngeal mask airway cuff can be seen on USG if the cuff is filled with fluid, but the fluid damages the cuff on subsequent autoclaving.[63] Airway obstruction due to a prevertebral hematoma after difficult central line insertion may be prevented by using USG for this procedure.[81] The larynx can be depicted from the luminal side by filling the larynx and the trachea above the cuff of the ETT with 0.9% saline to obtain sufficient tissue connection and to prevent the retention of air bubbles in the anterior commissure. The technique involves use of a thin-catheter high-frequency probe with a rotating mirror to spread the ultrasound ray, which produces a 360-degree image rectilinear to the catheter.[82,83] Three-dimensional, pocket-size USG devices are likely to move the boundaries for both the quality and the availability of USG imaging of the airway.

VI. LEARNING ULTRASONOGRAPHY

The following studies provide insight into what (and how little) is required to learn basic airway USG. After 8.5 hours of focused training comprising a 2.5-hour didactic course that included essential views of normal and pathologic conditions and three hands-on sessions of 2 hours each, physicians without previous knowledge of USG were able to competently perform basic general USG

examinations. The examinations were aimed at diagnosing the presence of pleural effusion, intra-abdominal effusion, acute cholecystitis, intrahepatic biliary duct dilation, obstructive uropathy, chronic renal disease, and deep venous thrombosis. In addition, the physicians correctly answered 95% of questions with a potential therapeutic impact.[3]

The USG experience needed to make a correct diagnosis is probably task specific. In other words, the basic skill required to detect a pleural effusion may be acquired in minutes and may then improve with experience.[84] A 25-minute instructional session, including both a didactic portion and hands-on practice, was given to critical care paramedics/nurses who were part of a helicopter critical care transport team. The instructional session focused solely on detection of the presence or absence of lung sliding, including secondary techniques such as power Doppler and M-mode USG. The participants' performance was studied on fresh ventilated cadavers. The presence or absence of lung sliding was correctly identified in 46 of 48 trials, for a sensitivity of 96.9% and a specificity of 93.8%. In a follow-up after 9 months, the presence or absence of lung sliding was correctly identified in all of 56 trials, resulting in a sensitivity and specificity of 100%.[85]

As mentioned earlier, residents given only 5 minutes of training were able to correctly identify esophageal intubation with 97% sensitivity when USG was performed dynamically, whereas the sensitivity was very poor when the examination was performed after the intubation.[52]

VII. CONCLUSIONS

Important structures relevant to airway management can be identified with the use of USG. These include a large part of the airway and adjacent structures from the mouth and tongue via the larynx and esophagus to the midtrachea, the pleural layers and their movement, the diaphragm, and the gastric antrum. Ultrasonography used dynamically, immediately before, during, and after airway interventions, gives real-time images highly relevant for several aspects of airway management. Esophageal intubation is detected without the need for ventilation or circulation, the cricothyroid membrane is identified before management of a difficult airway, ventilation is seen by observing lung sliding bilaterally, which is also the first choice for ruling out a suspected intraoperative pneumothorax, and percutaneous dilatational tracheostomy is facilitated by identifying the correct tracheal-ring interspace and depth from the skin to the tracheal wall.

VIII. CLINICAL PEARLS

- USG has many advantages for imaging the airway: It is safe, quick, repeatable, portable, and widely available and gives real-time dynamic images.

- USG must be used dynamically for maximum benefit and in direct conjunction with the airway management (immediately before, during, and after airway interventions).

- Direct observation can be made of whether an ETT is entering the trachea or the esophagus by placing the ultrasound probe transversely on the neck at the level of the suprasternal notch during intubation; in this way, intubation can be confirmed without the need for ventilation or circulation.

- The cricothyroid membrane (CTM) can easily be identified by USG prior to management of a difficult airway.

- Ventilation can be confirmed by observing lung sliding bilaterally.

- USG should be the first-choice diagnostic approach when a pneumothorax is suspected intraoperatively or during initial trauma evaluation.

- Percutaneous dilatational tracheostomy (PDT) can be improved by using USG for identifying the correct tracheal-ring interspace, avoiding blood vessels, and determining the depth from the skin to the tracheal wall.

- Numerous conditions that affect airway management can be diagnosed by preanesthetic USG, but it remains to be determined in which patients the predictive value of such an examination is high enough to recommend this as a routine approach to airway management planning.

Acknowledgments

Acta Anaesthesiologica Scandinavica, the Acta Anaesthesiologica Scandinavica Foundation, and Blackwell Publishing are acknowledged for Figures 3-1 through 3-11 and 3-14 through 3-16, which were first published in Kristensen MS: Ultrasonography in the management of the airway. *Acta Anaesthesiol Scand* 55:1155–1173, 2011.

I also thank Connie Jørgensen, MD, DMSc, Head of the Clinic for Fetal Medicine and Ultrasonography, Rigshospitalet, Copenhagen, Denmark, for illustrations and critical reading of the manuscript; Erik Sloth, MD, Phd, DMSc, Professor in Experimental Ultrasonography, Department of Anaesthesiology and Intensive Care Medicine, Aarhus University Hospital, Skejby, 8200 Aarhus N, Denmark, for illustrations and videos; Michael Friis-Tvede, MD, Rigshospitalet, Copenhagen, Denmark, for setting up the nonprofit home page for academic airway management (www.airwaymanagement.dk) and for incorporating the airway videos; Peter H. Cheng, MD, Director of Regional Anesthesia, Department of Anesthesiology, Kaiser Permanente Riverside Medical Center, Riverside, CA, USA, for illustrations and sparring; and Rasmus Hesselfeldt, MD, Rigshospitalet, Copenhagen, Denmark, for help in making the photos and videos.

SELECTED REFERENCES

All references can be found online at expertconsult.com.

1. Singh M, Chin KJ, Chan VWS, et al: Use of sonography for airway assessment: An observational study. *J Ultrasound Med* 29:79–85, 2010.
13. Gourin CG, Orloff LA: Normal head and neck ultrasound anatomy. In Orloff LA, editor: *Head and neck ultrasonography*, San Diego, 2008, Plural Publishing, pp 39–68.
25. Copenhagen University Hospital: Ultrasonography in airway management. Available at www.airwaymanagement.dk (accessed January 2011).
27. Lichtenstein DA, Mezière GA: Relevance of lung ultrasound in the diagnosis of acute respiratory failure: The BLUE protocol. *Chest* 134:117–125, 2008.
28. Sartori S, Tombesi P: Emerging roles for transthoracic ultrasonography in pleuropulmonary pathology. *World J Radiol* 2:83–90, 2010.
42. Lakhal K, Delplace X, Cottier J-P, et al: The feasibility of ultrasound to assess subglottic diameter. *Anesth Analg* 104:611–614, 2007.
61. Park SC, Ryu JH, Yeom SR, et al: Confirmation of endotracheal intubation by combined ultrasonographic methods in the emergency department. *Emerg Med Australas* 21:293–297, 2009.
68. Sustić A, Kovač D, Žgaljardić Z, et al: Ultrasound-guided percutaneous dilatational tracheostomy: A safe method to avoid cranial misplacement of the tracheostomy tube. *Intensive Care Med* 26:1379–1381, 2000.
79. Peris A, Tutino L, Zagli G, et al: The use of point-of-care bedside lung ultrasound significantly reduces the number of radiographs and computed tomography scans in critically ill patients. *Anesth Analg* 111:687–692, 2010.
85. Lyon M, Walton P, Bhalla V, Shiver SA: Ultrasound detection of the sliding lung sign by prehospital critical care providers. *Am J Emerg Med* 2011 Feb 17 [Epub ahead of print].

Chapter 4

Physics and Modeling of the Airway

D. JOHN DOYLE | KEVIN F. O'GRADY

I. THE GAS LAWS

A. Ideal Gases

Air is a fluid. Understanding the fundamentals of basic fluid mechanics is essential in grasping the concepts of airway flow. Because air is also a gas, it is important to understand the laws that govern its gaseous behavior. Gases are usually described in terms of pressure, volume, and temperature. Pressure is most often quantified clinically in terms of mm Hg (or torr), volume in mL, and temperature in degrees Celsius. However, calculations often require conversion from one set of units to another and therefore can be quite tedious. We have included a small section at the end of the chapter to simplify these conversions.

Perhaps the most important law of gas flow in airways is the ideal (or perfect) gas law, which can be written as follows[1]:

$$PV = nRT \tag{1}$$

where
P = pressure of gas (pascals or mm Hg)
V = volume of gas (m^3 or cm^3 or mL)
n = number of moles of the gas in volume V
R = gas constant (8.3143 J g-mol^{-1}·K^{-1}, assuming P in pascals, V in m^3)
T = absolute temperature (in kelvins or K; 273.16 K = 0° C)

One mole of gas contains 6.023×10^{23} molecules, and this quantity is termed Avogadro's number. One mole of an ideal gas takes up 22.4138 L at standard temperature and pressure (STP); standard temperature is 273.16 K, and standard pressure is 1 atmosphere (760 mm Hg).[1] Avogadro also stated that equal volumes of all ideal gases at the same temperature and pressure contain the same number of molecules.

The ideal gas law incorporates the laws of Boyle and Charles.[1] Boyle's law states that, at a constant temperature, the product of pressure and volume (P × V) is equal to a constant. Consequently, P is proportional to $1/V$ (P ∝ 1/V) at constant T. However, gases do not obey Boyle's law at temperatures approaching their point of liquefaction (i.e., the point at which the gas becomes a liquid).

Boyle's law concerns perfect gases and is not obeyed by real gases over a wide range of pressures (see Section II for a discussion of nonideal gases). However, at infinitely low pressures, all gases obey Boyle's law. Boyle's law does not apply to anesthetic gases and many other gases because of the van der Waals attraction between molecules (i.e., they are nonideal gases).

Charles' law states that, at a constant pressure, volume is proportional to temperature (i.e., V ∝ T at constant P). Gay-Lussac's law states that, at a constant volume, pressure is proportional to temperature (i.e., P ∝ T at constant V).[1] Often, these two laws are shortened for convenience to Charles' law. When a gas obeys both Charles' law and Boyle's law, it is said to be an ideal gas and obeys the ideal gas law.

In clinical situations, gases are typically mixtures of several "pure" gases. Quantifiable properties of mixtures may be determined using Dalton's law of partial pressures. Dalton's law states that the pressure exerted by a mixture of gases is the sum of the pressures exerted by the individual pure gases[1,2]:

$$P_{total} = P_A + P_B + P_C + \ldots + P_N \tag{2}$$

where P_A, P_B, and P_C are the partial pressures of pure ideal gases.

B. Nonideal Gases: The van der Waals Effect

Ideal gases have no forces of interaction, but real gases have intermolecular attraction, which requires that the pressure-volume gas law be rewritten as follows[1,2]:

$$\left(P + \frac{a}{V^2}\right) \times (V - b) = nRT \tag{3}$$

where
P = pressure of gas (pascals or mm Hg)
V = volume of gas (m^3 or cm^3 or mL)
n = number of moles of the gas in volume V
R = gas constant (8.3143 J g- mol^{-1}·K^{-1}, assuming P in pascals, V in m^3)
T = absolute temperature (K)
a and b = physical constants for a given gas

The values of *a* and *b* for a given gas may be found in physical chemistry textbooks and other sources.[1-5] This formulation, provided by van der Waals, accounts for intramolecular forces fairly well.

C. Diffusion of Gases

Clinically, diffusion of gases through a membrane is most applicable to gas flow across lung and placental membranes. The most commonly used relation to govern diffusion is Fick's first law of diffusion, which states that the rate of diffusion of a gas across a barrier is proportional to the concentration gradient for the gas. Fick's law may be expressed mathematically as follows[6]:

$$\text{Flux} = -D\frac{\Delta C}{\Delta X} \tag{4}$$

where
Flux = the number of molecules crossing the membrane each second (molecules/cm^2/s)
ΔC = the concentration gradient (molecules/cm^3)
ΔX = the diffusion distance (cm)
D = the diffusion coefficient (cm^2/s)

In general, the value of D is inversely proportional to the gas's molecular weight as well as intrinsic properties of the membrane.

Because gases partially dissolve when they come into contact with a liquid, Henry's law becomes important in some instances. It states that the mass of a gas dissolved in a given amount of liquid is proportional to the pressure of the gas at constant temperature. As a result, the gas concentration (in solvent) is equal to a constant × P (at constant T).[1]

D. Pressure, Flow, and Resistance

The laws of fluid mechanics dictate an intricate relationship among pressure, flow, and resistance. Pressure is defined as force per unit area. It is usually measured clinically in mm Hg or cm H_2O, but it is most commonly measured scientifically in pascals (Pa), or newtons of force per square meter (1 Pa = 1 N/m^2).

Flow (i.e., the rate of flow) is equal to the change in pressure (pressure drop or pressure difference) divided by the resistance experienced by the fluid. For example, if the flow is 100 mL/s at a pressure difference of 100 mm Hg, the resistance is 100 mm Hg/100 mL/s, or 1 mm Hg/mL/s. In laminar flow systems only, the resistance is constant, independent of the flow rate.[7,8]

An important formula that quantifies the relationship of pressure, flow, and resistance in laminar flow systems is given by the Hagen-Poiseuille equation. Poiseuille's law states that the fluid flow rate through a horizontal straight tube of uniform bore is proportional to the pressure gradient (ΔP), and the fourth power of the radius (π) and is related inversely to the viscosity of the gas (μ, in g/cm·s) and the length of the tube (L, in cm). This law, which is valid for laminar flow only, may be stated as follows[7,8]:

$$\Delta P = \frac{8 \mu L}{\pi^4} \times \text{Flow} \qquad (5)$$

See the discussion of laminar flow in Section II for further details.

When the flow rate exceeds a *critical velocity* (the flow velocity below which flow is laminar), the flow loses its laminar parabolic velocity profile, becomes disorderly, and is termed *turbulent* (Fig. 4-1). If turbulent flow exists, the relationship between pressure drop and flow is no longer governed by the Hagen-Poiseuille equation. Instead, the pressure gradient required (or the resistance encountered) during turbulent flow varies as the square of the flow rate. See the discussion of turbulent flow in Section II.

Viscosity, μ, characterizes the resistance within a fluid to the flow of one layer of molecules over another (shear characteristics).[7] Blood viscosity is influenced primarily by hematocrit, so that at low hematocrit blood flow is easier—that is, blood is more dilute. The critical velocity at which turbulent flow begins depends on the ratio of viscosity (μ) to density (ρ), which is defined as the *kinematic viscosity* (υ)—that is, $\upsilon = \mu/\rho$. (This is illustrated with an example in the section on turbulent flow).[7-9] The unit for viscosity is g/cm·s (poise). The typical unit for kinematic viscosity is cm^2/s.

The viscosity of water is 0.01 poise at 25° C and 0.007 poise at 37° C. The viscosity of air is 183 micropoise at 18° C. Its density (dry) is 1.213 g/L.[10]

Density is defined as mass per unit volume (g/cm^3 or g/mL). The density of water is 1 g/mL. The general relation for the density of a gas is given by the following equation:

$$D = D_0 \left(\frac{T_0 P}{T P_0} \right) \qquad (6)$$

where D_0 is a known density of the gas at temperature T_0 and pressure P_0, and D is the density of the gas at temperature T and pressure P. For dry air at 18° C and 760 mm Hg (atmospheric pressure), D = 1.213 g/L.[4]

The fall in pressure at points of flow constriction (where the flow velocity is higher) is known as the Bernoulli effect (Fig. 4-2).[7,8] This phenomenon is used in apparatus employing the Venturi principle, such as gas nebulizers, Venturi flowmeters, and some oxygen face masks. The lower pressure related to the Bernoulli effect sucks in (entrains) air to mix with oxygen.

One final consideration that is important in the study of the airway is Laplace's law for a sphere (Fig. 4-3). It states that, for a sphere with one air-liquid interface (e.g., an alveolus), the relation between the transmural pressure difference, surface tension, and sphere radius is described by the following equation[11]:

$$P = \frac{2T}{r} \qquad (7)$$

where
P = transmural pressure difference (dynes/cm^2; 1 dyne/cm^2 = 0.1 Pa = 0.000751 torr)
T = surface tension (dynes/cm)
R = sphere radius (cm)

The key point in Laplace's law is that the smaller the sphere radius, the higher the transmural pressure. However, real (in vivo) alveoli do *not* obey Laplace's law because of the action of pulmonary surfactant, which decreases the surface tension disproportionately compared with what is predicted on the basis of physical principles. When pulmonary surfactant is missing from the lungs, the lungs take on the behavior described by Laplace's law.

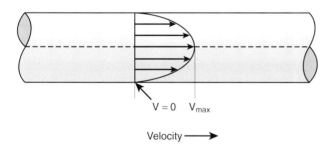

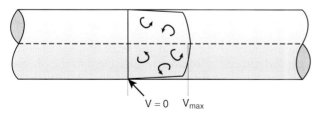

Figure 4-1 Laminar and turbulent flow. *Top,* Laminar flow in a long smooth pipe is characterized by smooth and steady flow with little or no fluctuations. The flow profile is parabolic in nature, with fluid traveling most quickly at the center of the tube and stationary at the edges. *Bottom,* Turbulent flow is characterized by fluctuating and agitated flow. Its flow profile is essentially flat, with all fluid traveling at the same velocity except at tube edges. *V,* Velocity.

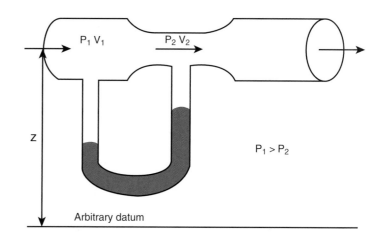

Figure 4-2   Bernoulli effect. **A,** Diagram shows fluid flow through a tube with varying diameters. At the point of flow constriction, fluid pressure is less than at the distal end of the tube, as indicated by the height of the manometer fluid column. This effect is described by the Bernoulli equation. In the case of a horizontal pipe, the distance between the centerline of the pipe and an arbitrary datum at two different points will be the same (Z). **B,** Venturi tube. The lower pressure caused by the Bernoulli effect entrains air to mix with oxygen. P, Pressure; V, velocity.

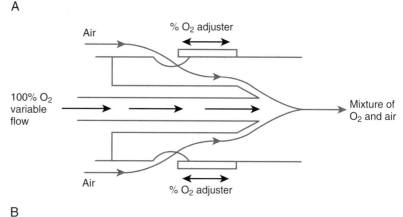

E. Example: Analysis of Transtracheal Jet Ventilation

Transtracheal jet ventilation (TTJV) has been used to oxygenate and ventilate patients who would otherwise perish because of a lost airway.[6] It is a temporizing measure that is used only until an airway can be secured. It is usually employed using equipment commonly available in the operating or emergency room and often using the 50-psi wall oxygen source.[6,12-14]

1. Analysis

The gas flow through a catheter depends on both the resistance of the catheter-connection hose assembly and the driving pressure applied to it. If the resistance of the assembly is R, the flow (F) from the catheter is $F = P_d/R$, where P_d is the pressure difference between the ends of the catheter-connection assembly. R itself certainly depends on F when the flow becomes turbulent, but the flow relationship still holds. However, P_d is very close to the driving pressure (P) applied to the ventilation catheter, because the lung offers little relative back pressure. (At back pressures greater than 100 cm H_2O, the lung is likely to burst, and P is often chosen to be 50 psi, or about 3500 cm H_2O.) Therefore, the flow relationship may be simplified to $F = P/R$.

Next, TTJV is applied through a sequence of "jet pulses," each resulting in a given tidal volume (e.g., 500 mL). Ignoring entrained air effects, the delivered tidal volume is equal to catheter flow × pulse duration. For a catheter flow of 30 L/min, a jet pulse lasting 1 second results in a tidal volume of 30 L/min × $\frac{1}{16}$ min = 0.5 L.

In a TTJV setup consisting of a 14-G angiographic catheter connected to a regulated oxygen source by a 4.5-foot polyvinyl chloride (PVC) tube of $\frac{7}{32}$-inch inner diameter (ID), for oxygen flows between 10 and 60 L/min, the resistance was found to be relatively constant between 0.6 and 0.8 psi/L/min.[15]

Many systems for TTJV choose 50 psi for convenience (50 psi being the oxygen wall outlet pressure), although a regulator is very often used to permit lower pressures. However, 50 psi may not be an optimal pressure choice for TTJV. Using the preceding data, the pressure required for TTJV for a tidal volume of 500 mL can be calculated. Assuming that the setup resistance is 0.7 psi/L/min and the desired flow rate is 30 L/min, the driving pressure should be 0.7 × 30 = 21 psi.

Similar analyses can be carried out for other arrangements derived from experiments to obtain resistance data.

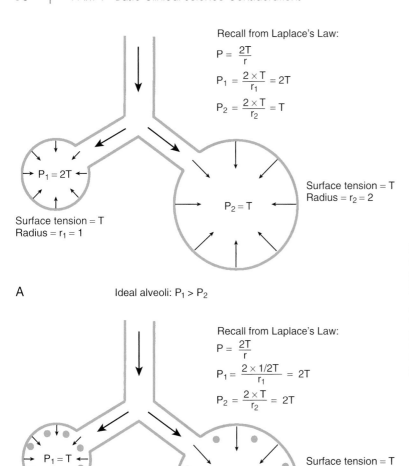

Recall from Laplace's Law:

$$P = \frac{2T}{r}$$

$$P_1 = \frac{2 \times T}{r_1} = 2T$$

$$P_2 = \frac{2 \times T}{r_2} = T$$

Surface tension = T
Radius = r_1 = 1

$P_1 = 2T$

$P_2 = T$

Surface tension = T
Radius = r_2 = 2

A   Ideal alveoli: $P_1 > P_2$

Recall from Laplace's Law:

$$P = \frac{2T}{r}$$

$$P_1 = \frac{2 \times 1/2T}{r_1} = 2T$$

$$P_2 = \frac{2 \times T}{r_2} = 2T$$

Surface tension = 1/2 T
Radius = r_1 = 1

$P_1 = T$

$P_2 = T$

Surface tension = T
Radius = r_2 = 2

B   Real alveoli: $P_1 = P_2$ with pulmonary surfactant

Figure 4-3 Laplace's law for a sphere. **A,** Laplace's law dictates that for two alveoli of unequal size but equal surface tension, the smaller alveolus experiences a larger intra-alveolar pressure than the larger alveolus. This causes air to pass into the larger alveolus and causes the smaller alveolus to collapse. **B,** Collapse of the smaller alveolus is prevented through the action of pulmonary surfactant. Surfactant serves to decrease alveolar surface tension in the smaller alveolus, which results in equal pressure in both alveoli. *P,* Transmural pressure difference; *r,* sphere radius.

II. GAS FLOW

A. Laminar Flow

In laminar flow, fluid particles flow along smooth paths in layers, or laminas, with one layer gliding smoothly over an adjacent layer.[7] Any tendencies toward instability and

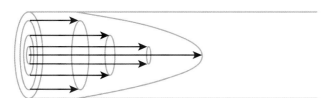

Figure 4-4 Laminar flow. Laminar gas flow through long straight tube of uniform bore has a velocity profile that is parabolic in shape, with the gas traveling most quickly at center of tube. Conceptually, it is helpful to view laminar gas flow as a series of concentric cylinders of gas, with the central cylinder moving most rapidly. (From Nunn JF: *Nunn's applied respiratory physiology,* ed 4, Stoneham, MA, 1993, Butterworth-Heinemann.)

turbulence are damped out by viscous shear forces that resist the relative motion of adjacent fluid layers. Under laminar flow conditions through a tube, the flow velocity is greatest at the center of the tube flow and zero at the inner edge of the tube (Fig. 4-4; see also Fig. 4-1). The flow profile has a parabolic shape. Under these conditions in a horizontal tube, the relation between flow, tube, and gas characteristics is given by the Hagen-Poiseuille equation (Equation 5), restated as follows[7-9]:

$$\dot{V} = \frac{\pi \Delta P r^4}{8 \mu L} \qquad (8)$$

where
$\dot{V}$ = flow rate (cm^3/s)
π = 3.1416
ΔP = pressure gradient (pascals)
r = tube radius (cm)
L = tube length (cm)
μ = gas viscosity (g/cm·s)

Typical units are shown in parentheses. The dot indicates rate of change: V represents volume, and $\dot{V}$ represents the *rate of change of volume*, or *flow rate*. Another way of looking at this concept is that, under conditions of laminar flow through a tube of known radius, the pressure difference across the tube is given by the following proportionality (which is also essentially the same as Equation 5):

$$\Delta \text{Pressure} \propto \frac{\text{Flow} \times \text{Viscosity} \times \text{Length}}{\text{Radius}^4} \quad (9)$$

The pressure gradient through the airway increases proportionately with flow, viscosity, and tube length but increases exponentially as the tube radius decreases.

The conditions under which flow through a tube is predominantly laminar can be estimated from *critical flow rates*. The critical flow is the flow rate below which flow is predominantly laminar in a given airflow situation.

1. Laminar Flow Example

Assume a tube of uniform bore that is 1 cm in diameter and 3 m in length. A pressure difference of 5 cm H_2O exists between the ends of the tube, and air is the fluid flowing through the tube. Assuming laminar flow, what flow rate should be expected?

ANSWER:

The relevant variables are expressed in the centimeter-gram-second (CGS) system of units:

r = 0.5 cm
L = 3000 cm
μ = 183 micropoise = 183×10^{-6} poise = 183×10^{-6} g/(cm·s)
ΔP = 0.5 cm H_2O = 490 dynes/cm^2

Using the Hagen-Poiseuille equation, the laminar flow is determined as follows:

$$\text{Flow} = \frac{\pi \times 490 \times (0.5)^4}{8 \times 183 \times 10^{-6} \times 3000} = 219.06 \text{ cm}^3/\text{s} \quad (10)$$

B. Turbulent Flow

Flow in tubes below the critical flow rate remains mostly laminar. However, at flows greater than the critical flow rate, the flow becomes increasingly turbulent. Under turbulent flow conditions, the parabolic flow pattern is lost, and the resistance to flow increases with flow itself. Turbulence may also be created where sharp angles, changes in diameter, and branches are encountered (Fig. 4-5). The flow-pressure drop relationship is given approximately by the following equation[7,8]:

$$V \propto \sqrt{\Delta P} \quad (11)$$

where
V = mean fluid velocity (cm/s)
ΔP = pressure (pascals)

1. Reynolds Number Calculation Example

The Reynolds number (Re) represents the ratio of inertial forces to viscous forces.[7,8,16] It is useful because it characterizes the flow through a long, straight tube of uniform bore. It is a dimensionless number having the following form:

$$\text{Re} = \frac{V \times D \times \rho}{\mu} = \frac{V \times D}{\nu} = \frac{2 \times \dot{V} \times \rho}{\pi \times r \times \mu} \quad (12)$$

where
Re = Reynolds number
$\dot{V}$ = flow rate (mL/s)
ρ = density (g/mL)
μ = viscosity (poise or g/cm·s)
r = radius (cm)
ν = kinematic viscosity (cm^2/s) = μ/ρ
D = diameter (cm)
V = mean fluid velocity (cm/s)

Typical units are shown in brackets. For tubes that are long compared with their diameter (i.e., length ÷ diameter > 0.06 × Re),[8] the flow is laminar when Re is less than 2000. For shorter tubes, flow is turbulent at Re values as low as 280.

When a tube's radius exceeds its length, it is an orifice; flow through an orifice is always turbulent. Under these conditions, the flow is influenced by the density rather than the viscosity of the fluid.[17] This characteristic explains why heliox (e.g., the mixture of 70% He and

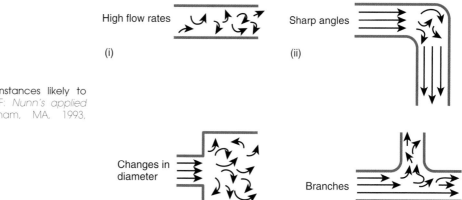

Figure 4-5 Turbulent flow. Four circumstances likely to produce turbulent flow. (From Nunn JF: *Nunn's applied respiratory physiology*, ed 4, Stoneham, MA, 1993, Butterworth-Heinemann.)

High flow rates (i)

Sharp angles (ii)

Changes in diameter (iii)

Branches (iv)

30% O_2) flows better in a narrow edematous glottis: as the following data suggest, helium has a very low density and thus presents less resistance to flow through an orifice.

	Viscosity at 20° C	Density at 20° C
Helium	194.1 micropoise	0.179 g/L
Oxygen	210.8 micropoise	1.429 g/L

How can one predict whether a given gas flow through an endotracheal tube (ETT) is laminar or turbulent? One approach is first to identify the physical conditions. For example, consider the case of an ETT with a 6-mm ID and a length of 27 cm through which 1 L/min of air is passing. In this setting,

L = 27 cm
r = 0.3 cm (size 6 mm ETT)
flow ($\dot{V}$) = 60 L/min = 1000 mL/s
viscosity (μ) = 183 micropoise = 183 $\times$ 10^{-6} g/cm·s (air at 18° C)
density (ρ) = 1.21 g/L = 0.001213 g/mL (dry air at 18° C)

With this information, one can calculate the Reynolds number:

$$Re = \frac{2 \times 1000 \times 0.001213}{\pi \times 0.3 \times 183 \times 10^{-6}} = 1.41 \times 10^4 \qquad (13)$$

Because this number greatly exceeds 2000, flow is probably quite turbulent.

C. Critical Velocity

The *critical velocity* is the point at which the transition from laminar to turbulent flow begins. This point is reached when Re becomes the critical Reynolds number, Re_{crit}. Critical velocity, the flow velocity below which flow is laminar, is calculated by the following equation[8]:

$$V_{crit} = V_c = \frac{Re_{crit} \times Viscosity}{Density \times Diameter} \qquad (14)$$

where Re_{crit} = 2000 for circular tubes.

As can be seen from this equation, the critical velocity is proportional to the viscosity of the gas and is related inversely to the density of the gas and the radius of the tube. (Viscosity has the dimensions of pascal-second (Pa $\times$ s), (equivalent to N $\times$ s/m^2, or kg/[m $\times$ s].)

The critical velocity at which turbulent flow begins depends on the ratio of viscosity to density, that is, μ/ρ. This ratio is known as the *kinematic viscosity*, υ, and has typical units of centimeters squared per second (cm^2/s). The actual measurement of viscosity of a fluid is carried out with the use of a viscometer, which consists of two rotary cylinders with the test fluid flowing between.

1. Critical Velocity Calculation Example

Using the same data as in the previous Reynolds number calculation, one can calculate the critical velocity at which laminar flow starts to become turbulent:

$$V_c = \frac{(2000) \times (183 \times 10^{-6} \text{ poise})}{(0.001213 \text{ g/cm}^3) \times (2 \times 0.3 \text{ cm})}$$
$$V_c = 502.8 \frac{\text{poise}}{(\text{g/cm}^3) \times \text{cm}} = 502.8 \frac{\text{cm}}{\text{s}} \qquad (15)$$

D. Flow Through an Orifice

Flow through an orifice (defined as flow through a tube whose length is smaller than its radius) is always somewhat turbulent.[17] Clinically, airway-obstructing conditions such as epiglottitis or swallowed obstructions are often best viewed as breathing through an orifice (Fig. 4-6). Under such conditions, the approximate flow across the orifice varies inversely with the square root of the gas density:

$$\dot{V} \propto \frac{1}{\sqrt{\text{Gas density}}} \qquad (16)$$

This is in contrast to laminar flow conditions, in which gas flow varies inversely with gas viscosity. The viscosity values for helium and oxygen are similar, but their densities are very different (Table 4-1). Table 4-2 provides useful data to allow comparison of gas flow rates through an orifice.[18]

1. Helium-Oxygen Mixtures

The low density of helium allows it to play a significant clinical role in the management of some forms of airway obstruction.[19-22] For instance, Rudow and colleagues described the use of helium-oxygen (heliox) mixtures in a patient with severe airway obstruction related to a large thyroid mass (see next section for clinical examples).[18]

The available percentage mixtures of helium and oxygen are typically 80:20 and 70:30. These mixtures are usually administered by a rebreathing face mask to patients who have an increased work of breathing due to airway pathology (e.g., edema) but for whom it is preferable to withhold endotracheal intubation at present.

Although the use of heliox mixtures in patients with upper airway obstruction has met with considerable success, the hope that this approach would also work well for patients with severe asthma has not been borne out. In a systematic review of seven clinical trials involving 392 patients with acute asthma, the authors cautioned that "existing evidence does not provide support for the

TABLE 4-1

Viscosity and Density Differences of Anesthetic Gases

	Viscosity at 300 K	Density at 20° C
Air	18.6 µPa $\times$ s	1.293 g/L
Nitrogen	17.9 µPa $\times$ s	1.250 g/L
Nitrous oxide	15.0 µPa $\times$ s	1.965 g/L
Helium	20.0 µPa $\times$ s	0.178 g/L
Oxygen	20.8 µPa $\times$ s	1.429 g/L

Data from Haynes WM: *CRC Handbook of chemistry and physics,* ed 91, Boca Raton, FL, 2010, CRC Press, and Streeter VL, Wylie EB, Bedford KW: *Fluid mechanics,* ed 9, New York, 1998, McGraw-Hill.

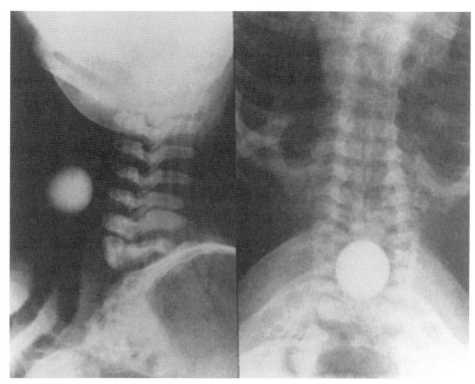

Figure 4-6 Airway obstruction. Anterior-posterior and lateral radiographs of 18-month-old infant who had swallowed a marble. The presence of this esophageal foreign body caused acute airway obstruction from extrinsic compression of the trachea. (From Badgwell JM, McLeod ME, Friedberg J: Airway obstruction in infants and children. *Can J Anaesth* 34:90, 1987.)

administration of helium-oxygen mixtures to emergency department patients with moderate-to-severe acute asthma."[23] A similar study noted that "heliox may offer mild-to-moderate benefits in patients with acute asthma within the first hour of use, but its advantages become less apparent beyond 1 hour, as most conventionally treated patients improve to similar levels, with or without it"; however, the authors suggested that its effect "may be more pronounced in more severe cases." They concluded that "there are insufficient data on whether heliox can avert endotracheal intubation, or change intensive care and hospital admission rates and duration, or mortality."[24]

2. Clinical Vignettes

Rudow and colleagues reported the following clinical illustration of heliox therapy.[18] A 78-year-old woman with both breast cancer and ophthalmic melanoma developed airway obstruction from a thyroid carcinoma that extended into her mediastinum and compressed her trachea. She had a 2-month history of worsening dyspnea, especially when positioned supine. On examination, inspiratory and expiratory stridor was present. The chest radiograph showed a large superior mediastinal mass and pulmonary metastases. A solid mass was identified on a thyroid ultrasound scan. Computed tomography revealed a large mass at the thoracic inlet and extending caudally. Clinically, the patient was exhausted and in respiratory distress.

A 78:22 heliox mixture was administered and provided almost instant relief, with improvements in measured tidal volume and oxygenation. Later, a thyroidectomy was carried out to alleviate the obstruction. For this procedure, topical anesthesia was applied to the airway and awake laryngoscopy and intubation were performed with the patient in the sitting position. After the airway was secured with the use of an armored tube, the patient was given a general anesthetic by intravenous induction.

TABLE 4-2				
Gas Flow Rates Through an Orifice				
	%	**Density (g/L)**	**(Density)$^{-1/2}$**	**Relative Flow**
Air	100	1.293	0.881	1.0
Oxygen	100	1.429	0.846	0.96
Helium (He)	100	0.179	2.364	2.68
He-oxygen	20/80	1.178	0.922	1.048
He-oxygen	60/40	0.678	1.215	1.381
He-oxygen	80/20	0.429	1.527	1.73

From Rudow M, Hill AB, Thompson NW, et al: Helium-oxygen mixtures in airway obstruction due to thyroid carcinoma. *Can Anaesth Soc J* 33:498, 1986.

Extubation after the surgery was performed without complication.

Another interesting clinical scenario was published by Khanlou and Eiger.[25] They presented the case of a 69-year-old woman in whom bilateral vocal cord paralysis developed after radiation therapy. Heliox was successfully used for temporary management of the resultant upper airway obstruction until the patient was able to receive a tracheostomy.

A final clinical vignette was reported by Polaner,[26] who used the laryngeal mask airway and an 80:20 heliox mixture to administer anesthesia to a 3-year-old boy with asthma and a large anterior mediastinal mass. Clinical management involved an unusual combination of management strategies: the child was kept in the sitting position, spontaneous ventilation with a halothane-in-heliox inhalation induction was used, and airway stimulation was minimized by use of the laryngeal mask airway. However, the author cautioned that cases such as these can readily take a deadly turn, noting that "one must, of course, always be prepared to intervene with either manipulations of patient position in the event of airway compromise (including upright, lateral, and prone) or more aggressive strategies, such as rigid bronchoscopy and even median sternotomy (in the case of intractable cardiovascular collapse), or to allow the patient to awaken if critical airway or cardiovascular compromise becomes evident at any time during the course of the anesthesia."[26]

E. Pressure Differences

From the analysis of equations governing laminar flow and turbulent flow, the pressure drop along the noncompliant portion of the airway is given approximately by the Rohrer equation[27]:

$$\Delta P = K_1 \dot{V} + K_2 \dot{V}^2 \qquad (17)$$

K_1 and K_2 are known as Rohrer constants. The physical interpretation of this equation is that airway pressure is governed by the sum of two terms:

1. Effects proportional to gas flow (laminar flow effects)
2. Effects proportional to the square of the gas flow (turbulent flow effects)

It can be seen that the lowest pressure loss across the airway (ΔP) would occur when $\dot{V}$ is small (i.e., with predominantly laminar flow). However, it is known that under conditions of laminar flow, K_1 is largely influenced by viscosity rather than density, and K_2 (the turbulent term) is influenced primarily by density and not viscosity.

F. Resistance to Gas Flow

When pressure readings are taken at each end of a horizontal tube with a fluid flowing through it, one notices that they are not identical: The pressure at the distal end of the tube is less than the pressure at the proximal end (with fluid flowing from the proximal to the distal end).

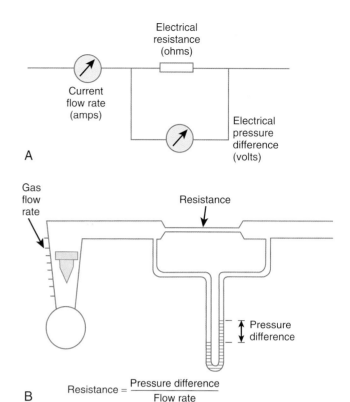

Figure 4-7 Analogy between laminar gas flow and flow of electricity through a resistor. **A,** Electrical flow rate (current) is measured in amperes; pressure difference (voltage) is measured in volts; resistance is measured in ohms and described by Ohm's law. **B,** Gas flow rate is measured as volume/second (e.g., mL/s); pressure difference is measured as force/area (e.g., dynes/cm²); resistance is described by Poiseuille's law. For gases, pressure difference = flow rate × resistance; for electricity, potential difference (voltage) = current × resistance. (From Nunn JF: *Nunn's applied respiratory physiology*, ed 4, Stoneham, MA, 1993, Butterworth-Heinemann.)

This pressure loss is attributable to frictional losses incurred by the fluid when in contact with the inside of the tube. This is analogous to heat losses incurred by resistors in an electrical circuit (Fig. 4-7).

Frictional losses are irreversible; that is, the energy lost cannot be recovered by the fluid and is mostly lost as heat. If the tube is not horizontal, there are additional pressure differences attributable to height differences. The most common relation that describes the flow in a tube is the Bernoulli equation, which is valid for both laminar and turbulent flow[8]:

$$\frac{V_1^2}{2g} + \frac{P_1}{\rho g} + Z_1 = \frac{V_2^2}{2g} + \frac{P_2}{\rho g} + Z_2 + h_f \qquad (18)$$

where
V = velocity (m/s)
g = gravitational constant (9.81 m/s² or 9.81 N/kg)
P = pressure (pascals or N/m²)
ρ = density of fluid (kg/m³)
Z = height from an arbitrary point (datum) (m)
h_f = frictional losses (m)

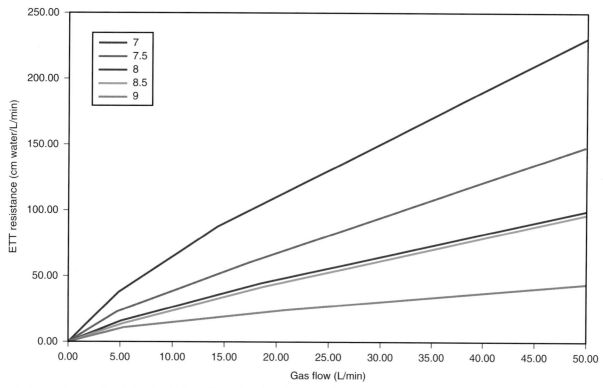

Figure 4-8   Dependence of endotracheal tube (ETT) on flow. The data provided by Hicks in Table 4-3 can be used to show that ETT resistance increases nonlinearly with flow (because of turbulence effects). For pure laminar flow, resistance would be constant, regardless of flow.

Typical units are shown in square brackets. Equation 18 is in units of meters and is termed "meters of head loss." This is typical of fluid mechanics equations. As mentioned previously, the Bernoulli equation is valid for both laminar and turbulent flow.

1. Endotracheal Tube Resistance

ETTs, like all tubes, offer resistance to fluid flow (Fig. 4-8). However, ETTs do not add external resistance to the normal airway; rather, they act as a substitute for the normal resistance of the airway from the mouth to the trachea, which accounts for 30% to 40% of normal airway resistance.[28] This is important because, although mechanical ventilators can overcome impedance to inspiratory flow during extended periods of artificial respiration, they do not augment passive exhalation. Resistance to exhalation through a long, small-diameter ETT, which is compounded by turbulence, can seriously constrain ventilation rate and tidal volume.[29,30]

The use of the ETT influences respiration in a number of ways. First, it decreases effective airway diameter and therefore increases the resistance to breathing. Resistance is further increased by the curved nature of the tube; resistance measurements are typically about 3% higher than if the tubes were straight.[31] Also, the passage from the mouth to the larynx is not a smooth curve and may create additional turbulence. Second, studies show that intubated patients experience decreased peak flow rates (inspiratory and expiratory), decreased forced vital capacity, and decreased forced expiratory volume in 1 second (FEV$_1$).[32] However, the tube may paradoxically increase peak flow rates during forced expiration by preventing dynamic compression of the trachea.[32] Finally, the tube may cause mechanical irritation of the larynx and trachea that may lead to a reflex constriction of the airway distal to the tube.[33]

The combination of tube and connector may cause higher resistance than the tube alone. Moreover, because of turbulence at component connections, the total resistance of a system is not necessarily the sum of the resistances of its component parts, especially if sharp-angled connectors are used (see Fig. 4-5).[25,34] In addition, humidified gases contribute to slightly higher resistances because of the increased density of moist gas, and the resistance of single-lumen tubes is generally lower than that of double-lumen tubes.[35]

The resistance associated with ETTs may be reduced by increasing the tube diameter, decreasing tube length, or decreasing the gas density (hence, the occasional use of heliox mixtures). It has been suggested that the presence of an ETT may double the work of breathing in chronically intubated adults and may lead to respiratory failure in some infants.[31] Therefore, it is important to use as large an ETT as is practical in patients who exhibit respiratory dysfunction.

ETT resistance can be measured in the laboratory using differential pressure and flow measurement techniques,[36,37] most commonly by the method of Gaensler and colleagues.[38] Theoretical estimates of resistance under laminar flow conditions can also be obtained by using the Poiseuille equation. In vivo measurements of ETT resistance are generally higher than in vitro measurements, perhaps because of secretions, head or neck position, tube deformation, or increased turbulence.[10,39]

Airway resistance may be established from first principles using Poiseuille's law if the gas flow is laminar. If gas flow is turbulent, resistance is no longer independent of material properties, and empirical measurements become the only feasible means of characterizing resistance. Intrinsic airway resistance is determined by measuring the transairway pressure—that is, the pressure drop between the airway opening and the alveoli. The following relationship applies[40]:

$$R = \frac{P_{airway} - P_{alveolar}}{\dot{V}} \qquad (19)$$

where
R = airway resistance (cm H_2O/L/s)
P_{airway} = proximal airway pressure (cm H_2O)
$P_{alveolar}$ = alveolar pressure (cm H_2O)
$\dot{V}$ = gas flow rate (L/s)

Typical units used are shown in parentheses.

In clinical practice, airway resistance is most easily determined by using a whole-body plethysmograph. However, this apparatus is unsuitable for critically ill patients. An alternative method of presenting airway resistance was provided by Hicks,[40] who used the following equation and constants:

$$\Delta P = a\dot{V}^b \qquad (20)$$

where
ΔP = pressure difference (cm H_2O)
$\dot{V}$ = gas flow (L/min)
a and b = empirical constants

The values for the coefficients *a* and *b* depend on tube size and are provided in Table 4-3.

Figure 4-8 depicts the effects of tube diameter and flow rate on ETT resistance. Notice that resistance is increased as a result of increasing turbulence caused by decreasing ETT diameter and increasing flow rate.

Clinically, the issue of ETT resistance is perhaps most important in pediatrics and during T-piece trials. In a laboratory study, Manczur and coworkers sought to determine the resistances of ETTs commonly used in neonatal and pediatric intensive care units.[41] They examined straight tubes with IDs of 2.5 to 6 mm and shouldered (Cole) tubes with ratios of ID to outer diameter ranging from 2.5/4 to 3.5/5 mm. Predictably, they found

that resistance increased as ETT diameter decreased. The resistances of the 6-mm ID ETTs were 3.1 and 4.6 cm H_2O/L/s at flows of 5 and 10 L/min, respectively, and the resistances of the 2.5-mm ID ETT were 81.2 and 139.4 cm H_2O/L/s, respectively. The authors reported that shortening an ETT to a length appropriate for the patient (e.g., shortening a 4.0-mm ID ETT from 20.7 to 11.3 cm) reduced resistance on average by 22%. They also noted that the resistance of a Cole tube was "about 50% lower than that of a straight tube with an ID corresponding to the narrow part of the shouldered tube."

Using an acoustic reflection research method, Straus and associates sought to study the influence of ETT resistance during T-piece trials by comparing the work of breathing in 14 successfully extubated patients at the end of a 2-hour trial and after extubation.[42] They found that work of breathing was identical in both groups and there was no significant difference between the beginning and the end of the T-piece trial. The work caused by the ETT amounted to about 11.0% of the total work of breathing, and the supralaryngeal airway resistance was significantly smaller than the ETT resistance. The authors concluded that "a 2 hr trial of spontaneous breathing through an ETT well mimics the work of breathing performed after extubation, in patients who pass a weaning trial and do not require reintubation."

III. WORK OF BREATHING

Breathing comprises a two-part cycle: inspiration and expiration. During normal breathing, inspiration is an active, energy-consuming process, and expiration is ordinarily a passive process in which the diaphragm and intercostal muscles relax (Figs. 4-9 and 4-10). However, expiration becomes an active process during forced expiration, such as during exercise or during expiration against a resistance load. Several studies have examined the work of breathing in various clinical settings.[43-48]

Considering only normal breathing, the work of breathing is given by the following formulas:

Work = force × distance
Force = pressure × area
Distance = volume ÷ area
Work = (pressure × area) × (volume/area) × pressure × volume

Because the air pressure in the lung varies with lung volume and pressure measurements are obtained distal to the end of the ETT, work may be expressed as follows[49]:

$$WORK_{INSPIRATION} = \int_{FRC}^{FRC+TV} P \, dV \qquad (21)$$

where
P = airway pressure (cm H_2O)
dV = (infinitesimal) volume of gas added to the lung (mL)
FRC = functional residual capacity of the lungs (mL)
TV = tidal volume breathed in during respiration (mL)

TABLE 4-3		
Coefficients for Airway Resistance Computations		
Tube	a	b
7.0	9.78	1.81
7.5	7.73	1.75
8.0	5.90	1.72
8.5	4.61	1.78
9.0	3.90	1.63

From Hicks GH: Monitoring respiratory mechanics. *Probl Respir Care* 2:191, 1989.

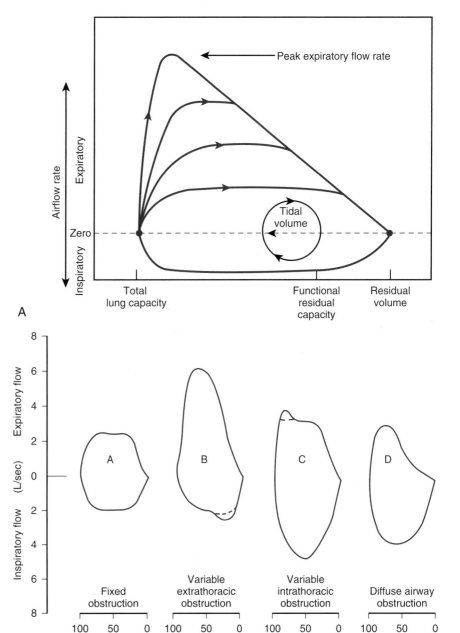

Figure 4-9 Flow-volume curves. **A,** A flow-volume curve consists of a plot of gas flow against lung volume. Four loops are shown, corresponding to four different levels of expiratory effort. Peak expiratory flow is effort dependent, but toward the end of expiration the curves converge (as flow is limited by dynamic airway collapse). From a diagnostic viewpoint, the expiratory portion of the loop is of more value than the inspiratory portion. **B,** Maximum inspiratory and expiratory flow-volume curves (flow-volume loops) in four types of airway obstruction. (**A,** From Nunn JF: *Nunn's applied respiratory physiology,* ed 4, Stoneham, MA, 1993, Butterworth-Heinemann; **B,** from Gal TJ: *Anesthesia,* ed 2, New York, 1986, Churchill Livingstone.)

When the pressure varies as a function of time, Equation 21 may be integrated in the following manner:

$$\text{LET } dV = \frac{dV}{dt} \times dt = \dot{V}\, dt \qquad (22)$$

Changing the limits of integration yields the following:

$$\text{WORK}_{\text{INSPIRATION}} = \int_{t_1}^{t_2} P(t)\, \dot{V}(t)\, dt \qquad (23)$$

where
t_1 = time at the beginning of inspiration (s)
t_2 = time at the end of inspiration (s)
P = pressure measured at a point of interest in the airway (e.g., at the tip of the ETT or at the carina) (cm H_2O)
$\dot{V}$ = flow (mL/s)

The preceding equation is cumbersome to integrate quickly. However, it is sometimes reasonable to assume that the pressure during inspiration remains fairly constant. Under these circumstances, integration of the original work equation during constant-pressure inspiration yields the following approximation:

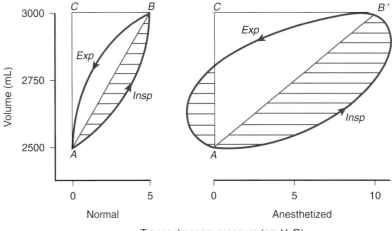

Figure 4-10 Work of breathing. Lung volume is plotted against transpulmonary pressure in a pressure-volume diagram for an awake ("Normal") patient and an anesthetized patient. The total area within the oval and triangles has the dimensions of pressure multiplied by volume and represents the total work of breathing. The hatched area to the right of lines *AB* and *AB'* represents the active inspiratory work necessary to overcome resistance to airflow during inspiration (*Insp*). The hatched area to the left of the triangle *AB'C* represents the active expiratory work necessary to overcome resistance to airflow during expiration (*Exp*) in the anesthetized subject. Expiration is passive in the normal subject because sufficient potential energy is stored during inspiration to produce expiratory airflow. The fraction of total inspiratory work necessary to overcome elastic resistance is shown by triangles *ABC* and *AB'C*. The anesthetized patient has decreased compliance and increased elastic resistance work (triangle *AB'C*) compared with the normal patient's compliance and elastic resistance work (triangle *ABC*). The anesthetized patient shown has increased airway resistance to both inspiratory and expiratory work. (From Benumof JL: *Anesthesia,* ed 2, New York, 1986, Churchill Livingstone.)

$$\text{WORK}_{\text{INSPIRATION}} = P_{\text{AVE}} \times TV \quad (24)$$

where

P_{AVE} = mean airway pressure during inspiration (cm H_2O)
TV = tidal volume of inspiration (mL)

During anesthesia, an ETT is often inserted, and additional energy is required to overcome the friction effects of the ETT. The added work of breathing presented by an ETT is given by the following equation:

$$\text{WORK}_{\text{ETT}} = \int_{\text{FRC}}^{\text{FRC+TV}} \Delta P \, dV \quad (25)$$

where ΔP is the pressure drop across the tube.

Often, the pressure gradient ΔP is relatively constant during inspiration, and therefore:

$$\text{WORK}_{\text{ETT}} = \Delta P \int_{\text{FRC}}^{\text{FRC+TV}} dV = \Delta P \times \Delta V \quad (26)$$

where

ΔP = pressure drop across ETT during inspiration (mm Hg)
ΔV = volume added to lungs = tidal volume (mL)

The total work done, measured in joules (kg × m²/s²), is as follows:

$$\text{WORK}_{\text{TOTAL}} = \text{WORK}_{\text{ETT}} + \text{WORK}_{\text{INSPIRATION}} \quad (27)$$

IV. PULMONARY BIOMECHANICS

A. The Respiratory Mechanics Equation

Approximately 3% of the body's total energy is required to maintain normal respiratory function.[11] Energy is required to overcome three main forces: (1) the elastic resistance of the lungs, which restores the lungs to their original size after inflation; (2) the force required to move the rib cage, diaphragm, and appropriate visceral contents; and (3) the dissipative resistance of the airway and any breathing apparatus.[50] The respiratory system is commonly modeled as the frictional airway R_L that is in series with the lung compliance C_L. Such a model is analogous to a resistor and capacitor in series that form a resistive-capacitive (R_C) circuit (Fig. 4-11).

A transmural (P_{TM}) pressure gradient exists between the airway at the mouth (i.e., at atmospheric pressure) and the pressure inside the pleural cavity. This pressure gradient is responsible for the lungs' "hugging" the thoracic cavity as the chest enlarges during inspiration. The presence of an external breathing apparatus causes a further pressure loss (P_{EXT}). The total pressure drop between the atmosphere and the pleural cavity is given by the respiratory mechanics equation and may be modeled as follows[50]:

$$P_{\text{TOTAL}} = P_{\text{EXT}} + P_{\text{TM}} = R_{\text{EXT}} \dot{V} + \frac{V}{C_L} + R_L \dot{V} \quad (28)$$

$$P_{\text{EXT}} = R_{\text{EXT}} \dot{V} \quad (29)$$

$$P_{\text{TM}} = \frac{V}{C_L} + R_L \dot{V} \quad (30)$$

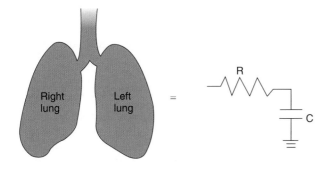

$$R = \text{Resistance} = \frac{\text{Pressure change}}{\text{Flow rate}}$$

$$C = \text{Compliance} = \frac{\text{Volume change}}{\text{Pressure change}}$$

Figure 4-11 Resistance-compliance (RC) model of the lungs. Resistance of lungs to airflow and natural ability to resist stretch (compliance) enable lungs to be modeled as an electrical circuit. A resistor of resistance R placed in series with a capacitor of capacitance C is a simple and convenient analogy on which to base pulmonary biomechanics.

where

P_{TOTAL} = pressure drop between atmosphere and pleural cavity

P_{EXT} = pressure drop across external breathing apparatus

P_{TM} = transmural pressure gradient

R_{EXT} = external apparatus resistance (e.g., an ETT)

$\dot{V}$ = dV/dt = gas flow rate into the lungs

C_L = lung compliance

R_L = airway resistance

V = volume of gas above the functional residual capacity (FRC) in the lungs

Thus, the pressure required to inflate the lungs depends on both lung compliance and gas flow rate. The time required to inflate the lungs is measured in terms of a pulmonary time constant. This time constant (t) is simply the product $R_L \times C_L$. However, determination of the time constant is not a trivial matter, and attention is now turned to that determination.

1. The Pulmonary Time Constant

Using the previous formula (Equation 29) in the case that no external resistance exists, one can show that, during passive expiration, the volume in the lungs in excess of FRC takes on the following form[51]:

$$V = V_0 e^{-t/\tau} \tag{31}$$

where V_0 is the volume taken in during inspiration and $\tau = R_L C_L$ is the time constant for the lungs.

Flow from the lungs is obtained by differentiating this equation with respect to time:

$$\dot{V} = \frac{dV}{dt} = V_0 \frac{d(e^{-t/\tau})}{dt} = V_0 e^{-t/\tau}\left(-\frac{1}{\tau}\right) = -\frac{V_0}{\tau}e^{-t/\tau} \tag{32}$$

Tau (τ) may be now estimated by dividing the preceding equation by the first one:

$$\frac{\dot{V}}{V} = \frac{V_0 e^{-t/\tau}\left(-\dfrac{1}{\tau}\right)}{V_0 e^{-t/\tau}} = -\frac{1}{\tau} \tag{33}$$

Therefore, τ can be estimated as the negative of the reciprocal of the average slope of the plot of flow ($\dot{V}$) against volume (V) during expiration. Another means of estimating τ is by taking the natural logarithm of the volume equation $V = V_0 e^{-t/\tau}$.

The value of τ can also be estimated as the negative of reciprocal of the average slope of the natural logarithm of the lung volume plotted against time.

$$\ln V = \ln(V_0) - \frac{t}{\tau} = \frac{d(\ln V)}{dt} = -\frac{1}{\tau} \tag{34}$$

2. Determination of Rohrer's Constants

A more complete approach to modeling the pressure-flow relationship of the respiratory system assumes that a single time constant τ may be inadequate to describe pulmonary biomechanics in some situations. The classical form of the equation,[27]

$$\frac{V}{\dot{V}} = -\tau = C_L \times R_L \tag{35}$$

can be changed to a more elaborate form of:

$$\frac{V}{\dot{V}} = -C_L(K_1 + K_2\dot{V}) \tag{36}$$

where K_1 and K_2 are known as Rohrer's constants and $(K_1 + K_2)$ is a form of R_L.

In this situation, the resistance of the pulmonary system is not assumed to be constant; rather, it is assumed to be flow dependent:

$$R = K_1 + K_2\dot{V} \tag{37}$$

When this equation is expressed in the following form,

$$\frac{V}{C_L\dot{V}} = -(K_1 + K_2\dot{V}) \tag{38}$$

K_1 and K_2 may be determined as the intercept and slope, respectively, of a plot of $V/C_L\dot{V}$ against $\dot{V}$.

3. Compliance

Pulmonary compliance measurements reflect the elastic properties of the lungs and thorax and are influenced by factors such as degree of muscular tension, degree of interstitial lung water, degree of pulmonary fibrosis, degree of lung inflation, and alveolar surface tension.[52] Total respiratory system compliance is given by the following calculation[40]:

$$C = \frac{\Delta V}{\Delta P} \tag{39}$$

where
ΔV = change in lung volume
ΔP = change in airway pressure

This total compliance may be related to lung compliance and thoracic (chest wall) compliance by the following relation:

$$\frac{1}{C_T} = \frac{1}{C_L} + \frac{1}{C_{Th}} \qquad (40)$$

where
C_T = total compliance (e.g., 100 mL/cm H_2O)
C_L = lung compliance (e.g., 200 mL/cm H_2O)
C_{Th} = thoracic compliance (e.g., 200 mL/cm H_2O)

The values shown in parentheses are some typical normal adult values that can be used for modeling purposes.[40] *Elastance*, the reciprocal of compliance, offers notational advantage over compliance in some physiologic problems. However, its use has not been popular in clinical practice.

Compliance may be estimated using the pulmonary time constant, τ. If a linear resistance of known value (ΔR) is added to the patient's airway, the time constant will change to τ', as follows[27]:

$$\tau' = (R_L + \Delta R) \times C_L = \tau + (C_L \times \Delta R) = \tau + \Delta \tau \quad (41)$$

Therefore, if ΔR is known and τ and τ' are determined experimentally, one can solve for C_L and then for R_L:

$$C_L = \frac{\tau' - \tau}{\Delta R} = \frac{\Delta \tau}{\Delta R} \qquad R_L = \tau \times \frac{\Delta R}{\Delta \tau} = \frac{\tau \times \Delta R}{\tau' - \tau} \quad (42)$$

B. An Advanced Formulation of the Respiratory Mechanics Equation

An alternative to the elementary respiratory mechanics equation may be used to describe the physical behavior of the lungs. The original formulation of this advanced respiratory mechanics equation was carried out by Rohrer during World War I, but the first completely correct formulation was devised by Gaensler and colleagues and has the following form[38]:

$$P = \frac{V}{C} + K_1 \dot{V} + K_2 \dot{V}^2 \qquad (43)$$

where
P = airway pressure
V = lung volume
$\dot{V}$ = gas flow rate into (out of) lung
C = compliance of the pulmonary system
K_1 and K_2 = empirical Rohrer's constants

This equation is more advanced than the elementary respiratory mechanics equation because it is able to account for flow losses attributable to turbulence. Because turbulent flow conditions are most likely to exist during anesthesia, the $\dot{V}^2$ term is very important in accurately quantifying the pressure losses of respiration. In addition, the advanced equation combines the resistance losses into the constants K_1 and K_2, which require only empirical determination.

V. ANESTHESIA AT MODERATE ALTITUDE

The parameters that govern the administration of anesthesia are altered slightly when the elevation above sea level is increased. Generally, a change in the atmospheric (or barometric) pressure is responsible for these differences. This section briefly examines the consequences of a moderate change in altitude.

The approximate alveolar gas equation is a useful tool in quantifying the differences that occur at higher elevations[53]:

$$P_{AO_2} = P_{IO_2} - \frac{P_{aCO_2}}{R} \qquad P_{IO_2} = (P_B - 47) \times F_{IO_2} \quad (44)$$

where
P_{AO_2} = alveolar oxygen tension
P_{IO_2} = inspired oxygen tension partial pressure
P_{aCO_2} = arterial carbon dioxide tension
R = 0.8 $\rightarrow$ gas exchange coefficient (CO_2 produced/O_2 consumed)
P_B = barometric pressure (760 mm Hg at sea level)
47 = water vapor pressure at 37° C
F_{IO_2} = fraction of inspired oxygen = 0.21 at all altitudes (room air)

All tensions are in mm Hg (torr).

A. Altered Partial Pressure of Gases

The effect of altitude is very apparent on the partial pressure of administered gases. The partial pressure of oxygen is given by $P_{IO_2} = (P_B - P_{H_2O}) \times 0.21$. At 1524 m (5000 ft) above sea level, P_{IO_2} is reduced to 128 mm Hg from 158 mm Hg at sea level, so that the maximum P_{aO_2} is about 83 mm Hg (assuming $P_{aCO_2} = 36$).[54] At 3048 m (10,000 ft), P_{IO_2} is 111 mm Hg, and the maximum P_{aO_2} is 65 mm Hg.[54] In order to counteract the effects of the hypoxia, ventilation is increased, so that at 5000 ft P_{aCO_2} = 36 mm Hg, and at 3048 m P_{aCO_2} = 34 mm Hg on average.[54] The effectiveness of nitrous oxide (N_2O) decreases with altitude because of an absolute reduction of its partial pressure (tension).

B. Oxygen Analyzers

There are five main types of oxygen analyzers: paramagnetic analyzers, fuel cell analyzers, oxygen electrodes, mass spectrometers, and Raman spectrographs. All respond to oxygen partial pressure (not concentration) so that the output changes with barometric pressure. At 1524 m, an analyzer set to measure 21% O_2 at sea level reads 17.4%. If these devices were to calculate the amount of oxygen in terms of partial pressure, the scale readings would reflect the true state of oxygen availability, but clinical practice dictates that a percentage scale be used anyway.

C. Carbon Dioxide Analyzers and Vapor Analyzers

Absorption of infrared radiation by gas is the usual analytic method used to determine the amount of CO_2 in a gas mixture, although other methods (e.g., Raman spectrographs) also work well. This type of method measures partial pressures, not percentages. To operate accurately, these machines must either be calibrated using known CO_2 concentrations at the correct barometric pressure or have the scale converted to read partial pressures.

Similar arguments apply to modern vapor analyzers, all of which respond to partial pressures, not concentrations, despite the fact that the output of these devices, by clinical custom, is usually calculated in percentages.

D. Vapors and Vaporizers

Practically speaking, the saturated vapor pressure of a volatile agent depends only on its temperature. At a given temperature, the concentration of a given mass of vapor increases as barometric pressure decreases, but its partial pressure remains unchanged. Similarly, the output of calibrated vaporizers is altered with changes in barometric pressure. Only the concentration of the vapor changes; the partial pressure remains the same, as does the patient's response at a given setting as compared with sea level. This assumes that the vaporizer characteristics do not change with altered density and viscosity of the carrier gases.

E. Flowmeters

Most flowmeters measure the drop in pressure that occurs when a gas passes through a resistance and correlate this pressure drop with flow. The pressure drop depends on gas density and viscosity. If the resistance is an orifice, resistance depends primarily on gas density. For laminar flow through a tube, viscosity determines resistance (Hagen-Poiseuille equation). Some flowmeters employ a floating ball or bobbin supported by the stream of gas in a tapered tube. The float is fluted so that it remains in the center of the flow. At low flow, the device depends primarily on laminar flow, and as the float moves up the tube, the resistance behaves progressively more like an orifice.

The density of a gas changes, of course, with barometric pressure, but the viscosity changes little, being primarily dependent on temperature. Gas flow through an orifice is inversely proportional to the square root of gas density: As the density falls, flow increases (orifice size being constant). Therefore, at high altitude, the actual flowmeter flow is greater than that indicated by the float position:

$$\text{Actual flow} = \text{Nominal flow} \times \sqrt{\frac{760 \text{ mm Hg}}{P_B}} \quad (45)$$

F. Flowmeter Calibration

The calibration of standard flowmeters, such as the Thorpe tube, depends on gas properties. Usually, a particular flowmeter is calibrated for a particular gas, such as oxygen or air. The factor used to convert nominal flow measurements to actual flow measurements is given by the following equation[53]:

$$k = \frac{\sqrt{\text{GMW}_A}}{\sqrt{\text{GMW}_B}} \quad (46)$$

where A is the gas for which the flowmeter was originally designed, B is the gas actually used, and GMW is the gram molecular weight of the gas in question.

A list of common anesthetic gases and their respective GMWs is presented in Table 4-4.

TABLE 4-4

Gram Molecular Weight (GMW) for Some Common and Anesthetic Gases

Name	Symbol	GMW
Hydrogen	H	1.00797
Helium	He	4.0026
Nitrogen (molecular)	N_2	28.0134
Oxygen (molecular)	O_2	31.9988
Neon	Ne	20.183
Argon	Ar	39.948
Xenon	Xe	131.30
Halothane	$CF_3CClBrH$	197
Isoflurane	$CF_2H\text{-}O\text{-}CHClCF_3$	184.5
Enflurane	$CF_2H\text{-}O\text{-}CF_2CFHCl$	184.5
Nitrous oxide	N_2O	44.013

1. Example Calculation 1

Determine the actual flow rate of a 70:30 heliox mixture if it is passed through an oxygen flowmeter that reads 10 L/min.

Answer:

$$\text{GMW}_{O_2} = 32 \text{ g/mol} \quad (47)$$

$$\text{GMW}_{\text{heliox}} = 0.3(32) + 0.7(4) = 12.4 \text{ g/mol} \quad (48)$$

The actual flow rate of heliox is given by the following equation:

$$\begin{aligned} \text{Actual flow rate} &= 10 \times \frac{\sqrt{\text{GMW}_{O_2}}}{\sqrt{\text{GMW}_{\text{heliox}}}} \\ &= 10 \times \frac{\sqrt{32}}{\sqrt{12.4}} = 16.1 \text{ L/min} \end{aligned} \quad (49)$$

2. Example Calculation 2

Determine the appropriate multiplier if oxygen is passed through an airflow meter.

Answer:

$$\begin{aligned} \text{Multiplier} &= \frac{\sqrt{\text{GMW}_{\text{AIR}}}}{\sqrt{\text{GMW}_{O_2}}} = \frac{\sqrt{0.21(32) + 0.79(28)}}{\sqrt{32}} \\ &= 0.95 \end{aligned} \quad (50)$$

G. Anesthetic Implications

At 10,000 ft, a 30% O_2 mixture has the same partial pressure as a 20% O_2 mixture at sea level.[54] In addition, the reduction in partial pressure of N_2O that occurs seriously impairs the effectiveness of the agent, and its administration may be of no benefit. The concept of minimum alveolar concentration (MAC) does not apply at higher altitudes and should be replaced by the concept of minimal alveolar partial pressure (MAPP) (Table 4-5). The use of this concept would eliminate many of the problems identified earlier.

VI. ESTIMATION OF GAS RATES

A. Estimation of Carbon Dioxide Production Rate

The carbon dioxide production rate ($\dot{V}_{CO_2}$) of a patient may be estimated in the following manner. The CO_2 production rate can be described as the product of the amount of CO_2 produced per breath and the number of breaths per minute (BPM), with typical units of mL/min. Therefore, $\dot{V}_{CO_2}$ may be expressed as follows:

$$\dot{V}_{CO_2} = CO_2 \text{ produced per breath} \times BPM \quad (51)$$

$$\dot{V}_{CO_2} = V_{CO_2} \times BPM \quad (52)$$

The amount of CO_2 produced per breath is calculated as follows:

$$V_{CO_2} = \int_{t=0}^{t=t_{end\ expiration}} C_{CO_2}(t) \times Q(t) \times \gamma dt \quad (53)$$

where
$C_{CO_2}(t)$ = capnogram signal (mm Hg)
$Q(t)$ = gas flow rate signal (mL/min)
γ = scaling factor to switch dimensions from mm Hg to concentration % = 100% ÷ 760 mm Hg = 0.1312

B. Estimation of Oxygen Consumption Rate

The oxygen consumption rate may be estimated similarly to $\dot{V}_{CO_2}$. The oxygen consumption rate can be expressed as the product of oxygen consumed per breath and the number of breaths per minute. Mathematically, this may be written as follows:

$$\dot{V}_{O_2} = O_2 \text{ consumed per breath} \times \text{number of} \atop \text{breaths per minute} \quad (54)$$

$$\dot{V}_{O_2} = V_{O_2} \times BPM \quad (55)$$

The amount of O_2 consumed per breath can now be expressed as follows:

$$V_{O_2} = \int_{t=0}^{t=t_{end\ expiration}} (P_{IO_2} - C_{O_2}) \times Q(t) \times \gamma dt \quad (56)$$

where
P_{IO_2} = inspiratory oxygen pressure = $(P_B - 47) \times F_{IO_2}$ (mm Hg)
C_{O_2} = oxygen signal (mm Hg)
$Q(t)$ = gas flow rate signal (mL/min)
γ = scaling factor = 0.1312

C. Interpretation of Carbon Dioxide Production and Oxygen Consumption Rates

The rates $\dot{V}_{O_2}$ and $\dot{V}_{CO_2}$ are linked by the respiratory exchange coefficient RQ ($RQ = \dot{V}_{CO_2}/\dot{V}_{O_2}$), which is governed largely by diet; some diets produce less CO_2 than others and have a smaller RQ). Typically, RQ = 0.8. $\dot{V}_{O_2}$ and $\dot{V}_{CO_2}$ both go up with increases in metabolism, which may be related to factors such as fever, sepsis, light anesthesia, shivering, malignant hyperthermia, and thyroid storm. Decreases in $\dot{V}_{CO_2}$ and $\dot{V}_{O_2}$ may also have many causes (e.g., hypothermia, deep anesthesia, hypothyroidism).

VII. MATHEMATICAL MODELING RELATED TO THE AIRWAY

A. Overview

In this section, the role of "ready-to-use" numeric analysis software for physiologic model building is discussed, using the respiratory system as a basis for discussion. This software is based on well-established physiologic principles, and it allows some "what if" physiologic questions

TABLE 4-5

Minimum Alveolar Concentration (MAC) at Various Altitude Levels and Comparative Values for Minimal Alveolar Partial Pressure (MAPP)

Agent	MAC (%)			MAPP	
	Sea Level	*5000 ft*	*10,000 ft*	*(kPa)*	*(mm Hg)*
Nitrous oxide	105.0	126.5	152.2	106.1	798.0
Ethyl ether	1.92	2.31	2.78	1.94	14.6
Halothane	0.75	0.90	1.09	0.76	5.7
Enflurane	1.68	2.02	2.43	1.70	12.8
Isoflurane	1.2	1.45	1.73	1.22	9.1

MAPP = MAC × 0.01 × 760 mm Hg.
Adapted from James MFM, White JF: Anesthetic considerations at moderate altitude. *Anesth Analg* 63:1097, 1984.

to be answered that could not have been answered in the past due to experimental complexity or ethical considerations. Because the model is based on simple equations accepted by the physiology community, the results obtained are directly credible, and many of the difficulties of direct experimentation are avoided.

The model concept is explored through a discussion of four oxygen transport problems, some of which are too complex in experimental design for empirical study to be practical. However, considerable insight can be obtained using numerical methods alone.

B. Background

Some physiologic systems are especially well suited to physiologic modeling. For example, physiologic modeling of the cardiopulmonary system may be performed to examine issues such as the determinants of pulmonary gas exchange. For instance, both Doyle and Viale and their coauthors have written custom software to explore the determinants of the arterial-alveolar oxygen tension ratio, and Torda has explored the determinants of the alveolar-arterial oxygen tension difference in a similar manner.[55-57] Before the common use of digital computers, graphic techniques were sometimes used for solving respiratory physiologic models. A well-known example is the early work by Kelman and colleagues on the influence of cardiac output (CO) on arterial oxygenation.[58] Central to the construction of such a mathematical model is the existence of a number of equations relating physiologic parameters. Examples of physiologic relationships in the respiratory system that are well described by equations include (1) the alveolar gas equation,[53,59] (2) the pulmonary shunt equation,[60] (3) the blood oxygen content equation,[60] and (4) various equations describing the oxyhemoglobin dissociation curve.[61-65]

C. Problems in Model Solving

Although many physiologic problems are readily solved by direct analytic methods, frequently their solution is hampered by nonlinearities, self-referencing (circular) equations, or other complexities. (An example of a nonlinearity is the equation $y = x^2$; an example of a self-referencing equation set is the equation pair $y = 1/x$; $x = y + 1$.) Experience has shown that early conventional spreadsheet programs were poorly equipped to solve systems of this kind because they were not generally designed for iterative equation-solving methods. Newer spreadsheets usually contain an iterative solver of some kind.

Some authors have applied successive approximation methods with custom-written software to solve equation sets of this kind.[55] However, this approach may involve considerable effort, even by experienced computer programmers. Furthermore, many physiologists have limited experience and training in writing computer programs. The next section describes how equation-solving computer programs can be used to advantage to solve complex physiologic modeling equations. TK SOLVER (Universal Technical Systems, Inc., Rockford, IL) is the equation-solver package used in most of the examples given here, but many other packages could also have been used.

D. Description of TK SOLVER

TK SOLVER (the TK stands for "tool kit") is a software package for equation solving.[2,26,47,66,67] Although intended primarily for engineering applications, TK SOLVER functions well in a variety of other application areas. On start-up, TK SOLVER displays 2 "sheets" or tables out of a total of 13. The Variable Sheet is presented on the bottom "window," and the Rule Sheet goes on the top. Equations are entered in the Rule Sheet using a built-in editor; the variables associated with the equations are then automatically entered in the variable sheet by TK SOLVER. Errors such as unmatched parentheses are automatically detected. Figure 4-12 shows sample Rule and Variable Sheets for a pulmonary exchange model.

Once the equations are entered, TK SOLVER is ready to find solutions. In some cases, the equation set can be solved in "direct-solver" mode, but complex equation sets usually must be solved in "iterative-solver" mode on the basis of initial guesses for all variables. A discussion of the methods used to obtain solutions has been presented by Konopasek and Jayaraman.[68] A book reviewing TK SOLVER from a user's viewpoint is also available.[69]

E. Example 1: Application of Mathematical Modeling to the Study of Gas Exchange Indices

Gas exchange indices are commonly used in anesthesia and critical care medicine to assess pulmonary function from an oxygen transport viewpoint. Although the determination of pulmonary shunt would be viewed by many as a gold standard preferable to any index, measurement of true pulmonary shunt requires pulmonary artery catheterization—a relatively expensive and risky procedure that is not always clinically warranted. Four gas exchange indices are in common use:

1. Alveolar-arterial oxygen tension difference ($P_{A_{O_2}} - Pa_{O_2}$)[57,69-71]
2. Arterial-alveolar oxygen tension ratio ($Pa_{O_2}/P_{A_{O_2}}$)[55,56,72-74]
3. Respiratory index (RI) = ($P_{A_{O_2}} - Pa_{O_2}$)/Pa_{O_2}[75,76]
4. $Pa_{O_2}/F_{I_{O_2}}$ ratio[34]

The importance of these indices and the controversies surrounding their clinical application are reflected in the many publications concerning their use and limitations.[34,66,77-79]

1. Analysis

The pulmonary shunt equation is used as a foundation upon which arterial oxygenation and gas exchange indices can be studied. It may be expressed as follows:

$$\frac{Qs}{Qt} = \frac{Cc'_{O_2} - Ca_{O_2}}{Cc'_{O_2} - C\bar{v}_{O_2}} \quad (57)$$

where
Q_s/Q_t = shunt fraction
Cc'_{O_2} = pulmonary end-capillary oxygen content
Ca_{O_2} = arterial oxygen content
$C\bar{v}_{O_2}$ = mixed venous oxygen content

```
========================== RULE SHEET ==============================
S  Rule
--------
    PaO2=PAO2-(Cav*(Z/(1-Z))-1.34*Hb*(ScO2-SaO2))/0.0031
    SaO2=PaO2^a/(PaO2^a+P50^a)
    ScO2=PAO2^a/(PAO2^a+P50^a)
    Cav=VO2/(10*CO)
    Sav=(Cav-0.0031*(PaO2-PvO2))/(1.34*Hb)
    SvO2=SaO2-Sav
    PvO2=P50*(SvO2/(1-SvO2))^(1/a)
    CaO2=1.34*Hb*SaO2+0.0031*PaO2
    CvO2=CaO2-Cav
    CcO2=1.34*Hb*ScO2+0.0031*PAO2

====================== VARIABLE SHEET ==========================
```

St	Input	Name	Output	Unit	Comment
	50	PAO2		mmHg	Alveolar Oxygen Tension
		PaO2	46.602925	mmHg	Arterial Oxygen Tension
		PvO2	29.722228	mmHg	Mixed Venous Oxygen Tension
		SaO2	.80944994	none	Arterial Saturation (%)
		ScO2	.83656560	none	End Pulmonary Capillary Saturation (%)
		SvO2	.56329721	none	Mixed Venous Saturation (%)
		Sav	.24615273	none	Arterio-Venous Saturation Difference
	250	vo2		ml/min	Oxygen Consumption
	5	co		L/min	Cardiac Output
	.1	z		none	Pulmonary Shunt Fraction
		Cav	5	vol%	Arterio-venous O2 Content Diff
	15	Hb		g/dl	Hemoglobin Concentration
	2.65	a		none	Hill's coefficient
	27	P50		mmHg	PO2 for 50% Saturation
		CaO2	16.414413	vol%	Arterial Oxygen Content
		CvO2	11.414413	vol%	Mixed Venous Oxygen Content
		CcO2	16.969968	vol%	End Pulmonary Capillary Oxygen Content

Figure 4-12 Sample TK SOLVER Rule Sheet (*top*) and Variable Sheet (*bottom*). In this case, equations relate factors that determine arterial oxygen tension (Pao$_2$). All variables are defined in comment section of variable sheet. The first equation in the Rule Sheet is from Torda and Doyle.[55,57] The second and third equations are from Hill.[64]

By algebraic manipulation of the shunt equation, it is possible to relate arterial oxygen tension to its influencing factors[55,57]:

$$Pao_2 = Pao_2 - \frac{Ca - \bar{v}o_2 \times \dfrac{\dfrac{Qs}{Qt}}{1-\dfrac{Qs}{Qt}} - 1.34 \times (Sc'o_2 - Sao_2) \times Hb}{0.0031} \quad (58)$$

where Pao$_2$ (mm Hg) is the alveolar oxygen tension; Ca$-\bar{v}$o$_2$ (vol%) is the arterial–mixed venous oxygen content difference (= Cao$_2$ – C$\bar{v}$o$_2$), Sc'o$_2$ is the pulmonary end-capillary fractional saturation, Sao$_2$ is the arterial oxygen saturation, and Hb is the blood hemoglobin concentration (g/dL). The full alveolar gas equation is used to determine Pao$_2$:

$$Pao_2 = (P_B - P_{H_2O}) \times Fio_2 - Paco_2 \times \left(Fio_2 + \frac{1-Fio_2}{R} \right) \quad (59)$$

where P$_B$ is the barometric pressure (assumed to be 760 mm Hg), P$_{H_2O}$ is the patient's water vapor pressure (assumed to be 47 mm Hg), Paco$_2$ is the arterial CO$_2$ tension (usually assumed to be 40 mm Hg), and R is the gas exchange ratio (assumed to be 0.8).

Equation 58 does not explicitly show the influence of P$_{50}$ (the oxygen tension corresponding to 50% hemoglobin saturation) on arterial oxygen tension; such influences are mediated indirectly, principally through the Sao$_2$ term. To make explicit the influence of Pao$_2$ and P$_{50}$ on Sao$_2$, we use the relationship given by Hill's equation[64]:

$$Sao_2 = \frac{Pao_2^n}{Pao_2^n + P_{50}^n} \quad (60)$$

where n is an empirical constant (usually taken as 2.65).

A similar expression relates Pao$_2$, P$_{50}$, and Sc'o$_2$.

The arterial oxygen tension (Pao$_2$), the alveolar-arterial oxygen tension difference (Pao$_2$ – Pao$_2$), and the arterial-alveolar oxygen tension ratio (Pao$_2$/Pao$_2$) can then be obtained using Equations 58, 59, and 60 for specific choices of physiologic variables. Unfortunately, Equation 58 is not easily solved because it requires the solution of two simultaneous nonlinear equations (i.e., equations 58 and 60). In the past, a custom, computer-based successive approximation method was employed to obtain a solution. This amounted to iteratively making successively more accurate estimates of PaO_2 levels that satisfied both of those equations. In the case of Doyle,[55] Equation 58 was solved in this way to an accuracy of 0.1 mm Hg for various values of Hb, $Ca-\bar{v}O_2$, FIO_2, $PaCO_2$, and Q_s/Q_t. The process is considerably simplified when TK SOLVER is used, as can be seen by examining the equation sheets presented in Figure 4-12.

F. Example 2: Theoretical Study of Hemoglobin Concentration Effects on Gas Exchange Indices

It is of both theoretical and clinical interest to know what changes in gas exchange indices might be expected with changes in Hb when other physiologic parameters are kept constant. Figure 4-13 shows the results of varying Hb under the following conditions:

Alveolar oxygen tension (PAO_2) = 100 mm Hg
Cardiac output (CO) = 5 L/min
Oxygen consumption ($\dot{V}O_2$) = 250 mL/min
Shunt fraction (Q_s/Q_t) = 0.1
P_{50} = 27 mm Hg

Based on this model, increasing Hb can be expected to improve both PaO_2 and the gas exchange indices under study. Such data would be almost impossible to obtain experimentally because of the difficulty of varying Hb independent of other physiologic factors such as CO.

G. Example 3: Modeling the Oxygenation Effects of P_{50} Changes at Altitude

It is well known that the oxyhemoglobin dissociation curve shifts in response to physiologic changes. Acidosis, hypercarbia, increased temperature, and increased levels of 2,3-diphosphoglycerate (2,3-DPG) all shift the curve to the right, reducing the affinity of hemoglobin for oxygen and thereby facilitating release of oxygen into tissues. Patients with chronic anemia, for example, have increased intraerythrocyte levels of 2,3-DPG and a right-shifted oxyhemoglobin curve.[80] Teleologically, this would also appear to be an appropriate response to high-altitude hypoxemia, but in fact the opposite is true: Animals that have successfully adapted to high-altitude hypoxemia have left-shifted curves,[81-83] as do Sherpas.[82,84] In the example that follows, computer modeling is used to develop a possible explanation for this finding.

It can be theorized that a left-shifted curve is beneficial in high-altitude hypoxemia because it increases arterial oxygen content by virtue of increasing pulmonary

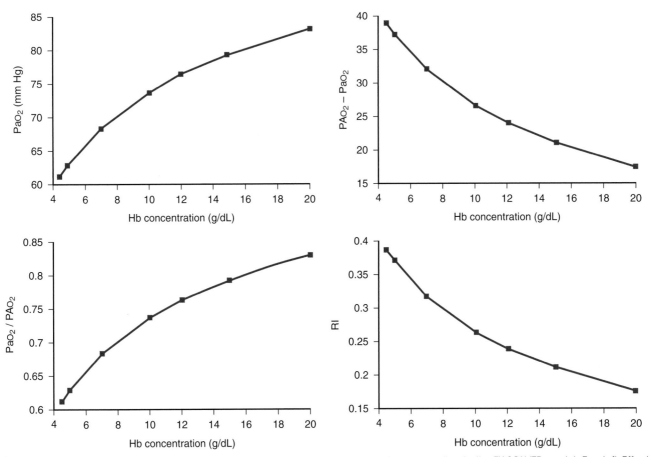

Figure 4-13 Effect of hemoglobin concentration (Hb) on various gas exchange indices according to the TK SOLVER model. *Top left,* Effect on arterial oxygen tension (*PaO₂*); *top right,* effect on alveolar-arterial oxygen tension difference (*PAO₂ – PaO₂*); *bottom left,* effect on arterial-alveolar oxygen tension ratio (*PaO₂/PAO₂*); *bottom right,* effect on the respiratory index (*RI*).

end-capillary oxygen content. The shunt equation described earlier (Equation 57) can be rearranged as follows:

$$Ca_{O_2} = Cc'_{O_2} - \frac{\dfrac{Qs}{Qt}}{1 - \dfrac{Qs}{Qt}} \times Ca\bar{v}_{O_2} \qquad (61)$$

This shows that, with a constant pulmonary shunt and constant arteriovenous oxygen content difference, increases in pulmonary end-capillary oxygen content will increase the arterial oxygen content.

Now, the pulmonary end-capillary oxygen content, Cc'_{O_2}, consists of two terms, the oxygen bound to hemoglobin and the oxygen dissolved in plasma:

$$Cc'_{O_2} = 1.34\,Hb\,Sc'_{O_2} + 0.0031\,P_{AO_2} \qquad (62)$$

where
Hb = hemoglobin concentration (g/dL)
Sc'_{O_2} = pulmonary end-capillary oxygen saturation
P_{AO_2} = alveolar oxygen tension (mm Hg)

P_{AO_2} is determined only by the alveolar gas equation and is independent of the position of the oxyhemoglobin curve.[60] Therefore, the dissolved oxygen portion of Cc'_{O_2} is also independent of the curve position. However, the Sc'_{O_2} term does vary with curve position, increasing with a left-shifted curve. Therefore, Cc'_{O_2} also increases with a left shift, taking on a maximum value of

$$[Cc'_{O_2}]_{max} = 1.34\,Hb + 0.0031\,P_{AO_2} \qquad (63)$$

This analysis demonstrates that a left-shifted curve increases arterial oxygen content by increasing pulmonary end-capillary oxygen content.

We now consider the effects of P_{50} changes in two situations.

1. In Situation A, a patient has high-altitude hypoxemia as a result of a P_{AO_2} of 50 mm Hg. With a CO of 5 L/min, an Hb of 15 g/dL, oxygen consumption ($\dot{V}_{O_2}$) of 250 mL/min, and a shunt fraction (Q_s/Q_t) of 0.1, it can be shown (Table 4-6) that Ca_{O_2} changes from 16.41 vol% with a P_{50} of 27 mm Hg to 18.44 vol% with a P_{50} of 18 mm Hg—a significant increase.
2. In Situation B, a patient has a large pulmonary shunt ($Q_s/Q_t = 0.4$), a normal P_{AO_2} (100 mm Hg), and other parameters as in situation A. In this case, Ca_{O_2} goes from 16.47 vol% with a P_{50} of 27 mm Hg to 16.87 vol% with a P_{50} of 18 mm Hg—an insignificant change (see Table 4-6).

Figure 4-14 illustrates this concept in more detail, showing the two examples for P_{50} values ranging from 10 to 50 mm Hg. The data provided in situations A and B and in Figure 4-14 were obtained by using the preceding mathematical computer model of the oxyhemoglobin dissociation curve. Hill's equation relating saturation, tension, and P_{50} was used in conjunction with Doyle's

TABLE 4-6

Oxygenation Effects of P_{50} Changes at Altitude

Oxygen Variable	Altitude Case*		Shunt Case	
	$P_{50} = 27$	$P_{50} = 18$	$P_{50} = 27$	$P_{50} = 18$
Pa_{O_2}	46.6	43.3	46.9	33.1
$P\bar{v}_{O_2}$	29.7	23.3	29.8	20.6
Sa_{O_2}	0.809	0.911	0.812	0.834
$S\bar{v}_{O_2}$	0.563	0.665	0.566	0.587
Sc'_{O_2}	0.837	0.937	0.970	0.989
Ca_{O_2}	16.41	18.44	16.47	16.87
Cv_{O_2}	11.41	13.44	11.47	11.87
Cc'_{O_2}	16.99	19.00	19.80	20.20

*Detailed figures for altitude case (Pa_{O_2} = 50 mm Hg) and for shunt case (Q_s/Q_t = 0.4). Other parameters are given in the text. Note that a shift from a P_{50} of 27 to a P_{50} of 18 significantly increases arterial oxygen content (Ca_{O_2}) in the altitude case but not in the shunt case.

equation for arterial oxygen tension and solved with the use of TK SOLVER.[55,64]

These two situations demonstrate that a leftward shift of the oxyhemoglobin dissociation curve significantly improves arterial oxygen content in the case of high-altitude hypoxemia but not in the case of a large shunt. This observation is consistent with the general finding of a right-shifted curve in patients, such as those with cyanotic heart disease, who have a right-to-left shunt.[62] In these cases, a left-shifted curve is not beneficial because only a trivial improvement in Cc'_{O_2} (and thus in P_{AO_2}) is obtained. Teleologically, it may be argued that in the presence of hypoxemia, at approximately equal arterial oxygen contents, the body prefers higher oxygen tensions (i.e., right shift), but if arterial oxygen content can be significantly improved, despite a decrease in oxygen tension, a left shift is preferred.

H. Example 4: Mathematical/Computer Model for Extracorporeal Membrane Oxygenation

Extracorporeal membrane oxygenation (ECMO) is sometimes used to treat respiratory failure that is refractory to more conservative measures.[16] Clinical experience with ECMO is limited, and even clinicians familiar with the therapy may disagree about its potential benefits in a particular clinical setting. This is especially true if the patient has a high CO (e.g., 20 L/min) and the ECMO pump is limited to much smaller flows (e.g., 5 L/min). In the example that follows, we describe how a computer model may be designed to facilitate management decisions for patients being considered for venovenous ECMO.

A mathematical model of the venovenous ECMO situation may be developed on the basis of the shunt equation,[56] the Hill model for the oxyhemoglobin dissociation curve,[57] Doyle's equation for arterial oxygen tension as a function of cardiorespiratory parameters,[58] and the schematic diagram for venovenous ECMO shown in Figure 4-15. The relevant equations are given in Figure 4-16. The model may be solved for various hypothetical clinical circumstances using an equation solver package. In this instance, we used EUREKA (Borland International, Scotts Valley, CA), a DOS-based

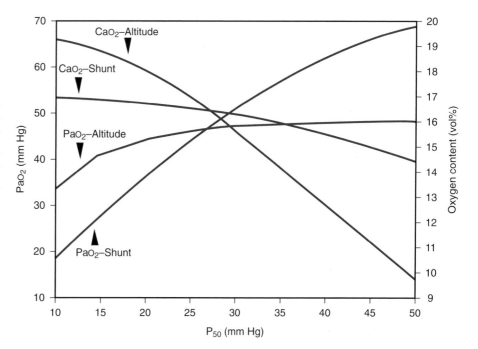

Figure 4-14 Arterial oxygen tension (Pao_2) and arterial oxygen content (Cao_2) as a function of oxygen tension corresponding to 50% hemoglobin saturation (P_{50}) for cases depicted in situations A (altitude hypoxemia) and B (shunt hypoxemia) in the text. Notice that a decrease in P_{50} (left-shifted curve) significantly increases oxygen content in the altitude case but not in the shunt case. (From Doyle DJ: Simulation in medical education: Focus on anesthesiology. *Can J Anaesth* 39:A89, 1992.)

commercial computer software package for solving systems of equations.

Some sample results are shown in Figure 4-17. The patient's parameters were as follows: CO = 5 L/min; $\dot{V}_{O_2}$ = 250 mL/min; Hb = 15 g/dL; Q_s/Q_t = 0.5; P_{AO_2} = 200 mm Hg. The oxygenator oxygen tension output was sufficient to result in complete hemoglobin saturation.

I. Discussion

Many questions in physiology are not easily answered by direct experimentation, either because it is impractical (or impossible) to control all the pertinent variables or because of ethical considerations. For example, in studying the influence of Hb on pulmonary gas exchange indices, it would be difficult to achieve rigorous experimental control of CO, total body oxygen consumption, and other variables. The modeling approach presented here offers several advantages:

1. It relies on well-established physiologic relationships (e.g., alveolar gas equation, pulmonary shunt equation).
2. It permits insight into physiologic issues not generally attainable in other ways.
3. It is inexpensive.
4. It potentially reduces the need to carry out animal experimentation.

Three drawbacks to the method exist:

1. It is no better than the equations on which it is based.
2. It may not be convincing to some physiologists who would be satisfied only by confirmatory experimental results.
3. Errors can occur in model building.

One potential difficulty with such modeling methods is that the results obtained depend critically on the equations used. If the equations are known from first principles (e.g., alveolar gas equation, pulmonary shunt equation), this is not an issue, but with empirical formulas, alternative equations may possibly produce different results. An example is the equation for the oxyhemoglobin dissociation curve, which has many competing formulations.[61-64] In that example, we used the formulation given by Hill.[64]

J. Utility

Where can such a model be useful? In a specific patient with severe adult respiratory distress syndrome and resulting severe hypoxemia, clinicians might be interested to know, for instance, how ECMO would be expected to improve oxygenation. From pulmonary artery catheterization and arterial blood samples, one can obtain the Hb concentration, CO, P_{50} level on the dissociation curve, arterial and mixed venous (arterial blood gas) measurements, and other data relevant to carrying out oxygen transport modeling.

On the basis of a model constructed for the time point when the data were gathered, one could explore, for example, the effect of augmenting CO and mixed venous oxygen tension in the ECMO situation. Without a model to describe this problem, the best that can be done is to fit empirical curves to experimental data. However, with a model, one can easily ask "what if" questions, such as, What happens when the ratio of pump oxygenator flow to CO is set at a particular value?.[80]

A good example is a question frequently asked in respiratory physiology: How does a patient's alveolar-arterial oxygen tension difference change with reduced

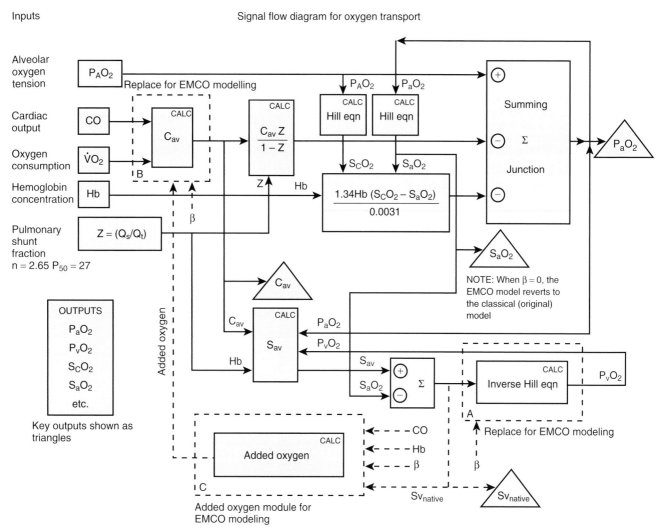

Inputs   Signal flow diagram for oxygen transport

Figure 4-15 β, Ratio of ECMO flow to cardiac output; C_{av}, arteriovenous oxygen content difference; *CO*, cardiac output; *Hb*, hemoglobin concentration (g/dL); P_{50}, oxygen partial pressure corresponding to 50 percent hemoglobin oxygen saturation; P_aO_2, arterial oxygen tension (mm Hg); P_AO_2, alveolar oxygen tension (mm Hg); P_vO_2, oxygen partial pressure for mixed venous blood; Q_s/Q_t, pulmonary shunt fraction (= Z); S_aO_2, arterial oxygen saturation; S_{av}, arteriovenous oxygen saturation content difference; S_CO_2, pulmonary end-capillary oxygen saturation; $\dot{V}O_2$, oxygen consumption; Sv_{native}, mixed venous oxygen saturation in the absence of ECMO support.

inspired oxygen tension? The first attempt at answering this question used pulse oximetry to infer arterial oxygen tension in volunteers subjected to controlled hypoxia by rebreathing.[81] A subsequent study took a more direct approach by cannulating the radial artery of elderly respiratory patient volunteers and drawing off serial arterial blood samples as the patients were subjected to hypoxemia in a hypobaric chamber.[83] Both of these studies were performed in 1974. The latter investigation was sufficiently invasive (and possibly risky) that many hospital ethics committees would not have approved it under current guidelines.

If more than one set of equations exist to describe a physiologic relationship, one can explore the effect of equation choice. However, if several equations exist and all do a good job of representing the underlying data, equation choice would not be expected to have a great influence on the results obtained. With modeling, one can obtain meaningful information about the interaction of several physiologic variables in a few days or even a few hours, provided that the relationships describing the

variables are available in equation form. By contrast, actual experimentation requires time, funds, and effort that may not always be available.

In fields such as oxygen transport, many relevant equations are simple, well-known physiologic principles written in equation form; examples include the alveolar gas equation, the pulmonary shunt equation, the oxyhemoglobin dissociation curve, and the definitions of oxygen transport parameters. To the extent that one accepts these physiologic principles, the results obtained should also be credible (provided that model design and implementation have been done correctly). In this respect, three issues exist:

1. How meaningful are the equations used? Are they a mathematical form of a well-known physiologic principle?
2. How accurate are the equations in describing the data on which they are based?
3. Has the model been appropriately designed and implemented?

```
alpha=2.65      ; Hill's constant
beta= 0.75        ; beta is the ratio of ECMO flow to cardiac output
CO=5              ; cardiac output
Hb=15             ; hemoglobin concentration
VO2=250           ; oxygen consumption
PAO2=200          ; alveolar oxygen tension
Z=0.6             ; pulmonary shunt
; P50=27          ; a resonable value for P50
; consider oxygen added to body by ECMO machine
; added02 = beta*CO*10*(1.34*Hb*(1-Sv02native))
Cav=(VO2 - (beta*CO*13.4*Hb*(1-Sv02native)))/(10*CO)
SvO2=SaO2 - (Cav - 0.0031*(PaO2-PvO2))/(1.34*Hb)
PaO2=PAO2 - (Cav*(Z/(1-Z)) - 1.34*Hb*(SAO2-SaO2))/0.0031
PaO2:=85
Sv02native:=0.7
Cav:=0.8
SAO2=PAO2^alpha / (PAO2^alpha + 27^alpha)  ; Hill's equation
SaO2=PaO2^alpha / (PaO2^alpha + 27^alpha)  ; Hill's equation
Pv02=27*(Sv02 /(1-Sv02))^(1/alpha)  ; augmented mixed-venous PO2
Pv02native=27*(Sv02native/(1-Sv02native))^(1/alpha)
Sv02native=(Sv02-beta)/(1-beta)    ; Sv02 entering ECMO
Pv02>=Pv02native
PAO2>PaO2 >0
Sv02>=Sv02native>0
Sv02native<1
```

Figure 4-16 Equations for venovenous extracorporeal membrane oxygenation (ECMO) model obtained by using EUREKA, an equation solver similar to TK SOLVER but somewhat easier to learn. The first seven lines indicate the values of physiologic parameters that are held constant. The next three lines are comments not used by EUREKA. Lines 11 through 13 and 17 through 21 list basic equations to be solved. Lines 14 through 16 provide initial estimates for EUREKA's iterative solver. Lines 22 through 25 give some physiologic constraints that cannot be violated (e.g., arterial oxygen tension must be less than alveolar oxygen tension). (EUREKA is also available in a shareware version known as Mercury, which runs under MS-DOS.) (Adapted from Doyle DJ: Computer model for veno-veno extracorporeal membrane oxygenation. *Can J Anaesth* 39:A34, 1992.)

K. Software

Several platforms exist to do such computations in the IBM-PC environment. TK SOLVER is still available (in a "Plus" form) from software distributors but does not have the market share of MATHCAD (PTC; Needham, MA), a widely available, popular mathematical modeling package with strong graphical features. MATHCAD has equation-solving features similar to those of TK SOLVER that would make it appropriate for mathematical model building. Another suitable package is Mercury, a shareware equation solver derived from EUREKA. All of these packages take some effort to master. In particular, the manner in which each package handles convergence to solution greatly affects ease of use and reliability. In general, the three packages mentioned (TK SOLVER, MATHCAD, and Mercury) work reasonably well with some effort. It is more difficult to do this modeling using ordinary computer spreadsheets (e.g., early releases of Lotus 1-2-3)—first, because it is somewhat awkward for working with equations, and second, because most spreadsheets are not set up to handle complicated iterative equation solving.

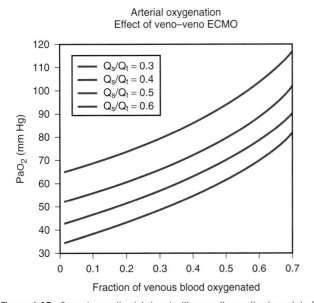

Arterial oxygenation
Effect of veno–veno ECMO

legend:
$Q_s/Q_t = 0.3$
$Q_s/Q_t = 0.4$
$Q_s/Q_t = 0.5$
$Q_s/Q_t = 0.6$

y-axis: PaO_2 (mm Hg)
x-axis: Fraction of venous blood oxygenated

Figure 4-17 Sample results obtained with a mathematical model of venovenous extracorporeal membrane oxygenation (*ECMO*) for various levels of relative flow through the ECMO oxygenator. Arterial oxygen tension (*Pao₂*) is plotted as a function of the fraction of venous blood passing through the ECMO oxygenator for various values of pulmonary shunt (*Qs/Qt, or Z*). (Adapted from Doyle DJ: Computer model for veno-veno extracorporeal membrane oxygenation. *Can J Anaesth* 39:A34, 1992.)

L. Computational Flow Diagrams

Mathematical modeling of complex physiologic systems can sometimes be facilitated by representing the relevant equations with the use of a computational flow diagram.

The concept is most easily understood by reviewing the examples mentioned previously.

Example 1. Computation of the alveolar-arterial oxygen tension gradient
Example 2. Computation of alveolar oxygen tension
Example 3. Computation of arterial oxygen tension
Example 4. Modeling the effects of venovenous ECMO

For those situations involving feedback (Examples 3 and 4), special iterative methods are necessary to obtain a solution. Not all spreadsheets are able to do this.

VIII. SELECTED DIMENSIONAL EQUIVALENTS

Discussions regarding physics in anesthesia may be confusing because of the variety of units used in the clinical literature. The list in Box 4-1 is a compilation of units and equivalents that one is likely to encounter.

IX. CONCLUSIONS

An understanding of a number of basic principles of physics can be very helpful in clinical airway management. This is especially true for the physics of fluid flow, such as the relationships between pressure, flow, and resistance under laminar and turbulent flow conditions.

In addition to the application of basic physics principles to airway situations, the application of mathematical methods and physiologic modeling can sometimes be enormously helpful in obtaining insights into complex physiologic systems related to the airway, such as the determination of arterial blood oxygenation under various conditions. In many cases, such modeling can produce results that would be extremely difficult to obtain by recourse to pure experimentation alone.

X. CLINICAL PEARLS

- An important formula that quantifies the relationship of pressure, flow, and resistance in laminar flow systems is given by the Hagen-Poiseuille equation. This law states that the fluid flow rate through a horizontal straight tube of uniform bore is proportional to the pressure gradient and the fourth power of the radius and is related inversely to the viscosity of the gas and the length of the tube. This law is valid for laminar flow conditions only.

- When the flow rate exceeds a *critical velocity* (the flow velocity below which flow is laminar), the flow loses its laminar parabolic velocity profile, becomes disorderly, and is termed *turbulent*. If turbulent flow exists, the relationship between pressure drop and flow is no longer governed by the Hagen-Poiseuille equation. Instead, the pressure gradient required (or the resistance encountered) during turbulent flow varies as the square of the gas flow rate. In addition, flow becomes inversely related to gas density rather than viscosity (as occurs with laminar flow).

- Clinically, airway-obstructing conditions such as epiglottitis or inhaled foreign bodies are often best modeled

| **BOX 4-1** | Selected Dimensional Equivalents |

Length
1 m = 3.2808 ft = 39.37 in
1 ft = 0.3048 m
1 m = 100 cm = 1000 mm = 1,000,000 μm = 10,000,000 Å = 10^{-3} km
1 km = 0.621 mi
1 in = 2.54 cm = 0.254 m

Volume
1 US gal = 0.13368 ft^3 = 3.785541 L
1 Imp gal = 4.546092 L
1 m^3 = 1000 L
1 mL = 1 cm^3

Mass
1 kg = 1000 g = 2.2046 lb_m = 0.068521 slugs
1 lb_m = 0.453592 kg
1 slug = 1 $lb_f \times s^2/ft$ = 32.174 lb_m

Force
1 lb_f = 4.448222 N = 4.448 × 10^5 dynes
1 N = 1 kg × m/s^2 = 10,000 dynes = 10,000 g × cm/s^2

Pressure
1 N/m^2 = 10 $dynes/cm^2$ = 1 Pa = 0.007501 mm Hg
1 atmosphere = 1013.25 millibars = 760 mm Hg = 101,325 Pa = 14.696 lb_f/in^2
1 cm H_2O = 0.735 mm Hg
1 lb_f/in^2 = 51.71 mm Hg
1 $dyne/cm^2$ = 0.1 Pa = 145.04 × 10^{-7} lb_f/in^2
1 bar = 10^5 N/m^2 = 14.504 lb_f/in^2 = 106 $dynes/cm^2$

Viscosity
1 kg/(m × s) = 1 N × s/m^2 = 0.6729 lb_m/(ft × s) = 10 poise

Energy
1 joule (J) = 1 kg × m^2/s^2
1 Btu = 778.16 ft × lb_f = 1055.056 J = 252 cal = 1.055 × 10^{10} ergs
1 cal = 4.1868 J

Power
1 watt (W) = 1 kg × m^2/s^3 = 1 J/s
1 hp = 550 ft × lb_f/s = 745.699 W

as breathing through an orifice. Under such conditions, the approximate flow across the orifice varies inversely with the square root of the gas density, in contrast to laminar flow conditions, in which gas flow varies inversely with gas viscosity. In such conditions, the low density of helium allows it to play a significant clinical role in the management of some forms of airway obstruction.

- Laplace's law predicts that for two alveoli of unequal size but equal surface tension, the smaller alveolus experiences a larger intra-alveolar pressure than the larger alveolus, causing the smaller alveolus to collapse. In real life, however, collapse of the smaller alveolus is prevented through the action of pulmonary surfactant, which serves to decrease alveolar surface tension in the smaller alveolus, resulting in equal pressure in both alveoli.

- One of the most important gas laws in physiology is the ideal (or perfect) gas law, $PV = nRT$ (where P = pressure of gas, V = volume of gas, n = number of moles of the gas in volume V, R = gas constant, and T = absolute temperature). This is the equation for ideal gases, which experience no forces of interaction. Real gases, however, experience intermolecular attraction (van der Waals forces), which requires that the pressure-volume gas law be written in a more complex form.

- Most flowmeters measure the drop in pressure that occurs when a gas passes through a known resistance and correlate this pressure drop to flow. When the resistance is an orifice, resistance depends primarily on gas density. Usually, a given flowmeter is calibrated for a particular gas, such as oxygen or air, with conversion tables available to provide flow data for other gases.

- Fick's law of diffusion, applicable to gas flow across lung and placental membranes, states that the rate of diffusion of a gas across a barrier is proportional to the concentration gradient for the gas and inversely proportional to the diffusion distance over which the gas molecules must travel.

- There are five main types of oxygen analyzers: paramagnetic analyzers, fuel cell analyzers, oxygen electrodes, mass spectrometers, and Raman spectrographs. All respond to oxygen partial pressure and not to oxygen concentration.

- The concept of minimum alveolar concentration (MAC) does not apply at higher altitudes and should be replaced by the concept of minimal alveolar partial pressure (MAPP).

- The pulmonary shunt equation is used as a foundation upon which arterial oxygenation and gas exchange indices can be studied. Calculation of pulmonary shunt requires the following information: (1) pulmonary end-capillary oxygen content, (2) arterial oxygen content, and (3) mixed venous oxygen content.

SELECTED REFERENCES

All references can be found online at expertconsult.com.
11. Sherwood L: *Human physiology: From cells to systems*, ed 2, St. Paul, MN, 1993, West Publishing.
20. Kemper KJ, Ritz RH, Benson MS, Bishop MS: Helium-oxygen mixture in the treatment of postextubation stridor in pediatric trauma patients. *Crit Care Med* 19:356–359, 1991.
23. Rodrigo GJ, Rodrigo C, Pollack CV, Rowe B: Use of helium-oxygen mixtures in the treatment of acute asthma: A systematic review. *Chest* 123:891–896, 2003.
25. Khanlou H, Eiger G: Safety and efficacy of heliox as a treatment for upper airway obstruction due to radiation-induced laryngeal dysfunction. *Heart Lung* 30:146–147, 2001.
26. Polaner DM: The use of heliox and the laryngeal mask airway in a child with an anterior mediastinal mass. *Anesth Analg* 82:208–210, 1996.
42. Straus C, Louis B, Isabey D, et al: Contribution of the endotracheal tube and the upper airway to breathing workload. *Am J Respir Crit Care Med* 157:23–30, 1998.
49. Bolder PM, Healy TE, Bolder AR, et al: The extra work of breathing through adult endotracheal tubes. *Anesth Analg* 65:853–859, 1986.
50. Davis PD, Kenny GNC: *Basic physics and measurement in anaesthesia*, ed 5, Philadelphia, 2003, Elsevier Health Science.
54. James MF, White JF: Anesthetic considerations at moderate altitude. *Anesth Analg* 63:1097–1105, 1984.
78. Herrick IA, Champion LK, Froese AB: A clinical comparison of indices of pulmonary gas exchange with changes in the inspired oxygen concentration. *Can J Anaesth* 37:69–76, 1990.

Chapter 5

Physiology of the Airway

WILLIAM C. WILSON | JONATHAN L. BENUMOF

I. NORMAL RESPIRATORY PHYSIOLOGY (NONANESTHETIZED)

Anesthesiologists require an extensive knowledge of respiratory physiology to care for patients in the operating room and the intensive care unit. Mastery of the normal respiratory physiologic processes is a prerequisite to understanding the mechanisms of impaired gas exchange that occur during anesthesia, during surgery, and with disease. This chapter is divided into two sections. The first section reviews the normal (gravity-determined) distribution of perfusion and ventilation, the major nongravitational determinants of resistance to perfusion and ventilation, transport of respiratory gases, and the pulmonary reflexes and special functions of the lung. In the second section, these processes and concepts are

The four zones of the lung

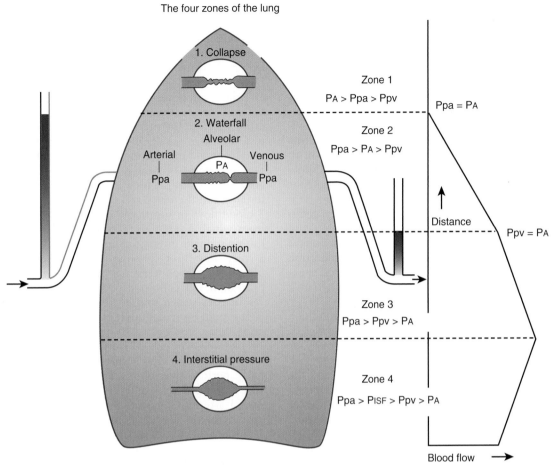

Figure 5-1 Schematic diagram showing the distribution of blood flow in the upright lung. In zone 1, alveolar pressure *(PA)* exceeds pulmonary artery pressure *(Ppa)*, and no flow occurs because the intra-alveolar vessels are collapsed by the compressing alveolar pressure. In zone 2, Ppa exceeds PA, but PA exceeds pulmonary venous pressure *(Ppv)*. Flow in zone 2 is determined by the Ppa-PA difference (Ppa – PA) and has been likened to an upstream river flowing over a dam. Because Ppa increases down zone 2 whereas PA remains constant, perfusion pressure increases, and flow steadily increases down the zone. In zone 3, Ppv exceeds PA, and flow is determined by the Ppa – Ppv difference, which is constant down this portion of the lung. However, transmural pressure across the wall of the vessel increases down this zone, so the caliber of the vessels increases (resistance decreases), and therefore flow increases. Finally, in zone 4, pulmonary interstitial pressure *(PISF)* becomes positive and exceeds both Ppv and PA. Consequently, flow in zone 4 is determined by the Ppa – PISF difference. (Redrawn with modification from West JB: *Ventilation/Blood flow and gas exchange*, ed 4, Oxford, 1970, Blackwell Scientific, 1970.)

discussed in relation to the general mechanisms of impaired gas exchange that occur during anesthesia and surgery.

A. Gravity-Determined Distribution of Perfusion and Ventilation

1. Distribution of Pulmonary Perfusion

Contraction of the right ventricle imparts kinetic energy to the blood in the main pulmonary artery. As this energy is dissipated in climbing a vertical hydrostatic gradient, the absolute pressure in the pulmonary artery (Ppa) decreases by 1 cm H_2O per centimeter of vertical distance up the lung (Fig. 5-1). At some height above the heart, Ppa becomes zero (i.e., equal to atmospheric pressure), and still higher in the lung, Ppa becomes negative.[1] In this region, then, alveolar pressure (PA) exceeds Ppa and pulmonary venous pressure (Ppv), which is very negative at this vertical height. Because the pressure outside the vessels is greater than the pressure inside the

vessels, the vessels in this region of the lung are collapsed, and no blood flow occurs; this is known as *zone 1* (PA > Ppa > Ppv). Because there is no blood flow, no gas exchange is possible, and the region functions as alveolar dead space, or wasted ventilation. Little or no zone 1 exists in the lung under normal conditions,[2] but the amount of zone 1 lung may be greatly increased if Ppa is reduced, as in oligemic shock, or if PA is increased, as in the application of excessively large tidal volumes (VT) or levels of positive end-expiratory pressure (PEEP) during positive-pressure ventilation.

Further down the lung, absolute Ppa becomes positive, and blood flow begins when Ppa exceeds PA (*zone 2*, Ppa > PA > Ppv). At this vertical level in the lung, PA exceeds Ppv, and blood flow is determined by the mean Ppa – PA difference rather than by the more conventional Ppa – Ppv difference (see later discussion).[3] In zone 2, the relationship between blood flow and alveolar pressure has the same physical characteristics as a waterfall flowing over a dam. The height of the upstream river (before reaching the dam) is equivalent to Ppa, and the height of the dam is equivalent to P_A. The rate of water flow over the dam is proportional to only the difference between the height of the upstream river and the dam ($Ppa - P_A$), and it does not matter how far below the dam the downstream riverbed (Ppv) is. This phenomenon has various names, including the waterfall, Starling resistor, weir (dam made by beavers), and sluice effect. Because mean Ppa increases down this region of the lung but mean P_A is relatively constant, the mean driving pressure ($Ppa - P_A$) increases linearly, and therefore mean blood flow increases linearly as one descends down this portion of the lung. However, respiration and pulmonary blood flow are cyclic phenomena. Therefore, absolute instantaneous Ppa, Ppv, and P_A are changing continuously, and the relationships among Ppa, Ppv, and P_A are dynamically determined by the phase lags between the cardiac and respiratory cycles. Consequently, a given point in zone 2 may actually be in either a zone 1 or a zone 3 condition at a given moment, depending on whether the patient is in respiratory systole or diastole or in cardiac systole or diastole.

Still lower in the lung, there is a vertical level at which Ppv becomes positive and also exceeds P_A. In this region, blood flow is governed by the pulmonary arteriovenous pressure difference, $Ppa - Ppv$ (*zone 3*, $Ppa > Ppv > P_A$), for here both these vascular pressures exceed P_A, and the capillary systems are thus permanently open and blood flow is continuous. In descending zone 3, gravity causes both absolute Ppa and Ppv to increase at the same rate, so the perfusion pressure ($Ppa - Ppv$) is unchanged. However, the pressure outside the vessels—namely, pleural pressure (Ppl)—increases less than Ppa and Ppv. Therefore, the transmural distending pressures ($Ppa - Ppl$ and $Ppv - Ppl$) increase down zone 3, the vessel radii increase, vascular resistance decreases, and blood flow consequently increases further.

Finally, whenever pulmonary vascular pressures (Ppa) are extremely high, as they are in a severely volume-overloaded patient, in a severely restricted and constricted pulmonary vascular bed, in an extremely dependent lung (far below the vertical level of the left atrium), and in patients with pulmonary embolism or mitral stenosis, fluid can transude out of the pulmonary vessels into the pulmonary interstitial compartment. In addition, pulmonary interstitial edema can be caused by extremely negative Ppl and perivascular hydrostatic pressure, such as may occur in a vigorously spontaneously breathing patient with an obstructed airway due to laryngospasm (most commonly) or upper airway masses (e.g., tumors, hematoma, abscess, edema), strangulation, infectious processes (e.g., epiglottitis, pharyngitis, croup), or vocal cord paralysis; with rapid reexpansion of lung; or with the application of very negative Ppl during thoracentesis.[4,5] Transuded pulmonary interstitial fluid can significantly alter the distribution of pulmonary blood flow.

When the flow of fluid into the interstitial space is excessive and the fluid cannot be cleared adequately by the lymphatics, it accumulates in the interstitial connective tissue compartment around the large vessels and airways and forms peribronchial and periarteriolar edema fluid cuffs. The transuded pulmonary interstitial fluid fills the pulmonary interstitial space and may eliminate the normally present negative and radially expanding interstitial tension on the extra-alveolar pulmonary vessels. Expansion of the pulmonary interstitial space by fluid causes pulmonary interstitial pressure (P_{ISF}) to become positive and to exceed Ppv (*zone 4*, $Ppa > P_{ISF} > Ppv > P_A$).[6,7] In addition, the vascular resistance of extra-alveolar vessels may be increased at a very low lung volume (i.e., residual volume); at such volumes, the tethering action of the pulmonary tissue on the vessels is also lost, and as a result, P_{ISF} increases positively (see later discussion of lung volume).[8,9] Consequently, zone 4 blood flow is governed by the arteriointerstitial pressure difference ($Ppa - P_{ISF}$), which is less than the $Ppa - Ppv$ difference, and therefore zone 4 blood flow is less than zone 3 blood flow. In summary, zone 4 is a region of the lung from which a large amount of fluid has transuded into the pulmonary interstitial compartment or is possibly at a very low lung volume. Both these circumstances produce positive interstitial pressure, which causes compression of extra-alveolar vessels, increased extra-alveolar vascular resistance, and decreased regional blood flow.

It should be evident that as Ppa and Ppv increase, three important changes take place in the pulmonary circulation—namely, recruitment or opening of previously unperfused vessels, distention or widening of previously perfused vessels, and transudation of fluid from very distended vessels.[10,11] Thus, as mean Ppa increases, zone 1 arteries may become zone 2 arteries, and as mean Ppv increases, zone 2 veins may become zone 3 veins. The increase in both mean Ppa and Ppv distends zone 3 vessels according to their compliance and decreases the resistance to flow through them. Zone 3 vessels may become so distended that they leak fluid and become converted to zone 4 vessels. In general, pulmonary capillary recruitment is the principal change as Ppa and Ppv increase from low to moderate levels, distention is the principal change as Ppa and Ppv increase from moderate to high levels, and transudation is the principal change when Ppa and Ppv increase from high to very high levels.

2. Distribution of Ventilation

Gravity also causes differences in vertical Ppl, which in turn causes differences in regional alveolar volume, compliance, and ventilation. The vertical gradient of Ppl can best be understood by imagining the lung as a plastic bag filled with semifluid contents; in other words, it is a viscoelastic structure. Without the presence of a supporting chest wall, the effect of gravity on the contents of the bag would cause the bag to bulge outward at the bottom and inward at the top (i.e., it would assume a globular shape). Inside the supporting chest wall, the lung cannot assume a globular shape. However, gravity still exerts a force on the lung to assume a globular shape; this force creates relatively more negative pressure at the top of the pleural space (where the lung pulls away from the chest wall) and relatively more positive pressure at the bottom of the lung (where the lung is compressed against the chest wall) (Fig. 5-2). The density of the lung determines the magnitude of this pressure gradient. Because the lung has about one fourth the density of water, the gradient of Ppl (in cm H_2O) is about one fourth the height of the upright

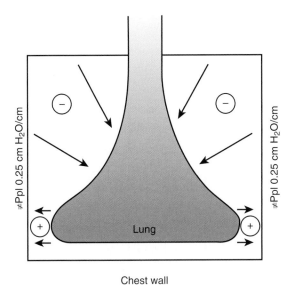

Figure 5-2 Schematic diagram of the lung within the chest wall showing the tendency of the lung to assume a globular shape because of gravity and the lung's viscoelastic nature. The tendency of the top of the lung to collapse inward creates a relatively negative pressure at the apex of the lung, and the tendency of the bottom of the lung to spread outward creates a relatively positive pressure at the base of the lung. Therefore, alveoli at the top of the lung tend to be held open and are larger at end-exhalation, whereas those at the bottom tend to be smaller and compressed at end-exhalation. Pleural pressure increases by 0.25 cm H_2O per centimeter of lung dependence.

lung (30 cm). Thus, Ppl increases positively by 30/4 = 7.5 cm H_2O from the top to the bottom of the lung.[12]

Because PA is the same throughout the lung, the Ppl gradient causes regional differences in transpulmonary distending pressure (PA – Ppl). Ppl is most positive (least negative) in the dependent basilar lung regions, so alveoli in these regions are more compressed and are therefore considerably smaller than the superior, relatively non-compressed apical alveoli. (The volume difference is approximately fourfold.)[13] If regional differences in alveolar volume are translated to a pressure-volume (compliance) curve for normal lung (Fig. 5-3), the dependent small alveoli are on the midportion, and the nondependent large alveoli are on the upper portion of the S-shaped compliance curve. Because the different regional slopes of the composite curve are equal to the different regional lung compliance values, dependent alveoli are relatively compliant (steep slope), and nondependent alveoli are relatively noncompliant (flat slope). Therefore, most of the VT is preferentially distributed to dependent alveoli which expand more per unit pressure change than the nondependent alveoli.

3. The Ventilation-Perfusion Ratio

Blood flow and ventilation (both shown on the left vertical axis of Fig. 5-4) increase linearly with distance down the normal upright lung (horizontal axis, reverse polarity).[14] Because blood flow increases from a very low value and more rapidly than ventilation does with distance down the lung, the ventilation-perfusion ratio ($\dot{V}A/\dot{Q}$,

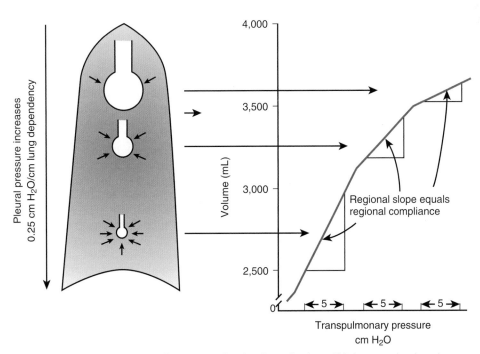

Figure 5-3 Pleural pressure increases by 0.25 cm H_2O every centimeter down the lung. This increase in pleural pressure causes a fourfold decrease in alveolar volume from the top of the lung to the bottom. The caliber of the air passages also decreases as lung volume decreases. When regional alveolar volume is translated to a regional transpulmonary pressure–alveolar volume curve, small alveoli are seen to be on a steep portion of the curve (large slope), and large alveoli are on a flat portion of the curve (relatively small slope). Because the regional slope equals regional compliance, the dependent small alveoli normally receive the largest share of the tidal volume. Over the normal tidal volume range the pressure-volume relationship is linear: lung volume increases by 500 mL, from 2500 mL (normal functional residual capacity) to 3000 mL. The lung volume values in this diagram are derived from the upright position.

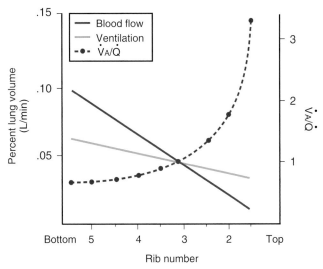

Figure 5-4 Distribution of ventilation and blood flow (left vertical axis) and the ventilation-perfusion ratio ($\dot{V}A/\dot{Q}$, right vertical axis) in normal upright lung. Both blood flow and ventilation are expressed in liters per minute per percentage of alveolar volume and have been drawn as smoothed-out linear functions of vertical height. The closed circles mark the $\dot{V}A/\dot{Q}$ ratios of horizontal lung slices (three of which are shown in Fig. 5-5). A cardiac output of 6 L/min and a total minute ventilation of 5.1 L/min were assumed. *(Redrawn with modification from West JB: Ventilation/Blood flow and gas exchange, ed 4, Oxford, 1970, Blackwell Scientific.)*

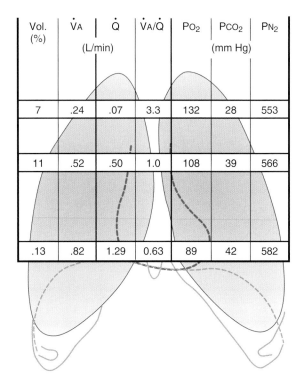

Vol. (%)	$\dot{V}A$	$\dot{Q}$	$\dot{V}A/\dot{Q}$	PO_2	PCO_2	PN_2
	(L/min)			(mm Hg)		
7	.24	.07	3.3	132	28	553
11	.52	.50	1.0	108	39	566
.13	.82	1.29	0.63	89	42	582

Figure 5-5 Ventilation-perfusion ratio ($\dot{V}A/\dot{Q}$) and the regional composition of alveolar gas. Values for regional flow ($\dot{Q}$), ventilation ($\dot{V}A$), partial pressure of oxygen (PO_2), and partial pressure of carbon dioxide (PCO_2) were derived from Figure 5-4. Partial pressure of nitrogen (PN_2) represents what remains from total gas pressure (760 mm Hg including water vapor, which equals 47 mm Hg). The percentage volumes *(Vol.)* of the three lung slices are also shown. When compared with the top of the lung, the bottom of the lung has a low $\dot{V}A/\dot{Q}$ ratio and is relatively hypoxic and hypercapnic. *(Redrawn from West JB: Regional differences in gas exchange in the lung of erect man. J Appl Physiol 17:893, 1962.)*

right vertical axis of Fig. 5-4) decreases rapidly at first and then more slowly.

$\dot{V}A/\dot{Q}$ best expresses the amount of ventilation relative to perfusion in any given lung region. For example, alveoli at the base of the lung are overperfused in relation to their ventilation ($\dot{V}A/\dot{Q} < 1$). Figure 5-5 shows the calculated ventilation ($\dot{V}A$) and blood flow ($\dot{Q}$), the $\dot{V}A/\dot{Q}$ ratio, and the alveolar partial pressures of oxygen (PA_{O_2}) and carbon dioxide (PA_{CO_2}) for horizontal slices from the top (7% of lung volume), middle (11% of lung volume), and bottom (13% of lung volume) of the lung.[15] PA_{O_2} increases by more than 40 mm Hg, from 89 mm Hg at the base to 132 mm Hg at the apex, whereas PCO_2 decreases by 14 mm Hg, from 42 mm Hg at the bottom to 28 mm Hg at the top. Therefore, in keeping with the regional $\dot{V}A/\dot{Q}$ ratio, the bottom of the lung is relatively hypoxic and hypercapnic compared with the top of the lung.

$\dot{V}A/\dot{Q}$ inequalities have different effects on arterial CO_2 tension (Pa_{CO_2}) than on arterial O_2 tension (Pa_{O_2}). Blood passing through underventilated alveoli tends to retain its CO_2 and does not take up enough O_2; blood traversing overventilated alveoli gives off an excessive amount of CO_2 but cannot take up a proportionately increased amount of O_2 because of the flatness of the oxygen-hemoglobin (oxy-Hb) dissociation curve in this region (see Fig. 5-25). A lung with uneven $\dot{V}A/\dot{Q}$ relationships can eliminate CO_2 from the overventilated alveoli to compensate for the underventilated alveoli. As a result, with uneven $\dot{V}A/\dot{Q}$ relationships, Pa_{CO_2}-to-Pa_{CO_2} gradients are small, and PA_{O_2}-to-Pa_{O_2} gradients are usually large.

In 1974, Wagner and colleagues described a method of determining the continuous distribution of $\dot{V}A/\dot{Q}$ ratios within the lung based on the pattern of elimination of a series of intravenously infused inert gases.[16] Gases of differing solubility are dissolved in physiologic saline solution and infused into a peripheral vein until a steady state is achieved (20 minutes). Toward the end of the infusion period, samples of arterial and mixed expired gas are collected, and total ventilation and total cardiac output ($\dot{Q}T$) are measured. For each gas, the ratio of arterial to mixed venous concentration (retention) and the ratio of expired to mixed venous concentration (excretion) are calculated, and retention-solubility and excretion-solubility curves are drawn. The retention- and excretion-solubility curves can be regarded as fingerprints of the particular distribution of $\dot{V}A/\dot{Q}$ ratios that give rise to them.

Figure 5-6 shows the types of distributions found in young, healthy subjects breathing air in the semirecumbent position.[17] The distributions of both ventilation and blood flow are relatively narrow. The upper and lower 9% limits shown (vertical interrupted lines) correspond to $\dot{V}A/\dot{Q}$ ratios of 0.3 and 2.1, respectively. Note that these young, healthy subjects had no blood flow perfusing areas with very low $\dot{V}A/\dot{Q}$ ratios, nor did they have

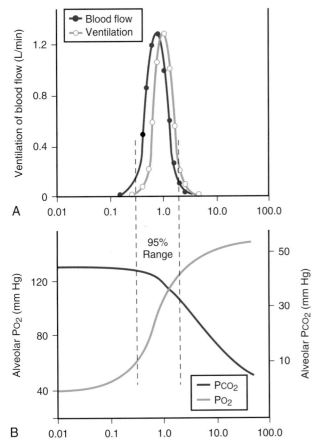

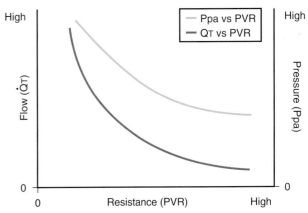

Figure 5-7 Passive changes in pulmonary vascular resistance *(PVR)* as a function of pulmonary artery pressure *(Ppa)* and pulmonary blood flow *(Q̇T)*: PVR = Ppa/Q̇T. As Q̇T increases, Ppa also increases, but to a lesser extent, and PVR decreases. As Q̇T decreases, Ppa also decreases, but to a lesser extent, and PVR increases. (Redrawn with modification from Fishman AP: Dynamics of the pulmonary circulation. In Hamilton WF, editor: *Handbook of physiology. Section 2: Circulation,* vol 2, Baltimore, 1963, Williams & Wilkins, p 1667.)

Figure 5-6   A, Average distribution of ventilation-perfusion ratios (V̇A/Q̇) in normal, young, semirecumbent subjects. The 95% range (between dashed lines) is 0.3 to 2.1. **B,** Corresponding variations in partial pressures of oxygen *(Po₂)* and carbon dioxide *(Pco₂)* in alveolar gas. (Redrawn from West JB: Blood flow to the lung and gas exchange. *Anesthesiology* 41:124, 1974.)

any blood flow to unventilated or shunted areas (V̇A/Q̇ = 0) or unperfused areas (V̇A/Q̇ = 8). Figure 5-6 also shows PAO₂ and PACO₂ in respiratory units with different V̇A/Q̇ ratios. Within the 95% range of V̇A/Q̇ ratios (i.e., 0.3 to 2.1), Po₂ ranges from 60 to 123 mm Hg, whereas the corresponding Pco₂ range is 44 to 33 mm Hg.

B. Nongravitational Determinants of Blood Flow Distribution

1. Passive Processes

a. CARDIAC OUTPUT

The pulmonary vascular bed is a high-flow, low-pressure system in health. As Q̇T increases, pulmonary vascular pressures increase minimally.[18] However, increases in Q̇T distend open vessels and recruit previously closed vessels. Accordingly, pulmonary vascular resistance (PVR) drops because the normal pulmonary vasculature is quite distensible (and partly because of the addition of previously unused vessels to the pulmonary circulation). As a result of the distensibility of the normal pulmonary circulation, an increase in Ppa increases the radius of the pulmonary vessels, which causes PVR to decrease (Fig. 5-7). Conversely,

the opposite effect occurs within the pulmonary vessels during a decrease in Q̇T. As Q̇T decreases, pulmonary vascular pressures decrease, the radii of the pulmonary vessels are reduced, and PVR consequently increases. The pulmonary vessels of patients with significant pulmonary hypertension are less distensible and act more like rigid pipes. In this setting, Ppa increases much more sharply with any increase in Q̇T because PVR in these stiff vessels does not decrease significantly due to minimal expansion of their radii.

Understanding the relationships among Ppa, PVR, and Q̇T during passive events is a prerequisite to recognition of active vasomotion in the pulmonary circulation (see Lung Volume). Active vasoconstriction occurs whenever Q̇T decreases and Ppa either remains constant or increases. Increased Ppa and PVR have been found to be "a universal feature of acute respiratory failure."[19]

Active pulmonary vasoconstriction can increase Ppa and Ppv, contributing to the formation of pulmonary edema, and in that way it has a role in the pathophysiology of adult respiratory distress syndrome (ARDS). Active vasodilation occurs whenever Q̇T increases and Ppa either remains constant or decreases. When deliberate hypotension is achieved with sodium nitroprusside, Q̇T often remains constant or increases, but Ppa decreases, and therefore so does PVR.

b. LUNG VOLUME

Lung volume and PVR have an asymmetric, U-shaped relationship because of the varying effect of lung volume on small intra-alveolar and large extra-alveolar vessels, which in both cases is minimal at functional residual capacity (FRC). FRC is defined as the amount of volume (gas) in the lungs at end-exhalation during normal tidal breathing. Ideally, this means that the patient is inspiring a normal VT, with minimal or no muscle activity or pressure difference between the alveoli and atmosphere at end-exhalation. Total PVR is increased when lung volume is either increased or decreased from FRC

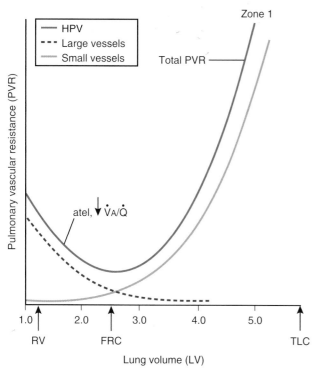

Figure 5-8 Total pulmonary vascular resistance *(PVR)* relates to lung volume as an asymmetric, U-shaped curve. The trough of the curve occurs when lung volume equals functional residual capacity *(FRC)*. Total PVR is the sum of the resistance in small vessels (increased by increasing lung volume *(LV)* and the resistance in large vessels (increased by decreasing LV). The end point for increasing LV toward total lung capacity *(TLC)* is the creation of zone 1 conditions, and the end point for decreasing LV toward residual volume *(RV)* is the creation of low ventilation-perfusion *(V̇A/Q̇)* and atelectatic *(atel)* areas that demonstrate hypoxic pulmonary vasoconstriction *(HPV)*. (Data fromr Bhavani-Shankar K, Hart NS, Mushlin PS: Negative pressure induced airway and pulmonary injury. *Can J Anaesth* 44:78, 1997; Berggren SM: The oxygen deficit of arterial blood caused by non-ventilating parts of the lung. *Acta Physiol Scand Suppl* 4:11, 1942; and Benumof JL: One lung ventilation: Which lung should be PEEPed? *Anesthesiology* 56:161, 1982.)

(Fig. 5-8).[20–22] The increase in total PVR above FRC results from alveolar compression of small intra-alveolar vessels, which results in an increase in small-vessel PVR (i.e., creation of zone 1 or zone 2).[23] As a relatively small mitigating or counterbalancing effect to the compression of small vessels, the large extra-alveolar vessels can be expanded by the increased tethering of interstitial connective tissue at high lung volumes (and with

spontaneous ventilation only—the negativity of perivascular pressure at high lung volumes). The increase in total PVR below FRC results from an increase in the PVR of large extra-alveolar vessels (passive effect). The increase in large-vessel PVR is partly due to mechanical tortuosity or kinking of these vessels (passive effect). In addition, small or grossly atelectatic lungs become hypoxic, and it has been shown that the increased large-vessel PVR in these lungs is also caused by an active vasoconstrictive mechanism known as hypoxic pulmonary vasoconstriction (HPV).[24] The effect of HPV (discussed in greater detail in "Alveolar Gases") is significant whether the chest is open or closed and whether ventilation is by positive pressure or spontaneous.[25]

2. Active Processes and Pulmonary Vascular Tone

Four major categories of active processes affect the pulmonary vascular tone of normal patients: (1) local tissue (endothelial- and smooth muscle–derived) autocrine or paracrine products, which act on smooth muscle (Table 5-1); (2) alveolar gas concentrations (chiefly hypoxia), which also act on smooth muscle; (3) neural influences; and (4) humoral (or hormonal) effects of circulating products within the pulmonary capillary bed. The neural and humoral effects work by means of either receptor-mediated mechanisms involving the autocrine/paracrine molecules listed in Table 5-1 or related mechanisms ultimately affecting the smooth muscle cell.[26] These four interrelated systems, each affecting pulmonary vascular tone, are briefly reviewed in sequence.

a. TISSUE (ENDOTHELIAL- AND SMOOTH MUSCLE–DERIVED) PRODUCTS

The pulmonary vascular endothelium synthesizes, metabolizes, and converts a multitude of vasoactive mediators and plays a central role in the regulation of PVR. However, the main effecter site of pulmonary vascular tone is the pulmonary vascular smooth muscle cell (which both senses and produces multiple pulmonary vasoactive compounds).[27] The autocrine/paracrine molecules listed in Table 5-1 are all actively involved in the regulation of pulmonary vascular tone during various conditions. Numerous additional compounds bind to receptors on the endothelial or smooth muscle cell membranes and modulate the levels (and effects) of these vasoactive molecules.

Nitric oxide (NO) is the predominant endogenous vasodilatory compound. Its discovery by Palmer and

TABLE 5-1

Local Tissue (Autocrine/Paracrine) Molecules Involved in Active Control of Pulmonary Vascular Tone

Molecule	Subtype	Site of Origin	Site of Action	Response
Nitric oxide	NO	Endothelium	Sm. muscle	Vasodilation
Endothelin	ET-1	Endothelium	Sm. muscle (ETA receptor)	Vasoconstriction
			Endothelium (ETB receptor)	Vasodilation
Prostaglandin	PGI_2	Endothelium	Endothelium	Vasodilation
Prostaglandin	$PGF_{2\alpha}$	Endothelium	Sm. muscle	Vasoconstriction
Thromboxane	TXA_2	Endothelium	Sm. muscle	Vasoconstriction
Leukotriene	LTB_4–LTE_4	Endothelium	Sm. muscle	Vasoconstriction

ETA receptor, ET-1 receptor located on the smooth muscle cell membrane; *ETB receptor*, ET-1 receptor located on the endothelial cell membrane; *Sm. muscle*, Pulmonary arteriole smooth muscle cell.

colleagues 25 years ago ended the long search for the so-called endothelium-derived relaxant factor (EDRF).[28] Since then, a massive amount of laboratory and clinical research has demonstrated the ubiquitous nature of NO and its predominant role in vasodilation of both pulmonary and systemic blood vessels.[29] In the pulmonary endothelial cell, L-arginine is converted to L-citrulline by means of nitric oxide synthase (NOS) to produce the small, yet highly reactive NO molecule.[30] Because of its small size, NO can diffuse freely across membranes into the smooth muscle cell, where it binds to the heme moiety of guanylate cyclase (which converts guanosine triphosphate to cyclic guanosine monophosphate [cGMP]).[31] cGMP activates protein kinase G, which dephosphorylates the myosin light chains of pulmonary vascular smooth muscle cells and thereby causes vasodilation.[31] NOS exists in two forms: constitutive (cNOS) and inducible (iNOS). cNOS is permanently expressed in some cells, including pulmonary vascular endothelial cells, and produces short bursts of NO in response to changing levels of calcium and calmodulin and shear stress. The cNOS enzyme is also stimulated by linked membrane-based receptors that bind numerous molecules in the blood (e.g., acetylcholine, bradykinin).[31] In contrast, iNOS is usually produced only as a result of inflammatory mediators and cytokines and, when stimulated, produces large quantities of NO for an extended duration.[31] It is well known that NO is constitutively produced in normal lungs and contributes to the maintenance of low PVR.[32,33]

Endothelin-1 (ET-1) is a pulmonary vasoconstrictor.[34] The endothelins are 21-amino-acid peptides that are produced by a variety of cells. ET-1 is the only family member produced in pulmonary endothelial cells, and it is also produced in vascular smooth muscle cells.[34] ET-1 exerts its major vascular effects through activation of two distinct G protein–coupled receptors (ETA and ETB). ETA receptors are found in the medial smooth muscle layers of the pulmonary (and systemic) blood vessels and in atrial and ventricular myocardium.[34] When stimulated, ETA receptors induce vasoconstriction and cellular proliferation by increasing intracellular calcium.[35] ETB receptors are localized on endothelial cells and some smooth muscle cells.[36] Activation of ETB receptors stimulates the release of NO and prostacyclin, thereby promoting pulmonary vasodilation and inhibiting apoptosis.[30] Bosentan, an ET-1 receptor antagonist, has produced modest improvement in the treatment of pulmonary hypertension.[37] The more selective ETA receptor antagonist, sitaxsentan, showed additional benefit in improving pulmonary hypertension.[38] However, both of these ET-1 receptor antagonists are associated with an increased risk of liver toxicity.[39] In summary, it appears that there is a normal balance between NO and ET-1, with a slight predominance toward NO production and vasodilation in health.

Similarly, various eicosanoids are elaborated by the pulmonary vascular endothelium, with a balance toward the vasodilatory compounds in health. Prostaglandin I_2 (PGI$_2$), now known as epoprostenol (previously known as prostacyclin), causes vasodilation and is continuously elaborated in small amounts in healthy endothelium. In contrast, thromboxane A_2 and leukotriene B_4 are elaborated under pathologic conditions and are thought to be involved in the pathophysiology of pulmonary artery hypertension (PAH) associated with sepsis and reperfusion injury.[26]

Therapeutically, epoprostenol has been used successfully to decrease PVR in patients with chronic PAH when infused or inhaled.[40,41] Currently, the synthetic PGI$_2$ (iloprost) is the most commonly used inhaled eicosanoid for reduction of PVR in patients with PAH.[41] Although most patients with chronic PAH are unresponsive to an acute vasodilator challenge with short-acting agents such as epoprostenol, adenosine, or NO,[42] long-term administration of epoprostenol has been shown to decrease PVR in these patients.[43] Furthermore, some patients with previously severe PAH have been weaned from epoprostenol after long-term administration, with dramatically decreased PVR and improved exercise tolerance.[42] The vascular remodeling required to provide such a dramatic reduction in PVR is probably the result of mechanisms besides simple local vasodilation, as predicted by Fishman in an editorial in 1998.[44] One such mechanism that appears to be important is the increased clearance of ET-1 (a potent vasoconstrictor and mitogen) with long-term epoprostenol administration.[45]

b. ALVEOLAR GASES

Hypoxia-induced vasoconstriction constitutes a fundamental difference between pulmonary vessels and all other systemic blood vessels (which vasodilate in the presence of hypoxia). Alveolar hypoxia of in vivo and in vitro whole lung, unilateral lung, lobe, or lobule of lung results in localized pulmonary vasoconstriction. This phenomenon is widely referred to as HPV and was first described more than 65 years ago by Von Euler and Liljestrand.[46] The HPV response is present in all mammalian species and serves as an adaptive mechanism for diverting blood flow away from poorly ventilated to better ventilated regions of the lung and thereby improving $\dot{V}_A/\dot{Q}$ ratios.[47] The HPV response is also critical for fetal development because it minimizes perfusion of the unventilated lung.

The HPV response occurs primarily in pulmonary arterioles of about 200 μm internal diameter (ID) in humans (60 to 700 μm ID in other species).[48] These vessels are advantageously situated anatomically in close relation to small bronchioles and alveoli, which permits rapid and direct detection of alveolar hypoxia. Indeed, blood may actually become oxygenated in small pulmonary arteries because of the ability of O_2 to diffuse directly across the small distance between the contiguous air spaces and vessels.[49] This direct access that gas in the airways has to small arteries makes possible a rapid and localized vascular response to changes in gas composition.

The O_2 tension at the HPV stimulus site (PsO_2) is a function of both PaO_2 and mixed venous O_2 pressure (P$\bar{v}O_2$).[50] The PsO_2-HPV response is sigmoid, with a 50% response when PaO_2, P$\bar{v}O_2$, and PsO_2 are approximately 30 mm Hg. Usually, PaO_2 has a much greater effect than P$\bar{v}O_2$ does because O_2 uptake is from the alveolar space to the blood in the small pulmonary arteries.[50]

Numerous theories have been developed to explain the mechanism of HPV.[46,51-53] Many vasoactive substances have been proposed as mediators of HPV, including leukotrienes, prostaglandins, catecholamines, serotonin, histamine, angiotensin, bradykinin, and ET-1, but none has been identified as the primary mediator. In 1992, Xuan proposed that NO has a pivotal role in modulating PVR.[54] NO is involved, but not precisely in the way that Xuan first proposed. There are multiple sites of O_2 sensing with variable contributions from the NO, ET-1, and eicosanoid systems (described earlier). In vivo, HPV is currently thought to result from the synergistic action of molecules produced in both endothelial cells and smooth muscle cells.[55] However, HPV can proceed in the absence of intact endothelium, suggesting that the primary O_2 sensor is in the smooth muscle cell and that endothelium-derived molecules modulate only the primary HPV response.

The precise mechanism of HPV is still under investigation. However, current data support a mechanism involving the smooth muscle mitochondrial electron transport chain as the HPV sensor (Fig. 5-9).[56] In addition, reactive oxygen species (possibly H_2O_2 or superoxide) are released from complex III of the electron transport chain and probably serve as second messengers to increase calcium in pulmonary artery smooth muscle cells during acute

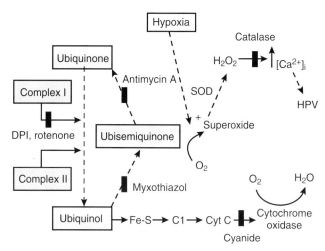

Figure 5-9 Schematic model of the mitochondrial O_2-sensing and effector mechanism probably responsible for hypoxic pulmonary vasoconstriction *(HPV)*. In this model, reactive O_2 species (ROS) are released from electron transport chain complex III and act as second messengers in the hypoxia-induced calcium *(Ca2$^+$)* increase and resultant HPV. The solid arrows represent electron transfer steps; solid bars show sites of electron chain inhibition. Normal mitochondrial electron transport involves the movement of reducing equivalents generated in the Krebs cycle through complex I or II and then through complex III (ubiquinone) and complex IV (cytochrome oxidase). The Q cycle converts the dual electron transfer in complex I and II into a single electron transfer step used in complex IV. The ubisemiquinone (a free radical) created in this process can generate superoxide, which in the presence of superoxide dismutase *(SOD)* produces H_2O_2, the probable mediator of the hypoxia-induced increased Ca2$^+$ and HPV. This process is amplified during hypoxia. Diphenyleneiodonium *(DPI)*, rotenone, and myxothiazol (not shown in figure) are inhibitors of the proximal portion of the electron transport chain. (From Waypa GB, Marks JD, Mack MM, et al. Mitochondrial reactive oxygen species trigger calcium increases during hypoxia in pulmonary artery myocytes. *Circ Res* 91:719, 2002.)

hypoxia.[57] However, alternative (less likely) mechanisms are still being investigated.[58] One alternative hypothesis suggests that smooth muscle microsomal reduced nicotinamide adenine dinucleotide phosphate (NADPH) oxidoreductase or sarcolemmal NADPH oxidase is the sensing mechanism.[58] Another, previously popular theory posited that voltage-sensitive potassium (K_V) channels were required for the HPV response. However, K_V channels are no longer believed to be obligate but instead are thought to be attenuators, because a study demonstrated that inhibition of K_V channels failed to inhibit the HPV response.[58]

In summary, HPV probably results from a direct action of alveolar hypoxia on pulmonary smooth muscle cells, sensed by the mitochondrial electron transport chain, with reactive O_2 species (probably H_2O_2 or superoxide) serving as second messengers to increase calcium and smooth muscle vasoconstriction. The endothelium-derived products serve to both potentiate (ET-1) and attenuate (NO, PGI_2) the HPV response. Additional mechanisms (humoral and neurogenic influences) may also modulate the baseline pulmonary vascular tone and affect the magnitude of the HPV response.

Elevated Pa_{CO_2} has a pulmonary vasoconstrictor effect. Both respiratory acidosis and metabolic acidosis augment HPV, whereas respiratory and metabolic alkalosis cause pulmonary vasodilation and serve to reduce HPV.

The clinical effects of HPV in humans can be classified under three basic mechanisms. First, life at high altitude or whole-lung respiration of a low inspired concentration of O_2 (FiO_2) increases Ppa. This is true for newcomers to high altitude, for the acclimatized, and for natives.[53] The vasoconstriction is considerable; in healthy people breathing 10% O_2, Ppa doubles whereas pulmonary wedge pressure remains constant.[59] The increased Ppa increases perfusion of the apices of the lung (through recruitment of previously unused vessels), which results in gas exchange in a region of lung not normally used (i.e., zone 1). Therefore, with a low FiO_2, Pa_{O_2} is greater and the alveolar-arterial O_2 tension difference and the ratio between dead space and tidal volume (V_D/V_T) are less than would be expected or predicted on the basis of a normal (sea level) distribution of ventilation and blood flow. High-altitude pulmonary hypertension is an important component in the development of mountain sickness subacutely (hours to days) and cor pulmonale chronically (weeks to years).[60] There is now good evidence that in both patients with chronic obstructive pulmonary disease (COPD) and those with obstructive sleep apnea (OSA), nocturnal episodes of arterial O_2 desaturation (caused by episodic hypoventilation) are accompanied by elevations in Ppa that can eventually lead to sustained pulmonary hypertension and cor pulmonale.[61]

Second, hypoventilation (low $\dot{V}_A/\dot{Q}$ ratio), atelectasis, or nitrogen ventilation of any region of the lung usually causes a diversion of blood flow away from the hypoxic to the nonhypoxic lung (40% to 50% in one lung, 50% to 60% in one lobe, 60% to 70% in one lobule) (Fig. 5-10).[62] The regional vasoconstriction and blood flow diversion are of great importance in minimizing transpulmonary shunting and normalizing regional $\dot{V}_A/\dot{Q}$ ratios during disease of one lung, one-lung anesthesia (see

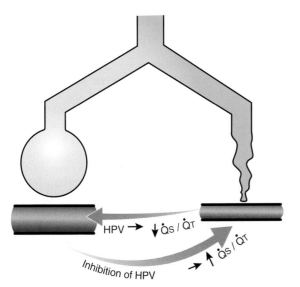

Figure 5-10 Schematic drawing of regional hypoxic pulmonary vasoconstriction (HPV); one-lung ventilation is a common clinical example of regional HPV. HPV in the hypoxic atelectatic lung causes redistribution of blood flow away from the hypoxic lung to the normoxic lung, thereby diminishing the amount of shunt flow ($\dot{Q}_S/\dot{Q}_T$) that can occur through the hypoxic lung. Inhibition of hypoxic lung HPV causes an increase in the amount of shunt flow through the hypoxic lung, thereby decreasing the alveolar oxygen tension (Pa_{O_2}).

Chapter 26), inadvertent intubation of a main stem bronchus, and lobar collapse.

Third, in patients who have COPD, asthma, pneumonia, or mitral stenosis but not bronchospasm, administration of pulmonary vasodilator drugs such as isoproterenol, sodium nitroprusside, or nitroglycerin inhibits HPV and causes a decrease in Pa_{O_2} and PVR and an increase in right-to-left transpulmonary shunting.[63] The mechanism for these changes is thought to be deleterious inhibition of preexisting and, in some lesions, geographically widespread HPV without concomitant and beneficial bronchodilation.[63] In accordance with the latter two lines of evidence (one-lung or regional hypoxia and vasodilator drug effects on whole-lung or generalized disease), HPV is thought to divert blood flow away from hypoxic regions

of the lung, thereby serving as an autoregulatory mechanism that protects Pa_{O_2} by favorably adjusting regional $\dot{V}_A/\dot{Q}$ ratios. Factors that inhibit regional HPV are extensively discussed elsewhere.[64,65]

c. NEURAL INFLUENCES ON PULMONARY VASCULAR TONE

The three systems used to innervate the pulmonary circulation are the same ones that innervate the airways: the sympathetic, parasympathetic, and nonadrenergic noncholinergic (NANC) systems.[26] Sympathetic (adrenergic) fibers originate from the first five thoracic nerves and enter the pulmonary vessels as branches from the cervical ganglia, as well as from a plexus of nerves arising from the trachea and main stem bronchi. These nerves act mainly on pulmonary arteries down to a diameter of 60 μm.[26] Sympathetic fibers cause pulmonary vasoconstriction through α_1-receptors. However, the pulmonary arteries also contain vasodilatory α_2-receptors and β_2-receptors. The α_1-adrenergic response predominates during sympathetic stimulation, such as occurs with pain, fear, and anxiety.[26] The parasympathetic (cholinergic) nerve fibers originate from the vagus nerve and cause pulmonary vasodilation through an NO-dependent process.[26] Binding of acetylcholine to a muscarinic (M_3) receptor on the endothelial cell increases intracellular calcium and stimulates cNOS.[26] NANC nerves cause pulmonary vasodilation through NO-mediated systems by using vasoactive intestinal peptide as the neurotransmitter. The functional significance of this system is still under investigation.[26]

d. HUMORAL INFLUENCES ON PULMONARY VASCULAR TONE

Numerous molecules are released into the circulation that either affect pulmonary vascular tone (by binding to pulmonary endothelial receptors) or are acted on by the pulmonary endothelium and subsequently become activated or inactivated (Table 5-2). The entire topic of nonrespiratory function of the lung is fascinating but beyond the scope of this chapter. Here, we highlight the effects that circulating molecules have on pulmonary vascular tone.

Although we understand the basic effect that various circulating factors have on pulmonary vascular tone, it is

TABLE 5-2

Effect of Compounds Passing Through Pulmonary Circulation

Molecule	Activated	Unchanged	Inactivated
Amines		Dopamine Epinephrine Histamine	5-Hydroxytryptamine Norepinephrine
Peptides	Angiotensin I	Angiotensin II Oxytocin Vasopressin	Bradykinin Atrial natriuretic peptide Endothelins
Eicosanoids	Arachidonic acid	PGI_2 PGA_2	PGD_2 PGE_1, PGE_2 $PGF_{2\alpha}$ Leukotrienes
Purine derivatives			Adenosine ATP, ADP, AMP

ADP, Adenosine diphosphate; *AMP*, adenosine monophosphate; *ATP*, adenosine triphosphate; *PG*, prostaglandin.
Modified from Lumb AB: Non-respiratory functions of the lung. In Lumb AB, editor: *Nunn's applied respiratory physiology*, ed 5, London, 2000, Butterworths, p 309.

unlikely that these compounds are modulators of pulmonary vascular tone in normal circumstances. However, they have marked effects during disease (e.g., ARDS, sepsis).

Endogenous catecholamines (epinephrine and norepinephrine) bind to both α_1- (vasoconstrictor) and β_2- (vasodilator) receptors on the pulmonary endothelium, but when elaborated in high concentration, they have a predominant α_1 (vasoconstrictor) effect. The same is true for exogenously administered catecholamines. Other amines (e.g., histamine, serotonin) are elaborated systemically or locally after various challenges and have variable effects on PVR. Histamine can be released from mast cells, basophils, and elsewhere. When histamine binds directly to H_1 receptors on endothelium, NO-mediated vasodilation occurs (as seen after epinephrine-induced pulmonary vasoconstriction). Direct stimulation of H_2 receptors on smooth muscle cell membranes also causes vasodilation. In contrast, stimulation of H_1 receptors on the smooth muscle membrane results in vasoconstriction. Serotonin (5-hydroxytryptamine) is a potent vasoconstrictor that can be elaborated from activated platelets (e.g., after pulmonary embolism) and can lead to acute severe pulmonary hypertension.[66]

Numerous peptides circulate and cause either pulmonary vasodilation (e.g., substance P, bradykinin, vasopressin [a systemic vasoconstrictor]) or vasoconstriction (e.g., neurokinin A, angiotensin). These peptides produce clinically detectable effects on PVR only when administered in high concentration, such as with exogenous administration or in disease.

Two other classes of molecules must be mentioned for completeness: eicosanoids (whose vasoactive effects were discussed earlier) and purine nucleosides (which are similarly highly vasoactive).[26] Adenosine is a pulmonary vasodilator in normal subjects, whereas adenosine triphosphate (ATP) has a variable normalizing effect, depending on baseline pulmonary vascular tone.[67]

3. Alternative (Nonalveolar) Pathways of Blood Flow Through the Lung

Blood can use several possible pathways to travel from the right side of the heart to the left without being fully oxygenated or oxygenated at all. Blood flow through poorly ventilated alveoli (regions of low $\dot{V}_A/\dot{Q}$ with an F_{IO_2} <0.3 have a right-to-left shunt effect on oxygenation) and blood flow through nonventilated alveoli (in atelectatic or consolidated regions, $\dot{V}_A/\dot{Q} = 0$ at all F_{IO_2} values) are sources of right-to-left shunting. Low-$\dot{V}_A/\dot{Q}$ and atelectatic lung units occur in conditions in which the FRC is less than the closing capacity (CC) of the lung (see "Lung Volumes, Functional Residual Capacity, and Closing Capacity").

Several right-to-left blood flow pathways through the lungs and heart do not pass by or involve the alveoli at all. The bronchial and pleural circulations originate from systemic arteries and empty into the left side of the heart without being oxygenated; these circulations constitute the 1% to 3% true right-to-left shunt normally present. With chronic bronchitis, the bronchial circulation may carry 10% of the cardiac output, and with pleuritis, the pleural circulation may carry 5% of the cardiac output.

Consequently, as much as a 10% or a 5% obligatory right-to-left shunt may be present, respectively, under these conditions.

Intrapulmonary arteriovenous anastomoses are normally closed, but in the presence of acute pulmonary hypertension, such as may be caused by a pulmonary embolus, they may open and result in a direct increase in right-to-left shunting. The foramen ovale is patent (PFO) in 20% to 30% of individuals but it usually remains functionally closed because left atrial pressure normally exceeds right atrial pressure. However, any condition that causes right atrial pressure to be greater than left atrial pressure may produce a right-to-left shunt, with resultant hypoxemia and possible paradoxical embolization. Such conditions include the use of high levels of PEEP, pulmonary embolization, pulmonary hypertension, COPD, pulmonary valvular stenosis, congestive heart failure, and postpneumonectomy states.[68] Even such common events as mechanical ventilation and reaction to the presence of an endotracheal tube (ETT) during the excitement phase of emergence from anesthesia have caused right-to-left shunting across a PFO and severe arterial desaturation (with the potential for paradoxical embolization).[69,70]

Transesophageal echocardiography has been demonstrated to be a sensitive modality for diagnosing a PFO in anesthetized patients with elevated right atrial pressure.[71] Esophageal to mediastinal to bronchial to pulmonary vein pathways have been described and may explain in part the hypoxemia associated with portal hypertension and cirrhosis. There are no known conditions that selectively increase thebesian channel blood flow. (Thebesian vessels nourish the left ventricular myocardium and originate and empty into the left side of the heart.)

C. Nongravitational Determinants of Pulmonary Compliance, Resistance, Lung Volume, Ventilation, and Work of Breathing

1. Pulmonary Compliance

For air to flow into the lungs, a pressure gradient (ΔP) must be developed to overcome the elastic resistance of the lungs and chest wall to expansion. These structures are arranged concentrically, and their elastic resistance is therefore additive. The relationship between ΔP and the resultant volume increase (ΔV) of the lungs and thorax is independent of time and is known as total compliance (C_T), as expressed in the following equation:

$$C_T \ (L/cm \ H_2O) = \Delta V \ (L)/\Delta P \ (cm \ H_2O) \qquad (1)$$

The C_T of lung plus chest wall is related to the individual compliance of the lungs (C_L) and of the chest wall (C_{CW}) according to the following expression:

$$1/C_T = 1/C_L + 1/C_{CW} \ [or \ C_T = (C_L)(C_{CW})/C_L + C_{CW}] \qquad (2)$$

Normally, C_L and C_{CW} each equal 0.2 L/cm H_2O; hence, $C_T = 0.1$ L/cm H_2O. To determine C_L, ΔV and the transpulmonary pressure gradient ($P_A - P_{pl}$, the ΔP for the lung) must be known; to determine C_{CW}, ΔV and the transmural pressure gradient (Ppl – $P_{ambient}$, the ΔP for the chest wall) must be known; and to determine C_T, ΔV and the transthoracic pressure gradient (PA – $P_{ambient}$, the ΔP for the lung and chest wall together) must be known. In clinical practice, only C_T is measured, which can be done dynamically or statically, depending on whether a peak or a plateau inspiratory ΔP (respectively) is used for the C_T calculation.

During a positive- or negative-pressure inspiration of sufficient duration, transthoracic ΔP first increases to a peak value and then decreases to a lower plateau value. The peak transthoracic pressure value is the pressure required to overcome both elastic and airway resistance (see "Airway Resistance"). Transthoracic pressure decreases to a plateau value after the peak value because with time, gas is redistributed from stiff alveoli (which expand only slightly and therefore have only a short inspiratory period) into more compliant alveoli (which expand a great deal and therefore have a long inspiratory period). Because the gas is redistributed into more compliant alveoli, less pressure is required to contain the same amount of gas, which explains why the pressure decreases. In practical terms, dynamic compliance is the volume change divided by the peak inspiratory transthoracic pressure, and static compliance is the volume change divided by the plateau inspiratory transthoracic pressure. Therefore, static C_T is usually greater than dynamic C_T, because the former calculation uses a smaller denominator (lower pressure) than the latter. However, if the patient is receiving PEEP, that pressure must first be subtracted from the peak or plateau pressure before thoracic compliance is calculated (i.e., compliance is equal to the volume delivered divided by the peak or plateau pressure – PEEP).

Alveolar pressure deserves special comment. The alveoli are lined with a layer of liquid. When a curved surface (a sphere or cylinder, such as the alveoli, bronchioles, and bronchi) is lined with liquid, a surface tension is created that tends to make the surface area that is exposed to the atmosphere as small as possible. Simply stated, water molecules crowd much closer together on the surface of a curved layer of water than elsewhere in the fluid. As lung or alveolar size decreases, the degree of curvature and the retractive surface tension increase.

According to the Laplace expression, shown in equation (3), the pressure in an alveolus (P, in dynes per square centimeter) is higher than ambient pressure by an amount that depends on the surface tension of the lining liquid (T, in dynes per centimeter) and the radius of curvature of the alveolus (R, in centimeters). This relationship is expressed in the following equation:

$$P = 2T/R \qquad (3)$$

Although surface tension contributes to the elastic resistance and retractive forces of the lung, two difficulties must be resolved. First, the pressure inside small alveoli should be higher than that inside large alveoli, a conclusion that stems directly from the Laplace equation (R in the denominator). From this reasoning, one would expect a progressive discharge of each small alveolus into a larger one until eventually only one gigantic alveolus

would be left (Fig. 5-11A). The second problem concerns the relationship between lung volume and transpulmonary ΔP (PA – Ppl). Theoretically, the retractive forces of the lung should increase as lung volume decreases. If this were true, lung volume would decrease in a vicious circle, with an increasingly progressive tendency to collapse as lung volume diminishes.

These two problems are resolved by the fact that the surface tension of the fluid lining the alveoli is variable and decreases as its surface area is reduced. The surface tension of alveolar fluid can reach levels that are well below the normal range for body fluids such as water and plasma. When an alveolus decreases in size, the surface tension of the lining fluid falls to an extent greater than the corresponding reduction in radius; as a result, the transmural pressure gradient (equal to 2T/R) diminishes. This explains why small alveoli do not discharge their contents into large alveoli (see Fig. 5-11B) and why the elastic recoil of small alveoli is less than that of large alveoli.

The substance responsible for the reduction (and variability) in alveolar surface tension is secreted by the intra-alveolar type II pneumocyte; it is a lipoprotein called *surfactant*, which floats as a 50-Å-thick film on the surface of the fluid lining the alveoli. When the surface film is reduced in area and the concentration of surfactant at the surface is increased, the surface-reducing pressure is increased and counteracts the surface tension of the fluid lining the alveoli.

2. Airway Resistance

For air to flow into the lungs, a pressure gradient (ΔP) must also be developed to overcome the nonelastic airway resistance (R_{AW}) of the lungs to airflow. The R_{AW} describes the relationship between ΔP and the rate of airflow ($\dot{V}$).

$$R \, (cm \, H_2O/L/sec) = \frac{\Delta P \, (cm \, H_2O)}{\Delta \dot{V} \, (L/sec)} \qquad (4)$$

The ΔP along the airway depends on the caliber of the airway and the rate and pattern of airflow. There are three main patterns of airflow. Laminar flow occurs when the gas passes down parallel-sided tubes at less than a certain critical velocity. With laminar flow, the pressure drop down the tube is proportional to the flow rate and may be calculated from the equation derived by Poiseuille:

$$\Delta P = \dot{V} \times 8 \, L \times \mu / \pi r^4 \qquad (5)$$

where ΔP is the pressure drop (in cm H_2O), $\dot{V}$ is the volume flow rate (in mL/sec), μ is viscosity (in poises), L is the length of the tube (in cm), and r is the radius of the tube (in cm).

When flow exceeds the critical velocity, it becomes turbulent. The significant feature of turbulent flow is that the pressure drop along the airway is no longer directly proportional to the flow rate but is proportional to the square of the flow rate according to equation (6) for turbulent flow:

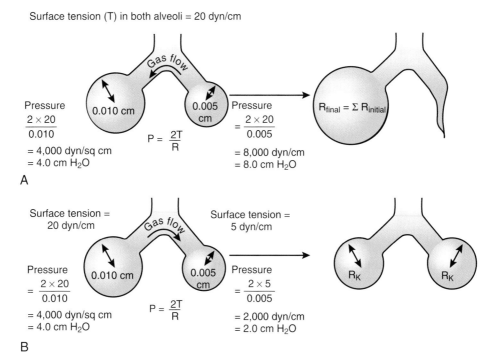

Figure 5-11 Relationship between surface tension (*T*), alveolar radius (*R*), and alveolar transmural pressure (*P*). The left side of the diagrams shows the starting condition, the right side shows the expected result in alveolar size (using the Laplace equation to calculate the starting pressure). In **A**, the surface tension in the fluid lining both the large and the small alveolus is the same (no surfactant). Accordingly, the direction of gas flow is from the higher-pressure small alveolus to the lower-pressure large alveolus, which results in one large alveolus ($R_{final} = \Sigma R_{initial}$). **B** shows the expected changes in surface tension when surfactant lines the alveolus (less tension in the smaller alveolus). The direction of gas flow is from the larger to the smaller alveolus until the two are of equal size and are volume stable (R_K). *K*, Constant; *ΣR*, sum of all individual radii.

$$\Delta P = \dot{V}^2 \rho f L / 4\pi^2 r^5 \qquad (6)$$

where ΔP is the pressure drop (in cm H_2O), $\dot{V}$ is the volume flow rate (in mL/sec), ρ is the density of the gas (or liquid), *f* is a friction factor that depends on the roughness of the tube wall, and r is the radius of the tube (in cm).[72] With increases in turbulent flow (or orifice flow, as described in the next paragraph), ΔP increases much more than $\dot{V}$ and therefore R_{AW} also increases more, as predicted by equation (4).

Orifice flow occurs at severe constrictions such as a nearly closed larynx or a kinked ETT. In these situations, the pressure drop is also proportional to the square of the flow rate, but density replaces viscosity as the important factor in the numerator. This explains why a low-density gas such as helium diminishes the resistance to flow (by threefold in comparison with air) in severe obstruction of the upper airway.

Because the total cross-sectional area of the airways increases as branching occurs, the velocity of airflow decreases in the distal airways; laminar flow is therefore chiefly confined to the airways below the main bronchi. Orifice flow occurs at the larynx, and flow in the trachea is turbulent during most of the respiratory cycle. By examining the components that constitute each of the preceding airway pressure equations, one can see that many factors can affect the pressure drop down the airways during respiration. However, variations in diameter of the smaller bronchi and bronchioles are particularly critical, because bronchoconstriction may convert laminar flow to turbulent flow and the pressure drop along the airways can become much more closely related to the flow rate.

3. Different Regional Lung Time Constants

Thus far, the compliance and airway resistance properties of the chest have been discussed separately. In the following analysis, pressure at the mouth is assumed to increase suddenly to a fixed positive value (Fig. 5-12) that overcomes both elastic and airway resistance and to be maintained at this value during inflation of the lungs.[73] The ΔP required to overcome nonelastic airway resistance is the difference between the fixed mouth pressure and the instantaneous height of the dashed line in Figure 5-12 and is proportional to the flow rate during most of the respiratory cycle.

The ΔP required to overcome nonelastic airway resistance is maximal initially but then decreases exponentially (see Fig. 5-12, A, hatched lines). The rate of filling therefore also declines in an approximately exponential manner. The remainder of the pressure gradient overcomes the elastic resistance (the instantaneous height of the dashed line in Fig. 5-12A) and is proportional to the change in lung volume. The ΔP required to overcome elastic resistance is minimal initially but then increases exponentially, as does lung volume. Alveolar filling ceases (lung volume remains constant) when the pressure

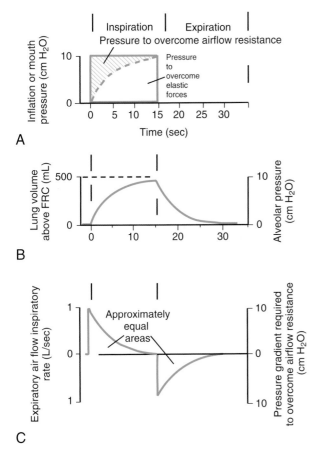

Figure 5-12 Artificial ventilation by intermittent application of constant pressure (square wave) followed by passive expiration. The pressure required to overcome airway resistance (*hatched lines* in **A**) and the airflow rate (in **C**) from equation (4) in the text are proportional to one another and decrease exponentially (assuming that resistance to airflow is constant). The pressure required to overcome the elastic forces (*height of the dashed line* in **A**) and lung volume **(B)** are proportional to one another and increase exponentially. Values shown are typical for an anesthetized supine paralyzed patient: total dynamic compliance, 50 mL/cm H_2O; pulmonary resistance, 3 cm H_2O/L/sec; apparatus resistance, 7 cm H_2O/L/sec; total resistance, 10 cm H_2O/L/sec; time constant, 0.5 seconds. *FRC,* Functional residual capacity. (Redrawn from Lumb AB: Artificial ventilation. In Lumb AB, editor: *Nunn's applied respiratory physiology,* ed 5, London, 2000, Butterworths, p 590.)

resulting from the retractive elastic forces balances the applied (mouth) pressure (see Fig. 5-12A, dashed line).

Because only a finite time is available for alveolar filling and because alveolar filling occurs in an exponential manner, the degree of filling obviously depends on the duration of the inspiration. The rapidity of change in an exponential curve can be described by its time constant τ, which is the time required to complete 63% of an exponentially changing function if the total time allowed for the function change is unlimited ($2\tau = 87\%$, $3\tau = 95\%$, and $4\tau = 98\%$). For lung inflation, $\tau = C_T \times R$; normally, $C_T = 0.1$ L/cm H_2O, $R = 2.0$ cm H_2O/L/sec, $\tau = 0.2$ sec, and $3\tau = 0.6$ sec.

When this equation is applied to individual alveolar units, the time taken to fill such a unit clearly increases as airway resistance increases. The time required to fill an alveolar unit also increases as compliance increases,

because a greater volume of air is transferred into a more compliant alveolus before the retractive force equals the applied pressure. The compliance of individual alveoli differs from top to bottom of the lung, and the resistance of individual airways varies widely depending on their length and caliber. Therefore, various time constants for inflation exist throughout the lung.

4. Pathways of Collateral Ventilation

Collateral ventilation is another nongravitational determinant of the distribution of ventilation. Four pathways of collateral ventilation are known. First, interalveolar communications (pores of Kohn) exist in most species; their number ranges from 8 to 50 per alveolus, and they may increase with age and with the development of obstructive lung disease. Their precise role has not been defined, but they probably function to prevent hypoxia in neighboring but obstructed lung units. Second, distal bronchiole-to-alveolus communications are known to exist (channels of Lambert); their function in vivo is speculative but may be similar to that of the pores of Kohn. Third, respiratory bronchiole–to–terminal bronchiole connections have been found in adjacent lung segments (channels of Martin) in healthy dogs and in humans with lung disease. Fourth, interlobar connections exist; the functional characteristics of interlobar collateral ventilation through these connections have been described in dogs,[74] and they have been observed in humans as well.[75]

5. Work of Breathing

The pressure-volume characteristics of the lung also determine the work of breathing (WOB). Because

$$\text{Work} = \text{Force} \times \text{Distance}$$
$$\text{Force} = \text{Pressure} \times \text{Area} \qquad (7)$$
$$\text{Distance} = \text{Volume/Area}$$

work is defined by the equation

$$\text{Work} = (\text{Pressure} \times \text{Area})(\text{Volume/Area}) = \text{Pressure} \times \text{Volume} \qquad (8)$$

and ventilatory work may be analyzed by plotting pressure against volume.[76] In the presence of increased airway resistance or decreased C_L, increased transpulmonary pressure is required to achieve a given V_T with a consequent increase in the WOB. The metabolic cost of the WOB at rest constitutes only 1% to 3% of the total O_2 consumption in healthy subjects, but it is increased considerably (up to 50%) in patients with pulmonary disease.

Two different pressure-volume diagrams are shown in Figure 5-13. During normal inspiration, transpulmonary pressure increases from 0 to 5 cm H_2O while 500 mL of air is drawn into the lung. Potential energy is stored by the lung during inspiration and is expended during expiration; as a consequence, the entire expiratory cycle is passive. The hatched area plus the triangular area ABC represents pressure multiplied by volume and is the WOB during one breath. Line AB is the lower section of the pressure-volume curve of Figure 5-13. The triangular

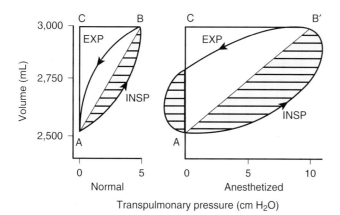

Figure 5-13 Lung volume plotted against transpulmonary pressure in a pressure-volume diagram for a healthy awake patient (Normal) and an anesthetized patient. The lung compliance of the awake patient (slope of line AB = 100 mL/cm H_2O) equals that shown for the small dependent alveoli in Figure 5-3. The lung compliance of the anesthetized patient (slope of line AB′ = 50 mL/cm H_2O) equals that shown for the medium midlung alveoli in Figure 5-3 and for the anesthetized patient in Figure 5-12. The total area within the oval and triangles has the dimensions of pressure multiplied by volume and represents the total work of breathing. The hatched areas to the right of lines AB and AB′ represent the active inspiratory work necessary to overcome resistance to airflow during inspiration *(INSP)*. The hatched area to the left of the triangle AB′C represents the active expiratory work necessary to overcome resistance to airflow during expiration *(EXP)*. Expiration is passive in the healthy subject because sufficient potential energy is stored during inspiration to produce expiratory airflow. The fraction of total respiratory work necessary to overcome elastic resistance is shown by the triangles ABC and AB′C. The anesthetized patient has decreased compliance and increased elastic resistance work (triangle AB′C) compared with the healthy patient's compliance and elastic resistance work (triangle ABC). The anesthetized patient represented in this figure has increased airway resistance to both inspiratory and expiratory work.

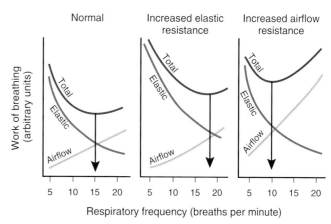

Figure 5-14 The diagrams show the work done against elastic and airflow resistance, both separately and summed to indicate the total work of breathing at different respiratory frequencies. The total work of breathing has a minimal value at approximately 15 breaths/min under normal circumstances. For the same minute volume, minimal work is performed at higher frequencies with stiff (less compliant) lungs and at lower frequencies when airflow resistance is increased. (Redrawn with modification from Lumb AB: Pulmonary ventilation: Mechanisms and the work of breathing. In Lumb AB, editor: *Nunn's applied respiratory physiology*, ed 5, London, 2000, Butterworths, p 128.)

area ABC is the work required to overcome elastic forces (C_T), whereas the hatched area is the work required to overcome airflow or frictional resistance (R). The second graph applies to an anesthetized patient with diffuse obstructive airway disease resulting from the accumulation of mucous secretions. There is a marked increase in both the elastic (triangle AB′C) and the airway (hatched area) resistive components of respiratory work. During expiration, only 250 mL of air leaves the lungs during the passive phase when intrathoracic pressure reaches the equilibrium value of 0 cm H_2O. Active effort-producing work is required to force out the remaining 250 mL of air, and intrathoracic pressure actually becomes positive.

The full WOB over time must include the ventilatory frequency. The following equation depicts the variables included in the WOB equation:

$$WOB = \dot{V}_E \times \frac{R_{AW}}{C_L} \qquad (9)$$

Evaluating each component in the WOB equation, $\dot{V}_E$ is the minute ventilation (rr × V_T) required to achieve a normal Paco$_2$. When patients have an increased CO_2 production (as occurs with fever) the $\dot{V}_E$, and hence the WOB, will need to be higher. When the dead space (either alveolar or anatomic) is increased, the $\dot{V}_E$ will

need to increase to achieve a normal Paco$_2$. Similarly, when airway resistance (R_{AW}) is increased, or compliance (C_L) is decreased, there will be a corresponding increase in the WOB.

Furthermore, for any constant minute volume, the work done against elastic resistance is increased when breathing is deep and slow. On the other hand, the work done against airflow resistance is increased when breathing is rapid and shallow. If the two components are summed and the total work is plotted against respiratory frequency, there is an optimal respiratory frequency at which the total WOB is minimal (Fig. 5-14).[77] In patients with diseased lungs in which elastic resistance is high (e.g., pulmonary fibrosis, pulmonary edema, infants), the optimal frequency is increased, and rapid, shallow breaths are favored. As with other muscles, respiratory muscles can become fatigued, especially with rapid, shallow breathing.[78] When airway resistance is high (e.g., asthma, obstructive lung disease), the optimal frequency is decreased, and slow, deep breaths are favored. Although the optimal frequency is slow (allowing a prolonged expiratory phase), a rapid, shallow breathing pattern also develops in these patients when fatigued and further exacerbates their primary (airway resistance) problem.[78]

6. Lung Volumes, Functional Residual Capacity, and Closing Capacity

a. LUNG VOLUMES AND FUNCTIONAL RESIDUAL CAPACITY

FRC is defined as the volume of gas in the lung at the end of a normal expiration when there is no airflow and P_A equals ambient pressure. Under these conditions, expansive chest wall elastic forces are exactly balanced by retractive lung tissue elastic forces (Fig. 5-15).[79]

The expiratory reserve volume is part of FRC; it is the additional gas beyond the end-tidal volume that can be

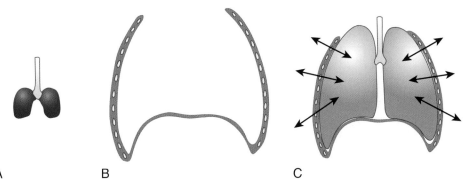

A   B   C

Figure 5-15   A, The resting state of normal lungs when they are removed from the chest cavity; that is, elastic recoil causes total collapse. **B,** The resting state of a normal chest wall and diaphragm when the thoracic apex is open to the atmosphere and the thoracic contents are removed. **C,** The lung volume that exists at the end of expiration is the functional residual capacity (FRC). At FRC, the elastic forces of the lung and chest walls are equal and in opposite directions. The pleural surfaces link these two opposing forces. (Redrawn with modification from Shapiro BA, Harrison RA, Trout CA: The mechanics of ventilation. In Shapiro BA, Harrison RA, Trout CA, editors: *Clinical application of respiratory care,* ed 3, Chicago, 1985, Year Book, p 57.)

consciously exhaled, resulting in the minimum volume of lung possible, known as residual volume. Therefore, FRC equals residual volume plus expiratory reserve volume (Fig. 5-16). With regard to the other lung volumes shown in Figure 5-16, V_T, vital capacity, inspiratory capacity, inspiratory reserve volume, and expiratory reserve volume can be measured by simple spirometry. Total lung capacity (TLC), FRC, and residual volume contain a fraction (residual volume) that cannot be measured by simple spirometry. However, if one of these three volumes is measured, the others can easily be derived, because the other lung volumes, which relate these three volumes to one another, can be measured by simple spirometry.

Residual volume, FRC, and TLC can be measured by any of three techniques: (1) nitrogen washout, (2) inert gas dilution (e.g., helium washin), and (3) total-body plethysmography. The first method, the nitrogen washout technique, is based on measuring expired nitrogen concentrations before and after the patient breathes pure O_2 for several minutes; the difference is the total quantity of nitrogen eliminated. If, for example, 2 L of N_2 is

eliminated and the initial alveolar N_2 concentration was 80%, the initial volume of the lung was 2.5 L. The second method, the inert gas dilution technique, uses the washin of an inert tracer gas such as helium. If 50 mL of helium is introduced into the lungs and, after equilibration, the helium concentration is found to be 1%, the volume of the lung is 5 L. The third method, the total-body plethysmography technique, uses Boyle's law ($P_1V_1 = P_2V_2$, where P_1 = initial pressure, V_1 = initial volume). The subject is confined within a gas-tight box (plethysmograph) so that changes in the volume of the body during respiration may be readily determined as a change in pressure within the sealed box. Although each technique has technical limitations, all are based on sound physical and physiologic principles and provide accurate results in normal patients. Disparity between FRC as measured in the body plethysmograph and as determined by the helium dilution method is often used as a way of detecting large, nonventilating air-trapped blebs.[80] Obviously, there are difficulties in applying the body plethysmograph to anesthetized patients.

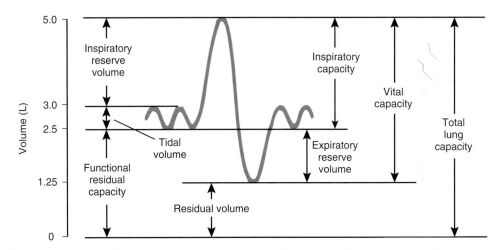

Figure 5-16   The dynamic lung volumes that can be measured by simple spirometry are tidal volume, inspiratory reserve volume, expiratory reserve volume, inspiratory capacity, and vital capacity. The static lung volumes are residual volume, functional residual capacity, and total lung capacity. Static lung volumes cannot be measured by simple spirometry and require separate methods of measurement (e.g., inert gas dilution, nitrogen washout, total-body plethysmography).

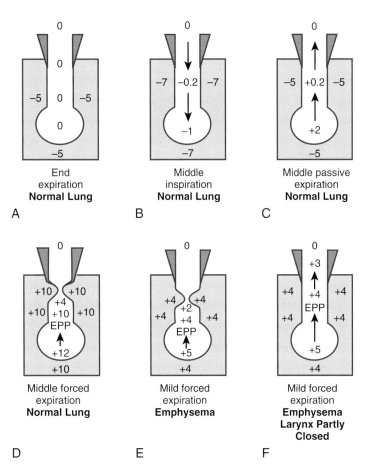

Figure 5-17 Pressure gradients across the airways. The airways consist of a thin-walled intrathoracic portion (near the alveoli) and a more rigid (cartilaginous) intrathoracic and extrathoracic portion. During expiration, the pressure from elastic recoil is assumed to be +2 cm H_2O in normal lungs (**A** through **D**) and +1 cm H_2O in abnormal lungs (**E** and **F**). The total pressure inside the alveolus is pleural pressure plus elastic recoil. The arrows indicate the direction of airflow. *EPP,* Equal pressure point. See text for explanation. (Redrawn with modification from Benumof JL: *Anesthesia for thoracic surgery,* ed 2, Philadelphia, 1995, Saunders, Chapter 8.)

b. AIRWAY CLOSURE AND CLOSING CAPACITY

As discussed earlier (see "Distribution of Ventilation"), Ppl increases from the top to the bottom of the lung and determines regional alveolar size, compliance, and ventilation. Of even greater importance to the anesthesiologist is the recognition that these gradients in Ppl may lead to airway closure and collapse of alveoli.

PATIENT WITH NORMAL LUNGS. Figure 5-17A illustrates the normal resting end-expiratory (FRC) position of the lung–chest wall combination. The distending transpulmonary ΔP and the intrathoracic air passage transmural ΔP are 5 cm H_2O, and the airways remain patent. During the middle of a normal inspiration (see Fig. 5-17B), there is an increase in transmural ΔP (to 6.8 cm H_2O) that encourages distention of the intrathoracic air passages. During the middle of a normal expiration (see Fig. 5-17C), expiration is passive; PA is attributable only to the elastic recoil of the lung (2 cm H_2O), and there is a decrease (to 5.2 cm H_2O) but still a favorable (distending) intraluminal transmural ΔP. During the middle of a severe forced expiration (see Fig. 5-17D), Ppl increases far higher than atmospheric pressure and is communicated to the alveoli, which have a pressure that is still higher because of the elastic recoil of the alveolar septa (an additional 2 cm H_2O).

At high gas flow rates, the pressure drop down the air passage is increased, and there is a point at which intraluminal pressure equals either the surrounding parenchymal pressure or Ppl; that point is termed the *equal pressure point* (EPP). If the EPP occurs in small intrathoracic air passages (distal to the 11th generation, the airways have no cartilage and are called *bronchioles*), they may be held open at that particular point by the tethering effect of the elastic recoil of the immediately adjacent or surrounding lung parenchyma. If the EPP occurs in large extrathoracic air passages (proximal to the 11th generation, the airways have cartilage and are called *bronchi*), they may be held open at that particular point by their cartilage. Downstream of the EPP (in either small or large airways), transmural ΔP is reversed (−6 cm H_2O), and airway closure occurs. Thus, the patency of airways distal to the 11th generation is a function of lung volume, and the patency of airways proximal to the 11th generation is a function of intrathoracic (pleural) pressure. In extrathoracic bronchi with cartilage, the posterior membranous sheath appears to give first by invaginating into the lumen.[81] If lung volume were abnormally decreased (e.g., because of splinting) and expiration were still forced, the caliber of the airways would be relatively reduced at all times, which would cause the EPP and point of collapse to move progressively from larger to smaller air passages (closer to the alveolus).

In adults with normal lungs, airway closure can still occur even if exhalation is not forced, provided that residual volume is approached closely enough. Even in patients with normal lungs, as lung volume decreases toward residual volume during expiration, small airways

(0.5 to 0.9 mm in diameter) show a progressive tendency to close, whereas larger airways remain patent.[82,83] Airway closure occurs first in the dependent lung regions (as directly observed by computed tomography) because the distending transpulmonary pressure is less and the volume change during expiration is greater.[32] Airway closure is most likely to occur in the dependent regions of the lung whether the patient is in the supine or the lateral decubitus position and whether ventilation is spontaneous or positive-pressure ventilation.[32,84,85]

PATIENTS WITH ABNORMAL LUNGS. Airway closure occurs with milder active expiration, lower gas flow rates, and higher lung volumes, and it occurs closer to the alveolus in patients with emphysema, bronchitis, asthma, or interstitial pulmonary edema. In all four conditions, the increased airway resistance causes a larger decrease in pressure from the alveoli to the larger bronchi, thereby creating the potential for negative intrathoracic transmural ΔP and narrowed and collapsed airways. In addition, the structural integrity of the conducting airways may be diminished because of inflammation and scarring, and therefore these airways may close more readily for any given lung volume or transluminal ΔP.

In emphysema, the elastic recoil of the lung is reduced (to 1 cm H_2O in Fig. 5-17 E), the air passages are poorly supported by the lung parenchyma, the point of airway resistance is close to the alveolus, and transmural ΔP can become negative quickly. Therefore, during only a mild forced expiration in an emphysematous patient, the EPP and the point of collapse are near the alveolus (see Fig. 5-17E). The use of pursed-lip or grunting expiration (the equivalents of partly closing the larynx during expiration), PEEP, and continuous positive airway pressure in an emphysematous patient restores a favorable (distending) intrathoracic transmural air ΔP (see Fig. 5-17F). In bronchitis, the airways are structurally weakened and may close when only a small negative transmural ΔP is present (as with mild forced expiration). In asthma, the middle-sized airways are narrowed by bronchospasm, and if expiration is forced, they are further narrowed by a negative transmural ΔP. Finally, with pulmonary interstitial edema, perialveolar interstitial edema compresses the alveoli and acutely decreases FRC; the peribronchial edema fluid cuffs (within the connective tissue sheaths around the larger arteries and bronchi) compress the bronchi and acutely increase closing volume.[86-88]

MEASUREMENT OF CLOSING CAPACITY. CC is a sensitive test of early small-airways disease and is performed by having the patient exhale to residual volume (Fig. 5-18).[89] As inhalation from residual volume toward TLC is begun, a bolus of tracer gas (e.g., xenon 133, helium) is injected into the inspired gas. During the initial part of this inhalation from residual volume, the first gas to enter the alveolus is the V_D gas and the tracer bolus. The tracer gas enters only alveoli that are already open (presumably the apices of the lung) and does not enter alveoli that are already closed (presumably the bases of the lung). As the inhalation continues, the apical alveoli complete filling and the basilar alveoli begin to open and fill, but with gas that does not contain any tracer gas.

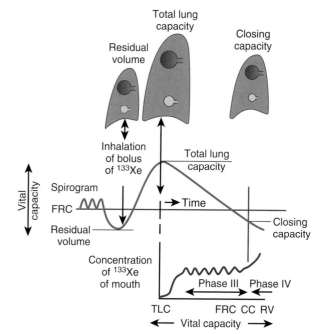

Figure 5-18 Measurement of closing capacity *(CC)* with the use of a tracer gas such as xenon 133 (*^{133}Xe*). The bolus of tracer gas is inhaled near residual volume *(RV)* and, because of airway closure in the dependent lung, is distributed only to nondependent alveoli whose air passages are still open. During expiration, the concentration of tracer gas becomes constant after the dead space is washed out. This plateau *(phase III)* gives way to a rising concentration of tracer gas *(phase IV)*, when there is once again closure of the dependent airways because the only contribution made to expired gas is by the nondependent alveoli with a high ^{133}Xe concentration. *FRC*, Functional residual capacity; *TLC*, total lung capacity. (Redrawn with modification from Lumb AB: Respiratory system resistance: Measurement of closing capacity. In Lumb AB, editor: *Nunn's applied respiratory physiology*, ed 5, London, 2000, Butterworths, p 79.)

A differential tracer gas concentration is thus established, with the gas in the apices having a higher tracer concentration than that in the bases (see Fig. 5-18). As the subject exhales and the diaphragm ascends, a point is reached at which the small airways just above the diaphragm start to close and thereby limit airflow from these areas. The airflow now comes more from the upper lung fields, where the alveolar gas has a much higher tracer concentration, which results in a sudden increase in the tracer gas concentration toward the end of exhalation (phase IV of Fig. 5-18).

Closing volume (CV) is the difference between the onset of phase IV and residual volume; because it represents part of a vital capacity maneuver, it is expressed as a percentage of vital lung capacity. CV plus residual volume is known as CC and is expressed as a percentage of TLC. Smoking, obesity, aging, and the supine position increase CC.[90] In healthy individuals at a mean age of 44 years, CC = FRC in the supine position, and at a mean age of 66 years, CC = FRC in the upright position.[91]

RELATIONSHIP BETWEEN FUNCTIONAL RESIDUAL CAPACITY AND CLOSING CAPACITY. The relationship between FRC and CC is far more important than consideration of FRC or CC alone, because it is this relationship that determines whether a given respiratory unit is normal or atelectatic

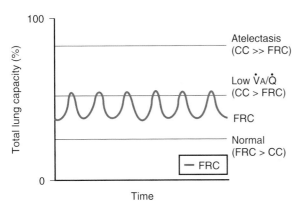

Figure 5-19 Relationship between functional residual capacity *(FRC)* and closing capacity *(CC)*. FRC is the amount of gas in the lungs at end-exhalation during normal tidal breathing, shown by the level of each trough of the sine wave tidal volume. CC is the amount of gas that must be in the lungs to keep the small conducting airways open. This figure shows three different CCs, as indicated by the three different straight lines. See the text for an explanation of why the three different FRC-CC relationships depicted result in normal or low ventilation-perfusion $(\dot{V}A/\dot{Q})$ relationships or atelectasis. The abscissa is time. *(Redrawn from Benumof JL: Anesthesia for thoracic surgery, ed 2, Philadelphia, 1995, Saunders, Chapter 8.)*

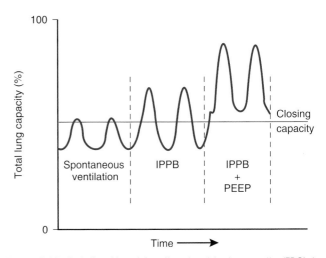

Figure 5-20 Relationship of functional residual capacity (FRC) to closing capacity (CC) during spontaneous ventilation, intermittent positive-pressure breathing *(IPPB)*, and IPPB with positive end-expiratory pressure *(IPPB + PEEP)*. See the text for an explanation of the effect of the two ventilatory maneuvers (IPPB and PEEP) on the relationship of FRC to CC. The abscissa is time.

or has a low $\dot{V}A/\dot{Q}$ ratio. The relationship between FRC and CC is as follows. When the volume of the lung at which some airways close is greater than the whole of VT, lung volume never increases enough during tidal inspiration to open any of these airways. As a result, these airways stay closed during the entire tidal respiration. Airways that are closed all the time are equivalent to atelectasis (Fig. 5-19). If the CV of some airways lies within VT, as lung volume increases during inspiration, some previously closed airways open for a short time until lung volume recedes once again below the CV of these airways. Because these opening and closing airways are open for a shorter time than normal airways are, they have less chance or time to participate in fresh gas exchange, a circumstance equivalent to a low-$\dot{V}A/\dot{Q}$ region. If the CC of the lung is below the whole of tidal respiration, no airways are closed at any time during tidal respiration; this is a normal circumstance. Anything that decreases FRC relative to CC or increases CC relative to FRC converts normal areas to low-$\dot{V}A/\dot{Q}$ and atelectatic areas,[83] which causes hypoxemia.

Mechanical intermittent positive-pressure breathing (IPPB) may be efficacious because it can take a previously spontaneously breathing patient with a low-$\dot{V}A/\dot{Q}$ relationship (in which CC is greater than FRC but still within VT, as depicted in Figure 5-20, right panel) and increase the amount of inspiratory time that some previously closed (at end-exhalation) airways spend in fresh gas exchange, thereby increasing $\dot{V}A/\dot{Q}$ (see Fig. 5-20, middle panel). However, if PEEP is added to IPPB, PEEP increases FRC to a lung volume equal to or greater than CC, thereby restoring a normal FRC-to-CC relationship so that no airways are closed at any time during the tidal respiration depicted in Figure 5-20 (left panel) (IPPB + PEEP). Thus, anesthesia-induced atelectasis (identified by crescent-shaped densities on computed tomography) in the dependent regions of patients' lungs has not been reversed with IPPB alone but has been reversed with IPPB plus PEEP (5 to 10 cm H_2O).[32]

D. Oxygen and Carbon Dioxide Transport

1. Alveolar and Dead Space Ventilation and Alveolar Gas Tensions

In normal lungs, approximately two thirds of each breath reaches perfused alveoli to take part in gas exchange. This constitutes the effective or alveolar ventilation ($\dot{V}A$). The remaining third of each breath takes no part in gas exchange and is therefore termed the total (or physiologic) dead space ventilation (VD). The relationship is as follows: alveolar ventilation ($\dot{V}A$) = frequency (f) (VT − VD). The physiologic (or total) dead space ventilation (VD$_{physiologic}$) may be further divided into two components: a volume of gas that ventilates the conducting airways, the anatomic dead space (VD$_{anatomic}$), and a volume of gas that ventilates unperfused alveoli, the alveolar dead space (VD$_{alveolar}$). Clinical examples of VD$_{alveolar}$ ventilation include zone 1, pulmonary embolus, and destroyed alveolar septa; such ventilation does not participate in gas exchange. Figure 5-21 shows a two-compartment model of the lung in which the anatomic and alveolar dead space compartments have been combined into the total (physiologic) dead space compartment; the other compartment is the alveolar ventilation compartment, whose idealized $\dot{V}A/\dot{Q}$ ratio is 1.0.

The VD$_{anatomic}$ varies with lung size and is approximately 2 mL/kg of body weight (150 mL in a 70-kg adult). In a normal healthy adult lying supine, VD$_{anatomic}$ and total VD are approximately equal to each other, because VD$_{alveolar}$ is normally minimal. In the erect posture, the uppermost alveoli may not be perfused (zone 1), and VD$_{alveolar}$ may increase from a negligible amount to 60 to 80 mL. Figure 5-21 illustrates that in a steady state, the volume of CO_2 entering the alveoli ($\dot{V}CO_2$) is equal to the volume of CO_2 eliminated in the expired gas, ($\dot{V}E$)

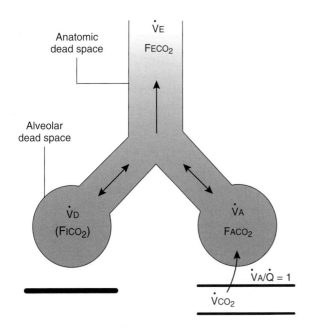

V_D = Total dead space
    = Anatomic + alveolar dead space

Figure 5-21 Two-compartment model of the lung in which the anatomic and alveolar dead space compartments have been combined into the total (physiologic) dead space ($\dot{V}_D$). F_{ACO_2} = alveolar CO_2 fraction; F_{ECO_2} = mixed expired CO_2 fraction; F_{ICO_2} = inspired CO_2 fraction; $\dot{V}_A$ = alveolar ventilation; $\dot{V}_{CO_2}$ = carbon dioxide production; $\dot{V}_E$ = expired minute ventilation. $\dot{V}_A/\dot{Q}$ = 1 means that ventilation and perfusion are equal in liters per minute. Normally, the amount of CO_2 eliminated at the airway ($\dot{V}_E \times F_{ECO_2}$) equals the amount of CO_2 removed by alveolar ventilation ($\dot{V}_A \times F_{ACO_2}$) because there is no CO_2 elimination from alveolar dead space (F_{ICO_2} = 0).

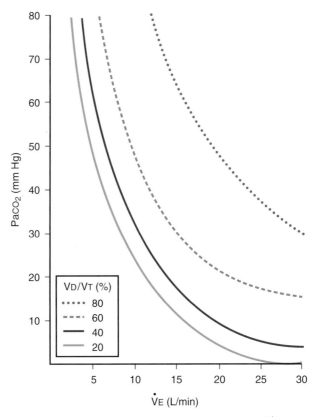

Figure 5-22 Relationship between minute ventilation ($\dot{V}_E$, *L/min*) and arterial partial pressure of carbon dioxide (P_{aCO_2}) for a family of ratios of total dead space to tidal volume (V_D/V_T). These curves are hyperbolic and rise steeply at low $\dot{V}_E$ values. See equation (10) in the text.

(F_{ECO_2}), where $\dot{V}_E$ = minute ventilation and F_{ECO_2} = fraction of expired CO_2. Thus, $\dot{V}_{CO_2} = (\dot{V}_E)(F_{ECO_2})$. However, the expired gas volume consists of alveolar gas, $(\dot{V}_A)(F_{ACO_2})$, and $\dot{V}_D$ gas, $(\dot{V}_D)(F_{ICO_2})$, where F_{ACO_2} and F_{ICO_2} are the alveolar and inspired fractions of CO_2, respectively. Thus, $\dot{V}_{CO_2} = (\dot{V}_A)(F_{ACO_2}) + (\dot{V}_D)(F_{ICO_2})$. Setting the first equation equal to the second equation and using the relationship, $\dot{V}_E = \dot{V}_A + \dot{V}_D$, subsequent algebraic manipulation, including setting P_{ACO_2} equal to P_{aCO_2}, results in the modified Bohr equation:

$$V_D/V_T = (P_{aCO_2} - P_{ECO_2})/P_{aCO_2} \qquad (10)$$

The CO_2 tension in expired gas, P_{ECO_2}, may be obtained by measuring exhaled CO_2 in a large (Douglas) bag or, more commonly, by using end-tidal CO_2 tension (P_{ETCO_2}) as a surrogate. In severe lung disease, physiologic V_D/V_T provides a useful expression of the inefficiency of ventilation. In a healthy adult, this ratio is usually less than 30%; that is, ventilation is more than 70% efficient. In a patient with COPD, V_D/V_T may increase to 60% to 70%. Under these conditions, ventilation is obviously grossly inefficient. Figure 5-22 shows the relationship between $\dot{V}_E$ and P_{aCO_2} for several V_D/V_T values. As $\dot{V}_E$ decreases, P_{aCO_2} increases for all V_D/V_T values. As V_D/V_T increases, a given decrease in $\dot{V}_E$ causes a much greater increase in

P_{aCO_2}. If P_{aCO_2} is to remain constant while V_D/V_T increases, $\dot{V}_E$ must increase more.

The alveolar concentration of a gas is equal to the difference between the inspired concentration and the ratio of the output (or uptake) of the gas to $\dot{V}_A$. Thus, for gas X during dry conditions, $P_{AX} = (P_{dry\ atm})(F_{IX}) \pm \dot{V}_X$ (output or uptake)/$\dot{V}_A$, where P_{AX} = alveolar partial pressure of gas X, F_{IX} = inspired concentration of gas X, $P_{dry\ atm}$ = dry atmospheric pressure = $P_{wet\ atm} - P_{H_2O} = 760 - 47 = 713$ mm Hg, $\dot{V}_X$ = output or uptake of gas X, and $\dot{V}_A$ = alveolar ventilation.

For CO_2, $P_{ACO_2} = 713(F_{ICO_2} + \dot{V}_{CO_2}/\dot{V}_A)$. Because $F_{ICO_2} = 0$ and using standard conversion factors:

$$P_{ACO_2} = 713[\dot{V}_{CO_2}\ (mL/min\ STPD)/\dot{V}_A \\ (L/min/BTPS)(0.863)] \qquad (11)$$

where BTPS = body temperature and pressure, saturated (i.e., 37° C, P_{H_2O} = 47 mm Hg) and STPD = standard temperature and pressure, dry. For example, 36 mm Hg = (713)(200/4000).

For O_2,

$$P_{AO_2} = 713[F_{IO_2} - \dot{V}_{O_2}\ (mL/min)/\dot{V}_A\ (mL/min)] \qquad (12)$$

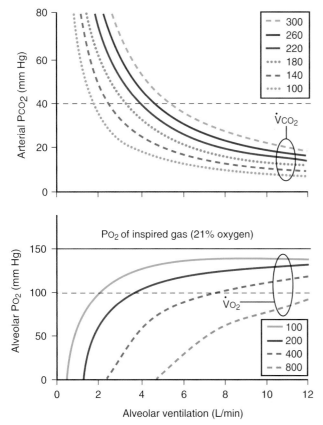

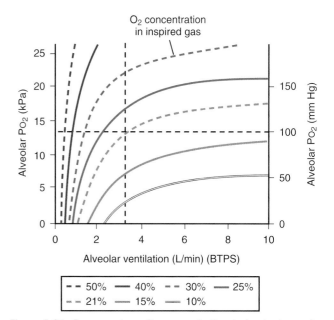

Figure 5-24 For any given O_2 concentration in inspired gas, the relationship between alveolar ventilation and alveolar O_2 tension (P_{AO_2}) is hyperbolic. As the inspired O_2 concentration is increased, the amount that alveolar ventilation must decrease to produce hypoxemia is greatly increased. *BTPS,* Body temperature, ambient pressure, saturated. (Redrawn from Lumb AB: Respiratory system resistance: Measurement of closing capacity. In Lumb AB, editor: *Nunn's applied respiratory physiology,* ed 5, London, 2000, Butterworths, p 79.)

Figure 5-23 *Top,* The relationship between alveolar ventilation and arterial carbon dioxide tension (P_{ACO_2}) for a group of different CO_2 production values ($\dot{V}_{CO_2}$). *Bottom,* The relationship between alveolar ventilation and alveolar oxygen tension (P_{AO_2}) for a group of different O_2 consumption values ($\dot{V}_{O_2}$). Values are derived from equations (10) and (11) in the text, and the curves are hyperbolic. As alveolar ventilation increases, P_{AO_2} and P_{ACO_2} approach inspired concentrations. Decreases in alveolar ventilation to less than 4 L/min are accompanied by precipitous decreases in P_{AO_2} and increases in P_{ACO_2}.

For example, 100 mm Hg = 713(0.21 - 225/3200).

Figure 5-23 shows the hyperbolic relationships expressed in equations (10) and (11) between P_{ACO_2} and $\dot{V}_A$ (see Fig. 5-22) and between P_{AO_2} and $\dot{V}_A$ for different levels of $\dot{V}_{CO_2}$ and $\dot{V}_{O_2}$, respectively. P_{ACO_2} is substituted for P_{ACO_2} because P_{ACO_2}-to-P_{aCO_2} gradients are small (as opposed to P_{AO_2}-to-P_{aO_2} gradients, which can be large). Note that as $\dot{V}_A$ increases, the second term on the right side of equations (11) and (12) approaches zero and the composition of the alveolar gas approaches that of the inspired gas. In addition, Figures 5-22 through Figure 5-24 show that, because anesthesia is usually administered with an oxygen-enriched gas mixture, hypercapnia is a more common result of hypoventilation than hypoxemia is.

2. Oxygen Transport

a. OVERVIEW

The principal function of the heart and lungs is supporting O_2 delivery to and CO_2 removal from the tissues in accordance with metabolic requirements while maintaining arterial blood O_2 and CO_2 partial pressures within a narrow range. The respiratory and cardiovascular systems are linked in series to accomplish this function over a wide range of metabolic requirements, which may increase 30-fold from rest to heavy exercise. The functional links in the O_2 transport chain are as follows: (1) ventilation and distribution of ventilation with respect to perfusion, (2) diffusion of O_2 into blood, (3) chemical reaction of O_2 with Hb, (4) total cardiac output of arterial blood, and (5) distribution of blood to tissues and release of O_2 (Table 5-3). The system is seldom stressed except at exercise, and the earliest symptoms of cardiac or respiratory diseases are often seen only during exercise.

The maximum functional capacity of each link can be determined independently. Table 5-3 lists these measured functional capacities for healthy, young men. Because theoretical maximal O_2 transport at the ventilatory step or at the diffusion and chemical reaction step (approximately 6 L/min in healthy humans at sea level) exceeds the O_2 transportable by the maximum cardiac output and distribution steps, the limit to O_2 transport is the cardiovascular system. Respiratory diseases would not be expected to limit maximum O_2 transport until functional capacities are reduced by 40% to 50%.

b. OXYGEN-HEMOGLOBIN DISSOCIATION CURVE

As a red blood cell (RBC) passes by the alveolus, O_2 diffuses into plasma and increases P_{AO_2}. As P_{AO_2} increases, O_2 diffuses into the RBC and combines with Hb. Each Hb molecule consists of four heme molecules attached to a globin molecule. Each heme molecule consists of glycine, α-ketoglutaric acid, and iron in the ferrous (Fe^{2+}) form. Each ferrous ion has the capacity to bind with one

TABLE 5-3

Functional Capacities and Potential Maximum O_2 Transport of Each Link in the O_2 Transport Chain in Normal Humans* at Sea Level

Link in Chain	Functional Capacity in Normal Humans	Theoretical Maximum O_2 Transport Capacity
Ventilation	200 L/min (MVV)	$0.030 \times$ MVV = 6.0 L O_2/min
Diffusion and chemical reaction		$DLO_2 = 6.1$ L O_2/min
Cardiac output	20 L/min	
O_2 extraction	75%	$0.16 \times$ Cardiac output = 3.2 L O_2/min
($CaO_2 - C\bar{v}O_2$ difference)	(16 mL O_2/100 mL or 0.16)	

*Hemoglobin = 15 g/dL; physiologic dead space in percentage of tidal volume = 0.25; partial alveolar pressure of oxygen >110 mm Hg.
From Cassidy SS: Heart-lung interactions in health and disease. *Am J Med Sci* 30:451–461, 1987.
$CaO_2 - C\bar{v}O_2$, Arteriovenous O_2 content difference; DLO_2, diffusing capacity of lung for oxygen; *MVV*, maximum voluntary ventilation.

O_2 molecule in a loose, reversible combination. As the ferrous ions bind to O_2, the Hb molecule begins to become saturated.

The oxy-Hb dissociation curve relates the saturation of Hb (rightmost y-axis in Fig. 5-25) to PaO_2. Hb is fully saturated (100%) by a PO_2 of approximately 700 mm Hg.

The saturation at normal arterial pressure (point a on upper, flat part of the oxy-Hb curve in Figure 5-25) is 95% to 98%, achieved by a PaO_2 of about 90 to 100 mm Hg. When PO_2 is less than 60 mm Hg (90% saturation), saturation falls steeply, and the amount of Hb uncombined with O_2 increases greatly for a given decrease in PO_2. Mixed venous blood has a PO_2 ($P\bar{v}O_2$) of about 40 mm Hg and is approximately 75% saturated, as indicated by the middle of the three points ($\bar{v}$) on the oxy-Hb curve in Figure 5-25.

The oxy-Hb curve can also relate the O_2 content (CO_2) (vol%, or mL of O_2 per dL of blood; see Fig. 5-25) to PO_2. Oxygen is carried both in solution in plasma (0.003 mL of O_2/mm Hg PO_2 per dL) and combined with Hb (1.39 mL of O_2/g of Hb), to the extent (percentage) that Hb is saturated. Therefore,

$$CO_2 = (1.39)(Hb)(\text{percent saturation}) + 0.003(PO_2) \quad (13)$$

For a patient with an Hb content of 15 g/dL, a PaO_2 of 100 mm Hg, and a $P\bar{v}O_2$ of 40 mm Hg, the arterial O_2 content (CaO_2) = $(1.39)(15)(1) + (0.003)(100)$ = $20.9 + 0.3 = 21.2$ mL/dL; the mixed venous O_2 content ($C\bar{v}O_2$) = $(1.39)(15)(0.75) + (0.003)(40) = 15.6 + 0.1 = 15.7$ mL/dL. Therefore, the normal arteriovenous O_2 content difference is approximately 5.5 mL/dL of blood.

Note that equation (13) uses the constant 1.39, which means that 1 g of Hb can carry 1.39 mL of O_2. Controversy exists over the magnitude of this number. Originally, 1.34 had been used,[92] but with determination of the molecular weight of Hb (64,458), the theoretical

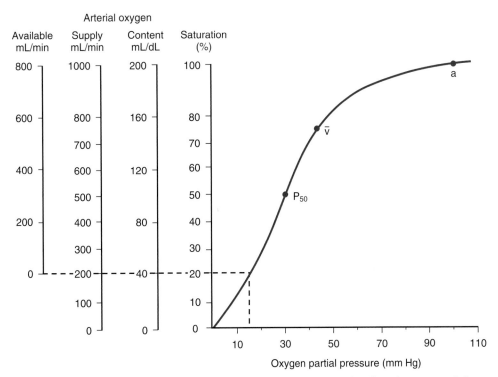

Figure 5-25 Oxygen-hemoglobin dissociation curve. Four different ordinates are shown as a function of oxygen partial pressure (the abscissa). In order from right to left, they are arterial O_2 saturation (%), O_2 content (mL of O_2/dL of blood), O_2 supply to peripheral tissues (mL/min), and O_2 available to peripheral tissues (mL/min), which is O_2 supply minus the approximately 200 mL/min that cannot be extracted below a partial pressure of 20 mm Hg. Three points are shown on the curve: *a*, normal arterial pressure; $\bar{v}$, normal mixed venous pressure; P_{50}, the partial pressure (27 mm Hg) at which hemoglobin is 50% saturated.

value of 1.39 became popular.[93] After extensive human studies, Gregory observed in 1974 that the applicable value was 1.31 mL O_2/g of Hb in human adults.[94] That the clinically measured $\bar{C}_{O_2}$ is lower than the theoretical 1.39 is probably due to the small amount of methemoglobin (MetHb) and carboxyhemoglobin (COHb) normally present in blood.

The oxy-Hb curve can also relate O_2 transport (L/min) to the peripheral tissues (see Fig. 5-25) to P_{O_2}. The term O_2 *transport* is synonymous with the term O_2 *delivery*. This value is obtained by multiplying the O_2 content by $\dot{Q}_T$ (O_2 transport = $\dot{Q}_T \times Ca_{O_2}$). To do this multiplication, one must convert the content unit of mL/dL to mL/L by multiplying by 10; subsequent multiplication of mL/L against $\dot{Q}_T$ in L/min yields mL/min. Thus, if $\dot{Q}_T$ = 5 L/min and Ca_{O_2} = 20 mL of O_2/dL, the arterial point corresponds to 1000 mL O_2/min going to the periphery, and the venous point corresponds to 750 mL O_2/min returning to the lungs, with $\dot{V}_{O_2}$ = 250 mL/min.

The oxy-Hb curve can also relate the O_2 actually available to the tissues (leftmost y axis in Fig. 5-25) as a function of P_{O_2}. Of the 1000 mL/min of O_2 normally going to the periphery, 200 mL/min of O_2 cannot be extracted because it would lower P_{O_2} below the level at which organs such as the brain can survive (rectangular dashed line in Fig. 5-25); the O_2 available to tissues is therefore 800 mL/min. This amount is approximately three to four times the normal resting $\dot{V}_{O_2}$. When $\dot{Q}_T$ = 5 L/min and arterial saturation is less than 40%, the total flow of O_2 to the periphery is reduced to 400 mL/min; the available O_2 is then 200 mL/min, and O_2 supply just equals O_2 demand. Consequently, with low arterial saturation, tissue demand can be met only by an increase in $\dot{Q}_T$ or, in the longer term, by an increase in Hb concentration.

The affinity of Hb for O_2 is best described by the P_{O_2} level at which Hb is 50% saturated (P_{50}) on the oxy-Hb curve. The normal adult P_{50} is 26.7 mm Hg (see Fig. 5-25).

The effect of a change in P_{O_2} on Hb saturation is related to both P_{50} and the portion of the oxy-Hb curve at which the change occurs.[95] In the region of normal Pa_{O_2} (75 to 100 mm Hg), the curve is relatively horizontal, and shifts of the curve have little effect on saturation. In the region of mixed venous P_{O_2}, where the curve is relatively steep, a shift of the curve leads to a much greater difference in saturation. A P_{50} lower than 27 mm Hg describes a left-shifted oxy-Hb curve, which means that at any given P_{O_2}, Hb has a higher affinity for O_2 and is therefore more saturated than normal. This lower P_{50} may require higher than normal tissue perfusion to produce the normal amount of O_2 unloading. Causes of a left-shifted oxy-Hb curve are alkalosis (metabolic and respiratory—the Bohr effect), hypothermia, abnormal fetal Hb, carboxyhemoglobin, methemoglobin, and decreased RBC 2,3-diphosphoglycerate (2,3-DPG) content. (The last condition may occur with the transfusion of old acid citrate-dextrose–stored blood; storage of blood in citrate-phosphate-dextrose minimizes changes in 2,3-DPG with time.[95]) A P_{50} higher than 27 mm Hg describes a right-shifted oxy-Hb curve, which means that at any given P_{O_2}, Hb has a low affinity for O_2 and is less saturated than normal. This higher P_{50} may allow a lower

tissue perfusion than normal to produce the normal amount of O_2 unloading. Causes of a right-shifted oxy-Hb curve are acidosis (metabolic and respiratory—the Bohr effect), hyperthermia, abnormal Hb, increased RBC 2,3-DPG content, and inhaled anesthetics (see later discussion).[95] Abnormalities in acid-base balance result in alteration of 2,3-DPG metabolism to shift the oxy-Hb curve to its normal position. This compensatory change in 2,3-DPG requires between 24 and 48 hours. Therefore, with acute acid-base abnormalities, O_2 affinity and the position of the oxy-Hb curve change. However, with more prolonged acid-base changes, the reciprocal changes in 2,3-DPG levels shift the oxy-Hb curve and O_2 affinity back toward normal.[95]

Many inhaled anesthetics have been shown to shift the oxy-Hb dissociation curve to the right.[96] Isoflurane shifts P_{50} to the right by 2.6 ± 0.07 mm Hg at a vapor pressure of approximately 1 minimum alveolar concentration (MAC) (1.25%).[97] On the other hand, high-dose fentanyl, morphine, and meperidine do not alter the position of the curve.

c. EFFECT OF $\dot{Q}_S/\dot{Q}_T$ ON ALVEOLAR OXYGEN TENSION

$P_{A_{O_2}}$ is directly related to $F_{I_{O_2}}$ in normal patients. $P_{A_{O_2}}$ and $F_{I_{O_2}}$ also correspond to Pa_{O_2} when there is little to no right-to-left transpulmonary shunt ($\dot{Q}_S/\dot{Q}_T$). Figure 5-26 shows the relationship between $F_{I_{O_2}}$ and Pa_{O_2} for a family of right-to-left transpulmonary shunts; the calculations assume a constant and normal $\dot{Q}_T$ and Pa_{CO_2}. With no $\dot{Q}_S/\dot{Q}_T$, a linear increase in $F_{I_{O_2}}$ results in a linear increase in $P_{A_{O_2}}$ (solid straight line). As the shunt is increased, the $\dot{Q}_S/\dot{Q}_T$ lines relating $F_{I_{O_2}}$ to Pa_{O_2} become progressively flatter.[98] With a shunt of 50% of $\dot{Q}_T$, an increase in $F_{I_{O_2}}$ results in almost no increase in Pa_{O_2}. The solution to the problem of hypoxemia secondary to a large shunt is not increasing the $F_{I_{O_2}}$ but rather causing a reduction in the shunt (e.g., PEEP, patient

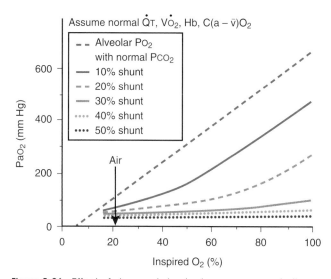

Figure 5-26 Effect of changes in inspired oxygen concentration on arterial oxygen tension *(Pa$_{O_2}$)* for various right-to-left transpulmonary shunts. Cardiac output *($\dot{Q}_T$)*, hemoglobin *(Hb)*, oxygen consumption *($\dot{V}_{O_2}$)*, and arteriovenous oxygen content differences *(C(a – v̄)$_{O_2}$)* are assumed to be normal. Pco$_2$, partial pressure of carbon dioxide; Po$_2$, partial pressure of oxygen.

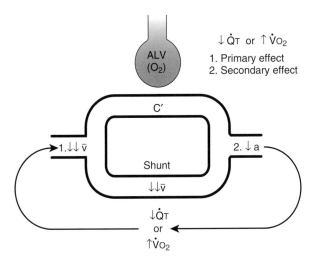

Figure 5-27 Effect of a decrease in cardiac output ($\dot{Q}T$) or an increase in oxygen consumption ($\dot{V}O_2$) on mixed venous and arterial oxygen content. Mixed venous blood ($\bar{v}$) either perfuses ventilated alveolar capillaries (*ALV*) and becomes oxygenated end-pulmonary capillary blood (c´), or it perfuses whatever true shunt pathways exist and remains the same in composition (i.e., desaturated). These two pathways must ultimately join together to form mixed arterial (*a*) blood. If $\dot{Q}T$ decreases or $\dot{V}O_2$ increases, or both, the tissues must extract more oxygen per unit volume of blood than under normal conditions. Thus, the primary effect of a decrease in $\dot{Q}T$ or an increase in $\dot{V}O_2$ is a decrease in mixed venous oxygen content. The mixed venous blood with a decreased oxygen content must flow through the shunt pathway as before (which may remain constant in size) and lower the arterial content of oxygen. Thus, the secondary effect of a decrease in $\dot{Q}T$ or an increase in $\dot{V}O_2$ is a decrease in arterial oxygen content.

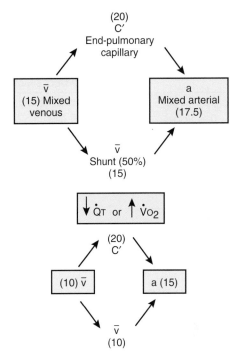

Figure 5-28 The equivalent circuit of the pulmonary circulation in a patient with a 50% right-to-left shunt. Oxygen content is in mL/dL of blood. A decrease in cardiac output ($\dot{Q}T$) or an increase in O_2 consumption ($\dot{V}O_2$) can cause a decrease in mixed venous oxygen content, from 15 to 10 mL/dL in this example, which in turn causes a decrease in the arterial content of oxygen, from 17.5 to 15.0 mL/dL. In this 50% shunt example, the decrease in mixed venous oxygen content was twice the decrease in arterial oxygen content.

positioning, suctioning, fiberoptic bronchoscopy, diuretics, antibiotics).

d. EFFECT OF $\dot{Q}T$ AND $\dot{V}O_2$ ON ARTERIAL OXYGEN CONTENT

In addition to an increased $\dot{Q}s/\dot{Q}T$, CaO_2 is decreased by decreased $\dot{Q}T$ (for a constant $\dot{V}O_2$) and by increased $\dot{V}O_2$ (for a constant $\dot{Q}T$). In either case, along with a constant right-to-left shunt, the tissues must extract more O_2 from blood per unit blood volume, and therefore, $C\bar{v}O_2$ must primarily decrease (Fig. 5-27). When blood with lower $C\bar{v}O_2$ passes through whatever shunt exists in the lung and remains unchanged in its $\dot{V}O_2$, it must inevitably mix with oxygenated end-pulmonary capillary blood (c´ flow) and secondarily decrease CaO_2. The amount of O_2 flowing per minute through any particular lung channel, as depicted in Figure 5-27, is a product of blood flow times the O_2 content of that blood. Thus, $\dot{Q}T \times CaO_2 = \dot{Q}c´ \times Cc´O_2 + \dot{Q}s \times C\bar{v}O_2$. With $\dot{Q}c´ = \dot{Q}T - \dot{Q}s$ and further algebraic manipulation,[99]

$$\dot{Q}s/\dot{Q}T = Cc´O_2 - CaO_2/Cc´O_2 - C\bar{v}O_2 \quad (14)$$

The larger the intrapulmonary shunt, the greater is the decrease in CaO_2, because more venous blood with lower $C\bar{v}O_2$ can admix with end-pulmonary capillary blood (c´) (see Fig. 5-37).[100,101] Therefore, the alveolar-arterial oxygen difference $P(A - a)O_2$ is a function both of the size of the $\dot{Q}s/\dot{Q}T$ and of what is flowing through the $\dot{Q}s/\dot{Q}T$—namely, $C\bar{v}O_2$—and $C\bar{v}O_2$ is a primary

function of $\dot{Q}T$ and $\dot{V}O_2$. Figure 5-28 shows the equivalent circuit of the pulmonary circulation in a patient with a 50% shunt, a normal $C\bar{v}O_2$ of 15 mL/dL, and a moderately low CaO_2 of 17.5 mL/dL. Decreasing $\dot{Q}T$ or increasing $\dot{V}O_2$, or both, causes a larger primary decrease in $C\bar{v}O_2$ to 10 mL/dL and a smaller but still significant secondary decrease in CaO_2 to 15 mL/dL; the ratio of change in $C\bar{v}O_2$ to change in CaO_2 in this example of 50% $\dot{Q}s/\dot{Q}T$ is 2:1.

If a decrease in $\dot{Q}T$ or an increase in $\dot{V}O_2$ is accompanied by a decrease in $\dot{Q}s/\dot{Q}T$, there may be no change in PaO_2 (i.e., a decreasing effect on PaO_2 is offset by an increasing effect on PaO_2) (Table 5-4). These changes sometimes occur in diffuse lung disease. However, if a decrease in $\dot{Q}T$ or an increase in $\dot{V}O_2$ is accompanied by an increase in $\dot{Q}s/\dot{Q}T$, PaO_2 may be greatly decreased (i.e., a decreasing effect on PaO_2 is compounded by another decreasing effect on PaO_2). These changes sometimes occur in regional ARDS and atelectasis.[102]

e. FICK PRINCIPLE

The Fick principle allows calculation of $\dot{V}O_2$ and states that the amount of O_2 consumed by the body ($\dot{V}O_2$) is equal to the amount of O_2 leaving the lungs ($\dot{Q}T$)(CaO_2) minus the amount of O_2 returning to the lungs ($\dot{Q}T$)($C\bar{v}O_2$):

$$\dot{V}O_2 = (\dot{Q}T)(CaO_2) - (\dot{Q}T)(C\bar{v}O_2) = \dot{Q}T(CaO_2 - C\bar{v}O_2)$$

Relationship Between Cardiac Output ($\dot{Q}_T$), Shunt ($\dot{Q}_S/\dot{Q}_T$), and Venous ($P\bar{v}_{O_2}$) and Arterial (Pa_{O_2}) Oxygenation

Changes	Clinical Situation
If $\dot{Q}_T \downarrow \rightarrow \downarrow P\bar{v}_{O_2}$ and $\dot{Q}_S/\dot{Q}_T = 0 \rightarrow Pa_{O_2}\downarrow$	Decreased cardiac output, stable shunt
If $\dot{Q}_T \downarrow \rightarrow \downarrow P\bar{v}_{O_2}$ and $\dot{Q}_S/\dot{Q}_T \downarrow \rightarrow Pa_{O_2} = 0$	Application of PEEP in ARDS
If $\dot{Q}_T \downarrow \rightarrow \downarrow P\bar{v}_{O_2}$ and $\dot{Q}_S/\dot{Q}_T \uparrow \rightarrow Pa_{O_2} \downarrow\downarrow$	Shock combined with ARDS or atelectasis

ARDS, Adult respiratory distress syndrome; *0,* no change; *PEEP,* positive end-expiratory pressure; ↓, decrease; ↑, increase.

Condensing the content symbols yields the usual expression of the Fick equation:

$$\dot{V}_{O_2} = (\dot{Q}_T)[C(a-\bar{v})_{O_2}] \qquad (15)$$

This equation states that O_2 consumption is equal to $\dot{Q}_T$ times the arteriovenous O_2 content difference $[C(a - \bar{v})O_2]$. Normally, (5 L/min)(5.5 mL)/dL = 0.27 L/min (see "Oxygen-Hemoglobin Dissociation Curve").

$$\dot{V}_{O_2} = \dot{V}_E(F_{IO_2}) - \dot{V}_E(F_{EO_2}) = \dot{V}_E(F_{IO_2} - F_{EO_2}) \qquad (16)$$

Similarly, the amount of O_2 consumed by the body ($\dot{V}_{O_2}$) is equal to the amount of O_2 brought into the lungs by ventilation ($\dot{V}_I$)(F_{IO_2}) minus the amount of O_2 leaving the lungs by ventilation ($\dot{V}_E$)(F_{EO_2}), where $\dot{V}_E$ is expired minute ventilation and F_{EO_2} is the mixed expired O_2 fraction: $\dot{V}_{O_2} = (\dot{V}_I)(F_{IO_2}) - (\dot{V}_E)(F_{EO_2})$. Because the difference between $\dot{V}_I$ and $\dot{V}_E$ is due to the difference between $\dot{V}_{O_2}$ (normally 250 mL/min) and $\dot{V}_{CO_2}$ (normally 200 mL/min) and is only 50 mL/min (see later discussion), $\dot{V}_I$ essentially equals $\dot{V}_E$.

Normally, $\dot{V}_{O_2} = 5.0$ L/min(0.21 − 0.16) = 0.25 L/min. In determining $\dot{V}_{O_2}$ in this way, $\dot{V}_E$ can be measured with a spirometer, F_{IO_2} can be measured with an O_2 analyzer or from known fresh gas flows, and F_{EO_2} can be measured by collecting expired gas in a bag for a few minutes. A sample of the mixed expired gas is used to measure P_{EO_2}. To convert P_{EO_2} to F_{EO_2}, one simply divides P_{EO_2} by dry atmospheric pressure: $P_{EO_2}/713 = F_{EO_2}$.

In addition, the Fick equation is useful in understanding the impact of changes in $\dot{Q}_T$ on Pa_{O_2} and $P\bar{v}_{O_2}$. If $\dot{V}_{O_2}$ remains constant (K) and $\dot{Q}_T$ decreases (↓), the arteriovenous O_2 content difference has to increase (↑):

$$\dot{V}_{O_2} = K = (\downarrow)\dot{Q}_T \, x(\uparrow)C(a-\bar{v})_{O_2}$$

The $C(a - \bar{v})_{O_2}$ difference increases because a decrease in $\dot{Q}_T$ causes a much larger and primary decrease in $C\bar{v}_{O_2}$ versus a smaller and secondary decrease in Ca_{O_2}, as follows[101]:

$$(\uparrow)C(a-\bar{v})_{O_2} = C(\downarrow a - \downarrow\downarrow \bar{v})_{O_2}$$

Thus, $C\bar{v}_{O_2}$ and $P\bar{v}_{O_2}$ are much more sensitive indicators of $\dot{Q}_T$ because they change more with

changes in $\dot{Q}_T$ than Ca_{O_2} (or Pa_{O_2}) does (see Figs. 5-27 and 5-37).

3. Carbon Dioxide Transport

The amount of CO_2 circulating in the body is a function of both CO_2 elimination and CO_2 production. Elimination of CO_2 depends on pulmonary blood flow and alveolar ventilation. Production of CO_2 ($\dot{V}_{CO_2}$) parallels O_2 consumption ($\dot{V}_{O_2}$) according to the respiratory quotient (RQ):

$$RQ = \frac{\dot{V}_{CO_2}}{\dot{V}_{O_2}} \qquad (17)$$

Under normal resting conditions, RQ is 0.8; that is, only 80% as much CO_2 is produced as O_2 is consumed. However, this value changes as the nature of the metabolic substrate changes. If only carbohydrate is used, the RQ is 1.0. Conversely, with the sole use of fat, more O_2 combines with hydrogen to produce water, and the RQ value drops to 0.7. CO_2 is transported from mitochondria to the alveoli in a number of forms. In plasma, CO_2 exists in physical solution, hydrated to carbonic acid (H_2CO_3), and as bicarbonate (HCO_3^-). In the RBC, CO_2 combines with Hb as carbaminohemoglobin (Hb-CO_2). The approximate values of H_2CO_3 ($H_2O + CO_2$), HCO_3^-, and Hb-CO_2 relative to the total CO_2 transported are 7%, 80%, and 13%, respectively.

In plasma, CO_2 exists both in physical solution and as H_2CO_3:

$$H_2O + CO_2 \rightarrow H_2CO_3 \qquad (18)$$

The CO_2 in solution can be related to P_{CO_2} by the use of Henry's law.[103]

$$P_{CO_2} \times a = [CO_2] \text{ in solution} \qquad (19)$$

where a is the solubility coefficient of CO_2 in plasma (0.03 mmol/L/mm Hg at 37° C). However, the major fraction of CO_2 produced passes into the RBC. As in plasma, CO_2 combines with water to produce H_2CO_3. However, unlike the slow reaction in plasma, in which the equilibrium point lies toward the left, the reaction in an RBC is catalyzed by the enzyme carbonic anhydrase. This zinc-containing enzyme moves the reaction to the right at a rate 1000 times faster than in plasma. Furthermore, almost 99.9% of the H_2CO_3 dissociates to HCO_3^- and hydrogen ions (H^+):

$$H_2O + CO_2 \xrightarrow[H_2CO_3 \rightarrow H^+ + HCO_3^-]{\text{carbonic anhydrase}} H_2CO_3 \qquad (20)$$

The H^+ produced from H_2CO_3 in the production of HCO_3^- is buffered by Hb ($H^+ + Hb \rightleftharpoons HHb$). The HCO_3^- produced passes out of the RBC into plasma to perform its function as a buffer. To maintain electrical neutrality within the RBC, chloride ion (⁻) moves in as HCO_3^- moves out (⁻ shift). Finally, CO_2 can combine with Hb in the erythrocyte (to produce Hb-CO_2). Again, as in HCO_3^- release, an H^+ ion is formed in the reaction of CO_2 and Hb. This H^+ ion is also buffered by Hb.

4. Bohr and Haldane Effects

Just as the percent saturation of Hb with O_2 is related to P_{O_2} (described by the oxy-Hb curve), so the total CO_2 in blood is related to P_{CO_2}. In addition, Hb has variable affinity for CO_2; it binds more avidly in the reduced state than as oxy-Hb.[95] The Bohr effect describes the effect of P_{CO_2} and $[H^+]$ ions on the oxy-Hb curve. Hypercapnia and acidosis both shift the curve to the right (reducing the O_2-binding affinity of hemoglobin), and hypocapnia and alkalosis both shift the curve to the left. Conversely, the Haldane effect describes the shift in the CO_2 dissociation curve caused by oxygenation of Hb. Low P_{O_2} shifts the CO_2 dissociation curve to the left so that the blood is able to pick up more CO_2 (as occurs in capillaries of rapidly metabolizing tissues). Conversely, oxygenation of Hb (as occurs in the lungs) reduces the affinity of Hb for CO_2, and the CO_2 dissociation curve is shifted to the right, thereby increasing CO_2 removal.

E. Pulmonary Microcirculation, Interstitial Space, and Fluid (Pulmonary Edema)

The ultrastructural appearance of an alveolar septum is depicted schematically in Figure 5-29.[104] Capillary blood is separated from alveolar gas by a series of anatomic layers: capillary endothelium, endothelial basement membrane, interstitial space, epithelial basement membrane, and alveolar epithelium (of the type I pneumocyte).

On one side of the alveolar septum (the thick, upper, fluid- and gas-exchanging side), the epithelial and endothelial basement membranes are separated by a space of variable thickness containing connective tissue fibrils,

elastic fibers, fibroblasts, and macrophages. This connective tissue is the backbone of the lung parenchyma; it forms a continuum with the connective tissue sheaths around the conducting airways and blood vessels. Thus, the pericapillary perialveolar interstitial space is continuous with the interstitial tissue space that surrounds terminal bronchioles and vessels, and both spaces constitute the connective tissue space of the lung. There are no lymphatics in the interstitial space of the alveolar septum. Instead, lymphatic capillaries first appear in the interstitial space surrounding terminal bronchioles, small arteries, and veins.[105]

The opposite side of the alveolar septum (the thin, down, gas-exchanging-only side) contains only fused epithelial and endothelial basement membranes. The interstitial space is greatly restricted on this side because of fusion of the basement membranes. Interstitial fluid cannot separate the endothelial and epithelial cells from one another. As a result the space and distance barrier to fluid movement from the capillary to the alveolar compartment is reduced; it is composed of only the two cell linings with their associated basement membranes.[106]

Between the individual endothelial and epithelial cells are holes or junctions that provide a potential pathway for fluid to move from the intravascular space to the interstitial space and finally from the interstitial space to the alveolar space (see Fig. 5-29). The junctions between endothelial cells are relatively large and are therefore termed "loose"; the junctions between epithelial cells are relatively small and are therefore termed "tight." Pulmonary capillary permeability is a direct function of, and essentially equivalent to, the size of the holes in the endothelial and epithelial linings.

To understand how pulmonary interstitial fluid is formed, stored, and cleared, it is necessary first to develop the concepts that (1) the pulmonary interstitial space is a continuous space between the periarteriolar and peribronchial connective tissue sheath and the space between the endothelial and epithelial basement membranes in the alveolar septum and (2) the space has a progressively negative distal-to-proximal ΔP.

The concepts of a continuous connective tissue sheath–alveolar septum interstitial space and a negative interstitial space ΔP are prerequisite to understanding interstitial fluid kinetics. After entering the lung parenchyma, both the bronchi and the arteries run within a connective tissue sheath that is formed by an invagination of the pleura at the hilum and ends at the level of the bronchioles (Fig. 5-30A). This results in a potential perivascular space between the arteries and the connective tissue sheath and a potential peribronchial space between the bronchi and the connective tissue sheath. The negative pressure in the pulmonary tissues surrounding the perivascular connective tissue sheath exerts a radial outward traction force on the sheath. This radial traction creates negative pressure within the sheath that is transmitted to the bronchi and arteries and tends to hold them open and increase their diameters.[106] The alveolar septum interstitial space is the space between the capillaries and alveoli (or, more precisely, the space between the endothelial and epithelial basement membranes) and is continuous with the interstitial tissue space that surrounds the larger

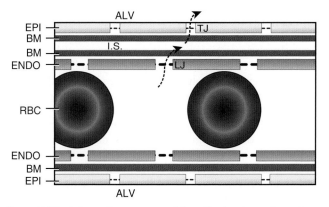

Figure 5-29 Schematic summary of the ultrastructure of a pulmonary capillary. On the upper side of the capillary, the endothelial *(ENDO)* and epithelial *(EPI)* basement membranes *(BM)* are separated by an interstitial space *(I.S.)*, whereas the lower side contains only fused ENDO and EPI BMs. The dashed arrows indicate a potential pathway for fluid to move from the intravascular space to the I.S. through loose junctions *(LJ)* in the endothelium and from the I.S. to the alveolar space *(ALV)* through tight junctions *(TJ)* in the epithelium. *RBC,* Red blood cell. (Redrawn from Fishman AP: Pulmonary edema: The water-exchanging function of the lung. *Circulation* 46:390, 1972.)

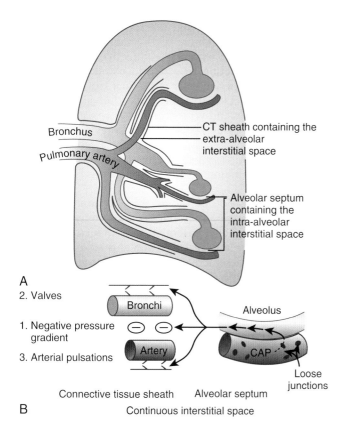

A

2. Valves

1. Negative pressure gradient

3. Arterial pulsations

Bronchi

Alveolus

Artery

CAP

Loose junctions

Connective tissue sheath   Alveolar septum

B   Continuous interstitial space

Figure 5-30 A, Schematic diagram of the concept of a continuous connective tissue sheath–alveolar septum interstitial space. The entry of the main stem bronchi and pulmonary artery into the lung parenchyma invaginates the pleura at the hilum and forms a surrounding connective tissue sheath. The connective tissue sheath ends at the level of the bronchioles. The space between the pulmonary arteries and bronchi and the interstitial space is continuous with the alveolar septum interstitial space. The alveolar septum interstitial space is contained within the endothelial basement membrane of the capillaries and the epithelial basement membrane of the alveoli. **B,** Schematic diagram showing how interstitial fluid moves from the alveolar septum interstitial space (no lymphatics) to the connective tissue interstitial space (lymphatic capillaries first appear). The mechanisms are a negative-pressure gradient (sump), the presence of one-way valves in the lymphatics, and the massaging action of arterial pulsations. *CAP,* Capillary. (Redrawn with modification from Benumof JL: *Anesthesia for thoracic surgery,* ed 2, Philadelphia, 1995, Saunders, Chapter 8.)

arteries and bronchi. Studies indicate that the alveolar interstitial pressure is also uniquely negative but not as much so as the negative interstitial space pressure around the larger arteries and bronchi.[107]

The forces governing net transcapillary–interstitial space fluid movement are as follows. The net transcapillary flow of fluid (F) out of pulmonary capillaries (across the endothelium and into the interstitial space) is equal to the difference between pulmonary capillary hydrostatic pressure (P_{inside}) and interstitial fluid hydrostatic pressure ($P_{outside}$) and the difference between capillary colloid oncotic pressure (π_{inside}) and interstitial colloid oncotic pressure ($\pi_{outside}$). These four forces produce a steady-state fluid flow (F) during a constant capillary permeability (K) as predicted by the Starling equation:

$$F = K[(P_{inside} - P_{outside}) - (\pi_{inside} - \pi_{outside})] \quad (21)$$

Box 5-1 Causes of Extremely Negative Pulmonary Interstitial Fluid Pressure ($P_{outside}$) in Pulmonary Edema

Vigorous spontaneous ventilation against an obstructed airway
  Laryngospasm
  Infection, inflammation, edema
  Upper airway mass (e.g., tumor, hematoma, abscess, foreign body)
  Vocal cord paralysis
  Strangulation
Rapid reexpansion of lung
Vigorous pleural suctioning (thoracentesis, chest tube)

K is a capillary filtration coefficient expressed in mL/min/mm Hg/100 g. The filtration coefficient is the product of the effective capillary surface area in a given mass of tissue and the permeability per unit surface area of the capillary wall to filter the fluid. Under normal circumstances and at a vertical height in the lung that is at the junction of zones 2 and 3, intravascular colloid oncotic pressure (≈ 26 mm Hg) acts to keep water in the capillary lumen; working against this force, pulmonary capillary hydrostatic pressure (≈ 10 mm Hg) acts to force water across the loose endothelial junctions into the interstitial space. If these were the only operative forces, the interstitial space and, consequently, the alveolar surfaces would be constantly dry and there would be no lymph flow. In fact, alveolar surfaces are moist, and lymphatic flow from the interstitial compartment is constant (≈ 500 mL/day). This can be explained in part by $\pi_{outside}$ (≈ 8 mm Hg) and in part by the negative $P_{outside}$ (-8 mm Hg).

Negative (subatmospheric) interstitial space pressure would promote, by suction, a slow loss of fluid across the endothelial holes.[108] Indeed, extremely negative pleural (and perivascular hydrostatic) pressure, such as may occur in a vigorously spontaneously breathing patient with an obstructed airway, can cause pulmonary interstitial edema (Box 5-1).[109] Relative to the vertical level of the junction of zones 2 and 3, as lung height decreases (lung dependence), absolute P_{inside} increases, and fluid has a propensity to transudate; as lung height increases (lung nondependence), absolute P_{inside} decreases, and fluid has a propensity to be reabsorbed. However, fluid transudation induced by an increase in P_{inside} is limited by a concomitant dilution of proteins in the interstitial space and therefore a decrease in $\pi_{outside}$.[110] Any change in the size of the endothelial junctions, even if the foregoing four forces remain constant, changes the magnitude and perhaps even the direction of fluid movement. Increased size of endothelial junctions (increased permeability) promotes transudation, whereas decreased size of endothelial junctions (decreased permeability) promotes reabsorption.

No lymphatics are present in the interstitial space of the alveolar septum. The lymphatic circulation starts as blind-ended lymphatic capillaries, first appearing in the interstitial space sheath surrounding terminal bronchioles and small arteries, and ends at the subclavian veins. Interstitial fluid is normally removed from the alveolar interstitial space into the lymphatics by a sump (pressure gradient) mechanism, which is caused by the presence of more negative pressure surrounding the larger arteries and bronchi.[3,111] The sump mechanism is aided by the presence of valves in the lymph vessels. In addition, because the lymphatics run in the same sheath as the pulmonary arteries, they are exposed to the massaging action of arterial pulsations. The differential negative pressure, the lymphatic valves, and the arterial pulsations all help propel the lymph proximally toward the hilum through the lymph nodes (pulmonary to bronchopulmonary to tracheobronchial to paratracheal to scalene and cervical nodes) to the central venous circulation depot (see Fig. 5-30B). An increase in central venous pressure, which is the backpressure for lymph to flow out of the lung, would decrease lung lymph flow and perhaps promote pulmonary interstitial edema.

If the rate of entry of fluid into the pulmonary interstitial space exceeds the capability of the pulmonary interstitial space to clear the fluid, the pulmonary interstitial space fills with fluid; the fluid, now under an increased and positive driving force (P_{ISF}), crosses the relatively impermeable epithelial wall holes, and the alveolar space fills. Intra-alveolar edema fluid also causes alveolar collapse and atelectasis, thereby promoting further accumulation of fluid and worsening right-to-left transpulmonary shunt.

II. RESPIRATORY FUNCTION DURING ANESTHESIA

Arterial oxygenation is impaired in most patients during anesthesia with either spontaneous or controlled ventilation.[112-117] In otherwise normal patients, it is generally accepted that the impairment in arterial oxygenation during anesthesia is more severe in elderly persons,[118,119] obese people,[120] and smokers.[121] In various studies of healthy young to middle-aged patients under general anesthesia, venous admixture (shunt) has been found to average 10%, and the scatter in $\dot{V}_A/\dot{Q}$ ratios is small to moderate.[119,122] In patients with a more marked deterioration in preoperative pulmonary function, general anesthesia causes considerable widening of the $\dot{V}_A/\dot{Q}$ distribution and large increases in both low-$\dot{V}_A/\dot{Q}$ (0.005 < $\dot{V}_A/\dot{Q}$ < 0.1) (underventilated) regions and shunting.[118,121,123] The magnitude of shunting correlates closely with the degree of atelectasis.[118,123]

In addition to these generalizations concerning respiratory function during anesthesia, the effect of a given anesthetic on respiratory function depends on the depth of general anesthesia, the patient's preoperative respiratory condition, and the presence of special intraoperative anesthetic and surgical conditions.

A. Anesthetic Depth and Respiratory Pattern

The respiratory pattern is altered by the induction and deepening of anesthesia. When the depth of anesthesia is inadequate (less than MAC), the respiratory pattern may vary from excessive hyperventilation and vocalization to breath-holding. As anesthetic depth approaches or equals MAC (light anesthesia), irregular respiration progresses to a more regular pattern that is associated with a larger than normal V_T. However, during light but deepening anesthesia, the approach to a more regular respiratory pattern may be interrupted by a pause at the end of inspiration (a "hitch" in inspiration), followed by a relatively prolonged and active expiration in which the patient seems to exhale forcefully rather than passively. As anesthesia deepens to moderate levels, respiration becomes faster and more regular but shallower. The respiratory pattern is a sine wave losing the inspiratory hitch and lengthened expiratory pause. There is little or no inspiratory or expiratory pause, and the inspiratory and expiratory periods are equivalent. Intercostal muscle activity is still present, and there is normal movement of the thoracic cage with lifting of the chest during inspiration.

The respiratory rate is generally slower and the V_T larger with nitrous oxide–narcotic anesthesia than with anesthesia involving halogenated drugs. During deep anesthesia with halogenated drugs, increasing respiratory depression is manifested by increasingly rapid and shallow breathing (panting). On the other hand, with deep nitrous oxide–narcotic anesthesia, respirations become slower but may remain deep. In the case of very deep anesthesia with all inhaled drugs, respirations often become jerky or gasping in character and irregular in pattern. This situation results from loss of the active intercostal muscle contribution to inspiration. As a result, a rocking boat movement occurs in which there is out-of-phase depression of the chest wall during inspiration, flaring of the lower chest margins, and billowing of the abdomen. The reason for this type of movement is that inspiration is dependent solely on diaphragmatic effort. Independent of anesthetic depth, similar chest movements may be simulated by upper or lower airway obstruction or by partial paralysis.

B. Anesthetic Depth and Spontaneous Minute Ventilation

Despite the variable changes in respiratory pattern and rate as anesthesia deepens, overall spontaneous $\dot{V}_E$ progressively decreases. In the normal awake response to breathing CO_2, an increasing end-tidal P_{CO_2} causes a linear increase in $\dot{V}_E$ (Fig. 5-31). The slope of the line relating $\dot{V}_E$ to the end-tidal CO_2 concentration (P_{CO_2}) in awake individuals is approximately 2 L/min/mm Hg. (In healthy individuals, the variation in the slope of this response is large.) Figure 5-31 shows that increasing the halothane concentration displaces the ventilation-response curve progressively to the right (i.e., at any end-tidal P_{CO_2}, ventilation is less than before), decreases the slope of the curve, and shifts the apneic threshold to a higher end-tidal P_{CO_2}.[124] Similar alterations are observed with narcotics and other halogenated anesthetics.[125] Figures 5-22 to 5-24 show that decreases in $\dot{V}_E$ cause increases in Pa_{CO_2} and decreases in Pa_{O_2}. The relative increase in Pa_{CO_2} caused by depression of $\dot{V}_E$ (<1.24 MAC) by halogenated anesthetics is desflurane = isoflurane > sevoflurane > halothane. At higher concentrations, desflurane causes increasing ventilatory depression, even

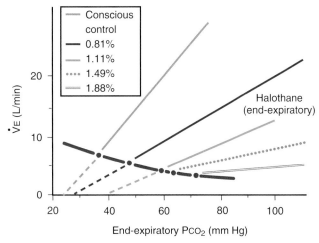

Figure 5-31 In conscious controls, increasing end-expiratory concentration of carbon dioxide (Pco_2, x-axis) increases pulmonary minute volume ($\dot{V}_E$, y-axis). The dashed line is an extrapolation of the CO_2 response curve to zero ventilation and represents the apneic threshold. Increases in end-expiratory anesthetic (halothane) concentration progressively diminish the slope of the CO_2 response curve and shift the apneic threshold to a higher Pco_2. The heavy line interrupted by dots shows the decrease in minute ventilation and the increase in Pco_2 that occur with increasing depth of anesthesia. (Redrawn with modification from Munson ES, Larson CP Jr, Babad AA, et al: The effects of halothane, fluroxene and cyclopropane on ventilation: A comparative study in man. *Anesthesiology* 27:716, 1966.)

more than isoflurane, and sevoflurane causes a degree of ventilatory depression similar to isoflurane.

C. Preexisting Respiratory Dysfunction

Anesthesiologists are frequently required to care for (1) patients with acute chest disease (pulmonary infection, atelectasis) or systemic diseases (sepsis, cardiac and renal failure, multiple trauma) who require emergency operations, (2) heavy smokers with subtle pathologic airway and parenchymal conditions and hyperreactive airways, (3) patients with classic emphysematous and bronchitic problems, (4) obese people susceptible to decreases in FRC during anesthesia,[126] (5) patients with chest deformities, and (6) extremely old patients.

The nature and magnitude of these preexisting respiratory conditions determine, in part, the effect of a given standard anesthetic on respiratory function. For example, in Figure 5-32, the FRC-CC relationship is depicted for normal, obese, bronchitic, and emphysematous patients. In a healthy patient, FRC exceeds CC by approximately 1 L. In the latter three respiratory conditions, CC is 0.5 to 0.75 L less than FRC. If anesthesia causes a 1-L decrease in FRC in a healthy patient, there is no change in the qualitative relationship between FRC and CC. In patients with special respiratory conditions, however, a 1-L decrease in FRC causes CC to exceed FRC and changes the previous marginally normal FRC-CC relationship to either a grossly low $\dot{V}_A/\dot{Q}$ or an atelectatic FRC-CC relationship. Similarly, patients with chronic bronchitis, who have copious airway secretions, may suffer more than other patients from an anesthetic-induced decrease in mucus velocity flow. Finally, if an

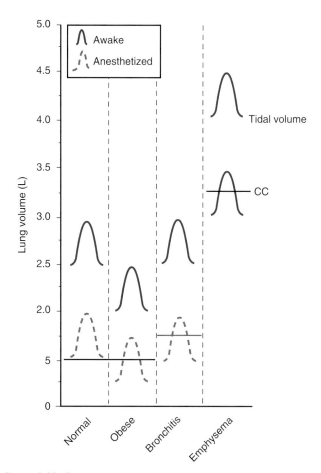

Figure 5-32 The lung volume (ordinate) at which tidal volume is breathed decreases (by 1 L) from the awake state to the anesthetized state. Functional residual capacity (FRC), which is the volume of gas existing in the lung at the end of a tidal breath, therefore also decreases (by 1 L) from the awake to the anesthetized state. In healthy, obese, bronchitic, and emphysematous patients, the awake FRC considerably exceeds the closing capacity (*CC*, horizontal lines), but the anesthetized state causes FRC to be less than CC. In healthy patients, anesthesia causes FRC to equal CC.

anesthetic inhibits HPV, the drug may increase shunting more in patients with preexisting HPV than in those without preexisting HPV. Thus, the effect of a standard anesthetic can be expected to produce varying degrees of respiratory change in patients who have different degrees of preexisting respiratory dysfunction.

D. Special Intraoperative Conditions

Some special intraoperative conditions (e.g., surgical position, massive blood loss, surgical retraction on the lung) can cause impaired gas exchange. For example, some of the surgical positions (i.e., the lithotomy, jack-knife, and kidney rest positions) and surgical exposure requirements may decrease $\dot{Q}_T$, cause hypoventilation in a spontaneously breathing patient, and reduce FRC. The type and severity of preexisting respiratory dysfunction, as well as the number and severity of special intraoperative conditions that can embarrass respiratory function, magnify the respiratory depressant effects of any anesthetic.

E. Mechanisms of Hypoxemia During Anesthesia

1. Equipment Malfunction

a. MECHANICAL FAILURE OF ANESTHESIA APPARATUS TO DELIVER OXYGEN TO THE PATIENT

Hypoxemia resulting from mechanical failure of the O_2 supply system (see Chapter 14) or the anesthesia machine is a recognized hazard of anesthesia. Disconnection of the patient from the O_2 supply system (usually at the juncture of the ETT and the elbow connector) is by far the most common cause of mechanical failure to deliver O_2 to the patient. Other reported causes of failure of the O_2 supply during anesthesia include the following: an empty or depleted O_2 cylinder, substitution of a nonoxygen cylinder at the O_2 yoke because of absence or failure of the pin index, an erroneously filled O_2 cylinder, insufficient opening of the O_2 cylinder (which hinders free flow of gas as pressure decreases), failure of gas pressure in a piped O_2 system, faulty locking of the piped O_2 system to the anesthesia machine, inadvertent switching of the Schrader adapters on piped lines, crossing of piped lines during construction, failure of a reducing valve or gas manifold, inadvertent disturbance of the setting of the O_2 flowmeter, use of the fine O_2 flowmeter instead of the coarse flowmeter, fractured or sticking flowmeters, transposition of rotameter tubes, erroneous filling of a liquid O_2 reservoir with N_2, and disconnection of the fresh gas line from machine to in-line hosing.[127–131] Monitoring of the inspired O_2 concentration with an in-line FIO_2 analyzer and monitoring of airway pressure should detect most of these causes of failure to deliver O_2 to the patient.[127–131]

b. IMPROPER ENDOTRACHEAL TUBE POSITION

Esophageal intubation results in almost no ventilation. Aside from disconnection, almost all other mechanical problems with ETTs (e.g., kinking, blockage of secretions, herniated or ruptured cuffs) cause an increase in airway resistance that may result in hypoventilation. Intubation of a main stem bronchus (see Chapter 7) results in absence of ventilation of the contralateral lung. Although potentially minimized by HPV, some perfusion to the contralateral lung always remains, and shunting increases and PaO_2 decreases. A tube previously well positioned in the trachea may enter a bronchus after the patient or the patient's head is turned or moved into a new position.[132] Flexion of the head causes the tube to migrate deeper (caudad) into the trachea, whereas extension of the head causes cephalad (outward) migration of the ETT.[132] A high incidence of main stem bronchial intubation after the institution of a 30-degree Trendelenburg position has been reported.[133] Cephalad shift of the carina and mediastinum during the Trendelenburg position caused the previously "fixed" ETT to migrate into a main stem bronchus. Main stem bronchial intubation may obstruct the ipsilateral upper lobe in addition to the contralateral lung.[134,135] Infrequently, the right upper bronchus or one of its segmental bronchi branches from the lateral wall of the trachea (above the carina) and may be occluded by a properly positioned ETT.

2. Hypoventilation

Patients under general anesthesia may have a reduced spontaneous VT for two reasons. First, increased WOB can occur during general anesthesia as a result of increased airway resistance and decreased CL. Airway resistance can be increased because of reduced FRC, endotracheal intubation, the presence of the external breathing apparatus and circuitry, and possible airway obstruction in patients whose tracheas are not intubated.[136–138] CL is reduced as a result of some (or all) of the factors that can decrease FRC.[89] Second, patients may have a decreased drive to breathe spontaneously during general anesthesia (i.e., decreased chemical control of breathing) (see Fig. 5-31).

Decreased VT may cause hypoxemia in two ways.[117] First, shallow breathing can promote atelectasis and cause a decrease in FRC (see "Ventilation Pattern [Rapid Shallow Breathing]").[40,139] Second, decreased $\dot{V}E$ decreases the overall $\dot{V}A/\dot{Q}$ ratio of the lung, which decreases PaO_2 (see Figs. 5-23 and 5-24).[117] This is likely to occur with spontaneous ventilation during moderate to deep levels of anesthesia, in which the chemical control of breathing is significantly altered.

3. Hyperventilation

Hypocapnic alkalosis (hyperventilation) can occasionally be associated with a decreased PaO_2 due to several indirect mechanisms: decreased $\dot{Q}T$ and increased $\bar{V}O_2$[140,141] (see "Decreased Cardiac Output and Increased Oxygen Consumption"),[99,101,140,141] a left-shifted oxy-Hb curve (see "Oxygen-Hemoglobin Dissociation Curve"), decreased HPV (see "Inhibition of Hypoxic Pulmonary Vasoconstriction"),[142] and increased airway resistance and decreased compliance (see "Increased Airway Resistance").[143] Although these theoretical causes of hypoxemia exist, they are seldom a major factor in the clinical realm.

4. Decrease in Functional Residual Capacity

The effect of decreased FRC on hypoxemia is very significant clinically. Induction of general anesthesia is consistently accompanied by a pronounced (15% to 20%) decrease in FRC,[32,83,144] which usually causes a decrease in compliance.[89] The maximum decrease in FRC appears to occur within the first few minutes of anesthesia,[32,145] and in the absence of any other complicating factor, FRC does not seem to decrease progressively during anesthesia. During anesthesia, the reduction in FRC is of the same order of magnitude whether ventilation is spontaneous or controlled. Conversely, in awake patients, FRC is only slightly reduced during controlled ventilation.[146] In obese patients, the reduction in FRC is far more pronounced than in normal patients, and the decrease is inversely related to the body mass index (BMI).[147] The reduction in FRC continues into the postoperative period.[148] For individual patients, the reduction in FRC correlates well with the increase in the alveolar-arterial PO_2 gradient during anesthesia with spontaneous breathing,[149] during anesthesia with artificial ventilation,[146] and in the postoperative period.[148] The reduced FRC can be restored to normal or above normal by the application of

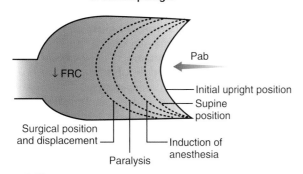

Figure 5-33 Anesthesia and surgery may cause a progressive cephalad displacement of the diaphragm. The sequence of events involves assumption of the supine position, induction of anesthesia, establishment of paralysis, assumption of several surgical positions, and displacement by retractors and packs. Cephalad displacement of the diaphragm results in decreased functional residual capacity (↓ FRC). Pab, Pressure of abdominal contents. (Redrawn with modification from Benumof JL: Anesthesia for thoracic surgery, ed 2, Philadelphia, 1995, Saunders, Chapter 8.)

PEEP.[82,150] The following discussion considers the most common causes of reduced FRC.

a. SUPINE POSITION

Anesthesia and surgery are usually performed with the patient in the supine position. With change from the upright to the supine position, FRC decreases by 0.5 to 1.0 L[32,83,144] because of a 4-cm cephalad displacement of the diaphragm by the abdominal viscera (Fig. 5-33). Pulmonary vascular congestion can also contribute to the decrease in FRC in the supine position, particularly in patients who experienced orthopnea preoperatively.

b. INDUCTION OF GENERAL ANESTHESIA: CHANGE IN THORACIC CAGE MUSCLE TONE

At the end of a normal (awake) exhalation, there is slight tension in the inspiratory muscles and no tension in the expiratory muscles. Therefore, at the end of a normal exhalation, there is a force tending to maintain lung volume and no force decreasing lung volume. After induction of general anesthesia, there is a loss of inspiratory tone and an appearance of end-expiratory tone in the abdominal expiratory muscles at the end of exhalation. The end-expiratory tone in the abdominal expiratory muscles increases intra-abdominal pressure, forces the diaphragm cephalad, and decreases FRC (see Fig. 5-33).[145,151] Thus, after the induction of general anesthesia, there is loss of the force tending to maintain lung volume and gain of the force tending to decrease lung volume. Indeed, Innovar (droperidol and fentanyl citrate) may increase tone in expiratory muscles to such an extent that the reduction in FRC with Innovar anesthesia alone is greater than that with Innovar plus paralysis induced by succinylcholine.[151,152]

With emphysema, exhalation may be accompanied by pursing the lips or grunting (i.e., with a partially closed larynx). An emphysematous patient exhales in either of these ways because both these maneuvers cause an expiratory retardation that produces PEEP in the intrathoracic air passage and decreases the possibility of airway closure and a decrease in FRC (see Fig. 5-17F). Endotracheal intubation bypasses the lips and glottis and can abolish the normally present pursed-lip or grunting exhalation in a patient with COPD and in that way contributes to airway closure and loss of FRC in some spontaneously breathing patients.

c. PARALYSIS

In an upright subject, FRC and the position of the diaphragm are determined by the balance between lung elastic recoil pulling the diaphragm cephalad and the weight of the abdominal contents pulling it caudad.[153] There is no transdiaphragmatic pressure gradient.

The situation is more complex in the supine position. The diaphragm separates two compartments of markedly different hydrostatic gradients. On the thoracic side, pressure increases by approximately 0.25 cm H_2O/cm of lung height,[38,154] and on the abdominal side, it increases by 1.0 cm H_2O/cm of abdominal height.[153] Therefore, in horizontal postures, progressively higher transdiaphragmatic pressure must be generated toward dependent parts of the diaphragm to keep the abdominal contents out of the thorax. In an unparalyzed patient, this tension is developed either by passive stretch and changes in shape of the diaphragm (causing an increased contractile force) or by neurally mediated active tension. With acute muscle paralysis, neither of these two mechanisms can operate, and a shift of the diaphragm to a more cephalad position occurs (see Fig. 5-33).[155] The latter position must express the true balance of forces on the diaphragm, unmodified by any passive or active muscle activity.

The cephalad shift in the FRC position of the diaphragm as a result of expiratory muscle tone during general anesthesia is equal to the shift observed during paralysis (awake or anesthetized patients).[145,156] The equal shift suggests that the pressure on the diaphragm caused by an increase in expiratory muscle tone during general anesthesia is equal to the pressure on the diaphragm caused by the weight of the abdominal contents during paralysis. It is quite probable that the magnitude of these changes in FRC related to paralysis also depends on body habitus.

d. LIGHT OR INADEQUATE ANESTHESIA AND ACTIVE EXPIRATION

Induction of general anesthesia can result in increased expiratory muscle tone,[151] but the increased expiratory muscle tone is not coordinated and does not contribute to the exhaled volume of gas. In contrast, spontaneous ventilation during light general anesthesia usually results in a coordinated and moderately forceful active exhalation and larger exhaled volumes. Excessively inadequate anesthesia (relative to a given stimulus) results in very forceful active exhalation, which can produce exhaled volumes of gas equal to an awake expiratory vital capacity.

As during an awake expiratory vital capacity maneuver, forced expiration during anesthesia raises intrathoracic and alveolar pressure considerably above atmospheric pressure (see Fig. 5-17). This increase in pressure results in rapid outflow of gas, and because part of the expiratory

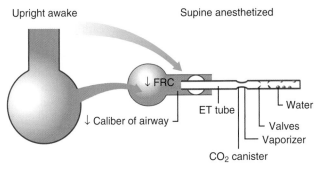

Figure 5-34 An anesthetized patient in the supine position has increased airway resistance as a result of decreased functional residual capacity *(FRC)*, decreased caliber of the airways, endotracheal intubation, and connection of the endotracheal tube *(ET)* to the external breathing apparatus and circuitry. ↓, Decreased. (Redrawn with modification from Benumof JL: *Anesthesia for thoracic surgery*, ed 2, Philadelphia, 1995, Saunders, Chapter 8.)

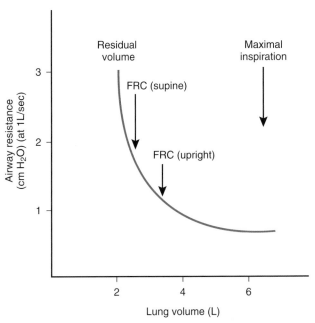

Figure 5-35 Airway resistance is an increasing hyperbolic function of decreasing lung volume. Functional residual capacity *(FRC)* decreases with a change from the upright to the supine position. (Redrawn with modification from Lumb AB: Respiratory system resistance. In Lumb AB, editor: *Nunn's applied respiratory physiology*, ed 5, London, 2000, Butterworths, p 67.)

resistance lies in the smaller air passages, a drop in pressure occurs between the alveoli and the main bronchi. Under these circumstances, intrathoracic pressure rises considerably above the pressure within the main bronchi. Collapse occurs if this reversed pressure gradient is sufficiently high to overcome the tethering effect of the surrounding parenchyma on the small intrathoracic bronchioles or the structural rigidity of cartilage in the large extrathoracic bronchi. Such collapse occurs in a normal subject during a maximal forced expiration and is responsible for the associated wheeze in both awake and anesthetized patients.[157]

In a paralyzed, anesthetized patient, the use of a subatmospheric expiratory pressure phase is analogous to a forced expiration in a conscious subject; the negative phase may set up the same adverse ΔP, which can cause airway closure, gas trapping, and a decrease in FRC. An excessively rapidly descending bellows of a ventilator during expiration has caused subatmospheric expiratory pressure and resulted in wheezing.[158]

e. INCREASED AIRWAY RESISTANCE

The overall reduction in all components of lung volume during anesthesia results in reduced airway caliber, which increases airway resistance and any tendency toward airway collapse (Fig. 5-34). The relationship between airway resistance and lung volume is well established (Fig. 5-35). The decreases in FRC caused by the supine position (≈ 0.8L) and induction of anesthesia (≈ 0.4L) are often sufficient to explain the increased resistance seen in a healthy anesthetized patient.[137]

In addition to this expected increase in airway resistance in anesthetized patients, there are a number of special potential sites of increased airway resistance, including the ETT (if present), the upper and lower airway passages, and the external anesthesia apparatus. Endotracheal intubation reduces the size of the trachea, usually by 30% to 50% (see Fig. 5-34). Pharyngeal obstruction, which can be considered to be a normal feature of unconsciousness, is most common. A minor degree of this type of obstruction occurs in snoring. Laryngospasm and obstructed ETTs (e.g., secretions,

kinking, herniated cuffs) are not uncommon and can be life-threatening.

The respiratory apparatus often causes resistance that is considerably higher than the resistance in the normal human respiratory tract (see Fig. 5-34).[89] When certain resistors such as those shown in Figure 5-34 are joined in series to form an anesthetic gas circuit, their effects are generally additive and produce larger resistance (as with resistance in series in an electrical circuit). The increase in resistance associated with commonly used breathing circuits and ETTs can impose an additional WOB that is two to three times normal.[136]

f. SUPINE POSITION, IMMOBILITY, AND EXCESSIVE INTRAVENOUS FLUID ADMINISTRATION

Patients undergoing anesthesia and surgery are often kept supine and immobile for long periods. In these cases, some of the lung can be continually dependent and below the left atrium and therefore in zone 3 or 4 condition. Being in a dependent position, the lung is predisposed to accumulation of fluid. Coupled with excessive fluid administration, conditions sufficient to promote transudation of fluid into the lung are present and result in pulmonary edema and decreased FRC.

When mongrel dogs were placed in a lateral decubitus position and anesthetized for several hours (Fig. 5-36), expansion of the extracellular space with fluid caused the P_{O_2} of blood draining the dependent lung to decrease precipitously to mixed venous levels (no O_2 uptake).[159] Blood draining the nondependent lung maintained its P_{O_2} for a period but declined after 5 hours in the presence of the extracellular fluid expansion. Transpulmonary shunting progressively increased. If the animals were turned every hour (and received the same fluid

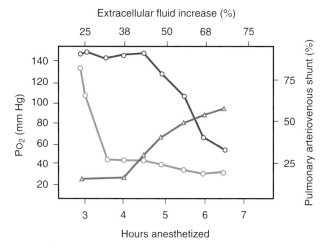

Figure 5-36 Mongrel dogs anesthetized with pentobarbital were placed in a lateral decubitus position and subjected to progressive extracellular fluid expansion. They had a marked decrease in the partial pressure of oxygen (Po₂) of blood draining the dependent lung *(yellow line)* and a smaller, much slower decrease in the Po₂ of blood draining the nondependent lung *(purple line)*. The pulmonary arteriovenous shunt rose progressively *(blue line)*. (Redrawn from Ray JF, Yost L, Moallem S, et al: Immobility, hypoxemia, and pulmonary arteriovenous shunting. *Arch Surg* 109:537, 1974.)

challenge), only the dependent lung, at the end of each hour period, suffered a decrease in oxygenation. If the animals were turned every half-hour and received the same fluid challenge, neither lung suffered a decrease in oxygenation.

In patients who undergo surgery in the lateral decubitus position (e.g., pulmonary resection, in which they have or will have a restricted pulmonary vascular bed) and receive excessive intravenous fluids, the risk of the dependent lung's becoming edematous is certainly increased. These considerations also explain, in part, the beneficial effect of a continuously rotating (side-to-side) bed on the incidence of pulmonary complications in critically ill patients.[160]

g. HIGH INSPIRED OXYGEN CONCENTRATION AND ABSORPTION ATELECTASIS

General anesthesia is usually administered with an increased FIO₂. In patients who have areas of moderately low $\dot{V}_A/\dot{Q}$ ratios (0.1 to 0.01), administration of FIO₂ greater than 0.3 adds enough O₂ into the alveolar space in these areas to eliminate the shunt-like effect that they have, and total measured right-to-left shunting decreases. However, when patients with a significant amount of blood flow perfusing lung units with very low $\dot{V}_A/\dot{Q}$ ratios (0.01 to 0.0001) have a change in FIO₂ from room air to 1.0, the very low $\dot{V}_A/\dot{Q}$ units virtually disappear, and a moderately large right-to-left shunt appears.[16,17,161] In these studies, the increase in shunting was equal to the amount of blood flow previously perfusing the areas with low $\dot{V}_A/\dot{Q}$ ratios during the breathing of air. Thus, the effect of breathing O₂ was to convert units that had low $\dot{V}_A/\dot{Q}$ ratios into shunt units. The pathologic basis for these data is the conversion of low $\dot{V}_A/\dot{Q}$ units into atelectatic units. The cause of the atelectatic shunting during O₂ breathing is presumably a large increase in O₂

uptake by lung units with low $\dot{V}_A/\dot{Q}$ ratios.[161,162] A unit that has a low $\dot{V}_A/\dot{Q}$ ratio during breathing of air will have a low PAO₂. When an enriched O₂ mixture is inspired, PAO₂ rises, and the rate at which O₂ moves from alveolar gas to capillary blood increases greatly. The O₂ flux may increase so much that the net flow of gas into blood exceeds the inspired flow of gas, and the lung unit becomes progressively smaller. Collapse is most likely to occur if FIO₂ is high, the $\dot{V}_A/\dot{Q}$ ratio is low, the time of exposure of the unit with low $\dot{V}_A/\dot{Q}$ to high FIO₂ is long, and C$\bar{v}$O₂ is low. Given the right $\dot{V}_A/\dot{Q}$ ratio and time of administration, an FIO₂ as low as 50% can produce absorption atelectasis.[161,162] This phenomenon is of considerable significance in the clinical situation for two reasons. First, enriched O₂ mixtures are often used therapeutically, and it is important to know whether this therapy is causing atelectasis. Second, the amount of shunt is often estimated during breathing of 100% O₂, and if this maneuver results in additional shunt, the measurement is hard to interpret.

h. SURGICAL POSITION

SUPINE POSITION. In the supine position, the abdominal contents force the diaphragm cephalad and reduce FRC.[83,145,151,156] The Trendelenburg position allows the abdominal contents to push the diaphragm further cephalad so that the diaphragm must not only ventilate the lungs but also lift the abdominal contents out of the thorax. The result is a predisposition to decreased FRC and atelectasis.[163] The decrease in FRC related to Trendelenburg position is exacerbated in obese patients.[147] Increased pulmonary blood volume and gravitational force on the mediastinal structures are additional factors that may decrease pulmonary compliance and FRC. In the steep Trendelenburg position, most of the lung may be below the left atrium and therefore in a zone 3 or 4 condition. In this condition, the lung may be susceptible to the development of pulmonary interstitial edema. Thus, patients with elevated Ppa, such as those with mitral stenosis, do not tolerate the Trendelenburg position well.[164]

LATERAL DECUBITUS POSITION. In the lateral decubitus position, the dependent lung experiences a moderate decrease in FRC and is predisposed to atelectasis, whereas the nondependent lung may have increased FRC. The overall result is usually a slight to moderate increase in total-lung FRC.[165] The kidney and lithotomy positions also cause small decreases in FRC above that caused by the supine position. The prone position may increase FRC moderately.[165]

i. VENTILATION PATTERN (RAPID SHALLOW BREATHING)

Rapid shallow breathing is often a regular feature of anesthesia. Monotonous shallow breathing can cause a decrease in FRC, promote atelectasis, and decrease compliance.[40,139,166] These changes with rapid shallow breathing are probably due to progressive increases in surface tension.[166] Initially, these changes may cause hypoxemia with normocapnia and may be prevented or reversed by periodic large mechanical inspirations, spontaneous sighs, PEEP, or a combination of these techniques.[166–168]

j. DECREASED REMOVAL OF SECRETIONS (DECREASED MUCOCILIARY FLOW)

Tracheobronchial mucous glands and goblet cells produce mucus, which is swept by cilia up to the larynx, where it is swallowed or expectorated. This process clears inhaled organisms and particles from the lungs. The secreted mucus consists of a surface gel layer lying on top of a more liquid sol layer in which the cilia beat. The tips of the cilia propel the gel layer toward the larynx (upward) during the forward stroke. As the mucus streams upward and the total cross-sectional area of the airways diminishes, absorption takes place from the sol layer to maintain a constant depth of 5 mm.[169]

Poor systemic hydration and low inspired humidity reduce mucociliary flow by increasing the viscosity of secretions and slowing the ciliary beat.[170–172] Mucociliary flow varies directly with body or mucosal temperature (low inspired temperature) over a range of 32° to 42° C.[173,174] High FIO_2 decreases mucociliary flow.[175] Inflation of an ETT cuff suppresses tracheal mucus velocity,[176] an effect that occurs within 1 hour, and apparently it does not matter whether a low- or high-compliance cuff is used. Passage of an uncuffed tube through the vocal cords and keeping it in situ for several hours does not affect tracheal mucus velocity.[176]

The mechanism for suppression of mucociliary clearance by the ETT cuff is speculative. In the report of Sackner and colleagues,[176] mucus velocity was decreased in the distal portion of the trachea, but the cuff was inflated in the proximal portion. Therefore, the phenomenon cannot be attributed solely to damming of mucus at the cuff site. One possibility is that the ETT cuff caused a critical increase in the thickness of the layer of mucus proceeding distally from the cuff. Another possibility is that mechanical distention of the trachea by the ETT cuff initiated a neurogenic reflex arc that altered mucous secretions or the frequency of ciliary beating.

Other investigators showed that when all the foregoing factors were controlled, halothane reversibly and progressively decreased but did not stop mucus flow over an inspired concentration of 1 to 3 MAC.[177] The halothane-induced depression of mucociliary clearance was probably due to depression of the ciliary beat, an effect that caused slow clearance of mucus from the distal and peripheral airways. In support of this hypothesis is the finding that cilia are morphologically similar throughout the animal kingdom. Inhaled anesthetics in clinical doses, including halothane, have been found to cause reversible depression of the ciliary beat of protozoa.[115]

5. Decreased Cardiac Output and Increased Oxygen Consumption

Decreased $\dot{Q}_T$ in the presence of constant O_2 consumption ($\dot{V}O_2$), increased $\dot{V}O_2$ in the presence of a constant $\dot{Q}_T$, and decreased $\dot{Q}_T$ concomitant with increased $\dot{V}O_2$ must all result in lower $C\bar{v}O_2$. Venous blood with lowered $C\bar{v}O_2$ then flows through whichever shunt pathways exist, mixes with the oxygenated end-pulmonary capillary blood, and lowers CaO_2 (see Figs. 5-27 and 5-28). Figure 5-37 shows these relationships quantitatively for several different intrapulmonary shunts.[100,101] The larger the intrapulmonary shunt, the greater the decrease in

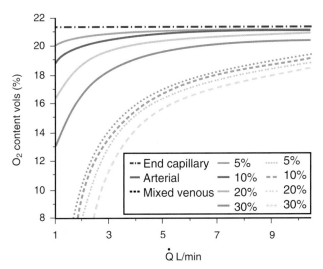

Figure 5-37 Effects of changes in cardiac output ($\dot{Q}$) on the O_2 content of end-pulmonary capillary, arterial *(solid lines)*, and mixed venous *(dashed lines)* blood for various transpulmonary right-to-left shunts. The magnitudes of the shunts are indicated by the percentages; the oxygen content of end-capillary blood is unaffected by the degree of shunting. Note that a given decrease in $\dot{Q}$ results in a greater decrease in the arterial content of O_2 with larger shunts. (Redrawn from Kelman GF, Nunn JF, Prys-Roberts C, et al: The influence of the cardiac output on arterial oxygenation: A theoretical study. *Br J Anaesth* 39:450, 1967.)

CaO_2, because more venous blood with lower $C\bar{v}O_2$ can admix with end-pulmonary capillary blood. Decreased $\dot{Q}_T$ may occur with myocardial failure and hypovolemia; the specific causes of these two conditions are beyond the scope of this chapter. Increased $\dot{V}O_2$ may occur with excessive stimulation of the sympathetic nervous system, hyperthermia, or shivering and can further contribute to impaired oxygenation of arterial blood.[178]

6. Inhibition of Hypoxic Pulmonary Vasoconstriction

Decreased regional PAO_2 causes regional pulmonary vasoconstriction, which diverts blood flow away from hypoxic regions of the lung to better ventilated normoxic regions. The diversion of blood flow minimizes venous admixture from the underventilated or nonventilated lung regions. Inhibition of regional HPV could impair arterial oxygenation by permitting increased venous admixture from hypoxic or atelectatic areas of the lung (see Fig. 5-9).

Because the pulmonary circulation is poorly endowed with smooth muscle, any condition that increases the pressure against which the vessels must constrict (i.e., Ppa) decreases HPV. Numerous clinical conditions can increase Ppa and therefore decrease HPV. Mitral stenosis,[179] volume overload,[179] low (but greater than room air) FIO_2 in nondiseased lung,[74] a progressive increase in the amount of diseased lung,[74] thromboembolism,[74] hypothermia,[180] and vasoactive drugs can all increase Ppa.[64] Direct vasodilating drugs (e.g., isoproterenol, nitroglycerin, sodium nitroprusside),[64,59] inhaled anesthetics,[65] and hypocapnia can directly decrease HPV.[64,142] Selective application of PEEP to only the nondiseased lung can selectively increase PVR in the nondiseased lung and may divert blood flow back into the diseased lung.[181]

7. Paralysis

In the supine position, the weight of the abdominal contents pressing against the diaphragm is greatest in the dependent or posterior part of the diaphragm and least in the nondependent or anterior part of the diaphragm. In an awake patient breathing spontaneously, active tension in the diaphragm is capable of overcoming the weight of the abdominal contents, and the diaphragm moves most in the posterior portion (because the posterior of the diaphragm is stretched higher into the chest, it has the smallest radius of curvature, and therefore it contracts most effectively) and least in the anterior portion. This circumstance is healthy because the greatest amount of ventilation occurs in areas with the most perfusion (posteriorly or dependently), and the least amount occurs in areas with the least perfusion (anteriorly or nondependently). During paralysis and positive-pressure breathing, the passive diaphragm is displaced by the positive pressure preferentially in the anterior, nondependent portion (where there is the least resistance to diaphragmatic movement) and is displaced minimally in the posterior, dependent portion (where there is the most resistance to diaphragmatic movement). This circumstance is unhealthy because the greatest amount of ventilation now occurs in areas with the least perfusion, and the least amount occurs in areas with the most perfusion.[156] However, the magnitude of the change in the diaphragmatic motion pattern with paralysis varies with body position.[156,182]

8. Right-to-Left Interatrial Shunting

Acute arterial hypoxemia from a transient right-to-left shunt through a PFO has been described, particularly during emergence from anesthesia.[70] However, unless a real-time technique of imaging the cardiac chambers is used (e.g., transesophageal echocardiography with color flow Doppler imaging),[71] it is difficult to document an acute and transient right-to-left intracardiac shunt as a cause of arterial hypoxemia. Nonetheless, right-to-left shunting through a PFO has been described in virtually every conceivable clinical situation that afterloads the right side of the heart and increases right atrial pressure. When right-to-left shunting through a PFO is identified, administration of inhaled NO can decrease PVR and functionally close the PFO.[183]

9. Involvement of Mechanisms of Hypoxemia in Specific Diseases

In any given pulmonary disease, many of the mechanisms of hypoxemia listed earlier may be involved.[117] Pulmonary embolism (air, fat, thrombi) (Fig. 5-38) and the evolution of ARDS (Fig. 5-39) are used to illustrate this point. A significant pulmonary embolus can cause severe increases in Ppa, and these increases can result in right-to-left transpulmonary shunting through opened arteriovenous anastomoses and the foramen ovale (possible in 20% of patients), pulmonary edema in nonembolized regions of the lung, and inhibition of HPV. The embolus can cause hypoventilation through increased dead space ventilation. If the embolus contains platelets, serotonin can be released, and such release can cause hypoventilation as a result of bronchoconstriction and pulmonary

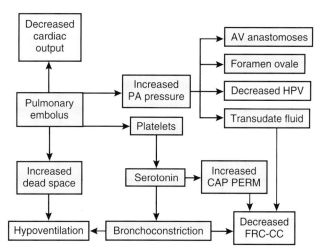

Figure 5-38 Mechanisms of hypoxemia during pulmonary embolism. See the text for an explanation of the pathophysiologic flow diagram. *AV,* Arteriovenous; *CAP PERM,* capillary permeability; *CC,* closing capacity; *FRC,* functional residual capacity; *HPV,* hypoxic pulmonary vasoconstriction; *PA,* pulmonary artery. (Redrawn with modification from Benumof JL: *Anesthesia for thoracic surgery,* ed 2, Philadelphia, 1995, Saunders, Chapter 8.)

edema as a result of increased pulmonary capillary permeability. Finally, the pulmonary embolus can increase PVR (by platelet-induced serotonin release,[4] among other mechanisms) and decrease cardiac output.

After major hypotension, shock, blood loss, sepsis, or other conditions, noncardiogenic pulmonary edema may occur and lead to acute respiratory failure or ARDS.[184] The syndrome can evolve during and after anesthesia and has the hallmark characteristics of decreased FRC and compliance and hypoxemia. After shock and trauma, plasma levels of serotonin, histamine, kinins, lysozymes, reactive oxygen species, fibrin degradation products, products of complement metabolism, and fatty acids all increase. Sepsis and endotoxemia may be present. Increased levels of activated complement stimulate neutrophils into chemotaxis in patients with trauma and

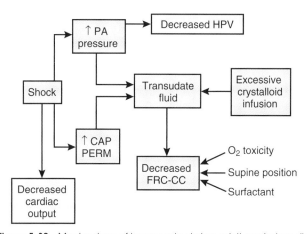

Figure 5-39 Mechanisms of hypoxemia during adult respiratory distress syndrome. See the text for an explanation of the pathophysiologic flow diagram. *CAP PERM,* Capillary permeability; *CC,* closing capacity; *FRC,* functional residual capacity; *HPV,* hypoxic pulmonary vasoconstriction; *PA,* pulmonary artery. (Redrawn with modification from Benumof JL: *Anesthesia for thoracic surgery,* ed 2, Philadelphia, 1995, Saunders, Chapter 8.)

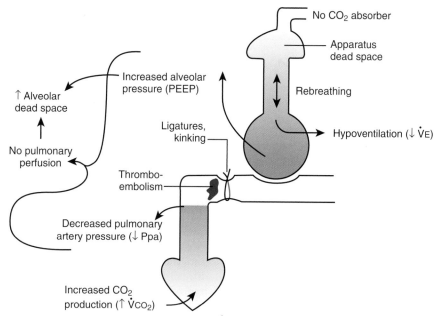

Figure 5-40 Schematic diagram of the causes of hypercapnia during anesthesia. An increase in carbon dioxide (CO_2) production $(\dot{V}_{CO_2})$ increases the arterial partial pressure of CO_2 (Pa_{CO_2}) with a constant minute ventilation $(\dot{V}_E)$. Several events can increase alveolar dead space: a decrease in pulmonary artery pressure *(Ppa)*, the application of positive end-expiratory pressure *(PEEP)*, thromboembolism, and mechanical interference with pulmonary arterial flow (ligatures and kinking of vessels). Most commonly in trauma, surgery, and critical care, hypovolemia due to hemorrhage or third spacing leads to increased alveolar dead space and consequently to increased Pa_{CO_2}. A decrease in $\dot{V}_E$ causes an increase in Pa_{CO_2} with a constant $\dot{V}_{CO_2}$. It is possible for some anesthesia systems to cause rebreathing of CO_2. Finally, the anesthesia apparatus may increase the anatomic dead space, and inadvertent switching off of a CO_2 absorber in the presence of low fresh gas flow can increase Pa_{CO_2}. ↑, increase; ↓, decrease. *(Redrawn with modification from Benumof JL: Anesthesia for thoracic surgery, ed 2, Philadelphia, 1995, Saunders, Chapter 8.)*

pancreatitis; activated neutrophils can damage endothelial cells. These factors, along with pulmonary contusion (if it occurs), can individually or collectively increase pulmonary capillary permeability. After shock, acidosis, increased circulating catecholamines and sympathetic nervous system activity, leukotriene and prostaglandin release, histamine release, microembolism (with serotonin release), increased intracranial pressure (with head injury), and alveolar hypoxia can occur and may individually or collectively (particularly after resuscitation) cause a moderate increase in Ppa. After shock, the normal compensatory response to hypovolemia is movement of a protein-free fluid from the interstitial space into the vascular space to restore vascular volume. Dilution of vascular proteins by protein-free interstitial fluid can cause decreased capillary colloid oncotic pressure. Increased pulmonary capillary permeability and Ppa along with decreased capillary colloid oncotic pressure results in fluid transudation and pulmonary edema. In addition, decreased $\dot{Q}_T$, inhibition of HPV, immobility, the supine position, excessive fluid administration, and an excessively high Fi_{O_2} can contribute to the development of ARDS.

F. Mechanisms of Hypercapnia and Hypocapnia During Anesthesia

1. Hypercapnia

Hypoventilation, increased dead space ventilation, increased CO_2 production, and inadvertent switching off of a CO_2 absorber can all cause hypercapnia (Fig. 5-40).

2. Hypoventilation

Patients spontaneously hypoventilate during anesthesia because it is more difficult to breath (abnormal surgical position, increased airway resistance, decreased compliance) and because they are less willing to breath (decreased respiratory drive due to anesthetics). Hypoventilation results in hypercapnia (see Figs. 5-22 and 5-23).

3. Increased Dead Space Ventilation

A decrease in Ppa, as during deliberate hypotension,[185] can cause an increase in zone 1 and alveolar dead space ventilation. An increase in airway pressure (as with PEEP) can also cause an increase in zone 1 and alveolar dead space ventilation. Pulmonary embolism, thrombosis, and vascular obliteration (e.g., kinking, clamping, blocking of the pulmonary artery during surgery) can increase the amount of lung that is ventilated but unperfused. Vascular obliteration can also increase dead space ventilation; this occurs with age $(V_D/V_T\% = 33 + age/3)$. Rapid, short inspirations may be distributed preferentially to noncompliant (short time constant for inflation) and badly perfused alveoli, whereas slow inspiration allows time for distribution to more compliant (long time constant for inflation) and better perfused alveoli. Thus, rapid, short inspirations may have a dead space ventilation effect.

The anesthesia apparatus increases total dead space (V_D/V_T) for two reasons. First, the apparatus simply increases the anatomic dead space. Inclusion of normal apparatus dead space increases the total V_D/V_T ratio from 33% to about 46% in intubated patients and to

Cardiovascular Response to Hypoxemia

Hemodynamic Variable O$_2$ Saturation (%)	Heart Rate	Systemic Blood Pressure	Stroke Volume	Cardiac Output	SVR	Predominant Response
>80	↑	↑	↑	↑	No change	Reflex, excitatory
60–80	↑ Baroreceptor	↓	No change	No change	↓	Local, depressant > reflex, excitatory
<60	↓	↓	↓	↓	↓	Local, depressant

SVR, Systemic vascular resistance; ↑, increase; ↓, decrease.

about 64% in patients breathing through a mask.[186] Second, anesthesia circuits cause rebreathing of exhaled gases, which is equivalent to dead space ventilation. The rebreathing classification by Mapleson during spontaneous ventilation with Mapleson circuits is A (Magill), D, C, and B. The order of increasing rebreathing (decreasing clinical merit) during controlled ventilation is D, B, C, and A. There is no rebreathing in system E (Ayre's T-piece) if the patient's respiratory diastole is long enough to permit washout with a given fresh gas flow (a common event) or if the fresh gas flow is greater than the peak inspiratory flow rate (an uncommon event).

The effects of an increase in dead space can usually be counteracted by a corresponding increase in the respiratory $\dot{V}_E$. If, for example, the $\dot{V}_E$ is 10 L/min and the V$_D$/V$_T$ ratio is 30%, alveolar ventilation is 7 L/min. If a pulmonary embolism occurred and resulted in an increase in the V$_D$/V$_T$ ratio to 50%, $\dot{V}_E$ would need to be increased to 14 L/min to maintain an alveolar ventilation of 7 L/min (14 L/min × 0.5).

4. Increased Carbon Dioxide Production

All causes of increased O$_2$ consumption also increase CO$_2$ production; these causes include hyperthermia, shivering, catecholamine release (light anesthesia), hypertension, and thyroid storm. If $\dot{V}_E$, total dead space, and $\dot{V}_A/\dot{Q}$ relationships are constant, an increase in CO$_2$ production results in hypercapnia.

5. Inadvertent Switching Off of a Carbon Dioxide Absorber

Many factors, such as patients' ventilatory responsiveness to CO$_2$ accumulation, fresh gas flow, circle system design, and CO$_2$ production, determine whether hypercapnia results from accidental switching off or depletion of a circle CO$_2$ absorber. However, high fresh gas flows (≥5 L/min) minimize the problem with almost all systems for almost all patients.

6. Hypocapnia

The mechanisms of hypocapnia are the reverse of those that produce hypercapnia. Thus, all other factors being equal, hyperventilation (spontaneous or controlled ventilation), decreased V$_D$ ventilation (e.g., change from a mask airway to an ETT airway, decreased PEEP, increased Ppa, decreased rebreathing), and decreased CO$_2$ production (e.g., hypothermia, deep anesthesia, hypotension) lead to hypocapnia. By far the most common mechanism of hypocapnia is passive hyperventilation by mechanical means.

G. Physiologic Effects of Abnormalities in Respiratory Gases

1. Hypoxia

The end products of aerobic metabolism (oxidative phosphorylation) are CO$_2$ and water, both of which are easily diffusible and lost from the body. The essential feature of hypoxia is the cessation of oxidative phosphorylation when mitochondrial P$_{O_2}$ falls below a critical level. Anaerobic pathways, which produce energy (ATP) inefficiently, are then used. The main anaerobic metabolites are hydrogen and lactate ions, which are not easily excreted. They accumulate in the circulation, where they can be quantified in terms of the base deficit and the lactate-pyruvate ratio.

Because the various organs have different blood flow and O$_2$ consumption rates, the manifestations and clinical diagnosis of hypoxia are usually related to symptoms arising from the most vulnerable organ. This organ is usually the brain in an awake patient and the heart in an anesthetized patient (see later discussion), but in special circumstances it may be the spinal cord (e.g., aortic surgery), kidney (e.g., acute tubular necrosis), liver (e.g., hepatitis), or limb (e.g., claudication, gangrene).

The cardiovascular response to hypoxemia is a product of both reflex (neural and humoral) and direct effects (Table 5-5).[187-189] The reflex effects occur first and are excitatory and vasoconstrictive. The neuroreflex effects result from aortic and carotid chemoreceptor, baroreceptor, and central cerebral stimulation, and the humoral reflex effects result from catecholamine and renin-angiotensin release. The direct local vascular effects of hypoxia are inhibitory and vasodilatory and occur late. The net response to hypoxia in a subject depends on the severity of the hypoxia, which determines the magnitude and balance between the inhibitory and excitatory components; the balance may vary according to the type and depth of anesthesia and the degree of preexisting cardiovascular disease.

Mild arterial hypoxemia (arterial saturation less than normal but still 80% or higher) causes general activation of the sympathetic nervous system and release of catecholamines. Consequently, the heart rate, stroke volume, $\dot{Q}_T$, and myocardial contractility—as measured by a shortened pre-ejection period (PEP), left ventricular ejection time (LVET), and a decreased PEP/LVET ratio—are increased (Fig. 5-41).[190] Changes in systemic vascular resistance (SVR) are usually slight. However, in patients under anesthesia with β-blockers, hypoxia (and hypercapnia when present) may cause circulating

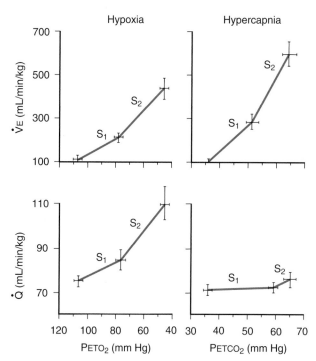

Figure 5-41 Changes in the minute ventilation and in the circulation of healthy awake humans during progressive isocapnic hypoxia and hyperoxic hypercapnia. *PETCO₂*, End-tidal Pco₂; *PETO₂*, end-tidal Po₂; *Q̇*, cardiac output; *S₁*, slope during the first phase of slowly increasing ventilation and/or circulation; *S₂*, slope during the second phase of sharply increasing ventilation and/or circulation; *V̇E*, expired minute ventilation. (Redrawn from Serebrovskaya TV: Comparison of respiratory and circulatory human responses to progressive hypoxia and hypercapnia. *Respiration* 59:35, 1992.)

catecholamines to have only an α-receptor effect, the heart may be unstimulated (even depressed by a local hypoxia effect), and SVR may be increased. Consequently, Q̇T may be decreased in these patients. With moderate hypoxemia (arterial O₂ saturation 60% to 80%), local vasodilation begins to predominate and SVR and blood pressure decrease, but the heart rate may continue to be increased because of a systemic hypotension-induced stimulation of baroreceptors. Finally, with severe hypoxemia (arterial saturation <60%), local depressant effects dominate and blood pressure falls rapidly; the pulse slows, shock develops, and the heart either fibrillates or becomes asystolic.

Significant preexisting hypotension converts a mild hypoxemic hemodynamic profile into a moderate hypoxemic hemodynamic profile and converts a moderate hypoxemic hemodynamic profile into a severe hypoxemic hemodynamic profile. Similarly, in well-anesthetized or sedated patients, early sympathetic nervous system reactivity to hypoxemia may be reduced and the effects of hypoxemia may be expressed only as bradycardia with severe hypotension and, ultimately, circulatory collapse.[191]

Hypoxemia can also promote cardiac dysrhythmias, which may in turn potentiate the already mentioned deleterious cardiovascular effects. Hypoxemia-induced dysrhythmias can be caused by multiple mechanisms; the mechanisms are interrelated because they all cause a decrease in the myocardial O₂ supply-demand ratio,

which in turn increases myocardial irritability. First, arterial hypoxemia can directly decrease the myocardial O₂ supply. Second, early tachycardia may result in increased myocardial O₂ consumption, and decreased diastolic filling time may lead to decreased myocardial O₂ supply. Third, early increased systemic blood pressure can cause an increased afterload on the left ventricle, which increases left ventricular O₂ demand. Fourth, late systemic hypotension may decrease myocardial O₂ supply because of decreased diastolic perfusion pressure. Fifth, coronary blood flow reserve may be exhausted by a late, maximally increased coronary blood flow as a result of maximal coronary vasodilation.[192] The level of hypoxemia that causes cardiac dysrhythmias cannot be predicted with certainty because the myocardial O₂ supply-demand relationship in a given patient is not known (i.e., the degree of coronary artery atherosclerosis may not be known). However, if a myocardial area (or areas) become hypoxic or ischemic, or both, unifocal or multifocal premature ventricular contractions, ventricular tachycardia, and ventricular fibrillation may occur.

The cardiovascular response to hypoxia includes a number of other important effects. Cerebral blood flow increases (even if hypocapnic hyperventilation is present). Ventilation is stimulated regardless of the reason for the hypoxia (see Fig. 5-41). The pulmonary distribution of blood flow is more homogeneous because of increased pulmonary artery pressure. Chronic hypoxia causes an increased Hb concentration and a right-shifted oxy-Hb curve (as a result of either an increase in 2,3-DPG or acidosis), which tends to raise tissue Po₂.

2. Hyperoxia (Oxygen Toxicity)

The dangers associated with inhalation of excessive O₂ are multiple. Exposure to high O₂ tension clearly causes pulmonary damage in healthy individuals.[193,194] A dose-time toxicity curve for humans is available from a number of studies.[193-195] Because the lungs of normal human volunteers cannot be directly examined to determine the rate of onset and the course of toxicity, indirect measures such as onset of symptoms have been used to construct dose-time toxicity curves. Examination of the curve indicates that 100% O₂ should not be administered for more than 12 hours, 80% O₂ for more than 24 hours, and 60% O₂ for more than 36 hours.[193-195] No measurable changes in pulmonary function or blood-gas exchange occur in humans during exposure to less than 50% O₂, even for long periods.[195] Nevertheless, it is important to note that in the clinical setting, these dose-time toxicity relationships are often obscured because of the complex multivariable nature of the clinical setting.[196]

The dominant symptom of O₂ toxicity in human volunteers is substernal distress, which begins as mild irritation in the area of the carina and may be accompanied by occasional coughing.[197] As exposure continues, the pain becomes more intense, and the urge to cough and to deep-breathe also becomes more intense. These symptoms progress to severe dyspnea, paroxysmal coughing, and decreased vital capacity when the Fio₂ has been 1.0 for longer than 12 hours. If excessive O2 is discontinued at this point, recovery of mechanical lung function usually occurs within 12 to 24 hours, but more than 24 hours may be required in some individuals.[195] As toxicity progresses, results of other pulmonary function studies such as compliance and blood gases show deterioration. Pathologically, in animals, the lesion progresses from tracheobronchitis (exposure for 12 hours to a few days), to involvement of the alveolar septa with pulmonary interstitial edema (exposure for a few days to 1 week), to pulmonary fibrosis of the edema (exposure for >1 week).[198]

Ventilatory depression can occur in patients who, by reason of drugs or disease, have been ventilating in response to a hypoxic drive. By definition, ventilatory depression that results from removal of a hypoxic drive through increasing the inspired O_2 concentration causes hypercapnia but does not necessarily produce hypoxia (because of the increased F_{IO_2}).

Absorption atelectasis was described earlier (see "High Inspired Oxygen Concentration and Absorption Atelectasis"). Retrolental fibroplasia, an abnormal proliferation of the immature retinal vasculature of a prematurely born infant, can occur after exposure to hyperoxia. Extremely premature infants are most susceptible to retrolental fibroplasia (i.e., those <1.0 kg in birth weight and <28 weeks of gestation). The risk of retrolental fibroplasia exists whenever F_{IO_2} causes Pa_{O_2} to be greater than 80 mm Hg for longer than 3 hours in an infant whose gestational age plus life age combined is less than 44 weeks. If the ductus arteriosus is patent, arterial blood samples should be drawn from the right radial artery; umbilical or lower-extremity Pa_{O_2} is lower than the Pa_{O_2} to which the eyes are exposed because of ductal shunting of unoxygenated blood.

The mode of action of O_2 toxicity in tissues is complex, but interference with metabolism seems to be widespread. Most importantly, many enzymes, particularly those with sulfhydryl groups, are inactivated by O_2-derived free radicals.[196] Neutrophil recruitment and release of mediators of inflammation occur next and greatly accelerate the extent of endothelial and epithelial damage and impairment of the surfactant systems.[196] The most acute toxic effect of O_2 in humans is a convulsive effect, which occurs during exposure to pressures in excess of 2 atmospheres (atm) absolute.

High inspired O_2 concentrations can be of use therapeutically. Clearance of gas loculi in the body may be greatly accelerated by the inhalation of 100% O_2. Inhalation of 100% O_2 creates a large nitrogen gradient from the gas space to the perfusing blood. As a result, nitrogen leaves the gas space and the space diminishes in size. Administration of O_2 to remove gas may be used to ease

intestinal gas pressure in patients with intestinal obstruction, to decrease the size of an air embolus, and to aid in the absorption of pneumoperitoneum, pneumocephalus, and pneumothorax.

3. Hypercapnia

The effects of CO_2 on the cardiovascular system are as complex as those of hypoxia. Like hypoxemia, hypercapnia appears to cause direct depression of both cardiac muscle and vascular smooth muscle, but at the same time it causes reflex stimulation of the sympathoadrenal system, which compensates to a greater or lesser extent for the primary cardiovascular depression (see Fig. 5-41).[189,192] With moderate to severe hypercapnia, a hyperkinetic circulation results with increased $\dot{Q}T$ and increased systemic blood pressure.[190] Even in patients under halothane anesthesia, plasma catecholamine levels increase in response to increased CO_2 levels in much the same way as in conscious subjects. Thus, hypercapnia, like hypoxemia, may cause increased myocardial O_2 demand (tachycardia, early hypertension) and decreased myocardial O_2 supply (tachycardia, late hypotension).

Table 5-6 summarizes the interaction of anesthesia with hypercapnia in humans; increased $\dot{Q}T$ and decreased SVR should be emphasized.[199,200] The increase in $\dot{Q}T$ is most marked during anesthesia with drugs that enhance sympathetic activity and least marked with halothane and nitrous oxide. The decrease in SVR is most marked during enflurane anesthesia and hypercapnia. Hypercapnia is a potent pulmonary vasoconstrictor even after the inhalation of 3% isoflurane for 5 minutes.[199]

Dysrhythmias have been reported in unanesthetized humans during acute hypercapnia, but they have seldom been of serious import. A high Pa_{CO_2} level is, however, more dangerous during general anesthesia. With halothane anesthesia, dysrhythmias frequently occur above a Pa_{CO_2} arrhythmic threshold that is often constant for a particular patient. Furthermore, halothane, enflurane, and isoflurane have been shown to prolong the QT_C interval in humans, thereby increasing the risk for torsades de pointes ventricular tachycardia, which in turn is notorious for decompensating into ventricular fibrillation.[201]

The maximum stimulatory respiratory effect is attained by a Pa_{CO_2} of about 100 mm Hg. With a higher Pa_{CO_2}, stimulation is reduced, and at extremely high levels, respiration is depressed and later ceases altogether. The P_{CO_2} ventilation-response curve is generally displaced to the right, and its slope is reduced by anesthetics and other depressant drugs.[202] With profound anesthesia, the

---

TABLE 5-6

Cardiovascular Responses to Hypercapnia (Pa_{CO_2} = 60–83 mm Hg) During Various Types of Anesthesia (1 MAC Equivalent Except for Nitrous Oxide)*

Anesthesia	Heart Rate	Contractility	Cardiac Output	Systemic Vascular Resistance
Conscious	↑↑	↑↑	↑↑↑	↓
Nitrous oxide	0	↑	↑↑	↓↓
Halothane	0	↑	↑	↓
Isoflurane	↑↑	↑↑↑	↑↑↑	↓

*The increase in the partial arterial pressure of carbon dioxide (Pa_{CO_2}) in conscious subjects was 11.5 mm Hg from a normal level of 38 mm Hg.
↑, <10% increase; ↑↑, 10–25% increase; ↑↑↑, >25% increase; 0, no change; ↓, <10% decrease; ↓↓, 10–25% decrease; ↓↓↓, >25% decrease; *MAC*, minimum alveolar concentration for adequate anesthesia in 50% of subjects.

response curve may be flat or even sloping downward, and CO_2 then acts as a respiratory depressant. In patients with ventilatory failure, CO_2 narcosis occurs when $PaCO_2$ rises to greater than 90 to 120 mm Hg. A 30% CO_2 concentration is sufficient for the production of anesthesia, and this concentration causes total but reversible flattening of the electroencephalogram.[203] As expected, hypercapnia causes bronchodilation in both healthy persons and patients with lung disease.[204] Quite apart from the effect of CO_2 on ventilation, it exerts two other important effects that influence the oxygenation of the blood.[117] First, if the concentration of nitrogen (or other inert gas) remains constant, the concentration of CO_2 in alveolar gas can increase only at the expense of O_2, which must be displaced. Thus, PAO_2 and PaO_2 may decrease. Second, hypercapnia shifts the oxy-Hb curve to the right, thereby facilitating tissue oxygenation.[95]

Chronic hypercapnia results in increased reabsorption of bicarbonate by the kidneys, which further raises the plasma bicarbonate level and constitutes a secondary or compensatory metabolic alkalosis. The decrease in renal reabsorption of bicarbonate in patients with chronic hypocapnia results in a further fall in plasma bicarbonate and produces a secondary or compensatory metabolic acidosis. In each case, arterial pH returns toward the normal value, but the bicarbonate ion concentration departs even further from normal.

Hypercapnia is accompanied by leakage of potassium from cells into plasma. Much of the potassium comes from the liver, probably from glucose release and mobilization, which occur in response to the rise in plasma catecholamine levels.[205] Because the plasma potassium level takes an appreciable time to return to normal, repeated bouts of hypercapnia at short intervals result in a stepwise rise in plasma potassium. Finally, hypercapnia can predispose the patient to other complications in the operating room; for example, the oculocephalic response is far more common during hypercapnia than during eucapnia.[206]

4. Hypocapnia

In this section, hypocapnia is considered to be produced by passive hyperventilation (by the anesthesiologist or ventilator). Hypocapnia can cause a decrease in $\dot{Q}T$ by three separate mechanisms. First, if it is present, an increase in intrathoracic pressure decreases $\dot{Q}T$. Second, hypocapnia is associated with withdrawal of sympathetic nervous system activity, and such withdrawal can decrease the inotropic state of the heart. Third, hypocapnia can increase pH, and the increased pH can decrease ionized calcium, which may in turn decrease the inotropic state of the heart. Hypocapnia with alkalosis also shifts the oxy-Hb curve to the left, which increases Hb affinity for O_2 and thus impairs O_2 unloading at the tissue level. The decrease in peripheral flow and the impaired ability to unload O_2 to the tissues are compounded by an increase in whole-body O_2 consumption as a result of increased pH-mediated uncoupling of oxidation from phosphorylation.[207] A $PaCO_2$ of 20 mm Hg increases tissue O_2 consumption by 30%. Consequently, hypocapnia may simultaneously increase tissue O_2 demand and decrease tissue O_2 supply. To have the same amount of O_2 delivery

to the tissues, $\dot{Q}T$ or tissue perfusion has to increase at a time when it may not be possible for it to do so. The cerebral effects of hypocapnia may be related to a state of cerebral acidosis and hypoxia because hypocapnia can cause a selective reduction in cerebral blood flow and also shifts the oxy-Hb curve to the left.[208]

Hypocapnia can cause $\dot{V}A/\dot{Q}$ abnormalities by inhibiting HPV or by causing bronchoconstriction and decreased CL. Finally, passive hypocapnia promotes apnea.

III. CONCLUSIONS

The primary purpose of the respiratory system is to facilitate gas exchange of O_2 and CO_2 in the alveoli. At the alveoli, O_2 combines with hemoglobin and is transported throughout the body by the circulatory system, while at the same time CO_2 which has been transported from the tissues is removed to be exhaled via the alveoli. These respiratory functions are achieved by coordinated action of the upper and lower airways, alveoli, pulmonary blood flow, respiratory muscles, and metabolic sensors, along with medullary and neural-based control centers.

The lungs also serve a number of very important nonpulmonary metabolic and humoral functions, as described in this chapter.

Ventilation is the process of bringing in O_2 rich air through the airways to the alveoli (inhalation), where gas exchange occurs; then, during exhalation, the O_2-depleted air (along with CO_2 produced in tissues) is returned to the external environment. The process of ventilation is tightly regulated by neural and non-neural mechanisms.

Perfusion relates to the quantity of blood flowing by the alveoli. Pulmonary perfusion is generally equal to cardiac output, unless shunts occur. Ventilation is closely coupled with perfusion of the alveoli. The interaction between ventilation and perfusion (ventilation-perfusion [$\dot{V}A/\dot{Q}$] relationship) ultimately determines the gas exchange in the lungs.

The transport of O_2 requires reversible binding of O_2 to Hb, which is then unloaded at the tissues. The O_2 flows through its concentration gradient to the extracellular space and cells. Intracellular concentrations of O_2 vary within the cell, with the mitochondrial PO_2 being very low compared to arterial and even mixed venous blood values. Furthermore, interaction of the circulatory system with the respiratory system adds another level of fine-tuning and complexity to the process of perfusion, ventilation, and ventilation-perfusion interaction.

Cardiac and respiratory functions are closely integrated with numerous feedback mechanisms designed to match ventilation with perfusion. The lungs and the heart are the only organs that receive the full $\dot{Q}T$. Accordingly, the lungs are anatomically well situated to perform many of the secondary (nonpulmonary) functions. The list of nonpulmonary functions continues to grow and includes filtering of metabolic products, conversion of important enzymes, and immune protection.

Pulmonary and nonpulmonary functions adapt to constantly changing needs of the body. Understanding the basic physiologic mechanisms involved in pulmonary and nonpulmonary functions of the lungs is the key to appreciating the pathophysiology of respiratory disorders and the rational management of respiratory function during resuscitation, perioperative management, and critical care.

IV. CLINICAL PEARLS

- The ventilated gas that participates in gas exchange is referred to as alveolar ventilation ($\dot{V}_A$). The amount of gas that is wasted is referred to as dead space ventilation (V_D). The aggregate total of dead space ventilation is referred to as the physiologic dead space ($V_{D_{physiologic}}$) and is divided into two subcomponents. The volume of gas that ventilates the conducting airways is called the anatomic dead space ($V_{D_{anatomic}}$), and the volume of gas that ventilates nonperfused alveoli is the alveolar dead space ($V_{D_{alveolar}}$).

- Ventilation-perfusion ($\dot{V}/\dot{Q}$) relationships are important in pulmonary gas exchange. At the top of the lung there is relatively high $\dot{V}/\dot{Q}$, whereas at the bottom, there is relatively low $\dot{V}/\dot{Q}$. However, most of the perfusion and most of the ventilation occur at the base, and perfusion is fairly well matched throughout the lung in normal, young, healthy individuals. Alveolar ventilation without perfusion results in alveolar dead space, and alveolar perfusion without ventilation results in a right-to-left transpulmonary shunt.

- The functional residual capacity (FRC) is the amount of gas in the lungs at end-exhalation during normal tidal breathing. The FRC is also equal to the sum of the expiratory reserve volume and the residual volume. The FRC has important clinical significance because it represents the major reservoir of oxygen in the body and is directly related to the time until desaturation after apnea. The FRC is also inversely proportional to the degree of low-$\dot{V}/\dot{Q}$ alveoli and shunt. For example, morbidly obese patients have low FRCs, tend to desaturate quickly, and have many more atelectatic alveoli and shunt units than normal, age-matched patients.

- Lung compliance (C_L, volume/pressure) is the inverse of elastance. C_L is bimodal: it is low at low lung volumes, highest at normal lung volumes (normal FRC), and low at very high lung volumes. The formula for compliance is analogous to the mathematical formula used to calculate capacitance in electronics.

- Factors that affect airway resistance include lung volume, bronchial smooth muscle tone, and the density/viscosity of the inhaled gas.

- Pulmonary vessels constrict in response to hypoxia, hypercarbia, and acidosis, whereas systemic vessels dilate when exposed to these factors.

- Clinically, the work of breathing (WOB) can be simplified to an equation, because it is directly related to the minute ventilation ($\dot{V}_E$) and airway resistance (R_{AW}) and inversely related to C_L (see Equation 9).

- Increased O_2 affinity shifts the oxygen-hemoglobin (oxy-Hb) dissociation curve to the left (i.e., increases the affinity of Hb for O_2, thus reducing P_{50}, the oxygen concentration at which Hb is 50% saturated), whereas decreased O_2 affinity shifts the oxy-Hb curve to the right (i.e., decreases Hb affinity for O_2 and thus increases P_{50}). The four primary processes that shift the oxy-Hb curve to the right are increased hydrogen ion concentration ($[H^+]$), increased carbon dioxide tension (P_{CO_2}), increased 2,3-diphosphoglycerate (2,3-DPG), and increased temperature.

- The Bohr effect refers to the effect of P_{CO_2} and $[H^+]$ ions on the oxy-Hb curve (i.e., increasing the propensity for O_2 to offload from Hb).

- The Haldane effect describes the shift in the CO_2 dissociation curve caused by oxygenation of Hb. Low P_{O_2} shifts the CO_2 dissociation curve to the left so that the blood is able to pick up more CO_2 (e.g., in capillaries of rapidly metabolizing tissues). Highly oxygenated Hb (as occurs in the lungs) reduces the affinity of Hb for CO_2, shifting the CO_2 dissociation curve to the right and thereby increasing CO_2 removal.

- CO_2 is transported in the blood primarily in three different forms: physically dissolved in blood, bound to amino groups of proteins (e.g., Hb) as carbamate compounds, and as bicarbonate ions.

SELECTED REFERENCES

All references can be found online at expertconsult.com.

 1. West JB, Dollery CT, Naimark A: Distribution of blood flow in isolated lung: Relation to vascular and alveolar pressures. *J Appl Physiol* 19:713, 1964.
 17. West JB: Blood flow to the lung and gas exchange. *Anesthesiology* 41:124, 1974.
 24. Benumof JL: Mechanism of decreased blood flow to the atelectatic lung. *J Appl Physiol* 46:1047, 1978.
 40. Bendixen HH, Bullwinkel B, Hedley-Whyte J, et al: Atelectasis and shunting during spontaneous ventilation in anesthetized patients. *Anesthesiology* 25:297, 1964.
 77. Lumb AB: Pulmonary ventilation: Mechanisms and the work of breathing. In Lumb AB, editor: *Nunn's applied respiratory physiology*, ed 5, London, 2000, Butterworths, p 128.
 112. Hedenstierna G: Gas exchange during anaesthesia. *Br J Anaesth* 64:507, 1990.
 117. Wilson WC, Shapiro B: Perioperative hypoxia: The clinical spectrum and current oxygen monitoring methodology. *Anesthesiol Clin North Am* 19:769, 2001.
 147. Pelosi P, Croci M, Ravagnan I, et al: The effects of body mass on lung volumes, respiratory mechanics, and gas exchange during general anesthesia. *Anesth Analg* 87:654, 1998.
 156. Froese AB, Bryan CA: Effects of anesthesia and paralysis on diaphragmatic mechanics in man. *Anesthesiology* 41:242, 1974.
 184. Ware LB, Matthay MA: Acute respiratory distress syndrome. *N Engl J Med* 342:1334, 2000.

Chapter 6

Airway Pharmacology

DAVID R. BALL | BARRY E. MCGUIRE

I. INTRODUCTION

Airway pharmacology is concerned with the effect of drug action on airway function, with relevance to anesthesia and critical care. We define a *drug* as a medicinal substance prescribed and administered with therapeutic intent. This definition excludes unprescribed substances consumed for social or recreational purposes. Drugs should be used rationally, with knowledge of *effect* (efficacy, the therapeutic intent) and *side effect* (toxicity). A measure of the safety margin between efficacy and toxicity is the *therapeutic ratio*, and the expected benefit should reasonably outweigh the risk. Drug selection should be a rational choice based on three principles:

1. *Pharmacodynamics:* concerned with drug action, both positive (efficacy) and negative (toxicity)

159

2. *Pharmacokinetics:* concerned with optimal delivery and removal of the drug from sites of action (the biophase)
3. *Pharmacoeconomics:* concerned with cost-effectiveness in the selection of drug.

In common with all forms of medical treatment, drug therapy carries risk, which should be considered and managed. Drug therapy must be viewed in context. Airway management involves the application of knowledge, skills, and attitudes. Drug administration is only one part of this process, used as part of an overall therapeutic plan. Use of drugs must be viewed within the context of this plan and individualized for a particular patient with a particular set of challenges.

This chapter offers a clinical perspective on airway pharmacology. It is divided into two parts. The first part reviews the actions of common anesthetic drugs on normal airway physiology. The second part reviews the use of drugs in managing the most common airway disorder, asthma, and its analog, intraoperative bronchospasm.

The effects of drugs on the upper airway (nares to glottis) and on the lower airway (glottis to terminal bronchioles) are integral to the practice of safe and effective airway management. Drug administration is often deliberate, either as a treatment for airway pathology or as part of an airway management plan for anesthesia. On occasion, however, there are unwanted effects that may contribute to airway compromise.

II. AIRWAY PHARMACOLOGY IN NORMAL AIRWAY PHYSIOLOGY

A. Clinical Issues

The relevance of airway pharmacology can be considered in relation to a number of clinically important issues.

1. Airway Patency

Maintenance of upper airway patency is critical to achieving adequate ventilation and is affected by a variety of drugs that influence motor tone or sensory feedback or both. Drugs may act directly (e.g., topically administered local anesthetics) or, more commonly, indirectly (e.g., analgesics, sedatives) by acting on the central nervous system (CNS) to compromise upper airway patency.

The lower airway behaves somewhat differently in response to changes in muscle tone, but the drug effects can also have an impact on ventilation and gas exchange.

2. Airway Protection

By similar direct and indirect mechanisms, drugs that are given to optimize the upper airway for airway management interfere with the generation of protective reflexes and thus affect a patient's ability to prevent aspiration.

3. Airway Reactivity

Because the irritability of the upper and lower airways is influenced by centrally-acting and locally-acting drugs used in anesthetic practice, skill in judgment of anesthetic depth is critical to safe airway management. Similarly, endotracheal intubation success is maximized and the risk of laryngeal trauma is minimized by drugs that provide nonreactive vocal cords and an open glottis.

4. Adverse Reactions

Drugs involved in airway management can result in a variety of unwanted sequelae, both local and systemic. These are considered in relation to specific drugs later in this chapter.

5. Optimizing Conditions for Instrumentation of the Airway

Airway management is most likely to be successful when conditions are ideal in terms of airway patency and reactivity. However, the potential reversibility of airway pharmacology must also be considered if the initial airway management plan proves unsuccessful. In this situation, a clinical decision may be taken to reverse the effects of the airway-active drugs as part of an airway rescue plan.

6. Management of the Obstructed Airway

Management of the obstructed airway is considered in Chapter 43.

B. Physiology of the Upper Airway

Physiology of the upper airway is considered in detail in Chapter 5. In the awake patient, airway patency is maintained by muscle tone in the head and neck, particularly the pharynx and tongue. The upper airway muscles are influenced by afferent information from a number of sources (Fig. 6-1), including receptors in the upper airway and lung that respond to changes in airway pressure and a variety of chemical and mechanical stimuli.

A number of nonpharmacologic factors influence the patency of the upper airway. These include the following.

1. Anatomy

Age, body habitus, and posture are all relevant factors. The increased amount of cervical adipose tissue in obesity decreases the volume of the upper airway. The influence of gravity on airway patency is such that tissues have a tendency to fall backward in the supine patient. Head-on-neck extension and jaw thrust move the hyoid bone

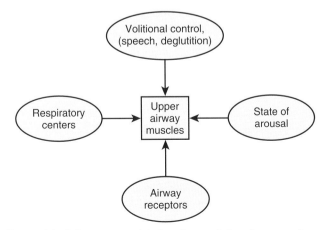

Figure 6-1 Influences modulating the activity of upper airway muscles.

and attached structures anteriorly, helping to relieve any obstruction.

2. Neuromuscular Function

Many of the upper airway muscles can be classed as either airway constricting or airway dilating. These muscles regulate upper airway function by regulating the shape of the upper airway, but their relationships are complex.

3. Autonomic Nervous System

Increased sympathetic nervous activity dilates the upper and lower airways. Sleep has the reverse effect, increasing upper airway resistance. General anesthesia blunts the sympathetic responses to noxious stimuli such as pain. Conversely, during exercise, neurogenic and chemical stimuli trigger dilation of the upper airway to cope with the increase in gas flow. The upper airway muscles, in conjunction with the diaphragm and chest wall muscles, respond to the stresses of hypoxia and hypercarbia to increase upper airway patency, in tandem with the increased ventilatory drive and improved lower airway function.

4. Voluntary Regulation of Airway Patency

Factors involving voluntary regulation of airway patency include speech and swallowing.

5. Disease

Malignancy, infection, neuromuscular disease, and obstructive sleep apnea can affect airway patency.

C. Effects of Drugs on the Airway

1. Direct Effect

Several types of drugs can be administered topically to the airway.

1. *Local anesthetics* attenuate the afferent limbs of the powerful reflexes that serve to protect the upper airway from aspiration of foreign material.
2. *Sympathomimetics*, such as epinephrine and phenylephrine, cause local vasoconstriction to minimize tissue vascularity or reduce edema.
3. *Volatile inhalational agents* cross the alveolar-capillary membrane to have an indirect effect on the respiratory tract via the CNS, but they also have direct effects, including bronchodilation and mucosal irritation.
4. *Bronchodilators* are commonly administered topically, as reviewed in the second part of this chapter.

2. Indirect Effect

Drugs that are administered intravenously (IV) as part of general anesthesia often affect the airway systemically.

1. *Sedatives and analgesics* affect central and peripheral neurologic pathways, largely motor but also sensory, to lessen muscle tone in the upper and lower airways and thereby affect patency and gas flow. Secondary effects on O_2 and CO_2 tension also affect airway tone.
2. *Neuromuscular blocking* (NMB) agents clearly affect skeletal muscle tone and have a major influence on airway management under general anesthesia.
3. *Lidocaine*, given intravenously, affects airway reactivity.
4. *Antihistamines*, used topically in the treatment of rhinitis, can be administered systemically to attenuate histamine-induced reflex bronchoconstriction.
5. *Antimuscarinics*, such as atropine, inhibit the parasympathetic nervous system to reduce salivary gland secretions and dry the upper airway. Upper airway tone is not significantly affected by this antiparasympathetic action, but lower airway resistance is reduced and airway reactivity is attenuated when drugs such as ipratropium bromide are given parenterally or are inhaled.
6. *Respiratory stimulants*, such as doxapram, are used occasionally to provoke spontaneous respiratory effort on cessation of general anesthesia. IV doxapram stimulates chemoreceptors in the carotid arteries, which in turn stimulate the respiratory center in the brainstem to increase respiratory muscle activity. Potentially serious side effects include cardiovascular instability and cerebral irritation.

III. DRUGS WITH A DIRECT EFFECT ON THE AIRWAY

A. Local Anesthetics

Local anesthetics produce a rapid, reversible depression of nerve conduction, particularly with regard to sensory nerves, by binding to sodium channels and interfering with their function, thereby preventing propagation of action potentials. Chemically, they usually consist of a lipophilic group connected to an ionizable group, typically a tertiary amine, by either an ester or an amide link (Fig. 6-2).

Local anesthetics are usually effective topically on airway mucosa. The clinical effect is to reduce airway reactivity. At the same time, there is a reduction in airway caliber and a reduction in the reflexes that protect against aspiration.

Topicalization of the upper airway is a common technique in the "awake" management of a difficult airway (DA), and it is also used during general anesthesia to facilitate upper airway instrumentation when NMB agents are being deliberately avoided. Topical local anesthesia is also used as an adjunct to general anesthesia in both upper airway and lower airway surgery.

Most local anesthetics are weak bases; they are formulated as chloride salts by combining them with acids to maximize their solubility. In plasma, they remain largely in the ionized or protonated form (BH^+) before converting to the non-ionized (lipophilic) form to penetrate the nerve. The proportion of the drug in non-ionized form depends on its acid dissociation constant (pKa): the lower the pKa (i.e., the closer to pH 7.4), the more "free base" (B) available to enter the nerve cell, and the more rapid the action. This relationship is defined by the Henderson-Hasselbalch equation:

$$\log[BH^+]/[B] = pKa - pH$$

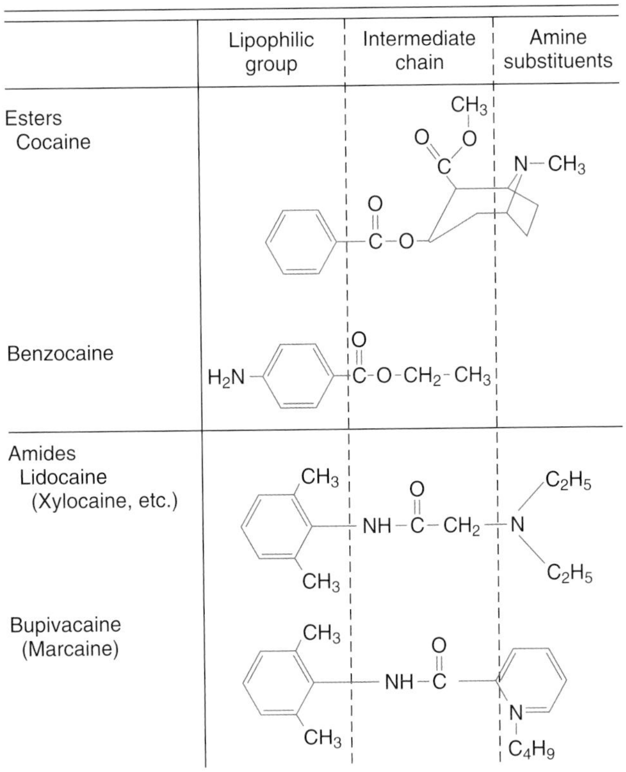

Figure 6-2 Structure of local anesthetics used for topical airway anesthesia.

1. Complications of Airway Local Anesthesia

In infected tissues, topical local anesthesia is often ineffective because of the lower pH of the tissues; this results in a relative increase in the ionized form of the drug, which will not enter the nerve. Alternative techniques may be required.

A reduction in upper airway patency has been demonstrated after topicalization of the airway.[1,2] This occurs because of the loss of afferent feedback and the resultant decrease in motor tone, which may lead to upper airway obstruction, particularly in an airway that is already compromised. Hence, care is needed when considering an awake airway management technique in a patient with evidence of upper airway narrowing.

Systemic toxicity is extremely rare in patients receiving local anesthesia for instrumentation or examination of the upper or lower airway. Most reports suggest that plasma lidocaine levels very rarely approach the reported toxic plasma concentration of 5 to 6 μg/mL. However, one study demonstrated near-toxic levels after gargling of large volumes of lidocaine.[3] Toxicity tends to involve the CNS with irritability or convulsions and the cardiovascular system with circulatory compromise. The safe maximum dose for airway administration for the most commonly used agent, lidocaine, is uncertain, but in one study in which patients received 9 mg/kg lidocaine, none had plasma concentrations in excess of 5 mg/mL.[4] However, the death of a healthy volunteer due to presumed lidocaine toxicity after topicalization for fiberoptic bronchoscopy has been reported in the literature, so some consideration of the dose administered is advisable.[5] The British Thoracic Society recommendation for the use of topical lidocaine with a flexible fiberoptic bronchoscope in adults is not to exceed 8.2 mg/kg.[6]

Topical lidocaine, particularly in higher doses, is an irritant to the upper airway and may stimulate unwanted reflexes. Other side effects include cardiotoxicity, allergy, and abuse potential.

2. Specific Local Anesthetic Agents

a. LIDOCAINE

Lidocaine is by far the most commonly used topical local anesthetic in airway management. It is available for upper airway use in formulations of 2% to 10%, with the 2% strength potentially lacking in potency for effective topicalization and the 10% having more potential for airway irritation. Duration of action is variable, anywhere from 15 and 90 minutes. There are few data concerning any dose-response relationship for intensity or duration of anesthesia. Case reports of toxicity from topical use are rare.

b. BUPIVACAINE

Bupivacaine has been used for topical airway anesthesia, but not commonly. It has the advantage of a more prolonged action but has a slower onset and an increased potential for toxicity compared with lidocaine.

c. BENZOCAINE

Benzocaine is available as a 20% solution for topical use and has a duration of action similar to that of lidocaine; although its toxic potential is low, it has a comparatively low potency. Absorbed benzocaine can produce methemoglobinemia with the potential to compromise O_2 transport.

d. COCAINE

Cocaine, available in solutions of 1% to 10%, provides excellent topical anesthesia and has the advantage of providing intense vasoconstriction, which is often desirable as part of topicalization of the nasal passages before intubation. However, concerns about sympathomimetic toxicity and abuse potential have reduced its use in recent years, particularly in children, since a fatality was reported.[7]

B. Sympathomimetics

The use of sympathomimetics to influence vascular blood flow in airway mucosal vessels is a technique that is commonly used in cases of acutely compromised upper airway in an attempt to reduce swelling. The most common agent used for this purpose is epinephrine, administered via a nebulizer.[8] Vasoconstrictors such as phenylephrine are also used electively to reduce the potential for bleeding during upper airway instrumentation (e.g., nasotracheal intubation).

Topical vasoconstrictors such as epinephrine can also be used to minimize systemic absorption of topical local anesthetics and thereby reduce toxicity, improve efficacy, and increase duration of action.[9] Unwanted effects of sympathomimetics are uncommon and largely relate to systemic absorption of the drug, which can result in an increase in cardiac work.

C. Inhaled Volatile Agents

Inhaled anesthetic agents have a number of direct effects. For example, all volatile agents cause bronchodilation (i.e., increase in the diameter of the lower airways). Isoflurane appears to have the most potent effect, whereas desflurane also has the potential to cause the reverse effect and induce airway constriction.[10]

Airway irritation with increased salivary, laryngeal, and bronchial secretions (caused by an increase in mucus production and a decrease in mucociliary flow rates) varies among agents, with sevoflurane and halothane being essentially nonirritant and isoflurane and desflurane being potential irritants. This stimulation of airway receptors also appears to be responsible for the tachycardia and hypertension observed when desflurane is administered in high concentrations. The depressed mucociliary function seen with volatile agents is likely to contribute to impaired clearance of secretions and potentially to postoperative respiratory complications. The concomitant use of IV opioids lessens the irritant effect of inhaled volatile agents such as desflurane.[11]

Inhibition of hypoxic pulmonary vasoconstriction results in ventilation-perfusion ($\dot{V}/\dot{Q}$) mismatch, with an increase in intrapulmonary shunt fraction.

IV. DRUGS WITH AN INDIRECT EFFECT ON THE AIRWAY

A. Sedatives and Upper Airway Patency

The effect of general anesthetic agents on the upper airway is crucial to the practice of safe airway management, largely in terms of airway patency but also in terms of airway reactivity and airway protection against aspiration. There is a decrease in muscle tone associated with the loss of wakefulness, and this is compounded by specific drug-induced inhibition of upper airway neural and muscle activity and suppression of protective arousal responses. These processes tend to narrow the airway lumen, leading to airway obstruction. The mechanism of the reduction in muscle electrical activity relates, in part, to depressed hypoglossal nerve activity that occurs in excess of a similar depressant effect on other respiratory muscles, such as the diaphragm or intercostal muscles, which are more resistant to this dose-dependent loss of muscle tone.[12] This reduction in hypoglossal nerve activity results in reduced tone in the muscles of the tongue and soft palate.

The differential suppression of respiratory muscles seems to vary among sedative agents, being less pronounced, for example, with ketamine than with other agents.[13] Ketamine also has an indirect effect on the lower airways, causing bronchodilation by inducing the release of endogenous catecholamines. However, the loss of muscle tone caused by sedatives may not only relate to a specific effect of motor nerves. The depressed state of arousal results in a reduction of inputs from the reticular activating system to these motor nerves. This theory is

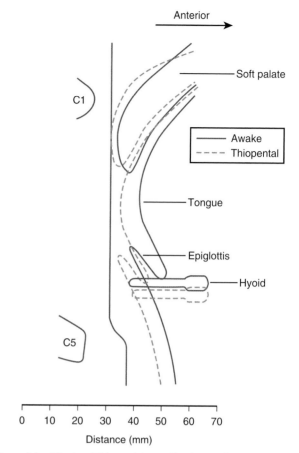

Figure 6-3 Effects of thiopental anesthesia on airway dimensions. Notice that the primary site of obstruction is at the level of the soft palate. (Modified from: Nandi PR, Charlesworth CH, Taylor SJ, et al: Effect of GA on the pharynx. *Br J Anaesth* 66:157, 1991.)

borne out by changes in upper airway patency demonstrated during natural sleep, which show similarities to those induced by sedative drugs.

Originally, the upper airway narrowing associated with anesthesia was attributed to a posterior shift of the base of the tongue. Evidence now suggests that the soft palate and, to a lesser extent, the epiglottis are more relevant (Fig. 6-3). One study using lateral radiography demonstrated that occlusion of the airway under general anesthesia occurred most consistently at the level of the soft palate and sometimes at the level of the epiglottis, but in no patient did the tongue base come into contact with the posterior pharyngeal wall.[14]

Despite the assumption that loss of upper airway patency relates to a reduction in tone of the surrounding muscles, a consistent relationship between electromyographic activity and upper airway resistance has not been demonstrated. Thiopental causes measurable changes in muscular activity, but the changes are inconsistent and do not correlate with the onset of airway obstruction.[15] Similarly, benzodiazepines increase upper airway resistance but again do not appear to have a consistent effect on genioglossus activity.[16] Therefore, airway obstruction under general anesthesia may not relate to a simple diminution of muscular activity but to a disruption of the normal coordination of muscle activity that provides overall control of upper airway function.

The phase of the respiratory cycle is also relevant to the patency of the upper airway during spontaneous ventilation under general anesthesia. In a study by Nandi and colleagues, the movement of the soft palate during expiration was similar to that during apnea. However, during attempted inspiration, there was a significant reduction in the airway lumen at all levels, with the tongue now reaching the posterior pharyngeal wall in some cases and thus contributing further to the airway obstruction.[14] This has relevance when one considers upper airway patency during anesthesia with or without muscle paralysis. The *dynamic* collapse of the upper airway that occurs during spontaneous inspiration anesthesia may be insignificant when pharmacologic paralysis is achieved. Similarly, the application of continuous positive airway pressure (CPAP) may also reduce this effect and help to maintain gas flow.

In summary, the increased collapsibility associated with anesthesia and sedation seems to be universal, regardless of whether the route of administration is inhalational or parenteral. Although this collapsibility lessens with decreasing anesthetic depth, the two do not necessarily have a linear relationship.[17,18] The extent of the upper airway narrowing may vary subtly among agents, but the only clinically relevant difference appears to be the described lesser effect with ketamine.

At a laryngeal level, the effect of general anesthesia is probably different. One study demonstrated that the width of the laryngeal vestibule increased after administration of thiopental and succinylcholine.[19]

B. Effect of Sedatives on Airway Reactivity and Airway Protection

Airway reflexes such as coughing, the expiration reflex, breath-holding, and laryngospasm are important in protecting the airway against contamination. These airway reflexes are usually obtunded by general anesthesia, although the exact relationship between specific agents and this suppression of activity has not been fully explored. Propofol, for example, has been shown to depress these reflexes,[20] but vigorous airway reflexes have been demonstrated under baseline propofol anesthesia, suggesting that the depression with propofol as a lone agent is relatively limited in moderate doses. Combination with fentanyl, however, appears to have a significant influence on lessening airway reflexes.[21]

C. Sedatives and the Potential to Produce Apnea

All sedatives have the potential to abolish respiratory drive, either transiently or for more prolonged periods, and this effect is largely dose dependent. This may be desirable during upper airway instrumentation, but it potentially may also contribute to life-threatening hypoxemia. Propofol, particularly if it is administered as a bolus, produces apnea extremely readily. Other IV sedative agents, such as thiopental and benzodiazepines, also do so, but less potently.

Inhalational agents have a lesser tendency to produce prolonged apnea, so inhalational induction of anesthesia

in a predicted difficult airway scenario remains a favored technique. Sevoflurane is the most commonly used agent now. It has a low blood-gas partition coefficient and is minimally irritating, which facilitates rapid, smooth induction of anesthesia to a depth that may be suitable to permit airway instrumentation. However, transient apnea can occur, as can airway obstruction, so the technique is not without complications.

D. Sedatives and the Lower Airway

All sedative agents that reduce muscular tone are likely to contribute to a reduction in a patient's functional residual capacity (FRC) and an increased work of breathing. Benzodiazepines appear not to have a significant effect on lower airway patency, despite causing an apparent relaxation of tracheal smooth muscle and potentially attenuating reflex bronchoconstriction. The effect of IV anesthetic agents on bronchial smooth muscle is also unlikely to be of clinical significance. In vitro data suggest that propofol has a direct relaxant action.[22] However, case reports and studies of IV induction agents used in asthmatics suggest that ketamine is the only agent with a significant bronchodilatory action. In contrast, volatile agents are fairly potent bronchodilators and have been used in the treatment of status asthmaticus.[23,24]

Multiple mechanisms contribute to the relaxation of smooth muscle produced by sedatives. These mechanisms involve both neural effects, predominantly relating to interference in vagal motor pathways that cause reflex bronchoconstriction, and direct effects on smooth muscle, such as attenuating increases in intracellular calcium. For example, bronchoconstriction caused by airway instrumentation is neurally mediated, whereas in anaphylaxis, the lower airway narrowing is caused by the release of inflammatory mediators. The latter is more likely to respond to a drug that has a *direct* effect on the airway smooth muscle.

E. Opioid Analgesics and the Airway

When fentanyl is combined with propofol, the depressant effect on upper airway reflexes is considerably more profound than with propofol alone, with the cough reflex being the most suppressed reflex and laryngospasm being the most resistant.[21] The central mechanisms for this depression of reflexes are unclear and are probably complex.

Muscle rigidity associated with opioid use has been described[25]; although rare, it may be the direct cause of a significant increase in lower airway resistance that can make ventilation extremely difficult. Others suggest that this rare phenomenon in fact has more to do with vocal cord closure than with decreased pulmonary compliance secondary to chest wall rigidity.[26] If the increase in airway resistance is truly linked to muscle rigidity, then its clinical manifestation is unpredictable and relates to many factors, including the opioid drug, its dose, its speed of administration, the effects of concomitant sedatives and muscle relaxants, and the age of the patient.

Short-acting narcotics are used at times in place of NMB agents, in combination with sedatives, to facilitate endotracheal intubation. However, upper airway conditions for airway instrumentation may be inferior, and the risks of arterial hypotension and laryngeal trauma may be higher.[27]

Remifentanil merits specific discussion because it is a relatively new drug in anesthesia and its use in facilitating safe and effective airway management is increasing. It is a potent, ultrashort-acting synthetic opioid that is administered typically by continuous infusion because it is immediately metabolized in the plasma. It causes profound respiratory depression and therefore is used clinically to successfully prevent spontaneous respiratory effort when assisted ventilation is the chosen mode of gas exchange. It also reduces muscle tone considerably and can be used to facilitate endotracheal intubation in the absence of NMB drugs.[28] Use of remifentanil to facilitate smooth extubation is well described, and for some anesthesiologists,[29] this technique has replaced deep general anesthesia extubation. Continuing remifentanil while discontinuing sedation results in a predominant effect of suppression of upper airway reflexes, in excess of any sedative effect. This allows extubation with good endotracheal tube (ETT) tolerance and a minimum of coughing. However, care is required when using the drug because of its potency. Apnea is likely and can even occur in a patient who is receiving remifentanil alone for conscious sedation.[30] As with other synthetic opioids, muscle rigidity is described but not common.[31]

The main effect of opioids on the lower airway is similar to that described earlier, namely reduced airway reactivity and attenuated reflex bronchoconstriction. Mechanisms of action are again a combination of a neural effect and a direct dose-dependent effect in relaxing airway smooth muscle. For example, there is evidence that morphine attenuates vagally mediated bronchoconstriction in asthmatics.[32] Opioid administration has been shown to cause histamine release, and there is also evidence that they cause an increase in tracheal smooth muscle tone, but neither effect has been associated with clinically demonstrable bronchoconstriction. A condition termed wooden chest syndrome has been described after administration of IV opioids, particularly if given at high dose; in this syndrome, thoracic and abdominal muscle rigidity apparently results in difficulty with assisted ventilation. The clinical significance of this finding is uncertain, but it has not restricted the use of these drugs worldwide.

F. Neuromuscular Blockade and the Airway

NMB agents have several properties that may affect airway function. They are used in clinical practice to facilitate endotracheal intubation by abolishing airway reflexes and to facilitate mechanical ventilation by eliminating spontaneous respiratory effort. Similar to the effects of sedative agents on the respiratory muscles, these drugs also demonstrate a differential effect, with the diaphragm and the adductor muscles of the larynx being more resistant to paralysis than some of the muscles affecting upper airway patency.[33] This relative sparing of the diaphragm permits the maintenance of respiratory effort even during complete paralysis of peripheral

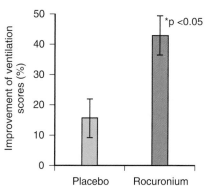

Figure 6-4 Efficacy of facemask ventilation in anesthetized patients with or without neuromuscular blockade. (From: Szabo TA, Spinale FG, et al: Neuromuscular blockade facilitates mask ventilation. *Anesthesiology* 109:A184, 2008.)

muscles. However, it also means that upper airway patency may be compromised at levels of paralysis that otherwise permit maintenance of normal spontaneous ventilation. Clinically, this is most relevant at extubation. A patient with residual NMB drug may maintain adequate ventilation with an artificial airway, such as an ETT or a supralaryngeal airway (SLA), in situ. After removal of the device, airway obstruction leading to hypoxemia may develop.

Removal of protective airway reflexes can have negative consequences if there is a risk of aspiration. Similarly, elimination of spontaneous respiratory effort may be deleterious if assisted ventilation cannot be delivered. Hence, care and experience are required for the safe use of NMB agents, and in certain clinical scenarios, it may be prudent to withhold them. However, the major clinical debate regarding their use seems to relate to their effect on upper airway patency. There is evidence that paralysis of the upper airway musculature *improves* upper airway patency. A recent study published data indicating that NMB using rocuronium facilitated bag-mask ventilation in anesthetized patients (Fig. 6-4).[34]

Another study on the physiologic comparison of spontaneous ventilation and positive-pressure ventilation (PPV) in laryngotracheal stenosis concluded that spontaneous ventilation creates a negative inspiratory extrathoracic intratracheal pressure that causes indrawing of the mobile tracheal segments, further narrowing the airway.[35] During expiration, there is positive intratracheal pressure, and a similar reduction in airflow does not occur. During PPV with muscle paralysis, however, a positive intraluminal pressure is created during inspiration that improves ventilation. Whether the conclusions of this paper can be extrapolated to the management of the upper airway under general anesthesia per se is uncertain, but several leading airway experts feel strongly that they should. The argument states that muscle relaxation makes upper airway management easier (and therefore safer) in terms of ventilation through a facemask or SLA and in terms of airway instrumentation, including intubation.[36,37]

Historically, there has been a fear that the prolonged effect of muscle paralysis during failing airway management under anesthesia contributes to severe hypoxic damage, but there does not appear to be any convincing evidence to support this supposition. The fear appears to relate to the loss of reversibility of the anesthetic technique, although it can never be certain whether the awakening of a patient during failing airway management is feasible before catastrophic desaturation occurs. The evidence suggests that, when faced with impossible bag-mask ventilation, very few anesthesiologists choose to discontinue the general anesthesia or avoid NMB.[38] Most choose to provide oxygenation by intubating the trachea or by ventilating through an SLA device or performing an emergency cricothyrotomy. If ventilation is possible but intubation has been unsuccessful, "wake up" is strongly advocated by discontinuing any sedative drugs while reestablishing muscular tone and respiratory drive and maintaining oxygenation.

Impaired neuromuscular transmission secondary to partial pharmacologic blockade, even to a degree insufficient to evoke respiratory symptoms, markedly impairs upper airway dimensions and function. This may be explained by an impairment of the balance between upper airway dilating forces and the negative intraluminal pressure generated during inspiration. The same effect does not appear to occur during expiration.[39] Furthermore, reflex glottic activity may be preserved, with a tendency toward coughing and laryngospasm, and it may also have a negative effect on gas flow. Complete muscular paralysis necessitating assisted PPV appears to have the reverse effect and increases upper airway patency.

The lower airway behaves differently under muscle paralysis, with a potential loss of airway patency when NMB agents are administered. This may relate to the loss of the subatmospheric intrapleural pressure that normally supports the intrathoracic bronchial tree. Therefore, whereas muscle paralysis may benefit upper airway patency, it may hinder lower airway patency. This can be clinically relevant during management of the scenarios of acute upper and lower airway obstruction.

Histamine release, caused by many of the muscle relaxants, tends to increase lower airway resistance, although clinically this is rarely significant. Some agents, such as atracurium and suxamethonium, are more likely to cause histamine release, although a relationship between these drugs and bronchoconstriction is not clear. Severe bronchoconstriction secondary to anaphylactoid or anaphylactic reactions is described for most muscle relaxants.

Monitoring of the degree of NMB during anesthesia involving muscle relaxants is indicated, but there are limitations with the available techniques. The degree of blockade is frequently monitored by the response of the adductor pollicis to stimulation of the ulnar nerve, although this muscle is more sensitive than the diaphragm to paralysis.[33] At present, monitoring methods that would reliably demonstrate the return of power required to maintain and protect the airway with an effective cough are lacking, and anesthesiologists tend to use a combination of monitoring and clinical assessment.

Reversal of nondepolarizing NMB before extubation and discontinuation of assisted ventilation is standard anesthetic practice. Use of a cholinesterase inhibitor, such as neostigmine, to flood the neuromuscular junction with acetylcholine and thereby restore neuromuscular function has traditionally been the only technique available for reversing the paralysis. These drugs could theoretically cause bronchospasm, but they appear to have no significant effect on airway resistance when combined with an anticholinergic drug such as atropine or glycopyrrolate. More importantly, inadequate reversal of the block, which is probably much more common than most anesthesiologists appreciate, can result in respiratory compromise, morbidity, and mortality.[40] A meta-analysis of current reports of NMB in anesthesia revealed a 41.3% incidence of residual paralysis.[41]

The recent introduction of sugammadex has provided an option for immediate and complete reversal of profound nondepolarizing NMB—when aminosteroid agents such as rocuronium or vecuronium have been used for muscle relaxation—to promote a rapid return of full muscle power and spontaneous respiratory effort. Sugammadex is a geometric donut with a lipophilic core and a hydrophilic periphery; it works in the plasma rather than the neuromuscular junction. The drug encapsulates rocuronium, binding it to its lipophilic core.

G. Other Drugs with Indirect Effect on the Upper Airway

IV lidocaine affects airway tone and reactivity, tending to relax smooth muscle and attenuate reflex bronchoconstriction such as that caused by intubation in asthmatics.[42] However, the effect is unpredictable, and reports of IV lidocaine's actually *causing* bronchoconstriction have been published.[43] Historically, IV lidocaine has been used to improve intubation and extubation conditions by reducing upper airway reactivity.

Administration of IV antihistamine (e.g., chlorpheniramine) reduces histamine-induced airway narrowing, largely affecting the lower airway via antagonism of the H_1 histamine receptors. Administration of such drugs is also recommended in the management of anaphylaxis, in which the upper airway may also be affected. Paradoxically, H_2 antagonists (e.g., ranitidine) may *increase* airway reactivity, although the mechanism of action is unclear.

V. AIRWAY PHARMACOLOGY FOR THE TREATMENT OF ASTHMA

Asthma (from the Greek, *asthma*, "panting"), as defined by the Global Initiative for Asthma (GINA),[44] is a "chronic inflammatory disorder of the airways in which many cellular elements play a role. The chronic inflammation is associated with airway hyperresponsiveness that leads to recurrent episodes of wheezing, breathlessness and coughing, particularly at night or in the early morning. These episodes are usually associated with widespread, but variable, airflow obstruction within the lung that is often reversible either spontaneously or with treatment."

A. Overview

The complex, recursive interplay of inflammation, hyperresponsiveness, and airflow limitation determines the

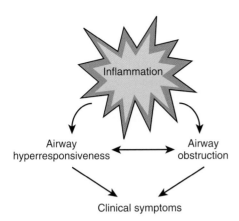

Figure 6-5 Interplay of airway inflammation, hyperresponsiveness, and obstruction. (Adapted from National Asthma Education and Prevention Program: Expert Panel Report III: Guidelines for the diagnosis and management of asthma. Summary report 2007. *J Allergy Clin Immunol* 120(Suppl 5):S94–S138, 2007.)

disease course, which over time produces structural airway changes, termed *remodeling*. There is presently greater recognition of the essentially inflammatory nature to asthma, with treatment directed at reducing this component over the long term as well as providing treatment to alleviate symptoms.[45] An idea of the interplay of these factors is shown in Figure 6-5.

1. Diagnosis

Asthma is a clinical diagnosis, based on the symptoms and signs. Symptoms are variable, with one or more of the following being present: wheeze, breathlessness, cough, and chest tightness.[46,47] None of these symptoms is specific to asthma. For example, wheeze is a function of any airway narrowing as a consequence of reduction of FRC. Signs of asthma include clinical verification by auscultation, spirometry, and lung function testing, which may include gas transfer measurements.[48]

There are no standard definitions for types of symptoms, nor for frequency or severity.[47]

2. Prevalence

Worldwide, asthma is estimated to affect more than 300 million people, 7% to 10% of the global population.[49] About 15 million daily adjusted life-years (DALYs) are lost each year, which places asthma 20th in the current disability ranking, similar to schizophrenia and diabetes. There are about 225,000 asthma deaths each year, amounting to 1 in 250 deaths from all causes.[50] In the United States, 7.3% of the population is diagnosed with asthma, and asthma accounted for 17 million physician consultations in 2006.[51] The worldwide prevalence of asthma is predicted to increase by another 100 million by 2025.[46]

3. Distribution

There are marked differences in national and geographic distribution. Although methodologic factors may confound accurate measurement, there is widespread agreement that asthma is a disease of industrialized nations.[46] Indoor aeroallergens, especially house dust mite[52]; tobacco smoking[53]; and obesity are some implicated factors.[54,55]

Genetic factors may contribute. Inheritance of an "asthmatic genotype" is complex with variable transmission.[56] *Atopy*, the development of immunoglobulin E (IgE) antibodies to specific allergens, is the strongest identifiable risk for developing asthma.[46,57,58] A family history of asthma, particularly on the maternal side, is a strong risk factor.[59] Other inheritable traits are the forced expiratory volume in 1 second (FEV_1) and response to drug therapies.[56]

Additionally, there are gender differences, with a higher incidence of asthma in prepubertal boys compared to girls.[60] In middle age, however, there is a higher incidence among women.

4. Pathology

The pathology of asthma is incompletely understood and is an area of active research.[61,62]

a. AIRFLOW LIMITATION

Airflow limitation results from a combination of bronchoconstriction, inflammatory edema, and hypersecretion of mucus with airway plugging. Blood vessel hyperemia may also narrow small airways.[63,64] These factors, either individually or collectively, narrow airways with impairment of respiratory gas exchange.

Mucus has a complex and variable structure. It is composed of long chains of mucin glycoproteins covalently cross-linked by disulphide bonds, polymerized DNA (from dead cells, particularly eosinophils), and polymerized (fibrous) F-actin together with a mixture of chemical mediators, modulators, and active, inactive, dead, or dying inflammatory cells[65] (Fig. 6-6).

Green sputum is common but is not always indicative of infection, rather resulting from an abundance of eosinophils.[66] When infection occurs, it is usually viral. Bacterial infection is uncommon.[67] Most asthma exacerbations attributed to infection are from viruses,[68] particularly rhinovirus.[69]

b. HYPERREACTIVITY

Hyperreactivity is an exaggerated defense response to potentially noxious stimuli such as inhaled allergens (aeroallergens). It results from a complex interplay of cells and signals, both chemical and neural.

c. INFLAMMATION

One crucial aspect of asthma is considered to be the relative dominance of pro-inflammatory over anti-inflammatory factors driven by a variety of cell types in complex, dynamic, and variable ways. CD4+ lymphocytes, particularly the T helper type 2 (Th2) subtype, are presently thought to have a key role, with a predominance of this population over the T helper 1 (Th1) group. Relative overactivity of the Th2 group, especially at crucial developmental (childhood) stages, with expression of inflammatory cytokines such as interleukin-4 (IL-4), IL-5, IL-9, and IL-13, is considered to play a pivotal role.[70]

The inflammatory cytokines recruit and activate mast cells and eosinophils, leading to cellular infiltration, the density of which is often linked to disease severity.[71] Some interleukins (IL-4 and IL-13) promote B-lymphocyte production of IgE in response to inhalation of allergens

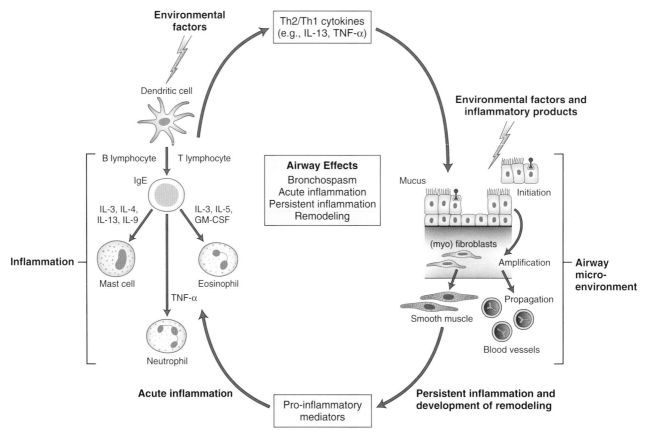

Figure 6-6 Factors limiting airflow in acute and persistent asthma. *GM-CSF,* Granulocyte-macrophage colony-stimulating factor; *IgE,* immunoglobulin E; *IL,* interleukin; *Th1* and *Th2,* helper T lymphocyte subtypes; *TNF-α,* tumor necrosis factor-α. (Adapted and redrawn from Holgate ST, Polosa R: The mechanisms, diagnosis and management of severe asthma in adults. *Lancet* 368:780–793, 2006.)

(aeroallergens). IgE binds to mast cell surface receptors, conferring immunologic memory and triggering release of mast cell contents (degranulation) when exposed to the specific aeroallergen.

A variety of substances such as histamine, proteases (including mast cell tryptase, a time-sensitive marker of degranulation), and cysteinyl-leukotrienes are released.[72] At least 100 mediators have been described.[73] Other stimuli, such as mechanical changes around these cells, may account for mast cell degranulation in response to cold-induced and exercise-induced asthma.[74]

Other cells, such as natural killer cells,[75] Th17 cells,[76] regulatory T cells,[77] dendritic cells,[78,79] macrophages,[80] mast cells,[81] and neutrophils, may be involved.[82] Neutrophil activity is associated with severe disease and sudden deterioration.[83]

d. REMODELING

Poorly controlled asthma may be complicated by anatomic changes in airway structure, which are often correlated to worsening of the disease[84] but may start before diagnosis.[85] A variety of cells are implicated in causing smooth muscle hypertrophy and hyperplasia, subepithelial fibrosis, angiogenesis, and mucus gland hyperplasia—collectively called the epithelial-mesenchymal trophic unit.

Recent attention has focused on the role of pulmonary blood flow in asthmatics, which is higher at rest compared with control subjects and increases during episodes of asthma enough to interfere with airflow.[86]

5. Treatment of Asthma

Major guidelines on treatment have been published by the National Asthma Education and Prevention Program (NAEPP) in the United States,[45] by GINA,[46] and by the British Thoracic Society in association with the Scottish Intercollegiate Guideline Network (SIGN) in the United Kingdom.[47] Management strategies for asthma in adults (including pregnant women), babies, and young children are covered. Treatment is broadly similar, but there are some differences in drugs chosen and doses used. Intensive care and intraoperative management of critical asthma generally lie outside the scope of these guidelines and therefore are covered in more detail in this chapter.

The guidelines specify two major treatment goals: relief of symptoms and risk reduction. Four treatment domains are described—assessment with monitoring, education, risk factor reduction, and drug treatment— covering therapies in four clinical states—episodic asthma, persistent asthma, exacerbation of asthma, and severe acute asthma.

The guidelines aim to provide common terms describing asthma, but other terms are often used within the literature in general, and definitions vary (Table 6-1). Of note is the term *status asthmaticus,* which refers to a life-threatening condition that mandates immediate

TABLE 6-1

Terms Describing the Severity of Acute Asthma

Descriptor	Features
Exacerbation, moderate	PF 50%-75% of predicted
Exacerbation, severe	PF 30%-50% of predicted, tachypnea (>25 breaths/min), tachycardia (>110 beats/min)
Life-threatening	Reduced GCS, systemic hypotension, "silent chest," hypoxemia
Near-fatal	As for life-threatening, plus arterial hypercarbia, need for ventilation
Brittle	Sudden, severe exacerbation or high PF variability to 50%-75% of predicted
Status asthmaticus	Either life-threatening or near-fatal

GCS, Glasgow Coma Score; *PF,* peak expiratory flow rate.

attention, treatment, or escalation of therapy. This term can be applied to severe asthmatic episodes that are resistant to orthodox therapy or require mechanical ventilation.

6. Routes of Drug Delivery

Three routes of drug delivery are available—inhaled, oral and parenteral—which are used alone or in combination.

Inhalation therapy offers the best potential for optimal delivery to the lungs with reduction in systemic side effects. The development and distribution of inhaler drugs and technologies have brought about major improvements in the prevention and treatment of asthma, so that most patients with access to treatment can lead an essentially normal life.

Drugs for inhalation require a dedicated device for delivery.[87] Three main types are available: dry-powder inhalers (DPI), pressurized metered-dose inhalers (pMDI), and nebulizers. All are designed to produce an aerosol for delivery to the lungs. An aerosol is a group of particles having a low settling volume. A practical measure is given by the mass mean aerodynamic diameter (MMAD), a product of mean diameter and square root density. Effective MMAD for therapeutic aerosols is between 0.5 and 5 μm.[88]

For lower values, the particles do not impact the airway and are exhaled. For larger values, impaction occurs in the upper airway,[89] with loss of efficacy and potential for local complications (e.g., oral candidiasis for inhaled glucocorticoids [IGCs])[90] and for systemic toxicity resulting from swallowing deposited drug. The aerosol dose reaching the lungs is called the *respirable mass.* Additional factors influencing drug response include patient compliance, inhalation technique, and the use of adjuncts to aid delivery from the device to the patient.

DPIs have no propellant; they require actuation by the patient with a high inspiratory flow (>40 L/min), and the drug can aggregate. This can be reduced by formulation with other powders, such as lactose, and by the use of baffles within the device to disaggregate the powder.

pMDIs contain drug with propellants, originally chlorofluorocarbons (CFC11 and CFC12). These chemicals contributed to atmospheric ozone depletion and have now been replaced by halogenated fluoroalkanes (HFA227 and HFA134A). Use of HFA as a propellant has allowed reduction of MMAD for steroids from 4 to 1 μm, which increases the respirable mass and allows dosage from the device to be reduced. pMDIs require breath actuation during inspiration with a sustained, but slow, inspiratory flow. Patient technique can be learned but is variable. The use of an adjunct, such as a spacer device with a face mask or mouthpiece, helps.[91] Devices with breath-actuated valves are superior. Selection of the face mask is important, and both size and seal must be considered. For small children, the dead space of some face masks is greater than their tidal volume (V_T).[92] If the face mask seal is poor, aerosol leakage considerably reduces efficacy.[93] Use of a mouthpiece produces superior drug delivery, compared with a face mask, but requires greater patient coordination.[94] Older spacing devices accumulated static charge that reduced aerosol delivery. Newer versions are "charge-reduced."[95]

Nebulizers vary in concept and design. The most common type is the jet nebulizer. It uses a high flow of driving gas through a narrow orifice, creating a Venturi effect, which draws the liquid drug into droplets that can be inhaled.[96] The aerosol produced is a mixture of droplet sizes (polydisperse). Compared with other devices, drug delivery is less efficient overall, with proportions of the drug lost as mist. In general, however, nebulizer therapy does not require patient technique, allows drug doses to be changed, and permits delivery in O_2.[87] Use of a patient mouthpiece, where possible, increases efficiency.[94]

Newer nebulizer devices that coordinate drug delivery with inspiration are now available.[97] pMDIs and nebulizers can be used to deliver drugs during anesthesia via breathing system and airway devices (e.g., an ETT).[98] Use in this setting is highly inefficient with, at best, only 10% of the administered drug reaching the lungs.[99] Most of the drug is deposited in the tubing or airway, termed *rain out.*[100] Delivery can be somewhat increased by actuating the pMDI during inspiratory flow,[99] prolonging inspiration, increasing V_T, and using wider ETTs.[101,102] For anesthesia, nebulization into the breathing system is superior to pMDI use.[102] Blockage of tubes by water lock must be avoided.

Oral medication is reserved for treatment of poorly responsive types of asthma, urgent treatment, and situations in which there are difficulties with inhalation therapy (e.g., poor technique due to age or illness). Oral formulations of inhaled drugs are used for severe disease (oral GCs) or when drugs that are available only for oral use (e.g., methylxanthines) are chosen.

Parenteral administration is reserved for severe and emergent treatment.

B. Drug Treatments for Asthma

Drug treatment for asthma is complex and changing. Currently, drugs are termed *relievers,* which provide symptomatic relief with β-adrenoceptor agonists (BA), or *controllers* (preventers), which reduce risk of disease exacerbation, such as GCs. Apart from the isolated use of a BA for symptom relief, combinations of these agents are

TABLE 6-2

Stepwise Approach to Asthma Management in Adults

Asthma Treatment Step	Drug Therapy
1. Mild intermittent asthma	SABA ± chromone
2. Regular controller therapy	SABA with IGC
3. Add-on controller therapy	LABA with IGC (LM and/or MX)
4. Therapy for persistent poor control	Increase IGC (increase LABA or add oral BA and/or LM and/or MX)
5. Therapy with continual or frequent systemic GC	Increase IGC (add alternative agents)

BA, β-agonist; *GC*, glucocorticoid; *IGC*, inhaled glucocorticoid; *LABA*, long-acting β-agonist; *LM*, leukotriene modifier; *MX*, methylxanthine; *SABA*, short-acting β-agonist.
For drugs listed in parentheses, consider addition of one or more agents.

used, with a variety of dose regimens and schedules. A stepwise approach is advised,[45-47] as outlined in Table 6-2. A suggested response to asthma exacerbation, with severity estimated by peak expiratory flow, is shown in Table 6-3.

For sustained control of asthma, a high degree of patient compliance is needed, which is problematic when the patient is very young or mentally or physically infirm. Indeed, the most common cause of "failed" treatment results from poor compliance or administration.[103]

Drug therapy for asthma is mainly based on modifications of natural substances that have been used since antiquity.[104] This section provides a description of the drugs used, followed by consideration of drug therapy for an additional and critical asthma-related state, intraoperative bronchospasm.

1. β-Adrenoceptor Agonists

BAs are the most potent and most widely used bronchodilators in clinical use. BAs bind to specific β-adrenoceptors.

TABLE 6-3

Drug Therapy for Asthma Exacerbation

Phase	Severity/Response	Treatment Options
A. First hour	If PF >60%	O₂ (aim for SpO₂ >90%), I SABA continuous
	If PF <60%	Move to phase B
B. Next hour	Moderate PF 60-80%	O₂, I SABA, I AC, O GC
	Severe PF <60%	O₂, I SABA, I AC, O/IV GC, IV Mg
C. Thereafter	Good PF >70%	O₂, IV SABA, I AC, O GC
	Incomplete PF <60%	O₂, I SABA, I AC, IV Mg, IV GC
	Poor PF <30%	O₂, I SABA, I AC, IV Mg; consider adding IV MX, IV SABA, IPPV

PF, Peak expiratory flow rate; *I AC*, inhaled anticholinergic; *I SABA*, inhaled short-acting β-agonist; *IPPV*, intermittent positive-pressure ventilation; *IV GC*, intravenous glucocorticoid; *IV Mg*, intravenous magnesium; *IV MX*, intravenous methylxanthine; *IV SABA*, intravenous short-acting β-agonist; *OGC*, oral glucocorticoid; *SpO₂*, oxygen saturation by pulse oximetry.

These are G protein-coupled receptors, members of a large protein family of cell-surface, transmembrane receptors that recognize extracellular signal molecules and activate a *signal transduction pathway* resulting in specific cellular responses to the received signal. BA binding results in a conformational (structural) change in the receptor, activating an associated G protein; the G protein detaches and stimulates a linked enzyme, adenylate cyclase, which converts adenosine triphosphate (ATP) to cyclic adenosine monophosphate (cAMP), the *second messenger*. cAMP enhances intracellular phosphorylation reactions catalyzed by specific protein kinases, particularly protein kinase A, resulting in reduced intracellular contractile processes. In the lung, this relaxes bronchial smooth muscle; decreases mast cell degranulation; inhibits a variety of cells, including lymphocytes, eosinophils, and neutrophils; and modulates vascular tone and mucociliary transport. cAMP is inactivated by the phosphodiesterase enzyme group.

The medicinal plant, *Ephedra*, yields ephedrine, which has been used in China as *Ma Huang* for more than 5000 years. Inhaled ephedrine was reported as a bronchodilator in 1910.[105] The in vitro bronchodilator effect of epinephrine (adrenaline) was reported in 1907, and it was first administered in clinical use as a nebulized solution by Percy Camps.[104]

Isoprenaline (isoproterenol), a synthetic agent with less significant cardiovascular effects, was introduced clinically in the 1940s and was a popular choice for the treatment of asthma.

Ahlquist demonstrated a rank order of potency for sympathomimetic agents, distinguishing α- from β-receptors, with further division into β₁ (heart) and β₂ (lung) receptors.[106]

Albuterol (salbutamol) was the first selective β₂-agonist, and it remains the most commonly used bronchodilator worldwide.[107,108] It is formulated as a racemic mixture of R and S forms. It has 29 times greater selectivity for β₂- than β₁-receptors. Subsequent side-chain modifications of the parent molecule have resulted in longer-acting agents, such as salmeterol and formoterol.[104]

a. PHARMACODYNAMICS

The therapeutic respiratory action of BA involves binding to membrane (β₂-subtype) adrenoreceptors on smooth muscle cell in the lung, which stimulates production of the second messenger catalyst, adenylate cyclase, and increases the intracellular concentration of cAMP.[109] The exact mechanism of action of cAMP remains unclear, but it probably decreases the intracellular calcium concentration and directly affects systems regulating the cellular contractile apparatus.[110,111] These effects produce bronchodilation. In addition, BA may also provide beneficial effects by modulating neurotransmission in the cholinergic and perhaps other neural systems, affecting the function of inflammatory cells, modulating bronchial blood flow, stimulating mucociliary transport, and influencing the composition of mucus secretions.[112] BA activity is enhanced by GCs.[113,114]

Selective agonists have varying degrees of selectivity for the β₂-adrenoreceptors, increasing their specificity for the lung and presumably decreasing undesired side effects, especially in the cardiovascular system. Like most other selective receptor agonists, however, these agents are *relatively* selective, with specificity decreasing as dose increases. *Mixed agonists* have effects on both β_1- and β_2-adrenergic receptors.

DURATION OF ACTION. One classification of BAs is by duration of action. *Short-acting agents* (<4 hours) are typified by isoproterenol (isoprenaline), which can be inhaled as a nebulized solution or given via pMDI. When it is nebulized, the adult dose is 0.5 mL of a 0.5% solution diluted in 2.5 mL of water. IV administration is not advised because of cardiovascular complications.[115]

Intermediate-acting BAs (4 to 6 hours) include albuterol (salbutamol), which is most often administered via pMDI in outpatients, with 1 puff delivering 90 µg of drug. The usual dose in ambulatory patients is 2 puffs given four times daily or immediately before exposure to exercise or other known stimuli. It is also available as a solution for nebulization, in tablet form (including a sustained-release preparation), and as a syrup for pediatric use.

The superiority of the R-isomer of albuterol (levalbuterol) compared to racemic (R and S) albuterol is controversial.[116] Some studies report that levalbuterol is as effective as racemic albuterol with less tremor and tachycardia, whereas others do not support this conclusion.[117-120]

Terbutaline is available as an aerosol inhaler or in tablets. Inhaled terbutaline is clinically equal to inhaled albuterol.[121] In the United States, it is the only selective β_2-agonist available for parenteral use, with the usual subcutaneous dose similar to that of epinephrine (0.25 to 0.5 mg SQ). When used in this way, its duration of action exceeds that of epinephrine, and it may have cumulative effects on repeated administration. The elimination half-life is approximately 6 hours. About 40% is converted in the liver to a sulfate conjugate. Both conjugate and unchanged drug are excreted by the kidneys.

Pirbuterol and metaproterenol also have intermediate duration of action.

Long-acting BAs (10 to 12 hours) include salmeterol and formoterol. These agents are now combined with an IGC and are administered twice a day for long-term control of asthma symptoms. The duration of action remains unexplained.[122] Bambuterol is the pro drug for terbutaline; it is activated by plasma cholinesterases, giving a longer duration of action. Use of long-acting BAs as monotherapy leads to tolerance or desensitization and a small increased risk of death.[123,124] Use of BAs alone is now contraindicated.[46]

An *ultralong-acting BA* (24 hours), indacaterol, was recently described.[125]

Epinephrine (adrenaline) is a potent inotrope and vasopressor with actions at α-, β_1-, and β_2-receptors. It can be given subcutaneously, intravenously, or via a pMDI or nebulizer. Nebulized epinephrine is not superior to other inhaled BAs.[126] The onset of action is rapid, making it often the first parenteral drug administered in an ambulatory emergency setting, to provide acute therapy until long-term measures can be instituted. The usual SQ dose is 0.4 mL of a 1:1000 solution in adults (0.005 mL/kg in pediatric patients), which may be repeated at 15-minute intervals. Side effects include hypertension, tachycardia, dysrhythmias, hyperglycemia, and acidosis. An IV dose regimen is described in the section on reactive management.

ADVERSE EFFECTS. Side effects complicate BA therapy. Acutely, they include dose-related tremor, nervousness, nausea, hypertension, tachycardia, and dysrhythmias. These effects are related to stimulation of adrenergic receptors in the cardiovascular system and are more prominent with mixed agonists, although they may also occur with selective BAs, especially at higher doses. Side effects of high-dose BA therapy include hypokalemia, which is increased with use of GCs and methylxanthines (MXs). Lactic acidosis often develops; it results from increased lipolysis and leads to liberation of free fatty acids, which inhibit oxidative metabolism.[127] MXs and GCs enhance β-receptor sensitivity to agonist activation and indirectly promote lactate production.[128] For chronic use, there are concerns regarding the safety of BA in the longer-term treatment of bronchospasm.[129]

Despite use of antiasthma medications in the last decades of the 20th century, the morbidity and mortality associated with asthma increased—a situation referred to as the *asthma paradox*.[130] Increased use of BAs has been implicated as one of the factors responsible. Studies have shown that therapy solely with β_2-agonists over treatment times ranging from 15 days to 1 year may actually enhance airway reactivity.[131-133] Others have found that regular use of inhaled BA bronchodilators is associated with an increased risk of death or near-death in asthmatics.[134,135]

It has been suggested that the chronic use of BAs may relieve symptoms without treating the underlying chronic inflammatory process that is apparently responsible for asthma.[130] This process can lead to irreversible thickening of the airway wall that ultimately worsens hyperreactivity. However, others have questioned this association.[136]

b. PHARMACOKINETICS

In general, BAs are cleared by a combination of hepatic conjugation reactions and renal excretion of unchanged drug. Albuterol is hydrolyzed by tissue esterases to inactive colterol. Additionally, hepatic conjugation with sulfate occurs.

Epinephrine, which is converted to metanephrine or normetanephrine, has an elimination half-time of a few minutes.

c. UTILITY

BAs are available in a variety of formulations, such as DPIs, nebulizer solutions, pMDIs, oral liquids, tablets, and IV preparations. BAs are used for reliever therapy by inhalation at all asthma treatment steps[45-47] (see Table 6-2). For step 1, use of an inhaled short-acting β-agonist (SABA) may be the only treatment needed. If two or more aerosol inhaler canisters are used per month, escalation to step 2 is advised.[46] For steps 2 and above, BAs are used as add-on therapies in combination with other agents.

Inhaler combinations of long-acting BAs with IGCs are often highly effective and may show synergistic activity.[137] These are now considered to be the most effective therapy available.[104]

BAs have utility for emergency treatment of asthma exacerbations of varying severity. Again, other agents should also be used, particularly a course of systemic GC, which is usually given by the oral route (50 mg/day prednisolone, or equivalent, for an adult) for 5 days without tapering the dose.[47,138,139] Nebulized ipratropium can also be added.[140,141]

For urgent cases, inhaled administration of BA is the reasonable choice, primarily with repeated doses of pMDI administered via a holding chamber, escalating to nebulized therapy. Repeated treatment at intervals of 15 to 30 minutes with doses of 5 to 10 mL/hr may be needed for adults.[47]

For severe acute asthma, administration of BA by continuous nebulization has efficacy equal to that of intermittent administration, with less tachycardia and hypokalemia.[142] IV BA is reserved for life-threatening asthma, usually together with nebulized BA.[47]

Sellers and Messahel used rapidly repeated IV salbutamol (albuterol) boluses for emergency treatment of acute severe asthma in seven patients (children and young adults).[143] All patients had received nebulized BA and systemic GC, and additionally two had received aminophylline by infusion. The dosage scheme was 5 µg/kg IV for children (250 µg for adults) given over 1 to 2 minutes, repeated every 2 minutes. The number of boluses given ranged from 2 to 7, and all were administered within 30 minutes. All patients showed clinical benefit.

An alternative to repeat bolus therapy was reported by Browne and Wilkins.[144] They used a single bolus of salbutamol 15 µg/kg (over 10 minutes), followed by an infusion of 1 to 5 µg/kg/min. For refractory cases, IV epinephrine, 0.35 to 0.7 mg/kg, may be given over 5 minutes, followed by an infusion of 0.5 to 2 µg/kg/min.

For the treatment of severe acute asthma in the emergency setting, the addition of MX to BA therapy is not generally advised.[145,146] A therapeutic response to MX in this setting is rare.[4]

2. Glucocorticoids

GCs are the most effective controllers of asthma, with no other drug treatment available matching their efficacy. Other names for these drugs include corticosteroids, glucocorticosteroids, and simply "steroids."

Solis-Cohen, a Philadelphia physician, demonstrated that "adrenal substance pills" were helpful in asthma.[147] This effect was originally attributed to epinephrine (adrenaline), but oral preparations of natural catecholamines (e.g., epinephrine) are inactivated in the gut, so it is likely that GCs were the effective components.[104]

Kendall and Reichstein independently isolated and synthesized cortisol (and adrenocorticotropic hormone [ACTH]), receiving the Nobel Prize (with Hench of the Mayo Clinic) for this work in 1950.[150] Boardley and colleagues reported rapid improvement in five asthma patients receiving ACTH,[148] and soon oral cortisone treatment gained widespread popularity for management of a wide variety of inflammatory illnesses, including asthma.[149] However, systemic side effects were common,

and inhaled cortisone was ineffective. After concerted efforts, a range of topical GC preparations were introduced for application to the skin (for eczema) and to the lungs. Topical efficacy, on either skin or lungs, is related to skin blanching, now called the MacKenzie test.[150]

The introduction of inhaled beclomethasone diproprionate, an effective drug with a high therapeutic index, heralded the era of IGC as the mainstay for asthma control.[151]

a. PHARMACODYNAMICS

GCs are anti-inflammatory agents that act mainly through alteration of nuclear DNA activity, a genomic effect by which the expression of target genes is activated or repressed. This is a highly complex and coordinated set of processes involving the production of an array of inflammatory and anti-inflammatory enzymes, receptors, cytokines, chemokines, and adhesion molecules.[152,153]

The overall effect of GC action is decreased inflammatory cell recruitment, survival, accumulation, and activity.[154,155] This takes hours to days to achieve. There are two types of GC receptors (α and β); both are intracellular. GC action is mediated by the α variant and inhibited by the β. GCs bind to the cytosolic α variant (not the β), with subsequent translocation of the complex into the nucleus, dimerization, and binding to specific domains of DNA—the glucocorticoid response elements (GREs) within promoter genes. The binding may result in activation or suppression of target gene transcription. Activation typically results in transcriptive and translative activity producing anti-inflammatory proteins.[156]

Suppression of gene activity results in decreased expression of inflammatory genes (switching off). This is achieved by action of the GC-receptor complex to activate histone deacetylase, an enzyme that removes acetyl groups from histone proteins involved in packing DNA. Deacetylation alters histone conformation, closing the associated DNA sequences and rendering the DNA less accessible for transcription.[157]

The β form of GC receptor (which does not bind with GC) can also bind to GREs, and this may provide an inhibitory pathway for overall GC activity.[158] Additionally, GC may enhance degradation of messenger RNA (mRNA) coding for inflammatory proteins, a post-transcriptional mechanism of anti-inflammatory regulation.[159,160]

GCs also enhance the actions of BA (and MX), explaining the synergistic therapeutic effects of these agents.[137] This is achieved by increased transcription of the β2-receptor genes,[161,162] protection from β2-receptor downregulation, and prevention of uncoupling of β2 receptors from their G proteins (which is promoted by some inflammatory mediators, such as IL-1), thereby sustaining β2 activity.[163,164] Reciprocally, BAs may increase GC activity by increasing translocation of GC receptor complexes into the nucleus.[165]

GCs have other nongenomic effects. These actions are rapid and are insensitive to blockers of gene transcription (e.g., actinomycin D) or protein synthesis (e.g., cyclohexidine).[159,166,167] These nongenomic actions have therapeutic import. Asthma is associated with an increase in pulmonary blood flow, and this may interfere with

TABLE 6-4

Equipotent Daily Doses of Inhaled Glucocorticoids

Drug	Low Dose (mg)	Medium Dose (mg)	High Dose (mg)
Beclomethasone diproprionate	200-500	>500-1000	>1000-2000
Budenoside	200-400	>400-800	>800-1600
Ciclesonide	80-160	>160-320	>320-1280
Flunisolide	500-1000	>1000-2000	>2000
Fluticasone propionate	100-250	>250-500	>500-1000
Mometasone furoate	200-400	>400-800	>800-1200
Triamcinolone acetate	400-1000	>1000-2000	>2000

airflow[63,64]; IGCs reduce this effect.[168,169] Additionally, reduction in lung hyperperfusion may prolong the bioavailability of inhaled BAs, which are cleared from the lung by the pulmonary circulation.[170]

Side effects of GC therapy are well known. Systemic therapy risks dose-dependent suppression of the hypothalamopituitary axis, osteoporosis, osteonecrosis, systemic hypertension, diabetes mellitus, obesity, skin thinning, myopathy, cataracts, and glaucoma.[46] For those patients who need systemic steroids to achieve asthma control (step 6), these complications are a serious risk, and this is the rationale for adding steroid-sparing therapies as outlined previously.

Inhalation therapy markedly reduces systemic toxicity but does not eliminate it.[171] IGC can be absorbed in two ways—from the lungs or after swallowing oropharyngeal deposited drug. Side effects are usually apparent with large doses (>400 µg/day budenoside or equivalent in an adult). Easy bruising, adrenal suppression, cataracts, and glaucoma have been described.[46] Local toxicity results in sore throat with oral candidiasis.[90]

b. PHARMACOKINETICS

With optimal technique, IGCs achieve rapid and efficient delivery to the airways. With poor technique, however, drug is deposited in the oropharynx, where it can be a local irritant or be swallowed.[90]

Oral GCs are usually rapidly absorbed and have a high volume of distribution. They are typically inactivated by the cytochrome group of enzymes, a set of heme-thiolate monooxygenases in liver microsomes.

c. UTILITY

IGCs are used as controller (preventer) medications at steps 2 through 4, and systemic (oral) GCs are used for step 5 (see Table 6-2). IGCs are currently the most effective anti-inflammatory therapy available. They reduce symptoms of asthma,[172] improve lung function[172] and quality of life,[172] and reduce airway reactivity.[172,173] The frequency and severity of exacerbations are reduced,[174] as is mortality.[175]

A wide variety of IGCs are available, either as a single formulation (pMDI or DPI) or in combination with a long-acting BA. Examples include beclomethasone (beclometasone) diproprionate, budenoside, fluticasone propionate, and mometasone furoate. Ciclesonide is a pro-drug that is activated in the lung by ester hydrolysis; its use aims to reduce oropharyngeal irritation and

systemic uptake of swallowed drug. The variety of IGCs has led to advice on standardization of IGC dosage as "budenoside equivalents" in low, medium, and high daily dose regimens,[46] as shown in Table 6-4.

Systemic GCs include prednisone, prednisolone, methylprednisone, methylprednisolone, betamethasone, dexamethasone, and hydrocortisone. These may be given by oral, IV, or intramuscular (IM) routes, with similar efficacies. Deflazacort and cortisone acetate are formulated for oral administration, and triamcinolone is reserved for intra-articular or IM use. The relative potencies of these drugs are shown in Table 6-5.

Oral GCs are used for treatment of exacerbation. Systemic drug should be given for "all but the mildest exacerbations"[46] for 5 days and may be stopped without tapering.[46] Oral GCs are usually effective but take at least 4 hours to produce clinical improvement. A usual single daily dose of methylprednisone, 60 to 80 mg, or hydrocortisone, 300 to 400 mg, in divided doses is advised.[46]

For patients who are unable to take or absorb oral medication and for those with life-threatening asthma, systemic (usually IV) administration is needed. Hydrocortisone, up to 4 mg/kg given three to four times a day (or equivalent) is used for life-threatening disease.

The rapid nongenomic effect of IGC in reducing lung hyperemia may have a therapeutic role in the treatment of exacerbation.[176,177] For example, one study showed equal efficacy of 3 mg nebulized fluticasone and 100 mg hydrocortisone in nonintubated patients with acute severe asthma.[178]

3. Methylxanthines

The MXs are a group of phosphodiesterase inhibitors. They include caffeine, present in coffee, and theophylline and theobromine, present in tea. Extracts have been used historically for treatment of respiratory disorders. In

TABLE 6-5

Equivalent Doses of Systemic Glucocorticoids

Glucocorticoid	Equivalent Dose
Prednisolone	5 mg
Betamethasone	750 µg
Cortisone acetate	25 mg
Deflazacort	6 mg
Dexamethasone	750 µg
Hydrocortisone	20 mg
Methylprednisolone	4 mg
Triamcinolone acetate	14 mg

1886, Henry Hyde Salter, a family physician in London, reported that drinking strong coffee on an empty stomach eased his asthma.[179] The solubility of MXs is low and is enhanced by the formation of complexes with other compounds; for example, aminophylline is a complex of theophylline and ethylenediamine. Before the widespread adoption of BA therapy, IV administration of a soluble MX was the standard first-line treatment for severe asthma.[104] Other preparations, such as salts of theophylline (e.g., oxytriphylline) and covalently modified derivatives (e.g., dyphylline), are available.

a. PHARMACODYNAMICS

MXs have multiple mechanisms of action, and the effects of clinical importance remain controversial.[180,181] Originally, they were thought to act as phosphodiesterase inhibitors. Phosphodiesterases are a group of enzymes, one action of which is inactivation of cAMP, the second messenger for adrenoceptor activation. Such inhibition increases intracellular cAMP, thereby enhancing adrenoceptor activity and resulting in bronchodilation.[182]

The phosphodiesterase isozymes 3 and 4 are implicated,[104] but the drug concentrations needed to demonstrate this effect in vitro may exceed those present at therapeutic levels in vivo.[183] Moreover, not all phosphodiesterase inhibitors are effective in asthma, and theophylline-induced relaxation of airway smooth muscle in vitro occurs without changes in intracellular cAMP levels.[184,185] Other mechanisms demonstrable in laboratory preparations, including antagonism of adenosine and stimulation of endogenous catecholamine release, also do not appear to be significant to the clinical action of theophylline.[186,187]

Some of the therapeutic actions of MXs may result from effects other than relaxation of smooth muscle. These drugs may improve mucociliary clearance, stimulate ventilatory drive,[184] and increase diaphragm contractility,[188,189] actions that may be beneficial in patients with reactive airways disease. MXs also have significant cardiovascular effects, including direct positive chronotropic and inotropic effects on the heart, reductions in preload and afterload, and diuresis, which may be beneficial in patients with cardiovascular disease.

There is increased evidence to support anti-inflammatory and immunomodulatory roles for MXs in asthma.[190,191] Theophylline increases the activity and number of suppressor T cells and reduces the activity of many inflammatory cells implicated in asthma.[192,193] More recently, MXs have been shown to stimulate histone deacetylase. The action of this nuclear enzyme results in reduced exposure of DNA elements to transcription, which may render inflammatory genes less active, an effect that is synergistic with GC.[194]

Because MXs have multiple systemic actions, side effects are common, mainly involving the CNS and the cardiovascular system.[195] CNS effects include stimulation, insomnia, and tremor, leading to convulsions at toxic plasma levels (considered to be >20 μg/mL). For the cardiovascular system, toxic levels may produce ventricular and atrial dysrhythmias. In addition to phosphodiesterase inhibition, adenosine receptor activation may be important.[104] Gastrointestinal disturbances ranging from epigastric discomfort to nausea and vomiting may also occur.

b. PHARMACOKINETICS

There are many MX formulations. Most vary the physical preparation of theophylline rather than chemical modification of it. Several forms of anhydrous theophylline are available in microcrystalline preparations to enhance rapid and reliable absorption. Sustained-release forms are also currently popular, providing dosing convenience and (perhaps) less fluctuation in blood levels. For IV administration, aminophylline (containing 85% anhydrous theophylline by weight) is used because of its greater aqueous solubility.

All MXs are eliminated primarily by hepatic metabolism. Plasma clearance varies widely even among healthy subjects, with the elimination half-life ranging from about 3 hours in children to 8 hours in adults.[196] The hepatic cytochrome P450 enzyme group (particularly CYP 1A2) clears MX. The activity of these enzymes may be enhanced, for example by smoking and by concurrent therapy with carbamazepine or rifampicin, leading to greater clearance. Conversely, the enzymes may be inhibited by drugs such as cimetidine and ciproxin, resulting in greater MX bioavailability. Disease states such as liver or cardiac failure alter clearance. Unpredicted changes in clearance may result in toxicity in critically ill patients, so measurement of plasma levels is important.

Regardless of the preparation chosen, plasma concentrations of theophylline should be monitored to ensure that levels are in the therapeutic range (5 to 20 μg/mL). For children receiving less than 10 mg/kg/day, monitoring is not considered necessary.[46]

c. UTILITY

With other therapeutic advances in the pharmaceutical treatment of asthma, some have questioned the continued role of MX in the management of reactive airways.[197] However, MXs still have a number of therapeutic roles, and it may become more popular again with increased recognition of the immunomodulatory and anti-inflammatory properties of these drugs.[198-200]

There are presently three main indications for MX use. First, for the relatively small group of patients who are unable to manage inhaler therapies, MXs may be used as primary controller therapy.[46]

Second, MXs have utility as add-on controller therapy to IGCs,[201-203] although the therapeutic effect is usually less than that achieved by adding long-acting BAs to IGCs.[204,205] When properly used, these drugs remain safe and effective for the chronic management of asthma and in some patients with chronic obstructive pulmonary disease (COPD).[206] With effective clinical support and plasma drug monitoring, adverse incidents are rare. One study of 36,000 patients receiving 225,000 prescriptions over 9 years reported that the incidence of hospital admission resulting from MX toxicity was less than 1 per 1000 patient-years.[207]

Third, for patients with severe exacerbation of asthma whose management is problematic, add-on therapy with IV aminophylline may be considered. This is not generally advised for all patients, and response to treatment in this situation is described as rare.[47,146] The initial loading dose is 5 mg/kg, administered over 30 minutes to minimize toxicity. This is followed by an infusion of 0.5 to 0.7 mg/kg/hr, which provides therapeutic levels in most patients. This loading dose and rate may need to be increased in smokers or decreased in severely ill patients and in those with liver disease or congestive heart failure. All dose recommendations are guidelines, and patients must be monitored with plasma theophylline concentrations (daily for the emergency patients).[47]

4. Leukotriene Modifiers

Leukotriene modifiers (LMs) include the cysteinyl-luekotriene-1 receptor antagonists (montelukast, pranlukast, and zafirlukast) and the 5-lipoxygenase inhibitor (5-LO), zileuton. They are inhibitors of arachidonic acid metabolites.

In 1938, Feldberg and Kelloway isolated substances with bronchoconstrictive and vasoactive properties from guinea pig lung perfused with cobra venom.[208] In 1960, these substances were shown to be released during anaphylactic shock and were named slow-reacting substance of anaphylaxis (SRS-A).[209] In 1979, Murphy and colleagues identified SRS-A as a mixture of lipids, later called leukotrienes—so named because they are produced by leucocytes and posses a carbon chain with three double-bonds.[104,210] Leukotrienes were later shown to have potent bronchoconstrictor properties when inhaled by asthmatics.[211] Inhibitory agents affecting this metabolic pathway, the first new class of drugs for asthma therapy in 30 years, were introduced into clinical practice in the 1990s.

a. PHARMACODYNAMICS

In response to pro-inflammatory stimuli directed toward various leucocytes (eosinophils, basophils, neutrophils, and macrophages), arachidonic acid is oxidized by 5-LO (with a membrane-bound helper protein called 5-lipoxygenase activating protein, or FLAP) to an unstable intermediate, leukotriene A_4 (LTA_4). This may be transformed into two types of derivatives, the cysteinyl-leukotrienes (cysLTs) LTC_4, LTD_4, and LTE_4, which are mainly produced by eosinophils and basophils, and LTB_4, from neutrophils and macrophages.

The cysLTs are formed in a sequential pathway involving initial conjugation of LTA_4 with the tripeptide glutathione to form LTC_4, which is exported out of the cell, where it rapidly changes to LTD_4 (by loss of a glutamyl residue) and to LTE_4 (by loss of a glycine residue). A number of variations in the enzymatic pathway exist. Genetic variation, or polymorphism, has been associated with aspirin-induced asthma (AIA).[212]

The cysLTs bind to a number of transmembrane-spanning G protein–coupled receptors found on a variety of leucocytes, smooth muscle cells, glandular epithelial cells, and endothelial cells. The target receptors are called cysLT1R and cysLT2R. Activation of cysLT1R (in the potency order $LTD_4 > LTC_4 > LTE_4$) results in bronchoconstriction, edema, and glandular secretion.[213-215] Activation of cysLT1R on fibroblasts may promote proliferation, a possible factor in airway remodeling and inflammatory cell recruitment.[216] CysLT2R activation has

effects on endothelial permeability and leucocyte activity.[217,218]

LTB_4 binds to the receptors BLT1R and BLT2R. BLT1R activation has been implicated in stimulation of T lymphocytes and mast cells.[219,220]

Montelukast (available in Europe and the United States), zafirlukast (in the United States), and pranlukast (in Japan) are cysLT1R antagonists that inhibit the effect of cysLTs only. Zileuton is a 5-LO inhibitor and therefore reduces formation of both cysLTs and LTB_4.

LMs are generally well tolerated, the most common complaints being abdominal discomfort, muscle weakness, and pain. Initial concerns that montelukast therapy was associated with mental disorder and suicidal ideation have not been supported.[221] Zileuton has been associated with liver toxicity, and liver function monitoring is advised.[222] There is an apparent association of LMs with Churg-Strauss syndrome,[223] but this may be related to the drugs' ability to spare steroid.[224,225]

b. PHARMACOKINETICS

LMs are given orally and are well absorbed after oral administration, which is an advantage. They are available in chewable formulations for pediatric use. Once-daily (montelukast), twice-daily (zafirlukast and pranlukast), and four-times-daily (zileuton) dosing is needed.

c. UTILITY

LMs may be used as controller medications in conjunction with other agents. They have a small, variable bronchodilator effect with anti-inflammatory activity and may reduce asthma exacerbations.[226-228] They may reduce cough[229] and may be useful for symptom control in viral-associated bronchospasm[230-233] and AIA.[234-236] When used alone as controller therapy, LMs are usually less effective than IGCs,[237] but when used in conjunction with IGCs, they can provide a steroid-sparing effect.[238]

LMs are not effective for management of acute asthma. A multicenter, randomized trial of high-dose zafirlukast performed in an emergency department showed only a small reduction in admissions in the treatment group.[239]

5. Anticholinergic Agents

Anticholinergic agents are muscarinic receptor antagonists (MRAs) that inhibit the action of the transmitter acetylcholine in the parasympathetic nervous system. Herbal preparations of jimson weed and thornapple (*Datura* spp.) containing atropine have been smoked in India for relief of respiratory symptoms, as have preparations of henbane (*Hyocyanamus muticus*) containing hyoscine (scopolamine) in Egypt.

Anticholinergic drugs are bronchodilators, pulmonary vasodilators, and inhibitors of tracheobronchial secretion. They lack anti-inflammatory action.[104] They also decrease salivary, gastric, and intestinal secretions. The parent agent is atropine. Other tropane alkaloids include hyoscine, ipratropium, oxtropium, glycopyrrolate, and tiotropium.

a. PHARMACODYNAMICS

Parasympathetic vagal efferent (autonomic motor) nerves form ganglia around large- and medium-diameter airways.[240,241] Postganglionic fibers supply bronchial smooth muscle, blood vessels, and mucus glands. Muscarinic receptors are located on the target cell membrane and are G protein–coupled receptors. Three types of muscarinic receptors are reported: M_1, M_2, and M_3.[242-244]

M_1 receptors are postjunctional within ganglia, facilitating transmission in parasympathetic pathways that innervate the airways, so antagonism of this effect should be beneficial. M_2 cholinergic receptors are also located within ganglia but are prejunctional (autoreceptors). Their activation decreases ganglionic transmission, inhibiting the release of acetylcholine from postganglionic nerves; antagonism of this effect may increase acetylcholine release and thus actually increase airway responsiveness.

M_3 receptors are located at postganglionic terminals at the effector sites; antagonism of their effects may be beneficial. The overall effect of MRAs depends on the balance of receptor activation, and those drugs with M_3 selectivity (e.g., tiotropium, glycopyrrolate) should therefore have greater utility.[104]

b. PHARMACOKINETICS

The parasympathetic nervous system is widely distributed and has multiple actions. MRAs with systemic activity produce many unwanted side effects, such as tachycardia, dysrhythmias, dry mouth, blurred vision, and confusion. MRA activity confined to the lung is optimal; inhalation therapy with minimal absorption is ideal.

Atropine (the prototypic muscarinic antagonist) and hyoscine may decrease airway resistance and attenuate airway reactivity when given parenterally or when inhaled, but systemic side effects have limited their use specifically as bronchodilators.

Ipratropium bromide is a quaternary ammonium derivative of tropane and is positively charged at physiologic pH. It is poorly absorbed from the lungs (<1%), does not readily cross the blood-brain barrier, and can be administered by inhalation at high dose and with minimal systemic side effects.[245,246] This and similar agents have slow onset times, up to 90 minutes.[247,248] Tiotropium, although not licensed for use in asthma, has a long duration of action, up to a week.[104]

c. UTILITY

Ipratropium is a clinically useful bronchodilator, but its slow onset limits efficacy as reliever medication, and BAs are first-line agents. Ipratropium may be useful as additive step-up therapy for patients with moderate impairment (FEV_1 50% to 70% predicted).[45] Ipratropium is available as a pMDI (18 μg/puff). The usual dose is 2 puffs given four times daily. For patients with COPD that includes a reversible component of bronchospasm, nebulized ipratropium may have benefits over BAs, including a longer duration of action and efficacy in some patients in whom BAs have little effect.[249]

In severe asthma, a combination of nebulized ipratropium and BA is superior to BA alone for adults and children.[250-252] A meta-analysis of 16 randomized, controlled trials comparing salbutamol and ipratropium versus salbutamol and placebo, showed reduction in hospital admission with improved lung function.[253] Multiple doses of ipratropium are superior to single use.[254]

Ipratropium may also be useful for treatment of bronchospasm induced by beta-blockers.[250] Tiotropium bromide is currently approved for bronchodilator therapy in COPD but not in asthma. In a recent trial in patients with moderately persistent asthma, tiotropium was reported to be equivalent to either doubling of the dose of inhaled beclomethasone or addition of inhaled salmeterol.[255] This finding shows therapeutic promise.

6. Chromoglycates (Chromones)

Cromolyn sodium, disodium cromoglycate, and nedocromil sodium are chromoglycates (chromoglicates) or chromones; they are clinically used as controller drugs with modest efficacy.[46] The parent compound, khellin, is derived from the medicinal plant, *Amni visnaga*, which is found around the eastern Mediterranean. They are useful only in the prevention of bronchospasm, not treatment.

a. PHARMACODYNAMICS

Cromolyn contains one chromone ring, nedocromil two. They are often called chromones, but nedocromil is structurally termed a pyranoquinolone. The first drug, cromolyn, was marketed as Intal (*in*hibitor of *al*lergy).[256] Chromolyn and nedocromil inhibit release of inflammatory mediators from various cell types associated with asthma, especially lung mast cells, particularly in response to airway irritants such as cold air or sulfur dioxide.[257,258]

The mechanism of action is not fully known, but two actions are proposed[104]: phosphorylation of a moesin-like membrane protein (a natural terminator of granule release) and inhibition of chloride-channel opening in response to mechanical (structural or osmotic) stresses imposed on mast cells.[74,259]

Side effects include oropharyngeal irritation and symptoms, such as cough, caused by the direct irritant effect of the powder. Serious complications (anaphylaxis) are very rare.

b. PHARMACOKINETICS

These drugs are poorly absorbed and are administered by inhalation of powdered drug via a pMDI. In the United States, chromolyn is also formulated for nebulization, but nedocromil is currently not marketed. In the United Kingdom, pMDI devices using HFA as propellant are available for both drugs. Absorbed drug is not significantly metabolized and is excreted in urine and bile.

c. UTILITY

Chromones are controller drugs, useful both as a single preventive treatment, when taken 15 minutes before exercise or exposure to antigens, and as therapy as an alternative to IGCs.[45,260,261] Efficacy in individual patients varies widely, and at present a therapeutic trial is the only way of determining which patients will benefit. The two drugs are equally effective in clinical use.[258] Neither agent has been studied as an adjunct to airway management in the perioperative period.

7. Alternative Agents

For refractory asthma, with relapse despite maximal therapies resorting to chronic or multiple courses of systemic GC, immune-suppressant and immune-modulating drugs have been used, as have novel inhalation therapies. These drugs may allow reduction of the systemic steroid dose, but they are generally limited by modest and variable response, by side effects such as opportunistic infection, and by uncertainty over long-term safety. In general, a 3- to 6-month trial is advised.[262,263] For some agents, treatment numbers have often been small and study design may be questionable.

Anti-IgE therapy with omalizumab is an option for those patients who need chronic systemic GC or multiple rescue courses.[264] Omalizumab is generally well tolerated.[265] In the United Kingdom, serum IgE levels higher than 700 IU/L need to be demonstrated.[47]

Methotrexate given for 3 months allows a 20% reduction in systemic steroid dose for about 60% of patients, but the risk-benefit ratio does not usually support its use.[266-268] Opportunistic infection is a risk, and there have been reports of *Pneumocystis* pneumonia.[266,269]

Cyclosporine, a lipophilic cyclic 11-residue peptide, also has steroid-sparing effects in about half of patients with severe asthma. The primary target is T cells. Cyclosporine binds to intracellular cyclophilins, forming a complex that inhibits a calcium/calmodulin-dependent phosphodiesterase and reducing transcription of a group of nuclear family proteins. This results in decreased cytokine production, particularly IL-2, but also IL-4 and IL-5. Cyclosporine may also promote apoptosis (cell death) of CD4+ T cells.[270] IL-1 production from monocytes and macrophages is also reduced.

A systematic review (of three trials) showed that cyclosporine reduces daily steroid use by 1 mg or less.[271] In one study of five children taking more than 10 mg of prednisone daily, cyclosporine allowed weaning of steroid in three children and small improvements in lung spirometry.[272] Cyclosporine has a narrow therapeutic index, and drug level testing is needed. Opportunistic infection, renal injury, and hypertension are the main side effects.

Tacrolimus is a fungal macrolide that has effects similar to those of cyclosporine.

Macrolide antibiotics have antimicrobial activity and also anti-inflammatory actions through reduction in the expression of IL-8, a neutrophil activator. Some asthma patients may be chronically infected with *Chlamydophila* or *Mycoplasma* susceptible to macrolide treatment.[273-275] In addition, some patients with severe asthma that is resistant to conventional treatment may have a neutrophilic disease process (as opposed to increased eosinophil activity) and may benefit from macrolide therapy.[276] However, a systematic review of the use of macrolides (clarithromycin, troleandomycin, and roxithromycin) in asthmatic patients and did not find enough evidence to form a meta-analysis.[277] Liver toxicity is a risk.

Gold therapy results in a small reduction in systemic steroid use. Proteinuria is a side effect.[278]

Colchicine is used to treat gout and familial Mediterranean fever with few side effects. A prospective, multicenter study of its use in patients with asthma did not show benefit of this drug over placebo.[279]

Hydroxychloroquine has established uses as an antimalarial agent and for connective tissue disease management. Retinopathy is the major risk. Its efficacy in asthma management is controversial, with conflicting reports of efficacy.[280,281]

Dapsone is an anti-inflammatory agent that is used in leprosy treatment. One small study showed therapeutic promise in asthma treatment, with a large steroid-sparing effect but complicated by anemia.[282] There are currently no published data from well-designed trials, leading to a conclusion that strong evidence supporting its use in asthma is lacking.[283]

Intravenous immunoglobulin has anti-inflammatory actions, but large trials have not supported its use in asthma, and side effects such as fever and urticaria are common.[284,285]

Antifungal therapy is another potential treatment of asthma. Environmental fungal exposure is virtually ubiquitous. Many asthma patients show IgE responses (sensitization) to common fungi such as the dermatophyte *Trichophyton*. This may be incidental to the overall disease process for asthma, or it may in certain patients be a major pathologic problem, called severe asthma with fungal sensitivity (SAFS).[286] In general, asthma severity is associated with specific IgE responses to *Trichophyton*; a trial in 2009 showed modest spirometric improvement during long-term antifungal treatment,[287] but this was not sustained on discontinuation of antifungal therapy.[288]

One disease, allergic bronchopulmonary aspergillosis, is characterized by lung colonization and major allergic response to the common fungus, *Aspergillus fumigatus*. Many of these patients have an asthma-like disease. Itraconazole is an effective antifungal treatment.[289]

Tumor necrosis factor α (TNF-α) is implicated in asthma.[290] *Anti-TNF-α agents* include etanercept, a soluble TNF-α receptor fusion protein that binds to TNF-α, as well as infliximab and golimumab, monoclonal antibodies that bind to TNF-α. Trials with etanercept,[291] infliximab, and golimumab have not supported their use.[292,293]

Interleukin antibody therapy is another potential treatment of asthma. IL-2 and its receptor, IL2R, are produced by Th2 cells in response to allergen exposure and stimulate sensitized Th2 proliferation. Monoclonal antibody to IL2R (daclizumab) inhibits this response. Intravenous daclizumab therapy resulted in small improvements in asthma control.[294]

IL-5 promotes eosinophil activation, and this is an important part of the disease process for a group of patients with eosinophilic asthma.[295] In this group, treatment with antibody to IL-5 (mepolizumab) has been shown to have clinical utility,[296] but not in the general asthma population.[297]

Heparin has anti-inflammatory and anti-eosinophilic properties.[298] Nebulized heparin may have therapeutic promise for asthma treatment.[299] Coagulopathy does not complicate therapy.

Nebulized lidocaine also has potential,[300] but the therapeutic effect remains controversial.[301]

The 2007 Expert Panel Report of the National Asthma Education and Prevention Program gave recommendations for use of alternative agents.[45] The report stated that "the data at present are insufficient" to recommend macrolide therapy. Moreover, the "current evidence does not support" the use of methotrexate, IL-4 receptor antibody, antibodies to IL-5 and IL-12, intravenous immunoglobulin, colchicine, troleandomycin, gold, or cyclosporine.

8. Investigative Drug Therapies

Investigative drug therapies provide an active and fast-changing area of research. It is uncertain which agents, if any, will be of practical patient benefit. As of early 2011, some drug targets include ADAM8 (a matrix metalloproteinase),[302] peroxisome proliferator-activated receptors (PPARs),[303] arginase,[304] and adenosine receptor.[305]

Nucleotide synthesis inhibitors (mycophenolate, leflunomide, and brequinar) may have clinical utility. They interfere with DNA replication, and lymphocytes are considered to be relatively more vulnerable.[262]

9. Other Agents

The mucolytic N-acetyl-L-cysteine (NAC), inhaled or ingested, has no proven efficacy in the management of asthma (or COPD or cystic fibrosis).[87] The aerosol form has a pH of 2.2, provokes airway secretions, and is an airway irritant.[306]

Other mucolytic agents have been used in the treatment of cystic fibrosis, including aerosol formulations of a DNase (dornase alfa) that hydrolyzes the DNA component of mucus. There are isolated reports of dornase delivered via a bronchoscope in status asthmaticus.[307] A newer agent, thymosin-β4, has hydrolytic activity for the fibrous form of actin in mucus.[65]

Antihistamines do not have clinical efficacy for asthma treatment.[46,104] It is ironic that the first isolated mediator in asthma, histamine,[308] is not amenable to blockade.

C. Anesthetic Management of Asthma

Given the worldwide prevalence of asthma, many patients present for surgery, planned or otherwise. A core feature of anesthetic practice is provision of airway control, often with instrumentation. Because asthmatic patients have, as a primary component of their disease, airway hyperreactivity, they are at risk for perioperative exacerbation, especially intraoperative bronchospasm (IOB). IOB develops when offensive factors (collectively termed *noxious stimuli*), such as airway instrumentation or surgery (e.g., incision, manipulation, traction) are greater than defensive factors provided by preoperative drug management or anesthetic technique. Surgery within major body cavities, especially cardiothoracic or abdominal surgery, is considered to pose a greater risk for IOB.[46]

Patients who do not have optimal control of their asthma and those who have a history of a previous perioperative exacerbation are also considered to be at risk for IOB.[100] Conversely, those patients with optimal control are not considered to pose an extra risk.[46]

Management is twofold—proactive and, if necessary, reactive. The proactive approach includes optimizing current therapies with provision of preventive strategies. The reactive approach involves therapies applied after IOB has developed.

1. Proactive Management: Prevention of Bronchospasm

The proactive strategy involves optimization and prevention. Each of these approaches is designed to reduce the risk of bronchospasm resulting from noxious intraoperative stimuli.

a. OPTIMIZATION

Optimization is best achieved with advice from a respiratory physician, so that treatment matches the disease severity. Compliance with prescribed medication should be confirmed. These interventions are practical for elective or scheduled surgery, if sufficient time is available. These opportunities are lost when urgent or emergent surgery is needed.

Smoking cessation 2 months before surgery is advised.[309] Control of gastroesophageal reflux is advised.[310] Patients with asthma have been reported to have three times the prevalence of reflux disease compared with patients without asthma. Long-term treatment, however, has not improved overall asthma control.[311,312]

b. PREOPERATIVE PREVENTION

Prevention includes preoperative and perioperative phases. Interventions are matched to the severity and stability of the disease. Preoperative prevention includes these options:

SYSTEMIC GLUCOCORTICOIDS. A preoperative course of systemic GC therapy (oral prednisolone, 40 to 60 mg/day for 5 days, or IV hydrocortisone, 100 mg three times daily) is advised for those patients with an FEV_1 less than 80% of predicted.[309] Treatment can be stopped without tapering (weaning the dose).[46]

For patients who have received systemic GC within the previous 6 months, a course of supplemental GC is advised (e.g., IV hydrocortisone 300 mg/day in divided doses) before surgery of intermediate or major intensity.[46] This can be stopped after 24 hours.[313]

BRONCHODILATORS. Short-acting inhaled bronchodilators are also advised.[309] pMDIs have efficacy equal to that of nebulized therapy provided technique is optimal. A preoperative combination of GC and BA is advised for patients with severe or brittle asthma and for those needing major surgery.[313,314]

GC and BA therapy, singly or combined, may result in electrolyte imbalances, particularly potassium and magnesium deficiencies. This should be anticipated and prevented by supplementation or corrected.[309]

ANXIOLYTICS. Fear (and pain) can be potent triggers for bronchospasm. Effective treatment with anxiolytics reduces this risk. Benzodiazepines do not provoke bronchoconstriction. There are reports of either no alteration in bronchial tone or decreased tone caused by direct effects in the lung (mediated by γ-aminobutyric acid [GABA] receptors) or by indirect effects in the CNS.[315-318]

Kil and associates reported no clinically measurable effect of oral midazolam 0.5 mg/kg on cardiorespiratory function in treated children with mild or moderate asthma who were presenting for dental extractions.[319] Benzodiazepines are therefore a reasonable choice. α_2-Agonists (dexmedetomidine or clonidine) provide dose-dependent sedation and bronchodilation with drying. These agents have therapeutic appeal but have not been formally investigated in the setting of perioperative asthma management.[100]

ANALGESICS. Multimodal analgesic regimens optimize pain relief before and after surgery. This approach avoids the use of single-analgesic therapy, which generally has restricted efficacy with increased risk of dose-dependent toxicity.

Naturally sourced opiates, such as morphine, have a traditionally considered capacity to provoke mast cell degranulation, but strong evidence for consistently provoking bronchospasm is lacking. Whereas morphine provokes degranulation from skin mast cells, it does not do this for mast cells in the lung.[320] Morphine may have bronchodilator effects in asthmatic patients.[321]

The use of nonsteroidal anti-inflammatory drugs (NSAIDs) for analgesia is traditionally controversial. They are generally considered safe to use in patients with well-controlled asthma and no known sensitivity.[322] The notable exception is in patients with AIA. This is a clinical syndrome of asthma that is worsened with aspirin and nasal polyposis, termed *Samter's triad*. Aspirin inhibits the cyclooxygenase pathway, diverting arachidonic acid metabolites into the lipoxygenase pathway and leading to an increase in cystLTs. Some estimate that up to 20% of asthmatics carry this risk.[323] AIA is associated with cigarette smoking.[324] Patients may have cross-reactivity with other NSAIDs, and referral to an allergy clinic has been advised.[325]

The general principles of anesthetic management for the asthmatic are the same as for any patient, namely protection of the patient from the stressors of surgical (and anesthetic) technique and provision of conditions amenable to successful surgery.

c. PERIOPERATIVE PREVENTION

Perioperative prevention involves a multimodal approach. List planning is important. Asthmatic patients should receive priority on a surgical list for two reasons: First, anxiety provoked by waiting can be reasonably reduced, and second, an early scheduled case allows more time for recovery during normal hospital hours.

A risk-benefit analysis of the available agents and techniques should be considered, and an individualized anesthetic plan (with an alternative) should be made for the induction, maintenance, and recovery phases. Agents and techniques implicated in a previous episode of bronchospasm should be avoided if possible. If these agents are deemed necessary, additional protective measures should be used.

A regional technique, either with sedation or with general anesthesia, may be appropriate. Systemic absorption (from a regional technique) of local anesthetic can attenuate bronchoconstriction. Shono and colleagues reported a case of a patient with asthma whose wheeze was reduced after extradural anesthesia with 2% lidocaine and returned after discontinuation of the drug.[326]

For general anesthesia, the principles of balanced anesthesia with hypnosis and reflex suppression apply. Induction is a time of risk. Combinations of synergistic agents, such as hypnotics with one or more opioids, benzodiazepines, α_2-agonists, or ketamine, can provide a smooth and sustained induction profile. Rapid administration of opioids has been reported to provoke the so-called rigid chest, even at low doses; this may, in part, result from laryngospasm.[26,327] These complications may be misinterpreted as bronchospasm. The antitussive effect of opioids is, however, reported to be therapeutic.[314]

Airway instrumentation is a risk factor for bronchospasm,[328] particularly with endotracheal intubation.[329] The effect of endotracheal intubation even in symptom-free asthmatics was shown in 10 volunteers who underwent the procedure with topical anesthesia. Intubation resulted in falls in FEV_1 in up to 50% of the subjects. This fall was attenuated in subjects receiving inhaled BA.[328] The response to mechanical stimuli is mediated by the parasympathetic nervous system and by direct local stimulation with release of mediators[330] such as neurokinin A and substance P from peripheral nerve terminals of C-fiber afferents.[331] Whereas endotracheal intubation is provocative, laryngeal mask airway insertion is not.[332]

INDUCTION. Preoperative anticholinergic therapy may protect against bronchospasm, and nebulized therapy has been reported to have utility.[333]

Inhaled lidocaine can attenuate airway reflexes in asthmatics and normal volunteers receiving inhaled histamine, but its efficacy is controversial.[300,301,334] A combination of topical lidocaine and BA has been used to attenuate reflexes for awake intubation in normal volunteers.[329] Lidocaine inhalation may provoke minor airway irritation, such as cough, breath-holding, or, more seriously, bronchospasm,[301,335-339] which can be attenuated with coadministration of IV lidocaine.[340] Lidocaine-provoked airway irritability can be reduced by anticholinergic or BA treatment.[336]

Propofol has been shown to have bronchodilator properties in animals and isolated human airway preparations.[22,341,342] Propofol is generally considered to be the most reasonable agent for induction,[343] superior to thiopental or etomidate.[20,344,345] Propofol modulates the slow inward calcium influx in smooth muscle and also reduces production of cytokines IL-1, IL-6, IL-8, and TNF-α. It is generally a bronchodilating agent,[346-348] but there are isolated reports of bronchospasm developing in association with propofol.[349] Formulations with preservatives are implicated, and those with irritable airways, such as smokers (and asthmatics), may be at greater risk.[350]

In contrast, thiopental may provoke bronchospasm when given to asthmatic patients. Wheeze was demonstrated in 48% of asthmatic patients receiving thiopental.[351]

Ketamine is a bronchodilator; it has a direct relaxant effect on airway smooth muscle through potentiation of catecholamines and inhibition of neutrally provoked bronchoconstriction.[348,352] Ketamine has been advised as an induction agent for asthmatic patients. In a case series of 40 patients with medically controlled asthma who received induction with ketamine, 26 patients had reduced bronchospasm.[353] For patients with severe asthma (persistent asthma or exacerbation) presenting for surgery, ketamine is advised as the hypnotic drug of choice for induction.[354] A case series of 5 patients with status asthmaticus needing emergency intubation reported rapid improvement of arterial CO_2 content after IV induction with ketamine.[355]

Ketamine may, however, provoke both upper and lower airway secretion. Prior administration of an anticholinergic (e.g., IV glycopyrrolate) is useful. Conventional induction doses of ketamine are associated with emergence delirium and dysphoria. These risks can be reduced by coadministration of a benzodiazepine. Ketamine has a slower induction course, which should be taken into account before proceeding to airway instrumentation.

Inhalational induction is an option for motivated patients. Sevoflurane is a reasonable choice. An inhalation induction with either isoflurane or desflurane causes initial upper airway irritation and may provoke coughing, breath-holding, and laryngospasm.[356]

Lidocaine, given systemically before instrumentation, may be bronchoprotective. In asthmatic volunteers, IV lidocaine (up to 2 mg/kg) reduced histamine bronchoprovocation. Groeben and colleagues showed that either IV lidocaine or inhaled albuterol reduced histamine-provoked wheeze and concluded that both agents should be used before induction of anesthesia.[357] This conclusion was not supported by another study of 60 asthmatic patients,[358] and bronchospasm after IV lidocaine has been reported.[43]

NMB agents without bronchoconstrictive properties should be chosen. Release of mast-cell histamine has been reported with atracurium, increasing airway resistance and provoking bronchospasm.[359,360] Mivacurium is also implicated.[361] Atracurium also enhances vagal activity, which may be involved in increases in bronchomotor tone.[362]

Suxamethonium increases airway resistance and sensitivity to acetylcholine in animal models.[363,364] There are rare case reports of suxamethonium associated with bronchospasm and anaphylaxis.[365-367]

NMB drugs that have activity at the M_2 receptor group, such as rapacuronium, pipecuronium, and gallamine, can provoke bronchoconstriction.[309,368] Rapacuronium, initially a promising, rapidly acting blocker, was withdrawn because of this problem.[369]

Vecuronium, rocuronium, cisatracurium, and pancuronium are considered reasonable choices,[370] but anaphylaxis[371]—albeit rare—is a risk.

MAINTENANCE. Airway gases and vapors should be warmed and humidified. Volatile agents are usually used for the maintenance phase of anesthesia. In general, these agents depress contractility of the smooth muscle of the lower airways and are potent bronchodilators. They reduce responses to bronchoconstricting stimuli in both humans and animals[10,372-376] and also reduce baseline airway resistance in animals.[10,372-377] Effects on baseline airway resistance in human subjects are more difficult to interpret because of confounding influences such as endotracheal intubation and decreases in lung volume associated with general anesthesia, but it appears that these agents may also reduce resting airway smooth muscle tone in humans.[378,379]

Multiple mechanisms contribute to the relaxation of airway smooth muscle produced by volatile anesthetics attenuating reflex bronchoconstriction, in part by depressing neural pathways that mediate these reflexes.[380-382]

Bronchodilation has been observed with the use of high-speed computed tomography.[383] The exception is desflurane, which lacks bronchodilator activity.[384] Whereas sevoflurane is a popular choice for maintenance anesthesia, its bronchodilating efficacy is presently uncertain.

Rooke and coworkers compared the bronchodilating effects of sevoflurane, isoflurane, and halothane, concluding that sevoflurane reduced airway resistance more than the others did.[385] However, Habre and colleagues studied the effect of sevoflurane anesthesia on children with or without asthma and concluded that respiratory resistance increased only in the asthmatic group[386] and could be prevented by preoperative salbutamol (albuterol) therapy.[387]

Sevoflurane anesthesia (in pigs) may increase the production of inflammatory mediators such as LC_4 and nitrogen oxides in the lungs.[388] Because tone in airway smooth muscle helps regulate the matching of ventilation to perfusion, suppression of normal airway smooth muscle tone may contribute to impaired gas exchange in the perioperative period with all volatile agents. Animal studies have shown that sevoflurane anesthesia (in rats) may result in impaired gas exchange within the lung as a result of changes in peripheral lung compliance.[389]

COMPLETION. Completion of surgery and anesthesia is a crucial time when airway reflexes return, although in a modified state. Removal of airway devices (especially ETTs), coupled with clearance maneuvers such as suction, is provocative. Options include airway interventions done during deep anesthesia, but these may compromise airway patency and protection and should be performed after a risk-benefit analysis. Changing an ETT for an SLA can permit satisfactory emergence conditions—the so-called bridge to extubation, described when one is weaning a patient with resolved status asthmaticus from invasive ventilator support in critical care.[390,391] IV lidocaine may attenuate airway irritation at this stage.[392]

REVERSAL. Reversal of NMB with neostigmine (a cholinesterase inhibitor) has the potential to provoke bronchospasm by enhancing acetylcholine concentration. When it is given with antimuscarinic agents (atropine or glycopyrrolate), there is no reported effect on airway resistance.[393] However, bronchospasm has been reported, and this is a risk for patients with renal impairment.[100,394] Some authors advise allowing NMB to wear off without recourse to reversal agents.[100,309] Sugammadex offers an alternative method for reversal of rocuronium.[395]

In the postoperative phase, warmed, humidified O_2 therapy, physiotherapy, incentive spirometry, and motivated mobilization are important factors. Restoration of optimal drug therapy is also important. A course of nebulized SABA may be helpful. Temporary noninvasive ventilation has been described.[100] Relief of pain and fear is a major goal.

2. Reactive Management: Treatment of Intraoperative Bronchospasm

IOB develops when the noxious stimuli of anesthetic or surgical techniques are not counteracted by planned protective anesthetic strategies. The reported incidence ranges from 1.7% to 16% of a general surgical patient population.[100] Isolated IOB may be the only recognized manifestation of anaphylaxis; it has been reported in 19% of patients subsequently shown to have anaphylaxis.[396] Recognized risk factors include reactive airways disease (asthma and COPD), tobacco smoking, and endotracheal intubation.[397] A gradation of severity can occur, from mild and transient to severe and sustained with threat to life. Critical IOB is an emergency and mandates immediate treatment. This is equivalent to the intensive care scenario of status asthmaticus,[346] from which much experience in management has been gained.

Treatment should be matched to severity, bearing in mind that the time course of IOB is variable and unpredictable. Escalation of drug therapies may be necessary. Rehearsed responses, with drugs available and doses calculated, are wise preemptive moves. A six-step reactive strategy outlines the necessary responses (Box 6-1).

a. RECOGNITION

Recognition is the first step. Vigilance is the key, with detection of change accomplished by use of clinical skills aided by appropriate use of monitors with suitably enabled alarms. Direct clinical examination of the patient, if possible, is important. Use of the human senses can yield vital information, confirming (or otherwise) a patient-centered problem.

Initial visible signs of IOB include rise in airway pressures, falls in delivered V_T, and decreased chest movement. Auscultation may reveal noisy breath sounds with expiratory wheeze predominating, but when IOB is severe, these signs are lost: *The "silent chest" is dangerous.* Auscultation of the expiratory limb of the breathing system may be helpful if the patient is isolated from direct examination.[100]

Bronchoconstriction results in an increase in airway resistance. If this increase is sufficient to increase the overall expiratory time constant beyond the maximal expiratory time, the lung relaxation volume cannot be reached, and inspiratory gas trapping ("breath stacking") occurs. Residual volume, FRC, and total lung volume are

increased,[398] and these effects may be directly visible. With critical IOB, pneumothorax can ensue. Barotrauma is associated with high inspiratory and plateau pressures during the respiratory cycle.[399] Whereas an inspiratory pressure greater than 50 cm H_2O is considered dangerous, it is not as indicative as plateau pressure.[400-402] Longer expiratory time and a lower V_T and rate are advised.[346] This results in hypercarbia but is far less dangerous than barotrauma resulting from attempts to "normalize" CO_2 tension.[402] Dynamic hyperinflation, termed *pulmonary tamponade* or a "tourniquet to the right heart," can compromise right ventricular function.[100,346,403] Cardiac arrhythmia may complicate the situation. It results from a combination of hypoxia, hypercarbia, acidosis, and sympathetic drive, either from the patient or due to drugs.[404] *These immediate concerns should be communicated to the team.*

b. REVIEW

It is important to exclude confounding causes of obstruction that can arise along the ventilatory pathway. Malfunction of the breathing system, such as internal blockage or external compression of the tubing, must be excluded. Valve and ventilator function must be assessed. An alternative breathing system can be used to exclude residual doubt, using hand ventilation to assess overall compliance.

Because wheeze can result from any cause of airway narrowing (i.e., any fall in FRC), other causes, such as airway plugging, pulmonary aspiration, and pneumothorax, should be directly considered and excluded. Appropriate depth of anesthesia must be confirmed, because anesthesia that is too light is a common cause of IOB.

c. REQUEST HELP

Severe IOB is complex, risky, uncertain, and dynamic.[405] Skilled help and support can make a real difference to outcome.

d. RESCUE

No single therapy can be reliably predicted to effectively treat IOB, especially when it is critical. A major distinction between IOB and severe asthma in awake, self-ventilating patients is the difference in bioavailability of inhaled drugs. Patients with IOB invariably have an airway device (face mask, SLA, or ETT) connected to a breathing system. The great majority of any aerosolized drug is deposited in this device, with only 3% to 9% of drug reaching the lung. This is about 10 times less efficient than administration in self-ventilating patients.[99,100] A combination of inhaled and IV drugs may confer additive or synergistic effect, and a number of drug interventions are available for use in an escalating sequence.

As for any scenario, especially an emergency, in which task saturation is a risk, safe drug selection and timing of use are crucially important. The therapeutic rescue options available are listed in the following paragraphs.

INCREASING ANESTHETIC DEPTH. Increasing the anesthetic depth is a simple approach. Additional doses of induction agent and opioid are used, or the inspiratory fraction of the volatile agent is increased.

USE OF A VOLATILE AGENT. A volatile agent may be used to increase the agent in use or to change to an alternative.[100] Diethyl ether,[406] halothane,[24,407,408] enflurane,[409] and isoflurane[410] have been used. Use of sevoflurane, either for induction or in conjunction with other agents,[411-413] has also been reported. Failures have been described (i.e., with isoflurane).[414] Desflurane is not regarded as a bronchodilator.[384]

INHALED BRONCHODILATORS. Inhaled short-acting bronchodilators are given, either as a nebulized solution (using an in-line nebulizer) or from a pMDI via an airway adaptor. Because most of the drug will deposit in the breathing system[99,309] (rain out), about 10 canister activations are initially used for an adult.[100]

INTRAVENOUS BRONCHODILATORS. The use of intravenous bronchodilators has received the most support in the management of severe asthma (in nonintubated patients).[415] Intravenous therapy is reported to be superior to the inhalational route.[416] Sellers and Massahel report giving 5 μg/kg IV albuterol to children, 250 μg to adults; the dose can be repeated.[143] Browne and Wilkins advised use of a single bolus of albuterol (salbutamol), 15 μg/kg over 10 minutes, followed by an infusion of 1 to 5 μg/kg/min.[144]

For refractory cases, parenteral epinephrine may be used. Cydulka and colleagues described the effective use of subcutaneous epinephrine in the emergency department.[417] For adults, they advise 0.3 mg SQ epinephrine every 20 minutes. Intramuscular doses for adults range from 0.5 to 1.0 mg. Intravenous epinephrine may also be given. Suggested doses for adults are 10 to 100 μg IV, repeated as needed. A suggested infusion scheme is 0.35 to 0.7 mg/kg IV epinephrine given over 5 minutes, followed by an infusion of 0.5 to 2 μg/kg/min.

These treatments produce profound cardiovascular stimulation with tachycardia and hypertension, alleviated by concurrent use of magnesium.[418] Lactic acidosis is a recognized complication of the treatment of severe asthma and IOB with high dose BAs.[127,128] Hypokalemia and hypomagnesemia complicate high-dose BA therapy.[47]

INTRAVENOUS GLUCOCORTICOIDS. Intravenous GC may provide delayed effect a number of hours later.[100,309,419]

INHALED GLUCOCORTICOIDS. Recognizing that GC can have therapeutic effect by nongenomic mechanisms, such as decreased airway hyperemia and mucosal edema,[168,169] nebulized IGCs may be useful.[346] One study showed equal efficacy of 3 mg nebulized fluticasone and 100 mg hydrocortisone in nonintubated patients with acute severe asthma.[420]

KETAMINE. Most experience with ketamine comes from anecdotal management of severe acute asthma or status asthmaticus.[414,421-426] Doses between 0.5 and 2 mg/kg IV are described, followed by an infusion of 0.5 to 2 mg/kg/hr. In a placebo-controlled, double-blind trial of 14 mechanically ventilated patients with bronchospasm, 7 patients received 1 mg/kg IV ketamine with improvement in oxygenation; CO_2 clearance was unchanged in the treated group but increased in the control group.[424] One study on use of 3 mg/kg/hr has been published.[426]

One investigation did not support superiority of ketamine in the treatment of severe acute asthma in awake patients. This was a randomized, double-blind study of 53 consecutive patients. The protocol was an IV bolus of 0.2 mg/kg ketamine, followed by an infusion of 0.5 mg/kg/hr. Dysphoric reactions in the first 9 recruits prompted the reduction of the bolus dose by half.[427]

MAGNESIUM. Intravenous magnesium therapy used in the treatment of severe acute asthma was found to be beneficial and safe,[428] based on the results of a multicenter, randomized, controlled trial in the emergency department giving 20 to 40 mg/kg IV over 10 minutes.[429] Tachycardia provoked by sympathetic stimulants is reduced, and NMB is prolonged.[418,430] Inhaled magnesium (sulfate) has been used therapeutically in the treatment of severe asthma,[431] but it can be an airway irritant. Other systematic reviews of inhaled and IV magnesium therapy have concluded that it can have therapeutic benefit.[432]

HELIUM-OXYGEN CARRIER GASES. Helium-oxygen (heliox) mixtures are not bronchodilators, and the potential for improvement in gas exchange and respiratory mechanics is limited to their duration of use. They improve transport of gases, vapors, and aerosols by sustaining laminar flow in breathing systems (including nebulizers) and airways,[433] but a major limitation is reduced inspiratory fraction of O_2.[47,100,346] Heliox mixtures have been used in the setting of severe acute asthma and status asthmaticus.[434-437] Use of heliox for critical IOB in ventilated patients is limited.[47,346,437] Systematic reviews have not provided firm evidence to support widespread use.[438,439]

NITRATES. There are sparse reports of the therapeutic use of nitroglycerin in severe IOB.[440-442]

LIDOCAINE. Intravenous lidocaine has been used to treat IOB.[443]

METHYLXANTHINES. MXs were used traditionally, but recent evidence does not support their general use for IOB, and response in the setting of severe acute asthma is rare.[47]

NEBULIZED FUROSEMIDE. Nebulized furosemide has been used in the management of acute asthma. Initial reports were encouraging,[444] but other studies have not supported this finding,[445-447] including a critical review.[448]

ANTIBIOTICS. Bacterial infection with acute asthma is rare.[67] Unless bacterial infection is clinically apparent, routine use of antibiotics is not supported.[449]

e. RESOURCES

As with any perioperative problem, timely provision of resources, including drugs, equipment, and people, can make all the difference.

f. RECOVERY

The place and time for recovery should be carefully considered, depending on IOB severity and response to treatment. Postoperative deterioration (biphasic effect) has been described in up to 20% of patients, especially those with bronchospasm associated with anaphylaxis.[450,451] Critical care admission is a realistic option.[100]

If the episode of IOB was unpredicted, testing for anaphylaxis should be considered.[371,452]

VI. CONCLUSIONS

Drugs can affect the upper and lower airways directly or indirectly to produce a variety of desirable and undesirable effects. Knowledge of the pharmacology of such drugs is essential to the safe practice of airway management for the conscious patient and for the patient requiring sedation or anesthesia. These drugs can be delivered locally to the respiratory tree or systemically, producing clinical effects on healthy airways (e.g., anesthesia) or therapeutic effects on diseased airways (e.g., bronchodilation).

Agents acting directly on the airway include local anesthetic agents, sympathomimetics, and bronchodilators. They are used to provide topical anesthesia and optimally dilated upper and lower airways but on occasion may produce unwanted effects such as airway irritability. Indirectly acting agents can influence the CNS and the musculoskeletal system to produce effects on airway patency, airway reactivity, and respiratory drive. These effects may optimize the upper airway and lower respiratory tract in terms of reactivity or patency. However, indirect deleterious effects, such as a loss of airway tone, loss of airway protective reflexes, and loss of respiratory drive, can result in airway-related morbidity or mortality.

This chapter began with a review of the effects of drugs for safe, effective anesthesia and sedation. Drug management for asthma, based on nationally devised guidelines, was then discussed, followed by therapies to prevent and treat perioperative bronchospasm.

VII. CLINICAL PEARLS

- Topical application of local anesthetic to the airway is unlikely to cause systemic toxicity, although the safe maximum dose is uncertain. Doses greater than 9 mg/kg may risk toxicity.

- Asthma is now recognized as an inflammatory disease of the airways, and the use of inhaled glucocorticoid (IGC) for prevention is a major therapeutic advance.

- General anesthesia for asthmatic patients requires optimization with inhaled β-agonist (BA) therapy, consideration of systemic GC therapy, and avoidance of triggering factors.

- Propofol and volatile agents, except desflurane, are bronchodilators.

- Intraoperative bronchospasm (IOB) results when airway stimulation, typically by instrumentation, is not countered by perioperative technique. A planned, rehearsed response is needed for safe and effective management.

SELECTED REFERENCES

All references can be found online at expertconsult.com.

14. Nandi PR, Charlesworth CH, Taylor SJ, et al: Effect of general anaesthesia on the pharynx. *Br J Anaesth* 66:157–162, 1991.
21. Taigato Y, Isono S, Nishino T: Upper airway reflexes during a combination of propofol and fentanyl anesthesia. *Anesthesiology* 88:1459–1466, 1998.
34. Szabo TA, Reves JG, Spinale FG, et al: Neuromuscular blockade facilitates mask ventilation. *Anesthesiology* 109:A184, 2008.
35. Nouraei SA, Giussani DA, Howard DJ, et al: Physiological comparison of spontaneous and positive-pressure ventilation in laryngotracheal stenosis. *Br J Anaesth* 101:419–423, 2008.
46. Bateman ED, Hurd SS, Barnes PJ, et al: Global strategy for asthma management and prevention: GINA executive summary. *Eur Respir J* 31:143–178, 2008.
87. Rubin BK: Air and soul: The science and application of aerosol therapy. *Respir Care* 55:911–921, 2010.
100. Woods BD, Sladen RN: Perioperative considerations for the patient with asthma and bronchospasm. *Br J Anaesth* 103:i57–i65, 2009.
104. Barnes PJ: Drugs for asthma. *Br J Pharmacol* 147:S297–S303, 2006.
309. Burburan SM, Xisto DG, Rocco PRM: Anaesthetic management in asthma. *Minerva Anestesiol* 73:357–365, 2007.
346. Marshall PS, Possick J, Chupp G: Intensive care unit management of status asthmaticus. *Clin Pulmon Med* 16:293–301, 2009.

Chapter 7

Physiologic and Pathophysiologic Responses to Intubation

AARON M. JOFFE | STEVEN A. DEEM

I. BACKGROUND

Laryngoscopy, endotracheal intubation, and other airway manipulations (e.g., placement of a nasopharyngeal or oropharyngeal supralaryngeal airway) are noxious stimuli that may induce profound changes in cardiovascular physiology, primarily through reflex responses. Although these responses may be of short duration and of little consequence in healthy individuals, serious complications can occur in patients with underlying coronary artery disease,[1,2] reactive airways,[3,4] or intracranial neuropathology.[5,6]

II. CARDIOVASCULAR RESPONSES DURING AIRWAY MANIPULATION

A. Cardiovascular Reflexes

The cardiovascular responses to noxious airway manipulation are initiated by proprioceptors responding to tissue irritation in the supraglottic region and in the trachea.[7] Located in close proximity to the airway mucosa, these proprioceptors consist of mechanoreceptors with small-diameter myelinated fibers, slowly-adapting stretch receptors with large-diameter myelinated fibers, and polymodal endings of nonmyelinated nerve fibers.[8] (The superficial location of these proprioceptors and their nerves explains why topical local anesthesia of the airway is such an effective means of blunting cardiovascular responses to airway interventions.) The glossopharyngeal and vagal afferent nerves transmit these impulses to the brainstem, which, in turn, causes widespread autonomic activation through the sympathetic and parasympathetic nervous systems. Bradycardia, often elicited in infants and small children during laryngoscopy or intubation, is the autonomic equivalent of the laryngospasm response. Although seen only rarely in adults, this reflex results from an increase in vagal tone at the sinoatrial node and is virtually a monosynaptic response to a noxious stimulus in the airway.

In adults and adolescents, the more common response to airway manipulation is hypertension (HTN) and tachycardia mediated by the cardioaccelerator nerves and sympathetic chain ganglia. This response includes widespread release of norepinephrine from adrenergic nerve terminals and secretion of epinephrine from the adrenal medulla.[9] Some of the hypertensive response to endotracheal intubation also results from activation of the renin-angiotensin system, including release of renin from the renal juxtaglomerular apparatus, which is innervated by β-adrenergic nerve terminals.

In addition to activation of the autonomic nervous system, laryngoscopy and endotracheal intubation result in stimulation of the central nervous system, as evidenced by increases in electroencephalographic (EEG) activity, cerebral metabolic rate, and cerebral blood flow (CBF).[10] In patients with compromised intracranial compliance, the increase in CBF may result in elevated intracranial pressure (ICP), which, in turn, may result in herniation of brain contents and severe neurologic compromise.

The effects of endotracheal intubation on the pulmonary vasculature are probably less well understood than the responses elicited in the systemic circulation. They are often coupled with changes in airway reactivity associated with intubation. Acute bronchospasm or a main stem bronchial intubation results in a marked maldistribution of perfusion to poorly ventilated lung units, causing desaturation of pulmonary venous blood and subsequent reduction in systemic arterial oxygen (O_2) tension. In addition, institution of positive end-expiratory pressure (PEEP) after endotracheal intubation causes a reduction in cardiac output related to impaired venous return to the left side of the heart from the pulmonary circulation. The impact of these changes can be profound in patients with severely compromised myocardial function or intravascular volume depletion.

B. Intubation in the Presence of Cardiovascular Disease

Myocardial ischemia results when there is an imbalance between myocardial O_2 supply and demand. In the presence of a stable O_2 content of whole blood (the product of hemoglobin concentration and saturation, with a minor contribution from dissolved O_2), the myocardial O_2 supply is almost entirely determined by coronary blood flow and distribution, because O_2 extraction at the cellular level is at or near maximum even under resting conditions.

The chief components on the demand side of the myocardial O_2 balance equation are beat frequency or heart rate (HR) and myocardial wall tension. Of the two, increases in HR are of greatest concern, because cardiac inotropism (contractility) subserves cardiac chronotropism (rate). Not only does tachycardia increase myocardial O_2 consumption per minute at constant wall tension, but elevations in rate effectively reduce the diastolic period. Because full diastolic relaxation may be impaired, a subsequent increase in resting wall tension will impair subendocardial blood flow, thereby reducing myocardial O_2 supply. Concomitantly, the rate of intraventricular pressure development in systole (dP/dT), a measure of myocardial contractility and another determinant of myocardial O_2 demand, will also increase.

It follows, then, that neuroendocrine responses to airway manipulation resulting in tachycardia and HTN may result in a variety of complications in patients with cardiac disease, myocardial ischemia chief among them. This set of circumstances is responsible for episodes of ischemic electrocardiographic ST-segment depression and increased pulmonary artery diastolic blood pressure (BP) that may be seen when intubation is performed in patients with arteriosclerosis; occasionally, these episodes presage the occurrence of a perioperative myocardial infarction.[2] However, short ischemic episodes (<10 minutes) evidenced by electrocardiographic ST-segment depression, such as those that may be experienced only during airway manipulation, have not been shown to correlate with postoperative myocardial infarction. In contrast, ST-segment changes of a single duration lasting longer than 20 minutes (mean SD 20 ± 30 minutes) or cumulative durations of longer than 1 hour (mean SD 1 ± 2 hours) do seem to be an important factor associated with adverse perioperative cardiac outcomes.[11,12]

Patients with aneurysmal disease of the cerebral and aortic circulation may also be at particular risk of complications related to a sudden increase in BP during airway instrumentation. Laplace's law defines the transmural wall tension of a blood vessel (the determinant of its likelihood of rupture) as the product of the pressure inside the vessel and its radius divided by the wall thickness. The presence of a thin-walled vascular aneurysm (higher transmural wall tension at baseline) combined with a sudden increase in intraluminal pressure can lead to rupture of the affected vessel and abrupt deterioration in the patient's status. Leaking aortic aneurysms are partially tamponaded by intra-abdominal pressure but can suddenly expand into the retroperitoneal space during arterial HTN. The results are significant blood loss and additional technical problems for the surgeon trying to resect the lesion and insert a vascular prosthesis.

C. Implications for Patients with Neurovascular Disease

Intracranial aneurysms and arteriovenous malformations (AVMs) often arise with a small "sentinel" hemorrhage that serves as a warning of worse things to come. During subsequent periods of elevated arterial BP, these lesions are likely to rebleed, resulting in sudden and permanent neurologic injury. Many neurosurgeons and interventional neuroradiologists attempt to stabilize cerebral aneurysms and AVMs soon after hospitalization in an effort to minimize the risk of rebleeding. This means that the patient presents for anesthesia at a time when the clot tamponading the aneurysm or AVM is particularly delicate, and a small increase in arterial transmural pressure could cause rerupture. One of the times at which this is most likely to occur is when the arterial BP and the HR are increased in response to endotracheal intubation.[5] Therefore, neurosurgical anesthesiologists pay meticulous attention to attenuating these responses during the course of anesthetic induction and endotracheal intubation.

D. Intubation in Patients with Neuropathologic Disorders

Reflex responses to endotracheal intubation are also a potential hazard to patients with compromised intracranial compliance resulting from neuropathologic processes such as intracranial mass lesions, brain edema, or acute hydrocephalus. Uncontrolled coughing can result in a marked increase in intrathoracic and intra-abdominal pressure that, in turn, increases cerebrospinal fluid pressure and may result in impairment of cerebral perfusion. In patients with impaired cerebral autoregulation (e.g., brain trauma, cerebrovascular accidents, neoplasms), the normal tendency for CBF to remain constant over the mean BP range of 50 to 150 mm Hg is impaired. When endotracheal intubation causes an increase in arterial BP, there is a marked increase in CBF and cerebral blood volume, which in turn can cause dangerous increases in ICP.[6] This effect is magnified by the fact that noxious stimuli, such as airway manipulation, result in increased CBF, which summates with the hypertensive BP response, occasionally causing profound increases in ICP (Fig. 7-1).

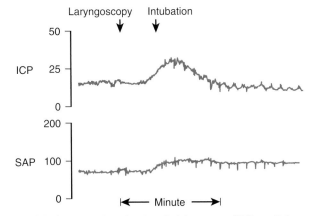

Figure 7-1 Increases in systemic arterial pressure *(SAP)* and intracranial pressure *(ICP)* in response to endotracheal intubation in a patient with a small brain tumor. Notice the minimal response to rigid laryngoscopy. There is a sustained increase in systemic arterial pressure but only a transient increase in ICP, which returns to normal as cerebrovascular autoregulation becomes operative. (From Bedford RF: Circulatory responses to tracheal intubation. *Probl Anesth* 2:201, 1988.)

E. Neuromuscular Blocking Drugs and Cardiovascular Responses

Neuromuscular blocking drugs (NMB) are often administered to optimize conditions for intubation. Accordingly, it is appropriate to consider the cardiovascular and cerebrovascular responses to the administration of these agents. Indeed, the hypertensive-tachycardic response to endotracheal intubation was not identified until NMB agents were introduced into clinical practice, because before that time intubation was performed only with the patient under such deep levels of anesthesia that relatively little cardiovascular response was generated.[13]

The depressor effects of benzylisoquinolinium relaxants (atracurium and mivacurium) are mediated by histamine release.[14] This effect could be viewed as a potential antagonist to the pressor response to laryngoscopy and endotracheal intubation. In the case of patients at risk for intracranial HTN, however, histamine-induced cerebral vasodilation may produce increases in ICP even as the BP falls.[15] By contrast, pancuronium, rocuronium, and, to a lesser extent, vecuronium may initiate a hyperdynamic cardiovascular state that can potentiate the cardiovascular responses seen after endotracheal intubation in lightly anesthetized patients. The faster onset of rocuronium (doses of up to 2 mg/kg have a 90% chance of providing perfect intubating conditions) are the reason for its current widespread use as an alternative to succinylcholine for rapid-sequence intubation (RSI) and in operations expected to last longer than 1 hour.[16]

Succinylcholine, or diacetylcholine, is associated with bradycardia in children, particularly when doses are repeated, but is a cardiovascular stimulant in adults. This phenomenon is often associated with activation of the EEG, and patients with brain tumors may sustain marked increases in ICP after succinylcholine administration if intracranial compliance is compromised and cerebrovascular autoregulation is impaired.[17] This has been shown in dogs to be a result of increased CBF related primarily to succinylcholine-induced increases in afferent muscle spindle activity at the time of fasciculation and secondarily to an elevated arterial carbon dioxide tension from fasciculation-induced carbon dioxide production.[18] The evidence to substantiate the clinical relevance of these findings is lacking, however. Whereas it has been reported that succinylcholine administered to patients with brain tumors may elevate ICP by a mean of 5 to 12 torr, cerebral perfusion pressure does not change significantly, and a negative effect on neurologic outcome has not been documented.[19,20] Additionally, this phenomenon can be prevented by pretreatment with defasciculating doses of nondepolarizing NMB drugs.[19] Further, when adequate ventilation is maintained, succinylcholine administered to intubated patients being treated for intracranial HTN of various causes or to those who have suffered severe head injuries caused by blunt trauma had no effect on ICP, cerebral perfusion pressure, or CBF.[21,22] As a result, succinylcholine is still considered a first-line agent for RSI in patients with acute head injury but is ideally used after pretreatment with a nondepolarizing agent and in the presence of slight hypocapnia.

F. Cardiopulmonary Consequences of Positive-Pressure Ventilation

Venous return is defined by the pressure gradient between the mean systemic pressure in the peripheral venous system and the mean right atrial pressure. An increase in mean intrathoracic pressure due to positive-pressure ventilation (PPV) may be transmitted to the thin-walled, compressible superior and inferior venae cavae, effectively elevating the downstream pressure for venous return and thereby reducing venous blood return to the right atrium. Because the left side of the heart can only pump what the right side delivers, cardiac output and subsequently arterial BP may fall with PPV. Patients with decreased intravascular volume may have an exaggerated hypotensive response as a result of this phenomenon.

Those with impaired myocardial reserve may also be sensitive to the effects of PPV. However, a failing heart may also benefit from the combined effects of decreased preload and decreased afterload. In other words, PPV, particularly PEEP or continuous positive airway pressure (CPAP), diminishes the transmural wall tension of the left heart by raising juxtacardiac pressures. One common clinical scenario is a patient who responds to intubation with a brisk increase in BP and then suddenly develops acute hypotension as PPV is instituted. In such a situation, volume expansion, positional changes, and judicious use of α-adrenergic agents such as phenylephrine may be needed.

It should also be noted that both hypoxemia and hypercapnia lead to a stress-induced catecholamine response, which may mask other potential causes of hypotension. This becomes readily apparent only after intubation in critically ill patients. Prophylactic volume expansion and the immediate availability of vasoactive infusions decrease severe hemodynamic collapse in this situation.[23]

III. PREVENTION OF CARDIOVASCULAR RESPONSES

A. Technical Considerations: Minimizing Stimulation of Airway Proprioceptors

As a general rule, cardiovascular responses to airway maneuvers can be minimized by limiting airway proprioceptor stimulation, starting with manipulation of the larynx itself. For instance, cricoid cartilage pressure with a posterior force of 4.5 kg is widely used to prevent regurgitation of gastric contents or to facilitate laryngeal visualization. In a double-blind study, cricoid pressure resulted in a significantly greater HR and BP response to endotracheal intubation than occurred in patients whose cricoid area was gently palpated.[24] This is a little-recognized effect of cricoid pressure that should be considered when estimating the risk-benefit ratio of this procedure in individual patients.

Laryngoscopy itself is a moderately stimulating procedure, and use of a straight blade (Miller blade) with elevation of the vagally innervated posterior aspect of the epiglottis results in significantly higher arterial BP than does use of a curved blade (Macintosh or

Corazzelli–London–McCoy [CLM]).[25] Newer video and optical laryngoscopes, which do not require alignment of the laryngeal axes for adequate visualization of the vocal cord inlet and subsequent intubation, have the potential to minimize the pressor response to airway manipulation by reducing the amount of force needed to displace oropharyngeal tissues and limiting cervical spine motion compared to traditional laryngoscopy with a Macintosh laryngoscope blade.[26] Nonetheless, reports documenting this advantage are few.

Use of the Pentax-AWS video laryngoscope (Pentax, Tokyo, Japan) has been reported to attenuate the hemodynamic response to endotracheal intubation after fentanyl/propofol induction when compared to either the GlideScope (Verathon, Bothell, WA) or the Macintosh laryngoscope (Fig. 7-2).[27] This finding is not universal. An earlier study comparing the Pentax-AWS to Macintosh laryngoscopy reported no significant differences in systolic BP, diastolic BP, or HR after intubation, and a separate study comparing the GlideScope and Macintosh laryngoscopy also failed to find significant differences in hemodynamic values at any point in the study.[28] None of these studies included patients with known cardiac disease or chronic HTN, who often have exaggerated pressor responses to stimulation; the newer airway devices may have greater value among this group compared with traditional laryngoscopy.

The act of passing an endotracheal tube (ETT) is far more hemodynamically stimulating than just laryngoscopy. Surprisingly, the use of a lighted intubation stylet fails to prevent hemodynamic stimulation when the ETT is advanced past the vocal cords.[29] Insertion of a conventional laryngeal mask airway (LMA) after induction of general anesthesia with thiopental or propofol and fentanyl has been shown to cause less cardiovascular and endocrine response than laryngoscopy or endotracheal intubation.[30-33] The LMA has the advantage of avoiding the vagally mediated infraglottic stimulation entailed by the use of a laryngoscope, thus enabling lighter levels of general anesthesia. Furthermore, because muscle relaxation is not required for airway control, spontaneously initiated ventilation is possible, with avoidance of the adverse hemodynamic consequences of PPV. In contrast, endotracheal intubation using the intubating LMA (iLMA) resulted in a hemodynamic and endocrine response similar to that resulting from direct laryngoscopy and intubation after propofol induction.[34] Therefore, if endotracheal intubation is necessary, there does not appear to be a hemodynamic advantage to instrumenting the airway with the iLMA.

Whatever the technique employed to manage the airway, it must be emphasized that the hypertensive-tachycardic response to intubation is a manifestation of insufficient anesthesia. Insofar as the pressor response can also be influenced by prolonged intubation time, rapid first-attempt success is also of particular importance.[7]

B. Topical and Regional Anesthesia

Topical anesthesia applied to the upper airway is effective in blunting hemodynamic responses to endotracheal intubation,[35,36] but it has almost invariably proved to be

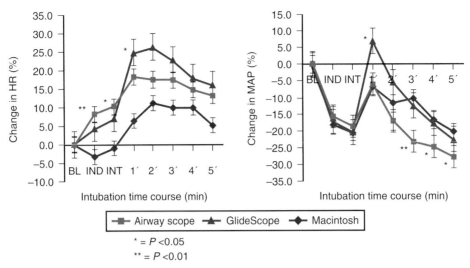

Figure 7-2 Percentage change from baseline in heart rate (HR, *left*) and mean arterial pressure (MAP, *right*) associated with endotracheal intubation using an Airway Scope, GlideScope, or Macintosh laryngoscope. Data values are presented as mean ± standard error. *$P < 0.05$ compared to Macintosh group. **$P < 0.01$ compared to Macintosh group. *BL,* Baseline; *IND,* 1 minute after induction; *INT,* at intubation; *1'* through *5',* minutes after endotracheal intubation. (From Tsai P, Chen B: Hemodynamic responses to endotracheal intubation comparing the airway scope, GlideScope, and Macintosh laryngoscopes. *Internet J Anesthesiol* 24(2), 2010.)

less effective than systemic administration of lidocaine. During general anesthesia, rigid laryngoscopy and instillation of lidocaine solution initiate the same adverse reflexes caused by placement of an ETT (Fig. 7-3).[37] Furthermore, a laryngotracheal spray of lidocaine solution may, in itself, produce profound cardiovascular

stimulation in adults, and in children it may produce the same sort of bradycardic response associated with endotracheal intubation.[38] If topical lidocaine is administered to the upper airway, there should be an intervening period of at least 2 minutes to allow initiation of anesthetic effect before airway instrumentation begins.[39]

Excellent topical anesthesia of the airway obtained before awake flexible fiberoptic intubation was responsible for reports suggesting that there was less cardiovascular stimulation after this procedure than after intubation with a rigid laryngoscope.[40] Later studies performed with patients under general anesthesia demonstrated no difference between the two modes of intubation with regard to hemodynamic impact, probably because the more profound stimulus results from placement of the ETT below the level of the glottis.[41-44]

Increasing the concentration of lidocaine used, and thus the total dose, also does not appear to mitigate this effect, although it may improve intubating conditions during awake flexible fiberoptic intubation.[45,46] Although both 2% and 4% lidocaine administered through an epidural catheter in the working channel of the flexible fiberoptic bronchoscope by a "spray-as-you-go" technique provided similar intubating conditions and hemodynamic profiles, the former resulted in a smaller overall dose, lower plasma levels, and therefore less chance for toxicity reactions.[46] Lower concentrations of lidocaine (1%) provided lower plasma levels and similar hemodynamics but appeared to provide less optimal intubating conditions than atomized 2% lidocaine when used for topical anesthesia before airway manipulation.[45]

In contrast to topical anesthesia of the airway, which appears to provide inconsistent benefit, regional nerve blocks involving the sensory pathways from the airway prevent hemodynamic responses to intubation. The superior laryngeal nerve (SLN) innervates the superior surface of the larynx, and the glossopharyngeal nerve innervates the oropharynx. Depositing local anesthetic on each

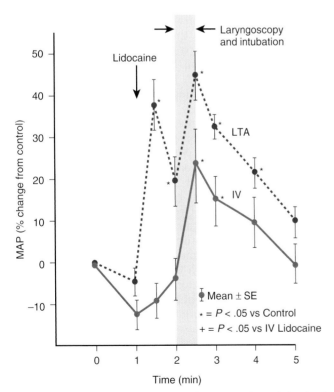

Figure 7-3 Mean arterial pressure *(MAP)* response to endotracheal intubation after either intravenous *(IV)* or intratracheal *(LTA)* lidocaine instillation. (From Hamill JF, Bedford RF, Weaver DC, Colohan AR: Lidocaine before endotracheal intubation: IV or laryngotracheal? *Anesthesiology* 55:578, 1981.)

cornu of the hyoid bone can block the SLN. Blockade of the glossopharyngeal nerve at the tonsillar pillars (sensory distribution above the level of the epiglottis) potentiates this effect by decreasing the stimulus of laryngoscopy.[47] The inferior surfaces of the larynx and trachea require topical anesthesia, however, because they are innervated by the recurrent laryngeal nerve and the vagus, which cannot be directly blocked. With the preceding combination, awake patients exhibit little response as the ETT is inserted.

Instillation of lidocaine via an ETT to prevent alterations in cerebrovascular hemodynamics in patients with severe head injury may be of some benefit. A dose of 1.7 mg/kg lidocaine instilled at body temperature given slowly (1 mL/sec) through a fine tube advanced to the end of the ETT but not in contact with the tracheal mucosa was reported to be efficacious in half of the patients treated.[48]

C. Inhalational Anesthetics

Defining the anesthetic dose requirement for effectively blocking (or even blunting) hemodynamic and ICP responses to endotracheal intubation has remained an elusive goal. Airway maneuvers are typically brief interventions that produce short-lived responses during a dynamic perioperative period, with drug concentrations rapidly fluctuating both in blood and at effect sites. Agents that are capable of preventing responses may also produce profound cardiovascular depression before and after the stimulation of endotracheal intubation. Accordingly, there are relatively few well-controlled dose-response studies, and those that are available often give information that is not useful for the clinical anesthesiologist.

For inhalational anesthetics, endotracheal intubation using doses in the range of the minimum alveolar concentration (1 MAC) resulted in marked cardiovascular stimulation during anesthesia with nitrous oxide (N_2O) supplemented with either halothane or morphine.[49] It should not be surprising that 1 MAC is insufficient, because it is known that approximately 1.5 to 1.6 MAC is needed to block the adrenergic and cardiovascular responses to a simple surgical skin incision (MAC-BAR).[50] The dose of anesthetic required to prevent coughing during endotracheal intubation with sevoflurane may exceed MAC by a factor of 2.86 in adults,[51] although this factor appears to be close to 1.3 in children.[52]

Accordingly, it appears that the dose of volatile anesthetic required to block the cardiovascular response to endotracheal intubation must be inordinately high, resulting in profound cardiovascular depression before endotracheal intubation.[53] From a cerebrovascular viewpoint, this approach is totally impractical, because high doses of volatile anesthetics cause cerebral vasodilation and marked increases in ICP in patients with compromised intracranial compliance. Furthermore, from a cardiovascular point of view, the arterial hypotension and reduced cerebral perfusion pressure before intubation would be entirely unacceptable for patients with cerebrovascular disease or brain injury.

D. Intravenous Agents

Propofol, barbiturates, and benzodiazepines are all associated with profound hypotension at doses that suppress the hemodynamic and ICP responses to intubation.[54-56] In the case of etomidate, the effective dose for blocking the cardiovascular response to intubation can be identified by a burst-suppression pattern on the cortical surface EEG, indicating fairly deep cerebral depression.[57] Because etomidate supports BP at such deep levels of anesthesia, it is probably the only contemporary agent that, by itself, can achieve suppression of cardiovascular responses without first producing undue arterial hypotension and compromise of coronary and cerebral perfusion.

Because it is clinically impractical to achieve sufficient anesthetic depth for preventing a hyperdynamic response to intubation solely with an intravenous (IV) or inhalational agent (etomidate excepted), a wide variety of anesthetic drug combinations, adjuvants, or both have been used in attempts to potentiate anesthetic effects while minimizing hemodynamic depression.

Opioids are the adjuvants most commonly administered in addition to other IV or inhaled agents to facilitate induction of anesthesia and subsequent airway manipulation. Their use in this capacity relates to their historical use as part of a N_2O-narcotic anesthetic often used in patients with marginal cardiac reserve. For example, Bennet and Stanley compared the cardiovascular responses after administration of N_2O-morphine 0.4 mg/kg versus N_2O-fentanyl 4 µg/kg 10 minutes before intubation. The HR, cardiac output, and systolic and mean BP were reduced compared to baseline and remained unaffected by intubation in the N_2O-fentanyl group, but these parameters were all significantly elevated compared with preanesthetic controls in the N_2O–morphine group.[58] Whereas the assumed potency of fentanyl in this study was 100 times that of morphine, the lack of effect of morphine suggests that, with respect to suppression of pressor responses to laryngotracheal manipulation, fentanyl is more than 100 times as potent.

As reported by Bennett and Stanley[58] and later by other investigators,[59] fentanyl may not achieve its peak central nervous system effect until 10 minutes after bolus IV injection. Fentanyl appears to provide blunting of hemodynamic responses in a graded manner: 2 µg/kg IV given several minutes before induction only partially prevented HTN and tachycardia during an RSI with thiopental and succinylcholine. In this situation, 6 µg/kg was considerably more effective.[60] Chen and coworkers reported almost complete suppression of hemodynamic response to intubation with both 11 and 15 µg/kg of IV fentanyl, whereas higher IV doses (30 to 75 µg/kg) allowed only a very occasional response to intubation.[61]

In doses that prevent hemodynamic response to intubation, however, fentanyl is not a short-acting agent, and the risk of prolonged postoperative respiratory depression must be weighed against the advantages of perioperative cardiovascular stability. With this risk in mind, it has been observed that pretreatment with 2 µg/kg IV fentanyl given 10 minutes before intubation during an infusion of propofol sufficient to reduce the Bispectral Index Score to 45 prevented a significant increase in HR or BP compared with awake preanesthetic values.[10] Similar results were observed when intubation was performed after administration of fentanyl, 2 μg/kg, and propofol bolus doses of 2.0 to 3.5 mg/kg.[10]

Fentanyl and propofol require 6.4 and 2.9 minutes, respectively, to achieve effect-site equilibrium after IV bolus administration.[10] Therefore, the common practice of administering 1 to 2 mL (50 to 100 μg) just before or almost simultaneously with other induction medications would not be expected to have any effect based on inadequate dose and inappropriate timing of administration. Rather, this may provide a more plausible explanation for hypotension during the minutes-long quiescent period between endotracheal intubation and actual surgical incision. It is strongly recommended that laryngoscopy and intubation be timed to coincide with the peak effect of these agents.

Opioids with shorter onset and offset times have some advantages over fentanyl for modulating circulatory responses to intubation. Alfentanil has a smaller steady-state distribution volume and shorter terminal elimination half-life than fentanyl.[62] Ausems and colleagues demonstrated that an alfentanil plasma concentration of 600 ng/mL effectively prevented hemodynamic responses to intubation during induction of N_2O anesthesia.[63] This was achieved by a 30-second infusion of alfentanil at 150 μg/kg. During this induction period, N_2O and succinylcholine were also administered. Only 5 of the 35 patients studied sustained an increase in HR or BP greater than 15% above preinduction values.

Remifentanil has been found to be highly effective in preventing hemodynamic responses to intubation, albeit always with the cost of impressive bradycardia or hypotension, or both, before and after airway manipulation.[64] Many studies have used vagolytic agents to avoid bradycardia, at the risk of an elevated HR response after intubation. Remifentanil's half-time for equilibration between blood and effect site is 1.3 minutes,[65] and it has a brief half-life of 3 to 5 minutes due to hydrolysis by tissue and blood esterases.[66] Typical remifentanil infusion rates used for blunting hemodynamic responses are 0.25 to 1.0 μg/kg/min in association with cautious propofol administration and nondepolarizing neuromuscular blockade.[67] For RSI with thiopental and succinylcholine, the optimal dose of remifentanil appears to be 1.0 μg/kg administered over 30 seconds, with laryngoscopy performed 1 minute after induction. A bolus dose of 1.25 μg/kg was associated with unsatisfactory bradycardia, whereas 0.5 μg/kg resulted in excessive cardiovascular stimulation.[68] This dosing recommendation is supported by another report that found remifentanil 1 μg/kg given over 30 seconds, followed by thiopental 5 mg/kg and rocuronium 1 mg/kg 100 seconds later, was more effective than lidocaine and esmolol in attenuating the hemodynamic response to RSI.[69]

IV lidocaine may also blunt hemodynamic and cerebrovascular responses to intubation. When given in a bolus of 1.5 mg/kg IV, it adds approximately 0.3 MAC of anesthetic potency.[70] Significant reductions in hemodynamic response to endotracheal intubation have been noted when lidocaine (3 mg/kg) was used as an adjunct to high-dose fentanyl anesthesia,[71] as well as during other light anesthetic techniques, such as thiopental-N_2O-O_2.[72] However, smaller doses of lidocaine (1.5 mg/kg) have not been consistently reported to be effective in reducing the hemodynamic response to laryngoscopy and endotracheal intubation.[73,74]

The general anesthetic properties of lidocaine tend to reduce cerebral metabolic rate for O_2 and CBF, thus lowering ICP in patients with compromised intracranial compliance.[75] Theoretically, these properties of lidocaine might be exploited to mitigate rises in ICP during airway manipulation in those patients with acute intracranial pathology or compromised intracranial compliance. However, only a single human study has been reported specifically evaluating the ability of IV lidocaine to blunt intubation-related elevations in ICP. Bedford and colleagues compared 1.5 mg/kg IV lidocaine with placebo in 20 patients diagnosed with brain tumor. When administered 2 minutes before intubation, lidocaine failed to prevent a rise in ICP from the preanesthesia baseline, although the increase was more modest than that observed with the placebo (−12.1 mm Hg; 95% confidence interval, −22.8 to −1.4 mm Hg; $P = 0.03$).[76] This dearth of direct benefit was underscored by a systematic review that also failed to identify any evidence that pretreatment with IV lidocaine before RSI consistently reduced ICP or positively affected neurologic outcome.[77] This review is now more than a decade old, but because no new direct evidence has been published in the interim, its conclusion remains valid.

With regard to the patient at risk for intracranial HTN, it is important that agents used to control cardiovascular responses to intubation also have a minimal adverse impact on ICP. Agents that act as cerebral vasodilators, such as volatile anesthetics, nitroglycerin, nitroprusside, or hydralazine, are generally avoided if there is a serious risk of intracranial HTN.

E. Nonanesthetic Adjuvant Agents

A final means for modifying the cardiovascular responses to endotracheal intubation is prophylactic administration of vasoactive substances that directly affect the cardiovascular system. This approach was introduced in 1960 by DeVault and associates, who found that pretreatment with phentolamine, 5 mg IV, prevented the hypertensive-tachycardic response to endotracheal intubation during a light barbiturate-succinylcholine anesthetic technique.[78] Since then, a large number of articles have appeared advocating the use of various vasodilators and adrenergic blocking agents as pretreatment before endotracheal intubation, including diltiazem, verapamil, and nicardipine[79-82]; hydralazine[83]; nitroprusside[84]; nitroglycerin[85]; labetalol[86]; esmolol[80,87-89]; and clonidine.[90,91] Virtually all of these agents appear to be somewhat effective when compared to placebo, particularly when used in high doses.

Esmolol is the best studied of the group. In a large, multicenter, placebo-controlled trial, esmolol at doses of 100 or 200 mg suppressed the hemodynamic response to endotracheal intubation, particularly when combined with a moderate-dose opiate.[87] However, esmolol doses of 200 mg were associated with a doubling of the incidence of hypotension compared to placebo. In another study, smaller doses of esmolol (1 mg/kg) had no effect on the hemodynamic response to laryngoscopy and intubation compared to placebo.[80] Most recently, the combination of lidocaine (1.5 mg/kg) and esmolol at a dose of 1 mg/kg effectively attenuated the pressor response to intubation but was not as effective as 1 µg/kg remifentanil.[69] Currently, the optimal use of any of these agents is undefined, although their use as adjuncts to RSI is reasonable taking into account evidence-based dosing recommendations for the situation.

IV. AIRWAY EFFECTS OF ENDOTRACHEAL INTUBATION

A. Upper Airway Reflexes

Because the upper airway protects the respiratory gas exchange surface from noxious substances, it is appropriate that the nose, mouth, pharynx, larynx, trachea, and carina have an abundance of sensory nerve endings and brisk motor responses. Anesthesiologists are especially familiar with the glottic closure reflex (laryngospasm), which is invariably encountered early in their training. The sneeze, cough, and swallow reflexes are equally important upper airway reflexes.

Afferent pathways for laryngospasm and the cardiovascular responses to endotracheal intubation are initiated by the glossopharyngeal nerve when stimulation occurs superior to the anterior surface of the epiglottis and by the vagus nerve when stimulation occurs from the level of the posterior epiglottis down into the lower airway. Because the laryngeal closure reflex is mediated by vagal efferents to the glottis, it is virtually a monosynaptic response, occurring primarily when a patient is lightly anesthetized as vagally innervated sensory endings in the upper airway are stimulated and conscious respiratory efforts cannot override the reflex.

B. Dead Space

Patients with severe chronic lung disease may find it easier to breathe after intubation or a tracheostomy. The improvement is most likely due to reduced dead space. The normal extrathoracic anatomic dead space, based on cadaver measurements, is between 70 and 75 mL.[92] The exact volume (V) of the ETT is easily calculated as that of a cylinder using the formula $V = r^2l$, where r is the radius of the tube and l is the length. For example, an ETT that has an 8-mm inner diameter (ID) of 25 cm and a length of 25 cm has a volume of 12.6 mL. Intubation would therefore result in a reduction in dead space of approximately 60 mL.

Tracheostomy tubes are shorter than oral ETTs and have an even smaller dead space, although the difference as a proportion of tidal volume (V_t) is negligible. In normal individuals, the reduction in dead space with insertion of a tracheostomy tube is negligible compared with the normal V_t, so there is little benefit. In a patient with severe restrictive lung disease such as in end-stage kyphoscoliosis, V_t may be as low as 100 mL and intubation can confer a major benefit. Similarly, patients with

emphysema who are changed from mouth breathing to tracheostomy demonstrate a reduction in minute volume required and a decrease in total body O_2 consumption, presumably due to a decreased work of breathing.[93] Most likely, the decreased volume required more than compensates for the slight increase in resistance.

The decreases in dead space described here refer only to the volume of the ETT alone and are applicable only during T-piece breathing. Any extensions or Y-pieces added to the breathing circuit and attached to the ETT must also be added to the total.

C. Upper Airway Resistance

Anesthesiologists are well aware that in most anesthetized patients, adequate ventilation can be maintained with an ETT as small as 6 mm ID in place. Intensivists caring for a patient with respiratory failure often insist that an ETT must have a minimum ID of 8 mm. These tube sizes are each appropriate for the clinical situations described. The high resistance of the 6 mm ETT is inconsequential for the low minute ventilation required under general anesthesia, but the high flow rates required for a patient with respiratory failure may render the resistance of a small ETT prohibitive.

The ETT creates a mechanical burden for a spontaneously breathing patient in the form of a fixed upper airway resistance; that is, it decreases airway caliber and increases resistance to breathing. Gas flow across an ETT is determined by the pressure difference across the tube and the resistance of the ETT. Gas flows whenever there is a pressure difference across the ETT, whether it is caused by subatmospheric pressure generated during spontaneous breathing or by positive pressure generated from a mechanical ventilator.

The apparent resistance of an ETT is influenced by the shape of the tube and by two types of friction: the friction among the gas molecules and the friction between the tube wall and the gas molecules.[94,95] Irregular surfaces created by secretions or by ridges from wire reinforcement may create greater friction and greater resistance.[96] ETTs and tracheostomies have a higher resistance than the normal upper respiratory tract.[97,98]

The relationship between pressure difference and flow rate depends on the nature of the flow: laminar, turbulent, or a mixture of the two. In an ETT, turbulent flow predominates. During turbulent flow, the measured resistance is not a constant but varies with the flow rate, becoming markedly higher at high flow rates. Instead of the laminar flow relationship of pressure being directly proportional to flow, the pressure required to move the gas through an ETT with turbulent flow is proportional to the square of the flow. The relationship can therefore be described by a parabolic curve, as in Figure 7-4. The apparent resistance of a tube is proportional to the fourth power of the radius during laminar flow (Poiseuille's law) but to the fifth power during turbulent flow. Assuming turbulent flow, the relative resistance of a 6-mm ETT versus an 8-mm ETT is $4^5/3^5$, or 4.2 times as great. However, because flow patterns are not entirely predictable, the exact respiratory pressure-flow relationships may not be predictable without empiric determination.

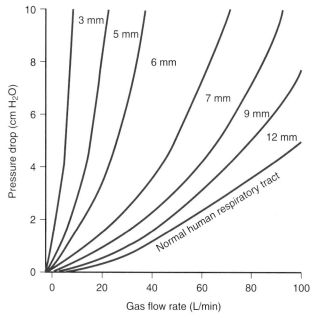

Figure 7-4 Pressure drop across endotracheal tubes of various sizes at flow rates ranging from 0 to 100 L/min. Note the wide disparity between 6- and 7-mm tubes as flow rate increases to the range typically seen in patients with respiratory failure. (Adapted from Nunn JF: *Applied respiratory physiology*, London, 1987, Butterworths.)

Such determinations are depicted in Figure 7-4. The slope of the pressure-flow graph is the apparent resistance. The parabolic shape of the graphs demonstrates the primarily turbulent nature of the flow through an ETT.

Although the resistance of the ETT may be several-fold greater than the resistance of the normal human upper airway, this is of relatively little consequence at low minute ventilation.[99] With a typical peak inspiratory flow of 25 to 30 L/min, approximately 0.5 cm H_2O pressure must be generated to overcome the resistance of the upper respiratory tract. This represents about 10% of the total work of breathing. Even a doubling or tripling of that resistance by placement of an ETT does not result in a clinically worrisome increase in the total work of breathing.[100]

As flow rates increase, however, flow becomes more turbulent and tube resistance may become a problem. For flow rates greater than 15 L/min, flow through any tube smaller than 10 mm ID becomes turbulent.[101] At the high flows required by patients in respiratory failure, the resistance of smaller tubes becomes prohibitive.[102] At the time of weaning patients with respiratory failure from mechanical ventilation, the importance of tube size often becomes a critical factor, with a common question being whether to change a 7-mm to a larger size. Note in Figure 7-4 that the pressure drop between 7-mm and 9-mm tubes is minimal at low inspiratory flows, but is considerable at flows of 60 L/min and higher.

Theoretically, the patient's native airway should have less resistance than any size ETT. However, a patient who has been intubated for an extended period may not have a normal upper airway. Indeed, some evidence suggests that work of breathing may actually increase after extubation, perhaps due to high upper airway resistance.[103,104] Therefore, if the patient is close to successful weaning, a reasonable approach may be to attempt extubation rather than to change ETTs, recognizing that the need for reintubation is a possibility. Alternatively, pressure support ventilation can be used to compensate for the added work of breathing through the smaller tube until extubation is warranted.[105]

Tracheostomy tubes have lower resistance than ETTs of comparable diameters because they are shorter. However, there is little, if any, difference in the work of breathing imposed by fresh tracheostomy tubes and ETTs of comparable ID.[106] On the other hand, tracheostomy does appear to decrease the work of breathing in patients who have undergone prolonged intubation and mechanical ventilation. This paradox may be explained by a reduction in the ID of an ETT over time, perhaps as a result of inspissated secretions or conformational changes.[107] This size reduction may explain the observation that patients being weaned from mechanical ventilation are sometimes more rapidly weaned after a tracheostomy is performed,[108] although it may also reflect the increased comfort of clinicians in discontinuing ventilatory support after the airway is secured.

D. Lower Airway Resistance

Bronchospasm after induction of anesthesia is a relatively uncommon but well-recognized event and is likely related to a reflex response to endotracheal intubation. Several studies provide some evidence regarding the frequency of bronchospasm. Tiret and associates studied complications at the time of induction of anesthesia and noted that bronchospasm accounted for 5.3% of fatal or near-fatal peri-induction complications.[109] The largest population was reported by Olsson, who found 246 cases of bronchospasm to have occurred out of a total of 136,929 anesthesia inductions, for an incidence of 1.7 per 1000.[110] However, the exact incidence undoubtedly depends substantially on the patient population.

The incidence of postintubation bronchospasm may be decreasing because of the increasing use of propofol as an induction agent (propofol being more effective than thiopental at preventing this complication). However, ventilation problems combined with hypoxia due to acute bronchospasm still represent important sentinel anesthesia events.[111]

Whereas the incidence of overt clinical bronchospasm is low, a reflex increase in airway resistance may occur much more often. Receptors in the larynx and upper trachea may cause large airway constriction distal to the tube, which in turn may extend to the smaller peripheral airways.[112] Support for this hypothesis comes from the work of Gal, who found an increase in lower airway resistance in a series of volunteers whose tracheas were intubated after topical anesthesia (Fig. 7-5).[113]

Bronchoconstriction also occurs after endotracheal intubation of normal subjects who have received thiopental/narcotic anesthesia.[114] In a series of patients pretreated before anesthesia with either a β-adrenergic

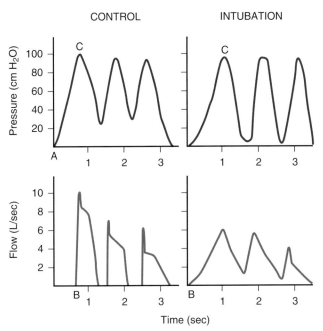

Figure 7-5 Pressure and flow curves (labeled *A* and *B*, respectively) generated during a burst of three successive coughs *(C)* by a volunteer before (control) and after endotracheal intubation. Notice that the flows and pressures generated are only modestly diminished after intubation. (From Gal TJ: How does tracheal intubation alter respiratory mechanics. *Probl Anesth* 2:191, 1988.)

agonist (albuterol) or an inhaled anticholinergic agent (ipratropium bromide), measured airway resistance after intubation was markedly lower compared with placebo treatment (Fig. 7-6).

Increases in airway resistance may result from changes in intrinsic smooth muscle tone, airway edema, or intraluminal secretions. These factors are, in turn, controlled by a series of intracellular and extracellular events,

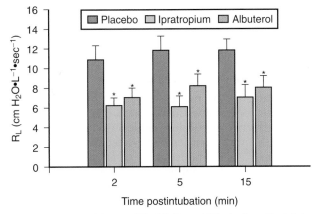

Figure 7-6 Lung resistance (*R*L) at 2, 5, and 15 minutes after intubation in patients pretreated with either a placebo, the β-adrenergic agonist albuterol, or the anticholinergic drug ipratropium bromide. Each of the drugs markedly diminished lung resistance for longer than 15 minutes after endotracheal intubation under thiopental-narcotic anesthesia. (From Kil HK, Rooke GA, Ryan-Dykes MA, et al: Effect of prophylactic bronchodilator treatment on lung resistance after tracheal intubation. *Anesthesiology* 81:43, 1994.)

including neural and hormonal factors. Rapid changes in airway caliber after airway instrumentation are thought to result largely from parasympathetic nervous system activation of airway smooth muscle.[115,116] Cholinergic innervation predominates in the larger central airways, with efferent nerves arising in the vagal nuclei of the brain stem and synapsing with ganglia in the airway walls. Postganglionic parasympathetic nerves release acetylcholine, activating muscarinic receptors on airway smooth muscle that lead to smooth muscle constriction. Such responses can be blocked via muscarinic blockade, using either systemic or inhaled anticholinergic agents.

Endotracheal intubation also may induce bronchospasm by causing coughing. A cough reduces lung volume, which in turn markedly increases bronchoconstriction in response to a stimulus.[117] In the patient with known reactive airways, prevention of coughing at the time of endotracheal intubation by use of either a deep level of anesthetic or a muscle relaxant may help to minimize the likelihood of bronchospasm.

E. Endotracheal Tube Resistance and Exhalation

In normal patients breathing at moderately elevated minute ventilation, exhalation is usually completed well before the next inhalation begins. By contrast, patients with obstructive airways disease may not complete full exhalation before the start of the next inhalation. In other words, inhalation begins before exhalation to functional residual capacity (FRC), resulting in persistent positive pressure in the alveoli. This phenomenon has been called auto-PEEP or dynamic hyperinflation, and it results in air trapping, elevated intrathoracic pressure, and hemodynamic compromise.[118]

Auto-PEEP most commonly occurs in patients with obstructive lung disease and high minute ventilation, but it may also rarely occur in patients with relatively normal airways who are ventilated at very high minute ventilation. This has been observed in patients with burns or sepsis, who may require as much as 30 to 40 L of minute ventilation. Under these circumstances, the resistance of the ETT may limit expiratory flow so that full exhalation does not occur. This has been demonstrated experimentally, with the magnitude of the auto-PEEP correlating directly with the resistance of the ETT.[119] Among patients under anesthesia, major resistance to exhalation caused by the ETT is of no consequence in routine cases and is only rarely seen in critically ill patients. However, low levels of auto-PEEP due to tube resistance probably occur frequently in patients with high minute ventilation[108] and during single-lung ventilation via a double-lumen ETT.

F. Functional Residual Capacity

The effect of endotracheal intubation on FRC has been a subject of considerable controversy. Intensivists are well aware of patients recovering from respiratory failure in whom oxygenation improved after extubation. The improvement has been attributed to "physiologic PEEP"— the presumption that a small positive pressure is normally created by the glottis and that this leads to breathing at a higher lung volume. The assumption is that an ETT removes the glottic barrier and may, therefore, lower lung volume. However, the existence of positive intratracheal pressure has never been documented, and in a study of volunteers who underwent awake intubation, no consistent change in FRC could be measured.[120-122]

By contrast, a different conclusion was reached in a series of patients who were studied just before and after extubation following recovery from respiratory failure. In this situation, both FRC and arterial oxygen tension (PaO_2) were found to increase after extubation, supporting the concept that the presence of an ETT decreases FRC.[123] Resolution of these disparate results was suggested by a rabbit study in which normal rabbits did not demonstrate a difference in oxygenation or tracheal pressure after intubation, but after respiratory failure was induced, endotracheal intubation worsened oxygenation.[124] These results suggest that the rabbits compensated for respiratory failure by using glottic closure to maintain a positive intratracheal pressure and that the effect of an ETT on FRC depends on that underlying respiratory state.

G. Cough

Although it is widely recognized that cough efficiency is reduced whenever an ETT is in place, it is a common observation that a disconnected ETT is likely to produce a plug of sputum whenever the patient is stimulated to cough. In awake intubation volunteers, peak airway flow was reduced but was still adequate to enable secretion clearance.[113] However, the ETT prevented collapse of the trachea by acting as a stent. Therefore, although secretions could be moved to the central airways, the ETT prevented maximum efficiency of expectoration. Large airway collapse is important for producing maximum force against secretions, and this explains why moving secretions from the trachea out through the ETT often requires the use of a suction catheter.

H. Humidification of Gases

Under normal circumstances, the upper airway warms, humidifies, and filters 7000 to 10,000 L of inspired air daily, adding up to 1 L of moisture to the gases. When the upper airway is bypassed by intubation, the gas must be warmed and humidified in the trachea if it is not adequately humidified before inhalation. In an anesthetized patient breathing dry gases, up to 10% of the average metabolic rate may be required to perform these tasks.[125] Delivery of cool, dry gases may also have a significant effect on mucociliary transport, a critical defense mechanism of the respiratory tract. Inhalation of unconditioned gas rapidly leads to abnormal mucosal ciliary motion, with subsequent encrustation and inspissation of tracheal secretions.[126,127] These changes occur as early as 30 minutes after intubation and, theoretically, may lead to an increase in postoperative complications in patients with limited chest excursion. Accordingly, assurance of adequate gas conditioning should be standard in all but very brief endotracheal intubations.

V. CONTROL AND TREATMENT OF THE RESPIRATORY RESPONSES TO AIRWAY INSTRUMENTATION

A. Preventing Upper Airway Responses

Cough and laryngospasm in response to intubation appear to be sound protective reflexes. Under most circumstances, the body needs to prevent further intrusion by a foreign body and to expel it from the airway. However, these responses can be troublesome during induction of anesthesia or at the time of extubation. Cough can lead to bronchospasm as lung volume is reduced, and it can also result in desaturation as the lung volume drops to residual volume. Laryngospasm may result in life-threatening abnormalities of blood gases. Consequently, anesthesiologists routinely try to prevent these responses with the use of medications delivered topically, via inhalation, or intravenously.

Inhibition of upper airway reflexes can certainly be accomplished by performing endotracheal intubation after the administration of NMB agents. However, both laryngeal and tracheal reflexes are difficult to inhibit by deep levels of general anesthesia alone.[128] When circumstances preclude the use of NMB agents, the clinician must give consideration to how best to prevent discomfort, gagging, coughing, and laryngospasm during endotracheal intubation: avoidance of endotracheal intubation, use of regional and topical anesthesia, very deep general anesthesia, or a combination of all modalities.

1. Technical Considerations: Minimizing Airway Stimulation

Although placement of an LMA is likely to be less noxious than direct laryngoscopy and endotracheal intubation, it remains a highly stimulating procedure. For example, Scanlon and colleagues found a 60% incidence of gagging, a 30% incidence of laryngospasm, and a 19% incidence of coughing when the LMA was placed after induction with thiopental 5 mg/kg.[129] Induction with propofol 2.5 mg/kg reduced these events by two thirds but did not ablate them. Therefore, instrumentation of the upper airway by any technique will illicit protective reflexes that must be obtunded with local or general anesthesia (or both).

2. Regional and Topical Anesthesia

The surfaces of the mouth and nose are easily anesthetized with topical anesthetic sprays or gels. Lidocaine is equally effective as cocaine and less toxic; it can be combined with a vasoconstrictor to give equivalent intubating conditions.[130-132] Administration of an antisialagogue 30 to 60 minutes before application of the topical anesthetic results in better anesthesia as well as better intubating conditions. The lack of secretions probably minimizes dilution of the applied anesthetic and also results in better intubating conditions.

The mouth and pharynx derive their sensory innervation from the trigeminal and glossopharyngeal nerves. The supraglottic larynx derives its sensory innervation from the SLN, a branch of the vagus, and intubation can be facilitated by blocking it bilaterally.[133] The nerve block relies on the consistent relationship of the SLN to the lateral horns of the hyoid bone. When combined with topical anesthesia of the nose or mouth and adequate anesthesia of the infraglottic larynx, the nerve block provides excellent intubating conditions, and most patients are able to accept an ETT without cough, gag, or laryngospasm. Equal success in blunting upper airway reflexes can be achieved by careful spraying of the larynx with topical anesthesia. A nasal trumpet helps ensure that solution reaches the larynx. Topical anesthesia spares the patient the need for two injections.

The infraglottic larynx derives sensory innervation from the recurrent laryngeal nerves, which run along the posterolateral surfaces of the trachea. Again, topical anesthesia rather than nerve block is the method of choice for obtunding reflexes. Injection of several milliliters of 4% lidocaine via the cricothyroid membrane routinely results in excellent blockade of sensation.

The efficacy of topical and nerve block anesthesia at suppressing airway reflexes during intubation is evident. Several studies have documented that topical anesthesia applied preoperatively (for brief cases) or intraoperatively can suppress cough and laryngospasm at the time of extubation.[134] A randomized study of patients undergoing tonsillectomy found that the incidence of stridor or laryngospasm at the time of extubation could be reduced from 12% to 3% by application of topical lidocaine at the time of intubation.[135] The LITA endotracheal tube (Laryngotracheal Instillation of Topical Anesthetic, Sheridan Corporation, Argyle, NY) contains a small channel that can be used to spray the upper airway while an ETT is in place. When this method was used to spray the ETT before extubation, coughs were reduced by more than 60%, and the severity of the coughing was decreased.[136]

The use of liquid, in the form of a lidocaine-bicarbonate mixture, rather than air to inflate the cuff of the ETT after intubation has also been reported to be effective in diminishing emergence phenomena.[137,138] Inflating the ETT cuff with 40 mg of lidocaine (2 mL of 2% solution) and then adding 3 to 7 mL of 8.4% sodium bicarbonate ($NaHCO_3$) until no cuff leak was present resulted in significant reductions in coughing, restlessness, and BP during emergence. In addition, sore throat complaints assessed at 15 minutes and at 1, 2, 3, and 24 hours postoperatively; postoperative dysphonia; and hoarseness after extubation were all reduced when compared to cuff inflation with air. When this technique was used, more than 50% of the original 40 mg of lidocaine still remained in solution at 2 hours after inflation of the cuff, and only about 75% was released even after 6 hours of surgery (Fig. 7-7).[137] Because standard 8.4% $NaHCO_3$ is a basic solution with a calculated pH of 7.8 (range 7 to 8.5), the addition of more than 2 mL of bicarbonate to the 2 mL of 2% lidocaine (calculated pH 6, range 5 to 7) already injected into the ETT cuff results in a solution with a pH 7.95 to 8.09; this leads to concern about tracheal mucosal damage from flash burn injury in the event of a cuff rupture. However, a direct comparison between solutions of 2 mL of 2% lidocaine with 8.4% versus 1.4% bicarbonate reported similar efficacy in reducing postoperative sore throat complaints and the occurrence of various

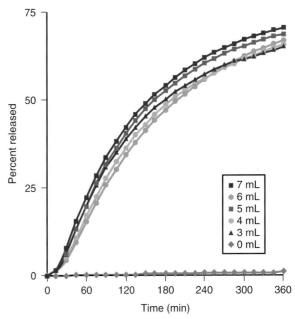

Figure 7-7 Percentage of lidocaine released in vitro as a function of time from an endotracheal tube (ETT) cuff filled with 40 mg lidocaine hydrochloride and additional 8.4% sodium bicarbonate solution equal to 0, 3, 4, 5, 6, or 7 mL. (From Estebe JP, Dollo G, Le Corre P, et al: Alkalinization of intracuff lidocaine improves ETT-induced emergence phenomena. *Anesth Analg* 94:227–230, 2002.)

emergence phenomena.[138] Therefore, in actual clinical practice, a favorable risk-benefit balance can be achieved by using the following combination in a 10-mL syringe: 5 mL 1% lidocaine, 1 mL 8.4% $NaHCO_3$ solution, and 4 to 5 mL of sterile diluent (J.P. Estebe, personal communication, 2010).

3. Intravenous Agents

Given a high enough dose, virtually all agents used as IV anesthetics will suppress the cough response to intubation. However, different agents appear to vary in their ability to inhibit upper airway reflexes when judged on the basis of equal potency in depressing consciousness and in depressing the cardiovascular system. Propofol/narcotic anesthesia may be adequate for intubating the trachea in some patients even without the use of muscle relaxants.[139] On the other hand, ketamine clinically appears to enhance laryngeal reflexes at doses that provide adequate anesthesia for surgery.

IV lidocaine is frequently used to prevent cough and laryngospasm at the time of intubation or extubation. Although the studies are not uniform in documenting efficacy, the preponderance of evidence supports the use of lidocaine.[140,141] Studies that did not document efficacy are sometimes flawed by the lack of documentation that adequate serum levels were reached. The maximal efficacy of IV lidocaine occurs 1 to 3 minutes after injection and requires a dose of 1.5 mg/kg or more. This corresponded to a plasma level in excess of 4 µg/mL.

The ability of IV lidocaine to suppress cough appears to be related to factors beyond induction of general anesthesia, because cough suppression occurs at levels routinely seen in awake patients being treated with the drug.

A comparison of the antitussive effects of lidocaine compared with meperidine and thiopental demonstrated that severe respiratory depression occurs with the latter drugs in achieving the same antitussive efficacy that can be achieved with lidocaine with virtually no respiratory depression.[142]

Whether IV lidocaine suppresses laryngospasm remains controversial. A study in which tonsillectomy patients were given 2 mg/kg of IV lidocaine and then extubated 1 minute later found suppression of laryngospasm.[143] Another study of tonsillectomy patients given 1.5 mg/kg of lidocaine found no clear effect.[144] A major difference in the latter study was the authors' design of not extubating the patient until swallowing had begun. This may have resulted in a significant difference in the anesthetic depth at which the children were extubated.

B. Preventing Bronchoconstriction

Bronchoconstriction results routinely after endotracheal intubation. In healthy subjects it appears to be of moderate degree, but the exaggerated response seen in patients with hyperactive airways can be life-threatening. Prevention or treatment of this response can be achieved with the use of topical or IV agents. Inhaled anesthetic agents also inhibit the response through direct absorption by smooth muscle or inhibition of reflexes.

Bronchospasm after intubation may be cholinergically mediated. Afferent parasympathetic fibers travel to bronchial smooth muscle and then produce bronchoconstriction by stimulating the M_3 cholinergic receptors on bronchial smooth muscle. In addition, stimulation of M_2 cholinergic receptors on airway smooth muscle potentiates bronchospasm by inhibiting β-adrenergic–mediated smooth muscle relaxation.[145]

1. Technical Considerations: Minimizing Airway Stimulation

Avoidance of endotracheal intubation is the most logical first step in terms of limiting airway irritation and bronchoconstriction. If general anesthesia is required, the LMA may be preferable to the ETT in terms of provocation of bronchospasm, but, as alluded to earlier, the LMA will not prevent coughing in the absence of NMB.[129] However, the LMA does appear to result in reduced lower airway resistance when compared with endotracheal intubation after induction of general anesthesia. This difference is assumed to result from induction of reversible bronchospasm by the ETT.[146,147] In addition, use of the LMA results in fewer pulmonary complications and improved pulmonary function when compared with endotracheal intubation in infants born prematurely with bronchopulmonary dysplasia and in adults without lung disease.[148,149]

2. Topical Anesthesia

The studies of Gal and Surratt demonstrated a doubling of lower airway resistance after endotracheal intubation of awake volunteers under topical anesthesia.[120] The bronchoconstrictive response must indeed be a powerful one if local anesthesia sufficient to permit volunteers to be intubated was not sufficient to prevent the reflex

bronchoconstriction. A study of awake fiberoptic intubation in asthmatics demonstrated a marked decrease in forced expiratory volume in 1 minute (FEV_1) after intubation. This decrease was somewhat mitigated by topical lidocaine although lidocaine was not as effective as albuterol in preventing the bronchoconstriction.[150] However, a lidocaine aerosol given to dogs before a challenge with inhaled citric acid did not attenuate the response to this irritant.[151] Because the aerosol itself produces a slight increase in lung resistance, the efficacy of the inhaled aerosol lidocaine may in part have been due to IV absorption of the drug. Given these considerations and the time required to administer the aerosol compared to the immediacy and efficacy of IV drugs or other inhaled drugs, aerosolized lidocaine is probably a poor choice for the attenuation of bronchoconstriction associated with endotracheal intubation.

3. Intravenous Agents

A variety of drugs have been studied for their bronchodilating properties. Although IV β-agonists clearly produce bronchodilation, there is no benefit to parenteral administration of these drugs rather than inhalational administration. Among anesthetic induction agents, considerable experimental evidence suggests that ketamine has both direct and indirect relaxant effects on airway smooth muscle through non–β-receptor mechanisms.[152-157] However, the clinical data supporting the use of ketamine for prevention or treatment of bronchospasm is largely anecdotal,[158] or in more rigorous trials unimpressive.[159-161] This may relate to reluctance to routinely use ketamine at high doses because of its side effects, including dysphoria and sympathetic stimulation, rather than a lack of benefit of the drug.

Propofol, midazolam, and etomidate all relax airway smooth muscle in vitro, although generally at higher site concentrations than would be used clinically.[162-166] In contrast, barbiturates may have direct bronchoconstricting effects.[167] Propofol may also have indirect effects on airway constriction, perhaps though inhibition of vagal tone.[157,168] Clinically, propofol has been shown to be superior to the barbiturates and to etomidate in reducing wheezing and airway resistance in both asthmatic and nonasthmatic subjects.[169-171] When asthmatics were induced with either thiopental, methohexital, or propofol at equipotent doses, none of the patients given propofol wheezed after endotracheal intubation, whereas both of the barbiturates resulted in a significant incidence of wheezing (Fig. 7-8).[169]

In animals, IV lidocaine has been reported to attenuate bronchoconstriction induced by a variety of experimental means.[172,173] In humans with bronchial hyperreactivity, IV lidocaine reduced the bronchoconstrictor response to histamine challenge and had an additive effect with albuterol in reducing this response.[174] However, a double-blind, placebo-controlled trial of IV lidocaine (1.5 mg/kg) or inhaled albuterol in asthmatics found that albuterol but not lidocaine prevented postintubation bronchoconstriction.[175] Although lidocaine may inhibit reflex-induced bronchospasm, it may also cause contraction of bronchial smooth muscle in the absence of reflex mechanisms. In a study of 15 asthmatics, IV lidocaine

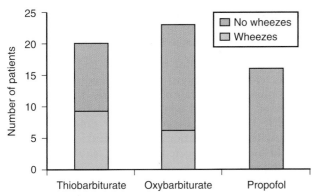

Figure 7-8 Incidence of wheezing after endotracheal intubation in asthmatics when induction was performed with either an oxybarbiturate, a thiobarbiturate, or propofol (*P* < 0.05 for either thiobarbiturate or oxybarbiturate versus propofol). (From Pizow R, Brown RH, Weiss YS, et al: Wheezing during induction of general anesthesia in patients with and without asthma: A randomized, blinded trial. *Anesthesiology* 81:1111, 1995.)

reduced airway diameter at total lung capacity assessed by computed tomography and resulted in significant decreases in FEV_1.[176] These untoward effects were underscored by a case report in which IV lidocaine 1.5 mg/kg administered to facilitate intubation was temporally associated with transient bronchospasm in a 17-month-old child with mild intermittent asthma.[177] A published best-evidence review also failed to find good evidence for use of IV lidocaine during intubation in patients with status asthmaticus.[178] Therefore, the evidence in support of IV lidocaine to prevent postintubation bronchospasm when used without the concomitant administration of an inhaled β-agonist is scant, and there is a potential risk of worsening airway resistance with its use. Therefore, the use of IV lidocaine for this indication cannot be endorsed.

4. Inhaled Agents

All of the volatile anesthetics have direct and perhaps indirect relaxant effects on airway smooth muscle in experimental models.[94,179-182] Although these agents have differences in potency in vitro, the clinical importance of these differences is unclear.[180,182,183] In adult patients, sevoflurane is more effective than isoflurane, desflurane, or halothane in reducing airway resistance after endotracheal intubation,[184-186] but does not prevent an increase in airway resistance after intubation of asthmatic children.[187] However, given the available data, sevoflurane is probably the volatile agent of choice, and desflurane is a poor choice for use in high-risk patients (Fig. 7-9).

There are no prospective, controlled studies comparing deep inhalation anesthesia to IV induction with bronchoprotective agents such as ketamine or propofol in high-risk patients. Achieving a deep plane of anesthesia with a bronchoprotective agent before intubation is likely the most important point in preventing severe bronchospasm in high-risk patients, rather than the choice of IV versus inhalation induction techniques.

Pretreatment of patients with inhaled β2-adrenergic agonists or an inhaled anticholinergic markedly reduced lung resistance following endotracheal intubation and should be used routinely in patients known to have bronchospasm.[114,188]

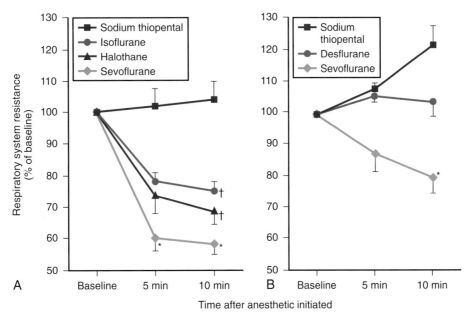

Figure 7-9 Respiratory system resistance (percent of baseline) during maintenance anesthesia. **A,** Isoflurane, halothane, and sevoflurane are compared with thiopental 0.25 mg/kg/min plus 50% nitrous oxide. *P* < 0.05 versus isoflurane, halothane, and thiopental. †*P* < 0.05 versus thiopental. **B,** Desflurane and sevoflurane are compared with thiopental 0.25 mg/kg/min. *P* < 0.05 versus desflurane and thiopental. (**A,** Adapted from Rooke GA, Choi JH, Bishop MJ: The effect of isoflurane, halothane, sevoflurane, and thiopental/nitrous oxide on respiratory system resistance after tracheal intubation. *Anesthesiology* 86:1294, 1997; **B,** From Goff MJ, Arain SR, Ficke DJ, et al: Absence of bronchodilation during desflurane anesthesia: A comparison to sevoflurane and thiopental. *Anesthesiology* 93:404, 2000.)

5. Choice of Neuromuscular Blocking Drug

The choice of muscle relaxants can influence bronchial tone after endotracheal intubation. Rapacuronium was withdrawn from the market after a number of reports of severe bronchospasm, most likely due to antagonism at the M_2 receptor.[189] Mivacurium releases significant amounts of histamine and leads to mast cell degranulation; it should be used extremely cautiously, if at all, in patients with a history of atopy or asthma.[190] Studies in France and Norway have suggested a high incidence of anaphylaxis with rocuronium, although this finding does not appear to be supported in literature from other countries.

VI. CONCLUSIONS

Airway manipulations of any kind can result in reflex-mediated changes in cardiopulmonary physiology. The type and depth of anesthesia provided must be individualized for the type of airway being used and the clinical situation for which it is required. Additionally, airway managers should be prepared to treat profound alterations in HR, BP, airways resistance, or ICP occurring during or immediately consequent to airway manipulation. Although these responses may be of short duration and of little consequence in healthy individuals, serious complications can occur in patients with underlying coronary artery disease, reactive airways, or intracranial neuropathology.

VII. CLINICAL PEARLS

- Laryngoscopy can induce bradycardia, by increasing vagal tone at the sinoatrial node, or HTN and tachycardia mediated by the cardioaccelerator nerves and sympathetic chain ganglia. The former is most common in infants and children, whereas the latter is typical for adolescents and adults.

- Laryngoscopy and intubation result in stimulation of the CNS and may increase cerebral blood flow (CBF), which may result in elevation of intracranial pressure (ICP) and brain herniation.

- Ischemic electrocardiographic changes lasting less than 10 minutes during airway manipulation have not been shown to correlate with postoperative myocardial infarction.

- Succinylcholine is associated with bradycardia in children, particularly when doses are repeated, but it is a cardiovascular stimulant in adults.

- Succinylcholine may directly elevate CBF and ICP, an effect that can be blunted by pretreatment with a nondepolarizing agent and strict maintenance of normocapnia.

- The application of cricoid pressure can result in greater HR and BP response to endotracheal intubation than when it is not used, and it should be considered when estimating the risk-benefit ratio of this procedure in individual patients.

- Fentanyl provides a graded response in blunting hemodynamic responses to intubation, with 2 µg/kg IV fentanyl given several minutes before induction only partially preventing hypertension and tachycardia during a rapid-sequence intubation (RSI).

- Fentanyl and propofol require 6.4 and 2.9 minutes, respectively, to achieve effect-site equilibrium after IV bolus administration. Therefore, the commonly observed practice of administering 1 to 2 mL of fentanyl (50 to 100 µg) just before or almost simultaneously with administration of other induction medications would not be expected to have any effect based on inadequate dose and inappropriate timing of administration.

- When given in a bolus of 1.5 mg/kg IV, lidocaine adds approximately 0.3 MAC of anesthetic potency, but it is not reliable at blunting the cardiovascular or airway response to laryngoscopy or intubation. Additionally, pretreatment with IV lidocaine before RSI does not consistently reduce ICP or positively affect neurologic outcome.

- For surgeries lasting longer than 2 hours, cough and throat complaints may be decreased by inflating the cuff of the ETT with a buffered solution containing 40 mg of lidocaine. This can be accomplished by using a 10-mL syringe containing 5 mL 1% lidocaine, 1 mL 8.4% $NaHCO_3$ solution, and 4 to 5 mL of sterile diluent and inflating the cuff until no leak is present.

- Propofol, midazolam, and etomidate are preferred to barbiturates for anesthetic induction in patients with known reactive airways and in those in whom acute bronchoconstriction is to be avoided.

SELECTED REFERENCES

All references can be found online at expertconsult.com.

12. Landesberg G, Mosseri M, Zahger D, et al: Myocardial infarction after vascular surgery: The role of prolonged stress-induced, ST depression-type ischemia. *J Am Coll Cardiol* 37:1839–1845, 2001.
18. Lanier W, Milde J, Michenfelder J: Cerebral stimulation following succinylcholine in dogs. *Anesthesiology* 64:551–559. 1986.
24. Saghaei M, Masoodifar M: The pressor response and airway effects of cricoid pressure during induction of general anesthesia. *Anesth Analg* 93:787–790, 2001.
32. Wood ML, Forrest ET: The haemodynamic response to the insertion of the laryngeal mask airway: A comparison with laryngoscopy and tracheal intubation. *Acta Anaesthesiol Scand* 38:510–513, 1994.
61. Chen CT, Toung TJK, Donham RT, et al: Fentanyl dosage for suppression of circulatory response to laryngoscopy and endotracheal intubation. *Anesthesiol Rev* 13:37–42, 1986.
69. Min JH, Chai HS, Kim YH, et al: Attenuation of hemodynamic responses to laryngoscopy and tracheal intubation during rapid sequence induction: Remifentanil vs. lidocaine with esmolol. *Minerva Anestesiol* 76:188–192, 2010.
73. Miller CD, Warren SJ: Intravenous lignocaine fails to attenuate the cardiovascular response to laryngoscopy and tracheal intubation. *Br J Anaesth* 65:216–219, 1990.
77. Robinson N, Clancy M: In patients with head injury undergoing rapid sequence intubation, does pretreatment with intravenous lignocaine/lidocaine lead to an improved neurological outcome? A review of the literature. *Emerg Med J* 18:453–457, 2001.
87. Miller DR, Martineau RJ, Wynands JE, et al: Bolus administration of esmolol for controlling the haemodynamic response to tracheal intubation: The Canadian Multicentre Trial. *Can J Anaesth* 38:849–858, 1991.
138. Estebe JP, Gentili M, Le Corre P, et al: Alkalinization of intracuff lidocaine: Efficacy and safety. *Anesth Analg* 101:1536–1541, 2005.

PART 2

The Difficult Airway: Definition, Recognition, and the ASA Algorithm

Chapter 8

Definition and Incidence of the Difficult Airway

SATYA K. RAMACHANDRAN | P. ALLAN KLOCK JR.

I. INTRODUCTION

The fundamental responsibility of an anesthesiologist is to ensure adequate gas exchange for the patient. Failure to maintain oxygenation for more than a few minutes can result in catastrophic anoxic injury. Data from closed claims of respiratory-related malpractice in 1990 reported brain damage or death in more than 85% of patients.[1] In the closed claims data from 2006, improvements in airway management techniques and monitoring standards had reduced the number of intubation-related claims,[2] but difficulties with airway management during emergence remained among the leading causes of serious perioperative problems. It has been estimated that the inability to successfully manage a difficult airway (DA) is responsible for as many as 30% of deaths directly attributable to anesthesia.[2]

In general, greater degrees of difficulty in maintaining airway patency are more likely to engender greater risk of brain damage or death. Before discussing the specific management of a DA, we must define the DA, classify the degrees of difficulty in maintaining a patent airway, and determine the incidence of each class or type of DA. In this discussion, it is assumed that a reasonably well-trained anesthesia provider always attempts to maintain airway patency.

II. DEFINITION AND CLASSIFICATION OF THE DIFFICULT AIRWAY

There are three common ways of maintaining airway patency and gas exchange. First, mask ventilation can deliver inspired gas via a mask that is sealed to the patient's face, while the natural airway from the face to the vocal cords is kept patent with or without external jaw thrust maneuvers or internal upper airway devices. Second, inspired gas can be delivered via a supraglottic airway device (SGA), such as a laryngeal mask airway (LMA; LMA North America, San Diego, CA). Third, with tracheal intubation, inspired gases are delivered via a tube that traverses the vocal cords, providing continuity from the respiratory circuit to the trachea.

The term *difficult airway* spans a spectrum of clinical situations (Fig. 8-1), from difficulty or inability to provide mask ventilation to difficulty or inability to intubate the trachea. The combined "cannot intubate, cannot ventilate" (CICV) scenario carries the highest risk of brain

DEFINITION OF DIFFERENT DEGREES OF A DIFFICULT AIRWAY

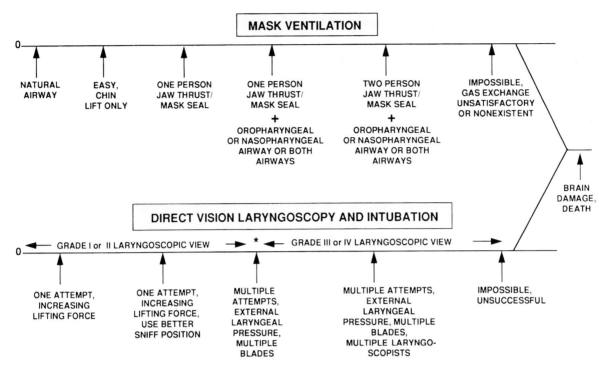

Figure 8-1 Conceptualization of a difficult airway. Difficult intubation refers to one or more of the following: difficult laryngoscopy, difficult video laryngoscopy, or difficult flexible bronchoscopic visualization. The widespread use of supraglottic airways has elevated them to immediate rescue devices in "cannot intubate, cannot ventilate" situations. The triad of difficult mask ventilation, difficult supraglottic airway placement, and difficult intubation increases the risk of hypoxic brain injury and death.

damage or death. To better describe the layers of difficulty, we have chosen several categories of difficult or impossible mask ventilation; difficult placement of, or ventilation via an SGA; difficult laryngoscopy; and difficult intubation using direct laryngoscopy, video laryngoscopy, or flexible bronchoscopy.

A. Difficult or Impossible Face Mask Ventilation

1. Causes of Difficult Mask Ventilation

There are two main causes of inadequate face mask ventilation. One is inability to establish an adequate seal between the face and the mask, which results in a leak of respiratory gas. The second cause is inadequate patency of the airway at the level of the nasopharynx, oropharynx, hypopharynx, larynx, or trachea. These conditions manifest as either inability to generate airway pressure that is adequate to drive gas into the lungs or inability to move gas into the lungs despite an adequate driving pressure.

2. Definition of Difficult Mask Ventilation

The simplest mask ventilation scale in contemporary literature was described by Han and colleagues in 2004 (Table 8-1).[3] In that scale, the progressive grades of difficulty are (1) ventilation by mask; (2) ventilation by mask with oral airway or other adjuvant with or without muscle relaxant; (3) difficult mask ventilation, defined as "inadequate, unstable, or requires two providers" with or

without muscle relaxant; and (4) impossible mask ventilation with an inability to mask ventilate with or without muscle relaxant.

Langeron and colleagues defined difficult face mask ventilation as "the inability of an unassisted anesthesiologist to maintain oxygen saturation >92%, as measured by pulse oximetry, or to prevent or reverse signs of inadequate ventilation during positive-pressure mask ventilation under general anesthesia."[4] In their study, mask

TABLE 8-1		
Han Mask Ventilation Scale and Incidence of Difficult Mask Ventilation		
Grade	Description	Incidence (*n*, [%])
1	Ventilated by mask	37,857 (71.3%)
2	Ventilated by mask with oral airway or other adjuvant with or without muscle relaxant	13,966 (26.3%)
3	Difficult ventilation (inadequate, unstable, or requiring two providers) with or without muscle relaxant	1,141 (2.2%)
4	Unable to mask ventilate with or without muscle relaxant	77 (0.15%)

From Han R, Tremper KK, Kheterpal S, O'Reilly M: Grading scale for mask ventilation. *Anesthesiology* 101:267, 2004.

ventilation was considered difficult if one or more of six criteria were present:

1. Inability for the unassisted anesthesiologist to maintain oxygen saturation >92% using 100% oxygen and positive-pressure mask ventilation
2. Important gas flow leak by the face mask
3. Need to increase gas flow to >15 L/min and to use the oxygen flush valve more than twice
4. No perceptible chest movement
5. Need to perform a two-handed mask ventilation technique
6. Change of operator required.

El-Ganzouri and coworkers defined difficult mask ventilation as the "inability to obtain chest excursion sufficient to maintain a clinically acceptable capnogram waveform despite optimal head and neck positioning and use of muscle paralysis, use of an oral airway, and optimal application of a face mask by anesthesia personnel."[5]

3. Incidence of Difficult Mask Ventilation

Two studies by Kheterpal and associates on difficult and impossible mask ventilation represent the largest investigations to date on the topic. The incidence of difficult mask ventilation was 1.4% in 22,660 patients and 2.2% in a subsequent study of 50,000 patients.[6,7] The incidence of impossible ventilation ranged from 0.15% to 0.16% in these two large studies. Langeron and colleagues reported a 5% incidence of difficult mask ventilation, with 1 of every 1502 patients impossible to ventilate with a face mask (0.07%).[4] In other large, prospective studies the incidence has ranged from 0.07% to 1.4%,[5,8,9] although this was not the primary outcome being assessed. In summary, difficult mask ventilation can be expected 1 or 2 times in every 100 anesthesias, and impossible mask ventilation 1 or 2 times in 1000 anesthesias.

Methods used to improve airway patency include the head-tilt, jaw-thrust, and chin-lift maneuvers as well as insertion of oral or nasal airways. If mask seal is poor, the practitioner may choose a different face mask, use a two-hand or two-person technique, insert bolsters between the alveolar ridge and the cheeks, or employ other methods to improve the interface between the face and the mask. When two persons are needed, ideally the primary anesthesiologist stands at the patient's head and initiates jaw thrust with the left hand at the angle of the left mandible and left-sided mask seal while the right hand compresses the reservoir bag. The standard position for the primary anesthesiologist appears in Figure 8-2. The secondary (helping) person stands at the patient's side, at the level of the patient's shoulder, facing the primary anesthesiologist. The right hand of the secondary anesthesiologist should cover the left hand of the primary anesthesiologist and contribute to left-sided jaw thrust and mask seal, and the left hand of the secondary person initiates right-sided jaw thrust and mask seal. In this way, all four hands are doing something important without interfering with one another, and there is almost no redundant effort. With this positioning, the secondary person can watch the monitors continuously, manipulate the larynx externally, and hand equipment to the primary anesthesiologist.

TWO-PERSON MAXIMUM MASK VENTILATION EFFORT

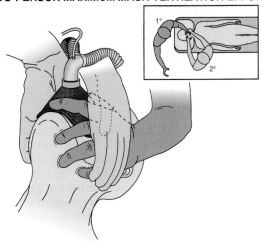

Figure 8-2 Optimal two-person mask ventilation effort. The primary anesthesiologist stands at the head of the patient and uses left and right hands in classic fashion. The secondary (helping) person stands facing the primary anesthesiologist at the level of the patient's shoulder and uses the right hand to help achieve left-sided jaw thrust and mask seal while the left hand achieves right-sided jaw thrust and mask seal.

B. Difficulties with Supraglottic Airway Devices

The last two decades have seen a phenomenal increase in the use of SGAs for elective and rescue purposes. Most studies of SGA devices describe first-attempt and overall success rates. Difficulties with the devices include failure of insertion, failure to form a clear passage to the trachea, and failure to form an effective seal in the airway.[10]

Most of the studies reporting difficulties with SGAs have focused on LMAs. Among these, the failure rate is 1% for the intubating and ProSeal models and 2% for the LMA classic and flexible models.[10]

1. Definition of Difficult Placement

Success rates after one, two, or three attempts are an accepted way to describe difficult SGA device placement. Other methods include time taken for successful placement, Likert-based difficulty scales (very easy, easy, or difficult), and secondary measures such as evidence of trauma during insertion.

2. Incidence of Success

For the ProSeal laryngeal mask airway (PLMA), first-attempt success rates range from 76% to 100% (mean, 87.3%), and overall insertion success rates range from 90% to 100% (mean, 98.4%).[11] One of the important rescue functions of the LMA is as a conduit for flexible bronchoscopic intubation. The inability to visualize vocal cords using a trans-LMA flexible bronchoscopic technique is a significant impediment to successful tracheal intubation. The incidence of difficult laryngeal visualization ranges from 0% to 26% with the PLMA.[11] Although it is possible that success rates with other SGA devices may differ, the inherent variability in success is an important learning point. Early recognition of unsuccessful placement and institution of alternative airway plans are essential to prevent morbidity from failure of an SGA device.

C. Difficult Direct Laryngoscopy

1. Laryngeal Visualization

The appearance of the laryngeal inlet on direct laryngoscopy is best described by the Cormack and Lehane grade of laryngeal view.[12] Difficult laryngoscopy is most commonly defined as presence of a grade 3 or 4 view on laryngoscopy.[6,7] Several maneuvers have been shown to improve the laryngeal view on laryngoscopy, but in general, poorer laryngeal views contribute progressively to greater difficulty in achieving successful tracheal intubation (Fig. 8- 3).[12-14] As the view worsens, increasing the

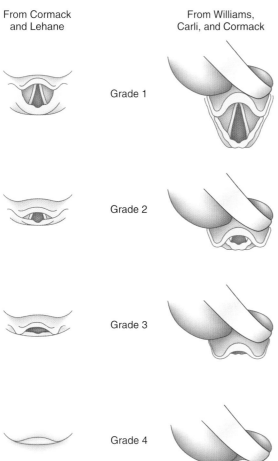

Laryngoscopic View Grading System

From Cormack and Lehane

From Williams, Carli, and Cormack

Grade 1

Grade 2

Grade 3

Grade 4

Figure 8-3 Four grades of laryngoscopic view. *Grade 1* is visualization of the entire laryngeal aperture; *grade 2* is visualization of just the posterior portion of the laryngeal aperture; *grade 3* is visualization of only the epiglottis; and *grade 4* is visualization of just the soft palate. It is assumed that care has been taken to get the best possible view of the vocal cords (see text for details). (Adapted from Cormack RS, Lehane J: Difficult tracheal intubation in obstetrics. *Anaesthesia* 39:1105, 1984; and Williams KN, Carli F, Cormack RS: Unexpected difficult laryngoscopy: A prospective survey in routine general surgery. *Br J Anaesth* 66:38, 1991.)

anterior lifting force with the laryngoscope blade, reinstituting the optimal sniff position, making multiple attempts, manipulating the larynx externally (see Chapter 17 and Fig. 17-10), or opting for alternative devices or laryngoscopists may be required to achieve intubation.

There is a learning curve for management of a DA, and a poor laryngeal view observed by an inexperienced laryngoscopist may easily be improved by a more experienced or skillful individual with perhaps a different blade. Although a severe grade 3 (epiglottis tip) or grade 4 (just soft palate) laryngoscopic view (see Fig. 8-3) may be overcome by the occasional successful "blind" intubation, these views more often render intubation impossible. Therefore, early recognition of a DA and immediate availability of skilled help and advanced equipment for airway management are essential components of DA management.

2. Incidence of Difficult Laryngeal Visualization

The incidence of difficult laryngoscopy or intubation in the general surgical population varies greatly depending on the laryngeal view, the individual study population, and the definition of a DA. A grade 2 or 3 laryngoscopic view requiring multiple attempts or blades (and presumably external laryngeal pressure) is relatively common and is found in 1% to 18% of cases (Table 8-2). Grade 3 laryngeal views result in a successful intubation at a rate of 1% to 4%. Intubation is unsuccessful in between 5 and 35 of every 10,000 patients, and the CICV scenario occurs in 0.01 to 2 patients per 10,000.

For studies of difficult laryngoscopy to be reliable and for the laryngoscopic grading system to be helpful, the reported grades must describe the best view that was obtained, which, in turn, depends on the best possible performance of laryngoscopy. The components of best performance of laryngoscopy consist of the optimal sniff position, good complete muscle relaxation, firm forward traction on the laryngoscope, and, if necessary, firm external laryngeal manipulation. For example, the application of external laryngeal pressure may reduce the incidence of a grade 3 view from 9% to between 5.4% and 1.3%.[9] In doubtful cases, the anesthesiologist, while performing laryngoscopy with the left hand, should quickly apply external pressure over the hyoid, thyroid, and cricoid cartilages with the right hand. The pressure point that affords the best laryngeal view can be determined in a matter of seconds.

Having found the position that gives the best view, the laryngoscopist should ask the assistant to carefully press on the same spot. Optimal external laryngeal manipulation by the assistant must be directed by the laryngoscopist, even if the assistant is fully trained. The best performance of laryngoscopy avoids awkward high-arm postures, positioning of the laryngoscope blade over the middle of the tongue, gripping of the laryngoscope at the junction of the handle and blade with rotation about a horizontal axis, choosing the wrong blade size or shape, and placing the blade incorrectly. Theoretically, if the components of best performance of laryngoscopy are used and the pitfalls are avoided, all laryngoscopists (novice and expert) should obtain almost the same laryngoscopic view.

TABLE 8-2

Incidence of Various Levels of Difficult Intubation

Degree of Difficulty with Intubation	RANGE OF INCIDENCE		
	n per 10,000	%	References
ETT intubation successful but multiple attempts and/or blades may be required; probable laryngoscopic grade 2 or 3	100-1800	1-18	9, 12
ETT intubation successful but multiple attempts and/or blades and/or laryngoscopists required; laryngoscopic grade 3	100-400	1-4	9, 14, 24
ETT intubation not successful; laryngoscopic grade 3 or 4	5-35	0.05-0.35	9, 12, 14
Cannot ventilate by mask, cannot intubate; transtracheal jet ventilation, tracheostomy, brain damage, or death	0.01-2.0	0.0001-0.02	9, 18, 19, 20, 23

ETT, Endotracheal tube.

D. Difficult Intubation During Direct Laryngoscopy

Unlike difficult mask ventilation and difficult laryngoscopy, there is no uniformly accepted method of classifying difficult intubation. The Intubation Difficulty Score (IDS) validated by Adnet and colleagues[15] describes a spectrum of intubation difficulty. The assessment variables for the IDS are number of additional attempts, number of additional operators, number of alternative intubation techniques used, Cormack-Lehane laryngeal view minus 1, need for excessive lifting force, need for laryngeal pressure, and vocal cord adduction. Each variable carries one point, and difficult intubation is defined as an IDS score greater than 5, indicating moderate to major difficulty, with infinity (∞) being assigned to an impossible intubation. Kheterpal and associates defined difficult intubation as intubation requiring more than three attempts by anesthesia attending staff to secure the airway with an endotracheal tube.[6,7]

1. Incidence of Difficult Intubation

The incidence of difficult intubation was 10.3% in a recent study of emergent tracheal intubations in a university hospital.[16] The incidence of failed tracheal intubation ranges from 0.05% to 0.35%; the low and high ends of this range are associated with elective surgical and obstetric patients, respectively. The incidence of failed intubation is approximately 8 times higher in the obstetric population than in others, with a 13-fold increase in the risk of death.[17]

2. Combined Difficult Mask Ventilation and Difficult Intubation

In one study, the incidence of combined difficult mask ventilation and difficult intubation was 0.37%.[6] Patients whose lungs were impossible to ventilate via mask had a risk for difficult intubation of 25%, significantly higher than that for the overall population. One in three patients with combined impossible mask ventilation and difficult intubation required an alternative intubation technique to secure the airway, with 10% of such patients requiring a surgical airway. Similarly, one of the significant findings in another study was that difficult mask ventilation conferred a fourfold greater risk for difficult intubation and a 12-fold greater risk of an impossible intubation.[5]

3. Impossible Mask Ventilation and Intubation

The incidence of CICV has been estimated to range from 0.01 to 2.0 cases per 10,000 patients.[17-20] In a recent study of 50,000 patients, Kheterpal and colleagues described the incidence as 3.75 per 10,000 patients.[7] Despite recent advances in airway devices and techniques, most busy hospitals encounter several such events every year, making it imperative to ensure that DA recognition and management remains a central tenet of anesthesiology education and training.

4. Variability in Incidence of Difficult Laryngoscopy and Difficult Intubation

Difficult direct laryngoscopy (a grade 3 or 4 laryngeal view) is synonymous with difficult intubation in most patients.[12] However, tracheal intubation and laryngoscopy have slightly differing skill requirements, which may contribute to variability in the occurrence of difficult laryngoscopy and difficult intubation. In one prospective study examining respiratory complications in 1005 patients whose tracheas were intubated, 3 patients had grade 4 laryngeal views. One of these patients was easy to intubate, one was "moderately difficult" to intubate, and one was "difficult" to intubate.[8] In the same study, among 68 patients with a grade 3 laryngoscopic view, 5 (7%) were difficult to intubate, 50 (74%) were moderately difficult, and 13 (19%) were easy to intubate.

Four relatively uncommon scenarios explain some of the discordance between difficult laryngoscopy and difficult intubation. First, some patients with a grade 3 view have a trachea that can be intubated on the first or second attempt if the distal end of the endotracheal tube is appropriately curved by a malleable stylet (hockey-stick shape) or if a small curved introducer is used (e.g., a gum elastic bougie). Second, grade 3 laryngoscopic views have been variously described as seeing only the palate and all of the epiglottis or as seeing only the palate and just the tip of the epiglottis.[21] The different attributes of grade 3 may respond differently to adjustments such as optimal external laryngeal pressure, and therefore they may differ initially and subsequently with respect to difficulty of tracheal intubation. Third, a grade 3 view with a curved blade placed in the vallecula (because of a long, floppy epiglottis) may become a grade 1 or 2 view if either a curved or straight blade is placed posterior to the epiglottis and lifted anteriorly.[22] Fourth, pathologic conditions

TABLE 8-3

Success Rates of Intubation with Video-Enabled Laryngoscopes in Patients with Non-difficult Airways

Device	Intubations	No. Patients	% Success	References
Storz VMac	1395	1400	99.6	29, 30, 45, 47, 49
Glidescope	1452	1495	97.1	26, 27, 28, 37, 38, 40, 41, 43, 45, 46, 47, 50
McGrath	432	440	98.2	31, 45, 47, 48, 51
Pentax AWS	1663	1669	99.6	32, 33, 34, 35, 36, 39, 40, 42, 43, 44, 46, 52

such as laryngeal web, laryngeal tumors, or tracheal stenosis may disassociate ease of laryngoscopy from difficulty of tracheal intubation.

5. Complications of Difficult Laryngoscopy and Difficult Intubation

Anesthesia in a patient with a DA can lead to direct airway trauma and morbidity from hypoxia and hypercarbia. Incidence of brain damage, cardiac arrest, and death related to airway disasters appears to be decreasing.[2,19,23] Directly mediated laryngovagal reflexes (airway spasm, apnea, bradycardia, arrhythmia, or hypotension) and laryngospinal reflexes (coughing, vomiting, or bucking) are the source of some morbidity. In general, DA management is more likely to be associated with use of physical force during laryngoscopy and more attempts to secure the airway; together, these increase the incidence of complications. Airway complications can range from minor (trivial or nuisance value) to major (life-threatening or fatal).

In a recent study on emergent tracheal intubations with a 10.8% incidence of difficult intubation, the complications seen in 4.2% of cases were aspiration, esophageal intubation, dental injury, and pneumothorax.[16] The independent predictors of complications in this study were multiple intubation attempts (odds ratio [OR], 6.7; 95% confidence interval [CI], 3.2 to 14.2), grade 3 or 4 laryngeal view (OR, 1.9; 95% CI, 1.1 to 3.5), general care floor location (OR, 1.9; 95% CI, 1.2 to 3.0), and emergency department location (OR, 4.7; 95% CI, 1.1 to 20.4).

In an earlier study, a 5% incidence of relatively minor upper airway complications (posterior pharyngeal and lip lacerations and bruises) was demonstrated with laryngoscopy and intubation in patients with normal airways. In patients with anticipated difficult intubation, the incidence of minor trauma increased to 17%.[24] In patients in whom tracheal intubation was actually found to be difficult (i.e., multiple attempts at laryngoscopy but ultimately successful), the incidence of upper airway complications was 63%.[24]

In previous studies of anesthetic cardiac arrests, the incidence of inability to ventilate after induction was 0.12 per 10,000 anesthesias, accounting for 12% of the preventable causes. However, in a large contemporary study of 50,000 patients undergoing anesthesia for surgery, no incidence of brain damage or death was noted.[7] This result validates the view that modern advances in preoperative airway assessment, patient monitoring, airway equipment, and techniques have significantly reduced severe morbidity due to a DA.

E. Difficult Video Laryngoscopy

Video laryngoscopes and optical laryngoscopes have been increasingly used in routine and DA management. In general, these devices provide a better laryngoscopic view than does direct laryngoscopy. It is important to note that an improved Cormack-Lehane laryngoscopic grade does not always guarantee successful intubation of the trachea.[25] Many of these devices use a highly angulated blade with a camera positioned to allow the user to "see around the corner" of the tongue. Whereas direct laryngoscopy creates a straight line between the operator's eye and the vocal cords, allowing straightforward intubation, highly curved video laryngoscopes maintain the natural curvature of the airway and require special techniques to pass a tube into the trachea.

An excellent review of video laryngoscope use in adult airway management has been published.[25] It pooled data from 27 studies in adult patients (Tables 8-3 and 8-4). The operators using the devices were different, and the criteria for successful intubation as well as the definition of a DA were inconsistently applied from study to study, so the reader should not make direct comparisons between the devices listed in these two tables. The tracheas of patients with normal airways were intubated between 97.1% and 99.6% of the time with these devices. There are fewer data for patients with DAs, but the rate of successful intubation varied from 95.8% to 100% with video-enabled devices.

F. Difficult Flexible Bronchoscopic Intubation

1. Definition of Difficult Flexible Bronchoscopic Intubation

Flexible bronchoscopic intubation skills are now considered essential for all practicing anesthesia providers. Although flexible bronchoscopic devices have enhanced patient safety, especially when DA management is

TABLE 8-4

Success Rates of Intubation with Video-Enabled Laryngoscopes in Patients with Predicted Difficult Airways

Device	Intubations	No. Patients	% Success	References
Storz Vmac	198	201	98.5	30, 31, 45, 49
Glidescope	113	118	95.8	26, 28, 38, 41, 45
McGrath	32	32	100	31, 45

anticipated, they are by no means fail-safe. A difficult or impossible flexible bronchoscopic intubation can broadly be described as inadequate laryngeal visualization with or without difficulty in advancing an endotracheal tube. The ease of laryngeal exposure was defined by Ovassapian as not difficult, moderately difficult (needing some manipulation of the fiberscope in all directions), or difficult (needing extensive manipulation of the bronchoscope in all directions with or without change in position).[53]

2. Incidence of Difficult or Failed Flexible Bronchoscopic Intubation

Inadequate laryngeal visualization is a result of several factors acting individually or in tandem: inexperienced operators, presence of blood or secretions, inadequate topical anesthesia, distorted airway anatomy, and equipment failure. Factors typically unaffected by direct laryngoscopy, such as the presence of a large, floppy epiglottis or small amounts of pharyngeal blood, could pose significant hurdles to successful flexible bronchoscopic intubation. The incidence of difficult laryngeal visualization has been reported to be 6.7% with orotracheal and 4.4% with nasotracheal awake flexible bronchoscopic intubation.[53] The incidence of difficult laryngeal visualization using orotracheal approach under general anesthesia was only 4.4%, reflecting differences in patient types, with distorted upper airway anatomy or a severely compromised airway typically being managed in an awake patient. The incidence of difficult flexible bronchoscopic intubation using an orotracheal approach was 29.1% in awake and 24.1% in anesthetized patients. In contrast, the incidence during nasotracheal intubation was markedly lower, at 6.0% in awake and 11.0% in anesthetized patients, reflecting important technical differences between the two approaches. Flexible bronchoscopic intubation failed in 1.4% of awake and 2.1% of anesthetized patients, with equal distribution of difficult visualization and inability to advance the endotracheal tube.[53]

III. CONCLUSIONS

Inability to adequately ventilate or oxygenate patients remains an important cause of anesthesia-related morbidity and mortality. It is incumbent on an anesthesia provider to ensure adequate gas exchange and oxygenation for his or her patient.

Difficult mask ventilation has been reported at a rate of 1 or 2 per 100 anesthesias, and impossible mask ventilation can be expected at a rate of 1 or 2 per 1000 anesthesias. The failure rate for SGA devices is approximately 2% for the classic and flexible LMAs and 1% for the intubating and ProSeal LMAs.

Fewer data exist regarding failure of video and optical laryngoscopy than for direct laryngoscopy, but the incidence of failed intubation with these devices ranges from 0.4% to 2.9% in patients with a normal airway and from 0% to 4.2% for patients with a DA.

Difficult laryngoscopy occurs at a rate of 1% to 18% of surgical cases, but most of these patients are successfully intubated. Unsuccessful intubation with direct laryngoscopy occurs at a rate of 5 to 35 per 10,000

anesthesias and the CICV scenario occurs at a rate of 0.01 to 2 per 10,000 anesthesias.

Because the incidence of serious airway problems occurs at a low rate, large populations must be examined to improve understanding of the causes and incidence of these events. Understanding of DA management will improve as data are collected from multicenter trials. If electronic medical and anesthesia records use common language and definitions, data can be pooled from multiple institutions, providing the resources for effective analysis of the serious problem of DA management. This will become increasingly important as advances in technology and techniques reduce the rate of DA management.

IV. CLINICAL PEARLS

- The inability to manage a difficult airway (DA) is responsible for a large proportion of deaths and morbidity directly attributable to anesthesia.

- Although it is important to have common definitions for common problems, the literature continues to report variable nomenclature related to DA management. It is important to have an understanding of the incidence of significant airway problems for the specialty to make advances in this area.

- Difficult mask ventilation has been reported at a rate of 1 to 2 per 100 anesthesias, and impossible mask ventilation can be expected at a rate of 1 to 2 per 1000 anesthesias.

- The failure rate for supraglottic airway (SGA) devices is approximately 2% for the classic and flexible laryngeal mask airways (LMAs) and 1% for the intubating and ProSeal LMAs.

- Fewer data exist regarding failure of video and optical laryngoscopes than for direct laryngoscopy, but the incidence of failed intubation with these devices ranges from 0.4% to 2.9% in patients with a normal airway and from 0% to 4.2% for patients with a DA.

- When difficult laryngoscopy is defined as a Cormack-Lehane grade 2 or 3 view requiring multiple attempts or blades, the reported incidence varies from 1% to 18% of surgical cases; however, most of these patients are successfully intubated.

- Unsuccessful intubation with direct laryngoscopy occurs at a rate of 5 to 35 per 10,000 anesthesias, and the "cannot intubate, cannot ventilate" (CICV) scenario occurs at a rate of 0.01 to 2 per 10,000 anesthesias.

- Large multicenter studies will be required to refine understanding of the incidence of serious airway problems.

SELECTED REFERENCES

All references can be found online at expertconsult.com.
1. Caplan RA, Posner KL, Ward RJ, Cheney FW: Adverse respiratory events in anesthesia: A closed claims analysis. *Anesthesiology* 72:828–833, 1990.

2. Cheney FW, Posner KL, Lee LA, et al: Trends in anesthesia-related death and brain damage: A closed claims analysis. *Anesthesiology* 105:1081–1086, 2006.

3. Han R, Tremper KK, Kheterpal S, O'Reilly M: Grading scale for mask ventilation. *Anesthesiology* 101:267, 2004.

4. Langeron O, Masso E, Huraux C, et al: Prediction of difficult mask ventilation. *Anesthesiology* 92:1229–1236, 2000.

5. el-Ganzouri AR, McCarthy RJ, Tuman KJ, et al: Preoperative airway assessment: Predictive value of a multivariate risk index. *Anesth Analg* 82:1197–1204, 1996.

7. Kheterpal S, Martin L, Shanks AM, Tremper KK: Prediction and outcomes of impossible mask ventilation: A review of 50,000 anesthetics. *Anesthesiology* 110:891–897, 2009.

12. Cormack RS, Lehane J: Difficult tracheal intubation in obstetrics. *Anaesthesia* 39:1105–1111, 1984.

25. Niforopoulou P, Pantazopoulos I, Demestiha T, et al: Video-laryngoscopes in the adult airway management: A topical review of the literature. *Acta Anaesthesiol Scand* 54:1050–1061, 2010.

Chapter 9

Evaluation and Recognition of the Difficult Airway

ALLAN P. REED

I. INTRODUCTION

The quest to forecast difficult airway (DA) management has spanned more than a half century. In that time, a plethora of scientific investigations, book chapters, editorials, lectures, and workshops have been devoted to this essential issue. In 1956, Cass and colleagues underscored the point and began the search for a simple beside test to determine whose airway will be difficult to manage.[1] As of this writing, such a test does not exist.[2] Practitioners apply multiple tests, none of which are accurate. Absent reliable data, airway managers depend on case reports and personal experience to formulate critically important airway management plans.[3]

The medical literature boasts an abundance of articles discussing predictors of difficult intubation (DI) but relatively few explaining predictors of difficult mask ventilation (DMV). Among all of them, practitioners seek to determine which criteria are dependable and which are not.[4] Having established a basis on which to predict DMV or DI or both, it becomes possible to select modes of airway management that optimize patients' safety and comfort.

Generally, failed endotracheal intubation occurs once in every 2230 attempts.[5] The average anesthesiologist in the United States has one failed intubation every other year. The incidence is small, but the potential consequences of DA management are of major importance. Failed ventilation accounted for 44% of intraoperative cardiac arrests reported by Keenan and Boyan.[6] Thirty-four percent of liability claims identified by Caplan and coauthors were based on adverse respiratory events,[7] of which three quarters were judged to be preventable.[8]

Radiographs and other imaging techniques have been advocated to predict DI but are too expensive and inconvenient to serve as routine screening tests. Highly specialized techniques such as acoustic reflectometry are of dubious reliability.[9] More quantitative, noninvasive measurements, such as those with the laryngeal indices caliper,[10] bubble inclinometer,[11] and goniometer, offer the potential for accurate measurements but have never found their way into clinical practice.

This chapter reviews the current state of the art regarding predictability of difficult mask airway management and difficult traditional laryngoscopy (DL). Historically, these procedures were performed with anesthesia face masks in the case of mask ventilation and with Macintosh or Miller blades in the case of laryngoscopy.

The ensuing discussion observes these limitations. The application of supralaryngeal airway devices and alternative intubation techniques are addressed in other chapters.

A history of DA is a strong predictor of future problems[12]; in my opinion, it is the single most reliable predictor of a DA. The contrapositive is not necessarily true, however. A history of problem-free airway management is suggestive of future ease but not a guarantee. Many factors that contribute to difficulty are progressive with time. Examples of such problems include rheumatoid arthritis and obesity. An airway history should be elicited from all patients. Review of prior anesthesia records is frequently helpful; they may describe previously encountered problems, failed therapies, and successful solutions.[13]

II. PROBLEMATIC VENTILATION BY TRADITIONAL FACE MASK

DMV occurs when a practitioner cannot provide sufficient gas exchange because of inadequate mask seal, large volume leaks, or excessive resistance to the ingress or egress of gas.[13] The incidence of DMV varies between 0.08% and 5%.[14,15] This wide range is probably related to conflicting definitions of DMV.[16] Impossible mask ventilation occurs in 0.07% to 0.16% of patients.[15,17] Risk factors for DMV include full beard, massive jaw, edentulous state, skin sensitivity (e.g., burns, epidermolysis bullosa, fresh skin grafts), facial dressings, obesity, age older than 55 years, and a history of snoring.[15] Other criteria that suggest the possibility of DMV include large tongue, heavy jaw muscles, history of obstructive sleep apnea (OSA), poor atlanto-occipital extension, some types of pharyngeal pathology, facial burns, and facial deformities[18] (Box 9-1).

Many types of pharyngeal problems can produce DMV, including lingual tonsil hypertrophy,[19] lingual tonsillar abscess, lingual thyroid,[20] and thyroglossal cyst.[21-24] Many abnormalities cannot be diagnosed by classic airway examination techniques. The presence of any one factor is suggestive of DMV, and as factors increase in number, the likelihood of difficulty increases. A greater than normal mandibulohyoid distance has been associated with OSA, the pathophysiology of which may be related to DMV.[25-27] Anesthetic technique could contribute to DMV. El-Orbany and Woehlck suggested that high-dose opioid–induced vocal cord adduction produces DMV.[28]

Traditional face mask airway management is generally safe and effective. In the unusual instances in which it is not, endotracheal intubation remains one fallback option. Although this scheme works well in most cases, approximately 15% of all DIs are also DMVs.[29] Some factors that predispose to DMV also contribute to DI; they include OSA, history of snoring, obese neck, and poor mandibular translation. Some 25% of impossible mask ventilation patients are also difficult to intubate. The overall incidence of impossible mask ventilation and DI is 1 in every 2800 patients.[30] Proposed predictors of impossible mask ventilation are listed in Box 9-2.

BOX 9-1   Risk Factors for Difficult Mask Ventilation

Obesity
Beards
Edentulousness
History of snoring
History of obstructive sleep apnea
Age older than 55 years
Large tongue
Poor temporomandibular joint translation
Skin sensitivity (burns, epidermolysis bullosa, fresh skin grafts)
Massive jaw
Heavy jaw muscles
Poor atlanto-occipital extension
Pharyngeal pathology
Lingual tonsil hypertrophy
Lingual tonsil abscess
Lingual thyroid
Thyroglossal cyst
Facial dressings
Facial burns
Facial deformities

III. PROBLEMATIC INTUBATION BY TRADITIONAL LARYNGOSCOPY

A. Sniffing Position

DI occurs when multiple attempts at endotracheal intubation are required.[13] The presence or absence of airway pathology does not influence its definition. Traditional laryngoscopy is performed to visualize the laryngeal opening. The observing laryngoscopist is situated outside the airway, above the patient's head. To see through the airway, light must travel from the glottic opening to the laryngoscopist's eye. Because light travels in straight lines, the technique requires an uninterrupted linear path between larynx and observer. Most of the manipulations performed attempt to satisfy this criterion.

The airway contains three visual axes. They are the long axes of the mouth, oropharynx, and larynx. In the neutral position, these axes form acute and obtuse angles with one another (Fig. 9-1). Light cannot bend around these angles under normal circumstances. To bring all three axes into better alignment, McGill suggested the "sniffing the morning air" position.[31] The true sniffing position has two components: cervical flexion and atlanto-occipital extension. Cervical flexion approximates the pharyngeal and laryngeal axes, and atlanto-occipital extension brings the oral axis into better alignment with the other two. Normal atlanto-occipital extension

---

BOX 9-2   Proposed Predictors of Impossible Mask Ventilation

Neck radiation changes
Beard
Male gender
Sleep apnea
Mallampati class III or IV

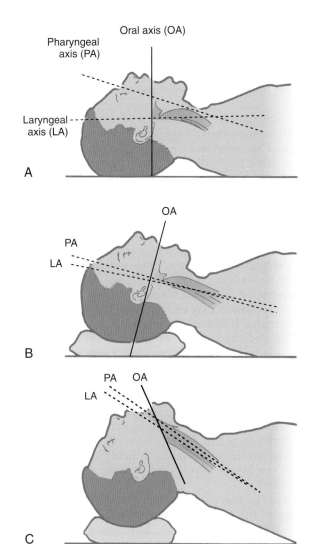

Figure 9-1 Visual axis diagram. **A,** Head in neutral position. None of the three visual axes align. **B,** Elevation of the head approximates the laryngeal and pharyngeal axes. **C,** Extension at the atlanto-occipital joint brings the visual axis of the mouth into better alignment with those of the larynx and pharynx. (From Stone DJ, Gal TJ: Airway management. In Miller RJ, editor: *Anesthesia*, ed 5, Philadelphia, 2000, Churchill Livingstone, p 1419.)

measures 35 degrees.[32] With optimal alignment of the airway's visual axes, it becomes possible to look through the airway into the laryngeal opening. A reduced atlanto-occipital gap or a prominent C1 spinous process impairs laryngoscopy[33,34] if vigorous attempts at extension are performed, because the trachea bows and the larynx is forced anteriorly.[33]

Inability to assume the sniffing position is a predictor of DI. Examples of problems that prevent the sniffing position are cervical vertebral arthritis, cervical ankylosing spondylitis, unstable cervical fractures, protruding cervical discs, atlantoaxial subluxation, cervical fusions, cervical collars, and halo frames. Morbidly obese patients sometimes have posterior neck fat pads that prevent atlanto-occipital extension.

The ability to achieve the sniffing position is easily tested. One simply has the patient flex the lower cervical vertebrae and extend at the atlanto-occipital joint. Pain, tingling, numbness, or inability to achieve these maneuvers predicts DI.[35] The benefits of the sniffing position have been dogma for more than 70 years, but Adnet and colleagues and Chou and Wu have questioned its utility.[36,37]

B. Mouth Opening

Mouth opening is important because it determines the available space for placing and manipulating laryngoscopes as well as endotracheal tubes.[38,39] A small mouth opening may not accommodate either. Mouth opening also provides room to see through the uppermost part of the airway. Mouth opening relies on the temporomandibular joint (TMJ), which has both a hingelike movement and a gliding motion. The gliding motion is known as *translation*. The hingelike movement allows the mandible to pivot on the maxilla. The more the mandible swings away from the maxilla, the bigger the mouth opening.

The adequacy of mouth opening is assessed by measuring the interincisor distance. An interincisor distance of 3 cm provides sufficient space for intubation, absent other complicating factors. This corresponds approximately to two finger breadths.[40] The two finger breadth test is performed by placing the examiner's second and third digits between the patient's central incisors. If they fit, there should be adequate room to perform laryngoscopy; if they do not fit, laryngoscopy may be difficult. Factors that interfere with mouth opening include masseter muscle spasm, TMJ dysfunction, and various integumentary aliments. Skin problems that adversely effect mouth opening include burn scar contractures and progressive systemic sclerosis. Masseter muscle spasm can be relieved by induction of anesthesia and administration of muscle relaxants. Mechanical problems at the TMJ remain unaltered by medications. Some patients demonstrate adequate mouth opening when awake but not after anesthesia induction.[41] The problem can often be relieved by pulling the mandible forward. A mouth opening that was sufficient for a previous anesthetic may not be so after temporal neurosurgical procedures.[42]

C. Dentition

Instrumentation of the airway places teeth at risk for damage. Multiple problems result from dental injury. Teeth may be dislodged or broken, leading to inability to chew, pain, and costly repair. Moreover, broken teeth can fall into the trachea, migrate to the lung, and predispose to abscesses. Poor dentition is at risk for damage as the mouth is opened and as the laryngoscope blade is employed. Teeth that can be extracted easily with digital pressure should probably be removed. During laryngoscopy in the presence of poor dentition, extra efforts are made to avoid placing pressure on maxillary incisors. This causes laryngoscopes to be manipulated into less than ideal positions for visualizing the larynx, resulting in poor visualization of the glottis.

Prominent maxillary incisors complicate laryngoscopy in another way. They protrude into the mouth and block the line of sight to the larynx. To overcome this problem, laryngoscopists must adjust their line of sight. This is done by bringing the observer's eye into a new position that is higher than the original one, so that the laryngoscopist looks tangentially over the protruding maxillary incisor. Two new points of observation exist in the adjusted line of sight and determine a new line of sight, one that brings the laryngoscopist's view to a more posterior laryngopharyngeal position. The result is a view that is posterior to the larynx. Consequently, the larynx is not visualized and a DL is produced. In much the same way, edentulous patients tend to be easy to intubate because the laryngoscopist can adjust the line of sight to a more advantageous angle.

D. Tongue

The tongue occupies space in the mouth and oropharynx. The base of the tongue lies close to the glottic aperture. During traditional direct laryngoscopy, the base of the tongue falls posteriorly, obstructing the line of sight into the glottis. Visualization of the larynx requires displacing the tongue base anteriorly so that the line of sight to the glottis is restored. The tongue is frequently displaced with a handheld rigid laryngoscope to which a Macintosh or Miller blade has been attached. These laryngoscopes push the tongue anteriorly, moving it from a posterior, obstructing position to a new anterior, nonobstructing position. The new position is within the *mandibular space*, the area between the two rami of the mandible. Even with the tongue maximally displaced into the mandibular space, visualization of the larynx is sometimes inadequate.

A normal-size tongue usually fits easily into a normal-size mandibular space. A large tongue fits poorly into a normal-size mandibular space. After filling the space, a large tongue still occupies some of the oropharyngeal airway and obstructs it. For this reason, a large tongue (macroglossia) is a predictor of DI. Similarly, a normal-size tongue fits poorly into a small mandibular space.[43] It, too, occupies some of the oropharyngeal airway, thereby obstructing the line of sight. Consequently, a small mandible (micrognathia) is a predictor of DI. In essence, a tongue that is large compared with the size of the mouth (oropharynx) and mandible takes up excessive space in the oropharynx and interferes with visualization.

The base of the tongue is located so close to the larynx that inability to adequately displace it anteriorly creates another problem. Because the base of the tongue hangs down over the larynx, the glottis is hidden from view. The glottic aperture is then anatomically anterior to the base of tongue—hence, the term *anterior larynx*. Under such circumstances, the larynx is anterior to the base of the tongue and cannot be seen because the tongue hides it. In this manner, glottic and supraglottic masses can create DI if they force the base of the tongue posteriorly. Some of the masses that may be encountered are lingual tonsils,[19,44] epiglottic cysts,[23] and thyroglossal duct cysts.

After the mandibular space is filled with the tongue, additional pressure on the laryngoscope blade lifts the mandible anteriorly. In this setting, mandibular displacement depends on the TMJ. In addition to its hingelike motion, the TMJ works in a gliding (translational) movement. It is the gliding motion that allows the mandible to slide anteriorly across the maxilla. If the joint does not translate, the mandible cannot be displaced anteriorly, and the tongue cannot be moved out of the line of sight.

Recognizing the implications of tongue size for successful laryngoscopy, Mallampati and colleagues[45] in 1985 and Samsoon and Young[5] in 1987 devised classification systems to predict DL utilizing this concept. Mallampati and Samsoon reasoned that a large tongue could be identified on visual inspection of the open mouth. Both classification systems relate the size of the tongue to the oropharyngeal structures identified. A normal-size tongue allows visualization of certain oropharyngeal structures. As the tongue size increases, some structures become hidden from view. Both investigators proposed systems that reasoned backward from this premise.

Application of the Mallampati or the Samsoon classification system is easy and painless. The patient is seated in the neutral position. The mouth is opened as wide as possible, and the tongue is protruded as far as possible. Phonation is discouraged because it raises the soft palate and allows visualization of additional structures.[46] The observer looks for specific anatomic landmarks: the fauces, pillars, uvula, and soft palate. The Mallampati classification system uses three groups and the Samsoon system uses four (Fig. 9-2). Both systems suggest that as tongue size increases, fewer structures are visualized and laryngoscopy becomes more difficult. Mallampati class tends to be higher in pregnant patients than in nonpregnant ones.[47]

Just as the size of tongue can be estimated, so too can the size of the mandible. The patient's head is extended at the atlanto-occipital joint. The mentum of the mandible and the thyroid cartilage are identified. The "Adam's apple" (thyroid notch) is the most superficial structure in the neck and serves as a good landmark for the thyroid cartilage. The vocal cords lie just caudad to the thyroid notch. The distance between the thyroid cartilage and the mentum (thyromental distance, or TMD) is measured in one of three ways: with a set of spacers, with a small pocket ruler, or with the observer's fingers. The normal TMD is 6.5 cm. A TMD greater than 6 cm is predictive of easy intubation, and a TMD of less than 6 cm is suggestive of DI.[48] If a ruler is not present at the bedside, practitioners can judge the TMD with their own fingers. The width of one's middle three fingers frequently approximates 6 cm, and the TMD can be compared with the fingers' span. In that way, clinically relevant approximations can be taken into account when examining patients for the purpose of predicting DI.

The ability to translate the TMJ is easily assessed before induction. The patient is simply asked to place the mandibular incisors (bottom teeth) in front of the maxillary incisors (upper teeth). Inability to perform this simple task usually results from one of two sources. First, the TMJ may not glide, predicting DI.[49] Second, some patients find it difficult to coordinate the maneuver, in which case there is no implication for DI.

The upper lip bite test was proposed as a modification of the TMJ displacement test.[50] The upper lip bite

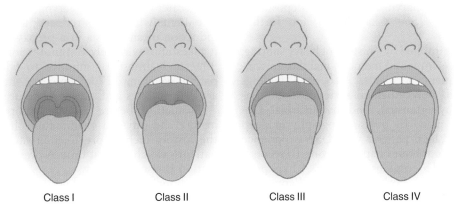

| Class I | Class II | Class III | Class IV |

Figure 9-2 Samsoon classification system. The oropharynx is divided into four classes on the basis of the structures visualized: *class I*—soft palate, fauces, uvula, pillars; *class II*—soft palate, fauces, uvula; *class III*—soft palate, base of uvula; *class IV*—soft palate not visible. (From Mallampati SR: Recognition of the difficult airway. In Benumof JL, editor: *Airway management: Principles and practice*, St. Louis, 1996, Mosby, p 132.)

test is performed by asking the patient to move the mandibular incisors as high on the upper lip as possible. The maneuver is similar to biting the lip. Contact of the teeth above or on the vermilion border is thought to predict adequate laryngoscopic views. Inability to touch the vermilion boarder with the mandibular teeth is thought to predict poor laryngoscopic views. Both the TMJ translation test and the upper lip bite test assess TMJ glide, which is an important consideration during laryngoscopy. Khan and coworkers confirmed the predictive importance of this maneuver.[51] Table 9-1 summarizes a quick, easy, bedside scheme for predicting DI.

IV. SPECIAL SITUATIONS

A. Morbid Obesity

The Centers for Disease Control and Prevention (CDC) defines morbid obesity (MO) in terms of body mass index (BMI). BMI is calculated as a ratio between weight in kilograms and height in meters squared:

$$BMI = Weight\ in\ kg/(Height\ in\ m)^2$$

A BMI of 20 to 25 kg/m² is normal, 25 to 30 kg/m² is overweight, 30 to 40 kg/m² is obese, and greater than 40 kg/m² indicates MO. Other definitions of MO have fallen into disfavor.

Patients with MO frequently develop upper airway obstruction, which may present as OSA. During normal inspiration, the diaphragm descends and the chest wall expands, resulting in creation of negative intrathoracic pressure (subatmospheric pressure). Negative intrathoracic pressure is transmitted along the entire airway, including the upper airway. Soft tissues are drawn into the airway as if it were imploding. Under normal circumstances, obstruction is prevented by contraction of three sets of dilator muscles. The tensor palatini prevents airway obstruction by the soft palate at the nasopharynx. The genioglossus pulls the tongue anteriorly to open the oropharynx. The hyoid muscles pull the epiglottis forward and upward to prevent obstruction at the laryngopharynx. In healthy young patients, these muscles prevent obstruction during sleep. As patients age, the dilator muscles become less efficacious and there is a tendency for partial obstruction to occur.

In patients with MO, adipose tissue deposits in the lateral pharyngeal walls. These deposits are not fixed to bone and are highly mobile. They protrude into the airway, narrowing it, and are drawn farther into the airway during periods of negative airway pressure, such as during inspiration. In these ways, reduced dilator

TABLE 9-1

Generally Accepted Predictors of Difficult Intubation

Criterion	Suggestion of Difficult Intubation
History of difficult intubation	Positive history
Length of upper incisors	Relatively long
Interincisor distance	Less than two finger breadths (<3 cm)
Overbite	Maxillary incisors override mandibular incisors
Temporomandibular joint translation	Inability to extend mandibular incisors anterior to maxillary incisors
Mandibular space	Small, indurated, encroached upon by mass
Cervical vertebral range of motion	Cannot touch chin to chest or cannot extend neck
Thyromental distance	Less than three finger breadths (<6 cm)
Mallampati-Samsoon classification	Mallampati III/Samsoon IV—relatively large tongue: uvula not visible
Neck	Short, thick

Adapted from American Society of Anesthesiologists Task Force on Difficult Airway Management: Practice guidelines for management of the difficult airway: An updated report. *Anesthesiology* 98:1269, 2003.

muscle function or pharyngeal adipose depositions predispose to OSA. (See Chapter 43 for further details.)

Clinically, OSA is implied by a history of heavy snoring, daytime somnolence, impaired memory, inability to concentrate, and frequent accidents. Associated findings include hypoxemia, polycythemia, systemic hypertension, pulmonary hypertension, and hypercarbia. Definitive diagnosis is made by polysomnography in sleep laboratories. During sleep, patients with OSA experience at least five episodes per hour of apnea lasting 10 seconds or longer or at least 15 episodes per hour of hypopnea (50% decrease in airflow). Both hypopnea and apnea are frequently associated with decreases in pulse oximetry of 4% or more. Risk factors for OSA are male gender, middle age or older, obesity, evening alcohol consumption, and drug-induced sleep.

Hypopnea or apnea occurs as the pharynx is obstructed. Partial obstruction leads to hypopnea and total obstruction produces apnea. Normally, dilator muscles prevent obstruction, but they do so less successfully with increasing age and obesity. As airflow to the alveoli diminishes, hypoxemia and possibly hypercarbia develop. Both result in enhanced sympathetic outflow, causing patients to awaken. In the awake state, dilator activity increases and airway patency is restored. Patients then fall asleep, and the cycle is repeated numerous times. Rapid-eye-movement sleep is achieved poorly, and patients remain tired during the day. Treatment frequently centers on application of continuous positive airway pressure (CPAP) during sleep, but not all patients tolerate the mask. Alternative therapies include oral appliances to move the tongue anteriorly and nocturnal administration of oxygen. Surgical options also exist, such as uvulopalatopharyngoplasty, genioglossus advancement, maxillomandibular advancement, and tracheostomy.

Although time to oxyhemoglobin desaturation is not a predictor of DI, it is an important consideration. The longer the time available to perform laryngoscopy, the greater the likelihood of success. Rapid hemoglobin desaturation limits that time and thereby reduces the chance of endotracheal intubation. A patient with MO and a BMI of 40 kg/m^2, breathing room air, who becomes apneic desaturates to an oxygen saturation in arterial blood (SaO$_2$) of 90% in approximately 1 minute, and to 60% in the next minute. In contrast, if the same patient is breathing 100% O$_2$ before induction of anesthesia, the SaO$_2$ takes approximately $2^1/_2$ minutes to fall to 90% and does not reach 60% for an additional $1^1/_2$ minutes.[51,52] The data show that successful oxygenation before induction of anesthesia extends the period of time until oxyhemoglobin desaturation takes place. Consequently, preoxygenation provides a longer period for laryngoscopy, which should increase the chances of successful intubation.

Preoxygenation may be thought of as denitrogenation. During preoxygenation, patients breathe 100% O$_2$. Air, which is mostly nitrogen, is washed out of alveoli and replaced with O$_2$. This process stores O$_2$ in all open alveoli, including those constituting the functional residual capacity (FRC). The more O$_2$ contained in the FRC, the more time before oxyhemoglobin desaturation and

the greater the period for laryngoscopy. Because the FRC in patients with MO is reduced, less O$_2$ is stored. After induction of anesthesia in a preoxygenated 70-kg adult, it takes approximately 8 minutes for the SaO$_2$ to fall to 90%, and almost 10 minutes to fall to 60%. For the patient weighing 127 kg, however, the comparable times are $2^1/_2$ minutes and almost 4 minutes.

Evaluation before airway manipulation requires a history and physical examination. Important aspects of the history include previous airway difficulties and the patient's weight at that time. A present-day airway examination is also necessary.

Although OSA pathology and pathophysiology predispose to DMV and DI, the true incidence of problems resulting from MO is undefined. The popularity of bariatric surgery has brought numerous patients with MO to the operating room. Because these patients receive face mask ventilation infrequently, there is little practical experience to refute classic teachings about such ventilation. It is reasonable to expect fat cheeks, a short immobile neck, a large tongue, and pharyngeal adipose deposits to complicate face mask ventilation.[53] Nevertheless, Brodsky and colleagues reported on a morbidly obese patient with a BMI of 43 kg/m^2 and OSA who was ventilated easily by face mask.[54] This experience serves to document the clinical findings of many practitioners. Along the same lines, considerable experience with laryngoscopy in patients with MO has developed. Absent findings to the contrary, most of these patients are easy to intubate. In other words, MO does not appear to be a strong independent predictor of DI.[54–57] The presence of other DI predictors implies potential problems.[58] Gonzalez and colleagues suggested that a neck circumference greater than 43 cm (19 inches) is such a predictor.[59] Pretracheal fat accumulation has been investigated as a predictor of DI, but the results have been conflicting.[60,61]

B. Pregnancy

Airway management is one of the most important factors contributing to maternal mortality.[62,63] (See Chapter 37 for further details.) Airway difficulties pose a risk of pulmonary aspiration and hypoxic cardiopulmonary arrest. Rocke and associates reported some degree of difficulty during intubation in almost 8% of full-term pregnant patients undergoing cesarean section.[55]

Pregnant patients usually are young and have full dentition. Prominent maxillary incisors obstruct the line of sight, as discussed previously, and many pregnant women present with reduced interincisor distances because of TMJ dysfunction or other etiologies. Reduced interincisor distances limit the space available for visualization and manipulation of instruments in the mouth.

Pregnant patients suffer from generalized soft tissue swelling. They all gain weight and often reach MO proportions. Short, fat necks tend to prevent achievement of the proper sniffing position, which impairs aligning the visual axes of the mouth, pharynx, and larynx. Redundant pharyngeal tissues may fall into the airway during traditional laryngoscopy, obstructing the line of sight. Tissue edema can produce so much mucosal swelling that landmarks, such as epiglottis and arytenoids, are hard to distinguish. The breasts may be so engorged that they interfere with placement of a laryngoscope handle.[64] As the space between mandible and chest diminishes, less room is available for the assistant's hand to provide cricoid pressure. In fact, the assistant's hand may take up space needed to open the mouth, thereby preventing adequate mouth opening. Sufficient mouth opening is required to see through the airway as well as to insert and manipulate equipment.

Tongue swelling produces macroglossia. Macroglossia prevents sufficient displacement into the mandibular space, so the line of sight is obstructed. It has been suggested that straining can exacerbate the Mallampati-Samsoon classification.[65]

Overzealous left lateral uterine displacement can tilt the torso and neck, altering the airway position in relation to the cervical spine. Cricoid pressure may exacerbate this problem by displacing the airway laterally, occluding it,[66] or angulating the larynx.

Swelling of the supraglottic airway interferes with face mask ventilation and complicates laryngoscopy and intubation. As the upper airway becomes edematous, it also becomes more friable. Instrumentation of such airways frequently leads to bleeding, which further complicates face mask ventilation and endotracheal intubation.[67]

Parturients, especially obese parturients, have reduced FRC.[68,69] All pregnant women experience an increase in O_2 consumption of approximately 20%. Consequently, periods of apnea, such as during laryngoscopy under general anesthesia, predispose to desaturation in these patients much more quickly than in their nonpregnant and nonobese counterparts.[70,71] Rapid oxyhemoglobin desaturation reduces the time available for laryngoscopy and detracts from the successful completion of intubation.

Other factors tend to impair successful laryngoscopy. Anxiety on the part of inexperienced physicians has led to intubation attempts before adequate conditions are achieved. Laryngoscopy under general anesthesia requires sufficient depth of anesthesia and profound muscle relaxation.[72,73] Absent one or both of these conditions, the chances of success are markedly reduced. The result is poor mouth opening, reduced interincisor distance, retching, vomiting, and aspiration. Well-intentioned, novice assistants degrade intubating conditions or fail to enhance them.[73] The *Report on Confidential Enquiries into Maternal Deaths in England and Wales* pointed to failure to provide cricoid pressure, poorly applied cricoid pressure, or release of cricoid pressure during a vomiting episode as major contributors to maternal morbidity and mortality.[62]

The application of cricoid pressure during active vomiting has been controversial. Sellick's original description of cricoid pressure called for release of the maneuver during vomiting episodes.[74] A single case report described an elderly woman who vomited during application of cricoid pressure and suffered an esophageal rupture.[75] Although other factors could have contributed to or caused the rupture in this patient, some have recommended relinquishing cricoid pressure during vomiting episodes on the basis of this occurrence. Sellick retracted his initial recommendation, and others have supported the maintenance of cricoid pressure during active vomiting,[76–78] believing that the risk of aspiration pneumonia is greater than the risk of esophageal rupture.[77,78] Furthermore, cricoid pressure sometimes pushes the entire neck posteriorly, resulting in forward flexion of the head on the neck. As a result, the advantages of the sniffing position are lost and laryngoscopy becomes more difficult. To correct this problem, bimanual cricoid pressure was suggested by Crowley and Giesecke.[79] To accomplish this maneuver, the assistant's left hand supports the patient's neck from underneath as the assistant's right hand places pressure on the cricoid cartilage.

C. Lingual Tonsil Hypertrophy

Over $11\frac{1}{2}$ years, Ovassapian and colleagues analyzed 33 cases of unanticipated DI. Before induction of anesthesia,[19] none of these patients was thought to pose a significant likelihood of difficulty on the basis of careful preanesthetic airway examinations. Of the 33 patients, 15 had normal airway examinations; 3 of those patients had BMIs of 31 to 40 kg/m². The remaining 18 patients presented with varying predictors of DI but were judged to be at low risk for poor laryngoscopic views. After induction, intubation turned out to be difficult in the hands of experienced attending anesthesiologists. All 33 patients subsequently underwent flexible fiberoptic pharyngoscopy for pharyngeal assessments, and all demonstrated lingual tonsil hypertrophy.

Lingual tonsils are lymph tissues located at the base of the tongue. They usually exhibit hypertrophy bilaterally but may do so unilaterally. Enlarged lingual tonsils can push the epiglottis posteriorly, obstructing the line of sight and preventing anterior displacement of the base of the tongue. They sometimes encroach on the vallecula, preventing optimal location of curved laryngoscope blades. They can distort the epiglottis so that it covers the glottic opening or is difficult to recognize. Not only do hypertrophied lingual tonsils prevent elevation of the base of the tongue from the line of sight, but they also have a tendency to bleed, complicating intubation even further.[80,81]

Lingual tonsil hypertrophy cannot be identified by classic airway examinations to predict DI. It is often asymptomatic, and its suggestive symptoms are nonspecific. They include sore throat, dysphagia, snoring, OSA, and sensations of fullness or lumps in the throat. Most patients have a history of palatine tonsillectomy or adenoidectomy.[44] Lingual tonsil hypertrophy has been associated with airway obstruction and OSA.[82–85] Other pharyngeal problems that can complicate laryngoscopy include acute lingual tonsillitis,[82] lingual tonsillar abscesses, lingual thyroids,[20] and thyroglossal cysts.[21–23] These structures reside at the base of the tongue, a location that is hidden from view during routine physical examination.

D. Burns

Thermal burns of the head and neck complicate airway management in several ways. (See Chapter 44 for further details.) Burn patients with coexisting airway problems experience approximately 50% greater mortality than burn patients without airway issues. Thermal damage to the upper airway results in massive swelling within 2 to 24 hours. Edematous mucosa encroaches on the airway lumen to create severe narrowing or even occlusion. A narrowed upper airway reduces the amount of air drawn into the lungs. An occluded upper airway prevents any O_2 from reaching the alveoli. Both effects result in hypoxia. As the mucosa swells, traditional laryngoscopy becomes difficult or impossible. So much edema can collect in the mucosa that landmarks may be unrecognizable. For these reasons, it is sometimes best to perform endotracheal intubation early in the care of burn patients, before swelling creates hypoxia and DI.[86]

Airway burns are suggested by the occurrence of fire in a closed space, stridor, hoarseness, dyspnea, singed nasal hairs, and carbonaceous material in the mouth, nares, or pharynx. The risk of airway compromise and DI in the near future is significant. Elective prophylactic intubation is indicated for such patients.

For those who survive the acute burn period, chronic airway problems occur frequently. Burn tissue heals by formation of scar, which is nonelastic. Scars over the face and neck limit mobility of the TMJ and cervical vertebrae. The result is a small mouth opening and inability to achieve the sniffing position. Scar release under local anesthesia may be helpful to restore mobility to these important joints and allow improved intubating conditions.

E. Acromegaly

The incidence of DI in acromegaly is four to five times higher than in the general population.[87] Acromegaly results from excess growth hormone, which is frequently produced by pituitary tumors. One screening test for acromegaly involves administration of 75 to 100 g of glucose. If plasma growth hormone concentrations do not fall after 1 to 2 hours, acromegaly is suspected. High plasma growth hormone levels may indicate acromegaly. Skull radiographs and computed tomographic scans showing an enlarged sella turcica suggest anterior pituitary adenoma.

Typical acromegalic features include enlarged nose, big tongue, thick mandible, full lips, elevated nasolabial folds, and prominent frontal sinuses. These patients appear to experience overgrowth of mucosa and soft tissues of the pharynx, larynx, and vocal cords.[88,89] Many experience OSA.[90,91] Early in the disease process, joint spaces may be widened, but later on arthritis develops and limits range of motion. This frequently occurs at the TMJ, resulting in a small mouth opening, and it may occur in cricoarytenoid joints. Overgrowth of tissues can produce vocal cord abnormalities, resulting in hoarseness or recurrent laryngeal nerve paralysis.

These features predispose to DMV and DL. Large tongues and epiglottides produce upper airway obstruction and make laryngoscopy difficult. Big mandibles increase the distance between teeth and vocal cords, necessitating longer laryngoscope blades. Thickened vocal cords and subglottic narrowing may require smaller tracheal tubes than would otherwise be selected. Nasal turbinate enlargement may obstruct the nasal airway and prevent passage of tubes. Dyspnea on exertion, stridor, or hoarseness may suggest laryngeal abnormalities that can complicate intubation. In addition to thick mandibles, acromegalics frequently present with long mandibles. Nonetheless, the resulting increased TMD has not been found to be associated with DL.[87]

F. Epiglottitis

Epiglottitis (supraglottitis) is caused by a potentially life-threatening infection that produces upper airway swelling and obstruction. Formerly, the most common etiology was *Haemophilus influenza* type B (HIB), and the disease usually occurred in children 2 to 8 years of age. Since the widespread use of HIB vaccine, epiglottitis is an unusual finding in the pediatric population, but it still occurs in immunosuppressed adults. Common presenting signs are sore throat and dysphagia. Other signs and symptoms include drooling, inspiratory stridor, high fever, rapid deterioration to respiratory distress, pharyngitis, tachypnea, cyanosis, lethargy, and tripod positioning. These patients are most comfortable sitting up, extending the neck, and leaning forward. The "muffled voice" is an infrequent finding.[92] Lateral radiographs of the neck classically demonstrate a swollen epiglottis. Mild adult forms may be treated with observation for exacerbation of respiratory function.[93–95] Severe cases with respiratory compromise require airway management, which usually means tracheal intubation and antibiotics.

Instrumentation of the airway in these cases can result in total airway obstruction and is contraindicated in the awake patient. Only deep general anesthesia is likely to protect against exacerbation of airway obstruction during intubation. Before induction of anesthesia, preparations are made for immediate tracheostomy if required. Intravenous access is obtained before or just after induction of anesthesia. Despite the fever, glycopyrrolate is administered to dry secretions, which are usually copious and hinder laryngoscopy. Inhalation induction with sevoflurane is begun in the sitting position. After loss of consciousness, patients are placed supine to deepen the level of anesthesia. Assisted ventilation by bag and mask is frequently necessary to maintain airway patency. Supraglottic swelling, copious secretions, and reactive upper airway combine to make mask ventilation and laryngoscopy difficult. Deep inhalation anesthesia allows high concentrations of inspired O_2. When appropriate, laryngoscopy and intubation are performed. Elective extubation usually takes place 2 to 4 days later.

G. Acute Submandibular Space Cellulitis

Acute cellulitis of the submandibular space (Ludwig's angina) can progress rapidly to a life-threatening situation. It generally begins as a mixed-flora infection around the mandibular molars. Aerobic and anaerobic pathogens are involved. The floor of the mouth swells and forces the tongue into the airway, creating upper airway obstruction. Extension to sublingual and hypopharyngeal areas produces tongue and pharyngeal swelling.[96,97] This mechanism is exacerbated in the supine position, and patients often cannot tolerate lying flat. Inability to assume the supine position precludes computed tomography, but the diagnosis can be confirmed with lateral neck soft tissue radiographs. Potential exists for infection to track down the airway and into the mediastinum, creating significant edema and swelling throughout the airway.

Submandibular cellulitis brings infection and edema fluid into the submandibular space, effectively reducing the area into which the tongue can be displaced during laryngoscopy. The swollen tongue fits poorly into the already reduced submandibular space, so that it cannot be elevated out of the line of sight during laryngoscopy. Swelling throughout the airway reduces space for visualization. It also distorts and hides landmarks needed for successful intubation. Many patients require awake tracheostomy under local anesthesia because traditional laryngoscopy fails to expose the larynx. Awake fiberoptic intubation may also be considered appropriate in these patients.

H. Rheumatoid Arthritis

Synovitis of the TMJ leads to reduced mandibular motion. Consequently, the mouth opening is small. This hampers laryngoscopy by limiting the amount of space available to insert a laryngoscope and endotracheal tube and impairing the manipulation of these devices once they are placed. Severe forms of Still's disease (juvenile rheumatoid arthritis) can involve the TMJ, leading to poor mandibular development (micrognathia). Micrognathia is probably related to a small mandibular space. The small mandibular space does not accommodate a normal size tongue during laryngoscopy. Consequently, the tongue is not displaced anteriorly out of the line of sight. It hangs down into the airway and obstructs visualization of the larynx.

Cervical spine arthritis limits the neck's range of motion. Consequently, patients can neither flex the lower cervical vertebrae nor extend the atlanto-occipital joint (sniffing position). Inability to perform these maneuvers prevents visual axis alignment of the mouth, pharynx, and larynx. Consequently, laryngoscopy may be difficult, and fiberoptic intubation may be considered. In addition, atlantoaxial subluxation and separation of the atlanto-odontoid articulation can result. The diagnosis is made by obtaining lateral neck radiographs. When separation occurs, the odontoid process is free to enter the foramen magnum and impinge on the spinal cord or vertebral arteries. Often the odontoid process is eroded, reducing the risk of spinal cord or vertebral artery compression. Cervical flexion deformities can render the neck totally immobile, impairing mask ventilation and laryngoscopy.

Cricoarytenoid arthritis may arise with hoarseness, pain on swallowing, dyspnea, stridor, and tenderness over the larynx. The arytenoids are edematous and fixed in adduction. Swelling may be so severe that the glottis is obscured.[98] The vocal cords move poorly,[99] which makes the larynx much more difficult to identify.[98]

V. RELIABILITY OF PREDICTION CRITERIA

Although intuitively it makes sense to perform and is consistent with best medical practices, airway evaluation frequently falls short of its intended goal.[13] Numerous rating systems based on recognized prediction criteria have been investigated. Most suffer from recurrent problems.[100]

The first problem is nomenclature. A standardized definition of the DA did not exist until 1993.[101] At that time, it was explained as a situation in which a conventionally trained anesthesiologist experienced difficulty with mask ventilation, difficulty with endotracheal intubation, or both. For years, individual investigators needed to establish their own definition of DI each time studies were conducted. Consequently, the end points of their work were not necessarily comparable to those of other investigations in the field. Multiple meanings of the term *DI* prevented comparative analysis of studies.

In 1993, the American Society of Anesthesiologists (ASA) Committee on Practice Guidelines for Management of the Difficult Airway offered a generally acceptable definition.[101] Ten years later, the definition was altered slightly, and DI now refers to any intubation that requires multiple attempts.[13] This is a good clinical definition, but it lacks the precision required for scientific investigation. For example, some practitioners may perform a single laryngoscopy and, on the basis of the view obtained, elect to forgo further attempts at laryngoscopy. Such cases may be handled with supraglottic ventilatory devices, regional anesthesia, or other techniques. This situation does not meet the definition of DI even though it would have if one more attempt at intubation had been made. *Failed intubation* may be an easier term to understand. A failed intubation exists when laryngoscopists give up and admit that traditional intubation will not be successful. The end point is clear and occurs with an incidence of 1 in 280 obstetric patients and 1 in 2230 among the general surgical population.[5]

The second problem is identifying features that predict DI. This is frequently accomplished by attempting to recognize characteristics found in patients who have proved to have DI. The problem with such an approach is the lack of information about the same characteristics in patients who have easy intubations. As Turkan and colleagues pointed out, we do not even know the normal values for many prediction criteria.[102] A better method is to apply multivariate analysis to populations of patients in a prospective manner. In that way, a single factor can be compared in difficult and easy intubations. Various rating systems have attempted to combine multiple predictors into a formula, but to date, none have been satisfactory.

The third problem is validating the tests once they are promulgated. Validation tests performed on the same population of patients used to identify them are misleading. Different sample populations are needed.

The fourth problem is experimental methods. Individual practitioners differ in many ways. Any given patient, on any given day, may be difficult to intubate for one laryngoscopist and not for another. Clinical practice has shown that a particular patient who is difficult to intubate in the hands of one laryngoscopist may be successfully intubated by another laryngoscopist. For this reason, experimental designs involving more than one laryngoscopist introduce a source of variation, which detracts from attempts to control experimental conditions. Relying on a single laryngoscopist obviates this problem but limits the number of patients who can be enrolled into a single study. Another source of experimental error is observer variation. Just as laryngoscopists differ, so do observers.[103,104] Observations performed by different experimenters are subject to variations and introduce another source of erroneous data. The best way to prevent this problem is to have all observations performed by a single experimenter. This, too, may limit the number of patients enrolled in a single study.

Statistical tests for assessing the usefulness of criteria involve sensitivity and positive predictive value. Sensitivity is the ratio of DI patients correctly identified compared with all the DI patients within the entire population of patients. For example, consider a population of patients in which five people are difficult to intubate. If a particular predictor of DI correctly identifies all five patients, its sensitivity is 100%. A sensitivity of 100% means that all the DI patients are identified by the test. If the test correctly identifies only two of the five patients, its sensitivity is 2/5, or 40%. Positive predictive value is the probability that DI patients identified by the test are, in fact, difficult to intubate. If the test predicts that five patients will be difficult to intubate and all five of those patients are difficult to intubate, the positive predictive value of the test is 100%. A positive predictive value of 100% means that if the test says that any particular patient will be difficult to intubate, that patient will be difficult to intubate. If the test predicts that 10 patients will be difficult to intubate but only 5 of them are in fact difficult to intubate, its predictive value is 5/10, 50%. Unfortunately, statistical tests such as sensitivity and positive predictive value, when applied to classic prediction criteria, have yielded disappointing results.[14,100]

In 1984, Cormack and Lehane described a grading system for comparing laryngoscopic views (Fig. 9-3).[105] Cormack-Lehane grade 1 views demonstrate the entire glottic opening. Grade 2 views show the posterior laryngeal aperture but not the anterior portion. Grade 3 views allow visualization of the epiglottis but not any part of the larynx. Grade 4 views allow the laryngoscopist to see the soft palate but not the epiglottis. Early evidence indicated a good correlation between Mallampati-Samsoon classes and laryngoscopic grades[5,45] (i.e., a higher Mallampati-Samsoon class predicted a correspondingly higher laryngoscopic grade for any given patient). This concept formed the basis for using Mallampati-Samsoon classes to predict DI. In 1992, Rocke and coworkers disproved that relationship.[55] They investigated several classic predictors of DI and demonstrated that none of them was a reliable predictor of DI (Fig. 9-4).

Classic prediction criteria essentially deal with surface anatomy. They screen for some factors that are associated with DI but fail to address others. Moreover, some potential problems are hidden from surface anatomy examinations. Glottic and supraglottic abnormalities such as

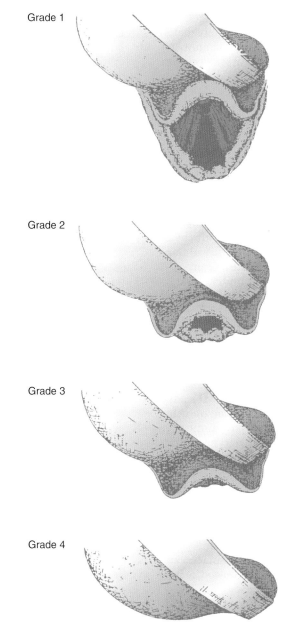

Figure 9-3 Cormack-Lehane grading system. Four laryngoscopic grades are identified: *grade 1*, most of the glottis is visible; *grade 2*, only the posterior extremity of the glottis is visible; *grade 3*, only the epiglottis is seen; *grade 4*, the epiglottis is not seen. (From Cormack RS, Lehane J: Difficult tracheal intubation in obstetrics. *Anaesthesia* 39:1105, 1984.)

lingual tonsil hypertrophy or epiglottic prolapse into the glottic opening cannot be diagnosed by standard physical examinations for predicting DI.[19,106,107] Pathophysiologic factors such as mobile TMJ discs or disc fragments can produce severely limited mouth opening after induction of anesthesia when none existed before.[106] Precise measurements of atlantoaxial motion sometimes fail to predict DI.[108] Supraglottic, glottic, or subglottic pathology may be unrecognized by standard tests but complicate intubation nonetheless.[109] As of this writing, no single factor reliably predicts DI. As more and more

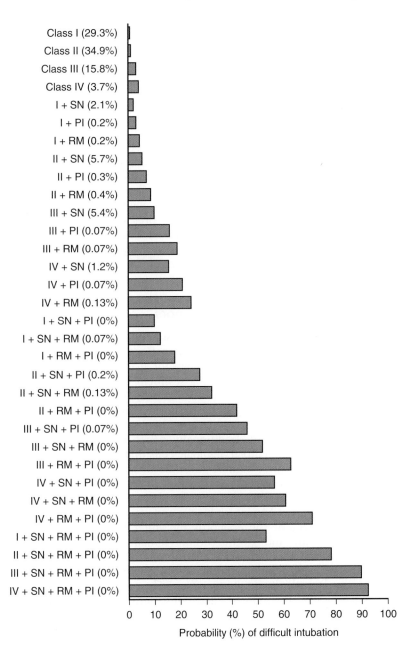

Figure 9-4 Probability of difficult intubation. Classes I-IV are mallampati-Samsoon classifications. *PI*, Protruding incisors; *RM*, receding mandible; *SN*, short neck. (From Rocke DA, Murray WB, Rout CC, Gouws E: Relative risk analysis of factors associated with difficult intubation in obstetric anesthesia. *Anesthesiology* 77:67, 1992.)

predictors of DI are found in the same patient at the same time, the likelihood of DI increases.[35,104,110–112]

VI. NONTRADITIONAL CONSIDERATIONS IN DIFFICULT AIRWAY PREDICTION

A. Imaging

Attempts at predicting DA management by imaging are not new. Standard radiographic films have been used to assess bony structures in an attempt to predict airway problems. However, they have been only minimally helpful. Charters took this concept to the next level; he advocated mathematical modeling, looking at relationships between bony structures.[113] One example is the minimal residual volume[114]: Insufficient volume between the rami of the mandible (i.e., the mandibular space) prevents sufficient anterior tongue displacement and forces the tongue inferiorly, where it drives the epiglottis against the posterior pharyngeal wall and prevents visualization of the larynx. Another example is lateral neck radiographs from which geometric calculations are made.[115] Radiography requires the use of large machines, specialty consultation by radiologists, moving patients to radiology suites, and considerable expense. These constraints are certainly not adaptable to screening large numbers of patients.

Other types of mathematical modeling include airway indices. Numerous indices have been promulgated. Despite the appeal of attaching numbers to criteria and performing calculations with these numbers, airway indices, such as those postulated by Wilson and Arne, have failed to accurately predict DI.[116] Newly created risk scores, such as the one offered by Eberhart and colleagues,[117] await independent validation. Interest in airway indices continues, in the hope that reliable predictions can be formulated based on bedside observations.

Among the most interesting of all mathematical models is computerized facial analysis.[118,119] Connor and Segal[119] are developing programs to assess facial images and predict difficulty of intubation. At present, they require high speed computers, substantial computing power, and network access. As impressive as this program appears, there are likely to be predictors of DI that are not included in their analysis.

B. Supraglottic and Glottic Tumors

Various types of imaging can diagnose supraglottic and glottic tumors. However, relatively few patients benefit from such studies. Most patients present for airway management without imaging. Airway assessment relies on the history and examination of surface anatomy. A history of voice changes, respiratory distress, snoring, and swallowing issues is nondescript and frequently absent when airway tumors are present. Traditionally, a high index of suspicion has prompted otolaryngologic consultation, but otherwise many of these tumors go undiagnosed. These masses can directly obstruct visualization of the larynx. They can occupy space in the vallecula, preventing optimal placement of Macintosh blades, and can interfere with displacement of the epiglottis by Miller blades.[23] Many supraglottic and glottic tumors remain undiagnosed and interfere with mask ventilation and intubation. The classic example is lingual tonsil hypertrophy. Enlarged lingual tonsils push the epiglottis posteriorly, preventing visualization of the glottis and obstructing mask ventilation.[120]

C. Radiation Changes

Traditional laryngoscopy relies on supple elastic laryngeal structures. After head and neck radiation, tissues sometimes become immobile and rigid. These postradiation changes can complicate laryngoscopy.

D. Arthritis

Arthritis is usually associated with joints in the extremities. It also affects laryngeal joints. Cricoarytenoid arthritis can impair Cormack-Lehane views. A related issue is ligament calcification. Stylohyoid ligament calcification can limit forward movement of the hyoid bone, thereby interfering with epiglottic displacement.[114]

E. Cancerous Goiter

In modern practice, thyroid goiters are usually removed before they grow very large. Goiters that bow the trachea generally leave the larynx in the midline. Even tracheomalacia rarely interferes with airway management. Nevertheless, cancerous goiter increases the risk of DI. It is postulated that laryngeal fibrosis extends from the cancer, diminishing soft tissue mobility.[121]

F. Offsetting Features

Individual predictors of DA management carry varying importance in different patients. In some circumstances, a given predictor may produce substantial difficulty, whereas in other situations, it may contribute little. Practitioners have observed this repeatedly. One reason may be offsetting features. One or more factors that contribute to DA management can be offset by others. Perhaps the best recognized example of this point is the edentulous maxilla.[122] Absence of upper teeth allows for such an advantageous line of sight that coexisting confounding issues may well be rendered clinically unimportant.

G. Interobserver Variation

In order to investigate factors that predict DA management and to apply that information clinically, it becomes important to agree on nomenclature and to standardize tests. If different investigators use varying definitions of terms, their findings cannot be compared. Once agreement has been reached among investigators, they must use the same end points in order to apply their findings. The wide range of reported sensitivity and specificity values among tests could relate to this fundamental issue. Interobserver variability confounds establishing specific tests as worthwhile and adversely affects their clinical use. Interobserver variability is especially well recognized for Mallampatti-Samsoon classification systems,[123] and it adversely affects other tests as well.

H. Anesthetic Technique

Optimal conditions for airway management are often dependent on adequate depth of anesthesia and sufficient muscle relaxation. If depth of anesthesia is inadequate for the level of stimulation or muscle relaxation is insufficient, airway management is frequently compromised. The combination of deep anesthesia and profound muscle relaxation provides the best conditions for manipulating the airway.

Patients with myasthenia gravis have undergone laryngoscopy and intubation without muscle relaxants, and this experience has been expanded into other realms, prompting more liberal avoidance of muscle paralysis during airway management. For very short periods of anesthesia, some practitioners are administering small induction doses of a hypnotic and large doses of short-acting opioid, while eliminating muscle relaxants. Such formulas allow for successful airway manipulation in most patients but risk problems.

During mask ventilation, partial or complete vocal cord adduction produces upper airway obstruction and interferes with ventilation as well as oxygenation. During laryngoscopy, passage of a tracheal tube between partially or completely adducted vocal cords may lead to problems, including vocal cord hematoma and laceration. These conditions can lead to hoarseness and altered voice quality on a temporary basis, and occasionally the changes can be permanent. For most patients, temporary voice changes are a nuisance, but for those who use their voice professionally, this complication becomes a major problem. For patients who experience permanent aphonia, these complications are major setbacks. More acutely, eliminating neuromuscular blockers from anesthetic induction and laryngoscopy increases the risk of DI or failed endotracheal intubation.[124]

VII. CONCLUSIONS

The first consideration in caring for patients is maintaining airway patency. In many cases, that is a hard goal to achieve. Predicting the DA is important because it allows appropriate management planning. It is hoped that heightened awareness and altered treatment strategies will prevent some of the untoward events associated with treatment in patients with DA.

At present, no single factor reliably predicts DI. Consequently, prediction of DI relies on various tests, the results of which are taken into account. After assimilating the data, practitioners assess the information and compare it with similar situations that have been encountered previously. In other words, clinical judgments are made on the basis of previous experience.

New tests are sorely needed. They should be painless to perform; patients do not tolerate discomfort for the sake of DA screening. The tests should be quick, should be simple to apply, and should require little or no equipment. Practitioners need to perform these tests on each patient. Complex procedures, cumbersome equipment, and difficult calculations will dissuade many physicians and nurses from using tests. They should be bedside procedures; it is impractical to send ambulatory surgery patients, day-of-admission surgery patients, or emergency patients to distant places for high-technology, expensive imaging studies. The tests should be objective, with little interexaminer variation,[16,103] and reproducible. They should be reliable.[14,112] High degrees of sensitivity and positive predictive value are crucial.

Classic prediction criteria deal primarily with surface anatomy and fail to address issues such as lingual tonsils, epiglottic cysts, and other soft tissue pathology. For this reason, despite outward appearances, a history of DI may be the most reliable predictor of future DIs. A history of prior DI is typically elicited in one of two ways—orally or in writing. Frequently, patients discuss prior intubation difficulties during the preanesthetic interview. Alternatively, this information may be discovered in old records of patients, in written letters, or through the Medic Alert National Registry (see Chapter 54). The Medic Alert Registry provides patients with bracelets and cards that identify their basic medical problem; more information is available through an emergency phone number provided to each registrant.

Until the ideal predictive criteria are discovered, practitioners will continue to rely on imperfect tests and identification of circumstances that are recognized as associated with DAs.

VIII. CLINICAL PEARLS

- No single test reliably predicts DMV or DL.

- Generally accepted predictors of DA management tend to have poor sensitivity and low positive predictive value.

- Proposed predictors of impossible facemask ventilation include neck radiation changes, beard, male gender, OSA, and Mallampati-Samsoon class III or IV.

- Recommended tests to predict DI include history of DI, protruding upper incisors, interincisor distance <3 cm, failed TMJ translation, small indurated mandibular space, limited cervical vertebral range of motion, TMD <6 cm, Mallampati-Samsoon Class III or IV, and short thick neck.

- The Cormack-Lehane views are as follows: grade I, entire glottic aperture visualized; grade II, posterior glottis visualized, but not the anterior portion; grade III, epiglottis visualized, but no part of the glottis; grade IV, soft palate visualized, but not the epiglottis.

- High-dose opioids sometimes produce vocal cord adduction leading to DMV and DI.

SELECTED REFERENCES

All references can be found online at expertconsult.com.

2. Shiga T, Wajima Z, Inoue T, et al: Predicting difficult intubation in apparently normal patients. *Anesthesiology* 103:429–437, 2005.
5. Samsoon GLT, Young JRB: Difficult tracheal intubation: A retrospective study. *Anaesthesia* 42:487–490, 1987.
7. Caplan RA, Posner KL, Ward RJ, et al: Adverse respiratory events in anesthesia: A closed claims analysis. *Anesthesiology* 72:828–833, 1990.
13. Practice guidelines for management of the difficult airway: An updated report by the American Society of Anesthesiologists Task Force on Management of the Difficult Airway. *Anesthesiology* 98:1269–1277, 2003. Erratum 10:565, 2004.
15. Langeron O, Masso E, Huraux C, et al: Prediction of difficult mask ventilation. *Anesthesiology* 92:1229–1236, 2000.
17. Kheterpal S, Han R, Tremper KK, et al: Incidence and predictors of difficult and impossible mask ventilation. *Anesthesiology* 105:885–891, 2006.
19. Ovassapian A, Glassenberg R, Randel GI, et al: The unexpected difficult airway and lingual tonsil hyperplasia: A case series and a review of the literature. *Anesthesiology* 97:124–132, 2002.
30. Kheterpal S, Martin L, Shanks AM, et al: Prediction of outcomes of impossible mask ventilation: A review of 50,000 anesthetics. *Anesthesiology* 110:891–897, 2009.
52. Benumof JL, Dagg R, Benumof R: Critical hemoglobin desaturation will occur before return to an unparalyzed state following 1 mg/kg of intravenous succinylcholine. *Anesthesiology* 87:979–982, 1997.
55. Rocke DA, Murray WB, Rout CC, et al: Relative risk analysis of factors associated with difficult intubation in obstetric anesthesia. *Anesthesiology* 47:67–73, 1992.
124. Lunstrom LH, Moller AM, Rosenstock C, et al: Avoidance of neuromuscular blocking agents may increase the risk of difficult tracheal intubation: A cohort study of 103,812 consecutive patients recorded in the Danish anaesthesia database. *Br J Anaesth* 103:283–290, 2009.

Chapter 10

The ASA Difficult Airway Algorithm: Analysis and Presentation of a New Algorithm*

ANSGAR M. BRAMBRINK | CARIN A. HAGBERG

I. INTRODUCTION

There is strong evidence that successful airway management in the perioperative environment depends on specific strategies. Suggested strategies from various subfields of medicine are now being linked together to form more comprehensive treatment plans or algorithms. The classic flow charts of this nature are the resuscitation algorithms that provide evidence-based guidance during cardiopulmonary resuscitation worldwide.

The purpose of the Algorithm on the Management of the Difficult Airway (DAA), published by the American Society of Anesthesiologists (ASA), is to facilitate management of the difficult airway (DA) and to reduce the likelihood of adverse outcomes. The principal adverse

outcomes associated with the DA include (but are not limited to) death, brain injury, cardiopulmonary arrest, unnecessary tracheostomy, airway trauma, and damage to teeth.

The original ASA DAA was developed over a 2-year period by the ASA Task Force on Guidelines for Management of the Difficult Airway.[1] The task force included academicians, private practitioners, airway experts, adult and pediatric anesthesia generalists, and a statistical methodologist. The algorithm was introduced by ASA as a practice guideline in 1993. In 2003, the ASA task force presented a revised algorithm that essentially retained the same concept but recommended a wider range of airway management techniques than was previously included, based on more recent scientific evidence and the advent of new technology.

This chapter presents and explains the ASA DAA and then provides a critical appraisal of the ASA algorithm based on recent evidence from the literature. This is followed by the presentation of a new, comprehensive

*Parts of this chapter are adapted and modified from a previous publication on a similar topic: Hagberg C, Lam N, Brambrink AM: Current concepts in airway management in the operating room: A new approach to the management of both complicated and uncomplicated airways. *Curr Rev Clin Anesth* 28:73–88, 2007.

airway management algorithm that provides an innovative and highly structured approach resembling the guidelines for cardiopulmonary resuscitation.

Both algorithms are concerned with the maintenance of airway patency at all times. Special emphasis is placed on an operating room setting, although the algorithm can be extrapolated to the intensive care unit, the ward, and the entire perioperative environment and beyond. Both algorithms are primarily intended for use by anesthesiologists or by individuals who deliver anesthetic care and airway management under the direct supervision of an anesthesiologist. The guidelines apply to airway management during all types of anesthetic care and anesthetizing locations, and to patients of all ages.

Both airway algorithms focus primarily on further improving patient safety during the perioperative period. Adherence to the principles of an airway management algorithm and widespread adoption of such a structured plan should result in a reduction of respiratory catastrophes and a decrease in perioperative morbidity and mortality.

II. THE ASA DIFFICULT AIRWAY ALGORITHM

A side-by-side comparison of the original (1993) and the updated (2003) versions of the ASA DAA is presented in Figure 10-1. The differences between the two algorithms are listed in Box 10-1. Certain aspects of the algorithm require further explanation.

A. Patient Evaluation and Risk Assessment

The ASA DAA begins with the most basic question of whether or not the presence of a DA is recognized (see Chapter 9). Recognizing the potential for difficulty leads to proper mental and physical preparation and an increased chance of a good outcome. In contrast, failure to recognize this potential results in unexpected difficulty in the absence of proper mental and, likely, physical preparation, with an increased chance for a catastrophic outcome.

Airway evaluation should take into account any characteristics of the patient that could lead to difficulty in the performance of (1) bag-mask or supraglottic airway ventilation, (2) laryngoscopy, (3) intubation, or (4) a surgical airway. Routine patient evaluation can be best structured as follows (see Chapter 9 for details):

1. Obtain an airway history to identify medical, surgical, and anesthetic factors that may indicate the presence of a DA.
2. Evaluate for systemic diseases (e.g., respiratory failure, coronary artery disease) that might place limits on awake intubation, such as increased fraction of inspired oxygen (FIO_2), or require special attention, such as prevention of sympathetic nervous system stimulation.
3. Examine previous anesthetic records, which can yield useful information about previous airway management.
4. Conduct a physical examination of the airway to detect physical characteristics that might indicate the presence of a DA (Table 10-1):
   - Maximal mouth opening with tongue extension and pharyngeal anatomy (e.g., uvula, tonsillar pillars)
   - Length of the submental space (mandible to hyoid) and the thyromental distance (mandible to thyroid notch)

| **Box 10-1** | **Differences between 1993 and 2003 ASA Management of the Difficult Airway Algorithms** |

1. *Difficult ventilation* is now listed first under item 1, "Assess the Likelihood and Clinical Impact of Basic Management Problems." Also, in the same category, *Difficult tracheostomy* was added.
2. A new item 2 was inserted: "Actively pursue opportunities to deliver supplemental oxygen throughout the process of difficult airway management."
3. When considering the relative merits and feasibility of basic management choices (item 3), awake intubation versus intubation attempts after induction of anesthesia should now be considered first, before noninvasive versus invasive techniques as the initial approach to intubation.
4. Use of the laryngeal mask airway (LMA) was incorporated into the algorithm in the awake induction limb and in both the nonemergency and emergency pathways for induction after general anesthesia (either as a ventilatory device or as a conduit for tracheal intubation).
5. The option for "One more intubation attempt" was removed.
6. Use of the rigid bronchoscope was added as an option for emergency noninvasive ventilation.

TABLE 10-1

Components of the Preoperative Airway Physical Examination

Airway Examination Component	Nonreassuring Findings
Length of upper incisors	Relatively long
Relation of maxillary and mandibular incisors during normal jaw closure	Prominent "overbite" (maxillary incisors anterior to mandibular incisors)
Relation of maxillary and mandibular incisors during voluntary protrusion of the jaw	Patient's mandibular incisors anterior to (in front of) mandibular incisors
Interincisor distance	<3 cm
Visibility of uvula	Not visible when tongue is protruded with patient in sitting position (e.g., Mallampati class III or IV)
Shape of palate	Highly arched or very narrow
Compliance of mandibular space	Stiff, indurated, occupied by mass, or nonresilient
Thyromental distance	<3 ordinary finger breadths
Length of neck	Short
Thickness of neck	Thick
Range of motion of head and neck	Patient cannot touch tip of chin to chest or cannot extend neck

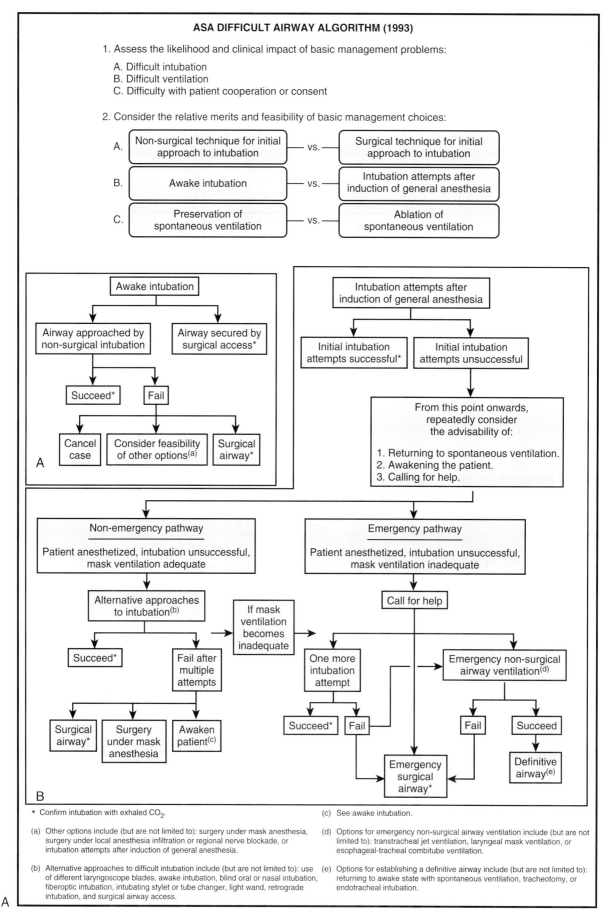

ASA DIFFICULT AIRWAY ALGORITHM (1993)

1. Assess the likelihood and clinical impact of basic management problems:

   A. Difficult intubation
   B. Difficult ventilation
   C. Difficulty with patient cooperation or consent

2. Consider the relative merits and feasibility of basic management choices:

   A. Non-surgical technique for initial approach to intubation — vs. — Surgical technique for initial approach to intubation

   B. Awake intubation — vs. — Intubation attempts after induction of general anesthesia

   C. Preservation of spontaneous ventilation — vs. — Ablation of spontaneous ventilation

A

Awake intubation

→ Airway approached by non-surgical intubation
→ Airway secured by surgical access*

Succeed* | Fail

Cancel case | Consider feasibility of other options[a] | Surgical airway*

Intubation attempts after induction of general anesthesia

→ Initial intubation attempts successful*
→ Initial intubation attempts unsuccessful

From this point onwards, repeatedly consider the advisability of:

1. Returning to spontaneous ventilation.
2. Awakening the patient.
3. Calling for help.

B

Non-emergency pathway

Patient anesthetized, intubation unsuccessful, mask ventilation adequate

Alternative approaches to intubation[b]

Succeed* | Fail after multiple attempts

Surgical airway* | Surgery under mask anesthesia | Awaken patient[c]

If mask ventilation becomes inadequate →

Emergency pathway

Patient anesthetized, intubation unsuccessful, mask ventilation inadequate

Call for help

One more intubation attempt

Succeed* | Fail

Emergency non-surgical airway ventilation[d]

Fail | Succeed

Emergency surgical airway* | Definitive airway[e]

* Confirm intubation with exhaled CO_2.

(a) Other options include (but are not limited to): surgery under mask anesthesia, surgery under local anesthesia infiltration or regional nerve blockade, or intubation attempts after induction of general anesthesia.

(b) Alternative approaches to difficult intubation include (but are not limited to): use of different laryngoscope blades, awake intubation, blind oral or nasal intubation, fiberoptic intubation, intubating stylet or tube changer, light wand, retrograde intubation, and surgical airway access.

(c) See awake intubation.

(d) Options for emergency non-surgical airway ventilation include (but are not limited to): transtracheal jet ventilation, laryngeal mask ventilation, or esophageal-tracheal combitube ventilation.

(e) Options for establishing a definitive airway include (but are not limited to): returning to awake state with spontaneous ventilation, tracheotomy, or endotracheal intubation.

A

Figure 10-1 A, The American Society of Anesthesiologists' difficult airway algorithm (ASA DAA), published in 1993.

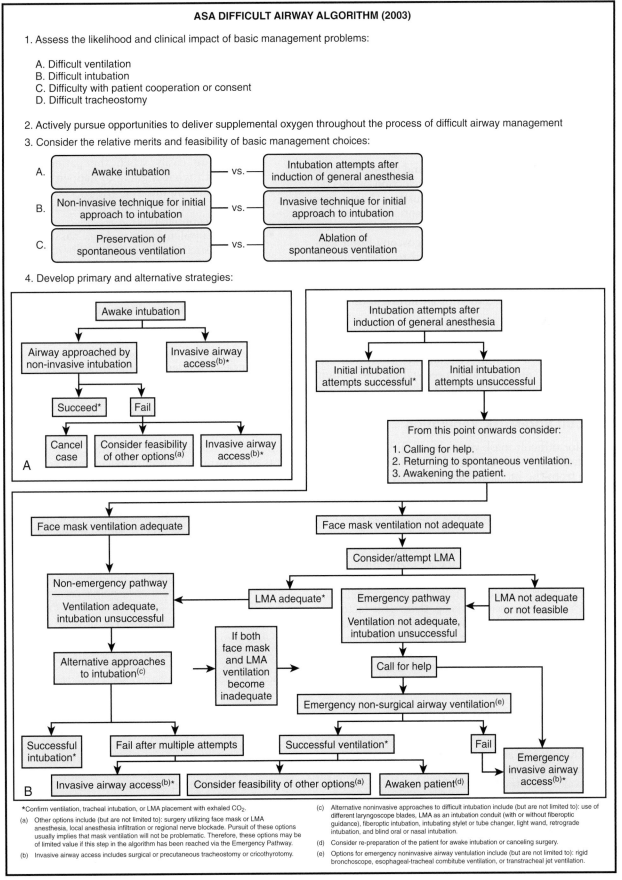

ASA DIFFICULT AIRWAY ALGORITHM (2003)

1. Assess the likelihood and clinical impact of basic management problems:

    A. Difficult ventilation
    B. Difficult intubation
    C. Difficulty with patient cooperation or consent
    D. Difficult tracheostomy

2. Actively pursue opportunities to deliver supplemental oxygen throughout the process of difficult airway management

3. Consider the relative merits and feasibility of basic management choices:

A.   Awake intubation —vs.— Intubation attempts after induction of general anesthesia

B.   Non-invasive technique for initial approach to intubation —vs.— Invasive technique for initial approach to intubation

C.   Preservation of spontaneous ventilation —vs.— Ablation of spontaneous ventilation

4. Develop primary and alternative strategies:

A

Awake intubation

→ Airway approached by non-invasive intubation
→ Invasive airway access[(b)]*

Airway approached by non-invasive intubation:
→ Succeed*
→ Fail

Succeed* → Cancel case
Fail → Consider feasibility of other options[(a)]
→ Invasive airway access[(b)]*

Intubation attempts after induction of general anesthesia

→ Initial intubation attempts successful*
→ Initial intubation attempts unsuccessful

Initial intubation attempts unsuccessful →

From this point onwards consider:

1. Calling for help.
2. Returning to spontaneous ventilation.
3. Awakening the patient.

B

→ Face mask ventilation adequate
→ Face mask ventilation not adequate

Face mask ventilation not adequate → Consider/attempt LMA

Consider/attempt LMA → LMA adequate*
LMA not adequate or not feasible

Face mask ventilation adequate →
Non-emergency pathway
_____
Ventilation adequate, intubation unsuccessful

LMA adequate* → (Non-emergency pathway)

Emergency pathway
_____
Ventilation not adequate, intubation unsuccessful

LMA not adequate or not feasible →

Non-emergency pathway → Alternative approaches to intubation[(c)]

If both face mask and LMA ventilation become inadequate →

Emergency pathway → Call for help
Call for help → Emergency non-surgical airway ventilation[(e)]

Alternative approaches to intubation[(c)] →
Successful intubation*
Fail after multiple attempts

Emergency non-surgical airway ventilation[(e)] →
Successful ventilation*
Fail

Fail after multiple attempts →
Invasive airway access[(b)]*
Consider feasibility of other options[(a)]
Awaken patient[(d)]

Fail → Emergency invasive airway access[(b)]*

---

*Confirm ventilation, tracheal intubation, or LMA placement with exhaled CO₂.

(a) Other options include (but are not limited to): surgery utilizing face mask or LMA anesthesia, local anesthesia infiltration or regional nerve blockade. Pursuit of these options usually implies that mask ventilation will not be problematic. Therefore, these options may be of limited value if this step in the algorithm has been reached via the Emergency Pathway.

(b) Invasive airway access includes surgical or precutaneous tracheostomy or cricothyrotomy.

(c) Alternative noninvasive approaches to difficult intubation include (but are not limited to): use of different laryngoscope blades, LMA as an intubation conduit (with or without fiberoptic guidance), fiberoptic intubation, intubating stylet or tube changer, light wand, retrograde intubation, and blind oral or nasal intubation.

(d) Consider re-preparation of the patient for awake intubation or canceling surgery.

(e) Options for emergency noninvasive airway ventulation include (but are not limited to): rigid bronchoscope, esophageal-tracheal combitube ventilation, or transtracheal jet ventilation.

B

Figure 10-1, cont'd B, The revised (2003) ASA DAA. (**A** from American Society of Anesthesiologists Task Force on Management of the Difficult Airway: Practice guidelines for management of the difficult airway: A report. *Anesthesiology* 78:597–602, 1993; **B** from Practice Guidelines for the Management of the Difficult Airway: An updated report by the American Society of Anesthesiologists Task Force on the Management of the Difficult Airway. *Anesthesiology* 98:1269–1277, 2003.)

- Side view to determine the ability to assume the "sniffing" position (flexion of the neck on the chest and extension of the head on the neck) and to identify maxillary overbite
- Nostril patency
- Length and thickness of the neck

Although each risk factor individually has a rather low positive predictive value for difficult intubation, when combined these factors can provide a gestalt for DA management.

The findings of the airway history and physical examination may be useful in guiding the selection of specific diagnostic tests and consultation to further characterize the likelihood or nature of the anticipated airway difficulty.[2]

An "awake look" using direct laryngoscopy (after adequate preparation) may be performed to assess intubation difficulty further. If an adequate view is obtained, endotracheal intubation may be performed, followed immediately by administration of an intravenous induction agent.

Presence of a pathologic factor or a combination of anatomic factors (large tongue size, small mandibular space, or restricted atlanto-occipital extension) indicates that the airway should be secured while the patient remains awake (awake techniques).

B. Difficult Bag-Mask Ventilation

The risk for difficult mask ventilation (DMV) is the first issue addressed in the most recent version of the DAA. Evidence from the literature[3] suggests that the incidence of DMV is 5% in the general adult population, that the presence of DMV is associated with difficult intubation, and that DMV is not accurately predicted by anesthesiologists.

Five independent criteria predict DMV (age >55 years, body mass index >26 kg/m^2, lack of teeth, presence of mustache or beard, and history of snoring), and the presence of two such risk factors indicates a high likelihood of DMV.[3] It is important to keep these risk factors in mind, because some of them can be reversed. For example, DMV may possibly be preventable by shaving a patient's beard, leaving dentures in place during bag-mask ventilation (BMV), and performing a workup and treating for possible obstructive sleep apnea.

C. Awake Tracheal Intubation

Awake intubation is generally more time-consuming for the anesthesiologist and a more unpleasant experience for the patient. However, if a difficult intubation is anticipated, awake endotracheal intubation is indicated for three reasons: (1) the natural airway is better maintained in most patients when they are awake (i.e., "no bridges are burned"); (2) the orientation of upper airway structures is easier to identify in the awake patient (i.e., muscle tone is maintained to keep the base of the tongue, vallecula, epiglottis, larynx, esophagus, and posterior pharyngeal wall separated from one another)[4,5]; and (3) the larynx moves to a more anterior position with the

induction of anesthesia and paralysis, which makes conventional intubation more difficult.[6]

Crucial to the success of endotracheal intubation while the patient is awake is proper preparation (see Chapter 11 for further details). Most intubation techniques work well in patients who are cooperative and whose larynx is nonreactive to physical stimuli. In general, the components of proper preparation for an awake intubation are the following:

- Psychological preparation (awake intubation proceeds more easily when the patient knows and agrees with what is going to happen)
- Appropriate monitoring (i.e., electrocardiography, noninvasive blood pressure monitoring, pulse oximetry, and capnography)
- Oxygen supplementation (e.g., nasal prongs, nasal cannula, suction channel of a fiberoptic bronchoscope [FOB], transtracheal catheter)[7-10]
- Vasoconstriction of the nasal mucous membranes (if performing nasal intubation)
- Administration of a drying agent
- Judicious sedation (keeping the patient in meaningful contact with the environment)
- Adequate airway topicalization (consider performance of bilateral laryngeal nerve blocks, blocking the lingual branch of the glossopharyngeal nerve and the superior laryngeal nerve)
- Aspiration prevention (see Chapter 12)
- Availability of appropriate airway equipment

Box 10-2 lists the suggested ASA guidelines for contents of a portable airway management cart.[11]

Box 10-2 Suggested Contents of the Portable Storage Unit for Difficult Airway Management

Important: The items listed here represent suggestions. The contents of the portable DA management cart should be customized to meet the specific needs, preferences, and skills of the practitioner and health care facility.

1. Rigid laryngoscope blades of alternative design and size from those routinely used; may include a rigid fiberoptic laryngoscope
2. Endotracheal tubes of assorted sizes
3. Endotracheal tube guides, such as semirigid stylets, ventilating tube changer, light wands, and forceps designed to manipulate the distal portion of the endotracheal tube
4. Laryngeal mask airways (LMAs) of assorted sizes; may include the Fastrach intubation LMA and the ProSeal LMA (LMA North America, San Diego, CA).
5. Fiberoptic intubation equipment
6. Retrograde intubation equipment
7. At least one device suitable for emergency nonsurgical airway ventilation, such as the esophageal-tracheal Combitube (Tyco Healthcare, Mansfield, MA), a hollow jet ventilation stylet, and a transtracheal jet ventilator
8. Equipment suitable for emergency surgical airway access (e.g., cricothyrotomy)
9. An exhaled carbon dioxide detector
10. A rigid ventilating bronchoscope

Box 10-3 Techniques for Difficult Airway Management

Important: This box lists commonly cited techniques in alphabetic order. It is not a comprehensive list, and no preference for a given technique or sequence of use is implied. Combinations of techniques may be employed. The techniques chosen by the practitioner depend on the specific needs, preferences, skills, and clinical constraints in the particular case.

Techniques for Difficult Intubation

Alternative laryngoscope blades
Awake intubation
Blind intubation (oral or nasal)
Fiberoptic intubation
Intubating stylet or tube changer
Invasive airway access
Laryngeal mask airway as an intubating conduit
Light wand
Retrograde intubation

Techniques for Difficult Ventilation

Esophageal-tracheal Combitube
Intratracheal jet stylet
Invasive airway access
Laryngeal mask airway
Oral and nasopharyngeal airways
Rigid ventilating bronchoscope
Transtracheal jet ventilation
Two-person mask ventilation

There are numerous methods to intubate the trachea or ventilate a patient (see Part Four of this text). Box 10-3 shows a list of the techniques contained within the ASA guidelines. The techniques chosen depend, in part, on the anticipated surgery, the condition of the patient, and the skills and preferences of the anesthesiologist. Based on recent evidence from the literature[12-14] considerations should also include the use of video laryngoscopy, despite the fact that this technique is not mentioned in the recent ASA algorithm, but likely will be included in future revisions of the guidelines.

Occasionally, awake intubation may fail owing to a lack of patient cooperation, equipment or operator limitations, or any combination thereof. An alternative route is chosen according to the precise cause of the failure:

- Surgery may be canceled (e.g., the patient needs further counseling, airway edema or trauma has resulted, different equipment or personnel is necessary).
- General anesthesia may be induced (the fundamental problem must be considered to be a lack of cooperation, and mask ventilation must be considered nonproblematic).
- Regional anesthesia may be considered (careful clinical judgment is required to balance risks and benefits; see Chapter 45).
- A surgical airway may be created (if the surgery is essential and general anesthesia is considered to be inappropriate until intubation is accomplished); this may be the best choice to secure the airway in patients with laryngeal or tracheal fracture or disruption, upper airway abscess, or combined mandibular-maxillary fractures.

D. Difficult Intubation in the Unconscious or Anesthetized Patient

Three typical scenarios require the anesthesiologist to manage a DA in an unconscious patient with a DA: (1) a comatose patient (e.g., secondary to trauma or intoxication); (2) a patient who absolutely refuses or cannot tolerate awake intubation (e.g., a child, a mentally retarded patient, an intoxicated and combative patient); and perhaps most commonly, (3) failure to recognize intubation difficulty on the preoperative evaluation. Of course, the preoperative airway evaluation is important even in the first and second situations, because the findings may dictate the choice of intubation technique. In all three of these situations, the patient may also have a full stomach.

All of the intubation techniques that are described for the awake patient[1,15] can be used in the unconscious or anesthetized patient without modification. However, direct laryngoscopy and fiberoptic laryngoscopy are likely to be more difficult in the paralyzed, anesthetized patient compared with the awake patient, because the larynx may move to a more anterior position, relative to other structures, as a result of relaxation of oral and pharyngeal muscles.[6] In addition and more importantly, orientation may be impaired because the upper airway structures can coalesce into a horizontal plane instead of separating out in a vertical plane.[4,5]

In the anesthetized patient whose trachea has proved difficult to intubate even with a video laryngoscope it is necessary to try to maintain gas exchange between intubation attempts (by mask ventilation) and, whenever possible, during intubation attempts through the use of (1) supplemental oxygen[11]; (2) positive-pressure ventilation via an anesthesia mask that incorporates a self-sealing diaphragm for entry of the FOB airway intubator (instead of the standard oropharyngeal airway)[5,16]; or (3) a laryngeal mask airway (LMA; LMA North America, Inc., San Diego, CA) as a conduit for the FOB (see Chapters 19 and 22).[17]

One must not continue with the same technique that did not work before. The amount of laryngeal edema and bleeding is likely to increase after every intubation attempt, particularly with the use of a laryngoscope or retraction blade. The most common scenario in the respiratory catastrophes in the ASA closed claims study was the development of progressive difficulty in ventilating by mask between persistent and prolonged failed intubation attempts. The final result was inability to ventilate by mask and provide gas exchange (see Chapter 55).[18]

For each additional attempt, consider modifications, such as improved sniffing position, external laryngeal manipulation, a new blade or new technique, or involvement of a much more experienced laryngoscopist. However, the number of intubation attempts should be limited and the following options should be considered: (1) awaken the patient and do the procedure another day; (2) continue anesthesia by mask or LMA ventilation; (3) perform a surgical airway (tracheostomy or cricothyrotomy) before the ability to ventilate the lungs by mask is lost (see Fig. 10-1).

If awakening the patient is not an option, for instance because surgery is emergent (e.g., cesarean section), and ventilation can be maintained via mask or LMA, surgery may be conducted as needed. Nevertheless, in some cases, the airway must be secured by a surgical airway (e.g., thoracotomy, intracranial-head-neck cases, cases in which the patient is in the prone position). If regurgitation or vomiting occurs at any time during attempts at endotracheal intubation in an anesthetized patient,

- Immediately apply Trendelenburg position.
- Turn the head, and perhaps the body, to the left.
- Suction the mouth and pharynx with a large-bore suction device.
- Try endotracheal intubation while the patient is in the lateral position (the tongue may be more out of the way, but this position is unfamiliar to most anesthesiologists).
- If the endotracheal tube (ETT) has been passed into the esophagus, it may be left there; this may allow decompression of the stomach, and it identifies the esophagus during subsequent intubation attempts (the disadvantage is that it interferes with satisfactory mask seal).
- After securing the airway, consider tracheal suctioning, mechanical ventilation, positive end-expiratory pressure, fiberoptically guided saline lavage, steroids, antibiotics (see Chapter 35).

E. The "Cannot Intubate, Cannot Ventilate" Scenario

In rare cases, it is impossible either to ventilate the lungs of a patient by mask or to intubate the trachea. This "cannot intubate, cannot ventilate" (CICV) scenario is an immediately life-threatening situation, and an alternative ventilation procedure must be performed. Established rescue methods are the LMA, Combitube (Tyco Healthcare, Mansfield, MA), transtracheal jet ventilation (TTJV), rigid bronchoscope, and, ultimately, cricothyrotomy.

The development of the LMA was a major advance in the management of difficult intubation and difficult ventilation scenarios. The LMA is suggested as a ventilation device or a conduit for a flexible FOB,[19,20] and the Fastrach intubating LMA (ILMA) may also be utilized.[10,17,21] The LMA and the Combitube are supraglottic ventilatory devices and are not helpful if the airway obstruction is located at or below the glottic opening.[22] Use of the rigid bronchoscope may be required to establish a patent airway because it allows ventilation even past an obstruction at these levels. If immediately available, TTJV is relatively easy to perform and can be life-saving.[23] However, it carries significant risks such as subcutaneous emphysema (if the upper airway is not patent or the catheter is not entirely tracheal) and barotrauma (too forced ventilation or proximal airway obstruction)[24] The techniques mentioned can provide time until definitive airway management by tracheal intubation (via direct, fiberoptic, or retrograde technique) or by formal tracheostomy can be performed.[25,26] Future research will determine the role of the new rigid video laryngoscopes in the rescue of the "cannot intubate, cannot ventilate" scenario.

Ultimately, a cricothyrotomy may be necessary, but fewer than 50% of anesthesiologists feel competent to perform one.[27] Nevertheless, when one is faced with a failed airway, preparations for a surgical airway must begin immediately, and once the decision is made, it is essential to use an effective technique (see Chapters 30 and 31). Despite limited familiarity with the procedure, the risks of an invasive rescue technique must be weighed against the risks of hypoxic brain injury or death.[28]

F. Extubation of a Patient with a Difficult Airway

Extubation of the patient with a DA should be carefully assessed and performed. The anesthesiologist should develop a strategy for safe extubation of these patients, depending on the type of surgery, the condition of the patient, and the skills and preferences of the anesthesiologist. Additional considerations include the following:

- Awake extubation versus extubation before return of consciousness
- Clinical symptoms with the potential to impair ventilation (e.g., altered mental status, abnormal gas exchange, airway edema, inability to clear secretions, inadequate return of neuromuscular functions)
- Airway management plan if the patient is not able to maintain adequate ventilation
- Short-term use of a ventilating tube exchanger (TE) or jet stylet (can be used for ventilation and guided reintubation)

The ideal method of extubation of a patient with a DA is gradual, step by step, and reversible at any time. Extubation over a ventilating TE or jet stylet closely approximates this ideal.[16] The equipment that should be immediately available for the extubation of a DA includes that necessary for intubation of the DA (see Chapter 50).[29]

G. Follow-up Care of a Patient with a Difficult Airway

The presence and nature of the airway difficulty should be documented in the medical record. The intent of this documentation is to guide and facilitate the delivery of future care. Aspects of documentation that may prove helpful include the following:

- Description of the airway difficulties, which should distinguish between difficulties with mask ventilation and those with tracheal intubation
- Description of the airway management techniques used, which should indicate the beneficial or detrimental role of each technique in management of the DA
- Information given the patient (or responsible person) concerning the airway difficulty that was encountered. The intent of this communication is to assist the patient (or responsible person) in guiding and facilitating the delivery of future care. The information conveyed may include, for instance, the presence of a DA, the apparent reasons for the difficulty, and implications for future care.

The provider should also strongly consider dispensing or advising a Medic-Alert bracelet for the patient (see

Chapter 54). Finally, the anesthesiologist should evaluate and observe the patient for potential complications of DA management, such as airway edema, bleeding, tracheal or esophageal perforation, pneumothorax, and aspiration.

III. SUMMARY OF THE ASA ALGORITHM

Difficulty in managing the airway is the single most important cause of major anesthesia-related morbidity and mortality.

Successful management of a DA begins with recognition of the potential problem. All patients should be examined for their ability to open their mouth widely, the structures visible on mouth opening, the size of the mandibular space, and the ability to assume the sniffing position.

If there is a good possibility that intubation or ventilation by mask, or both, will be difficult, the airway should be secured while the patient is still awake rather than after induction of general anesthesia. For a successful awake intubation, it is essential that the patient and the provider be properly prepared.

When the patient is properly prepared, any one of a number of intubation techniques is likely to be successful. If the patient is already anesthetized or paralyzed and intubation is found to be difficult, many repeated forceful attempts at intubation should be avoided, because laryngeal edema and hemorrhage will progressively develop, and the ability to ventilate the lungs by mask may consequently be lost.

After several unsuccessful attempts at intubation, it may be best to awaken the patient; administer regional anesthesia, if appropriate (see Chapter 45); proceed with the case using mask or LMA ventilation; or perform a semielective tracheostomy. If the ability to ventilate by mask is lost and the patient's lungs cannot be ventilated, LMA ventilation should be instituted immediately. If LMA ventilation does not provide adequate gas exchange, either TTJV or a surgical airway should be instituted immediately.

Tracheal extubation of a patient with a DA over a jet stylet permits a controlled, gradual, withdrawal from the airway that is reversible in that ventilation and reintubation are possible at any time.

Four concepts emerge from the preceding discussion—four very important, take-home messages on the ASA DAA. These are presented in Box 10-4.

IV. PROBLEMS WITH THE ASA ALGORITHM AND LIKELY FUTURE DIRECTIONS

The strength of the ASA DAA is twofold. First, it is very thorough and complete with respect to the options available when an anesthesiologist encounters a DA. Second, it emphasizes the need for and importance of an organized approach to airway management.[30]

On the other hand, the algorithm has several deficiencies that diminish its application in clinical practice.

> **Box 10-4**   **ASA Difficult Airway Algorithm Take-Home Messages**
>
> 1. If suspicious of trouble → Secure the airway awake
> 2. If you get into trouble → Awaken the patient
> 3. Have plans B and C immediately available and in place = think ahead
> 4. Intubation choices → Do what you do best

- Although it is intended to apply to all patients of all ages, there are certain populations of patients in which further considerations are necessary. Examples include pediatric patients (see Chapter 36), obstetric patients (see Chapter 37), nonfasted patients, and patients with obstruction at or below the level of the vocal cords.[31]
- The algorithm's clinical end point is successful intubation, but endotracheal intubation may not be necessary, and successful ventilation may suffice.
- The algorithm is fairly complex, allowing a wide choice of techniques at each stage, and its multiplicity of pathways may limit its clinical usefulness in guiding day-to-day practice.[32] Unlike the algorithm used in advanced life support (ACLS) guidelines, for example, the ASA DAA is not binary in nature.[33]
- Somewhat vague terminology is used in its definitions of difficult tracheal intubation and difficult laryngoscopy. Definitions of optimal-best attempts at conventional laryngoscopy, mask ventilation, and difficult laryngoscopy or intubation are important because they provide an end point at which the practitioner should stop using a particular approach (limiting risk) and move on to something that has a better chance of working (gaining benefit).
- The algorithm mentions ablation of spontaneous ventilation with muscle relaxants but does not discuss the great clinical management implications of muscle relaxants that have different durations of action.
- Although the algorithm advises confirmation of endotracheal intubation, the usefulness of capnography for this purpose is limited during cardiac arrest, which is not an uncommon consequence of the CICV scenario; the esophageal detector device is not similarly limited (see Chapter 32).
- The algorithm does not provide a definitive flow chart for extubation of the DA that incorporates the use of a device that can serve as a guide for expedited reintubation or ventilation, if necessary.
- The role of regional anesthesia in patients with a DA requires further clarification (see Chapter 45).
- The algorithm does not include the use of rigid video laryngoscopy which has dramatically changed the day-to-day clinical practice in recent years and has been shown to be able to rescue failed direct laryngoscopy, particularly in the DA.[12,13]

Several of the issues mentioned need more in-depth discussion, including the definition of difficult endotracheal intubation, the optimal-best attempt at laryngoscopy, the optimal-best attempt at mask ventilation, and the best muscle relaxant to use.

A. Terminology in the ASA Difficult Airway Algorithm

The original publications that introduced the ASA algorithm and provided basic terms that define a DA were relatively vague in their terminology[1]:

- *Difficult mask ventilation*: "It is *not* possible for the anesthesiologist to provide adequate face mask ventilation due to one or more of the following problems: inadequate mask seal, excessive gas leak or excessive resistance to the ingress or egress of gas."
- *Difficult laryngoscopy*: "Not being able to visualize any portion of the vocal cords after multiple attempts at conventional laryngoscopy."
- *Difficult intubation*: "When tracheal intubation requires multiple attempts in the presence or absence of tracheal pathology."
- *Failed intubation*: "Placement of the tracheal tube fails after multiple intubation attempts" (0.05% of surgical patients and 0.13% to 0.35% in obstetric patients).

These definitions do not identify a specific Cormack-Lehane grade to characterize larynx visibility, and they do not state a specific number of attempts; therefore, on both counts, they can be interpreted differently by individual practitioners. Also, there is no mention of adjuvants such as positioning and use of appropriate equipment to aid laryngoscopy, ventilation, and intubation. Such information would allow the anesthesiologist to proceed in a new direction at certain junctures, knowing that continuing the same maneuvers would accomplish diminishing returns.

In the same vein, it is important to define "attempt" in an airway management algorithm——for example, as physical placement and removal of the laryngoscope blade. Moreover, an ideal airway management algorithm should define and use the "optimal-best attempt" as the unit, because optimizing the conditions for the various maneuvers has clearly been shown to have a profound effect on successful intubation.

B. Definition of Optimal-Best Attempt at Conventional Laryngoscopy

Difficulty in performing endotracheal intubation is the end result of the difficulties that occurred during laryngoscopy, which depends on the operator's level of expertise, the patient's characteristics, and circumstances. The problem with multiple repeated attempts at conventional laryngoscopy is the creation of laryngeal edema and bleeding, which impair mask ventilation and subsequent endotracheal intubation attempts, thereby creating a CICV situation. Therefore, it is imperative that the anesthesiologist makes his or her optimal-best attempt at laryngoscopy as early as possible, under the best circumstances, which is usually the first or second attempt. If the optimal-best attempt fails twice, an alternative plan should be activated as the next step, so that no further risk is incurred from additional attempts without likely benefit.

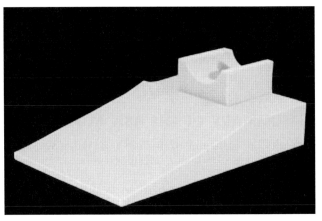

Figure 10-2 Troop Elevation Pillow with additional foam head rest. (Courtesy of Mercury Medical, Clearwater, FL.)

An *optimal-best attempt at conventional laryngoscopy* is defined as having the following characteristics[34,35]:

1. Performed by a reasonably proficient anesthesiologist with at least 3 years of experience (*Rationale:* If such an experienced anesthesiologist is having difficulty in visualizing the glottis, no other anesthesiologist or surgeon needs to or should attempt the same maneuver)
2. With the patient in the optimal "sniffing" position (*Rationale:* No attempt is wasted because the position was suboptimal; slight flexion of the neck on the head and severe extension of the head on the neck aligns the oral, pharyngeal, and laryngeal axes into a straight line; positioning devices are necessary in the obese patient [Fig. 10-2])
3. Using the appropriate type and length of blade (*Rationale:* Macintosh-type blades work best in patients with little upper airway room, and Miller-type blades are ideal for patients who have small mandibular space, anterior larynx, large incisors, or a long, floppy epiglottis). Based on most recent literature, a rigid video laryngoscope should be considered at least for the second attempt, if immediately available.
4. Using the appropriate blade length (*Rationale:* Patients' airways vary in size, and optimal fit of the blade to the airway allows the best possible pressure application to lift the epiglottis directly or indirectly)
5. Having a low threshold for using optimal external laryngeal manipulation (OELM) or backward upward rightward pressure (BURP) (Fig. 10-3) (*Rationale:* Both maneuvers can frequently improve the laryngoscopic view by at least one entire grade and should be an inherent part of laryngoscopy and an instinctive reflex response to a poor laryngoscopic view)

With this definition and no other confounding factors, an optimal-best attempt at laryngoscopy may be achieved on the first attempt, and no more than three attempts should be required (e.g., wrong blade, wrong length).

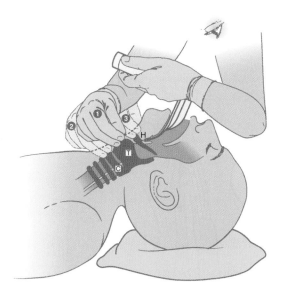

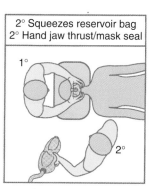

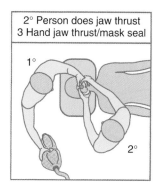

Two-person mask ventilation

2° Person does jaw thrust
3 Hand jaw thrust/mask seal

2° Squeezes reservoir bag
2° Hand jaw thrust/mask seal

Figure 10-4   Optimal mask ventilation. *Left,* Two-person effort when second person knows how to perform jaw thrust; *right,* two-person effort when second person can only squeeze the reservoir bag.

Figure 10-3   *Determining optimal external manipulation (OELM) with the free (right) hand. OELM should be an inherent part of laryngoscopy and is performed when the laryngoscopic view is poor. Ninety percent of the time, the best view is obtained by pressing over the thyroid cartilage (T, hand position 1) or the cricoid cartilage (C, position 2); pressing over the hyoid bone (H, position 3) may also be effective.*

C. Definition of Optimal-Best Attempt at Conventional Mask Ventilation

If the patient cannot be intubated, gas exchange is dependent on mask ventilation. If the patient cannot be ventilated by mask, a CICV situation exists, and immediate resuscitation maneuvers must be instituted. Because each of the acceptable responses to a CICV situation has its own risks, the decision to abandon mask ventilation should be made after the anesthesiologist has made an optimal-best attempt at mask ventilation.

An *optimal-best attempt at conventional mask ventilation* is defined as having the following characteristics[34,35]:

1. Performed by a reasonably proficient anesthesiologist with at least 3 years of experience (*Rationale:* as above)
2. With the patient in the optimal sniffing position (*Rationale:* as above)
3. Using two-person BMV with the most proficient anesthesiologist holding the mask and the less proficient anesthesiologist squeezing the bag (Fig. 10-4) (*Rationale:* Usually this leads to a far better mask seal, better jaw thrust, and therefore higher tidal volume than can be achieved with one person in a difficult-to-mask patient)
4. Using appropriately sized oropharyngeal or nasopharyngeal airway devices that have been inserted correctly (*Rationale:* This provides a canal for airflow through the soft tissue of the upper airway; establishes and improves tidal volume)

If mask ventilation is very poor or nonexistent, even with a vigorous two-person effort in the presence of large artificial airways, this constitutes a classic CICV scenario, and the team needs to start potentially life-saving plan B (see Fig. 10-1).

D. Options for the CICV Scenario

Both the LMA and the Combitube have been shown to work well to rescue airway emergencies.[17,36,37] The ASA DAA does not dictate the order of preference of these devices in the CICV situation, but the following considerations must be taken into account: (1) the anesthesiologist's own experience and level of comfort in the use of these methods, (2) the availability of these devices, (3) the type of airway obstruction (upper versus lower), and (4) the benefits and risks involved.

The ProSeal LMA usually forms a better seal than the LMA-Classic and provides improved protection against aspiration.[38-48] When properly positioned, the Combitube allows ventilation with a higher seal pressure than the LMA-Classic, protects against regurgitation,[49] and allows further attempts at intubation while the esophageal cuff protects the airway.[50] The Combitube has been successfully used in difficult intubation and CICV situations,[49,51-55] including ventilation failure with an LMA.[56]

Both the LMA and the Combitube are supraglottic ventilatory devices (Fig. 10-5). They cannot solve a truly glottic problem (e.g., spasm, massive edema, tumor, abscess) or a subglottic problem.[37] If an obstacle is suspected to exist in the glottic or subglottic area, the ventilatory mechanism (e.g., ETT, TTJV, rigid ventilating bronchoscope, surgical airway) needs to be positioned below the level of the lesion. The ASA DAA does not discriminate between the obstructed and the unobstructed airway, and this is a critical weakness of the algorithm.

E. Determinants of the Use of Muscle Relaxants for Difficult Airway Management

Muscle relaxants have different characteristics regarding time of onset and duration that significantly determine their advantages and disadvantages in the context of airway management (Table 10-2). The key elements in the choice of a nondepolarizing muscle relaxant are whether mask ventilation will be adequate and what rescue plan has been determined. For instance, with the induction of general anesthesia in an uncooperative

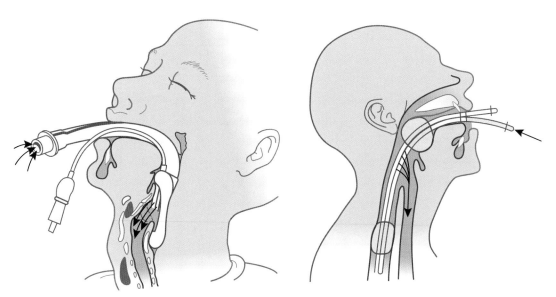

Figure 10-5 The laryngeal mask airway *(left)* and the Combitube *(right)* are supraglottic ventilatory devices.

patient who has a DA, the anesthesiologist should consider the relative merits of preservation of spontaneous ventilation versus use of muscle relaxants. Alternatively, if a small dose of succinylcholine (0.5 to 0.75 mg/kg) is used, good intubating conditions can be achieved within 75 seconds for about 60 seconds, allowing an early-awaken option if the ETT cannot be placed. In contrast, use of succinylcholine during DA management may not be the best choice if mask ventilation is considered possible and the alternative plan of action is FOB.[5]

Moreover, endotracheal intubation can be successfully accomplished without the use of any muscle relaxant, and this option should be considered in certain situations.[57,58] Another consideration is that in most patients, prior administration of a small dose of a nondepolarizing neuromuscular blocker may slightly diminish the duration of action of succinylcholine,[59] and therefore the time to spontaneous recovery of airway reflexes may be shortened.

Experts are debating whether a second dose of succinylcholine should be provided during a cannot-intubate situation when the patient resumes spontaneous ventilation. We believe that this practice is appropriate if the chance of successful endotracheal intubation is high (i.e., a fairly good laryngoscopic grade at the initial attempt) and laryngoscopy is difficult because of incomplete paralysis. A second dose of succinylcholine may also be appropriate when mask ventilation is possible, the laryngoscopist is highly skilled, and a simple change in either the patient's

position or the type of laryngoscope is necessary for final success. Glycopyrrolate at a dose of 0.2 to 0.4 mg should be administered in conjunction with the repeated dose of succinylcholine in order to prevent a bradycardic response.

F. Summary

In summary, the ASA DAA has worked well over the past decade. In fact, there has been a very dramatic decrease (30% to 40%) in the number of respiratory-related malpractice lawsuits, brain damage, and deaths attributable to anesthesia since 1990 (Fig. 10-6).[60] However, a number of issues have emerged that indicate that the algorithm can be improved, as discussed earlier. Consideration of these issues should make the algorithm still more clinically specific and functional. Nonetheless, the DAA provides excellent guidelines for anesthesiologists in their clinical decision-making for patients with DAs. Successful management in these cases is key to reducing the risk of anesthesia-related morbidity and mortality.

V. INTRODUCTION OF A NEW COMPREHENSIVE AIRWAY ALGORITHM

Based on the reasoning presented to this point, currently available evidence from the literature, and a plethora of clinical experience, we created a new and comprehensive algorithm for airway management with the intent of

TABLE 10-2

Advantages and Disadvantages of Muscle Relaxants with Different Durations of Action

Muscle Relaxant	Advantages	Disadvantages
Succinylcholine	Permits the awaken option at the earliest time possible	A period of poor ventilation (spontaneous or with positive pressure) may occur as the drug wears off Does not permit a smooth transition to plan B (e.g., use of a fiberoptic bronchoscope) and so on
Nondepolarizing	Permits a smooth transition to plan B and so on, provided mask ventilation is adequate	Does not allow awaken option at an early time

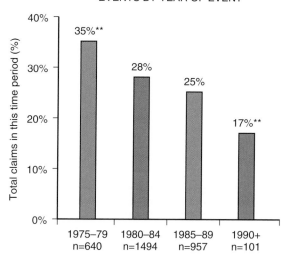

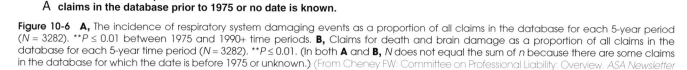

RESPIRATORY SYSTEM DAMAGING
EVENTS BY YEAR OF EVENT

** *P* ≤.01 between 1975 and 1990+ time periods; N = 3282
Claims for respiratory system damaging events as a proportion
of all claims in the database for each 5-year time period.
**Note: N does not equal the sum of n as there are some
claims in the database prior to 1975 or no date is known.**

A

CLAIMS FOR DEATH AND BRAIN
DAMAGE BY YEAR OF EVENT

**P ≤.01 between 1975 and 1990+ time periods; N = 3282
Claims for death and brain damage as a proportion of all
claims in the database for each 5-year time period.

B

Figure 10-6 A, The incidence of respiratory system damaging events as a proportion of all claims in the database for each 5-year period (*N* = 3282). *******P* ≤ 0.01 between 1975 and 1990+ time periods. **B,** Claims for death and brain damage as a proportion of all claims in the database for each 5-year time period (*N* = 3282). *******P* ≤ 0.01. (In both **A** and **B,** *N* does not equal the sum of *n* because there are some claims in the database for which the date is before 1975 or unknown.) (From Cheney FW: Committee on Professional Liability: Overview. *ASA Newsletter* 58:7-10, 1994.)

improving patient safety during the perioperative period. This new airway algorithm includes several subalgorithms that address the various potential clinical scenarios and suggest clear procedures and readily available equipment to solve the problem.

Most recently we incorporated the use of video laryngoscopy into the new comprehensive airway algorithm based on new evidence that strongly supports its role either as primary device or as first rescue device during the management of a difficult airway.[12,13]

The *main algorithm* comprises all the necessary information for routine airway management. It is supplemented with four subalgorithms (A through D) that describe maneuvers and instruments necessary to solve various DA scenarios and are organized in an escalating manner according to the immediate threat of the respective scenario. In addition, a fifth subalgorithm (E) suggests a standardized approach for extubation of these patients.

- *Subalgorithm A* = cannot ventilate, cannot intubate (CICV)
- *Subalgorithm B* = can ventilate but cannot intubate via laryngoscopy
- *Subalgorithm C* = ventilation established through a subglottic airway, further management options
- *Subalgorithm D* = surgical airway management
- *Subalgorithm E* = extubation of a patient with a known or suspected DA

Extubation of these patients carries significant risks and requires a systematic approach. To our knowledge, this new airway algorithm is the only algorithm that provides

a specific paradigm to address extubation of the patient with a DA.

A. The Main Algorithm

This algorithm (Fig. 10-7) is intended for and limited to elective surgery in the operating room and does not include airway trauma and crash intubations. As with the ASA algorithm, the crux of management of the DA lies in its recognition (Box 10-5). If difficulties are anticipated, surgery under regional anesthesia may be considered. However, there are anesthetic, surgical, and patient factors that may render the option of regional anesthesia for surgery inappropriate (Box 10-6). If regional anesthesia is considered appropriate and successful anesthesia is achieved, then surgery may proceed. However, if regional anesthesia fails, then the option for an awake airway technique or inhalation induction should be considered. Similarly, if regional anesthesia is not an appropriate option for surgery, then the performance of an awake intubation or inhalation induction is recommended.

The choice of awake versus asleep spontaneous ventilation depends on the experience of the anesthesiologist and the patient's level of cooperation. In general, the awake technique is the safest technique. However, in some patients (e.g., children; mentally retarded or incapacitated patients; aggressive, intoxicated, or delirious patients), an awake technique may not be possible. Additionally, in patients with cervical spine pathology who are at risk for neurologic injury, extreme caution should be exercised during an awake technique, and precautions should be undertaken to prevent any cervical movement.

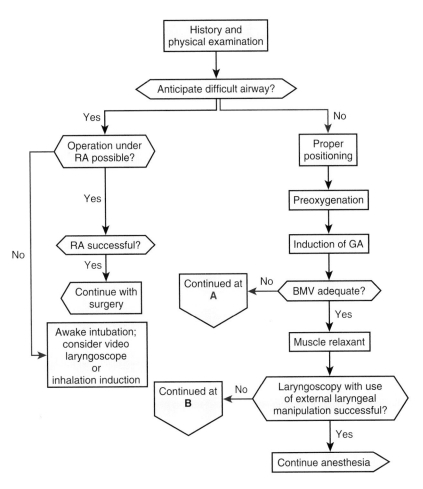

Figure 10-7 The main algorithm for airway management. *BMV,* Bag-mask ventilation; *GA,* general anesthesia; *RA,* regional anesthesia. (Courtesy of Ansgar Brambrink, MD, and Carin Hagberg, MD.)

Box 10-5 | Individual Predictors of Difficult Airway Management*

History

Congenital/acquired syndromes, malignancy, trauma, or disease states affecting the airway (e.g., diabetes, obstructive sleep apnea)
Recent difficult intubation
Prior surgery involving the larynx or neck

Physical

Facial hair (beard or mustache)
Prominent protruding teeth or dentures
Micrognathia
Limited mouth opening <4 cm
Inability to protrude mandible
Mallampati class III or IV
Thyromental distance <6 cm
Hyomental distance <4 cm
Sternomental distance <12 cm
Limited range of motion of neck <80°
Neck circumference >60 cm
Body mass index (BMI) >30 kg/m^2
Upper airway obstruction
Presence of blood or vomitus in oropharynx
Tracheal deviation

*Includes predictors of difficult mask ventilation, difficult laryngoscopy, difficult intubation, and surgical airway.

Failure of an awake technique usually falls into three categories: oversedation, obscuration of vision (by blood or secretions), and technical difficulties. If the patient is oversedated, airway issues may become complicated. If optimal attempts at BMV are successful, then Pathway B may be followed. However, if optimal attempts at BMV fail, the anesthesiologist should quickly proceed to Pathway A. If difficulty occurs with any of the awake fiberoptic techniques as a result of blood, mucus, or secretions such that adequate visualization is not possible, a blind technique may be considered (see "Bloody Airways.") Additionally, more invasive techniques, such as a surgical airway or retrograde intubation may be performed.

1. The Nonpredicted Difficult Airway

Although projected difficulties with airway management may not be present, making an optimal-best attempt at ventilation and intubation is paramount. First, even the best airway assessment will not detect 100% of DAs, as is evident from the literature. Second, the optimal-best attempt allows the anesthesiologist to follow the algorithm quickly and appropriately. Third, when the first attempt is the optimal-best attempt, this allows a greater margin of safety before patient decompensation begins. Fourth, making the first attempt the optimal-best attempt minimizes repeated attempts at airway manipulation,

Box 10-6 Factors Influencing the Choice of Regional Anesthesia (RA) in Patients with a Difficult Airway (DA)

Anesthesiologist

Expertise in both RA and DA management
Enough preoperative time to perform RA technique
Appropriate RA technique for surgical procedure
Prepared for alternative plans for DA management

Patient

Informed consent
Cooperative and calm
Adequate intravenous access
Hemodynamically stable
Ability to tolerate sedation, if required
Ability to communicate with anesthesiologist throughout procedure
No history of claustrophobia
Dependable and reliable
Willing and able to supplement RA with local anesthetics
Cooperative with primary and alternative plans for DA management

Surgical Procedure

Nonemergent
Appropriate duration
Patient position allows airway access during surgery
Procedure can be interrupted
Limited or moderate blood loss

Support

Equipment, including a DA cart with specialized devices and airway adjuncts
Staff (additional experienced anesthesiologists and operating room nurses)

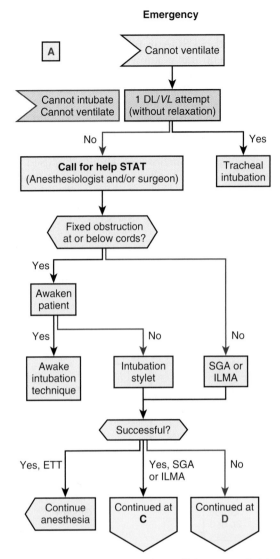

Figure 10-8 Pathway A: cannot ventilate, cannot intubate. *DL,* Direct laryngoscopy; *ETT,* endotracheal tube; *ILMA,* intubating laryngeal mask airway; *SGA,* supraglottic airway; *VL,* video laryngoscopy.

which may lead to greater morbidity. Therefore, the algorithm emphasizes proper positioning and the use of external laryngeal pressure even in patients without predicted airway difficulty.

After proper positioning, preoxygenation, and induction of general anesthesia, adequacy of BMV should be assessed. (An exception may be made for patients who undergo a rapid-sequence induction). If BMV is deemed adequate, intermediate- or long-acting muscle relaxants can be given to aid direct laryngoscopy. Liberal use of external laryngeal manipulation to optimize the laryngoscopist's view of the glottic opening is recommended. If BMV is inadequate despite optimal positioning and placement of an oropharyngeal or nasopharyngeal airway, then the "emergency situation," Pathway A, should be followed.

If direct laryngoscopy is successful, then surgery may proceed. However, if direct laryngoscopy is unsuccessful and BMV is adequate, then the "elective measures," Pathway B, should be followed. In performing a rapid-sequence induction, a short-acting muscle relaxant is usually given after induction of general anesthesia without checking BMV adequacy; therefore, if the anesthesiologist fails to intubate after induction, he or she should proceed directly to Pathway B and continue along the algorithm based on the initial laryngoscopic view.

2. New Algorithm Pathways

a. PATHWAY A

The CICV scenario is an emergency situation in which the optimal-best attempt at ventilation and intubation has failed (Fig. 10-8). If muscle relaxants have not been administered, then one further laryngoscopy attempt, preferably using a video laryngoscope if available, or a conventional direct laryngoscope.[12,13] without muscle relaxation can be made (preferably by another experienced anesthesiologist). If tracheal intubation fails, assistance should be summoned. Thereafter, the algorithm alerts the anesthesiologist to the difference in airway management with respect to the possibility of a fixed obstruction (e.g., tumor, vocal cord paralysis) at or below the cords.

If the patient has no known obstruction at or below the cords, a supraglottic airway (SGA) may help establish ventilation. If ventilation is inadequate via an SGA, then a surgical airway (Pathway D) should be performed. If an

SGA does establish adequate ventilation, then Pathway C is recommended, in which endotracheal intubation is performed with an SGA in place.

If the patient has a known fixed obstruction at or below the cords, then use of an SGA would be inappropriate. Ventilation attempts with an SGA would most likely be unsuccessful. If awakening the patient is a valid option, an awake intubation technique should be performed. If awakening the patient is not an option, an intubating stylet in combination with a video laryngoscope or a rigid bronchoscope should be used. These devices, unlike an SGA, allow the provider to establish a conduit beyond the obstructed area. Again, if these approaches are unsuccessful, rapid progression to a surgical airway via Pathway D is advised.

b. PATHWAY B

Pathway B (Fig. 10-9) is derived from a situation where oxygenation and ventilation are adequate but a definitive

airway has not been established. After calling for assistance and repeating laryngoscopy, using a video laryngoscope, if available, the management is divided based on the grade of glottic view. If a Cormack-Lehane grade 2B or 3 laryngoscopic view is visualized, an intubating stylet, or special laryngoscopic blade or video laryngoscope can be helpful. If this is successful, surgery may proceed. However, if the attempt is not successful, then adequacy of BMV must be reassessed, especially if BMV has not been attempted previously (i.e., rapid-sequence induction). If BMV is adequate, then further elective measures may be considered. If a grade 4 laryngoscopic view is observed, a retrograde technique may be considered or the anesthesiologist may proceed directly to SGA or ILMA, depending on the availability of equipment and the expertise of the anesthesiologist. However, if BMV is inadequate, then it is likely inappropriate to perform a fiberoptic intubation (FOI) or retrograde intubation. Instead, the anesthesiologist should recognize this as an emergent situation and immediately attempt SGA or ILMA.

c. PATHWAY C

Pathway C (Fig. 10-10) represents a situation in which the patient is anesthetized and oxygenation and ventilation are adequate via an SGA. The decision to intubate depends on the answer to the question, "Is endotracheal intubation necessary for the surgical procedure?" If the answer is "No," surgery may continue with an SGA. If the answer is "Yes," FOI through the SGA with an Aintree Intubation Catheter (Cook Critical Care, Bloomington, IN) may be performed. Alternatively, if an ILMA or CTrach (LMA International, Singapore) was inserted as the SGA, intubation via these devices is appropriate. However, if intubation attempts fail, it would be appropriate to awaken the patient and perform an awake intubation.

d. PATHWAY D

In Pathway D (Fig. 10-11), all attempts to oxygenate and ventilate the patient have been unsuccessful. A surgical airway is crucial, and in patients older than 6 years of age, the cricothyroid membrane (CTM) remains the window to the airway. However, if the patient is younger than 6 years old, the CTM is not well developed, and TTJV or the performance of a surgical tracheostomy is advised.

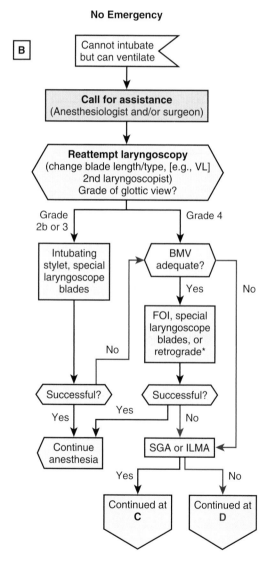

Figure 10-9 Pathway B: can ventilate, but cannot intubate via laryngoscopy. *FOI,* Fiberoptic intubation; *ILMA,* intubating laryngeal mask airway; *SGA,* supraglottic airway; *VL,* video laryngoscopy.

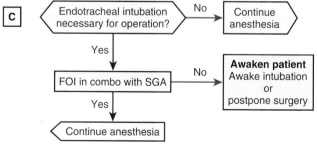

Figure 10-10 Pathway C: ventilation established through a subglottic airway, further management options. *FOI,* Fiberoptic intubation; *SGA,* supraglottic airway.

All Attempts to Oxygenate Unsuccessful, Mask Ventilation Impossible

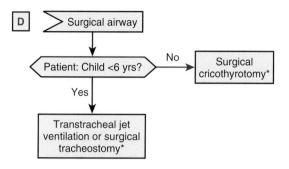

* Obtain surgeon's assistance, but without unnecessary delay, if possible

Figure 10-11 Pathway D: surgical airway management.

e. PATHWAY E

After a secure airway has been established, there will come a time when extubation is necessary. Consultants of the ASA Task Force on Management of the Difficult Airway,[5] as well as the Canadian Airway Focus Group, recommended a preformulated strategy for extubation of the DA.[61] Extubation strategies are discussed in detail in Chapter 50. Extubation strategies for the DA include, but are not limited to, bronchoscopic examination under general anesthesia through an SGA, substitution of an ETT with an SGA, and extubation over a TE.

Pathway E (Fig. 10-12) is an extubation algorithm in which a TE used is for patients who underwent multiple attempts at direct laryngoscopy or for whom alternative rescue devices were used. It should also be used for patients with a known or suspected DA who have undergone successful intubation. If the patient has met the extubation criteria (Box 10-7), one of the aforementioned extubation strategies can be used. A TE may be placed and the ETT removed over it, leaving the TE in the trachea. If ventilatory parameters and oxygenation are adequate, the TE can then be removed, provided there is no evidence of laryngeal edema or respiratory difficulty. The length of time for which these catheters are left in place is most commonly 30 to 60 minutes, although durations as long as 72 hours have been reported in the literature. Clinical judgment should be used according to the particular situation.

If minute ventilation, tidal volume, or oxygen saturation is inadequate, passive insufflation of oxygen or jet ventilation may improve the situation. If improvement does not occur or fails to be persistent, reintubation over a TE using direct laryngoscopy or video laryngoscopy is necessary. However, reintubation over the TE may not be successful for various reasons (e.g., kinked TE, wrong size TE, accidental TE removal, ETT catching at the arytenoids). If reintubation is unsuccessful, the TE should be removed and BMV adequacy ascertained. If BMV is adequate, the provider can attempt to establish an airway via Pathway B in a semielective fashion. If BMV is inadequate, the situation has become emergent, and one should continue rapidly down Pathway A.

Extubation of Patients with a Difficult Airway*

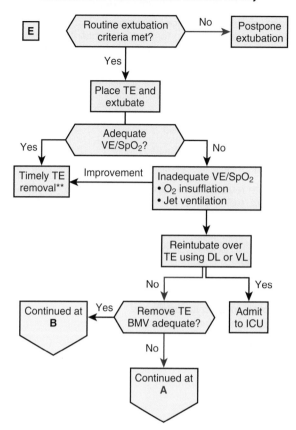

* Multiple attempts at DL or use of alternative device because of expected difficulty performing DL

**If there is no evidence of laryngeal edema or respiratory difficulty

Figure 10-12 Pathway E: a standardized approach for extubation of a patient with a known or suspected difficult airway. *BMV,* Bag-mask ventilation; *DL,* direct laryngoscopy; *ICU,* intensive care unit; *SpO₂,* peripheral oxygen saturation by pulse oximetry; *TE,* tube exchanger; *VE,* ventilation; *VL,* video laryngoscopy.

B. Shortcomings of the New Airway Algorithm

This new comprehensive algorithm is designed for use by anesthesiologists dealing with patients who are to undergo surgery. It is not designed for crash intubations or disrupted airways. It is not an attempt to encompass all airway situations. Rather, it focuses on airway issues in the operating room and guides the practitioner more thoroughly than other algorithms do in that setting.

To simplify the flow of decision making, the situations of failed awake technique and bloody airways are covered in this chapter text rather than in the actual algorithm. Also, a bloody airway can occur at any time in any pathway.

Some airway management algorithms attempt to cover all airway scenarios. They may mention several devices (e.g., Combitube, lighted stylets, ILMA, fiberoptic techniques) without clarification as to their limitations and, more importantly, when they are not appropriate or contraindicated. Blind nasal intubation may be promoted without consideration of disrupted airways and the

---

Box 10-7 Routine Extubation Criteria

Awake, alert, able to follow commands
• Sustained eye opening for pediatric patients or patients unable to understand commands

Vital signs stable
• Blood pressure, pulse rate, temperature
• Respiratory rate ≤30 breaths/min
• O_2 saturation

Protective reflexes returned
• Gag
• Swallow
• Cough

Adequate reversal of neuromuscular blockade
• TOF 4/4, sustained tetany at 50 Hz
• Strong hand grip
• Unassisted head lift (>5 sec)

Arterial blood gases reasonable with FiO_2 40%
• pH > 7.30
• PaO_2 ≥ 60 mm Hg
• $PaCO_2$ < 50 mm Hg

Respiratory mechanics adequate
• Tidal volume > 5 mL/kg
• Vital capacity > 15 mL/kg
• NIF > –20 cm H_2O

For patients at risk for laryngeal edema, consider cuff leak test and airway inspection
• FOB evaluation

FiO_2, Fraction of inspired oxygen; *FOB,* fiberoptic bronchoscopy; *NIF,* negative inspiratory force; *$PaCO_2$,* carbon dioxide tension; *PaO_2,* oxygen tension; *TOF,* train-of-four stimulation.

possibility of converting a clean airway to a bloody airway. Airway trauma may not be covered (and is also not covered in this algorithm). Finally, in other airway algorithms, the rapidly emerging and highly promising technology of video laryngoscopy is not considered and there is a lack of guidelines for using the SGA as a conduit for intubation.

C. Bloody Airways

If blood appears in the airway as a result of awake or asleep intubation techniques, direct visualization through a FOB may be technically challenging. In these cases, a video laryngoscopy plus high-volume oral-pharyngeal suction or a "blind" technique may be more useful. Three commonly used "blind" techniques are lightwand intubation, ILMA, and retrograde intubation.

D. Summary

The new comprehensive algorithm presented here streamlines the various airway management decisions, allowing the airway provider to focus on using rather than choosing airway devices. It emphasizes that the first attempt should be the best attempt and distinguishes supraglottic from nfraglottic obstruction. Also, it provides for the first time a systematic and evidence-based role for video laryngoscopy in management of the difficult airway.

Additionally, it clearly delineates pathways for intubation via an SGA, for airway issues encountered during awake fiberoptic intubations, and for extubation. Furthermore, these guidelines address issues such as bloody airways, as well as exclusion criteria for regional and awake techniques. Although this algorithm does not include crash intubations and disrupted airways, it focuses on airway issues in the operating room in great detail.

VI. CONCLUSIONS

Specific strategies can be linked together to form more comprehensive treatment plans or algorithms. The first comprehensive airway algorithm was introduced by the ASA in 1993, and after two revisions this algorithm has now provided guidance for more than 15 years. Yet, several shortcomings of the ASA algorithm can be identified. In this chapter, we present a new comprehensive airway management algorithm that eliminates some of the critical weaknesses of the predecessor ASA DAA. Based on its binary character, similar to that of ACLS algorithms, this new airway algorithm provides immediate direction in critical situations.

As the practice of airway management becomes more advanced, anesthesiologists must become both knowledgeable and proficient in the use of various airway devices and techniques. Although no airway algorithm can be practiced in its entirety on a regular basis, anesthesiologists need to incorporate alternative devices and techniques into their daily practice so that they can develop the confidence and skill required for their successful use in the emergent setting. All of the equipment described should be available for regular practice, and a DA cart or portable unit should be located near every anesthetizing location. Finally, appropriate follow-up and communication should be performed so that future caretakers will not unwittingly reproduce the same experience and risk.

VII. CLINICAL PEARLS

• There is strong evidence demonstrating that successful airway management in the perioperative environment depends on the specific strategies used. The purpose of the American Society of Anesthesiologists Algorithm on the Management of the Difficult Airway (ASA DAA) is to facilitate management of the difficult airway (DA) and to reduce the likelihood of adverse outcomes.

• We are presenting a new comprehensive airway management algorithm that is organized like the BLS/ACLS algorithms in a binary fashion and eliminates some of the weaknesses of the ASA DAA.

• Based on most recent evidence, video laryngoscopy emerges as a superior alternative for primary management of the difficult airway and as an excellent rescue device for failed DL in such circumstance.

• Recognizing the potential for difficulty leads to proper mental and physical preparation and increases the chance of a good outcome.

- Airway evaluation should take into account any characteristics of the patient that could lead to difficulty in the performance of (1) bag-mask or supraglottic airway ventilation, (2) laryngoscopy, (3) intubation, or (4) a surgical airway.

- In the anesthetized patient whose trachea has proved to be difficult to intubate, it is necessary to try to maintain gas exchange by mask ventilation between intubation attempts and also during intubation attempts, whenever possible.

- The most common scenario in the respiratory catastrophes reported in the ASA closed claims study was the development of progressive difficulty in ventilating by mask between persistent and prolonged failed intubation attempts; the final result was inability to ventilate by mask or to provide gas exchange.

- The Laryngeal Mask Airway (LMA) and the Combitube are supraglottic ventilatory devices and are not helpful if the airway obstruction is located at or below the glottic opening.

- Extubation of the patient with a DA should be carefully assessed and performed, and the anesthesiologist should develop a strategy for safe extubation of these patients (depending on the type of surgery, the condition of the patient, and the skills and preferences of the anesthesiologist).

- The presence and nature of the airway difficulty should be documented in the medical record.

- If blood appears in the airway as a result of awake or asleep intubation techniques, direct visualization through a fiberoptic bronchoscope may be technically challenging. In such situations, a blind technique may be more useful.

- Although no airway algorithm can be practiced in its entirety on a regular basis, anesthesiologists need to incorporate alternative devices and techniques into their daily practice so that they can develop the confidence and skill required for their successful use in the emergent setting.

SELECTED REFERENCES

All references can be found online at expertconsult.com.

1. American Society of Anesthesiologists Task Force on Management of the Difficult Airway: Practice guidelines for management of the difficult airway: A report. *Anesthesiology* 78:597–602, 1993.
2. Hagberg CA, Ghatge S: Does the airway examination predict difficult intubation? In Fleisher L, editor: *Evidence-based practice of anesthesiology*, Philadelphia, 2004, Elsevier Science, pp 34–46.
3. Langeron O, Masoo E, Huraux C, et al: Prediction of difficult mask ventilation. *Anesthesiology* 92:1229–1236, 2000.
5. Practice Guidelines for the Management of the Difficult Airway: An updated report by the American Society of Anesthesiologists Task Force on the Management of the Difficult Airway. *Anesthesiology* 98:1269–1277, 2003.
10. Mark L, Foley L, Michelson J: Effective dissemination of critical airway information: The Medical Alert National Difficult Airway/Intubation Registry. In Hagberg CA, editor: *Airway management: Principles and practice*, ed 2, Philadelphia, 2007, Mosby.
17. Benumof JL: Laryngeal mask airway: Indications and contraindications. *Anesthesiology* 77:843–846, 1992.
18. Caplan RA, Posner KL, Ward RJ, et al: Adverse respiratory events in anesthesia: A closed claims analysis. *Anesthesiology* 72:828–833, 1990.
27. Ezri T, Szmuk P, Warters RD, et al: Difficult airway management practice patterns among anesthesiologists practicing in the United States: Have we made any progress? *J Clin Anesth* 15:418–422, 2003.
32. Heidegger T, Gerig HJ, Ulrich B, et al: Validation of a simple algorithm for tracheal intubation: Daily practice is the key to success in emergencies—An analysis of 13,248 intubations. *Anesth Analg* 92:517–522, 2001.
60. Cheney FW: Committee on Professional Liability: Overview. *ASA Newsletter* 58:7–10, 1994.

PART 3

Preintubation-Ventilation Procedures

Chapter 11

Preparation of the Patient for Awake Intubation

CARLOS A. ARTIME | ANTONIO SANCHEZ

I. BACKGROUND

A. History

He sat in bed supporting himself with stiffened arms; his head was thrown forward, and he had the distressed anxiety so characteristic of impending suffocation depicted on his countenance. His inspirations were crowing and laboured.… He complained of intense pain … and begged that something should be done for his relief.

The preceding quotation is from Dr. Macewen's 1880 account in the *British Medical Journal* of the first awake endotracheal intubation and describes a patient suffering from glottic edema. The patient underwent an awake manual endotracheal intubation using a metallic endotracheal tube (ETT). This technique was performed without benefit of anesthesia and without topical or regional blocks, sedatives, or analgesics. The ETT was kept in place with the patient in an awake state for 36 hours.[1] Although one may perceive this as brutal, Dr. Macewen was aware, more than 130 years ago, that despite the patient's discomfort, the safest method for securing the airway was to perform an awake intubation (AI) rather than to provide comfort at the risk of further compromising the airway. Since that time, there have been countless reports of successful AI for management of the difficult airway (DA).[2-5]

B. Awake Intubation in Management of the Difficult Airway

The DA is defined as "the clinical situation in which a conventionally trained anesthesiologist experiences difficulty with mask ventilation, difficulty with endotracheal intubation, or both."[6,7] The American Society of Anesthesiologists (ASA) Closed Claims Study in 1990 found that 34% of injury cases in the Closed Claims database involved respiratory events.[8] The ASA formed the Task Force on Management of the Difficult Airway (TFMDA) in 1992 and sought to establish guidelines to facilitate the management of the DA and reduce the likelihood of adverse outcomes.[6] The task force constructed an algorithm to assist the anesthesiologist in devising a strategy for management of the DA (see Chapter 10). In this algorithm, one of the primary management choices for the anesthesiologist is the decision whether to perform AI or to attempt intubation after induction of general anesthesia.[6] In 2002, the practice guidelines were updated and the choice of AI remained an important component of the recommendations.[7]

C. Indications for Awake Intubation

The ASA algorithm stresses the concept that formulation of a strategy for intubation should include the feasibility of three basic options: (1) AI versus intubation after induction of general anesthesia, (2) noninvasive versus invasive (surgical) techniques, and (3) preservation versus ablation of spontaneous ventilation.[7] It is the opinion of most of the consultants of the TFMDA, and has been expressed in the literature,[2,3,5-7,9-11] that the safest method for a patient who requires endotracheal intubation and has a DA is for that patient to undergo AI for the following reasons:

1. Patency of the airway is maintained by upper pharyngeal muscle tone.
2. Spontaneous ventilation is maintained.
3. A patient who is awake and well topicalized is easier to intubate, because the larynx moves to a more anterior position after induction of anesthesia compared with the awake state.
4. The patient can still protect his or her airway from aspiration.
5. The patient is able to monitor his or her own neurologic symptoms (e.g., the patient with potential cervical pathology).[2,5,9]

General indications for AI are compiled in Box 11-1. There are no absolute contraindications to AI other than patient refusal, a patient who is unable to cooperate (such as a child, a mentally retarded patient, or an intoxicated, combative patient), or a patient with a documented true allergy to all local anesthetics.[9]

II. THE PREOPERATIVE VISIT

In this section, the focus is placed on elective patients, for whom there is time for airway evaluation and meaningful communication. In the setting of an emergency—which in itself should increase the probability of airway

---

BOX 11-1 Indications for Awake Intubation

1. Previous history of difficult intubation
2. Anticipated difficult airway based on physical examination:
   Small mouth opening
   Receding mandible/micrognathia
   Macroglossia
   Short, muscular neck
   Limited range of motion of the neck (rheumatoid arthritis, ankylosing spondylitis, prior cervical fusion)
   Congenital airway anomalies
   Morbid obesity
   Pathology involving the airway (tracheomalacia)
   Airway masses (malignancy of the tongue, tonsils, or larynx; large goiter; mediastinal mass)
   Upper airway obstruction
3. Unstable cervical spine
4. Trauma to the face or upper airway
5. Anticipated difficult mask ventilation
6. Severe risk of aspiration
7. Severe hemodynamic instability
8. Respiratory failure

From Kopman AF, Wollman SB, Ross K, et al: Awake endotracheal intubation: A review of 267 cases. *Anesth Analg* 54:323–327, 1975; Thomas JL: Awake intubation: Indications, techniques and a review of 25 patients. *Anaesthesia* 24:28–35, 1969; Bailenson G, Turbin J, Berman R: Awake intubation: Indications and technique. *Anesth Prog* 14:272–278, 1967.

---

difficulty, especially with a patient in extremis[9]—the physician may not have time, nor can he or she be expected to be able to perform the detailed investigation of the airway described here.

A. Reviewing Old Charts

Whenever possible, previous anesthesia records should be examined because they may provide useful information.[7,12] Obviously, the most important records are those involving intubation, especially the most recent ones. Other records documenting ease of mask ventilation and tolerance of drugs are also valuable. One should be alert for evidence of reactions to local anesthetics and of apnea with minimal doses of opioids. Another reason for checking as many anesthesia records as possible, including the surgical procedure involved, is that the last intubation may have been routine but the three previous ones may have been difficult, or the last intubation may have been routine but the operation then performed may have rendered the airway difficult.

When reading through a chart, one should focus on four important features:

1. Degree of difficulty of the endotracheal intubation (the difficulty encountered and the method used)
2. Positioning of the patient during laryngoscopy (sniffing position, use of a ramp)
3. Equipment used (even if the intubation was performed routinely in one attempt, a Bullard blade or a fiberoptic bronchoscope [FOB], neither of which requires alignment of the three axes, may have been used)

TABLE 11-1

Incidence of Recall among Patients Undergoing Awake Intubation (AI)

Reference	Number of AIs	Complete Amnesia	Partial Recall	Unpleasant Memories
Kopman, et al[2]	249	213	19	17
Thomas[5]	25	6	14	5
Mongan & Culling[17]	40	25	5	0
Ovassapian, et al[18]	129	89	37	3
Total	443	343 (77%)	75 (17%)	25 (6%)

4. Whether the technique that was used previously is a familiar one (one should not attempt to learn a new technique on a DA)

After the medical records have been reviewed, the preoperative interview should address the possibility of events that may have occurred since the last anesthesia, such as weight gain, laryngeal stenosis from previous airway intervention, facial cosmetic surgery (e.g., chin implants), worsening temporomandibular joint disorder, or worsening rheumatoid arthritis.

B. The Patient Interview

Dorland's Medical Dictionary defines "empathy" as the intellectual and emotional awareness and understanding of another person's thoughts, feelings, and behaviors, even those that are distressing and disturbing. Although the anesthesiologist may participate in 1000 operations per year, few patients undergo more than five in a lifetime.[13] The patient's perception of empathy from the physician is the cornerstone of the patient's acceptance of an AI. Empathy helps the interviewer establish effective communication, which is important for accurate diagnosis and management.[14] Two facets of medical education limit the clinician's development of empathy: the traditional format of interviewing training and the social ethos of medical training and medical practice, which stresses clinical detachment.[14,15] With empathy and the ability to communicate it, the physician can perform the interview in a more patient-oriented rather than disease-oriented fashion, resulting in better data gathering and better patient compliance.[16]

After the anesthesia practitioner has made the decision that AI is necessary, communication with the patient and psychological preparation is of the utmost importance to maximize the odds for a successful AI.[9] One should in a careful, unhurried manner describe to the patient conventional intubation contrasted with AI. Focusing on the fact that the former is easier and less time-consuming but that the latter is safer in light of the patient's own anatomy or condition, one must communicate to the patient that the knowledgeable, caring physician is willing to take extra measures to ensure the patient's safety. Recommendations should be presented to the patient with conviction but at the same time allowing the patient the option of the conventional method of intubation as a last resort.[10]

Complications of AI should also be presented, including local anesthetic toxicity, airway trauma, discomfort, recall, and failure to secure the airway. Patients' recall after AI using different methods of sedation, analgesia, or local anesthetics has not been studied in a controlled fashion. Although episodes of explicit awareness during general anesthesia are rare, the incidence of recall during AI with minimal levels of sedation is likely to be higher.[13] In a review of 443 cases of AI (four studies) in which various combinations of sedation and analgesia were used (Table 11-1), a mean of 17% of the patients had partial recall and 6% had recall with unpleasant memories.[2,5,17,18]

If a patient refuses AI, the anesthesiologist may discuss the case with the primary care physician or the surgeon, or both, in order to recruit their help to convince the patient of the importance of cooperation. If this and subsequent discussion with the patient are unsuccessful, the anesthesiologist should document these efforts in the chart.

III. PREOPERATIVE PREPARATIONS

The preparation of the patient for AI begins, as discussed, with the patient interview, followed by appropriate premedication (discussed later). Additional preparation for AI includes assembling the necessary equipment and arranging in advance for needed assistance.

A. Transport

The acuteness and urgency of the case must be considered when arranging transport to the operating room (OR). In some cases, the airway needs to be secured at once (e.g., the patient in extremis who warrants a bedside emergency airway procedure). In other cases, there is an urgent need for intubation but with sufficient time to transport the patient to the OR with supplemental oxygen (O_2) and appropriate monitors (electrocardiogram [ECG], pulse oximeter, and noninvasive blood pressure monitoring), accompanied by the anesthesiologist, surgeon, or both. Finally, there may be no requirement for immediate attention, and the patient can be transported routinely to the OR. In the elective scenario, supplemental O_2 should be provided, if appropriate (high-dose O_2 may be detrimental in some patients, such as those who rely on hypoxic respiratory drive),[13] and position should be considered (e.g., the patient who is morbidly obese may experience dramatic physiologic changes when supine and should be transported in a wheelchair or on a gurney in a semirecumbent position.).[19,20]

B. Staff

According to the TFMDA guidelines, there should be "at least one additional individual who is immediately available to serve as an assistant in difficult airway management."[7] Whenever possible, it is preferable to have a second member of the anesthesia care team who can assist in the monitoring, ventilation, and pharmacotherapy of the patient, as well as providing an extra set of hands during fiberoptic intubation (FOI). For patients in extremis and those who refuse AI, a surgeon trained in performing a surgical airway should be available with a tracheostomy/cricothyrotomy tray, ready to perform an emergency surgical airway, if necessary.

C. Monitors

During AI, the routine use of ECG, pulse oximetry, noninvasive blood pressure monitoring, and capnography is required as part of standard basic intraoperative monitoring. Depending on the complexity of the surgery and the patient's condition, invasive hemodynamic monitoring (i.e., arterial line) may need to be placed before AI. Indications for this procedure include hemodynamic instability, severe ischemic or valvular heart disease, and a patient for whom hypertension and tachycardia are potentially dangerous (e.g., the patient with aortic dissection or intracerebral aneurysm).

D. Supplemental Oxygen

Administration of supplemental O_2 should be considered throughout the process of DA management.[7] Arterial hypoxemia has been well documented during bronchoscopy, with an average decrease in arterial oxygen tension (PaO_2) of 20 to 30 mm Hg in patients breathing room air, and has been associated with cardiac dysrhythmias.[21] In addition, sedation administered to supplement topicalization for AI may result in unintended respiratory depression or apnea.

Studies have shown that either traditional preoxygenation (≥3 minutes of tidal volume [V_T] ventilation) or fast-track preoxygenation (i.e., four vital-capacity breaths in 30 seconds) is effective in delaying arterial desaturation during subsequent apnea.[7] Daos and colleagues showed that the use of supplemental O_2 delayed circulatory arrest resulting from local anesthetic toxic effects in animals.[22]

In the interest of improving patient safety, therefore, adequate preoxygenation and the use of supplemental O_2 throughout airway management (including sedation, topicalization, intubation, and extubation) is encouraged in all patients undergoing AI.[7]

In addition to the standard methods of supplemental O_2 delivery (nasal cannula or face mask), other opportunities include, but are not limited to, delivering O_2 through the suction port of a flexible fiberoptic bronchoscope (FFB),[9] delivering O_2 through an atomizer or nebulizer during topicalization, and elective transtracheal jet ventilation (TTJV) in a patient in extremis.[9,23,24]

Modified from Practice guidelines for management of the difficult airway: an updated report by the American Society of Anesthesiologists Task Force on Management of the Difficult Airway: Practice guidelines for management of the difficult airway. *Anesthesiology* 98:1269–1277, 2003.

E. Airway Equipment

Consultants of the TFMDA strongly agreed that "preparatory efforts enhance success and minimize risk to the patient" (i.e., lead to fewer adverse outcomes).[7] The concept of preassembled carts for emergency situations is not new; examples include "crash carts" for cardiac arrest and malignant hyperthermia carts. The task force recommends that every anesthetizing location should have readily available a portable storage unit that contains specialized equipment for DA management. Suggested contents of this portable unit are listed in Box 11-2.

There are many techniques that can be used to secure the airway in the awake patient. Direct laryngoscopy, video laryngoscopy, intubating laryngeal mask airways (iLMAs), FFB, rigid fiberoptic laryngoscopy, retrograde intubation, lighted stylets, and blind nasal intubation have all been used successfully to perform AI.[2,25-30] No matter which technique is selected, all of the necessary equipment should be prepared ahead of time and readily available when needed. The practitioner should also have several backup modalities in mind, and the required equipment available, in case the initial technique used is ineffective.

TABLE 11-2

Pharmacologic Characteristics of Anticholinergic Drugs

Drug	Tachycardia	Antisialagogue Effect	Sedation
Atropine	+++	++	+
Glycopyrrolate	++	+++	0
Scopolamine	+	+++	+++

0, No effect; +, minimal effect; ++, moderate effect; +++, marked effect.
Adapted from Morgan GE Jr, Mikhail MS, Murray MJ: *Clinical anesthesiology*, ed 3, New York, 2002, McGraw-Hill, p 208.

IV. PREMEDICATION AND SEDATION

Once the preoperative visit is concluded and the patient has agreed to proceed with AI, premedication is commonly employed to alleviate anxiety, provide a clear and dry airway, protect against the risk of aspiration, and enable adequate topicalization of the airway. The agents most commonly used in the preparation for AI include antisialagogues, mucosal vasoconstrictors, aspiration prophylaxis agents, and sedatives/hypnotics.

A. Antisialagogues

One of the most important goals of premedication for AI is drying of the airway. Secretions can obscure the view of the glottis, especially when FFB is used. In addition, secretions can prevent local anesthetics from reaching intended areas, resulting in failed sensory blockade, or they can wash away and dilute local anesthetics, diminishing their potency and duration of action.

The medications most often used for their antisialagogic properties are the anticholinergics.[31] These drugs inhibit salivary and bronchial secretions by their antimuscarinic effects. Because they only prevent formation of new secretions and do not eliminate secretions that are already present, anticholinergics should be administered at least 30 minutes before topicalization. The anticholinergics used in clinical practice are atropine, glycopyrrolate, and scopolamine. A summary of their pharmacologic properties is presented in Table 11-2.

1. Atropine

Atropine (0.4 to 0.6 mg IV or IM) has a rapid onset after intravenous (IV) administration of 1 minute; the onset after intramuscular (IM) dosing is 15 to 20 minutes. Atropine produces only a mild antisialagogic effect, but it causes significant tachycardia because of its potent vagolytic effects. As such, it is not an ideal drug for use in drying the airway. As a tertiary amine, it easily crosses the blood-brain barrier and causes mild sedation. It may occasionally cause delirium, especially in elderly patients.

2. Glycopyrrolate

Glycopyrrolate (0.2 to 0.3 mg IV or IM) has an onset after IV dosing of 1 to 2 minutes; the onset after IM dosing is 20 to 30 minutes. The duration of its vagolytic effect after IV dosing is 2 to 4 hours; its antisialagogic effect lasts longer. Glycopyrrolate is devoid of central nervous system effects because its quaternary amine structure prevents passage through the blood-brain barrier. Its pharmacologic profile makes it the drug of choice as a premedicant for AI.

3. Scopolamine

Scopolamine (0.4 mg IV or IM) has an onset of 5 to 10 minutes after IV dosing and 30 to 60 minutes after IM. The duration of action is about 2 hours after IV dosing and 4 to 6 hours after IM dosing. In addition to being a very effective antisialagogue, scopolamine has very potent central nervous system effects, with sedative and amnestic properties. In some patients, however, this may lead to restlessness, delirium, and difficulty waking after short procedures. Because it is the least vagolytic of the anticholinergics in clinical use, it may be the drug of choice for patients in whom tachycardia is contraindicated.

B. Nasal Mucosal Vasoconstrictors

The nasal mucosa and nasopharynx are highly vascular. When a patient requires nasal AI, adequate vasoconstriction is essential, because bleeding can make FOI extremely difficult. One agent commonly used for this purpose is 4% cocaine, which has vasoconstrictive as well as local anesthetic effects (see later discussion). An alternative to cocaine is a 3:1 mixture of 4% lidocaine and 1% phenylephrine, which yields a solution of 3% lidocaine with 0.25% phenylephrine.[32] When these agents are applied with cotton swabs or pledgets to the nasal area, adequate anesthesia and vasoconstriction can be achieved in 10 to 15 minutes, facilitating nasal AI. Alternatively, vasoconstrictive nose sprays may be administered to the patient before local anesthetic topicalization. Phenylephrine 0.5% and oxymetazoline 0.05% sprays are available. They should be administered 15 minutes before attempted nasal intubation.

C. Aspiration Prophylaxis

A percentage of patients requiring AI may need prophylaxis against aspiration pneumonitis because of the presence of risk factors such as a full stomach, symptomatic gastroesophageal reflux disease, hiatal hernia, presence of a nasogastric tube, morbid obesity, diabetic gastroparesis, or pregnancy.[33,34]

Preoperative administration of a nonparticulate antacid, such as sodium citrate, provides effective buffering of gastric acid pH.[35] Total gastric volume is increased, but this effect is offset by an increase in the pH of gastric fluid so that, if aspiration occurs, morbidity and mortality are significantly lower.[36] One disadvantage of sodium citrate is the potential to cause emesis due to its unpleasant taste.

1. Histamine Receptor Blockers

Histamine (H_2) receptor blockers are selective and competitive antagonists that block secretion of hydrogen ion

(H^+) by gastric parietal cells and also decrease the secretion of gastric fluid. With IV administration of cimetidine 300 mg, famotidine 20 mg, or ranitidine 50 mg, peak effects are achieved within 30 to 60 minutes, increasing gastric pH and decreasing gastric volume.[37,38] Of the three, ranitidine is probably the drug of choice because it has fewer adverse effects, greater efficacy, and a longer duration of action.[39,40]

2. Proton Pump Inhibitors

Proton pump inhibitors (PPIs), such as pantoprazole and omeprazole, have not been shown to be as effective as H_2 blockers at increasing gastric pH and decreasing gastric volume.[41,42] PPIs may have a role in aspiration prophylaxis for the patient on chronic H_2 blocker therapy.[43]

3. Metoclopramide

Metoclopramide is a dopamine antagonist that stimulates motility of the upper gastrointestinal tract and increases lower esophageal sphincter tone. The net effect is accelerated gastric emptying with no effect on gastric pH. The standard adult dose is 10 mg IV. Metoclopramide can precipitate extrapyramidal symptoms and should be avoided in patients with Parkinson's disease.[34] For patients at high risk for aspiration, antacids, H_2 blockers, and metoclopramide may be used alone or in combination.

D. Sedatives/Hypnotics

Depending on the clinical circumstance, IV sedation may be useful in allowing the patient to tolerate AI by providing anxiolysis, amnesia, and analgesia. Benzodiazepines, opioids, hypnotics, α_2-agonists, and neuroleptics can be used alone or in combination.[25] It is important that these agents be carefully titrated to effect, because oversedation can render a patient uncooperative and make AI more difficult.[9] Spontaneous respiration with adequate oxygenation and ventilation should always be maintained.[25] Care should be taken in the presence of critical airway obstruction, because awake muscle tone is sometimes necessary in these patients to maintain airway patency.[44] Avoidance of oversedation is also important in the patient with a full stomach, because an awake patient can protect his or her own airway in the chance of regurgitation.[9]

1. Benzodiazepines

Benzodiazepines, via their action at the γ-aminobutyric acid (GABA)–benzodiazepine receptor complex, have hypnotic, sedative, anxiolytic, and amnestic properties.[45] They have also been shown to depress upper airway reflex sensitivity,[46] a property that is desirable for AI. Benzodiazepines are frequently used to achieve sedation for AI in combination with opioids,[47] and they are used for their amnestic and anxiolytic effects when other sedatives (e.g., dexmedetomidine, ketamine, remifentanil) are chosen as the primary agent.[48,49] Three benzodiazepine receptor agonists are commonly used in anesthesia practice: midazolam, diazepam, and lorazepam.[45]

a. MIDAZOLAM

Because of its more rapid onset and relatively short duration, midazolam is the most commonly used agent.

Sedation with midazolam is achieved with doses of 0.5 to 1 mg IV repeated until the desired level of sedation is achieved. The IM dose is 0.07 to 0.1 mg/kg. Onset is rapid, with peak effect usually achieved within 2 to 3 minutes of IV administration. The duration of action is 20 to 30 minutes, with termination of effect primarily a result of redistribution. Although recovery is rapid, the elimination half-life is 1.7 to 3.6 hours, with increases noted in patients with cirrhosis, congestive heart failure, or morbid obesity; in the elderly; and in patients with renal failure. It is extensively metabolized by the liver and renally eliminated as glucuronide conjugates.[45,50]

b. DIAZEPAM AND LORAZEPAM

Diazepam has a slightly slower onset and longer duration of action than midazolam and has been shown to be a less potent amnestic.[45,50,51] It can cause pain on IV injection and has the added risk of thrombophlebitis.[25] Lorazepam provides the most profound sedating and amnestic properties; however, it is more difficult to use, because these effects are slower in onset and longer lasting than with either midazolam or diazepam.[25,45]

c. PRECAUTIONS

Care must be used when using benzodiazepines in combination with other sedative drugs. The pharmacologic effects of benzodiazepines are augmented synergistically by other medications used for sedation, including opioids and α_2-agonists.[52] Propofol has been shown to increase the plasma concentration of midazolam by decreasing distribution and clearance.[53] Systemic absorption of local anesthetics used for airway topicalization may also lead to potentiation of the sedative/hypnotic effects of midazolam.[54]

The primary adverse effect of oversedation with benzodiazepines is respiratory depression, which may lead to hypoxemia or apnea.[45] Flumazenil, a specific benzodiazepine antagonist, may be used to reverse the sedative and respiratory effects of benzodiazepines if a patient becomes too heavily sedated. It is given in incremental IV doses of 0.2 mg, repeated as needed to a maximum dose of 3 mg. Because it has a half-life of 0.7 to 1.8 hours, resedation can be a problem if flumazenil is being used to reverse high doses or longer-acting benzodiazepines, and patients should be monitored carefully in those circumstances. Flumazenil is generally safe and devoid of major side effects.[55,56]

2. Opioids

Opioids, by way of their agonist effect on opioid receptors in the brain and spinal cord, provide analgesia, depress airway reflexes, and prevent hyperventilation associated with pain or anxiety. These properties make them a useful addition to the sedating regimen for AI. Although any opioid receptor agonist could theoretically be used for this purpose, the synthetic phenylpiperidine class of opioids—fentanyl, sufentanil, alfentanil, and remifentanil—are best suited to the task. These drugs are particularly useful due to their rapid onset, relatively short duration of action, and ease of titration.[57]

a. FENTANYL

Analgesic doses range from 0.5 to 2 µg/kg IV. Onset is rapid, within 2 to 3 minutes. Duration of a single bolus dose is roughly 30 to 60 minutes. The duration is relatively short because fentanyl is redistributed to a large peripheral compartment rather than rapidly eliminated. Hence, the duration of effect after cessation of a prolonged infusion is markedly longer, due to redistribution to the central compartment from the peripheral compartment. Fentanyl is widely used in anesthesia practice, and it seems to be the most commonly used opioid for AI.[47,58]

b. SUFENTANIL

Sufentanil is 7 to 10 times more potent than fentanyl and has a similar pharmacokinetic profile after a single bolus dose. The primary difference is a significantly faster recovery, compared with fentanyl, after prolonged infusion.[59] Sedative doses are 5 to 20 µg IV in adult patients. Its use in combination with midazolam and droperidol for AI has been reported.[60]

c. ALFENTANIL

Compared with fentanyl and sufentanil, alfentanil has an even quicker onset (1.5 to 2 minutes). It is approximately 1/70 as potent as fentanyl; however, because of rapid plasma to effect-site equilibration, comparatively smaller doses are needed to achieve a similar peak effect. Because smaller doses are needed relative to its potency, recovery from a single bolus of alfentanil is faster than with the other agents of this class, potentially making alfentanil the drug of choice when a transient peak effect after a single bolus is desired, as in AI.[59] Sedative doses range from 10 to 30 µg/kg IV.[57] In patients premedicated with oral diazepam, alfentanil 20 µg/kg IV significantly improved fiberoscopic conditions and attenuated the hemodynamic effects of awake nasal FOI. Moderate respiratory depression was noted without overt apnea or hypoxia.[61]

d. REMIFENTANIL

Remifentanil is an ultrashort-acting opioid that is unique compared with the other short-acting agents in that it is metabolized by nonspecific plasma esterases, with a half-life of 3 minutes. It undergoes no redistribution and therefore has no context sensitivity. Its potency approximates that of fentanyl.[62] Several studies have shown the effectiveness and safety of remifentanil sedation for AI as a single agent,[48,49,63] as well as in combination with midazolam or propofol.[64-68] Dosing is usually weight-based.

Several different remifentanil dosing strategies have been described in the literature for AI, with infusion rates ranging between 0.06 and 0.5 µg/kg/min, with or without an initial bolus of 0.5 to 1.5 µg/kg.[48,63,64,67] Studies using target-controlled infusions for AI have shown that the mean effect-site concentration of remifentanil needed for AI is 2 to 3 ng/mL.[49,65,66,68] The dosing strategy described by Atkins and Mirza,[62] a bolus of 0.5 µg/kg followed by an infusion of 0.1 µg/kg/min, uses the Minto pharmacokinetic model and rapidly achieves a target site concentration of 2 to 2.5 ng/mL. The infusion can subsequently be titrated by 0.025 to 0.05 µg/kg/min in 5-minute intervals to achieve adequate sedation.

e. PRECAUTIONS

The most serious adverse effect of opioids is respiratory depression leading to overt apnea. Opioids reduce the stimulatory effect of carbon dioxide (CO_2) on ventilation while increasing the apneic threshold and the resting end-tidal CO_2. Factors that increase susceptibility to opioid-induced respiratory depression include old age, obstructive sleep apnea, and concomitant administration of central nervous system depressants.

Naloxone, an opioid antagonist, can be used to restore spontaneous ventilation in patients after an opioid overdose. Onset after IV administration is rapid, within 1 to 2 minutes, and the duration of action is 30 to 60 minutes. Naloxone should be administered in boluses of 0.04 to 0.08 µg IV boluses every 2 to 3 minutes. Doses of 1 to 2 µg/kg will restore adequate spontaneous ventilation in most cases while preserving adequate analgesia. Potential complications of naloxone administration are reversal of analgesia, tachycardia, hypertension, and, in severe cases, pulmonary edema or myocardial ischemia. Because of the relatively short duration of action of naloxone, one should carefully monitor for recurrence of respiratory depression, especially when it is used to reverse longer-acting opioids such as morphine or hydromorphone. In those situations, an intramuscular dose of 2 times the required IV dose or a continuous IV infusion (2.5 to 5 µg/kg/hr) should be considered.[57]

Chest wall rigidity leading to ineffectual bag-mask ventilation is commonly cited as a potential adverse effect of opioids, particularly fentanyl, sufentanil, alfentanil, and remifentanil. Opioids do have the potential to cause muscle rigidity, but clinically significant rigidity usually occurs only after an opioid dose sufficient to cause apnea, because the patient loses consciousness.[57] Studies in intubated patients and patients with tracheostomies have shown that decreases in pulmonary compliance due to chest wall rigidity are not sufficient to explain an inability to maintain bag-mask ventilation after a large dose of opioid,[69,70] and fiberoscopic examination of the vocal cords during induction with sufentanil has shown that vocal cord closure is the primary cause of difficult ventilation after opioid-induced anesthesia.[71] Careful titration to prevent overdose is perhaps the best way to prevent rigidity-associated difficult ventilation. Should it occur, treatment with naloxone or neuromuscular blocking agents is effective.[72,73]

3. Intravenous Anesthetics

a. PROPOFOL

Propofol (2,6-diisopropylphenol) is the most frequently used IV anesthetic today.[45] Its primary effect is hypnosis, which results from an unclear mechanism; however, there is evidence that a significant portion of this hypnotic effect is mediated by interaction with GABA receptors. Propofol has a rapid onset of approximately 90 seconds, with rapid recovery (4 to 5 minutes after an induction dose) as a result of both elimination and redistribution. It attenuates airway responses in induction doses via an unclear mechanism and provides a smooth induction with few excitatory effects. Although it is frequently used as an induction agent in doses of 1.5 to 2.5 mg/kg IV, intermittent doses of approximately 0.25 mg/kg IV or a continuous IV infusion of 25 to 75 µg/kg/min provides an easily titratable level of sedation with rapid recovery.

The use of propofol in AI is well described both as a single agent and in combination with remifentanil.[26,65,68] Target-controlled infusion studies have shown that the effective plasma concentration of propofol to facilitate AI is 1 to 2 µg/mL.[26,65,68] Care should be taken if the patient has a critical airway, because propofol causes reduction of V_t and an increase in respiratory frequency at sedative doses. At sufficiently elevated plasma concentrations, propofol can lead to apnea. Other common adverse effects are a decrease in arterial blood pressure and pain on injection. An additional benefit of propofol is its antiemetic properties.

b. DEXMEDETOMIDINE

Dexmedetomidine is a centrally acting, highly selective α_2-adrenoreceptor agonist with several properties that make it well suited for use in AI.[74-77] It has sedative, analgesic, anxiolytic, antitussive, and antisialagogue effects while causing minimal respiratory impairment, even at high doses. Compared with clonidine, it is 8 to 10 times more specific for the α_2- versus the α_1-adrenergic receptor and has a shorter half-life (2 to 3 hours). Dexmedetomidine sedation provides unique conditions in which the patient is asleep but is easily arousable and cooperative when stimulated. It is approved for continuous IV sedation in intubated and mechanically ventilated patients and for sedation in nonintubated patients undergoing surgical or other procedures.

There are several reports of dexmedetomidine sedation in awake FOI,[77-80] including a phase IIIb Food and Drug Administration (FDA) study specifically for this indication.[81] Dosing for AI is a 1 µg/kg load over 10 minutes, followed by a continuous infusion of 0.2 to 0.7 µg/kg/hr. Some patients may require higher maintenance doses.[82,83] A reduced loading dose of 0.5 µg/kg and a reduction in the maintenance infusion should be considered in elderly patients (age >65 years) and in those with hepatic or renal impairment.[84] For AI, dexmedetomidine is usually combined with airway topicalization, although its successful use as a sole agent without local anesthetics has been reported.[78] Although lowering of bispectral index scores (BIS) and partial amnesia have been reported with its use,[85,86] dexmedetomidine is not a reliable amnestic and is frequently combined with midazolam to decrease the incidence of recall.[79,87]

Dexmedetomidine can cause adverse hemodynamic effects including bradycardia, hypotension, and hypertension. During the loading dose, hypertension and bradycardia can occur due to stimulation of peripheral postsynaptic α_{2B}-adrenergic receptors, resulting in vasoconstriction. Central α_{2A}-mediated sympatholysis eventually leads to bradycardia, hypotension, and decreased cardiac output.[88] The bradycardic effect can be mitigated by pretreatment with an anticholinergic (e.g., glycopyrrolate) or by combining the dexmedetomidine with

ketamine for its cardiostimulatory properties.[79,89] Caution should be used in patients with depressed systolic function.[84]

c. KETAMINE

Ketamine[45] is a phencyclidine derivative and N-methyl-D-aspartate (NMDA) antagonist that produces *dissociative anesthesia*, which manifests clinically as a cataleptic state with eyes open and many reflexes intact, including the corneal, cough, and swallow reflexes. Ketamine-induced anesthesia is associated with amnesia, nystagmus, and the potential for hallucinations and other undesirable psychological reactions. Benzodiazepines are commonly administered to attenuate or treat these reactions; dexmedetomidine has also been shown to reduce the incidence and severity of ketamine-induced postanesthesia delirium.[90] Ketamine has an opioid-sparing effect and produces analgesia that extends well into the postoperative period, because plasma levels required for analgesia are considerably lower than those required for loss of consciousness. Usual doses for sedation range from 0.2 to 0.8 mg/kg IV, with peak plasma levels occurring after less than 1 minute and a duration of hypnosis of 5 to 10 minutes. At these doses, minute ventilation, V_t, FRC, and the minute ventilation response to CO_2 are maintained. Although airway reflexes and upper airway skeletal muscle tone are preserved, airway protection remains necessary in patients who are at risk for aspiration.

Ketamine increases blood pressure, heart rate, cardiac output, and myocardial O_2 consumption via a centrally mediated stimulation of the sympathetic nervous system. Ketamine is a direct myocardial depressant, however, and in patients with depleted catecholamine stores (e.g., the patient in shock), it may cause hypotension.[91] Its use in AI has been described in combination with benzodiazepines and dexmedetomidine.[2,89,92] Patients receiving ketamine sedation should always be pretreated with an antisialagogue, because ketamine causes increased airway secretions that can lead to upper airway obstruction or make FOI difficult.

d. DROPERIDOL

Droperidol, a butyrophenone, is a neuroleptic medication occasionally used in anesthesia practice for its sedative and antiemetic properties.[10,45] Its mechanism of action is antagonism of dopamine receptors in the central nervous system; it also interferes with GABA-, norepinephrine-, and serotonin-mediated neuronal activity. In combination with fentanyl, it produces a state of hypnosis, analgesia, and immobility classically referred to as *neuroleptanalgesia*. In combination with a hypnotic or nitrous oxide, droperidol and fentanyl produce general anesthesia (*neuroleptanesthesia*), not unlike the dissociative state produced by ketamine. Neuroleptanalgesia has been used for AI with favorable results.[2,93,94] In this state, patients may experience extreme fear and apprehension despite appearing outwardly calm; droperidol is also a poor amnestic. For this reason, benzodiazepines should be administered for anxiolysis and amnesia.

Doses for neuroleptanalgesia range from 2.5 to 5 mg IV; the antiemetic dose is 0.625 to 1.25 mg. Onset is in 20 minutes, with a half-life of about 2 hours. Side effects include mild hypotension due to peripheral α-adrenergic blockade, dysphoria, and extrapyramidal symptoms. Droperidol can also cause QT prolongation, especially in larger doses. This has led to an FDA "black box" warning concerning the risk for potentially fatal torsades de pointes. As a result, droperidol should not be administered to patients with a prolonged QT interval (>440 msec for males, >450 msec for females), and ECG monitoring should be performed during and for 2 to 3 hours after treatment.[95]

V. TOPICALIZATION

Topicalization of the airway with local anesthetics should, in most cases, be the primary anesthetic for AI; many times, it is all that is needed.[9] When using local anesthetics, it is important to be familiar with the speed of onset, duration of action, optimal concentration, signs and symptoms of toxicity, and maximum recommended dosage of the drug chosen.[96] The rate and amount of topical local anesthetic absorption vary depending on the site of application, the concentration and total dose of local anesthetic applied, the hemodynamic status of the patient, and individual patient variation.[97] Local anesthetic absorption is more rapid from the alveoli than from the tracheobronchial tree, and more rapid from the tracheobronchial tree than from the pharynx. The most commonly used agents for topical anesthesia of the airway are lidocaine and cocaine.

Although AI with airway topicalization is considered the safest method of airway management for the patient with a DA, it is not without risk. Local anesthetic toxicity is a real concern; death due to lidocaine toxicity of a healthy volunteer undergoing bronchoscopy has occurred.[98,99] In addition, total airway obstruction during topical anesthesia in a nonsedated patient with a critical airway has been reported. This was postulated to have been caused by dynamic airway obstruction related to loss of upper airway tone as a result of topicalization.[100]

A. Lidocaine

Lidocaine, an amide local anesthetic, is the most commonly used agent for airway topicalization.[101,102] It is available in various concentrations (1% to 10%) and in preparations including aqueous and viscous solutions, ointments, gels, and creams. For infiltration and minor nerve blocks, 1% to 2% lidocaine is commonly used; for topical anesthesia, the concentration used is 2% to 4%. Lidocaine is an excellent choice for airway anesthesia because of its reasonably rapid onset of 2 to 5 minutes and its high therapeutic index. Its duration of action is 30 to 60 minutes after topical application or infiltration; addition of epinephrine extends the duration to 2 to 3 hours when used for infiltration. It is hepatically metabolized with a half-life of 90 minutes; care should be taken in patients with hepatic failure.

The maximum recommended dosage for infiltration of lidocaine without epinephrine is 5 mg/kg of lean body mass. For topicalization of the airway, the maximum dose is less well established. The British Thoracic Society recommends a maximum dose of 8.2 mg/kg,[103] based on

a study by Langmack and associates.[104] Studies of plasma concentration after nebulization of 6 mg/kg of lidocaine showed peak plasma levels an order of magnitude lower than the toxic plasma level of 5 μg/mL.[105] Other studies using total doses as high as 10.5 mg/kg in obese patients failed to demonstrate signs or symptoms of lidocaine toxicity.[106] Early symptoms of lidocaine toxicity include euphoria, dizziness, tinnitus, confusion, and a metallic taste in the mouth. Signs of severe lidocaine toxicity include seizures, respiratory failure, loss of consciousness, and circulatory collapse. In asthmatics, lidocaine has been reported to precipitate bronchoconstriction by a nonhistamine-mediated mechanism.[107]

B. Cocaine

Cocaine, a naturally occurring ester anesthetic, is used primarily for anesthesia of the nasal mucosa when the nasal route is planned for AI.[108] It has a vasoconstrictor property that makes it particularly useful for this application, because the nose is highly vascularized and bleeding can make FOI impossible. It is available commercially as a 4% solution (each drop containing 3 mg), and can be applied to the nasal mucosa using cotton pledgets or cotton-tipped swabs. The maximum recommended dosage for intranasal application is 1.5 mg/kg. After topical application of cocaine to the nasal mucosa, peak plasma levels are achieved in 30 to 45 minutes, and the drug persists in the plasma for 5 to 6 hours.

Cocaine is primarily metabolized by plasma pseudocholinesterase; it also undergoes slow hepatic metabolism and is excreted unchanged by the kidney. The signs and symptoms of cocaine toxicity include tachycardia, cardiac dysrhythmia, hypertension, and fever. Severe complications include convulsions, respiratory failure, coronary spasm, cardiac arrest, stroke, and death. It must be used with caution in patients with hypertension, coronary artery disease, hyperthyroidism, pseudocholinesterase deficiency, or preeclampsia, and in those patients taking monoamine oxidase inhibitors.

C. Other Local Anesthetics

Benzocaine is a water-insoluble ester-type local anesthetic agent that is mainly useful for topical application. The onset of action is rapid (<1 minute), and the effective duration is 5 to 10 minutes. Benzocaine is most commonly available as a 20% aerosol spray that is easily applied to the oropharyngeal mucosa. The limiting factor in benzocaine use is the potential development of clinically significant methemoglobinemia. In some patients, this can occur with as little as 1 to 2 seconds of spraying.[109] The risk increases by almost 20-fold when benzocaine exposure is repeated within 1 week. Although most patients tolerate benzocaine airway topicalization without any adverse effects, it is not possible to identify in advance those patients who are at risk for significant methemoglobinemia. Some have advocated for the cessation of benzocaine use across the board.[110] Symptoms of early methemoglobinemia toxicity can be seen with methemoglobin levels of 5% and include cyanosis, tachycardia, and tachypnea. As levels increase to 20% to 30%, patients may develop chest pain, ischemic changes on ECG, hypotension, altered mental status, syncope, or coma. The most severe cases have led to neurologic hypoxic injury, myocardial infarction, and death. Should symptomatic methemoglobin occur, treatment is with methylene blue 1 to 2 mg/kg IV given over 5 minutes.[110,111]

Tetracaine is an amide local anesthetic agent with a longer duration of action than lidocaine or cocaine. It is available as 0.5% to 1% solutions for local use. It is metabolized through hydrolysis by plasma cholinesterase. Tetracaine is rapidly absorbed from the respiratory and gastrointestinal tract when used to anesthetize the airway, and aerosol doses as small as 20 mg have been shown to precipitate toxicity.[112] Severe toxic reactions after tetracaine overdose include convulsions, respiratory arrest, and circulatory collapse.[113] Fatalities have been reported with topical application of tetracaine 100 mg used to anesthetize mucous membrane.[114] These issues have limited its use as a primary local anesthetic for airway topicalization.

Cetacaine is a topical application spray containing 14% benzocaine, 2% tetracaine, and 2% butyl aminobenzoate (a local anesthetic similar to benzocaine). Like 20% benzocaine spray, this combination produces rapid airway anesthesia, but with a prolonged duration of action compared to benzocaine alone. The risk of methemoglobinemia is still a consideration, and cases of severe toxicity have been reported.[115,116]

EMLA cream (eutectic mixture of local anesthetic) contains 2.5% lidocaine and 2.5% prilocaine and is considered a topical anesthetic for use on intact skin. Although the manufacturer does not recommend its use on mucosal surfaces because of faster systemic absorption, it has been employed safely as a topical anesthetic for AI. Larijani and colleagues described 20 adult patients who underwent awake FOI using 4 g of EMLA applied over the upper airway. The measured peak plasma concentrations of lidocaine or prilocaine did not reach toxic levels, and methemoglobin levels did not exceed normal values (1.5%).[117]

Benzonatate, an oral antitussive chemically similar to ester-type local anesthetics, has also been used for airway topicalization. The dose used is 200 mg; the capsules are pierced with a needle, and the patient is instructed to crush the capsules with the teeth or to hold the capsules in the back of the mouth. Oropharyngeal anesthesia is quickly obtained. In a study by Mongan and Culling, intubating conditions using benzonatate were comparable to those achieved with topical benzocaine and superior laryngeal nerve blocks, with no adverse effects noted.[17]

D. Application Techniques

1. Atomizers

A common method for applying local anesthetic to the airway is with an atomizer. One system for local anesthetic atomization involves the use of a standard DeVilbiss atomizer with the bulb removed. The atomizer reservoir is filled with 2% to 4% lidocaine. O_2 tubing is connected from the atomizer to an O_2 cylinder with a flow rate of 8 to 10 L/min. A bleed hole is cut in the O_2

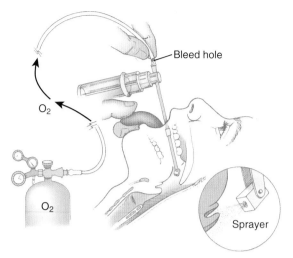

Figure 11-1 Atomizer connected to an oxygen tank. A bleed hole is made near the operator's hand to allow intermittent spraying. Inset shows the tip of the atomizer as it is angulated to spray toward the glottic opening. (From Difficult Airway: Teaching Aids. Irvine, University of California, Department of Anesthesia.)

tubing; this allows for intermittent application of the local anesthetic when a thumb is placed over the hole in the tubing. The atomizer spray is directed toward the soft palate and posterior pharynx to topicalize the mucosa (Fig. 11-1). Any residual anesthetic agent in the oropharynx should be suctioned out to reduce absorption from the gastrointestinal tract. Disposable plastic atomizers are available for this purpose as well (Fig. 11-2). The device is attached to an O_2 tank, and the phalange is depressed to deliver the local anesthetic solution to the oropharyngeal mucosa. A disadvantage with these methods is the difficulty of controlling the exact amount of local anesthetic administered.

Alternatively, the MADjic Mucosal Atomization Device (Wolfe Tory Medical, Inc., Salt Lake City, UT) is an inexpensive, disposable, latex-free device that, when attached to a Luer fitted syringe containing local anesthetic, can be used to dispense a fine mist to the oropharyngeal or nasal mucosa (Fig. 11-3). The tubing is

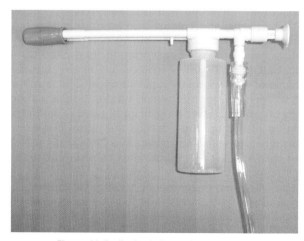

Figure 11-2 Typical disposable atomizer.

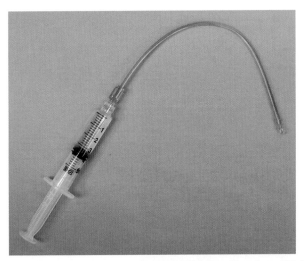

Figure 11-3 MADjic Mucosal Atomization Device. (Courtesy of Wolfe Tory Medical, Inc., Salt Lake City, UT).

malleable, allowing for delivery of local anesthetic to deeper pharyngeal structures and to the glottis. Because a syringe is used, a known amount of local anesthetic can be administered.

2. Nebulizers

Nebulizers may be used to apply local anesthetic to the airway. The advantages of this technique include ease of application and safety. A standard mouthpiece-type nebulizer (Fig. 11-4) can topicalize the oropharynx and trachea. If nasal cavity anesthesia is needed, a facemask-type nebulizer (Fig. 11-5) can be used; the patient is instructed to breathe in through the nose. This approach is especially advantageous for patients with increased intracranial pressure (ICP), open eye injury, or severe coronary artery disease.[118] Foster and Hurewitz compared the administration of lidocaine using two different modalities (nebulizer-atomizer combination and atomizer alone) in patients undergoing bronchoscopy.[119] They found that the nebulizer-atomizer combination was more efficacious, resulting in a reduction of the dose required to anesthetize the upper airway. A typical dose of lidocaine used in a standard nebulizer is 4 mL of 4% lidocaine. This results in a total dose of 160 mg of lidocaine, which is well within the safe dosage range. Studies using

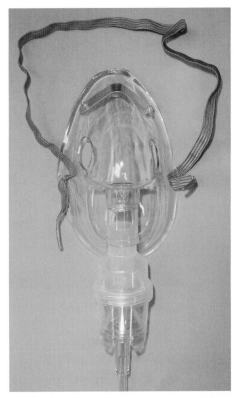

Figure 11-5 Typical facemask-type nebulizer.

6 mg/kg of 10% lidocaine showed that peak plasma concentrations are much lower than would be expected if all the lidocaine had been absorbed—evidence that some of the local anesthetic is lost during exhalation.[105]

3. "Spray-As-You-Go"

In addition to using a nebulizer or an atomizer to anesthetize the vocal cords and trachea, a technique termed "spray-as-you-go" through the FFB can be performed. The technique is noninvasive and involves injecting local anesthetics through the suction port of the FOB. Two methods have been described. The first requires attaching a triple stopcock (Fig. 11-6) to the proximal portion of

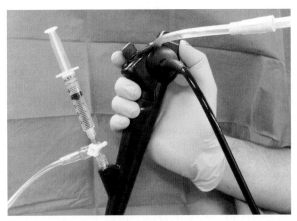

Figure 11-6 "Spray-as-you-go" technique. An oxygen hose and a triple stopcock are attached to the suction port of a flexible fiberoptic bronchoscope with syringe attached containing local anesthetic.

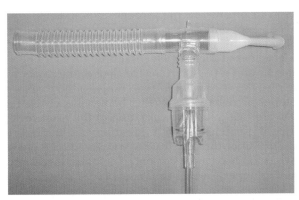

Figure 11-4 Typical mouthpiece-type nebulizer.

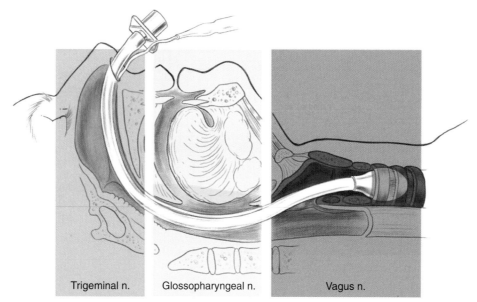

Trigeminal n.   Glossopharyngeal n.   Vagus n.

Figure 11-7 Innervation of the upper airway. (From Brown D, editor: *Atlas of regional anesthesia*, ed 2, Philadelphia, 1999, Saunders.)

the suction port to connect O_2 tubing from a regulated O_2 tank set to flow at 2 to 4 L/min. Under direct vision through the bronchoscope, targeted areas are sprayed with aliquots of 0.2 to 1.0 mL of 2% to 4% lidocaine. The physician then waits 30 to 60 seconds before advancing to deeper structures and repeating the maneuver. The flow of O_2 allows higher delivery of a higher fraction of inspired oxygen (FIO_2), keeps the FOB lens clean, disperses mucous secretions away from the lens, and aids in nebulizing the local anesthetic. The second method involves passing a multiorifice epidural catheter (0.5- to 1.0-mm inner diameter [ID]) through the suction port of an adult FOB.[120] These techniques are especially useful in patients who are at risk for aspirating gastric contents because the topical anesthetic is applied only seconds before the intubation is accomplished, allowing the patient to maintain airway reflexes as long as possible.

VI. NERVE BLOCKS

Because of the multitude of nerves innervating the airway (Fig. 11-7), there is no single anatomic site where a physician can perform a nerve block and anesthetize the entire airway. Even though topicalization of the mucosa serves to anesthetize the entire airway adequately in most patients, some require supplementation to ablate sensation in the nerve endings that run deep to the mucosal surface, such as the periosteal nerve endings of the nasal turbinates and the stretch receptors at the base of the tongue, which are involved in the gag reflex. Some studies have shown superior patient comfort and hemodynamic stability when a combined regional block technique was used rather than nebulized local anesthetic.[121] The following nerve blocks are remarkable for their ease of performance, their minimal risk to the patient, and their speed of onset. Nerve blocks are applied to the nasal cavity and nasopharynx,[4,12,102,122-127] the oropharynx,[12,102,122,128-134] the larynx,[9,12,25,102,113,122,128,135-140] and the trachea and vocal cords.[12,25,102,113,122,141]

A. Nasal Cavity and Nasopharynx

1. Anatomy

Most of the sensory innervation of the nasal cavity is derived from two sources: the sphenopalatine ganglion and the anterior ethmoidal nerve. The sphenopalatine ganglion (pterygopalatine, nasal, or Meckel's ganglion) is a parasympathetic ganglion that is located in the pterygopalatine fossa (Fig. 11-8A), posterior to the middle turbinate. Its sensory root is derived from sphenopalatine branches of the maxillary nerve, cranial nerve (CN) V_2. As they pass through the sphenopalatine ganglion, these sensory branches form the greater and lesser palatine nerves, which provide sensory innervation to the nasal cavity as well as the roof of the mouth, soft palate, and tonsils. The anterior ethmoidal nerve (see Fig. 11-8B) is one of the sensory branches of the ciliary ganglion, which is located within the orbital cavity and inaccessible to nerve blocks. It provides sensory innervation to the anterior portion of the nasal cavity.

2. Nasal Pledgets or Nasopharyngeal Airways

Regardless of which technique is used to anesthetize the nasal cavity, the nares should first be inspected for a deviated septum by using a nasal speculum and asking the patient to breathe deeply through each individual naris while the opposite naris is occluded. Patency can also be determined by using bayonet forceps to place cotton pledgets soaked in either 4% cocaine or 4% lidocaine with epinephrine 1:200,000 along the floor of the nasal cavity. The pledgets are advanced posteriorly to the level of the posterior nasopharyngeal wall. The benefits of this technique are that initial topicalization of the nasal cavity is achieved, the angle of ETT insertion can be predicted, and dilation of the nasal cavity is initiated. The pledgets are then followed by placement of nasopharyngeal airway (nasal trumpet) coated in 2% to 4% viscous lidocaine (a 34-F nasal trumpet predicts easy passage of a 7.0-mm ID ETT).[4,102]

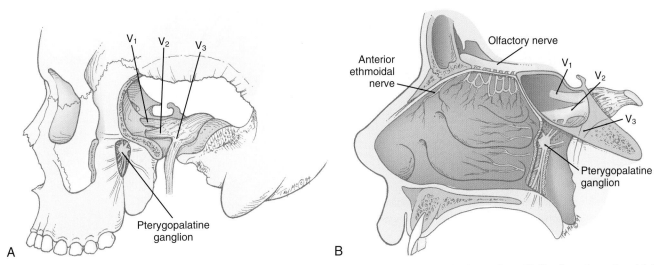

Figure 11-8 **A,** Left lateral view of the skull with temporal bone removed depicting the trigeminal ganglion with the three branches (V_1 to V_3) of the trigeminal nerve. V_2 is the major contributor to the sphenopalatine (pterygopalatine) ganglion, shown as it sits in the pterygopalatine fossa. **B,** Left lateral view of the right nasal cavity depicting the anterior ethmoidal nerve, olfactory nerve, and the trigeminal nerve (V_1 to V_3). The pterygopalatine ganglion lies just beneath the mucosal surface on the caudad surface of the sphenoid sinus and forms the roof of the pterygopalatine fossa. (From Difficult Airway: Teaching Aids. Irvine, University of California, Department of Anesthesia.)

3. Sphenopalatine Nerve Block

a. ORAL APPROACH

With the patient in the supine position, the physician stands facing the patient on the contralateral side of the nerve to be blocked. Using the nondominant index finger, the physician identifies the greater palatine foramen. It is located on either side of the roof of the mouth between the second and third maxillary molars, approximately 1 cm medial to the palatogingival margin, and can usually be palpated as a small depression near the posterior edge of the hard palate. In approximately 15% of the population, the foramen is closed and inaccessible. A 25-G spinal needle, bent 2 to 3 cm proximal to the tip to an angle of 120 degrees, is inserted through the foramen in a superior and slightly posterior direction to a depth of 2 to 3 cm. An aspiration test is performed to ascertain that the sphenopalatine artery has not been cannulated, and 1 to 2 mL of 2% lidocaine with epinephrine 1:100,000 is injected. The epinephrine is used as a vasoconstrictor for the sphenopalatine artery, which runs parallel to the nerves, to decrease the incidence of epistaxis. The injection of the local anesthetic should be performed in a slow, continuous fashion (preventing acute increases in pressure within the fossa) to decrease sympathetic stimulation.[123-125,127]

This block anesthetizes the greater and lesser palatine nerves as well as the nasociliary and nasopalatine nerves, which also contribute to the sensory innervation of the nasal cavity. Complications include bleeding, infection, nerve trauma, intravascular injection of local anesthetic, and hypertension. Pain on insertion of the needle can be avoided by application of 2% viscous lidocaine with a cotton-tipped applicator for 1 to 2 minutes before the block is applied. See Figures 11-9 and 11-10.

b. NASAL APPROACH

Two noninvasive nasal approaches to the sphenopalatine ganglion have been described, both of which take advantage of the ganglion's shallow position beneath the nasal mucosa. The first involves the application of long cotton-tipped applicators soaked in either 4% cocaine or 4% lidocaine with epinephrine 1:200,000 over the mucosal surface overlying the ganglion (Fig. 11-11A). The applicator is passed along the upper border of the middle turbinate at an angle of approximately 45 degrees to the hard palate and directed posteriorly until the upper posterior

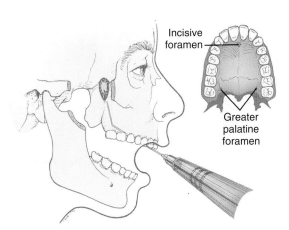

Figure 11-9 Inferior view of the hard palate showing location of the greater palatine foramen. Right lateral view of the head with zygomatic arch and coronoid process of the mandible removed to expose the sphenopalatine ganglion, with angulated spinal needle in place. (From Difficult Airway: Teaching Aids. Irvine, University of California, Department of Anesthesia.)

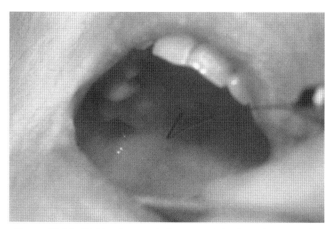

Figure 11-10 Right sphenopalatine nerve block, oral approach.

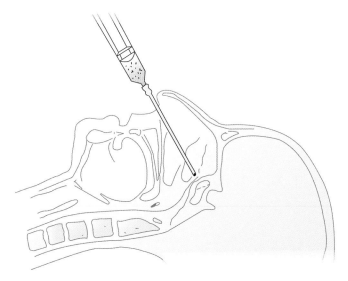

Figure 11-12 Left lateral view of the right nasal cavity. Angiocatheter with syringe angled at 45 degrees to the hard palate is aimed at the sphenopalatine ganglion. (Modified from Boudreaux AM: Simple technique for fiberoptic bronchoscopy. *Am Soc Crit Care Anesthesiol* 6:8, 1994.)

wall of the nasopharynx (sphenoid bone) is reached. The applicator is then left in place for 5 to 10 minutes. The second method involves using the plastic sheath of a 20-G angiocatheter placed along the same path (Fig. 11-12). An anesthetic solution (4 mL of 3% lidocaine/0.25% phenylephrine) is then rapidly injected. About 2 minutes should be allowed for the anesthetic to take effect.[4,122,123,126]

4. Anterior Ethmoidal Nerve Block

The anterior ethmoidal nerve is blocked by insertion of a long cotton-tipped applicator, soaked in either 4% cocaine or 4% lidocaine with epinephrine 1:200,000, parallel to the dorsal surface of the nose until it meets the anterior surface of the cribriform plate

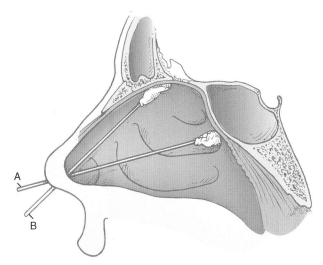

Figure 11-11 Left lateral view of the right nasal cavity, showing long cotton-tipped applicators soaked in local anesthetic. *A,* Applicator angled at 45 degrees to the hard palate with cotton swab over mucosal surface overlying the sphenopalatine ganglion. *B,* Applicator placed parallel to the dorsal surface of the nose, blocking anterior ethmoidal nerve. (From Difficult Airway: Teaching Aids. Irvine, University of California, Department of Anesthesia.)

(see Fig. 11-11B). The applicator is held in position for 5 to 10 minutes.[126]

B. Oropharynx

1. Anatomy

The somatic and visceral afferent sensory fibers of the oropharynx are supplied by a plexus derived from the vagus (CN X), facial (CN VII), and glossopharyngeal (CN IX) nerves. The glossopharyngeal nerve (GPN) emerges from the skull through the jugular foramen and passes anteriorly between the internal jugular and carotid vessels, traveling along the lateral wall of the pharynx. It supplies sensory innervation to the posterior third of the tongue via the lingual branch and to the vallecula, the anterior surface of the epiglottis, the posterior and lateral walls of the pharynx, and the tonsillar pillars. Its only motor innervation in the pharynx is to the stylopharyngeus muscle, one of the muscles of deglutition.

In most patients, topicalization of the mucosa of the oropharynx is sufficient to allow instrumentation of the airway. In some, however, the gag reflex is so pronounced that topicalization alone may be insufficient for AI. The afferent limb of the gag reflex arises from stimulation of deep pressure receptors found in the posterior third of the tongue, which cannot be reached by the diffusion of local anesthetics through the mucosa. There are various measures for minimizing this problem: instructing the patient to breathe in a nonstop panting fashion, avoiding pressure on the base of the tongue by performing a nasal intubation, administering opioids, and performing blockade of the GPN. The GPN block is easy to perform and is highly effective in abolishing the gag reflex and decreasing the hemodynamic response to laryngoscopy, including awake laryngoscopy. Several different approaches have been described.

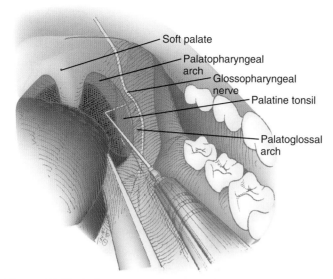

Figure 11-13 Left glossopharyngeal nerve block, posterior approach. A 25-G spinal needle bent at a right angle (or a tonsillar needle) is placed behind the midportion of the palatopharyngeal fold. (From Difficult Airway: Teaching Aids. Irvine, University of California, Department of Anesthesia.)

2. Glossopharyngeal Nerve Block

a. POSTERIOR APPROACH (PALATOPHARYNGEAL FOLD)

The classic intraoral approach to the GPN block involves injecting local anesthetic at the base of the posterior tonsillar pillar (palatopharyngeal fold).[102,128,129] Because of the proximal location of the nerve targeted, this technique has the potential to block both the sensory fibers (pharyngeal, lingual, and tonsillar branches) and the motor branch innervating the stylopharyngeus muscle.

After adequate topicalization of the oropharynx, the patient is placed in a semireclined position with the physician facing the patient on the ipsilateral side of the nerve to be blocked. The patient's mouth is opened wide. With a tongue depressor held in the nondominant hand, the tongue is displaced caudad and medially, exposing the soft palate, uvula, palatoglossal arch, tonsillar bed, and palatopharyngeal arch (Figs. 11-13 and 11-14). This

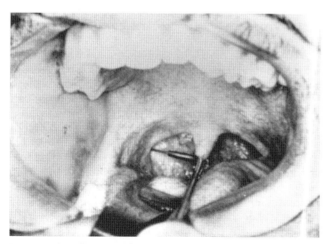

Figure 11-14 Right glossopharyngeal nerve block, posterior approach.

maneuver stretches both the palatopharyngeal arch and the palatoglossal arch, making them more accessible. A Macintosh size 3 laryngoscope blade may also be useful for retraction, because it provides additional light. The dominant hand holds a 23-G tonsillar needle attached to a syringe. Alternatively, a 22-G, 9-cm spinal needle with the distal 1 cm of the needle bent at a 90-degree angle may be used. The needle is inserted submucosally into the caudad portion of the posterior tonsillar pillar. After an attempt to aspirate blood, 5 mL of 0.5% to 1% lidocaine is slowly injected. If blood is aspirated or the patient complains of headache during injection, the needle should be removed and repositioned. The procedure is repeated on the contralateral side.

Because of the proximity of the GPN at this location to the internal carotid artery, care must taken to avoid intra-arterial injection, which could result in headache or seizure. Hypopharyngeal swelling and mucosal bleeding may occur. Tachycardia may also result from blockade of the afferent nerve fibers of the GPN that arise from the carotid sinus.[133]

b. ANTERIOR APPROACH (PALATOGLOSSAL FOLD)

The lingual branch of the GPN provides sensory innervation to the posterior third of the tongue and is the afferent limb of the gag reflex. The anterior approach, which isolates this branch as it passes medial to the base of the anterior tonsillar pillar, is easier and is better tolerated by the patient because it requires less exposure.[9,130-132]

The patient is placed in the sitting position with the physician facing the patient on the contralateral side of the nerve to be blocked. The patient's mouth is opened wide with the tongue protruded. With the nondominant hand, the physician uses a tongue blade or a Macintosh size 3 laryngoscope blade to displace the tongue medially, forming a gutter or trough along the floor of the mouth between the tongue and the teeth. The gutter ends in a cul-de-sac formed by the base of the palatoglossal arch (also known as the anterior tonsillar pillar), which is a U- or J-shaped structure that starts at the soft palate and runs along the lateral aspect of the pharynx. A 25-G spinal needle is inserted 0.25 to 0.5 cm deep at the base of the palatoglossal arch, just lateral to the base of the tongue, and an aspiration test is performed (Figs. 11-15 and 11-16). If air is aspirated, the needle has been advanced too deeply (i.e., the tip has advanced all the way through the palatoglossal arch) and should be withdrawn until no air can be aspirated; if blood is aspirated, the needle should be redirected more medially. Two mL of 1% to 2% lidocaine is injected, and the procedure is repeated on the contralateral side.

Although this block is targeted at the lingual branch of the GPN, studies using methylene blue dye have shown that, in some cases, retrograde submucosal tracking of local anesthetic occurs, blocking more proximal branches of the GPN (i.e., pharyngeal and tonsillar branches). Serious complications are rare for this approach, although one study reported that 91% of patients undergoing this procedure experienced oropharyngeal discomfort for at least 24 hours after the procedure.[134]

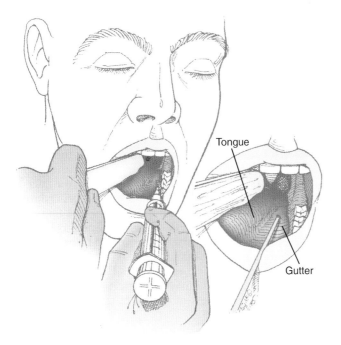

Figure 11-15 Left glossopharyngeal nerve block, anterior approach. The tongue is displaced medially, forming a gutter (glossogingival groove), which ends distally in a cul-de-sac. A 25-G spinal needle is placed at the base of the palatoglossal fold. (From Difficult Airway: Teaching Aids. Irvine, University of California, Department of Anesthesia.)

c. EXTERNAL APPROACH (PERISTYLOID)

The external approach is most useful when the patient's mouth opening is insufficient to allow adequate visualization to perform one of the intraoral blocks.[102,129] The patient is placed supine with the head in a neutral position. The styloid process is located by identifying the midpoint of the line between the mastoid process and the angle of the jaw. A skin wheal with local anesthetic is made at this location, and a 22-G spinal needle is advanced perpendicularly to the skin until the styloid process is contacted. Depending on the patient's habitus, this should occur at a depth of 1 to 2 cm. The needle is then redirected posteriorly, and as soon as contact is lost

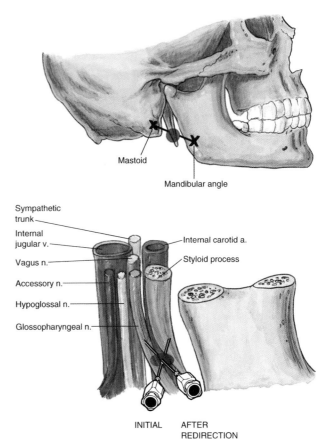

Figure 11-17 Glossopharyngeal nerve block, peristyloid approach. A 22-G spinal needle is inserted to contact the styloid process. It is then redirected posteriorly, putting the tip of the needle near the glossopharyngeal nerve. (From Brown D, editor: *Atlas of regional anesthesia*, ed 2, Philadelphia, 1999, Saunders.)

with the styloid process, 5 to 7 mL of 0.5% to 1% lidocaine is injected after a negative aspiration for blood (Fig. 11-17). The procedure is then repeated on the opposite side. Similar precautions should be taken for the peristyloid approach as for the posterior approach because of the proximity of the GPN at this anatomic location to both the internal carotid artery and the internal jugular vein.

C. Larynx

1. Anatomy

Sensory innervation of the larynx is supplied by the superior laryngeal nerve (SLN), a branch of the vagus nerve. The SLN originates from the ganglion nodosum and descends deep to the carotid artery. It then courses anteriorly, and at the level of the cornu of the hyoid bone it branches into the external and internal branches. The external branch supplies motor innervation to the cricothyroid muscle, which functions to tighten and elongate the vocal cords. The internal branch of the SLN contains sensory fibers that are distributed to the base of the tongue, vallecula, epiglottis, aryepiglottic folds, arytenoids, and glottis down to the level of the vocal cords. It passes medially between the greater cornu of the hyoid bone and the superior cornu of the thyroid cartilage and

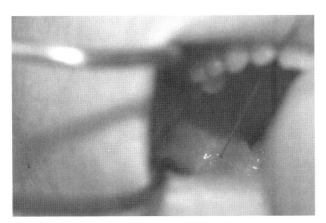

Figure 11-16 Right glossopharyngeal nerve block, anterior approach. (From Difficult Airway: Teaching Aids. Irvine, University of California, Department of Anesthesia.)

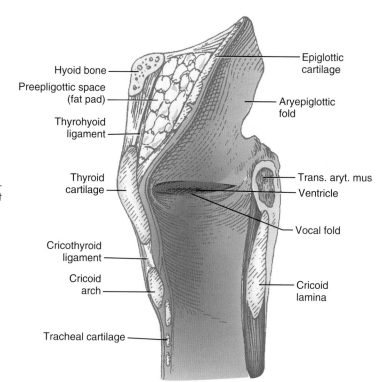

Figure 11-18 Midsagittal view of the larynx showing the pre-epiglottic space containing fat pad and thyrohyoid ligament (see Fig. 11-19).

pierces the thyrohyoid membrane along with the superior laryngeal artery and vein. The nerve then lies in the paraglottic space, a closed space bounded by the thyrohyoid membrane laterally and the laryngeal mucosa medially, where it ramifies (Figs. 11-18 and 11-19).

Blockade of the SLN produces dense anesthesia of the hypopharynx and upper glottis, including the vallecula and the laryngeal surface of the epiglottis. In combination with oropharyngeal topical anesthesia with or without a GPN block, this allows adequate airway anesthesia for a variety of AI techniques, including direct laryngoscopy. In the external approach, local anesthetic is injected into the paraglottic or pre-epiglottic space, targeting the nerve soon after it pierces the thyrohyoid ligament. The internal approach targets the nerve as it courses submucosally in the region of the pyriform recess.

2. Superior Laryngeal Nerve Block

a. EXTERNAL APPROACH

In the external approach,[5,102,113,128,135,136] the patient is placed in the supine position, head slightly extended, with the physician standing on the side to be blocked. The two main anatomic structures that are useful to identify are the hyoid bone and the superior cornu of the thyroid cartilage. The hyoid bone lies above the thyroid cartilage. It is identified by deep palpation; this can be uncomfortable to the patient and is difficult in patients who have a short or thick neck. Because it does not articulate with any other bones, the hyoid is freely movable, which helps in its identification. The greater cornu of the hyoid is the most lateral aspect of the bone that can be palpated. One side can be made more prominent by displacing the contralateral side toward the side

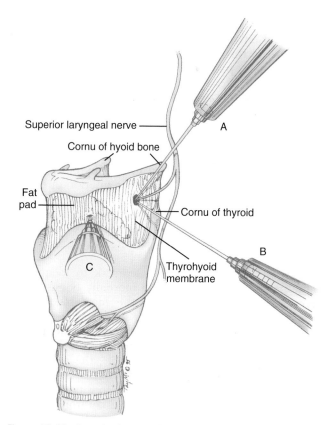

Figure 11-19 Superior laryngeal nerve block, external approach using as a landmark the greater cornu of the hyoid bone (A), the superior cornu of the thyroid cartilage (B), or the thyroid notch (C). (From Difficult Airway Teaching Aids. Irvine, University of California, Department of Anesthesia.)

being blocked. The superior lateral cornu of the thyroid cartilage can be identified by palpating the superior thyroid notch ("Adam's apple") and tracing the upper edge of the thyroid cartilage laterally until the most lateral aspect is identified. Three techniques using different landmarks have been described (see Fig. 11-19). Using 1% to 2% lidocaine, satisfactory sensory blockade is achieved within 5 minutes, with a success rate of 92% to 100%.[136]

GREATER CORNU OF THE HYOID. After identifying the greater cornu of the hyoid, the physician uses the non-dominant index finger to depress the carotid artery laterally and posteriorly. With the dominant hand, a 25-G needle is "walked off" the cornu of the hyoid bone (see *A* in Fig. 11-19) in an anterior-inferior direction, aiming toward the middle of the thyrohyoid membrane. A slight resistance is felt as the needle is advanced through the membrane, usually at a depth of 1 to 2 cm (2 to 3 mm deep to the hyoid bone). The needle at this point has entered the pre-epiglottic space. Aspiration through the needle should be attempted. If air is aspirated, the needle has gone too deep and may have entered the pharynx; it should be withdrawn until no air can be aspirated. If blood is aspirated, the needle has cannulated the superior laryngeal artery or vein or the carotid artery; the needle should be directed more anteriorly. After satisfactory needle placement is achieved, 2 to 3 mL of local anesthetic is injected as the needle is withdrawn. The block is repeated on the opposite side. An ultrasound-guided technique for this approach has been described and may be beneficial for patients with abnormal neck anatomy.[138]

SUPERIOR CORNU OF THE THYROID. A similar technique to the one previously described uses the superior lateral cornu of the thyroid as the landmark. The benefit of this technique is that, in many patients, this structure is easier and less painful to palpation than the hyoid bone. A 25-G needle is walked off the cornu of the thyroid cartilage (see *B* in Fig. 11-19) in a superior-anterior direction, aiming toward the lower third of the thyroid membrane. The same precautions as before are taken, and the local anesthetic solution is injected as the needle is withdrawn. The block is repeated on the opposite side.

THYROID NOTCH. The easiest landmark to identify in many patients, especially in the morbidly obese, is the thyroid notch (Adam's apple), the most medial and superficial aspect of the thyroid cartilage. The thyroid notch is palpated, and the upper border of the thyroid cartilage is traced laterally for approximately 2 cm (see *C* in Fig. 11-19). With a 25-G needle, the thyrohyoid ligament is pierced just above the thyroid cartilage at this location, and the needle is advanced in a posterior and cephalad direction to a depth of 1 to 2 cm from the skin. The tip of the needle is then in the pre-epiglottic space, which normally contains the terminal branches of the internal branch of the SLN imbedded in a fat pad (see Fig. 11-18). After an aspiration test, the entire volume of local anesthetic is injected into the pre-epiglottic space, and the needle is withdrawn. The block is repeated on the opposite side. An added benefit of this approach

is the decreased likelihood of blocking the motor branch of the SLN.

b. INTERNAL APPROACH

A noninvasive SLN block can be performed by applying local anesthetic to the pyriform recess. At this anatomic location, the internal branch of the SLN lies submucosally, and blockade is possible by diffusion of concentrated local anesthetic.[25,113] After adequate topicalization of the oropharynx, the patient is placed in the sitting position with the physician standing on the contralateral side of the nerve to be blocked. The patient's mouth is opened widely with the tongue protruded. The tongue is grasped with the nondominant hand using a gauze pad and gently pulled anteriorly, or it is depressed with a tongue blade. With the dominant hand, a Krause forceps holding a sponge soaked in 4% lidocaine is advanced over the lateral posterior curvature of the tongue along the downward continuation of the tonsillar fossa (Fig. 11-20). The tip of the forceps is advanced until it cannot be advanced any farther (Fig. 11-21); at that point, the handle of the forceps should be in a horizontal position and the tip should be resting in the pyriform recess. The position of the tip of the forceps may be checked by palpating the neck lateral to the posterior-superior aspect of the thyroid cartilage. The forceps are kept in this position for 5 minutes or longer, and then the process is repeated on the opposite side. This approach requires a considerable length of time and is limited to those patients who can open their mouths sufficiently wide.

3. Cautions, Complications, and Contraindications

When performing a SLN block from an external approach, care should be taken to avoid insertion of the needle into the thyroid cartilage, to preclude the possibility of injecting the local anesthetic at the level of the vocal cords, which could cause laryngeal edema and airway

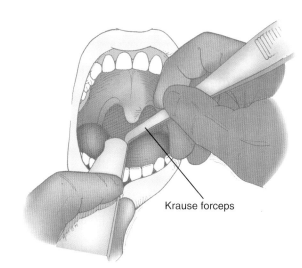

Figure 11-20 Superior laryngeal nerve block, internal approach. A Krause forceps is advanced over the tongue toward the pyriform sinus. (From Difficult Airway Teaching Aids, Irvine, University of California, Department of Anesthesia.)

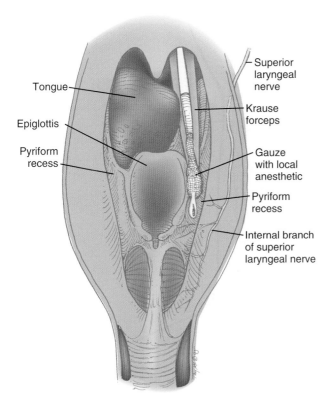

Figure 11-21 Superior laryngeal nerve block, internal approach. Posterior view of the larynx showing tip of Krause forceps at the level of the pyriform sinus. (From Difficult Airway: Teaching Aids. Irvine, University of California, Department of Anesthesia.)

Labels in figure: Tongue; Epiglottis; Pyriform recess; Superior laryngeal nerve; Krause forceps; Gauze with local anesthetic; Pyriform recess; Internal branch of superior laryngeal nerve

D. Trachea and Vocal Cords

1. Anatomy

The sensory innervation of the trachea, inferior larynx, and vocal cords is supplied by the recurrent (inferior) laryngeal nerves, branches of the vagus nerve. The right recurrent laryngeal nerve (RLN) originates at the level of the right subclavian artery; the left originates at the level of the aortic arch, distal to the ligamentum arteriosum. Both ascend along the tracheoesophageal groove to supply sensory innervation to the tracheobronchial tree up to and including the vocal cords, as well as supplying motor nerve fibers to the intrinsic muscles of the larynx (except the cricothyroid muscle). Because the sensory and motor fibers run together, nerve blocks cannot be performed because they would result in bilateral vocal cord paralysis and complete airway obstruction.

The alternative is topicalization of the mucosa. In addition to the use of a nebulizer, atomizer, or "spray-as-you-go" technique, topicalization of the trachea may be achieved by translaryngeal (transtracheal) injection. Although this technique does not provide a nerve block in the strictest sense, it is invasive and bears risks similar to those of other airway nerve blocks. In one study comparing transtracheal injection, "spray-as-you-go" topicalization through an FFB, and nebulization, transtracheal injection was most preferred by patients and bronchoscopists.[142] Tracheal topicalization is also of particular benefit in cases in which a neurologic examination is required after intubation, because it makes the presence of an ETT more comfortable.

2. Translaryngeal (Transtracheal) Anesthesia

a. POSITIONING AND LANDMARKS

The ideal position for translaryngeal anesthesia is the supine position with the neck in extension. In this position, the cervical vertebrae push the trachea and cricoid cartilage anteriorly and displace the strap muscles of the neck laterally. As a result, the cricoid cartilage and the structures above and below it are easier to palpate. The thyroid cartilage (Adam's apple) is palpated at midline and followed caudally until a depression and a firm ring of tissue are identified. These are the cricothyroid groove and the cricoid cartilage, respectively. Overlying the cricoid groove is the cricothyroid membrane.

b. TECHNIQUE

The physician should stand at the side of the patient with the dominant hand closest to the patient. The patient is asked not to talk, swallow, or cough until instructed. The midline of the cricothyroid membrane is identified as the needle insertion site. The index and middle finger of the nondominant hand can be used to mark this spot and stabilize the trachea (Fig. 11-22). Using a tuberculin syringe or a 25-G needle, the physician raises a small skin wheal. A 20-G angiocatheter attached to a 5- to 10-mL syringe containing 3 to 5 mL saline is used. The needle is advanced through the skin perpendicularly or slightly caudally while aspirating. When air is freely aspirated, the sheath of the angiocatheter is advanced slightly, the needle is removed, and a syringe containing 3 to 5 mL of

obstruction. The carotid artery should be identified and displaced posteriorly to minimize the risk of intravascular injection; even small amounts (0.25 to 0.5 mL) of local anesthetic injected into the carotid artery can induce seizures.

Hypotension and bradycardia have also been associated with SLN blockade. A number of possible causes of this reaction have been postulated, including (1) vasovagal reaction related to painful stimulation, (2) digital pressure on the carotid sinus, (3) excessive manipulation of the larynx causing vasovagal reaction, (4) large doses of or accidental intravascular administration of local anesthetic drugs, and (5) direct neural stimulation of the branch of the vagus nerve by the needle.[139] It is recommended that anticholinergics be administered before the block is performed.

Complications of the external approach also include hematoma and rupture of the ETT cuff in patients already intubated. Pharyngeal puncture and subsequent aspiration of air may occur and is generally a benign occurrence; the needle should be withdrawn until no more air is aspirated before local anesthetic is injected.

Contraindications to the external approach include local infection, local tumor growth, and coagulopathy. Although the position is not universally accepted, some have advocated avoidance of SLN anesthesia in patients who are at high risk for aspiration.[140]

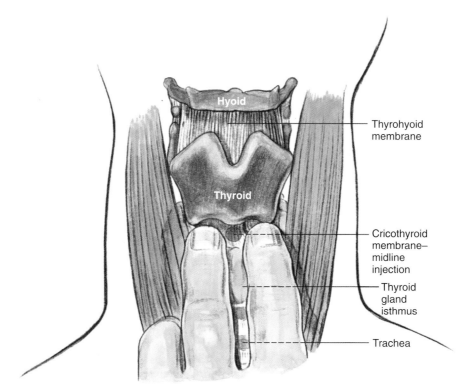

Figure 11-22 Translaryngeal anesthesia, anatomic landmarks. (From Brown D, editor: *Atlas of regional anesthesia*, ed 2, Philadelphia, 1999, Saunders.)

2% to 4% lidocaine is carefully attached to the catheter sheath that has been left in place. Aspiration of air is reconfirmed, the patient is warned to expect vigorous coughing, and the local anesthetic is injected rapidly during inspiration (Fig. 11-23). The sheath of the angio-catheter may be left in place until the intubation is complete in case more local anesthetic is needed and to decrease the likelihood of subcutaneous emphysema. Coughing helps to nebulize the local anesthetic so that the inferior and superior surfaces of the vocal cords can be anesthetized along with the tracheobronchial tree and inferior larynx. Anesthesia of the epiglottis, vallecula, tongue, and posterior pharyngeal wall are possible but unreliable. The success of translaryngeal anesthesia has been found to be as high as 95% and is attributed to both topicalization of the airway and systemic absorption.

This technique may be performed using a standard 20- or 22-G needle. This may, however, increase the risk of airway injury from the sharp metal bevel as the patient coughs. If this technique is used, care should be taken to remove the needle immediately after injection of the local anesthetic. This technique has also been described using a 25-G needle, but this is not recommended, because it introduces the risk of needle breakage as a result of movement of the cricoid cartilage cephalad when the patient coughs.[141]

c. CAUTIONS, COMPLICATIONS, CONTRAINDICATIONS

The tip of the needle should never be aimed in a cephalad direction, to avoid laryngeal trauma and to ensure adequate spread of local anesthetic below the vocal cords. Because this procedure eliminates the patient's ability to

protect the airway from aspiration, it should not be performed in patients who are at high risk for aspiration. Coughing elicited by this block may result in increased heart rate, mean arterial blood pressure, ICP, and intra-ocular pressure. As a result, it is contraindicated in patients with elevated ICP or open globe, and care should be taken in patients with significant cardiac disease. It is also relatively contraindicated in patients with cervical instability, although its routine use in these patients has been described without complications.[143] Transtracheal injection should be avoided in patients with local tumor or large goiter.

Potential complications are similar to those described for retrograde intubation (see Chapter 20). They include subcutaneous and intratracheal bleeding, infection, subcutaneous emphysema,[144] pneumomediastinum, pneumothorax, vocal cord trauma, and esophageal perforation. These complications are rare, as was illustrated by a review of 17,500 cases of translaryngeal puncture that showed an incidence of complications of less than 0.01%.[141]

VII. CONCLUSIONS

Once the decision to perform an AI has been made, the physician has many choices to make regarding the mode of preparation and the technique to be used. Regardless of the indication for AI, these clinical situations involve greater risk than a standard anesthetic technique. Safety should be the primary concern. Sedation should generally be a supplement to, rather than a substitute for, topical anesthesia of the airway. As long as the patient is awake,

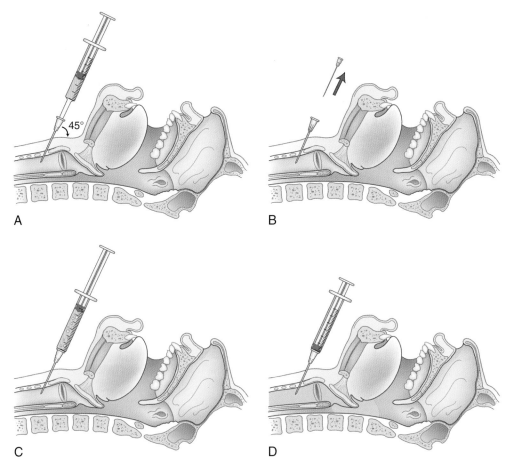

Figure 11-23   Translaryngeal anesthesia (midsagittal view of the head and neck). **A,** The angiocatheter is inserted at the cricothyroid membrane, aimed caudally. An aspiration test is performed to verify the position of the tip of the needle in the tracheal lumen. **B,** The needle is removed from the angiocatheter. **C,** The syringe containing local anesthetic attached, the aspiration test is repeated. **D,** Local anesthetic is injected, resulting in coughing and nebulization of the local anesthetic (*shaded area*). (From The Retrograde Cookbook. Irvine, University of California, Department of Anesthesia.)

cooperative, maintaining the airway, and spontaneously ventilating, no bridges have been burned. It is important that the physician be comfortable with the techniques used for topicalization and intubation; during management of a critical airway is not the time to learn a new technique. There should be a detailed backup plan in place in the event that the primary technique planned is unsuccessful. With the proper planning, patient preparation, and technique, AI is an invaluable tool for management of the DA.

VIII. CLINICAL PEARLS

- When faced with a difficult airway (DA), awake intubation (AI) is the gold standard for airway management.

- Preparation begins with a careful history and physical examination and a detailed discussion of the procedure with the patient.

- The goals of premedication are to alleviate anxiety, provide a clear and dry airway, protect against the risk of aspiration, and enable adequate topicalization.

- Sedation may be accomplished with benzodiazepines, opioids, or intravenous hypnotics, either alone or in combination; these agents must be titrated carefully to maintain cooperation and adequate ventilation.

- Adequate topicalization of the airway with local anesthetics is the key to a successful AI.

- If airway topicalization is insufficient, airway nerve blocks may be employed to supplement airway anesthesia.

- There are many choices involved when preparing for AI. Safety should be the primary consideration.

SELECTED REFERENCES

All references can be found online at expertconsult.com.
2. Kopman AF, Wollman SB, Ross K, et al: Awake endotracheal intubation: A review of 267 cases. *Anesth Analg* 54:323–327, 1975.
5. Thomas JL: Awake intubation: Indications, techniques and a review of 25 patients. *Anaesthesia* 24:28–35, 1969.
7. Practice guidelines for management of the difficult airway: An updated report by the American Society of Anesthesiologists Task Force on Management of the Difficult Airway. *Anesthesiology* 98:1269–1277, 2003. Erratum 10:565, 2004.

9. Benumof JL: Management of the difficult adult airway, with special emphasis on awake tracheal intubation. *Anesthesiology* 75:1087–1110, 1991.

18. Ovassapian A, Krejcie TC, Yelich SJ, et al: Awake fibreoptic intubation in the patient at high risk of aspiration. *Br J Anaesth* 62:13–16, 1989.

25. Reed AP: Preparation of the patient for awake flexible fiberoptic bronchoscopy. *Chest* 101:244–253, 1992.

45. Reves JG, Glass PSA, Lubarsky DA, et al: Intravenous nonopioid anesthetics. In Miller RD, editor: *Miller's anesthesia*, ed 6, Philadelphia, 2005, Elsevier Churchill Livingstone, pp 317–378.

57. Fukuda K: Intravenous opioid anesthetics. In Miller RD, editor: *Miller's anesthesia*, ed 6, Philadelphia, 2005, Elsevier Churchill Livingstone, pp 379–438.

102. Simmons ST, Schleich AR: Airway regional anesthesia for awake fiberoptic intubation. *Reg Anesth Pain Med* 27:180–192, 2002.

126. Hagberg CA: Airway blocks. In Chelly JE, editor: *Peripheral nerve blocks: A color atlas*, ed 3, Philadelphia, 2008, Lippincott Williams & Wilkins, pp 177–184.

Chapter 12

Aspiration Prevention and Prophylaxis: Preoperative Considerations

MARK D. TASCH | OLIVIER LANGERON

I. PERIOPERATIVE ASPIRATION

The pulmonary aspiration of gastric contents has generated a body of research and recrimination that might seem disproportionate to its reported incidence. Aspiration pneumonitis is an anesthetic complication whose consequences can be formidable but whose prevention would seem, at least in theory, to be readily attainable. The desire to minimize risks long ago led to rituals of fasting that were later challenged, at least with respect to fluids. Any experience with aspiration and its dire sequelae may, however, inspire rigid adherence to conservative nil per os (NPO) standards and avid administration of prophylactic preoperative medications.

A. Incidence

The statistical incidence of perioperative aspiration has been examined in long-term case reviews. A multicenter, prospective study of almost 200,000 operations performed in France found the overall incidence of clinically apparent aspiration to be 1.4 per 10,000 anesthesias.[1] Leigh and Tytler's 5-year survey of almost 110,000 anesthesias found 6 cases of aspiration requiring unplanned critical care.[2] Warner and colleagues retrospectively reviewed more than 215,000 general anesthesias and found an incidence of aspiration of 3.1 per 10,000 cases.[3]

Olsson and associates examined the records of more than 175,000 anesthesias administered at one hospital over more than 13 years and reported an incidence of aspiration of 4.7 per 10,000.[4] Kallar and Everett's multicenter survey of more than 500,000 outpatient anesthesias found the incidence of aspiration to be 1.7 per 10,000.[1]

In their 1999 review of 133 Australian cases, Kluger and Short reported that the incidence of passive regurgitation was three times that of active vomiting and that a majority of aspiration episodes accompanied anesthesias delivered by face mask or laryngeal mask airway (LMA). Thirty-eight percent of those who aspirated developed radiographic infiltrates, more often in the right lung than in the left. The authors also noted that "a recurring theme in many incidents was one of inadequate anaesthesia leading to coughing/straining and subsequent regurgitation/vomiting."[5] In their 1999 survey of pediatric aspiration, Warner and coauthors also wrote that "nearly all cases of pulmonary aspiration ... occurred in patients who gagged or coughed during airway manipulation or during induction of anesthesia."[6]

Several authors have observed that only about 50% or fewer of the episodes of perioperative aspiration occur during anesthetic induction and intubation, perhaps because concern is less heightened at other times.[1-9] These potentially catastrophic events also take place before induction (when the unguarded patient may be excessively sedated), during anesthesia maintenance, and during or after emergence and extubation.

B. Consequences

When aspiration does occur, the subsequent clinical course can range from benign to fatal. Olsson and colleagues reported that 18% of patients who aspirated perioperatively required mechanical ventilatory support, and 5% died. All those who died had a poor preoperative physical status.[4] Warner and coworkers reported that 64% of patients did *not* manifest coughing, wheezing, radiographic abnormalities, or a 10% decrease in arterial oxygen saturation (Sao_2) from preoperative room air values during the first 2 hours after aspiration. Such patients who remained asymptomatic for 2 hours developed no respiratory sequelae. Of the patients who did manifest signs or symptoms of pulmonary aspiration within 2 hours after the event, 54% required mechanical ventilatory support for 6 hours or longer, and 25% were ventilated for more than 24 hours. Approximately 50% of those ventilated for 24 hours or longer died, generating an overall mortality rate of less than 5% of all aspirations.[3]

Mortality rates resulting from perioperative pulmonary aspiration have ranged from less than 5% to more than 80% in other reports.[10,11] In the studies of Warner and Olsson and their coworkers, there were no deaths in healthy patients undergoing elective surgery.[3,4] In their 1999 survey of 133 perioperative aspirations in Australia, Kluger and Short wrote that "the deaths following aspiration events occurred in sicker patients ... although mortality can occur in healthy, younger patients."[5] Reviewing more than 85,000 Scandinavian anesthesias, Mellin-Olsen and associates noted that only 3 of 25 patients who aspirated developed serious morbidity, 2 of whom endured a prolonged course of illness but all of whom survived.[8] In general, most healthy patients who aspirate only gastric fluid can expect to survive without residual respiratory impairment, albeit sometimes after a stormy postoperative course.

C. Risk Factors

1. Demographic

Published surveys have associated some characteristics of patients or circumstances with an increased incidence of aspiration. Warner and colleagues noted that the relative risk of aspiration was more than four times higher for emergency surgeries compared with elective surgeries. A higher American Society of Anesthesiologists (ASA) physical status classification was also associated with a higher risk of aspiration. The incidence of aspiration increased from 1.1 per 10,000 elective anesthesias in ASA class I patients to 29.2 per 10,000 emergency anesthesias in ASA class IV and V patients. Contrary to conventional wisdom, "Age, gender, pregnancy ... concurrent administration of opioids, obesity ... experience ... of anesthesia provider, and types of surgical procedure were not independent risk factors for pulmonary aspiration. ... The most common predisposing condition in all patients was gastrointestinal obstruction."[3] Borland and coauthors

also wrote that "aspiration occurred significantly more often in patients with greater severity of underlying illness."[12]

Olsson and colleagues found that children and elderly persons were more likely than patients of intermediate ages to aspirate perioperatively.[4] Statistically, the risk of aspiration was more than three times higher in emergency surgeries than in elective operations. The incidence of aspiration was increased more than sixfold when surgery was performed at night rather than during daylight hours. More recent studies of both adult and pediatric cases have confirmed an impressive increase in the incidence of perioperative aspiration in emergency operations,[6,8] but Borland and coauthors found this increase to be only "marginally significant."[12]

In Kallar and Everett's outpatient survey,[1] aspiration occurred most frequently in patients younger than 10 years of age. They also reported, "In patients with no other identifiable risk factors, 67% of aspirations occurred after difficulties in airway management or intubation."[1] In the study of Olsson and colleagues, 15 of 83 aspirations occurred in patients with no known risk factors.[4] In 67% (10/15) of these cases, aspiration accompanied airway problems. In contrast to Kluger and Short's findings,[5] no patient aspirated while intubated. Although regional techniques are often favored for patients at increased risk for aspiration, elderly patients, in particular, have been reported to vomit and aspirate during subarachnoid anesthesia. Hypotension resulting from neuraxial sympathectomy can induce nausea and vomiting, and supplemental analgesics and sedatives given during lengthy operations can seriously obtund protective airway reflexes.[4,13,14]

Patients who are likely to have gastric contents of increased volume or acidity, elevated intragastric pressure, or decreased tone of the lower esophageal sphincter (LES) are traditionally considered to be at increased risk for perioperative pulmonary aspiration (Boxes 12-1 and 12-2).[10,15] As discussed later, pregnancy combines several of these likely risk factors. Although a lengthy NPO period before elective surgery is intended to minimize the volume of gastric contents, up to 90% of fasted patients have a gastric fluid pH level lower than 2.5.[11] Recent ethanol ingestion or hypoglycemic episodes stimulate gastric acid secretion, whereas tobacco inhalation temporarily lowers LES tone. LES tone has also been found to be reduced by gastric fluid acidity, caffeine, chocolate, and fatty foods.[11]

BOX 12-1 Risk Factors for Aspiration of Gastric Contents

Regurgitation or vomiting
Hypotension in awake patient
Opioids in awake patient
Increased intragastric volume and pressure
Decreased lower esophageal barrier pressure
Incompetent laryngeal protective reflexes
Neurologic disease
Neuromuscular disease
Central nervous system depressants
Advanced age or debility

BOX 12-2 Factors That Increase Intragastric Volume and Pressure

Increased gastric filling
Air inflation during mask ventilation
Increased gastric acid production
Gastrin
Histamine$_2$ (H$_2$) receptor stimulation
Recent ethanol ingestion
Recent hypoglycemic episode
Decreased gastric emptying
Intestinal obstruction
Diabetic gastroparesis
Opioids
Anticholinergics
Sympathetic stimulation (pain and anxiety)

Surgical outpatients have traditionally been thought to carry gastric contents of expanded volume and reduced pH, possibly because of preoperative anxiety. Clinical studies, however, have not consistently confirmed this expectation.[1] Furthermore, Hardy and associates contradicted several conventional notions by finding that neither gastric content volume nor pH correlated with preoperative anxiety, body mass index (BMI), ethanol or tobacco intake, or reflux history.[15]

2. Obesity

Obese patients were traditionally thought to pose a relatively high risk for aspiration because of their greater gastric fluid volume and acidity, intragastric pressure, and incidence of gastroesophageal reflux (GER).[16] This assumption has been challenged. In 1998, Harter and colleagues studied 232 fasted, nondiabetic surgical patients who had received no relevant preoperative medication. Using conventional arbitrary criteria, they found that only 27% of obese patients, compared with 42% of the nonobese, had gastric contents of high volume and acidity. Grading obesity by BMI, they also found no association between degree of obesity and gastric fluid volume or pH.[16] The presumed sluggishness of gastric emptying in obese patients has also been denied. Verdich and coworkers reported that obese and lean patients did not differ in rate of gastric emptying during the first 3 hours after a test meal.[17] Lower esophageal pressure has also been shown not to differ significantly between obese and nonobese patients.[16]

On the other hand, the laryngoscopic challenges that arise with corpulence, along with the association between airway difficulties and aspiration episodes, appear to increase the risk of aspiration in obese patients regardless of their gastrointestinal motility. Clinical studies have both confirmed and denied a demonstrable increase in the incidence of difficult intubation (DI) in the obese.[18–21] In a review of the topic, Freid noted that "obese patients … develop oxygen desaturation faster than the nonobese, and the safe apneic period is reduced from more than five minutes to less than two to three minutes in the preoxygenated state." Importantly, he observed that "far more morbidity occurs owing to hypoxemia during difficult or failed intubation than from aspiration."[7]

3. Systemic Diseases

Patients with connective tissue, neurologic, metabolic, or neuromuscular disease may be imperiled by esophageal dysfunction or laryngeal incompetence. Progressive systemic sclerosis and myotonia dystrophica have been specifically mentioned in case reports.[22–24] Hardoff and coworkers found that "gastric emptying time in patients with Parkinson's disease was delayed compared with control volunteers [and] was even slower in patients treated with levodopa."[25] Advanced age may be associated with attenuated cough or gag reflexes.

Long-standing diabetes mellitus is commonly considered to delay gastric emptying and may also compromise LES function.[26] Several authors have reported a high incidence of gastroparesis and prolonged mean gastric emptying times, at least for solid foods, in diabetic patients compared with control subjects.[27–30] Impairment of gastric motility was usually found to correlate with findings of autonomic neuropathy but not with peripheral neuropathy or with indices of glycemic stability.

4. Pregnancy

Pregnancy imposes a constellation of potential risk factors. The enlarging uterus increases intragastric pressure by compressing the stomach, physically delays gastric emptying by pushing the pylorus cephalad and posteriorly, and promotes GER by altering the angle of the gastroesophageal junction. Progesterone decreases the tone of the LES, and excess gastrin, produced by the placenta, promotes gastric acid secretion.[26,31,32] The alterations in physique that are typical of late pregnancy can interfere with laryngoscopy and endotracheal intubation. Laryngeal and upper airway edema is also common in the parturient and can be exaggerated by preeclampsia.[33]

Studies of gastric emptying in pregnancy have produced somewhat inconsistent results. Wong and colleagues found that water was readily cleared from the stomachs of nonobese, nonlaboring parturients at term and wrote that "recent studies of gastric emptying in nonlaboring term women … suggest that gastric emptying is not delayed during pregnancy."[34] Chiloiro and coworkers found that gastric emptying time did not become slower with the progress of gestation but that total orocecal transit time did.[35] A more common clinical concern is the parturient in labor. Scrutton and associates reported that laboring patients who consumed a light solid meal had significantly greater gastric volumes than those allowed only water.[36] Although pain, in any circumstance, is thought to delay gastric emptying, Porter and coauthors stated that "pain does not appear to be the sole cause of gastric slowing in late labour since [there was] a similar delay in women in late labour who had received either epidural local anesthetic alone or no analgesia."[37]

5. Pain and Analgesics

Pain and its treatment are considered to be risk factors for aspiration, notably in patients presenting with trauma. As stated by Crighton and colleagues, "circulating catecholamines have an inhibitory effect on gastric emptying, and noradrenaline release in response to painful stimuli may cause inhibition of gastric tone and emptying."[38]

Patients with spinal cord or brain injuries have also been shown to manifest delayed gastric emptying of both liquid and solid contents.[39–41]

Administration of opioids to alleviate pain is an essential act of kindness but may further impair gastrointestinal function. Opioid receptors can be found throughout the gastrointestinal tract; human and animal studies suggest that there are central and peripheral mechanisms by which these drugs retard gastric emptying.[42] Even modest intravenous doses of morphine demonstrably prolong gastric transit times in clinical studies.[38,43–45]

Neuraxial opioids can also prolong gastric emptying. In obstetric anesthesia, Kelly and associates "conclude[d] that the administration of fentanyl 25 mg intrathecally delays gastric emptying in labor compared with both extradural fentanyl 50 mg with bupivacaine and extradural bupivacaine alone."[46] Older reports indicated that epidural fentanyl boluses of 50 or 100 mg would retard gastric emptying. On the other hand, the addition of fentanyl (2 or 2.5 mg/mL) to dilute bupivacaine for epidural infusion during labor was not found to affect gastric motility.[37,47]

6. Positioning

Agnew and colleagues continuously monitored esophageal and tracheal pH in thoracotomy patients "considered to be at low risk of GER." Twenty-eight percent of their patients not treated with a histamine$_2$ (H$_2$)-receptor antagonist were found to have acid reflux into the esophagus while in the lateral decubitus position, and almost 8% had acid in the trachea. Although the authors did not correlate clinical outcomes with their findings, they did advise that patients undergoing thoracotomy be considered for routine preoperative aspiration chemoprophylaxis.[48]

D. Pathophysiology

When gastric contents enter the lungs, the resultant pulmonary pathology depends on the nature of the material aspirated (Box 12-3). Food particles small enough to enter the distal airways induce a foreign body reaction of inflammation and eventual granuloma formation. The aspiration of particulate antacids produces the same adverse response.[32,49] Acid aspiration induces an inflammatory response that begins within minutes and progresses over 24 to 36 hours.[49,50] In 1940, Irons and Apfelbach wrote that the "characteristic microscopic changes are intense engorgement of the alveolar capillaries, ... edema, and hemorrhage into the alveolar spaces.... Another outstanding characteristic is the extensive desquamation of the lining of the bronchial tree."[51] Other authors have also described hemorrhagic pulmonary edema, intense inflammation, and derangement of the pulmonary epithelium.[50,52] The membranous epithelial cells that produce surfactant are damaged or destroyed by the acid and replaced by granular epithelial cells.[14] As surfactant production fails, lung units progressively collapse. Fibrin and plasma leak from the capillaries into the pulmonary interstitium and alveoli, producing the noncardiogenic pulmonary edema often referred to as adult (or acute) respiratory distress syndrome (ARDS).[14,50,53,54] With effective supportive care, the acute inflammation can diminish, and epithelial regeneration can begin, within 72 hours.

The clinical features of aspiration pneumonitis have been well described for more than 60 years. Even earlier, in 1887, Becker referred to bronchopneumonia as a postoperative complication related to the inhalation of gastric contents.[51] Hall, in 1940, published the first description of gastric fluid inhalation in obstetric patients. He distinguished between the aspiration of solid material, which could quickly kill by suffocation, and the aspiration syndrome produced by gastric fluid, for which he coined the term *chemical pneumonitis*.[55] Mendelson, in 1946, described the clinical features of 66 cases of peripartum aspiration observed from 1932 to 1945. Solid food produced airway obstruction, which was quickly fatal in two instances. Otherwise, wheezing, rales, rhonchi, tachypnea, and tachycardia were prominent.[56] (Subsequent reports have not found wheezing to be so universal a manifestation, occurring in about one third of aspirations.) When present, wheezing is thought to result from bronchial mucosal edema and from a reflex response to acidic airway irritation.[11,50,57]

Refractory hypoxemia can ensue almost immediately as bronchospasm, airway edema or obstruction, and alveolar collapse or flooding increase the effective intrapulmonary shunt fraction (Box 12-4). The awake patient may experience intense dyspnea and may cough up the pink, frothy sputum characteristic of pulmonary edema.[11,32,50] More modest aspirations may not become clinically evident for several hours.[32,58,59]

Hemodynamic derangements can also demand therapeutic attention. As the alveolar-capillary membrane loses its integrity, plasma leaks out of the pulmonary vasculature. If the leak becomes a flood, the loss of circulating fluid volume can produce hemoconcentration,

---

BOX 12-3 Pathophysiology of Aspiration

Particulate aspiration
Airway obstruction
Granulomatous inflammation
Acid aspiration
Neutrophilic inflammation
Hemorrhagic pulmonary edema
Destruction of airway epithelium
Loss of type I alveolar cells
Loss of surfactant
Alveolar instability and collapse
Disruption of alveolar-capillary membrane
Plasma leakage from pulmonary capillaries
Noncardiogenic pulmonary edema
Hypovolemia

BOX 12-4 Aspiration and Hypoxemia

Upper airway obstruction
Increased lower airway resistance
Obstruction by airway debris
Airway edema
Reflex bronchospasm
Alveolar collapse and flooding

hypotension, tachycardia, and even shock.[11,32] Pulmonary vasospasm may also contribute to right ventricular dysfunction.[11]

The radiographic evidence of pulmonary aspiration may become evident promptly, if aspiration is massive, or after a delay of several hours. There is no pattern on the chest roentgenogram that is specific for aspiration. The distribution of infiltrates depends on the volume of material inhaled and the patient's position at the time of the event. Because of bronchial anatomy, aspiration occurring in the supine patient affects the right lower lobe most commonly, the left upper lobe least often.[11,32] If pulmonary aspiration is not complicated by secondary events, improvement in symptoms can be anticipated within 24 hours, although the radiographic picture may continue to worsen for another day.[32]

E. Determinants of Morbidity

1. pH and Volume of Aspirate

In his 1946 report, Mendelson undertook to determine the relationship between gastric fluid acidity and pulmonary morbidity. When liquid containing hydrochloric acid (HCl) was instilled into rabbits' tracheas, the animals developed a syndrome "similar in many respects to that observed in the human following liquid aspiration,"[56] with cyanosis, dyspnea, and pink, frothy sputum. On the other hand, when neutral liquid was instilled into the trachea, the rabbits endured a brief symptomatic period, "but within a few hours they [were] apparently back to normal, able to carry on rabbit activities uninhibited."[56] (Mendelson maintained a discreet silence about the nature of these uninhibited rabbit activities.)

Since Mendelson's report, numerous attempts (and assumptions) have been made to define the "critical" volume and pH of gastric contents required to inflict significant damage on the lungs. Such neatly defined threshold values may be illusory objects of desire rather than features of clinical reality. Nonetheless, almost all researchers in the field of aspiration pneumonitis have made some use of critical values to define the success or failure of drug therapies in the modification of gastric contents.

In 1952, Teabeaut injected HCl solutions of different volumes and acidities into rabbits' tracheas. He found that solutions with a pH higher than 2.4 caused a relatively benign tissue response similar to that induced by the intratracheal injection of water. As the pH of the injectate was reduced from 2.4 to 1.5, a progressively more severe tissue reaction was elicited. At pH 1.5, the damage was maximal and equal to that found at lower pH values.[60] From this study stemmed the popular concept of the pH value of 2.5 as a threshold for chemical pneumonitis.

The determination of a critical volume of gastric contents required to produce severe aspiration pneumonitis has been even more contentious than that of a critical pH. Two teams of investigators each found that, in dogs, pulmonary injury became independent of pH as the volume of aspirate was increased from 0.5 to 4.0 mL/kg.[11] A preliminary experiment by Roberts and Shirley, involving gastric fluid instillation into the right main stem bronchus of a single monkey, long ago led to the acceptance, in some quarters, of 0.4 mL/kg as the volume of gastric fluid that places a subject at risk for development of aspiration pneumonitis.[61-63] Subsequent researchers challenged this number. James and colleagues demonstrated that aspirate volumes as low as 0.2 mL/kg could induce pulmonary injury if the pH of the aspirate were reduced to 1.09.[64] On the other hand, Raidoo and coworkers, also studying monkeys, found that the aspiration of 0.4 to 0.6 mL/kg of fluid with a pH of 1.0 produced mild or moderate pulmonary injury, and 0.8 to 1.0 mL/kg at pH 1.0 produced severe pneumonitis, with a 50% mortality rate (3/6) at 1.0 mL/kg.[61]

Clearly, the volume of aspirate that is considered hazardous depends on how much morbidity or pathology must be produced to be considered significant. Arguments have also been made concerning the experimental instillation of gastric fluid into one lung versus both lungs and the reliability of gastric fluid volume measurements. In addition, even if a critical volume for aspiration pneumonitis could be reliably determined, it cannot be known how much fluid must be present in the stomach in order to deposit this critical volume into the lung or lungs.[61,65] However, studies of therapeutic interventions must have criteria for defining success or failure, and threshold values for gastric fluid volume and pH are typically employed, regardless of their validity.

2. Particulate Matter

Volume and acidity are not, of course, the only determinants of sequelae when gastric contents enter the lungs. Since the report of Bond and coworkers in 1979, it has been appreciated that gastric fluid containing particulate antacids can produce severe aspiration pneumonitis, even at near-neutral pH, with wheezing, pulmonary edema, and hypoxemia requiring mechanical ventilatory support.[66] Animal studies confirmed that nonparticulate gastric acid and particulate antacid solutions have similar potentials for pulmonary mischief if aspirated.[58] Although blood and digestive enzymes do not appear to induce chemical pneumonitis, feculent gastric contents with a high bacterial density readily produce pneumonitis and death in animals. (Acidic gastric contents are normally sterile.) Another study demonstrated that the mucus present in the gastric fluid of dogs with intestinal obstruction produced diffuse small airway obstruction and pulmonary injury when aspirated.[11]

II. PREVENTION OF ASPIRATION

The clinical challenges of perioperative pulmonary aspiration are prevention, prophylaxis, and treatment. Ideally, gastric contents can be physically prevented from entering the lungs in the first place. Should prevention fail, pharmacologic prophylaxis may modify the volume and character of gastric contents so that they inflict minimal damage on the lungs. Least desirably, aspiration pneumonitis can require intensive medical treatment and ventilatory support.

The nonpharmacologic means of keeping gastric contents out of the lungs are preoperative fasting, gastric decompression, and optimal airway management.

A. Preoperative Fasting

The most common means of keeping gastric contents out of the lungs is to minimize the volume of such contents through preoperative fasting. However, both the utility and the necessity of adhering to traditional NPO regimens for clear liquids have been challenged. As noted by Sethi and coauthors, "the stomach can never be completely empty even after a midnight fast since it continues to secrete gastric juices."[67] The issue has been studied in both pediatric and adult surgical patients and has become particularly contentious and emotional regarding obstetric anesthesia.

1. Pediatric Patients

Conventional preoperative fasting can impose physical and emotional discomfort on children and their parents and may be difficult to enforce reliably in outpatients. Dehydration in infants and hypoglycemia in neonates may also result from prolonged NPO times.[1,10] The normal stomach can empty 80% of a clear liquid load within 1 hour after ingestion. Whereas the stomach continues to secrete and reabsorb fluid throughout NPO time, ingested clear liquids are completely passed into the duodenum within 2.25 hours.[68] Several researchers have therefore sought to demonstrate that children may safely be allowed to drink clear liquids until just 2 to 3 hours before elective surgery.

Van der Walt and Carter, as well as other groups, determined that healthy infants could drink limited volumes of clear liquids 3 to 4 hours before surgery with no effect on gastric content volumes.[69] Splinter and colleagues found that healthy infants could drink clear liquids ad libitum until 2 hours before anesthetic induction without altering gastric fluid volume or pH. (Gastric fluid pH was quite variable, and mean pH was less than 2.5 in all groups of patients studied, regardless of NPO time.) On the other hand, milk or formula intake on the morning of surgery (4 to 6 hours before induction) was associated with the presence of curds in many of the gastric aspirates. This was considered to represent an unacceptable risk of particulate aspiration. The authors therefore concurred with previous recommendations that infants not be allowed milk or formula on the morning of surgery.[70]

More recently, Cook-Sather and associates studied 97 healthy infants undergoing elective surgery and found that gastric fluid volume was not increased when the fasting time for formula was reduced from 8 hours to either 6 or 4 hours.[71] Schreiner and colleagues compared the gastric contents of children subjected to conventional preoperative fasting (mean NPO time, 13.5 hours) with those of children permitted clear liquids until 2 hours before anesthetic induction (mean NPO time, 2.6 hours). Gastric fluid volumes actually tended to be somewhat smaller in the children allowed to drink clear liquids up to 2 hours preoperatively, and almost all children in both groups had gastric content pH values of 2.5 or less.[72] Sandhar and coauthors, studying children 1 to 14 years old, also found that clear liquid ingestion 2 to 3 hours preoperatively did not significantly increase the mean volume of gastric contents and did not increase the number of patients with gastric contents more voluminous than 0.4 mL/kg.[68] Reports by Splinter, Moyao-Garcia, Maekawa, and Gombar and their colleagues all concluded that permitting children to drink nonparticulate fluids 2 to 3 hours before surgery had either no effect or a small beneficial influence on the quantity and acidity of their gastric contents.[73–76]

Ingestion of clear liquids alone therefore appears to pose no demonstrable hazard if taken no later than 2 hours before anesthesia by children without gastrointestinal pathology. However, solid or semisolid foods are not cleared from the stomach as rapidly as clear liquids. Meakin and associates found that a light breakfast of biscuits or orange juice with pulp, taken 2 to 4 hours before induction, did increase the volume of gastric aspirate in healthy children compared with those who had fasted for 4 hours or longer. In all fasted children, and in almost all of the fed children, the gastric content pH was 2.5 or less.[77] Hyperosmolar glucose solutions are also associated with delayed gastric emptying.[68]

In 1999, the ASA issued the report of its Task Force on Preoperative Fasting, which included practice guidelines. These guidelines were intended to apply to healthy patients who have no known relevant risk factors or injuries and are scheduled for elective surgery. Within these limitations, the ASA Task Force "support[ed] a fasting period for clear liquids of two hours for all patients [and] a fasting period for breast milk of four hours for both neonates and infants" while considering it "appropriate to fast from intake of infant formula for six or more hours."[78]

2. Adult Patients

In adult surgical patients, too, considerable evidence has demonstrated that clear liquid intake within 2 to 3 hours of anesthetic induction does not increase the risk of gastric acid aspiration. It is important to note that these studies typically involved healthy, nonpregnant, nonobese patients who were free of known gastrointestinal pathology, were not receiving opioids or other medications known to interfere with gastric emptying, and were undergoing elective surgery. The results of such studies cannot, therefore, be reliably applied to any other groups of patients.[79–82]

With adults, as with children, the basic arguments favoring relaxed NPO regimens for clear liquids involve their normally rapid gastric clearance. More than 90% of a 750-mL bolus of isotonic saline was found to pass from the normal stomach within 30 minutes.[83] After 2 hours of fasting, the fluid in the stomach primarily represents the acid secreted by the stomach itself. Exogenous clear liquids tend to dilute endogenous gastric acid and may even accelerate gastric emptying.[65,72,81] Solids, lipids, and hyperosmotic liquids are thought to delay gastric emptying, and their intake would therefore be considered ill advised before anesthetic induction.[65]

Several researchers have sought to correlate these theoretical considerations with clinical situations. Maltby and colleagues studied outpatients who were either kept NPO from the previous midnight or given 150 mL of water 2.5 hours before anesthetic induction. Although the mean gastric pH did not differ significantly between the two groups, the mean gastric volume was significantly less in the patients who drank than in those who fasted.[83] Read and Vaughan similarly found that permitting patients to drink water ad libitum until 2 hours before surgery had no impact on gastric volume or pH but did decrease preanesthetic anxiety. Many patients had gastric pH values less than or equal to than 2.5, regardless of the time elapsed since fluid intake.[84]

Phillips and colleagues also determined that patients who were allowed to drink clear liquids until 2 hours before surgery had gastric volume and pH values similar to those of patients who fasted for 6 hours. Other studies have also confirmed that the ingestion of 150 mL of (pulp-free) orange juice, coffee, tea, or apple juice 2 to 3 hours before surgery has no detrimental effect on gastric pH or volume in surgical outpatients.[81] (Since the publication of these reports, one can only wonder how many hours of presurgical time have been consumed in speculation regarding the pulp content of orange juice that patients have admitted to consuming.)

The safety of clear liquid ingestion before surgery does not, of course, imply that solid food may also be taken with impunity. In an early study, Miller and coworkers compared 22 adults kept NPO overnight before surgery with 23 adults permitted a light breakfast (one slice of buttered toast and tea or coffee with milk) on the morning of surgery (mean NPO time, 3.8 hours). The two groups were found not to differ significantly in mean volume or median pH of gastric contents or in the percentage of patients with a gastric pH lower than 3.0.[80] Soreide and coauthors reported that the particulate elements of a light breakfast had not completely exited after 4 hours.[85] Reflecting a consensus of clinical comfort, the aforementioned ASA Task Force recommended a 6-hour preoperative fast following a "light meal" and a fast of 8 hours or longer "for a meal that included fried or fatty foods or meat."[78]

3. Pregnant Patients

As preoperative NPO standards became more relaxed, strenuous debate arose over the necessity of adhering to conventional NPO regimens for patients in labor. Obstetricians, nurse-midwives, and psychologists joined the fray. On the one hand, anesthesiologists have long recognized that advanced gestation increases the risk of gastric content aspiration. On the other hand, proponents of liberalizing oral intake for parturients cited the infrequency of aspiration pneumonitis in modern practice, the futility of fasting in ensuring an empty stomach, and the detrimental effects of fasting on maternal and fetal well-being. The fashionable battle cry of "patient autonomy" was also heard.

Elkington cited a Washington state survey (1977-1981) in which none of 36 maternal deaths resulted from anesthetic complications and a North Carolina survey (1981-1985) in which only 1 of 40 maternal deaths resulted from aspiration. He did not advocate uninhibited feeding of patients in labor but rather recommended that, "For otherwise uncomplicated parturients, a nonparticulate diet should be allowed as desired."[86]

Ludka and Roberts referred to a Michigan survey (1972-1984) showing that only 1 of 15 maternal deaths (0.82 per 100,000 live births) resulted from the

aspiration of gastric contents, that no deaths were related to regional anesthesia, and that "failure to secure a patent airway was the primary cause of anesthesia-related maternal deaths."[87] They cited other studies indicating that women who ate during labor were less ketotic, required less analgesic medication and oxytocin, and had more active fetuses and neonates with higher Apgar scores than women who fasted during labor. They also "found that laboring women self-regulated intake. Once active labor began, women usually preferred liquids."[87]

Regarding the inevitability of a full stomach in the parturient, Kallar and Everett referred to an ultrasound study in which almost two thirds of patients in labor had solid food in the stomach, regardless of how long they had fasted.[1] Elkington cited a report that approximately 25% of parturients were "at risk" for aspiration pneumonitis, regardless of the duration of fasting, and that prolonged fasting was actually associated with increased gastric fluid volume at a lower pH.[86] Broach and Newton contended that "administration of narcotics, not labor itself, appears to be the major factor in delaying stomach emptying."[88] In a recent review, de Souza and associates wrote the following: "It has now been proven that pregnancy by itself does not delay gastric emptying. Many investigators using different modalities have confirmed this finding. Obese term pregnant patients have also been found to have normal gastric emptying. We emphasize that these findings apply only to patients who are not in labor."[89]

McKay and Mahan stated that, "among many factors that can be linked to the occurrence of aspiration, the most important appears to be faulty administration of obstetric anesthesia." They questioned "whether parturients should be kept … on restricted liquid intake to protect them from what appears to be the basic problem: inadequate anesthesia practices."[90] The apparent implication was that the parturient should eat, drink, and be merry, for if she should aspirate, only poor anesthetic care would be to blame.

On the other hand, Chestnut and Cohen cited the Report on Confidential Enquiries into Maternal Deaths in England and Wales 1982-1984, which found that 7 of 19 anesthesia-associated maternal deaths resulted from aspiration of gastric contents into the lungs, and an ASA review of closed malpractice claims in which "maternal aspiration was the primary reason for 8% of all claims against anesthesiologists for obstetric cases." The authors argued that "These data hardly suggest that the risk of maternal aspiration is remote."[91]

In his reply to McKay and Mahan, Crawford observed that "most of the deaths from aspiration prior to the mid-1950s … were due to asphyxia, caused by respiratory obstruction with solid or semisolid material—since that time, with introduction of a firm dietary regimen for labor, only 2 of the 146 deaths noted have been in that category." Furthermore, he contended, "There is inevitably an incidence of cesarean section and of general anesthesia in every obstetric population…. In an obstetric population the incidence of failed or difficult intubation is roughly one in 300."[92]

In the work of Scrutton and colleagues, permitting parturients a "light diet" (as opposed to water only) had no effect on the course of labor or the neonatal Apgar scores but did increase the volume of gastric contents and of vomitus. They stated that "the presence of undigested food particles in the vomitus is probably of greater importance [than low pH] as a cause of mortality [and] would not support the policy of encouraging women to eat any solid food once in labour particularly when isotonic drinks appear to offer an adequate calorific alternative."[36] In their review, Ng and Smith concluded that "there is insufficient evidence to clarify changes in risk in the first 24 hours of the postpartum period, when operative procedures are common."[93]

Obviously, the pregnant patient with a difficult airway cannot always be avoided, nor can general anesthesia for cesarean section, no matter how aggressively regional anesthesia is promoted. Regardless of gastric fluid volume or acidity, the presence of solid food imparts the immediate hazard of asphyxiation. Mendelson warned that "misinformed friends and relatives often urge the patient to ingest a heavy meal early in labor before going to the hospital."[56] Crawford concluded, "Grafting good anesthetic technique upon poor preparation of a patient for anesthesia is unjustifiable—there is an essential symbiosis between the two if safety is to be ensured."[92]

B. Preinduction Gastric Emptying

When a patient who is at increased risk for aspiration presents for surgery, the stomach can be emptied, at least in part, by an orogastric or a nasogastric (NG) tube. Some patients, of course, already have such tube placed for gastric decompression, particularly if intestinal obstruction has been diagnosed. In such cases, the anesthesiologist must decide whether to remove the gastric tube before induction. If gastric decompression has not been attempted, the anesthesiologist may wish to do so while the patient's protective airway reflexes remain intact.

It has long been argued that the presence of a gastric tube interferes with the sphincter function of the gastroesophageal junction and promotes GER by acting as a "wick."[94] The presence of a foreign body in the pharynx could also interfere with laryngoscopy. These considerations would favor removal of the gastric tube before induction. However, in an early study by Satiani and colleagues, the incidence of "silent" GER was found to be 12% in anesthetized patients without an NG tube and 6% in patients with an NG tube in place (a statistically insignificant difference).[95] Hardy wrote that "a nasogastric tube need not be withdrawn before induction of anesthesia. The tube can act as an overflow valve" and provide "a venting mechanism whereby pressure cannot build up in the stomach."[96]

Dotson and associates prospectively studied the effect of NG tube size on GER in normal subjects. Attempts were made to provoke GER with a device that elevated abdominal pressure stepwise to 100 mm Hg. In this report, GER "was not detected at any level of abdominal pressure regardless of the presence or size of a nasogastric tube."[97] Salem and colleagues had previously demonstrated that "cricoid pressure is effective in sealing the esophagus around an esophageal tube against an intraesophageal pressure up to 100 cm H_2O."[98] They also

advocated the utility of an NG tube as a "blow-off valve" for increased intragastric pressure during induction.[98] The presence of an NG tube, while allowing gastric decompression, may also hold open the LES.[11,99]

Vanner and Asai advised that an NG tube already inserted "should be [suctioned and] left in place [for anesthetic induction], since its presence does not reduce the efficacy of cricoid pressure."[9] On the other hand, Brock-Utne contended that "the recommendation that a nasogastric tube should be left *in situ* during a rapid sequence technique induction is not supported by the evidence. Clinicians who have seen aspiration of gastric contents with an nasogastric tube *in situ* will, no doubt, remove the nasogastric tube before anesthetic induction."[100] None of these writings addressed the usually surgical decision concerning which patients should have NG tubes placed before entering the operating room.

Some of the studies just cited would seem to indicate that an NG tube, already inserted, can be safely left in place during induction and may even have a protective benefit. Gastric decompression during surgery could also reduce the risk of regurgitation and aspiration in the postanesthetic period.[96] The necessity and the utility of NG tube insertion just before induction are not so well defined. The benefits of awake gastric decompression depend, in part, on how completely the stomach can thereby be emptied. The primary drawback is patient discomfort.

Several authors have studied the thoroughness of gastric emptying attainable by gastric tube suctioning, usually in the context of comparing different methods for estimating gastric residual volume. Ong and coauthors reported, as early as 1978, that the volume of fluid obtained by orogastric suctioning correlated poorly with the gastric residual volume calculated by a dilution method, "the volume aspirated being frequently much less than the volume calculated."[101] They concluded that "aspiration through a gastric tube will not empty the stomach completely." Mechanical decompression of the stomach before induction might therefore be of limited reliability and thus provide a false sense of security.[101] Taylor and associates studied 10 obese patients in whom gastric contents were first aspirated through a 16-F multiorificed Salem Sump tube, then "completely" removed by a gastroscope. "The blind aspirated volume underestimated true total gastric volume by an average of 14.7 mL, [which] was statistically significant.... The residual content volume left in the stomach after blind aspiration varied from 4 mL to 23 mL,"[102] a maximal discrepancy far less than that found by Ong and coworkers in 42 patients.[101]

Hardy and colleagues measured the volume of gastric fluid aspirated through an 18-F Salem Sump tube in 24 patients, then directly inspected the stomach and measured the volume of fluid remaining. The residual volume that eluded orogastric suctioning ranged from 0 to 13 mL. The authors concluded "that the volume of aspirated gastric fluid … is a very good estimate of the volume present in the stomach at the time of induction" and that gastric tube suctioning "could also be suitable to empty the stomach of its liquid contents prior to anaesthesia."[103]

It can be argued that any reduction in intragastric volume and pressure before anesthetic induction is desirable and should therefore be attempted. On the other hand, as Satiani and colleagues conceded, "particulate matter [is] impossible to evacuate through the lumen of an ordinary nasogastric tube."[95] Salem and associates concluded that "placement of a nasogastric tube before anesthetic induction seems to be indicated only in patients with overdistention of the stomach."[98] Although obvious enteric obstruction is conventionally treated with gastric decompression before anesthetic induction, not every emergency or at-risk patient is subjected to NG tube insertion while awake. There is currently no consensus to dictate preinduction placement of a gastric tube in any set of patients without intestinal obstruction. In any case, gastric decompression in no way substitutes for proper perioperative management of the airway.

C. Rapid-Sequence Induction and Cricoid Pressure

For the patient whose stomach is assumed to be full, the anesthesiologist must first decide whether to secure the airway before or after anesthetic induction. Awake intubation with topical anesthesia of the airway and varying degrees of sedation can always be considered. Without meticulous explanation and preparation, the patient's enthusiasm for this technique is unlikely to match the practitioner's.

If anesthetic induction is to precede endotracheal intubation, the standard protective maneuver for 5 decades has been rapid-sequence induction (RSI) with cricoid pressure. The traditional components of this technique include preoxygenation and denitrogenation of the lungs, rapid administration of anesthetic induction and neuromuscular blocking agents with brief onset times, cricoid pressure, no manual ventilation by mask, and (one hopes) endotracheal intubation immediately after consciousness and neuromuscular transmission have been obtunded. As El-Orbany and Connolly wrote, this sequence "has achieved a status close to being a standard of care for anesthesia induction in patients with full stomachs. Despite the technique's widespread use, there is still no agreement on how it should best be performed."[104] The practice of RSI has generated contention regarding both cricoid pressure and obligatory apnea between induction and intubation.

Abstention from positive-pressure ventilation (PPV) during RSI rests on the fear that the resulting gastric insufflation will increase the likelihood of regurgitation and aspiration of gastric contents before endotracheal intubation. The preservation of adequate oxygenation despite apnea is, of course, crucial. As noted by El-Orbany and Connolly, "Currently, some experts strongly recommend the routine use of PPV ... in certain [RSI] situations. Hypoxemia can develop in obese, pregnant, pediatric, and critically ill patients ... even after adequate administration of oxygen ... because of their low functional residual capacity."[104] Fifty years ago, Ruben and colleagues demonstrated that "manual ... ventilation did not result in gastric insufflation when airway pressures were kept <15 cm H_2O. ... With the application of

cricoid pressure, no gastric insufflation occurred even when the inflating pressure was increased to 45 cm H_2O."[105] Of course, if the patient becomes hypoxemic, manual ventilation becomes mandatory.

The utility of cricoid pressure has been challenged on many fronts. As described by Sellick in 1961, "The manoeuver consists in temporary occlusion of the upper end of the oesophagus by backward pressure of the cricoid cartilage against the bodies of the cervical vertebrae.... Extension of the neck and application of pressure on the cricoid cartilage obliterates the oesophageal lumen at the level of the body of the fifth cervical vertebra.... Pressure is maintained until intubation and inflation of the cuff of the endotracheal tube is completed."[106] Kopka, Herman, and colleagues noted that cricoid pressure was used as early as 1774 to avert regurgitation related to gastric distention with air during resuscitation from drowning.[107,108] In Sellick's original report of 26 high-risk cases, 23 patients neither vomited nor regurgitated at any time near induction, and in the other 3 cases the "release of cricoid pressure after intubation was followed immediately by reflux into the pharynx of gastric or oesophageal contents, suggesting that in these three cases cricoid pressure had been effective."[106]

Although the LES has received considerable attention with regard to the pharmacology and pathophysiology of GER, there is also effective sphincter tone at the upper end of the esophagus. As described by Vanner and colleagues, "The upper oesophageal sphincter is formed mainly by the cricopharyngeus, a striated muscle situated behind the cricoid cartilage. The muscle tone of the cricopharyngeus creates a sphincter pressure which prevents regurgitation in the awake state."[109] These authors found that general anesthesia with neuromuscular blockade reduced the upper esophageal sphincter pressure from 38 mm Hg (while awake) to 6 mm Hg, a pressure that would typically permit passive regurgitation. Although cricoid pressure could exceed the normal awake level of upper esophageal sphincter pressure, in only half of their study patients was it applied firmly enough to do so.[109]

Other authors have noted the inconsistency with which Sellick's maneuver is applied. As Stept and Safar wrote in 1970, "The attempt to close the esophagus by pressing the cricoid cartilage against the cervical vertebrae is rarely applied with proper timing, namely, starting with the onset of unconsciousness and continuing until the tracheal cuff is inflated."[110] In their study of simulated cricoid pressure, Meek and coauthors reported that target pressures could be sustained with a flexed arm for a mean of only 3.7 to 6.4 minutes and with an extended arm for 7.6 to 10.8 minutes.[111]

A rising chorus of skepticism concerning the efficacy of cricoid pressure has been heard. In their reviews, Kluger and Short[5] and Thwaites and colleagues[112] cited reports of lethal aspiration occurring despite Sellick's maneuver. The former authors specifically questioned the "almost unerring faith in the efficacy of this manoeuvre."[5] In their prospective investigation of emergency intubations in critically ill patients, Schwartz and associates reported that "twelve patients had an unexplained infiltrate that probably resulted from aspiration.... Nine of the twelve patients had cricoid pressure applied during airway management."[113] Specifically addressing medico-legal arguments, Jackson contended that "there is no scientific validation for the commonly held belief that 'improper application of cricoid pressure might explain any failures' to prevent aspiration."[114]

Although it is largely accepted that cricoid pressure limits the incidence of passive regurgitation, "it cannot be expected to prevent regurgitation during coughing, straining, or retching."[9] Sellick himself warned against applying cricoid pressure to a patient who is actively vomiting, lest the resulting increased pressure injure the esophagus.[106] In addition, the maneuver itself can induce gagging and even vomiting in the awake patient.[9] Ralph and Wareham reported a case in which "rupture of the oesophagus occurred during the application of cricoid pressure at induction of anaesthesia when the patient vomited." Fatal mediastinitis ensued.[115]

It has also become more widely acknowledged that cricoid pressure can interfere with both pulmonary ventilation and endotracheal intubation. Hocking and associates reported that "cricoid pressure produced a reduction in tidal volume (V_T) and an increase in peak inspiratory pressure" in 50 female patients given mechanical ventilation by mask with an oral airway. Although the changes in pressure and volume were not large, "Complete airway obstruction resulted on three occasions, all with cricoid pressure applied."[116] Saghaei and Masoodifar, in their study of 80 healthy anesthetized adults, found that bimanual cricoid pressure induced decreases in V_T with significant increases in peak inspiratory pressure, blood pressure, and heart rate.[117] Hartsilver and Vanner reported similar findings, concluding that "the degree of airway obstruction is related to the force applied to the cricoid cartilage. Therefore, if it is difficult to ventilate via a facemask, the amount of cricoid pressure should be reduced."[118]

Cricoid pressure can also impede ventilation through an LMA. Asai and colleagues reported that standardized cricoid pressure reduced the success rate of LMA ventilation from 100% (22/22) to 14% (3/22). Under fiberoptic visualization, the 18 LMAs that had been properly positioned became displaced when cricoid pressure was applied.[119] Similarly, Harry and Nolan stated that cricoid pressure reduced the success rate of endotracheal intubation through an intubating LMA from 84% to 52%.[120] Using fiberoptic visualization by LMA, MacG Palmer and Ball noted that cricoid pressure commonly caused cricoid deformation or occlusion, vocal cord closure, and impairment of ventilation, especially in women.[121]

The application of cricoid pressure may either improve or impede conventional laryngoscopy. According to Vanner and coauthors, standard cricoid pressure usually facilitated the exposure of the glottis, and "cricoid pressure in an upward (cephalad) and backward direction was more likely to give a better view at laryngoscopy than the standard technique."[122] In a substantial minority of their patients, however, cricoid pressure had either no impact or a detrimental effect on laryngoscopy. Hillman and colleagues reported that "the change in laryngoscopic view with increasing cricoid pressure fell into one of four broad patterns: little change (11/40), gradual

deterioration (10/40), improvement at low force followed by deterioration [at high force] (9/40), [and] improvement at high force (10/40).... [I]n some individuals, a force close to that currently recommended may cause a complete loss of the glottic view."[123] Other authors have contended that cricoid pressure tends to interfere with intubation with lightwand or fiberoptic techniques.[124,125] On the other hand, Riad and Ansari found that "application of cricoid pressure during induction of anaesthesia for elective caesarean section neither prolongs the time nor interferes with ease of endotracheal intubation using Airtraq [a disposable optical laryngoscope]."[126] In a randomized study of 700 adult surgical patients, Turgeon and colleagues concluded that "cricoid pressure applied by trained personnel does not increase the rate of failed intubation."[127]

MacG Palmer and Ball concluded that "Orthodox application of cricoid pressure may ... be directly implicated in the 'can't intubate, can't ventilate' scenario."[121] In their review of the current practice of RSI, Thwaites and coworkers sharpened the point of their critique by reminding us "that hypoxia can kill rapidly, while aspiration only might occur and only might kill."[112] Although Sellick's maneuver remains a conventional element of aspiration prevention, many authors now assert that it should not be slavishly pursued to the detriment of gas exchange and airway securement.

III. MEDICAL PROPHYLAXIS OF ASPIRATION

A. Gastroesophageal Motility

Although preparation of the patient (rational NPO strategy and perhaps gastric suctioning) and airway management are the twin pillars of aspiration prevention, pharmacologic prophylaxis has been promoted as adjunctive to patients' safety. Because gastric contents must first pass through the esophagus before entering the pharynx and trachea, the LES has become a locus of attention. As described by Ciresi, the LES "consists of functionally but not anatomically specialized smooth muscle, about 2-4 cm in length, just proximal to the stomach. The sphincteric muscle maintains closure of the distal esophagus through a mechanism of tonic contraction ... accompanied by a zone of intraluminal high pressure."[128] Normally, a cholinergic reflex loop acts to increase LES pressure when intragastric or intra-abdominal pressure rises.[4] The pressure gradient between the LES and the stomach, referred to as the *barrier pressure*, is responsible for preventing GER (Boxes 12-5 and 12-6).[13,129,130]

LES function is modulated by neurohumoral influences. Cholinergic stimulation increases LES tone, whereas dopaminergic and adrenergic stimulations reduce it.[13,24,129] β-Adrenergic agents and theophylline reduce LES pressure and promote GER, often with symptomatic heartburn in awake patients. β-Adrenergic blockade elevates LES pressure.[131] Anticholinergics attenuate LES tone and impair the efficacy of medications given to increase LES barrier pressure.[1,26,58,132,133] Although prochlorperazine raises LES pressure (presumably by an antidopaminergic effect), promethazine lowers LES pressure because of its anticholinergic properties.[13] Among the wide variety of other drugs that may reduce LES tone are benzodiazepines, opioids, barbiturates, dopamine, tricyclic antidepressants, calcium channel blockers, nitroglycerin, and nitroprusside.[1,26] Although succinylcholine-induced fasciculations can elevate intra-abdominal pressure, LES tone concurrently rises, and the barrier pressure is maintained or increased.[1,13] Apart from pharmacologic influences, Rabey and colleagues demonstrated that "barrier pressure may be reduced after insertion of an LMA during anesthesia with spontaneous ventilation."[130]

In many cases, agents that increase LES contractility also promote forward passage of gastric contents, and the factors that attenuate LES tone also retard gastric emptying. This correlation compounds pharmacologic opportunities for either protection or mischief. Opioids and anticholinergics inhibit gastrointestinal motility, increasing the volume of gastric contents available for vomiting or regurgitation.[133,134] Although pain and anxiety delay gastric emptying through sympathetic stimulation, the administration of an opioid for analgesia can further retard the propulsion of gastric contents into the duodenum.[26,129]

1. Metoclopramide

Gastroprokinetic drugs are now available to promote gastric emptying while simultaneously enhancing LES barrier pressure. Metoclopramide is the prototypical agent in this category. The mechanisms of action proposed for metoclopramide include central antidopaminergic activity and prolactin stimulation as well as peripheral blockade of dopamine receptors and stimulation of cholinergic function in the upper gastrointestinal tract. Although metoclopramide retains its gastrokinetic effect in vagotomized subjects, atropine has been shown to interfere with this activity.[128,135] Metoclopramide both

raises LES contractility and barrier pressure and accelerates gastric emptying. The latter effect is achieved by intensifying gastric longitudinal muscle contraction while relaxing the gastroduodenal sphincter and increasing the coordination of gastrointestinal peristalsis. Metoclopramide has no effect on gastric acid secretion.[58,128]

Metoclopramide has been extensively investigated as a chemoprophylactic agent for aspiration pneumonitis in children and in adults. Several original studies of patients given metoclopramide, in a dose of 10 or 20 mg either orally (PO) or intravenously (IV), demonstrated the drug's utility in reducing gastric residual volume.[58,136,137] Gonzalez and Kallar wrote that "metoclopramide 10 mg PO or IV, in combination with Bicitra or an H_2-receptor antagonist, provides the most effective control of gastric volume and pH."[58] Given PO, metoclopramide has an onset of action that reportedly varies from 30 to 60 minutes, with a duration of action of 2 to 3 hours.[58] Ciresi found that metoclopramide at either 10 or 20 mg IV could reliably empty the stomach within 10 to 20 minutes.[128] Manchikanti and coworkers reported that metoclopramide 10 mg IV reduced the increase in gastric volume that followed ingestion of sodium citrate and citric acid (Bicitra) but did not interfere with Bicitra's antacid activity.[136] Metoclopramide was also found to reduce the volume of gastric contents in pediatric trauma patients.[138]

Other researchers found metoclopramide to be less uniformly effective, especially in the context of opioid coadministration or the recent ingestion of a solid meal.[132] Christensen and colleagues demonstrated no influence of metoclopramide 0.1 mg/kg on the gastric pH or volume of healthy pediatric patients.[139] As a perioperative antiemetic, metoclopramide was shown to be inconsistently useful.[132] Side effects attributed to metoclopramide have included somnolence, dizziness, and faintness. These problems may surface more frequently in elderly or severely ill patients.[58,128] Extrapyramidal reactions are a more serious problem but reportedly occur in only 1% of subjects.[128] Deehan and Dobb reported on a patient with traumatic brain injury in whom metoclopramide 10 mg IV twice induced a severe rise in intracranial pressure associated with increased cerebral blood flow.[140]

Metoclopramide has also been investigated in obstetric anesthesia. The drug has been shown to increase LES tone in pregnant women and therefore may be a useful prophylactic agent before cesarean section.[132,135] However, studies of gastric emptying in parturient women have provided less consistent results. Metoclopramide was shown to accelerate gastric emptying in patients undergoing scheduled or urgent cesarean section.[135,137] On the other hand, Cohen and associates examined 58 healthy parturients after an overnight fast and found that metoclopramide, 10 mg IV, had no significant effect on mean gastric volume or pH or on the proportion of patients with a gastric content volume exceeding 25 mL. They suggested that the drug might be more useful in the emergency setting for patients with active labor, recent food intake, pain, and anxiety.[135] Maternal metoclopramide administration does produce detectable and variable neonatal blood levels of the drug but without reported effects on Apgar scores or neurobehavioral test results.[135,141]

2. Erythromycin

Erythromycin is a macrolide antibiotic that has been in common use for more than 50 years. Given intravenously, it has been shown to improve gastric motility in patients with diabetic gastroparesis. Enteral feedings with erythromycin also pass more quickly through the stomach than control feedings. This action is thought to arise from the stimulation of motilin receptors in gastric smooth muscle.[142] Boivin and associates demonstrated that intravenous "erythromycin increased gastric emptying in a dose-response manner.... [N]ausea and stomach cramping were associated with the 3.0 mg/kg dose of erythromycin; drowsiness was associated with metoclopramide [10 mg]."[143] The potential applicability of these findings to perioperative aspiration prophylaxis is interesting but unproved.

B. Reduction of Gastric Acid Content

Chemoprophylaxis of aspiration pneumonitis can also include the inhibition of gastric acid secretion or the neutralization of HCl already in the stomach. The former should eventually increase the pH and reduce the volume of gastric contents but has no effect on acidic fluid already in place. The latter should elevate gastric fluid pH but may also increase gastric fluid volume. The aspiration of particulate antacids can pose hazards equivalent to those of gastric acid inhalation, as previously described. In 1982, Eyler and colleagues demonstrated severe pulmonary pathology in rabbits resulting from aspiration of a commercial particulate antacid.[144] Oral antacid prophylaxis should therefore include only soluble, nonparticulate agents.

1. Neutralization of Gastric Acid

The clear antacid solutions most commonly studied are sodium citrate (0.3 molar solution) and Bicitra. The pH of sodium citrate solutions typically exceeds 7.0, whereas that of Bicitra is 4.3.[136] Manchikanti and associates compared surgical outpatients given Bicitra 15 or 30 mL PO with a matched control group. All patients studied were nonobese and NPO for at least 8 hours. Of the control patients, 88% had a gastric content pH of 2.5 or less, in contrast to 32% of those given Bicitra 15 mL and only 16% of those given Bicitra 30 mL.[136]

Sodium citrate has been evaluated as a sole prophylactic agent in a variety of surgical settings, with inconsistent results. Kuster and colleagues found that sodium citrate 30 mL, taken shortly before elective surgery, resulted in gastric fluid pH values greater than 3.5 in 95% of patients.[145] Colman and coworkers administered 15 or 30 mL of sodium citrate to 30 parturient women before emergency cesarean section. All 15 patients given 30 mL sodium citrate and 14 of 15 given 15 mL had gastric pH values of 2.5 or higher.[146] In other reports, however, sodium citrate failed to alter gastric fluid pH in surgical patients. In a 0.3 molar solution, 30 mL may be more consistently effective than 15 mL, but it may still not have prolonged effects in patients with rapid gastric emptying.[13,147,148] Antacid prophylaxis may therefore be adequate at the induction of anesthesia but inadequate at

the time of awakening. Larger volumes of sodium citrate can induce nausea and vomiting or diarrhea.[136]

2. Inhibition of Gastric Acid Secretion

a. H₂-RECEPTOR BLOCKADE

Gastric acid production is strongly modulated by the action of H_2 receptors. H_2-receptor blockade inhibits basal acid secretion as well as that stimulated by the presence of gastrin or food. Both H_2 antagonists and anticholinergic agents block the neural stimulation of gastric acid secretion.[128] However, this beneficial anticholinergic effect is overridden by the inhibition of gastrointestinal motility, so that gastric volume is not reduced and gastric pH is elevated only inconsistently.[58] Although H_2 antagonists do not delay gastric emptying, their inhibition of acid secretion tends to correlate inconsistently with both the timing and the magnitude of maximal drug concentration in the plasma.[93] Various H_2 antagonists have been evaluated in both surgical and obstetric settings, with different doses and routes of administration, and with and without other prophylactic medications, to produce an expansive volume of findings.

CIMETIDINE. Given before elective surgery, a variety of cimetidine regimens can ensure that most patients have gastric fluid volume or pH values, or both, in the safe range, as defined by the investigators. These usually effective regimens include cimetidine 300 mg PO at bedtime followed by 300 mg PO or intramuscularly (IM) on the morning of surgery; cimetidine 300 to 600 mg PO given 1.5 to 2 hours preoperatively; and cimetidine 200 mg IV given 1 hour before surgery. In one study, cimetidine most reliably produced gastric content safety when combined with preoperative metoclopramide.[1] The reliability of oral cimetidine is generally improved if the drug is administered both the night before and on the morning of anesthesia.[11]

A gastric fluid pH of 2.5 or lower has been found in 5% to 35% of patients treated with single 300-mg doses of cimetidine given PO, IM, or IV in different studies. Significant elevation of gastric pH requires 30 to 60 minutes to become evident after the IV administration of cimetidine and 60 to 90 minutes after IM or PO dosing. Effective inhibition of gastric acid secretion persists for 4 to 6 hours.[58,132] Papadimitriou and colleagues administered cimetidine 400 mg IV to 20 patients facing emergency surgery. Compared with 10 such patients given placebo treatment, those receiving cimetidine were found to have significantly lower mean gastric acidity, but the range of pH values was 1.6 to 7.2.[149]

Cimetidine chemoprophylaxis has also been evaluated in obstetric anesthesia. In a study of 100 patients undergoing emergency cesarean section, cimetidine 200 mg IM was administered when surgical delivery was decided upon, followed by oral intake of a 0.3-molar solution of sodium citrate 30 mL just before induction. None of these patients had a gastric fluid pH lower than 2.7, and only 1 of 100 had a gastric fluid pH lower than 3.0.[90] Cimetidine administered in this fashion would most likely reduce gastric acidity by the time of extubation, whereas sodium citrate would be required to neutralize the acid already present.

Although cimetidine has a well-established record of safety when administered for perioperative aspiration prophylaxis, there are potential and observed side effects. The rapid IV infusion of large doses (e.g., 400 to 600 mg) has reportedly induced both hypotension and dangerous ventricular dysrhythmias.[129,132] Smith and colleagues advised that IV cimetidine be infused over at least a 10-minute period.[150] Other side effects sporadically associated with cimetidine include confusion, dizziness, headaches, and diarrhea, although these have not been reported to occur with single-dose preoperative administration.[128,129,132]

Cimetidine competitively inhibits the hepatic mixed-function oxidase system (cytochrome P450 enzyme) and also reduces hepatic perfusion.[129,131,132] As a result, cimetidine may elevate the blood concentrations of other drugs that are cleared by the liver, including warfarin, propranolol, diazepam, theophylline, phenytoin, meperidine, bupivacaine, and lidocaine. Clinically, this seems to be a greater concern with long-term use than with one- or two-dose administration.[128,132,146]

RANITIDINE. After cimetidine, ranitidine emerged as the next option for H_2 blockade. Ranitidine is considered to exert little or no inhibition of hepatic enzymes, has a longer duration of action (6 to 8 hours) than cimetidine, and has an efficacy greater than or equal to that of the original H_2 blocker. Effective onset times for the two drugs appear to be similar.[1,58,132,146,151] Smith and coauthors reported that ranitidine 50 mg, given IV over 2 minutes to 20 critically ill patients, led to variable, transient reductions in mean arterial pressure and systemic vascular resistance. These hemodynamic effects occurred less frequently and were of lesser degree and duration than those resulting from cimetidine 200 mg, similarly administered. Previous sporadic case reports associated significant bradycardia with the IV administration of either cimetidine or ranitidine.[150]

In the study of adult surgical outpatients by Maltby and colleagues, ranitidine 150 mg PO, given 2.5 hours before anesthetic induction, significantly decreased gastric residual volume and significantly increased gastric fluid pH compared with placebo. In no patient was there the conventional (but arbitrary) at-risk combination of gastric pH lower than 2.5 and gastric volume greater than 25 mL.[83] McAllister and associates treated adult patients with a single oral dose of ranitidine 300 mg, given 2 hours before surgery, and found both a significant increase in mean gastric fluid pH and a significant decrease in mean gastric fluid volume compared with placebo treatment. Noting the occasional patient with gastric fluid pH lower than 2.5, the authors cautioned that "it is unsafe to assume that H_2 antagonists will always eliminate the risk of acid aspiration pneumonitis."[152] Single-dose IV administration of ranitidine, 40 to 100 mg, has also been found to reliably generate gastric fluid pH values greater than 2.5 in adults, manifesting a greater efficacy than that of cimetidine 300 mg IV.[1]

Sandhar and coworkers evaluated the efficacy of a single oral dose of ranitidine, 2 mg/kg, given 2 to 3 hours before surgery to patients aged 1 to 14 years. Although ranitidine significantly reduced both the volume and the acidity of gastric contents compared with placebo, 6 of 44 children receiving ranitidine did have gastric fluid pH values of 2.5 or lower.[68] These findings confirmed those of a similar study of Goudsouzian and Young,[153] although other authors have not demonstrated such a consistent reduction in gastric fluid volume.[1,83]

Papadimitriou and associates compared ranitidine 150 mg IV with cimetidine 400 mg IV and with placebo given 1 hour before anesthetic induction to emergency surgical patients. Ranitidine and cimetidine caused similar reductions in gastric volume and acidity; only the reductions in acidity were statistically significant. Although the mean pH values in the cimetidine and ranitidine groups were similar, only ranitidine consistently produced safe gastric pH values (all of which were 5.0 or higher).[149] Vila and colleagues, evaluating H_2 antagonists in morbidly obese surgical patients, concluded that ranitidine was superior to cimetidine in elevating gastric fluid pH.[154] A literature review cited by Gonzalez and Kallar also found that ranitidine more reliably ensured that gastric fluid pH would exceed 2.5 than did cimetidine, although neither agent consistently reduced gastric fluid volume into the range considered safe by study authors.[58]

The effect of PO ranitidine (150 mg, given 2 to 3 hours before the scheduled time of surgery) with or without PO metoclopramide (10 mg, given 1 hour before surgery) and/or sodium citrate (30 mL on call to the operating room) on gastric fluid volume and pH was measured in 196 elective surgical inpatients. Although no combination guaranteed a safe combination of fluid volume and pH, a single oral dose of ranitidine was statistically as effective as triple prophylaxis.[155] In pediatric patients, both Gombar and Maekawa and their colleagues showed that PO ranitidine (either 2 mg/kg or 75 mg) effectively elevated gastric fluid pH with no appreciable effect on gastric volume.[76,156] In his study of the IV administration of these drugs 15 minutes before anesthetic induction, Hong concluded that "prophylactic ranitidine (50 mg IV) and metoclopramide (10 mg IV) may be an easy and useful method to decrease the volume while increasing the pH of gastric contents."[157]

Ranitidine has also been evaluated for prophylactic use in obstetric anesthesia. Rout and colleagues evaluated the efficacy of ranitidine 50 mg IV given to laboring patients when cesarean section was decided upon. A control group received no H_2-antagonist therapy, but all patients were given 30 mL of 0.3-molar sodium citrate shortly before induction. At the time of induction, 4% of those given only sodium citrate had a gastric fluid volume greater than 25 mL along with a pH lower than 3.5, compared with 2.3% of those given both citrate and ranitidine ($P = 0.05$).[151] At the time of extubation, 5.6% of those given only sodium citrate were considered to be at risk by the preceding criteria, compared with only 0.3% of those given both citrate and ranitidine ($P < 0.05$). In a recent *Cochrane Database Systems Review*, Paranjothyand coworkers concluded that, although "the quality of the evidence was poor, … the findings suggest that the combination of antacids plus H_2 antagonists is superior to antacids alone in increasing gastric pH [in patients undergoing caesarean section]. When a single agent is used, antacids alone are superior to H$_2$ antagonists."[158]

OTHERS. A voluminous body of evidence thus documents the general safety and efficacy of preoperative cimetidine and ranitidine in ameliorating the acidity and volume of gastric contents. Newer agents, such as famotidine (10 mg PO) and nizatidine, have also been evaluated, with generally favorable results.[154,159] Wajima and colleagues reported that nizatidine 300 mg PO was uniformly effective in maintaining gastric content pH above 2.5 and volume below 25 mL when given 2 hours before surgery.[160]

On the basis of the presumably high ratio of benefit to risk, H$_2$-blocking agents have been recommended for surgical patients who have an increased likelihood of inhaling gastric contents.[1,65] However, given the infrequency of perioperative aspiration pneumonitis, documentation of the actual clinical benefit of such practice has yet to be provided. In the review by Warner and coauthors of more than 215,000 general anesthesias in adults, 35 patients with acknowledged risk factors did aspirate perioperatively. Of these 35, 17 had been given prophylactic medication. In this small sample, aspiration prophylaxis produced no discernible difference in the incidence of pulmonary complications.[3] In general, the routine preoperative use of H$_2$ antagonists is not considered either essential or cost-effective. As stated by Kallar and Everett, "It has yet to be proven that prophylaxis against acid aspiration changes morbidity or mortality in healthy patients having elective surgery."[1]

b. PROTON PUMP INHIBITION

Proton pump inhibitors (PPIs) constitute a newer class of agents for the suppression of gastric acid production. Acetylcholine, histamine, and gastrin all stimulate HCl secretion by the gastric parietal cell. Although these agonists stimulate different populations of receptors, their mechanisms of action all eventually result in the formation of cyclic adenosine monophosphate (cAMP). cAMP activates the proton pump, H$^+$,K$^+$-adenosine triphosphatase (H$^+$,K$^+$-ATPase), which exchanges intraluminal potassium ions for intracellular hydrogen ions. Hydrogen ions are thereby secreted from the parietal cell into gastric fluids.[68,152] Omeprazole, the prototype PPI, is actually a pro-drug that is absorbed in the small intestine and is activated in the highly acidic milieu of the gastric parietal cell. Activated omeprazole then remains in the parietal cell for up to 48 hours, inhibiting the proton pump in a prolonged manner.[141,161-163] Inhibition of gastric acid secretion can be nearly complete, with no discernible side effects. A single dose of omeprazole, 20 to 40 mg, reduces gastric acidity for up to 48 hours. On the other hand, PPIs are characterized by variable first-pass metabolism with resulting inconsistencies in the plasma concentration after any given oral dose. As is the case with H$_2$ antagonists, there is also an unpredictable relationship between peak plasma concentration and peak inhibition of gastric acid production.[93]

Omeprazole has been evaluated as a preoperative agent for the chemoprophylaxis of aspiration pneumonitis. Bouly and colleagues gave omeprazole 40 mg PO to healthy patients either the evening before or 2 hours before elective surgery. Although mean gastric fluid pH was significantly higher with omeprazole treatment than with placebo, 6 of 30 patients receiving omeprazole had gastric fluid pH values lower than 2.5 at the time of induction. Omeprazole significantly reduced gastric fluid volume compared with placebo.[161]

Omeprazole has also been evaluated in obstetric anesthesia. In a study by Orr and associates, all 15 patients who received omeprazole and also metoclopramide 20 mg IM at least 20 minutes before elective cesarean section had gastric fluid pH values greater than 2.5, both on induction and at extubation. When omeprazole 80 mg PO was given only on the morning of elective cesarean section, 2 of 33 patients had a gastric fluid pH lower than 2.5 at induction, 1 of whom also had a gastric fluid volume greater than 40 mL. All gastric fluid pH values were greater than 2.5 at extubation. Of 16 patients who also received metoclopramide 20 mg IM at least 20 minutes before elective cesarean section, 2 still had gastric fluid pH values lower than 2.5 (with gastric fluid volumes less than 25 mL) on induction, but all gastric fluid pH values exceeded 2.5 at extubation.[141]

In general, the PPIs have been found most effective when given in two doses, one on the night before and one on the morning of surgery.[93] Given the dwindling proportion of patients hospitalized before elective surgery, however, two-dose regimens for chemoprophylaxis would seem somewhat impractical. Furthermore, Nishina and coauthors reported that a single preoperative oral dose of ranitidine was more effective in reducing gastric acid content than two-dose regimens of rabeprazole or lansoprazole.[164] On the other hand, Pisegna and colleagues found that "pantoprazole (40 mg IV) decreased gastric acid output and volume, and increased pH within 1 hour of dosing. Effects were sustained for up to 12 hours following single-dose administration."[165]

IV. CONCLUSIONS

It is clearly best to prevent gastric contents of any volume or pH from entering the trachea. Although this ideal may not always be attainable, even by the most skillful of clinicians, its likelihood would appear to be favored by optimal preparation of patients and a carefully executed, well-designed plan for anesthetic induction and airway management. The place of awake induction and gastric emptying in high-risk cases is influenced by patients' characteristics and practitioners' experience and confidence. Although RSI with cricoid pressure remains a standard prophylactic maneuver, it is now recognized that airway management and effective ventilation may mandate its modification, or even discontinuation, in certain circumstances.

An impressive array of pharmacologic agents can now be employed to promote antegrade gastric emptying, inhibit GER, and reduce the acid content of gastric fluids. These drugs have an established record of safety and offer the reasonable expectation of rendering gastric fluid less threatening to the lungs. However, because of the low incidence of clinically significant perioperative aspiration, it may not be possible to demonstrate statistically that the use of these agents actually improves patients' outcomes. In reference to gastric prokinetic drugs, antacids, and inhibitors of acid secretion, the ASA Task Force concluded that "the routine preoperative use of [such medications] in patients who have no apparent increased risk for pulmonary aspiration is not recommended."[78] Chemoprophylaxis is only an adjunct to and not a substitute for otherwise sound clinical practice. It is, of course, less desirable to have aspirated and survived than never to have aspirated at all.

V. CLINICAL PEARLS

- Regurgitation and aspiration can result from "light" anesthesia, coughing, and gagging in the patient not intubated.

- About half of all cases of perioperative aspiration occur at times other than anesthetic induction.

- Patients manifesting no evidence of respiratory impairment for 2 hours after a known or suspected aspiration episode are highly unlikely to become significantly symptomatic later.

- Delayed gastric emptying in diabetic patients correlates with the presence of autonomic, but not peripheral, neuropathy.

- Both pain and opiates significantly retard gastric emptying.

- Aspiration of particulate antacids can induce a severe granulomatous pneumonitis.

- Ingestion of clear liquids 2 to 3 hours before anesthetic induction does not appear to increase the risk of gastric content aspiration in patients with no gastrointestinal pathology.

- Cricoid pressure can compromise ventilation by either mask or LMA and can either facilitate or interfere with direct laryngoscopy.

- Nonparticulate antacids rapidly raise gastric fluid pH in most patients, with an inconsistent duration of action.

- H_2 antagonists more reliably reduce gastric fluid acidity than gastric fluid volume.

- Metoclopramide reduces gastric fluid volume in most patients without consistently affecting gastric fluid pH.

SELECTED REFERENCES

All references can be found online at expertconsult.com.

3. Warner MA, Warner ME, Weber JG: Clinical significance of pulmonary aspiration during the perioperative period. *Anesthesiology* 78:56–62, 1993.

7. Fried EB: The rapid sequence induction revisited: Obesity and sleep apnea syndrome. *Anesthesiol Clin North Am* 23:551–554, 2005.

56. Mendelson CL: The aspiration of stomach contents into the lungs during obstetric anesthesia. *Am J Obstet Gynecol* 52:191, 1946.

78. American Society of Anesthesiologists Task Force on Preoperative Fasting: Practice guidelines for preoperative fasting and the use of pharmacologic agents to reduce the risk of pulmonary aspiration: Application to healthy patients undergoing elective procedures. *Anesthesiology* 90:896–905, 1999.

89. de Souza DG, Doar LH, Mehta SH, et al: Aspiration prophylaxis and rapid sequence induction for elective cesarean delivery: Time to reassess old dogma? *Anesth Analg* 110:1503–1505, 2010.

92. Crawford JS: How can aspiration of vomitus in obstetrics best be prevented? Commentary: Setting the record straight. *Birth* 15:230–235, 1988.

93. Ng A, Smith G: Gastroesophageal reflux and aspiration of gastric contents in anesthetic practice. *Anesth Analg* 93:494–513, 2001.

104. El-Orbany M, Connolly LA: Rapid sequence induction and intubation: Current controversy. *Anesth Analg* 111:1318–1325, 2010.

106. Sellick BA: Cricoid pressure to control regurgitation of stomach contents during induction of anaesthesia. *Lancet* 2:404, 1961.

158. Paranjothy S, Griffiths JD, Broughton KH, et al: Interventions at caesarean section for reducing the risk of aspiration pneumonitis (review). *Cochrane Database Syst Rev* (1):CD004943, 2010.

Chapter 13

Preoxygenation

ANIS S. BARAKA | M. RAMEZ SALEM

I. HISTORICAL PERSPECTIVE

In 1948, Fowler and Comroe demonstrated that inhalation of 100% oxygen (O_2) resulted in a very rapid increase of arterial oxyhemoglobin saturation (SaO_2) to between 98% and 99%, but that attainment of the last 1% to 2% was a much slower process.[1] They also observed that the rate of increase was attenuated in patients with pulmonary emphysema or pulmonary artherosclerosis.[1] In 1955, Hamilton and Eastwood showed that "denitrogenation" was 95% complete within 2 to 3 minutes in subjects breathing normally from a circle anesthesia system with 5 L/min O_2.[2] Dillon and Darsi, in the same year, observed significant arterial oxyhemoglobin desaturation during apnea after anesthetic induction with sodium thiopental and recommended that induction of anesthesia and endoscopy should be preceded by O_2 administration for 5 minutes.[3] Six years later, Heller and Watson found that 3 to 4 minutes of O_2 breathing was necessary in patients before anesthetic induction, whereas adequate oxygenation could be accomplished with the use of manual ventilation in 30 seconds.[4] With the introduction of the rapid-sequence induction and intubation (RSI) technique in the 1950s in patients at risk for aspiration of gastric contents, preoxygenation became a component of the technique.[5,6] Preoxygenation was emphasized by Sellick when he introduced cricoid pressure into clinical practice in 1961,[7] and it was also recommended before RSI in pediatric patients in the 1970s.[8]

Preoxygenation before anesthetic induction and intubation became a widely accepted maneuver designed to increase O_2 reserves and thereby delay the onset of arterial oxyhemoglobin desaturation during apnea. Various techniques and regimens have been advocated to ensure adequate preoxygenation. For many years, tidal volume breathing (TVB) of O_2 for 3 to 5 minutes has been commonly practiced.[2,3] Gold and colleagues challenged the need for 3 minutes of TVB by demonstrating that 4 deep breaths within 0.5 minutes (4 DB/0.5 min) and TVB for 5 minutes using a semiclosed circle absorber system were equally effective in increasing arterial oxygen tension (PaO_2).[9] Although some investigators corroborated their findings,[10,11] others showed that TVB for 3 minutes provided better preoxygenation and longer protection against hypoxemia during apnea than 4 DB/0.5 min.[12-15] Later investigations suggested that the use of extended deep breathing (8, 12, and 16 deep breaths in 1.0, 1.5, and 2.0 minutes, respectively) could produce maximal preoxygenation comparable to that achieved with TVB for 3 minutes and could also delay the onset of apnea-induced oxyhemoglobin desaturation.[16,17]

Regardless of the technique used, preoxygenation has become an integral component of the RSI technique, and it is particularly important if manual ventilation is not desirable, if difficulty with ventilation or endotracheal intubation is anticipated, and in patients with oxygen transport limitations. Because the "cannot intubate, cannot ventilate" (CICV) situation is largely unpredictable, the desirability of maximal preoxygenation is theoretically present for all patients.[18]

The original American Society of Anesthesiologists' (ASA) difficult airway (DA) algorithm made no mention of preoxygenation. In an updated report by the ASA Task Force on Management of the DA (2003), the topic of "facemask preoxygenation before initiating management of the difficult airway" was added.[19] "Routine" preoxygenation has become a new "minimum standard" of care, not only during induction of anesthesia, but also during emergence from anesthesia and tracheal extubation.[20-22]

II. BODY OXYGEN STORES

Oxygen is carried in the blood in two forms: the greater portion is in reversible chemical combination with hemoglobin (Hb), and the smaller part is dissolved in plasma.[23] The ability to carry large amounts of O_2 in Hb is important, because without it, the amount carried in the plasma would be so small that the cardiac output would need to be increased more than 20 times to yield an adequate O_2 flux.[23] The amount of chemically bound O_2 is directly related to the concentration of Hb and how saturated the Hb is with O_2. Arterial O_2 content (Cao_2) can be calculated from the following equation:

$$Cao_2 = Hb \times 1.36 \times Sao_2 + Pao_2 \times 0.003$$

where
1.36 = estimated mass volume of O_2 that can be bound by 1 g of normal Hb
Sao_2 = arterial oxyhemoglobin saturation (when fully saturated, Sao_2 = 100%)
Pao_2 = arterial partial pressure of oxygen
0.003 = solubility coefficient of O_2 in human plasma

The Cao_2 with an Hb concentration of 15 g/dL is approximately 20 mL of O_2 per 100 dL of blood. In addition, approximately 0.3 mL of O_2/100 dL blood is in physical solution. This amount of dissolved O_2 normally accounts for only 1.5% of the total O_2, but its contribution increases when Pao_2 is increased (dissolved O_2 is linearly related to Pao_2). The venous O_2 content ($C\bar{v}o_2$) when there is a mixed venous O_2 tension ($P\bar{v}o_2$) of 40 mm Hg and mixed venous oxyhemoglobin saturation ($S\bar{v}o_2$) of 75% can be calculated accordingly.

Hb uptake and release of O_2 are regulated by a pattern demonstrated by the familiar oxyhemoglobin dissociation curve, which is a plot of Sao_2 as a function of Pao_2. The sigmoid shape of the curve reflects the fact that the four binding sites on a given Hb molecule interact with each other.[23] When the first site has bound a molecule of O_2, the binding of the next site is facilitated, and so forth. The result is a curve that is steep up to a Po_2 of 60 mm Hg and becomes more shallow thereafter, approaching 100% saturation asymptotically. At a Po_2 of 100 mm Hg, the normal arterial value, 97% of the hemes have bound O_2; at 40 mm Hg, a typical value for ($P\bar{v}o_2$) in a resting person, the saturation declines to about 75%. The shape

of the oxyhemoglobin dissociation curve has important physiologic implications. The flatness of the curve above a Po_2 of 80 mm Hg ensures a relatively constant Sao_2 despite wide variations in alveolar O_2 pressure. The steep portion of the curve between 20 to 60 mm Hg permits unloading of O_2 from Hb at relatively high Po_2 values, which favors the delivery of large amounts of O_2 into the tissues by diffusion.

The O_2-binding properties of Hb are influenced by a number of factors, including pH, Pco_2, and temperature.[23] These factors cause shifts of the oxyhemoglobin dissociation curve to the right or left without changing the slope of the curve. For example, an increase in temperature or a decrease in pH, such as may occur in active tissues, decreases the affinity of Hb for O_2 and shifts the oxyhemoglobin dissociation curve to the right. As a result, a higher Po_2 is required to achieve a given saturation, which facilitates unloading of O_2 at the tissue. To quantify the extent of a shift of the oxyhemoglobin dissociation curve, the so-called P_{50} is used—that is, the Po_2 required for 50% saturation. The P_{50} of normal adult Hb at 37° C and normal pH and Pco_2 is 26 to 27 mm Hg.

Despite its great importance, O_2 is a very difficult gas to store in a biologic system. In subjects breathing air, O_2 stores are small (Table 13-1).[23,24] The relatively steep oxyhemoglobin dissociation curve and the small O_2 stores imply that factors affecting Pao_2 produce their full effects very quickly. This is in contrast to CO_2, for which the large size of the stores buffers the body against rapid changes. Therefore, in a subject breathing air, a pulse oximeter probably gives an earlier indication of hypoventilation than does CO_2 measurement. In contrast, in a subject breathing a high fraction of inspired O_2 (Fio_2), CO_2 measurement gives an earlier indication of hypoventilation.[23]

The amounts of body O_2 in the various storage sites of a person breathing air are increased with breathing 100% of O_2 (Fig. 13-1; see also Table 13-1).[23,24] The maximal increase of O_2 stores occurs in the functional residual capacity (FRC). Storage of O_2 in the tissue is rather difficult to assess, but assuming that Henry's law applies and the partition coefficient for gases approximates the gas-water coefficients, breathing O_2 for 3 minutes significantly increases tissue O_2 stores.[24]

TABLE 13-1

Body O_2 Stores (in mL) during Room Air and 100% O_2 Breathing

Storage Site	Room Air	100% O_2
In the lungs (FRC)	450	3000
In the blood	850	950
Dissolved in tissue fluids	50	100
In combination with myoglobin	200?	200
Total	1550	4250

FRC, Functional residual capacity; O_2, oxygen.
From Nunn JF, editor: *Nunn's applied respiratory physiology*, ed 4, Oxford, 1993, Butterworth-Heinemann, p 288.

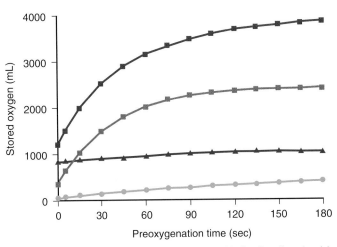

Figure 13-1 Variation in volume of O_2 stored in the functional residual capacity *(blue)*, the blood *(red)*, the tissue *(turquoise)*, and the whole body *(purple)* with duration of preoxygenation. (From Campbell IT, Beatty PCW: Monitoring preoxygenation. *Br J Anaesth* 72:3–4, 1994.)

III. PHYSIOLOGY OF APNEA AND APNEIC MASS-MOVEMENT OXYGENATION

During apnea, the total body O_2 consumption ($\dot{V}O_2$) remains fairly constant at about 250 mL/min. Consequently, the alveolar O_2 concentration (PAO_2) decreases rapidly as a result of the depletion of the diminishing O_2 stores in the lungs. If the airway becomes obstructed, O_2 removal will generate a substantial and immediate negative pressure, contributing to a further decrease of PaO_2. Although the PaO_2 falls in direct relation to PAO_2, SaO_2 remains greater than 90% as long as the Hb can be reoxygenated in the lungs.[25-28] SaO_2 starts to decrease only after the lung O_2 stores are depleted and the PaO_2 is lower than 60 mm Hg. It is for this reason that oximetry is not the best "physiologic means," compared with PaO_2, for predicting the onset of hypoxemia. However, because it detects decreases in SaO_2 before other clinical signs, oximetry is an invaluable clinical monitor that adds to the safety of anesthetic management.[27] Critical oxyhemoglobin desaturation may be defined as SaO_2 less than or equal to 80%; for patients with SaO_2 less than 80%, the range in the rate of decrease is 20% to 40% per minute during apnea.[29]

Preoxygenation followed by O_2 insufflation during subsequent apnea maintains SaO_2 by apneic diffusion oxygenation.[25,26] In the apneic adult, the $\dot{V}O_2$ averages 230 mL/min, whereas the output of CO_2 to the alveoli is limited to about 21 mL/min and the remaining CO_2 production (approximately 90%) is buffered within the body tissues. The lung volume initially decreases by the net gas exchange ratio of 209 mL/min. Therefore, a pressure gradient is created between the upper airway and the alveoli, and if the airway is patent, this results in a mass movement of O_2 down the trachea into the alveoli. Conversely, CO_2 is not exhaled because of this mass movement of O_2 down the trachea, and the alveolar CO_2 concentration ($PACO_2$) shows an initial rise of about 8 to

16 mm Hg during the first minute and a subsequent fairly linear rise of about 3 mm Hg/min.[30]

Fraioli and colleagues emphasized the importance of the ratio of FRC to body weight during apneic diffusion and demonstrated that patients with a low FRC/body weight ratio could not tolerate apnea for more than 4 minutes, whereas those with a high FRC/body weight ratio (>53.3 ± 7 mL/kg) maintained PaO_2 at 90% of the control value.[25] Some studies demonstrated that with a patent airway and an FIO_2 of 1, SaO_2 can be maintained at greater than 90% for up to 100 minutes with apneic oxygenation.[25,26]

The success of apneic mass-movement oxygenation depends on airway patency to allow O_2 to move into the apneic lungs. In the presence of air obstruction, not only does the lung gas volume decrease rapidly, but the intrathoracic pressure also decreases at a rate that is dependent on $\dot{V}O_2$ and thoracic compliance, subsequently leading to a marked fall in PaO_2. When airway obstruction is relieved, rapid flow of O_2 into the lungs occurs, and with high FIO_2, rapid reoxygenation resumes.[27]

Apneic mass-movement oxygenation can be achieved by preoxygenation followed by insufflation of O_2 through a nasopharyngeal or oropharyngeal cannula or through a needle inserted in the cricothyroid or cricotracheal membrane. This provides at least 10 minutes of adequate oxygenation in healthy apneic patients whose airways are unobstructed and therefore has many practical applications.[31] In patients who are difficult to intubate or ventilate, pharyngeal O_2 insufflation (or tracheal insufflation, in cases of upper airway obstruction) may allow additional time for laryngoscopy and endotracheal intubation.[31-33] This can be advantageous in patients who have decreased O_2 reserves, such as children, pregnant women, obese patients, and patients with adult respiratory distress syndrome (ARDS).[30,32] The combination of preoxygenation and apneic diffusion oxygenation can be used during bronchoscopy and can provide the otolaryngologist with adequate time for glottic surgery unimpeded by the presence of the endotracheal tube (ETT) or by the patient's respiratory movements.[33]

During apneic diffusion oxygenation via an open airway, the increase in time to Hb desaturation achieved by increasing the FIO_2 from 0.9 to 1.0 is greater than that caused by increasing the FIO_2 from 0.21 to 0.9. Increasing the FIO_2 from 0.9 to 1.0 more than doubles the time to desaturation[34] (Fig.13-2).

IV. EFFICACY AND EFFICIENCY OF PREOXYGENATION

Studies of preoxygenation have focused on measurements of indices reflecting its efficacy and efficiency.[18] Measurements of alveolar O_2,[14,35,36] alveolar N_2,[37] or PaO_2 reflect the efficacy of preoxygenation, whereas the decline of SaO_2 during apnea is indicative of its efficiency.[9,16,18,37,38]

The SaO_2 may be misleading as a guide to alveolar denitrogenation. A saturation of 100% measured by pulse oximetry (SpO_2) is most definitely not a reason to stop denitrogenation and may occur well before the lungs are

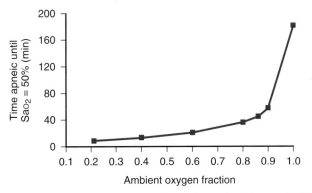

Figure 13-2 The time (duration of apnea) required to reach 50% Sao_2 with an open airway exposed to various ambient O_2 fractions. (From McNamara MJ, Hardman JG: Hypoxaemia during open-airway apnoea: A computational modelling analysis. *Anaesthesia* 60:741–746, 2005.)

adequately denitrogenated. Conversely, failure of SpO_2 to increase substantially during denitrogenation does not necessarily indicate failure of preoxygenation or lack of its value; patients with substantial pulmonary shunting may achieve excellent pulmonary O_2 reservoirs while remaining hypoxemic.[39]

A. Efficacy of Preoxygenation

Preoxygenation increases the alveolar O_2 and decreases the alveolar N_2 in a parallel fashion (Fig. 13-3).[37,40] It is the washout of N_2 from the lungs that is the key to achieving preoxygenation.[37,40] The terms *preoxygenation* and *denitrogenation* have been used synonymously to describe the same process, although a change in focus from preoxygenation to denitrogenation has been suggested.[37]

With normal lung function, the O_2 washin and nitrogen washout (the reverse of the washin) are exponential functions; therefore, the rate of preoxygenation (or denitrogenation) is governed by the time constant (τ) of the exponential curves. This constant is the same for both washin and washout curves and is proportional to the ratio of alveolar ventilation ($\dot{V}A$) to FRC. Because the O_2 flow used for $\dot{V}A$ is delivered via an anesthesia circuit, preoxygenation occurs in two sequential stages according to the time constant, which is the time required for a flow through a container (volume) to equal the capacity. These two stages are

1. Washout of the anesthesia circuit by O_2 flow

$$\tau = \frac{\text{Size of the circuit}}{O_2 \text{ flow}}$$

2. Washout of the FRC by alveolar ventilation

$$\tau = \frac{\text{FRC}}{\dot{V}A}$$

After 1 τ, the O_2 concentration of FRC will be increased by approximately 63% of its original value; after 2 τ, to 86%; after 3 τ, to 95%; and after 4 τ, to about 98% of its original value.

In order to hasten denitrogenation, it is advisable to washout (flush) the anesthesia circuit by a high O_2 flow before applying the face mask to the patient. On preoxygenation of the patient, an O_2 flow per minute that eliminates rebreathing should be used. Therefore, three steps are required to enhance preoxygenation:

1. The anesthesia circuit is flushed by a high O_2 flow.
2. A nonleaking face mask is used to avoid air entrainment.
3. An O_2 flow of 5 L/min is required for TVB, and a flow of 10 L/min is necessary for the deep breathing.

It should be noted that the time spent instructing the patient about the procedure, flushing the circuit,

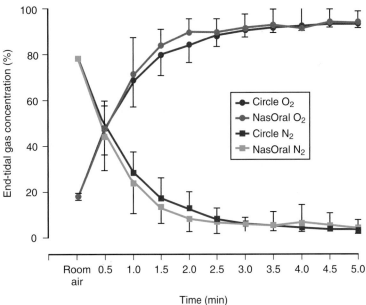

Figure 13-3 Comparison of mean end-tidal O_2 and N_2 concentrations obtained at 30-second intervals during 5-minute periods of spontaneous tidal volume oxygenation using the circle absorber and NasOral systems in 20 volunteers. Data are shown as mean ± SD. (From Nimmagadda U, Salem MR, Joseph NJ, et al: Efficacy of preoxygenation with tidal volume breathing: Comparison of breathing systems. *Anesthesiology* 93:693–698, 2000.)

positioning the face mask tightly with or without head straps, and turning on the O_2 flow may prolong the time to achievement of maximal preoxygenation.

The end points of maximal alveolar preoxygenation or denitrogenation have been defined as an end-tidal O_2 concentration (EtO_2) of approximately 90% and an end-tidal nitrogen concentration (EtN_2) of 5%.[15,35,36] In an adult with a normal FRC and $\dot{V}_{O_2}$, an EtO_2 greater than 90% means that the lungs contain more than 2000 mL of O_2 (8 to 10 times the $\dot{V}_{O_2}$).[27] Because of the obligatory presence of CO_2 and water vapor in the alveolar gas, an EtO_2 greater than 97% cannot be easily achieved. Factors affecting the efficacy of preoxygenation include FIO_2, duration of breathing, and the $\dot{V}_A$/FRC ratio (Box 13-1).

1. Fraction of Inspired Oxygen

The main reasons for failure to achieve an FIO_2 close to 1.0 are a leak under the face mask,[14,18,41-43] rebreathing of exhaled gases, and the use of systems incapable of delivering a high O_2 concentration, such as resuscitation bags.[40] Even the presence of minor leaks may not be fully compensated for by increasing the fresh gas flow (FGF) or by increasing the duration of preoxygenation. Bearded patients, edentulous patients, patients with sunken cheeks, the presence of nasogastric tubes, use of a wrong face mask size, improper use of head straps, and use of systems allowing air entrainment under the face mask are all common factors causing leaks between the face mask and the patient's head resulting in lower FIO_2. Clinical end points indicative of a sealed system are movement of the reservoir bag in and out with inhalation and exhalation, presence of a normal capnogram and end-tidal CO_2, ($EtCO_2$), and measurements of inspired and $EtCO_2$ values.[18]

There is reluctance among some anesthesiologists to use preoxygenation routinely because the mask presents discomfort to the patient and some patients find preoxygenation objectionable. There is clearly marked overestimation of the patient's discomfort by the anesthesiologist. In fact, patients' discomfort during preoxygenation is not more than the discomfort during other procedures such as the placement of intravenous lines.[44,45] It is our experience that patients accept a tight-fitting mask if the procedure is explained beforehand and they are told that "it is important to fill the tank with oxygen."

Although anesthetic circuits can deliver 100% O_2 concentration, the FIO_2 can be influenced by the type of breathing, the level of FGF, and the duration of breathing.[17] In a study involving volunteers that compared preoxygenation techniques using a semiclosed circle absorber with varying FGF in the same subjects, it was found that with TVB, inspired O_2 concentration was 95% with FGF of 5 L/min and increased to 98% with FGFs of 7 and 10 L/min. However, with deep breathing, the inspired O_2 concentration was only 88% at 5 L/min, 91% at 7 L/min, and 95% at 10 L/min FGF (Fig. 13-4).[17] These findings imply that increasing the FGF from 5 to 10 L/min has little impact on increasing FIO_2 during TVB but has a noticeable effect during deep breathing.[17] Because of the breathing characteristics of the circle system, the minute ventilation during deep breathing may exceed the FGF, resulting in rebreathing of exhaled gases (N_2) and consequently decreasing the FIO_2; in contrast, during TVB,

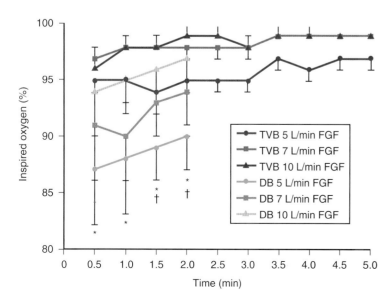

Figure 13-4 Comparison of tidal volume breathing (TVB) and deep breathing (DB) preoxygenation techniques on inspired O_2 using 5, 7, and 10 L/min fresh gas flow (FGF). *Significant difference (*P* < .05) between 5, 7, and 10 L/min FGF; †significant difference (*P* < .05) from deep breaths at 0.5 and 1.0 minute. (From Nimmagadda U, Chiravuri SD, Salem MR, et al: Preoxygenation with tidal volume and deep breathing techniques: The impact of duration of breathing and fresh gas flow. *Anesth Analg* 92:1337–1341, 2001.)

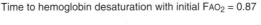

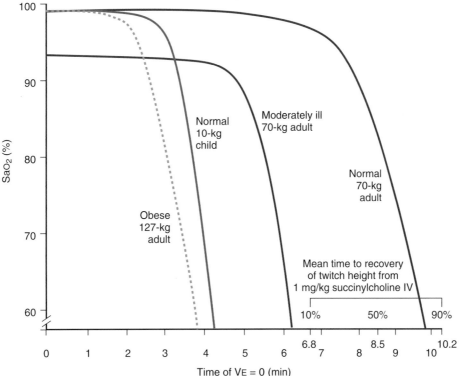

Figure 13-5 Arterial oxyhemoglobin saturation (*Sao₂*) versus time of apnea in an obese adult, a 10-kg child (low functional residual capacity (FRC) and high oxygen consumption (V̇o₂)), and in a moderately ill adult, compared with a healthy adult. *FAo₂*, Fractional alveolar oxygen concentration; *VE*, expired volume. (From Benumof JL, Dagg R, Benumof R: Critical hemoglobin desaturation will occur before return to unparalyzed state from 1 mg/kg succinylcholine. *Anesthesiology* 87:979–982, 1997.)

rebreathing of exhaled gases is negligible, and increasing the FGF from 5 to 10 L/min would have only a slight effect on F_{IO_2}.[12,17]

2. Duration of Breathing, Functional Residual Capacity, and Alveolar Ventilation

Sufficient time is needed to accomplish maximal preoxygenation. With an F_{IO_2} close to 1, most healthy adult patients can reach the target level of Et_{O_2} greater than or equal to 90% (or $Et_{N_2} \leq 5\%$) within 3 to 5 minutes of TVB. The half-time for exponential change in fraction of alveolar O_2 concentration (F_{AO_2}) with a step change in F_{IO_2} for a nonrebreathing system is given by the equation, $F_{AO_2} = 0.693 \times V_{FRC}/\dot{V}_A$. ($V_{FRC}$ is volume of functional residual capacity). With a V_{FRC} of 2.5 L, the half-times are 26 seconds when $\dot{V}_A = 4$ L/min and 13 seconds when $\dot{V}_A = 8$ L/min.[18] Therefore, most of the O_2 that can be stored in the lungs may be brought in by hyperventilation with an F_{IO_2} of 1.0 for a shorter period of time than that needed with TVB.[18] This is the basis for the deep breathing techniques, which have been introduced as an alternative to TVB.[9,18]

Changes in $\dot{V}_A$ and FRC can have a marked effect on the rate of rise in Et_{O_2} (and decrease in Et_{N_2}) during preoxygenation. Because of their increased $\dot{V}_A$ and decreased FRC, Et_{O_2} rises faster in pregnant women than in nonpregnant women.[14,46,47] Similarly, preoxygenation can be accomplished faster in infants and children than in adults.[48,49]

B. Efficiency of Preoxygenation

Preoxygenation can markedly delay arterial oxyhemoglobin desaturation during apnea. In healthy individuals breathing air, desaturation to 70% can occur within 1 minute, whereas with adequate preoxygenation, desaturation occurs after 5 minutes. The delay in desaturation during apnea depends on the efficacy of preoxygenation, the capacity for O_2 loading, and $\dot{V}_{O_2}$ (see Box 13-1). Patients with a decreased capacity for O_2 loading (decreased FRC, Pa_{O_2}, Ca_{O_2}, or cardiac output) or with increased $\dot{V}_{O_2}$, or both, desaturate much faster during apnea than healthy patients do.[18,29,42,50-52] The main difference in the rate of apnea-induced oxyhemoglobin desaturation after different preoxygenation techniques is observed between Sa_{O_2} levels of 100% and 99%.[18,27,29,34,50] This range represents the flat portion of the oxyhemoglobin dissociation curve. When O_2 reserves are depleted, rapid desaturation occurs regardless of the technique of preoxygenation and is similar to that observed in patients breathing air.

Farmery and Roe developed a computer model describing the rate of oxyhemoglobin desaturation during apnea.[50] This model was found to agree reasonably well with actual data from patients whose weight and degree of normalcy and preoxygenation were reliably known (Fig. 13-5).[29,50] Because it would be dangerous to obtain data in time to marked oxyhemoglobin desaturation in humans, this model is uniquely useful for analysis of oxyhemoglobin desaturation below 90%.[29,50]

Tidal Volume Breathing
Traditional tidal volume breathing (3-5 min)
One vital capacity breath followed by tidal volume breathing

Deep Breathing
Single vital capacity breath
Four deep breaths (4 inspiratory capacity breaths)
Eight deep breaths (8 inspiratory capacity breaths)
Extended deep breathing (12-16 inspiratory capacity breaths)
One vital capacity breath followed by deep breathing

Preoxygenation and an Additional Maneuver
Preoxygenation and continuous positive airway pressure (CPAP)
Preoxygenation and O_2 insufflation
Preoxygenation and bi-level positive airway pressure (BiPAP)

As the preapnea FAO_2 is progressively decreased from 0.87 to 0.8, 0.7, 0.6, 0.5, 0.4, 0.3, and 0.13 (air) in a healthy 70-kg patient, the apnea time to 60% SaO_2 is progressively decreased from 9.9 to 9.31, 8.38, 7.30, 6.37, 5.40, 4.40, 3.55, and 2.8 minutes, respectively.[29,50] Figure 13-5 shows that for a healthy 70-kg adult, a moderately ill 70-kg adult, a healthy 10-kg child, and an obese 127-kg adult, 80% SaO_2 is reached after 8.7, 5.5, 3.7, and 3.1 minutes, respectively, whereas 60% SaO_2 is reached at 9.9, 6.2, 4.23, and 3.8 minutes, respectively.[18,29]

V. TECHNIQUES OF PREOXYGENATION

Two main techniques are used: TVB and deep breathing (Box 13-2).

A. Tidal Volume Breathing

The traditional TVB has proved to be an effective preoxygenation technique. To ensure maximal preoxygenation, the duration of TVB should be 3 minutes or longer in adults, and an FIO_2 near 1 should be maintained (see Box 13-2 and Fig. 13-3). Various anesthetic systems (circle absorber,[9-12] Mapleson A,[14,53-55] Mapleson D,[13-15,54,55] and nonrebreathing systems) and FGFs ranging from 5 to 35 L/min have been used successfully.[2,14,15,43,54,55] However, the circle absorber system (the system most commonly used in the operating room) with an FGF as low as 5 L/min is just as effective.[40] Increasing the FGF from 5 to 10 L/min has little effect in enhancing preoxygenation during TVB in normal subjects (Fig. 13-6).[40]

B. Deep Breathing Techniques

Based on the assumption that alveolar denitrogenation can be achieved rapidly by deep breathing, Gold and colleagues introduced the 4 DB/0.5 min method of preoxygenation.[9] They showed that the PaO_2 after 4 DB/0.5 min was no different from the PaO_2 after TVB for 3 minutes. Although a few studies corroborated their findings,[10,11] other investigations showed that 3 minutes of TVB provided better preoxygenation (Fig.13-6) and longer protection against hypoxemia during apnea than the 4 DB/0.5 min method did, particularly in pregnant women, patients with morbid obesity (MO), and elderly patients.[12-15]

There are two main reasons why the 4 DB/0.5 min method is inferior to TVB. First, if the ventilation in 0.5 minutes is much greater than the O_2 inflow rate, rebreathing of exhaled nitrogen must occur, which decreases FIO_2. Nimmagadda and colleagues confirmed that 4 DB/0.5 min provided suboptimal preoxygenation in volunteers; no

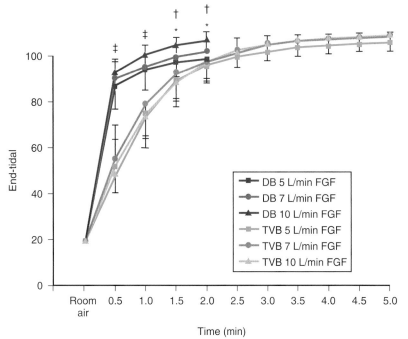

Figure 13-6 Comparison of tidal volume breathing (TVB) and deep breathing (DB) preoxygenation techniques on end-tidal O_2 using 5, 7, and 10 L/min fresh gas flow (FGF). *Significant difference ($P < .05$) from DB at 5 and 7 L/min FGF; †significant difference ($P < .05$) from DB at 0.5 and 1.0 minute; ‡significant difference ($P < .05$) from TVB. (From Nimmagadda U, Chiravuri SD, Salem MR, et al: Preoxygenation with tidal volume and deep breathing techniques: The impact of duration of breathing and fresh gas flow. *Anesth Analg* 92:1337-1341, 2001.)

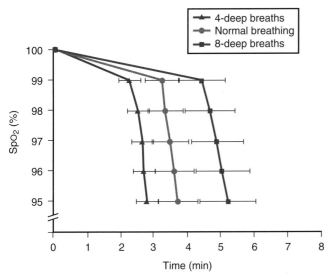

Figure 13-7 Mean times to reach percentage decrease in hemoglobin saturation during apnea after three different preoxygenation techniques. *SpO₂,* O₂ saturation from pulse oximetry. (From Baraka AS, Taha SK, Aouad MT, et al: Preoxygenation: Comparison of maximal breathing and tidal volume breathing techniques. *Anesthesiology* 91:612–616, 1999.)

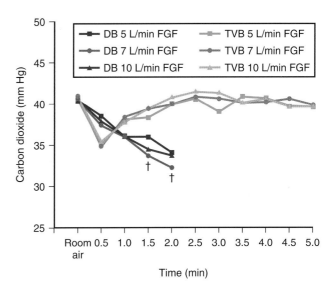

Figure 13-8 Effect of the deep breathing technique on end-tidal carbon dioxide tension using 5, 7, and 10 L/min fresh gas flow *(FGF). DB,* Deep breathing; *TVB,* tidal volume breathing. †Significant difference (*P* < .05) from deep breaths at 0.5 and 1.0 minute. (From Nimmagadda U, Chiravuri SD, Salem MR, et al: Preoxygenation with tidal volume and deep breathing techniques: The impact of duration of breathing and fresh gas flow. *Anesth Analg* 92:1337–1341, 2001.)

subject achieved an EtO_2 value of 90% or better (see Fig. 13-6).[17] Another possible reason why patients preoxygenated with 4 DB/0.5 min desaturate faster is that the tissue and venous compartments need longer than 0.5 minutes to fill with O_2.[18,24] Probably, these compartments have the capability of storing additional O_2 above that contained while breathing room air.[17,18] Such stored O_2 increases in an exponential fashion. It is possible that the 4 DB/0.5 min technique leads to rapid arterial oxygenation without substantial increase in the tissue O_2 stores and hence results in more rapid desaturation during subsequent apnea than would a longer period of preoxygenation with TVB.[18] Because the 4 DB/0.5 min technique yields submaximal preoxygenation, it should be reserved for emergency situations when time is limited.[17]

To optimize the deep breathing method of preoxygenation, investigators have focused on (1) extending the duration of deep breathing to 1, 1.5, and 2 minutes (to allow 8, 12, and 16 deep breaths, respectively) and (2) using high FGF (≥10 L/min).[16,17] These maneuvers result in maximal preoxygenation (evidenced by higher EtO_2, PaO_2, and lower EtN_2) and improved efficiency (delayed onset of oxyhemoglobin desaturation during apnea) compared with the original 4 DB/0.5 min method.[16,17] An investigation suggested that preoxygenation using 8 deep breaths in 1.0 minute at an FGF of 10 L/min is associated with slower oxyhemoglobin desaturation than that using 4 DB/0.5 min or TVB for 3 min (Fig. 13-7).[16] Several explanations were given for this finding, including leftward shift of the oxyhemoglobin dissociation curve secondary to hyperventilation-induced reduction in $PaCO_2$ (Fig. 13-8) and the occurrence of several extra deep breaths during anesthetic induction.[18,56]

The use of maximal exhalation before any preoxygenation maneuver has been suggested.[32,57] In a healthy

subject with an FRC of 3 L, forced exhalation to the residual volume decreases the lung volume to approximately 1.5 L. A 50% reduction of the FRC leads to 50% reduction in the time constant of the O_2 washin (N_2 washout) curve.[58] The influence of prior maximal exhalation on preoxygenation using TVB or deep breathing has been studied.[59] TVB after maximal exhalation resulted in a more rapid rise in EtO_2 during the first minute than did TVB without prior maximal exhalation. However, the time required to reach maximal preoxygenation (EtO_2 ≥90%) was the same (2.5 minutes) with or without maximal exhalation before TVB (Fig. 13-9).[59] During deep breathing, the time courses of preoxygenation with and without prior maximal exhalation were identical. Apparently, the decrease in FRC resulting from maximal exhalation is minor in comparison with the level of $\dot{V}A$ associated with deep breathing. Regardless of whether prior maximal exhalation was used, 1.5 minutes of deep breathing was still required to reach an EtO_2 of 90% or greater. Therefore, prior maximal exhalation confers little or no additional practical benefit to preoxygenation.[59]

It has been demonstrated that preoxygenation using the single vital capacity breath (SVCB) technique can provide within 30 seconds a PaO_2 comparable to that achieved by TVB for 3 minutes (Fig. 13-10).[60] This technique is basically a triphasic process. The first phase consists of forced exhalation to the residual volume, which minimizes lung N_2 content and the subsequent dilution of incoming O_2. The second phase is deep inspiration to expand the lungs to their total capacity, with a consequent maximal increase in PaO_2. The third phase consists of holding the chest in full inspiratory position, which may allow gas movement from the compliant alveoli to the less compliant alveoli (pendelluft maximization), because the time constants of filling between alveoli are

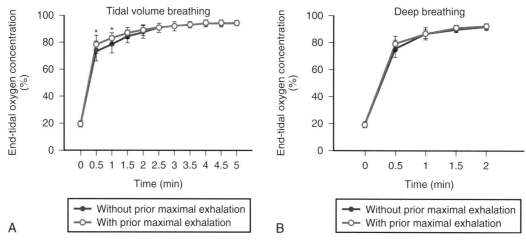

Figure 13-9 A, Comparison of end-tidal O_2 concentration values (mean ± SD) over 5-minute periods during simulated preoxygenation using tidal volume breathing (TVB) technique after maximal exhalation (*blue* ○) versus TVB without prior maximal exhalation (*purple* ●). *Statistically significant difference (*P* < .05) between techniques (TVB with or without prior maximal exhalation) at that time period. **B,** Comparison of end-tidal O_2 concentration values (mean ± SD) over 2-minute periods during simulated preoxygenation using deep breathing technique after maximal exhalation (*blue* ○) versus deep breathing without prior maximal exhalation (*purple* ●). (From Nimmagadda U, Salem MR, Joseph NJ, Miko I: Efficacy of preoxygenation using tidal volume and deep breathing techniques with and without prior maximal exhalation. *Can J Anesth* 54:448–452, 2007.)

not uniform.[60] The SVCB technique can optimize pre-oxygenation, especially when it is used for fast induction of inhalation anesthesia.[60]

VI. BREATHING SYSTEMS FOR PREOXYGENATION

Mapleson suggested that the degree of rebreathing during spontaneous respiration is less with the Mapleson A system than with the Mapleson D system.[61] Such difference of rebreathing between the anesthesia systems can affect the efficacy of preoxygenation. When using the Mapleson A or the circle system for preoxygenation by TVB, an O_2 flow of 5 L/min can adequately preoxygenate the patient within 3 minutes, whereas an O_2 flow of 10 L/min is required to achieve a similar EtO_2 with the

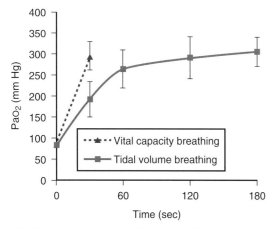

Figure 13-10 The mean arterial O_2 tension (*Pao₂*) achieved after preoxygenation by the single vital capacity breath technique (▲) compared with that achieved by the traditional preoxygenation technique (■). (From Baraka A, Haroun-Bizri S, Khoury S, et al: Single vital capacity breath for preoxygenation. *Can J Anaesth* 47:1144–1146, 2000.)

Mapleson D system.[54,55] In contrast, when deep breathing is used, an O_2 flow of 10 L/min is required irrespective of the anesthesia circuit.[55]

A system designed specifically for preoxygenation has gained some popularity in Europe (NasOral; LogoMed GambH, Windhagen, Germany).[62,63] The NasOral system is a nonrebreathing system that delivers O_2 from a 3.3-L reservoir bag to a small nasal mask, with exhalation occurring by the oral route using a mouthpiece.[40,62,63] One-way valves in the nasal mask and the mouthpiece ensure unidirectional flow (Fig. 13-11). The FGF is adjusted to the individual ventilation to maintain an inflated reservoir bag.[62,63] Investigations have shown that the semiclosed circle absorber and NasOral systems are equally effective in achieving oxygenation despite their different characteristics (see Fig. 13-3).[40] Accordingly, there is little justification for the additional cost of this device for use in the operating room, where the circle absorber can be used for preoxygenation and the administration of anesthesia.[40]

In the critical care setting, resuscitation bags are commonly used for preoxygenation. However, their effectiveness differs markedly during spontaneous respiration.[40] Some, because of their design, cannot deliver high FIO_2 despite an FGF of 15 L/min or greater (Fig. 13-12).[40] Resuscitation bags can be categorized into two groups depending on the type of valve mechanism. Disk-type valve systems use single or multiple disks to allow fresh gas to flow to the subject (and seal the exhalation port) during inspiration. The disk returns to its former position and opens the exhalation port during exhalation (Fig. 13-13). Because the disk valve function is not dependent on compression of the reservoir bag, this type of resuscitation bag functions equally well during manual and spontaneous ventilation and therefore can be used for preoxygenation.[40,64,65]

Resuscitation bags using duckbill inspiratory valves function differently during manual and spontaneous

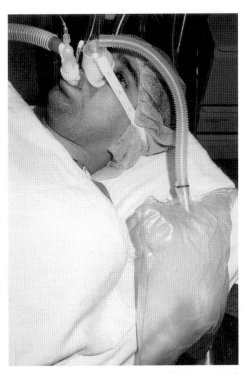

Figure 13-11 The NasOral system uses a small nasal mask for inspiration of O_2 from a reservoir bag. Exhalation occurs through a mouthpiece. One-way valves in the nasal mask and the mouthpiece ensure unidirectional flow. (From Nimmagadda U, Salem MR, Joseph NJ, et al: Efficacy of preoxygenation with tidal volume breathing: Comparison of breathing systems. *Anesthesiology* 93:693–698, 2000.)

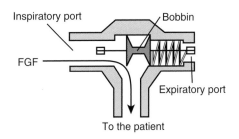

Inspiratory phase

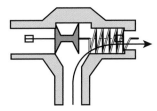

Expiratory phase

Figure 13-13 Diagram of a typical disk valve in a disk-type resuscitation bag. During inhalation *(top)*, the piston seals the exhalation port and allows fresh gas to flow to the patient. During exhalation *(bottom)*, the fresh gas port is sealed by the piston while gas is allowed to flow to the exhalation port. *FGF*, Fresh gas flow. (From Moyle JTB, Davey A, editors: *Ward's anaesthetic equipment*, London, 1998, WB Saunders, p 190.)

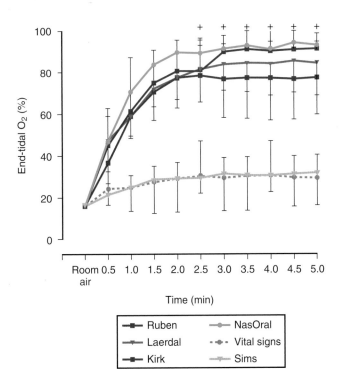

Figure 13-12 Comparison of mean end-tidal O_2 concentrations obtained at 30-second intervals during 5-minute periods of spontaneous tidal volume oxygenation using the NasOral system and five different resuscitation bags in 20 volunteers. Data shown as mean ± SD. ⁺Significant difference (*P*, < .01) between systems. (From Nimmagadda U, Salem MR, Joseph NJ, et al: Efficacy of preoxygenation with tidal volume breathing: Comparison of breathing systems. *Anesthesiology* 93:693–698, 2000.)

ventilation.[40,65] During manual ventilation, gas is forced through the valve base, opening the duckbill valve and delivering fresh gas to the patient's lungs. The force generated also seals the valve base to the exhalation port. During exhalation, the valve base returns to its former position, and exhaled gases are vented to the exhalation port (Fig. 13-14). Mills and colleagues found that duckbill-type resuscitation bags, without one-way exhalation valves to prevent air entrainment, showed variability in delivered O_2 concentration during spontaneous respiration.[65] These findings were confirmed by Nimmagadda and associates, who showed that some duckbill resuscitation bags cannot deliver a high FIO_2 during spontaneous ventilation even if a high FGF is used.[40] In the absence of a one-way valve on the exhalation port, generation of sufficient negative pressure to open the duckbill valve becomes impossible. During inspiration, the unsealed valve base allows room air to enter through the exhalation port and mix with O_2 from a partially open duckbill valve (see Fig. 13-14). With the addition of a one-way valve on the exhalation port, duckbill-type resuscitation bags (Laerdal and Kirk) can reliably deliver an FIO_2 greater than 0.9 with an FGF of 15 L/min. This valve seals the exhalation port during inspiration and allows the patient to generate sufficient negative pressure to open the duckbill valve, permitting O_2 to flow without dilution[40] (see Fig. 13-14).

The NasOral system has several advantages over resuscitation bags when used for preoxygenation: (1) It provides better preoxygenation than all available resuscitation bags because of a higher FIO_2 and reduced apparatus dead space (see Fig. 13-12), (2) It is economical when O_2 tanks are used because it requires an FGF comparable to the subject's minute ventilation; (3) It can provide apneic oxygenation through the nasal mask during laryngoscopy

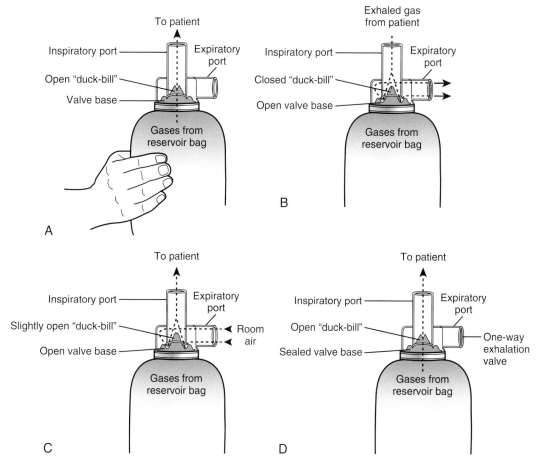

Figure 13-14 Schematic diagrams of a duckbill-type resuscitation bag during inspiration by manual ventilation **(A)**, exhalation by manual or spontaneous ventilation **(B)**, spontaneous inspiration without a one-way exhalation valve **(C)**, and spontaneous inspiration with a one-way exhalation valve **(D)**. (From Nimmagadda U, Salem MR, Joseph NJ, et al: Efficacy of preoxygenation with tidal volume breathing: Comparison of breathing systems. *Anesthesiology* 93:693–698, 2000.)

and orotracheal intubation, if needed. Disadvantages of the NasOral system are that it requires the patient's cooperation to use the mouthpiece and that the system cannot be used for positive-pressure ventilation.[40]

The inability of a resuscitation bag to deliver a high FIO_2 may have serious consequences during RSI in the critical care setting or during transport of the spontaneously breathing, critically ill patient.[40] Clinicians should ascertain that the resuscitation bags used for preoxygenation in their institutions are capable of delivering a high FIO_2 during spontaneous ventilation.[40]

VII. SPECIAL SITUATIONS

Investigations have highlighted risk factors for the rapid development of hypoxemia during apnea. These factors are additive and include a reduced FRC, inadequate denitrogenation, hypoventilation prior to apnea, increased VO_2, and airway obstruction.[34,39] Patients with a combination of these risk factors should be considered to be at high risk for hypoxemia during apnea.

A. Pregnant Patients

Because pregnant women are at high risk for pulmonary aspiration, RSI is desirable whenever general anesthesia

is administered to these patients. Maximal preoxygenation can be achieved faster in pregnant than in nonpregnant women because of the increased $\dot{V}A$ and decreased FRC.[11,14,47] However, during apnea, pregnant women become hypoxemic more rapidly because of the limited O_2 stores in their small FRC and increased $\dot{V}O_2$.[46] This can be further compounded by pregnancy-associated airway changes which can add to delay in securing the airway.[27] From the fifth month of pregnancy, the FRC decreases to 80% of that in the nonpregnant state, while the $\dot{V}O_2$ increases by 30% to 40%. In pregnant women, preoxygenation can be accomplished by TVB for 3 minutes or by deep breathing for 1 minute or longer before anesthetic induction. A combination of both techniques may also be used. Because of the increased $\dot{V}A$ during pregnancy, an O_2 flow of 10 L/min or higher is necessary (using the circle absorber) during TVB or deep breathing.[66] However, the 4 DB/0.5 min technique should be used only in emergency situations when time is limited.

The influence of preoxygenation in the supine position versus the 45-degree head-up position on the duration of apnea leading to a decrease in SpO_2 to 95% has been investigated.[46] The average time for SpO_2 to reach 95% was shorter in pregnant than in nonpregnant patients (173 versus 243 seconds) in the supine position.[46] Use of

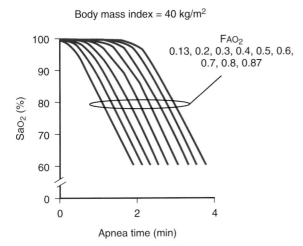

Figure 13-15 Diagram comparing the mean time to apnea-induced oxyhemoglobin desaturation during apnea in a morbidly obese patient at different alveolar O_2 fraction (Fao$_2$) values. Sao_2, Arterial oxyhemoglobin saturation. (From Benumof JL: Obesity, sleep apnea, the airway and anesthesia, 53rd Annual ASA Refresher Course Lectures, Park Ridge, IL, American Society of Anesthesiologists, 2002.)

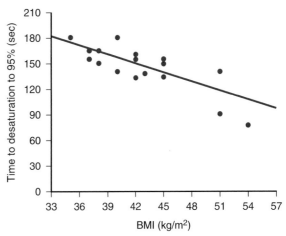

Figure 13-16 Correlation between time required for desaturation to 95% in seconds and body mass index (BMI) in kg·m^{-2} during apnea after preoxygenation in morbidly obese patients. The time to desaturation is inversely related to the body mass index: $R^2 = 0.66$ ($P < 0.05$). (From Baraka AS, Taha SK, Siddik SM, et al: Supplementation of preoxygenation in morbidly obese patients using nasopharyngeal O_2 insufflation. Anaesthesia 62:769–773, 2007.)

the head-up position resulted in an increase in desaturation time in nonpregnant patients but had no effect in pregnant patients.[46] It is possible that the gravid uterus prevents descent of the diaphragm in the upright position and therefore does not allow the expected increase in FRC.

B. Morbidly Obese Patients

MO is associated with a more rapid decrease in SpO_2 during apnea after induction of anesthesia.[10,53,67-70] This is particularly hazardous because MO complicated by obstructive sleep apnea may be associated with an increased risk of difficult intubation (DI) and difficult mask ventilation (DMV).

The more rapid hemoglobin desaturation in the patient with MO is attributed to increased $\dot{V}O_2$ associated with a decreased FRC (Fig. 13-15). The supine position further decreases the FRC due to the cephalad displacement of the diaphragm by the abdominal contents. Anesthetic induction results in an additional reduction of the FRC. Whereas the FRC of nonobese patients decreases by 20% after induction of anesthesia, it decreases by 50% in MO patients. The tidal volume of the patient with MO may fall within the closing capacity, resulting in atelectasis, with a subsequent increase in intrapulmonary shunting.

In the patient with MO, the time required for SpO_2 to fall to 90% during apnea after preoxygenation with TVB for 3 minutes is significantly reduced compared to the time in nonobese patients (Fig. 13-16).[29,70] In one study, the time to desaturation (Sao_2 = 90%) for patients of normal weight was 6 minutes after preoxygenation, but for those with MO it was 2.7 minutes.[67] A significant negative correlation between body mass index (BMI) and time to oxyhemoglobin desaturation has been described (see Fig. 13-15).[70] The head-up position (25 degrees) during preoxygenation in MO patients has been shown to prolong the time of desaturation by about 50

seconds.[69] The application of continuous positive airway pressure (CPAP) has been suggested to optimize preoxygenation in these patients, based on the assumption that CPAP will increase the FRC.[71] However, clinical observations showed that it did not delay the onset of desaturation, because the FRC returns to pre-CPAP levels once the patient is anesthetized and the CPAP mask is removed.[71]

It has been shown that nasopharyngeal O_2 insufflation after preoxygenation in patients with MO delays the onset of oxyhemoglobin desaturation during the subsequent apnea by apneic diffusion oxygenation.[70] In the critically ill MO patient with respiratory failure, traditional preoxygenation without or even with subsequent nasopharyngeal O_2 insufflation may not increase the FRC O_2 store and improve Sao_2 before, during, or after endotracheal intubation. This may be attributed to atelectasis and decreased FRC with marked intrapulmonary shunting. In this situation, the use of noninvasive bi-level positive airway pressure (BiPAP) can improve alveolar recruitment with a consequent decrease in intrapulmonary shunting.[72] BiPAP preoxygenation can achieve a notable increase in Sao_2 associated with less hypercarbia, compared with the traditional technique of preoxygenation.[72]

C. Elderly Patients

Several changes during aging may influence the period of preoxygenation needed in elderly patients and the subsequent time to oxyhemoglobin desaturation.[13,15,36] On one hand, the basal $\dot{V}O_2$ declines with age (from 143 mL/min/m^2 in a male aged 20 years to 124 mL/min/m^2 in a male aged 60 years), so the demand for O_2 is less; on the other hand, changes in lung function make O_2 uptake less efficient. The closing volume increases with age, leading to less efficient denitrogenation and a longer period of preoxygenation. The reduction of O_2 demand

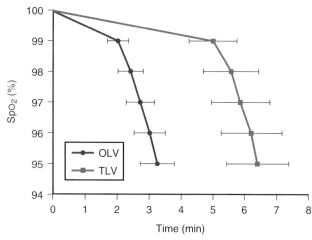

Figure 13-17 Diagram comparing the mean time to apnea-induced oxyhemoglobin desaturation from pulse oximetry O_2 saturation (SpO_2) of 100% down to 95% after two-lung ventilation (TLV) versus one-lung ventilation (OLV). (From Baraka A, Aouad M, Taha S, et al: Apnea-induced hemoglobin desaturation during one-lung vs two-lung ventilation. *Can J Anaesth* 47:58-61, 2000.)

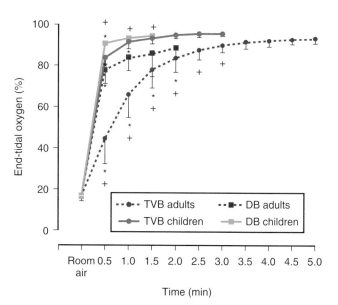

Figure 13-18 Comparison of the effects of tidal volume breathing (TVB) and deep breathing (DB) preoxygenation techniques on end-tidal O_2 in adults and children. *Significant difference from all other time periods. †significant difference ($P, < .01$) between adults and children. (From Salem MR, Joseph NJ, Villa EM, et al: Preoxygenation in children: Comparison of tidal volume and deep breathing techniques (abstract). *Anesthesiology* 97:A1247, 2001.)

in elderly patients does not compensate fully for the less efficient O_2 uptake, because the mean times to 93% desaturation in elderly patients are approximately one half of those reported for equivalent preoxygenation periods in young patients. Reliable preoxygenation can be achieved with extended TVB (>3 minutes) or deep breathing for longer than 1 minute.

D. Patients with Lung Disease

Patients with ARDS have decreased FRC, increased intrapulmonary shunting, and increased $\dot{V}O_2$; therefore, interruption of ventilation can result in rapid oxyhemoglobin desaturation. During thoracic surgery, the time to desaturation after one-lung ventilation is almost one half the time after two-lung ventilation (Fig. 13-17).[73] This can be attributed to collapse of the nonventilated lung with a consequent decrease of the FRC O_2 store; the rate of oxyhemoglobin desaturation may be further exaggerated by the associated intrapulmonary shunting.[73] A similar decrease of the safety margin may occur in patients with lung disease characterized by decreased FRC or increased intrapulmonary shunting or both. In these patients, maximal preoxygenation should precede interruption of ventilation or tracheobronchial suction.

E. Pediatric Patients

Because of their smaller FRC and increased metabolic requirements, children are at increased risk for developing faster oxyhemoglobin desaturation than in adults whenever there is an interruption of their O_2 delivery.[48,74-80] The younger the child, the faster is the onset of hypoxemia.[45,74-80] With a satisfactory mask fit, the efficacy of preoxygenation depends on the age and the duration and type of breathing.[48,80,81] Studies in children have demonstrated that maximal preoxygenation can be reached faster than in adults. With TVB, an EtO_2 of 90%

or greater is reached within 60 to 100 seconds in almost all children.[48,49,80] Among those in the first year of life, it is reached in 36 seconds (range, 20 to 60 seconds); between 3 and 5 years age, it is reached in 50 seconds (range, 30 to 90 seconds), and in those older than 5 years, it is reached in 68 seconds (range, 30 to 100 seconds).[80] Deep breathing in children results in faster preoxygenation than TVB and also faster preoxygenation than deep breathing in adults (Fig. 13-18).[49] Optimal preoxygenation can be accomplished in children with the use of deep breathing for 30 seconds.[49]

Several factors affect the onset of apnea-induced oxyhemoglobin desaturation after preoxygenation in children. These include the efficacy of preoxygenation, the child's age (or weight), the presence of disease, and the composition of gases in the lungs. Some studies have examined the time required for SpO_2 to decrease from 100% to 95% (Fig. 13-19)[76,77]; others have targeted a level as low as 90%.[75,78,81] In a comparison of three groups of children who breathed 100% O_2 at TVB for 1, 2, and 3 minutes before apnea, the times needed for SpO_2 to decrease from 100% to 98%, 95%, and 90% were shorter in those who had breathed O_2 for 1 minute.[81] On the basis of these findings, 2 minutes of preoxygenation with TVB in children seems to provide maximum benefit and allows at least 2 minutes of safe apnea.[81] In a 1-month-old infant, the rate of decline in PaO_2 during apnea is three times more rapid than in an adult.[82] The times for SpO_2 to decrease from 100% to 95% and to 90% are shorter in younger children than in older children. Most infants reach an SpO_2 of 90% in 70 to 90 seconds (see Fig. 13-19).[75] This duration is shortened in the presence of upper respiratory infection.[76] The benefit of preoxygenation is greater in the older child than that in the infant.[82]

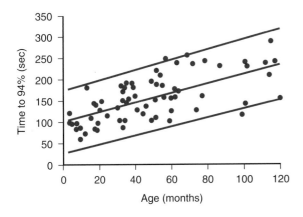

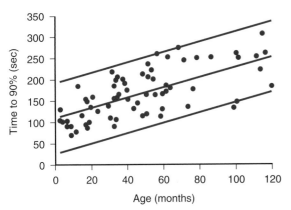

Figure 13-19 Relationship between desaturation times to 94% *(top)* and to 90% *(bottom)* versus age with a prediction interval of 95 (*P* < .001). (From Dupeyrat A, Dubreuil M, Ecoffey C: Preoxygenation in children (letter). *Anesth Analg* 79:1027, 1994.)

In an 8-year-old, the time after the onset of apnea to 90% SaO$_2$ is 0.47 minutes without preoxygenation but slightly longer than 5 minutes with preoxygenation.[82]

Although the time for desaturation is mainly dependent on the O$_2$ content of the lungs at the start of apnea, other gas components may play a role. If 60% nitrous oxide (N$_2$O) in O$_2$ is used, the time for SpO$_2$ to decrease to 95% is shortened to approximately one third,[77] but it is still longer than the time observed after air-O$_2$ breathing and maintains the same delivered O$_2$ concentration.[77] This can be explained by the second-gas effect. Compared with N$_2$ in case of air-O$_2$ breathing, N$_2$O continues to dissolve into the blood and is carried away from the lungs, resulting in an increase in the PaO$_2$ and hence delaying the onset of desaturation.[77]

It should be emphasized that the apnea-desaturation studies were performed in healthy children with a patent airway. The presence of cardiac or respiratory disease or airway obstruction could lead to faster desaturation during apnea.[77] Premature infants are usually given a low FIO$_2$ using an air-O$_2$ mixture because of fear of retinopathy. Oxyhemoglobin desaturation occurs very quickly in these infants even after a short period of apnea. Transiently increasing the FIO$_2$, limiting apnea to very short periods, and close monitoring are important

considerations.[83] The respiratory rate in preterm infants is 30 to 60 breaths/min. Rapid respirations tend to maintain their FRC by not allowing time to complete exhalation. Slow respirations and apnea result in marked decrease of FRC and fast desaturation after apnea.[83]

F. Tracheobronchial Suctioning

Tracheobronchial suctioning to remove secretions is a commonly practiced maneuver in anesthetized and critically ill patients. Although the effects of suctioning are usually mild, they on occasion can have serious consequences.[84-93] Cardiovascular collapse and even death as a consequence of severe hypoxemia associated with suctioning were recognized as early as the 1950s.[84] Traditionally, tracheobronchial suctioning requires disconnection of the ETT from the anesthesia machine or the ventilator. A catheter is then introduced inside the ETT or tracheostomy tube, and suction is performed. This common method is referred to as open endotracheal suctioning (OES).[94] The mechanisms of acute hypoxemia after OES are twofold.[90,92,94] First, disconnection dilutes the FIO$_2$ with air and induces massive loss of FRC, especially in patients with acute lung injury.[90,92,94] Second, the high negative pressure required for removal of secretions contributes to further dilution of FIO$_2$ and decrease in FRC, which results in atelectasis, fall in lung compliance, and intrapulmonary shunting.[86,93]

The effects of OES can be severe in patients with limited O$_2$ reserves, when large suction catheters are used, with prolonged suctioning, and when selective bronchial suctioning is performed.[86,89-95] Especially vulnerable is the infant, because a suction catheter may occupy a large part of the lumen of a small ETT.[86,95] Studies in infants have consistently demonstrated a sharp fall in pulmonary compliance with prolonged suctioning and when large catheters are used.[86] Infants ventilated at constant volumes had increases in transpulmonary pressure after tracheal suctioning ranging from 15% to 60%, whereas in infants ventilated with pressure-preset ventilators, tidal volumes fell by 25% to 70% (Fig. 13-20).[86] Failure of tidal volumes to return to the pre-suctioning level was observed for periods as long as 30 minutes[86] (Fig. 13-21).

In adult patients with acute lung injury, OES induces an 18% decrease in PaO$_2$ and an increase in PaCO$_2$ of 8%[94] (Fig. 13-22). The maximum impairment appears within 1 minute after suctioning is begun and persists for 15 minutes after the end of suctioning. A 70% reduction in PaO$_2$ has been observed in some patients.[94] Decreases in S$\overline{v}$O$_2$ are commonly observed during OES in critically ill patients.[91] The rise in PaCO$_2$ may explain why OES is frequently associated with an increase in intracranial pressure in patients with severe head injury.[94,96] A collapsed lung, as a consequence of suctioning, may remain collapsed for hours or even days, unless high pressures or high volumes are used to reinflate the lungs.[86] Collapsed alveoli begin to open at an airway pressure of 18 to 23 cm H$_2$O, and frequently an inflation pressure of 25 cm H$_2$O or higher is desirable.[86] Impairment in oxygenation after OES can be attenuated by prior maximal preoxygenation

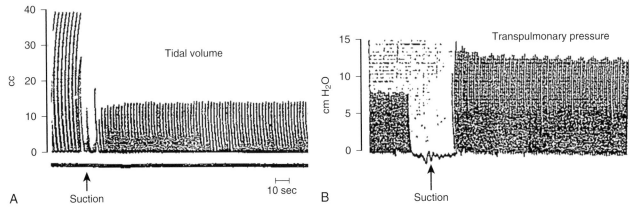

Figure 13-20 A, Effect of tracheal suctioning on tidal volume in an infant ventilated with a Bird respirator set to produce a peak transpulmonary inflation limit of 11 cm H_2O. **B,** Effect of tracheal suctioning on transpulmonary pressure in an infant ventilated at a constant tidal volume of 20 mL. (From Brandstater B, Muallem M: Atelectasis following tracheal suction in infants. *Anesthesiology* 31:468–473, 1969.)

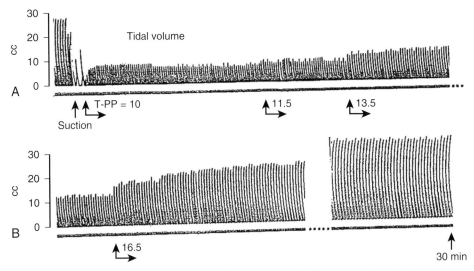

Figure 13-21 Tidal volume record from an infant ventilated with a Bird respirator. **A,** After tracheal suctioning, re-expansion of the lungs did not occur at low transpulmonary pressures. Little expansion occurred when the transpulmonary pressure was 13.5 cm H_2O. **B,** At 16.5 cm H_2O, re-expansion progressed until it was complete after 30 minutes. *T-PP,* Trans-pulmonary pressure. (From Brandstater B, Muallem M: Atelectasis following tracheal suction in infants. *Anesthesiology* 31:468–473, 1969.)

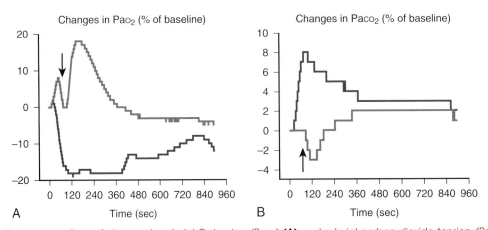

Figure 13-22 Continuous recordings of changes in arterial O_2 tension *(Pao$_2$)* **(A)** and arterial carbon dioxide tension *(Paco$_2$)* **(B)** from the beginning (time 0) to 15 minutes after endotracheal suctioning in nine patients undergoing at random open and closed-circuit endotracheal suctioning. Pao$_2$ and Paco$_2$ were sampled every second in each patient, and the mean curves are presented. *Red lines* represent open suctioning, whereas *blue lines* represent closed-circuit suctioning followed by a recruitment maneuver. Arrows indicate the beginning of the recruitment maneuver. (From Lasocki S, Lu Q, Sartorius A, et al: Open and closed-circuit endotracheal suctioning in acute lung injury: Efficiency and effects on gas exchange. *Anesthesiology* 104:39–47, 2006.)

and by using a postsuctioning maneuver consisting of a multiple number of high tidal volumes.

In the critical care setting, closed-circuit endotracheal suctioning (CES) has been advocated to prevent hypoxemia resulting from ventilator disconnection.[94,97-99] Two methods are used. In one, suctioning is performed via a swivel adapter positioned at the proximal tip of the ETT; and in the other, total CES is done with a catheter continuously placed between the ETT and the Y-piece of the ventilator circuit.[93,94] Because neither method requires disconnection, the loss of lung volume and hypoxemia are much less compared with OES, and the effect of suctioning becomes dependent only on the negative suction pressure.[93]

There is evidence that OES is more efficient than CES for secretion removal.[94] Several mechanisms contribute to this difference. First, during OES, the airway pressure is zero, whereas in CES it is positive, especially if positive end-expiratory pressure (PEEP) is used. Second, during CES, the positive pressure from the ventilator fills the suction catheter with gas and tends to blow secretions distally. Third, disconnection from the ventilator during OES induces a sudden decrease in expiratory lung volume, and bronchial secretions may be entrained proximally with the expiratory gas flow, thereby facilitating secretion removal. The problem of decreased secretion removal with CES can be corrected by increasing the negative suction pressure from -200 cm H_2O to -400 cm H_2O, which enhances suctioning efficiency without further impairment of gas exchange.[94]

1. Guidelines for Suctioning

Suctioning may be divided into three stages: the presuctioning stage, the suctioning procedure, and the postsuctioning maneuvers. The strategies may depend on the method used.

a. OPEN ENDOTRACHEAL SUCTIONING

1. *The Presuctioning Stage*: Before suctioning, the patient's cardiovascular and respiratory status are optimized, and appropriate monitoring is continued. An additional dose of a muscle relaxant, opioid, or intravenous lidocaine may be given. The patient's oxygenation should be maximized by using an FIO_2 of 1 for several minutes. An indication of the efficacy of oxygenation is an EtO_2 close to 90%. Other respiratory parameters may be adjusted to enhance O_2 delivery. Suction equipment and sterile supplies should be checked. The choice of appropriate suction catheter size is important. The outer diameter (OD) of the catheter should be approximately 60% of the inner diameter (ID) of the ETT (e.g., 16 F for an 8.0-mm ETT, 14 F or for a 7.5-mm ETT). In infants, a slightly larger suction catheter with an OD 70% of the ID of the ETT may be used.

2. *The Suctioning Procedure*: After disconnection from the anesthesia machine or the ventilator, the suction catheter is introduced into the ETT and advanced until resistance is felt and is then withdrawn about 2 cm. Negative pressure of -50 to -200 cm H_2O is applied intermittently for 2 to 4 seconds by occluding the side hole located at the proximal end of the

catheter with the operator's thumb. Intermittent suctioning may be continued (up to 20 seconds), during which the catheter is gently rotated and withdrawn. If additional suctioning is required, a recruitment maneuver (with high FIO_2) should be performed before suctioning is repeated.

3. *Postsuctioning Maneuvers*: After suctioning, the patient is reconnected to the ventilator and a recruitment maneuver is performed while administering high FIO_2 immediately.[92,94] The most common maneuver is tidal volumes set at twice the baseline value, provided that the airway pressure does not exceed 25 to 50 cm H_2O (depending on the existing lung pathology). The numbers of these high tidal volumes can vary from 2 to 20 breaths. In anesthetized healthy patients, 3 large TVBs are adequate. A study in ARDS patients showed that 2 consecutive sustained inflations lasting 20 seconds with an interval of 1 minute in between reversed the OES-induced decrease in PaO_2 and lung volume.[100]

b. CLOSED-SYSTEM ENDOTRACHEAL SUCTIONING

In CES, the suction catheter is introduced via the swivel adapter or the sealed system. The same suctioning procedure described for OES is used. Negative pressure of -200 cm H_2O may be applied for up to 20 seconds. To enhance removal of secretions, -400 cm H_2O may be used. Although the deterioration in gas exchange is markedly reduced with CES, it is probably beneficial to use a recruitment maneuver immediately after suction.

G. "Routine" Preoxygenation Before Induction, During Recovery from Anesthesia, and in Critically Ill Patients

Preoxygenation is mandatory in the context of RSI, and it is arguably so in an additional range of scenarios. Imperative preoxygenation is indicated in those patients who cannot tolerate a fall in PO_2, such as those with ischemic heart disease, and in patients with low PaO_2, such as those with lung disease or right-to-left shunt. Because conditions such as the DI-DMV scenarios are unpredictable and many adverse reactions (e.g., drug-induced anaphylaxis, hypotension, hypoventilation) can occur, "routine" preoxygenation offers identifiable safety benefits during anesthetic induction.[20-22] However, "routine" preoxygenation must be used as an adjunct rather than an alternative to a sequence of fundamental preoperative precautions that minimize adverse sequelae.[21]

Recovery from anesthesia and extubation have received limited critical safety measures compared with attention to the identification and management of potential DI, despite the observation that airway complications are more likely to be associated with extubation than intubation.[101-103] The ASA Task Force on Management of the DA recommended that each anesthesiologist must have a preformulated strategy for extubation of the DA and an airway management plan for dealing with postextubation hypoventilation.[19] Even routine discontinuation of anesthesia and tracheal extubation can be complicated with hypoxemia, hypoventilation, and loss of airway patency because of the residual effects of anesthetics and incomplete reversal of neuromuscular block.[104,105] These effects can result in decreased functional activity of the pharyngeal muscles, leading to upper airway obstruction and a fivefold increase in the risk of aspiration; and they can affect the contractions of the respiratory muscles, resulting in hypoventilation and inability to cough effectively.[104,105] They can also obtund the hypoxic drive by the peripheral chemoreceptors.[105] In addition, adequate oxygenation before reversal of neuromuscular block is essential to ensure safe reversal and to minimize neostigmine-induced cardiac arrhythmias.[106] Accordingly, "routine" preoxygenation before reversal of neuromuscular blockade and extubation is recommended to improve the margin of safety, given the potential of unpredictable airway and ventilation problems.

In critically ill, hemodynamically unstable patients, preoxygenation is less effective in raising PaO_2. Whereas in a healthy patient, preoxygenation ($FIO_2 = 1$) typically raises the PaO_2 from 80 to 400 mm Hg, the increase in hemodynamically unstable patients is from 67 to 107 mm Hg only.[107] Multiple factors limit the rise in PaO_2, including inability to provide high FIO_2, increased VO_2, blood loss, anemia, stress, hypoventilation, acidemia, hypermetabolic state, older age, cardiopulmonary disease, and airway obstruction.[107] This limitation implies that the time available to safely perform airway management maneuvers is rather limited in critically ill patients. Nevertheless, preoxygenation enhances the safety of these patients requiring emergency intubation. Findings from a recent swine hemorrhagic shock model confirm that FIO_2 does influence the rate of apneic desaturation.[108] A fivefold increase in time until critical desaturation can be achieved with preoxygenation compared with breathing of room air.[108]

VIII. CONCLUSIONS

Oxygenation before anesthetic induction and endotracheal intubation has become an accepted maneuver designed to increase O_2 reserves and thereby delay the onset of arterial oxyhemoglobin desaturation during apnea. It is particularly important when manual mask ventilation is undesirable and when difficulty with ventilation or endotracheal intubation is anticipated. Because the CICV situation is largely unpredictable, maximal preoxygenation is desirable in all patients. It is also essential in patients who have a decreased capacity for O_2 loading (decreased FRC, PaO_2, or cardiac output) or an increased VO_2 or both. Preoxygenation should be considered when maneuvers that deplete the O_2 reserves, such as suctioning, one-lung ventilation, or apneic oxygenation, are performed.

In the operating room, maximal preoxygenation can be accomplished in most patients with the commonly used anesthetic systems—either TVB for 3 to 5 minutes or deep breathing for 1.0 to 1.5 minutes. Elderly patients and patients with pulmonary disease may require longer periods of preoxygenation, whereas pediatric patients may need a shorter time. Except in children, the 4 DB/0.5 min technique provides submaximal preoxygenation and therefore should be reserved for emergency situations when time is limited. When deep breathing is used, an FGF of 10 L/min or greater is necessary; otherwise, rebreathing of exhaled gases occurs, leading to decreased inspired O_2 concentration. During preoxygenation, it is important that a tight-fitting mask be used to prevent air entrainment and that the reservoir bag be fully inflated. Almost all patients accept mask preoxygenation if the procedure and its importance are explained to them beforehand.

Clinical end points indicative of maximal preoxygenation are movement of the reservoir bag in and out with each inspiration and exhalation, presence of a normal capnographic tracing, and a near-normal $EtCO_2$ throughout the period of preoxygenation. Monitoring of O_2 or N_2, or both, to ensure a target level of EtO_2 90% or higher or an ENO_2 5% or lower is desirable, if available.

"Routine" preoxygenation with 100% O_2 is considered a "safety" measure during anesthetic induction and emergence from anesthesia and in critically ill patients requiring emergency airway management. However, it must be used as an adjunct rather than an alternative to a sequence of fundamental precautions that minimize adverse sequelae.

IX. CLINICAL PEARLS

- The principal stores of body O_2 are increased with breathing 100% O_2; the maximal increase occurs in the functional residual capacity (FRC).

- The end points of maximal preoxygenation or denitrogenation have been defined as EtO_2 of 90% or higher and EtN_2 5% or lower.

- An O_2 saturation of 100% on pulse oximetry (SpO_2) should not be a reason to stop preoxygenation; conversely, failure of SpO_2 to increase substantially does not necessarily indicate failure of preoxygenation.

- During apneic diffusion oxygenation via an open airway, the increase in time to hemoglobin desaturation achieved by increasing the fraction of inspired oxygen (FIO_2) from 0.9 to 1.0 is greater than that caused by increasing the FIO_2 from 0.21 to 0.9.

- In most patients, maximal preoxygenation can be accomplished by using tidal volume breathing (TVB) for 3 minutes or longer with a fresh gas flow (FGF) of 5 L/min or deep breathing for 1.5 minutes (FGF of 10 L/min) with the circle absorber.

- In the critical care setting, clinicians should ascertain that the resuscitation bags used for preoxygenation before rapid-sequence intubation (RSI) are capable of delivering high FIO_2 during spontaneous ventilation.

- Patients with decreased O_2 stores or increased VO_2 or both—including morbidly obese patients, children, pregnant women, critically ill patients, patients with ARDS, patients undergoing one-lung ventilation, and those patients with airway obstruction—develop faster arterial oxyhemoglobin desaturation during apnea.

- Preoxygenation in the head-up position in morbidly obese patients prolongs the time of oxyhemoglobin desaturation.

- "Routine" preoxygenation is recommended, not only before anesthetic induction, but also before and during reversal of neuromuscular blockade, emergence from anesthesia, and extubation. It is also recommended before interruption of ventilation and tracheobronchial suctioning and before emergency intubation in the critically ill.

- Routine preoxygenation must be used as an adjunct rather than an alternative to a sequence of fundamental precautions that minimize adverse sequelae.

SELECTED REFERENCES

All references can be found online at expertconsult.com.

17. Nimmagadda U, Chiravuri SD, Salem MR, et al: Preoxygenation with tidal volume and deep breathing techniques: The impact of duration of breathing and fresh gas flow. *Anesth Analg* 92:1337–1341, 2001.

18. Benumof JL: Preoxygenation: Best method for both efficacy and efficiency [editorial]. *Anesthesiology* 91:603–605, 1999.

24. Campbell IT, Beatty PCW: Monitoring preoxygenation. *Br J Anaesth* 72:3–4, 1994.

29. Benumof JL, Dagg R, Benumof R: Critical hemoglobin desaturation will occur before return to unparalyzed state from 1 mg/kg succinylcholine. *Anesthesiology* 87:979–982, 1997.

34. McNamara MJ, Hardman JG: Hypoxaemia during open-airway apnoea: A computational modeling analysis. *Anaesthesia* 60:741–746, 2005.

40. Nimmagadda U, Salem MR, Joseph NJ, et al: Efficacy of preoxygenation with tidal volume breathing: Comparison of breathing systems. *Anesthesiology* 93:1–7, 2000.

42. Drummond GB, Park GR: Arterial oxygen saturation before intubation of the trachea. *Br J Anaesth* 54:987–992, 1984.

46. Baraka AS, Hanna MT, Jabbour SI, et al: Preoxygenation of pregnant and nonpregnant women in the head-up versus supine position. *Anesth Analg* 75:757–759, 1992.

50. Farmery AD, Roe PG: A model to describe the rate of oxyhemoglobin desaturation during apnoea. *Br J Anaesth* 76:284–291, 1996.

69. Dixon BJ, Dixon JB, Carden JR, et al: Preoxygenation is more effective in the 25° head-up position than in the supine position in severely obese patients. *Anesthesiology* 102:1110–1115, 2005.

PART 4

The Airway Techniques

Chapter 14

Oxygen Delivery Systems, Inhalation Therapy, and Respiratory Therapy

ARTHUR J. TOKARCZYK | STEVEN B. GREENBERG | JEFFERY S. VENDER

I. INTRODUCTION

Many patients suffer from acute and chronic dysfunction of the pulmonary system. Management of the surgical and critical care patient requires an understanding of pulmonary pathophysiology and the appropriate prophylactic and therapeutic techniques. Oxygen (O_2) therapy is one of the most commonly employed medical interventions. An understanding of O_2 delivery systems and devices is essential for optimal care. Bronchial hygiene has become a cornerstone in prophylactic care of the perioperative surgical patient, and these techniques may restore normal pulmonary physiology in patients with compromised function. Many medications that are specifically intended to treat pulmonary pathophysiology can be delivered by inhalation therapy with greater efficiency and less toxicity than oral or parenteral methods.

This chapter reviews the various procedures and techniques used in the respiratory care of patients.

II. OXYGEN THERAPY

A. Indications

O_2 is one of the most common therapeutic substances used in the practice of critical care medicine. O_2 therapy may improve outcomes of patients undergoing surgery. Use of O_2 concentrations greater than 50% FiO_2 has reduced the incidence of wound infections in patients undergoing colorectal or spinal surgery.[1-4] This section reviews some of the indications, goals, and modes of O_2 therapy in the adult patient.

> **BOX 14-1** Calculation of Arterial Oxygen Content
>
> $$Cao_2 = Sao_2 \times Hg \times 1.34 + Pao_2 \times 0.0031$$
>
> Cao_2 = arterial O_2 content (mL/dL)
> Hg = hemoglobin (g/dL)
> 1.34 = O_2-carrying capacity of hemoglobin
> Pao_2 = arterial partial pressure of O_2 (mm Hg)
> 0.0031 = solubility coefficient of O_2 in plasma

Treatment or prevention of hypoxemia is the most common indication for O_2 therapy, and the final goal of effective treatment is avoidance or resolution of tissue hypoxia. Tissue hypoxia exists when delivery of O_2 is inadequate to meet the metabolic demands of the tissues. O_2 content (Box 14-1) depends on the arterial partial pressure of O_2 (Pao_2), the hemoglobin concentration of arterial blood, and the saturation of hemoglobin with O_2. O_2 delivery (Do_2) is calculated by multiplying cardiac output (liters per minute) by the arterial O_2 content. Do_2 is measured in milliliters of O_2 per minute, and for a 70-kg, healthy patient, it is approximately 1000 mL/min (Box 14-2).

Hypoxia may result from a decrement of any of the determinants of Do_2, including anemia, low cardiac output, hypoxemia, or abnormal hemoglobin affinity (e.g., carbon monoxide toxicity) out of proportion to demand. Hypoxia may also arise from a failure of O_2 use at the tissue level (e.g., microvascular perfusion defect of shock) or at the cellular level (e.g., cyanide poisoning).

Aerobic metabolism requires a balance between Do_2 and O_2 consumption. Inspiration of enriched concentrations of O_2 may increase the Pao_2, the percentage of saturation of hemoglobin, and the O_2 content, thereby augmenting Do_2 until the underlying cause of the hypoxia can be corrected (e.g., transfusing the anemic patient, reversing cardiac dysfunction). The clinical situation in which O_2 therapy is most effective, however, is in the treatment of hypoxemia.

Hypoxemia may be defined as a deficiency of O_2 tension in the arterial blood, typically defined as a Pao_2 value less than 80 mm Hg. The most common perioperative causes of hypoxemia include decreased alveolar O_2 tension (e.g., ventilation-perfusion mismatch, hypoventilation) and capillary shunt (e.g., atelectasis). Less common causes of perioperative hypoxemia include decreased mixed venous O_2 content ($C\bar{v}o_2$) and diffusion defect.

Mismatch of ventilation and perfusion ($\dot{V}/\dot{Q}$) is essentially an uncoupling of alveolar blood supply and ventilation. In an area of low $\dot{V}/\dot{Q}$, hypoxemia results when mixed venous blood flowing past the alveolar-capillary membrane (ACM) takes away O_2 molecules faster than ventilation to the alveolus can replace them. The resultant partial pressure of O_2 in the alveolus (Pao_2) is too low to oxygenate the blood flowing past it. In a true intrapulmonary shunt, the ventilation decreases to zero, with $\dot{V}/\dot{Q} = 0$. Anatomic shunt occurs when blood flows from the right side of the heart to the left side without traversing the pulmonary capillaries. A small percentage of physiologic shunt results from bronchial and thebesian circulation. True intrapulmonary shunts cause hypoxemia that is poorly responsive to O_2 therapy. Therapy for "oxygen-refractory" hypoxemia is aimed at reducing the shunt. Different levels of shunting, such as low-ventilation areas, often cause blood to flow through capillaries adjacent to alveoli that do not participate in ventilation. Atelectasis is a common cause of this type of shunt. Respiratory therapy, such as tracheobronchial toilet, to remove mucous plugging of a lobar bronchus or adjusting an endotracheal tube (ETT) that has advanced into a main stem bronchus, may be effective at reversing causes of relative shunt. Positive airway pressure therapy can reduce intrapulmonary shunting in certain disease states associated with a diffuse reduction in functional residual capacity.

In a situation that is the opposite of a high $\dot{V}/\dot{Q}$ ratio, a portion of ventilation does not participate in gas exchange. Dead space ventilation occurs when the perfusion becomes zero, and the $\dot{V}/\dot{Q}$ ratio approaches infinity. Anatomic dead space is an area of the lungs that does not participate in gas exchange, such as the larger airways. Physiologic dead space is the total dead space that contributes to elevated $\dot{V}/\dot{Q}$ ratio. Dead space ventilation does not contribute significantly to hypoxemia unless perfusion is significantly disrupted, as occurs in a pulmonary embolus.

Hypoventilation causes hypoxemia when an increase in alveolar carbon dioxide (CO_2) displaces the O_2 molecules and decreases Pao_2, as demonstrated in the alveolar gas equation:

$$Pao_2 = Fio_2(P_{atm} - Ph_2o) - Paco_2/RQ$$

Clinical entities associated with low Pao_2 values include chronic obstructive pulmonary disease (COPD), asthma, retained secretions, sedative or narcotic administration, acute lung injury syndrome, and early or mild pulmonary edema. Inspiration of enriched concentrations of O_2 under these circumstances increases Pao_2, which increases the O_2 gradient across the ACM, resulting in faster equilibration of mixed venous blood exposed to the ACM and a higher pulmonary venous, left atrial, left ventricular, and arterial Po_2.

Even small increases in inspired O_2 tension can affect hypoxemia when caused by low Pao_2. Drug-induced

---

> **BOX 14-2** Calculation of Oxygen Delivery
>
> $$Do_2 = Cao_2 \times CO \times 10$$
>
> Cao_2 = arterial O_2 content per 100 mL of blood mL/dL. This value is approximately 20 mL/dL in the normal adult with a hemoglobin of 15 g/dL.
> CO = cardiac output (L/min). This value is approximately 5 L/min in the healthy, 70-kg adult.
> Do_2 = O_2 delivery (mL/min). This value is approximately 1000 mL/min in the healthy, 70-kg adult.

alveolar hypoventilation resulting in hypoxemia on room air is exquisitely sensitive to increases in inspired O_2 concentration. Appropriate initial management of patients with alterations in mental status includes the use of O_2 therapy as long as ventilatory needs are also monitored.

Cases of hypoxemia caused by true shunt or $\dot{V}/\dot{Q}$ mismatch share a common phenomenon, which is exaggerated by a decreased mixed venous hemoglobin saturation (low $S\overline{v}O_2$). Because hemoglobin saturation is the major determinant of O_2 content in blood, a low $S\overline{v}O_2$ leads to a low venous O_2 content ($C\overline{v}O_2$). Low $C\overline{v}O_2$ causes hypoxemia by worsening the hypoxemic effect of any existing shunt or areas of low $\dot{V}/\dot{Q}$ by presenting more desaturated blood to the left atrium. Decreased $C\overline{v}O_2$ arises from low O_2 delivery (e.g., low cardiac output, anemia, hypoxemia) or increased O_2 consumption (e.g., high fever, increased minute ventilation and work of breathing).

The consequences of untreated hypoxemia include tachycardia, acidosis, and increased myocardial O_2 demand, as well as increased minute volume and work of breathing. By treating hypoxemia, supplemental O_2 restores homeostasis and greatly decreases the stress response and its attendant cardiopulmonary sequelae.

B. Oxygen Delivery Systems

With the exception of anesthetic breathing circuits, virtually all O_2 delivery systems are nonrebreathing. In nonrebreathing circuits, the inspiratory gas is not made up in any part by the exhaled tidal volume (V_T), and the only CO_2 inhaled is that in any entrained room air. To avoid rebreathing, exhaled gases must be sequestered by one-way valves, and inspired gases must be presented in sufficient volume and flow to satisfy the high peak flow rates and minute ventilation demonstrated in critically ill patients. Inspiratory entrainment of room air or the use of inspiratory reservoirs (including the anatomic dead space of the nasopharynx, oropharynx, and non–gas-exchanging portion of the bronchial tree) and one-way valves typifies nonrebreathing systems and defines them as two groups.[5-7] Low-flow systems depend on inspiration of room air to meet inspiratory flow and volume demands. High-flow systems attempt to provide the entire inspiratory demand. High-flow systems use reservoirs or very high flow rates to meet the large peak inspiratory flow demands and the exaggerated minute volumes found in many critically ill patients.

1. Low-Flow Oxygen Systems

A low-flow, variable-performance system depends on room air entrainment to meet the patient's peak inspiratory and minute ventilatory demands that are not met by the inspiratory gas flow or O_2 reservoir alone. Low-flow devices include the nasal cannula, simple face mask, partial rebreathing mask, nonrebreathing mask, and tracheostomy collar. Low-flow systems are characterized by the ability to deliver high and low values of FIO_2. The FIO_2 becomes unpredictable and inconsistent when these devices are used for patients with abnormal or changing ventilatory patterns.[8] Low-flow systems produce FIO_2

TABLE 14-1

Example 1: V_T Is Decreased to 500 mL

Cannula	6 L/min	V_T, 500 mL	
Mechanical reservoir	None	I/E ratio = 1:2	
Anatomic reservoir	50 mL	Rate = 20 breaths/min	
100% O_2 provided/sec	100 mL	Inspiratory time = 1 sec	
Volume inspired O_2			
Anatomic reservoir	50 mL		
Flow/sec	100 mL		
Inspired room air (0.20 × 350 mL)	70 mL		
O_2 inspired	220 mL		

$$FIO_2 = \frac{200\,mL\ O_2}{500\,mL\ V_T} = 0.44$$

FIO_2, Fraction of inspired oxygen; I/E ratio, inspiration/expiration ratio; V_T, tidal volume.

values of 21% to 80%. The FIO_2 may vary with the size of the O_2 reservoir, O_2 flow, and the patient's ventilatory pattern (e.g., V_T, peak inspiratory flow, respiratory rate, minute ventilation). With a normal ventilation pattern, these devices can deliver a relatively predictable and consistent FIO_2 level.

Low-flow systems do not mean low FIO_2 values. With changes in V_T, respiratory rate, O_2 reservoir size, and so on, the FIO_2 can vary dramatically at comparable O_2 flow rates. The following examples are theoretical mathematical estimates of an FIO_2 produced by a low-flow system (e.g., nasal cannula) in two clinical conditions.

The example for estimation of FIO_2 from a low-flow system is based on the standard normal patient and ventilatory pattern. Several assumptions are used for the FIO_2 calculation. The anatomic reservoir for a nasal cannula consists of nose, nasopharynx, and oropharynx, and it is about one third of the entire normal anatomic dead space (including trachea). For example, 150 mL ÷ 3 = 50 mL; assume a nasal cannula O_2 flow rate of 6 L/min (100 mL/sec), V_T of 500 mL, respiratory rate of 20 breaths/min, inspiratory (I) time of 1 second, and expiratory (E) time of 2 seconds. If the terminal 0.5 second of the 2-second expiratory time has negligible gas flow, the anatomic reservoir (50 mL) completely fills with 100% O_2, assuming an O_2 flow rate of 100 mL/sec. Using the preceding normal variables, the FIO_2 is calculated for a patient with a 500 mL and a 250 mL V_T (Tables 14-1 and 14-2).

TABLE 14-2

Example 2: If V_T Is Decreased to 250 mL

Volume inspired O_2	
Anatomic reservoir	50 mL
Flow/sec	100 mL
Inspired room air (0.20 × 100 mL)	20 mL
O_2 inspired	170 mL

$$FIO_2 = \frac{170\,mL\ O_2}{250\,mL\ V_T} = 0.68$$

FIO_2, Fraction of inspired oxygen; V_T, tidal volume.

The preceding 50% variability in F_{IO_2} at 6 L/min of O_2 flow clearly demonstrates the effects of a variable ventilatory pattern. In general, the larger the V_T or faster the respiratory rate, the lower the F_{IO_2}. The smaller the V_T or lower the respiratory rate, the higher the F_{IO_2}.

Low-flow O_2 devices are the most commonly employed O_2 delivery systems because of simplicity, ease of use, familiarity, economics, availability, and acceptance by patients. In most clinical situations (see "High-Flow Oxygen Systems" and "High-Flow Devices"), these systems should be initially employed.

2. High-Flow Oxygen Systems

High-flow, fixed-performance systems are nonrebreathing systems that provide the entire inspiratory atmosphere needed to meet the peak inspiratory flow and minute ventilatory demands of the patient. The flow rate and reservoir are essential to meet the patient's peak inspiratory flow. Flows of 30 to 40 L/min (or three to four times the measured minute volume) are often necessary. High-flow devices include aerosol masks and T-pieces that are powered by air-entrainment nebulizers or air-O_2 blenders and Venturi masks (see "Oxygen Delivery Devices"). Regardless of the patient's respiratory pattern, high-flow systems are expected to deliver predictable, consistent, and measurable high and low F_{IO_2} values. High-flow systems also can control the humidity and temperature of the delivered gases. The primary limitations of these systems are cost, bulkiness, and patients' tolerance.

There are two primary indications for high-flow O_2 devices:

1. Patients who require a consistent, predictable, minimal F_{IO_2} to reverse hypoxemia but prevent respiratory compromise due to excessive O_2 delivery (see "Complications")
2. The patient with increased minute ventilation and abnormal respiratory pattern who needs predictable and consistent high F_{IO_2} values

C. Oxygen Delivery Devices

1. Low-Flow Devices

a. NASAL CANNULAS

Because of their simplicity and the ease with which patients tolerate them, nasal cannulas are the most frequently used O_2 delivery devices. The nasal cannula consists of two prongs, with one inserted into each naris, that deliver 100% O_2. To be effective, the nasal passages must be patent, but the patient need not breathe through the nose. The flow rate settings range from 0.25 to 6 L/min. The nasopharynx serves as the O_2 reservoir (Fig. 14-1). Gases should be humidified to prevent mucosal drying if the O_2 flow exceeds 4 L/min. For each 1 L/min increase in flow, the F_{IO_2} is assumed to increase by 4% (Table 14-3).

An F_{IO_2} of 0.24 to 0.44 can be delivered predictably if the patient breathes at a normal minute ventilation rate with a normal respiratory pattern. Increasing flows to more than 6 L/min does not significantly increase the F_{IO_2} above 0.44 and is often poorly tolerated by the patient.

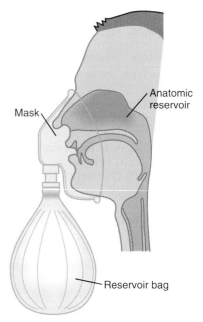

Figure 14-1 The three reservoirs of low-flow oxygen therapy. (From Vender JS, Clemency MV: O_2 delivery systems, inhalation therapy, and respiratory care. In Benumof JL, editor: *Clinical procedures in anesthesia and intensive care,* Philadelphia, 1992, JB Lippincott, pp 63–87.)

The components of a nasal cannula are nasal cannula prongs, delivery tubing, and an adjustable, restraining headband. Additional equipment includes an O_2 flowmeter to provide controlled gas delivery from a wall outlet; a humidification system increases patients' comfort at higher flows (≥4 L/min).

Procedurally, the initiation of O_2 therapy should be preceded by a review of the chart and documentation of the O_2 concentration and device ordered. If a humidifier (typically prefilled, single-use, disposable) is used, it should be filled to the appropriate level with sterile water and connected to the flowmeter. The nasal prong should be secured in the patient's naris and the cannula secured around the patient's head by a restraining strap.

Avoidance of undue cutaneous pressure is essential. Gauze may be needed to pad pressure points around the cheeks and ears during prolonged use. The flowmeter should be adjusted to the prescribed liter flow to attain the desired F_{IO_2} (see Table 14-3).

TABLE 14-3	
Approximate F_{IO_2} Delivered by Nasal Cannula	
Flow Rate (L/min)	**Approximate F_{IO_2}[*]**
1	0.24
2	0.28
3	0.32
4	0.36
5	0.40
6	0.44

F_{IO_2}, Fraction of inspired oxygen.
[*]Based on normal ventilatory patterns.

Although nasal cannulas are simple and safe, several potential hazards and complications exist. O_2 supports combustion, and any type of O_2 therapy is a fire hazard. Nasal trauma from prolonged use of or pressure from the nasal prongs can cause tissue damage. With poorly humidified, high gas flows, the airway mucosal surface can become dehydrated. This mucosal dehydration can result in mucosal irritation, epistaxis, laryngitis, ear tenderness, substernal chest pain, and bronchospasm.[5,7,9] Because this is a low-flow system, the FIO_2 can be inaccurate and inconsistent, leading to the potential for underoxygenation or overoxygenation. Overoxygenation may induce respiratory distress in patients with severe COPD by reversing protective hypoxic pulmonary vasoconstriction, depressing ventilation, and minimizing the Haldane effect (see "Complications"). Underoxygenation potentiates any problems associated with hypoxemia.

b. SIMPLE FACE MASK

To provide a higher FIO_2 value than that provided by nasal cannula with low-flow systems, the size of the O_2 reservoir must increase (see Fig. 14-1). A simple face mask consists of a mask with two side ports. The mask serves as an additional O_2 reservoir of 100 to 200 mL. The side ports allow room air entrainment and exit for exhaled gases. The mask has no valves. An FIO_2 of 0.40 to 0.60 can be achieved predictably when patients exhibit normal respiratory patterns. Gas flows greater than 8 L/min do not significantly increase the FIO_2 above 0.60 because the O_2 reservoir is filled. A minimum flow of 5 L/min is necessary to prevent CO_2 accumulation and rebreathing. The delivered O_2 value depends on the ventilatory pattern of the patient, similar to the situation with nasal cannulas.

The equipment needed is identical to that used for nasal cannula O_2 administration. The only difference is the use of a face mask. The predicted FIO_2 can be estimated from the O_2 flow rate (Table 14-4). Appropriate mask application is needed with all masks to maximize the FIO_2 and the patient's comfort. The mask should be positioned over the nasal bridge and the face, restricting O_2 escape into the patient's eye, which can cause ocular drying and irritation. If FIO_2 values above 0.60 are required, a partial rebreathing mask, nonrebreathing mask, or high-flow system should be employed. All O_2 devices that deliver higher values of FIO_2 increase the potential of O_2 toxicity (see "Complications").

c. PARTIAL REBREATHING MASK

To deliver an FIO_2 level of more than 60% with a low-flow system, the O_2 reservoir system must be increased (see

TABLE 14-4
Approximate FIO_2 Delivered by Simple Face Mask

Flow Rate (L/min)	FIO_2*
5–6	0.4
6–7	0.5
7–8	0.6

FIO_2, Fraction of inspired oxygen.
*Based on normal ventilatory patterns.

TABLE 14-5
Approximate FIO_2 Delivered by Mask with Reservoir Bag

Flow Rate (L/min)	FIO_2*
6	0.6
7	0.7
8	0.8
9	0.8+
10	0.8+

FIO_2, Fraction of inspired oxygen.
*Based on normal ventilatory patterns.

Fig. 14-1).[7] A partial rebreathing mask adds a reservoir bag with a capacity of 600 to 1000 mL. Side ports allow entrainment of room air and the exit of exhaled gases. The distinctive feature of this mask is that the first 33% of the patient's exhaled volume fills the reservoir bag. This volume is derived from the anatomic dead space and contains little CO_2. During inspiration, the bag should not completely collapse. A deflated reservoir bag results in a decreased FIO_2 because of entrained room air. With the next breath, the first exhaled gas (which is in the reservoir bag) and fresh gas are inhaled—accounting for the name *partial rebreather*. Fresh gas flows should be 8 L/min or greater, and the reservoir bag must remain inflated during the entire ventilatory cycle to ensure the highest FIO_2 and adequate CO_2 evacuation. An FIO_2 of 0.60 to 0.80 or more can be delivered with this device if the mask is applied appropriately and the ventilatory pattern is normal (Table 14-5). This mask's rebreathing capacity allows O_2 conservation and may be useful during transportation, when O_2 supply may be limited. Complications with partial rebreathing O_2 delivery systems are similar to those with other mask devices with low-flow systems.

d. NONREBREATHING MASK

A nonrebreathing mask (Fig. 14-2) is similar to a partial rebreathing mask but adds three unidirectional valves. One valve is located on each side of the mask to permit the venting of exhaled gases and to prevent room air entrainment. The third unidirectional valve is situated between the mask and the reservoir bag and prevents exhaled gases from entering the bag.

The bag must be inflated throughout the ventilatory cycle to ensure the highest FIO_2 and adequate CO_2 evacuation. Typically, the FIO_2 level is 0.80 to 0.90. Fresh gas flow is usually 15 L/min (range, 10 to 15 L/min). If room air is not entrained, an FIO_2 value approaching 1.0 can be achieved. If fresh gas flows or reservoir volume do not meet ventilatory needs, many masks have a spring-loaded tension valve that permits room air entrainment if the reservoir is evacuated. This spring valve is often called a *safety valve*. The spring valve tension should be checked periodically. If such a valve is not present, one of the unidirectional valves on the mask should be removed to allow room air entrainment if needed to meet ventilatory demands. This may be required to meet the increased inspiratory drive of critically ill patients. If the total ventilatory needs are met without room air entrainment, the rebreathing mask performs like a high-flow system. The operational application of a nonrebreathing mask is

Nonrebreathing oxygen mask

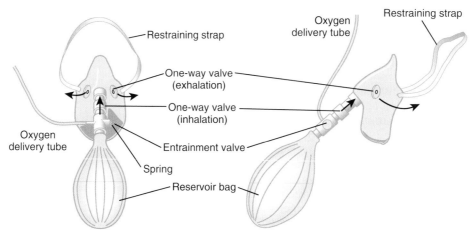

Figure 14-2 A nonrebreathing oxygen mask. In addition to the exhalation valve, the mask has a one-way inhalation valve. (From Vender JS, Clemency MV: Oxygen delivery systems, inhalation therapy, and respiratory care. In Benumof JL, editor: *Clinical procedures in anesthesia and intensive care,* Philadelphia, 1992, JB Lippincott.)

similar to that of other mask devices. To optimize the system, the mask should fit snugly (without excessive pressure) to avoid air entrainment around the mask, which would dilute the delivered gas and lower the FIO_2. If the mask fit is appropriate, the reservoir bag responds to the patient's inspiratory efforts. The high flows often employed increase the potential for several problems. Gastric distention, cutaneous irritation, and distention of the venting valves in the open position allowing room air entrainment can occur with excessive gas flows.

e. TRACHEOSTOMY COLLARS

Tracheostomy collars are used primarily to deliver humidity to patients with artificial airways. O_2 may be delivered with these devices, but as with other low-flow delivery systems, the FIO_2 is unpredictable, inconsistent, and dependent on ventilatory pattern due to the limited reservoir volume. The consistency of delivered FIO_2 by tracheostomy also depends on the patient breathing entirely through the tracheostomy. Cuff deflation or tube fenestration allows entrainment of air through the upper airways, and this may alter the concentration of delivered O_2.

2. High-Flow Devices

a. VENTURI MASKS

High-flow systems have flow rates and reservoirs large enough to provide the total inspired gases reliably. Most high-flow systems use gas entrainment at some point in the circuit to provide the flow and FIO_2 needs. Venturi masks entrain air by the Bernoulli principle and constant pressure-jet mixing.[10] This physical phenomenon is based on a rapid velocity of gas (e.g., O_2) moving through a restricted orifice. This action produces viscous shearing forces that create a decreased pressure gradient (subatmospheric) downstream relative to the surrounding gases. The pressure gradient causes room air to be entrained

until the pressures are equalized. Figure 14-3 illustrates the Venturi principle.

Altering the gas orifice or entrainment port size causes the FIO_2 value to vary. The O_2 flow rate determines the total volume of gas provided by the device. It provides predictable and reliable FIO_2 values of 0.24 to 0.50 that are independent of the patient's respiratory pattern. These masks come in two varieties:

1. A fixed FIO_2 model, which requires specific inspiratory attachments that are color coded and have labeled jets that produce a known FIO_2 with a given flow
2. A variable FIO_2 model (Fig. 14-4), which has a graded adjustment of the air entrainment port that can be set to allow variation in delivered FIO_2

To use any air entrainment device properly to control the FIO_2, the standard air-O_2 entrainment ratios and minimum recommended flows for a given FIO_2 level must be used (Table 14-6). The minimum total flow requirement should result from entrained room air added to the fresh O_2 flow and equal three to four times the minute ventilation. This minimal flow is required to meet the patient's peak inspiratory flow demands. As the desired FIO_2 increases, the air-O_2 entrainment ratio decreases with a net reduction in total gas flow. The higher the desired FIO_2, the greater the probability of the patient's needs exceeding the total flow capabilities of the device.

Venturi masks are often useful when treating patients with COPD who may develop worsening respiratory distress and dead space ventilation with supplemental increases in O_2 fraction.[11,12] The Venturi mask's ability to deliver a high flow with no particulate H_2O makes it beneficial in treating asthmatics, in whom bronchospasm may be precipitated or exacerbated by aerosolized H_2O administration.

Several specific concerns regarding the application of a Venturi mask must be recognized to provide

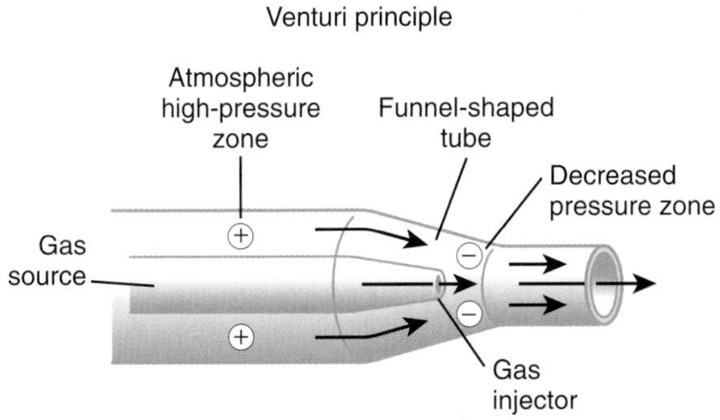

Venturi principle

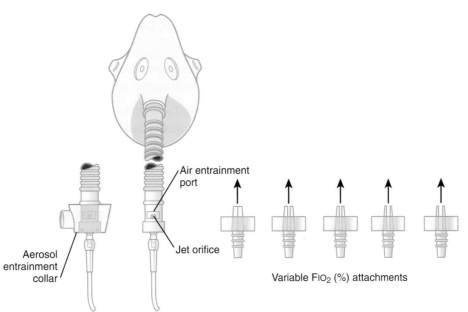

Figure 14-3 Application of the Venturi principle. (From Vender JS, Clemency MV: Oxygen delivery systems, inhalation therapy, and respiratory care. In Benumof JL, editor: *Clinical procedures in anesthesia and intensive care*, Philadelphia, 1992, JB Lippincott.)

TABLE 14-6

Approximate Air Entrainment Ratio and Gas Flow (FIO_2)

FIO_2 (%)	Ratio	Recommended O_2 Flow (L/min)	Total Gas Flow to Port (L/min)*
24	25.3:1	3	79
26	14.8:1	3	47
28	10.3:1	6	68
30	7.8:1	6	53
35	4.6:1	9	50
40	3.2:1	12	50
50	1.7:1	15	41

FIO_2, Fraction of inspired oxygen.
*Varies with manufacturer.

appropriate function. Obstructions distal to the jet orifice can produce back pressure and an effect referred to as Venturi stall. When this occurs, room air entrainment is compromised, causing a decreased total gas flow and an increased FIO_2. Occlusion or alteration of the exhalation ports can also produce this situation. Aerosol devices should not be used with these devices. Water droplets can occlude the O_2 injector. If humidity is needed, a vapor-type humidity adapter collar should be used.

b. HIGH-FLOW NASAL CANNULAS

High-flow nasal cannulas have been developed that can provide humidified gas flows up to 50 L/min while achieving 72% to 100% FIO_2.[13] Consistent delivery of humidification is also maintained at 72% to 99.9% relative humidity through the use of specialized nasal cannulas,[14] larger tubing, high-flow humidifiers, and O_2 blenders. These high-flow nasal cannulas can generate moderate levels of continuous positive airway pressure (CPAP) in nasal- and mouth-breathing patients.[15] It does not require a face mask, unlike most other high-flow systems, and this affords patients the opportunity to verbally communicate and eat in a normal manner.

Two types of high-flow cannulas are available for adults: the High Flow Adult Cannula (Salter Labs, Arvin, CA) and the Nasal High Flow (Fisher & Paykel Healthcare, New Zealand). Both can achieve high relative humidity and high FIO_2 values. The High Flow Adult Cannula appears similar to a regular nasal cannula. Key differences include larger, three-channel tubing that is colored green; an enlarged reservoir at the prongs; and flow rates up to 15 L/min. The Nasal High Flow employs small-diameter corrugated tubing throughout the length of the supply tubing to achieve flow rates up to 50 L/min.

Venturi mask and variable FIO_2 attachment

Figure 14-4 Graded air entrainment by the Ventimask provides specific FIO_2 levels through the jet orifices. (From Vender JS, Clemency MV: Oxygen delivery systems, inhalation therapy, and respiratory care. In Benumof JL, editor: *Clinical procedures in anesthesia and intensive care*, Philadelphia, 1992, JB Lippincott.)

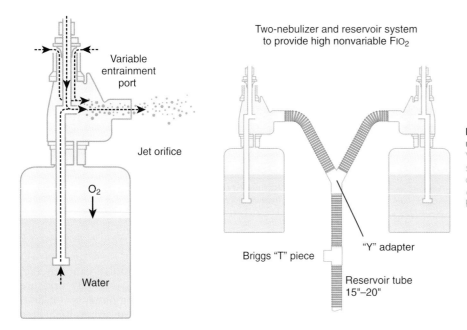

Two-nebulizer and reservoir system
to provide high nonvariable FIO_2

Variable
entrainment
port

Jet orifice

O_2

Water

Briggs "T" piece

"Y" adapter

Reservoir tube
15"–20"

Figure 14-5 Single-unit and double (tandem)-unit mechanical aerosol systems. (From Vender JS, Clemency MV: Oxygen delivery systems, inhalation therapy, and respiratory care. In Benumof JL, editor: *Clinical procedures in anesthesia and intensive care,* Philadelphia, 1992, JB Lippincott.)

c. AEROSOL MASKS AND T-PIECES WITH NEBULIZERS OR AIR-OXYGEN BLENDERS

Large-volume nebulizers and wide-bore tubing are optimal for delivering FIO_2 levels greater than 0.40 with a high-flow system. Aerosol masks, in conjunction with air entrainment nebulizers or air-O_2 blenders, deliver consistent and predictable FIO_2 levels, regardless of the patient's ventilatory pattern. A T-piece is used in place of an aerosol mask for patients with an artificial airway.

Air entrainment nebulizers can deliver FIO_2 of 0.35 to 1.00 and produce an aerosol. The maximum gas flow through the nebulizer is 14 to 16 L/min. As with the Venturi masks, less room air is entrained with higher FIO_2 values. As a result, total flow at high FIO_2 values is decreased. To meet ventilatory demands, two nebulizers may feed a single mask to increase the total flow, and a short length of corrugated tubing may be added to the aerosol mask side ports to increase the reservoir capacity (Fig. 14-5). If the aerosol mist exiting the mask side ports disappears during inspiration, room air is probably being entrained, and flow should be increased.

Circuit resistance can increase as a result of water accumulation or kinking of the aerosol tubing. The increased pressure at the Venturi device decreases room air entrainment, increases the FIO_2 level, and decreases total gas flow. If a predictable FIO_2 level of more than 0.40 is desired, an air-O_2 blender should be used. Air-O_2 blenders can deliver consistent and accurate FIO_2 values from 0.21 to 1.0 and flows of up to 100 L/min with humidification. The higher flows tend to produce excessive noise through the large-bore tubing. Air-O_2 blenders are recommended for patients with increased minute ventilation who require a high FIO_2 level and in whom bronchospasm may be precipitated or worsened by a nebulized H_2O aerosol. With an artificial airway, a 15- to 20-inch reservoir tube should be added to the Briggs T-piece (Hudson, RCI, Temecula, CA) to prevent the potential of entraining air into the system.

D. Humidifiers

Humidity is the water vapor in a gas. When air is 100% saturated at 37° C, it contains 43.8 mg of H_2O/L. The amount of water vapor a volume of gas contains depends on the temperature and water availability. The vapor pressure exerted by the water vapor is equal to 47 mm Hg. Alveolar gases are 100% saturated at 37° C. When the inspired atmosphere contains less than 43.8 mg of H_2O/L or has a vapor pressure of less than 47 mm Hg, a gradient exists between the respiratory mucosa and the inhaled gas. This gradient causes water to leave the mucosa and to humidify the inhaled gas.

Room air that has a relative humidity of 50% at 21° C has a relative humidity of 21% at 37° C. Under normal conditions, the lungs contribute about 250 mL of H_2O per day to maximally saturate inspired air.[7]

The administration of dry O_2 lowers the water content of the inspired air. The upper respiratory tract filters, humidifies, and warms inspired gases. Nasal breathing is more efficient than oral breathing for conditioning inspired gases. The use of an artificial airway bypasses the nasopharynx and oropharynx, where a significant amount of warming and humidification of inspired gases are accomplished. As a result, O_2 administration and the use of artificial airways increase the demand on the lungs to humidify the inspired gases.

The increased demand ultimately leads to mucosal drying, inspissated secretions, and decreased mucociliary clearance, which can eventually result in bacterial infections, mucous plugging, atelectasis, and pneumonia. To prevent these complications, a humidifier or nebulizer should be used to increase the water content of the inspired gases.

Indications for humidity therapy include high-flow therapeutic gas delivery to nonintubated patients, delivery of gases through artificial airways, and reduction of airway resistance in asthma. Low flows (1 to 4 L/min) usually do not need humidification except in specific individuals, but all O_2 delivered to infants should be humidified.

A humidifier increases the heated or unheated water vapor in a gas. This can be accomplished by passing gas over heated water (heated passover humidifier); by fractionating gas into tiny bubbles as gas passes through water (bubble diffusion or jet humidifiers); by allowing gas to pass through a chamber that contains a heated, water-saturated wick (heated wick humidifier); and by vaporizing water and selectively allowing the vapor to mix with the inspired gases (vapor-phase humidifier). Other variations of humidification systems exist but are beyond the scope of this chapter.[16]

Bubble humidifiers can be used with nasal cannulas, simple face masks, partial and nonrebreathing masks, and air-O_2 blenders. They increase the relative humidity of gas from 0% to 70% at 25° C, which is approximately equal to 34% at 37° C.[17,18] Large-volume bubble-through humidifiers are available for use with ventilator circuits or high-gas-flow delivery systems.

A heated humidifier may be used when delivering dry gases to patients with ETTs because it allows delivery of gases with an increased water content and relative humidity exceeding 65% at 37° C. When heated humidifiers are used, proximal airway temperature should be monitored to ensure a gas temperature that allows maximum moisture-carrying capacity but prevents mucosal burns.

Heat and moisture exchangers (HMEs) are simple, small humidifier systems designed to be attached to an artificial airway. The HMEs are often referred to as an *artificial nose*. The efficiency of these devices is quite variable, depending on the HME design, V_T, and atmospheric conditions. HMEs are typically used for short-term ventilatory support and for humidification during anesthesia. Several contraindications include use in neonatal and small pediatric patients; copious secretions; significant spontaneous breathing, in which the patient's V_T exceeds the HME specifications; and large-volume losses through a bronchopleural fistula or leakage around the ETT.[16]

A nebulizer increases the water content of the inspired gas by generating aerosols (small droplets of particulate water) that become incorporated into the delivered gas stream and then evaporate into the inspired gas as it is warmed in the respiratory tract. There are two basic kinds of nebulizers: pneumatic and electric. Pneumatic nebulizers operate from a pressured gas source and are jet or hydrodynamic. Electric nebulizers are powered by an electrical source and are referred to as *ultrasonic*. There are several varieties of both types of nebulizers, and they depend more on design differences than on the power source. A more in-depth discussion of nebulizers is available elsewhere.[7,9] The resultant humidity ranges from 50% to 100% at 37° C, depending on the device used. If heated, the relative humidity of the gas can exceed 100% at 37° C. Air entrainment nebulizers are used in conjunction with aerosol masks and T-pieces.

Aerosol therapy can be used for three general purposes. First, aerosol therapy increases the particulate and molecular water content of the inspired gases. The aerosol increases the water content of desiccated and retained secretions, enhancing bronchial hygiene. This does not alleviate the need for systemic hydration. Second, delivery of medications is a primary indication for aerosol therapy. For example, β_2-agonists, corticosteroids, anticholinergics, and antiviral-antibacterial agents (see "Inhalation Therapy") may be delivered to patients' airways by aerosol therapy. Third, aerosol therapy can be employed for sputum induction. The success of aerosol therapy depends on appropriate application and proper technique of administration.

The aerosol generated by the nebulizer can precipitate bronchospasm of hyperactive airways.[5,7] Prophylactic bronchodilator therapy should be employed before or during the aerosol treatment. Fluid accumulation and overload have been reported. These problems are more common in treating pediatric patients and with continuous ultrasonic rather than intermittent or jet therapy. Dry secretions are hydrophilic and can swell because of the absorbed water content. If secretions swell, they can obstruct airways. Mobilization of secretions limits this problem. Aerosol therapy for drug delivery has been reported to precipitate the same side effects as systemic drug delivery. Therapeutic aerosols have been implicated in nosocomial infections.[19] Cross-contamination between patients must be avoided.

E. Manual Resuscitation Bags

Manual resuscitation bags are used primarily for resuscitation and manual ventilation of ventilator-dependent patients. These bags can deliver an F_{IO_2} of more than 0.90 and V_T values up to 800 mL when O_2 flows to the bag are 10 to 15 mL/min. Factors that promote the highest F_{IO_2} level include the use of an O_2 reservoir, connection to an O_2 source, and slow rates of ventilation that allow the bag to refill completely. Positive end-expiratory pressure (PEEP) valves should be used for patients who require more than 5 cm H_2O of PEEP. The clinician should be aware of different capabilities among various resuscitation bags in the delivery of maximum F_{IO_2}.[20-22]

F. Complications

Complications related to O_2 delivery can be divided into two groups: complications related to the O_2 delivery systems (see sections that discuss the specific devices) and pathophysiologic complications related to O_2 therapy. Pathophysiologic complications related to O_2 therapy can lead to serious consequences. The three major complications encountered in adults are hypoventilation, absorption atelectasis, and O_2 toxicity.

O_2 therapy must be used appropriately in patients with severe COPD because of a risk of developing respiratory distress. Conventional teaching of hypoxic drive theory and excessive O_2 delivery have not been consistently supported in the literature.[11,23] Disturbances in $\dot{V}/\dot{Q}$ develop in patients with COPD, and through hypoxic pulmonary vasoconstriction, the perfusion is then redistributed to areas of higher O_2 tension. In the presence of low O_2 tension, pulmonary arterioles constrict, resulting in increased vascular resistance. This results in shunting of blood flow to areas of higher O_2 tension. Increasing mixed venous or alveolar O_2

tension can reverse this shunting and worsen $\dot{V}/\dot{Q}$ matching.[12,24]

In addition to regional ventilation disturbances, patients with severe COPD typically have a chronically elevated $PaCO_2$ value, a normal pH, and a PaO_2 level that usually is less than 60 mm Hg. The patient may become desensitized to ventilatory stimulation from changes in $PaCO_2$ because an increased $PaCO_2$ is compensated by an increased bicarbonate ion concentration in the arterial blood and in the cerebral spinal fluid. Instead, the chemoreceptors in the aortic and carotid bodies stimulate ventilation. They are sensitive to PaO_2 values less than 60 mm Hg. When worsening hypoxemia is treated with supplemental O_2, the goal is to raise the PaO_2 to the patient's chronic level. Although many patients will demonstrate an initial decrease in respiratory rate with hyperoxia, the minute ventilation soon normalizes.[24] By means of the Haldane effect, deoxygenated hemoglobin binds to and reduces dissolved CO_2. By displacing the CO_2 from hemoglobin, the elevated O_2 concentration reverses the compensatory mechanism of the Haldane effect.[25]

Absorption atelectasis occurs when high alveolar O_2 concentrations cause alveolar collapse. Nitrogen, already at equilibrium, remains within the alveoli and "splints" alveoli open. When high FIO_2 values are administered, nitrogen is washed out of the alveoli, which are then filled primarily with O_2. In areas of the lungs with reduced $\dot{V}/\dot{Q}$ ratios, O_2 is absorbed into the blood faster than ventilation can replace it. The affected alveoli become smaller and smaller and eventually collapse with increased surface tension. Progressively higher fractions of inspired O_2 greater than 0.50 cause absorption atelectasis in healthy individuals. FIO_2 values of 0.50 or greater may precipitate this phenomenon in patients with decreased $\dot{V}/\dot{Q}$ ratios.

The third pathophysiologic complication of O_2 therapy, O_2 toxicity, becomes clinically important after 8 to 12 hours of exposure to a high FIO_2 level.[26] O_2 toxicity probably results from direct exposure of the alveoli to a high FIO_2 level. Healthy lungs appear to tolerate FIO_2 values of less than 0.6. In damaged lungs, FIO_2 values of more than 0.50 can result in a toxic alveolar O_2 concentration. Because most O_2 therapy is delivered at 1 atm barometric pressure, the FIO_2 and the duration of exposure become the determining factors in the development of most clinically significant O_2 toxicity.

The mechanism of O_2 toxicity is related to the significantly higher production of O_2 free radicals, including superoxide anions (O_2^-), hydroxyl radicals (OH^-), hydrogen peroxide (H_2O_2), and singlet O_2. These radicals affect cell function by inactivating protein sulfhydryl enzymes, disrupting DNA synthesis, and disrupting the cell membrane integrity by lipid peroxidation. Vitamin E, superoxide dismutase, and sulfhydryl compounds promote normal, protective free radical scavenging within the lung. During periods of lung tissue hyperoxia, these protective mechanisms are overwhelmed, and toxicity results.[27]

The classic clinical manifestations of O_2 toxicity include cough, substernal chest pain, dyspnea, rales, pulmonary edema, progressive arterial hypoxemia, bilateral pulmonary infiltrates, decreasing lung compliance, and atelectasis. These signs and symptoms are nonspecific, and O_2 toxicity is frequently difficult to distinguish from severe underlying pulmonary disease. Often, only subtle progression of arterial hypoxemia heralds the onset of pulmonary O_2 toxicity.

Classic O_2 toxicity in animal models occurs in two distinct phases. The early or exudative phase, observed during the first 24 to 48 hours, is characterized by the capillary endothelial thinning and vacuolization,[28] destruction of type I pneumocytes, and development of interstitial and intra-alveolar hemorrhage and edema. The late or proliferative phase, which begins after 72 hours, is characterized by reabsorption of early infiltrates, hyperplasia, proliferation of type II pneumocytes, and increased collagen synthesis. When O_2 toxicity progresses to the proliferative stage, permanent lung damage may result from scarring, fibrosis, and proliferation of type II pneumocytes.[28]

The best treatment for O_2 toxicity is preventing it from occurring altogether. O_2 therapy should be directed at improving oxygenation with the minimum FIO_2 needed to obtain an arterial oxygenation (SaO_2) of more than 90%. Inhalation treatments and raised expiratory airway pressure may be useful adjuncts in improving pulmonary toilet, decreasing $\dot{V}/\dot{Q}$ mismatch, and improving arterial oxygenation. These therapies may be used to maintain adequate oxygenation at an FIO_2 of 0.50 or less.

III. TECHNIQUES OF RESPIRATORY CARE

The provision of adequate pulmonary gas exchange is implicit in our teaching and management of respiratory care. For optimal gas exchange to occur, the airways must be maintained clear of foreign material (e.g., secretions). The various therapeutic techniques available are aimed at the mobilization and removal of pulmonary secretions. Therapies are intended to optimize breathing efficiency.

Respiratory therapy aimed at the patient with impaired pulmonary function can improve several outcome measures. Using common physiotherapy techniques such as postural drainage, vibration, percussion, and suction on critically ill patients can lead to decreases in intrapulmonary shunt. The lining of the lungs secretes a mucous layer that usually moves toward the larynx at a rate of 1 to 2 cm/min by ciliary motion. This mucous layer is responsible for transporting foreign particles from the lungs to the larynx. Critically ill patients have many factors contributing to the presence of increased secretions. Alterations in the mucociliary escalator system related to smoking, stress, high FIO_2 levels, anesthesia, foreign bodies in the trachea (e.g., ETT), tracheobronchial diseases, and abnormalities in mucus production are all recognized contributors to retention of airway secretions. To help compensate for these deficiencies, the patient must be able to generate an adequate cough. Critically ill patients and individuals with an artificial airway often do not have an adequate cough. If any of these problems is present, there is an increased tendency to retain secretions.

Retained secretions promote several potential complications. Occlusion of the airway promotes ventilation-perfusion inequalities. This produces a progressively worse hypoxemia that is less responsive to O_2 therapy (see indications in "Oxygen Delivery Systems"). Retained secretions and distal airway occlusion promote an increased incidence of postobstructive pneumonia. Retained secretions increase the patient's work of breathing because of an increased airway resistance associated with the airway inflammation and partial airway occlusion. Reduced pulmonary compliance results from atelectasis and reduced lung volumes.

Many of the fundamental practices of respiratory care are aimed at the provision of optimal airway care, tracheobronchial toilet, and the prevention and management of retained secretions. Because dehydration is a common cause of retained secretions, adequate hydration and humidification of gas delivery are essential. Humidity and aerosol therapy are discussed in the Oxygen Delivery Systems section of this chapter. The remainder of this section addresses other techniques commonly employed in respiratory care, including airway suctioning, chest physical therapy, and incentive spirometry. Intermittent positive-pressure breathing (IPPB) is discussed separately because it is used for the promotion of tracheobronchial toilet and the delivery of medications (see "Inhalation Therapy").

A. Suctioning

Airway suctioning is commonly employed in respiratory care to promote optimal tracheobronchial toilet and airway patency in critically ill patients. Because of the perceived simplicity and limited complications, airway suctioning is frequently employed. If proper indications and technique are not appreciated, however, the potential for significant complications exists.

1. Indications

Suctioning of the airway should not be done without appropriate clinical indications. The audible (auscultatory) or visible presence of airway secretions is the most common indication. Increasing peak inspiratory pressures in mechanically ventilated patients are often indicative of retained secretions. Routine prophylactic suctioning is unwarranted except in neonates, in whom the small airway diameters can be acutely obstructed by a small accumulation of secretions.

In addition to removal of secretions, suction catheters are employed as aids in evaluating airway patency. If an artificial airway appears to be occluded, an attempt to pass a suction catheter can help assess airway patency. Causes of artificial airway occlusion include mucous plugging, foreign body obstructions, kinking, and cuff herniations. If the suction catheter cannot be passed and ventilation is obstructed, the artificial airway may require replacement. Bronchoscopic evaluation may assist the clinician in the evaluation of the airway. Provision of airway suctioning depends on an appreciation of the available equipment, the appropriate techniques, and the potential complications.

2. Equipment

Numerous commercial suction catheters exist.[5,7,29] The ideal catheter is one that optimizes secretion removal and minimizes tissue trauma. Specific features of the catheters include the material of construction, frictional resistance, size (length and diameter), shape, and position of the aspirating holes. An opening at the proximal end of the catheter to allow the entrance of room air, neutralizing the vacuum without disconnecting the vacuum apparatus, is ideal. The proximal hole should be larger than the catheter lumen. Tracheal suctioning can occur only with occlusion of this proximal opening. The conventional suction catheter has side holes and end holes (Fig. 14-6).

The length of the typical catheter should pass beyond the distal tip of the artificial airway. The diameter of the suction catheter is very important. The optimal catheter diameter should not exceed one half of the internal diameter of the artificial airway. A catheter that is too large can produce an excessive vacuum and evacuation of gases distal to the tip of the airway, promoting atelectasis because of inadequate space for entrainment of air around the suction catheter. If the catheter is too small, removal of secretions can be compromised.

3. Technique

The technique of suctioning is important for the optimal removal of secretions and limitation of complications. This is a sterile procedure necessitating appropriate care in handling the catheter. Gloves and hand washing are necessary unless a closed system is employed. Other necessary equipment includes a vacuum source, sterile rinsing solution, AMBU O_2 system, and lavage solution. The optimal vacuum pressure should be adjusted for the patient's age.

Before suctioning, the patient should be preoxygenated by increasing the FIO_2 to 100% or by manual ventilatory assistance. Preoxygenation minimizes the hypoxemia

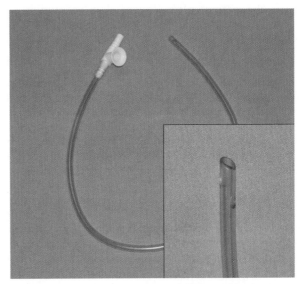

Figure 14-6 A conventional suction catheter has side and end holes. *Inset,* Enlarged view of the beveled tip and dual side holes.

induced by circuit disconnection and application of the suction vacuum. After preoxygenation, the sterile catheter is advanced past the distal tip of the artificial airway without the vacuum. When the catheter can no longer easily advance, it should be slightly withdrawn, and intermittent vacuum pressure should be applied while the catheter is removed in a rotating fashion. This technique reportedly reduces mucosal trauma and enhances secretion clearance. The vacuum (suction) time should be limited to 10 to 15 seconds, and discontinuation of ventilation and oxygenation should not exceed 20 seconds. After removal of the catheter, reoxygenation and ventilation are essential. Throughout the procedure, the patient's stability and tolerance should be monitored. If signs of distress or dysrhythmias develop, the procedure should be immediately discontinued and oxygenation and ventilation reestablished. Suctioning is repeated until secretions have been adequately removed. After airway suctioning, oropharyngeal secretions should be suctioned and the catheter should be disposed.

Optimization of secretion removal necessitates adequate hydration and humidification of delivered gases. Occasionally, secretions can become quite viscous. Instillation of 5 to 10 mL of sterile normal saline can aid removal.

In critically ill patients, using a closed system or swivel adapter to allow simultaneous suctioning and ventilation limits the consequences of airway disconnection, minimizes the loss of PEEP, and enhances sterility. These disposable systems are usually more costly but are used for up to 72 hours.

When an artificial airway is absent, nasotracheal suctioning techniques are employed. These techniques are technically less effective and more difficult than oral suctioning without an artificial airway and have the potential for additional complications. After appropriate lubrication, the catheter is inserted into a patient's nasal passage (often through a previously placed nasopharyngeal airway). The catheter is advanced into the larynx. Breath sounds from the proximal end of the catheter are often used as an audible guide. On the catheter's entry into the larynx, the patient often coughs. The vacuum is connected, and suctioning of the trachea is accomplished as previously described.

4. Complications

Complications of suctioning can be significant.[7,30] Although the suction vacuum is used to remove secretions, it also removes O_2-enriched gases from the airway. If inappropriately applied and monitored, suctioning can produce significant hypoxemia. The use of arterial O_2 monitors (e.g., pulse oximetry) can often help detect alterations in SaO_2, heart rate, and the presence of dysrhythmias.

Cardiovascular alterations are common. Dysrhythmias and hypotension are the most frequent cardiac complications. Arterial hypoxemia (and eventually myocardial hypoxia) and vagal stimulation from tracheal suctioning are recognized precipitory causes of cardiovascular complications. Coughing induced by stimulation of the airway can reduce venous return and ventricular preload. Avoidance of hypoxemia, prolonged suctioning (>10 seconds),

and appropriate monitoring and sedation help reduce the incidence and significance of these complications.[31]

Inappropriate suction catheter size can produce excessive evacuation of gas distal to the artificial airway because of inadequate space for proximal air entrainment. This leads to hypoxemia and atelectasis. It is best avoided by reducing the catheter size to less than one half of the internal diameter of the airway. Presuctioning and postsuctioning auscultation of the lungs helps detect significant atelectasis. After suctioning, several hyperinflations of the lungs can help reinflate atelectatic lung segments.

Mucosal irritations and trauma are common with frequent suctioning. The incidence and severity of trauma depend on the frequency of suctioning; technique; catheter design; absence of secretions, allowing more direct mucosal contact; and amount of vacuum pressure applied. Blood in the secretions is usually the first sign of tissue trauma. Meticulous technique is essential to limit this common complication. Airway reflexes can be irritated by direct mechanical stimulation. Wheezing resulting from bronchoconstriction can necessitate bronchodilator therapy. Nasotracheal suctioning can induce several additional complications, such as nasal irritation, epistaxis, and laryngospasm. Laryngospasm can be life-threatening if it is not recognized and appropriately managed.

B. Chest Physical Therapy

Chest physical therapy techniques are an integral part of respiratory care. Chest physical therapy plays an important role in the provision of bronchial hygiene and optimization of ventilation. The mucociliary escalator systems and cough can be aided by adjunctive techniques.

1. Postural Drainage and Positional Changes

The fundamental goal of postural drainage is to move loosened secretions toward the proximal airway for eventual removal. Pulmonary drainage takes advantage of the normal pulmonary anatomy and gravitational flow. Flow of secretions is optimized by liquefaction (see "Humidifiers").

The primary indications for pulmonary drainage are malfunctioning of normal bronchial hygiene mechanisms and excessive or retained secretions.[7,9,32,33] In patients with ineffective lung volumes and cough, pulmonary drainage can be used prophylactically to prevent accumulation of secretions. Clinical conditions that typically benefit from pulmonary drainage include bronchiectasis, cystic fibrosis (CF), COPD, asthma, lung abscess, spinal cord injuries, atelectasis, pneumonia, and healing after thoracic and abdominal surgery.

To administer postural drainage appropriately, the practitioner must be able to understand the location of the involved lung segments and the proper position to optimize drainage into the proximal airway. The lungs are divided into lobes, segments, and subsegments, and fluid drainage is directed centrally to the hilum (Table 14-7).

Precise anatomic descriptions of the various pulmonary subsegments and positions are beyond the scope of this chapter. The large posterior and superior basal

TABLE 14-7

Lung Segments

Right Side	Left Side
Upper Lobe	**Upper Lobe**
Apical	Apical-posterior
Posterior	Anterior
Anterior	
Middle Lobe	**Lingula**
Lateral	Superior
Medial	Inferior
Lower Lobe	**Lower Lobe**
Superior	Superior
Medial basal	Anteromedial basal
Anterior basal	Lateral basal
Lateral basal	Posterior basal
Posterior basal	

segments of the lower lobe are commonly involved in hospital patients with atelectasis and pneumonia. In the typical hospital patient, these segments are most gravity dependent, causing stasis of secretions (Fig. 14-7).

Appropriate positioning of the patient can enhance gravitational flow. This therapy also includes turning or rotating the body around its longitudinal axis. Newer critical care beds have this feature incorporated into their design and function. Commonly employed positions for postural drainage are demonstrated in Figure 14-8.

Postural drainage should be done several times each day. For optimal results, postural drainage should follow humidity treatments and other bronchial hygiene therapies. Postural drainage should precede meals by 30 to 60 minutes, and the duration of treatment continues as long as the patient tolerates the therapy and may last up to 1 hour in certain patient populations (e.g., CF patients).

Postural drainage can produce physiologic and anatomic stresses that are potentially detrimental to specific patients.[34] Alterations in the cardiovascular system from abrupt changes in position are well recognized. Hypotension, dysrhythmias, or congestive heart failure that is due to changes in preload can be induced by positional change. $\dot{V}/\dot{Q}$ relationships are altered by changes in position. When pulmonary drainage occurs in the uppermost position, blood preferentially flows to the gravity-dependent, nondiseased segments, improving the ventilation-perfusion relationships. The head-down position, which is commonly used, is best avoided in patients with intracranial disease. Decreased venous return from the head can increase intracranial pressure.

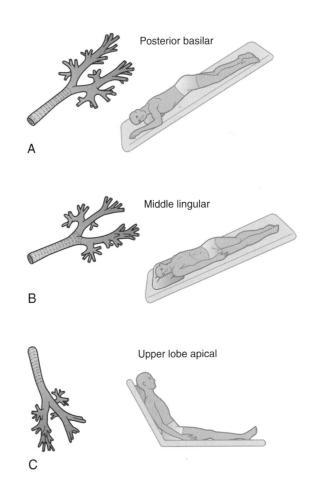

Dependent lung segments

Posterior basilar segments

A Semi-upright position

Apical segments

B Supine position

Figure 14-7 Lung segments typically are at risk for retained secretions, atelectasis, and pneumonia due to body position during convalescence. **A,** Posterior basilar segment of the lower lobe. **B,** Apical segment of the lower lobe. (From Vender JS, Clemency MV: Oxygen delivery systems, inhalation therapy, and respiratory care. In Benumof JL, editor: *Clinical procedures in anesthesia and intensive care,* Philadelphia, 1992, JB Lippincott.)

Posterior basilar

A

Middle lingular

B

Upper lobe apical

C

Figure 14-8 Common position for optimizing postural drainage of the posterior basilar **(A),** middle lingular **(B),** and upper lobe apical segments **(C).** (From Vender JS, Clemency MV: Oxygen delivery systems, inhalation therapy, and respiratory care. In Benumof JL, editor: *Clinical procedures in anesthesia and intensive care,* Philadelphia, 1992, JB Lippincott.)

The prone position has been demonstrated to improve oxygenation in patients with acute respiratory distress syndrome. The placement of critically ill patients in the prone position can be done without significant morbidity despite the presence of multiple sites of vascular access and intubation. The improvement in oxygenation probably depends on recruitment of collapsed alveoli, more evenly distributed pleural pressure gradients, and caudad movement of the diaphragm.[35]

Continuous rotational therapy employs dedicated intensive care unit beds that slowly and continuously rotate the patient along a longitudinal axis. The theory is that rotation of patients prevents gravity-dependent airway closure or collapse, worsening of pulmonary compliance and atelectasis, and pooling of secretions and subsequent pulmonary infection caused by long-term immobilization.[36] The use of rotational therapy may lead to a significantly lower incidence of patients diagnosed with pneumonia compared with patients cared for on conventional beds.[37]

Continual assessment of patients' tolerance during the procedure is necessary. Vital signs, oxygenation monitoring, general appearance, level of consciousness, and subjective comments by the patient are all part of the appraisal process.

2. Percussion and Vibration Therapy

Percussion and vibration therapy are used in conjunction with postural drainage to loosen and mobilize secretions that are adherent to the bronchial walls.[7,38] Percussion involves a manually produced, rhythmic vibration of varying intensity and frequency. In a clapping motion (cupped hands), a blow is delivered during inspiration and expiration over the affected area while the patient is in the appropriate position for postural drainage (Fig. 14-9).

Mechanical energy is produced by compression of the air between the cupped hand and the chest wall. Proper percussion should produce a popping sound (similar to striking the bottom of a ketchup bottle). Proper force and rhythm can be accomplished by placing the hands not farther than 5 inches from the chest and then alternating flexing and extending of the wrists (similar to a waving motion). The procedure should last 5 to 7 minutes per affected area.

Like all respiratory care, percussion therapy should not be performed without a medical order. Therapy should not be performed over bare skin, surgical incisions, bone prominences, kidneys, and female breasts or with hard objects. If a stinging sensation or reddening of the skin develops, the technique should be reevaluated. Special care must be given to the fragile patient. Fractured ribs, localized pain, coagulation abnormalities, bone metastases, hemoptysis, and empyemas are relative contraindications to percussion therapy.

Vibration therapy is used to promote bronchial hygiene in a fashion similar to chest percussion. Manually or mechanically (Fig. 14-10) gentle vibrations are transmitted through the chest wall to the affected area during exhalation. Vibration frequencies in excess of 200/min can be achieved if the procedure is done correctly. In patients

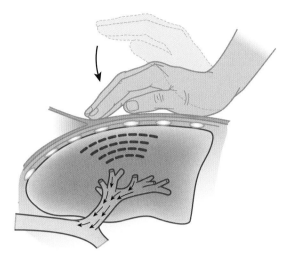

Figure 14-9 Typical hand position for chest percussion therapy. The hand is cupped and positioned about 5 inches from the chest, and the wrist is flexed. The hand strikes the chest in a waving motion. (From Vender JS, Clemency MV: Oxygen delivery systems, inhalation therapy, and respiratory care. In Benumof JL, editor: *Clinical procedures in anesthesia and intensive care*, Philadelphia, 1992, JB Lippincott.)

receiving IPPB, all chest physical therapy procedures should be performed during the IPPB.

3. Incentive Spirometry

In the 1970s, alternative methods for prophylactic bronchial hygiene were developed to replace the more costly and controversial use of IPPB. Incentive spirometry (IS) was developed after several techniques using expiratory maneuvers (e.g., blow and glove bottles) and CO_2-induced hyperventilation were found to be clinically ineffective or to cause other risks.[5,7,9]

IS was developed with an emphasis on sustained maximal inspiration (SMI). IS provides a visual goal or incentive for the patient to achieve SMI. Normal, spontaneous breathing patterns have periodic hyperinflations

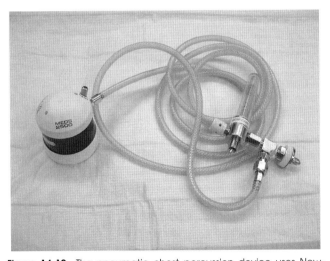

Figure 14-10 The pneumatic chest percussion device uses Newton's third law of motion to assist the respiratory therapist in controlling percussion intensity. Therapists control the pulse intensity by how firmly they press the device. The device provides percussion without the need for clapping. It is less fatiguing for the therapist and may be more comfortable for the patient than manual percussion.

that prevent the alveolar collapse associated with shallow tidal ventilation breathing patterns. Narcotics, sedative drugs, general anesthesia, cerebral trauma, immobilization, and abdominal or thoracic surgery can promote shallow tidal ventilation breathing patterns. Complications from this breathing pattern include atelectasis, retained secretions, and pneumonia.

The physiologic principle of SMI is to produce a maximal transpulmonary pressure gradient by generating a more negative intrapleural pressure. This pressure gradient produces alveolar hyperinflation with maximal airflow during the inspiratory phase.[39]

The indications for IS and SMI are primarily related to bronchial hygiene. These techniques should be employed perioperatively in surgical patients at an increased risk for pulmonary complications. IS involves the patient in his or her care and recovery, which can be psychologically beneficial while also being cost advantageous relative to the equipment and personal costs associated with other forms of respiratory care (e.g., IPPB).

The goals of IS and SMI therapy are to optimize lung inflation to prevent atelectasis, to optimize the cough mechanism by providing larger lung volumes, and to provide a baseline standard to assess the effectiveness of therapy or detect the onset of acute pulmonary disease (indicated by a deteriorating performance). To achieve these goals, patient instruction and supervision are preferred. Preoperative education enhances the effectiveness of postoperative bronchial hygiene therapy (e.g., IS, SMI). Appropriate instruction for proper breathing techniques can help produce an effective cough mechanism.

Various clinical models of incentive spirometers are available.[9] The devices vary in how they function, guide the therapy, or recognize the achievements. Each manufacturer provides instructions for use that should be followed. The devices are aimed at generating the largest inspiratory volumes during 5 to 15 seconds. The actual device used or rate of flow is not as important as the frequency of use and the attainment of maximal inspiratory volumes and sustained inspiration. Maximal benefit with most devices can be achieved only with user education.

The administration of IS and SMI therapy necessitates a physiologically and psychologically stable patient. The patient's cooperation and motivation are very important. For the therapy to be optimally effective, the patient should be free of acute pulmonary distress, have a forced vital capacity of more than 15 mL/kg, and have a spontaneous respiratory rate of less than 25 beats/min. Ideally, the patient should not require a high F_{IO_2} level. Therapy should be done hourly while the patient is awake. Typically, the patient should do four or five SMIs at a 30- to 60-second interval to prevent fatigue or hyperventilation. The patient should be coached to inspire slowly while attaining maximal inspiratory volumes.

Significant complications are not associated with IS and SMI therapy. The only relative contraindications are patients who are uncooperative, physically disabled with acute pulmonary disease, or unable to generate minimum volumes for lung inflation (e.g., 12 to 15 mL/kg).

Although the use of IS is widespread throughout the United States, many reviews cast doubts on the superiority of IS in reducing postoperative pulmonary complications over other methods of postoperative respiratory care.[40] Meta-analyses suggest that IS does not prevent pulmonary complications in patients undergoing coronary artery bypass grafting (CABG) or upper abdominal surgery.[41-43]

C. Intermittent Positive-Pressure Breathing

In the past 40 years, few respiratory care therapies have been as controversial as IPPB.[5,7,9] Objective data assessing therapeutic benefit relative to cost and alternative therapies have been less than confirmatory.[44,45] Numerous conferences have been sponsored by medical organizations to evaluate literature supporting and opposing IPPB. The inconclusive result of these efforts has significantly reduced the use of IPPB in contemporary clinical practice. IPPB has been largely replaced with other forms of noninvasive positive-pressure ventilation (PPV), such as CPAP and bi-level positive airway pressure (BiPAP). This section is intended to define IPPB, discuss its indications, and describe the technique of administration and potential side effects and complications. An extensive historical and in-depth analysis of IPPB controversies is beyond the scope of this section.

1. Indications

IPPB is the therapeutic application of inspiratory positive pressure to the airway and is distinctly different from intermittent PPV or other means of prolonged, continuous ventilation. The clinical indications for IPPB have evolved over the lifetime of this therapy and include the need to provide a large V_T with resultant lung expansion, provide for short-term ventilatory support (although this has been replaced with noninvasive PPV), and administer aerosol therapy.[46] The fundamental basis and primary goal of IPPB is to provide a larger V_T to the spontaneously breathing patient in a physiologically tolerable manner. If this goal is achieved, IPPB could be employed to improve and promote the cough mechanism, to improve distribution of ventilation, and to enhance delivery of inhaled medications.

Bronchial hygiene can be compromised in patients with a reduced or inadequate cough mechanism. An adequate vital capacity (VC; 15 mL/kg) is necessary to generate the volume and expiratory flow needed to produce an effective cough. Although IPPB can increase V_T significantly, effectiveness still depends on the pressure and flow patterns generated and on an understanding of cough technique. If cough is improved, the clinician can indirectly see the benefit of IPPB for removal of secretions and for limiting complications associated with this problem.

The increased V_T produced by IPPB can be used to improve the distribution of ventilation. As in most respiratory care therapies, the efficacy depends on the patient's underlying condition, selection of patients, optimal technique, and frequency of application. Continual assessment of the therapy is mandatory. Theoretically, if ventilation increases, atelectasis can be prevented or treated.

In patients who are unable to provide an adequate inspiratory volume, IPPB can enhance drug delivery and distribution. When the patient is capable of an adequate cough and spontaneous deep breath, a hand nebulizer should be as efficacious as IPPB. IPPB is rarely used solely for delivery of medication.

2. Administration

The effectiveness of IPPB depends on the individual administering the therapy.[9] It is incumbent for that individual to understand the appropriate operation, maintenance, and clinical application of the mechanical device employed; to select the appropriate patient; to provide the necessary education to the patient to optimize the effort; to assess the effectiveness relative to goals and indications; and to identify complications or side effects associated with the therapy.

The generic device uses a gas pressure source, a main control valve, a breathing circuit, and an automatic cycling control. Typically, IPPB is delivered by a pressure-cycled ventilator. Positive pressure (e.g., 20 to 30 cm H_2O) is used to expand the lungs. To be effective, the increase in V_T from the IPPB treatment must exceed the patient's limited spontaneous VC by 100%. A prolonged inspiratory effort to the preset pressure limit should be emphasized. Therapy is typically 6 to 8 breaths/min, lasting 10 minutes.

Keys to successful therapy include machine sensitivity to the patient's inspiratory effort; a tight seal between the machine and patient because these are pressure-limited devices; a progressive increase in the inspiratory pressure as tolerated by the patient in an effort to achieve a desired exhaled volume; and a cooperative, relaxed, and well-educated patient.

The physiologic side effects and complications associated with IPPB are well described in the literature.[9] Hyperventilation and variable oxygenation can result from IPPB therapy. Hypocarbia (resulting in a respiratory alkalosis) due to an increased V_T and respiratory frequency can produce altered electrolyte concentrations (e.g., K^+), dizziness, muscle tremors, and tingling and numbness of the extremities. Proper instruction to the patient and a 5 to 10 minute rest period after therapy can minimize this problem. Hypoxemia and hyperoxia caused by inaccurately delivered F_{IO_2} can be a concern in patients with severe COPD.

The use of IPPB can increase mean intrathoracic pressure, resulting in a decreased venous return. As with other forms of PPV, a decreased venous return (preload) can produce a decreased cardiac output and subsequent vital sign changes (hypotension or tachycardia). The patient may be unable to coordinate breathing patterns with IPPB and therefore develop auto-PEEP with resultant increase in work of breathing and elevation of intrathoracic pressures. In addition to cardiovascular changes, IPPB can impede venous drainage from the head. This is a potential but limited concern in patients with increased intracranial pressure if IPPB is appropriately administered in the sitting position.

Barotrauma is a concern with all forms of PPV. The exact etiologic mechanism of PPV in the development of pneumothorax and ruptured lobes is unclear. PPV results in increased intrapulmonary volume and pressure, but the same conditions tend to promote a better cough

mechanism that causes sudden marked changes in pressure and lobe rupture. Before proceeding with an IPPB treatment, any chest pain complaints must be evaluated to rule out barotrauma.

Other reported complications include gastric insufflation and secondary nausea and vomiting, psychological dependency, nosocomial infections, altered airway resistance, and adverse reactions to medications administered through the IPPB system. The incidence and significance of these adverse effects are often the result of inappropriate administration, noncompliance by the patient, selection of inappropriate patients, and simple lack of attention to detail.

There are few definite contraindications to IPPB.[47] Relative contraindications to IPPB are focused on its lack of documented efficacy. Untreated pneumothorax is a definite contraindication to IPPB. Relative contraindications include elevated intracranial pressures (>15 mm Hg), hemodynamic instability, esophageal and gastric conditions such as recent surgery or fistulas, and recent intracranial surgery. Good clinical contraindications are lack of a definite indication for IPPB or an available, less expensive alternative therapy.

D. Noninvasive Ventilation

Administration of positive pressure by noninvasive means, such as a face mask, nasal mask, or helmet, avoids the adverse events associated with endotracheal intubation (e.g., pneumonia, airway trauma). Noninvasive ventilation (NIV) is a cornerstone of treatment for COPD exacerbations and cardiogenic pulmonary edema, but a full discussion of NIV is beyond the scope of this chapter. Its use in the perioperative period is gaining acceptance and warrants discussion.

CPAP is the application of the same level of positive airway pressure through the entire respiratory cycle. The subsequent increase in intrathoracic and alveolar pressure supports patency of the airway, prevents alveolar collapse and atelectasis, maintains functional residual capacity, and decreases the work of breathing. PPV also reduces afterload by decreasing left ventricular transmural pressure and supporting left ventricular output. BiPAP adds pressure support above the level of CPAP during the inspiratory phase. With the addition of pressure support, CPAP is the baseline pressure during exhalation and is defined as PEEP. Pressure support allows for larger V_T and VC values, recruitment of atelectatic alveoli, increased ventilation, and improved oxygenation.

1. Indications

Perioperative NIV use can be viewed as prophylactic or therapeutic.[48] Prophylactic use of NIV involves administration of NIV after extubation to patients at risk for respiratory distress (e.g., cardiac, thoracic, or abdominal surgery, obstructive sleep apnea, COPD, congestive heart failure). Data continue to emerge regarding the potential beneficial use of perioperative CPAP in reducing postoperative pulmonary complications in patients undergoing cardiothoracic and abdominal surgery.[49,50] The therapeutic use of NIV in the perioperative setting may aid in reducing symptoms of respiratory distress, hypoxemia, or hypoventilation. Further studies need to validate NIV for prophylactic and therapeutic use in a broader patient population.

2. Limitations

NIV requires that patients are cooperative with therapy, spontaneously ventilating, and able to protect their airway. It is most effective when a proper seal is achieved around the airway to minimize air leak. The use of high levels of positive pressure above 25 cm H_2O increases the risk of gastric insufflation and therefore limits its use in this circumstance. Patients with copious secretions may not be ideal candidates for NIV due to a constant requirement for bronchial hygiene.

IV. INHALATION THERAPY

Inhalation therapy is often used synonymously with the term *respiratory care*. In a general context, inhalation therapy can be thought of as the delivery of gases for ventilation and oxygenation, as aerosol therapy, or as a means of delivering therapeutic medications.

Therapeutic aerosols have been employed in the treatment of pulmonary patients with bronchospastic airway disease, COPD, and pulmonary infection. The basic goals of aerosol therapy are to improve bronchial hygiene, humidify gases delivered through artificial airways, and deliver medications. The first two goals are discussed earlier in this chapter.

The advantages of delivering drugs by inhalation include the following: easier access, rapid onset of action, reduced extrapulmonary side effects, reduced dosage, coincidental application with aerosol therapy for humidification, and general psychological support with treatment.[5,7,9] In the nonintubated patient, aerosol therapy necessitates the patient's cooperation and skilled help. The equipment is a potential source of nosocomial infections.[19] Aerosol therapy has many of the same disadvantages as humidification. Although drug use is often reduced, precise titration and dosages are difficult to ascertain because of variable degrees of drug deposition in the airway.

The following sections provide an overview of inhalation pharmacology and discuss the basic principles, devices for medication delivery, and specific pharmacologic agents that are employed. A more comprehensive topic review and specific drug information are available in reference texts.[48-50]

A. Basic Pharmacologic Principles

The pharmacology of inhalation therapy necessitates a brief review. A *medication* is a drug that is given to elicit a physiologic response and is used for therapeutic purposes. Undesired responses (side effects) are also produced. The medication can interact with receptors by direct application (topical effect) or absorption into the bloodstream.

Various routes of pharmacologic administration are used for respiratory care. Subcutaneous, parenteral, gastrointestinal, and inhalation administrations are commonly employed in the management of pulmonary diseases. Inhalation therapy employs the increased surface area of the lung parenchyma as a route of medication administration. This necessitates the drug reaching the alveolar and tracheobronchial mucosal surfaces for systemic capillary absorption.

Although inhaled medications can have topical effects, the primary reasons for the inhalation of medications are convenience, a safe method for self-administration, and maximal pulmonary benefit with reduced side effects. If the drug depends on systemic absorption, the drug's distribution and blood concentration are important. Blood concentration is altered by several mechanisms, such as dosage, route of administration, absorption, metabolism, and excretion. Alteration in liver and kidney function can produce unexpected drug levels and side effects.

If multiple drugs are employed for respiratory care, drug interactions can occur. Potentiation is the result of one drug with limited activity changing the response of another drug; synergism results when two drugs with similar action produce a greater response than the sum of the individual responses. If the response to the two drugs is the sum of the responses to the individual medications, they are additive. Tolerance necessitates increasing drug levels to elicit a response, and tachyphylaxis results in the inability of larger doses to produce the expected response.

The nomenclature for drug dosages should be understood. Two common methods for expressing drug dosage are ratio strength (drug dilutions) and percentage strength (percentage solutions). A solution is a homogeneous mixture of two substances. A solute is the dissolved drug, and a solvent is the fluid in which the drug is dissolved. A gram of water equals 1 mL of water, and 1 g equals 1000 mg. Ratio strength is expressed in terms of parts of solute in relation to the total parts of solvent (or grams of solute per grams of solvent). A 1:1000 solution is 1 g of a drug in 1000 g of solvent (1000 mg/1000 mL [1 mg/mL]). Percentage strength is expressed as the number of parts of solute in 100 parts of solvent (or grams of solute per 100 g of solvent). A 1% solution is 1 g of drug in 100 g of solvent.

B. Aerosolized Drug Delivery Systems

Therapeutic aerosols are commonly employed in respiratory care. Inhalation delivery of drugs can often produce therapeutic drug effects with reduced toxicity. The effectiveness of aerosols is related to the amount of drug delivered to the lungs. The pulmonary deposition of aerosolized drugs is a result of drug sedimentation that is due to gravity, inertial impact that is due to airway size, and directional change of airflow and kinetic energy.[7] Aerosol delivery also depends on particle size, pattern of inhalation, and degree of airway obstruction. Particle size should be smaller than 5 μm; otherwise, the particles may become trapped in the upper airway rather than following airflow into the lungs. Aerosol particles that can traverse artificial airways (e.g., ETT) are usually less than 2 μm in diameter. Particles less than 2 μm are deposited in peripheral airways. Particles less than 0.6 μm in diameter are often exhaled before reaching their site of action.

The ideal pattern of inhalation should be large volume, slow inspiration (5 to 6 seconds), and accentuated by an inspiratory hold (10 seconds). This breath-holding enhances sedimentation and diffusion. Faster inspiratory inflows increase deposition of particles on oropharyngeal and upper airway surfaces. If airway obstruction is significant, adequate deposition of drugs may be compromised. If the obstruction is not relieved, larger dosages or increased frequency of administration may be necessary. Application of the aerosol early in inspiration allows deeper penetration into the lungs, whereas delivery of medications at the back end of the breath enhances application to slower filling lung units. Concerns are raised in areas of the lung with poor ventilation related to airflow obstruction or low compliance. There are several methods for delivering aerosolized medications to the patient: jet nebulizers, pressurized metered-dose inhalers (MDIs), dry-powder inhalers (DPIs), ultrasonic nebulizers, and IPPB.

DPIs and pressurized MDIs are the most common delivery systems because of their low cost and ease of use. The MDI is a convenient, self-contained, and commonly employed method of aerosolized drug delivery (Figs. 14-11 and 14-12).[5,9] These prefilled drug canisters are activated by manual compression and deliver a predetermined unit (metered) of medication. Appropriate instruction is necessary for optimal use.[51] With the canister in the upside-down position, the device should be compressed only once per inhalation. A slow maximal inspiration with a breath-hold is typically recommended. It is imperative that the tongue not obstruct flow, but it is controversial whether the device should be placed in the mouth or held several centimeters from the lips with the mouth wide open. Concerns about excessive oral deposition of large particles must be offset against consistency of administration when the device is held away from the mouth. Other issues regarding use of MDIs include ideal lung volume for actuation, time of inspiratory hold, and inspiratory flow rate. If multiple doses are prescribed, an interval of several minutes between puffs is advisable. Most pharmaceutical manufacturers recommend 1 to 2 minutes between doses. However, studies have not shown

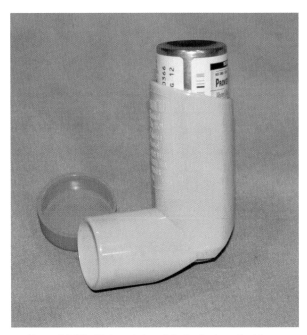

Figure 14-12 Metered-dose inhaler for handheld use.

any consistent difference in pulmonary function in extending the time interval between doses.[52,53]

MDI drug delivery is associated with several problems. Manual coordination is necessary to activate the canister. Arthritis can cause difficulty, as can misaiming the aerosol. Pharyngeal deposition can lead to local abnormalities (e.g., oral candidiasis from aerosolized corticosteroids). Systemic effects that are caused by swallowing the drug can be reduced if the pharynx is rinsed after inhalation to reduce pharyngeal deposition.[5] Newer MDI devices have been designed to reduce some of these problems. Several spacing devices are available as extensions to MDIs. Spacers are designed to eliminate the need for hand-breath coordination and reduction of large-particle deposition in the upper airway.

The gas-powered nebulizers can be handheld or placed in line with the ventilatory circuit (Fig. 14-13).[5,9] The handheld devices are typically employed for more acutely ill individuals and as an alternative to an MDI. The full handheld system uses a nebulizer, a pressurized gas

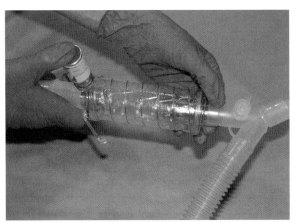

Figure 14-11 Metered-dose inhaler and circuit inspiratory limb spacer (Aero Vent). (Courtesy of Monaghan Medical, Plattsburgh, NY.)

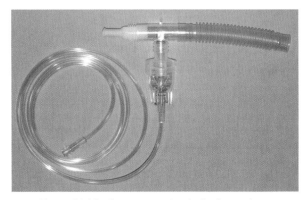

Figure 14-13 Gas-powered nebulization system.

source, and a mouthpiece or face mask. Patients' cooperation is not required, and high doses of drugs can be delivered. Disadvantages include expense and decreased portability.

These systems are more expensive, cumbersome, and often less efficient than MDIs. Supervision is usually necessary for appropriate drug preparation and administration. Typically, the drug is diluted in saline. The drug is usually more concentrated because most of the drug is never aerosolized or is lost during exhalation. Only the drug that is inspired can reach the lung.

The total volume to be nebulized is usually 3 mL (see "Pharmacologic Agents") at gas flows of 6 to 8 L/min (flow is device dependent). The treatment time is usually 5 to 10 minutes. During the course of treatment, the patient's vital signs and subjective tolerance must be monitored. Aerosolization of medication for drug delivery is different from aerosol therapy for humidification (see "Humidifiers").

The MDI and the gas-powered nebulizers can be used in line with an artificial airway or ventilator circuit, or both (see Figs. 14-11 and 14-13) The drug delivery system is positioned in the inspiratory limb and as proximal to the artificial airway as possible. With this configuration, drug delivery is equivalent between MDI and nebulizer.[54] In-line drug delivery is usually less efficient in ventilated patients than in spontaneously breathing, nonintubated patients because of the breathing pattern, drug deposition on the ETT, and airway disease.[55]

C. Pharmacologic Agents

Numerous drugs are used in the management of pulmonary diseases. Inhaled medications offer advantages over intravenous or oral administration. These include more specific targeting to the site of action and resulting lower doses limiting systemic side effects. Nebulized (aerosolized) drug delivery is commonly employed to improve mucociliary clearance (mucokinetics) and to relieve bronchospastic airway disease. The major drugs employed for inhalation therapy can be categorized by their ability to affect these two issues. Certain anti-inflammatory, antiasthmatic, antifungal, antiviral, and antibacterial drugs are given by aerosol. The following sections review some of the commonly employed aerosolized drugs but are not meant to be a comprehensive review of respiratory pharmacology. All listed dosages are meant to be representative for adult patients (if needed, specific product literature should be referred to before use).

1. Mucokinetic Drugs

Mucokinetic drugs are employed to enhance mucociliary clearance. These agents can be classified according to their mechanism of action. Hypoviscosity agents are the most commonly employed mucokinetic agents. Saline, sodium bicarbonate, and alcohol have been used to affect mucus viscosity by disrupting the mucopolysaccharide chains that are the primary components of mucus. The other category of mucokinetic aerosol agents is made up of the mucolytics. The following sections offer a synopsis of the various drugs in these two groups.[56]

a. HYPOVISCOSITY AGENTS

Saline is the most commonly employed mucokinetic agent. It can be used as a primary drug or a solvent. The mechanism of action is reduction of viscosity by dilution of the mucopolysaccharide strands. The indication for use is thick, tenacious mucous secretions. The typical concentration is 0.45% to 0.9% of sodium chloride (NaCl). The two major side effects associated with aerosolized saline are overhydration and the promotion of bronchospasm in patients with hyperactive airway disease (especially in newborns).

Hypertonic saline (HTS) is able to encourage osmosis of water from the interstitium and alveoli into mucus and act as a cough stimulant. HTS may induce bronchospasm, and inhaled bronchodilators are employed to mitigate the associated bronchospastic effects. Because the mechanism depends on migration of water from the alveolar tissue, HTS has an additional theoretical benefit of reducing adventitial edema. With repeated use, hypovolemia may follow repeated administration.

Alcohol (ethyl alcohol and ethanol) decreases the surface tension of pulmonary fluid. The typical concentration is 30%, and the dosage is 4 to 10 mL.[57] The primary indication is pulmonary edema. This agent should be administered by side-arm nebulization or IPPB but not as a heated aerosol. The contraindication is a hypersensitivity to alcohol or its derivative. Side effects include airway irritation, bronchospasm, and local dehydration.

b. MUCOLYTIC AGENTS

Thickened secretions are problematic for the intubated patient or patient with chronic pulmonary disease. Secretions can directly obstruct the airways, predispose the patient to obstructive pneumonia, and become a nidus for infection. Vigorous suctioning intended to clear the burden of secretions can cause direct injury to the airways. As a result, altering the rheologic properties of tenacious secretions encourages the return of normal pulmonary function.

Acetylcysteine 10% (Mucomyst) is an effective mucolytic. The mechanism of action is lysis of the disulfide bonds in mucopolysaccharide chains, reducing the viscosity of the mucus. The indication is for management of viscous, inspissated, mucopurulent secretions. The actual effectiveness in the treatment of mucostasis is inconclusive, and each individual must be monitored to determine the benefit of therapy. The usual dosage is 2 to 5 mL every 6 hours.[54] Hypersensitivity is a contraindication. In general, acetylcysteine is relatively nontoxic. Side effects include unpleasant taste and odor, local irritation, inhibition of ciliary activity, and bronchospasm. For these reasons, pretreatment with a bronchodilator is recommended. Other reported side effects include nausea and vomiting, stomatitis, rhinorrhea, and generalized urticaria. Acetylcysteine is incompatible with several antibodies. The drug should be avoided or used with extreme caution in patients with bronchospastic airway disease. Other special concerns are a need for refrigeration, reactivity with rubber, and its limited use after opening (96 hours).[58]

Mesna (mistabron) is a thiol-containing compound that can lyse the disulfide bonds on mucoproteins, and it has been shown to support thinning of secretions.[59] In addition to the direct mucolytic activity, Mesna is a hypertonic solution and may reduce viscosity of secretions by a second mechanism. As for acetylcysteine, studies of Mesna have been unable to demonstrate conclusive benefit of secretion clearance or improvement in lung compliance despite concomitant bronchodilator adminstration.[59] When given by nebulizer, 1 mL of Mesna is combined with a bronchodilator, such as albuterol or salbutamol. It can also be administered as a bolus of 600 mg (3 mL) through the ETT. It usually is well tolerated, with bronchospasm and hypersensitivity as possible side effects.

Recombinant human DNase (rhDNase) promotes lysis of DNA that is present in the secretions of patients with CF or infected secretions. The abundance of DNA increases the viscosity of these secretions. A few reports and retrospective analyses have shown rhDNase to improve secretion clearance and atelectasis.[60] The increased cost of rhDNAse limits its widespread use in clinical practice.

2. Bronchodilators and Antiasthmatic Drugs

Acute and chronic bronchospastic airway diseases afflict many individuals. Many drugs that vary primarily by their mechanism of action and route of delivery are available to manage this problem. The following sections deal only with aerosolized drugs that are commonly employed in the therapy of bronchospastic airway disease (Table 14-8).[16,61,62] The drugs are grouped by their mechanism of action: sympathomimetics, anticholinergics, corticosteroids, and cromolyn. A comprehensive review of these drugs, the various mechanisms for bronchodilation, and the management of specific pathophysiologic problems is beyond the scope of this chapter.

a. SYMPATHOMIMETICS

Sympathomimetics include the β-adrenergic agonists and methylxanthines (not available in aerosol). The rhDNase-adrenergic agents couple to the β_2-adrenoreceptor through the G protein α subunit to adenylate cyclase, which results in an increase in intracellular cyclic adenosine monophosphate (cAMP), which leads to activation of protein kinase A. Activated protein kinase A inhibits phosphorylation of certain muscle proteins that regulate smooth muscle tone and inhibits release of calcium ion from intracellular stores. Responses of sympathomimetic drugs usually are classified according to whether the effects are α, β_1, or β_2. The β_2 receptors are responsible for bronchial smooth muscle relaxation. The common side effects associated with β-adrenergic agonists result from their additional β_1 and α effects. The β_1 effects cause an increase in heart rate, dysrhythmias, and cardiac contractility; α effects increase vascular tone. Potent β_2 stimulants can produce unwanted symptoms: anxiety, headache, nausea, tremors, and sleeplessness. Prolonged use can lead to receptor downregulation and reduced drug response. Ideally, the more pure the β_2 response, the better the therapeutic benefit relative to side effects. The

following sympathomimetics are commonly employed in clinical practice.[5,7,39,58]

Albuterol (Ventolin, Proventil) is a sympathomimetic agent available in an MDI. It has a strong β_2 effect with limited β_1 properties. Its β_2 duration of action is approximately 6 hours.

Racemic epinephrine 2.25% (Vaponephrine) is a mixture of levo and dextro isomers of epinephrine. It is a weak β and mild α drug. The α effects provide mucosal constriction. In the aerosol form, this drug acts as a good mucosal decongestant. The drug has minimal bronchodilator action. Cardiovascular side effects are limited. Typical dosage is 0.5 mL (2.25%) in 3.5 mL of saline, given as frequently as every hour in adult patients. Racemic epinephrine is commonly mixed with 0.25 mL (1 mg) of dexamethasone or budesonide for the management of post-extubation swelling and croup (see "Antiallergy and Asthmatic Agents").

Isoproterenol (Isuprel) is the prototype pure β-adrenergic bronchodilator. Bronchodilation depends on adequate blood levels. In addition, isoproterenol is a pulmonary and mucosal vascular dilator. This causes an increased rate of absorption, higher blood levels, and increased β_1 side effects. The side effects can be quite significant and often reduce the use of this agent in patients with cardiac disease; dysrhythmias, myocardial ischemia, palpitations, and paradoxical bronchospasm can occur. If the pulmonary vasculature vasodilates to areas of low ventilation, the potential to augment ventilation-perfusion mismatch and increase intrapulmonary shunt exists. Typical dosage is 0.25 to 0.5 mL (0.5%) in 2 to 2.5 mL of saline. The effect lasts 1 to 2 hours. Isoproterenol is also available as an MDI.

Newer inhaled β-adrenergic drugs include salmeterol, pirbuterol, and bitolterol (a catecholamine). Salmeterol can be administered as an oral inhalation powder twice a day 50 μg. Pirbuterol acetate is usually administered through a pressurized MDI (200 μg). Bitolterol can be provided as a pressurized MDI or a solution. Salmeterol was the first long-acting adrenergic bronchodilator approved for use in the United States. Its duration of action is about 12 hours, with an onset of about 20 minutes and a peak effect occurring in 3 to 5 hours. It is particularly useful in patients with nocturnal asthma because of its longer duration of action. The prolonged effect of some of the newer bronchodilators results from their increased lipophilicity (Table 14-9).

b. ANTICHOLINERGIC AGENTS AND ANTIBIOTICS

Anticholinergic drugs play an increasing role in the management of bronchospastic pulmonary disease but have been found more effective as maintenance treatment of bronchoconstriction in COPD. These drugs inhibit acetylcholine at the cholinergic receptor site, reducing vagal nerve activity. This produces bronchodilation (preferentially in large airways) and a reduction in mucus secretion. Major side effects include dry mouth, blurred vision, headache, tremor, nervousness, and palpitations.

Ipratropium bromide (Atrovent) is a commonly used anticholinergic. Its effects are primarily on the muscarinic receptors of bronchial smooth muscle. It is available as an MDI. The standard dosage is 34 μg taken four times

TABLE 14-8

Aerosolized Bronchodilators and Antiasthmatic Drugs

Type of Drug (Mechanism)	Method	Dose*
Sympathomimetics (β_2-Agonists; increase in cyclic AMP)		
Short-Acting Beta Agonists		
Albuterol (Ventolin, Proventil)	MDI/Neb	2 puffs (90 µg/puff) q4hr prn
Levalbuterol hydrochloride (Xopenex)	Neb	0.63–1.25 mg nebulized solution q6–8hr
Pirbuterol acetate (Maxair)	MDI	2 puffs (200 µg/puff) q4hr prn
Racemic epinephrine	Neb	0.25 mL in 3.5 mL
Long-Acting Beta Agonists		
Salmeterol xinafoate (Serevent)	DPI	1 puff (50 µg) bid
Formoterol fumarate (Foradil)	DPI	1 capsule (12 µg) by Aerolizer inhaler bid
Anticholinergics (Cholinergic blockers; increase β stimulation)		
Ipratropium bromide (Atrovent)	MDI/Neb	2 puffs (17 µg/puff) qid 17 µg (0.02%) qid
Tiotropium bromide (Spiriva)	DPI	1 capsule inhaled (18 µg) by HandiHaler qd
Anti-Inflammatories		
Inhaled Corticosteroids (Anti-inflammatory; inhibit leukocyte migration; potentiate β agonists)		
Beclomethasone acetate (Vanceril, Beclovent)	MDI	1–4 puffs (40 µg/puff) bid
Flunisolide (AeroBid)	MDI	2–4 puffs (250 µg/puff) bid
Triamcinolone acetonide (Azmacort)	MDI	2–8 puffs (100 µg/puff) bid
Budesonide (Pulmicort)	DPI/Neb	1–4 puffs (200 µg/puff) bid 0.25 mg/2 mL bid 0.5 mg/2 mL bid
Fluticasone propionate (Flovent)	MDI	44, 110, or 220 µg; up to a maximum of 880 µg/day
Mometasone furoate (Asmanex)	DPI	1–2 puffs (220 µg/puff) qd
Combination Products		
Albuterol sulfate/ipratropium bromide (Combivent)	MDI/Neb	2 puffs (0.09 mg/0.018 mg/puff) qid 1 vial (3 mg/0.5 mg) qid
Fluticasone propionate/salmeterol Xinafoate (Advair)	DPI	100, 250, or 500 µg/50 µg; 1 puff bid

AMP, Adenosine monophosphate; *bid,* twice per day; *DPI,* dry-powder inhaler; *MDI,* metered-dose inhaler; *Neb,* nebulizer; *qd,* once per day; *qid,* four times per day.
*Dosages may vary; references to specific drug inserts are recommended.

per day (17 µg/puff). Hypersensitivity to the drug is a contraindication. Caution should be exercised in patients with narrow-angle glaucoma. Tiotropium is a long-acting anticholinergic agent that has shown to improve lung function and reduce exacerbations of COPD with once-daily dosing.[63] The dosage is 2 puffs of an 18-µg capsule taken once daily using the supplied DPI. The side effects

TABLE 14-9

Onset and Duration of Commonly Used Bronchodilators

Drug	Onset (min)	Peak (min)	Duration (hr)
Isoproterenol*	2–5	5–30	1–2
Isoetharine*	2–5	15–60	1–3
Bitolterol*	3–5	30–60	5–8
Albuterol	15	30–60	3–8
Pirbuterol	5	30	5
Salmeterol	20	180–300	12

*A catecholamine.

are similar to ipratropium bromide, with most common symptoms being dry mouth and upper respiratory tract infections. Rarely, inhaled anticholinergic drugs have been associated with paradoxical bronchospasm.

Antibiotics are also delivered by an inhalational route. Aerosolized tobramycin is used in patients with CF, and ribavirin is employed in children against respiratory syncytial virus. Pentamidine can be employed as prophylaxis against *Pneumocystis (carinii) jiroveci.* However, the support for the general use of nebulized antibiotics in ventilator-associated pneumonia (VAP) is inconclusive. As a result, the addition of nebulized antibiotics is reserved for multidrug-resistant organism pneumonia refractory to first-line therapy. The use of aerosolized gentamycin or vancomycin, in addition to systemic antibiotics, for treatment of tracheobronchitis led to quicker resolution of pneumonia, decreased bacterial resistance, and less recurrence of VAP.[64] Nebulized polymyxins (e.g., colistin) allow focused delivery of antibiotics that were historically underutilized because of significant nephrotoxicity with systemic administration. The evidence for the use of nebulized colistin is promising but remains inconclusive. When added to a regimen of systemic antibiotics in patient with multidrug-resistant gram-negative bacteria, nebulized colistin has shown to be beneficial for treatment of pneumonia without systemic side effects.[65]

c. ANTIALLERGY AND ASTHMATIC AGENTS

The two main groups of aerosolized agents for treating allergies and asthma are cromolyn and corticosteroids. These drugs are often used concomitantly with other medications.

Newer mediator antagonists include zafirlukast, montelukast, and zileuton. Zafirlukast and montelukast work as leukotriene receptor antagonists and selectively inhibit leukotriene receptors LTD_4 and LTE_4. Leukotrienes are produced by 5-lipoxygenase from arachidonic acid and stimulate leukotriene receptors to cause bronchoconstriction and chemotaxis of inflammatory cells. As with cromolyn sodium, these agents should not be used for acute asthmatic attacks but rather for long-term prevention of bronchoconstriction.[62]

Corticosteroids are commonly used for maintenance therapy in patients with chronic asthma.[66,67] The mechanism of action is attributed to their anti-inflammatory properties, reducing leakage of fluids, inhibiting migration of macrophages and leukocytes, and possibly blocking the response to various mediators of inflammation. Corticosteroids have been reported to potentiate the effects of the sympathomimetic drugs.[9] Systemic and topical side effects can occur with inhaled corticosteroids. These effects include adrenal insufficiency, acute asthma episodes, possible growth retardation, and osteoporosis. Local effects include oropharyngeal fungal infections and dysphonia. Adrenal suppression is usually not a concern with doses below 800 µg/day.

Beclomethasone dipropionate (Vanceril, Beclovent) is an aerosolized corticosteroid that is highly active topically and that has limited systemic absorption or activity. The typical dosage is 1 to 4 puffs (40 µg/puff) taken two times per day. Hoarseness, sore throat, and oral candidiasis are reported side effects. The risk of candidiasis can be minimized with oral rinse after drug administration, and candidiasis can be managed with topical antifungal drugs. Mild adrenal suppression is reported with high doses, and caution is advised when switching from oral to inhaled corticosteroids.

The preceding pharmacologic agents are representative of those commonly employed by aerosol in respiratory care. Appropriate pharmacologic management necessitates assessing response to therapy. Objective and subjective relief of symptoms and improvement in pulmonary function while minimizing side effects of these drugs are the endpoints of good inhalation therapy. Effective inhalation therapy involves relief of symptoms, improvement in pulmonary function, and minimizing drug side effects.

V. CONCLUSIONS

Oxygen therapy, bronchial hygiene, and inhalation therapy are some of the interventions available to the physician in order to improve pulmonary function.

Oxygen delivery systems attempt to prevent rebreathing of exhaled air and can be differentiated based on the ability to maintain near-consistent oxygen delivery. Low-flow oxygen systems entrain room air to meet the patient's ventilatory demands, but inspired oxygen concentration becomes unpredictable with changes in ventilatory patterns. High-flow systems have high flows rates and attempt to provide a reliable oxygen concentration despite variations in minute ventilation. Humidification is added to these oxygen delivery systems to prevent cooling and drying of the respiratory tract.

Other modalities may be required to correct specific or more significant derangements of pulmonary function. Airway suctioning is often employed to clear secretions and optimize tracheobronchial toilet. Chest physical therapy, including postural drainage and percussion therapy, can assist mucociliary action to mobilize secretions. Incentive spirometry attempts to optimize lung inflation and prevent atelectasis, although it requires patient teaching and cooperation. Noninvasive positive pressure ventilation increases intrathoracic and alveolar pressure to prevent atelectasis, maintain functional residual capacity, maintain airway patency, and decrease the work of breathing.

Inhalation therapy delivers therapeutic medications and aerosols to humidify the airway or elicit a physiologic response. The MDI, nebulizer, and DPI can be used to deliver medications to the airways. Mucokinetic agents can decrease the viscosity of secretions, and include hypertonic saline and mucolytics. The β-adrenergic agonists, methylxanthines, and anticholinergics produce bronchodilation, albeit by different mechanisms. Corticosteroids, leukotriene receptor antagonists, and mast cell stabilizers are often used in prevention or management of bronchospasm due to asthma or allergic stimuli.

Most patients with mild pulmonary dysfunction may require only increasing inspired oxygen concentration, whereas more significant dysfunction requires understanding pulmonary physiology and choosing appropriate therapy. In the perioperative setting, hypoxemia is most commonly caused by ventilation-perfusion mismatch, hypoventilation, and capillary shunt. If left untreated, hypoxemia can cause tachycardia, acidosis, increased myocardial oxygen demand, and an increased work of breathing.

VI. CLINICAL PEARLS

- Hypoxemia may be defined as a deficiency of O_2 tension in the arterial blood, typically defined as a PaO_2 less than 80 mm Hg. The most common perioperative cause of hypoxemia is capillary shunt (atelectasis).

- A low-flow, variable-performance system depends on room air entrainment to meet the patient's peak inspiratory and minute ventilatory demands that are not met by the inspiratory gas flow or O_2 reservoir alone.

- High-flow, fixed-performance systems are nonrebreathing systems that provide the entire inspiratory atmosphere needed to meet the peak inspiratory flow and minute ventilatory demands of the patient. To meet the patient's peak inspiratory flow, the flow rate and reservoir are very important. Flows of 30 to 40 L/min (or four times the measured minute volume) are often necessary.

- O_2 therapy must be used appropriately in patients with severe chronic obstructive pulmonary disease (COPD) due to a risk of developing respiratory distress. Disturbances in ventilation and perfusion develop in patients with COPD, and through hypoxic pulmonary vasoconstriction, the perfusion is redistributed to areas of higher O_2 tension. Increasing mixed venous or alveolar O_2 tension can reverse this shunting and worsen $\dot{V}/\dot{Q}$ matching.

- O_2 toxicity becomes clinically important after 8 to 12 hours of exposure to a high F_{IO_2} level. O_2 toxicity may result from direct exposure of the alveoli to a high F_{IO_2} level. Healthy lungs appear to tolerate F_{IO_2} levels of less than 0.6. In damaged lungs, F_{IO_2} levels greater than 0.50 may result in a toxic alveolar O_2 concentration.

- Airway suctioning is commonly employed in respiratory care to promote optimal tracheobronchial toilet and airway patency in critically ill patients. Because of the perceived simplicity and limited complications, airway suctioning is frequently employed.

- Percussion and vibration therapy are used in conjunction with postural drainage to loosen and mobilize secretions that are adherent to the bronchial walls.[17,48] Percussion involves a manually produced, rhythmic vibration of varying intensity and frequency.

- Normal, spontaneous breathing patterns have periodic hyperinflations that prevent the alveolar collapse associated with shallow tidal ventilation breathing patterns. Narcotics, sedative drugs, general anesthesia, cerebral trauma, immobilization, and abdominal or thoracic surgery can promote shallow tidal ventilation breathing patterns. Incentive spirometry (IS) is commonly employed in the postoperative period to encourage patients to generate a maximal tidal volume breath. However, IS has yet to be proved to reduce postoperative pulmonary complications.

- Perioperative noninvasive ventilation (NIV) is both a prophylactic and therapeutic modality. Prophylactic use of NIV has emerged as a measure to reduce postoperative pulmonary complications in patients undergoing cardiothoracic and abdominal. Therapeutic use of NIV in the perioperative setting may aid in reducing symptoms of respiratory distress, hypoxemia, or hypoventilation.

- The metered-dose inhaler (MDI) and the gas-powered nebulizers may be used with an artificial airway or ventilator circuit, or both. The drug delivery system is positioned in the inspiratory limb as proximal to the artificial airway as possible. This position makes drug delivery equivalent between MDI and nebulizer.

Acknowledgements

Portions of the text are from Vender JS, Clemency MV: Oxygen delivery systems, inhalation therapy, respiratory care. In Benumof JL, editor: *Clinical procedures in anesthesia and intensive care*, Philadelphia, JB Lippincott, 1992, pp 63–87.

SELECTED REFERENCES

All references can be found online at expertconsult.com.
5. Kacmarek RM, Stoller JK, editors: *Current respiratory care*, Toronto, 1988, BC Decker.
7. Shapiro BA, Kacmarek RM, Cane RD, et al: *Clinical application of respiratory care*, ed 4, St Louis, 1991, Mosby.
48. Jaber S, Chanques G, Jung B: Postoperative noninvasive ventilation. *Anesthesthesiology* 112:453–461, 2010.
54. Dolovich MB, Ahrens RC, Hess DR, et al: Device selection and outcomes of aerosol therapy: Evidence-based guidelines: American College of Chest Physicians/American College of Asthma, Allergy, and immunology. *Chest* 127:335–371, 2005.

Chapter 15

Nonintubation Management of the Airway: Airway Maneuvers and Mask Ventilation

ERIC C. MATTEN | TORIN SHEAR | JEFFEREY S. VENDER

I. OVERVIEW

Maintaining a patent airway is the first principle of resuscitation and life support. It is an essential skill for those caring for anesthetized or critically ill patients. Clinicians working in a hospital setting should be competent in the essentials of airway management.

Too frequently, inexperienced personnel believe airway management necessitates intubation of the trachea. This chapter reviews the tools and skills for nonintubation airway management and discusses airway management techniques. Endotracheal intubation and pharyngeal intubation (e.g., laryngeal mask airways [LMAs]) are discussed elsewhere in this textbook. The topic of airway management can be divided into the establishment and maintenance of a patent airway and ventilatory support. Airway patency is achieved by manipulating the head and

neck in ways that maximize the native airway or by using artificial airway devices. Ventilatory support techniques control the composition of gases that the patient breathes and allow manual respiratory assistance.

A. Upper Airway Anatomy and Physiology

Nonintubation airway management seeks to produce patency to gas flow through the oropharynx, nasopharynx, and larynx without the use of artificial airway devices that extend into the laryngopharynx or trachea. A thorough understanding of upper airway anatomy and physiology is necessary to appreciate the therapeutic maneuvers and devices employed in airway management (Fig. 15-1). More detailed reviews of airway anatomy are found elsewhere in this book and in various atlases and texts.[1-3]

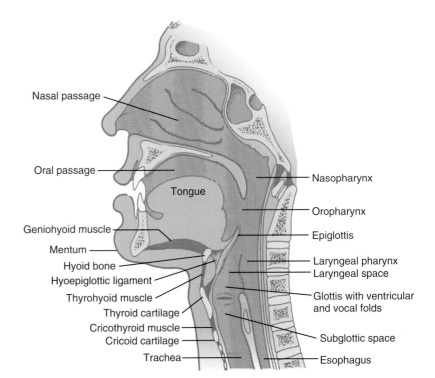

Figure 15-1 Normal anatomy of the airway and surrounding structures is demonstrated in a lateral view of the head and neck in the neutral position. Notice the right-angle geometry of the muscular connections from the mentum to the cricoid cartilage: mentum, geniohyoid muscle, hyoid bone, thyrohyoid muscle, thyroid cartilage, cricothyroid muscle, and cricoid cartilage. This line can be straightened by extending the head at the neck and anteriorly displacing the jaw, pulling the epiglottis and tongue away from the posterior wall of the airway.

Labels in figure: Nasal passage; Oral passage; Tongue; Geniohyoid muscle; Mentum; Hyoid bone; Hyoepiglottic ligament; Thyrohyoid muscle; Thyroid cartilage; Cricothyroid muscle; Cricoid cartilage; Trachea; Nasopharynx; Oropharynx; Epiglottis; Laryngeal pharynx; Laryngeal space; Glottis with ventricular and vocal folds; Subglottic space; Esophagus

Gas passes from outside the body to the larynx through the nose or mouth. If through the nose, ambient gas passes through the nares, choanae, and nasopharynx (where it is warmed and humidified). The humidified gas then traverses the oropharynx and hypopharynx (also called laryngopharynx) on its way to the larynx. If through the mouth, the oropharynx and hypopharynx are traversed before entering the glottis. Nasal passages can be obstructed by choanal atresia, septal deviation, mucosal swelling, or foreign material (e.g., mucus, blood). Entry to the oropharynx can be blocked by the soft palate lying against the posterior pharyngeal wall. The pathway of gas by either route can be restricted by the tongue in the oropharynx or the epiglottis in the hypopharynx. These are sites of potential pharyngeal collapse.[4-7] Airway manipulation and devices can remedy these causes of obstruction. Laryngeal obstruction related to spasm, however, must be treated by positive airway pressure, deeper anesthesia, muscle relaxants, or endotracheal intubation.

Laryngeal closure is accomplished by the intrinsic or extrinsic muscles of the larynx. Tight closure, as seen in laryngospasm, results from contraction of the external laryngeal muscles, which force the mucosal folds of the quadrangular membrane into apposition (Fig. 15-2). Muscle groups also extend from the thyroid cartilage to the hyoid and cricoid cartilages. When they contract, the interior mucosa and soft tissue (ventricular and vocal folds) are forced into the center of the airway, and the thyroid shield is deformed (compressed inward), providing a spring to reopen the airway rapidly after these muscles relax.[8] The larynx closes at the level of the true cords by action of the intrinsic muscles of the larynx during phonation, but this closure is not as tight as the laryngospasm described earlier.

Opening of the pharynx and larynx is achieved by elongating and unfolding the airway from the hyoid to the cricoid cartilage.[8] Several muscle groups tether the various airway structures to one another to form a functional airway apparatus. When the head is tilted, the chin and mandible are displaced forward on the temporomandibular joint. This produces maximum stretch at the hyoid-thyroid-cricoid area. The hyoid bone is pulled in an anterior direction along with the epiglottis and base of the tongue, which opens the oropharynx. The ventricular and vocal folds flatten against the sides of the thyroid cartilage, opening the laryngeal airway.[8]

The inferior and middle constrictors close the superior part of the esophagus (cervical sphincter) to prevent regurgitation. Muscle relaxants open the airway by relaxing the intrinsic and extrinsic laryngeal muscles that close the airway, but they also relax the pharyngeal constrictors, potentially permitting regurgitation and aspiration of gastric contents. Balancing airway patency and airway protection represents the major dilemma of airway management without, and while placing, an endotracheal tube (ETT).

B. Upper Airway Obstruction

Upper airway obstruction is a common airway emergency necessitating nonintubation airway manipulation and airway devices. Soft tissue obstructions may occur at the level of the pharynx, hypopharynx, or larynx. Recognition of upper airway obstruction is an essential clinical skill that depends on observation, suspicion, and clinical data.

1. Pharyngeal Obstruction

The causes of soft tissue upper airway obstruction at the level of the pharynx include loss of pharyngeal muscle

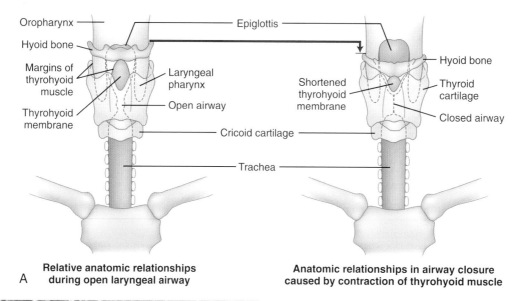

A   **Relative anatomic relationships during open laryngeal airway**

Anatomic relationships in airway closure caused by contraction of thyrohyoid muscle

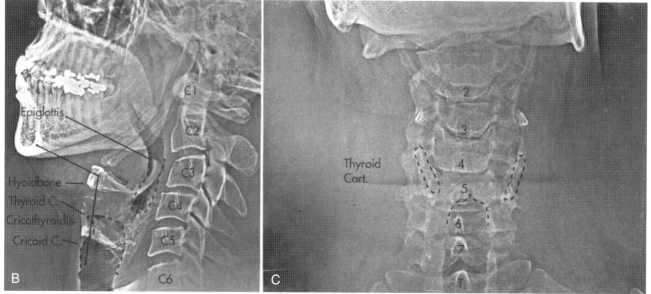

Figure 15-2 Laryngeal closure. Schematic frontal views **(A)** of the airway at the larynx show a patent airway *(left)* with a centrally located air column and the hyoid bone superior to the thyroid shield. Obliteration of the air column *(right)* is caused by apposition of the ventricular and vocal folds, and approximation of the hyoid bone to the thyroid cartilage is caused by contraction of the thyrohyoid muscle. Lateral **(B)** and frontal **(C)** xerograms were obtained during Valsalva-induced laryngeal closure. In the lateral view, notice the thyrohyoid approximation. An abrupt airway cutoff (with lack of an air column within the thyroid shield) can be seen at the C4-5 level in the frontal view.

tone resulting from central nervous system dysfunction (e.g., anesthesia, trauma, stroke, coma), anatomic and passive airway abnormalities as seen in obstructive sleep apnea, expanding space-occupying lesions (e.g., tumor, mucosal edema, abscess, hematoma), and foreign substances (e.g., teeth, vomitus, foreign body).

In patients susceptible to obstructive sleep apnea, the geometry of the pharynx can be altered during normal sleep.[9] Although it is usually oval with the long axis in the transverse plane, the pharynx in patients with obstructive sleep apnea is round or oval with the long axis in the anterior-posterior plane (the lateral walls are thickened).[10,11] This obstruction can often be treated effectively with nasal continuous positive airway pressure and with intraoral devices that advance the mandible as much as the jaw thrust maneuver.[12-14]

2. Hypopharyngeal Obstruction

Hypopharyngeal obstruction has been investigated by placing a nasal fiberscope at the level of the soft palate in anesthetized subjects.[15] The epiglottis and the glottic opening can be seen, recorded, and analyzed. The percentage of glottic opening (POGO) seen from this view can be determined. Typically, airflow increases and snoring decreases as POGO increases. However, a POGO of 100% has been documented with airway occlusion, and a POGO of 0% has been documented with no stridor and no obvious impairment to ventilation. Although less than perfect, these evaluations do support the potential for airflow restriction at the hypopharynx and are consistent with the cause being the epiglottis obstructing the airway.

3. Laryngeal Obstruction

Laryngeal obstruction is most often related to increased muscle activity from attempted vocalization or a reaction to foreign substances, such as secretions, vomitus, foreign bodies, and tumors. Obstruction of the laryngeal aperture by a foreign body can directly inhibit airflow. Alternatively, the presence of secretions or blood in the airway can cause laryngospasm. Treatment includes removal of foreign substances and, in the case of laryngospasm, positive-pressure ventilation (PPV) with or without muscle relaxation.

4. Clinical Recognition of Upper Airway Obstruction

Airway obstruction can be partial or complete. Partial upper airway obstruction is recognized by noisy inspiratory or expiratory sounds. The tone of the sounds depends on the magnitude, cause, and location of the obstruction. Snoring is the typical sound of partial airway obstruction in the oropharynx or hypopharynx, and it can be heard during inspiration and expiration. Stridor or crowing suggests glottic (laryngeal) obstruction or partial laryngospasm, and it is heard most often during inspiration. In addition to audible clues, signs and symptoms of hypoxemia or hypercarbia should alert the clinician to the possibility of an airway obstruction.

Complete airway obstruction is a medical emergency that requires immediate attention. Signs of complete obstruction in the spontaneously breathing individual are inaudible breath sounds or the inability to perceive air movement; use of accessory neck muscles; sternal, intercostal, and epigastric retraction with inspiratory effort; absence of chest expansion on inspiration; and agitation.

II. NONINTUBATION APPROACHES TO ESTABLISH AIRWAY PATENCY

Prevention and relief of airway obstruction are the focus of this chapter. The preceding information on airway anatomy and airway obstruction constitutes essential background for understanding airway maneuvers. When possible, rapid, simple maneuvers should take precedence in the management of this problem.

When the muscles of the floor of the mouth and tongue relax, the tongue may cause soft tissue obstruction by falling back onto the posterior wall of the oropharynx. It is also possible for the epiglottis to overlie and obstruct the glottic opening or to seal against the posterior laryngopharynx. This effect can be exaggerated by flexing the head and neck or opening the mouth, or both (Fig. 15-3), because the distance between the chin and the thyroid notch is relatively short in the flexed position. Any intervention that increases this distance straightens the mentum-geniohyoid-hyoid-thyroid line and therefore elevates the hyoid bone further from the pharynx. The elevated hyoid then secondarily elevates the epiglottis through the hyoepiglottic ligament, potentially alleviating the obstruction.

A. Simple Maneuvers for the Native Airway

Two well-described, simple maneuvers can lengthen the anterior neck distance from the chin to the thyroid notch: head tilt-chin lift and jaw thrust.

1. Head Tilt-Chin Lift

The head tilt-chin lift is accomplished by tilting the head back on the atlanto-occipital joint while keeping the mouth closed (teeth approximated) (Fig. 15-4). This technique may be augmented by elevating the occiput 1 to 4 inches above the level of the shoulders (sniffing position) as long as the larynx and posterior pharynx stay in their original position. The head tilt-chin lift is the simplest and first airway maneuver used in resuscitation, but it should be used with extreme caution in patients with suspected neck injuries.

In some patients, the cervical spine is stiff enough that elevating the head into the sniffing position also elevates the C4-5 laryngeal area, leaving the airway unimproved. In children younger than 5 years, the upper cervical spine is more flexible and can bow upward, forcing the posterior pharyngeal wall upward against the tongue and epiglottis and exacerbating an obstruction. A child's airway is usually best maintained by leaving the head in a more neutral position than that described for an adult.

2. Jaw Thrust

The jaw thrust maneuver more directly lifts the hyoid bone and tongue away from the posterior pharyngeal wall by subluxating the mandible forward onto the sliding part of the temporomandibular joint (mandibular advancement) (Fig. 15-5). The occluded teeth normally prevent forward movement of the mandible, and the thumbs must depress the mentum while the fingers grip the rami of the mandible and lift it upward. This results in the mandibular teeth protruding in front of the maxillary teeth (after the mouth opens slightly). In practice, the insertion of a small airway sometimes makes this procedure easier because it separates the teeth, allowing the mandible to more easily slide forward. In most people, the mandible is readily drawn back into the temporomandibular joint by the elasticity of the joint capsule and masseter muscles. Consequently, this position can be difficult to maintain with one hand.

In up to 20% of patients, the nasopharynx is occluded by the soft palate during exhalation when the airway muscles are relaxed. If the mouth and lips are also closed, exhalation is impeded. In these cases, the mouth must be opened slightly to ensure that the lips are parted. When the head tilt-chin lift, jaw thrust, and open mouth maneuvers are done together, it is known as the *triple airway maneuver* (see Fig. 15-5). The triple airway maneuver is the most reliable manual method to achieve patency of the native upper airway (Box 15-1).

3. Heimlich Maneuver

Airway maneuvers can aid in establishing and maintaining airway patency, but they do not relieve an obstruction due to foreign material lodged in the upper airway. Foreign body obstruction should be suspected after a witnessed aspiration when the patient cannot speak,

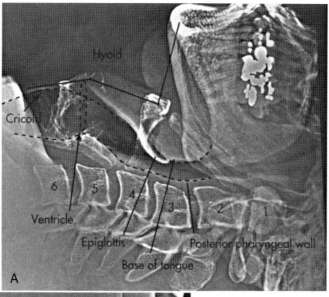

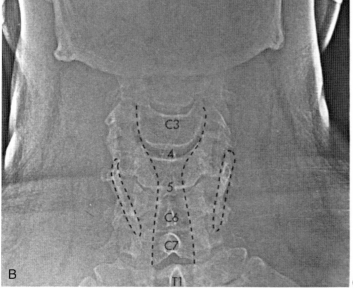

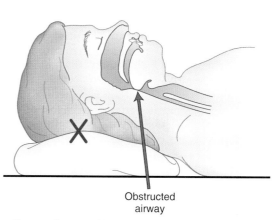

Obstructed
airway

Tongue in apposition to posterior pharyngeal wall

Figure 15-3 **A,** Lateral xerogram of the head and neck in the neutral position in an awake and supine patient shows the mentum is directly anterior to the hyoid bone, the base of the tongue and the epiglottis are close to the posterior pharyngeal wall, and the thyroid and cricoid cartilages are at the C5-6 level. Notice that an oropharyngeal airway could easily touch the tip of the epiglottis, pushing it downward. **B,** Frontal view of the same patient shows the air column within the thyroid shield with its narrowest site at the level of the vocal cords (C5-6). **C,** Diagram of a patient with a flexed neck shows the tongue in apposition to the posterior pharyngeal wall.

when spontaneous ventilation is absent, or when PPV remains difficult after routine airway maneuvers have been performed. A Heimlich maneuver (subdiaphragmatic abdominal thrusts) is recommended when coughing or traditional means, such as back blows, are unable to relieve complete airway obstruction due to foreign material (Fig. 15-6 and Box 15-2). The goal is to increase intrathoracic pressure sufficiently to simulate a cough. Alternatively, a forceful chest compression in the manner of a rapidly executed bear hug (for upright patients) or a sternal compression (for supine patients) can also be effective. In emergency situations, the failure of one technique to relieve an obstruction should not preclude additional attempts using the various alternatives.

B. Artificial Airway Devices

When simple airway maneuvers, such as those described previously, are inadequate to establish upper airway patency, it is often necessary to employ artificial airway devices. The next sections address some of the more commonly available devices and discuss techniques for insertion, indications, contraindications, and complications.

1. Oropharyngeal Airways

An oropharyngeal airway (OPA) is the most commonly used device to provide a patent upper airway. OPAs are manufactured in a wide variety of sizes from neonatal to large adult, and they are typically made of plastic or

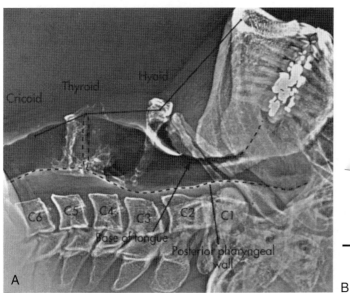

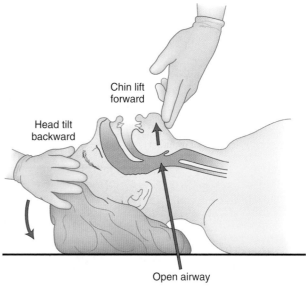

Figure 15-4 **A,** Lateral xerogram of the head and neck shows the extended position (head tilt) in an awake and supine patient (compare with Fig. 15-3A). The mentum is superior to the hyoid bone, the base of the tongue and the epiglottis are farther from the posterior pharyngeal wall, and the thyroid and cricoid cartilages are at the C4-5 level. The hyoid bone has been raised and elevated from C3-4 to C2-3. **B,** Diagram of the head tilt-chin lift maneuver.

rubber (Fig. 15-7). They should be wide enough to make contact with two or three teeth on each of the mandible and maxilla, and they should be slightly compressible so that the pressure exerted by a clenched jaw is distributed over all of the teeth while the lumen remains patent. OPAs are frequently designed with a flange at the buccal (proximal) end to prevent swallowing or over insertion. They also feature a distal semicircular section to follow the curvature of the mouth, tongue, and posterior pharynx so that the tongue is displaced anteriorly (concave side against the tongue). An air channel is often provided to facilitate oropharyngeal suctioning.

The most commonly used OPA in adults is the Guedel Airway (see Fig. 15-7). It has a plastic elliptical tube with a central lumen reinforced by a harder inner plastic tube at the level of the teeth and by plastic ridges along the pharyngeal section. Because the airway is completely enclosed (other than the proximal and distal ends), redundant oral and pharyngeal mucosae cannot occlude or narrow the lumen from the side. Its oval cross section allows the four central incisors to make contact with it during masseter spasm.

The Ovassapian Airway has a large anterior flange to control the tongue and a large opening at the level of the teeth (open posteriorly) to allow a flexible fiberoptic bronchoscope and ETT to be passed through it and later disengaged from the airway (see Fig. 15-7). Consequently, it is often employed during fiberoptic intubations to aid in maintaining upper airway patency.

BOX 15-1 **Simple Maneuvers for the Native Airway**

Head Tilt-Chin Lift

Procedure: With the patient supine, place one hand on the forehead and the first two fingers of the other hand on the underside of the chin. Simultaneously exert upward traction on the chin while tilting the forehead gently backward to extend the head on the atlanto-occipital joint.

Indications: Soft tissue upper airway obstruction

Contraindications: Cervical spine fracture, basilar artery syndrome, infants

Complications: Neck soreness, pinched cervical nerve roots

Jaw Thrust

Procedure: From above the patient's head, place the thumbs on the chin and the fingers behind the angle of the jaw bilaterally. Simultaneously open, lift, and displace the jaw forward, subluxating the mandible anteriorly on the temporomandibular joint.

Indications: Soft tissue airway obstruction when a head tilt-chin lift is contraindicated (e.g., fractured neck) or ineffective

Contraindications: Fractured or dislocated jaw, awake patient

Complications: Jaw dislocation, dental injury

Triple Airway Maneuver

Procedure: Perform the head tilt-chin lift followed by a jaw thrust maneuver. Maintain the mouth in an open position after subluxating the mandible during the jaw thrust.

Indications: Expiratory obstruction after a head tilt-chin lift and jaw thrust

Contraindications: Same as for a head tilt-chin lift and jaw thrust

Complications: Same as for a head tilt-chin lift and jaw thrust

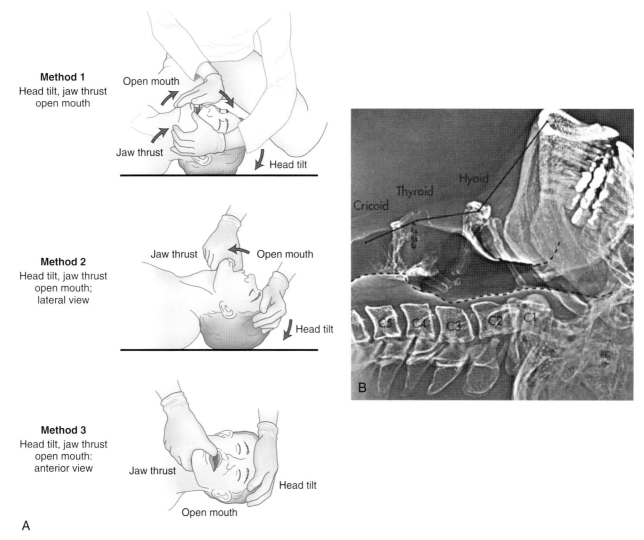

Method 1
Head tilt, jaw thrust
open mouth

Open mouth

Jaw thrust

Head tilt

Method 2
Head tilt, jaw thrust
open mouth;
lateral view

Jaw thrust

Open mouth

Head tilt

Method 3
Head tilt, jaw thrust
open mouth:
anterior view

Jaw thrust

Head tilt

Open mouth

A

B

Cricoid Thyroid Hyoid

C5 C4 C3 C2 C1

Figure 15-5 The triple airway maneuver includes the head tilt-chin lift, jaw thrust, and open mouth. **A,** Diagrams show three methods of performing the maneuver: (1) the head extended on the atlanto-occipital joint, (2) the mouth opened to take the teeth out of occlusion, and (3) the mandible lifted upward, forcing the mandibular condyles anteriorly at the temporomandibular joint. **B,** Lateral xerogram of the head and neck show the extended position with jaw protrusion (compare with Figs. 15-3A and 15-4A). Notice that the mandibular incisors protrude beyond the maxillary incisors and that the mandibular condyles are subluxated anteriorly from the temporomandibular joint.

BOX 15-2 The Heimlich Maneuver

Procedure: In the upright patient, wrap both arms around the chest with the right hand in a closed fist in the low sternal-xiphoid area and the left hand on top of the fist. With a rapid, forceful thrust, compress upward, increasing subdiaphragmatic pressure and creating an artificial cough.

Indication: Complete upper airway obstruction by a foreign body with impending asphyxia

Contraindications: Partial airway obstruction, fractured ribs (relative), cardiac contusion (relative)

Complications: Fractured ribs or sternum, trauma to liver, spleen, or pancreas

---

Use of an OPA seems deceptively simple, but the device must be used correctly. The patient's pharyngeal and laryngeal reflexes should be depressed before insertion to avoid worsening obstruction due to airway reactivity. The mouth is opened, and a tongue blade is placed at the base of the tongue and drawn upward, lifting the tongue off of the posterior pharyngeal wall (Fig. 15-8A). The airway is then placed so that the OPA is just off the posterior wall of the oropharynx, with 1 to 2 cm protruding above the incisors (see Fig. 15-8B). If the flange is at the teeth when the tip is just at the base of the tongue, the airway is too small, and a larger size should be inserted. A jaw thrust is then performed as described previously to lift the tongue off of the pharyngeal wall while the thumbs tap down the airway the last 1 to 2 cm so that the curve of the OPA lies behind the base of the tongue (see Fig. 15-8C). The mandible is then allowed to reduce back into the temporomandibular joint, and the mouth is inspected to ensure that neither the tongue nor the lips are caught between the teeth and the OPA.

An alternative method of placement is to insert the airway backward (convex side toward the tongue) until the tip is close to the pharyngeal wall of the oropharynx. It is then rotated 180 degrees so that the tip rotates and sweeps under the tongue from the side (see Fig. 15-8D). This method is not as reliable as the tongue blade–assisted technique described earlier, and it has the added risk of causing dental trauma in patients with poor dentition.

If the upper airway is not patent after the placement of an OPA, the following situations must be considered. With an OPA that is too small, the pronounced curve may impinge on the base of the tongue, or the tongue may obstruct the native airway distal to the OPA. If a larger OPA still results in obstruction, the curve might have brought the distal end into the vallecula or the OPA might have pushed the epiglottis into the glottic opening or posterior wall of the laryngopharynx. In the lightly anesthetized or awake patient, this stimulation causes coughing or laryngospasm. The best treatment for this problem is to withdraw the OPA 1 to 2 cm. A topical anesthetic spray or a water-soluble local anesthetic lubricant reduces the chance of laryngeal activity, but it should be used judiciously or avoided in patients thought to be at increased risk for aspiration.

Two major complications can occur with the use of OPAs: iatrogenic trauma and airway hyperreactivity. Minor trauma, including pinching of the lips and tongue, is common. Ulceration and necrosis of oropharyngeal structures from pressure and long-term contact (days) have been reported.[16] These problems necessitate intermittent surveillance during extended use. Dental injury can result from twisting of the airway, involuntary clenching of the jaw, or direct axial pressure. Dental damage is most common in patients with periodontal disease, dental caries, pronounced degrees of dental proclination, and isolated teeth.

Airway hyperactivity is a potentially lethal complication of OPA use, because oropharyngeal and laryngeal reflexes can be stimulated by the placement of an artificial airway. Coughing, retching, emesis, laryngospasm, and bronchospasm are common reflex responses. Any OPA that touches the epiglottis or vocal cords can cause these responses, but the problem is more common with larger OPAs. Initial management is to partially withdraw the OPA. If an anesthetic is being administered, deepening the plane of anesthesia (most easily accomplished with an intravenous agent) is often effective in blunting airway hyperreactivity. In cases of laryngospasm, it may be necessary to apply mild positive airway pressure and, in trained hands, to cautiously administer small doses of succinylcholine to achieve resolution.

2. Nasopharyngeal Airways

The nasopharyngeal airway (NPA) is an alternative airway device for treating soft tissue upper airway obstruction. When in place, an NPA is less stimulating than an OPA and therefore better tolerated in the awake, semicomatose, or lightly anesthetized patient. In cases of oropharyngeal trauma, a nasal airway is often preferable to an oral airway. NPAs are pliable, bent cylinders made of soft plastic or rubber in variable lengths and widths (Fig. 15-9). A flange (or moveable disk) prevents the outside

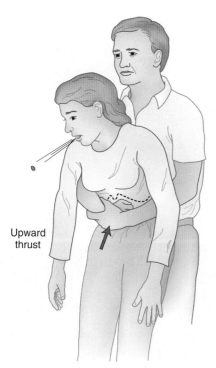

Figure 15-6 Heimlich maneuver. An airway obstructed by a laryngeal foreign body is opened by compressing the lungs through external pressure on the abdomen, forcing the diaphragm cephalad. An alternative method creates this "external cough" by compressing the thorax directly.

Upward thrust

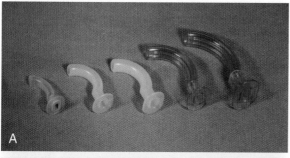

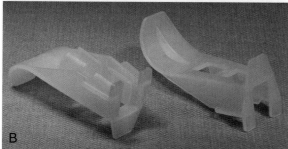

Figure 15-7 Oropharyngeal airways. **A,** Guedel Airways in sizes from neonatal to large adult. **B,** The Ovassapian Airway has a large anterior flange to control the tongue. The airway is open posteriorly (including no posterior flange) so that an endotracheal tube can be inserted with a flexible fiberoptic scope and the assembly later separated.

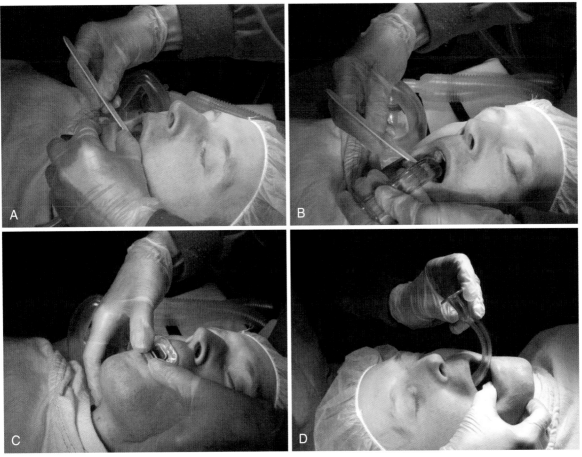

Figure 15-8 Techniques for insertion of an oropharyngeal airway: standard technique **(A–C)** and alternative technique **(D)** without a tongue blade. **A,** The tongue blade is placed deep into the mouth and depresses the tongue at its posterior half. The tongue is then pulled forward in an attempt to pull it off the back wall of the pharynx. **B,** The airway is then inserted with the concave side toward the tongue until the tube is just off the posterior wall of the oropharynx with 1 to 2 cm protruding above the incisors. The tongue blade is then removed. **C,** A jaw thrust is performed while the thumb taps the airway into place. After the jaw is allowed to relax, the lips are inspected to ensure they are not caught between the teeth and airway. **D,** In an alternative technique, the airway is placed in a reverse manner (convex side toward tongue) and then spun 180 degrees into place so that the lower section of the airway rotates between the tongue and posterior pharyngeal wall.

end from passing beyond the nares, thereby controlling the depth of insertion. The concavity is meant to follow the superior side of the hard palate and posterior wall of the nasopharynx. The tip of the airway is beveled to aid in following the airway and minimizing mucosal trauma as it is advanced through the nasopharynx. A narrow NPA is often desirable to minimize nasal trauma but may be too short to reach behind the tongue. As an alternative, an ETT of the same diameter may be cut to the appropriate length to provide a longer airway. A 15-mm adapter should be inserted in the cut end of the ETT to prevent migration of the proximal end beyond the naris (see Fig. 15-9).

Before insertion of an NPA, the nares should be inspected to determine their size and patency and to evaluate for the presence of nasal polyps or marked septal deviation. Vasoconstriction of the mucous membranes can be accomplished with cocaine (which has the added benefit of providing topical anesthesia) or phenylephrine drops or spray. This can also be accomplished by soaking cotton swabs in either of these solutions and then

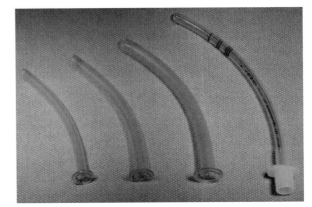

Figure 15-9 Nasopharyngeal airways. A flange prevents the outside end from passing beyond the nares, controlling the depth of insertion. Alternatively, an endotracheal tube may be cut down to provide a longer airway, with its 15-mm adapter reinserted in the cut end.

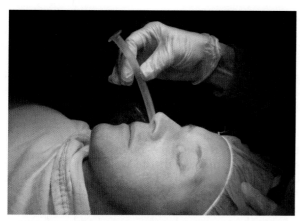

Figure 15-10 Insertion of a nasopharyngeal airway. The airway is oriented with its concave side toward the hard palate and inserted straight posteriorly. Gripping the airway near the top allows the tube to bend if there is resistance to passage. If it is gripped too close to the naris, the clinician can generate sufficient force to shear off a turbinate.

inserting them into the naris (with careful attention to removing the swabs before insertion of the NPA). The NPA is typically lubricated with a water-based lubricant (with or without a water-soluble local anesthetic) and then gently but firmly passed with the concave side parallel to the hard palate through the nasal passage until resistance is felt in the posterior nasopharynx (Fig. 15-10).

When there is resistance to passage, it is sometimes helpful to rotate the NPA 90 degrees counterclockwise, bringing the open part of the bevel against the posterior nasopharyngeal mucosa. As the tube makes the bend (indicated by a relative loss of resistance to advancement), it should be rotated back to its original orientation. If the NPA does not advance with moderate pressure, there are three management options: attempt placement of a narrower tube, redilate the naris, and attempt placement in the other naris. If the tube does not pass into the oropharynx, the clinician may withdraw the tube 2 cm and then pass a suction catheter through the nasal airway as a guide for advancement of the NPA. If the patient coughs or reacts as the NPA is inserted to its full extent, it should be withdrawn 1 to 2 cm to prevent the tip from touching the epiglottis or vocal cords. If the patient's upper airway is still obstructed after insertion, the NPA should be checked for obstruction or kinking by passing a small suction catheter. If patency of the NPA is confirmed, it is possible that the NPA is too short and the base of the tongue is occluding its tip. In this case, a 6.0 ETT can be cut at 18 cm to provide a longer airway.

Indications for an NPA include relief of upper airway obstruction in awake, semicomatose, or lightly anesthetized patients; in patients who are not adequately treated with OPAs; in patients undergoing dental procedures or with oropharyngeal trauma; and in patients requiring oropharyngeal or laryngopharyngeal suctioning. The contraindications (absolute or relative) include known nasal airway occlusion, nasal fractures, marked septal deviation, coagulopathy (risk of epistaxis), prior transsphenoidal hypophysectomy or Caldwell-Luc procedures, cerebrospinal fluid rhinorrhea, known or suspected basilar skull fractures, and adenoid hypertrophy.

The complications of NPAs consist of failure of successful placement, epistaxis due to mucosal tears or avulsion of the turbinates, submucosal tunneling, and pressure sores. Epistaxis often becomes evident when the NPA is removed, thereby removing the tamponade. It is usually self-limited. Bleeding from the nares usually is attributable to anterior plexus bleeding, and it is treated by applying pressure to the nares. If the posterior plexus is bleeding (with blood pooling into the pharynx), the physician should leave the NPA in place, suction the pharynx, and consider intubating the trachea if the bleeding does not stop promptly. The patient may be positioned on his or her side to minimize the aspiration of blood. An otolaryngology consultation may be necessary to further treat posterior plexus bleeding. The management of submucosal tunneling into the retropharyngeal space is to withdraw the airway and obtain otolaryngology consultation.

III. NONINTUBATION APPROACHES TO VENTILATION: MASK VENTILATION

In some cases, ventilation may still be inadequate despite a patent airway. Ventilatory assistance can be achieved through several alternatives other than intubation. Standard cardiopulmonary resuscitation courses have long taught the effectiveness of mouth-to-mouth and mouth-to-nose ventilation. Mouth-to-artificial-airway ventilation using a disposable face mask overcomes many of the sanitary objections to the previous techniques. More sophisticated approaches to ventilatory assistance (as in the course of anesthesia care) typically include the use of bag-mask-valve systems. Ventilation of a patient typically requires a sealed interface between the patient and a delivery system that supplies airway gases and can be pressurized. For nonintubation ventilation, this seal is on the skin of the face (face mask techniques) or in the hypopharynx (LMA). The most reliable seal, allowing high positive-pressures, is in the trachea through endotracheal intubation, but it is achieved at the expense of increased airway and hemodynamic reflex activity. The remainder of this chapter reviews nonintubation ventilation by face mask and discusses the factors that must be considered when choosing an airway technique.

A. Face Mask Design and Techniques for Use

The face mask is typically the starting point for linking a positive-pressure generating device to a patient's airway. Although face masks have different materials, shapes, types of seal, and degrees of transparency, all are composed of three main parts: a body, a seal (or cushion), and a connector (Fig. 15-11). The body is the main structure of the mask and the primary determinant of the mask's shape. Because the body rises above the face, all masks increase ventilatory dead space. However, this is rarely clinically significant for spontaneous or controlled ventilation. The seal is the rim of the mask that contacts the patient's face. The most common type of seal is an air-filled cushion rim. The connector is at the top of the body and provides a 22-mm female adapter for adult and large

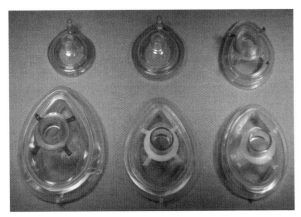

Figure 15-11 Assorted sizes of disposable, transparent face masks. The smallest masks have a 15-mm male adapter, and the larger sizes have a 22-mm female adapter to allow them to be connected to a standard breathing circuit or resuscitator bag.

pediatric masks or a 15-mm male adapter for small pediatric and neonatal masks to connect to a standard breathing circuit. A collar with hooks allows a retaining strap to be attached to hold the mask to the patient's face (Fig. 15-12). The precise application of the straps (crossed or uncrossed) is a matter of preference and is usually the result of a trial-and-error process to find the best seal for each individual patient.

Disposable, single-use, transparent plastic masks are the most common style. They are made with a high-volume, low-pressure cushion that seals easily to a variety of face shapes. The cushion may be factory sealed or have a valve that allows for the injection or withdrawal of air to alter the cushion's volume. They have little or no chin curve, however, which can sometimes make it difficult to maintain a patent airway.

The proper use of a face mask depends on establishing the best compromise between the adequacy of the seal to the patient's face and the patency of the upper airway. Successfully balancing these two factors is fundamental to providing adequate ventilation and inhalation

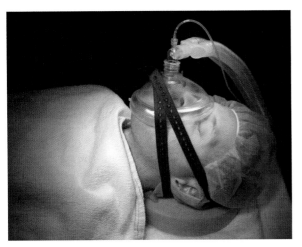

Figure 15-12 Use of a retaining strap to help seal the face mask to the patient's face. The precise application of the straps (crossed or uncrossed) is a matter of preference.

anesthesia. The mask should comfortably fit the hand of the user and the face of the patient. If the mask is too long, the face can be elongated 1 to 2 cm by placing an OPA. If the mask is too short, it can be moved 1 to 2 cm cephalad along the bridge of the nose to make a good seal at the patient's chin. When this is done, careful attention is required to avoid ocular trauma.

Several methods are described for holding the mask, but regardless of the precise method chosen, close monitoring for leaks is necessary. Traditionally, the user's left hand grips the mask with the thumb and index finger around the collar (Fig. 15-13). The left side of the mask fits into the palm, with the hypothenar eminence extending below the left side of the mask. If it does not, the mask may be too large for the user's hand, and a smaller mask should be tried. The problem with a mask that is too large for the user is that the hypothenar eminence cannot pull the patient's cheek against the left side of the mask to maintain a seal if pronation is necessary to seal the right side. The patient may require a large mask in which case retaining straps are usually necessary to achieve a satisfactory seal throughout.

The user's middle finger can be placed on the mask or the patient's chin, depending on the span of the user's hand, the size of the mask and face, and the ease of the fit. The proximal interphalangeal joints of the fingers and the distal interphalangeal joint of the thumb should be at the midline of the mask. This allows the pads of the fingers to put pressure on the right side of the mask. The nasal portion of the mask is sealed by downward pressure of the user's thumb. To seal the chin section, the mandible is gripped with the user's fourth and fifth fingers, and the wrist is rotated so as to pull the mandible up into the mask with the fingers while pushing the bridge of the mask down with the thumb. This action of lifting the face up to the mask is critical to avoid obstructing the upper airway by simply applying downward pressure to seal the mask to the patient's face. To seal the left side, gather the patient's left cheek against the side of the mask with the hypothenar eminence. The right side is then sealed by pronating the user's forearm while pressing the ends of the thumb, index finger, and possibly middle finger onto the right side of the mask.

The sides of the mask are somewhat malleable to adjust to wide or narrow faces. In edentulous patients, the cheeks are often too hollow to allow for an adequate seal. Edentulous patients also lose vertical dimension to their faces that can be restored with an oral airway. In rare situations, dentures may be left in place to allow a better mask fit (though with the associated risk of dislodgement with consequent airway obstruction by this foreign body). Alternatively, a large mask can be used so that the chin fits entirely within the mask with the seal on the caudal surface of the chin. In this configuration, the cheeks fit within the sides of the mask, and the sides seal along the lateral maxilla and mandible. These maneuvers to make a difficult mask fit possible are often best sidestepped by endotracheal intubation or the use of an LMA, based on clinical judgment (see "Choosing an Airway Technique"). Mask retaining straps can be placed below the occiput and connected to the mask collar to assist the seal, but care should be taken to ensure that

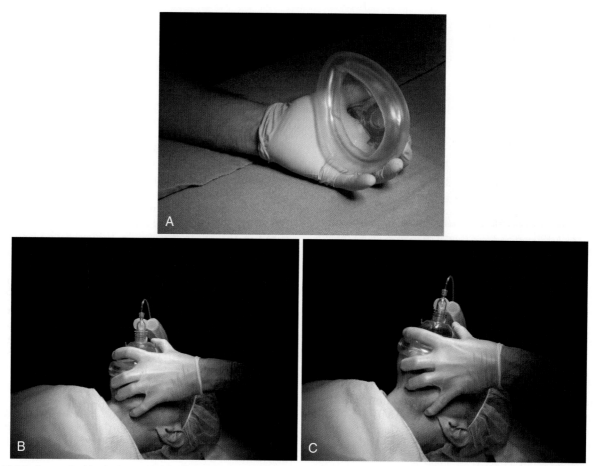

Figure 15-13 Suggested techniques for holding and supporting a face mask. **A,** In the proper hand grip of the face mask, the thumb and index finger encircle the collar while the hypothenar eminence extends below the left side of the mask. **B,** In the side view of the standard one-handed application of the face mask, the thumb and first finger (or first two) encircle the collar of the mask while the remaining fingers pull the mandible up into the mask while gently extending the head. **C,** During the one-handed mask grip with concurrent jaw thrust, notice how the little finger is located at the angle of the jaw, pulling backward and upward to maintain the jaw thrust (subluxation). Because of the increased span of the hand, only the first finger is on the mask while the middle and ring fingers pull the mandible up into the mask and extend the head.

the tension on the straps is no more than necessary to achieve a seal.

B. Controlled Ventilation by Face Mask

1. Anesthesia Circle System

Use of a face mask is a simple and reliable method of airway management for assisted spontaneous ventilation and controlled ventilation of patients during routine anesthesia care. When used as part of an anesthesia circle system, a face mask is used to seal a patient's airway to allow delivery of a precise composition of respiratory gases and inhaled anesthetics. This includes preoxygenation with spontaneous ventilation, controlled ventilation before endotracheal intubation, rescue ventilation when endotracheal intubation is unsuccessful or not feasible, and spontaneous or controlled ventilation during inhaled general anesthesia by mask alone.

Controlled ventilation by mask is relatively contraindicated in patients at increased risk for aspiration of gastric contents. Problems include the presence of a full stomach, hiatus hernia, esophageal motility disorders, and pharyngeal diverticula. When there is a likelihood of gas insufflating the stomach (e.g., mask ventilation requiring high airway pressures), an adverse patient position (usually any position other than supine), or inability to easily reach the head of the patient, use of a mask for PPV must be done cautiously. Mask ventilation is also relatively contraindicated when there is a need to avoid the head and neck manipulation that may be necessary to maintain the airway. The inability to sustain adequate assisted or spontaneous ventilation is a relative contraindication to further use of a face mask.

Use of a face mask is associated with several potential complications. A poor mask fit or seal can result in gas leaks that prevent the maintenance of positive airway pressure and contaminate the operating room environment with anesthetic gases. Pressure from a malpositioned mask, especially with the use of restraining straps, can potentially cause skin, nerve, and ocular injury. Gastric distention and aspiration constitute the most

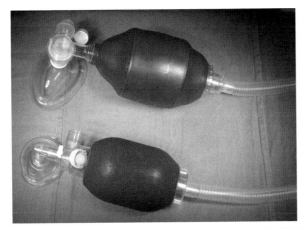

Figure 15-14 Adult and pediatric sizes of air-mask-bag unit (AMBU). The AMBU is a portable, self-inflating, easy-to-use system for the delivery of positive-pressure ventilation. It can be used with a face mask, laryngeal mask airway, or endotracheal tube.

serious (and potentially lethal) complication of PPV by mask.

2. Resuscitator Bags

The air-mask-bag unit (AMBU) was described in 1955 by Henning Ruben (Fig. 15-14).[17] The AMBU provides an alternative means of controlled ventilation to the standard anesthesia circle system. The bag can be used with a face mask, LMA, or ETT. Its main advantages are that it is self-inflating and readily portable, but it lacks the "feel" (airway compliance and resistance) that the clinician has with a circle system, and it requires a compressed oxygen source to deliver oxygen concentrations above that of room air. Although there are various types of AMBU systems in use, all incorporate one-way valves to allow PPV and to prevent rebreathing. AMBUs are an excellent choice for portable, easy-to-use systems for the delivery of PPV and supplemental oxygen outside of the operating room environment.

C. Determining the Effectiveness of Mask Ventilation

The effectiveness of mask ventilation should be judged by careful attention to and frequent reassessment of exhaled tidal volume, chest excursion, presence and quality of breath sounds, pulse oximetry, and capnography (when available). Capnography is considered the best indicator of adequate ventilation, assuming the patient has adequate cardiac output. In the absence of cardiac output (i.e., cardiac arrest), no carbon dioxide (CO_2) is returned to the lungs, and minimal CO_2 is measured in the expired gases. In this case, the presence of breath sounds and chest excursion are the best indicators of adequate ventilation.

The mask seal should be sufficient to permit a positive pressure of 20 cm H_2O with minimal leak. Positive airway pressure should be limited to 25 cm H_2O to minimize insufflating the stomach, which increases the chance of regurgitation and aspiration. If the patient cannot be ventilated with 25 cm H_2O of positive pressure, the physician should evaluate for upper airway obstruction, decreased pulmonary compliance, and increased airway resistance.

Occasionally, it is sufficiently difficult to maintain an adequate mask seal and patent upper airway with one hand that the patient's safety is best served with the assistance of a second operator. In this case, the mask and airway are controlled with the first operator's two hands (one on each side of the face mask) while the second operator ventilates the patient by squeezing the bag (Fig. 15-15). This maneuver can be done from the side of the patient and from above the head. Because this usually is not a stable situation, an alternative airway technique (e.g., placement of an LMA or ETT) usually should be employed.

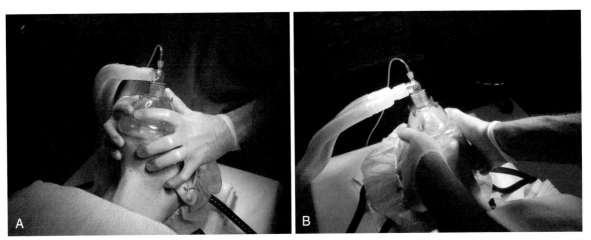

Figure 15-15 Two-hand control of a face mask. In both scenarios, a second provider must ventilate the patient. **A,** In the view of two-hand control of a face mask from above the patient, notice how the lower fingers on both hands apply a jaw thrust while the thumbs seal the mask to the face. **B,** In the view of two-hand control of a face mask from the side of the patient, the person ventilating the patient has improved access to the head as the airway is maintained from the patient's side. This arrangement is beneficial if the ventilating provider is preparing to perform laryngoscopy.

IV. NONINTUBATION AIRWAY MAINTENANCE IN SPECIFIC CLINICAL SCENARIOS

Airway maintenance without endotracheal intubation is a necessity of the practice of anesthesia, respiratory care, emergency medicine, and critical care. Occasionally, nonintubation techniques are preferable because they avoid the autonomic and airway reflexes (e.g., tachycardia, hypertension, coughing) that accompany endotracheal intubation. However, this approach is not well suited to prolonged periods of PPV. Three situations requiring airway maintenance without endotracheal intubation that deserve special mention are sedation anesthesia, transitional periods surrounding endotracheal intubation, and induction and maintenance of a general anesthetic by mask airway.

A. Sedation Anesthesia

When the painful stimuli of surgery have been largely ablated by regional, neuraxial, or local anesthetic infiltration, sedation anesthesia is used to allay anxiety or minimize discomfort related to patient positioning. Mild sedation during which the patient can converse typically does not require special airway management, although supplemental oxygen by nasal cannula is often used.

Moderate sedation to the point of somnolence or stertor generally requires intervention to ensure the adequacy of ventilation. A chin lift or jaw thrust maneuver can result in increased patient awareness and clearing of the stertor, reassuring the anesthetist that the patient is not overly sedated. If stertor returns, turning the head 45 degrees to one side or the other may help relieve the upper airway obstruction. A moderately sedated patient often allows a face mask (attached to a circle system) to lie over the nose and mouth, permitting monitoring of ventilation by capnography and providing a means to deliver supplemental oxygen. With moderate sedation, placement of an OPA is usually not advised because this level of stimulation may induce retching or other protective airway reflexes.

The use of deep sedation (often bordering on general anesthesia) has become an increasingly common part of modern anesthesia practice. This technique routinely requires airway support using a combination of nonintubation airway maneuvers and artificial airway devices to provide supplemental oxygen and to monitor ventilation. Given the ease with which this can transition into general anesthesia, deep sedation should be performed only by providers who are experienced in caring for patients under general anesthesia and who are facile in placing the advanced airway devices (e.g., LMAs and ETTs) that this often requires.

B. Transitional Airway Techniques for Endotracheal Intubation and Extubation

Before intubation of the trachea, the patient usually has received a neuromuscular blocker or, in the case of cardiopulmonary arrest, has no muscle tone. The larynx is open, and laryngospasm is not a consideration. The previously discussed techniques of airway maintenance are usually sufficient to permit controlled manual ventilation by face mask.

Airway maintenance from endotracheal extubation to smooth, spontaneous ventilation can be complicated by upper airway obstruction and by a reactive larynx capable of spasm. In these cases, the timing of extubation is an important consideration. Extubation can occur at a deep plane of anesthesia (with minimal airway reactivity) or during very light anesthesia (almost or fully awake) when there is full control of reflex activity. The patient extubated during the intermediate period may be at increased risk for laryngospasm.

Post-extubation upper airway obstruction is treated in the manner described earlier, with the following caveat. If an OPA is in place, it should not be removed with excessive force because lateral stresses may dislodge teeth. The anesthesiologist should wait for jaw relaxation or open the jaw with firm pressure on the mandibular ramus between the clenched teeth and the buccal mucosa. Post-extubation laryngospasm can be treated (as previously described) with PPV by mask, with reinduction of general anesthesia, or by the judicious administration of small doses of neuromuscular blockers. If spontaneous ventilation remains inadequate after extubation, the practitioner should consider performing laryngoscopy to investigate the cause and potentially reintubate the patient.

C. General Anesthesia by Mask Airway

Regardless of whether induction of general anesthesia is accomplished by intravenous or inhalational route, the most important feature of mask airway management during the maintenance of anesthesia is monitoring the progress of the operation and the status of the airway. Increasing levels of stimuli must be anticipated and the anesthetic deepened before their occurrence, usually by increasing the concentration of inhaled anesthetic. Failure to match the anesthetic depth to the intensity of the surgical stimuli can easily result in laryngospasm in patients who have not been administered neuromuscular blockers.

Fatigue of the anesthesiologist is a common problem in administering general anesthesia by mask if the operation is long and the airway is difficult to manage. There are many ways to minimize fatigue. Adjusting the height of the operating room table so that the patient's head is at a level between the anesthesiologist's waist and shoulders, while keeping the left arm and elbow tucked against the side helps to reduce shoulder and elbow strain. Use of a retaining strap can lessen reliance on the forearm muscles to maintain an adequate mask seal. The length of time for which general anesthesia by face mask can be safely administered depends in great part on the ease of maintaining the airway and mask seal.

1. Intravenous Induction

In the case of general anesthesia by mask airway after intravenous induction, the anesthesia workspace should be prearranged in the standard manner. Equipment for intubation should always be readily available, as should various artificial airway devices, in case difficulty is encountered in mask ventilation of the native airway. All drugs expected to be used should be predrawn into labeled syringes. Premedication with a combination of an anxiolytic (e.g., midazolam), narcotic analgesic (e.g., fentanyl), and antisialogogue (e.g., glycopyrrolate) may be done at the discretion of the anesthesiologist.

Preoxygenation is then performed in the usual fashion, typically followed by an induction dose of intravenous anesthetic (most commonly propofol, but any potent, short-acting sedative or amnestic may be used successfully). This frequently results in apnea (particularly if the patient had been premedicated with a narcotic analgesic), which then mandates that the anesthesiologist manually ventilate the patient. During this period of controlled ventilation by mask, increasing concentrations of inhalation anesthetic are titrated to achieve the desired depth of anesthesia. Ventilation is best controlled until incision, when the increased stimulation is often sufficient to promote spontaneous ventilation. Attempts to achieve spontaneous ventilation before the onset of surgical stimulation usually require a decrease in the depth of anesthesia, and the patient often is too lightly anesthetized when the procedure begins. After the patient resumes spontaneous ventilation, the levels of inhalational anesthetic and narcotic analgesic can be titrated to achieve balanced anesthesia. If upper airway obstruction occurs at any time during this sequence, it should be managed as described in "Nonintubation Approaches to Establish Airway Patency."

2. Inhalation Induction

Inhalation induction of general anesthesia by mask is most commonly performed in children to avoid the discomfort and difficulty of placing an intravenous catheter in an awake patient. In an adult, inhalation induction is often considered when maintaining spontaneous ventilation is paramount (e.g., airway tumors, anterior mediastinal masses with airway compromise).

The first approach to inhalation induction is to preoxygenate the patient with 100% oxygen and then rapidly increase the inhaled concentration of volatile anesthetic to maximum levels. This is most commonly done with sevoflurane, because it is associated with a minimal degree of airway irritation (compared with desflurane), and its vaporizer can be set to deliver up to 8% inspired concentration (approximately 4 times the minimum alveolar concentration [4 MAC]). This approach frequently works well in young children who are unable to be coached through a slower induction, but it is associated with more bradycardia and coughing.

The second approach, which tends to be effective in older children and adults, involves preoxygenating the patient and then slowly introducing the inhalation agent in an incremental fashion while coaching the patient through the sensations experienced with increasing levels of anesthetic. As the patient nears the second stage of anesthesia (heralded by uneven respirations and agitation), it is common to rapidly increase the concentration of the volatile agent (and introduce up to 70% nitrous oxide) to more quickly achieve a deeper plane of anesthesia. After a sufficient depth of anesthesia is obtained, the concentration of inhalation anesthetic (and intravenous narcotic) can be titrated as described earlier.

V. CHOOSING AN AIRWAY TECHNIQUE

Choosing an airway technique for conducting general anesthesia is just as important a medical decision as choosing the drugs and doses to be used. It is based on a risk-benefit analysis of various factors related to the patient, the surgical procedure, the surgeon, and the anesthesiologist involved. The three commonly employed airway techniques that are compatible with a semiclosed or closed breathing system and allow for assisted or controlled ventilation are face mask, LMA, and endotracheal intubation. They vary in their ability to seal the airway, maintain airway patency, and free the hands of the anesthetist. They are associated with different degrees of patient stimulation and potential complications (Box 15-3).

VI. CONCLUSIONS

Nonintubation management of the airway by face mask continues to be a vital skill in the care of anesthetized and critically ill patients. Although its use as the primary airway management technique has largely been supplanted by the LMA, it remains an essential part of other approaches to airway management as a transitional technique during induction and emergence or as a back-up plan when other techniques fail. With the increasing use of moderate to deep procedural sedation in the operating room, the anesthesiologist is frequently required to employ nonintubation airway maneuvers and artificial airway devices to provide supplemental oxygen and to monitor and support ventilation. Understanding the advantages, disadvantages, and limitations of various airway management techniques continues to be a cornerstone of a safe and effective practice of anesthesia.

VII. CLINICAL PEARLS

• An understanding of nonintubation ventilation is critical for the safe management of the airway. It can be applied to many clinical scenarios as a primary management technique or a rescue technique.

• A thorough understanding of upper airway anatomy and physiology is necessary to appreciate the therapeutic maneuvers and devices employed in airway management.

• Airway obstruction can be partial or complete. Partial upper airway obstruction is recognized by noisy inspiratory or expiratory sounds (e.g., snoring). Complete airway obstruction is a medical emergency that requires immediate attention. Signs include inaudible breath sounds; use of accessory neck muscles; sternal, intercostal, and epigastric retraction with inspiratory effort; absence of chest expansion on inspiration; and agitation.

BOX 15-3   Airway Management Choices

Face Mask with Oropharyngeal Airway

Indications: Ventilation preceding endotracheal intubation, failed endotracheal intubation, awake or lightly sedated patient requiring a high inspired oxygen concentration

Advantages: Can be done on an awake patient, does not require neuromuscular blocking agents, minimally stimulating to the patient

Disadvantages: Requires constant attention (left hand of anesthesia provider is continuously on the patient's face or mask), gastric insufflation common if ventilatory pressures frequently exceed 20 cm H_2O, minimal protection from aspiration of regurgitated gastric contents

Contraindications: Known increased risk of vomiting or regurgitation, known significant airway obstruction, surgical duration to exceed 60 minutes, adverse patient position (any position other than supine)

Complications: Aspiration risk highest of the three techniques, lip or dental trauma, inadequate airway patency (laryngospasm, upper airway obstruction), facial pressure injury (nerve injury from fingers or retaining straps)

Laryngeal Mask Airway

Indications: Failed endotracheal intubation, difficult mask ventilation

Advantages: Does not require neuromuscular blocking drugs (return to spontaneous ventilation typically faster than with endotracheal intubation), generally smoother emergence than with endotracheal intubation, frees the hands of the anesthesia provider (after placement)

Disadvantages: Cannot reliably generate more than 30 cm H_2O of positive pressure, typically requires general anesthetic for placement, does not prevent laryngospasm, risk of atelectasis with extended duration (>2 hours), minimal protection from aspiration of regurgitated gastric contents

Contraindications: Known increased risk of vomiting or regurgitation, known significant airway obstruction, high positive ventilatory pressures required (e.g., laparoscopy)

Complications: Regurgitation and aspiration, laryngospasm, inadequate placement and inadequate ventilation, lingual nerve injury, pharyngeal trauma

Endotracheal Tube Airway

Indications: Increased risk of vomiting or regurgitation, high airway pressures anticipated, inaccessibility of airway during the procedure, need for prolonged controlled ventilation

Advantages: Most secure airway, seals the trachea from the upper airway (lowest risk of aspiration of gastric contents), can remain in place for extended duration (days), can generate the highest inspiratory pressures, laryngospasm not possible after placement

Disadvantages: Most difficult to place of the three techniques, most stimulating to the patient during placement (nociceptive response to tracheal foreign body), coughing during and after extubation and emergence, usually requires neuromuscular blocking drugs to place, can lead to death if esophageal misplacement unrecognized

Contraindications: Unavailability of capnography (relative), significant morbidity from possible minor voice changes (e.g., professional singer) (relative)

Complications: Coughing and straining at emergence and extubation, post-extubation laryngospasm, hypertension/tachycardia, bronchospasm, hoarseness, unrecognized esophageal intubation

---

- Two simple maneuvers can relieve upper airway obstruction by lengthening the anterior neck distance from the chin to the thyroid notch: head-tilt-chin lift and jaw thrust.

- When simple airway maneuvers fail to establish upper airway patency, it is often necessary to employ artificial airway devices, such as oropharyngeal airways and nasopharyngeal airways.

- Ventilatory assistance can be achieved through several alternatives other than intubation and typically include bag-mask-valve systems.

- To achieve adequate ventilation using a mask, the user's left hand grips the mask with the thumb and index finger around the collar. The left side of the mask fits into the palm, with the hypothenar eminence extending below the left side of the mask. To improve airway patency, a chin lift is performed using the middle or ring finger of the left hand. Proper sizing of the mask and continuous observation for leaks are crucial.

- The effectiveness of mask ventilation should be judged by careful attention to and frequent reassessment of many factors: exhaled tidal volume, chest excursion, presence and quality of breath sounds, pulse oximetry, and capnography (when available).

SELECTED REFERENCES

All references can be found online at expertconsult.com.

4. Haponik EF, Smith PL, Bohlman ME, et al: Computerized tomography in obstructive sleep apnea. Correlation of airway size with physiology during sleep and wakefulness. *Am Rev Respir Dis* 127:221–226, 1983.

5. Issa FG, Sullivan CE: Upper airway closing pressures in obstructive sleep apnea. *J Appl Physiol* 57:520–527, 1984.

7. Rama AN, Tekwani SH, Kushida CA: Sites of obstruction in obstructive sleep apnea. *Chest* 122:1139–1147, 2002.

8. Fink BR, Demarest RJ: *Laryngeal biomechanics*, Cambridge, Mass, 1978, Harvard University Press.

9. Benumof JL: Obesity, sleep apnea, the airway and anesthesia. *Curr Opin Anaesthesiol* 17:21–30, 2004.

10. Schwab RJ, Gefter WB, Hoffman EA, et al: Dynamic upper airway imaging during awake respiration in normal subjects and patients with sleep disordered breathing. *Am Rev Respir Dis* 148:1385–1400, 1993.

11. Schwab RJ, Gupta KB, Gefter WB, et al: Upper airway and soft tissue anatomy in normal subjects and patients with sleep-disordered breathing. Significance of the lateral pharyngeal walls. *Am J Respir Crit Care Med* 152:1673–1689, 1995.

13. Pitsis AJ, Darendeliler MA, Gotsopoulos H, et al: Effect of vertical dimension on efficacy of oral appliance therapy in obstructive sleep apnea. *Am J Respir Crit Care Med* 166:860–864, 2002.

15. Meier S, Geiduschek J, Paganoni R, et al: The effect of chin lift, jaw thrust, and continuous positive airway pressure on the size of the glottic opening and on stridor score in anesthetized, spontaneously breathing children. *Anesth Analg* 94:494–499, 2002.

17. Ruben H: A new nonrebreathing valve. *Anesthesiology* 16:643–645, 1955.

Chapter 16

Indications for Endotracheal Intubation

PAUL A. BAKER | ARND TIMMERMANN

I. INTRODUCTION

Endotracheal intubation is placement of an endotracheal tube (ETT) into the trachea as a conduit for ventilation or other lung therapy. The benefits of endotracheal intubation are shown in Box 16-1. Historically, endotracheal ventilation arose as a means of resuscitation by a tracheostomy and progressed with the development of the ETT, which provided protection of the lungs from aspiration. The eventual discovery of inhalation anesthesia facilitated surgical applications requiring a secure airway, controlled ventilation, and lung therapy. This chapter reviews these primary indications for endotracheal intubation in the context of resuscitation, prehospital airway management, emergency medicine, intensive care, and anesthesiology.

II. ENDOTRACHEAL INTUBATION FOR RESUSCITATION

In 1543, Andreas Vesalius, a Belgian anatomist, was probably the first to perform endotracheal intubation by inserting a cane tube through a tracheostomy into the trachea of a pig. This landmark development allowed controlled ventilation and laid the foundation for subsequent advances in resuscitation. Endotracheal intubation for human resuscitation was first performed in 1754 by an English surgeon, Benjamin Pugh, who orally intubated an asphyxiated neonate with his *air pipe*. This was followed in 1788 by Charles Kite, another English surgeon, who reported the use of his curved metal cannula, which he introduced blindly into the trachea of several drowning victims from the river Thames.[1]

Endotracheal intubation remains the gold standard for maintaining an airway and providing ventilation in patients requiring cardiopulmonary resuscitation (CPR).[2] Although alternative ventilation techniques have been successfully used, including bag-mask ventilation and supralaryngeal airway (SLA) devices, and there is no evidence to support any specific technique for airway maintenance and ventilation during CPR,[2] there are many advantages of endotracheal intubation during resuscitation. Endotracheal intubation provides ventilation during continuous chest compressions without interruption,[3] protection against aspiration, minimal gastric inflation, and a clear airway for effective ventilation (particularly in the presence of low lung compliance and high resistance). Disadvantages include unrecognized esophageal or endobronchial intubation,[4] prolonged intubation attempts, ETT dislodgement, and hyperventilation. These problems are particularly prevalent among inexperienced practitioners.

The best airway technique for resuscitation depends on the patient's needs and clinical circumstances, the availability of appropriate equipment, and the skill of the rescuer.[2,5] Solutions to these problems involve training in airway management, appropriate selection of airway devices, and patient monitoring.

Endotracheal intubation for resuscitation of the newborn is indicated if bag-mask ventilation has been prolonged or is ineffective or if chest compressions are indicated. Care and experience is required to avoid trauma and esophageal intubation. Endotracheal intubation may also be indicated for tracheal obstruction due to meconium or other causes in nonvigorous infants when suction is required; however, routine intubation and suctioning of vigorous infants born through meconium liquor are not recommended.[6,7]

Drowning victims who suffer cardiopulmonary arrest require early reversal of hypoxemia and airway protection, ideally with a cuffed ETT.[8] A range of ventilation techniques has been suggested for victims of drowning. Endotracheal intubation has the advantage of providing a clear secure airway with positive-pressure ventilation

---

BOX 16-1   Benefits of Endotracheal Intubation

1. A patent airway by oral, nasal or tracheal routes
2. Controlled ventilation with up to 100% oxygen
3. Ventilation with high airway pressure
4. Airway protection from aspiration
5. Removal of secretions
6. Lung isolation
7. Administration of medication including anesthetic gases

(PPV) in the presence of low lung compliance and high airway resistance.

Airway management for electrocution may require early endotracheal intubation if there are electric burns around the face and neck causing soft tissue edema and airway obstruction.[8] Chapter 44 provides further details.

III. ENDOTRACHEAL INTUBATION FOR PREHOSPITAL CARE

Emergency endotracheal intubation in the prehospital environment often occurs in unfavorable conditions on patients who can be critically ill with shock, cardiopulmonary arrest, traumatic brain injury (TBI), airway trauma, or uncorrected respiratory failure. There are no prospective, controlled trials comparing basic and advanced prehospital management of adult trauma patients, but the benefit of endotracheal intubation has been described in several studies.[9-11] Some evidence suggests that clinical outcomes of children who have had prehospital endotracheal intubation by paramedics are no better than outcomes of children who have only received bag-mask ventilation.[12] Another study of children, however, indicates that prehospital endotracheal intubation performed by a helicopter-transport medical team is safe and effective, but complications of this procedure performed by emergency medical service paramedics was unacceptably high.[13]

Prehospital endotracheal intubation is recommended by the international Brain Trauma Foundation guidelines for all patients with a Glasgow Coma Scale (GCS) score of 8 or less.[14] Early treatment of hypoxia, normoventilation, and prevention of aspiration are associated with improved outcomes in this group of patients.[10] Despite these recommendations, compliance is low, and some clinical data have shown an association between early intubation and increased mortality.[15-17]

The increased mortality associated with prehospital intubation may be caused by suboptimal intubation performance and hyperventilation.[18] Endotracheal intubation is significantly more difficult to manage in the prehospital setting. In a study of 1106 prehospital endotracheal intubations by anesthesia-trained emergency physicians, trauma patients were more often associated with difficult airway management and failed intubation than nontrauma patients.[19] In this study, the difficult airway occurred in 14.8% of prehospital intubations compared with an estimated incidence of 1% to 4% in the operating room.[20] This has prompted some to suggest techniques such as SLAs or alternatives to direct laryngoscopy should be used for prehospital airway management, particularly by less experienced personnel.[5,21]

Controlled ventilation improves the outcome of TBI, but prehospital control of P_{ACO_2} is inconsistent. In a randomized, controlled trial of prehospital ventilated TBI patients, normoventilation occurred in only 12.9% when capnography was not used, compared with 57.5% for the monitored group.[22] Although capnography is commonly used and recommended to confirm correct ETT placement and monitor mechanical ventilation, the P_{ETCO_2} is not a reliable indicator of P_{ACO_2}. Arterial blood gas monitoring may improve the quality of prehospital mechanical ventilation, particularly for patients who require tight control of P_{ACO_2} or patients needing lengthy transportation.[23]

IV. ENDOTRACHEAL INTUBATION FOR EMERGENCY MEDICINE

Management of the airway in the emergency department (ED) is often a fine balance between urgency and risk. The time to evaluate the patient, examine the airway, and prepare an airway plan can be limited because the patient is deteriorating or in extremis. The patient is often physiologically unstable, at risk for aspiration, uncooperative, or unconscious but in need of urgent attention. Managing the airway in the presence of a potentially unstable cervical spine is common. Medical history is often incomplete or unobtainable. Preoperative airway assessment may not be possible in the ED.[24] Such risks must be tempered by the urgency of the clinical situation.

In the ED, the urgency of many clinical situations means that the benefits of endotracheal intubation outweigh the risks. The benefits of endotracheal intubation for emergency medicine patients are the same as those for elective surgical patients: provision of a secure airway, controlled ventilation, airway protection, and removal of secretions. The risks of endotracheal intubation in critically ill patients include hemodynamic instability, esophageal intubation, pneumothorax, and pulmonary aspiration.[25] These risks make it essential that medical personnel, skilled in airway management and using suitable airway equipment, are available to attend the patient. Risks are heightened when airway management is required away from the operating room and when multiple endotracheal intubation attempts are made.[26,27] In a study observing more than 2500 endotracheal intubation attempts outside the operating room, Mort calculated the increased relative risk for more than two intubation attempts for hypoxemia, regurgitation of gastric contents, aspiration of gastric contents, bradycardia, and cardiac arrest and showed a significant increase in these complications with repeated laryngoscopic attempts.

The indications for endotracheal intubation often relate to clinical urgency. If the patient is in cardiorespiratory arrest, for example, or near arrest with absent muscle tone and loss of protective airway reflexes, endotracheal intubation in the ED becomes an emergency. In this situation, immediate direct laryngoscopy and oral intubation with a cuffed ETT, without adjunct drugs, is indicated.

Urgent endotracheal intubation is indicated for a range of situations involving the trauma patient, when the airway may be at immediate or potential risk, or the patient's medical condition requires urgent airway management. These patients may be managed with a rapid sequence induction (RSI) and endotracheal intubation. RSI with preoxygenation followed by induction of anesthesia with a potent anesthetic agent (etomidate, propofol, ketamine, or thiopentone) and a rapid- and short-acting muscle relaxant (succinylcholine) is the gold standard technique for oral endotracheal intubation in the ER. RSI has a high success rate and is the main back-up procedure when other oral or nasal intubation techniques fail and require rescue, which occurs in up to 2.7% of emergency intubations.[28] The use of cricoid pressure for RSI is debatable and may compromise airway management.[29,30] Urgency may be assessed clinically from signs of respiratory distress and impending fatigue (Box 16-2).

Other medical conditions may justify a more conservative approach to airway management, depending on the progress of medical treatment, including anaphylaxis, burns, asthma, laryngotracheobronchitis, or acute epiglottis. These patients may require endotracheal intubation if the clinical situation deteriorates or if the progress of the condition is likely to deteriorate. Airway management for unconscious patients with drug overdose is often managed without endotracheal intubation.

RSI is contraindicated if the patient has a mouth opening that is impossible or severely limited and in patients with intrinsic pathology of the larynx, trachea, or distal airway. This includes patients presenting with stridor after a penetrating neck injury and patients in respiratory distress with a mediastinal mass. Restricted mouth opening can result from angioedema, Ludwig's angina, an immobile mandible, cervical spine pathology, a wired jaw, or airway distortion.[31] These patients may require alternative intubation techniques and may benefit from a collaborative multidisciplinary approach to airway management.[32]

Awake intubation with a flexible fiberoptic bronchoscope is promoted for cooperative, stable patients with a known or suspected difficult airway.[33] This technique is inappropriate in the ED for the rapidly deteriorating patient, especially when performed by inexperienced practitioners. Endotracheal intubation may also be warranted for the unstable emergency patient requiring a secure and safe airway during transfer for computed tomography or magnetic resonance imaging in the radiology department or to the intensive care unit (ICU).

V. ENDOTRACHEAL INTUBATION FOR INTENSIVE CARE

The most common indications for endotracheal intubation in the ICU are acute respiratory failure, shock, and neurologic disorders.[34] Endotracheal intubation is indicated for controlled ventilation of a patient with refractory hypoxemia, often in the presence of multiple organ failure. Predictors of hypoxemic respiratory failure appear in Box 16-3.

The decision to intubate is usually made on clinical grounds and based on the expected prognosis of the patient's condition. Clinical signs (see Box 16-2) or evolving deterioration in objective criteria (Table 16-1) may support this decision.

Urgent intubation in the ICU may be required immediately for apnea, airway obstruction, reintubation, or cardiopulmonary arrest. If the patient is unconscious, without airway reflexes, or paralyzed, endotracheal intubation can proceed without pharmacologic support.

RSI, commonly used in the ED, may not be as applicable for the unstable ICU patient. Preoxygenation of the patient with limited respiratory reserve is compromised by decreased functional residual capacity (FRC) and increased dead space.[35] Commonly used induction agents can adversely affect the unstable patient. In these situations, a non-RSI technique with sedation and local anesthetic may be used.

Noninvasive ventilation techniques have become increasingly popular over the past 20 years, with development of clear indications and a range of masks and interfaces. Indications include patients with cardiogenic pulmonary edema and exacerbations of chronic obstructive pulmonary disease (COPD). Noninvasive ventilation is contraindicated for respiratory arrest or patients who are unable to be mask ventilated.[36] Relative contraindications for noninvasive ventilation that favor endotracheal intubation are listed in Box 16-4.

The incidence of airway mishaps in the ICU involving endotracheal intubation is relatively low. In a study of 5046 intubated ICU patients, the airway accident rate was 0.7%. Accidents were less common with ETTs than with tracheostomies.[37] Self-extubation is the most common ETT accident, with rates of up to 16%. With strict clinical monitoring and in-service education, this rate can be reduced to 0.3%. After unplanned extubation, reintubation rates range from 14% to 65%.[38]

BOX 16-2 Signs of Respiratory Distress and Impending Fatigue

1. Look of anxiety (frowning)
2. Signs of sympathetic overactivity (dilated pupils, forehead sweat)
3. Dyspnea (decreased talking)
4. Use of accessory muscles (holds head off pillow)
5. Mouth opens during inspiration (licking of dry lips)
6. Self-PEEP (pursed lips, expiratory grunting, groaning)
7. Cyanosed lips
8. Restlessness and fidgeting (apathy and coma)

PEEP, Positive end-expiratory pressure.
Data from references 61 to 64.

BOX 16-3 Predictors of Hypoxemic Respiratory Failure

1. No or minimal rise in the ratio of PaO_2 to FIO_2 after 1 to 2 hours
2. Patients older than 40 years
3. High acuity illness at admission (simplified acute physiology score > 35)[65]
4. Presence of acute respiratory distress syndrome (ARDS)
5. Community acquired pneumonia with or without sepsis
6. Multiorgan failure

Adapted from Nava S, Hill N: Non-invasive ventilation in acute respiratory failure. *Lancet* 374:250–259, 2009.

TABLE 16-1

Objective Quantitative Criteria for Endotracheal Intubation

RESPIRATORY FUNCTION		Acceptable Range	Possible Intubation, Chest PT, Oxygen, Drugs, Close Monitoring	Possible Intubation, Probable Intubation, and Ventilation
Category	Variable			
Mechanics	Vital capacity (mL/kg)	67-75	65-15	<15
	Inspiratory force (cm H_2O)	75-100	50-25	<25
Oxygenation	$PaO_2 - PaO_2$ (mm Hg) room air	<38	38-55	>55
	$FIO_2 = 1.0$	<100	100-450	>450
	PaO_2 (mm Hg) room air	<72	72-55	<55
	$FIO_2 = 1.0$	>400	400-200	<200
Ventilation	Respiratory rate (breaths/min)	10-25	25-40 or <8	>40 or <6
	$PaCO_2$ (mm Hg)	35-45	45-60	<60

$PaO_2 - PaO_2$, Alveolar-arterial partial pressure of oxygen difference; $PaCO_2$, arterial partial pressure of carbon dioxide; PaO_2, arterial partial pressure of oxygen; FIO_2, inspired concentration of oxygen; *PT*, physical therapy.
Adapted from Pontpoppidan H, Geffin B, Lowenstein E: Acute respiratory failure in the adult: 2. *N Engl J Med* 287:743–752, 1972.

In addition to mechanical ventilation, endotracheal intubation facilitates other types of respiratory therapy. Patients with moderate to severe carbon monoxide poisoning benefit from 100% oxygen. This concentration of oxygen in normobaric conditions is most reliably achieved through an ETT. Other therapy through an ETT includes synthetic surfactant for premature newborns with established respiratory distress syndrome (RDS). Nitric oxide is administered to adults, infants, and neonates receiving mechanical ventilation to treat acute lung injury, acute respiratory distress syndrome (ARDS), and RDS. Heliox is a blend of oxygen and helium gas used to improve gas flow to patients with airway narrowing such as in asthma. Use of the ETT as a route for emergency drug administration during CPR is no longer recommended due to unpredictable plasma concentrations and the reliability of the intraosseous route.[2]

Clearing secretions by suctioning through the ETT is important to maintain ventilation by avoiding atelectasis and consolidation. Suctioning is associated with a number of complications such as hypoxemia, cardiovascular instability, elevated intracranial pressure, atelectasis, infection, and trauma to the airway. Evidence-based recommendations for endotracheal suctioning of adult intubated intensive care patients are provided in Box 16-5.[39]

VI. ENDOTRACHEAL INTUBATION FOR ANESTHESIA

Significant improvements to the design of the ETT have been historically precipitated by evolving surgical techniques. Upper airway surgery performed in the early 19th century led to an increase in postoperative pneumonia cases caused by aspiration of surgical debris. In 1878, William Macewen first used an ETT in anesthesia for a patient with a tumor of the base of the tongue.[40] Macewen was also concerned with preventing aspiration, and in 1880, he developed a metal ETT with a sponge collar that he introduced blindly through the mouth for endotracheal intubation. In 1888, O'Dwyer designed a curved metal cannula with a conical end to provide a laryngeal seal. This device helped raise intratracheal pressure to avoid pulmonary collapse during thoracic surgery. In 1895, Alfred Kirstein performed awake direct laryngoscopy with the *autoscope*.[41] This primitive instrument was the precursor of other laryngoscopes developed by Jackson and others, aiding application of the ETT. World War I precipitated a demand for plastic surgery of the head and neck, which led to oral and nasal ETT designs with pharyngeal or tracheal cuffs by Rowbotham and Magill. Anesthetic management for thoracic surgery

BOX 16-4   Relative Contraindications to Noninvasive Ventilation and Indications for Endotracheal Intubation

1. Medically unstable
2. Agitated and uncooperative
3. Unable to protect the airway
4. Swallow is impaired
5. Excessive secretions that are not being adequately managed
6. Multiple organ failure (two or more organs)
7. Recent upper airway or upper gastrointestinal surgery
8. Failed noninvasive ventilation

Adapted from Nava S, Hill N: Non-invasive ventilation in acute respiratory failure. *Lancet* 374:250–259, 2009.

BOX 16-5   Recommendations for Endotracheal Suctioning of Intubated Adult Patients in Intensive Care

1. Suction no longer than 15 seconds.
2. Perform continuous rather than intermittent suctioning.
3. Avoid saline lavage.
4. Provide hyperoxygenation before and after suctioning.
5. Provide hyperinflation combined with hyperoxygenation routinely.
6. Always use an aseptic technique.
7. Use closed or open suction systems.

Adapted from Pedersen CM, Rosendahl-Nielsen M, Hjermind J, et al: Review. Endotracheal suctioning of the adult intubated patient—What is the evidence? *Intensive Crit Care Nurs* 25:21–30, 2009.

led to the next advance in ETT design with the introduction of the first endobronchial tubes in 1932 by Gale and Waters.[1] By this time, the technique of endotracheal intubation was established, prompting the statement by Macintosh that "the ability to pass an ETT under direct vision was the hallmark of a successful anesthesiology."[42]

Endotracheal intubation is used extensively in modern anesthesia for elective and emergency indications as a primary and a rescue airway. Patient characteristics and surgical indications often dictate the appropriateness of an ETT. Elective endotracheal intubation is indicated for patients requiring anesthesia for major surgery when controlled ventilation, resuscitation, airway access, patient positioning, and duration of surgery are factors in the overall airway plan. Specialized ventilation tubes are used for specific indications. Examples include thoracic surgery requiring lung isolation, laryngeal surgery requiring microlaryngoscopy or laser treatment, and nasal intubation for limited mouth opening, oral surgery, and maxillofacial surgery.

Endotracheal intubation may occur when the primary surgical plan changes. An example is conversion of a diagnostic procedure such as bronchoscopy to a lung resection. Occasionally, complications arise during simple anesthesia that necessitate endotracheal intubation during resuscitation, such as major hemorrhage, anaphylaxis, or malignant hyperthermia.

SLAs rival the oral ETT for routine airway management in the fasted elective patient. Limitations of the SLA include the inability to provide a nasal airway, the volume of the SLA in the oral cavity, and inadequate PPV due to a disrupted airway, low lung compliance, or high airway resistance. These are important considerations when choosing a suitable airway device. Second generation laryngeal masks with improved cuff seal and gastric drainage tubes have extended the application of the SLA.[43] Procedures that previously were only considered suitable for endotracheal intubation such as laparoscopic surgery,[44] prone position,[45,46] surgery in obese patients,[47,48] prolonged surgery,[49] tonsillectomy,[50] and craniotomy in sedated patients can now be managed with an SLA in experienced hands with close monitoring of airway quality.[51] Selection of an SLA as a ventilation device should be based on case selection with careful individual patient assessment.

Safe airway management should always include a plan B for failed mask or SLA ventilation. Conversion of the airway to endotracheal intubation may occur as plan B after inadequate mask or SLA ventilation. Impossible mask ventilation during anesthesia has an incidence of 0.15% and is associated with neck changes from irradiation, male gender, sleep apnea, a Mallampati III or IV score, and the presence of a beard.[52] In a study by Kheterpal of 53,041 operations that included an attempt at mask ventilation, 77 patients proved impossible to ventilate (0.15%). Of those 77 patients, 19 (25%) were also difficult to intubate, but 15 of the patients were intubated. Ultimately, 74 of the 77 impossible mask ventilation cases were intubated,[52] reinforcing the value of endotracheal intubation for failed ventilation.

The American Society of Anesthesiologists (ASA) *Practice Guidelines for Management of the Difficult Airway* recommend awake intubation for the patient with a known difficult airway.[33] This usually involves endotracheal intubation with a flexible fiberoptic bronchoscope, but other techniques have been described, including retrograde awake intubation,[53] submental awake intubation,[54] awake intubating LMA,[55] and awake lightwand intubation.[56] The outcome of each technique is a secure airway with an ETT.

Endotracheal intubation is regarded as the gold standard for protection against aspiration of gastric contents in anesthetized patients.[57] However, evaluation of the cuff seal is important because of the risk of fluid draining past the cuff. This particularly applies to high-pressure, low-volume cuffs.[58] Evidence evaluating the relative risk of an ETT or SLA for pulmonary aspiration is limited. An analysis of the relative risk in 65,712 procedures found that the use of an LMA was not associated with an increased risk of pulmonary aspiration compared with an ETT.[59]

VII. CONCLUSIONS

The benefits of endotracheal intubation apply to patients in many clinical situations. Although recent developments of SLAs have provided a useful alternative, particularly for day surgery procedures or for inexperienced practitioners in emergency situations, endotracheal intubation remains the first choice in many situations. The limiting factors for the safe application of this important technique are the skill of the practitioner, the use of patient monitoring, and an understanding of the indications for endotracheal intubation. The ability to safely perform endotracheal intubation remains one of the most important skills for airway specialists.

VIII. CLINICAL PEARLS

- The best airway technique for resuscitation depends on the patient's needs and clinical circumstances, the availability of appropriate equipment, and the skill of the rescuer.[2,5]

- Prehospital endotracheal intubation improves outcome for all patients with a GCS score of 8 or less, with early treatment of hypoxia, normoventilation, and prevention of aspiration, and it is recommended by the international Brain Trauma Foundation guidelines.[10]

- The increased mortality associated with prehospital intubation may be caused by suboptimal intubation performance and hyperventilation.[18]

- Elective endotracheal intubation is indicated for patients requiring anesthesia for major surgery when controlled ventilation, resuscitation, airway access, patient positioning, and duration of surgery are factors in the overall airway plan.

- SLAs rival the oral ETT for routine airway management in the fasted elective patient, but limitations of the SLA include inadequate PPV (particularly in the presence of a disrupted airway, low lung compliance, or high airway resistance), the volume of the SLA in the oral cavity, and the inability to provide a nasal airway.

- Endotracheal intubation protects against aspiration of gastric contents in anesthetized patients[57]; however, the use of a LMA is not associated with an increased risk of pulmonary aspiration compared with an ETT.[59]

- Endotracheal intubation facilitates various types of respiratory therapy, including mechanical ventilation, 100% O_2 for carbon monoxide poisoning, nitric oxide, surfactant, Heliox, and suctioning.

- Risks of endotracheal intubation are heightened when airway management is required away from the operating room and when multiple endotracheal intubation attempts are made.[26,27,60]

- The limiting factors for the safe application of endotracheal intubation are the skill of the practitioner, the use of patient monitoring, and an understanding of the indications for endotracheal intubation. The ability to safely perform endotracheal intubation remains one of the most important skills for the airway specialist.

SELECTED REFERENCES

All references can be found online at expertconsult.com.
1. White GM: Evolution of endotracheal and endobronchial intubation. *Br J Anaesth* 32:235–246, 1960.
4. Timmermann A, Russo SG, Eich C, et al: The out-of-hospital esophageal and endobronchial intubations performed by emergency physicians. *Anesth Analg* 104:619–623, 2007.
10. Winchell RJ, Hoyt DB: Endotracheal intubation in the field improves survival in patients with severe head injury. Trauma Research and Education Foundation of San Diego. *Arch Surg* 132:592–597, 1997.
15. Franschman G, Peerdeman SM, Greuters S, et al: Prehospital endotracheal intubation in patients with severe traumatic brain injury: Guidelines versus reality. *Resuscitation* 80:1147–1151, 2009.
25. Schwartz DE, Matthay MA, Cohen NH: Death and other complications of emergency airway management in critically ill adults. A prospective investigation of 297 tracheal intubations. *Anesthesiology* 82:367–376, 1995.
34. Jaber S, Amraoui J, Lefrant JY, et al: Clinical practice and risk factors for immediate complications of endotracheal intubation in the intensive care unit: A prospective, multiple-center study. *Crit Care Med* 34:2355–2361, 2006.
36. Nava S, Hill N: Non-invasive ventilation in acute respiratory failure. *Lancet* 374:250–259, 2009.
39. Pedersen CM, Rosendahl-Nielsen M, Hjermind J, et al. Endotracheal suctioning of the adult intubated patient—What is the evidence? *Intensive Crit Care Nurs* 25:21–30, 2009.
52. Kheterpal S, Martin L, Shanks AM, et al: Prediction and outcomes of impossible mask ventilation: A review of 50,000 anesthetics. *Anesthesiology* 110:891–897, 2009.
59. Bernardini A, Natalini G: Risk of pulmonary aspiration with laryngeal mask airway and tracheal tube: Analysis on 65,712 procedures with positive pressure ventilation. *Anaesthesia* 64:1289–1294, 2009.

Chapter 17

Laryngoscopic Orotracheal and Nasotracheal Intubation

JAMES M. BERRY | STEPHEN HARVEY

Creation
Our very breath, pre-language of the lingus,
Unspoken and unseen, lies all around us;
It tunnels through a darkened path to bring us
Before the guarded gates that would confound us:
Dentition, palate, epiglottic folds
Are navigated as the case is started
And followed through to cartilage that holds
The two true cords, those gleaming pillars, parted;
Here human hands, left trembling with creation,
Are re-creating life as it began,
Beginning with the step of intubation,
The God-breathed breath of life blown into man.

Stephen Harvey

I. A SHORT HISTORY OF ENDOTRACHEAL INTUBATION

As we participate in the 21st century practice of medicine, it is useful to recollect the origin and development of some of the techniques commonly used for airway management. It is remarkable that modern airway techniques are less than 50 years old but are derived from physiologic experiments done primarily in the 18th and 19th centuries. Skilled airway management is a central pillar of the practice of anesthesiology, resuscitation, and critical care, and an appreciation of the evolution and development of airway techniques can improve our understanding and application of these essential skills.

Cannulation of the trachea, or *aspera arteria*, as it was called by Robert Hooke,[1] was initially described as a technique for positive-pressure ventilation (PPV):

... the Dog being kept alive by the Reciprocal blowing up of his Lungs with Bellowes, and they suffered to

subside, for the space of an hour or more, after his Thorax had been so display'd, and his Aspera Arteria cut off just below the Epigolotis, and bound on upon the nose of the Bellows

The use of tracheal cannulation for the administration of anesthetics and provision of a patent airway was first reported in 1858 by John Snow in *On Chloroform and Other Anaesthetics*,[2] in which he described a tracheostomy and cannulation for the administration of chloroform in a spontaneously breathing rabbit. The first human use of tracheostomy for anesthesia and protection against aspiration was reported by Trendelenburg in 1869, and it also was accompanied by spontaneous ventilation.[3] In the next 10 years, numerous investigators developed nonsurgical techniques and apparatus for cannulation of the trachea for surgical (ear, nose, throat) or medical (diphtheria) indications. Matas was among the first to advocate the use of PPV through a tracheal cannula to avoid the catastrophic consequences of pneumothorax for a spontaneously ventilating patient during thoracotomy.[5]

Endotracheal anesthesia came into its own during and immediately after World War I because of the volume of facial and mandibular injuries treated in England, especially at the hospital in Sidcup. In 1936, I.W. Magill wrote one of many descriptive treatises on intubation in anesthesia[5]:

The maintenance of a free airway has long been recognized as a first principle in general anesthesia and the danger of complete laryngeal obstruction has always been obvious. On the other hand, the cumulative effects of partial respiratory obstruction have, in the past, been frequently overlooked and it is not improbable that many of the surgical difficulties, postoperative complications, and even fatalities attributed to the anesthetic agent have been primarily due to an imperfect airway. It may be said without exaggeration that in remedying this defect endotracheal anesthesia has proved as great a factor in the advances of anesthesia as the discovery of new drugs or the development of improved apparatus.

Immediately thereafter, Magill inserts a caveat:

… owing to the ease of control it affords, there is a tendency towards its employment in every operation, regardless of other considerations. This tendency is to be deprecated, especially in the teaching of students. The novice should learn airway control by simple methods in the first instance, for he may be called to administer an anesthetic in circumstances in which artificial devices are not available. Moreover, as the method involves instrumentation, which is not devoid of the risk of trauma, even though it may be slight, intubation should only be attempted when the necessity for it has been considered carefully.

The historical lesson here is that, no matter how routine endotracheal intubation becomes, it is still an invasive procedure with nontrivial risks and significant complications. It should be used for specific indications and only after careful consideration of the balance of risks to and benefits for the patient.

II. LARYNGOSCOPIC OROTRACHEAL INTUBATION

The conventional orotracheal route is the simplest and most direct approach to tracheal cannulation. Done under direct laryngoscopic vision, this technique is the easiest and most straightforward for the purposes of administering general anesthesia, ventilation of critically ill patients, and cardiopulmonary resuscitation. The vocal cords are visualized with the aid of a handheld laryngoscope, and the endotracheal tube (ETT) is introduced and positioned in the trachea under continuous direct observation. After confirmation of correct placement, the tube is secured in place and ventilation assisted or controlled as indicated.

A. Preparation and Positioning

Box 17-1 lists the basic materials required for conventional orotracheal intubation. The materials are grouped according to the temporal sequence of events. All items are required for routine intubation, dealing with common difficulties, or preventing complications. Redundancy is the key in preparing for a critical event, such as endotracheal intubation. All essential equipment (e.g., laryngoscope handles, ETTs) should have readily available back-up counterparts in case of unexpected failure. An assortment of laryngoscope blades, both straight (Miller) and curved (Macintosh), should be available.

BOX 17-1 Basic Equipment for Endotracheal Intubation

Preoxygenation and Ventilation
1. Oxygen (O_2) source
2. Ventilation bag or anesthesia circuit (for positive-pressure ventilation)
3. Appropriately sized face mask
4. Appropriately sized oropharyngeal and nasopharyngeal airways
5. Tongue blade

Endotracheal Tubes
6. Appropriately sized endotracheal tubes (at least twp)
7. Malleable stylet
8. Syringe for tube cuff, 10 mL
9. Jelly and/or ointment, 4% lidocaine (Xylocaine)

Drugs
10. Intravenous anesthetics and muscle relaxants (ready to administer)
11. Reliable, free-flowing intravenous infusion (some pediatric exceptions)
12. Topical anesthetics and vasoconstrictors (for nasotracheal intubation)

Laryngoscopy
13. Working suction apparatus with tonsil tip
14. Assortment of Miller blades with functioning battery handle
15. Assortment of Macintosh blades with functioning battery handle
16. Bolsters (folded sheets, towels) for positioning of head and shoulders

Fixation of the Endotracheal Tube
17. Tincture of benzoin
18. Appropriate tape or tie
19. Stethoscope
20. End-tidal carbon monoxide ($ETCO_2$) monitor
21. Pulse oximeter

The proper sequence of events before laryngoscopy should be followed:

1. Adequate access to the head of the bed or table is essential. Removal of side rails and headboard (if outside the operating room) ensures freedom of movement; confirming that the bed or table is locked in position prevents unnecessary and stress-inducing pursuit of the patient around the room. The height of the surface should be adjusted to the level of the laryngoscopist's chest. An experienced aide should be in constant attendance to provide items such as suction lines, airways, tubes, and drugs to the primary laryngoscopist, as well as to apply optimal external laryngeal manipulation (OELM), as needed.

2. The patient must be properly positioned before laryngoscopy. Patients who are uncooperative, agitated, or otherwise mobile may require rapid and efficient positioning after sedation. Pads or rolls should be prepared in advance and be readily at hand.

Head and neck position and the axes of the head and neck upper airway

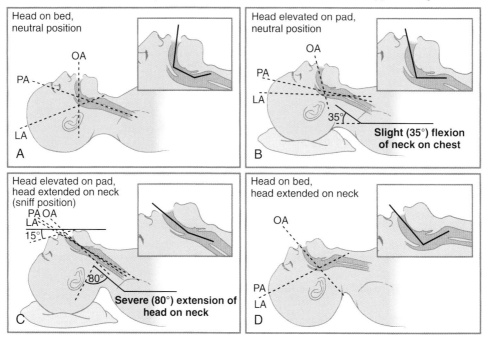

Figure 17-1 Schematic diagrams show the alignment of the oral axis *(OA)*, pharyngeal axis *(PA)*, and laryngeal axis *(LA)* in four different head positions. Each head position is accompanied by an *inset* that magnifies the upper airway (oral cavity, pharynx, and larynx) and superimposes *(bent bold line)* the continuity of these three axes within the upper airway. **A,** The head is in the neutral position with a marked degree of nonalignment of the LA, PA, and OA. **B,** The head is resting on a large pad that flexes the neck on the chest and aligns the LA with the PA. **C,** The head is resting on a pad (which flexes the neck on the chest). Concomitant extension of the head on the neck brings all three axes into alignment (sniffing position). **D,** Extension of the head on the neck without concomitant elevation of the head on a pad, which results in nonalignment of the PA and LA with the OA. (From Benumof JL, editor: *Airway management: principles and practice,* St. Louis, 1996, Mosby, p 263.)

The earliest attempts at laryngoscopy used the classic positioning of full extension. Described by Jackson in 1913, this position required full extension of the head and neck on a flat surface.[6] After 20 years, he amended his view to one that supported the contemporary *sniffing position* of flexion at the neck and extension at the head.[7] This was accomplished by supporting the head on a pillow that was at least 10 cm thick. Numerous investigators have examined radiographs of subjects to determine the optimal positioning for orotracheal access. Various theoretical models of positioning for intubation have been proposed. For the past 60 years, the three-axis theory has proposed that the oral, pharyngeal, and laryngeal axes should be brought into approximate alignment to best facilitate orotracheal visualization and intubation (Fig. 17-1). Proposed by Bannister and MacBeth in 1944, this model presumes that laryngoscopy is done in the midline (two-dimensional model) and that laryngeal axis alignment is necessary for proper intubation.[8] This idea has been challenged by the work of Adnet and colleagues in imaging studies and clinical comparisons.[9-11]

Adnet's conclusion, however, has been questioned at length.[12] Greenland and colleagues reexamined the issue, finding "the sniffing position the most favorable for direct laryngoscopy" as determined by magnetic resonance imaging (MRI).[13] This perspective has been corroborated by evidence indicating 9 cm as the optimal pillow height.[14] Others have advocated for an *extension-extension position*, in which the head and neck are extended by lowering the head of the table 30 degrees, proposing that direct laryngoscopy requires less axial force in this position than in the sniffing position.[15] Whether the lower cervical spine is flexed, extended, or neutral, the extension of the atlanto-occipital joint remains the critical factor for optimal positioning. The reasonable option in view of conflicting evidence (and patients' variability) is to position the patient with the occiput on a pad (traditional sniffing position) and be prepared to remove the pad (convert to simple extension) if the initial laryngoscopy becomes inadequate (Fig. 17-2).

Obese patients often require more extensive padding (planking) starting at the midpoint of the back to the head to assume an optimal position for laryngoscopy. Occasionally, it is necessary to place towels and blankets under the scapula, shoulders, nape of the neck, and head to flex the neck on the chest (see Figs. 17-1B and 17-2) and extend the head on the neck (see Figs. 17-1C and 17-2). In this instance, the purpose of the scapula, shoulder, and neck support is to give the head room so that it may be extended on the neck. When in doubt, the final assessment of the position should be from a lateral view of the patient, because only a lateral view enables precise assessment of the chest, neck, face, and head axes (see Figs. 17-1C and 17-2).

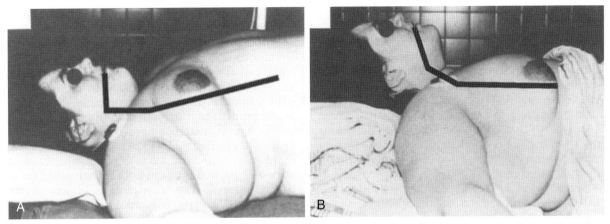

Figure 17-2 **A,** In some obese patients, placing the head on a pillow does not result in the sniffing position; in the obese patient shown and as illustrated by the overlying *bold black line*, the oral and laryngeal axes are perpendicular to one another, the neck is not flexed on the chest, and the head is not extended on the neck at the atlanto-occipital joint. **B,** In the same patient, placing support (e.g., blankets, towels) under the scapula, shoulders, nape of the neck, and head results in a much better sniffing position; the oral, pharyngeal, and laryngeal axes form only a slightly bent curve, the neck is flexed on the chest, and the head is extended on the neck at the atlanto-occipital joint. (From Benumof JL, editor: *Airway management: Principles and practice*, St. Louis, 1996, Mosby, p 264.)

B. Preoxygenation

Instrumentation of the airway may be done on an awake, spontaneously breathing patient. This sometimes is the safest and most prudent approach, but most commonly, laryngoscopy and intubation are performed on an anesthetized and (usually) apneic patient. Because this requires some finite period of time, the patient is at risk for arterial desaturation and hypoxic injury. Preoxygenation is done before laryngoscopy to minimize this risk.

Administration of 100% oxygen (O_2) through a tight-fitting face mask may occur by means of the patient's spontaneous respirations or by PPV by a bag-mask unit. In either case, adequate ventilation must occur to "wash out" alveolar nitrogen (N_2) and fill the lungs with O_2. The goal is to fill the alveoli used in normal tidal breathing and the remaining alveoli and airways constituting the functional residual capacity (FRC). This additional O_2 serves as a reservoir to delay the onset of arterial hypoxia for as long as 5 minutes. A number of guidelines have been proposed to accomplish this potentially lifesaving goal.

Depending on the minute ventilation of the patient (spontaneous or assisted), the time to complete effective preoxygenation varies from 1 to 5 minutes; although in an awake and cooperative patient, this may be mostly accomplished with three or four full, vital capacity (VC) breaths.[16,17] Work has documented the increased efficacy of eight full breaths in about 60 seconds, with times to desaturation approaching those of the more traditional 3- to 5-minute preoxygenation.[18] A higher minute ventilation level leads to more rapid and complete preoxygenation. Measures of the adequacy of preoxygenation include real-time gas analysis of expired O_2 concentration (goal = 95%) and analysis of expired N_2 (goal < 5%). Essential to either of these measurements is the presence of a capnograph waveform with a plateau reflecting the expected alveolar carbon dioxide (CO_2) concentration. This documents the presence of an effective seal of the

circuit-bag system to the patient's airway and the effective delivery of 100% O_2. The use of an air-mask-bag unit (AMBU) without an expiratory valve may not provide optimal preoxygenation.[19]

The effectiveness of preoxygenation in preventing hypoxia during laryngoscopy is significantly reduced in the morbidly obese patient. Even with the most careful preoxygenation, the duration of apnea before the onset of hypoxia is one half of the duration seen in patients with normal body weight. This situation is attributed to the considerable reduction in FRC and VC in the obese patient and to the additional reduction attributable to the cephalad diaphragmatic shift related to supine positioning.[20] This places morbidly obese patients at significantly increased risk for injury if any difficulty with ventilation or intubation is encountered.

Pharyngeal insufflation of O_2 can significantly prolong the safe duration of apnea. In a typical adult, approximately 250 mL/min of O_2 is transferred from the lungs into the bloodstream, while only 200 mL/min of CO_2 enters the lungs from the bloodstream (respiratory quotient = 0.8). This alveolar gas deficit causes alveolar pressures to become slightly subatmospheric. If the airway is patent, there is a net flow of gas from the pharynx into the alveoli (apneic oxygenation). If, after adequate preoxygenation, the pharynx is filled with O_2, the onset of hypoxia is delayed because O_2, rather than air, is drawn into the lungs by this mechanism. Pharyngeal insufflation may be conveniently achieved by passing a catheter into the pharynx through a nasopharyngeal airway and attaching an O_2 source at 2 to 3 L/min. Alternatively, some laryngoscopes have a side port suitable for attachment of O_2 tubing. When preoxygenation is followed by pharyngeal insufflation as previously described, in normal but apneic patients, the O_2 saturation from pulse oximetry [SpO_2] remains equal to 98% for 10 or more minutes (although at the end of 10 minutes the arterial carbon dioxide tension [$PaCO_2$] may be expected to be about 80 mm Hg).[21]

C. Laryngoscopy

The purpose of direct laryngoscopy is to provide adequate visualization of the glottis to allow correct placement of the ETT with the minimum effort, elapsed time, and potential for injury to the patient. Considerable effort has been expended to develop laryngoscopic techniques and equipment to facilitate this important procedure. Although this textbook outlines numerous techniques for tracheal cannulation, the facilitative use of direct laryngoscopy is by far the most common technique.

Two basic types of laryngoscope blades are the curved blade (Macintosh) and the straight blade with a curved tip (Miller).[22,23] They are designed for right hand–dominant use; the laryngoscope is held in the left hand while the right hand manipulates the ETT. Historically, either hand (or both) could be initially used, shifting the laryngoscope to the left hand while the right hand manipulated the tube. Both blade styles include a flange on the left side of the blade for lateral retraction of the tongue and contain a light-emitting area (bulb or fiberoptic tip). Each blade has a channel with an open right side for visualization of the larynx and for insertion of the ETT (Figs. 17-3 to 17-10). Despite numerous modifications

and variations, they are all lighted, handheld retractors for oropharyngeal soft tissues.

Although contact with the upper incisors from the laryngoscope blade should be avoided, some patients with limited mouth opening, front caps, or obvious decay are at risk for damage by even the most innocuous, transient trauma. If the possibility of incisor trauma exists, it seems prudent to provide some protection for the upper teeth. Several materials have been used in the past to guard the upper teeth: a folded strip of lead (introduced by Magill and now obsolete), folded tape, cardboard or alcohol wipe, or a purpose-built mouth guard (as used in contact sports). The disadvantage of any of these is that they occupy a few millimeters of the available mouth opening, reducing the available aperture for laryngoscopy.

Two methods are used to open the mouth and facilitate the introduction of the blade. First, extension of the head on the neck (by pressure from the right hand at the vertex) causes the lips to part and the mouth to open (see Fig. 17-4). Alternatively, the thumb of the right hand can press down on the right lower molar teeth, and the index finger of the right hand can simultaneously press up on the right upper molar teeth (scissors maneuver) (see Fig. 17-5).

Conventional Laryngoscopy with a Curved Blade

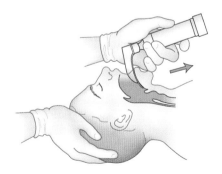

A   Insert the laryngoscope blade into the right side of the mouth

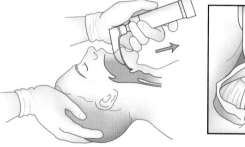

B   Advance the laryngoscope blade toward the midline of the base of the tongue by rotating wrist

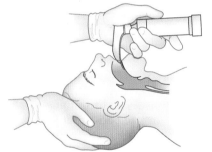

C   Approach the base of the tongue and lift the blade forward at a 45° angle

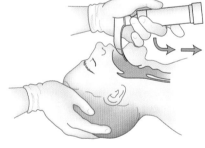
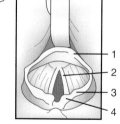

D   Engage the vallecula and continue to lift the blade forward at a 45° angle

Figure 17-3 Schematic diagrams show how to perform laryngoscopy with a Macintosh blade (curved blade). **A,** As shown in lateral and frontal views, the laryngoscope blade is inserted into the right side of the mouth so that the tongue is to the left of the flange. **B,** In the lateral view, the blade is advanced around the base of the tongue, in part by rotating the wrist so that the handle of the blade becomes more vertical *(arrows)*. **C,** In the lateral view, the handle of the laryngoscope is lifted at a 45-degree angle *(arrow)* as the tip of the blade is placed in the vallecula. **D,** In the lateral view, continued lifting of the laryngoscope handle at a 45-degree angle results in exposure of the laryngeal aperture. The epiglottis (1), vocal cords (2), cuneiform part of arytenoid cartilage (3), and corniculate part of arytenoid cartilage (4) are identified in the frontal view. (From Benumof JL, editor: *Airway management: Principles and practice.* St. Louis, 1996, Mosby, p 267.)

Figure 17-4   The mouth can be opened wide by extending the head on the neck with the right hand while the small finger and medial border of the left hand simultaneously push the anterior aspect of the mandible in a caudad direction (extraoral technique). As the blade approaches the mouth, it should be directed toward the right side of the mouth. Gloves should be worn during laryngoscopy because the hands may come in contact with patient's secretions. (From Benumof JL, editor: *Airway management: Principles and practice,* St. Louis, 1996, Mosby, p 265.)

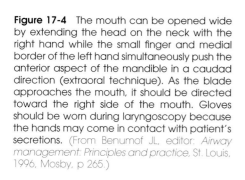
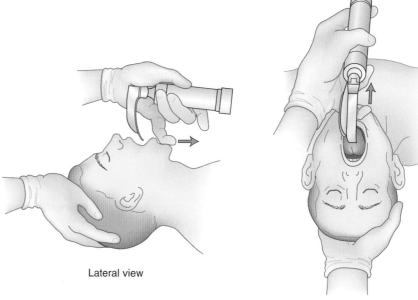

Lateral view

Frontal view

The laryngoscope blade is inserted into the right side of the mouth (see Fig. 17-3A). During the insertion of the laryngoscope, the patient's lower lip should be pulled away from the lower incisors (with the right hand or by an assistant) to prevent injury to the lower lip by entrapment of the lower lip between the laryngoscope blade and the lower incisor teeth. The blade is simultaneously advanced forward toward the base of the tongue and the tip directed centrally toward the midline so that the tongue is completely displaced to the left side of the mouth by the flange of the laryngoscope blade (see Fig. 17-3B). After the blade has been applied to the base of the tongue, the laryngoscope is lifted to expose the epiglottis (see Fig. 17-3C). During this process, the left wrist should remain straight, with all lifting done by the left shoulder and arm. If the laryngoscopist follows a natural inclination to radial-flex the wrist further, thereby using the laryngoscope like a lever whose fulcrum is the upper

incisor or gum, injury is likely to result. With the patient properly positioned, the direction of force necessary to lift the mandible and tongue and expose the glottis is along an approximately 45-degree straight line above the long axis of the patient. The best aid for inexperienced laryngoscopists learning laryngoscopy may be a 10-pin bowler's wrist brace, which immobilizes the wrist.

After the epiglottis is visualized, the next step depends on the type of laryngoscope blade being used. If the blade is curved (Macintosh), the tip should be placed in the vallecula (space between the base of the tongue and the pharyngeal surface of the epiglottis) (see Fig. 17-3D). Subsequent forward and upward movement of the blade tenses the hyoepiglottic ligament, causing the epiglottis to move upward like a trapdoor, first exposing the arytenoid cartilages and then allowing more and more of the glottic opening and vocal cords to come into view (see Fig. 17-3D).

Figure 17-5   The mouth can be opened wide by pressing the thumb of the right hand on the right, lower, posterior molar teeth in a caudad direction while the index finger of the right hand simultaneously presses on the right, upper, posterior molar teeth in a cephalad direction (intraoral technique). Gloves should be worn during laryngoscopy because the hands may come into contact with patient's secretions. (From Benumof JL, editor: *Airway management: Principles and practice,* St. Louis, 1996, Mosby, p 266.)

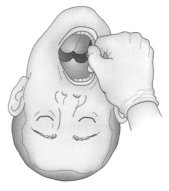
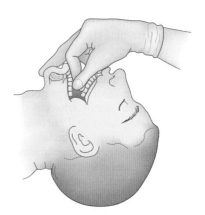

Frontal view

Lateral view

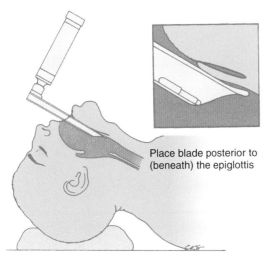

Place blade posterior to (beneath) the epiglottis

Figure 17-6 Conventional laryngoscopy with a straight blade. A straight laryngoscope blade (Miller blade) should be passed underneath the laryngeal surface of the epiglottis. The handle of the laryngoscope then should be elevated at a 45-degree angle, similar to the lifting that takes place with the use of a curved laryngoscope blade. (From Benumof JL, editor: *Airway management: Principles and practice*, St. Louis, 1996, Mosby, p 268.)

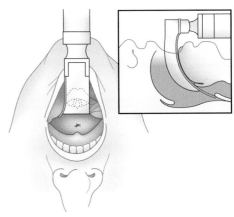

Figure 17-7 Insertion of the laryngoscope blade too deeply into the pharynx may result in elevation of the entire larynx so that the opening of the esophagus rather than the glottic aperture is visualized. The esophagus is located just to the right of the midline and posteriorly, and the esophageal opening is round and puckered with no structure around it. (From Benumof JL, editor: *Airway management: Principles and practice*, St. Louis, 1996, Mosby, p 268.)

The ability to identify the epiglottis and then lift anteriorly to reveal progressively more of the glottic aperture has led to a convenient system for grading the laryngoscopic view of any patient.[24,25] A grade I laryngoscopic view consists of visualization of the vocal cords in their entirety. A grade II laryngoscopic view is visualization of the posterior portion of the laryngeal aperture (arytenoid cartilages) but not any portion of the vocal cords. A grade III laryngoscopic view is visualization of the epiglottis but not the posterior portion of the laryngeal aperture, and a grade IV laryngoscopic view is visualization of the soft palate but not the epiglottis. This grading system is necessarily subjective and skill dependent, but it does correlate somewhat with difficult intubation.

If the blade is straight (Jackson, Wisconsin, or Miller blades), the tip should extend just behind (posterior to) or beneath the laryngeal surface of the epiglottis (see Fig. 17-6). As with a curved laryngoscope blade, subsequent forward and upward movement of the straight blade (exerted along the axis of the handle, not by pulling back on the handle) exposes the glottic opening (see Fig. 17-6).

The use of a curved blade is thought to be less stimulating to the patient and possibly less traumatic to the epiglottis for two reasons. First, the tip of a curved blade does not normally touch the epiglottis. Second, the pharyngeal surface of the epiglottis is innervated by the glossopharyngeal nerve, whereas the superior laryngeal nerve supplies the laryngeal surface of the epiglottis. Stimulation of the laryngeal surface of the epiglottis is thought to predispose to laryngospasm and bronchospasm more than stimulation of the pharyngeal surface of the epiglottis. Curved blades are thought to be less traumatic to the teeth and to provide more room for passage of the ETT through the oropharynx. However, straight blades provide a better view of the glottis in a patient with a long, floppy epiglottis or an anterior larynx. Straight blades are preferred in infants, pediatric patients, and patients with an anterior larynx. Use of a longer blade (curved or straight) is more appropriate in very large patients and patients with a very long thyromental distance.

Four major common problems are encountered in performing laryngoscopy. First, with either laryngoscope blade, inserting the blade too deeply into the pharynx may elevate the entire larynx so that the opening of the esophagus is visualized rather than the glottic aperture (see Fig. 17-7). Insertion of a curved blade too far into the vallecula and continued rotation of the handle to the vertical may push the epiglottis down over the glottic opening, resulting in limited exposure of the larynx (see Fig. 17-8). The tracheal and esophageal openings are usually easily distinguished. The esophagus is located just to the right of the midline and more posteriorly, and the esophageal opening is round and puckered, with no

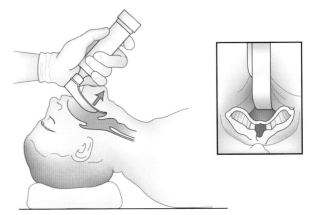

Figure 17-8 Insertion of the laryngoscope blade too deeply into the vallecula may push the epiglottis down over the laryngeal aperture, diminishing exposure of the vocal cords. (From Benumof JL, editor: *Airway management: Principles and practice*, St. Louis, 1996, Mosby, p 267.)

Figure 17-9   The tongue should be to the left of the laryngoscope blade. **A,** The flange on the laryngoscope blade should keep the tongue completely to the left side of the mouth. If this is accomplished, the tongue does not obstruct the view of the vocal cords. The tracheal rings on the anterior aspect of the trachea are evident. **B,** If the tongue slips over the laryngoscope blade and occupies part of the right side of the mouth, the view of the vocal cords is obscured by the part of the tongue that is on the right side of the mouth. (From Benumof JL, editor: *Airway management: Principles and practice*, St. Louis, 1996, Mosby, p 269.)

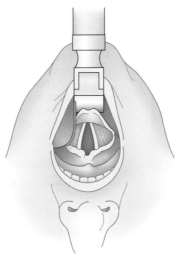
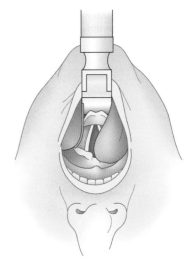

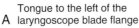

A   Tongue to the left of the laryngoscope blade flange

B   Tongue on both sides of the laryngoscope blade will obscure the laryngeal aperture

structures around it. The glottis is located in the midline, has a triangular shape, and contains the prominent knobs of the arytenoids posteriorly and the pale white true vocal cords bilaterally.

Second, it is important to keep the tongue completely to the left side of the mouth with the flange of the laryngoscope blade. Many difficult or failed intubations result from the tongue protruding over the flange of the blade toward the right side of the mouth, obstructing a clear path through which the vocal cords must be visualized and the ETT passed (see Fig. 17-9B). Vision is obscured further when the ETT occupies part of the view. With a partially obstructed (tunnel) view the endoscopist can partially visualize but not instrument the larynx. All of the tongue must be to the left of the blade (Fig. 17-9A).

Third, in an effort to keep the tongue to the left, the blade tip may be displaced to the right of the midline. This position obscures the view of the epiglottis and may precipitate trauma and bleeding from friable tissue in the tonsillar bed. Especially with the use of the straight blade, the shaft of the blade can be to the right of midline (over the right molars), but the tip must reside exactly in the midline of the hypopharynx. An assistant may be useful in retracting the right cheek and enlarging the space to the right of the blade, facilitating visualization of the larynx, and introduction of the ETT.

Fourth, in barrel-chested, obese, or large-breasted patients, it may be difficult initially to insert the blade of a laryngoscope correctly into the mouth and avoid obstruction to movement of the handle of the laryngoscope by the chest wall. In these patients, further initial neck extension or a 45-degree rotation of the laryngoscope handle to the right permits easier introduction of the blade of the laryngoscope into the mouth. Alternatively, a short laryngoscope handle (designed for this situation) may be used instead of the full-length handle.

The use of OELM can significantly improve the laryngoscopic view. For example, routine use of OELM may reduce the incidence of a grade III view from 9% to between 1.3% and 5.4%.[26] Although backward, upward, and rightward pressure (BURP) placed on the thyroid cartilage is typically the most useful OELM, it is best for the laryngoscopist to determine what form of external manipulation is optimal. This can best be accomplished using his or her right hand when it becomes free after the patient's head is properly positioned (extended) and mouth fully opened (see Fig. 17-10).

D. Endotracheal Tube

Insertion of the ETT is frequently easy after the vocal cords are exposed and the tongue is out of the way (see Fig. 17-9A). However, endotracheal intubation is often problematic even if the vocal cords are visualized. Adult tracheas readily accept ETTs with 7- to 10-mm internal diameters (IDs) (see Chapter 36 for pediatric sizes). If it is thought that fiberoptic bronchoscopy (FOB) will be necessary subsequently for diagnosis or therapy, an 8-mm or larger ETT should be used. If it is thought that the space between the upper and lower teeth will be small, allowing the cuff of the tube to come in contact with the teeth, the distal part of the tube and cuff should be lubricated to facilitate orotracheal intubation and protect the cuff from tearing. In the case of limited mouth opening, air should be evacuated from the cuff to allow as low a profile as possible. The tip of the ETT should be introduced into the far right corner of the mouth and passed along an axis that intersects the line of the laryngoscope blade at the glottis. In this manner, the tube does not block the view of the vocal cords down the channel of the blade. The common error of trying to use the laryngoscope blade as a midline guide, through which the tube is passed, violates this principle, obscures vision, and is a significant source of difficulty for the inexperienced laryngoscopist. The tube tip is passed through the cords, stopping 2 cm after the tube cuff completely passes

**Determining optimal external layngeal
manipulation with free (right) hand**

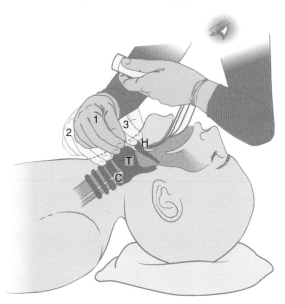

Figure 17-10 Optimal external laryngeal manipulation (OELM) to improve the laryngoscopic view is determined by the laryngoscopist by quickly pressing in the cephalad and posterior directions with the right hand over the thyroid (T) (1), which is most common. The cricoid (C) (2), and the hyoid cartilages (H) (3). If the laryngoscopic view is critically improved by this maneuver, the laryngoscopist can use an assistant's hands or fingers as an extension of his or her own right hand to reproduce the OELM. (From Benumof JL, editor: Airway management: Principles and practice, St. Louis, 1996, Mosby, p 268.)

through the vocal cords. Alternatively, when the external tube markings at the level of 22 to 24 cm reach the lower incisors, the tip of the tube is at the midtrachea.[7] The laryngoscopist must not take his or her eyes off the laryngeal aperture until the cuff disappears just beyond the vocal cords. The most common cause of inadvertent esophageal intubation is failure to clearly see the tube pass through the cords (and inspect it in situ after placement). The arytenoid cartilages frequently displace the tube tip posteriorly into the esophagus unless care is taken to pass the tip anteriorly and squarely into the tracheal lumen.

The use of a stylet may be valuable in controlling the direction of passage of an ETT. By providing increased rigidity and malleability, it allows more control of the tube. However, the ETT cannot be readily reshaped after it is introduced past the teeth. Insertion of an ETT through the mouth allows only two degrees of free movement: depth of insertion and rotation of the tip. The direction of the tube tip can be changed only by rotation. The ETT should be inserted as far to the right lateral aspect of the mouth as possible to facilitate the motion of the tip through torque applied to the connector end of the ETT. When speed of intubation is important (e.g., in a patient with a full stomach), an ETT should always be equipped with a stylet. A stylet should be easily malleable and well lubricated (although plastic-coated stylets may be adequately slippery) and not extend beyond the tip of the tube. Occasionally, a curved, styleted ETT impinges on the anterior tracheal wall as it is being

inserted and after passage through the vocal cords. In these circumstances, after the ETT tip is through the vocal cords, the stylet should be withdrawn, which returns the tip of the ETT to its inherent flexibility and permits further passage distally.

After placement of the ETT, the laryngoscope is removed from the mouth, and the cuff of the tube is inflated to a cuff pressure of 22 to 32 cm H_2O. If a cuff pressure gauge is unavailable, the tube is inflated until moderate tension is felt in the pilot balloon to the cuff. The tube should then be connected to a source of PPV and held in place with one hand. The hand holding the ETT in place should be securely resting against the cheek (as a temporary fixation) until the ETT is secured to prevent any sudden movement from dislodging the ETT.

E. Verification of Correct Placement

The next, most important task is to determine definitively that the tube has been inserted into the trachea rather than the esophagus (Box 17-2). This issue is extensively discussed in Chapter 16, and only a brief summary of the signs of endotracheal intubation is given here. Helpful but not absolute signs of endotracheal intubation consist of breath sounds in the axillary chest wall, lack of breath sounds over the stomach, lack of gastric distention, chest rise with inspiration, large exhaled tidal volumes (V_T), the sound of air exiting from the ETT when the chest is compressed, and appropriate compliance of a reservoir bag during hand ventilation. A progressive decrease in SpO_2 may indicate failure to intubate the trachea, but it is a very late sign of esophageal intubation (especially on 100% O_2), and it may also indicate bronchospasm, endobronchial intubation, aspiration, kinking of the tube, machine or equipment malfunction, or merely the normal response delay inherent in pulse oximetry.

More reliable signs of endotracheal intubation are the presence of a normal CO_2 waveform (capnogram) and rapid expansion of a large rubber tracheal indicator bulb (see Chapter 16). Cardiac arrest (when no CO_2 is excreted), severe bronchospasm, or kinking or plugging of the ET may prevent the appearance of CO_2 in the exhaled gas (false-negative finding), and CO_2 may appear if the tip of the tube is proximal to but near the larynx (false-positive finding). The self-inflating bulb has high sensitivity and specificity in normal patients, but it has a significant false-negative rate in obese patients.[27]

The only absolutely reliable methods of definitively determining endotracheal intubation are direct observation of the ETT going through the vocal cords and the use of FOB. Direct visualization of the tube lying in the glottic opening may be enhanced by displacing the tube posteriorly, which may pull the glottic opening posteriorly and into a better view. FOB allows visualization of the cartilaginous rings of the trachea and the tracheal carina but is not an accepted practice for routine determination of correct tube placement.

If a CO_2 waveform, breath sounds, and chest movement are lacking, the anesthesiologist should remove the ETT, ventilate the patient with a mask-bag system several times with 100% O_2, and attempt endotracheal intubation again after inspecting the used tube for defects or plugs in the lumen. Changes in the shape or curvature of the ETT and in the position of the head and neck, as well as the need for anterior tracheal pressure, should be considered and coordinated during the period of mask ventilation.

The next task is to ascertain that the tip of the ETT is above the carina. This is done by observing equal expansion of both hemithoraces and by stethoscopic examination for breath sounds throughout both peripheral lung fields. However, hearing uniform breath sounds throughout all lung fields does not guarantee correct tube position. If there is any question about a possible main stem bronchus intubation, the physician should retract the tube about 1 cm at a time and reexamine the breath sounds (stopping before complete withdrawal above the vocal cords). In one study, an insertion depth of 20 to 21 cm in adult women and 22 to 23 cm in adult men resulted in no incidence of main stem bronchial intubation.[28] Simultaneous palpation of pulsed pressures in the cuff in the suprasternal notch and the pilot balloon of the cuff is another simple way of determining the location of the tube in the trachea. FOB is another, but complex, way of determining the location of the tube in the trachea. Outside the operating room, it is always advisable to confirm ETT position by chest radiography. Ideally, the tip of the tube should be 2 to 4 cm above the carina at the clavicular (midtracheal) level.

When the ETT is placed and during taping of the tube, the marking of the ETT at the level of the teeth should be noted for reference should the tube become displaced.

F. Securing the Endotracheal Tube

After the depth of the ETT at the tooth level has been confirmed, the tube should be tightly secured in place. This is important to prevent accidental extubation and to minimize tube movement within the airway. Taping the tube to the facial skin with adhesive tape is the most common method of securing the ETT.

The skin of the maxilla should be considered the primary source of fixation for an orotracheal tube because it is less mobile and therefore less likely to allow excessive motion of the tube within the airway. The tube then lies along the palate and is less likely to be displaced by the tongue of a conscious patient. The fixation of the tube in place can be improved by having the lateral ends of the tape completely encircle the neck; however, the risk of restriction of venous return from the head (especially with intracranial pathology) requires careful consideration. Application of tincture of benzoin to the skin before the tape is applied helps provide a stronger bond between the tape and skin. In case of prolonged intubation, changing the tape and reapplying it to a new area on the face every 2 days helps prevent maceration of the skin.

In patients with beards or in whom the adhesive tape fails to stick to the skin, the tube can be tied into the place with a length of umbilical tape that is knotted around the tube and then encircles the neck. Adhesive tape may be used over the umbilical tape for added security. A surgical face mask, reversed so that the ties are in front and the mask at the occiput, can serve as a reasonable, temporary means of fixation. Another reliable method of securing an orotracheal tube is to wire the tube to a tooth. One or two layers of adhesive tape are wrapped around the tube at the level of the upper incisor teeth. Stainless steel wire (25 to 28 gauge) is passed around an upper incisor tooth and twisted around the tape on the ETT. In anesthetized patients, a suture may be passed through the gum and then around a ring of adhesive tape on the ETT (as with wire) or through the wall of the ETT and then tied to the tube. A bite block, rolled gauze, or an oropharyngeal airway (used in most endotracheal intubations for general anesthesia) should be placed between the teeth to prevent the patient from biting down and occluding the lumen of an oral tube. Numerous commercial products are available to attempt to improve the stability, patient's comfort, and convenience of stabilizing and immobilizing an orotracheal tube.

III. LARYNGOSCOPIC NASOTRACHEAL INTUBATION

Nasotracheal intubation usually is a more difficult procedure than orotracheal intubation. However, nasal tubes are thought to be better tolerated than oral tubes, and nasal tubes have been considered the tube of choice for medium-term mechanical ventilation. The issue of nasotracheal tubes contributing to the development of sinusitis and pneumonia has been investigated, and existing evidence has not demonstrated an association.[29] Nonetheless, the use of nasotracheal intubation for longer-term ventilation has been declining in favor of orotracheal intubation or early tracheostomy. The use of nasotracheal tubes is currently confined to surgical procedures requiring free access to the oropharynx (e.g., dental procedures, mandibular fixation) and to some pediatric procedures in which stability and security of the tube are of overwhelming concern (usually because of proximity to the surgical field).

The ETT is inserted into a nostril (preferably the right) and then passed through the nasal cavity and nasopharynx to the oropharynx. After the tube has been passed into the oropharynx, it can be guided into the glottis under conventional direct laryngoscopic vision, or it can be grasped by a Magill forceps and directed into the glottis. Nasotracheal intubation is accompanied by a transient bacteremia, and endocarditis prophylaxis should be used in susceptible patients.

A. Preparation

Before insertion of the single-lumen nasotracheal tube, the nasal mucosa should be sprayed with a vasoconstrictor drug. Vasoconstriction of blood vessels in the nasal mucosa minimizes bleeding related to the unavoidable trauma, and it increases the diameter of the nasal passages by constricting (shrinking) the nasal mucosa. Softening the tip of the nasotracheal tube by soaking it in a warm saline solution may decrease the incidence of mucosal damage and bleeding. The naris selected should be the one that the patient thinks is the most patent (because of the significant incidence of septal deviation in patients). However, if both nares offer equal resistance, the right naris should be chosen because the bevel of the nasotracheal tube, when introduced through the right naris, more easily passes the vocal cords (Fig. 17-11).

The question of potential trauma to the turbinates by the open bevel of the tube and the best orientation of the bevel in passing the turbinates has not been resolved. There is a risk that the tube tip, in passing the inferior turbinate, may strike and damage or avulse the turbinate. In the worst case, the turbinate may be dislodged and occlude the lumen of the tube, causing epistaxis and complete tube obstruction. Care must be taken to pass the tube along the floor of the nose below the inferior turbinate and to avoid any excessive force in advancing the tube. Other measures may include preliminary vasoconstriction, lubrication of the tube, gentle rotation as the tube is advanced, and evacuation of all air from the cuff to minimize its effective diameter. Efforts to rationalize the direction of the bevel as it passes the turbinate have not been demonstrated to change the incidence of this complication.

In most adults, tubes with a 7.0 to 7.5 mm ID pass easily through the nares. Other prelaryngoscopic maneuvers described under direct-vision orotracheal intubation (positioning of the head, suctioning, and preoxygenation) should be performed for direct-vision nasotracheal intubation. The nasotracheal tube should be lubricated and passed through the nose in one smooth, posterior, caudad, medially directed movement until resistance to forward movement significantly decreases as the tube enters the oropharynx (usually at a distance of 15 to 16 cm). Significant resistance should be overcome not by force but by withdrawal, rotation, and reinsertion of the ETT. Difficult passage should prompt the selection of the opposite nostril or of a smaller tube.

The pathway that the nasotracheal tube takes should be visualized as lying on its side. The curve of the ETT

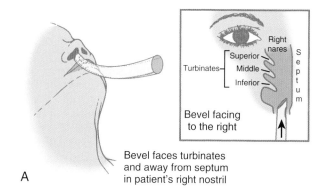

Bevel faces turbinates
and away from septum
in patient's right nostril

A

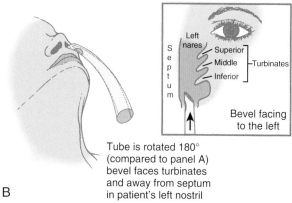

Tube is rotated 180°
(compared to panel A)
bevel faces turbinates
and away from septum
in patient's left nostril

B

Figure 17-11 Insertion of a nasotracheal tube into the nares. **A,** When the nasotracheal tube is passed into the right naris, the bevel should be facing to the right toward the turbinates *(inset)*. In this way, the tip of the tube is against the septum, and the risks of catching the tip of the tube on a turbinate and tearing or dislocating it are minimized. In this orientation, the concavity of the tube is pointing anteriorly. **B,** When the nasotracheal tube is passed into the left naris, the bevel should be facing to the left toward the turbinates *(inset)*. In this way, the tip of the tube is against the septum, and the risks of catching the tip of the tube on a turbinate and tearing or dislocating it are minimized. In this orientation the concavity of the tube is pointing posteriorly. *(From Benumof JL, editor: Airway management: Principles and practice, St. Louis, 1996, Mosby, p 273.)*

should be aligned to facilitate passage along this curved course. As the tube passes through the nose into the nasopharynx, it must be directed inferiorly to pass through the pharynx. In making this turn, it may strike against the posterior nasopharyngeal wall and resist any attempt to push it further. The tube should be pulled back a short distance, and the patient's head should be extended further to facilitate attempts to pass this point smoothly and atraumatically. If this is not performed and the tube is forced, the mucosal covering of the posterior nasopharyngeal wall may be torn, and the tube may be passed into the submucous tissues. This false passage is accompanied by a boggy feeling and by complete obstruction of the tube lumen.

B. Laryngoscopy

The laryngoscopy for nasotracheal intubation is identical to that described for orotracheal intubation.

C. Endotracheal Intubation

After the tube is in the oropharynx, the tip of the tube must be aligned with the glottic opening. This requires that the tip of the tube be visible in the hypopharynx. The tube should be advanced or withdrawn until this is the case. A combination of tube rotation and repositioning of the head may allow clear passage of the tube tip into the trachea, but it is likely that the tube will require guidance using Magill forceps held in the intubator's right hand.

The advantage of the design of these forceps is that when the grasping ends are parallel to the long axis of the ETT, the handle is outside the right side of the mouth and at a right angle to the long axis of the tube. Because the handle is outside the right side of the mouth, it is away from the line of sight. As the forceps are grasped parallel to the long axis of the tube, a backhand motion of the right hand passes the ETT toward the glottic opening (Fig. 17-12). The intubator can have the larynx exposed by the laryngoscope held in the left hand, the tube in full view, a means (using the forceps) of manipulating the alignment of the ETT, and a means of advancing the tube. However, it is often desirable to have an assistant advance the proximal end of the ETT so that the intubator is free to guide the tube into the larynx without having to pull it with the Magill forceps. The tip of the tube should be grasped to guide it into the trachea; grasping the cuff area is likely to lead to cuff trauma and possible damage. The addition of a small amount of air into the ETT cuff should center the tube within the glottis, and as the ETT is advanced, the cuff deflates.

In some patients, as the ETT enters the trachea, the tube's anterior curvature may direct it against the anterior tracheal wall and interfere with passage past this point. To resolve this difficulty, the head must be lifted (flexed) slowly as the ETT is advanced. A nasotracheal tube should be advanced until the cuff is 2 cm below the vocal cords or until the external markings are 24 to 25 cm for women and 26 to 27 cm for men (3 cm more than for oral ETTs) at the nares. The tube's correct placement must be verified as in any intubation (see "Verification of Correct Placement"), but this is particularly critical with nasotracheal intubations because the relation to external tube markings and the location of the tip are not as firmly established as for orotracheal intubations. If nasal bleeding occurs, it is probably wise to leave the ETT in place to provide tamponade. If the bleeding is severe, the ETT can be retracted and the cuff inflated to provide better tamponade.

D. Securing the Endotracheal Tube

The nasotracheal tube can be secured with adhesive tape as described for orotracheal intubation. A nasotracheal tube can be secured by a suture through the nasal septum and then tied, after being tightly wound around an adhesive band on the tube or passed through the wall of the tube by a needle and then tied.

IV. CONCLUSIONS

The art of laryngoscopic endotracheal intubation is one of infinite variety and unpredictability. We treat a diverse population of patients with many disease processes, and when their pathology includes airway abnormalities, gaining control of the airway can be a life-threatening or lifesaving process. Ongoing study and practice of airway techniques are the only protection we have in the intrinsically hazardous field of airway management. Mastery of the art begins with a mastery of the fundamentals. Although practiced by a wide variety of health professionals, laryngoscopic intubation is an extraordinarily complex and continually evolving branch of anesthesiology and critical care.

V. CLINICAL PEARLS

- Redundancy is the key to adequate preparation. All essential equipment (laryngoscopy handles and ETTs) should have back-up counterparts readily available in case of unexpected failure.

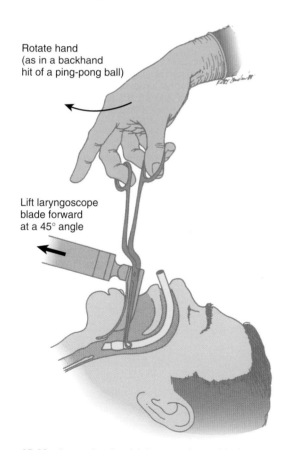

Guiding a nasotracheal tube into the larynx using a Magill forceps

Rotate hand (as in a backhand hit of a ping-pong ball)

Lift laryngoscope blade forward at a 45° angle

Figure 17-12 A nasotracheal tube can be guided under direct vision (laryngoscopic control) through the laryngeal aperture with a Magill forceps by rotating the hand as when using a backhand motion to hit a ping pong ball. The Magill forceps should grab the nasotracheal tube proximal to the cuff of the ETT. (From Benumof JL, editor: *Airway management: Principles and practice,* St. Louis, 1996, Mosby, p 275.)

- Proper positioning is essential to successful intubation. Atlanto-occipital extension is the most critical component of positioning. The sniffing position (with the occiput elevated 9 cm) may provide a more favorable laryngoscopic view.

- Preoxygenation delays the onset of hypoxemia by denitrogenating the lungs and filling the functional residual capacity (FRC) with O_2. The benefit of preoxygenation is limited in morbidly obese patients due to a decrease in FRC and an exaggerated cephalad diaphragmatic shift related to supine positioning.

- Although numerous techniques for tracheal cannulation exist, direct laryngoscopy is by far the most common technique.

- The tip of the laryngoscopic blade is inserted into the right side of the mouth and advanced toward the midline base of the tongue, displacing the tongue to the left side of the mouth. Lifting of the laryngoscopist's arm at a 45-degree angle from the long axis of the patient without moving the wrist exposes the epiglottis while minimizing risk of injury to the airway. The tip of a curved blade is inserted into the vallecula, thereby tensing the hypoepiglottic ligament, lifting the epiglottis, and exposing the arytenoids and glottic opening. The tip of a straight blade is extended beneath the laryngeal surface of the epiglottis, and subsequent upward and forward movement of the blade exposes the glottic opening.

- The use of a curved blade is thought to be less stimulating and less traumatic to the teeth and epiglottis than a straight blade, and it may provide more room for passage of the ETT through the oropharynx. A straight blade may provide a better view in a patient with a long epiglottis or anterior larynx.

- The use of optimal external laryngeal manipulation (OELM) can significantly improve the laryngoscopic view.

- It is essential to confirm endotracheal intubation by auscultation of breath sounds, chest wall excursion, lack of gastric sounds or distention, large exhaled V_T value, and a normal capnogram finding.

- The most common cause of inadvertent esophageal intubation is failure to clearly visualize the ETT pass through the vocal cords.

- Depths of 20 to 21 cm for women and 22 to 23 cm for men can safeguard against endobronchial intubation during orotracheal intubation.

- The ETT must be tightly secured to prevent inadvertent extubation or tube movement within the airway.

- Because nasotracheal intubation is thought to be better tolerated and has not been shown to be associated with an increased incidence of sinusitis, it is preferred over orotracheal intubation for medium-term mechanical ventilation. The nasal mucosa should be pretreated with a vasoconstrictor drug to facilitate nasotracheal intubation and to minimize the risk of trauma. Gentle head flexion may assist in the passage of a nasotracheal tube as it contacts the anterior tracheal wall.

SELECTED REFERENCES

All references can be found online at expertconsult.com.
6. Jackson C: *Bronchoscopy, oesophagoscopy, and gastroscopy*, ed 3, Philadelphia, 1934, WB Saunders.
8. Bannister FB, MacBeth RG: Direct laryngoscopy and tracheal intubation. *Lancet* 2:651, 1944.
9. Adnet F, Baillard C, Borron SW, et al: Randomized study comparing the "sniffing position" with simple head extension for laryngoscopic view in elective surgery patients. *Anesthesiology* 95:836–841, 2001.
13. Greenland KB, Edwards MJ, Hutton NJ, et al: Changes in airway configuration with different head and neck positions using magnetic resonance imaging of normal airways: A new concept with possible clinical applications. *Br J Anaesth* 105:683–690, 2010.
17. Gold MI, Duarte I, Muravchick S: Arterial oxygenation in conscious patients after 5 minutes and after 30 seconds of oxygen breathing. *Anesth Analg* 60:313–315, 1981.
20. Jense HG, Dubin SA, Silverstein PI, O'Leary-Escolas U: Effect of obesity on safe duration of apnea in anesthetized humans. *Anesth Analg* 72:89–93, 1991.
21. Teller LE, Alexander CM, Frumin MJ, Gross JB: Pharyngeal insufflation of oxygen prevents arterial desaturation during apnea. *Anesthesiology* 69:980–982, 1988.
23. Miller RA: A new laryngoscope. *Anesthesiology* 2:317–320, 1941.
24. Cormack RS, Lehane J: Difficult tracheal intubation in obstetrics. *Anaesthesia* 39:1105–1111, 1984.
25. Wilson ME, Spiegelhalter D, Robertson JA, Lesser P: Predicting difficult intubation. *Br J Anaesth* 61:211–216, 1988.

Chapter 18

Blind Digital Intubation

CHRIS C. CHRISTODOULOU | ORLANDO R. HUNG

I. HISTORY

Although it was probably first described by Herholdt and Rafn in 1796 for the management of drowning victims,[1] blind digital orotracheal intubation did not receive much attention in the medical literature until its revival in emergency medicine and prehospital care by Stewart in the mid-1980s.[2,3] Notable publications over the years have portrayed the technique as an acceptable, if not preferable, alternative to standard laryngoscopic endotracheal intubation, particularly when the standard technique is contraindicated, has failed, or is not possible because of a lack of equipment.

In 1880, Macewen described the technique utilizing a curved metal tube in awake patients,[4] and Sykes[5] recommended routine use of the digital technique in anesthetic practice in the 1930s. Siddall and Lanham relegated the technique to last-ditch efforts following the failure of conventional intubation methods.[3,6,7] The technique has been described in neonatal resuscitation and as an adjunct in blind nasotracheal intubation.[8-10]

Currently, there is widespread variation in awareness, expertise, and application of the technique in anesthesia, emergency medicine,[11,12] and prehospital care. Although advances in airway management equipment and expertise have made obsolete the routine use of blind digital orotracheal intubation, it remains a valuable skill in some situations, especially in the emergency setting or under circumstances in which the anesthesiologist cannot be positioned at the head of the patient,[3] rendering laryngoscopic intubation impossible.

II. INDICATIONS

The use of the digital technique is neither aesthetically pleasing, easily accomplished, nor entirely safe. Placing the fingers far enough down a patient's throat to elevate the epiglottis and guide an endotracheal tube (ETT) into the trachea has implications related to selection of patients and the manual dexterity and anatomic features of the anesthesiologist.

The technique has received some popularity in the prehospital care environment, where difficult positioning of the patient, poor lighting conditions, disrupted anatomy, potential cervical spine instability, and unknown status regarding infectious disease are the norm. Digital intubation is ordinarily used when other maneuvers have failed or are likely to fail and when alternative equipment is unavailable or not functional.

Successful digital intubation demands that the patient be unconscious, both for the patient to tolerate the intense oropharyngeal stimulus and to prevent bite injuries to the anesthesiologist. Neuromuscular blockade facilitates the technique, although it is relatively contraindicated in patients with anatomically difficult or disrupted airways. Digital intubation may be indicated in the following scenarios:

1. When equipment required to undertake alternative techniques is unavailable or not functional.
2. When positioning of the patient or the anesthesiologist prevents conventional intubation.
3. When other methods have failed or are likely to fail and the skill and experience of the anesthesiologist make the digital technique a reasonable alternative.
4. In the presence of potential or actual cervical spine instability when the anesthesiologist selects the digital technique on the basis of the risk-benefit analysis. Although there is no evidence to suggest that the use of digital intubation alters the neurologic outcome of a patient, there may be less cervical spine motion during intubation with the digital technique compared with conventional laryngoscopic orotracheal intubation without in-line stabilization.

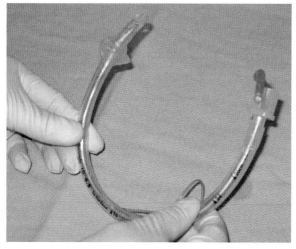

Figure 18-1 With the stylet in place, the distal half of the endotracheal tube is bent to a U shape.

5. When adequate visualization of the airway to allow conventional intubation is not possible because of the presence of copious secretions, blood, or vomitus in the oropharynx or traumatic disruption of the upper airway anatomy.

III. TECHNIQUE OF DIGITAL INTUBATION

A. Preparation

As with any intubation technique, preparation involves assembling the necessary equipment and personnel, including emergency drugs and adequate suction, to optimize success and preserve ventilation and oxygenation. An appropriately sized ETT is selected. The use of a stiff but malleable stylet improves maneuverability during the intubation. Lubrication of the stylet with a water-soluble lubricant ensures easy retraction after the tip of the ETT is placed in the glottic opening. The stylet is then inserted into the ETT so that the distal end of the stylet is at the level of the Murphy eye. With the stylet

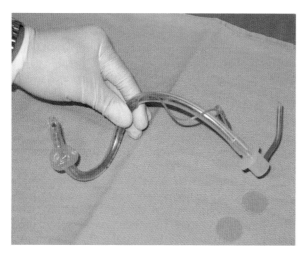

Figure 18-2 The proximal half of the endotracheal tube is bent 90 degrees toward the dominant side of the anesthesiologist.

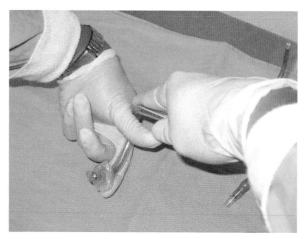

Figure 18-3 Final configuration of the styletted endotracheal tube (SETT) allows improved control of the ETT with both hands. During the intubation, the index finger of the dominant hand can help advance the ETT while the index and middle fingers of the nondominant hand guide the tip of the ETT into the glottis.

in place, the distal half of the styletted ETT unit (SETT) is bent into a "U" configuration (Fig. 18-1). The proximal half of the SETT is then bent approximately 90 degrees toward the dominant side of the ETT to allow manipulation of the SETT by the dominant hand during intubation (Figs. 18-2 and 18-3). The degree of bend should be individualized and is dependent on the anesthesiologist's experience.

The tip of the ETT should be well lubricated with a water-soluble lubricant. In the uncommon event that the intubation is performed in an awake patient, especially an uncooperative patient, a bite block should be placed between the patient's molars on one side to minimize the risk of injury to the anesthesiologist's fingers.

B. Positioning

The patient should be supine with the head in a slight sniffing position, as for laryngoscopic intubation. The anesthesiologist stands (or kneels if the patient is on the ground) beside the patient so that his or her nondominant side is closest to the patient. An assistant can help to facilitate the intubating procedure.

C. Technique

Pulling the tongue forward by an assistant facilitates palpation of the epiglottis, thus improving the success rate for digital intubation. The patient's mouth is opened, and the tongue is grasped gently by the assistant with a piece of gauze (Fig. 18-4). Traction on the tongue moves the epiglottis slightly cephalad, enhancing its palpability and facilitating placement of the tip of the ETT into the glottic opening. The anesthesiologist then inserts the index and middle fingers of the nondominant hand into the oral cavity and slides the palm down along the surface of the tongue (Fig. 18-5). The tip of the middle finger touches the tip of the epiglottis, which is then directed anteriorly (Fig. 18-6). The ease of palpating and lifting the epiglottis depends on the length of the

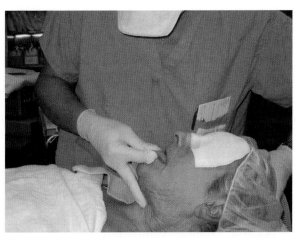

Figure 18-4 The tongue is grasped gently by an assistant with a piece of gauze. Traction on the tongue moves the epiglottis slightly cephalad, enhancing its palpability and facilitating the placement of the tip of the endotracheal tube into the glottic opening. An upward (cephalad) and backward (posterior) pressure applied anteriorly to the larynx by the assistant may help the anesthesiologist to feel the epiglottis during digital intubation.

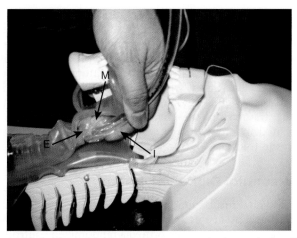

Figure 18-6 View of the larynx of a mannequin demonstrating the guidance of the endotracheal tube into the glottic opening by the tip of the index (I) and middle (M) fingers of the nondominant hand. The fingers are advanced to the point at which the middle finger is able to palpate the tip of the epiglottis (E) and push it anteriorly. Gloves should be worn at all times when performing the technique on patients.

anesthesiologist's fingers, the height of the patient, the anatomy of the oropharynx, and the presence or absence of teeth.

Once the epiglottis is identified and directed anteriorly, the SETT is inserted through the corner of the mouth. The SETT glides along the groove between the middle and index fingers on the palmar surface of the nondominant hand (see Fig. 18-3). While firm anterior pressure is maintained against the epiglottis with the middle finger, the SETT is advanced slowly into the glottic opening by the dominant hand. The index finger may be used to guide the tip of the SETT into the glottic opening (see Fig. 18-6).

The ETT should be stabilized while the stylet is withdrawn, and the ETT is then slowly advanced into the trachea. During the intubation, the SETT should never be advanced forcefully against resistance. Accurate placement is confirmed by conventional techniques, such as auscultation and carbon dioxide detection. Occasionally, the tip of the epiglottis cannot be palpated. An upward

(cephalad) and backward (posterior) pressure applied anteriorly to the larynx by an assistant may be helpful (see Fig. 18-4). As an alternative, the index and middle fingers of the nondominant hand may be used to keep the SETT in the midline while tissue movement in the anterior neck is observed during gentle rocking of the SETT back and forth in an attempt to locate the glottic opening.

An alternative technique described by Cook begins with placement of the index and middle finger tips of the nondominant hand in the hypopharynx, posterior to the larynx.[13] The ETT held in the dominant hand is then passed into the pharynx. The volar surfaces of the fingers serve as a "basketball backstop" to guide the ETT held in the dominant hand through the glottic opening. If required, the index finger of the nondominant hand may be flexed to help guide the ETT through the glottis.

D. Tracheal Introducer–Assisted Digital Intubation

A recent case report highlighted the use of a tracheal introducer (commonly known as "bougie") in facilitating a digital intubation technique in a patient with an unanticipated difficult airway after direct laryngoscopy attempts were unsuccessful.[14] A SunMed ETT Introducer (SunMed, Largo, FL) was first guided into the trachea using the digital technique. Tracheal clicks were used to confirm successful placement of the introducer in the trachea. The ETT was then guided into the trachea using the introducer as conduit.

The advantage of this technique is that it is easier to advance a tracheal introducer through the glottic opening and then railroad the ETT into the trachea than it is to place a SETT in the trachea. The tracheal introducer has a small outer diameter and is easily manipulated with the fingers to enable passage through the vocal cords. In addition, the clicks that are felt as the tracheal introducer advances over the tracheal rings, combined with

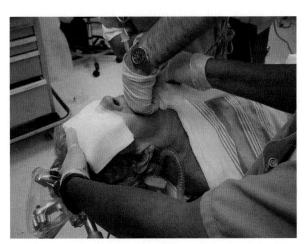

Figure 18-5 The index and middle fingers of the nondominant hand are inserted into the mouth with the palm facing down.

"hold-up," will assist in confirmation of tracheal place-ment. ("Hold-up" is the inability to advance the tracheal introducer beyond the lower bronchial tree. Esophageal placement of the tracheal introducer typically meets with no resistance, particularly when no anatomical abnormal-ity exists.) The SETT, which combines the ETT with the malleable stylet, is rigid and perhaps more likely to cause blunt trauma to the airway structures, especially if repeated manipulation is necessary for successful entry into the trachea.

E. Neonatal Digital Intubation

Blind digital intubation in neonates has not gained wide-spread acceptance as a primary technique of intubation. Moura and associates performed a randomized controlled trial comparing laryngoscopic intubation with the digital method in neonates.[15] They found that neonatal digital intubation had a higher success rate and a shorter intuba-tion time. A single experienced anesthesiologist was responsible for performing all the procedures, and this was identified as a study limitation.

Neonatal digital intubation has been used in several third-world countries where experience with and access to standard laryngoscopes are limited.[8] Hancock and Peterson used the blind digital intubation technique in neonatal resuscitation and accidental extubation situa-tions.[16] The anesthesiologist uses the gloved index finger of the nondominant hand to identify the epiglottis and glottic opening. The index finger is then used to guide the ETT through the glottic opening. The thumb of the nondominant hand can be used to apply external cricoid pressure. A SETT is recommended. The fifth finger of the nondominant hand can be used in very small neonates.

Advantages of the blind digital technique in neonates include reduced lip and gum trauma, controlled palpa-tion of anatomic landmarks, and easy access to the airway in various transport scenarios without the need to adjust lines and monitoring equipment in unstable patients. The technique can also be used to confirm accidental extuba-tion of the trachea. Caution should be exercised when airway pathology is suspected. Blind digital intubation of neonates and infants can be considered in situations in which other direct visualization techniques have failed.

F. Combined Techniques

The technique of blind digital intubation has been com-bined with the BAAM Whistle (Beck Airway Airflow Monitor, Great Plains Ballistics, Lubbock, TX) and the Endotrol tube (Mallinckrodt Medical, Argyle, NY) to facilitate endotracheal intubation in several situations after failure of direct laryngoscopy.[17,18] The BAAM device was initially developed to facilitate the teaching of blind nasotracheal intubation techniques under spontaneous ventilation. The BAAM produces a whistling sound of slightly different pitches during inspiration and expira-tion if the ETT is positioned within the air column leaving or entering the trachea. The device has also been shown to be effective in guiding nasotracheal tube place-ment in situations in which external cardiac massage is being applied.[18]

The Endotrol tube's unique design allows the anesthe-siologist to bend the distal tip anteriorly by pulling on a plastic wire that runs along the concave curvature of the ETT. This motion allows better alignment of the distal tip of the tube with the glottic opening.

In fiberoptic intubation, it can be difficult to advance the ETT into the trachea. Asai and colleagues reported use of the digital technique to help guide a 39-F double-lumen tube off the flexible fiberoptic bronchoscope and into the trachea of a patient undergoing an anterior tho-racic laminectomy procedure.[19] The anatomy of the patient's airway and that of the anesthesiologist's hand are key determinants in deciding which technique should be used in a given situation.

Light-guided endotracheal intubation using the Trach-light (Laerdal Medical, Wappingers Falls, NY) can be difficult in patients who have a long and floppy epiglot-tis.[20] This difficulty can be overcome by using the com-bined light-guided digital intubating technique. During the intubation, the middle finger of the nondominant hand can be used to lift the epiglottis off the posterior wall of the pharynx to allow the ETT with the Trachlight to go underneath the epiglottis into the glottic opening. The light glow at the anterior neck can be used to confirm the correct placement of the ETT tip into the glottis. During the past several years, we have performed more than 20 intubations using this combined light-guided digital intubating technique. The lightwand-guided intu-bation technique has also been described in newborns and infants with difficult airways.[21]

Digital assistance for nasotracheal intubation has been reported in the pediatric population to facilitate atrau-matic passage of the tube behind the soft palate and entrance into the trachea.[22] However, this technique has not been systematically studied in a randomized con-trolled trial.

IV. CASE HISTORY

Blind digital intubation is a relatively simple technique that can be learned easily. The following case history serves to illustrate the role of digital intubation in the emergency airway management of a patient whose trachea could not be intubated by the conventional method.

A call was received by the 911 center of a large, urban Emergency Medical Services (EMS) system reporting a "man not breathing" at a downtown hotel. A mobile intensive care unit from the nearest ambulance station was dispatched immediately. When it arrived 3 minutes later, the EMS team was directed to the top floor of the hotel, where a wedding reception was in progress. On the floor of a small washroom, the 120-kg patient was found in cardiac arrest, pulseless, and not breathing. According to the history given by relatives, the patient had chest pain while dancing after a large meal. He went into the washroom and collapsed.

Cardiopulmonary resuscitation (CPR) with bag-mask ventilation was performed immediately. Vomiting ensued, obscuring the laryngoscopic view of the paramedic who was attempting orotracheal intubation using a Macintosh laryngoscope. Suctioning was attempted with a portable suction unit, but so much vomitus was present that the collecting bottle of the suction unit filled rapidly and further suctioning was not possible in clearing the upper airway. "Quick-look" paddles revealed asystole.

While chest compressions and bag-mask ventilation continued, attempts at intravenous access were successful. Second and third attempts at direct laryngoscopic intubation resulted in esophageal placement, readily recognized by the paramedic team.

It became clear that further attempts at direct visualization of the airway would not be successful because of the large amount of vomitus in the oropharynx. A decision was made to place the ETT using the tactile (digital) method. An ETT with a 7.5-mm inner diameter was used. A physician carried out a digital intubation through the vomitus and secretions and was successful on the first attempt, as confirmed by colorimetric CO_2 detection. Ventilation and suctioning were performed through the ETT, and the patient's color improved. CPR continued during transport to a local hospital.

In another case, the editor of this book, who is director of advanced airway management at a Houston hospital, successfully performed blind digital intubation of a 51-year-old gentleman who had a history of insulin-dependent diabetes, hypertension, obesity, and peptic ulcer disease. An anesthesiologist was called emergently when this patient sustained a cardiac arrest in the intensive care unit after massive bleeding from a perforated gastric ulcer. When she arrived at the bedside, CPR was in progress. Although a Yankauer suction was immediately available and was being used, there was a continuous profuse stream of blood coming into the patient's oropharynx. While waiting for a cricothyrotomy kit to become available, she performed blind digital intubation and the airway was successfully secured with a size 8.0 ETT. The patient was resuscitated, and CPR was discontinued.

V. LIMITATIONS

Digital intubation in uncooperative patients is generally difficult. The more alert the patient is, the less likely it is that digital intubation will be tolerated or successful. Patients with limited mouth opening, carious or prominent dentition, a small mouth, or a large tongue, as well as very tall patients, can be predictably difficult to intubate regardless of the method employed, including the digital method. With practice, however, digital intubation has been shown to be an effective alternative method of intubation.[18]

The risk of injury to the anesthesiologist from the patient's teeth and body fluids can be minimized by selecting unconscious or paralyzed patients or by placing a bite block between the patient's molars. In our experience, double gloving provides a wider margin of safety in protection against barrier interruption, injury from teeth, and the potential for disease transmission.

As with other techniques of intubation, complications such as trauma to the upper airway can occur during digital intubation. However, trauma can be minimized by advancing the ETT gently during the intubation. Other potential complications of digital intubation, including esophageal intubation, can be minimized by a good technique, gentle manipulation, and use of tracheal placement confirmation techniques such as CO_2 detection.

Digital intubation is a "blind" technique and therefore is relatively contraindicated in patients with upper airway abnormalities resulting from infectious diseases, neoplasms, foreign bodies, caustic or thermal burns, or anaphylaxis.

VI. CONCLUSIONS

Digital intubation is seldom the method of first choice in securing a definitive airway. However, it offers an alternative that, in the event of failure of conventional techniques, may prove life-saving. Successful digital intubation depends largely on the anesthesiologist's preparation, experience, and skill.

VII. CLINICAL PEARLS

- Blind digital intubation should be considered as an airway management technique when alternative options are either unavailable or not functional.

- The technique may be considered in situations in which positioning for conventional intubation is not possible or soiling of the airway limits visualization of the larynx and glottis inlet.

- Universal infectious disease precautions must be taken at all times, and the patient's level of consciousness and state of paralysis must always be kept in mind.

- Pulling the tongue forward by an assistant during the technique facilitates traction on the epiglottis, thereby improving the overall chance of successful intubation.

- Blind digital intubation may be facilitated by the use of a tracheal introducer or bougie that produces confirmatory tracheal clicks before railroading of the ETT.

- Various intubation devices and techniques (e.g., BAAM whistle, Endotrol ETT, Trachlight, nasotracheal intubation, double-lumen ETT intubation) may be combined and facilitated by blind digital intubation.

- Successful ETT placement in the trachea after blind digital intubation should be confirmed with carbon dioxide detection devices.

- Experience with blind digital intubation in elective settings with patients who are anesthetized and paralyzed will enhance the clinician's skill acquisition and confidence in performance of the technique.

SELECTED REFERENCES

All references can be found online at expertconsult.com.
2. Stewart RD: Tactile orotracheal intubation. *Ann Emerg Med* 13:175–178, 1984.
5. Sykes WS: Oral endotracheal intubation without laryngoscopy: A plea for simplicity. *Curr Res Anesth Analg* 16:133, 1937.

10. Korber TE, Henneman PL: Digital nasotracheal intubation. *J Emerg Med* 7:275–277, 1989.
13. Cook RT Jr: Digital endotracheal intubation. *Am J Emerg Med* 10:396, 1992.
14. Rich JM: Successful blind digital intubation with a bougie introducer in a patient with an unexpected difficult airway. *Proc Bayl Univ Med Cent* 21:397–399, 2008.
15. Moura JH, da Silva GA: Neonatal laryngoscope intubation and the digital method: A randomized controlled trial. *J Pediatr* 148:840–841, 2006.
16. Hancock PJ, Peterson G: Finger intubation of the trachea in newborns. *Pediatrics* 89:325–327, 1992.
17. Cook RT, Jr, Polson DL: Use of BAAM with a digital intubation technique in a trauma patient. *Prehosp Disaster Med* 8:357–358, 1993.
21. Xue FS, Liu JH, Zhang YM, et al: The lightwand-guided digital intubation in newborns and infants with difficult airways. *Paediatr Anaesth* 19:702–704, 2009.
22. Mahajan R, Kumar S, Kumar Batra Y: Digital assistance of nasotracheal intubation: Another way to prevent trauma during nasotracheal intubation. *Paediatr Anaesth* 17:703, 2007.

Chapter 19

Fiberoptic and Flexible Endoscopic-Aided Techniques

KATHERINE S. L. GIL | PIERRE AUGUSTE DIEMUNSCH

I. INTRODUCTION AND HISTORICAL BACKGROUND

In addition to covering fundamental and advanced aspects of flexible fiberoptic/endoscopic airway management, this chapter focuses on exciting current inventions in airway equipment, related devices, and techniques.

The purpose of this chapter is threefold:

1. Incorporate recent airway management developments for integration with flexible endoscopes.
2. Impart knowledge concerning flexible endoscopic techniques and tips for airway use.
3. Increase the likelihood that readers might achieve a level of expertise in flexible endoscopic intubation and airway management.

Historically, a wide variety of devices have been employed to visualize the airway in living human subjects. Manuel Garcia, a singing instructor, ingeniously used mirrors to reflect sunlight in 1854, allowing him to examine his own moving vocal cords. He was considered the "first laryngoscopist" after a presentation to the Royal Society of Medicine.[1] Using a blind digital technique, William Macewen completed the first endotracheal intubation under anesthesia as well as the first awake intubation for surgery and anesthesia in 1878.[2] On hearing of an accidental intratracheal insertion in 1895, Alfred Kirstein used an esophagoscope that incorporated a proximal light source and spatula-like area to perform the first "direct" laryngoscopy.[3]

Bronchoscopy history began to develop in 1887, when Gustav Killian extracted a foreign body from a farmer's respiratory tract with a rigid bronchoscope. Chevalier Jackson modified this rigid bronchoscope by inclusion of a distal tungsten light bulb and suction channel in 1904, resulting in the significantly greater likelihood of successful endotracheal intubation.[4]

Finally, a remarkable development took place in 1966. Shigeto Ikeda proposed his ideas for construction of a flexible fiberoptic bronchoscope (FOB) to two companies, Machida Endoscope and Olympus.[5] Meanwhile, in 1967, Peter Murphy ingeniously used a choledochoscope for endotracheal intubation.[6] In 1968, the Machida company at last produced an extremely "bendable," guided FOB, which featured an eyepiece for seeing images transmitted along 15,000 glass fibers that were 14 μm in diameter. Clinically, Ikeda's technique was to insert this very flexible instrument through a rigid bronchoscope. Later that year, Olympus produced a more maneuverable FOB with a working channel that allowed the application of cytology brushes. Ikeda's new FOB pictures of the distal airway, presented at the International Congress on Disease of the Chest in Copenhagen, were instantaneously news-making revelations. He was able to demonstrate a stand-alone FOB insertion method for endotracheal intubation in many countries, and he published his experiences in 1971.[7]

Initially many clinicians advanced FOB use for diagnostic purposes, for ordinary intubation procedures, and, eventually, for airway management in patients with very challenging airways.[8-12] The inherent characteristic of FOB superiority forged its involvement as an instrument of first choice in difficult intubation (DI) cases, cervical spine risk scenarios, and as a diagnostic and therapeutic tool for patients with hypoxemia, high airway pressure, pulmonary tumors, infection, foreign bodies, airway stenosis, obstructive sleep apnea, tracheomalacia, and many more wide-ranging abnormalities.

Raj advocated the role of FOB assistance in double-lumen tube (DLT) placement[11] while Ovassapian further delineated its advantages in one-lung isolation in 1987.[13] Through FOB use, Benumof compared bronchial insertions of right and left DLTs to explain why the relationship of bronchial anatomy to DLT construction inevitably resulted in less successful right-sided DLT positioning.[14] In the 1980s, the Asahi Pentax Company's integration of the FOB with a preexisting invention, the charge-coupled device (CCD), permitted video monitor viewing of the airway and heightened its educational and clinical benefits.[15] FOB construction creativity has continued to evolve, with sizes available for all types of patients, many featuring full-color imaging and a working suction/injection channel. Light-emitting diodes (LED) and micro video complementary metal-oxide semiconductor chips (CMOS) for transmission capability have also been implemented.

Most recently, some flexible bronchoscopes have targeted the idea of being "single-use patient contact instruments," either as a reusable FOB with a disposable, sheath-like protective barrier or as an entirely disposable "non-fiberoptic" flexible bronchoscope.

Although universal acceptance of FOB use for intubation was somewhat slow for many years, Ovassapian and colleagues were leading and effective pioneers in the educational promotion of its use through workshop training and simulation, eventually popularizing this astonishingly effective technique.[16] Currently, the FOB resides worldwide within all algorithms for DI, and there is a clear, growing tendency to use this technique in combination with other recent advances as a multimodal approach to difficult airway (DA) management.

II. FLEXIBLE FIBEROPTIC AND NON-FIBEROPTIC BRONCHOSCOPE DESIGN AND CARE

FOBs and non-fiberoptic flexible bronchoscopes (non-FOBs) are available from a number of manufacturers, including Olympus, Pentax, Karl Storz, Ambu, and Vision Sciences. For simplicity, all "scopes" will be referred to as FOBs, unless indicated. Most FOBs are very expensive and quite delicate. Knowledge of their functionality and care is paramount to prevent damage and loss of clinical availability. Repair costs may reach more than $1000 per instrument per month in teaching hospitals in the United States but can drop to almost one-fiftieth of that with diligent care and training.

A. Fiberoptic Bronchoscope Design

Variations in design may seem endless, but all flexible endoscopes have certain commonalities. Differences are described later in this chapter. There are three main parts: handle, insertion tube, and flexible tip (Fig. 19-1).

At the end of the handle is either a battery-operated light source, which allows for more portability, or an optical cable connection to an external light source. The proximal "visual section" of the handle is the location of an eyepiece and lens, a video output adaptor, or an actual video screen with an integrated camera (depending on the model). FOBs with a CCD or CMOS camera chip at the tip have a wide-angle image and a higher resolution of the picture transmitted, compared with older models, which have a narrower field of view and less optical detail (Fig. 19-2). This makes video fiberscope deployment useful clinically, particularly in teaching.

Many FOBs have a visible black notch in the eyepiece at the 12-o'clock position to aid with orientation. Near the handle, an adjustable focusing ring or diopter can be

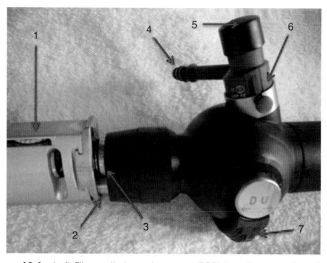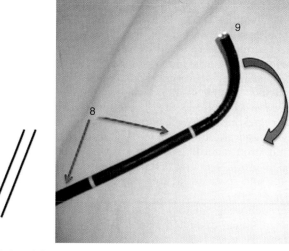

Figure 19-1 *Left,* Fiberoptic bronchoscope (FOB) handle (control section) design. *1,* Focus adjusting ring; *2,* light source connection; *3,* video output connection; *4,* suction port; *5,* valve; *6,* working channel; *7,* angulation control lever. *Right,* FOB insertion tube leading to flexible tip: *8,* Insertion tube; *9,* flexible tip.

fine-tuned to sharpen the image. Some models have a venting ethylene oxide sterilization cap nearby.

The handle is attached to the insertion tube (i.e., the section that goes into the patient). The tube's outer diameter (OD) determines the minimum internal diameter (ID) of the endotracheal tube (ETT) into which the FOB can easily pass. Insertion tubes average 50 to 65 cm in length and are surrounded by a flexible inner stainless steel mesh and a flexible outer, water-impermeable plastic wrap.

Four specific components travel inside the insertion tube along the FOB length (Fig. 19-3). The first allows the transmission of light going toward the tip by way of one or two light guide bundles constructed of noncoherent glass fibers. A high degree of light intensity is focused on the proximal light guide bundle, but heat filters or reflecting mirrors prevent injury to the insertion tube components.

The eyepiece lens in the handle and the objective lens of the FOB tip are perpendicular to the longitudinal axis of the insertion tube, enabling the second tube

component to transmit identical patient images from the distal lens to the proximal one. This component involves 10,000 to 50,000 glass fibers, as low as 8 to 9 μm in diameter, which are arranged in coherent bundles to transmit the image to the visual section in a completely spatially oriented state. (By comparison, human hairs are 17 to 180 μm in diameter.) A secondary glass cladding layer surrounds each strand to reflect light internally and maintain intensity by preventing external absorption or reflection of light from the lateral surface of each fiber. The glass fibers are extremely sensitive to damage. Although many thousands of fibers might seem expendable, when one is broken, a black dot becomes visible within the transmitted image. Excessive FOB bending, dropping, or external pressure (e.g., by teeth) can quickly

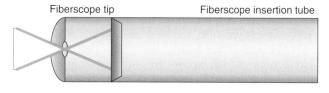

Fiberscope tip   Fiberscope insertion tube

Legend:

▷ Field of view

◍ Lens

▮ CCD chip

✕ Light rays of image entering fiberscope

Figure 19-2 Fiberoptic tip mechanics: Field of view. Insertion tip transmission of light through a lens to the charge-coupled device *(CCD)* chip.

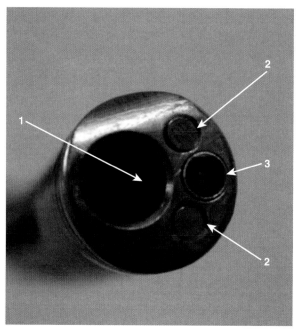

Figure 19-3 Fiberoptic tip components. *1,* Working channel; *2,* two angulation wires; *3,* cladded fiberoptic-lighted bundle.

add up to many dozens of black spots, rendering significant impairment of FOB visual acuity and necessitating costly repair.

On the back of the handle is a bending or angulation lever. Through an up or down movement of the thumb, it causes pulling on the third insertion tube component located along the sagittal plane, the two angulation wires. This initiates movement of the FOB tip in the opposite direction (i.e., down or up, respectively) by as much as 240 to 350 degrees (see Fig. 19-1). These delicate wires can also be broken with excessive pressure, including lever motion if the FOB tip is still within the ETT lumen.

The last component is termed the working channel; it is 1.2 to 2.8 mm in diameter and runs the length of the FOB from the suction or working port on the handle to the FOB tip. When the working port is attached to suction or oxygen tubing, the nearby spring valve can be opened by index finger pressure to allow suctioning or oxygen administration. Alternatively, a syringe with local anesthetic or other medication can be attached to the working port (also called the suction port) or to the biopsy/injection port below the handle (present in some models). When drugs are being given, the operator must make sure the suction is off so that the medication actually goes forward.

The FOB tip or bending section is hinged and has an objective lens (approximately 2 mm in diameter) with a fixed focal point and a short field of view (75 to 120 degrees) (see Figs. 19-1 to 19-3).

Many models are available in sizes from premature infant to large adult and with varying fields of view, video monitors, closed-valve systems, and other features (Table 19-1).

B. Fiberoptic Bronchoscope Cleaning

Almost half a million bronchoscopies are performed per year in the United States.[17] Whenever any equipment is

TABLE 19-1

Comparison of Specifications of Flexible Fiberoptic and Endoscopic Intubating Devices

Models	Unique Qualities	Light Source	External Diameter (mm)	Working Channel (mm)	Working Length (cm)	Tip Field-of-View Range (degrees)	Up/Down Range of Motion (degrees)
Olympus							
LFV	Fib; CCD	Electric	4.1	1.2	60	120	120/120
LF-DP, LF-GP, LF-TP	Fib	Battery/electric	3.1-5.2	1.2-2.6	60	90	120-180/120-130
LF-P	Fib; neonate	Electric	2.2	—	60	75	120/120
MAF-GM, TM	Fib; built-in screen; camera	Battery	4.1-5.2	1.5-2.6	60	90	120-180/120-130
BF-XP60, BF-3C40, BF-MP60, BF-P60, BF-IT60, BF-XT40	Fib; designed for therapeutic applications	Electric	2.8-5.9	1.2-3	Up to 55-60	90-120	180/130
Other BF models	Some have CCD; often for therapeutic applications (including intubation); one autoclavable model						
Pentax							
F1-7BS, F1-7RBS	Fib; neonate; eyepiece; CVS	Battery	2.4	—	60	95	130/130
F1-9BS, F1-10BS, F1-13BS, F1-16BS	Fib; eyepiece; CVS	Battery/electric	3.1-5.1	1.2-2.6	60	90-95	130-160/130
F1-9RBS, F1-10RBS, F1-13RBS, F1-16RBS	Fib; eyepiece; CVS	Battery/electric	3.1-5.1	1.2-2.6	60	90-95	130-160/130
EB-1570K, EB-1970K	Fib; CCD; CVS	Electric	5.1-6.3	2.0-2.8	60	120	180-210/130
Karl Storz							
K.S. 1130 AB, K.S 11302 BD, K.S. 11301 BN	Fib; CCD	Battery/electric	2.8-5.0	1.2-2.3	50-65	80-110	120-160/120-160
Ambu							
Ambu aScope	CMOS; no suction; disposable	Battery	5.3	0.8	63	80	120/120
Vision Sciences							
BRS-4000	Fib; disposable EndoSheath with suction	Battery	Insertion tube, 1.5-2.1+ Channel, 5.2-5.8	1.5-2.1	57	90	215/135
BRS-5000	Fib; disposable EndoSheath with suction		Insertion tube, 1.5-2.1+ Channel, 5.2-5.8	1.5-2.1	57	120	215/135

CCD, Charge-coupled device; *CMOS*, complementary metal-oxide semiconductor; *CVS*, closed-valve system (allows fluid injection without siphoning into the suction); *Fib*, fiberoptic.

reused between patients, there is always a concern for avoiding the transmission of communicable diseases. Although there have not been any reports of infection or cross-contamination caused by fiberoptic intubation for elective or emergency purposes, sporadic references testify to instances of infection or contamination after flexible bronchoscopic procedures such as bronchial washings or bronchoscopic lavage. Between the years 2000 and 2007, the American Association for Respiratory Care (AARC), American College of Chest Physicians (AACP), American Association for Bronchology and Interventional Pulmonology (AABIP), and Association for Professionals in Infection Control (APIC) issued guidelines and consensus statements to assist in the prevention of FOB-associated infection or contamination.[18-20]

Since the 1970s, sources of contamination have included a number of factors: sentinel patients, contaminated water, inadequate sterilization technique (due to insufficient quality or quantity of sterilizing solution), repeated use of cleaning fluid or brushes, automated endoscope reprocessors, and FOB instruments with design errors or damage.[21-24] Valves and working channels are usually the most suspect areas for ineffective FOB sterilization. Multiple organisms have been found, including *Pseudomonas aeruginosa*, non-tuberculosis mycobacteria, *Serratia marcescens*, *Mycobacterium tuberculosis, Stenotrophomonas maltophilia*, *Legionella pneumophila, Rhodotorula rubra*, *Klebsiella* species, *Proteus* species, and fungi.[21,25-28]

When an FOB is being used for patient management, involved clinical sites automatically fall under the aegis of mandatory universal precautions. Constant vigilance in FOB care and high-level disinfection are imperative. Once used, an FOB should be directly handed off to trained assistants or placed in a vertical holding tube (e.g., ProShield, Seitz Technical Products, Avondale, PA) for rapid pickup. Holding tubes should be long enough to handle FOBs up to 65 cm in length; they prevent damage and contamination that might occur from contact with other equipment or people.

Disinfection may take up to 45 min (Fig. 19-4). The assistant should carefully insert a cleaning brush into portals entering the working channel. The brush must be advanced fully along the compete span of this conduit to effect early removal of secretions according to the instructions of the manufacturer and the health care organization.

Next, the FOB has to be diligently inspected for any damage, tears, indentations, or abnormalities along its entire length. A leak test to detect holes in the insertion tube sheath is essential at this point, and failures necessitate sending the FOB for repairs without any further sterilization.

The suction ports and biopsy ports (if present) need to be disassembled from the rest of the FOB. All nondisposable parts must be gently placed in glutaraldehyde, peracetic acid, orthophthaldehyde, hydrogen peroxide gas plasma, or other manufacturer-indicated sterilization solution, and the working channel must be syringe-flushed with this disinfectant conforming to manufacturer and health care organization instructions.[29-31]

After completion of the specified sterilization time, all parts must be removed to prevent caustic damage to the

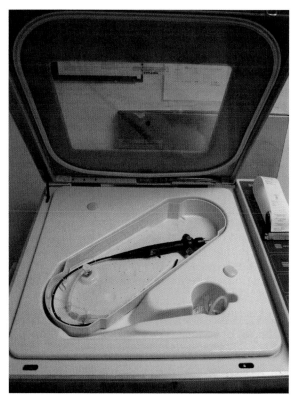

Figure 19-4 Steris machine for sterilization of a fiberoptic bronchoscope. The working channel is flushed out before being carefully placed within the sterilizer.

instrument. The FOB should be gently washed and thoroughly rinsed with sterile water, including flushing of the working channel to prevent toxicity from residual chemicals.[32] It is mandatory to dry the channel by suctioning or purging with 70% alcohol and compressed air for a time period in keeping with manufacturer and health care organization instructions.

Most bacteria, fungi, and viruses are susceptible to these sterilization processes, including human immuno-deficiency virus (HIV) and hepatitis. FOBs that have been used in patients with contagious diseases (e.g., tuberculosis) may require a lengthy ethylene oxide sterilization and aeration procedure for up to 24 hours, with the venting cap secured to the venting connector. In the case of suspected prion infection (Creutzfeldt-Jakob or variants), it is best to avoid bronchoscopy if possible, because the sterilization process for most medical instruments would be damaging.[18-20,33]

Presently, routine surveillance cultures have not been recommended by the AARC, AACP, AABIP, or APIC because of lack of criteria to determine testing frequency, relevance when positive results occur, indeterminate courses of action, and costs of testing procedures.[18-20]

During all handling and sterilization techniques, keeping the FOB as straight as possible is extremely important to avoid damage. Once the device has been cleaned, it is preferable to store it suspended by its handle in a moderately lighted, climate- and humidity-controlled, safe location. Close proximity to radiation should be avoided because of deleterious effects on the FOB material.[34]

C. Disposable Flexible Bronchoscopes

Because efforts toward the production of a truly auto-clavable FOB (e.g., Bronchosteril endoscope, Andromis, Geneva, Switzerland) did not lead to a widely accepted device, other solutions aimed at a simplified approach to the prevention of cross-contamination were developed.

1. Sheathed Fiberoptic Bronchoscope

Vision Sciences, Inc. (Orangeburg, NY) has produced two adult-sized, channel-less FOBs for use with a clear, durable, snugly fitting, presterilized flexible, thermoplastic, elastomer EndoSheath that incorporates its own 1.5- to 2.1-mm working channel. The disposable sheath potentially prevents transmission of organisms and may increase FOB availability by requiring no down-time for sterilization. It might also reduce costs in centers where economic factors limit the purchase of more than a minimum number of bronchoscopy systems or limit the availability of sterilization equipment or personnel.[35,36]

2. Non-fiberoptic Flexible Bronchoscope

The Ambu aScope (Ambu A/S, Ballerup, Denmark) is a fully disposable, sterile, battery-operated non-FOB with a small (0.8-mm) working channel capable of drug instillation but not suctioning. It has a CMOS chip, a steering button to flex the tip, and a distal LED (Fig. 19-5). Images are transmitted along a cable within the insertion tube and transferred to a small portable monitor by way of a video connection cable at the handle. In its early version, this non-FOB had a timing mechanism allowing it to function for a maximum of 30 minutes during an 8-hour period starting from the initial power startup. A more recent version of this device comes without these time limitations. The monitor can be used for 150 intubations and is connected to an external monitoring system. Apart from routine use of this instrument, a particular advantage may occur in patients with highly contagious disease (e.g., Creutzfeldt-Jakob), in immunosuppressed patients, or in situations in which cheaper devices may be beneficial (e.g., where economic factors limit purchases or where FOB is seldom used).[37,38]

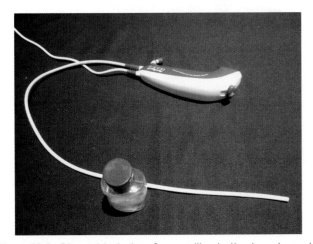

Figure 19-5 Disposable Ambu aScope with a button lever to angle the tip down or up.

III. RATIONALE FOR FIBEROPTIC INTUBATION

Airway management failure is a leading cause of patient morbidity and mortality in closed claims analyses.[39] During the period 1999 to 2005, failed intubation or DI was the cause of 2.3% of the 2211 anesthesia-related deaths in the United States.[40] With rigid laryngoscopes (RLs), DI was reported to have a frequency ranging from 1% to 13%.[41-45] Shiga and colleagues performed a meta-analysis of studies on 50,760 patients and estimated the average occurrence of difficult intubation to be 5.8%,[46] with a range of 4.5% to 7.5% overall[47,48] and an even greater incidence in obstetric or obese patients.[49-51] Anesthesia Associates, Inc. (AincA), San Marcos, CA Benumof's estimate of "cannot intubate, cannot mask-ventilate" scenario was verified by Heidegger and associates at 0.007%,[52,53] whereas Kheterpal and coworkers showed the incidence of impossible mask ventilation to be 0.15% in a prospective series of 53,041 patients.[54]

FOB intubation has always had a place in these scenarios, but this simple technique seems formidable to many. However, despite the increasing availability of less expensive intubating supraglottic airways (SGAs), lighted stylets, video laryngoscopes (VLs), and optical laryngoscopes (OLs), an explosion of improved laryngoscopic views, and greater intubating success rates, there is still a definite need for FOB intubation. A survey of American anesthesiologists by Rosenblatt and colleagues revealed a strong preference for FOB intubation for DA patients.[55] Avarguès and associates' survey of French anesthetists in 1999 revealed that 64% of responders expressed the need for more training in FOB intubation.[56] Furthermore, FOB use was mentioned twice in the revised 2003 DA algorithm by a panel of experts who formulated the American Society of Anesthesiologists (ASA) Practice Guidelines for Difficult Airway Management.[57] In a 2009 review of the existing algorithms for DA management, Frova and Sorbello affirmed that FOB is universally recognized as the gold standard in the awake, sedated, or anesthetized "difficult to intubate" patient.[58]

Finally and more practically, there have been numerous cases in which older devices and even the most recently developed airway management devices have proved to be inadequate. FOB employment and assistance steadfastly facilitates the execution of successful intubations, often rescuing these failures, either alone or as part of a multimodal approach to the DA.[59,60]

The FOB has a number of unique, wide-ranging characteristics:

- Its flexible, gliding attributes allow FOB skimming along the most twisted of DA obstacle courses while still posting the highest success rates for intubation.
- During intubation, the FOB is the device least likely to result in any cervical spine motion.[61]
- The FOB can be used for intubation in any body position, via oral or nasal routes, in all age groups.
- Under excellent local airway anesthesia, FOB intubation is associated with negligible hemodynamic changes.
- The FOB has multiple diagnostic capabilities for determining abnormal anatomy, assisting with

implementation of other airway devices, and trouble-shooting ventilatory problems.

A. Indications for Flexible Fiberoptic or Endoscopic Intubation

Although many anesthesiologists routinely carry out FOB intubation on all of their patients, most tend to adhere to specific indications. There is no hard or fast rule for "awake" versus "asleep" fiberoptic intubation. An awake approach is usually chosen to lessen significant patient risk in comparison to other methods, especially rigid laryngoscopy. The awake approach may be more advisable in cases of a very difficult airway or with a somewhat difficult airway in a patient with intolerant comorbidities endangered by the trauma or hypoxemia of non-FOB techniques (e.g., critical coronary artery disease). A list of indications for flexible airway endoscopy is presented in Box 19-1.

B. Contraindications: Absolute, Moderate, and Relative

The most important contraindication to FOB use may well be lack of skill of the endoscopist (i.e., FOB operator) due to inadequate training or inadequate maintenance of formerly acquired skills. Any lack of a trained assistant or of available, ready to use, proper equipment may also negate FOB plans. There are few other contraindications to FOB use. These may involve situations in

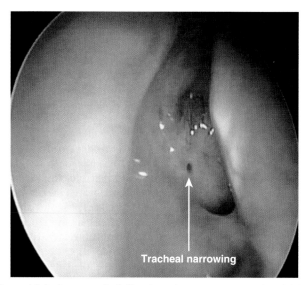

Figure 19-6 Severe subglottic stenosis appears as a pinpoint tracheal opening.

which harm to the instrument may occur (e.g., uncooperative patients), cases in which FOB use is extremely likely to be unsuccessful (e.g., patients with known near-total upper airway obstruction [Fig. 19-6]), or rare instances in which another technique may pose less risk for airway management (e.g., patients who have massive facial trauma with excessive bleeding might do better with a tracheostomy). Contraindications for awake and asleep FOB intubation are listed in Boxes 19-2 and 19-3, respectively.

Box 19-1	**Indications for Use of Flexible Fiberoptic or Endoscopic Intubation**

1. Routine intubation
2. Difficult intubation (DI)
   a. History of prior DI
   b. Suspected DI from patient history or physical examination
   c. Rescue of failed intubation attempt
   d. Intubating patients with preexisting Combitube or Rüsch EasyTube
3. Prevention of cervical spine motion in at-risk patients
4. Avoidance of traumatic oral or nasal effects of intubation (e.g., loose teeth, nasal polyps)
5. Avoidance of aspiration in high-risk patients
6. Diagnostic purposes
   a. Trouble-shooting high airway pressures
   b. Trouble-shooting hypoxemia
   c. Observation for airway pathology (e.g., stenosis, tracheomalacia, vocal cord paralysis)
   d. Removal of airway pathology (e.g., secretions)
7. Therapeutic uses beyond planned FOB intubation
   a. Endotracheal tube exchange
   b. Assistance with airway placement (e.g., SGA, retrograde intubation, etc.)
   c. Positioning of double-lumen tubes or bronchial blockers
   d. Positioning of endotracheal tubes at specific depths
   e. Intratracheal observation of initial tracheostomy instrument entry

FOB, Fiberoptic bronchoscope; *SGA*, supraglottic airway device.

Box 19-2	**Contraindications for Awake FOB Techniques**

1. Absolute contraindications
   a. A completely wild, uncooperative patient
   b. Lack of endoscopist skill, assistance, or equipment
   c. Near-total upper airway obstruction unless for diagnostic purposes
   d. Massive trauma (but, if retrograde intubation is chosen, FOB may help; see text)
2. Moderate contraindications
   a. Relatively uncooperative patient
   b. Obstructing or obscuring blood, fluid, anatomy, or foreign body in the airway that might inhibit success
   c. Very small entry space
3. Relative contraindications
   a. Concern for vocal cord damage that might be caused by blind ETT passage over the FOB
   b. With some perilaryngeal masses, blindly advancing the ETT can "cork out" or seed the tumor (this situation should be discussed with the ENT specialist, if possible)
   c. Documented or suspected nonconventional infectious agents, agents resistant to multiple drugs, or infectious diseases in the absence of a single-use device

ENT, Ear, nose, and throat; *ETT*, endotracheal tube; *FOB*, fiberoptic bronchoscope.

1. Absolute contraindications
   a. Lack of endoscopist skill, assistance, or equipment
   b. Near-total upper airway obstruction unless for diagnostic purposes
   c. Massive trauma (but, if retrograde intubation was chosen, FOB may help; see text)
2. Moderate contraindications
   a. Too high an aspiration risk or too difficult an airway
   b. Inability to tolerate even a short period of apnea
   c. Obstructing or obscuring blood, fluid, anatomy, or foreign body in the airway that might inhibit success
   d. Very small entry space
3. Relative contraindications
   a. Concern for vocal cord damage that might be caused by blind ETT passage over the FOB
   b. With some perilaryngeal masses, blindly advancing the ETT can "cork out" or seed the tumor (this situation should be discussed with the ENT specialist, if possible)
   c. Documented or suspected nonconventional infectious agents, agents resistant to multiple drugs, or infectious diseases in the absence of a single-use device

ENT, Ear, nose, and throat; *ETT,* endotracheal tube; *FOB,* fiberoptic bronchoscope.

IV. EQUIPMENT

A. Fiberoptic and Non-fiberoptic Bronchoscope Model Details

FOB specifications and characteristics have been presented in Table 19-1. Some models have eyepieces or video attachments. Others have varying degrees of portability. Sizes and ranges of view are also variable, from the smallest infant to the largest adult size. In 2010, Olympus developed a unique MAF-GM system; it features a lithium rechargeable battery-operated FOB with a fixed, rotatable video screen by the handle—all totally immersible for sterilization. Its CCD camera has a memory card and an xD chip for still photography and video recording.

B. Fiberoptic Bronchoscope Cart

Preparation for highly useful FOB techniques is important to increase the likelihood of success. The incorporation of an FOB cart as a movable asset capable of rapid transport to operating rooms, specialty units, or floors is ideal for routine or emergency use. Contents need to be arranged logically in a readily available design so that the composition and organization will be uniform across the facility in the event that more than one cart is needed for an institution. All airway specialists must be familiar with the contents of the FOB cart and know how to have it transported to required patient sites without delay. Preferably, the cart should have two widely separated tubular structures for hanging a clean FOB and, later, a used one (Fig. 19-7). Typically, the FOB cart will also

have a light source, a video monitor (ideally), endoscopy masks, bronchoscopy swivel adapters, oral intubating airways, bite blocks, atomizers, tongue blades, cotton-tipped swabs, gauze, soft nasal airways, and local anesthetics (e.g., 2% and 4% lidocaine, 2% lidocaine gel or paste).

In addition to clinical use, FOB carts can be used for institutional continuous education programs and teaching workshops. All carts should be organized and upgraded by the anesthesiology team.

Optionally, an FOB cart setup could also be incorporated as part of a more complete DA cart that includes items needed to follow the DA algorithm. Among other items, a DA cart should contain a VL and screen, SGAs, intubating SGAs, ETT introducer/exchangers,[62,63] and percutaneous airway rescue sets.

C. Ancillary Equipment

1. Bronchoscopy Swivel Adapters and Endoscopy Masks

Bronchoscopy adapters and endoscopy masks are often used in asleep or awake patients for FOB examination, intubation, diagnosis, or therapy.

Bronchoscopy swivel adapters have the capacity to rotate when placed between the ventilating system and a mask, SGA, or ETT. They look like elbow adapters but are equipped with a "flip-cap port" covering a diaphragm with a central opening (Fig. 19-8). This permits passage

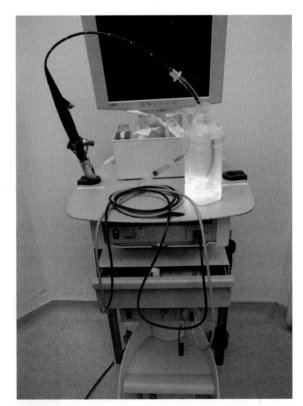

Figure 19-7 Mobile fiberoptic cart with a video screen and supplies underneath. The fiberoptic bronchoscope (FOB) is braced in the clean container on the left, and a holding tube for the used FOB is located on the right. The FOB insertion section lies within an endotracheal tube in a warm saline solution.

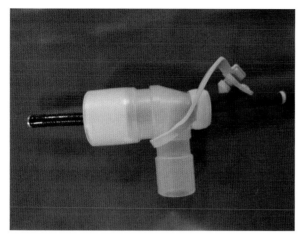

Figure 19-8 Bronchoscopy swivel adapter with a snug fiberoptic bronchoscope diaphragm opening that allows ventilation without leaking.

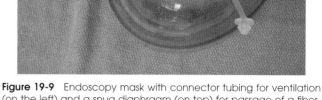

Figure 19-9 Endoscopy mask with connector tubing for ventilation (on the left) and a snug diaphragm (on top) for passage of a fiberoptic bronchoscope within an endotracheal tube.

of an FOB with virtually no leak during use of the continuous ventilation system on a patient.

Endoscopy masks differ from regular masks by having at least one larger additional opening whose function is similar to that of a bronchoscopy swivel adapter port (Fig. 19-9). The opening permits both FOB and ETT passage for intubation during continuous mask ventilation. Some masks have recessed one-way, valve-like openings for FOB and ETT entry.

2. Intubating Oral Airways

Intubating oral airways (IOAs) are often used in unconscious patients or in the topically anesthetized oropharynx of awake patients to act as a conduit through which an FOB is inserted for oral intubation (Fig. 19-10). It is

extremely useful when an assistant holds the IOA midline throughout the intubation procedure. These airways should not be jammed fully into the patient if they seem too large for smaller mouth openings. If no IOA is used secondary to inadequate mouth opening or endoscopist preference, a bite block should be placed between the molars or incisors to prevent FOB injury.

The ideal IOA would have the following advantages: It would protect the FOB from damage caused by the patient's teeth or jaws, shield the FOB from the tongue and soft tissues, have an ideal length to form a path leading to the glottis, allow passage of an adequate-sized ETT, permit maneuverability of the ETT and FOB within it, possess a breakaway quality for easy removal after intubation, and have the ability to assist with mask

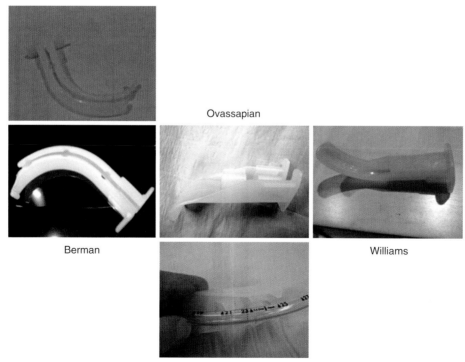

Ovassapian

Berman

Williams

Figure 19-10 From left to right, Berman, Ovassapian, and Williams intubating oral airways.

ventilation as needed. In a truly ideal world, this ideal IOA would provoke no gag reflex, even without local anesthesia (LA).

Most studies comparing characteristics of different IOA involve non-DA.[64] No IOA is ideal, and some have disadvantages: Sizes may be too great for patients with small mouth openings; their construction may cause palate or other tissue discomfort or trauma during placement; they may lead the FOB astray (off midline); ETT cuffs may catch and tear on them; and their removal may be slightly intricate. All IOAs are disposable except for the aluminum-made Patil-Syracuse (Anesthesia Associates, Inc. (AincA), San Marcos, CA) oral airway.

The Berman intubating pharyngeal airway (Teleflex Medical Research, Triangle Park, NC) admits ETTs of 8.5 mm or smaller diameter and comes in various adult, child, and neonatal sizes. Its full-length tubular shape does not permit FOB maneuvering, but it has a wide slit the length of its side for breaking away from the ETT after intubation. If kept midline, it provides a better lead to the glottis, assuming its length is appropriate.[65] If the length is too long, its distal end is usually found in the vallecula; pulling it out 1 to 2 cm may rectify that situation. Lateral breaking away of this airway from the ETT can be difficult, particularly if periglottic ETT impingement has occurred.

The proximal half of the Ovassapian fiberoptic intubating airway (Teleflex Medical Research Triangle Park, NC) has a channel that permits passage of an ETT with a diameter of 9 mm or less. This channel has flexible lateral walls and an opening posteriorly for easy ETT removal. The distal half of the airway has a wide, flat, curved area designed to keep the tongue and soft tissues away from the FOB. Its flatness makes it easier to keep it in the midline, and its openness permits free FOB movement throughout its length. Once the FOB is near the carina and the ETT enters between the teeth, this IOA can be partially broken away to avoid tearing the ETT cuff on its corners. FOB orientation during passage through the device can be assisted by drawing a line with a marker lengthwise down the middle of the concave surface of the IOA.[66]

The Williams airway intubator (Williams Airway Intubator LTD, Calgary, Canada) has two adult sizes that allow passage of an ETT of 8.5 mm diameter or smaller. Proximally, it has a circumferentially closed channel and a distally curved section with a scalloped opening on the lingual surface. The distal area permits free FOB movement. As long as this airway is kept midline and its length is appropriate, it may be the best guide to the larynx.[67] If it is too long, visualization can be problematic. There may be a concern for more frequent cuff damage with ETT sizes larger than 7.0 mm when using the smaller size of this IOA. For removal, the ETT has to be disengaged from the 15-mm ETT connector. The enclosed channel part should have been liberally prelubricated to accomplish easier ETT release. Sometimes removal can be difficult.[68]

3. Short, Soft Nasopharyngeal Airways

Two techniques have described use of nasopharyngeal airways (NPAs) during FOB intubation. A method to simplify nasal FOB intubation by using a lengthwise, laterally cut NPA for breakaway capability was reported by Lu and colleagues (Fig. 19-11).[69] The lubricated, modified NPA is gently inserted into one nostril. Afterward, the lubricated FOB is guided through this NPA with the idea that the FOB tip will lead directly toward the glottis. After the FOB has entered just above the carina, the NPA is stripped away, and the ETT is railroaded over the FOB into the trachea.

A second advantage of NPA use is its role during FOB intubation in oxygen administration and as a conduit for inhalation anesthesia administration (most commonly in pediatric patients).[70,71] This is particularly advantageous when FOB intubation is preferred to be undertaken unhurriedly in spontaneously breathing patients who need extra anesthesia. An NPA (often with a Murphy eye–type hole cut distally) is placed in one nostril and attached to a breathing circuit by a 15-mm ETT adapter while the FOB intubation procedure is completed orally or nasally through the opposite nostril.[72]

4. Endotracheal Tubes

Regular polyvinylchloride (PVC) ETTs are used for most FOB intubations. However, the most distal ETT tip area can get caught on the arytenoids, especially the right, causing difficulty for passage into the trachea. Other

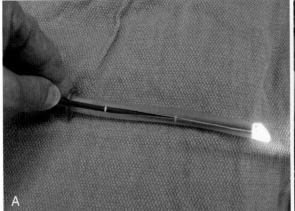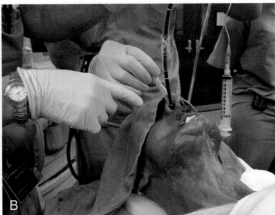

Figure 19-11 A, A cut breakaway nasopharyngeal airway (NPA). **B,** Once the carina is visualized, the breakaway NPA is removed from the fiberoptic bronchoscope to allow passage of an endotracheal tube.

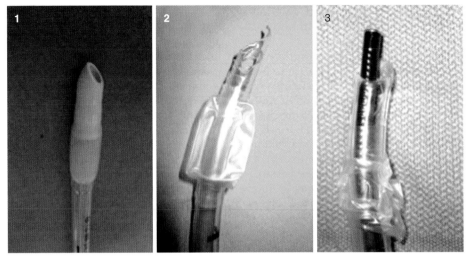

Figure 19-12 Comparison of curved-tipped versus straight-tipped endotracheal tubes: *1*, Fastrach (LMA North America, San Diego, CA); *2*, Parker (Parker Medical, Englewood, CO); *3*, polyvinylchloride (PVC) type.

centrally-curved, soft-tip ETTs have been reported to have greater success rates of passage.[73-75] However, Joo and coworkers demonstrated no difference in insertion success rate or number of manipulations required during awake FOB intubation when these two types of ETTs were compared, so long as the correct orientation of the common PVC ETT tip was made. The orientation required during insertion is that in which the Murphy eye of the ETT faces anteriorly with respect to the patient's body, to avoid arytenoid contact. This represents a 90-degree counterclockwise rotation of the ETT from the normal ETT direction used during rigid laryngoscopy (Fig. 19-12).[76]

V. CLINICAL TECHNIQUES OF FIBEROPTIC INTUBATION

A. Oral Fiberoptic Intubation of the Conscious Patient

FOB intubation techniques tend to be more successful in "awake" circumstances for a number of reasons, even though the airways can be very challenging. In the conscious patient, several factors contribute to this success: The preservation of muscular tone avoids obstructive soft tissue collapse; spontaneous ventilation is more likely to dilate airway structures; and the ability to deep breathe on command can sometimes reveal obscured airway passages.

During awake FOB intubation, the patient's state of consciousness may vary from completely awake to arousable with moderate stimulation (level 3 or 4 on the Ramsay scale) (Box 19-4).

Patients should have an awake FOB intubation under any of the following circumstances: anticipated very difficult intubation, a high likelihood of difficult mask ventilation and intubation, a DA with comorbidities likely to result in adverse effects if intubation is not easily accomplished, and after a failed asleep intubation (using any device). Application of excellent local airway anesthesia before endoscopy significantly decreases the odds of hemodynamic changes, severe coughing, laryngospasm, and failure.

1. Equipment, Monitoring, and Drug Availability

A preexisting intravenous route for drug administration is preferable, although intramuscular medication may be necessary for uncooperative patients until an intravenous line is established.

Unless emergency circumstances dictate otherwise, very strongly recommended standard equipment should include a full FOB cart, an ordinary airway cart, a checked oxygen delivery system, two available suctions (one for the FOB, the other for airway suctioning), monitors (blood pressure, electrocardiography, pulse oximetry, and capnography), drugs (local anesthetics, vasoconstrictors, sedatives, narcotics, reversal agents for these drugs, and possibly inhalation agents), and perhaps target-controlled infusion devices. If the patient's airway is anticipated to be very risky for ordinary awake FOB intubation, the DA cart should be present as well, for safety backup. Under any circumstances, if an FOB intubation is perceived as not going smoothly, the DA cart should be summoned to the site. This is particularly true if the patient has any difficulty breathing.

2. Psychological Preparation of the Patient

Psychological preparation of a patient is a basic step that is easily achieved with an explanatory, reassuring, and professional discussion. The following subjects can be emphasized: benefits of using the FOB method in relation

Box 19-4 Ramsay Sedation Scale
1. Patient is anxious and agitated, restless, or both.
2. Patient is cooperative, oriented, and tranquil.
3. Patient responds to commands only.
4. Patient exhibits brisk response to light glabellar tap or loud auditory stimulus.
5. Patient exhibits a sluggish response to light glabellar tap or loud auditory stimulus.
6. Patient exhibits no response.

to the patient's indications for the technique, probable amnesia for the procedure, effects of sedation versus respiratory depression, and the experience of the endoscopist. LA can be described as sprays, as injections with very tiny needles, and so on. The patient should be informed about any unpleasant taste, and a comparison with tonic water may be helpful. Advanced notice of enlisting patient aid during the process should be mentioned, such as gargling, swallowing, taking deep breaths, or exhaling completely, if needed. Oral intubating airways do not need to be mentioned, but their presence can be depicted as sensing a piece of plastic like a whistle in the mouth. Detailing similarities to other, more pleasant LA procedures; mentioning that a professional familiar with LA is involved; and alluding to actual FOB and ETT passage as being painless under LA (even with no sedation), can give a good frame of reference. Describing the expectation that patients will not notice much difference between sedation and general anesthesia (GA) can alleviate patient fears if sedation is not a concern and GA is planned after intubation.

Only oxygen is given if airway endangerment is a concern (i.e., no sedative or narcotic). Certainly, those patients for whom no sedation or extremely little sedation is advisable must be prepared to understand why. Explaining safety and how cooperation makes the process easier, faster, and less worrisome is beneficial.[77] Hypnosis has been used for FOB use, but special training is required.

3. Rationale for Pharmacologic Therapy

Supplemental oxygen is highly recommended but is not mandatory except in cases of a compromised airway.

If any topical intraoral anesthetic is planned, an anti-sialogogue is given 15 to 20 minutes beforehand to allow sufficient onset time, unless contraindicated. These agents minimize dilution of LAs, formation of a secretion barrier between LAs and the mucosa, and washing away of topical agents down the esophagus. In addition, they reduce the volume of secretions or blood that might obscure the optics of the FOB. Because of lesser degrees of tachycardia and side effects, glycopyrrolate (3 μg/kg) may be preferable to atropine (6 μg/kg) except in children.

Use of sedatives, narcotics, and LA agents depends on the urgency and respiratory status of the patient's situation. Sedatives may be titrated before the procedure for noncompromised patients. The most popular short-acting, amnestic anxiolytic is midazolam (15 to 30 μg/kg). Diazepam (35 to 70 μg/kg) and lorazepam (30 μg/kg) are alternatives that have much longer durations of action. Narcotics are only administered sparingly if the patient is in pain or if a painful or uncomfortable maneuver is anticipated (e.g., an injection).

B. Respiratory Monitoring Methods

The concern for respiratory events, especially after sedative and narcotic administration, has made continuous pulse oximetry a mandatory constant in addition to various monitoring schemes.

One solution involves surveillance by nasal cannula, using a side port for detection of end-tidal carbon dioxide

pressure (P_{ETCO_2}) detection and setting alarm parameters for P_{ETCO_2} and respiratory rate. There are several drawbacks. First, many FOB operators frown upon this method. Their concern is particularly valid when ETT passage is difficult. They do not want to get into a frantic disconnection of the P_{ETCO_2} sampling tubing from the nasal cannula and then go through a subsequent reconnection to the ventilatory system to verify correct ETT placement, through the presence of P_{ETCO_2}. Second, endoscopists complain that this monitoring draws away their attention if they are constantly having to look at the respiratory screen while performing airway maneuvers. Third, alarms may be erroneous when patients breathe through the mouth and not the nose.

Respiratory rate monitoring is also possible on electrocardiographic equipment that measures impedance during thoracic excursion. The drawback to this method is that waveforms are not always reliable, particularly with large body habitus, lack of thoracic impedance, and placement of electrocardiographic leads away from the chest.

C. Sedation and Analgesia

As vital as the pharmacologic approach is, a quiet, peaceful, and stress-free atmosphere is of paramount importance when performing an awake FOB intubation. Any external pressure from non-airway experts must be gently but firmly excluded. Other personnel should be advised of the reasoning for the procedure and a realistic waiting time until completion of airway management.

As the FOB process is about to begin, sedation may continue to be titrated with caution. Sedatives tend to be more associated with dysphoria and patient combativeness than narcotics, which can be used to offset discomfort and airway reflexes. In addition to respiratory depression, sedatives and narcotics are associated with increased collapse of airway soft tissues, aspiration, and laryngospasm. One must be on guard for obstruction during sedation, even at low dosages.

Many combinations have been used with expert care, including midazolam (1 to 2 mg) for amnesia and sedation and fentanyl (0.7 to 1.5 μg/kg) for analgesia and antitussive effects. Other agents commonly used include ketamine (0.025 to 0.15 mg/kg) for sedation and analgesia, a combination of ketamine and propofol, propofol (25 to 75 μg/kg/min) for sedation, and remifentanil (0.05 to 0.01 μg/kg bolus followed by 0.03 to 0.05 μg/kg/min infusion) for analgesia.

Ketamine produces less respiratory depression but is longer acting and has no known reversal therapy in humans. One study on ketamine/xylazine use in primates showed reversal with atipamezole (Antisedan), an α-adrenergic antagonist, but because xylazine is a clonidine analogue, it is difficult to say whether the ketamine alone would be reversed to the same extent.[78]

Dexmedetomidine (0.7 to 1.0 μg/kg bolus over 10 minutes followed by 0.5 to 1.0 μg/kg/hr infusion) is associated with hypnosis, amnesia, analgesia, and less respiratory depression. It has been used and titrated so that the patient remains responsive to verbal command. In animal studies, dexmedetomidine has been shown to be reversible by atipamezole, but no human studies are available.[79]

The most appropriate way to administer precisely titrated sedation seems to be with target-controlled infusion. The technique described for nasal FOB intubation has valid principles for oral approaches. Propofol and remifentanil have been studied most extensively.[80] Mean target plasma concentrations for propofol and remifentanil were 1.3 μg•mL^{-1} (standard deviation [SD], 0.2 μg•mL^{-1}) and 3.2 ng•mL^{-1} (SD, 0.2 ng•mL^{-1}), respectively. Rai and colleagues found no difference in patient satisfaction between the two but reported better FOB intubation conditions and a higher incidence of recall with remifentanil than with propofol.[81] Similar results were found by Cafiero and coworkers.[82] In patients with cervical trauma, a remifentanil effect site concentration as low as 0.8 ng•mL^{-1} proved to be effective for awake FOB intubation.[83] The very short induction and recovery times with remifentanil may represent a major advantage. Nevertheless, the possibility of increased thoracic wall rigidity and laryngospasm should be kept in mind.[84]

D. Local Anesthesia Purposes and Preparedness

Ideally, LA application is performed to achieve an excellent state of airway anesthesia to prevent discomfort, psychological distress, hemodynamic changes, and lack of cooperation. When it is appropriately executed, FOB intubation is made markedly easier and more successful. If the patient still has secretions in spite of antisialogogue action, wiping the tongue or directing the patient to suck on gauze can be helpful to soak up excess saliva. Before administration of LA, the relevant anatomy, drug concentrations, appropriate and maximum dosages, time of onset, toxicity, and alternative techniques must be known. Drugs and full resuscitation equipment must be readily available for treatment of toxic reactions. The systemic effects of two or more local anesthetics are additive, and consideration has to be given to the age and size of the patient, the site of application, and combinations of local anesthetics planned. In particular, the tracheobronchial tree is known to have very rapid systemic absorption of these agents. Vasoconstrictors have little effect on duration of action or prevention of toxicity from topical oropharyngeal anesthetics.

1. Innervation of Orotracheal Airway Structures

Cranial nerve IX, the glossopharyngeal nerve (GPN), supplies sensory innervation to the soft palate, the posterior third of the tongue, the tonsils, and most of the pharyngeal mucosa.[85,86] Some fibers also supply the lingual surface of the epiglottis.[87] This nerve controls the afferent component of the gag reflex. Cranial nerve V, the trigeminal, gives sensory supply to the anterior two thirds of the tongue but this area rarely needs anesthesia.

Cranial nerve X, the vagus, also forms part of the pharyngeal plexus, giving motor function to the soft palate and pharyngeal muscles. The superior and inferior laryngeal branches of the vagus carry out sensory supply to the laryngopharynx. The superior laryngeal nerve has an internal division that supplies sensory innervation to the base of the tongue, vallecula, epiglottis, piriform recesses, supraglottic mucosa, and the laryngeal vestibule above the vocal cords. Its external division provides motor control to the adductors/tensors, the cricothyroid muscle, and the cricopharyngeal part of the inferior constrictor of the pharynx. The inferior branch of the vagus, the recurrent laryngeal nerve, receives sensory input below the vocal cords, including the subglottic mucosa.

2. Topical Orotracheal Anesthesia Techniques

Determination of what technique is needed for local airway anesthesia depends on the intended approach for FOB intubation. Relative and perhaps absolute contraindications to these techniques include infection in the area, inability to determine anatomy, lack of patient cooperation, and any comorbidity such as coagulopathy or documented allergy that would pose an unwarranted risk. For a completely insensate oral approach, anesthesia must be provided to some of the soft palate, posterior tongue, posterior wall of the pharynx, vallecula, periglottic area, larynx, and trachea.

LA of the airway can be performed without sedation and should be the method of choice if patients have significant airway compromise. If possible, however, it is more desirable to give sedation before any deep pharyngeal/laryngeal anesthesia, to mask the choking feeling that many patients may experience and avoid this potentially distressing sensation. The bitter taste of the LAs can be somewhat masked by the use of mint strips.

a. GLOSSOPHARYNGEAL ANESTHESIA

In advance of performing a GPN nerve block, give instructions to the patient that he or she may be requested to take deep breaths, gargle, or swallow. It is helpful to vocally mimic gargling so that the patient understands this directive. While pressure is applied on the lateral tongue surface with a tongue depressor, the operator shifts the tongue medially and sprays the LA during inspiration at the anterior tonsillar pillar (Fig. 19-13). After waiting a number of seconds for patient recovery, the process is repeated on the opposite side, then once more on both sides.

Advantages include a lower likelihood of provoking gagging and greater cooperation when the tongue pressure is initiated laterally, compared with a midline approach. Also, inhaling and gargling are more likely to maximize anesthetic spread, as opposed to coughing the aerosol at the endoscopist. Optional methods include using a 3-mL syringe of 3% lidocaine on a MADgic atomizer (LMA North America, San Diego, CA) or Exactacain spray (benzocaine 14%, butamben 2%, tetracaine hydrochloride 2%), or alternatively, by touching the pillars for 5 seconds with a swab or pledget soaked in LA. An uncommon and not recommended technique is to actually inject the area with the LA. This last method is fraught with danger to the endoscopist (from biting) and to the patient due to the chance of hematoma formation or toxicity secondary to injection into a very vascular area.

b. ALTERNATIVE METHODS OF INTRAORAL ANESTHESIA

Alternative methods of intraoral anesthesia may anesthetize not only the GPN distribution but also the laryngeal

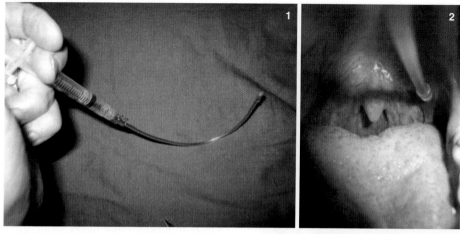

Figure 19-13 *1,* Flexible memory of MADgic atomizer. *2,* Glossopharyngeal nerve block in tonsillar fossa.

area or even the trachea as drugs are either inhaled or aspirated. With the atomized technique, lidocaine solution is applied via the MADgic to the palate, tonsillar pillars, vallecula, epiglottis, and larynx during deep inspiration by bending the stylet-like applicator in whatever curve is needed.

In the "lollipop" method of LA, 3 cm of lidocaine paste is placed on both sides of one end of a tongue depressor. The operator puts this end on the middle of the patient's tongue and advises the patient to keep the depressor held in place between the teeth. For the "toothpaste" method, the gel is placed directly down the middle of the tongue, while the tongue tip is held with gauze (Fig. 19-14). In these latter two instances, the lidocaine is left to dissolve over 5 to 10 minutes.

With the gargle method, a "slurry" or 4 mL viscous lidocaine is gargled continuously for 5 minutes. Finally, the Tessalon Perle (benzonatate) method involves keeping the Perle in the middle of the tongue so that it dissolves. If the Perle does not start to dissolve within a few minutes, it can be bitten slightly to permit leakage of the drug.

c. SUPERIOR LARYNGEAL NERVE BLOCK

The superior laryngeal nerve (SLN) block is advantageous for patients who have limited intraoral cooperation (e.g., perhaps only allowing a quick peritonsillar spray), for those who have no possible oral cavity entry (i.e., requiring nasopharyngeal FOB intubation), or as a rescue method after a failed internal SLN attempt when coughing or hemodynamic changes from sprays are undesirable.

Two techniques are available for the external neck approach to bilateral SLN block. In the simpler technique, attach a 10-mL syringe with 6 mL of 1% lidocaine to a 21- or 22-G needle as an injection system (Video 19-1). Clean the neck area with antiseptic solution and locate both hyoid cornua (Fig. 19-15). Keep the forefinger of the nondominant hand by one cornu for visual reference, and hold the syringe dart-like near the needle hub while advancing the needle perpendicularly toward that cornu. Once bone is felt, shift the nondominant hand to brace against the neck and hold the system near the hub. Aspirate the syringe gently; if no blood returns, inject 3 mL slowly. Repeat the process on the other side.

The second external approach to SLN block is more complex and takes longer to perform. The same system is used to hit the cornu. Then the operator walks off anteromedially and caudally 0.1 to 0.4 cm and feels the click of going through the thyrohyoid membrane at a depth of 1 to 2 cm.[88] The needle is then braced, and the remainder of the technique is identical. The block has to be repeated on the other side.

Internal anesthetization of the SLN can be accomplished by previously mentioned intraoral techniques including spraying toward the "imagined larynx." An uncommon method involves putting pressure in the piriform fossa with a gauze soaked in local anesthetic; the gauze is held in place by a curved clamp for 10 minutes.

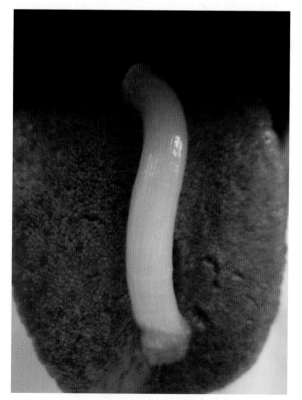

Figure 19-14 Glossopharyngeal nerve block and internal superior laryngeal nerve block. Five percent lidocaine is used for the toothpaste technique of intraoral anesthesia.

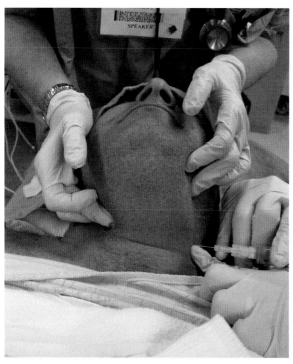

Figure 19-15 Superior laryngeal nerve block. The assistant holds pressure on the right hyoid cornu while the operator directs the local anesthetic 22-G needle at the left hyoid cornu.

Trouble-Shooting

1. The cervical collar is in the way: Open the collar on one side of the neck and flip its anterior portion over to the other side. Perform both blocks and close the collar when finished.
2. The hyoid is hard to feel with only one hand: It will be more prominent if an assistant presses gently against the opposite hyoid cornu toward the operator's finger on the side being blocked.
3. Blood is aspirated: The system has to be withdrawn slightly, redirected, and braced until aspiration is negative. (This is particularly important to prevent intracarotid arterial injection and seizures.)
4. Bone is felt but injection is not possible: The needle tip is probably in the periosteum. Using two hands, brace the system constantly, and imperceptibly withdraw 1 mm at a time until negative aspirations are followed by the ability to inject. Excessive distance during withdrawal can cause failure.

d. TRANSTRACHEAL BLOCK

If a collar is in place, locate the cricothyroid area through the anterior collar opening or by flipping the anterior part laterally, as described previously (Video 19-2). Apply antiseptic, and mark the area before refastening the collar. Straddle the trachea with two digits of the nondominant hand. With the dominant hand, direct a 10-mL syringe containing 4 mL of 4% lidocaine attached to a 21- or 22-G needle as a system, aiming posteriorly in the cricothyroid space while aspirating gently (Fig. 19-16). Shift the other hand to keep the system braced on the neck, if possible, and help guide it until many air bubbles are freely obtained. At this point, brace or encircle the system

firmly while the dominant thumb is poised to inject. Instruct the patient to breathe in gently and exhale gently but maximally. When exhalation is at completion, rapidly inject the anesthetic. As the LA enters the trachea, the patient may cough, but because exhalation has taken place, a quick breath must be taken to initiate any more cough, and this will help spread the anesthetic. Usually more coughing ensues. By bracing against the neck (or collar) and encircling the system, one need not worry about excessive needle penetration, removal, or breakage even if the patient's neck moves quite a bit. The system can be removed when finished.

According to Todd, concern about coughing in patients with cervical spine risk is unfounded, because patients cough periodically and those coughing during transtracheal blockade have never been shown to develop secondary neurologic damage.[89] Some clinicians prefer using a 20-G angiocatheter in lieu of the needle. They perform the technique in a similar fashion, but after air is aspirated they advance the catheter 0.5 to 1 cm, brace the catheter, remove the needle and syringe, disconnect the syringe, connect the syringe to the catheter, aspirate the catheter for air, and proceed in as previously described. The benefit of the needle technique is that it is faster, it is less likely to provoke more coughing caused by hitting the posterior tracheal wall (particularly when the catheter is threaded in too far), and it is more successful (because the needles are shorter, less flexible, and, even if pulled out of the trachea, can be advanced easily). In contrast, with a catheter coming out of the trachea, the needle would have to be reinserted with it, or the angiocatheter would have to be entirely replaced if the plastic is damaged.

Trouble-Shooting

1. The cricothyroid space is impossible to feel: A cricotracheal injection is acceptable.
2. More than a tiny wisp of blood is aspirated: Remove the system and refill the syringe with fresh local anesthetic to avoid injecting blood into the respiratory system.
3. The hyoid bone seems very close to the cricothyroid space: Reassess anatomy or abandon the technique to prevent vocal cord damage.

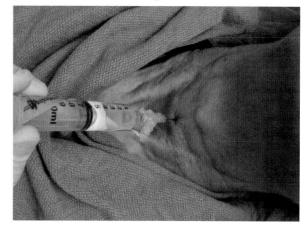

Figure 19-16 Transtracheal block. The operator braces his or her hand on the patient's chest while aspirating for air through the cricothyroid membrane.

4. The patient is at very high risk for aspiration: To maintain the patient's protective reflexes, avoid transtracheal anesthesia. Instead, use the "spray as you go" technique (discussed later) on the visualized vocal cords. Rapidly insert the FOB, and follow immediately with ETT passage and cuff inflation.

The combination of the three blocks described (GPN, SLN, and transtracheal) provides the quietest airway. Any order can be chosen, but usually the oropharynx is anesthetized first because it requires more cooperation on the part of the patient. The external neck approach to the SLN would be next if needed, followed by the transtracheal block, in order to have the procedure that elicits the most patient reaction (i.e., coughing) come last.

e. AEROSOL METHOD

The advantage of the aerosol method is that nebulized local anesthetic can be administered without needling and without much cooperation if given by mask. If it works, it is the best method to avoid coughing. This may take up to 15 minutes with some aerosols but can be faster with others such as the Aeroneb Go nebulizer (Dangan, Galway, Ireland). Nebulized lidocaine (5 mL, 4%) can be given via a mouthpiece for oral approaches. Instruct the patient to inhale only through the mouth until nebulization is complete (i.e., to prevent dilution of inhaled anesthetic from breathing through the nose). More cooperation is necessary for success, and the patient needs constant observation to ensure that instructions are actually being followed.

f. "SPRAY AS YOU GO" TECHNIQUE

The "spray as you go" method is used for patients who have partial or no pharyngeal, superior laryngeal, or transtracheal anesthesia. The operator uses an adult FOB with working channels of 2 to 2.5 mm and directs an assistant to give a quick pulse of 1 mL of 2% to 4% lidocaine (4 mL total), when areas with insufficient anesthesia are approached. If the working channel diameter is small (≤1 mm), this permits smaller incremental doses of LA administration (0.2 mL) to jet out as a spray. Do not employ simultaneous suction, because anesthetic will be lost in the suction.

Patients are more likely to react and cough after these pulses, and the FOB view may be obscured for some seconds, after which the FOB can be advanced until another unanesthetized area is reached.[90] An interesting method to avoid the obscured view is to attach a syringe containing local anesthetic to an epidural catheter (0.5 to 1 mm ID, single distal hole) and pass it through a three-way stopcock attached at the FOB injection port through the working channel. On the second stopcock port, attach the suction tubing for easy use by a simple turn. Extend the catheter tip 1 cm beyond the FOB tip so that as LA is injected, the spray goes a farther distance away, causing less visual disturbance to the FOB. Taping the proximal epidural at the working channel port area keeps its tip a fixed distance.

3. Local Anesthetic Drug Choices

LA dosing for various airway blocks is listed in Table 19-2. Toxicities of these injectable drugs have been described elsewhere, but with regard to the airway, some considerations need clarification.

Nydahl and colleagues demonstrated that 20 mL of 2% lidocaine gel in the nasopharynx was mostly swallowed in the stomach. Only one eighth of the described toxic blood level of an equal amount of injected drug resulted. Doubling the volume to 40 mL was equivalent to producing less than one third of the toxic level.[91]

Higher dosing and routes are most significant and should depend on a patient's height and size. Woodall and associates reported symptoms attributable to local anesthetic in 36% of 200 healthy subjects (anesthesiologists attending an FOB course).[92] Local anesthetics used

TABLE 19-2		
Oropharyngeal Local Anesthesia		
Drug	**Form**	**Appropriate Blocks**
Lidocaine	Pacey's paste (slurry): 7 mL 2% solution + 7 mL 2% viscous in two syringes with 3 mL air each + sweetener (mix back and forth via three-way stopcock); should be swished intraorally in 2 aliquots	
	2-4% solution	All blocks except as listed below
	1% solution	Preferred for SLN neck blocks
	4% solution	Preferred for transtracheal blocks
	2% viscous lidocaine	Intraoral or nasopharyngeal
	2-5% gel/ointment/paste	Intraoral
Exactacain (benzocaine, butamben, tetracaine HCl)	Metered spray	Intraoral
Cetacaine (benzocaine, tetracaine HCl, butamben, benzalkonium chloride)	Spray	Intraoral
Hurricaine (benzocaine)	Spray	Intraoral
Tessalon Perle (benzonatate)	200-mg capsule	Intraoral

SLN, Supralaryngeal nerve.

included nebulized lidocaine (200 mg or 5 mL 4%), nasopharyngeal lidocaine (100 mg or 2 mL 5%), and "spray as you go" lidocaine (600 mg or the equivalent of 15 mL 4%). The maximum dose in their study, 9 mg/kg lidocaine, was somewhat higher than the average dose of 5 mg/kg cited for performance of the described blocks in this chapter whose total dosage is 370 mg (i.e., GPN, 150 mg; SLN, 60 mg; and transtracheal, 160 mg).

Exactacain spray is a metered anesthetic with a six-spray maximum limit in adults to reduce the risk of toxicity. Each spray delivers 9.3 mg of benzocaine. Onset is within 30 seconds, and the duration is 30 to 60 minutes. Care must be taken to avoid use in patients with ester allergies or if the possibility of methemoglobinemia is likely due to patient comorbidities or concomitant drug therapy. Methemoglobinemia is more often associated with unlimited, continuous spraying of the Cetacaine spray (benzocaine 14.0%, butyl aminobenzoate 2.0%, tetracaine hydrochloride 2.0%) or Hurricaine spray (benzocaine 20%), which deliver 28 mg of benzocaine in a 0.5-second spray.[93-95] According to Khorasani and colleagues, dosing can be variable with these agents due to the orientation of the container to the patient during spraying or fluctuations in LA canister volume.[94] Between 1950 and 2005, only 26 of 126 total reported methemoglobinemia cases were related to endotracheal intubation. Transesophageal echocardiography was the procedure with the most frequent association, with a documented incidence of 0.115%.[95] Some sources consider this to be an underestimation. Because of recent Exactacain straw applicator connection manufacturing changes, care must be taken to use the same straws that come with the local anesthetic canister or to hold them securely while spraying, to prevent "popping off" of straws into a patient.[96]

A general plan of patient preparation is itemized in Box 19-5. Steps that are inappropriate for any specific patient should be eliminated or changed.

E. Fiberoptic Orotracheal Technique

1. Three Successive Directions for Fiberoptic Guidance

Airway specialists are remarkably familiar with the upper airway configuration as routinely observed during direct laryngoscopy. On the other hand, the different axes successively followed by the structures involved during FOB intubation, and their reciprocal spatial organization, are less a matter of emphasis in the classic teaching programs. Moreover, many sketches or drawings in medical textbooks are inaccurate, showing the upper airways as a regularly curved line joining the oropharynx or nasopharynx to the carina. This is obviously misleading, because three successive directions must be followed in the supine patient in order to reach the trachea through the nasal or the oral route.[97] These successive directions are (1) downward to the posterior wall of the oropharynx or nasopharynx, (2) upward to the anterior commissure of the vocal cords, and (3) downward again into the laryngeal and tracheal lumen to the carina.

Box 19-5	**General Plan of Patient Preparation for Awake FOB Intubation**

1. Check FOB equipment.
   - Choose FOB diameter closest in size to ETT diameter (have lubricant available if very close).
   - Plug in electrical outlet, turn on light source, and adjust according to FOB instructions.
   - Test lever and FOB tip motion, clarity, and focus by looking at printing on a nearby object.
   - Use defogger or insert FOB into warm irrigation bottle.
   - Place tested ETT in warm irrigation bottle, choosing at least one-half size smaller if a difficult airway is present.
2. Obtain history and physical examination and discuss the plan with the patient (psychological preparation).
3. Administer antisialogogue.
4. Administer sedative and insert an intravenous line if none is present.
5. Administer sodium citrate if aspiration risk is present.
6. Monitor the patient.
7. Lower the bed maximally.
8. Administer oxygen by cannula.
9. Position patient supine (ideally), or sitting for patients who are unable to lie flat, with the intention of facing the patient during endoscopy (note that anatomy will be inverted in the latter case). See obesity concerns discussed in the text.
10. Titrate sedative/narcotic while local airway anesthesia is applied.

ETT, Endotracheal tube; *FOB,* fiberoptic bronchoscope.

Oral FOB entry is usually midline but a retro-molar entry is possible in some patients with limited openings. When one is performing an FOB intubation via the oral route, it can be difficult to stay in the median sagittal plane, and this problem gets worse when obstructive flaccidity of the pharynx is present. The difficulty can be overcome with the use of a special airway (e.g., the Ovassapian device), help from an assistant, or FOB intubation through a supraglottic airway such as a laryngeal mask airway (LMA; LMA North America, San Diego, CA).

During the second phase of the fiberscope progression, in the upward direction to the anterior commissure of the vocal cords, the posterior part of the glottic aperture comes into view. In the absence of anatomic distortions, the temptation to push the fiberscope unswervingly in this direction should be resisted. It may be better to continue toward the anterior commissure of the cords, keeping the tip of the device in a sharp anterior path (by pushing down with the thumb on the button of the handle). Only when the anterior commissure is approached should the tip be angled correctly downward, toward the middle of the lumen of the larynx. This maneuver aligns the fiberscope with the anatomic axis of the larynx successively in its supraglottic and infraglottic segments, avoiding contact damage to the mucosa and arytenoid cartilages (Fig. 19-17).

2. Practical Application

Preparation before the FOB procedure should follow in sequence while adjustments are made depending on

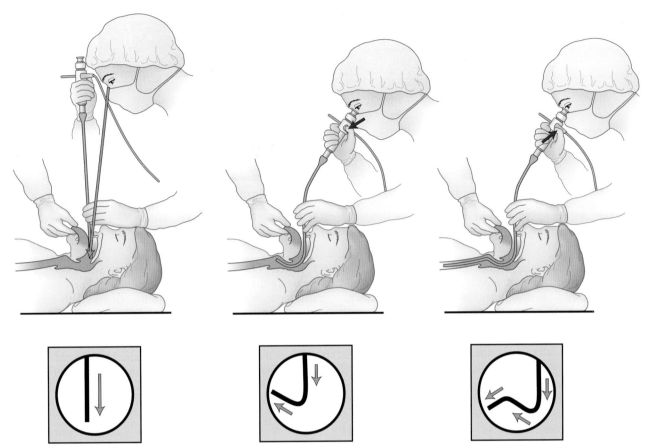

Figure 19-17   Three directions in the anatomic approach to fiberoptic intubation *(left to right)*: downward into the pharynx, upward through the vocal cords, and downward into the trachea.

individual patient concerns: equipment preparation, patient preparation, antisialogogues, sedatives, narcotics, local anesthetics, monitoring, and nasal cannula oxygen (if permitted; see Box 19-5). If there are not enough people available for assistance, the thumb-control port of the suction may be sealed ahead of time with tape, to make it a one-handed tool, which may help in the midst of a busy FOB procedure. The bed or table is moved to its lowest setting while keeping the patient supine. Use a stepstool to keep the FOB straight, if needed; in the case of a sitting, dyspneic patient approach the FOB procedure by facing the patient.

Employ the back-up bed position at whatever height makes the patient's comfort of breathing better. Traditionally, endoscopists like to "ramp" overweight patients up with many blankets under the upper thorax, neck, and head regions to align the airway when using RL, to decrease soft tissue encroachment on the airway. Rao and colleagues compared ramping with elevating the back of the bed until the patient's external auditory meatus is at the level of the sternal notch (Fig. 19-18).[98] There was no difference between the two methods in demographics, time to intubation, grade of glottic view, or number of RL attempts until intubation was successful. There was a significant difference in the added time and effort needed to position patients with blankets and then to remove blankets (and most likely in laundering cost, at 75¢ per blanket, although this was not mentioned in the

study). By extrapolation, elevating the back of the bed or using a reverse Trendelenburg position to align the external auditory meatus with the sternal notch may facilitate FOB intubation in obese patients with less wasted resources.

Once oropharyngeal LA is accomplished, many FOB operators direct patients to close their eyes, placing a surgical towel loosely on the upper face as a barrier to avoid injury to the eyes (e.g., from stray liquid agents). The towel can also serve to promote sedation by preventing patient observation of needles and instruments. After the remainder of the airway anesthesia has been completed, gently suction the oropharynx, curving anteriorly and caudally toward the larynx in the midline with a soft suction catheter if the mouth opening is limited, or with a Yankauer suction catheter. If the patient gags, GPN anesthesia is lacking, whereas if coughing occurs, SLN anesthesia is inadequate. This can be rescued by administering the appropriate block, or by using the "spray as you go" technique. Another benefit of suctioning is to remove secretions or blood out of the viewing path of the FOB.

Have an assistant hold the tip of the patient's tongue with gauze by grasping its anterior and posterior surfaces and extending it carefully so as not to cause tearing of the frenulum linguae. This lifts the tongue off the palate and elevates the epiglottis (Fig. 19-19). Apply 2 cm of 5% lidocaine paste to the distal lingual side of the IOA

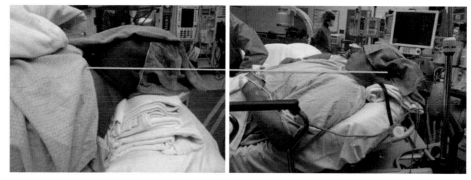

Figure 19-18 Comparison of positions for intubation in patients with increased body mass index. *Left,* Ramping with multiple blankets, which need to be situated and then removed after intubation. *Right,* More simplistic back-up bed position. Reverse Trendelenberg or back-up positions are used to align the external auditory meatus with the sternal notch *(blue line)*. Following intubation, the bed is easily returned to normal.

before gently positioning it, but only if using an Ovassapian or Berman type of airway. The assistant should hold the IOA midline during endoscopy to prevent deviation from the path to the larynx.[99] Alternatively, use a bite block (e.g., BiteGard [Gensia Automedics, San Diego, CA]) placed between the premolars to protect the FOB from dental trauma (Fig. 19-20).

Slide the lubricated ETT completely up the FOB, and either tape the connecter there or hold the ETT syringe with a little finger. Many FOB operators recommend holding the FOB handle in the nondominant hand, because thumb movement of the lever or forefinger depression of the suction valve are not as intricate movements as directing the FOB tip with the dominant hand.

Control FOB progress into the mouth and keep it midline by using the dominant hand's thumb and first two fingers, similar to holding a pen. The fourth and fifth fingers are placed on the patient's upper lip or cheek. This precise anchorage allows for firm stabilization of the FOB to prevent tremulous movement of the view and also prevents eye injuries caused by a stray little finger while the endoscopist's visual concentration is fixed on the screen or through the eyepiece during advancement. Old-school teaching used the hands in reversed roles, and many still prefer this idea.

To keep the FOB straight and prevent bending damage, rest the hand holding the FOB handle high on that extremity's ipsilateral shoulder to lessen fatigue.

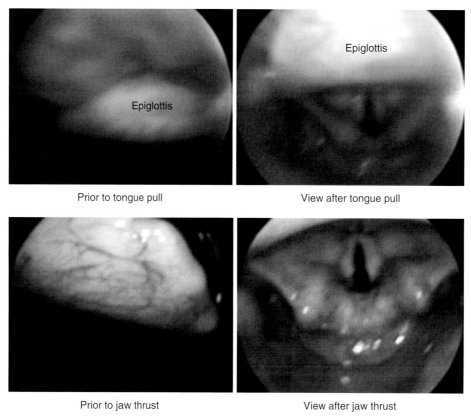

Prior to tongue pull

View after tongue pull

Prior to jaw thrust

View after jaw thrust

Figure 19-19 Effects of tongue pull and jaw thrust on epiglottic and glottic views.

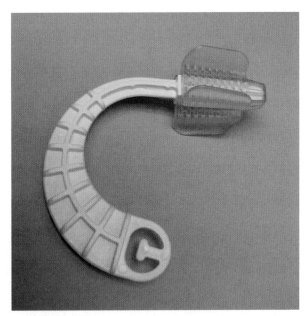

Figure 19-20 BiteGard for dental and fiberoptic bronchoscope protection is inserted between the premolars.

Alternatively, hold the instrument vertically straight adjacent to the patient. The patient's head and neck normally stay in a neutral position.

Insert the FOB into the patient's mouth, following the IOA while keeping the demarcation between the color of the IOA and the color of the mucosa in the center of view. Use the lever to look up or down and turn the FOB as a unit to look left or right, always keeping recognizable structures along the desired path in the center of view. Go around unwanted obstacles, such as secretions. If urgency is not a factor, slowly feed the FOB 6 to 8 cm, past the palate and past the uvula, and use the lever to look for the epiglottis, glottis, and tracheal rings. Stop two to three rings above the carina. If nothing is recognizable along the way, back up and look around with slow lever motion until structures are familiar, then proceed again. Do not provoke coughing by getting too close to the carina, which is unlikely to be anesthetized.

Hold the scope immobile and slide the ETT forward with the Murphy eye oriented anteriorly if using a PVC ETT, to prevent it from getting hung up on the arytenoid. Statistically, it gets caught on the right side most often.[100] Do not let the FOB go forward as the ETT advances toward the back of the oropharynx. At this point, look at the patient to judge when the ETT may be near the larynx. Ask the patient to take some deep breaths so that the vocal cords open more widely to admit the ETT. Time the breathing, and when ready, quickly push the ETT forward. After judging that it has gone beyond the vocal cords, look at the FOB tracheal view again, and slide the ETT until it ends up two to three rings above the carina and has just passed the FOB tip. Inflate the ETT, stabilize it, and remove the FOB. Put the FOB in the used vertical holder, or hand it in a straight fashion to an assistant. Attach the ventilating system while checking for P_{ETCO_2}, tape the ETT, and continue whatever patient care is anticipated next.

For very difficult airway and ETT insertions, it is worthwhile to check placement with the FOB after taping and patient positioning, which may be a source of ETT dislodgement.

Trouble-Shooting

1. The tongue extended preoperatively, but now, just before FOB insertion, it cannot be fished out for a tongue pull: Have the assistant firmly apply a large suction tubing to the tongue and slowly draw it out enough so that it can be grasped with the gauze. An alternative, especially for larger tongues, is to snag it with a clamp (e.g., ring forceps) or, rarely, with a large-diameter suture.
2. The patient has excessive oropharyngeal secretions or blood, and visualization with the FOB is almost impossible:
   - Have an assistant suction the oropharynx, even continuously if necessary. If possible, use an IOA. If not, insert the FOB midline between the fingers of an assistant at the entry point into the mouth. Keep the tip straight while it goes into the mouth a distance equal to two thirds of the distance from the mouth to the ear. Have someone turn off the room lights, and use the FOB similar to a lightwand. With lever manipulation, angle the tip forward and use transillumination to advance the FOB until an extremely bright pretracheal glow is seen. If the light appears off to one side of the neck, retract the FOB slightly and move it away from that side. If the light glow is anterior but less strong and resistance is felt, the tip may be in the submental area. Retract it slightly and redirect it posteriorly. If the glow is very dim, entry into the esophagus is most likely. Again, retract and angle anteriorly until the pretracheal glow brightens. At the glottis, the FOB entry into the trachea is exceedingly bright and visual optics may return. If not, suction via the FOB and continue forward until trachea or carina reaction is observed or those structures are visualized. An epidural catheter could be inserted for confirmatory P_{ETCO_2} monitoring.
   - An alternative approach is to insert an IOA or any SGA to seal the periglottic area. One with a gastric access tube may be the best choice. Then the ventilating lumen should be suctioned clear of secretions or blood and tested for P_{ETCO_2}. The FOB can be passed through it for intubation, knowing that there is less chance of continued soiling of the FOB or the airway.
   - Another alternative is to have a long (≥ 80 cm) guidewire with a few centimeters extending from the FOB tip that is nestled within an ETT just short of the ETT's distal end. Secure the wire proximally. With ongoing oropharyngeal suctioning, the FOB may stay clear of the soiling fluids, and the wire may be directed into the trachea. Once the wire is at least 8 cm into the trachea, the FOB and then the ETT can quickly be advanced, with rapid cuff inflation to prevent aspiration.
   - Lastly, a retrograde-FOB assisted intubation may be successful (see "Retrograde Incubation").
   - At some point, consider a surgical airway.

3. The optics are not clear; maybe the FOB is fogged: For an unclear view, try turning the focus dial. For fogging, touch the FOB tip on mucosa to clear it (Video 19-3). For secretions, suction with the FOB or use a suction catheter in the oropharynx, or both. Otherwise, FOB removal and cleaning of the tip may be the last choice. To clean, do not jab the FOB tip into anything, because delicate fibers can be broken. Hold the tip still but quite tightly near the very end, and gently wipe with alcohol.

4. It is impossible to look to the left or right because the lever only moves the FOB tip up and down: To look left, loosen the grip on the distal FOB insertion section between the thumb and two fingers while simultaneously rotating the handle section counter-clockwise, to avoid torque. To look right, turn the handle section clockwise in a similar fashion. Alternatively, rotate both hands equally in the same direction.

5. The FOB cannot get under the epiglottis because it is stuck on the posterior pharynx: Ask the assistant to pull the tongue out farther and perform a jaw thrust maneuver to lift the epiglottis (see Fig. 19-19).[101] Try moving the FOB more caudally or laterally, to get under the epiglottis.

6. The patient keeps gagging or coughing as the FOB advances: Consider repeating the LA blocks or use the "spray as you go" method.

7. After the FOB enters the trachea, the patient gets agitated and desaturates: In a compromised patient with tracheal stenosis or obstructive pathology, this may be the result of inadequate room around the FOB for the patient to breathe. The intubation process should be sped up, and the FOB should be removed as soon as possible. Be especially wary of starting oxygen insufflation through the working channel in this situation, in case not enough tidal volume can be expelled around the FOB. This sequence of events could precipitate the development of a pneumothorax.

8. The FOB is above the carina, but the ETT will not enter the trachea: Try not to jam the ETT, because it is advancing blindly and could damage perilaryngeal structures. Withdraw the ETT 1 to 2 cm, turn it 180 degrees counter-clockwise, and advance it rapidly after asking for a deep breath. If this is unsuccessful, rotate the ETT 180 degrees clockwise and repeat. If it is still not passing, repeat the other way. Try giving jaw thrust or even releasing jaw thrust. Use cricoid pressure, or neck flexion.[85] Finally, a rescue may be effected by removing the FOB and trying a smaller ETT; using a centrally curved, soft-tip ETT; inserting an Aintree Intubation Catheter (Cook Medical Inc., Bloomington, IN) on a pediatric FOB; or using a nasopharyngeal approach.

9. While using a pediatric FOB in an adult patient, tracheal rings were seen; the ETT went in, the FOB was removed, and the ETT was attached to the ventilator, but there was no PETCO2, breath sounds, or chest movement: The tip of the FOB must end up within 2 to 3 cm of the carina in an adult, particularly if a pediatric FOB is being used. If it is only partially down the trachea, pressure against the ETT as it pushes forward in the periglottic area against tissue (e.g., arytenoid) may divert it into the esophagus or bend it back into the oropharynx and cause "flippage." Flippage may occur when a stiff ETT tip indents into the somewhat flexible insertion section of the FOB as the ETT is diverted into the esophagus or pharynx, causing the short entry of the FOB to flip out of the trachea.

10. A centrally curved, soft-tip ETT was partially inserted into the oropharynx of an adult patient; next, the FOB was inserted through the ETT, and the tip of the adult FOB was positioned 2 to 3 cm above the carina; the ETT was then railroaded over the FOB, but in spite of all maneuvers, it will not pass through the glottis: If time and resources are available, look in the oropharynx with another FOB to diagnose the problem. If the FOB crossed through the Murphy eye, the ETT will never advance into the trachea. Trying to force the ETT forward may cause serious FOB damage and injure the patient. Occasionally, when this happens, the FOB might not even be able to be withdrawn easily, particularly if forceful moves were already made. Strong attempts at removing an FOB stuck in the ETT may result in severe damage due to "sharper" Murphy eye edges digging into the outer plastic wrap of the FOB. If any significant resistance occurs in this "ETT insertion first" type of scenario, remove both devices simultaneously.

11. More than just a few drops of blood are in the trachea after a transtracheal injection: Do not give positive-pressure ventilation (PPV). Attach the oxygen system, and suction the ETT. To avoid coughing, give sedative agents and, if desired, muscle relaxants before suctioning.

F. Nasal Fiberoptic Intubation of the Conscious Patient

The patient must be questioned regarding prior coagulation status or anticoagulant therapy, nasal abnormalities, trouble breathing through either side of the nose, and any previous surgery in the area (e.g., recent transsphenoidal surgery). Psychological preparation, monitoring, and pharmacologic therapy concerns are similar to those for oral FOB intubation. Any one-sided nasal pathology should be avoided. If there is a deviated septum, the larger nasal passage should be selected, to steer clear of situations in which the FOB can easily enter the trachea, but the ETT cannot traverse the nasopharyngeal passage.

1. Innervation of Nasopharyngeal Airway Structures

Cranial nerve V, the trigeminal, supplies sensation to the anterior half of the nasopharynx by its first branch. The second branch of the trigeminal nerve forms part of the sphenopalatine ganglion, innervating some of the anterior, superior, and central regions.[85,86] Cranial nerve IX, the GPN, supplies parasympathetic innervation, while the carotid plexus supplies sympathetics.[102] Cranial nerve VIII, the facial nerve, has parasympathetic function and forms part of the sphenopalatine ganglion to assist in control of nasopharyngeal reflexes.

2. Topical Nasopharyngeal Local Anesthetic Techniques

A completely insensate nasotracheal FOB intubation approach would involve anesthetization of the nasopharynx, posterior wall of the pharynx, periglottic area, larynx, and trachea. Techniques that work well include a triple combination of nasal, SLN, and transtracheal LA; use of a face mask nebulizer, and the "spray as you go" technique. When administering nonaerosolized agents, apply them to both nasal passages whenever possible in order to find the largest pathway. Another benefit to anesthetizing both passages may result in cases in which it is impossible to complete FOB or ETT entry on one side: there will be no delay due to suddenly having to anesthetize the other route.

Besides anesthetization, the nose requires the addition of a vasoconstrictor to decrease the likelihood of epistaxis (see Table 19-2). Dip four Q-tip swabs into solutions of cocaine or a vasoconstrictor mixed with local anesthetic. Swab insertion gives the FOB operator an idea of the caliber of each nasal passage. Apply a single swab to the outermost part within the nostril. Push it inward with a forefinger, perpendicularly to the plane of the face, until slight resistance is met (Video 19-4). Put the next swab in the opposite nostril, and continue alternating insertion of swabs parallel to previous ones. By the time the last swab is placed, the initial insertions will have caused some vasoconstriction, and slight swab pressure will push each one in further. If desired, midway through the process, spray 0.2 mL of solution with a 20-G angiocatheter (needle removed) in three different directions within each nostril. Continue this process until all swabs are at the back of the nasopharynx. This method uses a total of 2 mL (80 mg) of cocaine. If the possibility of tachycardia is a concern, apply a mixture of lidocaine and a vasoconstrictor instead of cocaine, with swabs positioned as described. Some FOB operators recommend another technique, using lidocaine gel and phenylephrine as a coating on short nasal airways to gauge nasal passage size. Any excess drug that is not absorbed usually drips back to anesthetize the posterior pharyngeal wall.

As an alternative, spray the mixture twice in each nostril, but only in an upright patient. Spraying in supine patients can result in overdoses if the spray becomes a stream. Several case reports have been published in which application of topical phenylephrine or a potent vasoconstrictor resulted in dangerous hypertension. Beta-blocking agents administered in this circumstance may promote the occurrence of pulmonary edema and should be avoided, according to the New York State guidelines on the topical use of phenylephrine in the operating room.[103]

For nasotracheal intubation under GA, vasoconstrictors are very useful to prevent epistaxis.

3. Vasoconstrictors and Local Anesthetic Drug Choices

Drugs are listed in Box 19-6.

Box 19-6 Nasopharyngeal Drug Therapy Before Intubation Using a Fiberoptic Bronchoscope

Vasoconstriction

Phenylephrine 0.5% spray
Oxymetazoline 0.05% spray

Local anesthesia

Lidocaine 2-4% spray, gel, viscous, paste

Both Vasoconstriction and Local Anesthesia

Cocaine 4% with a maximum dose of 1.5 mg/kg[104]
Mixture of 2-4% lidocaine (3 mL) + 0.5% phenylephrine (1 mL) or 0.05% oxymetazoline (1 mL)

G. Fiberoptic Nasotracheal Technique

Because of the relative narrowness of the nasal passage, an ETT at least one-half size smaller than would be chosen for the oral route should be selected, depending on the patient's history or size. Some endoscopists erroneously think that inserting progressively larger nasal airways or "trumpets" can mechanically "dilate the passage." However, Adamson and coworkers reported that use of this method caused increased trauma, hemorrhage, and delay of intubation.[104]

Pre-block preparation is similar to that for the oral approach, although antisialogogues are not quite as important if intraoral LA is not planned. The well-lubricated FOB can initially be introduced in one of three ways: (1) by itself for a distance of 12 to 15 cm, (2) within a lubricated short nasal airway that is designed to break away, or (3) after a well-lubricated ETT is first partially inserted into the posterior nasopharynx. After inserting the FOB, steer it to follow the dark conduits or openings of the nasal passage until the epiglottis is seen. As a substitute technique, insert the breakaway nasal airway or partially insert the ETT before FOB entry. This will virtually lead the FOB tip directly toward the larynx. Avoid the "ETT before the FOB" technique in coagulopathic patients and in situations in which bleeding is more likely to occur.

After locating the larynx and entering through the glottis, the remainder of the procedure, including depth of FOB passage, orientation of the Murphy eye, and ETT railroading to the correct depth, is similar to that for oral FOB intubation.

Whether the ETT is inserted before the FOB or after it, direct its leading edge along the septum. Through the left nostril, one may insert the ETT in the usual fashion until the back of the nasopharynx is reached. Through the right side, however, the concave surface of the ETT should face cephalad until the ETT tip reaches the back of the nasopharynx. At this point, the ETT is rotated 180 degrees to align the concavity anteriorly. This may help to prevent evisceration of the turbinates.

A proactive method to avoid trauma is to insert, as a unit, a lubricated and slightly protruding nasogastric or suction tube that almost fills up the lumen of the ETT. This prevents scooping or cutting into tissues by the firm, leading ETT edge. Another option is to use a centrally curved, soft-tip ETT.

Trouble-Shooting

1. The plan was to partially insert the ETT first, but it does not want to pass: Be gentle and do not exert force. Try the other side. If that does not work, try alternative methods listed previously.
2. Partially inserting the ETT caused epistaxis (no FOB yet): Inflate the ETT cuff to tamponade the area, or externally pinch the nose for 5 to 10 minutes. If blood is welling out of the nostril but no blood trickles into the back of the pharynx (i.e., there is no choking, swallowing, or continual need for suctioning), try pulling the deflated ETT a little and reinflating the balloon at what may be the site of injury. To prevent additional trauma, try not to remove the ETT unless blood keeps entering into the back of the pharynx regardless of the number of times these maneuvers were engaged.

H. Oral or Nasal Fiberoptic Intubation of the Unconscious Patient

1. Under Routine General Anesthesia

Eyes should always be protected in unconscious patients before any airway manipulation. If mask ventilation is expected to be easy under GA before surgery, a purely elective FOB procedure can always be used to intubate patients if consciousness is not required. This form of achieving intubation is very acceptable. It is considered ethical not to inform the patient of this plan because it is one normally used by many patient caregivers.[105] In some circumstances, "asleep" FOB intubation may have specific indications (e.g., a patient with extensive anterior dental work).

Preparation should include administration of an antisialogogue, complete FOB equipment readiness, premedication, monitoring, and positioning. If the surgery dictates a preference for nasotracheal intubation, nasal vasoconstrictor sprays should be applied while the patient is awake and in the sitting position. Because tissue laxity can obscure the airway in comparison to awake states, a smaller-sized ETT should be used. Positive-pressure face mask oxygenation is standard after induction and muscle relaxant delivery until the drugs have taken effect. At that point, lift the mask off the patient's face while the assistant performs a tongue pull, places the IOA, or gives a jaw thrust as needed. Insert the FOB and intubate as described previously. If desired, direct someone to keep track of passing time (Video 19-5; see also Video 19-3).

Trouble-Shooting

1. The technique is not succeeding: Careful monitoring and awareness of 2 to 3 minutes' passage of time, even in the case of technical difficulty, should keep the situation under control. If unsuccessful, always reinstitute face mask ventilation and decide whether the problem is caused by anatomic difficulty, being off-midline, insufficient assistance, or a lack of equipment. Think about giving more anesthetic before another attempt, or use an alternative intubation plan (e.g., intubation with another device). Frequently, combination FOB techniques should be considered (see "Combination Techniques").

2. After Rapid-Sequence Induction

Although they are not common, scenarios may arise in which patients with high aspiration risk have a DA but are not candidates for the awake intubation technique. An FOB can also be used electively after induction of GA in patients who are too young to understand or in uncooperative patients. In the former situation, the steps involved in an awake FOB intubation might cause an unwanted degree of psychic trauma, whereas in the latter case, the primary concern is risk to the patient or even to the FOB due to fighting or biting. Because of the risk of aspiration or airway loss, only a very experienced endoscopist, who expects a very high chance of success, should embark upon this procedure from the start under GA. Otherwise, initiation of this method during GA is inappropriate, and it is an especially poor choice for patients with very difficult airways.

If the decision is made to proceed, have two operable suctions attached, one on the FOB and the other on a Yankauer or soft suction tubing in case of regurgitation. Choose a smaller-sized ETT. If not contraindicated, preoperative preparation is identical to that used for rapid-sequence GA, with inclusion of an antisialogogue, clear oral antacid, histamine H_2-blocker, and/or gastric motility–inducing agent. After induction and cricoid pressure applied as originally explained by Sellick,[106] use the FOB intubation technique with good assistance. Once the FOB nears the carina, the ETT should be inserted quickly and the cuff inflated immediately.

Sometimes, asleep FOB intubation may be selected as a rescue tactic for patients who have incurred failed intubation with another device. Early use of an FOB for intubations that have gone awry is much less likely to cause the devastation that can result from repeated failed RL attempts.

Trouble-Shooting

1. The epiglottis and periglottic areas are easily seen, but the glottis is very small with closed vocal cords, and the FOB cannot enter: Check the nerve stimulator for degree of muscle relaxation. If this is insufficient and laryngospasm is suspected, spray down the FOB with 4% lidocaine. If the patient is relaxed, ask the assistant to slowly decrease the cricoid pressure to see if things improve, because this pressure can be associated with impaired glottic visualization. If regurgitation occurs, another assistant should suction the oropharynx, and pressure may need to be reinstituted, with a tentative release tried later.

I. Fiberoptic Intubation in Unconscious, Unanesthetized Patients

For emergency FOB intubation in unconscious, unanesthetized patients, ideally all equipment is available. The approach must be speeded up, however. Three important caveats must be considered before FOB technique in this situation: a full stomach must be assumed, cricoid pressure must be employed, and the most experienced FOB endoscopist should perform the procedure. More descriptive directions may be required for assistants, who are likely to be less experienced in these urgent cases.

VI. COMBINATION TECHNIQUES

Whether the patient is awake or under GA, an FOB can be combined with ancillary devices and laryngoscopy instruments to accomplish intubation. FOB combinations have practical utility in realizing improved airway control, assisting in diagnostic and therapeutic efforts, and rescuing failed intubations. In many combination techniques, physical maneuvers (tongue pull and jaw thrust) are very advantageous.

Elective use of an FOB combination with other airway management equipment has a very high rate of success with the added luxury of planning. This may be extraordinarily beneficial in the most difficult airway predicaments. As an illustration, a Fastrach intubating laryngeal mask airway (LMA North America) may be desirable to seal off the laryngeal area from blood and accomplish ventilation in a patient who is difficult to mask ventilate, difficult to intubate, and has significant intraoral bleeding. This intubating airway has a moderately high success rate for blind insertion of its ETT (90% to 96.2% with ≤3 attempts or adjusting maneuvers).[107-109] Its use in combination with an FOB, however, can change a blind technique to a more controlled visual one, with a greater chance of success.[110]

Examples of diagnostic abilities of an FOB often become evident in patients who have undergone prolonged spinal surgery in the prone position. If such a patient's airway pressure rises intraoperatively, FOB examination through a bronchoscopy swivel adapter can be used to determine the cause (e.g., secretions, endobronchial intubation, a kinked ETT). A therapeutic role periodically occurs at the end of this type of surgery. A degree of indecision as to how well the patient might fare after extubation (due to length of surgery and airway edema) can be remedied by the therapeutic capability of combination use of an FOB with an Aintree catheter through the existing ETT. The Aintree is left as an "airway stent" and then secured in place after the ETT and FOB have been removed. Should the patient appear to be failing the extubation trial, an ETT-fitted FOB is reinserted down the Aintree for reintubation.

A common failed intubation scenario occurs in a morbidly obese patient with redundant intraoral tissues who is undergoing GA and laryngoscopy with an RL that reveals a Cormack-Lehane grade 3 view. Intubation failure despite the use of an intubation guide catheter can result in a deteriorating situation after multiple attempts due to tissue trauma, and it is made notably worse if mask ventilation becomes problematic. Attempts at FOB rescue by itself might be difficult. In combination, however, the RL can be used to elevate tissues out of the way of the FOB in order to obtain the best laryngoscopic view by RL, even if it only reveals the epiglottis. This can offer a much easier route for the FOB to follow to achieve the goal of intubation.

Finally, combining multiple approaches to manage the DA is just another illustration of the general concept of multimodal therapy, in contrast to monotherapy. Multimodal therapy is used in the everyday practice of health caregivers, such as when different classes of drugs are used to provide an overall "tailored" anesthetic, or when combinations of various analgesics are used for chronic pain control. The multimodal approach to the airway, unduly disregarded for a long time, seems to be increasingly accepted as the drawbacks of individual airway devices or techniques become more obvious and the failures of each, when used alone, are more frequently reported.[111]

A. Superficial Airway Devices and Flexible Fiberoptic Bronchoscopes

1. Combination with Endoscopy Masks

Very often the FOB-endoscopy mask combination can help to obtain either the objective of anatomic airway examination or actual airway control. These masks may have one or more openings for simultaneous FOB and ETT passage. A model that seals around both is ideal. Be cautious of models having a port that seals only around an FOB, because ETT insertion can result in a leak to the atmosphere with inability to ventilate the patient.

Preparation for use of the FOB-endoscopy mask combination during GA is the same as detailed earlier. The ETT, with its 15-mm connector removed, is placed over the FOB. Keep the connector in a secure spot. After induction, insert an IOA and strap the mask in place with 100% oxygen while an assistant holds the mandible to prevent obstruction. If no muscle relaxant is used, the patient should be relatively deeply asleep to prevent laryngospasm when the larynx is touched. This can be treated by instilling LA in a "spray as you go" technique. With muscle relaxation, the patient does not have to be as deeply anesthetized, but the assistant must be competent enough to maintain positive-pressure mask ventilation.

Insert the ETT-loaded FOB sequentially through the port, IOA, and trachea for subsequent intubation (Fig. 19-21). After ETT intubation, remove the FOB and mask and join the ETT to the ventilation system. If patient

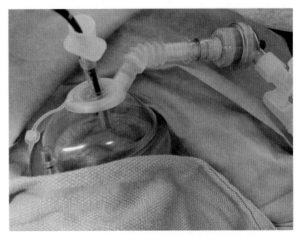

Figure 19-21 Combination of a fiberoptic bronchoscope with an endotracheal tube through an endoscopy mask.

conditions warrant urgent ventilation, institute it through the ETT after removal of the FOB. Retire the mask at any time thereafter. One advantage of using this technique for an elective case is that it affords more time for endoscopy, particularly if surgery will not be delayed because the incision site is at the other end of the body.

These masks can also provide a supplementary method for administering oxygen during awake FOB intubation in a patient who is so respiratory-compromised that a nasal cannula might be insufficient. Administer nasal cannula oxygen during mask-lifting periods while LA is being given. After LA administration and airway suctioning, follow the same FOB-endoscopic mask steps detailed earlier.

If an FOB and an ETT are inserted simultaneously into the endoscopy mask port at the beginning of the procedure, FOB manipulation is not a significant problem in the straight forward-aiming oral route to the larynx. For nasotracheal intubation, it is better not to insert both initially, because the ETT might limit FOB maneuverability in entering the nasopharynx. During simultaneous insertion, this transpires when the exiting direction the FOB takes from the ETT is at odds with the entry into the nasal passage. In this case, insert the FOB well ahead of the ETT until the carina is located, and then advance the tube.

2. Combination with Swivel Adapters

A bronchoscopy swivel adapter for FOB examination or intubation can be placed between the ventilation circuit and an ordinary face mask, an SGA, or an ETT.

For intubation purposes, the combined use of an FOB and a swivel adapter can be undertaken under GA or oxygen-enrichment conditions similar to those for FOB-endoscopy mask use. With the patient under GA, insert a pediatric FOB within an Aintree intubation catheter (ID 4.7 mm, OD 6.3 mm) through the swivel adapter port while the patient is breathing spontaneously or being mask ventilated (Fig. 19-22). Once the FOB enters the trachea and nears the carina, slide the Aintree over it until it is two to three rings above the bifurcation. Hold the Aintree securely while noting the depth of insertion, and take out the FOB. Remove the Aintree connector to

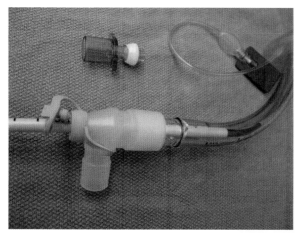

Figure 19-22 Combination of a fiberoptic bronchoscope with an Aintree catheter through a swivel adapter.

extract the mask, SGA, or old ETT. Then, slide a lubricated ETT-loaded FOB through the Aintree and down the trachea, stopping again near the carina. Pass the ETT farther down over the Aintree until the ETT tip lies 2 to 3 cm above the bifurcation. While firmly holding the ETT, remove the FOB and the Aintree. Reconnect the ETT to the ventilation circuit.

Optionally, apply ventilation via the Aintree 15-mm connector when the device is first placed if urgent respiratory assistance is needed or to confirm P_{ETCO_2} return before attempted ETT passage. This is also an alternative method to ventilate patients in cases where the ETT fails to enter the trachea.

3. Combination Using Short, Soft Nasal Airways

The role of the breakaway soft nasal airway in facilitation of awake FOB intubation was detailed earlier (see "Fiberoptic Nasotracheal Technique"), and the principle can be transferred to generate similar results in patients under GA.

In addition, soft nasal airways may serve a very different function, as a conduit for GA gases while FOB intubation is pursued. In this technique, attach the anesthesia machine to a 15-mm ETT connector inserted into an intact nasal airway in a spontaneously breathing, very deeply anesthetized patient for the FOB manipulation. When the NPA method is used, considerable amounts of anesthetic gases are lost to the atmosphere, which is less than ideal. Nevertheless, it is the best choice in many cases. For example, an NPA is more commonly chosen for pediatric patients, who are prone to desaturate rapidly when intubation attempts are made during stoppages in mask ventilation. For nasotracheal intubation, it is not unusual to see this technique used on one nostril, with a breakaway NPA for intubation on the opposite side. During total intravenous anesthesia, the NPA only supplies oxygen.

B. Supraglottic Airways and Flexible Fiberoptic Bronchoscopes

The original LMA for ventilation had obvious airway management benefits from its inception, particularly for difficult mask ventilation and for DI. This device has saved countless lives and is rightfully prominently embedded in the ASA DA algorithm. It can be used in patients who are unconscious, awake with local airway anesthesia, or under GA. Since its development, dozens of SGA and intubating SGA devices have been invented. The idea of performing FOB intubation through the LMA was spawned by the knowledge that, when seated properly, this SGA had to be situated around the glottis and could provide a pathway for an ETT. The combination of FOB-SGA for ETT intubation has been successfully tried with numerous SGA brands (Fig. 19-23).

The FOB has also been combined with this sort of airway for trouble-shooting SGA insertion problems (e.g., high airway pressures, leak), as described earlier. The combination can also be used for assistance in accomplishing placement of the SGA itself, by having the FOB just recessed within the airway's "bowl" as the SGA is advanced into the oropharynx.

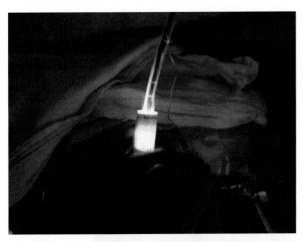

Figure 19-23   Intubating with the combination of a fiberoptic bronchoscope within an Ambu Aura-i intraoperatively.

1. Combination with SGA and Multiple Endotracheal Tube Techniques

If an FOB-SGA combination technique is being used for intubation, ascertain first that the desired lubricated ETT size is able to traverse through the SGA. Of course, the ETT must also be appropriate in size for the FOB. Many SGA have indicators for the maximum tolerated ETT size, and the larger ones permit entry of an adult-sized FOB. For smaller SGAs, a pediatric FOB and a smaller ETT are better choices. With the LMA brand, alignment of the bevel of the ETT in a transverse plane or preemptive cutting of the epiglottic deflectors will avoid situations in which the FOB tip and the ETT tip straddle an aperture bar. ETT sizes usually must be smaller.

Induce GA and position the SGA. While administering 100% oxygen, in a spontaneously breathing, deeply anesthetized patient or a ventilated, muscle-relaxed patient, try to obtain an optimal PETCO2 waveform with good chest excursions. Disconnect the SGA from the circuit, and slide the ETT-loaded FOB down the SGA until the glottis is visualized. Place the FOB tip near the carina and advance the ETT. Remove the FOB and confirm ETT placement with PETCO2. Remove the 15-mm ETT connector, and use a smaller ETT as a push rod (similar to the Fastrach pusher rod). With the pusher, keep the first ETT steady, and slide the SGA out until the first ETT can be grasped in the oropharynx. Then remove the second ETT and SGA and connect the first ETT to ventilate the patient.

Trouble-Shooting

1. The only ETT that could pass is small and too short, prompting concern that its cuff will lodge between the vocal cords:
   - An option is to cut and discard a 4-cm section of the tubular end of the SGA, allowing for deeper ETT insertion. Push the ETT deeper, using a one-size-smaller ETT, impinging it in the first one's proximal end like a pusher rod. After pushing in 4 to 5 cm, hold the ETT system steady and withdraw the SGA. After seeing the first ETT in the oropharynx, continue with the same technique described earlier.

   - Alternatively, consider wedging a larger ETT circumferentially around the first ETT's proximal end. Then employ the same technique.
   - A very much longer Micro Laryngeal Tube (Rüsch Incorporated, Duluth, GA) (26 to 33 cm long, cuff sizes equivalent to an 8-mm ETT) is a better option. The SGA can be extracted over the Micro Laryngeal Tube with no need for a second ETT. Also, remember that SGA removal is not mandatory; simply leave it in place and deflate its cuff.

2. Combination with SGA and Aintree Catheters

As detailed earlier, intubate with an Aintree-loaded FOB via an SGA. Fix the Aintree, and remove the FOB and SGA. Complete the intubation with the ETT-loaded FOB via the Aintree (Fig. 19-24A).

3. Combination with SGA and Guidewires

Similarly, thread a long guidewire (110 to 145 cm long, 0.38 to 0.97 mm diameter) through the working channel of the FOB far into the trachea by way of the SGA (see Fig. 19-24B). While holding the wire in place, extract both FOB and SGA. Subsequently, thread the near end of the wire through the FOB tip, up the working channel of an ETT-loaded FOB. Use the FOB to visually follow the wire into the trachea for completion of ETT intubation.

4. Concerns

There are some limitations to FOB and SGA combinations:

- Correct SGA placement is not successful in 100% of cases.
- The ETT may not fit or pass through the SGA, so the combination must be prechecked.
- Not all lubricants are equally adept at lubricating the ETT. Viscous lidocaine, Exactacain, and Neosporin (polymyxin B sulfate, neomycin sulfate, bacitracin zinc) ointment achieve a far greater degree of "slickness" than common surgical lubricants.
- Compare the length of the ETT with the length of the SGA, because the distance from the periglottic opening of the SGA to the vocal cords may be 3.5 cm or more. Inattention to lengths may produce a "too short" ETT picture. Trying to cut a 4-cm section of a SGA tube to avert this problem (as mentioned earlier) may lead to problems: the SGA connector may not separate easily from its original seat within the SGA tube, or it may have a poor fit when plugged into the cut-off SGA section.

C. Intubating Supraglottic Airways and Flexible Fiberoptic Bronchoscopes

Reports of FOB intubation through the LMA prompted the development of the Fastrach. This silicon-covered, steel-body, intubating SGA comes in three sizes for patients weighing more than 30 pounds and has a moveable epiglottis deflector bar. Its dedicated centrally curved, soft-tip ETT more readily traverses the glottic aperture in comparison to PVC ETTs.

A number of intubating SGA models have now been manufactured. The Ambu Aura-i (Ambu, Glen Burnie,

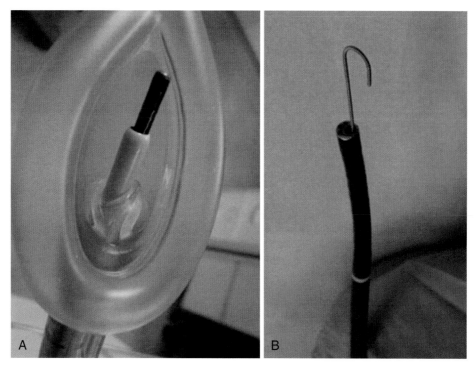

Figure 19-24 *A,* Combination of a fiberoptic bronchoscope (FOB), Aintree catheter, and ETT in a laryngeal mask airway. *B,* The guidewire is shown within the working channel of the FOB.

MD) is a soft, rounded PVC SGA available in infant to large adult sizes. It was designed with less of a J-curve, and on its bite block area the maximum ETT size able to pass through it is clearly labeled.

Intubating SGAs were originally designed to act as conduits with high success rates for blind passage of an ETT into the trachea. They are more aptly designed for this purpose than most SGA devices, because larger ETTs can be deployed. When used with an FOB in a similar fashion to FOB-SGA combinations, their intubation success rate soars (Fig. 19-25). In a study by Erlacher and associates, 180 patients were intubated blindly through CobraPLUS (Pulmodyne, Indianapolis, IN), air-Q (Trudell Medical Marketing Limited, London, Ontario, Canada), and Fastrach devices with success rates of 47%, 57%, and 95%, respectively.[112] Of the approximately 60 patients for whom blind intubation failed when these intubating SGAs were used alone, FOB insertion for intubation was attempted; the overall success rate for the FOB-intubating SGA combination was greater than 98%.

D. Combination with Rigid Laryngoscopes

Occasionally, when an FOB is used as the sole airway device, impediments may prevent entry into the glottis; examples include a nonmobile or floppy, posteriorly directed epiglottis and upper airway edema. An RL can assist in lifting the mandible and moving obstructing tissues out of the way to improve the route for the FOB (Fig. 19-26). The FOB-RL technique requires at least two people: two endoscopists, or one endoscopist and a very knowledgeable assistant. The assistant must be able to hold the RL immobile after it has been placed optimally or to manage the FOB controls.[110,113] The clinical

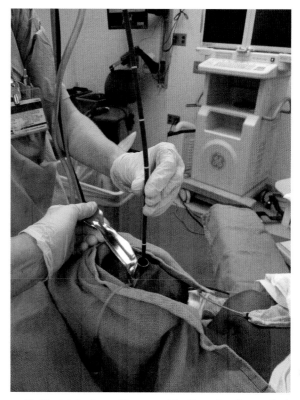

Figure 19-25 Intubating with a combination of a fiberoptic bronchoscope through a Fastrach.

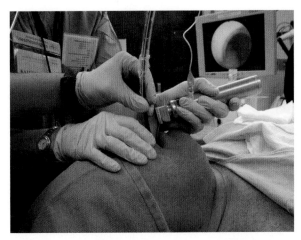

Figure 19-26 Fiberoptic intubation assisted by a rigid laryngoscope with video view of the trachea.

situation, together with the knowledge and technical abilities of the personnel involved, dictate who handles the RL and who directs the FOB tip or completes glottic insertion of the FOB or both. Successful FOB-aided controlled tracheal extubation and reintubation using the RL-FOB combination has been reported in intensive care unit patients.[114]

A possible, but not proven, advantage may be reduced nociceptive stress of intubation in response to lower RL blade pressure at the base of the tongue during use of FOB-RL combinations.

1. Nonsoiled Airway Situation

Use the RL to visualize the airway toward the glottis as much as possible, while moving blocking structures out of the way. Ensure that the RL is fixed in place. Before FOB insertion, suction the airway as needed. Endeavor to use the visual features of the ETT-loaded FOB to advance its tip by hand under the epiglottis, toward the larynx, for entry into the trachea and intubation. During maneuvers, direct the assistant to hold the RL steady or to manage the FOB controls.

2. Soiled Airway Situation

If it is impossible to use the visual features of the FOB due to soiling, obtain the best overall view with the RL. Direct an assistant to manage the controls. While holding the RL steady, advance the FOB tip under the epiglottis by looking directly in the mouth, similar to inserting an ETT. Do so by using the light from the RL, not the optical system of the FOB. Once the FOB tip is beyond the epiglottis, monitor its progress by using the FOB visual capability, and advance the insertion section while instructing the assistant to move the tip up or down. Continue until the glottic aperture is reached, while holding the RL firmly in place. When necessary, clear the FOB tip by touching it on mucosa or requesting the assistant to suction the patient, or both. After the trachea has been entered, insert the FOB tip near the carina and ask the assistant to railroad the ETT. Considerable cooperation is important.

Alternatively, after the best view is obtained with the RL, direct the assistant to hold the RL fixed. Introduce the FOB as far as possible under direct vision next to the RL (again, similar to inserting an ETT). Once further insertion under direct vision is impossible, monitor via the FOB and handle the controls until trachea and carina are secured. Then railroad the ETT.

E. Combination with Video Laryngoscopes or Optical Laryngoscopes

VLs and OLs are amazing devices that have a firmly rooted place in airway management and definitely should be part of the DA algorithm. Many can give stunning images due to options such as wide-angle camera capability, exceptionally clear optics, and video monitoring. Their learning curves are very fast. In most patients, the 60-degree angulation design with video or optical mirror capability improves Cormack-Lehane views of the larynx by one to two grades over those seen with the RL.[115-117] VL devices will most heavily impact what is now obviously an inferior device for airway management—the RL—and will result in continual declining use of that instrument.[118]

Despite superior visual capabilities, these devices can have failures in diverse airway cases.[117-119] It is unlikely that VL will replace FOB use because of the very nature of FOB—the flexibility to conform to intricate airway pathology. The VL can optimize laryngoscopy but does not share the FOB's second most desirable property, the ability to mechanically guide the direction of an ETT into the trachea to a specific end point. Clinicians may be delighted by the improved images from the VL, but they also are disappointed periodically when it remains impossible to intubate a patient despite "a perfect laryngeal view." Many such failures have been reported with all types of VLs and OLs.[59,119] In addition, pharyngeal perforation (palate or tonsillar pillars) may rarely result from the ETT tip during VL use. The cause is simple to understand. Whereas the ETT is initially advanced under direct vision, at some point it is pushed ahead blindly until it is finally seen again on the video screen.[120-122] Care taken to directly observe the ETT hugging the tongue and curving it centrally and caudally within the airway greatly lessens this possibility. This type of trauma is unlikely with an FOB system in which the ETT slides over its insertion section.

Even the FOB has limitations compared to VL devices. FOBs have a more narrow-angled field of view, a shorter focal distance, a greater possibility of obscured optics if the airway is soiled, an inability to open the airway, and a degree of inability to maintain a midline position in the pharynx while advancing toward the glottis.[123]

Ideal circumstances combine an FOB with a VL to employ the strengths of both techniques. Having both FOB and VL screens available would be a situation of truly superior airway management. With this combination, the VL is used to keep the oropharynx open and lift tissues away from the glottis and epiglottis during oropharyngeal or nasopharyngeal FOB intubation. The VL view of the FOB position and the simultaneous FOB view of pharyngeal and later laryngeal anatomy permits better FOB control and a greater range of vision. This combination of an FOB with a VL assists in reaching and entering the larynx by reducing unwanted FOB movements in lateral directions.

VLs can also help diagnose FOB problems. In many cases, the FOB-VL technique provides visualization of the passage of the ETT over the fiberscope into the glottic area, aiding in the resolution of ETT "hang ups" at the arytenoid and other passage difficulties. The combined technique does have a drawback in that it requires both an endoscopist and a very knowledgeable assistant, but management of DI may necessitate two operators in any event. Indeed, use of the combination of FOB and VL has been shown to be advantageous and has been reported in DA patients.[124]

Another virtue of the FOB-VL combination is that it permits the use of a VL to fully observe FOB manipulation by trainees. This can enhance instruction and maximize learning experiences.[125]

1. Non–Channel-Loading Devices and Fiberoptic Bronchoscopes

The type and number of personnel and the technique involved with combination of an FOB and a non–channel-loading device are similar to those of the combined FOB-RL method. Situate FOB and VL video screens, if available, near one another. After GA induction, attempt laryngoscopy with the VL until the best view is achieved. While holding the VL in place, direct the tip of the FOB under the epiglottis and toward the glottis (Fig. 19-27). Instruct the assistant to control the FOB tip. When the tip is beyond the view of the VL, use the FOB view. Continue to advance the insertion section, and after locating the tip near the carina, ask the assistant to railroad the ETT as described previously. Alternatively, after the VL attempt, have the assistant fix the VL in place. Take over total control of the FOB to locate the glottis, trachea, and carina and complete ETT passage.

In the event of a soiled airway, the FOB-VL combination can be used in a fashion somewhat similar to the FOB-RL methods under soiled conditions.

Trouble-Shooting
1. The brightness of the VL is making the FOB view excessively "whited out": Dim the brightness of the VL model, if it possesses this feature, to prevent excessive

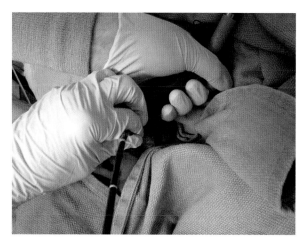

Figure 19-27 Intubating with a combination of a fiberoptic bronchoscope and a GlideScope video laryngoscope.

glare when viewing through the FOB (Fig. 19-28). If the VL model does not have this capability, power it off after the FOB insertion if this problem arises. Power it back on intermittently to monitor FOB and ETT progress.

2. It is impossible to get the FOB tip under the epiglottis, even when directly looking into the mouth to position it: The FOB tip may be too flimsy to execute this maneuver. Observe the VL view of the FOB, gently advance the ETT just past the FOB tip, and snake the ETT under the epiglottis. Request a tongue pull or jaw thrust, or both. If successful, advance the FOB and complete the intubation.

2. Channel-Loading Devices and Fiberoptic Bronchoscopes

Visualization of the larynx may be perfect with the channel-loading type of VL or OL and yet result in failure of ETT intubation. In this scenario or even if insufficient visualization occurs, the VL may be used to open an airway path. Insert the FOB within an ETT either in the channel or next to the device. Direct it toward the glottis if it seems easy to do so, or use the FOB-VL techniques detailed earlier (Fig. 19-29).

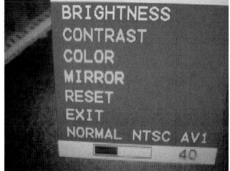

Controlled VL brightness permits good FOB viewing

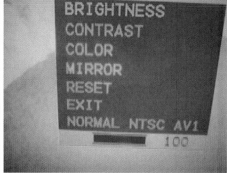

Excessive VL brightness may impair FOB viewing

Figure 19-28 Controlled brightness with the GlideScope video laryngoscope *(VL)* prevents glare during combined fiberoptic bronchoscopic *(FOB)* viewing.

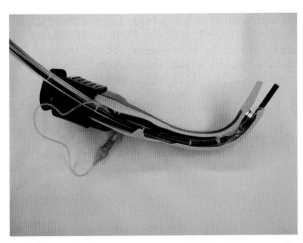

Figure 19-29 Combination of a fiberoptic bronchoscope with an endotracheal tube within an Airtraq optical laryngoscope.

VII. SPECIAL FLEXIBLE FIBEROPTIC BRONCHOSCOPE USES

Attempts at airway control may be undertaken by using equipment in a suboptimal manner, with little assurance of having good outcomes. Here, FOB assistance can increase the rate of success. In these instances, the FOB is most likely to avoid esophageal instrumentation, which is especially ideal if this structure is at a greater risk than usual. Also, it is often a preferred technique in patients with cervical spine risk.

Before embarking on these procedures, make sure that a sufficient number of aware personnel, monitoring equipment, and emergency airway equipment are readily available in the vicinity. This is particularly important in DA patients and in those who are unable to tolerate short periods of apnea. Have alternative management plans in mind, and consider marking off the area of the cricothyroid membrane, applying antiseptic solution, and draping a sterile towel on the neck, in readiness for surgical access.

A. Endotracheal Tube Exchange

Patients may require exchange of an existing ETT for a number of reasons: (1) incorrect ETT size, (2) ETT obstruction, (3) cuff leakage, (4) requirements for a specialty type of tube (e.g., preformed ETT), (5) preference for a regular ETT in place of a preexisting specialty tube, or (6) the need for an alternative route for ETT intubation (e.g., a nasal ETT in place of an oral one).

Commonly, an RL has been used to observe the old ETT within the glottis, placement of a new ETT nearby, and the exchange itself, as an assistant simultaneously withdraws the old ETT and a new one is inserted in its place. On the other hand, a Cook Airway Exchange Catheter (Cook Medical) has been used to blindly carry out this process. However, these two methods are not always successful in DA situations, which become fraught with airway losses, morbidity, and mortality. Use of an FOB to facilitate this exchange can provide a more controlled, successful completion of the goal.

In addition to the following, multiple combination techniques and the usual intubation maneuvers (e.g., jaw

thrust) may be beneficial. Also, spraying local anesthetic in the periglottic/glottic area minimizes reactivity and hemodynamic changes. Preoxygenation and use of positive end-expiratory pressure, as indicated, are required for at least 10 minutes unless the situation is urgent.

1. FOB-Aintree method: Pass an FOB within an Aintree catheter into the old ETT to carry out the exchange. When just above the carina, remove the FOB while bracing the Aintree. Remove the old ETT from around the secured Aintree. Insert a new ETT-loaded FOB down the Aintree until just above the carina. Situate the new ETT, and extract the FOB and Aintree from the patient.

2. FOB-wire method: Thread a wire into the working channel of the FOB until it projects 2 to 3 cm beyond the tip. Slide both into the old ETT, and remove everything except for the wire. Pass an ETT-loaded FOB along the wire by inserting the end projecting out of the oropharynx into the working channel at the FOB tip. Advance the FOB to the precarina area, and railroad the ETT into the patient.

3. FOB-ETT or FOB-wire side-by-side method (especially if a different route of ETT intubation is needed): Insert an ETT-loaded FOB under visual control into the trachea along the anterior commissure next to the preexisting ETT. When the FOB tip reaches the old cuff, deflate it to ease FOB passage until it rests two to three rings above the carina. Constantly observing the carina through the FOB, withdraw the old ETT and advance the new one.[126] Alternatively, insert a wire projecting from the loaded FOB, 8 to 10 cm into the trachea (deflate cuff for passage, if needed). Remove the old ETT, follow the wire toward the carina, and proceed with intubation.

Trouble-Shooting

1. The FOB cannot enter the trachea beside the old ETT: Keep the FOB tip next to the glottic opening so that as the old ETT is slowly withdrawn, the tip can quickly be tucked into the glottis. Note that a combination with a RL may assist in this procedure by opening the pathway.

2. Too many tracheal secretions by the old ETT are preventing FOB visualization: Deflate the old ETT and give two PPV breaths to blow secretions out of the peri-ETT region above its cuff. Reinflate the cuff, suction the secretions, and reattempt the exchange procedure.

B. Preexisting Combitube or Rüsch EasyTube and Intubation

There are a number of reasons for removal of a Combitube (Tyco Healthcare, Mansfield, MA) or a Rüsch Easy-Tube (Teleflex Medical, Research Triangle Park, NC) in exchange for an ETT. First, these devices are available only in very large sizes, which have a limited timeline for remaining in a patient because of concerns regarding direct pressure effects on esophageal or airway structures. Second, suctioning of the trachea for pulmonary toilet can be difficult because of the intra-oropharyngeal obstruction that is normally inherent with the presence of these devices. Moreover, studies have shown that a Combitube has a 5% chance of being placed in the trachea during blind insertion.

FOB assistance in performing endotracheal intubation should be undertaken before the Combitube is removed, to prevent regurgitation and aspiration. Ovassapian and colleagues found that the bulkiness of these types of tubes often created obstacles to manipulation of the FOB. Nevertheless, the exchange success rate was relatively high because the Combitube often caused a lifting up of the epiglottis, making FOB targeting easier.[127]

When an ETT is needed, prepare to exchange these in-dwelling tubes by loading an FOB according to desired ETT, Aintree, or wire combination technique. After maximal oxygenation, partially deflate the oropharyngeal Combitube or EasyTube cuff to allow passage of the loaded FOB into the oropharynx for subsequent exchange. Proceed with FOB placement by using the methods previously described for ETT exchange (see "Endotracheal Tube Exchange").

C. Trouble-Shooting Blind Nasotracheal Intubation

In the case of a spontaneously breathing patient with abnormal obstructive nasopharyngeal or oral pathology, traversing next to nasal abnormalities may cause visual confusion during FOB use. If the patient is able to breathe well through one passage, it is possible to succeed by slow, gentle insertion of a nasal ETT in a mode similar to that used for blind nasal intubation (i.e., feeding it forward while listening to breath sounds). As the sounds increase greatly in volume, insert the FOB through the ETT to enable visual localization of the entrance into the trachea, and continue with the intubation process.

If the nasopharyngeal opening is too small for FOB and ETT admission together, put the FOB in the opposite nasal passage. From this vantage point, insert the ETT into the other nostril. Observe its course as an assistant pushes it forward, and help the assistant to steer it by giving advice about turning the ETT or moving the patient's head and neck.

D. Use of the Fiberoptic Bronchoscope as a Lightwand

A lightwand is a malleable, lighted, stylet-like device that is inserted into a lubricated ETT for blind intubation. An example is the Bovie Aaron Surch-Lite (Bovie Medical Corporation, Clearwater, FL). It is bent at a 45- to 90-degree angle within the ETT while its tip is kept just within but near the ETT tip. Both are placed centrally as a unit into the oropharynx while the patient's mandible is lifted. The room lights are turned off, and the unit is directed toward the glottis. A very bright pretracheal transillumination is sought in the neck, indicating imminent entry into the glottis. Successful intubation rates approach 90%.

When used identically in a darkened room, an FOB may improve the success rate of intubation, but its tip does not need to lie within the ETT, because this is a visually controlled technique.[128] In comparison to the lightwand, with which extension beyond the ETT is not advised, the flexibility of the FOB is unlikely to cause trauma, and there is no worry about thermal injury (which, in reality, is also unlikely with the lightwand). This technique can be advantageous in two ways. First, when one is assisting someone in directing an FOB with no video monitor available, rather than constantly interrupting the operator's view to personally look down the eyepiece to survey nearby anatomy, one should look for FOB transillumination in the neck to prompt advice as to the direction in which the operator should lead the FOB. Second, FOB transillumination may be very useful in patients with soiled airways that interfere with FOB visual reconnaissance. In such cases, transillumination can be used through the soiled surroundings, with the hope that at some point the view will clear to confirm anatomic structures.

E. Double-Lumen Tube or Bronchial Blocker Assistance

Very frequently, lung isolation is accomplished with a DLT by auscultation of the ipsilateral side of the chest during one-lung ventilation and repeated auscultation during ventilation of the opposite side.[129] Periodically, there may be a desire to ensure the correct location of the DLT initially during insertion, or a doubt may arise about its correct placement. The FOB is uniquely suited to aid in the initial alignment or to diagnose proper positioning of the DLT. In addition, the FOB is particularly appropriate to direct the placement of bronchial blockers.

1. Double-Lumen Tube

For a left-sided DLT placement, load a lubricated pediatric FOB down the bronchial lumen of a tested, lubricated DLT. After induction of GA and positive-pressure mask ventilation with 100% oxygen, insert an IOA with careful monitoring to keep the patient appropriately anesthetized during manipulations. Pass the FOB into the trachea until it is above the carina, remove the airway, and slide in the DLT. After seeing the DLT within the trachea, feed the FOB tip into the left bronchus. Continue sliding the DLT until it also ends up within the left bronchus (resistance is felt). Inflate the tracheal cuff, remove the FOB, and ventilate the patient. Attach a swivel adapter to permit continuous respiration. Check left bronchial positioning by inserting the FOB via the adapter down the tracheal lumen. Position the FOB tip to observe the carina and left bronchial area. Inflate the left bronchial cuff. If the inflated cuff is barely bulging out of the left bronchus, the DLT should be secured at this depth. Otherwise, move the DLT in or out until this end point is reached. Use an identical technique (but on the opposite side) to place a right-sided DLT. Note that for a smaller DLT, a pediatric-sized FOB may prevent excessive airway pressures from the FOB's obstructing bulk within the lumen during observation.

Trouble-Shooting

1. During surgery, it is apparent that the bronchial position is incorrect: Observe down the tracheal lumen. Deflate both cuffs, and withdraw the DLT over the

FOB until the carina is identified. Reinsert the DLT into the bronchus. Again, check its position by using the FOB in the tracheal lumen.

2. Bronchial Blocker

Induce GA and intubate the patient's trachea. Pass a preshaped bronchial blocker, with the FOB following alongside it for direction, through the port of a swivel adapter during continuous ventilation. An alternative technique, especially for right-sided blockade due to the high takeoff of the first bronchial branch, is to use a 6- or 8-F, styleted Fogarty venous embolectomy catheter with a 10-mL inflatable balloon. Using a prebent shape, this can be inserted through the ETT next to the FOB and directed into the bronchus.

The Arndt blocker (Cook Medical) (9 F, 75 cm long) comes with a three-port adapter for the ventilatory system, FOB, and bronchial blocker. Insert the FOB down the middle of this adapter to catch the blocker loop on its tip. Insert both, and after entering into the targeted bronchus, disengage the loop to leave the blocker and slowly withdraw the FOB until blocker inflation within the bronchus is in the optimal position.

F. Retrograde Intubation

In some cases, the FOB or other devices for intubation may fail due to abnormal anatomy or airway soiling. Retrograde intubation can be a rescue in these circumstances. This technique utilizes passage of a guidewire through a cricothyroid/thyrotracheal needle or angiocatheter that is directed cephalad. The wire exits the mouth or nose or is fished out with a clamp. The object of this technique is to slide a Teflon guide catheter down the wire to lead an ETT around it into the trachea while the wire is under tension at the neck insertion site and the end is projecting from the 15-mm ETT connector. It is not always successful because of the wire's acute angle and hang-ups at the glottis.

An FOB can be used for rescuing the retrograde technique if placement of the wire is successful but the ETT will not enter the trachea as a result of discordant diameter sizes of the ETT and the wire. The diameter of the FOB can act like a bridge between the ETT and the wire. After passing and securing the wire by the retrograde method, thread the cephalad end of the wire into the working channel at the FOB tip until it exits near the handle. Slide the FOB along the tensed wire into the periglottic area under visual control toward the wire's tracheal entry. Ask for a release of wire tension at the neck and continue the FOB journey toward the carina. At that point, remove the wire and railroad the ETT. An FOB-retrograde combination may be the easiest and most successful technique to pursue any time a retrograde intubation technique is considered.

VIII. RARELY RECOMMENDED: OXYGEN INSUFFLATION VIA BRONCHOSCOPE

Previously, oxygen insufflation at 3 to 5 L/min via the FOB working channel in adults during intubation was proposed to supply supplementary oxygen, clear secretions, and prevent fogging.[52,130,131] Benumof described this technique but recommended that it had to be used very cautiously.[52] If flow of oxygen into the patient exceeds gaseous escape into the atmosphere, serious barotrauma may occur. An FOB squeezing by a significant airway obstruction during endoscopy can limit the egress of gases and result in a pneumothorax. Pneumothorax has also been reported in children and in an infant when flows of 3 to 5 L/min were used.[132,133] Adult flow rates are excessive for tiny pediatric airways. Acute cervical, facial, and thoracic emphysema were reported in one patient.[134] Gastric rupture with subsequent mortality has been documented. It is most likely to occur when oxygen flow is directed into the esophagus or into an area that is unrecognizable (which could be the esophagus).[135-137] Ovassapian and Mesnick declared this to be a technique that should not be recommended.[138] More acceptable during FOB use is the supply of oxygen via nasal cannula, mask, or a catheter in the mouth. FOB oxygen insufflation definitely should not be employed if the flows are too high for the patient's airway diameter, the FOB tip is down the esophagus, or the tip is in an unidentified area.

In spite of these cautions, oxygen insufflation through the FOB may be of value in certain select cases.[139] There are some reports in which its use may have been very beneficial. Hung and colleagues[140] reported a case of a patient undergoing craniotomy in the prone position who had a pin system holding the neck flexed. Intraoperatively, the ETT was totally dislodged. Because of a very enlarged tongue and neck flexion, FOB nasotracheal reintubation was chosen. The patient was placed in reverse Trendelenburg position with a left-sided tilt, and the endoscopist, while sitting on the floor, used intermittent FOB oxygen insufflation throughout the intubation period. The patient was given passive high-flow oxygen by mask. The oxygen saturation remained greater than 90% during the ordeal, which required less than 6 minutes. Would any FOB endoscopist not have used oxygen insufflation in similar circumstances?

IX. FIBEROPTIC INTUBATION IN INFANTS AND CHILDREN

One could say that the indications and entire production of FOB endoscopy in infants and children is the same as for adults except smaller—but that would ignore the major difference in these two patient groups and would be far too simplistic. Flexible fiberoptic intubation of infants and children is a necessary option that must be readily available, particularly for patients in whom this type of airway management is vital. As with adult patients, confidence and competence are easily attainable through clinical practice and knowledge of pediatric concerns. Otherwise, uncertainty and fear may prevail and make the challenge of airway management cases a dreaded disaster. FOB sizes exist in a broad range to service patients as small as premature infants. These FOB models can assist with intubation using ETTs as small as 2.5 mm ID (see Table 19-1). Be aware that the smallest FOB may lack working channels, if the OD is less than 3.1 mm.

Indications for FOB use in infants and children are almost identical to those for adults but are expanded to embrace numerous congenital syndromes and hereditary diseases (Box 19-7). For these special pediatric conditions, many undertakings of FOB endoscopy have been addressed in the literature. Scores of anomalies may have wide-ranging anatomic or systemic effects in this patient population.[141-143] Some have greater effects on localized regions of the airway system and symptomatology. These and acquired pathologic states or trauma can result in DA, aspiration, reactive airways, cough, bronchospasm, and declining respiratory function.

Sleep apnea and increased secretions often figure prominently, and these patients may be more sensitive to drugs and more likely to develop post-extubation failure. Some abnormalities occur more frequently within certain subsets. Altman and colleagues found that 37% of patients with congenital syndromes also had multiple airway abnormalities.[142] Laryngeal abnormalities were three times more common than tracheal ones. Twenty-eight percent of these patients had gastroesophageal reflux. The most common symptom was stridor, in 74%, followed by significant episodes of cyanosis, apnea, and failure to thrive. Nineteen percent of the patients required a tracheostomy for airway management.

Regarding airway control in patients with these problems, mask ventilation may be difficult, and insertion of oral airways may worsen the situation if there is buckling of the tongue posteriorly or if a long epiglottis is folded downward.[143] Patients with noncompressible or nondisplaceable tongues due to lingual enlargement, smaller oropharyngeal access, small mandibles, or cervical spine limitations can be extremely poorly suited to rigid laryngoscopy and, to a lesser extent, video laryngoscopy. Considering the low profile, flexibility, and conformity of FOBs to unpredictable airways, it is often justifiable to consider that an FOB may be the best choice for problematic pediatric cases.

A. Oral Fiberoptic Intubation of the Conscious Pediatric Patient

The approach to oral FOB intubation of more mature or older conscious pediatric patients is very similar to that for adults. With less mature patients, and particularly with younger ones, the differences in monitoring, drugs, psychological preparation, equipment, and technique are striking.

1. Equipment, Monitoring, and Drug Availability

Standard monitoring, capnography, an FOB cart, full airway equipment, oxygen, suctioning equipment, sedatives, opiates, local anesthetics, and vasoconstrictors must be present unless circumstances dictate otherwise. Reversal agents for sedatives or narcotics should be immediately on hand. In the pediatric patient, drugs can be given intravenously, intramuscularly, intranasally, orally, or rectally. Uncommonly, some patients may need inhalation agents until the intravenous line is established. In some cases, a DA cart may be necessary.

2. Psychological Preparation of the Patient

For older children, psychological preparation is useful, and the presence of guardians may contribute to patient cooperation and understanding. For younger ones, preparation may be impossible.

3. Rationale for Pharmacologic Therapy

Antisialogogues, sedatives, and narcotics may be administered after dosing considerations in addition to observation of clinical effects. Before FOB instrumentation, antisialogogues should be given either intravenously, as soon as that route is established, or intramuscularly. Short-acting sedatives or narcotics are preferred because of the propensity for younger pediatric patients to desaturate when obstruction or respiratory depression occurs. Patient fears due to immaturity or lack of intellectual understanding often increase drug resistance until significant respiratory deterioration transpires.

Ketamine is especially suited for infants, small children, and mentally handicapped patients, but transient apnea of less than 60 seconds duration has been reported.[145] In the patient with DA or respiratory compromise, however, ketamine may be advantageous because respiratory function tends to be adequate with fewer adverse breathing difficulties, as demonstrated by Hostetler and colleagues.[144] Prior administration of antisialogogues will offset ketamine's effect in increasing upper airway secretions, occasionally to the point of inciting laryngospasm or causing interference with FOB endoscopy. As a reminder, the airway should be suctioned before FOB instrumentation. During FOB endoscopy, no difficulties due to increased airway reactivity have been documented with this drug.[145]

Drug dosages used for pediatric patients are listed (Table 19-3). Maintenance of spontaneous ventilation together with a degree of sedation or analgesia (or both) is the objective, unless contraindicated.

TABLE 19-3

Pediatric Drug Dosages Assisting Fiberoptic Intubation

Drug	Dosage
Atropine	0.02 mg/kg IV or IM
Glycopyrrolate	0.004 mg/kg IV or IM
Fentanyl	0.5 µg/kg IV increments
Ketamine	0.5 mg/kg IV increments (4-5 mg/kg IM if lesser airway difficulty)
Ketamine	2 mg for each 1 mL propofol infused as a propofol drip at 50-200 µg/kg/min
Midazolam	10-20 µg/kg IV increments
Propofol	0.5-2.0 mg/kg IV bolus; infused as a drip at 50-200 µg/kg/min
Remifentanil	infused as an IV drip at 0.05-0.1 µg/kg/min

Dexmedetomidine and propofol are titratable sedatives that are advantageous for quick onset and rapid awakening. Less respiratory depression and more analgesia make dexmedetomidine the more attractive of the two, although it would be an off-label.

4. Anatomic Specifics of Pediatric Airway Structures

Anatomic differences between the airways of the adult, child, and infant are described in Chapter 36. In pediatric patients, the tongue is relatively larger, the larynx is more rostral, and the vocal cords are more inclined.[146] In contrast to adults, the larynx in newborns is not only relatively smaller in comparison to their bodies but softer and more sensitive. The shape is funnel-like, and as a result the cricoid cartilage is at the narrowest point. As the infant ages, the larynx descends in a caudad direction toward the final adult location (Table 19-4).[143]

The infantile omega-shaped epiglottis is floppier, longer, and tubular in comparison to that of adults. It is often directed posteriorly, although variations can occur. Innervation of the airway is similar to that in adults, except that the left recurrent laryngeal nerve takes a relatively longer course around the aortic arch and, therefore, may be more prone to pathology.

5. Topical Orotracheal Anesthesia Techniques

LA techniques can make FOB use a very quiet, efficient procedure for awake intubation. Even under GA, this technique is useful as a method for reducing hemodynamic responses and reflexes that are particularly prone to occur in pediatric patients. Techniques for local airway anesthesia are very similar in the pediatric population and in adults with some exceptions, mostly involving younger patients.

TABLE 19-4

Changing Levels of the Larynx from Fetus to Puberty

Age	Spinal Level (Cervical Vertebrae)
Fetus	C2 and C3
Newborn	C4
Age 6 years	C5
Puberty	C6-C7

For transtracheal anesthesia, the cricothyroid area is much smaller and harder to palpate in infants younger than 6 months of age. In addition, needling of very small tracheas should be avoided, because any drops of blood within the trachea would compromise the airway to a much greater extent than in larger patients. One should also be wary of any needling in the neck for the external approach to the SLN. In the smallest patients and those with the most difficult airways, intra-arterial injection is more likely because of the closer proximity of relatively miniature structures, even if tiny needles are used. Intra-oral techniques may work well for patients who are able to cooperate. Aerosolized techniques tend to be most effective when patients have a history of using inhalers and can relate to the idea of breathing in medicines.

6. Local Anesthetic Drug Choices

These patients are smaller, and dosages must be tapered down accordingly. Drugs containing benzocaine must not be administered to infants because of concerns for methemoglobinemia. They should probably be avoided also in small children weighing less than 40 kg, because the spray method of delivery increases the complexity of gauging drug dosages accurately.

Suggested dosages for aerosolized lidocaine should be reviewed before administration (Table 19-5).

7. Positioning of Infants and Small Children

Usually, the head and neck can remain in neutral position. In some cases, a slight extension of the neck with a towel under the upper thorax may be useful if the head is large and tends to produce neck flexion in the supine position.

The table or bed height should be adjusted to a low but appropriate level to keep the FOB relatively straight. In some cases, a stepstool may be of value. Infants can be swathed in a towel or sheet with sufficient length for one end and then the other to be wrapped over the baby's arm and stuffed under the body. No restriction of ventilation results from this restraining method, in contrast to an entire body wraparound.

8. Endotracheal Tubes: Uncuffed Versus Cuffed

The choice of an uncuffed ETT for patients younger than 8 years of age has been a tradition for decades owing to various apprehensions. One concern was that a smaller-ID, high-volume, low-pressure, cuffed ETT would have to be

TABLE 19-5

Aerosolized Lidocaine: Suggested Dosing According to Weight

Weight (kg)	Volume of 4% Lidocaine (mL)	Volume of Saline (mL)
10-14	0.5	2
15-19	1.0	2
20-24	1.5	3
25-29	2.0	4
30-34	2.5	0
35-39	3.0	0
40-44	3.5	0
≥45	4.0	0

selected, rather than an uncuffed ETT, because of the added width of the deflated cuff within the trachea. Downsizing the ETT prompted a worry that there might be increased resistance to ventilation. However, because the trachea is relatively large for the pediatric body habitus, this should not be a factor as long as an ETT size is chosen appropriately for the patient's age and dimensions.[147] Another worry was that cuff pressure might result in a higher incidence of subglottic ischemia and stenosis.[148,149] Particularly in tiny patients, there was a concern that although the tip of the ETT was within their tracheas, the cuff might remain between the vocal cords.

More recent literature, which includes extensive comparisons of morbidities and outcomes in surgical and intensive care unit patients, may be starting to refute some of these ideas.[150-153] Weiss and associates studied two groups of patients undergoing surgery with a cuffed ETT (Microcuff PET with distance markings [Microcuff GmbH, Weinheim, Germany]) versus an uncuffed ETT (multiple brands). Among the 2246 children with ASA class I or II physical status (mean age <2 years), there was a 15 times lower incidence of repeat laryngoscopy in the cuffed ETT group and, of course, less trauma.[151] The most common cause for repeat laryngoscopy was an initial ETT that was too large or too small. The incidence of stridor between the two groups was almost identical (4.4% and 4.7%, respectively).

An added advantage of cuffed ETT use is better aspiration protection, better seal pressure for ventilation, and less atmospheric contamination during GA. There are still a number of factors that are of concern, however. Longer outcome models are needed with improved pediatric ETT design to eliminate the intraglottic inflated cuff worry and higher ETT costs. If cuffed ETTs are used, intra-cuff pressures should be monitored to a limit of 20 to 25 cm H_2O.[154]

B. Fiberoptic Orotracheal Technique

FOB intubation of infants and children uses similar procedures, techniques, and aiding maneuvers (e.g., tongue pull) as in adults. It requires an assistant and equipment appropriate to body habitus. The patient should receive an antisialogogue before any instrumentation. An IOA such as the VBM Bronchoscope Airway (VBM Medical, Noblesville, IN) can be used. It is produced in newborn and child sizes. This airway initially is three-quarters enclosed with an open side. In its distal half, it gives way to a completely curved and open, spatula-like area, somewhat similar to the Ovassapian fiberoptic intubating airway. A bite block is another choice, with the endoscopist's inserting hand gently resting on the patient's face to keep the FOB midline.

If necessary for oxygen administration, endoscopy masks (e.g., VBM) are available in infant and child sizes (see Fig. 19-21). The advantage of the central endoscopy port of a mask is accessibility in children to both oral and nasal FOB approaches. A regular mask with a bronchoscopic swivel adapter can also be employed. Supplementary oxygen "blow-by" or a nasal cannula is another option.

Place an IOA or brace the hand to facilitate keeping the FOB midline, which is a critical step in dealing with the differences associated with smaller structures in pediatric patients. Hold the FOB and insert it as described previously for adults. For either oral or nasal intubation in younger patients, it is almost always advised to introduce the FOB before the ETT, because if part of the smaller ETT precedes FOB entry into the oropharynx, its size may limit full FOB maneuverability. As always, one should strive to keep recognizable structures in the middle of the view during insertion.

C. Two-Stage Fiberoptic Intubation

Some patients have airways that are too small to admit an FOB. In these cases, intubation can be carried out in two stages. First, thread a guidewire from an airway exchange catheter set (e.g., Cook Pediatric Airway Exchange Catheter [PAEC]) through the working channel of the FOB. The PAEC is available in sizes as small as 8 F (2.7 mm) with a length of 83 cm. Allow only up to 1.0 cm of the wire to exit beyond the FOB tip as the scope is introduced into the oropharynx. When the glottis is visualized, advance the wire into the trachea for a distance approximating the length to the carina. Remove the FOB. For the second stage, use the Cook catheter setup to pass an appropriately sized ETT over the wire, in a manner similar to the ETT exchange technique previously described.

D. Nasal Fiberoptic Intubation of the Conscious Pediatric Patient

Attention should be paid to history and to examination for any nasal anomalies.

Warming the ETT to soften it and pretreatment with phenylephrine or oxymetazoline may help stave off nosebleeds. Antisialogogue, sedative or narcotic, and LA dosages need to be appropriate for the patient's size. A breakaway NPA may be used in older patients.

In the nasopharynx, introduction of the ETT before the FOB heightens anxiety about provoking epistaxis. Hypertrophied adenoids are common between the ages of 2 and 6 years, and they are more susceptible to the trauma of a blind ETT entry. Epistaxis must be seriously avoided, because of the greater degree of difficulty presented by any blood in the small airways of these very small patients.

This technique is similar to that for adults in regard to preparation, except that administration of the anticholinergic (antisialogogue) should absolutely be carried out as a preventative against bradycardia before instrumentation in younger patients. Endoscopy masks and swivel adapters are much more amenable to nasal entry of the FOB in pediatric patients compared with adults, because their noses are closer to their mouths.

Trouble-Shooting

1. The FOB cannot pass through the intended ETT: A technique similar to that described for trouble-shooting blind nasotracheal intubation may be used. Insert the FOB through one nostril and the ETT through the other.[155] While observing the ETT and airway through the FOB, advise the assistant how to move the ETT,

head, and neck to achieve endotracheal intubation. This technique may require one FOB operator and one or more experienced assistants to perform all the maneuvers.

E. Oral or Nasal Fiberoptic Intubation of the Unconscious Pediatric Patient

1. Patient Under Routine General Anesthesia

Again, the patient's eyes should always be protected and an anticholinergic agent given. LA of the airway to limit the reflexes should be considered if the patient is cooperative enough. Full equipment preparation, as described previously, is imperative. This should include two suctions if there is any threat of regurgitation. Older patients may be approached with the same techniques used in adults.

If difficult mask or laryngeal airway management is not anticipated, induce GA and perform mask ventilation with 100% oxygen. Among volatile anesthetics, sevoflurane is popular for its less irritating qualities. With the patient under deep anesthesia with spontaneous respiration or lighter GA with muscle relaxant, remove the mask and execute the FOB intubation as previously described. To ward off laryngospasm, muscle relaxants are advantageous if the patient is too uncooperative to attempt local airway anesthesia preoperatively. However, if spontaneous ventilation is more desirable, 2% to 4% lidocaine may be used on the vocal cords in a "spray as you go" technique. Even if a patient has not reacted to more superficial instrumentation, this may prevent glottic closure as a result of FOB touching of the vocal cords. If intubation is not quickly performed, it is important to remember that this technique of lifting the mask can lead to rapid desaturation in some patients, particularly smaller ones and those at higher risk. For this reason, promptly return to mask ventilation between brief periods of instrumentation.

An alternative is to perform simultaneous mask ventilation and intubation using an endoscopy mask or bronchoscopic swivel adapter. Very good assistance with patient ventilation is needed to ensure safety with this method.

Another possibility is to use an SGA or an intubating SGA. In some cases, pressure from the SGA may direct an epiglottis posteriorly to obscure the laryngeal opening. This can impair correct seating of these perilaryngeal airways or inhibit blind attempts at ETT passage. An FOB can assist with SGA placement, and the FOB-SGA combination for intubation is more likely to result in successful insertion of the ETT. The combination also is more likely to avert trauma from blind attempts near delicate airway structures in very young patients. The pediatric setting is another example of the usefulness of the multimodal approach to the DA.

2. General Anesthesia Using Short, Soft Nasopharyngeal Airways

A breakaway NPA may be used in older children to assist FOB passage, as detailed earlier.

The method of administering anesthesia with an NPA during FOB intubation has also been described

previously. This is a more common technique for younger pediatric patients.[156-158] For this technique, adapt an NPA by cutting a Murphy eye–type hole near the distal end and insert the NPA into one nostril.[159] Connect the anesthetic circuit to a 15-mm adapter within the NPA to supply inhalation anesthesia to the spontaneously breathing patient. Meanwhile, proceed with FOB intubation orally or nasally. Alternatively, insert an ETT into one nasal passage and use that for continued anesthetization while executing either oral or nasal intubation through the opposite nostril.

X. ADVANTAGES OF FLEXIBLE FIBEROPTIC BRONCHOSCOPES

It is a universally documented fact that the FOB can be used to perform all aspects of patient intubation for routine airway control before any surgery. The FOB has a long history of having the greatest success of any non-surgical technique for DA management, and for rescue of failed airway management by other devices, because of its innate ability to enter through very limited oral or nasal openings, glide along aberrant structures, and follow the contour of the airway in patients with any body position, body habitus, or age. Its multimodal ability to be combined with many other airway devices, including surgical ones, is incomparable. These three unique characteristics prove that the FOB is the most superior of all nonsurgical methods for airway control. It is not surprising then, that the FOB can be life-saving and life-altering as a result of its rescue capabilities and capacity to ward off surgical airway takeovers. In extreme situations, its use can accomplish safe intubation and allow GA for operations on patients for whom airway control would otherwise be impossible, even surgically, such as those with severe ankylosing spondylitis (Fig. 19-30).

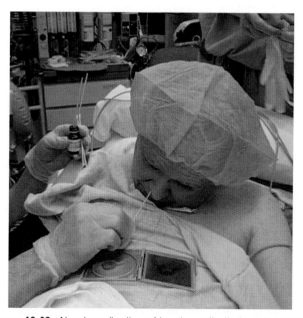

Figure 19-30 Nasal application of local anesthetic in anticipation of awake fiberoptic intubation in a patient with severe "chin on chest" ankylosing spondylitis, ideally managed with the use of a fiberoptic bronchoscope. (Used with permission.)

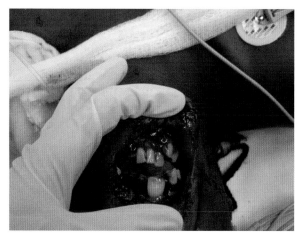

Figure 19-31 Fiberoptic nasotracheal intubation is planned for a patient with multiple loose and displaced teeth secondary to an automobile injury.

A. Most Accurate Confirmation of Respiratory Tract Endotracheal Intubation

No other airway management device provides the same degree of certainty of respiratory tract intubation as the FOB, because it is the only instrument that yields detailed visualization of respiratory tract anatomy. Also, FOB use assists and confirms DLT and bronchial blocker placement.

B. Less Patient Trauma or Side Effects

In combination with excellent LA, patients can be intubated with almost no cardiovascular stimulation. Whether the FOB is used to intubate the trachea under LA or under GA, it is the most likely airway instrument to prevent damage to airway structures, especially those most at risk (Fig. 19-31).

C. Minimal Cervical Spine Motion

It has been well documented (Box 19-8) that FOB intubation and blind nasal intubation are associated with the least amount of cervical spine motion during cineradiography, compared with other intubation techniques. Of course, the former is more advantageous, because FOB intubation is a visual technique with a higher success rate and lower propensity for trauma. It is extremely popular in the cervical spine risk setting compared with other carefully performed intubation methods involving a minimum of cervical motion; however, neither of these two techniques has been shown to be safer or more likely to prevent secondary neurologic deficits (Fig. 19-32).

D. Diagnostic Capabilities

The FOB is a multifunctional device with excellent diagnostic capabilities. It is used to investigate vocal cord motion (e.g., detecting recurrent laryngeal nerve injury), tracheal motion (e.g., detecting tracheomalacia after thyroidectomy), high airway pressures, presence of secretions, infection sites, endobronchial intubation, problems with single-lung ventilation (e.g., high takeoff of right upper lobe), foreign bodies, site entry during tracheostomies, malpositioned SGA, folded-over epiglottis, intratracheal or pharyngeal pathology, and other scenarios. It is also useful to assess the quality of a bronchial or tracheal suture and to permit evaluation of the airway status in burned patients.

E. Therapeutic Capabilities

Aside from the capability to assist in successful placement or adjustment of numerous pieces of airway equipment, the FOB can be therapeutic in other ways. It is used for exact positioning of an ETT to bypass obstructive pathology. Changes in oxygenation can be investigated to determine whether endobronchial intubation is a factor, and the FOB can assist with ETT repositioning. The FOB is therapeutic for removal of blood, secretions, or foreign bodies and for exchanging endotracheal or tracheostomy tubes.

Box 19-8	**Cervical Spine Risk and Airway Management: Literature Support***

Todd M: Cervical spine mechanics, instability and airway management. Ovassapian Memorial Lecture. Presented at the Society for Airway Management Annual Meeting, Chicago, September 2010.

Wong DM, Prabhu A, Chakraborty S, et al: Cervical spine motion during flexible bronchoscopy compared with the Lo-Pro GlideScope. *Br J Anaesth* 102:424–430, 2009.

Crosby E: Considerations for airway management for cervical spine surgery in adults. *Anesthesiol Clin* 25:511–533, 2007.

Crosby E: Airway management in adults after cervical spine trauma. *Anesthesiology* 104:1293–1318, 2006.

Brimacombe J, Keller C, Künzel K, et al: Cervical spine motion during airway management: A cinefluoroscopic study of the posteriorly destabilized third cervical vertebrae in human cadavers. *Anesth Analg* 91:1274–1278, 2000.

Crosby T: Tracheal intubation in the cervical spine injured patient (editorial). *Can J Anaesth* 39:105–109, 1992.

Meschino A, Devitt H, Koch J, et al: The safety of awake tracheal intubation in cervical spine injury. *Anesthesiology* 39:114–117, 1992.

Suderman V, Crosby T, Lui A: Elective oral tracheal intubation in cervical spine-injured adults. *J Anaesth* 38:785–789, 1991.

Crosby E, Lui A: The adult cervical spine: Implications for airway management. *Can J Anaesth* 37:77–93, 1990.

Graham J: Complications of cervical spine surgery: A five-year report on a survey of the membership of the Cervical Spine Research Society by the Morbidity and Mortality Committee. *Spine* 14:1046–1050, 1989.

Grande CM, Barton CR, Stene JK: Appropriate techniques for airway management of emergency patients with suspected spinal cord injury. *Anesth Analg* 67:714–715, 1988.

*Suggested reading for a more in-depth determination of at-risk cervical spine considerations with regard to airway management.

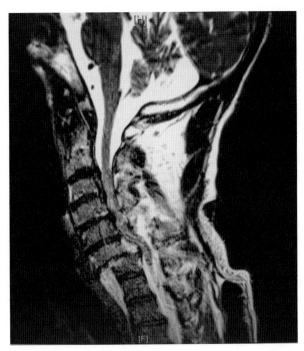

Figure 19-32 Patients with cervical spine risk are least in danger of cervical motion if a fiberoptic bronchoscope is used for intubation.

XI. DISADVANTAGES AND COMPLICATIONS OF FLEXIBLE FIBEROPTIC BRONCHOSCOPES

This section details only problems related to FOB technique, not those common to all airway control methods (e.g., endobronchial intubation) or LA, which are discussed elsewhere.

A. Unsuccessful Intubation

Although success rates of intubation with FOB intervention are high, failures do occur from a variety of causes. During intubation, the FOB enters into the trachea and the ETT is railroaded over it in a blind fashion. At times, the ETT can get hung up, usually on the right arytenoid, and not pass. If the Murphy eye faces anteriorly, there is a much greater chance of successful intubation. However, failure can transpire occasionally even if the Murphy eye is directed correctly. For additional success, a centrally curved, soft-tip ETT may be the answer.[160] Another solution to this situation is simultaneous use of video laryngoscopy, which allows observation of the passage of the ETT over the FOB near the laryngeal structures to resolve potential conflicts between the ETT bevel and airway structures.

Disparate diameters between the FOB and the ETT is another source for impeding ETT passage. Choosing an FOB diameter closer to that of the ETT or using an Aintree bridge lessens this possibility.

With greater degrees of diameter disparity, flippage is more likely to occur as a cause of failed FOB intubation. When the FOB is advanced into the trachea only a short distance and forceful pressure is exerted on the ETT

caught in the periglottic area, the ETT can get even more stuck. The pressure may finally be released through a wayward movement of the ETT into the esophagus. The transmitted pressure of the ETT in the interim may cause pressure on the very flexible FOB, resulting in the insertion section's being flipped out of the trachea. Keeping a long length of the insertion section within the trachea by ensuring that the FOB tip is just above the carina decreases the likelihood of this problem, as does diminishing the disparity between the FOB and ETT diameter.

Another cause for difficulty may result if the ETT is advanced first, part way into the pharynx, and the FOB is passed into the ETT. The FOB may exit out the Murphy eye and prevent successful ETT intubation even though a great view of the carina is evident (Fig. 19-33). Passage of the FOB first obviates this complication, but if passing the ETT first is desired, careful observation and slow FOB passage down the ETT, while being on guard to this possibility, will preclude an adverse result.

Rarely, the FOB enters a wide-open esophagus that is mistaken for the trachea. Identifying what seem to be tracheal rings is not enough to prevent this error. The esophagus may seem to have indentation-like rings, particularly in pediatric patients, in whom structures are in closer proximity. This is also more likely to occur when thick secretions or fogging is present. Identifying the carina provides more definitive proof that the FOB is in the correct system.

The FOB tends to be at a disadvantage in any soiled airway because of the small diameter of the viewing tip, which is more easily obscured as it makes its journey forward through confounding elements. Use of an FOB in these conditions is not completely contraindicated, but success is less likely. Combinations with other devices (e.g., an SGA) may overcome these difficulties.

B. Worsening Respiratory Tract Obstruction

Patients who have preexisting narrowing or obstructive pathology in their upper airways may have difficulty when any non-hollow object is placed in the area. To ward off effects of near or total obstruction once the FOB enters the respiratory tract, FOB manipulation must be speedy and careful.

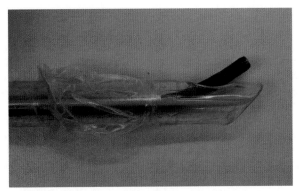

Figure 19-33 Flexible fiberoptic bronchoscope tip exiting from the Murphy eye on an endotracheal tube; this scenario will prevent intubation.

C. Fragility and Expense

FOB instruments are very delicate and frequently very expensive. Repairs for major teaching centers equipped with full systems, an FOB video screen, and other features can run into thousands of dollars per month. Tapping the FOB tip on cleansing pads, bending the shaft, using the angulation lever to move the tip within an ETT, compressive damage from being bitten or being pinched by a slammed drawer, and dropping the instrument must be avoided. Forcing an FOB through an ETT can shear off outer fabrics or cause kinking. If this damage is very extreme, it could cause ETT obstruction, and the FOB may be permanently stuck within it.

An added expense is cleaning the devices and paying for assistants to clean them. The question of which type of system, disposable or nondisposable, would be cheaper depends on how many usages are involved. Obviously, if very few FOB actions are being undertaken, disposables would be cheaper, but another factor to consider is that success rates are more likely to drop the fewer times FOB technique is used on patients. These concerns affect the choice between a classic FOB and a disposable "chip on the tip" endoscope.

To keep costs to a minimum, an FOB does not need to be stroked or talked to, but it does need to be babied. Constant education and conscientious use are the main requisites that can keep repair costs down—in the range of only a few hundred dollars per scope per year!

D. System Bulk and Storage Space Requirements

The FOBs are lengthy, with long handle parts in addition to insertion sections of approximately 60 cm. For anything beyond an Olympus MAF Airway Mobilescope (Olympus America, Center Valley, PA), an Ambu aScope, or a fiberscope with eyepiece only, an entire system is quite bulky. It may involve a video monitoring tower, light source setup, and areas to hang clean and used instruments (see Fig. 19-7). Adequate storage space often requires logistic help in situating the FOB systems among patients, personnel, and other equipment needed for patient care.

E. Complications

Many expert endoscopists can perform FOB intubation in less than 30 seconds. In comparison to other techniques, however, FOB intubation usually requires slightly more time in routine airway cases. As the period of apnea lengthens, oxygen desaturation is more likely to occur. Close monitoring and rapid correction should stave off any untoward events.

FOB intubation performed under GA only can precipitate hemodynamic changes similar to those observed with rigid laryngoscopy or video laryngoscopy.[161] This may be secondary to the FOB endoscopist's manipulation of the ETT in response to tube impingement during passage or to pain caused by tongue pull or jaw thrust. Preemptive therapy is useful. Vigilance and prompt responsive therapy should avoid complications.

Postoperative sore throat, dysphonia, and dysphagia after FOB intubation in non-DA patients have an identical incidence to that after rigid laryngoscopy. This might be related to the manipulation and to ETT impingement on perilaryngeal structures, particularly if the ETT is vigorously pushed. Gentle technique, optimal ETT usage, and avoidance of forceful actions minimize these effects.

XII. OTHER CAUSES OF FAILURE WITH FIBEROPTIC BRONCHOSCOPES

A. Inexperience

The number one cause of FOB intubation failure is inexperience due to insufficient training and practice with lack of attention to detail in performing the correct steps to execute flawless FOB procedures. To achieve the greatest degree of success, indications and contraindications must be followed. A proactive low threshold for FOB use is important when considering either a DA associated with comorbidities, which could be adversely affected by airway management problems, or just an exceedingly difficult airway. Indiscriminate use of an RL in these circumstances could worsen an already bleak picture, and if FOB attempts are to follow, hopes of success may soon spiral downward.

B. Lack of Assistance

An inadequate number of personnel and poor understanding of what they will be required to perform prevents everyone from functioning as a cohesive unit. Competent assistance with clear direction can turn FOB management into a simple, triumphant procedure.

C. Lack of Preparation

Inferior preparation of patients, equipment, and personnel doom FOB use to difficulty, if not failure. Psychological preparation, equipment, antisialogogues, sedatives, narcotics, and local anesthetics must be optimized and individualized for each patient. Untrained personnel must understand the techniques of tongue pull, jaw thrust, keeping the airway in the midline, and injecting LA through the FOB.

D. Insufficient Trouble-Shooting and Adaptability

An Indian proverb states, "If you live in the river you should make friends with the crocodile." In other words, a frame of mind to adapt to changing conditions and attempt trouble-shooting will eliminate problems as they arise. Have a number of plans available for any possibility. For example, defoggers can be useful on a distal FOB tip, but it might be the eyepiece lens that needs treatment if fogging is occurring proximally due to warm exhaled breath around the FOB operator's mask.[162] One should especially consider multimodal approaches and enlist more than one assisting action to help with techniques.

E. Inadequacy of Local Anesthesia

Obviously, insufficient LA is a hindrance. To avert difficulty, LA levels should be tested; for example, suctioning the oropharynx toward the larynx tests both GPN (gagging) and SLN (coughing) blocks. If one of these is inadequate, the block can be repeated or the "spray as you go" technique can be used. A tongue depressor can be used for testing the GPN, but this lacks the advantage of clearing secretions or blood. Absence of cough during a transtracheal injection should make the adequacy of the technique suspect. A repeat injection of only 1 mL of the LA can be used to test for cough. If the patient coughs, it is likely that the drug was not injected in the correct area the first time, and the remainder of the dose should be given. If no cough occurs, it is probably unnecessary and perhaps dangerous to give the rest. Good LA prevents gagging, vomiting, coughing, and laryngospasm, which can impede laryngeal visualization and intubation. It also prevents hemodynamic responses to the FOB.

F. Failure to Remember Airway Device Combinations

The combination option should be high on the priority list for rescue of difficult FOB intubation or other airway device techniques. The multimodal approach is most likely to impact airway control in patients with upper airway bleeding, secretions, or edema and those with periglottic or periepiglottic pathology.

G. Discordance in Fiberoptic Bronchoscope and Endotracheal Tube Diameter

Impingement problems with discordance between the FOB and ETT diameter size have been described and can be avoided with better selection of the FOB or ETT and use of an Aintree catheter (Fig. 19-34). Make sure that the lubricated FOB easily traverses the ETT to prevent

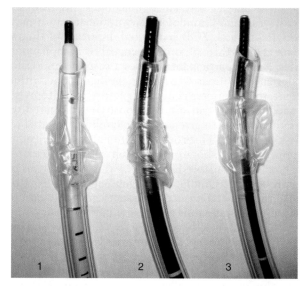

Figure 19-34 Diameter differences should be minimized: *1,* pediatric fiberoptic bronchoscope (FOB) within Aintree within endotracheal tube (ETT); *2,* adult FOB within ETT; *3,* pediatric FOB within ETT.

intussusception of its outer cover. Initial insertion with the FOB rather than the ETT usually improves its maneuverability.

XIII. LEARNING FIBEROPTIC INTUBATION

It has been more than 50 years since Shigeto Ikeda catapulted airway control, from use of a steel, 1940s-style RL to use of a sleek video-emitting FOB. FOBs have consistently been used to rescue patients from failures of that 1940s device, but the opposite is rarely true in competent hands. A wealth of studies and case reports in the most difficult of situations have described superiority of the FOB. Thanks to this instrument, surgeries have not been cancelled, teeth have not been knocked out, slashing of necks with subsequent scarring has been avoided, complications have not come to pass, and lives have been saved.

How is it, then, that patient caregivers in airway management, whether in the fields of anesthesiology, emergency medicine, or critical care medicine, are still reluctant and insufficiently resolved to master this technique? A technique with which a novice can be successful 95% of the time on the first attempt at FOB intubation after 10 cases, while averaging 91 seconds to completion?[163] A technique that 94% of respondents in 2007, from 23 medical schools, characterized as a basic residency skill?[107] Fortunately, as medical care advances, more professionals have realized the value of the unique, multifaceted qualities of the FOB.

Learning FOB intubation should not be just a technical skills endeavor. It should be integrated into a broader frame of airway management that emphasizes technical skills as well as decision-making strategy. Strategy acquisition will lead to appropriate decisions in stressful situations and the ability to act as a team leader in emergency and nonemergency settings.

A. Understanding the Fiberoptic Bronchoscope: Resources

Priorities in becoming a totally competent airway management specialist must be set. Although the FOB may seem formidable, it is not. Familiarity with its delicate construction and function will breed enlightenment. Like video games or golf, FOB use requires practice.

Box 19-9 presents a personal quotation that was authored by Dr. Ovassapian for use at the Annual Meeting of the ASA Basic Adult Fiberoptic Laryngoscopy Workshop and has been cited at every ASA Basic Adult Flexible Fiberoptic Intubation Workshop since 2007.

Getting to know and become friends with the FOB offsets any reluctance toward it. This can be achieved through in-service training (equipment representatives are excellent resources to assist clinicians), digital video discs, videos, on-line sources such as YouTube.com, textbooks, journal articles, and FOB workshops. Internet resource sites are listed in Silos and Bolliger's article on educational resources for bronchoscopy with small summaries concerning their content and even a star rating system for the value of each Web site.[164] These resource sites include the following (all accessed May 2012):

http://www.bronchoscopy.org/education/BiEducEB_.asp

http://www.bronchoscopy.org/education/BiEducArt_vw_.asp

http://www.bronchoscopy.org/education/BiEducStep_.asp

http://www.thoracic-anesthesia.com/?page_id=2

http://www.lumen.luc.edu/lumen/MedEd/medicine/pulmonar/procedur/bronchd.htm

Many of these resources are instructional and have free downloads, and some are even fun to watch.

B. Handling the Fiberoptic Bronchoscope

Practicing on an intubation mannequin is a fairly interesting experience, and attending a fiberoptic workshop is always worthwhile. Practice in these arenas will overcome the suspicion that lack of manual dexterity and insufficient competence in this technique can rule the professional lives of airway specialists, whether in the intensive care unit, emergency room, or operating room.

1. Practice with Dexterity Models and Simulators

Many dexterity models are available commercially to exercise hand-eye coordination and optical recognition. There is research evidence that higher benefits are derived from practice with these models than from didactic lectures. Some are free, whereas others cost thousands of dollars (Video 19-6).

This type of learning is based on the concept of "part or partial task training," which involves the deconstruction of a complex psychomotor task —FOB intubation— into several elementary tasks. An example of one part learned through simulation would be to follow precisely the three directions of entering the oropharynx, traversing the larynx, and advancing into the trachea (i.e., downward, upward, and downward again). Subsequently, the acquisition of multiple partial tasks results in integration of all the different acquired steps.[165]

How much practice is needed? Participants usually find that intubating head models are very straightforward, very easy, and hardly challenging. Whatever dexterity model is chosen, the end point for practice is when FOB maneuvers are carried out as intended, without excessive back-pedaling or repeats. Then it is time to move on to live subjects.

a. HIGH-FIDELITY INANIMATE AIRWAY MODELS

Expensive, human-looking models are available that mimic the airway down to the level of the first bronchi to aid in FOB training. The CLA Broncho Boy series (CLA, Coburg, Germany) has models that simulate pathology. One model even has a fluorescing bronchial tree. The Laerdal Airway Management Trainer (Laerdal Medical, Wappingers Falls, NY) is similarly designed but can simulate multiple DAs (e.g., tongue obstruction, laryngospasm) through its accompanying computer and computer program.

b. PAPIER MACHÉ RESPIRATORY TRACT MODEL

On the cheaper side, Di Domenico and coworkers made a wire and papier maché model of the respiratory tract for FOB practice that was used successfully by participants to gain fiberoptic dexterity.[166]

c. PURELY COMPUTER-BASED BRONCHOSCOPY SIMULATORS

A computer-generated model was developed to improve understanding of the most distant airway anatomy, FOB technique, and dexterity. Diemunsch developed the Virtual Fiberoptic Intubation (VFI) program (Fig. 19-35).[167] This system anatomically presents clinical scenarios, with and without multiple types of airway pathology, for which FOB use can be practiced easily on a personal computer. To give a better understanding of overall anatomic structures, three separate images are available for simultaneous review: a transparent reconstructed image derived by virtue of computed tomography or magnetic resonance imaging scans, the scans themselves, and simulated airway anatomy imagery through which an FOB is directed. Insertion of the FOB can be chosen through oropharyngeal or nasopharyngeal routes. As the participant chooses a scenario and follows predesigned motions to advance the fiberscope within a patient, the computer-generated picture of anatomy seen by the fiberscope can simultaneously be compared with the other images to give an understanding of spatial relationships. The VFI program eliminates the need for expensive and elaborate simulation setups, takes up no space, and is available in compact disc form at no cost from Karl Storz GmbH, Tuttlingen, Germany.

Alternatively, computer-based integrated endoscopic manipulation simulators are somewhat expensive systems that use simple, face-like models for FOB entry and practice with bronchoscopes. A computer-based interface aids in training, and the system can act as a testing site for competency; examples include the National Taiwan University Endoscopic Simulation Study Group (NTUSEC) computer-based bronchoscopy simulator and the AccuTouch bronchoscope simulation system (Immersion

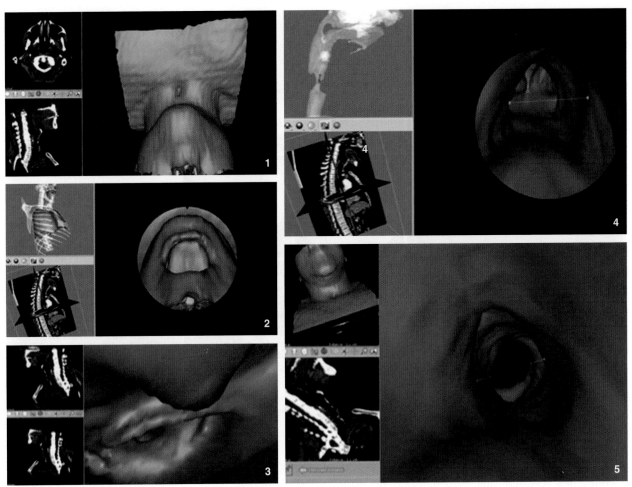

Figure 19-35   Virtual Fiberoptic Intubation (VFI) images: *1,* comparison with radiologic scans; *2,* transparent anatomic and radiologic comparison with pharyngeal entry; *3,* posterior nasopharyngeal view of uvula above and posterior larynx below; *4,* carina comparison with imaging planes; *5,* intratracheal view.

Medical, Gaithersburg, MD).[168-170] Surprisingly, Chandra and coworkers demonstrated that training on the costly AccuTouch simulator did not bring additional benefits compared with training on a low-cost, low-fidelity model consisting of three wooden panels with holes ("Choose The Hole") into which the trainee is asked to insert the FOB in different directional combinations.[171]

d. COMMERCIAL DEXTERITY MODEL

Dexter (Dexter Endoscopy, Wellington, New Zealand) is an expensive semi- or non-anatomic, modular training system featuring multiple paths, bifurcations, conduits, and maps by which an FOB can be directed to improve dexterity.

e. GIL 5-MINUTE FIBEROPTIC DEXTERITY MODEL

The Gil dexterity model has no computer, costs little, and requires only 5 minutes for anyone to make (Fig. 19-36). If rusty FOB dexterity skills need refurbishing, this cheap dexterity model can be constructed quickly from pieces of readily available materials (i.e., tape, pieces of ventilation hose, ETTs, and suction tubing).[172] Tape the elements down in a "dexterity course layout," and cover the layout with a towel. Practice for 10 minutes before the patient arrives in the care area. Remember that on

the model, insertion of the FOB between the simulated vocal cords under the towel is no challenge; the dexterity challenge comes in choosing a bronchus for the FOB and aiming for one of multiple tubing targets. Difficulty can be added by moving the simulated bronchi sideways or placing something under them to produce a slight misalignment with the simulated trachea or the targets. The indicated steps for model construction are presented in Video 19-7.

2. Practice with Intubation Mannequins

Very expensive intubation mannequins such as SimMan (Laerdal Medical) afford much more realistic anatomic structures to search through and to search for, compared with intubating heads. Many pathologic states are programmable for added challenge and dexterity practice. They can be used for a variety of airway techniques such as FOB combination methods and insertion of bronchial blockers.

3. Practice with Patients

Whereas practice on mannequins is interesting, there is nothing like the astonishing reality of using an FOB to see vibrant, living, anatomically amazing tissues in a living patient. The easiest approach is to examine the airway of

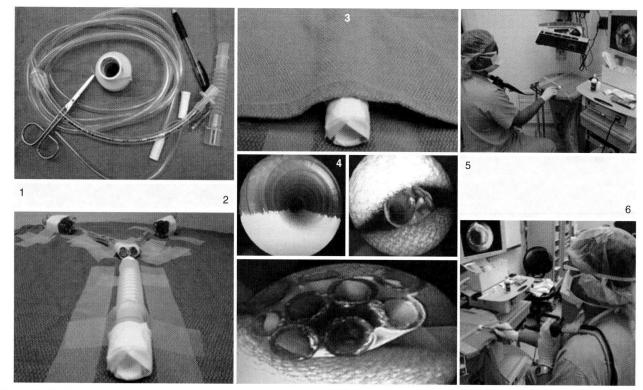

Figure 19-36 Gil 5-Minute Dexterity Model: *1,* simple discarded or inexpensive materials for model construction; *2,* model shown to trainee with "trachea" leading to "carina" leading to two sets of targets; *3,* covered model; *4,* fiberoptic views seen—flexible corrugated tubing "trachea" with "membranous" posterior tape, "carina," and one set of suction tubing "targets"; *5,* trainee visualizing one set of targets, with correct hand position and care of the fiberoptic bronchoscope evident; *6,* trainee successfully entering chosen target.

a patient under GA. The survey of trainees by McNarry and colleagues revealed that 82.7% found no ethical concern in performing FOB intubation in patients under GA without the patient's prior knowledge or consent to performing this task.[105] This attitude is most likely related to the influence of many anesthesiologists who use FOB for most patients who require intubation in the operating room as a standard of practice, secondary to its high rate of success and minimal trauma.

Simple initial goals during FOB use in patients with a "normal" airway under GA provide the visual reality and dexterity practice that will one day be required in more difficult situations. It is important to select younger, healthier patients with surgical sites distant from the airway and to have no one pressing for a hurried approach to intubation. Discussing a plan for expanding FOB experience alleviates the concerns of nearby colleagues and personnel and enlists their concurrence in a quest to become proficient. One or more FOB techniques could be tried in the following scenarios.

a. AN ALREADY INTUBATED PATIENT

Use the FOB to examine airway anatomy in a sufficiently anesthetized or paralyzed patient. Examine all structures within the oropharynx, including the glottis. With extreme gentleness, while using the smallest lubricated FOB available, inspect the nasopharynx down to the larynx if possible. Do not use vasoconstrictors, because this exposes a patient to a drug that is unwarranted for a pure examination technique. Definitely do not pass the FOB down the nasal passage if even the slightest resistance occurs.

b. AN ANESTHETIZED PATIENT WITH AN ENDOSCOPY MASK OR SWIVEL ADAPTER

Use an FOB to examine and perhaps even intubate patients, but make sure they are deeply anesthetized or that someone is assisting them if muscle relaxant is being used. Some pressure-assist ventilators can carry out this function. Make sure that ventilation and vital signs are observed.

c. A PATIENT UNDER GENERAL ANESTHESIA WHO HAS HIGH AIRWAY PRESSURE, LOW SATURATION, OR A NEED TO CHECK FOR CORRECT SUPRAGLOTTIC AIRWAY POSITION, ENDOBRONCHIAL INTUBATION, OR ONE-LUNG ISOLATION

An FOB can be used for examination down the ETT to check for obstruction, secretions, and endobronchial intubation, as well as SGA and DLT positioning, as described previously. The use of an FOB in these cases adds to experience that can be translated to eventual successful FOB intubation and use.

d. A PATIENT WHO NEEDS A GENERAL ANESTHESIA AND INTUBATION

Inform the staff that, to provide experience, the patient will be anesthetized and mask-ventilated with 100% oxygen, and 2 minutes will be taken to perform FOB laryngoscopy while an assistant helps with maneuvers and watches ventilation and vital signs and someone is looking at the clock. A video screen helps gain the cooperation of others, because direct observation improves their understanding. After 2 minutes, if the trachea is entered, railroad the ETT. If the trachea is not entered, use the usual fall-back intubation technique (e.g., RL). Make sure to decide whether more anesthetic agent or mask ventilation (or both) is necessary for this attempt.

e. A PATIENT WHO NEEDS AWAKE FOB INTUBATION

Perform all facets of this technique as detailed earlier. The technique of awake FOB intubation definitely requires patient consent and is not one recommended for developing experience or dexterity. However, after one has performed at least 20 FOB intubations on patients under GA, the awake approach can be taken with a good degree of confidence in patients with relatively normal airway anatomy. If an operator with a greater degree of FOB expertise is available, that person's assistance would be beneficial to heighten the learning experience in these circumstances and ensure a high likelihood of success.

XIV. ASSESSING PROFICIENCY

A. Instruction

Trainee proficiency cannot be expected to take place unless participants have experienced very adequate and thorough teaching. Instruction in FOB use must include imparting knowledge of FOB mechanics, patient preparation, and FOB technique. Model and dexterity practice must be encouraged.

Instructors in clinical areas need to choose less problematic patients for novice trainees and should emphasize the delicacy of the equipment and correct procedures. The situation in all cases can be optimized, but this is especially so in the case of novices or trainees with DA patients. It is helpful to plan on carrying out adjunct maneuvers, such as tongue pull and jaw thrust, and on keeping the FOB or IOA in the midline.

The use of a video monitor, visible to all personnel, is extremely advantageous to facilitate instruction. If only an eyepiece is available, consideration should be given to turning the lights off after FOB insertion and observing trainee movements of the FOB via transillumination in the neck, similar to a lightwand. Otherwise, if the trainee is uncertain of the anatomy being observed, the instructor might have to periodically look through the eyepiece, while the trainee braces the FOB, to supply instruction.

If video monitoring is not available, many endoscopists choose the nasotracheal route as a good method for an initial attempt, because it tends to lead the trainee most easily to the epiglottis and larynx. Vasoconstriction is mandatory. Passage through a lubricated, breakaway NPA or a partially inserted, lubricated ETT will virtually direct the FOB tip toward the glottis within seconds.

As mentioned earlier, Johnson and Robert's studies in first-year residents who were novices to FOB use showed that they were successful in 50% of their first 5 cases, in 90% of their next 5 cases, and in 100% of their final 5 cases.[163] After 10 cases, the average time to successful FOB intubation was 90 seconds or less. This fast learning curve correlated with the marked improvement exhibited after 10 nasotracheal intubation cases by emergency room trainees, as reported by Delaney and Hessler.[173]

B. Assessing Planning and Technique

Proficiency evaluation for trainees must include appropriate appreciation of a number of factors: the indications for and contraindications to FOB use, the ability to inform patients properly, complete equipment preparation, monitoring, positioning, use of assistants, and administration of drugs such as antisialogogues, sedatives, narcotics, and local anesthetics. Some of this knowledge can be gauged through written testing or clinical observation.

The method usually described to assess residency proficiency in actual FOB use is simplistic recording of the total number of FOB experiences. Nevertheless, as described in Dr. Ovassapian's quotation (see Box 19-9), the performance of 50 FOB experiences is estimated to provide competence with the technique and the ability to perform FOB intubation independently. His opinion was that 15 to 20 of these practice experiences should be asleep FOB intubations, and 15 to 20 should be awake FOB intubations. Competency of FOB use in DA cases is more difficult to determine, but Dr. Ovassapian also documented that use of the FOB for the myriad of purposes and techniques described in this chapter could lead one to the expert level of 100 or more FOB cases by the end of residency.[162]

Besides determining proficiency by pure numbers, the quality of the FOB intubations has been evaluated in several studies. Proposed items to be recorded for this determination include success or failure, time needed to achieve the FOB intubation, a validated global rating scale, and a performance checklist, as described by Chandra and associates.[171]

XV. INTRODUCING FIBEROPTIC INTUBATION INTO ONE'S OWN PRACTICE

Lack of FOB training or rusty skills in this technique are obstacles that can easily be eliminated whether one works in a teaching hospital or in private practice. Considering role reversal: Would any airway management professional in the fields of emergency medicine, anesthesiology, or critical care medicine prefer to be a patient in the hands of someone lacking FOB intubation skills? In spite of knowing that all airway specialists regard their patients as having the highest priority, there are still factors that prompt some hesitancy in the use of FOB techniques.

One factor is time. There is a concern (particularly in private practice) that too much time will be needed to perform an FOB technique. Perhaps the realization that far more time may be spent on unsuccessful airway management using non-FOB methods would change negative thinking toward FOB use—to say nothing of the vast difference that might develop in costs resulting from subsequent patient complications.

Of significant concern here is the idea that other health personnel might harass anyone trying to become more experienced. Gaining FOB experience is not really

Box 19-10	Steps to Introduce Fiberoptic Intubation Techniques into a Practice

Step 1: Go to the Web sites, and read the literature; DVDs and videos are also available.

Step 2: Attend workshops on use of fiberoptic bronchoscopes (FOBs) or use the FOB representatives to provide in-service training, or both.

Step 3: Practice on mannequins and dexterity models.

Step 4: Have all equipment prepared ahead of time.

Step 5: Look for proper prospects—healthy, young patients undergoing general anesthesia whose surgical sites are far removed from the airway.

Step 6: Use the FOB to examine and to observe normal anatomy in anesthetized patients, not plastic models.

Step 7: Emphasize the fact that experience equals safety by enlisting surgery, nursing, and technical colleagues.

a long trek. For most airway management professionals, it can be one of their best journeys, and the success obtained in a particularly vital patient rescue while averting disaster will make an endoscopist soar to the highest peaks. To begin the journey, however, steps must be taken (Box 19-10).

Emphasize to all colleagues and ancillary personnel the desire to gain experience and become an expert to avoid trauma, cost, and anxiety in difficult, uncontrolled cases. Maintain a self-imposed time limit of 2 to 3 minutes for FOB intubation, to be followed by routine alternatives if unsuccessful. Success usually follows within a short time span! Communication, preparation, and time limits for reverting to an alternative plan will ensure that impressions of the FOB approach are positive and professional, no matter the outcome. Lack of any of these points raises concern and may present a bad impression. Avoid this by all means.

XVI. SKILL RETENTION

Psychomotor skills can deteriorate with infrequent FOB use. Dexterity models, mannequins, and FOB workshops should be utilized frequently if patient practice is not possible. Voluntary enrollment in a systematic program, such as the one developed by Dr. K. Gil in the framework of the ASA Annual Meeting's Basic Fiberoptic Workshop, is a structured way to ensure success. Fundamentally, however, real patient practice is crucial to maintaining skills. A good method is to designate a certain day of the week or twice a month as "Fiberoptic Day." Planning a set pattern in which FOB use must take place on a particular day will become a routine, and expectations to gain experience will not surprise colleagues or assistants.

XVII. CONCLUSIONS

Airway loss is a two-word phrase that chills the hearts of all health-related professionals. Closed claims analysis and numerous reviews reveal the importance of the capability to perform all techniques of airway management.[174,175] The superiority of FOB use for patient safety cannot be denied. Nor can the training needed to develop

expertise and the cost, maintenance, and space requirements be ignored. With developments in microchip camera technology and video transmission, both costs and equipment bulk are beginning to decrease.

The costs of FOB purchase and maintenance should be balanced in relation to the cost of a failed intubation or lost airway and subsequent injury to cardiac, neurologic, or other systems. The expense of airway management failure and resulting complications may vastly exceed the cost of one FOB system. There is no question that the role and value of FOB techniques are secured. As proof of its importance, every single printed airway management text in anesthesiology, critical care, or emergency medicine places an extremely high value on this technique, making it a required skill with a place in the armamentarium of every professional airway management caregiver in each of these fields.

XVIII. CLINICAL PEARLS

- A proactive low threshold for use of the fiberoptic bronchoscope (FOB) is important when considering a difficult airway. Indiscriminate use of a rigid laryngoscope (RL) in these circumstances could worsen an already bleak picture, and if FOB attempts are to follow, hopes of success may soon spiral downward.

- FOB instruments are very delicate and frequently very expensive. Yet it is important to consider the balance of FOB purchase and maintenance costs in relation to the expense of a failed intubation or lost airway with subsequent injury to cardiac, neurologic, or other systems.

- When any topical intraoral anesthetic is planned, an antisialogogue (glycopyrrolate) should be administered 15 to 20 minutes beforehand. Supplemental oxygen is highly recommended. Use of sedatives, narcotics, or local anesthetics is dependent on the urgency of the patient's situation and respiratory status. Proper topicalization should prevent discomfort, psychological distress, hemodynamic changes, and lack of cooperation.

- After laryngeal entry, three directions must be followed successively in the supine patient to reach the trachea through the nasal or the oral route: downward to the posterior wall of the oropharynx or nasopharynx, upward to the anterior commissure of the vocal cords, and downward again into the laryngeal and tracheal lumen to the carina.

- The number one cause of FOB intubation failure is inexperience due to insufficient training and practice. Getting to know the FOB will offset any reluctance toward it. This can be achieved with understanding and practice involving indications, contraindications, and handling of the FOB.

- Inferior preparation of patients, equipment, and personnel doom FOB use to difficulty, if not failure. Psychological preparation, equipment, antisialogogues, sedatives, narcotics, and local anesthetics must be optimized and individualized for each patient. Untrained personnel must understand the techniques of tongue pull, jaw thrust, keeping the intubating oral airway in the midline, and injecting local anesthetic through the FOB.

- Rarely, the FOB enters a wide-open esophagus that is mistaken for the trachea. Identifying what seem to be tracheal rings is not enough to prevent this error. Identifying the carina provides more definitive proof of the location of the FOB.

- The option of combined use of an FOB with other airway devices should be high on the priority list for rescue of difficult FOB intubation or other types of difficult intubations. The multimodal approach is most likely to impact airway control in patients with upper airway bleeding, secretions, or edema and those with periglottic or periepiglottic pathology.

- One situation in which the FOB tends to be at a disadvantage is in any soiled airway, because of the small diameter of the viewing tip. Combinations with other devices such as a supraglottic airway (SGA) may overcome these difficulties.

- Patients who have preexisting narrowing or obstructive pathology in their upper airways may have difficulty when any non-hollow object is placed in the area. To ward off effects of near or total obstruction once the FOB enters the respiratory tract, FOB manipulation must be speedy and careful.

Acknowledgment

This chapter was undertaken with the specific intention of expanding on the vision that many others have had while contributing to education in the service of patient care. Although the entire substance of the material in this chapter has been researched thoroughly and is unique, we are pleased to retain a number of the topics in fond remembrance of Dr. Andranik Ovassapian, as can be noted in the chapter he co-authored with Dr. Mellissa Wheeler in the first and second edition of this textbook. We are particularly appreciative of the magnitude of Dr. Ovassapian's experience and instruction of countless airway management specialists throughout his career.

SELECTED REFERENCES

All references can be found online at expertconsult.com.

13. Ovassapian A, Schrader SC: Fiber-optic aided bronchial intubation. *Semin Anesth* 6:133, 1987.
33. Culver DA, Minai OA, Gordon SM, Mehta AC: Infection control and radiation safety in the bronchoscopy suite. In Wang KP, Mehta AT, Turner JF, editors: *Flexible bronchoscopy*, ed 2, Malden, MA, 2004, Wiley-Blackwell, pp 9–22.
42. Crosby ET, Cooper RM, Douglas MJ, et al: The unanticipated difficult airway with recommendations for management. *Can J Anaesth* 45:757–767, 1998.
46. Shiga T, Wajima Z, Inoue T, Sakamoto A: Predicting difficult intubation in apparently normal patients: A meta-analysis of bedside screening test performance. *Anesthesiology* 103:429–437, 2005.
53. Heidegger T, Gerig H, Ulrich B, Kreienbühl G: Validation of a simple algorithm for tracheal intubation: Daily practice is the key to success in emergencies—An analysis of 13,248 intubations. *Anesth Analg* 92:517–522, 2001.
64. Atlas G: A comparison of fiberoptic-compatible oral airways. *J Clin Anesth* 16:66–73, 2004.
69. Lu GP, Frost EA, Goldiner PL: Another approach to the problem airway [letter]. *Anesthesiology* 65:101–102, 1986.
105. McNarry AF, Dovell T, Dancey FM, Pead ME: Perception of training needs and opportunities in advanced airway skills: A survey of British and Irish trainees. *Eur J Anaesthesiol* 24:498–504, 2007.
171. Chandra DB, Savoldelli GL, Joo HS, et al: Fiberoptic oral intubation: The effect of model fidelity on training for transfer to patient care. *Anesthesiology* 109:1007–1013, 2008.
174. Mort TC: Emergency tracheal intubation: Complications associated with repeated laryngoscopic attempts. *Anesth Analg* 99:607–613, 2004.

Chapter 20

Retrograde Intubation Techniques

ANTONIO SANCHEZ

I. HISTORY

The first reported case of retrograde intubation (RI) was by Butler and Cirillo in 1960.[1] The technique involved passing a red rubber catheter cephalad through the patient's previously existing tracheostomy. When the catheter exited the oral cavity, it was tied to the endotracheal tube (ETT), allowing it to be pulled into the trachea.

The first person to perform RI as presently practiced was Waters, a British anesthesiologist in Nigeria.[2] In 1963, he reported treating patients who had cancrum oris, an invasive gangrene that deforms the oral cavity, severely limiting mouth opening. His technique involved passing a standard Tuohy needle through the cricothyroid membrane (CTM) and feeding an epidural catheter cephalad into the nasopharynx. He "fished" the catheter out of the nasopharynx through the nares, using a hook he devised. The epidural catheter was then used as a stylet to guide the ETT through the nares and into the trachea.

Over the ensuing years, RI did not gain clinical acceptance because of its invasiveness and the potential for complications from the CTM puncture. After 1964, when fiberoptic technology became available, RI was irregularly but occasionally discussed in the literature.[1-165] In 1993, RI was designated as part of the anesthesiologist's armamentarium by the American Society of Anesthesiologists (ASA) Difficult Airway (DA) Task Force.[3]

The term *retrograde intubation*, used by Butler and Cirillo, is a misnomer.[4] The technique is actually a translaryngeal guided intubation, but for historical reasons we continue using the name retrograde intubation.

II. INDICATIONS

The RI technique has been used both in the hospital setting and in prehospital mobile units (in the field).[5,6] It has been employed with both anticipated and unanticipated DAs[2,5-20]; after failure to intubate by conventional means (direct laryngoscopy,[6,9,11] blind nasal intubation,[10,11] bougie,[13,21] laryngeal mask airway [LMA], and fiberoptic laryngoscopy[18,22-24]); and in both humans and animals.[25,26] In the literature, including my own experience (31 patients), there have been approximately 807 cases (670 patients and 137 cadavers) in which RI was used as a means of securing the airway. Although in most cases RI has been used to place a single-lumen ETT, one case report described placement of a double-lumen ETT through RI.[7]

A wide variety of airway diseases have necessitated RI (Box 20-1). RI has been most frequently associated with limited range of motion of the neck (153 trauma victims with potential cervical spine injury), and its use has been reported in facial trauma. It has been employed in both adults and pediatric patients with success (Box 20-2).

Not all reports have described the amount of time required to perform the technique, but in one study involving emergency medical service personnel (paramedics and registered nurses) using training mannequins, the average time was 71 seconds (range, 42 to 129 seconds).[27] Barriot and Riou described 13 patients with maxillofacial trauma who could not be intubated in the field using direct laryngoscopy (six attempts; average time, 18 minutes).[5] Intubation was subsequently performed in these patients on the first RI attempt, with an average time of less than 5 minutes. An additional 6 patients were intubated in less than 5 minutes when RI

was used as the initial method of choice. Slots and colleagues reported a modified technique using a Mini-Trach II set on 20 cadavers with an average time for intubation of 6.7 seconds (range, 3 to 10 seconds); it was subsequently used on an emergency basis on 3 patients with an average time of 10 seconds. The investigators concluded that the RI technique was a rapid, efficacious method for intratracheal intubation of trauma patients, especially patients with maxillofacial trauma.[28]

Historical indications for RI are the following:

1. Failed attempts at laryngoscopy, LMA, or fiberoptic intubation (FOI)
2. Urgent establishment of an airway where visualization of the vocal cords is prevented by blood, secretions, or anatomic derangement in scenarios in which ventilation is still possible
3. Elective use when deemed necessary in clinical situations such as unstable cervical spine, maxillofacial trauma, or anatomic anomaly

III. CONTRAINDICATIONS

Contraindications to RI have been cited, often anecdotally (Box 20-3). Most are relative contraindications and can be divided into four categories: unfavorable anatomy, laryngotracheal disease, coagulopathy, and infection.

A. Unfavorable Anatomy

Because in most cases RI is performed above or below the cricoid cartilage, absolute lack of access to this region, as in patients with severe flexion deformity of the neck, poses a contraindication if not an impossibility.[29,30] For the same reason, the patient with nonpalpable landmarks,[31-33] obesity,[34] overlying malignancy,[32] or large thyroid goiter should be approached cautiously.[32] Shantha reported a case of RI in a patient with a large thyroid goiter.[35] After failure of conventional intubating methods (including FOI), the surgeons dissected down to the CTM and subsequently passed the catheter cephalad. Thirteen cases of RI have been reported in obese patients without major complications.[12,18,34,36]

B. Laryngotracheal Disease

Theoretically, laryngotracheal stenosis may contraindicate RI because narrowing of the trachea or larynx could be made worse by either the needle puncture or the catheter.[2,31] However, RI has been used in patients with laryngeal cancer,[37] epiglottitis,[38] and laryngeal edema resulting from burn injuries.[16,24] It should not be used if laryngeal tracheal stenosis is present directly under the intended puncture site.

C. Coagulopathy

Preexisting bleeding diathesis should be considered a relative contraindication.[31,32,39-44] Although there is a potential for bleeding, the CTM is considered to be a relatively avascular plane (see later discussion). A small, self-limited hematoma was reported in a patient who underwent a coronary artery bypass grafting with intraoperative heparin and postoperative disseminated intravascular coagulation.[9]

D. Infection

RI in the presence of preexisting infection over the puncture site or in the path of the puncture, as in pretracheal abscess or Ludwig's angina, could result in transmittal of bacterial flora into the trachea and should be avoided. This, again, should be considered a relative contraindication, because transtracheal aspiration is performed to obtain a sputum sample in patients with pneumonia despite the possibility of pretracheal abscess (see "Complications").[31,32,43,45-47]

IV. ANATOMY

The performance of RI requires basic anatomic knowledge of the cricoid cartilage (Fig. 20-1) and the structures above and below it to minimize complications and failure. Indeed, regardless of the intubation technique planned, the cricoid cartilage and CTM should be identified preoperatively in every patient.[48] Cartilage and membrane, vascular structures, and the thyroid gland are relevant anatomic structures.

A. Cartilage and Membrane

The cricoid cartilage has the shape of signet ring (see Fig. 20-1). It consists of a broad, flat, posterior plate called the *lamina* and a narrow, convex, anterior structure called the *arch*.[49,50] In most cases the cartilage can be easily palpated by identifying the thyroid notch and running a finger down the midline in a caudad direction until a rigid, rounded structure is encountered. The vertical height of the arch is 0.5 to 0.7 cm (Fig. 20-2).[50] The CTM connects the superior border of the arch to the inferior border of the thyroid cartilage and measures approximately 1 cm in height and 2 cm in width.[49,51] The lateral borders are the paired cricothyroid muscles.[45] The cricotracheal ligament connects the inferior border of the arch to the upper border of the first tracheal ring and measures 0.3 to 0.6 cm in height.[52] The distance between the inferior border of the thyroid cartilage and the vocal cords varies with gender but is approximately 0.9 cm.[53]

B. Vascular Structures

There are paired major blood vessels above and below the cricoid cartilage: the cricothyroid artery and the superior thyroid artery (Fig. 20-3).

The cricothyroid artery,[50,51,53-55] a branch of the superior thyroid artery, runs along the anterior surface of the CTM, usually close to the inferior border of the thyroid cartilage. In some cases, the cricothyroid arteries anastomose in the midline and give rise to a descending branch

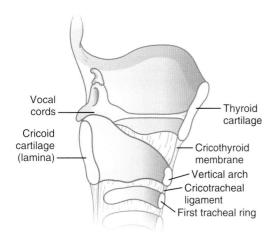

Figure 20-1 Anatomy of the cricoid cartilage. Midsagittal view of the larynx and trachea. (From Sanchez AF: *The retrograde cookbook,* Irvine, 1993, University of California, Department of Anesthesia.)

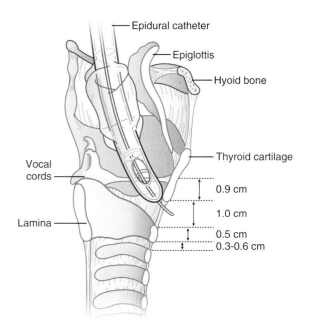

Figure 20-2 Midsagittal view of the larynx and trachea showing the distance between the vocal cords and the upper border of the first tracheal ring. Only a small portion of the Murphy eye of the endotracheal tube is below the vocal cords. (From Sanchez AF: *The retrograde cookbook,* Irvine, 1993, University of California, Department of Anesthesia.)

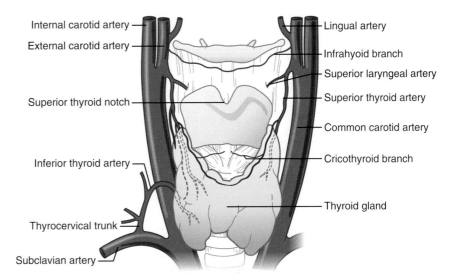

Figure 20-3 Vascular anatomy above and below the cricoid cartilage. (Modified from Naumann H, editor: *Head and neck surgery*, Philadelphia, 1984, WB Saunders.)

that feeds the middle lobe of the thyroid gland when present. On the basis of dissections that I have performed on cadavers, the cricothyroid artery becomes insignificant in size as it approaches the midline. No major venous plexus could be found mentioned in the literature, and none was found in my own dissections.

The anterior branch of the superior thyroid artery runs along the upper border of the thyroid isthmus to anastomose with its counterpart from the opposite side.[50,53-55] The inferior thyroid artery also anastomoses with the superior thyroid artery at the level of the isthmus. The arteries are remarkable for their large size and frequent anastomoses. In fewer than 10% of the population, an unpaired thyroid artery ascends ventral to the trachea (from either the aortic arch or the brachiocephalic artery) to anastomose at the level of the isthmus. It is usually small but may be very large. A rich venous plexus is formed in and around the isthmus.

C. Thyroid Gland (Isthmus, Pyramidal Lobe)

The isthmus of the thyroid gland (see Fig. 20-3) is rarely absent and generally lies anterior to the trachea between the first and fourth tracheal rings (usually between the second and third), although there are many variations. Its size and vertical height vary; the average vertical height and depth are 1.25 cm. Extending from the isthmus, the highly vascular pyramidal lobe (Fig. 20-4) is well developed in one third of the population. It is found more frequently on the left of the midline and may extend up to the hyoid bone (the upper continuation is usually thyromuscular).[25,49,50,54,55]

V. PHYSIOLOGY

Sympathetic stress responses—increased heart rate, blood pressure, intraocular pressure, and intracranial pressure and elevated catecholamine levels—have been reported with laryngoscopy, endotracheal intubation, coughing, translaryngeal local anesthesia, laryngotracheal anesthesia, and FOI. Therefore, concern is appropriate when performing RI in patients with coronary artery disease,

elevated intraocular pressure, or elevated intracranial pressure.[29,30,56-62] It is reasonable to argue, however, that RI, performed skillfully, is not more stimulating than any other technique for managing the airway.

No apparent significant changes in hemodynamics were reported in multiple case reports of patients with cardiac disease (congenital anomalies, ischemic coronary artery disease, valvular disease, pericarditis, and congestive heart failure) who underwent RI, both awake with topical anesthesia and under general anesthesia.[9,11,15,17,38,63-68] Casthely and colleagues reported on 25 patients with DA due to rheumatoid arthritis who underwent open heart surgery (coronary artery bypass graft and valve replacement).[9] The patients had invasive monitors (Swan-Ganz catheters and peripheral arterial lines) placed preoperatively. The initial 24 patients underwent a cardiac induction of anesthesia (diazepam 10 mg, fentanyl 25 to 30 µg/kg, and pancuronium 0.1 mg/kg) before rigid laryngoscopy followed by RI. Comparison of hemodynamic responses to rigid laryngoscopy (Macintosh and Miller blades) versus RI demonstrated that the former approach was more stressful (Table 20-1). Patient 25

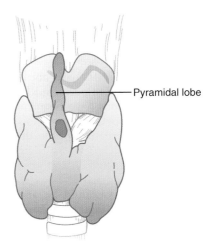

Figure 20-4 Pyramidal lobe of the isthmus. (Modified from Naumann H, editor: *Head and neck surgery*, vol 4, Philadelphia, 1984, WB Saunders.)

TABLE 20-1
Hemodynamic Effects of Retrograde Intubation

	Laryngoscopy	Retrograde Intubation
HR	Increase	No change from baseline
MAP	Increase	No change from baseline
CI	Decrease	No change from baseline
PCWP	Increase	No change from baseline
ECG	3-mm ST depression	No change from baseline

CI, Cardiac index; *ECG*, electrocardiogram (ST segment changes in lead V5); *HR*, heart rate; *MAP*, mean arterial pressure; *PCWP*, pulmonary capillary wedge pressure.
Modified from Casthely PA, Landesman S, Fynaman PN: Retrograde intubation in patients undergoing open heart surgery. *Can Anaesth Soc J* 32:661, 1985.

underwent RI before induction of anesthesia after application of topical anesthesia with no significant hemodynamic response.

Two case reports documented patients with a previous history of DA and intracranial pathology (pseudotumor cerebri and intracranial tumor with elevated intracranial pressure) who underwent elective, awake RI after topical anesthesia with no evidence of further increase in intracranial pressure.[8,14] I myself, unmedicated except for topical lidocaine, underwent awake RI with no significant hemodynamic changes.[48]

VI. TECHNIQUES

A. Preparation

1. Positioning

The ideal position for RI is the supine sniffing position with the neck hyperextended.[69,70] In this position, the cervical vertebrae push the trachea and cricoid cartilage anteriorly and displace the strap muscles of the neck laterally. As a result, the cricoid cartilage and the structures above and below it are easier to palpate. RI can also be performed with the patient in a sitting position,[48] which may be the only position in which some patients can breathe comfortably. Potential cervical spine injury or limited range of motion of the cervical spine may necessitate RI with the neck in a neutral position, which is a well-documented practice (see Box 20-1).

2. Skin Preparation

Although most documented RIs have not been elective, every effort should be made to perform RI using aseptic technique. Recommendations have been made for prophylactic antibiotics in diabetic or immunocompromised patients, who may be more susceptible than others to infection.[71]

3. Anesthesia

If time permits, the airway should be anesthetized to prevent sympathetic stimulation, laryngospasm, and discomfort. In the literature, many different combinations of techniques have been described:

1. Translaryngeal anesthesia during intravenous sedation or general anesthesia[2,8-10,16,18,72]
2. Translaryngeal anesthesia with superior laryngeal nerve block[5,6,73]
3. Translaryngeal anesthesia with topicalization of the pharynx (aerosolized or sprayed)[7,14,74,75]
4. Glossopharyngeal nerve block and superior laryngeal nerve block with nebulized local anesthetic[17]

(Refer to Chapter 11 for a detailed description of neural blockade of the airway.)

In my own experience,[48] an awake RI can be performed using translaryngeal anesthesia (4 mL 2% lidocaine) supplemented with topicalization (nebulized or sprayed local anesthetics) of the pharynx and hypopharynx. Special caution should be exercised when performing the translaryngeal anesthesia, because coughing, grunting, sneezing, or swallowing causes the cricoid cartilage to travel cephalad, with the potential for breaking the needle in the trachea.[76,77] To avoid this, one can insert a 20-G angiocatheter and remove the needle before injecting the local anesthetic.

4. Entry Site

The transtracheal puncture for RI can be made either above or below the cricoid cartilage. The CTM is relatively avascular and has less potential for bleeding (see "Anatomy"). The disadvantages of the CTM are that initially only 1 cm of ETT is actually placed below the vocal cords, and the angle of entry of the ETT into the trachea is more acute. An initial puncture performed at the cricotracheal ligament or lower affords the added advantage of allowing the ETT to travel in a straighter path as well as allowing a longer initial length of ETT below the vocal cords. The disadvantage is that this site (below the cricoid cartilage) has more potential for bleeding (although none has been reported). Both entry sites have been used successfully. In cadaver studies, the success rate for RI was higher with less vocal cord trauma when the cricotracheal ligament rather than the CTM was used. Vocal cord trauma has not been reported in living patients.[78,79]

B. Classic Technique

The classic technique of RI is performed percutaneously using a standard 17-G Tuohy needle and epidural catheter.

After positioning (Fig. 20-5), skin preparation, and anesthesia, a right hand–dominant person should stand on the right side of the supine patient. The left hand is used to stabilize the trachea by placing the thumb and third digit on either side of the thyroid cartilage. The index finger of the left hand is used to identify the midline of the CTM and the upper border of the cricoid cartilage.

Because the Tuohy needle is blunt, a small incision through the skin and subcutaneous tissue with a no. 11 scalpel blade is recommended. Because of the significant force required to perforate the skin and the CTM, there is a risk of perforating the posterior tracheal wall as well. This has been verified in cadaver studies with the use of a fiberoptic bronchoscope (FOB).[34]

The right hand then grasps the Tuohy needle and saline syringe like a pencil (using the fifth digit to brace

Figure 20-5 Classic technique. Midsagittal view of the head and neck. (From Sanchez AF: *The retrograde cookbook*, Irvine, 1993, University of California, Department of Anesthesia.)

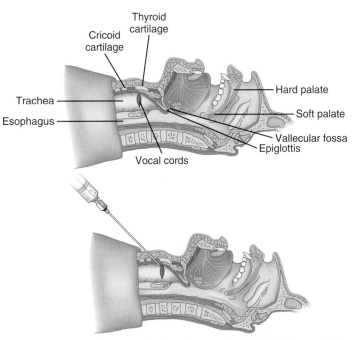

Figure 20-7 Classic technique. The angle of the Tuohy needle is changed to 45 degrees with the bevel pointing cephalad, again verifying position by aspirating air. (From Sanchez AF: *The retrograde cookbook*, Irvine, 1993, University of California, Department of Anesthesia.)

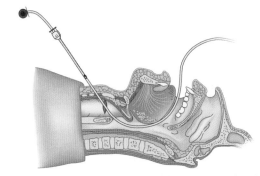

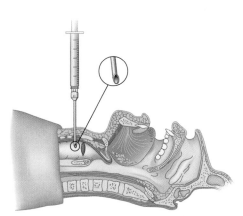

Figure 20-6 Classic technique. Standard no. 17 Tuohy needle (with saline-filled syringe) is advanced (with bevel pointing cephalad) through the cricothyroid membrane at a 90-degree angle, trying to stay as close as possible to the upper border of the cricoid cartilage. Entrance into the trachea is verified by aspiration of air. (From Sanchez AF: *The retrograde cookbook*, Irvine, 1993, University of California, Department of Anesthesia.)

Figure 20-8 Classic technique. An epidural catheter is advanced through the vocal cords and into the pharynx. During this time, the patient is asked to stick the tongue out or tongue can be pulled out manually. Most of the time, the epidural catheter comes out of the mouth on its own. The Tuohy needle is then withdrawn to the caudal end of epidural catheter. (From Sanchez AF: *The retrograde cookbook*, Irvine, 1993, University of California, Department of Anesthesia.)

the right hand on the patient's lower neck) and performs the puncture, aspirating to confirm placement in the lumen of the airway (Figs. 20-6 and 20-7).

Once the Tuohy needle is in place, the epidural catheter is advanced into the trachea (Fig. 20-8). When advancing the epidural catheter, it is important to have the tongue pulled anteriorly to prevent the catheter from coiling up in the oropharynx. The catheter usually exits on its own from either the oral (Fig. 20-9) or the nasal cavity. A hemostat should then be clamped to the catheter at the neck skin line to prevent further movement of the epidural catheter. If the catheter has to be retrieved from the oropharynx, my preferred instrument is a nerve hook (V. Mueller NL2490, Baxter, Deerfield, IL). Magill forceps have been used, but these were designed to grasp large structures such as an ETT and may not grip the relatively small catheter (the distal tips of the forceps do not completely occlude); in addition, they may traumatize the pharynx. Arya and associates described an innovative atraumatic method of retrieving catheters from the oral pharynx in patients with limited mouth opening. They used a "pharyngeal loop" that they devised from a ureteral guidewire that was threaded through a 3-mm uncuffed polyvinyl chloride ETT and doubled up to form a loop.[80]

Originally, the catheter was threaded through the main distal lumen (beveled portion) of the ETT. Bourke and Levesque modified the technique by threading the

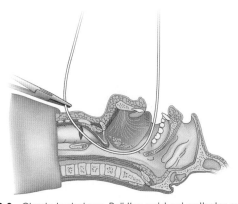

Figure 20-9 Classic technique. Pull the epidural catheter out of the mouth to an appropriate length; then clamp a hemostat flush with the skin. (From Sanchez AF: *The retrograde cookbook*, Irvine, 1993, University of California, Department of Anesthesia.)

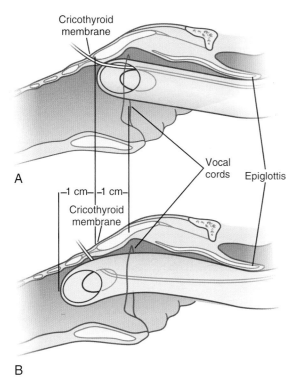

Figure 20-10 Classic technique. Cross section of larynx and trachea with endotracheal tube (ETT) and catheter guide passing through the cricothyroid membrane. **A,** Catheter passes through end of ETT, and 1 cm of ETT passes the cords. **B,** The catheter exits the side hole, allowing 2 cm of ETT to pass beyond the vocal cords. (From Sanchez AF: *The retrograde cookbook*, Irvine, 1993, University of California, Department of Anesthesia.)

catheter through the Murphy eye (Fig. 20-10), reasoning that this would allow an additional 1 cm of ETT to pass through the cords.[81] Lleu and coworkers,[78,79] in cadaver studies, showed that using the cricotracheal ligament as the puncture site in combination with threading the epidural catheter through the Murphy eye enhanced success compared with the original technique.

When the ETT is being advanced over the epidural catheter (Figs. 20-11 through 20-13), a moderate amount

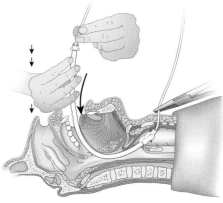

Figure 20-12 Classic technique. When the endotracheal tube (ETT) reaches the cricothyroid membrane (CTM), it is important to maintain pressure *(small arrows),* forcing the ETT into the oropharynx *(large arrow)* to cause continuing pressure against the CTM with the tip of the ETT. Moderate tension is still maintained on the epidural catheter. (From Sanchez AF: *The retrograde cookbook*, Irvine, 1993, University of California, Department of Anesthesia.)

of tension should be employed.[13,40] Excessive tension pulls the ETT anteriorly, making it more likely to be caught up against the epiglottis, vallecula, or anterior commissure of the vocal cords. If there is difficulty in passing the opening of the glottis, the ETT can be rotated 90 degrees counterclockwise or exchanged for a smaller tube.[13,23,34]

Ideally, one would like to verify that the ETT is below the vocal cords before removing the epidural catheter (Fig. 20-14; see Fig. 20-13). The methods of verification are the following:

1. By direct vision, using the FOB (see "Fiberoptic Technique")
2. If the patient is breathing spontaneously, by listening to breath sounds through the ETT
3. By capnography, using a fiberoptic elbow adapter connected to a capnograph[82]
4. By luminescent techniques using a light wand[83]

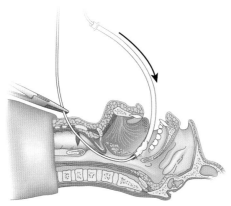

Figure 20-11 Classic technique. Thread a well-lubricated endotracheal tube (ETT) over the epidural catheter. Maintain a moderate amount of tension on the epidural catheter *(arrow)* as you advance the ETT forward; you will feel a small click as the ETT travels through the vocal cords. (From Sanchez AF: *The retrograde cookbook*, Irvine, 1993, University of California, Department of Anesthesia.)

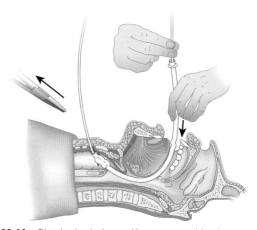

Figure 20-13 Classic technique. Have an assistant remove the hemostat *(large arrow)* while pressure is maintained *(small arrow)* to push the endotracheal tube up against the cricothyroid membrane. (The epidural catheter may be cut flush with the hemostat before hemostat is removed.) (From Sanchez AF: *The retrograde cookbook*, Irvine, 1993, University of California, Department of Anesthesia.)

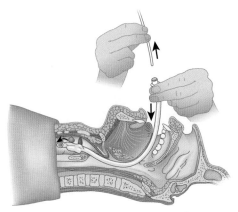

Figure 20-14 Classic technique. Simultaneously remove epidural catheter as you advance the endotracheal tube (ETT) *(straight arrows)*. The tip of the ETT will drop from its position up against the cricothyroid membrane to the midtrachea *(curved arrow)*. Advance the ETT to the desired depth. (From Sanchez AF: *The retrograde cookbook*, Irvine, 1993, University of California, Department of Anesthesia.)

C. Guidewire Technique

The modified technique using a guidewire was developed because the flexible epidural catheter is prone to kinking.[4,7,13-15,19,23-25,31-33,38,39,59-63,72-74,84-91] Equipment consists of an 18-G angiocatheter, a J-tip guidewire with 0.038 inch outer diameter (OD) and 110 to 120 cm in length, and a guide catheter (Fig. 20-15).

Use of a guidewire offers the following advantages:

1. The J tip tends to be less traumatic to the airway.[24,39,74,87]
2. Retrieval of the guidewire from the oral or nasal cavity is easier.[33,74,87]
3. The guidewire is less prone to kinking.[92]
4. The guidewire can be used with the FOB (see "Fiberoptic Technique").
5. The guidewire is easy to handle.[32,73,87]
6. The technique takes less time to perform than the classic technique.[27,33]

Discrepancy between the external diameter of the guidewire and the internal diameter (ID) of the ETT allows a "railroading" effect to occur, with the tip of the ETT catching peripherally on the arytenoids or vocal cords instead of going straight through the cords. Sliding the guide catheter over the guidewire from above (antegrade) when it has exited the mouth or nose increases the external diameter of the guidewire,[82] and use of the guide catheter in combination with a smaller-diameter ETT allows the ETT to enter the glottis in a more centralized position with respect to the glottic opening.

Various types of antegrade guide catheters have been used: FOBs (described in the next section), nasogastric tubes,[34,93] suction catheters,[34,94] plastic sheaths from Swan-Ganz catheters,[88] Eschmann stylets,[13] and tube changers.[24,89] The Cook Critical Care retrograde guidewire kit (Cook Incorporated, Bloomington, IN) contains a tapered antegrade guide catheter, which is my choice of antegrade guide catheter (see Fig. 20-15) and is used here to describe the basic guidewire and antegrade guide catheter technique.

The guidewire and antegrade guide catheter technique is as follows. The trachea is identified (Figs. 20-16 to 20-18) with the syringe and 18-G angiocatheter. The J wire is then fed through the intratracheal catheter (Fig. 20-19) until it passes out the mouth (Fig. 20-20). The guidewire is clamped at the neck skin line, and the tapered antegrade guide catheter is fed over the guidewire (Fig. 20-21) until the antegrade guide catheter reaches the CTM (Fig. 20-22). The ETT is then fed over the antegrade guide catheter (Figs. 20-23 and 20-24) and the antegrade guide catheter is removed (Fig. 20-25). The standard Cook RI set has been modified to include a tapered antegrade guide catheter with distal sideports and Rapi-Fit adapters (Arndt Airway Exchange Catheter) to allow oxygenation and ventilation of the patient and to facilitate placement of an ETT.

Three other modifications have been reported using guide catheters. First, the guidewire is removed when the guide catheter abuts against the CTM (see Fig. 20-21). The guide catheter alone is then advanced farther into the trachea and used as a stylet for the ETT.[88,72,89] Second,

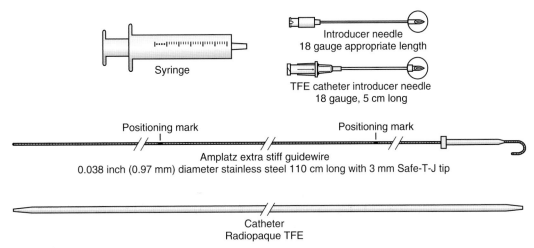

Syringe

Introducer needle
18 gauge appropriate length

TFE catheter introducer needle
18 gauge, 5 cm long

Positioning mark   Positioning mark

Amplatz extra stiff guidewire
0.038 inch (0.97 mm) diameter stainless steel 110 cm long with 3 mm Safe-T-J tip

Catheter
Radiopaque TFE

Figure 20-15 Guidewire technique. Retrograde kit TFE (Teflon guide catheter). (From Cook Incorporated, Bloomington, IN.)

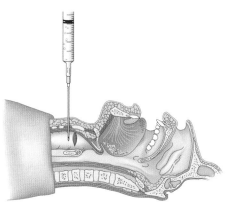

Figure 20-16 Guidewire technique. The angiocatheter (18 G) is placed at 90-degree angle to the cricothyroid membrane, aspirating for air to confirm position. (From Sanchez AF: *The retrograde cookbook*, Irvine, 1993, University of California, Department of Anesthesia.)

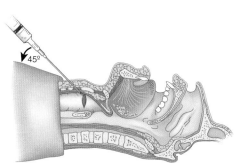

Figure 20-17 Guidewire technique. The angle of the angiocatheter is changed to 45 degrees, again aspirating air to confirm position. (From Sanchez AF: *The retrograde cookbook*, Irvine, 1993, University of California, Department of Anesthesia.)

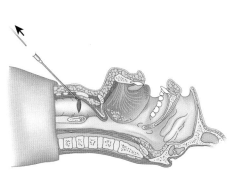

Figure 20-18 Guidewire technique. Advance the sheath of angiocatheter cephalad, and remove the needle. (From Sanchez AF: *The retrograde cookbook*, Irvine, 1993, University of California, Department of Anesthesia.)

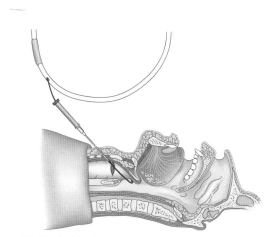

Figure 20-19 Guidewire technique. Advance the J-tip guidewire through the angiocatheter sheath. (From Sanchez AF: *The retrograde cookbook*, Irvine, 1993, University of California, Department of Anesthesia.)

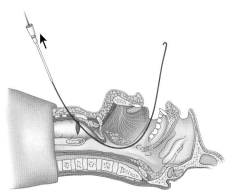

Figure 20-20 Guidewire technique. Retrieve the end of the guidewire from the mouth as in classic technique. Remove the angiocatheter *(small arrow)*. (From Sanchez AF: *The retrograde cookbook*, Irvine, 1993, University of California, Department of Anesthesia.)

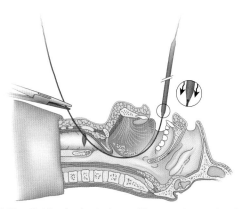

Figure 20-21 Guidewire technique. Clamp a hemostat flush with neck skin, and advance the tapered tip of the guide catheter *(inset)* over the guidewire into the mouth. (From Sanchez AF: *The retrograde cookbook*, Irvine, 1993, University of California, Department of Anesthesia.)

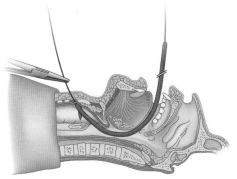

Figure 20-22 Guidewire technique. Advance the guide catheter to the cricothyroid membrane. (From Sanchez AF: *The retrograde cookbook*, Irvine, 1993, University of California, Department of Anesthesia.)

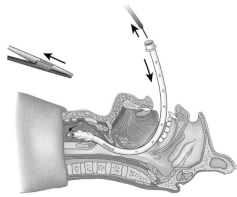

Figure 20-25 Guidewire technique. Remove the wire and catheter as in classic technique, except that the guidewire and guide catheter are removed simultaneously. (From Sanchez AF: *The retrograde cookbook*, Irvine, 1993, University of California, Department of Anesthesia.)

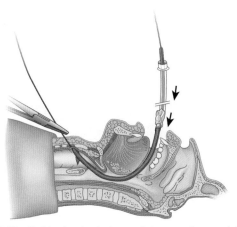

Figure 20-23 Guidewire technique. Advance the endotracheal tube (ETT) over the entire structure *(arrows)*. Use an ETT that has an inner diameter of 6.0 to 7.0 mm. The size of the ETT is dictated by the external diameter of the guide catheter. (From Sanchez AF: *The retrograde cookbook*, Irvine, 1993, University of California, Department of Anesthesia.)

an RI is performed with the bare guidewire (or epidural catheter) alone. When the ETT abuts the CTM, the guide catheter is advanced through the ETT from above (antegrade), passing distally to the carina.[11] The guidewire is then removed, and the guide catheter is again used as a stylet for the ETT. In my opinion, the best results from a blind RI are obtained by using the cricotracheal ligament as a puncture site and the technique in which the guide catheter is passed over the guidewire. Third, an LMA has been used as conduit for the exit of the guidewire; a jet stylet is then placed over the guidewire, and both LMA and guidewire are removed, leaving the jet stylet as a guide catheter for the ETT. The benefits of this technique include a longer time for ventilation and the ability to place a larger ETT than the LMA would have accommodated.[95]

D. Fiberoptic Technique

The FOB is a versatile tool for the anesthesiologist,[54] but like RI, has its limitations. In some cases, the combination of two techniques, when previously either technique alone has failed, allows achievement of tracheal intubation.[14,15,19,34,38,63,73,82] The combination of RI with direct laryngoscopy or RI using FOB can improve the chance of successful intubation.[14,15,19,38,63,73] The advantages of passing an FOB antegrade over a guidewire placed by RI are as follows:

1. The OD of the guidewire and the ID of the suction port of the FOB form a tight fit that prevents railroading between the two cylinders, allowing the FOB to follow a straight path through the vocal cords without being caught on anatomic structures.
2. The FOB acts as a large antegrade guide catheter (see "Guidewire Technique") and prevents railroading of the ETT.
3. When the FOB has passed over the wire through the vocal cords, it can be advanced freely beyond the puncture site to the carina, which eliminates

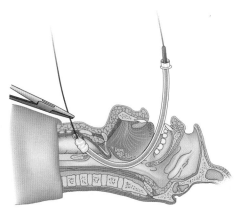

Figure 20-24 Guidewire technique. Advance the endotracheal tube through the vocal cords and up against the cricothyroid membrane. (From Sanchez AF: *The retrograde cookbook*, Irvine, 1993, University of California, Department of Anesthesia.)

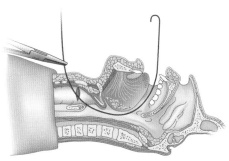

Figure 20-26 Fiberoptic technique. The guidewire is placed as in the guidewire technique and pulled out to appropriate length to accommodate the fiberoptic bronchoscope (hemostat in place). (From Sanchez AF: *The retrograde cookbook*, Irvine, 1993, University of California, Department of Anesthesia.)

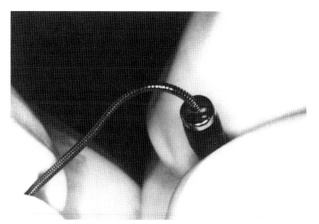

Figure 20-28 Fiberoptic technique. Close-up view of J tip being fed into suction port of fiberoptic bronchoscope. (From Sanchez AF: *The retrograde cookbook*, Irvine, 1993, University of California, Department of Anesthesia.)

the problem of distance between vocal cords and puncture site.

4. Use of the FOB allows placement of the ETT under direct vision.
5. The FOB can be used by less experienced operators.
6. Oxygen can be delivered continuously through the FOB with the guidewire still in place (see "Pediatrics").

Preparation of the FOB should be completed before RI is initiated. The rubber casing from the proximal portion of the suction port must be removed (to allow the guidewire to exit from the FOB handle), and the FOB should be armed with the appropriate-sized ETT (6.5 to 7.0 mm ID). The RI is performed using the guidewire technique (Fig. 20-26), and the FOB is then passed antegrade over the guidewire like a guide catheter (Figs. 20-27 through 20-30). Once the tip of the FOB abuts the CTM (Fig. 20-31), there are the following options:

1. *Option 1:* Remove the guidewire distally (Fig. 20-32) or proximally (through the fiberoptic handle) and, after advancing under direct vision to

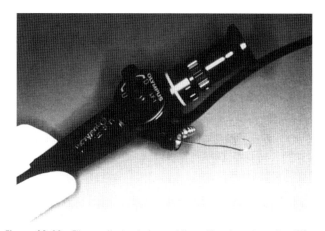

Figure 20-29 Fiberoptic technique. J tip exiting from handle of fiberoptic bronchoscope. (From Sanchez AF: *The retrograde cookbook*, Irvine, 1993, University of California, Department of Anesthesia.)

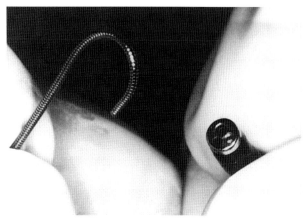

Figure 20-27 Fiberoptic technique. Close-up view of J tip of guidewire and distal tip of fiberoptic bronchoscope. (From Sanchez AF: *The retrograde cookbook*, Irvine, 1993, University of California, Department of Anesthesia.)

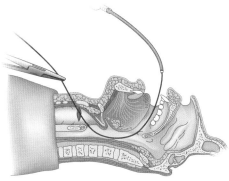

Figure 20-30 Fiberoptic technique. Begin advancing the fiberoptic bronchoscope (armed with the endotracheal tube) over the guidewire. (From Sanchez AF: *The retrograde cookbook*, Irvine, 1993, University of California, Department of Anesthesia.)

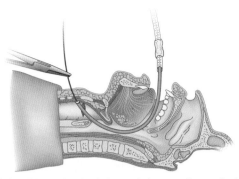

Figure 20-31 Fiberoptic technique. Advance fiberoptic broncho-scope to the cricothyroid membrane. (From Sanchez AF: *The retro-grade cookbook*, Irvine, 1993, University of California, Department of Anesthesia.)

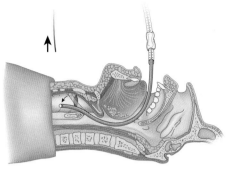

Figure 20-33 Fiberoptic technique. Remove the guidewire from the cricothyroid membrane *(straight arrow)*. The tip of the fiberoptic bronchoscope then drops into midtracheal position *(curved arrow)*. (From Sanchez AF: *The retrograde cookbook*, Irvine, 1993, University of California, Department of Anesthesia.)

the carina, intubate (Figs. 20-33 and 20-34). Removal of the guidewire distally is less likely to dislodge the FOB from the trachea, but anecdotal reports suggest that removal proximally should decrease the incidence of infection resulting from oral contaminants.[71,96]

2. *Option 2:* Instead of removing the guidewire, allow it to relax caudad into the trachea, advance the FOB below the cricoid cartilage, and then remove the guidewire. This allows a greater length of the FOB in the trachea before the guidewire is removed.

3. *Option 3:* Remove the guidewire proximally only until it is seen through the FOB to have popped out of the CTM and into the trachea; then advance the guidewire through the FOB to the carina. The FOB can then be advanced antegrade over the guidewire to the carina. (Caution: Be sure both ends of the guidewire are floppy.)

4. *Option 4:* Tobias used a fiberoptic technique that did not make use of the suction port of the FOB.[19] A standard RI was performed, feeding the guide-wire or epidural catheter first through the main lumen (bevel) of the ETT and immediately exiting out of the Murphy eye. The ETT was then advanced to the level of the CTM (Fig. 20-35). At this time, the FOB was advanced proximally through the ETT to the level of the carina. The retrograde guidewire was then removed, and a standard FOI was performed.

(My own preference is for option 3.)

The combination of FOB and RI is the easiest to perform of all the RI techniques. The disadvantages are that it requires more equipment (not readily available in cases of emergency) and more preparation time and may not be suitable in certain conditions (e.g., an airway with large amounts of blood or secretions).

E. Silk Pull-Through Technique

Various pull-through techniques have been described using epidural catheters,[39,97] central venous pressure catheters,[67] monofilament sutures,[75] and Fogarty catheters[98]; the silk technique is also a pull-through technique.[34,36,48] The basic principle involves advancing the epidural catheter retrograde as in the classic technique, attaching it to a length of silk, attaching the length of silk to the tip of the ETT, and then using the catheter-silk combination to pull the ETT into the trachea. The silk technique offers the following advantages:

1. The necessary equipment is readily available in the operating room.
2. The silk is intimately attached to the ETT, eliminating railroading.
3. Multiple attempts at intubation are allowed without having to repeat the procedure (CTM puncture) if it fails initially.

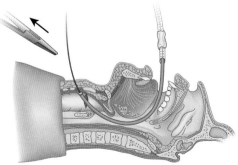

Figure 20-32 Fiberoptic technique. Have an assistant remove the hemostat *(arrow)*. (From Sanchez AF: *The retrograde cookbook*, Irvine, 1993, University of California, Department of Anesthesia.)

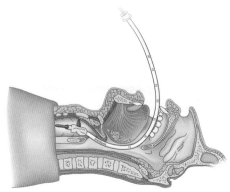

Figure 20-34 Fiberoptic technique. Continue as for a standard fiberoptic intubation. (From Sanchez AF: *The retrograde cookbook*, Irvine, 1993, University of California, Department of Anesthesia.)

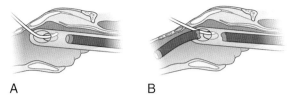

Figure 20-35   Fiberoptic technique. **A,** Midsagittal view of the larynx with the tip of the endotracheal tube (ETT) at the level of the crico-thyroid membrane. The fiberoptic bronchoscope (FOB) is advanced through the main lumen of the ETT. **B,** The FOB is advanced to the level of the carina before the guidewire is removed. (Modified from Tobias R: Increased success with retrograde guide for endotracheal intubation (letter). *Anesth Analg* 62:366, 1983.)

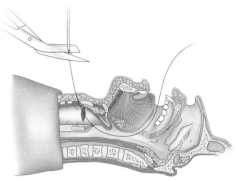

Figure 20-37   Silk pull-through technique. Pull the epidural catheter caudad until the silk suture exits the skin above the cricothyroid membrane; then cut off the epidural catheter. (From Sanchez AF: *The retrograde cookbook,* Irvine, 1993, University of California, Department of Anesthesia.)

4. Oxygen can be delivered through the ETT using a standard anesthesia circle system, and in-line capnography can be used to verify placement of the ETT.

5. If necessary, postoperative reintubation can be accomplished using the silk, which is left in place until the time of discharge from the recovery room.

The silk technique employs the principles and equipment of the classic technique, with the addition of a length of silk suture (3-0 nylon monofilament may also be used). Once the epidural catheter (which is used only to place the silk) is out of the oral or nasal cavity, the silk suture is tied to the cephalad end of the catheter (Fig. 20-36), and the silk is pulled antegrade through the CTM (Fig. 20-37). The epidural catheter is cut off and discarded (see Fig. 20-37), and the cephalad end of the silk is tied to the Murphy eye (Fig. 20-38). The silk suture is then used to pull the ETT gently into the trachea (Fig. 20-39). If a floppy epiglottis causes obstruction, one can deliberately intubate the esophagus; as the ETT is being gently withdrawn from the esophagus, tension applied simultaneously to the distal end of the silk pops the tip of the ETT anteriorly, lifts up the epiglottis, and allows the ETT to enter the larynx. When the ETT abuts against the CTM, the tension on the silk suture is released and the ETT is passed further to enter the trachea (Fig. 20-40). If a nasal intubation is required, a urologic

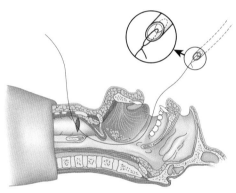

Figure 20-38   Silk pull-through technique. Tie the suture to the Murphy eye as shown *(inset).* Have an assistant pull the patient's tongue forward. Begin pulling the suture with one hand while the opposite hand holds the endotracheal tube (ETT) steady and in midline. At all times maintain tension on the suture while advancing the ETT. (From Sanchez AF: *The retrograde cookbook,* Irvine, 1993, University of California, Department of Anesthesia.)

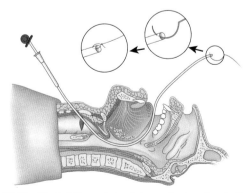

Figure 20-36   Silk pull-through technique. Proceed as in the classic technique. After the epidural catheter has exited the oral cavity, tie it to a 3-0 noncutting silk suture (30-inch length), as shown in the insets. (From Sanchez AF: *The retrograde cookbook,* Irvine, 1993, University of California, Department of Anesthesia.)

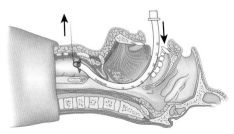

Figure 20-39   Silk pull-through technique. Simultaneously pull the silk caudad *(arrow at throat)* as you advance the endotracheal tube *(arrow at oral cavity)* with the opposite hand. Advance the endotracheal tube to the cricothyroid membrane. (From Sanchez AF: *The retrograde cookbook,* Irvine, 1993, University of California, Department of Anesthesia.)

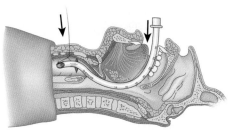

Figure 20-40 Silk pull-through technique. Release the suture, and with the opposite hand advance the endotracheal tube (ETT) to the desired depth. The suture partially retracts *(arrow at throat)* into the trachea as the ETT is advanced *(arrow at oral cavity)* past the cricothyroid membrane. The remaining suture is secured to the neck with transparent dressing. On extubation, the silk is left in place as a precaution, should reintubation be required. The suture is removed in the recovery room on the patient's discharge by cutting it flush with the skin and pulling it out of the oral cavity. (From Sanchez AF: *The retrograde cookbook*, Irvine, 1993, University of California, Department of Anesthesia.)

catheter can be used to cause the epidural catheter to exit the nasal rather than the oral cavity (Figs. 20-41 through 20-44).

In practice, it may be difficult to suture the silk onto the epidural catheter. A small learning curve is required not to allow any slack on the silk until the CTM is reached and to gauge properly the fine balance between pulling on the silk and simultaneously advancing the ETT. The technique is easy, and because the silk can be left in place with no discomfort for the duration of the anesthesia and after extubation, emergent reintubation can be accomplished. I have had two occasions to reintubate in the recovery room using this technique; both patients had suffered maxillofacial trauma, had initially been intubated awake using the retrograde silk technique, and had arch bars placed in the operating room.

VII. PEDIATRICS

In pediatric patients, the physician is faced with the formidable problems of small anatomic structures that are difficult to palpate, immature anatomic structures such as anterior larynx and narrow cricoid cartilage, congenital anomalies, and pathologic disorders that intimately affect

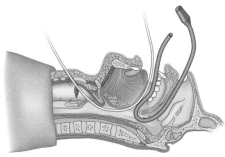

Figure 20-42 Silk pull-through technique. The tip of the urologic catheter is retrieved from the oral cavity. (From Sanchez AF: *The retrograde cookbook*, Irvine, 1993, University of California, Department of Anesthesia.)

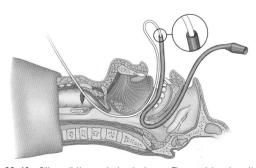

Figure 20-43 Silk pull-through technique. The epidural catheter is fed into the urologic catheter *(inset)* and may be tied together. (From Sanchez AF: *The retrograde cookbook*, Irvine, 1993, University of California, Department of Anesthesia.)

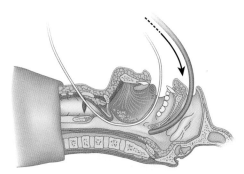

Figure 20-41 Silk pull-through technique. With the epidural catheter already in place, a 16-F red rubber urologic catheter is advanced through the nose *(arrow)*. (From Sanchez AF: *The retrograde cookbook*, Irvine, 1993, University of California, Department of Anesthesia.)

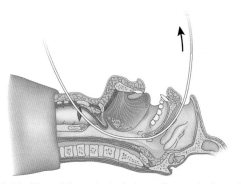

Figure 20-44 Silk pull-through technique. The urologic catheter is removed *(arrow)* so that the epidural catheter exits the nose. The epidural catheter can now be used as a nasotracheal guide. (From Sanchez AF: *The retrograde cookbook*, Irvine, 1993, University of California, Department of Anesthesia.)

the airway (e.g., acute epiglottitis). Because the pediatric airway is different, concerns have been raised about whether RI is indicated or contraindicated in infants.[69,70,74,99] Some have claimed that RI is dangerous but without citing any clinical supportive evidence.[99] The number of articles and case reports in the medical literature on the subject of RI in the pediatric population is limited.[2,10,11,16,20,34,38,40,69,70,73,74,81,99]

RI has been used with both anticipated and unanticipated pediatric DA, primarily after failure of conventional intubating techniques (blind nasal intubation, direct laryngoscopy, or FOI). The technique used is the same as in the adult, but a higher incidence of difficulties has been reported, including problems in cannulating the ETT and inability to pass the ETT through the glottic opening.[11,73,100]

In some cases, combined techniques have offered more success than blind RI. In one case report of a 16-year-old patient with acute epiglottitis, intubation was accomplished only by RI combined with rigid laryngoscopy; the retrograde catheter marked a path through an otherwise completely distorted anatomy.[38] The largest pediatric series with the highest success rate was reported by Audenaert and colleagues[73]; in that series, RI was performed for 20 pediatric patients, aged 1 day to 17 years, with DAs primarily resulting from congenital anomalies (Table 20-2). The authors' preferred approach, a combination of FOI with retrograde guidewire, offers the following advantages:

1. Higher success rate
2. Faster intubation
3. Ability to insufflate oxygen through the suction port of the FOB with the guidewire in place (Table 20-3)
4. No hanging up of the ETT in the glottis
5. No need to rely on anatomic landmarks to guide the FOB into the trachea
6. Less requirement for experience to manage the FOB

No major complications were reported, and the technique was considered a valuable addition to pediatric airway management.[73]

Przybylo and Stevenson described a unique method of managing the airway in a pediatric patient for closure of a tracheocutaneous fistula. The patient was a 4-year-old girl with severe micrognathia and limited temporomandibular joint motion and mouth opening who required a tracheostomy in the neonatal period for upper airway obstruction. Attempts at oral-nasal FOI were unsuccessful; the FOB was passed through the existing tracheocutaneous fistula in a cephalad direction, into the nasal cavity, and the FOB was then used as a stylet for nasal intubation.[101]

VIII. COMPLICATIONS AND CAUTIONS

Although it has been demonstrated that transtracheal needle puncture is safe and associated with only minor complications (Box 20-4), numerous potential complications of RI have been cited in the literature (Box 20-5). Documented complications of RI are relatively few, and most were self-limited (Box 20-6). The most common

---

BOX 20-4 Translaryngeal Anesthesia (Complications)

17,500 Reported Cases

2 Broken needles
2 Laryngospasms
4 Soft tissue infections

Modified from Gold MI, Buechel DR: Translaryngeal anesthesia: A review. *Anesthesiology* 20:181, 1959.

BOX 20-5 Potential Complications of Retrograde Intubation

Esophageal perforation
Hemoptysis
Intratracheal submucosal hematoma with distal obstruction
Laryngeal edema
Laryngospasm
Pretracheal infection
Tracheal fistula
Tracheitis
Vocal cord damage

From Sanchez AF: *The retrograde cookbook*, Irvine, 1993, University of California, Department of Anesthesia.

BOX 20-6 Reported Complications of Retrograde Intubation

Self-Limited

Bleeding
    Puncture site, 8
    Peritracheal hematoma, 1
    Epistaxis, 2
Subcutaneous emphysema, 4
Pneumomediastinum, 2
Breath holding, 1
Catheter traveling caudad,* 4

Not Self-Limited

Trigeminal nerve trauma, 1
Incorrect placement (pharyngeal), 1
Pretracheal abscess, 1
Pneumothorax, 1
Loss of hook,† 2

From Sanchez AF: *The retrograde cookbook*, Irvine, 1993, University of California, Department of Anesthesia.
*Refers to catheter traveling in a caudad direction toward the lungs instead of cephalad toward the oral cavity.
†Refers to Dr. Waters' technique of retrieving catheter from nasopharynx using a self-made hook (Waters DJ: Guided blind endotracheal intubation: For patients with deformities of the upper airway. *Anaesthesia* 18:158, 1963).

TABLE 20-2

Summary of Clinical Approaches to Pediatric Patients with Airways Difficult to Manage Clinically*

Case No.	Age	Weight (kg)	Primary/Surgical Diagnosis	Airway Problems[†]	Scope	Tube ID (mm)	Rationale or Failed Means of Endotracheal Intubation[‡]
1	1 day	2.9	Congenital anomalies/omphalocele	Micrognathia, nonvisualization	AUR-8	3.0	A, D
2	6 mo	4.5	Congenital anomalies/bilateral radial club hand	Nonvisualization	AUR-8	3.0	D
3	7 mo	5.7	Amyoplasia/congenital hip dislocation	Micrognathia, nonvisualization, limited mouth opening	AUR-8	4.0	A, D, F[§]
4	8 mo	6.8	Amyoplasia/clubfoot	Micrognathia, limited mouth opening, nonvisualization	AUR-8	4.0	A, D
5	10 mo	4.9	Pierre Robin syndrome/cleft palate	Micrognathia, nonvisualization	AUR-8	3.5	A, D
6	11 mo	7.8	Arthrogryposis/clubfoot	Klippel-Feil, micrognathia	AUR-8	4.0	A
7	15 mo	8.0	Undiagnosed congenital anomalies/congenital hip dislocation	Nonvisualization	AUR-8	4.0	D
8	24 mo	13.2	Hurler's syndrome/bone marrow transplant	Short neck, large tongue, limited neck motion, nonvisualization	AUR-8	4.0	A, D
9	26 mo	11.4	Camptomelic dysplasia/cervical fusion	Cervical spine abnormalities and instability, limited motion of neck, mouth	AUR-8	3.0	A, C
10	3 yr	11.2	Hallermann-Streiff syndrome/ophthalmologic procedures	Narrowed trachea, micrognathia, malar hypoplasia, microstomia, nonvisualization	AUR-8	4.5	A, D
11	5 yr (6 yr)	15.1 (16.9)	Escobar syndrome (multiple pterygium)/orthopedic and plastic procedures	Klippel-Feil, brevicollis, limited mouth and neck motion, nonvisualization	LF-1	5.0	A, D
12	6 yr	11.3	Multiple congenital anomalies/infantile scoliosis	Micrognathia, cervical hemivertebra, limited mouth opening, nonvisualization	LF-1	5.0	H, A, D, R, F[§]
13	7 yr	17.1	Spondyloepiphyseal dysplasia congenital/C1-2 subluxation	C-spine abnormalities	LF-1	5.5	C
14	7 yr (7 yr)	15.9 (17.1)	Schwartz-Jampel syndrome/C2-3 subluxation	Microstomia, limited neck and mouth motion, C-spine abnormalities	LF-1	5.0	A, C
15	9 yr	14	Cerebral palsy/congenital hip dislocation	Nonvisualization	AUR-8	5.5	D
16	12 yr	22	Escobar syndrome (multiple pterygium)/scoliosis	Klippel-Feil, brevicollis, limited mouth, neck motion, micrognathia nonvisualization	LF-1	5.5	A, D, L
17	12 yr	15.2	Undiagnosed congenital progressive neuromuscular disease/extreme cervicothoracolumbar fixed lordosis for release and fusion	Extreme fixed cervicothoracic lordosis, micrognathia nonvisualization	AUR-8	5.0	A, D
18	14 yr	51	Juvenile rheumatoid arthritis/joint fusion	Limited motion, neck and mouth	LF-1	5.5	H, A
19	15 yr	71	Juvenile rheumatoid arthritis/phalangeal replacements	Limited motion, neck and mouth	LF-1	6.0	H, A
20	17 yr	74	Trauma/cervical spine and facial fractures	Facial fractures, in cervical traction, unstable cervical spine	LF-1	7.5	C

AUR-8 urethroscope (Circon ACMI, Stamford, CN); *ID,* inner diameter of endotracheal tube; *LF-1* tracheal intubation fiberscope (Olympus, Center Valley, PA).

*Case numbers have been assigned for reference and convenience only. The tracheas of patients 11 and 14 were each intubated twice with retrograde-assisted fiberoptic technique.

[†]*Nonvisualization* refers to failure to expose the cords or arytenoid cartilages with direct laryngoscopy. On all occasions on which the AUR-8 scope was used, the 22-G catheter and 0.018-inch wire were also used. Likewise, when the LF-1 scope was used, the 20-G catheter and 0.025-inch wire were used.

[‡]This column reveals a few patients in whom this technique was used primarily, usually for cervical spine consideration (C) or when the airway was known to be extremely difficult by history or previous experience (H) or by preoperative assessment (A). Direct laryngoscopy (D), fiberoptic laryngoscopy (F), light wand (L), and retrograde alone (R) techniques were attempted unsuccessfully where so noted.

[§]Use of a Bullard rigid fiberoptic laryngoscope afforded an excellent view of the vocal cords, but owing to limited mouth opening the endotracheal tube could not be properly positioned.

Modified from Audenaert SM, Montgomery CL, Stone B: Retrograde-assisted fiberoptic tracheal intubation in children with difficult airways. *Anesth Analg* 73:660, 1991.

TABLE 20-3

Flow Measurement of Various Fiberscopes*

Scope (Mfgr.)	Outer Scope Diam. (mm)	Inner Lumen Diam. (mm)	Working Length (cm)	Maximum Tip Flexion (degrees)	Scope Configuration	Max. O_2 Flow (L/min)
AUR-8 (Circon ACMI, Stamford, CN)	2.7	0.8	37	140	Straight	9.4 ± 0.1
					90-degree curve and 90-degree tip flexion	9.4 ± 0.0
					90-degree curve with 0.018-inch wire in place	4.37 ± 0.01
LF-1 (Olympus, Center Valley, PA)	3.8	1.2	60	120	Straight	18.1 ± 0.2
					90-degree curve and 90-degree tip flexion	17.9 ± 0.1
					90-degree curve with 0.025-inch wire in place	12.4 ± 0.1
BF-1 (Olympus, Center Valley, PA)	5.9	2.8	55	100	Straight	159 ± 5
					90-degree curve and 90-degree tip flexion	152 ± 1
					90-degree curve with 0.035-inch wire in place	145 ± 1

*Flow measurements represent mean ± SD; *Mfgr.*, manufacturer.
From Audenaert SM, Montgomery CL, Stone B: Retrograde-assisted fiberoptic tracheal intubation in children with difficult airways. *Anesth Analg* 73:660, 1991.

complications were bleeding and subcutaneous emphysema.[5,6,9,20,31,37,39,40,92]

A. Bleeding

Insignificant bleeding (4 to 5 drops of blood) has been observed with CTM puncture during RI.[40,92] Even a patient who had received heparin intraoperatively and had postoperative disseminated intravascular coagulation experienced only a small, self-limited hematoma after the procedure.[9] Controversy exists with respect to making the puncture below the cricoid cartilage because of a greater potential for bleeding.[2,39,79] Three studies involving 57 patients who underwent RI with punctures at the cricotracheal ligament or between the second and third tracheal rings showed no evidence of major bleeding.[6,20,39] There are, however, scattered reports of severe hemoptysis after transtracheal needle puncture with resultant hypoxia, cardiorespiratory arrest, dysrhythmias, and death.[41,44,102-104] Two patients had epistaxis after nasal intubation (no vasoconstricting agent was used).[25,40] The following measures have been suggested to decrease the potential for bleeding:

1. Avoid RI in patients with bleeding diathesis.
2. Apply pressure to the puncture site for 5 minutes.
3. Apply pressure dressing to the puncture site for 24 hours.
4. Maintain patient in the supine position for 3 to 4 hours after puncture.

B. Subcutaneous Emphysema

Subcutaneous emphysema localized to the area of a transtracheal needle puncture site is common but self-limited.[6,20,30,42,76,82,102-108] In severe cases, air may track through the fascial planes of the neck, leading to tracheal compression with airway compromise, pneumomediastinum, and pneumothorax.[29,30,29,30,42,44,77,106,108,109] Accumulation of air occurs gradually (1 to 6 hours) after a transtracheal puncture.[42,106] Severe subcutaneous emphysema has been attributed to use of a large-bore needle, multiple CTM punctures, and exposure of the puncture site to persistent elevated intratracheal pressure (coughing, grunting, or sneezing). In addition, pneumomediastinum has been reported in patients who underwent transtracheal puncture with a needle and was attributed to elevated endotracheal pressure (paroxysmal coughing and sneezing).[41-43] When the patient has been intubated by the retrograde technique, elevated peak inspiratory pressure (PIP) and elevated end-expiratory pressure (PEEP) should not increase the likelihood of these complications intraoperatively, because the puncture site is located above the ETT cuff, so that the area of the initial puncture site is not exposed to high pressure. Lee and coauthors reported on a patient with a history of noncardiogenic pulmonary edema and atelectasis who, after RI, received 7.5 cm H_2O with PEEP with no complications (PIP values were not reported).[65]

C. Other Complications

Other reported self-limited complications were breath holding and travel of the catheter (a straight, flexible guidewire) caudally.[20,40,84]

Complications that were not self-limited were as follows:

1. Trigeminal nerve trauma,[12] which the author suspected was due to multiple laryngoscopies
2. Guidewire fracture, in which wire had to be surgically removed[64]
3. Loss of hook (the type that was originally used by Waters and is no longer used)[2,40,100]

4. Pneumothorax, which necessitated use of a chest tube[42]
5. Pretracheal abscess in diabetic patients after multiple punctures at the CTM requiring incision and drainage[71]

IX. CONCLUSIONS

The anesthesia care provider is charged with the responsibility for securing the airway. In most cases, this can be accomplished with the use of conventional techniques, but in a small number of cases these techniques cannot be successfully applied to the clinical problem at hand. No method, including RI, offers 100% success; therefore, it is wise to have multiple available options and to be facile with alternative techniques for intubation.

RI has been a particularly useful alternative in difficult intubations after multiple manipulations that have caused bleeding, in facial injuries in which bleeding is already present, and in patients with limited neck movement and mouth opening. The technique is easy to learn, requires little equipment, and in practiced hands is a rapid, safe, and effective method for intubating the trachea.

International awareness (in multiple specialties) of the value of RI in selected clinical settings has increased.[110,111] In my opinion, RI is a valuable additional airway management technique and should be included as part of the armamentarium of health care providers involved in the care of seriously injured or ill patients.

X. CLINICAL PEARLS

- Have the equipment readily available!

- Know your anatomy and practice daily: During your daily patient airway evaluation, make sure to palpate and note the location of the arch of the cricoid cartilage on every patient (important for RI and for emergency cricothyrotomy).

- Positioning of the patient and, more importantly, positioning of the anesthesiologist should be practiced on the mannequin until it becomes second nature.

- The initial puncture site through the cricothyroid membrane (CTM) should be as close to the upper border of the arch of the cricoid cartilage as possible. This allows for a longer length of the ETT to be below the vocal cords before removal of the guidewire (preventing the ETT from buckling backward into the esophagus).

- Use an ETT with smaller inner diameter (6.5 to 7.0 mm ID) to prevent "railroading." I believe many of the failures are caused by the use of a large ETT that gets caught on the arytenoids (similar to the problem found during FOIs).

- Although it is more time consuming and more cumbersome to perform, the silk pull-through technique is my method of choice because it addresses most of the challenges encountered (railroading , potential need to perform multiple attempts, and ability to reintubate the patient postoperatively).

Acknowledgments

This writing is dedicated to my daughter, Danielle. Special thanks to Mrs. Debi Quilty, Mrs. Norma Claudio, and Elsie Vindiola for their research assistance and to Tay McClellan for her outstanding medical illustrations.

SELECTED REFERENCES

All references can be found online at expertconsult.com.

14. Gupta B, McDonald JS, Brooks HJ: Oral fiberoptic intubation over a retrograde guidewire. *Anesth Analg* 68:517, 1989.
27. Van Stralen DW, Rogers M, Perkin RM, et al: Retrograde intubation training using mannequin. *Am J Emerg Med* 13:50, 1995.
33. Stern Y, Spitzer T: Retrograde intubation of the trachea. *J Laryngol Otol* 105:746, 1991.
35. Shantha TR: Retrograde intubation [letter]. *Br J Anaesth* 55:855, 1983.
37. Guggenberger H, Lenz G, Heumann H: Success rate and complications of a modified guided blind technique for intubation in 36 patients. *Anaesthesist* 36:703, 1987.
52. Shantha TR: Retrograde intubation using the subcricoid region. *Br J Anaesth* 68:109, 1992.
73. Audenaert SM, Montgomery CL, Stone B: Retrograde-assisted fiberoptic tracheal intubation in children with difficult airways. *Anesth Analg* 73:660, 1991.
95. Arndt GA, Topp J, Hannah J, et al: Intubation via the LMA using a Cook retrograde intubation kit. *Can J Anaesth* 45:257, 1998.
132. Latto IP, Rosen M: Management of difficult intubation. In Latto IP, Rosen M, editors: *Difficulties in tracheal intubation*, Philadelphia, 1984, Baillière Tindall.
136. Linscott MS, Horton WC: Management of upper airway obstruction. *Otolaryngol Clin North Am* 12:351, 1979.
152. Sanchez AF: Retrograde intubation. *Anesthesiol Clin North Am* 13:439, 1995.

Chapter 21

Intubating Introducers, Stylets, and Lighted Stylets (Lightwands)

JEANETTE SCOTT | ORLANDO R. HUNG

I. INTRODUCTION

The procedure of placing an endotracheal tube (ETT) in the trachea for ventilation and oxygenation is more than a thousand years old. It was first performed on pigs by the Persian physician, Avicenna, between 980 and 1037 AD.[1,2] Blind digital intubation in humans was first described in 1796 by Herholdt and Rafn in a resuscitation protocol for drowning victims.[3] In 1880, Macewen described blind digital intubation in awake patients using a curved metal tube.[4] However, modern methods of laryngoscopic endotracheal intubation did not emerge until early in the 20th century, after the introduction of a flexible metal tube by Kuhn[5] and of the laryngoscope by Jackson.[6]

Over the years, direct laryngoscopic intubation has been shown to be an effective, safe, and relatively easy technique. In fact, using a laryngoscope to obtain line of sight to the laryngeal inlet has become the standard method of endotracheal intubation in the operating room, the intensive care unit, and the emergency department. However, even in the hands of experienced laryngoscopists, accurate and prompt placement of the ETT remains a significant challenge in some patients. This is particularly true in "unprepared" patients and in patients requiring emergency intubation. With any standard laryngoscope, obtaining line of sight to the patient's larynx can prove difficult in the presence of specific anatomic variations such as a receding mandible, prominent upper incisors, a restricted mouth opening, or limited movement of the cervical spine. It has been estimated that 1% to 3% of surgical patients have a so-called difficult airway (DA), making laryngoscopic intubation problematic and sometimes impossible.[7] In the obstetric population, the incidence of failed laryngoscopic intubation has been reported to be 0.05% to 0.35%.[8] Many predictors of difficult laryngoscopy (DL) have been suggested in the literature,[9,10] but the sensitivity and specificity of these tests remain relatively low.[11-13] Therefore, all clinicians must be prepared to deal with the prospect of both anticipated and unanticipated DLs.

Given that direct laryngoscopic visualization of the glottis may not be possible, especially in a timely manner during emergency situations, a number of devices have been developed to enable the clinician to pass the ETT "blindly" into the trachea. During the last few decades, the use of intubating guides such as stylets and introducers and light-guided intubation based on the principle of transillumination have proved to be effective, safe, and simple approaches. This chapter briefly reviews the principles and techniques of these alternative intubation procedures.

Many types of intubating guides and lighted stylets have been commercially available for many years. Where possible, this chapter focuses on devices that have been proven to be effective and safe in the medical literature. However, the concepts and techniques discussed here may be applicable to other similar devices.

II. INTUBATING INTRODUCERS AND STYLETS

A. History

Intubating guides or introducers were first reported in the late 1940s. In 1949, Macintosh described "the use of a gum elastic introducer as an aid to passing endotracheal tubes" (Fig. 21-1) as follows[14]:

> This projects some 2-3 inches beyond the distal end of the tube, and since it is malleable the curve can be shaped to facilitate its introduction through the cords. Once the tip of the introducer lies within the trachea, the ETT slides over it, easily, into position. This device has proved of real worth on rare occasions, when, for one reason or another, it has not been possible to obtain a view of the vocal cords. Provided the epiglottis can be seen, it has been possible to direct the curved introducer posterior to it, and then through the underlying glottis. The ETT now follows into position.

B. The Eschmann Introducer

Use of an introducer in this fashion did not become widespread until the development of the Eschmann Introducer (EI) by Venn in 1973. Venn's design has several key features. First, it is relatively long at 60 cm (Fig. 21-2), allowing one to place the introducer between the cords before "railroading" the ETT over its distal end. It has been suggested that a naked introducer affords better dexterity and tactile sensation to the user compared with an introducer on which an ETT has been preloaded.[15] Second, the EI has a coudé tip (a 40-degree bend) for "hooking" under the epiglottis. The material from which the EI is made—a combination of a polyester core and resin covering—no doubt has contributed to its success.[15] The EI is malleable, firm enough to direct, yet flexible enough to yield on contact. Furthermore, it is a multiuse device that can be sterilized between uses. The EI is commonly referred to as a "gum elastic bougie" despite not being made of gum, having no elastic properties, and not being a "bougie" at all (a bougie being a dilating device).[16,17] The EI is currently sold under the name "Portex Venn Introducer" (Smiths Medical, UK.)

Although an EI can be used to direct the ETT toward an "anterior" or narrow larynx, its real strength lies as a tool to facilitate intubation when the laryngeal aperture cannot be seen during laryngoscopy (e.g., Cormack-Lehane grade 3 view).[18] If the epiglottis cannot be visualized at all (i.e., Cormack-Lehane grade 4 view), we do not recommend use of the EI, because the likelihood of successful intubation with the EI is unacceptably low. In cases in which the epiglottis can be seen, the coudé tip can be hooked under the epiglottis and the EI advanced blindly through the glottis. The success of this maneuver is improved if the EI has been preshaped into a curve.[19] As the introducer is advanced further, the tracheal "clicks" are felt approximately 90% of the time if the EI is correctly placed,[20] whereas no "clicks" will be observed if the EI has been advanced into the esophagus. We

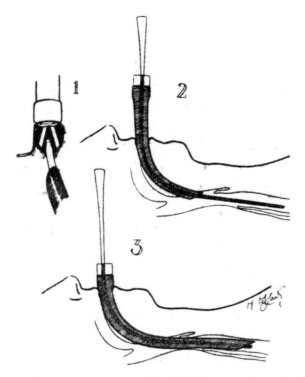

Figure 21-1 Images from Macintosh's 1949 paper demonstrating use of a "long gum-elastic catheter" as "a guide to aid intubation." (From Macintosh RR: An aid to oral intubation. *Br Med J* 1:28, 1949.)

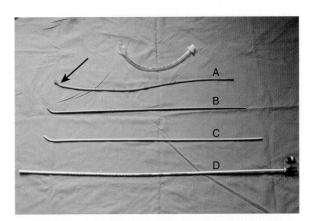

Figure 21-2 Tracheal introducers. *A*, The Eschmann Introducer, or EI, commonly known as the "gum elastic bougie," with a J (coudé) tip (*arrow*), (currently sold as "Portex Venn Introducer," Smiths Medical, UK). *B*, The hollow Frova Intubation Introducer. The optional rigid internal cannula has been removed, and one of the two ventilation ports can be seen near its tip (Cook Inc., Bloomington, IN). *C*, The single-use Endotracheal Tube Introducer (Sun Med, Largo, FL). *D*, The Cook Airway Exchange Catheter (Cook Inc., Bloomington, IN).

believe that "clicks" are more likely to be perceived if, once the tip of the EI is through the cords, the introducer is advanced at a shallow angle relative to the patient. This maneuver is intended to ensure that the tip of the introducer will contact the cartilaginous rings on the anterior tracheal wall as it advances, producing the "clicking" sensation. One can imagine that "clicks" are less likely to be felt if the only contact between the trachea and the EI is the coudé bend in the introducer that is sliding along the posterior tracheal wall, or even along the trachealis muscle.

Additional clues to confirm correct tracheal placement include the perception that the EI slightly deviates to the right as it advances into the right main bronchus and a "hold up" felt at the 30- to 35-cm mark as the EI becomes lodged in a distal airway (reportedly a 100% reliable sign).[20] In contrast, if the EI is placed in the esophagus, the entire EI could be advanced without encountering any resistance, although theoretically it would be possible for a pharyngeal pouch to hold up the introducer if one were present.[21] Some authors have cautioned against the use of the hold-up sign, believing that it increases the risk of airway trauma. If clicks are felt, then the hold-up test is not required.[20]

After tracheal placement, the ETT is advanced distally over the EI into the trachea. A jaw lift-jaw thrust by the nondominant hand of the clinician or by a laryngoscope will facilitate the advancement of the ETT over the EI by elevating the tongue and epiglottis. If difficulty persists while the ETT is being advanced, rotating the ETT 90 degrees counterclockwise will turn its bevel posteriorly and minimize the risk of catching on the structures of the glottic opening.[22] After intubation, the position of the ETT is confirmed by conventional methods such as measurement of the end-tidal carbon dioxide concentration ($EtCO_2$) and auscultation.

The EI is long enough to be useful for nasal intubations and can also be used to place supralaryngeal airways (SLAs) or double-lumen tubes.[23] The long length of the EI enables it to be used as an airway exchange device; it can be placed down the lumen of a correctly placed ETT or SLA, which can then be removed over the introducer and discarded before a new airway is "railroaded" in its place. During the whole maneuver, the EI remains within the trachea, thereby guiding correct placement of the new airway. After the EI is removed, as always, the position of the new airway should be confirmed with the use of standard methods.

C. Other Types of Intubating Guides

Many intubating guides of different sizes, shapes, lengths, and materials have been developed. All of the designs serve a function similar to that of the EI, but many have some additional features. Some are single-use devices that were designed after concern was raised regarding the possibility of prion transfer between patients with multiuse airway equipment. However, there is growing skepticism about whether disease transfer from reused but sterilized medical instruments poses any tangible risk to patients, whereas the risk to patients from the use of suboptimal airway equipment with limited clinical

evaluation is very real. Clinicians should be wary of new equipment and always insist on using only instruments that have proved to be effective and safe.[24]

1. Frova Intubation Introducer

The Frova Intubation Introducer (Cook Inc., Bloomington, IN) is a single-use introducer, firmer than the EI, that has a 35-degree coudé tip, two side ports, and a hollow lumen (see Fig. 21-2). It comes with a Rapi-Fit connector that connects directly to standard ventilatory equipment, such as the bag of an air-mask-bag unit (AMBU) or an anesthetic circuit, enabling the Frova to also serve as a conduit for O_2 delivery or ventilation. This requires extreme caution however, because high-pressure source ventilation via the narrow lumen may result in severe barotrauma. The Frova may be connected to an esophageal detection device so that one can confirm correct placement before "railroading" the ETT.[25] The rigid, removable internal cannula is designed to increase the stiffness of the Frova; it has limited clinical indication and may increase the risk of trauma. The Frova introducer has two sizes: a 65-cm-long blue adult version for ETTs with greater than 5.5 mm inner diameter (ID) and a 33-cm-long yellow pediatric version for ETTs with 3.0 to 5.0 mm ID. First-pass success rates with the Frova introducer are similar to those with the EI and are substantially better than those of the similarly shaped Portex introducer.[26] It is presumed that this success is due to the increased malleability of the EI and the Frova, which enables preshaping of the device, compared with the Portex introducer.[26]

2. Endotracheal Tube Introducer

The Endotracheal Tube Introducer (Sun Med, Largo, FL) is an example of a single-use version of the EI (see Fig. 21-2). It is similar to the EI in size and shape but 10 cm longer (i.e., 70 cm long). Like the Frova, it is stiffer than the EI. There are 10-cm markings on the top of the Sun Med introducer to indicate the depth of insertion. Although it is marketed as a single-use, disposable device, resterilization is possible.

3. Parker Flex-It Directional Stylet

The Schroeder Oral/Nasal Directional Stylet, also known as the Parker Flex-It Directional Stylet (Parker Medical, Englewood, CO), is a disposable articulating stylet that requires no bending before intubation. Inserting the stylet into an ETT allows the clinician to elevate the tip of the ETT by wrapping all four fingers around the proximal ETT and using the base of thumb to depress the proximal end of the stylet (Fig. 21-3). Although the stylet is suitable for both oral and nasal intubation, it has been reported to be somewhat awkward to use, and the curvature created is not at the tip but rather over the distal half of the tube.[27] However, it has been reported to be effective for difficult intubations (DIs) as well as for blind intubations.[28]

The effectiveness of intubating guides in patients with a DA has been well established.[29-31] Most of these studies used the EI. With only a few exceptions, there are currently few data to support the use of the newer introducers for endotracheal intubation, particularly in patients with a history of DA. It should be emphasized that most of these new intubating guides and stylets are disposable

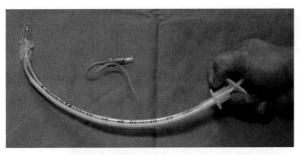

Figure 21-3 The Schroeder Directional Stylet can be used to elevate the tip of the endotracheal tube (ETT) by wrapping all four fingers around the proximal ETT and using the base of thumb to depress the proximal end of the stylet.

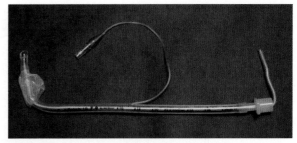

Figure 21-4 An endotracheal tube (ETT). The stylet remains "straight to cuff," at which point the ETT can be bent to the desired angle, resembling a hockey stick.

and designed for single-use. In contrast, the EI is more cost-effective because it is reusable.

D. Tube Exchangers

Although the EI can be used as a tube exchanger, several devices have been created especially for this purpose.

1. Cook Airway Exchange Catheter

The Cook Airway Exchange Catheter (CAEC; Cook Critical Care, division of Cook Inc.) is a hollow, flexible, straight tube that is designed as a tube exchanger for patients with a DA. The CAEC can be used to ventilate patients under difficult circumstances through the inner lumen and the distal ports after fitting the provided adaptor at the proximal end (see Fig. 21-2).

2. Sheriden Tube Exchanger

The Sheriden Tube Exchanger (Sheriden Catheter Corp., Oregon, NY) serves a similar function as the CAEC.

E. Stylets

A stylet is a plastic-coated metal rod that can be placed inside the lumen of an ETT before intubation to stiffen or preshape the ETT. Unlike the EI and other introducers, the stylet should not protrude past the tip of the ETT, so as to avoid unnecessary trauma. Water-based lubricant should be used, and easy passage of the stylet in and out of the ETT should be demonstrated before use. The "best" shape for a stylet-shaped ETT depends on the clinician's preference and the patient's position and anatomy. However, Levitan and colleagues showed that the line of sight to the larynx can be improved if the stylet remains "straight to cuff,"[32] at which point the ETT can then be bent to the desired angle (i.e., shaped like a hockey stick) (Fig. 21-4). An angle of 35 degrees or less reduces the risk of traumatic injury.[32] Once the ETT has passed through the vocal cords, the stylet should be withdrawn as the ETT is advanced into the trachea.

In a randomized trial, Gataure and associates compared the efficacy of the EI with that of the malleable stylet in 100 patients with simulated DL (Cormack-Lehane grade 3 view) under general anesthesia. The EI group had a success rate of 96% after two attempts, compared with 66% in the stylet group.[33]

F. Complications

Despite long-standing and widespread use, complications caused by ETT introducers, tube exchangers, and stylets are rare. To date, there have been only half a dozen case reports of pharyngeal, laryngeal, or tracheal perforation during airway manipulation that may have been caused by introducers or stylets.[34,35] Reports of trauma during airway management frequently come from cases in which multiple attempts at securing the airway occurred and multiple devices were used, making it difficult to attribute damage to a single device. Because of their firmer material, single-use ETT introducers exert more pressure at the tip compared with the multiuse EI.[26] Whether this corresponds to greater risk of airway trauma remains unknown.[25] However, as with all airway devices, undue force should always be avoided. Holding an ETT introducer close to the coudé tip (i.e., with Magill's forceps) increases the pressure exerted at the tip and therefore is not recommended.

After endotracheal intubation, all introducers and stylets should be inspected to ensure that no part of the device has been left behind. One report described a case in which the tip of an EI became detached and lodged in a patient's airway,[36] and in a similar case, plastic coating peeled off a stylet, blocking the ETT.[37] An unusual case report described the involution of an ETT at its tip while the EI was being withdrawn, which caused the EI to lodge firmly within the ETT and necessitated removal of both instruments.[38] Routine generous lubrication of intubating guides should reduce the likelihood of such events.

G. Clinical Utility

Intubating introducers, stylets, and tube exchangers have been used successfully to facilitate endotracheal intubation for many decades. In particular, the EI is a cheap, reliable, and familiar tool in the hands of anesthesia practitioners and, more recently, those of emergency physicians and in the prehospital setting.[39-42] Although the popularity of these nonvisual intubating techniques may decrease because of the improved glottic view afforded by the new video laryngoscopes, studies report the efficacy and usefulness of stylets and introducers to assist videoscopic intubation,[43-48] suggesting that these instruments will remain a mainstay of intubating adjuncts.

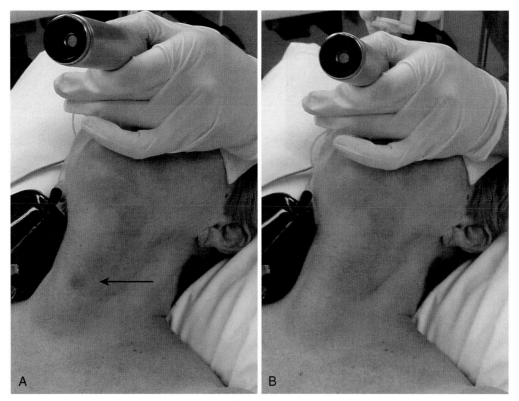

Figure 21-5 **A,** When the tip of the endotracheal tube (ETT) with the lighted stylet is placed at the glottic opening under direct laryngoscopy, a well-defined, circumscribed glow (*arrow*) in the anterior neck just below the thyroid prominence can be readily seen. **B,** If the tip of the ETT is in the esophagus, the transmitted glow is diffuse and cannot be readily detected under ambient lighting conditions.

III. LIGHTED STYLETS

A. History

Macintosh and Richards are frequently credited with being the first to use a lighted stylet for orotracheal intubation. In 1957, they reported the use of a lighted introducer to assist the placement of an ETT in the trachea under direct vision using a laryngoscope.[49] However, they did not describe the technique whereby transillumination of the soft tissues of the neck is used to guide the placement of the ETT. This transillumination technique was likely first described by Yamamura and colleagues, who reported the use of a lighted stylet for nasotracheal intubation in 1959.[50]

Modern lighted stylets use the principle of transillumination of the soft tissues of the anterior neck to guide the tip of the ETT into the trachea. This method takes advantage of the anterior (superficial) location of the trachea relative to the esophagus. When the tip of the ETT with the lighted stylet enters the glottic opening, a well-defined, circumscribed glow can be readily seen slightly below the thyroid prominence (Fig. 21-5A). However, if the tip of the ETT is in the esophagus, the transmitted glow is diffuse and cannot be readily detected under ambient lighting conditions (see Fig. 21-5B). If the tip of the ETT is placed in the vallecula, the light glow is diffuse and appears slightly above the thyroid prominence. Using these landmarks and principles, the clinician can guide the tip of the ETT easily and safely into the trachea without the use of a laryngoscope.

Despite its potential clinical advantages, intubation using a lighted stylet (lightwand) did not receive widespread popularity until a commercial intubating device became available. During the past 30 years, several versions of a lighted stylet have been introduced, including the Fiberoptic Lighted-Intubation Stilette (Benson Medical Industries Inc., Markham, Ont., Canada), the Flexilum (Concept Corporation, Clearwater, FL), the Tubestat (Concept Corporation), and the Fiberoptic Lighted Stylet (Fiberoptic Medical Products, Inc., Allentown, PA) (Fig. 21-6). Over the years, these devices have proved to be effective and safe in placing the ETT both orally and nasally.[51-53] Despite favorable results and growing experience with the technique of light-guided intubation,[51-54] early commercial lighted stylets had some limitations. These included: (1) poor light intensity; (2)

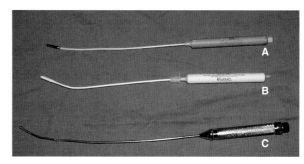

Figure 21-6 Some commercially available lighted stylets. *A,* Flexilum. *B,* Tubestat. *C,* Fiberoptic Lighted-Intubation Stilette.

short length, which limited the use of the lighted stylet device to short or cut ETTs; (3) absence of a connector to secure the ETT to the lighted-stylet device; (4) rigidity of the lighted stylet, which hampered use of the devices for other intubating techniques, including light-guided nasal intubation; and (5) single-use design in most lighted stylets, which increased the cost of intubation.

To address the shortcomings of these existing devices, the Trachlight (Laerdal Medical Corp., Wappingers Falls, NY) was introduced in 1995. The Trachlight was longer than its predecessors and incorporated an improved light source and a more flexible wand portion of the device. These features added flexibility, broadened the utility of the device for both oral and nasal intubation, made intubation easier, and permitted evaluation of the position of the tip of the ETT after intubation. To date, the Trachlight has been the most popular and best studied of the lighted stylets. Although the Trachlight is no longer manufactured, a new, similar version of this lighted stylet is being developed. We have had considerable experience with the Trachlight, and one of us (OH) was a key player in its design and development. Much of what follows reflects this experience and partiality toward the Trachlight. Nevertheless, the concept and principles of intubation using transillumination are applicable to all other lighted stylets.

B. Trachlight

The Trachlight consists of three parts: a reusable handle, a flexible wand, and a retractable metal wire stylet (Fig. 21-7). The power control circuitry and 3 AAA batteries are encased within the handle. The stylet or "wand" consists of a durable, flexible plastic shaft with a bright light bulb affixed at the distal end. Enclosed within the wand is a stiff but malleable, retractable wire stylet. This stylet may well be the most important feature of this device, because it significantly improves its ease of use.

A major feature of the Trachlight is its improved light source, which in most cases permits intubation under

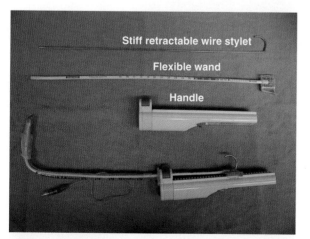

Figure 21-7 The Trachlight consists of three parts: a handle, a flexible wand, and a stiff retractable wire stylet. With the Trachlight placed inside the endotracheal tube (ETT), the ETT-TL unit is bent at a 90-degree angle just proximal to the cuff of the tube in the shape of a field-hockey stick.

ambient lighting conditions. After 30 seconds of illumination, the light bulb blinks to minimize heat production and provide a convenient reminder of elapsed time. Because the tip of the stylet is encased within the ETT, and because of the efficient heat-exchange capacity of the upper airway mucosa, it is extremely unlikely that heat from the bulb would cause any thermal injury during intubation. An animal study confirmed that there were no histopathologic changes after use of the Trachlight.[55]

The flexible wand can be adjusted to any length deemed clinically appropriate by means of a plastic connector that slides along the Trachlight handle. The same connector is used to attach or completely detach the wand from the handle. An optional retractable wire stylet within the wand adds stiffness and malleability. Once the handle, wand, and wire stylet are connected as a unit, the lubricated wand is placed inside an ETT, and the ETT is firmly secured to the Trachlight by means of a clamp on the Trachlight handle. To avoid unnecessary trauma, the wand should not protrude beyond the tip of the ETT. Final adjustments to wand length can be made by using the handle's sliding plastic connector.

For standard orotracheal intubation, the retractable wire stylet is best used to shape the ETT into the form of a field-hockey stick (see Fig. 21-7). This configuration directs the bright light of the bulb against the anterior wall of the larynx and trachea. In addition, the hockey-stick configuration enhances maneuverability during intubation and facilitates placement of the ETT through the glottic opening. However, this is an awkwardly shaped object to advance into the trachea. Therefore, once the tip of the ETT-Trachlight (ETT-TL) unit has passed through the glottic opening, the wire stylet should be retracted by approximately 10 cm. This makes the distal end of the ETT-TL unit pliable and enables advancement into the trachea safely and without difficulty.

The glow emitted from the Trachlight can be seen to migrate down the patient's neck and may be used to confirm correct placement of the ETT. When the glow reaches the sternal notch, the tip of the ETT is located about halfway between the vocal cords and the carina.[56] The clamp securing the ETT to the Trachlight is released, and the Trachlight is removed, leaving the ETT in place.

C. Lighted-Stylet Intubation: Detailed Technique

1. Preparation

The importance of preparation, a frequently overlooked or rushed step, cannot be overstated. Proper preparation will make the use of lighted stylets much easier and increase the likelihood of successful intubation.

The Trachlight wand has an internal wire stylet that is best lubricated using silicone fluid (Endoscopic Instrument Lubricant AE-1, ACMI, Southborough, MA). This ensures its easy retraction during intubation. With the internal wire stylet in place, the clinician attaches the wand to the handle. As with any standard stylet, the outside of the flexible wand should be well lubricated with a water-soluble lubricant to facilitate ready removal after tracheal placement of the ETT. Once the wand is inserted into the ETT, a clamp firmly attaches the ETT to the Trachlight handle. The length of the wand can be easily adjusted by sliding the wand along the handle, and the light bulb is placed close to, but not protruding beyond, the tip of the ETT.

With the Trachlight in place, the ETT-Trachlight (ETT-TL) unit is bent at a 90-degree angle just proximal to the cuff of the tube, similar to a field-hockey stick. The degree of bend should be individualized to the patient, but the 90-degree bend usually makes the intubation considerably easier and is our preference for most orotracheal intubations. When the tip of the ETT is in the glottic opening, the 90-degree bend projects the maximum light intensity toward the surface of the skin, producing a well-defined, circumscribed exterior glow through the soft tissues of the neck. In contrast, if the Trachlight is bent to 45 degrees, the maximum light intensity will be directed down the trachea, and the glow will not be so readily seen. For obese patients and patients with short necks, a more acute bend (>90 degrees) provides better transillumination. The exact point at which to make the bend in the Trachlight has been debated, although it is our experience that 6.5 to 8.5 cm is suitable for most patients. A study by Chen and colleagues suggested that the bent length of the Trachlight should be adjusted according to the patient's thyroid prominence-to-mandibular angle distance (TMD) after demonstrating that a shorter bent length (6.5 cm) was more suitable for patients with a shorter TMD (<5.5 cm).[57] It stands to reason that the shape of the Trachlight should be individualized to the patient's anatomy.

Finally, the tip of the ETT should be coated with a water-soluble lubricant to facilitate its passage into the trachea.

2. Positioning

In the hospital setting, the clinician usually stands at the head of the table or bed. It is also possible to use the Trachlight from the front or side of the patient, making it a useful tool in the prehospital environment. Depending on the clinician's height, it may be advisable to lower the table or to use a footstool to allow maximal visualization of the anterior neck of the patient during intubation. In contrast to the technique for laryngoscopic intubation, the patient's head and neck should be in a neutral or relatively extended position, not in the "sniffing" position. The epiglottis is in close contact with the posterior pharyngeal wall when the head is in the sniffing position, making it more difficult for the Trachlight to pass posterior to the epiglottis. In contrast, the epiglottis is lifted off the posterior pharyngeal wall when the head is extended, facilitating entrance of the ETT into the glottic opening.

3. Control of Ambient Light

Compared with its predecessors, the light emitted by the Trachlight is extremely bright, with a directed beam that enhances soft tissue transillumination of the neck. In most cases, endotracheal intubation can be performed easily under ambient lighting conditions. In a large clinical study, endotracheal intubation using the Trachlight was successfully performed under ambient light in 85% of the cases.[58] In very thin patients and in children, it is possible to mistakenly interpret an esophageal intubation as an intratracheal placement, although the glow generated from inside the esophagus is more diffuse in character. Dimming of the room lights should be done only when absolutely necessary, such as in the case of an obese patient or a patient with a thick neck. In the emergency department or prehospital setting where control of the ambient lighting is not possible, it may be helpful to shade the neck with a towel or hand.

4. Technique of Intubation

a. OROTRACHEAL INTUBATION

As with other intubation techniques, proper denitrogenation should precede airway manipulation. Full muscle relaxation is recommended, if clinically appropriate. In a study of 176 patients, Masso and colleagues showed that muscle relaxation is associated with a lower failure rate, decreased intubation time, and fewer attempts when performing lighted-stylet orotracheal intubation.[59] When the patient is under anesthesia and lying supine, the tongue falls posteriorly, pushing the epiglottis against the posterior pharyngeal wall (Fig. 21-8). In order to have a clear passage to the glottic opening during intubation, it is necessary for the clinician to grasp the jaw or mandible and lift it upward using the thumb and index finger of the nondominant hand (Fig. 21-9). This lifts the tongue and epiglottis away from the posterior pharyngeal wall to facilitate placement of the tip of the ETT posterior to the epiglottis and into the glottic opening. The nondominant hand must be kept close to the corner of the mouth to ensure an unobstructed path in the midline for the lighted stylet.

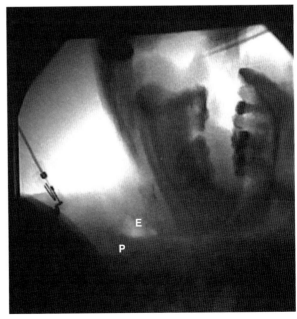

Figure 21-8 Lateral radiographic view of the upper airway of an anesthetized patient shows that the tongue falls posteriorly, pushing the epiglottis (E) against the posterior pharyngeal wall (P).

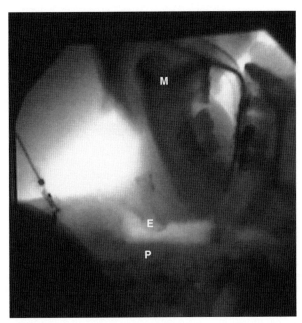

Figure 21-9 Lateral radiographic view of the upper airway of an anesthetized patient shows that a jaw lift, or mandible (M) lift, can elevate the tongue and the epiglottis (E) off the posterior pharyngeal wall (P), providing an open passage for the endotracheal tube-Trachlight (ETT-TL) unit to enter the glottic opening.

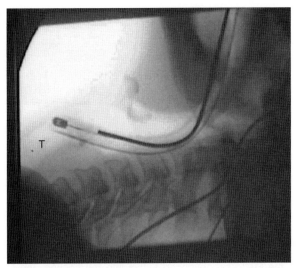

Figure 21-10 Lateral radiographic view of the upper airway of an anesthetized patient shows that when the tip of the endotracheal tube-Trachlight (ETT-TL) unit is placed at the glottic opening, the ETT cannot be advanced readily into the trachea (T) because of the preshaped hockey-stick configuration of the Trachlight.

With the Trachlight switched on, the ETT-TL unit is grasped by the dominant hand and inserted into the midline of the oropharynx. The midline position of the ETT-TL is maintained while the device is advanced gently along an imaginary arc in the sagittal plane, thereby moving the light source closer to the larynx. Commonly seen, but ill-advised, is the practice of enthusiastically placing the ETT-TL within the oropharynx while looking for a glow in the anterior neck. Such gross unsupervised movement of the ETT-TL increases the risk of pharyngeal trauma. Instead, under visual guidance, the ETT-TL should be able to be placed and angled so that the tip is very close to the larynx before transillumination of the neck tissues is sought. The ETT-TL should always be manipulated gently.

Once satisfied that the tip of the ETT-TL is close to the larynx, the clinician looks to see a glow in the anterior neck. The dominant hand can then be used to slowly rotate the Trachlight slightly to the right or left. These movements are exaggerated at the tip of the ETT-TL. By watching the transillumination in the patient's neck moving from side to side, the degree of rotation required to ensure that the tip of the Trachlight is exactly midline can be established. Once it is in the midline, a faint glow seen above the laryngeal prominence indicates that the tip of the ETT-TL is located in the vallecula. A jaw lift or a retraction of the tongue[60] helps to elevate the epiglottis and enhance passage of the ETT-TL under the epiglottis, and "rocking" the handle backward advances the tip of the lighted stylet toward the vocal cords. When the tip of the ETT-TL enters the glottic opening, a well-defined, circumscribed glow can be seen in the anterior neck slightly below the laryngeal prominence (see Fig. 21-5A). However, the ETT-TL cannot be readily advanced

into the trachea because of the preshaped hockey stick configuration of the Trachlight (Fig. 21-10).

Retraction of the stiff internal wire stylet approximately 10 cm makes the distal portion of the ETT-TL unit more pliable, allowing advancement into the trachea with reduced risk of trauma (Fig. 21-11). Advancement of the pliable ETT-TL unit into the trachea before removal of the Trachlight improves the success rate of intubation. This is analogous to the successful placement of an intravenous cannula by advancing the angiocath together with the needle a few millimeters into the vein after the needle tip has entered the vein. This ensures that the catheter is inside the vein before the needle is removed from the angiocath. The glow from the ETT-TL can be seen migrating down the neck. When the glow

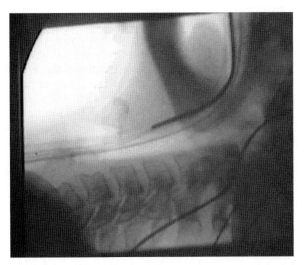

Figure 21-11 Lateral radiographic view of the upper airway of an anesthetized patient shows that with the stiff internal wire stylet (S) retracted approximately 10 cm, the distal endotracheal tube-Trachlight (ETT-TL) unit becomes more pliable, allowing easy advancement of the ETT into the trachea.

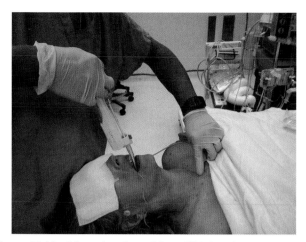

Figure 21-12 After retraction of the stiff internal wire stylet, the endotracheal tube-Trachlight (ETT-TL) unit becomes pliable, permitting the ETT to be advanced further into the trachea. The ETT is advanced until the glow is at the sternal notch.

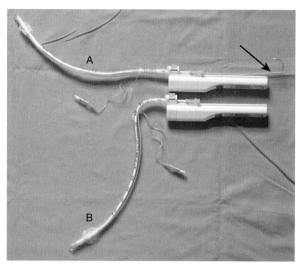

Figure 21-13 If a nasal RAE endotracheal tube (ETT) is used, the stiff internal wire stylet (arrow) of the Trachlight can be retracted halfway (approximately 15 cm) to allow unbending of the proximal curvature of the nasal RAE ETT (A) or its complete removal (B).

begins to disappear at the sternal notch (Fig. 21-12), the tip of the ETT is approximately 5 cm above the carina in the average adult.[61]

After release of the locking clamp, the Trachlight can be removed from the ETT. The ETT cuff is inflated, and correct ETT placement is confirmed by standard means, such as chest auscultation and capnography. Although structural damage to the Trachlight during intubation would be an unlikely event, it is good practice to examine the Trachlight for structural integrity after intubation lest a foreign body be inadvertently left in the airway.

Occasionally, the circumscribed glow cannot be readily seen in the anterior neck due to anatomic features such as morbid obesity or a short neck. Neck extension, as described earlier, may be helpful. Placement of a support under the shoulders may further assist neck extension.[62] Retraction of the breast or chest wall tissues caudally together with indentation of the tissues around the trachea by an assistant enhances transillumination of the soft tissues in the anterior neck. Dimming of the ambient light is required only in some occasions.

After retraction of the internal wire stylet, the tip of the tube and lighted stylet can sometimes be difficult to advance. This may occur because the tip of the ETT-TL is caught at the vestibular folds of the cords, or the tip may abut the anterior wall of the larynx or trachea. Such a hold-up can usually be overcome by rotating the ETT-TL sideways 90 degrees or more to the right or left side of the head. The tip of the ETT will then be pointing to the side or downward, disengaging the hold-up and allowing ready entrance of the ETT into the trachea. Alternatively, the clinician may grasp the anterior larynx with the nondominant hand with an upward lift to help the tip of the ETT come off the vestibular folds or tracheal ring.

b. NASOTRACHEAL INTUBATION

Light-guided nasotracheal intubation using the Trachlight is particularly useful when guided or "blind" nasal intubation is indicated, such as in emergency situations in patients with a limited mouth opening and cervical

spine instability. Although similar to Trachlight oral intubation, Trachlight nasal intubation differs in a few important ways.

Complete removal of the internal stiff wire stylet from Trachlight makes the ETT-TL unit pliable enough for atraumatic nasotracheal intubation. If a nasal Ring-Adair-Elwyn (RAE) ETT is used, the internal stiff wire stylet of the Trachlight can be retracted halfway (about 15 cm). This "unbends" the proximal curvature of the nasal RAE ETT (Fig. 21-13), making lighted-stylet nasal intubation with a RAE ETT easier.

Application of a vasoconstrictor nasal spray to the nasal mucosa before intubation may minimize bleeding. If time permits, the ETT-TL should be immersed in warm sterile water or saline to soften the ETT and further reduce the risk of mucosal damage during nasal intubation. Water-soluble lubricant is applied to the nostril to facilitate entry of the ETT-TL through the nose.

As with oral Trachlight intubation, the head is placed in a neutral or extended position, not the sniffing position. The Trachlight is switched on once the tip of the ETT-TL has been advanced into the oropharynx, positioned in the midline, and advanced gently using the light glow as a guide. A jaw-lift maneuver is necessary to lift the epiglottis from the posterior pharyngeal wall (Fig. 21-14). However, without the stiff internal wire stylet in situ, difficulty may be encountered controlling the tip of the ETT during blind nasal intubation. In particular, because of the natural curvature of the ETT, the tip commonly goes posteriorly into the esophagus. Various maneuvers may help. To bring the tip of the ETT anteriorly during intubation, it is sometimes necessary to flex the neck of the patient while advancing the ETT-TL slowly. If flexing of the neck is contraindicated, inflating the ETT cuff completely with 20 cc of air will help to elevate the ETT tip and align it with the glottis during intubation.[63] Alternatively, an ETT with a controllable tip (the Endotrol tube by Mallinckrodt Critical Care, Inc., St. Louis) can be used for nasotracheal intubations and

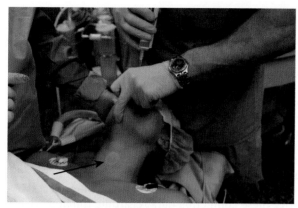

Figure 21-14 During nasotracheal intubation using the Trachlight, the jaw is grasped and lifted upward by the nondominant hand. This elevates the tongue and epiglottis away from the posterior wall of the pharynx to facilitate placement of the tip of the endotracheal tube (ETT) into the glottic opening. When the ETT-Trachlight (ETT-TL) unit enters the glottic opening, a well-defined, circumscribed glow will be seen in the anterior neck just below the thyroid prominence (arrow).

directed toward the glottis.[64] In some difficult circumstances, nasotracheal intubation can be performed effectively and safely with the internal stiff wire stylet in place.[65,66] Although there can be an increased risk of nasal trauma with the wire stylet in place, this technique may be associated with fewer head-neck manipulations and perhaps better control of the tip of the ETT.

D. Clinical Utility of Lighted Stylets

1. Routine Use

Endotracheal intubation using a lighted stylet is easy to learn. The Trachlight has a learning curve of 10 to 30 intubations.[67,68] Once mastered, the Trachlight is quick to use. A large study involving 950 elective surgical patients demonstrated Trachlight intubation to be statistically significantly faster than direct laryngoscopic intubation (15.7 ± 10.8 versus 19.6 ± 23.7 seconds, respectively),[58] although such a small time difference is unlikely to be clinically significant. In the same study, the Trachlight appeared to compare favorably with the conventional laryngoscopic technique with regard to effectiveness and failure rate. There was a 1% failure rate with the Trachlight, and 92% of intubations were successful on the first attempt, compared with a 3% failure rate and an 89% success rate on first attempt using a standard laryngoscope. There were significantly fewer traumatic events and sore throats in the Trachlight group compared with laryngoscopy patients. Tsutsui and Setoyama reported similar findings in a study with 511 patients.[69] Trachlight intubation appeared to be highly effective (99%), with successful intubation after one attempt in most cases (93%). Unsuccessful intubation, even after three attempts, occurred in 3 patients (1%).

Other lighted stylets have been less well studied. However, in 1991, a letter to the editor reported on 1200 TubeStat intubations in one institution over a 2-year period. In that series, the TubeStat was used without laryngoscopic assistance. Although most intubations were

undertaken with the patient under general anesthesia, some were performed with topical anesthesia in anticipation of a probable DA. The authors reported that the TubeStat had a high success rate after failed laryngoscopic intubation and a low failure rate when used as a first-choice device. They concluded that "in the majority of elective cases, TubeStat intubation is our method of choice."[70]

2. Difficult Airway

The Trachlight has also proved to be useful for nasal or oral intubation in patients with anticipated or unanticipated DAs.[71] During the development of the Trachlight, a study reported on its clinical utility in 265 patients with DAs. Group 1 (n = 206) had a documented history of DA or anticipated DA, whereas group 2 (n = 59) were anesthetized patients with an unanticipated failed laryngoscopic intubation. In group 1, intubation was successful in all but 2 of the patients, with a mean (±SD) time to intubation of 25.7 ± 20.1 seconds. The tracheas of these 2 patients (1 morbidly obese patient weighing 220 kg and 1 patient with severe flexion deformity of the cervical spine) were intubated successfully using a flexible fiberoptic bronchoscope (FFB). Orotracheal intubation with the Trachlight was successful in all patients in group 2, with a mean time to intubation of 19.7 ± 13.5 seconds. Apart from minor mucosal bleeding (mostly from nasal intubation), no serious complications were observed in any of the study patients.

Other investigators have also reported successful use of the Trachlight for tracheal placement in patients with a DA. These reports have included patients with a history of limited mouth opening,[72] severe burn contractures,[73] pediatric tongue-flap surgery,[74] Pierre-Robin syndrome,[75] other pediatric craniofacial abnormalities,[76] and patients with DA and cardiac conditions.[77]

The Trachlight can also be used for patients with cervical spine abnormalities. In a randomized crossover trial of 36 healthy patients, Turkstra and associates compared cervical spine motion produced by Macintosh laryngoscopy, the Glidescope video laryngoscope, and the Trachlight when manual in-line stabilization was applied.[78] Using fluoroscopic video, these investigators showed that the Glidescope and Trachlight methods of intubation produced roughly half as much cervical spine motion as Macintosh laryngoscopy. This study, and another by Huang,[79] found Trachlight intubation to be considerably faster than Glidescope intubation in healthy anesthetized patients with simulated in-line cervical spine stabilization. In Huang's randomized study of 60 patients, time to intubate was 15 ± 5 seconds in the Trachlight group and 33 ± 9 seconds in the Glidescope group (P < 0.05).[79] In a more recent prospective, randomized crossover trial of 20 patients, the Trachlight produced as little cervical spine motion as intubation using an FFB in anesthetized, paralyzed adults with a normal cervical spine.[80] A prospective, randomized trial of 148 patients with cervical spine abnormalities compared airway management with the Trachlight versus the Fastrach laryngeal mask airway (LMA), an intubating LMA (iLMA). The Trachlight was found to be considerably quicker (23 ± 9 versus 71 ± 24 seconds) and more reliable (97.3% versus 73.0%

successful intubations after a maximum of two attempts) than the iLMA in this patient population.[81]

The utility of lighted stylets for the management of predicted DA is not limited to the Trachlight. In 2009, Rhee and coworkers randomly assigned 60 patients with high Mallampati scores (class III or IV) to receive endotracheal intubation using either the standard laryngoscope or the Surch-Lite lighted stylet (Aaron Medical Industries, St. Petersburg, FL). The rate of successful endotracheal intubation was significantly higher in the Surch-Lite group after one attempt (97%, versus 80% in the direct laryngoscopy group), and Surch-Lite intubation was also significantly quicker (12 ± 6 versus 17 ± 12 seconds, respectively).[82]

3. Hemodynamic Effects

Although many studies have reported on the comparative hemodynamic changes associated with Trachlight intubation and laryngoscopic intubation, the results have been inconsistent. Several studies involving only a small number of patients (26 to 60) showed that there were no statistical differences in the hemodynamic changes occurring after endotracheal intubation using either the lighted stylet or the laryngoscope.[83-87] However, most of these studies did not perform a power analysis to determine the appropriate sample size for the study, thereby running the risk of having a type II error. Although the study by Siddiqui and colleagues comparing conventional laryngoscopy to the Trachlight and the Glidescope was properly powered to detect changes in blood pressure and heart rate, there was no significant difference in these parameters between the groups.[86] One study did not include a standardized general anesthetic technique.[83]

These findings were not consistent with the results of other studies that showed lower hemodynamic responses after endotracheal intubation using a lighted stylet compared to a laryngoscope.[69,88-90] In one large study ($n = 511$), Tsutsui and Setoyama reported that Trachlight intubation was associated with less elevation of the blood pressure during intubation, compared with laryngoscopic intubation.[69] During the development of the Trachlight, a study involving 450 elective surgical patients showed that the increases in mean arterial pressure (MAP) and heart rate occurring after intubation were significantly less with the Trachlight than with laryngoscopy.[88] However, the anesthetic technique used in this study was not standardized. In a study by Rhee and associates of 60 patients with high Mallampati scores (class III and IV), those patients who received direct laryngoscopy had significantly higher increases in MAP and heart rate after intubation than did those in the Surch-Lite lighted-stylet group.[82]

In a small study ($n = 40$), Nishikawa and coworkers showed that the lighted-stylet technique significantly attenuated hemodynamic changes after intubation in normotensive patients, compared with the laryngoscopic technique.[89] However, they did not find any significant difference in hemodynamic changes between the two techniques in patients with hypertension. These results were in direct contrast to the findings of another comparative study of the hemodynamic changes using three intubating techniques: a Macintosh laryngoscope, a Trachlight, and an iLMA in 75 patients.[90] The

investigators in that study reported that both the iLMA and the Trachlight attenuated the hemodynamic stress response to endotracheal intubation, compared with the Macintosh laryngoscope, in hypertensive but not in normotensive patients.

In a randomized, controlled trial of 80 patients with coronary artery disease, Montes and colleagues compared hemodynamic responses to intubation with the Trachlight versus direct-vision laryngoscopy.[91] Although the results were not significantly different, the Trachlight group tended to have lower blood pressure and heart rate during the intubation period.[91] Clearly, future studies involving large numbers of patients are necessary to clarify these conflicting data regarding the hemodynamic stimulation associated with endotracheal intubation using a lighted stylet.

4. Pediatric Use

The pediatric Trachlight has been used both orally and nasally,[92] including in patients with a DA.[74,93] In 2008, Xue and coworkers published a case series of four children with craniofacial abnormalities who were unable to be intubated via direct laryngoscopy (all children had Cormack-Lehane grade 4 views) or with a FFB.[76] The tracheas of these four children were intubated successfully within 30 seconds using the Trachlight. The small body of published pediatric Trachlight experience suggests that some adjustments to technique may be necessary. Suggestions include the following[76]:

1. The Trachlight should be bent to 60 to 80 degrees instead of the usual 90 degrees to better suit pediatric anatomy.
2. The distance before the bend in the Trachlight should reflect the short length of the pediatric airway.
3. Because of the small distances involved, transillumination must be expected soon after insertion of the Trachlight.
4. The Trachlight glow is so readily seen through the relatively small amount of tissue in a child that transilllumination from the esophagus can more easily be mistaken for that from the trachea, although experience will enable the clinician to tell the difference.

5. Synergy with Direct Laryngoscopy

Endotracheal intubation can fail with the Trachlight as well as with the laryngoscope. However, in an early study of 950 patients, all Trachlight failures were resolved with direct laryngoscopy.[58] Similarly, all failures of direct laryngoscopy were resolved with Trachlight. These results suggest that a success rate approaching 100% can be achieved in endotracheal intubation by combining the two methods.

The techniques can even be used simultaneously, which may be particularly useful for unanticipated DL (e.g., patients with a Cormack-Lehane grade 3 laryngoscopic view).[18] While maintaining the grade 3 view with a standard laryngoscope in situ, the clinician can use an ETT-TL with a 90-degree bend. Under direct laryngoscopy, the tip of the ETT-TL can be "hooked" under the epiglottis. If the tip of the ETT is placed at the glottic opening, a well-defined, circumscribed glow can be seen in the anterior neck slightly below the laryngeal prominence. If a glow is not seen, the ETT-TL should be repositioned until a glow can be seen in the anterior neck. Since the development of the Trachlight, we have recorded more than a dozen failed intubations using either the Trachlight or a laryngoscope, but in each of these failures, endotracheal intubation was successful using the laryngoscope together with the Trachlight. Others have also reported the successful use of this combined technique. In one study, the investigators successfully performed endotracheal intubation in all 350 study surgical patients with a simulated DA using the laryngoscope together with the Trachlight.[94]

6. Use with Other Airway Devices

In addition to its use with the laryngoscope, the Trachlight has been combined successfully with other intubating techniques. These include intubation through the LMA-Classic,[95,96] through the iLMA,[97] with the Bullard laryngoscope,[98,99] and with a retrograde intubating technique.[100]

7. Percutaneous Tracheotomy

The Trachlight can be used to identify the intratracheal position of the tip of the ETT during percutaneous tracheostomy.[101] This simple technique can help to avoid puncturing the ETT or the cuff, thus ensuring adequate ventilation and oxygenation during the percutaneous tracheotomy. This technique is also inexpensive and minimizes the risk of damaging equipment such as the FFB. If it is used properly, it is possible that this simple, light-guided technique can also be used to accurately determine when the tip of the ETT is above the surgical tracheotomy site as the tube is pulled back during surgical tracheotomy.

E. Limitations

Although the Trachlight and other lighted stylets have been demonstrated to be effective and safe for oral and nasal intubation, the technique requires transillumination of the soft tissues of the anterior neck without visualization of the laryngeal structure. Therefore, it should not be used in patients with known abnormalities of the upper airway, such as tumors, polyps, infection (e.g., epiglottitis, retropharyngeal abscess), or trauma of the upper airway, or if there is a foreign body in the upper airway. In these cases, other alternatives using direct laryngoscopy or fiberoptic intubation (FOI) should be considered. The lighted stylets should also be used with caution in patients in whom transillumination of the anterior neck may not be adequate, such as patients who are grossly obese or who have limited neck extension. Intuitively, this light-guided technique should not be attempted with an awake, but potentially uncooperative patient unless a bite block is used to prevent damage to the device or injury to the clinician.

F. Complications

Since its introduction in 1995, the Trachlight has been used extensively in many countries. Although there is a potential risk of damage to the glottic opening during endotracheal intubation using a "nonvisualizing"

intubating technique, there have been very few case reports of complications.

In 2001, Aoyama and colleagues reported that the epiglottis of a patient was partially pushed into the laryngeal inlet, along with the ETT, after Trachlight intubation.[102] To investigate the potential risk of laryngeal damage during Trachlight intubation. Hung and colleagues placed an FFB in the nasopharynx. They reported that during orotracheal placement of the ETT using the Trachlight, structures around the glottic opening, including the epiglottis and the arytenoids, could be transiently displaced. In some instances, the epiglottis was pushed into the glottic opening. Usually, the epiglottis spontaneously returned to the correct position. The authors suggested that there are potential risks of laryngeal damage in addition to downfolding of the epiglottis during ETT placement using the Trachlight, but such occurrences have not been observed to cause permanent damage, and the reduction in the incidence of sore throat in patients undergoing Trachlight intubation compared to laryngoscopic intubation suggests that such occurrences are of little clinical significance.[58]

Subluxation of the cricoarytenoid cartilage occurs rarely but was reported in a study using an older version of a lighted stylet (Tubestat).[103] However, with correct use of the retractable wire stylet, the risk of damaging the arytenoid cartilage during Trachlight intubation is low.

In 2008, Zhang and associates reported a case in which the part of the silicon sheath that protects the Trachlight wand and bulb broke from the Trachlight unit during intubation and was left behind within the lumen of the ETT.[104] This is the only such published case involving the Trachlight, although there have been four similar case reports of instrument disarticulation with other lightwand devices.[105-107] In Zhang's case, "the wand was withdrawn from the ETT with some difficulty."[104] Softening the ETT before intubation by placing it in warm saline makes it more malleable, and lubricating the wand with a water-based lubricant makes disengaging the Trachlight from the ETT unit much easier. These steps, together with the mindset that undue force should always be avoided, will likely reduce any structural damage to the Trachlight. Nevertheless, it is good practice to always examine the Trachlight after intubation for structural integrity.

Noguchi and colleagues reported that application of 8% xylocaine in a pump spray as a lubricant for the Trachlight resulted in disappearance of the print markings of the wand.[108] However, lidocaine jelly and glycerin showed no effect on the print marks. The investigators suggested that lidocaine pump spray should not be used as a lubricant on the Trachlight wand.

Although the lighted stylet has been shown to be an effective and safe intubating device, its potential risks and complications, as well as its indications, must be kept in mind.

IV. CONCLUSIONS

Occasional DL has led to the development of many alternative techniques for placing an ETT. Use of an intubating guide such as the reusable and malleable EI or "gum elastic bougie" has been shown to be a safe, effective, and quick method of guiding the ETT into the trachea when the laryngeal aperture cannot be well seen under direct vision using a laryngoscope. Use of the EI is well supported by many reports and 40 years of clinical use. Some newer, single-use ETT introducers, such as the Frova, have also performed well in studies, although they tend to be stiffer and less malleable than the EI. The longer and larger-diameter ETT exchangers are introducers specifically designed to be securely placed in the trachea so that ETTs can be "railroaded" over the top of the exchanger. Because they are hollow, they can also be used as temporary conduits for oxygen delivery and ventilation. ETT exchangers are useful when a secure airway should be changed or temporarily removed but direct-vision laryngoscopy is likely to be difficult. Stylets, the plastic-coated metal rods that enable stiffening and reshaping of an ETT before intubation, have been used for many years but are not well studied. Limited evidence suggests that these stylets are not as effective as introducers when used for the management of DAs.

Transillumination of the soft tissues of the neck using a lighted stylet has been shown to be an effective intubation technique for decades. Although there are many versions of lighted stylets, the Trachlight is the best studied and has incorporated many design modifications to facilitate both oral and nasal intubation in awake and anesthetized patients. It has been demonstrated to be an effective and safe intubating device in a large variety of surgical patients, including those with documented DAs. However, lighted stylets should not be used in patients with anatomic abnormalities or distortions of the upper airway. As with any intubation technique, regular use and practice with these intubating devices will improve performance and may also reduce the likelihood of complications.

V. CLINICAL PEARLS

- The Eschmann Introducer (EI) is best used when the epiglottis can be seen under direct laryngoscopy (Cormack-Lehane grade 3 view); the coudé tip can be hooked under the epiglottis and the EI advanced blindly through the glottis. The success of this maneuver is improved if the EI has been preshaped into a curve.

- If "clicks" are felt on blind advancement of the EI into the trachea, the potentially more traumatic "hold-up sign," though reliable, need not be sought.

- To facilitate the advancement of the ETT over the EI after tracheal placement, the tongue and epiglottis should be elevated by a jaw lift, or preferably by a laryngoscope.

- During blind nasotracheal intubation, inflating the ETT cuff completely with 20 cc of air can help to elevate the ETT tip and align it with the glottic opening, facilitating tracheal placement.

- In order to have a clear passage to the glottic opening during lightwand intubation, it is necessary for the clinician to perform a jaw lift, which will elevate the tongue and epiglottis away from the posterior pharyngeal wall to facilitate placement of the tip of the ETT posterior to the epiglottis and into the glottic opening.

- Although the lightwand has been demonstrated to be effective and safe for endotracheal intubation, the technique requires transillumination of the soft tissues of the anterior neck without visualization of the laryngeal structure. Therefore, a lightwand should not be used in patients with known abnormalities of the upper airway, such as tumors, polyps, infection, or trauma of the upper airway.

SELECTED REFERENCES

All references can be found online at expertconsult.com.

13. Karkouti K, Rose D, Wigglesworth D, Cohen M: Predicting difficult intubation: A multivariable analysis. *Can J Anesth* 47:730–739, 2000.
18. Cormack RS, Lehane J: Difficult tracheal intubation in obstetrics. *Anaesthesia* 39:1105–1111, 1984.
27. Levitan R, Ochroch EA: Airway management and direct laryngoscopy: A review and update. *Crit Care Clin* 16:v, 373–388, 2000.
32. Levitan RM, Pisaturo JT, Kinkle WC, et al: Stylet bend angles and tracheal tube passage using a straight-to-cuff shape. *Acad Emerg Med* 13:1255–1258, 2006.
57. Chen TH, Tsai SK, Lin CJ, et al: Does the suggested lightwand bent length fit every patient? The relation between bent length and patient's thyroid prominence–to–mandibular angle distance. *Anesthesiology* 98:1070–1076, 2003.
71. Hung OR, Pytka S, Morris I, et al: Lightwand intubation: II. Clinical trail of a new lightwand to intubate patients with difficult airways. *Can J Anaesth* 42:826–830, 1995.
78. Turkstra TP, Craen RA, Pelz DM, Gelb AW: Cervical spine motion: A fluoroscopic comparison during intubation with lighted stylet, GlideScope, and Macintosh laryngoscope. *Anesth Analg* 101:910–915, table of contents, 2005.
86. Siddiqui N, Katznelson R, Friedman Z: Heart rate/blood pressure response and airway morbidity following tracheal intubation with direct laryngoscopy, GlideScope and Trachlight: A randomized control trial. *Eur J Anaesthesiol* 26:740–745, 2009.
100. Hung OR, al-Qatari M: Light-guided retrograde intubation. *Can J Anaesth* 44:877–882, 1997.

Chapter 22

Laryngeal Mask Airway

CHANDY VERGHESE | GABRIEL MENA | DAVID Z. FERSON | ARCHIE I.J. BRAIN

I. INTRODUCTION

The laryngeal mask airway (LMA, LMA Company, Henley, England) is a supraglottic airway device developed by Archie Brain, a physician and honorary consultant anesthetist of the Royal Berkshire Hospital, Reading, England. It was introduced into clinical practice in 1988. In the first paper on the LMA,[1] Brain described the device as "an alternative to either the endotracheal tube (ETT) or the face-mask with either spontaneous or positive-pressure ventilation (PPV)." Twenty years and more than 200 million safe uses later, the LMA has significantly improved the comfort and safety of airway management worldwide. Many authorities in anesthesia consider the LMA to be the most important development in airway management in the past 50 years.

While experimenting with different shapes and materials for the LMA, Brain recognized the importance of studying, understanding, and incorporating into its design the anatomic and physiologic principles that govern the oropharyngolaryngeal complex. This effort resulted in an effective airway device that is minimally intrusive. Realizing that one LMA model could not fulfill all clinical needs, Brain introduced three additional models of the LMA from 1993 to 2003: the flexible LMA (FLMA), the Fastrach intubating laryngeal mask airway (ILMA), and the ProSeal LMA (PLMA). These models represent only a fraction of the potentially useful clinical designs that have originated from Brain's research.

The LMA is a minimally invasive device designed for airway management in the unconscious patient. An inflatable mask is fitted with a tube that exits the mouth to

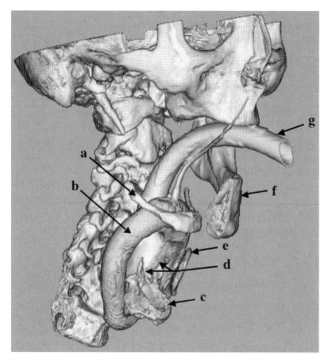

Figure 22-1 Three-dimensional radiologic reconstruction of the human airway with the laryngeal mask airway (LMA) in situ: hyoid bone (a); LMA's cuff (b); cricoid ring (c); arytenoid cartilages (d); thyroid cartilage (e), which is digitally partially removed to demonstrate the position of the LMA; mandible (f), which is digitally partially removed to demonstrate the position of the LMA; and the LMA's shaft (g). The LMA's cuff forms a seal with the periglottic tissues and provides a continuous connection between the natural airway and the device.

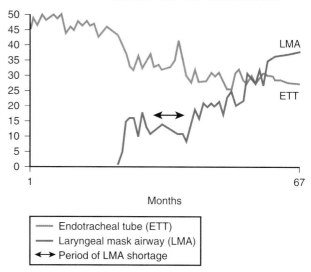

Figure 22-2 Harold Wood Hospital (England) data show the percentage of cases managed with an endotracheal tube (ETT) or laryngeal mask airway (LMA) from June 1986 through November 1991. Use of the ETT has significantly declined in favor of the LMA in the United Kingdom.

permit ventilation of the lungs. The mask fits against the periglottic tissues, occupying the hypopharyngeal space and forming a seal above the glottis instead of within the trachea (Fig. 22-1). Originally produced as a single, general-purpose design in a range of sizes, it is currently made in various forms to satisfy different requirements.

The LMA is a supraglottic airway management device. A substantial body of literature, while supporting the wisdom of exercising caution when learning to use the supraglottic approach, provides ample evidence of a wide range of uses that go beyond those originally postulated.[2] For example, the LMA is becoming increasingly popular outside the operating room, as evidenced by its endorsement by the European Resuscitation Council and the American Heart Association.[3] Its more exotic uses include the adoption of the Fastrach ILMA, which is the intubating form of the LMA, by the National Aeronautics and Space Administration (NASA) as part of its emergency medical kit for space travel. A literature search indicates that the later varieties of the LMA, including the FLMA, ILMA,[4] and PLMA,[5] may be more appropriate tools for specific uses than the original LMA.

More than 2000 scientific articles have described the impact of the LMA on modern anesthesia, and a full review is beyond the scope of a single chapter. Our aim instead is to provide an overview of the LMA's uses worldwide. After a historical review and comments regarding the correct LMA insertion technique, we explore the principal uses of each LMA model, discuss

possible problems, and offer suggestions for getting the best results from each device. We describe the evolution of the LMA's use in patients with difficult-to-manage airways and provide the current recommendations for LMA use from the American Society of Anesthesiologists (ASA) difficult airway algorithm.[6]

II. HISTORY AND DEVELOPMENT

In 1988, the definitive device, now referred to as the LMA Classic, was released commercially in the United Kingdom. Although the LMA was rapidly adopted there, it was not until 1991 that the U.S. Food and Drug Administration permitted release of the device in the United States and then only with the stricture that "the LMA is not a replacement for the endotracheal tube." Because the LMA was at that time a very unconventional way of managing the airway, this caution was understandable. Nevertheless, it resulted in a somewhat slower acceptance of the concept of "masking the larynx" in the United States than in the United Kingdom, where the LMA was purchased by every health authority within 2 years of its launch, resulting almost immediately in a reduction in ETT use (Fig. 22-2).

A. From Idea to First Prototype

Brain is often asked how the idea of the LMA first arose. Like many before him, he thought that a supraglottic approach would be less traumatic than intubation and therefore more desirable, provided the method could be easier to control and more reliable than the face mask. Other inventors had mainly explored the oral and pharyngeal spaces above the larynx,[7-12] but the LMA was the

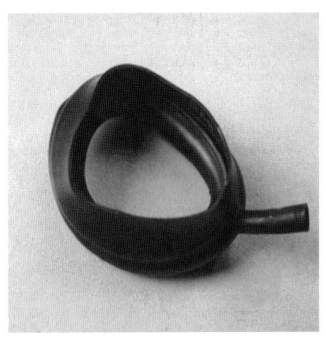

Figure 22-3 The Goldman dental nose piece was used to develop the early cuffs for the laryngeal mask airway prototypes. The central portion of the mask was cut out to allow attachment of the tube.

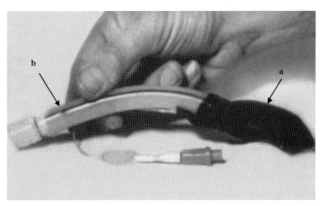

Figure 22-4 The early laryngeal mask airway (LMA) prototype was made of a Goldman dental nose piece modified to form a cuff (a) and a diagonally cut endotracheal tube (b). The two pieces were glued together to form the first LMA to be tested clinically.

first device to encircle the periglottic tissues in the hypopharynx with a mask. The idea was conceived in early 1981, and later that year, Brain began providing dental anesthesia at the outpatient clinic of the Royal London Hospital. At that time, a device known as the Goldman dental nose piece was being used for airway maintenance during dental extractions in anesthetized patients. It was a reusable, vulcanized rubber mask that could be detached from its rigid base for cleaning (Fig. 22-3). The mask was designed to fit over the nose, leaving the mouth free for surgical access. Noticing a certain similarity between the contours around the nose and those around the glottis, Brain wondered if the Goldman mask could be modified to fit over the larynx. Placing a device over the larynx would short-circuit the upper airway passages, perhaps eliminating some of the problems associated with maintaining their patency under anesthesia.

Because the Goldman mask was scheduled to be discontinued in favor of a disposable version, Brain was able to obtain samples for experimentation. Using an acrylic adhesive, he glued a diagonally cut, 10-mm Portex ETT to the rubber mask's attachment flange, which he had to draw across the mask aperture into the midline to form a base (Fig. 22-4). Figure 22-5 is a 1981 photograph of the inventor as he is about to insert one of the resulting prototypes into his anesthetized pharynx to test the validity of his hypothesis. In his diary, he recorded an absence of any complications, despite having repeated the experiment four times. This observation, combined with a broadly worded institutional review board approval, provided the justification for subsequent extensive clinical investigations, which occupied him for the next 7 years. During this time, he built many prototypes, which he used in approximately 7000 patients.[13] He also kept extensive notes in private diaries to record his

progress but published only a small number of cases, because he believed there was little point in presenting data concerning an invention that was not ready for production.

B. Early Publications

The first article about the LMA, published in the *British Journal of Anaesthesia* in 1983, presented data from only 23 patients and received little attention.[1] A second description 2 years later in *Anaesthesia* was subtitled "Development and Trials of a New Type of Airway" and detailed the LMA's use in 118 patients, although it also reported that Brain and colleagues had gained experience

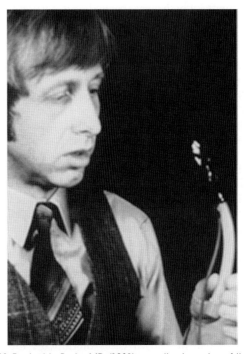

Figure 22-5 Archie Brain, MD (1981), was the inventor of the laryngeal mask airway (LMA). He is shown about to insert one of the LMA prototypes into his anesthetized pharynx to test his hypothesis that a supraglottic device was effective, safe, and much less invasive than the endotracheal tube.

in more than 500 cases.[14] On the basis of this experience and a case report published the previous year in *Archives of Emergency Medicine*,[15] Brain and colleagues felt justified in concluding that "the laryngeal mask may have a valuable role to play in all types of inhalational anesthesia, while its proven value in some cases of difficult intubation indicates that it may contribute to the safety of general anesthesia."[14]

In the same issue of *Anaesthesia*, Brain presented further evidence of the potential usefulness of the device in cases of difficult intubation, but there was still no response to these claims from the profession, perhaps because no product was available for independent assessment.[16] However, he had given one of his prototypes to a visiting American anesthesiologist, Ronald Katz, a physician and chairman of the anesthesiology department at the University of California–Los Angeles. Katz provided the first independent description of the LMA based on his experience with this prototype, writing in *Wellcome Trends in Anesthesiology* in October 1985 and again in February 1986.[17,18] The second article provided the first published image—reproduced from one of the inventor's transparencies—of the glottis seen fiberoptically through the LMA prototype and mentioned the potential of the device to overcome intubation problems. American awareness of the LMA preceded its availability in the United States by 6 years.

C. From Handmade Models to Clinical Use

There were three reasons why the LMA took so long to become clinically available: the initial lack of commercial interest, which meant there were no models available for others to use; the solitary nature of the LMA's development, which was carried out virtually single-handedly by a clinician who continued to work with largely homemade equipment until the first commercial prototypes were made in early 1988; and the complexity of the airway anatomy, which made it hard to design a device that was safe and effective. One advantage of the long development process was that the considerable clinical history that the inventor accumulated between 1981 and 1988 guided the development of the LMA, and the first factory-made models required little modification. They were produced in Gary, Indiana; tested by Brain; and then demonstrated to colleagues at the Royal East Sussex Hospital, Hastings, United Kingdom, in April 1988. Colin Alexander, the chairman of the anesthesiology department at the Royal East Sussex Hospital, immediately authorized the LMA's use in his department and published his experience in a letter ("Use your Brain") in *Anaesthesia* that year.[19] He concluded that the device "should be considered whenever the indication for tracheal intubation does not include protection of the airway from gastric contents." Meanwhile, a few colleagues who had been given prototypes by Brain (one person built his own) continued to explore the LMA's use in known cases of difficult intubation, with encouraging results.[13]

Arguably, the most influential clinical study using Brain's hand-built prototypes was not published until 1989, after the commercial form of the device had become available. Brodrick and colleagues studied 100 cases in which the patients breathed spontaneously.[20] Eighteen anesthesiologists took part in the study and recorded a "clear and unobstructed airway in 98% of cases," but obstruction on initial placement of the LMA occurred in 10 cases and "appeared to be as a result of downfolding of the epiglottis." A stainless steel introducer tool with a handle similar to that of the Fastrach ILMA and a blade fitting into a slot in the distal anterior end of the LMA's mask had been designed to overcome this problem. An aperture in the blade into which the epiglottis fit caused the epiglottis to be drawn upward as the tool was removed from the patient's pharynx. This insertion tool was used successfully in these cases, but fears that it could cause trauma led to it being abandoned in the commercial form of the LMA. Brodrick is often quoted in support of limiting the use of the LMA to spontaneously breathing patients. However, because the LMAs used by Nunn's group were prototypes, only a size 3 device was available for use in 72 men and 28 women (weight not recorded). Given the possibility that the LMA's size was less than optimal, it is not surprising that eight patients could not be ventilated using positive pressure without unacceptable leaks and that the mean leak pressure was 17 cm H_2O, similar to that recorded by Brain 6 years earlier.[13]

In addition to the information accumulated in his clinical work, study of the anatomy and physiology of the larynx and pharynx guided Brain throughout development of the LMA. As the work progressed, he struggled to achieve a balance in simplicity, efficacy, and safety. In designing a device that fit into the lower pharynx, measures favoring efficacy tended to counteract those favoring simplicity. Improving the seal, for example, required more complex construction to avoid potential trauma related to high mucosal pressures. Likewise, an effort to make the device easier to insert led to the development of an insertion tool, which was determined by Brain to be potentially unsafe and therefore abandoned, despite the efficacy it demonstrated.[13] Ultimately, the solutions chosen were compromises. For example, Brain realized that seals with a leak pressure much higher than 20 cm H_2O were rarely necessary in practice and that an inadequate seal often could be overcome by using a more appropriately sized device, using a better fixation technique, or giving a more appropriate anesthetic. To make insertion of the LMA maximally reliable and minimally traumatic, a technique gradually evolved that was based on the swallowing mechanism. Unfortunately, he underestimated the difficulty of teaching others to master such a subtle technique, which is virtually impossible to learn without direct, hands-on demonstration and guidance.[21] As a result, many articles in the LMA literature suggest variant insertion methods, most of which had already been tried and rejected by Brain for being unreliable or traumatic.

Despite these difficulties, the history of the LMA since its first commercial launch is essentially a story of steady expansion in use around the world. Availability, cost, and user education have governed the speed at which the various forms of the LMA have been accepted. Figure 22-2 demonstrates data collected by the anesthesiology department of Harold Wood Hospital, a typical general hospital near London, on the influence of the LMA Classic in the first 3 years of its availability and on the use of the ETT and the face mask. The dip in the curve representing LMA use indicates a period when it was commercially unavailable. These data show that use of the ETT almost immediately declined in favor of the new method of airway management, and they illustrate the rapid growth of LMA use in the United Kingdom. They also cast some doubt on the widely held view that the popularity of the LMA in the United Kingdom has been due to the more frequent use of the face mask there than in the United States.

As new models of the LMA have become available, countries with different anesthesia traditions have responded to them with various degrees of enthusiasm. In all cases, however, use of the LMA has steadily increased (personal communication, LMA International SA, March 2004).

III. LARYNGEAL MASK AIRWAY INSERTION TECHNIQUE

The LMA occupies a potential space that is shared by the respiratory and alimentary tracts, which are subject to the control and coordination of several complex reflexes. Although anesthesiologists do not need a detailed knowledge of the specific reflexes to use the LMA, they do need to understand the basic concept behind the recommended insertion technique, which ensures the greatest success and results in the fewest complications. Physiologically, the alimentary tract is capable of accepting (i.e., swallowing) or rejecting (i.e., vomiting) liquids or solids in the form of food. In contrast, the respiratory tract mobilizes defensive responses (e.g., coughing, laryngospasm, bronchospasm) only when invaded by liquids or solids (e.g., an ETT). When inserted correctly, the LMA does not stimulate the respiratory tract defenses because the device forms an end-to-end seal against the periglottic tissues.

Investigations using magnetic resonance imaging (MRI) to assess the effect of the LMA on the anatomy of the airway may help to explain the reliability of the device. A study by Shorten and coworkers of 46 adults requiring sagittal MRI views of the head and neck compared the anatomic differences in awake, sedated, and anesthetized patients.[22] With an LMA in place, the epiglottic angle was more than twice as great with respect to the posterior pharyngeal wall in the anesthetized group as it was in the sedated or awake group. This had no apparent effect on ventilatory function in most patients, probably due to the depth of the LMA bowl, which the inventor found to be a critical dimension when experimenting with different design ideas during the 1980s. The recommended standard insertion technique evolved slowly as Brain gained experience, and it was not until he had been inserting LMAs for almost 10 years that he realized that his technique was becoming more and more similar to the physiologic act of swallowing food. When he realized this, it was a simple matter to study this mechanism more closely and make allowances for the fact that in the anesthetized patient, this reflex is partially or completely abolished. The following key points emerged:

1. *Correct mask deflation is important.* The purpose of chewing food is to form a soft, atraumatic paste that can easily be passed through the pharynx and esophagus. At the onset of swallowing, this paste (i.e., food bolus) is pressed by the tongue into the hard palate. The pressure generated is distributed widely over the palatal surface, so there is no localized high-pressure point, which would give the sensation of a sharp object and lead to rejection instead of swallowing. Brain realized that to imitate the sensation of a soft food bolus, he needed to deflate the mask so that it presented an elastic, hollow shape. When this shape was pressed into the dome of the palate, the hollow form would need to be inverted. The pressure required by inserting the finger to achieve this would cause the outer rim of the mask to act like a gentle spring, producing the desired effect of spreading pressure smoothly over the entire posterior surface of the mask. This spring effect cannot be achieved without deflating the mask to a vacuum pressure of about −40 cm H_2O. Only in this way was it possible to prevent the pointed distal end of the mask bowl from transmitting an irritating localized pressure point as it was pressed into the oropharyngeal curve. Partial mask inflation could not achieve this aim, however, because the soft distal end of the mask rolled backward, allowing the pointed tip of the mask bowl to scratch the palatal surface. Deflating the mask such that it followed the curvature of the palate had the same disadvantage, because it made the pointed end even more prominent. Inserting a fully inflated mask introduced excessive bulk, which created the possibility of tearing the cuff against the teeth and was physiologically equivalent to swallowing too large a bolus of food, which could lead to the rejection reflex.

2. *The deflated mask must be lubricated if the oral cavity is not already wet.* There is a parallel with swallowing because lubrication is a key part of deglutition. Because the mask is slid against the palate, it makes sense to apply a bolus of lubricant to the distal hollowed posterior surface of the mask immediately before insertion. Water-soluble jelly is a good substitute for oral secretions. It is not necessary or desirable to spread the lubricant over the whole surface of the mask before insertion.

3. *Flatten the mask against the hard palate.* Initially during swallowing, the tongue flattens the softened food bolus against the hard palate; during the first step in LMA insertion, the mask, correctly prepared to impart a sensation similar to that of a soft food bolus, is flattened by pressing it against the hard palate. Placing the index finger on the airway tube at its junction with the mask under the deflated proximal rim of the cuff is the best way to impart the necessary force.

4. *Cranioposterior movement of the index finger.* In swallowing, the bolus of food is advanced into the pharynx, esophagus, and stomach through precise coordination of several muscle groups, beginning with the tongue. During LMA insertion, the clinician must use her or

his index finger to advance the mask in the craniopos-terior direction, imitating the action of the tongue. This allows a completely deflated tip to slide smoothly along the hard palate, soft palate, and posterior pharyngeal wall while minimizing the contact of the mask with anterior structures such as the base of the tongue, epiglottis, and laryngeal inlet. The finger must continue to push in a cranioposterior direction even though the anatomy forces the mask and the finger to move caudally. The finger must never consciously be directed caudally and should be inserted to its fullest extent until resistance is felt as the mask tip enters the upper esophageal sphincter (UES). It is anatomically impossible to perform this action correctly without extending the proximal metacarpophalangeal joint of the index finger and flexing the wrist.

5. *Widening the oropharyngeal angle is the first role of the nondominant hand.* Cadaveric work demonstrates that if the head of the supine subject is pushed by the supinated hand in a caudal direction, head extension, neck flexion, and mouth opening are simultaneously achieved. This maneuver widens the oropharyngeal angle to greater than 90 degrees in the normal subject and draws the larynx away from the posterior pharyngeal wall. Both effects facilitate LMA insertion. The nondominant hand should therefore maintain firm caudal pressure on the occiput from the start of insertion until the mask has passed behind the tongue.

6. *Removal of the index finger is the second role of the nondominant hand.* To prevent the mask sliding out of position after it is fully inserted, the nondominant hand should move from behind the head to grasp the proximal end of the LMA before the index finger is removed. As the index finger is removed, the mask is held steady, or if it has not been fully inserted, it can be pressed further into position by the nondominant hand.

7. *The mask is inflated.* As the mask is inflated, its increased bulk and the relatively large radius of the airway tube cause it to slide cranially. It can be shown anatomically that this results in loss of contact between the mask tip and the UES. However, the LMA should not be held in place during inflation because this can result in the distal end of the mask stretching the UES. All LMAs should be inflated to a pressure of less than 60 cm H_2O; pressures above this have been found to cause discomfort in awake volunteers.

8. *Device fixation restores stability of the seal against the UES.* The distal end of the tube is again pressed into the curve of the hard palate to reestablish firm contact between the proximal end of the device and the UES. While this pressure is maintained, adhesive tape is applied to the maxilla on one side of the patient's face and passed over and under the tube in a single loop before fixing to the opposite maxilla. This form of fixation ensures stability of the device and is likely to afford maximum protection in the event of unexpected regurgitation, and it reduces the incidence of gastric insufflation during PPV.*

---

*One study involving 108 patients showed that a malpositioned LMA was 26 times more likely to be associated with gastric insufflation.[171]

The basic insertion technique is identical for all LMA models. Unfortunately, misunderstanding of and a lack of commitment to mastering this technique are widespread, as reflected in the multiplicity of insertion methods advocated in the literature and the common belief that a failure rate of 10% is acceptable. When variant insertion techniques are used, the failure rate is about fivefold higher than it is with the standard insertion technique. The risk of complications, such as laryngeal or pharyngeal trauma and pulmonary aspiration, probably increases even more than the failure rate when the standard insertion technique is not used. The use of variant insertion techniques also may hinder or prevent the user from acquiring the skills necessary for advanced clinical applications of the LMA. As shown in several reports, use of the standard insertion technique results in a reliable airway, a minimal stress response, and an extremely low risk of complications, probably because the LMA's position in relation to the respiratory and alimentary tracts is optimal when the standard insertion technique is used. The manuals for the LMA Classic, the FLMA, the Fastrach ILMA, and the PLMA offer step-by-step instructions on the recommended insertion technique.[23]

IV. CLASSIC LARYNGEAL MASK AIRWAY

A. Basic Uses

1. Indications for Use

Indications for LMA use have evolved since its invention. Although it has long been accepted that success rates for establishing an airway with the LMA tend to be high, even in relatively unskilled hands, it is equally clear that there is more to the art of using the LMA than getting it into place. Indications have steadily expanded as the device's popularity has spread. Just as complications tend to diminish with increasing user experience, so the more confident and more adept user seems to find applications for the LMA that might previously have seemed inappropriate. Using the LMA for airway maintenance during atrial septal defect repair in children, for example, would no doubt strike many American anesthesiologists as highly unconventional, just as it would have alarmed the inventor had it been suggested he try this in 1988.[24]

The problem of defining indications for the LMA is perhaps best resolved by recommending that, as with any skill, it is best to start at a simple level and progress gradually to more complex uses. What are appropriate basic uses for the LMA? Broadly speaking, any nonemergency case requiring general anesthesia in a patient in the supine position who has an ASA classification of I (ASA I) or II and in whom the surgeon is performing a routine, short procedure that does not involve the alimentary or respiratory tract would constitute an appropriate basic use. In practice, such cases are likely to be found in the ambulatory setting and include simple orthopedic, urologic, superficial, or gynecologic procedures. Although it involves external manipulation of the bowel, inguinal canal surgery also falls within this category.

2. Inherent Teaching Difficulties: A Vicious Circle

The learning curve for correct LMA insertion extends beyond the often cited 10 to 15 uses by one or two orders of magnitude.[25] For the anesthesiologist who is just starting to get used to the LMA, an important advantage of confining its use to simple cases is that they represent the greater part of the surgical caseload in many locations, and there are many opportunities for learning and practice. Most anesthesiology residents, however, start out in a teaching hospital, where the case-load tends to be weighted more heavily toward long and complex procedures for which LMA use would be inappropriate in any but the most experienced hands. For this reason, it is common to hear experienced U.K. and U.S. consultant anesthesiologists complain that newly appointed colleagues, who have spent the greater part of their training years in teaching hospitals, appear to have only the most rudimentary concept of LMA use. It is, unfortunately, the same academic colleagues who carry out many of the studies that make up the core of evidence-based knowledge for the LMA. This represents a vicious circle that is not easy to break, particularly at a time when there is increasing pressure on the medical profession to justify all clinical activity by reference to proven techniques. A suggested way out of this impasse is outlined subsequently.

3. Graduating from Simple to Specialized Uses of the Laryngeal Mask Airway

The safety of the patient must be the guiding principle when deciding whether someone is qualified to perform specialized uses of the LMA. A clinician whose first-time insertion success rate is 90% or less should not be considered adequately trained to progress beyond the simplest procedures in ASA I patients. Davies and colleagues reported a success rate of 94% in the first 10 cases in which naval medical trainees used the LMA for the first time in ASA I anesthetized patients.[26] The insertion success rate depends on the types of cases routinely encountered, and the preceding generalization applies to clinicians in an average peripheral hospital that performs a broad range of common procedures.

Those who wish to gain greater expertise in the use of the LMA, but whose practice is based in specialized centers that lack suitable simple cases, can consider the practice of inserting an LMA routinely at the start of a case and then switching to the preferred airway technique before the surgery. Brain found this to be a useful strategy in the teaching hospital environment. Its justification is that the skills acquired could be life-saving in the event of an airway emergency. If the LMA has been inserted successfully and the patient subsequently proves impossible to intubate, the clinician has an already proven way of at least maintaining oxygenation while other strategies are considered. Alternatively, if the clinician has been unable to use the LMA successfully in a certain patient, time is not wasted in trying to use it after a subsequent failed intubation in this patient.

B. Specialized Uses

1. Procedures Outside the Operating Room

a. RADIOLOGY AND MAGNETIC RESONANCE IMAGING

The potential advantages of the LMA in investigative imaging were first described in a letter to *Anaesthesia* from Glasgow, Scotland, in 1990.[27] The investigators pointed out that the LMA permitted hands-free control of the airway in patients who needed to be kept immobile for prolonged periods, a situation often necessitating general anesthesia in restless or young patients. To improve its performance and durability, the LMA's valve later was fitted with a small, stainless steel spring, which unfortunately interfered with MRI of the head and neck. However, LMAs equipped with valves made of nonferrous material were subsequently made available for use in this situation. Stevens and Burden, in a letter to *Anaesthesia* in 1994, commented that they had used the LMA Classic with the modified, nonmetallic valve in more than 500 small children undergoing MRI and that it had proved safe and reliable.[28] They also presented an MRI image demonstrating that the FLMA could not be used for investigations involving the head and neck because the tube contained a wire, which obliterated the image of the surrounding area.

Goudsouzian and associates were the first Americans to report the efficacy of the LMA during MRI, using the images obtained during investigations in 28 children to comment on the position of the device when inserted by residents in training.[29] Despite poor user skills (21% of attempts resulted in a failure to insert, 21% of the cases required more than one insertion attempt, 82% had a downward deflection of the epiglottis, and 7% had oropharyngeal misplacement), satisfactory ventilatory parameters were maintained in all of the children. The safety of the LMA, even in less than fully skilled hands, is a powerful argument for its use in areas remote from the operating room. Van Obbergh and colleagues, working in Brussels, Belgium, presented results from somewhat more experienced users.[30] The LMA was used during MRI in 100 consecutive procedures in children that were carried out using propofol. The position of the LMA was not recorded, but only 16% of the cases required more than one insertion attempt, there were no failures to insert, and oxygen saturation values of 99.1% or above were maintained in all of the children. Ventilation was manually assisted using an Ayre T-piece.

b. RADIATION THERAPY

Grebenik and coworkers were the first to describe the use of the LMA in pediatric radiation therapy in their study of 25 children who underwent a total of 312 courses of radiation therapy under anesthesia.[31] The children were between 3 weeks and 3 years old, and eight of them were anesthetized once daily for 20 or more consecutive days. In each case, the LMA was left in place until the protective reflexes returned. The absence of complications suggests that the LMA may be appropriate for procedures requiring frequent, repeated use of anesthetics in children.

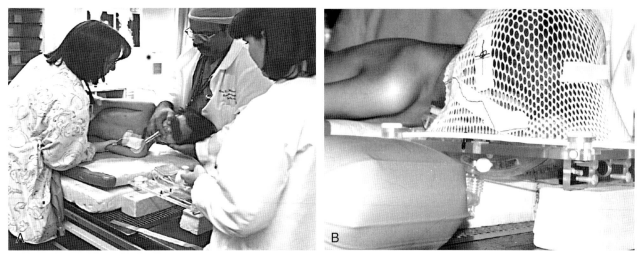

Figure 22-6 Use of the laryngeal mask airway (LMA) in a child undergoing a series of radiation treatments at the University of Texas M.D. Anderson Cancer Center in Houston. **A,** Propofol is used to induce general anesthesia, and after the LMA is inserted, the child is placed in a prone position. **B,** Continuous intravenous infusion of propofol is used as the sole anesthetic agent during radiation treatment while the child is breathing spontaneously through the LMA. This allows more rapid turnover of patients and more efficient use of the radiation therapy suite.

A major advantage of the LMA over the ETT in children receiving radiation therapy on a daily basis during a 4- to 6-week course of treatment is that the LMA does not invade the trachea. The risk of tracheal ulcerations, granulation tissue, and subsequent tracheal stenosis associated with repeated intubations with an ETT is eliminated. The LMA causes much less stimulation than does an ETT; anesthesia requirements for the LMA are significantly lower. For example, at the University of Texas M.D. Anderson Cancer Center in Houston, all children undergoing radiation therapy receive an intravenous infusion of propofol as the sole anesthetic agent during their treatment. The LMA is frequently used for airway management, and spontaneous respiration is preserved (Fig. 22-6). This allows more rapid turnover of patients and more efficient use of the radiation therapy suite.

c. DIAGNOSTIC AND SHORT THERAPEUTIC PROCEDURES IN CHILDREN

The LMA can be very useful during short diagnostic, therapeutic, and minor surgical procedures performed in children in the hospital's procedure room or in the operating room. These procedures include spinal puncture with or without intrathecal therapy, bone marrow aspirations, insertion or removal of a central line or a Port-a-Cath, and minor biopsies (Fig. 22-7). Most children tolerate these procedures well under deep intravenous sedation with propofol and local anesthesia with maintenance of spontaneous respiration. However, some children develop respiratory depression or airway obstruction during deep sedation. In those children, the LMA can be an excellent and much less invasive alternative to endotracheal intubation, resulting in a clear airway without resorting to general anesthesia and muscle relaxation.

d. CARDIOLOGY

The LMA can be useful in patients undergoing transesophageal echocardiography (TEE). TEE is an invasive procedure, and many patients experience significant discomfort or are unable to tolerate TEE under topical anesthesia. In the cardiology clinic setting, TEE is usually performed with topical anesthesia consisting of spraying the oropharynx with a local anesthetic (e.g., 4% lidocaine or 20% benzocaine), with or without sedation.[32,33] However, a significant number of patients experience discomfort during the procedure, and many cannot tolerate the insertion of the probe, even after sedation.[34,35] Because topical anesthesia and light sedation do not completely abolish the gag reflex, deep sedation or general anesthesia may be necessary for patients with highly sensitive reflexes in the upper airway and pharynx. A possible solution for patients who cannot tolerate the

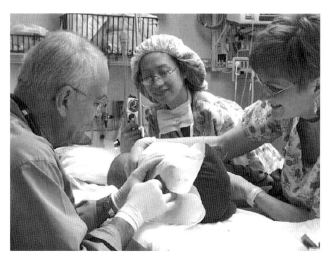

Figure 22-7 Lumbar spinal tap and intrathecal therapy performed on a small child at the University of Texas M.D. Anderson Cancer Center in Houston. Continuous infusion of propofol is used to achieve deep sedation. The laryngeal mask airway (LMA) is used to maintain the open airway, and the child is allowed to breathe spontaneously. The LMA is less invasive than the tracheal tube, and less medication is required to tolerate the device.

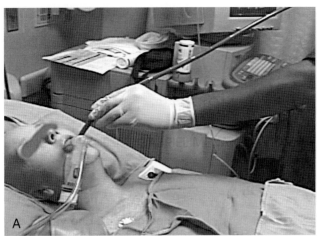
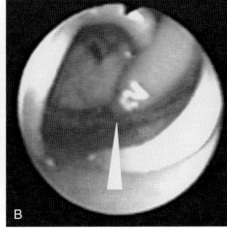

Figure 22-8 Use of the laryngeal mask airway (LMA) during transesophageal echocardiography (TEE) at the University of Texas M.D. Anderson Cancer Center in Houston. The LMA is inserted after TEE placement. **A,** The LMA does not interfere with TEE examination. **B,** Fiberoptic view through the LMA shows the TEE probe (arrowhead) inside the LMA bowl.

insertion of the TEE probe with topical anesthesia and light sedation is deep sedation with propofol. The LMA can be used to maintain the airway in patients undergoing TEE examination during deep sedation with propofol.[36] The LMA can easily be inserted with the TEE probe in place, and the presence of the LMA does not interfere with the manipulation of the probe (Fig. 22-8).

The LMA can be a better alternative than endotracheal intubation in patients undergoing cardioversion in whom face mask ventilation is difficult or inadequate. The minimal hemodynamic stimulation associated with insertion of the LMA, which contrasts with a significant hemodynamic response during endotracheal intubation, offers a great advantage in patients with cardiovascular disease.[37]

2. Head and Neck Surgery

Most of the applications of the LMA in procedures involving the head and neck are done with the FLMA. However, a unique advantage of using the LMA Classic in these patients is the access to the larynx that the device allows (Fig. 22-9), which is particularly useful for diagnostic evaluation of the larynx and trachea and during neodymium:yttrium-aluminum-garnet (Nd:YAG) laser surgery. It is difficult to manage the airway using an ETT in patients who require Nd:YAG laser treatment of lesions located in the vocal cords or the proximal part of the trachea because the ETT limits access to these lesions. There also is a high risk of a laser-induced airway fire when an ETT is used. In contrast, the LMA provides an unobstructed view of the surgical field and virtually eliminates the risk of airway fire (Fig. 22-10).

Head and neck surgery is associated with the risk of bruising or otherwise traumatizing nerves that control the motor functions of the larynx. The LMA can be useful in evaluating the function of the vocal cords at the conclusion of neck dissection and thyroid and parathyroid surgery.[38] While the patient is still under general anesthesia, the LMA is inserted behind the ETT and inflated. The anesthesiologist then removes the ETT, and

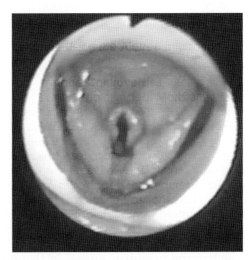

Figure 22-9 View of the larynx through a fiberscope placed coaxially through the optimally positioned laryngeal mask airway. The epiglottis is not downfolded, and the tip of the mask lies behind the larynx, occluding the upper esophageal sphincter.

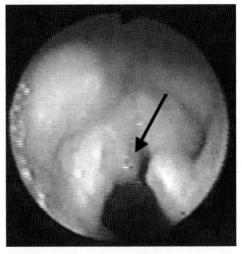

Figure 22-10 Fiberoptic view through the laryngeal mask airway of the left vocal cord lesion (arrow). This type of lesion would be very difficult to treat with the Nd:YAG laser if an endotracheal tube were used.

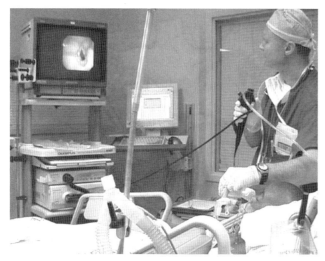

Figure 22-11 A child was admitted to the intensive care unit after brainstem surgery at the University of Texas M.D. Anderson Cancer Center in Houston. Using deep sedation with propofol, the laryngeal mask airway (LMA) was inserted behind the endotracheal tube (ETT). After successful LMA insertion, the ETT was removed to allow visualization of the vocal cords and evaluation of their function in a spontaneously breathing child. This helped the intensivist and the surgeon determine whether the patient would be able to maintain the airway postoperatively.

the patient is allowed to breathe spontaneously. As the patient emerges from general anesthesia, a fiberoptic bronchoscope (FOB) is inserted through the lumen of the LMA to observe the function of the vocal cords. At M.D. Anderson Cancer Center, this technique has become an important diagnostic tool to detect the functional status of the nerves providing motor function to the larynx and has allowed the anesthesiologists and surgeons to make more informed decisions about the postoperative airway management of their patients. Similarly, patients undergoing brainstem surgery in the area that involves the lower cranial nerves, which control the pharynx and larynx, can be evaluated fiberoptically through the LMA in the intensive care unit. This helps the intensivist and the surgeon determine whether the patient will be able to maintain her or his airway postoperatively (Fig. 22-11).

3. Pulmonary Medicine and Thoracic Surgery

a. BRONCHOSCOPY IN CHILDREN AND ADULTS

Physicians in the fields of thoracic surgery and pulmonary medicine have shown interest in the LMA because of the unique access it provides to the larynx and respiratory tree. Diagnostic fiberoptic laryngoscopy and FOB can be performed readily through the LMA in patients under general anesthesia or under topical anesthesia with sedation.[39-41] Maekawa and colleagues, in a 1991 letter to *Anesthesiology* describing the use of a size 1 LMA as a conduit for FOB with a 3.6-mm flexible endoscope in two children (ages 2 and 8 months), listed four advantages. First, the LMA tube is much larger (5-mm internal diameter) than the corresponding ETT, permitting the use of a larger bronchoscope, which gives a better view than that obtained through the 2- to 2.5-mm

bronchoscope normally required to fit through the ETT in this age group. Second, the use of the LMA permitted examination of the larynx, including vocal cord movement and the part of the trachea normally occupied by the ETT. Third, the larger-diameter LMA airway tube permits easy ventilation, which permits uninterrupted observation. Fourth, not using an ETT may be valuable in cases of laryngeal or tracheal stenosis that may be made worse by the passage of the ETT.[42]

In a letter to *Anesthesiology*, Theroux and associates described the use of the size 1 LMA as a conduit for intubation in a 2.5-kg baby with Schwarz-Jampel syndrome who could not be intubated by other means.[43] The uncuffed ETT was advanced over a 2.2-mm bronchoscope, which was easily passed into the trachea through the LMA. In 1997, Mizikov and coworkers reported their experience of using FOB through the LMA in 45 children: 15 diagnostic cases, 22 cases of lavage, 7 cases of foreign body removal, and 1 case of electrocoagulation of an adenoma.[44] Total intravenous anesthesia and PPV were used in all cases. Patients' ages ranged from neonatal to 15 years. They used the Olympus BF3C20 bronchoscope (3.6-mm diameter) with the size 1 LMA, and the Olympus BFP30 (5-mm diameter) was used with the size 2 LMA. The epiglottis was within the mask in 96.5% of cases but was not associated with significant airway obstruction in any case.

b. LASER SURGERY OF THE TRACHEA

In 1992, Slinger and colleagues provided a detailed account of a difficult case of palliative laser resection of a severely obstructing distal tracheal mass.[45] The airway was initially managed using a size 4 LMA, through which a 6-mm Olympus FOB was passed by a swivel connector to apply the laser. Spontaneous ventilation with propofol-isoflurane anesthesia was used. After 120 minutes, 50% of the tracheal lumen had been restored, at which point it was decided to convert to rigid bronchoscopy so that the surgeon could remove larger pieces of tissue by forceps, thereby facilitating the procedure. The physicians repeated this approach in two less severe cases without complications. They pointed out that the laser is not likely to burn the silicone LMA tube if it is switched on only when in the trachea. However, they stressed that use of the rigid bronchoscope remained the gold standard for such cases.

c. TRACHEOBRONCHIAL STENT PLACEMENT

Another advantage of using the LMA in patients with pathology involving the tracheobronchial tree is evident during stent placement using fiberoptic guidance.[46] The LMA's shaft permits use of a 6-mm FOB and provides a larger cross-sectional area than does a 9-mm ETT, which is usually employed during stent placement. The LMA allows better ventilation during stent placement than does an ETT in patients who already have compromised respiratory function. In patients who have an obstruction high in the trachea, the LMA is much better than an ETT because it allows placement of the stent without the risk of extubating the patient (Fig. 22-12).

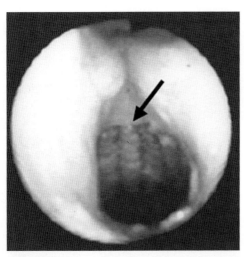

Figure 22-12   Fiberoptic view of the tracheal stent *(arrow)* placed high in the trachea (1.5 cm below the vocal cords) through the laryngeal mask airway (LMA). The LMA's shaft permits use of a 6-mm fiberoptic bronchoscope and provides a bigger cross-sectional area than a 9-mm endotracheal tube (ETT), allowing better ventilation during stent placement than the ETT in patients who already have compromised respiratory functions.

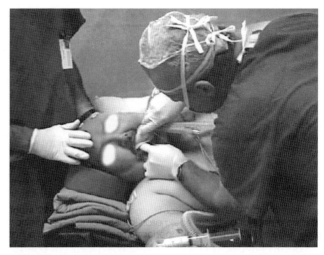

Figure 22-13   Insertion of the ProSeal laryngeal mask airway (PLMA) into a patient undergoing craniotomy with awake intraoperative speech mapping. The anesthesiologist is facing the patient and uses his thumb to insert the PLMA into the patient.

4. Neurosurgery

The hemodynamic stability associated with LMA use may be beneficial during induction in patients undergoing neurosurgical repair of an intracranial aneurysm and in patients with increased intracranial pressure. Silva and Brimacombe reported that hypertension, coughing, and bucking, all of which are common during emergence from general anesthesia with an ETT, were prevented in neurosurgical patients by replacing the ETT with the LMA at the end of the procedure.[47] The insertion and use of the LMA in patients under general anesthesia have been associated with minimal changes in intracranial pressure.[48] This characteristic may be particularly useful during ventriculoperitoneal shunt placement in children, adults, and patients who have suffered a traumatic brain injury.

Other uses for the LMA in neurosurgical patients include awake craniotomy and stereotactic procedures in children and adults. In an awake craniotomy, eloquent areas of the brain are mapped and monitored intraoperatively by stimulating the cerebral cortex with an electrical current. This direct electrical stimulation of the cerebral cortex greatly increases the risk of focal or generalized seizures. Airway management using a face mask and endotracheal intubation during generalized seizures can be very difficult because the patient is usually lying on her or his side, giving the anesthesiologist limited access to the airway, and the patient's head is fixed by metal pins and a frame to provide a stable surgical field and allow the use of modern intraoperative image guidance. However, an experienced and skilled anesthesiologist can easily insert the LMA into such patients, allowing ventilation and oxygenation in this potentially difficult clinical situation (Fig. 22-13).[49]

Stereotactic biopsies can be performed in children using the LMA. Anesthesia is induced with propofol in the radiology suite, and the LMA is inserted (Fig. 22-14).

Local anesthetic is then injected to anesthetize the skin before pins for the stereotactic frame are applied. During continuous infusion of propofol, an MRI is obtained while the child breathes spontaneously through the LMA. While asleep, the child is transported to the operating room for the stereotactic biopsy. This technique provides optimal comfort for the children and excellent operating conditions for the radiologists and surgeons.

V. FLEXIBLE LARYNGEAL MASK AIRWAY

Many operations, particularly procedures performed on the head and neck, require the anesthesiologist and surgeon to share access to the airway. Traditionally, special ETTs that have a spiral coil built into them to increase the flexibility of the tube and to prevent kinking have been used to allow the surgeon to manipulate the ETT

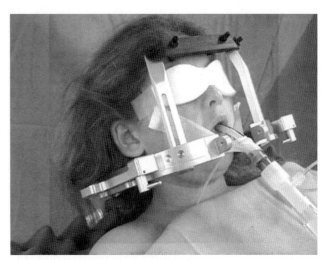

Figure 22-14   A young child undergoing stereotactic biopsy at the University of Texas M.D. Anderson Cancer Center in Houston. Anesthesia is induced with propofol in the radiology suite, and the laryngeal mask airway is inserted.

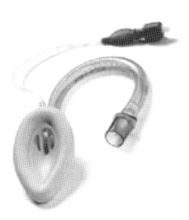

Figure 22-15 The flexible laryngeal mask airway (FLMA), which was introduced into clinical practice in 1994, has a spiral coil built into the shaft to increase the flexibility of the tube and to prevent kinking. This allows the surgeon to manipulate the FLMA's shaft during the surgery and to have good access to the operating field. The FLMA has been used successfully in patients undergoing a variety of head, neck, eye, and oral operations.

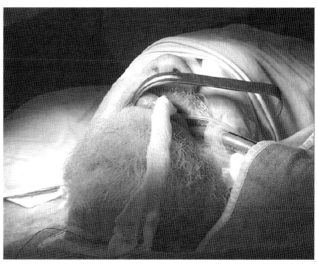

Figure 22-16 The flexible laryngeal mask airway (FLMA) was used in a patient undergoing oral surgery. Because the FLMA causes less hemodynamic stimulation than the endotracheal tube, it is safer to use in patients with severe atherosclerotic heart disease.

during surgery to gain access to the operating field. To make an LMA specifically for head and neck procedures, a similar spiral coil was incorporated into the LMA's shaft, creating the FLMA (Fig. 22-15), which was introduced into clinical practice in 1994. The FLMA has since been used successfully in patients undergoing a variety of head and neck procedures.

A. Tonsillectomy and Adenoidectomy

Several investigators have reported the successful use of the FLMA during tonsillectomies and adenoidectomies. The main advantages of using the FLMA for these procedures are better tolerance of the FLMA by the patients, fewer adverse airway events during emergence and on extubation, and less blood soiling of the airway because of the shielding of the larynx by the LMA's cuff. Williams and Bailey reported that when the FLMA was used in children during adenotonsillectomies,[50,51] there was little soiling of the trachea with blood. In contrast, when an uncuffed ETT was used, blood was almost always present in the trachea, causing coughing on emergence. At the end of surgery, there were also fewer episodes of airway obstruction in the FLMA group than in the ETT patients. This is probably because the FLMA was better tolerated by the patients, allowing extubation when the airway reflexes were less obtunded and the patients were able to maintain an open airway. Fiani and coworkers demonstrated in a randomized study of patients undergoing elective tonsillectomies that fewer complications such as laryngospasm, bleeding, bronchospasm, and desaturation occurred in the FLMA group than in the ETT group.[52]

The FLMA is useful during ear and nose surgery, such as tympanoplasty, myringoplasty, rhinoplasty, septoplasty, and nasal polypectomy.[50,53-58] As reported by Watcha and colleagues, the LMA provided better oxygen saturation and better surgical conditions in pediatric patients

undergoing myringoplasties than did the face mask.[59] Although in other studies the FLMA and the ETT were equally effective in adult patients undergoing nasal surgery, there was less blood in the trachea and fewer airway events during emergence in the FLMA group.[54,59]

B. Dental and Oral Surgery

The FLMA has been useful during dental procedures and oral surgery in children and adults (Fig. 22-16).[60,61] For example, George and Sanders,[62] in a comparison of the FLMA with the nasal mask during dental procedures in children, reported significantly fewer instances of airway obstruction, oxygen desaturation, and cardiac dysrhythmias in children in the FLMA group. Other oral surgeries in which the FLMA has been used successfully include repair of a cleft palate,[63-65] glossopexy,[66] removal of a tongue tumor,[67] and fixation of mandibular fractures after failed endotracheal intubation.[68]

C. Ophthalmologic Procedures

Patients with increased intraocular pressure who are undergoing intraocular procedures are frequently at higher risk for injury from sudden pressure changes during laryngoscopy and endotracheal intubation.[69] Coughing and bucking on the ETT during emergence from general anesthesia can be detrimental and may cause suture rupture.[70] The benefits of using the FLMA for eye surgery include less change in the intraocular pressure during induction and emergence from general anesthesia and less hemodynamic stimulation.[71,72] The FLMA has been particularly useful during cataract surgery, trabeculectomy, and vitroretinal surgery.[73] Use of the device has also benefited children undergoing strabismus repair, gonioscopy, nasolacrimal duct probing, eyelid repair, scleral and conjunctival procedures, and foreign body removal.[74]

VI. LARYNGEAL MASK AIRWAY USE IN PATIENTS WITH DIFFICULT-TO-MANAGE AIRWAYS

One of the most important tasks of an anesthesiologist is to provide ventilation and oxygenation for the patient during surgery. This requires establishing and maintaining a patent airway during the course of anesthesia. As reported in 1990 in a closed claims study published by the ASA, airway-related problems were among the leading causes of major morbidity and mortality directly related to anesthesia.[75] This study laid the groundwork for the development of the ASA difficult airway algorithm, which established pathways for the care of patients with difficult-to-manage airways.[76] Although the algorithm provides an organized approach to airway management based on preoperative findings, it does not constitute a foolproof system. Many patients still prove difficult to intubate by means of conventional laryngoscopy, even when the preoperative interview and physical examination do not yield any signs of potential difficulty. Airway swelling may ensue quickly after multiple intubation attempts. Although face mask ventilation in these patients might have been adequate initially, it may soon become difficult, creating the very dangerous and potentially life-threatening situation of inadequate oxygenation.

During the past 10 years, the LMA has received much attention because it can be effective in patients who are difficult to intubate by conventional laryngoscopy and difficult to ventilate with a face mask. The success of the LMA in these patients results from its design. The LMA fits into the potential space of the pharynx much like a hand fits into a glove. In contrast to rigid laryngoscopy, insertion of the LMA does not rely on direct visualization of the larynx. Many factors that are associated with difficult rigid laryngoscopy (e.g., Mallampati class III and IV, Cormack-Lehane grade 3 and 4 views) do not affect the insertion of and ventilation through the LMA.[77,78]

A. Classic Laryngeal Mask Airway

The potential of the LMA for the emergency and nonemergency management of patients with difficult airways was appreciated shortly after its invention. In February 1983, an early prototype was used successfully by Brain in a 114-kg man undergoing laparotomy who could not be intubated. However, the first publication describing the LMA as a possible solution to airway management problems in emergency situations did not appear in the scientific literature until 1984.[79] By 1985, the LMA had been used successfully in five adults in whom difficult intubation was anticipated, and in October 1987, it was used for the first time in cases of failed pediatric intubation.[13] In 1989, Allison and McCrory used fiberoptic guidance for endotracheal intubations,[80] and in 1991, McCrirrick and Pracilio first reported an awake intubation through the LMA.[81] Numerous case reports appeared describing airway management with the LMA in several clinical situations, including adult and pediatric patients with cervical spine pathology, including cervical spine instability[12,81-84]; morbid obesity[85]; micrognathia and

macrognathia[86,87]; Klippel-Feil syndrome[88]; Treacher Collins syndrome[89]; Pierre Robin syndrome[90]; Goldenhar's syndrome[91]; Hurler's syndrome[92]; Down syndrome[93]; or unexpected failed intubation associated with difficult face mask ventilation.[94,95]

A major step in recognizing the LMA's potential in the management of airway emergencies took place in 1993, when it was incorporated into the Practice Guidelines for Management of the Difficult Airway by the ASA Task Force on Management of the Difficult Airway.[76] Not enough data were available then to appreciate fully the LMA's role in difficult airway situations. By 1996, the reported experience with the LMA had substantially increased, and Jonathan Benumof, who participated in the development of the ASA algorithm, assessed the LMA's potential in a difficult airway scenario.[96] His recommendations were that the LMA should be considered as originally recommended in the emergency pathway of the algorithm and in four additional situations: during awake intubation as an aid to endotracheal intubation, as a definite airway in nonemergency situations, as an aid to tracheal intubation in anesthetized patients, and as an aid to tracheal intubation after the airway is established in emergency situations. In his review, Benumof concluded, "With multiple uses and multiple places of use, the LMA is an important option within the ASA difficult airway algorithm. More importantly, the clinical record of LMA use in 'cannot intubate, cannot ventilate' situations has been excellent, and in patients whose lungs cannot be ventilated because of the supraglottic obstruction and whose trachea cannot be intubated due to unfavorable anatomy (but not periglottic pathology), the LMA should be immediately available and considered as the first treatment of choice."[96] In 2003, Benumof's recommendations fully materialized in the Practice Guidelines for Management of the Difficult Airway that was updated by the ASA Task Force on Management of the Difficult Airway.[6] Essentially, depending on the user's level of expertise, the LMA can be used in any place in the algorithm.

B. Fastrach Intubating Laryngeal Mask Airway

In 1983, while developing the LMA, Brain conducted a fiberoptic investigation that revealed the LMA's potential as a guide for endotracheal intubation. The same year, he developed a prototype LMA and used it to intubate blindly three patients using a 9-mm ETT (Fig. 22-17). However, the development of an intubating LMA was not revisited by Brain until 1994. In response to clinicians' growing demands for a device that had the same ventilatory properties as the LMA Classic but would serve as a better conduit for intubation, he designed the Fastrach ILMA (LMA North America, San Diego, CA), which was introduced in 1997 (Fig. 22-18).

The ILMA is designed to facilitate blind or fiberoptically guided endotracheal intubations without the need to move the cervical spine during intubation. Available only in adult sizes, the ILMA consists of an anatomically curved, stainless steel tube with a 13-mm internal diameter that is connected firmly at its distal end to the laryngeal mask. The angle of the metal shaft was carefully

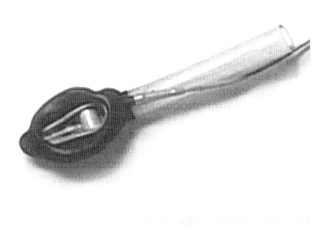

Figure 22-17 A prototype of the intubating laryngeal mask was built and used by Archie Brain in 1983. It was used to blindly intubate three patients who had a history of difficult intubation with a 9-mm-ID tracheal tube.

designed using measurements from sagittal MRI images to fit well into the oral and pharyngeal space while keeping the head and neck in a neutral position. Proximally, the metal shaft forms a standard 15-mm connector for the anesthesia circuit, and a rigid guiding handle serves to insert the device, eliminating the need to insert fingers into the mouth, and to stabilize and direct the device during intubation attempts. The two bars at the aperture of the LMA Classic have been replaced in the ILMA by a single, movable epiglottic elevating bar that pushes the epiglottis out of the way and allows smooth and unobstructed passage of the ETT as it emerges from the distal end of the ILMA's metal shaft (Fig. 22-19). This shaft can accommodate an ETT up to 8.5 mm in diameter. The shaft of the ILMA is shorter than that of the LMA Classic, eliminating the need for longer ETTs in patients with long necks.

The ILMA was first described by Brain and coworkers in 1997 in the *British Journal of Anaesthesia*.[97] In the same

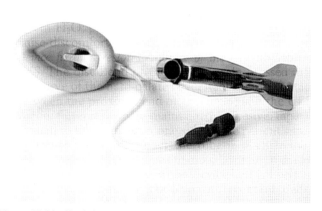

Figure 22-18 The intubating laryngeal mask airway (ILMA) was introduced in 1997. It consists of the mask, which has the same shape as the LMA Classic, and the 13-mm internal diameter, stainless steel shaft, which can accommodate an endotracheal tube with an internal diameter up to 8.5 mm.

issue, there were two separate reports by Brain and Kapila and their colleagues[98,99] of early clinical experience with the ILMA. Unfortunately, Kapila's report described results obtained 3 years earlier using a more primitive prototype of the ILMA and created some confusion regarding the technique of intubation through the device. At the same time, early versions of the ILMA instruction manual included recommendations for use based on these early prototypes. Subsequently, the results from a large study that evaluated the effectiveness of the ILMA in patients with different types of difficult-to-manage airways rendered most of these earlier recommendations irrelevant by demonstrating that the only technique that improved the rate of blind intubation through the ILMA was Chandy's maneuver (Chandy Verghese, Royal Berkshire Hospital, Reading, England, personal communication, January 1998).[100]

Chandy's maneuver consists of two steps that are performed sequentially. The first step, which is important for establishing optimal ventilation, is to rotate the ILMA slightly in the sagittal plane using the metal handle until the least resistance to bag ventilation is achieved. The second step of Chandy's maneuver is performed just before blind intubation and consists of using the metal handle to lift slightly (but not tilt) the ILMA away from the posterior pharyngeal wall. This facilitates the smooth passage of the ETT into the trachea (Fig. 22-20). Ferson and colleagues assessed the effectiveness of the ILMA in 254 patients, including patients with Cormack-Lehane grade 4 views, immobilized cervical spines, and airways distorted by tumors, surgery, or radiation therapy and patients wearing stereotactic frames.[100] Insertion of the ILMA was accomplished in three attempts or fewer in all patients. The overall success rates for blind and fiberoptically guided intubations were 97% and 100%, respectively. This represents the largest analysis examining the use of the ILMA in patients with difficult-to-manage airways and demonstrates that the ILMA may be a particularly valuable tool in the emergency or elective airway management of patients in whom other techniques have failed and in the treatment of patients with immobilized cervical spines.

The ILMA can be used as an intubating tool in patients with normal airways. In a study conducted by Brain and colleagues, the hemodynamic response to the ILMA was similar to the response to the LMA Classic; in patients with compromised cardiovascular systems the ILMA could be a less stimulating alternative to rigid laryngoscopy for intubation of the trachea.[98,101] Using the ILMA in patients with normal airways allows clinicians to develop good skills and familiarity with the device before using it in emergency situations.

VII. PROSEAL LARYNGEAL MASK AIRWAY

The PLMA (LMA North America, San Diego, CA) (Fig. 22-21) was designed by Brain with the principal objective of providing a separate conduit to permit gastric fluids to bypass the glottis. He thought such a device was needed because even in fasted patients, the anesthesiologist can never be completely certain that the stomach is empty.

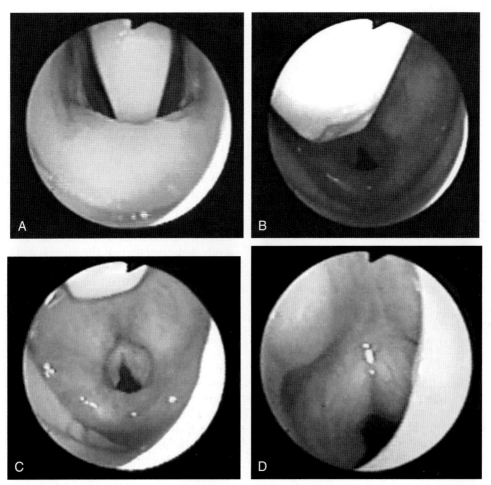

Figure 22-19   Fiberoptic view of intubation through the intubating laryngeal mask airway (ILMA). **A,** Epiglottic elevating bar (EEB) as seen from inside the shaft. **B,** The tip of the endotracheal tube (ETT), as it advances through the LMA Fastrach, pushes the EEB upward. **C,** This movement of the EEB lifts the epiglottis out of the way. **D,** It also provides a clear passage for the ETT through the vocal cords.

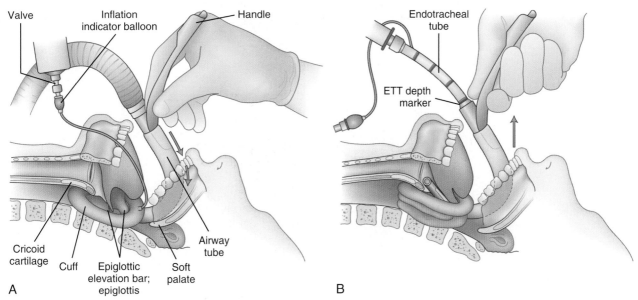

Figure 22-20   Chandy's maneuver consists of two steps that are performed sequentially. **A,** The first step is important for establishing optimal ventilation. The intubating laryngeal mask airway (ILMA) is rotated slightly in the sagittal plane using the metal handle until the least resistance to bag ventilation is achieved. **B,** The second step is performed just before blind intubation. The metal handle is used to lift slightly (but not tilt) the ILMA away from the posterior pharyngeal wall. This facilitates the smooth passage of the endotracheal tube *(ETT)* into the trachea.

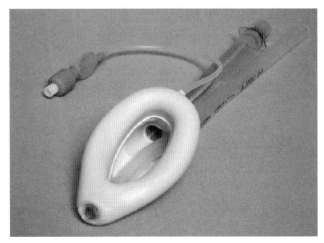

Figure 22-21 The ProSeal laryngeal mask airway (PLMA) was designed to separate the respiratory and gastrointestinal tracts and to provide a better seal around the glottis and allow positive-pressure ventilation in a more reliable manner than the LMA Classic.

The PLMA permits access to the stomach using standard gastric tubes, provides a more reliable seal around the glottis, reduces the leakage of inspired gases into the stomach, provides a more comfortable fit within the pharynx, facilitates the use of mechanical ventilation, and permits the diagnosis of incorrect LMA placement.

The LMA Classic may or may not block the esophagus, depending on how precisely it is positioned in the hypopharynx. Realizing this, Brain developed insertion and fixation techniques to ensure correct positioning, but these recommendations are widely ignored or unknown to most users, who continue to choose their own favored insertion techniques and methods of fixation. It therefore comes as no surprise that there are cases of aspiration in the LMA literature, although they are rare.[102] In the PLMA, the drain tube opening at the distal tip of the mask ensures that if the tip is not correctly placed against the UES, inflation of the reservoir bag causes some of the gas to be diverted back up the drain tube, providing measurable evidence of inadequate device placement. The PLMA instruction manual further details the diagnostic functions made possible by the drain tube.[103]

PLMA, which will soon be available in the same range of sizes as the LMA Classic (excluding size 6), has several important differences. The adult sizes are fitted with a posterior extension to the cuff that expands to a relatively small degree when inflated within the confined space of the pharynx, as demonstrated radiologically (Fig. 22-22). Similar images in which the cuff is inflated excessively demonstrate that the presence of the posterior cuff, although probably increasing the seal pressure by about 10%, introduces two dangers that must be guarded against. One is the possibility of herniating the cuff bowl forward toward the glottis, thereby causing partial or complete blockage of the delicate drain tube and compromising the airway (Fig. 22-23). Second, overinflation may cause the mask to slide proximally, reducing the efficacy of its seal against the UES. If the drain tube is blocked and its opening is simultaneously moved away from contact with the UES, the major advantages of the device are lost because there is no longer any guarantee that a seal exists against the UES, although the seal may appear to be excellent. The PLMA is therefore a more sophisticated device than the LMA Classic, and instructions for its use must be followed carefully.

Pediatric sizes of the PLMA feature the drain tube but no posterior cuff. The relatively larger airway and drain tube configuration required for optimal functioning in

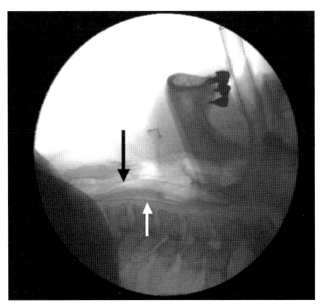

Figure 22-22 Lateral neck radiograph with the ProSeal laryngeal mask airway (PLMA) in place. When inflated correctly with a pressure up to 60 cm H$_2$O, the posterior cuff of the mask expands only slightly (*white arrow*). This ensures the patency of the gastric drain tube (*black arrow*).

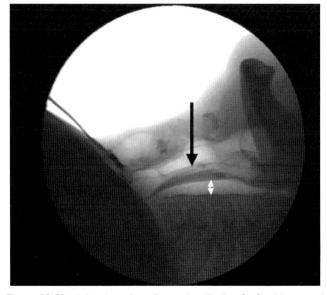

Figure 22-23 Lateral neck radiograph with the ProSeal laryngeal mask airway (PLMA) in place. If the cuff is inflated with excessive volume, exceeding a pressure of 60 cm H$_2$O, the gastric drain tube can be partially or completely occluded (*black arrow*) by the bowl of the mask that is pushed toward the glottis by the overinflated cuff (*white double arrow*).

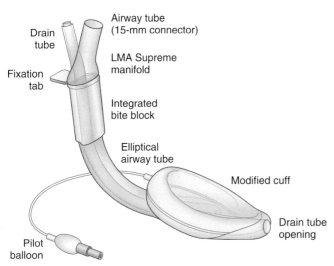

Figure 22-24   The LMA Supreme has a manifold with an integral bite block, an anatomically shaped airway tube enclosing a drain tube, a modified cuff through which the drain tube passes, and a cuff inflation line with pilot balloon.

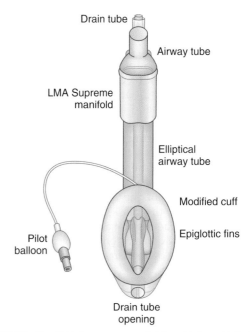

Figure 22-25   The LMA Supreme manifold and integral bite block is at the proximal end of the device. Two tubes project from the manifold. The 15-mm-diameter airway tube is designed to be connected to the airway circuit. The narrower tube is the proximal end of the drain tube.

the pediatric anatomy result in a wider device angle when viewed laterally. If a posterior cuff were added, the angle would become critically large, causing the device to slide proximally out of the pharynx as it is inflated. Halaseh and colleagues reported their experience with the PLMA in 3000 elective cesarean sections in a single center and using a method of insertion that allowed a rapid establishment of a patent airway together with gastric drainage.[104]

VIII. SUPREME LARYNGEAL MASK AIRWAY

After several years of continuous research, Brain designed the LMA Supreme (Intavent, Direct, Maidenhead, United Kingdom) as a single-use laryngeal mask airway device with gastric access. The intent was to combine some of the desirable features of the ILMA, such as ease of insertion, without the need for the insertion of the fingers into the oropharynx, and the PLMA, which offers higher seal pressures with a gastric tube access to permit drainage from and access to the stomach, and it provides confirmatory evidence of correct or incorrect device placement.

The LMA Supreme has a manifold with an integral bite block, an anatomically shaped airway tube enclosing a drain tube, a redesigned inflatable cuff (through which the drain tube passes), and a cuff inflation line with pilot balloon (Figs. 22-24 and 22-25). The LMA Supreme manifold and integral bite block is at the proximal end of the device. Two tubes project from the manifold. The standard 15-mm diameter airway tube is designed to be connected to the airway circuit. The narrower tube is the proximal end of the drain tube.[104,105]

The fixation tab is a rectangular structure molded onto the manifold at right angles, and it projects over the patient's upper lip. It is designed to facilitate easy insertion and fixation of the LMA Supreme after insertion and inflation of its cuff. The fixation tab was found in early pilot studies to act as a visual guide to correct size

selection. After fixation of the device and inflation of the cuff to a pressure of 60 cm H$_2$O, the fixation tab should be 1.5 to 2 cm from the upper lip. If the fixation tab is less than this distance, the size chosen may be too small, and if it is more than 3.0 cm from the upper lip, the size chosen may be too large (see Figs. 22-24 and 22-25).

Extending distally from the manifold is the flattened, semirigid airway tube, which has an elliptical cross section and an integral bite block at its proximal end. The airway tube ends distally at the laryngeal inlet. The elliptical shape of the airway tube is intended to facilitate insertion in patients with reduced interdental space without requiring the insertion of fingers into the mouth. After it is in place, the flattened shape and stiffness of the airway tube also helps to minimize accidental rotation. The airway tube is much stiffer than that of the PLMA, but it is intended to bend with movements of the head and neck, unlike the completely rigid metallic airway tube of the ILMA. Patented lateral grooves on the airway tube of the LMA Supreme prevent it from kinking and occluding when bent, no matter how much it is flexed (see Figs. 22-24 and 22-25).

The drain tube runs from its rigid proximal end on the manifold through the middle of the airway tube and continues along the posterior surface of the cuff to the distal end of the cuff. At the distal end, it terminates as a centrally placed orifice designed to face into the opening of the UES, when the device is correctly inserted. The drain tube equalizes the pressure at the UES and atmosphere. In addition to venting gastrointestinal gases and liquids, the drain tube also serves as a conduit for the passage of a well-lubricated gastric tube (up to 16 F) into the stomach. The drain tube functions as a continuous clinical monitoring tool during PPV, indicating whether the LMA Supreme is correctly positioned immediately after insertion and warning the user if the device becomes displaced from its optimal position during use. Incorrect positioning of the LMA Supreme results in a poor airway seal and an audible leak of delivered gases through the drain tube (see Figs. 22-24 and 22-25).

The modified shape and enlarged surface area of the inflatable cuff enhances the anatomic fit of the device into the pharynx, permitting higher glottic seal pressures than the LMA Classic and LMA Unique. The distal cuff is over-molded to strengthen the tip and prevent it from folding over during insertion. Two fin-shaped structures extend on either side of the drain tube where it passes through the bowl of the mask, designed to prevent the epiglottis from obstructing the airway (see Figs. 22-1 and 22-2). The cuff has a conventionally placed inflation line terminating in a pilot balloon and one-way valve for mask inflation and deflation.

The technique for LMA Supreme insertion described in the study by Balog and coworkers is similar to that recommended in the instruction manual.[74] The device was deflated to a vacuum using a 50-mL syringe and correctly shaped at the distal tip by compressing between finger and thumb during deflation to form a thin wedge. Insertion was performed with the head and neck in the semi-sniffing position. Complete extension is not required for successful insertion.[105,106]

In a prospective, descriptive study on the use of the LMA Supreme for airway management in 205 adult patients undergoing elective orthopedic surgery in the prone position, the investigators were able to demonstrate that first-pass success was achieved in 184 insertions.[107] Regurgitation of gastric contents through the LMA drainage tube was observed in 205 patients. There were no cases of clinically relevant aspiration. Sharma and colleagues concluded that the LMA Supreme was a useful device for airway management in patients anesthetized in the prone position and for possible airway management with PPV, with or without neuromuscular block.[107] No patient had to be turned to the supine position because of an airway problem during anesthesia. Brimacombe and coworkers demonstrated in 40 adult patients that maintenance of anesthesia is feasible in the prone position when the LMA Supreme was inserted by experienced users.[108]

The PLMA and LMA Supreme offer the additional advantages of higher glottic seal pressures than the LMA Classic, providing a separate conduit for passive passage of gastric contents and allowing the passage of a lubricated gastric tube through the drain tube to access liquid and gaseous gastric contents. The advantages of a higher glottic seal pressure, easy access to the stomach,[105] ease of insertion in the supine, lateral, and prone positions, efficacy for PPV, and as a reliable and noninvasive airway during the recovery phase from general anesthesia support its use in this form of surgery.

In a well-designed, randomized, prospective study comparing the safety and efficacy of the LMA Supreme with the PLMA in elective ambulatory procedures, Seet and associates included 99 patients and concluded that although the LMA Supreme has lower oropharyngeal leak pressures than the PLMA, the first attempt insertion success rate was higher for the LMA Supreme.[109] It is a safe, efficacious, and easy to use disposable supraglottic airway device suitable for elective ambulatory procedures.[109] The higher first-attempt success rate may make the LMA Supreme a more suitable choice as an airway rescue device.

The higher intracuff pressures demonstrated for the PLMA may be related to the cuff material. The PLMA is made from silicone, and the LMA Supreme is constructed from polyvinyl chloride.[106] Mucosal pressures are lower than pharyngeal perfusion pressure over the inflation range for the PLMA.[110]

Eschertzhuber and colleagues found a lower leak pressure with the size 4 LMA Supreme than with the size 4 PLMA in 93 healthy, female patients.[106] However, there was no significant difference in leak pressure with the LMA Supreme and PLMA in two other studies by Verghese and Ramaswamy[105] and Hosten and coworkers.[111] A literature review of the oropharyngeal leak pressure of the supreme LMA and the PLMA showed conflicting results. A prospective, randomized, crossover study of 36 female patients using a size 4 Supreme or the PLMA showed no difference in the oropharyngeal leak pressure (28.6 versus 28.5 cm H_2O, $P = 0.91$).[105] Hosten and associates conducted a prospective, randomized, controlled trial enrolling 60 patients (men and women) and comparing the Supreme with the Proseal.[111] Various LMA sizes (sizes 3 through 5) were used according to body weight. The leak pressures were also found to be similar for the Supreme and ProSeal groups at intracuff pressures of 60 cm H_2O (26.1 versus 26.9 cm H_2O).[111] However, muscle relaxants were given to 13 of 60 patients, which might have confused the results. The application of neuromuscular blocking agents can result in a decreased leak pressure of the PLMA and may have influenced the accuracy of measurement.[112] The lower oropharyngeal leak pressure for the LMA Supreme may be related to the less elastic properties of polyvinyl chloride.

Cuff pressures are not directly related to leak pressures. The materials play a major role in the compliance and elasticity of the device, as do the volume and elasticity of the patient's oropharyngeal anatomy, but it is also essential that the device is correctly located in the hypopharynx and that it remains securely fixed in position. The fact that leak pressures have been found by some to be lower in the LMA Supreme may be due to material differences, but it could also reflect positioning and subsequent movement of the airway after insertion.[113]

IX. DISPOSABLE LARYNGEAL MASK AIRWAYS

Infection is a perennial risk to health care workers and patients. The risk of infection in hospitals seems to be about as intractable a problem as iatrogenic disease. Newer antimicrobial agents encourage the emergence of resistant organisms just as more powerful therapeutic tools offer new opportunities for human error in their application. Although laryngeal masks have never been proved to be a source of infection transmission, the continuing uncertainty surrounding the size of the population of Creutzfeldt-Jakob disease carriers and the risk of transmission of the infectious agent through the tonsillar bed, together with the difficulties in ensuring effective device sterilization against small virus-like particles, have led to increased interest in disposable airway equipment, particularly in some European countries. The U.K. Department of Health required surgeons and anesthesiologists to use disposable equipment for tonsillectomies but reversed this decision when the use of poorly designed disposable surgical instruments was implicated in the death of a patient. In London's main otolaryngologic hospital, the Royal Throat, Nose, and Ear Hospital, the reusable FLMA had for some years been used in approximately 90% of tonsillectomies (Paul Bailey, personal communication, March 2004), and substitution with the disposable ETT was believed to be a retrospective step. Accordingly, the Department of Health agreed to fund the cost of treating the reusable FLMA as a single-use item, pending the availability of a disposable version of the device.

The lessons learned from this experience were that we should be wary of rushing to embrace disposable forms of an established device until we are sure that their function is equivalent and that the avoidance of a theoretical risk of low probability (e.g., transmission of prion infection associated with tonsillectomy) should not take precedence over the avoidance of known risks (e.g., imposition of untried and unfamiliar equipment for an operation, the safety of which depends on skill, training, and well-established techniques).

All pediatric and adult sizes of the disposable LMA (LMA Unique; LMA North America) have been subjected to a rigorous series of tests to confirm that their function is equivalent to that of the reusable silicone device.[114,115] This has not been easy to accomplish because vinyl plastic materials lack the elasticity of silicone, and this tends to affect the insertion and seal characteristics of the LMA. It is likely that the plastic disposable LMAs will be found to be less appropriate for PPV than the LMA Classic. However, this limitation may be regarded as academic because the PLMA is specifically designed for use with positive pressure.

X. EXCHANGE USING THE AINTREE INTUBATION CATHETER

When an LMA is placed after a difficult intubation or difficult ventilation by face mask, the anesthesiologist must determine whether the airway should be secured by an ETT for the surgical procedure. The Aintree intubating catheter (AIC, Cook Critical Care, Bloomington, IN) is a semirigid, 560-mm-long tube with internal and external diameters of 47 and 70 mm, respectively.[116,117] It was designed to enable fiberoptically guided intubation of the trachea through a supraglottic airway device. The technique permits fiberoptic instrumentation of the airway while oxygenation and ventilation take place around the fiberscope through the airway device. Use of the AIC through the LMA Classic and the PLMA have been reported when conventional tracheal intubation has failed.[118-122]

The PLMA may offer additional benefits over the LMA Classic when using the AIC because of its larger airway bowl and the absence of aperture bars at the distal end of the airway tube. The deeper bowl of the PLMA and the absence of bars may allow improved access to the larynx compared with the LMA Classic and improve passage of the AIC during insertion.[123,124] The PLMA is not as easy to insert as the LMA Classic, and it has a slightly smaller internal diameter through which an AIC can easily pass.

Clinical studies have reported less than 30 intubations with the LMA Classic or the cuffed oropharyngeal airway (COPA). Both reports were executed by the inventors of the device and between them involved only three operators. On a manikin study comparing the use of AIC over the LMA Classic and the PLMA using the fiberscope, Blair and colleagues found no significant difference between the devices with regard to ease of advancement of the fiberscope or the view of the vocal cords with the AIC.[125] The study concluded that in a manikin, fiberoptically guided intubation through a PLMA was at least as easy and reliable as through the LMA Classic.[125] The technique of exchanging an LMA over an AIC has only been described in humans during difficult airway situations and found as case reports in the literature.

XI. PROBLEMS AND CONTROVERSIES

The occurrence of problems and complications associated with the use of the LMA appears to be inversely proportional to the experience and skill level of the operator. Most adverse events associated with LMA are probably the result of incorrect use of the device or inappropriate selection of patients. Some of the advanced clinical applications of the device (e.g., PPV with the LMA) have been considered controversial. However, as their experience and skill with the LMA advance, many clinicians find it to be a very useful tool in situations that they had previously considered to be problematic. The skill level and experience of the clinician, not the type of application, should guide the use of the LMA. In the following sections, we address the controversies regarding the LMA's use and discuss reported problems and complications and ways to manage them when they occur.

A. Oropharyngolaryngeal Morbidity

Any foreign body that comes into contact with airway structures can cause complications. The LMA passes through and occupies anatomic areas from the oral cavity to the hypopharynx. Structures that are at high risk for injury from supraglottic airways, including the LMA, are mucous membranes, soft tissues of the pharynx and larynx, salivary glands, nerves and blood vessels of the neck, laryngeal cartilages, and bones of the neck. When injury occurs, it usually manifests in minor complaints such as a dry mouth or sore throat.[126] These problems usually resolve quickly and have no long-term sequelae. However, more serious complications, such as hypoglossal and lingual nerve palsy, trauma to the epiglottis and larynx, dysarthria, dysphonia, and tongue cyanosis related to vascular compression, have been reported.[127-133]

1. Sore Throat

Sore throat, dry throat, pharyngeal erythema, and minor pharyngeal abrasions have been reported with the LMA. The published incidence of sore throat varies between 0% and 70%.[126,132] Initially, it was not clear why the incidence of sore throat varied so much. Factors that may affect the incidence include the insertion technique, duration of the procedure, type of lubricant, type of ventilation (i.e., spontaneous or controlled), and intracuff pressure.[134-137] Of these, the only variable that has been shown to reduce the incidence of sore throat reliably is lowering the intracuff pressure.[138] Overinflation of the LMA's cuff is a common practice when the size of the device is too small for a given patient and the practitioner encounters a significant leak while attempting assisted ventilation or PPV. The overinflated cuff becomes stiff and exerts high local pressure on tissues, especially those surrounding bony structures, such as the hyoid bone and cervical spine. Nitrous oxide diffuses through the silicone walls of the LMA, increasing the pressure inside the cuff.[139] This can be remedied by monitoring the intracuff pressure and periodically withdrawing the gas from the LMA's cuff. Based on Brain's unpublished research in awake volunteers, the maximum pressure inside the LMA's cuff should not exceed 60 cm H_2O because higher pressure causes discomfort, presumably because of stretching of the constrictor muscles. Appropriate LMA size selection combined with a good insertion technique and low intracuff pressure reduces significantly the incidence of postoperative sore throat.

2. Vascular Compression and Nerve Damage

Although rare, compression of the blood vessels of the tongue that leads to tongue cyanosis has been observed after LMA insertion.[130] This complication is likely to occur when the LMA is not inserted deeply enough or when the LMA's cuff is overinflated. The blood vessels of the tongue or the lingual nerve can be compressed by malpositioning of the LMA's shaft on the lateral side of the tongue, as found in cadaveric research. Similarly, if during LMA insertion the cuff is partially or fully inflated, the device frequently lies higher than when the correct insertion technique is used. Malpositioning of the LMA can compress the lingual or hypoglossal nerve, resulting in transient or prolonged nerve palsy. The hypoglossal nerve, which supplies all of the intrinsic and all but one of the extrinsic muscles of the tongue, is particularly vulnerable to injury at the point where the nerve loops anteriorly, close to the greater cornu of hyoid bone, and then runs along the lateral surface of the hyoglossal muscle and above the posterior border of the mylohyoid muscle before dividing into several branches that supply tongue muscles. To avoid these complications, the anesthesiologist should select the appropriate LMA size, use the standard insertion technique, and ensure that the intracuff pressure is no higher than 60 cm H_2O.

B. Risk of Aspiration

Aspiration during general anesthesia has an overall incidence of 1.4 to 6.5 per 10,000 cases and a mortality rate of 5%.[140-143] In a study of 215,488 anesthesia cases, Warner and coworkers reported that the incidence of aspiration was 2.6 per 10,000 patients undergoing elective surgery and 11 per 10,000 patients undergoing emergency procedures.[144] The mortality rate was 0.14 per 10,000 patients with an ASA physical status classifications III through V. The study by Warner and colleagues did not include patients whose airways were managed using the LMA.[144]

The LMA does not reliably protect against aspiration and should not be used electively in patients who are at high risk for this complication. However, most users do not adhere to the recommended insertion or fixation techniques when using the LMA, which are designed to optimize the seal of the distal end of the device against the UES. Nonetheless, a meta-analysis of the literature on the LMA by Brimacombe and Berry revealed that the overall incidence of pulmonary aspiration with the LMA is approximately 2 per 10,000 patients.[145] Eighteen cases of suspected pulmonary aspiration during LMA use have been found by meta-analysis, and only 10 of these were confirmed radiographically. In only three patients did the aspiration warrant ventilatory support, which lasted 1 to 7 days. None of the patients who aspirated through the LMA suffered any long-term effects. Most of these patients had one or more factors predisposing them to aspiration, including emergency surgery in an unfasted patient, a difficult airway, obesity, a steep Trendelenburg position with intra-abdominal insufflation, and previous gastric surgery. Although the meta-analysis study contained only reports published through September 1993, a subsequent analysis of 11,910 LMA anesthesia cases by Verghese and Brimacombe yielded an even smaller incidence of aspiration (0.84 per 10,000).[146]

A study by Bernadini and Natalini compared the risk of pulmonary aspiration in patients whose lungs were mechanically ventilated through an LMA airway (35,630 procedures) or ETT (30,082 procedures).[147] Three cases of pulmonary aspiration occurred with the LMA and seven with the ETT. No deaths were related to pulmonary aspiration. The incidence and outcome of pulmonary aspiration detected in this study were similar to those previously reported. The adjusted odds ratio (OR) for pulmonary aspiration with the LMA was determined to be 1.06 (95% confidence interval [CI], 0.20 to 5.62). Unplanned surgery (OR = 30.5; 95% CI, 8.6 to 108.9) and male sex (OR = 8.6, 95% CI, 1.1 to 68) were associated with an increased risk of aspiration and age younger than 14 years with a reduced risk (OR = 0.21; 95% CI, 0.07 to 0.64). There were contraindications and exclusions to the use of the LMA, but in this selected population, use of an LMA was not associated with an increased risk of pulmonary aspiration compared with an ETT.

Even allowing that critical events in anesthesia are frequently under-reported, the absence of admissions to intensive care units for ventilatory support indicates that aspiration with the LMA is rare. Nevertheless, the anesthesiologist must always be meticulous about selecting patients appropriately, using the correct insertion technique to obtain the optimal LMA position, paying attention to the appropriate depth of anesthesia, and maintaining constant vigilance during surgery. If regurgitation or aspiration occurs despite all of these measures, the following plan of action should be implemented:

1. Do not attempt to remove the LMA because a significant amount of regurgitant fluid may be trapped behind its cuff. The cuff shields and protects the larynx from the trapped fluid, and removing the LMA may worsen the situation.
2. Temporarily disconnect the circuit to allow drainage of the fluid while tilting the patient's head down and to the side.
3. Suction the LMA, and administer 100% oxygen to the patient.
4. Ventilate the patient manually using low gas flows and small tidal volumes to minimize the risk of forcing fluid from the trachea into the small bronchi.
5. Use a large FOB to evaluate the tracheobronchial tree, and suction any remaining fluid.
6. If aspiration below the vocal cords is confirmed, consider intubating the patient with an ETT, and institute appropriate treatment protocols.

The risk of aspiration with an LMA is likely to be significantly reduced with the PLMA, which incorporates a drainage tube into the LMA design, warns of an inadequate UES seal, and permits more reliable PPV than does the LMA Classic.

C. Positive-Pressure Ventilation

When the first independent trial of the LMA was carried out, only a size 3 was available, and the correct fixation technique for ensuring an adequate seal against the UES had not been developed.[148] When used in large patients, the device was not very reliable for applying PPV. Because the LMA concept was new, it was prudent for clinicians initially to limit the use of the LMA to patients who were breathing spontaneously. Even now, PPV should be considered an advanced use of the LMA, and clinicians should practice and gain experience using the LMA in patients who are breathing spontaneously before attempting controlled ventilation. However, after the LMA was introduced commercially in a range of sizes, first for adults and then for children, many LMA users found that after they became experienced, the LMA could be effective during PPV.[73] Devitt and colleagues compared the effectiveness of the LMA with that of the ETT in 48 patients and demonstrated that PPV (range, 15 to 30 cm H_2O) through the LMA was adequate and comparable to that achieved through the ETT.[149] Epstein and associates studied the effectiveness of the LMA with controlled ventilation in children 3 months to 17 years old and concluded that the device performed effectively and reliably.[150] In another study, Epstein and coworkers established that the airway seal pressures (25.9 to 31.2 cm H_2O) were well maintained with the LMA in children.[151]

Two large clinical studies of more than 7000 patients led by Verghese and Van Damme established that the LMA was as effective as the ETT for controlled ventilation.[114,152] Van Damme's study also assessed the airway seal pressures and demonstrated that at 15 cm H_2O or less pressure, leaks occurred with the LMA in only 2.7% of patients. Subsequently, Verghese reported his experience of using the LMA successfully in 5236 patients undergoing a variety of surgical procedures under general anesthesia and PPV.[147]

The following principles should be considered when using the LMA with PPV:

1. *Selection of patients*: Most patients with normal lung compliance who have fasted can be mechanically ventilated effectively with the LMA.
2. *Size selection*: Select the largest LMA size appropriate for the patient, which prevents a tendency to compensate for inadequate seal pressure by overinflating the cuff.
3. *Insertion technique*: Carefully follow the correct insertion technique to ensure optimal positioning of the LMA in the airway.
4. *Fixation technique*: Use the correct method of taping the LMA. This ensures proper contact between the LMA's tip and the esophagus and prevents gastric insufflation.
5. *Auscultation*: Always auscultate over the stomach to ensure that gastric insufflation is not taking place.
6. *Ventilatory parameters*: Limit tidal volumes to 8 mL/kg, and control the end-tidal carbon dioxide by adjusting the respiratory rate.
7. *Treatment of inadequate tidal volume*: Maintain an adequate level of anesthesia for the particular surgical procedure.

If leaking occurs when using the LMA for PPV, investigate the cause, and try to correct the situation. If the device has been correctly fixed in place and remains correctly inflated, the problem usually is caused by the need for more relaxant or deeper anesthesia.

D. Use for Prolonged Procedures

The maximum duration for which the LMA can be safely used is not well established, but a limit of 2 hours was suggested soon after the LMA became widely available for clinical use.[82] This recommendation was based on the possible increased risk of aspiration or pharyngeal morbidity. Subsequent reports demonstrated that in the hands of experienced users, the LMA can be safely used during procedures lasting up to 8 hours.[153,154] In rare circumstances, the LMA has been used in the intensive care arena to provide effective respiratory support for 10 to 24 hours with no evidence of adverse effects.[155] The PLMA, which is designed for PPV and has a gastric drainage tube to minimize the risk of aspiration, may be best suited for prolonged procedures.[156] Regardless of the model used, clinicians must remain vigilant and provide adequate anesthesia to their patients, minimizing the risks of complications. If nitrous oxide is administered to the patient, the anesthesiologist should remember that this gas diffuses into the LMA's cuff, increasing intracuff pressure. During prolonged LMA use, close monitoring of the intracuff pressure is recommended. To minimize the risk of mucosal ischemia associated with high intracuff pressures, hourly removal of a few milliliters of air from the cuff is considered a prudent practice.[157]

E. Use in Nonsupine Positions

Use of the LMA in patients in other than the supine position should be considered an advanced technique.[158-163] An alternative plan is necessary in case the device dislodges from its original position during the procedure. Because of the risk of LMA dislodgment in patients in nonsupine positions, consider inducing general anesthesia and inserting the LMA after the patient has been positioned for the procedure. This ensures the feasibility of inserting the LMA at any time during the procedure. If insertion cannot be performed successfully, reconsider whether the LMA should be used in that patient. The LMA insertion technique in patients in the lateral or prone position is significantly different from the insertion technique in supine patients. Using a thumb to insert the LMA may be the most useful method in patients positioned prone or laterally.[164] An advantage of using the LMA in patients in the prone position is that they are able to position themselves comfortably before induction of general anesthesia, potentially reducing the incidence of back problems.[165]

F. Device Problems

Before its clinical release, the LMA was subjected to rigorous testing to ensure compliance with the medical industry standards. However, some complications have been reported, including separation of the LMA cuff from the shaft,[166,167] fragmentation of the device inside the patient,[168] kinking of the LMA's shaft,[169] and failure to inflate or deflate the cuff.[170,171] Most of these complications are related to use of the device beyond the manufacturer's recommendations and to use of the wrong chemicals for sterilization and coating the device with silicone lubricants, which are not recommended for the LMA. Strict adherence to the manufacturer's instructions for cleaning, sterilization, and use should always be followed, including not exceeding the recommended 40 uses per device. Instructions from the manufacturer's manual should be followed if a malfunction occurs. With the introduction of the disposable LMA models, the number of device problems linked to overuse and wrong sterilization techniques may be eliminated, but all LMAs should be inspected and tested before use to ensure optimal performance and safety.

XII. CONCLUSIONS

When the LMA was first introduced, it was considered to be an alternative to the face mask. However, its clinical applications have exceeded the original recommendations and benefit patients undergoing operations in all surgical and anesthetic subspecialties. Modern surgical techniques often are much less invasive than traditional operations, and many patients undergo procedures in day surgical centers. The LMA is much less stimulating to patients than the ETT and is considered the first choice for diagnostic and minimally invasive surgical procedures. The LMA has been effective and frequently life-saving in patients with difficult-to-manage airways. A study by Combes and colleagues demonstrated that the ILMA and gum elastic bougie were the most frequently used and most successful techniques in patients with unexpected difficult intubation in the operating room.[172]

The LMA has unequivocally established the precedence that the supraglottic approach to airway management is feasible and preferred in many clinical situations. This has created an interest on the part of the medical industry in developing other supraglottic airways. Although this represents a healthy exploration of different clinical approaches to airway management, clinicians should be careful when inserting these devices into their patients because there are no separate standards or regulations guiding the safety and efficacy of supraglottic airways. The responsibility for any complications from these devices rests with the clinicians using them. The American Society for Testing and Materials and the U.S. Food and Drug Administration recently developed standards and regulations for supralaryngeal airways. These standards can guide the development of airway devices, which we hope will have the same record of safety as the LMA.

XIII. CLINICAL PEARLS

- Learn and follow the correct maneuvers for precise insertion and fixation of each of the LMA devices as thoroughly described by Brain. Extensive research has demonstrated that using the proper insertion and fixation techniques leads to higher success rates for insertion and less troubleshooting.

- Optimal results on placement of all LMA types are achieved when the tip of the LMA is delivered to the upper esophageal sphincter (UES).

- Anesthesiologists must understand the advantages and disadvantages of using the LMA.

- Ventilation through the LMA when intubation and face mask ventilation have failed may be a life-saving procedure.

- Proper patient population selection, appropriate LMA selection, adequate size selection, proper attention to the adequate depth of anesthesia (especially when the patient is not paralyzed), and maintenance of an intracuff pressure no higher than 60 cm H_2O (44 mm Hg) enhance the safety and efficacy of all LMAs.

SELECTED REFERENCES

All references can be found online at expertconsult.com.
105. Verghese C, Ramaswamy B: LMA Supreme—A new single-use LMA with gastric access: A report on its clinical efficacy. *Br J Anaesth* 101:405–410, 2008.

106. Eschertzhuber S, Brimacombe J, Hohlrieder M, Keller C: The Laryngeal Mask Airway Supreme—A single use laryngeal mask airway with an esophageal vent: A randomised, cross-over study with the Laryngeal Mask Airway ProSeal in paralysed, anaesthetised patients. *Anaesthesia* 64:79–83, 2009.

107. Sharma V, Verghese C, McKenna PJ: Prospective audit on the use of the LMA-Supreme for airway management of adult patients undergoing elective orthopedic surgery in the prone position. *Br J Anaesth* 105:228–232, 2010.

109. Seet E, Rajeev S, Firoz T, et al: Safety and efficacy of laryngeal mask airway Supreme versus laryngeal mask airway ProSeal: A randomised controlled trial. *Eur J Anaesthesiol* 27:602–607, 2010.

111. Hosten T, Gurkan Y, Ozdamar D, et al: A new supraglottic airway device: LMA-Supreme, comparison with LMA ProSeal. *Acta Anaesthesiol Scand* 53:852–857, 2009.

Chapter 23

Non–Laryngeal Mask Airway Supraglottic Airway Devices

TIM M. COOK | CARIN A. HAGBERG

I. INTRODUCTION

Nothing is more fundamental to the practice of general anesthesia than the maintenance of a clear upper airway. The choice of device depends on several factors, including access to the airway, duration of surgery, and risk factors for aspiration. After placement, the cuffed ETT provides a secure airway and protects against aspiration, but placement and removal of an ETT require training and judgment. Although ETTs typically are used without incident, complications ranging from trivial to life-threatening can occur.[1]

Advanced airway management depends on many airway devices, several of which have been included in the American Society of Anesthesiologists (ASA) difficult airway algorithm.[2] The Classic laryngeal mask airway (LMA Classic, LMA North America, San Diego, CA) was introduced into clinical practice in 1988. Since then and particularly in the past 10 years, there has been an explosion of supraglottic airway devices (SADs) designed to compete with the LMA Classic, especially single-use devices. The introduction of single-use devices has been driven by concern about the sterility of cleaned, reusable devices (e.g., elimination of proteinaceous material, risk of transmission of prion disease) and the inability to recycle the device enough to be cost-effective. More than 20 manufacturers produce single-use LMs. Other designs of SADs have been introduced, and they are the main focus of this chapter.

II. NOMENCLATURE

The term *supraglottic airway device* (SAD) is used to describe a group of airway devices designed to establish and maintain a clear airway during anesthesia. SADs have several roles, including maintenance of the airway during spontaneously breathing or controlled-ventilation anesthesia, airway rescue after failed intubation or out of the hospital, use during cardiopulmonary resuscitation, and use as a conduit to assist difficult tracheal intubation. Brimacombe recommended that the term *extraglottic airway* be used, because many of these devices have components that are infraglottic (i.e., hypopharynx and upper esophagus).[3] This textbook describes all airway devices that have a ventilation orifice or orifices above the glottis as *supraglottic* and those that deliver anesthetic gases or oxygen below the vocal cords (e.g., transtracheal jet ventilation, cricothyrotomy) as *infraglottic*. Other terms and acronyms include supraglottic airway (SGA), extraglottic airway device (EAD), and periglottic airway device (PAD), but SAD is more widely accepted and is used in this chapter.

Brimacombe and Miller suggested there should be a classification system for this increasingly complex family of devices. Miller[4] described three main sealing mechanisms: cuffed perilaryngeal sealers, cuffed pharyngeal sealers, and cuffless, anatomically preshaped sealers. Further subdivision can be made by considering whether the device is single use or reusable and whether protection from aspiration of gastric contents is offered. The practical value of this type of classification is uncertain. Chapters 22 and 27 review the LMA, its variants, and the Combitube.

The acronym *LMA* is a protected term and should be used to refer to any laryngeal mask airway produced by the manufacturers of the LMA Classic (LMA North America and associated international companies). The acronym *LM* refers to a laryngeal mask manufactured by anyone other than the original manufacturers.

First-generation SADs are devices that can be considered simple airway tubes. They include the LMA Classic, a flexible LMA (LMA Flexible), and all LMs. They also include the Laryngeal Tube and the Cobra perilaryngeal airway (CobraPLA). They may or may not protect against aspiration in the event of regurgitation, but they are not specifically designed to lessen this risk.

Second-generation SADs have been designed with safety in mind, and they incorporate design features that aim to reduce the risk of aspiration.[5] They include the ProSeal LMA (PLMA), i-gel, LMA Supreme, Laryngeal Tube Suction II (LTS-II), disposable version of the LTS (LTS-D), the Streamlined Liner of the Pharynx Airway (SLIPA), and the Baska mask. The efficacy of several of these designs has not been proven.

III. LIMITATIONS OF THE CLASSIC LARYNGEAL MASK AIRWAY

Prior to 1988, choices of airway devices essentially were limited to the face mask and endotracheal tube (ETT). The LMA Classic was designed by Archie Brain in the United Kingdom in the early 1980s, and it was introduced into anesthetic practice in 1988. Its introduction revolutionized airway management (Fig. 23-1). It was soon recognized to be a suitable device to use for many cases that previously were managed with a face mask or an ETT, because the LMA Classic had many advantages over both devices.[6] It has been used in approximately 200 million episodes of anesthesia globally. More than 2500

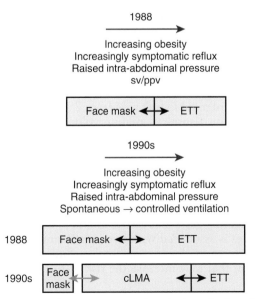

Figure 23-1 Evolution of airway choices before (*top*) and after (*bottom*) the introduction of the LMA Classic in 1988. *cLMA,* LMA Classic; *ETT,* endotracheal tube; *ppv,* positive-pressure ventilation; *sv,* spontaneous ventilation.

studies on the device have been published. The LMA Classic is considered the benchmark against which other SADs are judged. A 2008-2009 UK census found that 56% of all episodes of general anesthesia were delivered with a SAD as the primary airway,[7] and 90% of the devices were LMAs and LMs.

When correctly placed, the mask lies with its tip behind the cricoid cartilage at the esophageal inlet, with the airway orifice facing anteriorly and the cuff encircling the laryngeal inlet. The lateral cuff lies against the piriform fossa, and the upper cuff is located at the base of the tongue. The mask is held in a stable position by the hypopharyngeal constrictor muscles laterally and the cricopharyngeus muscle inferiorly. Inflation of the mask cuff produces a low-pressure seal around the larynx.

Limitations of the LMA include problems with controlled ventilation, airway protection, access through the airway for intubation, reusable design, and absence of a bite block. The first two limitations limit the case mix for which the LMA Classic is suitable.

A. Problems with Controlled Ventilation

The LMA Classic performs well during spontaneous ventilation, but it is so widely used during controlled ventilation that this is no longer considered an advanced use. The LMA Classic is an alternative to anesthesia with a face mask or an ETT. Its introduction has transformed the routine practice of anesthesia, and face mask anesthesia has become uncommon. However, the LMA Classic is not suitable for all cases, and good case selection is the key to successful use.

The LMA Classic usually seals the pharynx with a pressure of 16 to 24 cm H_2O, and this airway leak pressure is rarely above 30 cm H_2O. This relatively low-pressure seal means that when positive pressure is applied to the LMA Classic, gas leakage is common. Studies have shown a 5% failure rate for achieving an expired tidal volume of 10 mL/kg,[8] an audible leak in 48% of patients when ventilating to peak pressures of 17 to 19 cm H_2O, and a detectable leak rate as high as 90%, with an 8% failure rate for adequate ventilation.[9,10] Devitt and colleagues applied increasing peak airway pressures while ventilating through an LMA Classic. They found that as the airway pressure rose from 15 to 30 cm H_2O, the incidence of audible leak rose from 25% to 95%, and the leak fraction ([inspired minute volume–expired minute volume]/inspired minute volume) rose from 13% to 27%.[11] As the airway pressure increased, the incidence of airway leak into patients' stomachs rose from 2% to 35%. These findings indicate that the LMA Classic has a relatively low-pressure airway (pharyngeal) seal and that as higher airway pressures are applied, there is a risk of loss of ventilating gases and gastric inflation. Loss of ventilating gases is associated with hypoventilation, loss of anesthetic agent, and environmental pollution, and gastric inflation that may increase the risk of regurgitation.

B. Problems with Airway Protection

Several factors affect the risk of and protection against aspiration during use of a SAD. A device with a good pharyngeal seal minimizes the risk of air leak into the esophagus during positive-pressure ventilation, especially if airway pressures rise. A correctly positioned drain tube that is not obstructed by mucosa can vent gas entering the upper esophagus and minimize the risk of gastric inflation. If regurgitation does occur, a correctly positioned drain tube can vent liquid (and solids if large enough) so that it bypasses the oral cavity and alerts the anesthesiologist to the occurrence of regurgitation.

Several factors determine whether regurgitant fluid can enter the glottis: the seal between the tip of the SAD and the upper esophagus (i.e., esophageal seal), the bulk of the SAD in the hypopharynx and oral cavity, the pharyngeal seal, and perhaps the presence of a sump. Reliable placement of a gastric tube through a SAD enables stomach emptying and reduces the risk of regurgitation and aspiration. Many protective factors depend on correct positioning of the SAD. A device that is reliably placed in the correct position is likely to provide better protection. A malpositioned device likely disrupts the pharyngeal and esophageal seals, may displace or obstruct the drain tube, and may lead to high airway pressures during positive-pressure ventilation. The ability to check correct device position (e.g., PLMA) is another benefit. Among available SADs, the ProSeal LMA has the most evidence for protection against regurgitation and aspiration.

The LMA Classic is not regarded as providing protection against aspiration of regurgitated gastric contents and is contraindicated for patients who are not fasted or who may have a full stomach. The LMA Classic has a pharyngeal seal that is usually in the range of 16 to 24 cm H_2O. Its tip obturates the upper esophagus, and it has an esophageal seal of 40 to 50 cm H_2O, but it has no drain tube.[12] Despite this design, cadaver work shows the LMA Classic protects the glottis from regurgitant esophageal fluid considerably more efficiently than the unprotected airway.[13]

Soon after the introduction of the LMA Classic, several small studies raised concerns about the ability of the LMA Classic to protect the airway from regurgitant matter and therefore from pulmonary aspiration. Early concerns were raised that the LMA Classic, sitting at the back of the throat, might stimulate a swallowing reflex, especially during light planes of anesthesia, leading to relaxation of the upper and lower esophageal sphincters and increasing the risk of regurgitation and aspiration. A physiologic study recorded a fall in the lower esophageal barrier pressure of 4 cm H_2O during LMA Classic anesthesia, compared with a 2 cm H_2O rise during face mask anesthesia.[14] A study using swallowed methylene blue capsules demonstrated a 25% incidence of soiling of the inner portion of the LMA Classic on removal, and a small study reported a 2% incidence of aspiration, which occurred during spontaneous and controlled ventilation.[15,16]

As experience has accumulated, the evidence of a fundamental problem with aspiration has been reevaluated. Until 2004, 16 years after its introduction, there were no published reports of fatal aspiration during use of an LMA Classic. In 2004, Keller and colleagues published a series of three cases of serious morbidity, including one death from aspiration during LMA Classic anesthesia.[17] Each case had risk factors for aspiration, and on reviewing all 20 published reports of aspiration during use of an LMA Classic, the investigators found identifiable risk factors in 19 of 20 cases. In the accompanying editorial, Asai listed more than 40 factors that increased the risk of aspiration.[18] Several large studies have shown a low rate of aspiration; Verghese and Brimacombe reported a series of 11,910 uses (40% with controlled ventilation, 19% during intra-abdominal surgery, and 5% with a duration longer than 2 hours).[19] Insertion success rate was 99.8%, the incidence of airway-related critical incidents was 0.16% during spontaneous ventilation and 0.14% during controlled ventilation, and there was one case of aspiration. Bernardini and Natalini reported three aspirations in a series of 35,630 LMA Classic uses for controlled ventilation (1 of 11,877).[20] In an editorial, Sidaras and Hunter[21] estimated an incidence of confirmed pulmonary aspiration during LMA Classic use of 1 in 11,000, and Brimacombe and Berry's meta-analysis calculated a risk during elective surgery of 1 case in 4300 operations.[6] This is similar to the rate of aspiration reported by Warner and colleagues in a study of 214,000 patients predating use of the LMA, in which aspiration occurred in 1 in 4000 elective operations.[22]

Although the risk of aspiration is relatively low in expert hands, this rate is achieved primarily by careful and appropriate case selection, expert insertion, and meticulous management of the airway after insertion. The Fourth National Audit Project of the Royal College of Anaesthetists and Difficult Airway Society (NAP4) in the United Kingdom studied major airway complications of 2.9 million episodes of general anesthesia and found that aspiration was the most common cause of airway-related deaths.[1] One third of these complications occurred during maintenance with a LM or LMA in place, and for many of the patients, the risk of aspiration made this unwise.

Aspiration remains a significant cause of morbidity and mortality during anesthesia, and all anesthesiologists should consider the patient's risk for aspiration before selecting the appropriate airway device. In making that selection, they should consider the degree of protection provided by the airway device, particularly when using a SAD.

C. Problems with Accessing the Airway for Intubation

The LMA Classic sits over the vocal cords in more than 90% of cases and may be used as a conduit for intubation, but several factors limit the ease of this application.[23] The internal lumen of the device is relatively narrow, limiting the size of ETT that can be passed. Size 4 and 5 LMA Classic devices accommodate most manufacturers' cuffed ETTs with internal diameters (IDs) of 6.0 and 6.5 mm, respectively. A tube of adequate length must be used to exit the LMA Classic and reach the midtrachea; an ETT of approximately 29 cm can be placed through a size 5 LMA Classic. Across the distal end of the airway tube are two flexible bars forming a grill that prevents the tongue from impeding insertion and the epiglottis from

causing obstruction after placement; these bars may act as an impediment to intubation through an LMA Classic. The angle at which an ETT exits the mask of the LMA Classic means that blind insertion frequently leads to esophageal intubation. Brimacombe reported blind intubation with an ETT through the LMA Classic to have a first-time success rate of 52% and overall success rate of 59%.[24] Use of a bougie is less successful (32% of first attempts and 45% overall), and even fiberoptically guided techniques have a failure rate of 18%. After intubation has been achieved, removal of the LMA Classic without displacement of the ETT is cumbersome. Overall, direct intubation through the LMA Classic is a far from ideal technique.

The technique is dramatically improved if an Aintree intubation catheter (AIC, Cook Critical Care, Bloomington, IN) is used.[25] The hollow AIC (ID of 4.6 mm, external diameter [ED] of 7.0 mm, length of 46 cm) is placed over a fiberscope, the scope and AIC are negotiated through the LMA Classic into the midtrachea, and the fiberscope then is removed, followed by removal of the LMA Classic. Care must be taken to ensure the AIC is not advanced too far, especially if gases are passed through it, as this risks barotraumas. This technique can be performed with or without the use of a Bodai adapter (Sontek Medical, Lexington, MA). The Bodai adapter allows oxygen and gas administration through the attached breathing circuit during exchange of the LMA to an ETT. The AIC remains in place, and a suitably sized lubricated ETT is then advanced over the catheter. Although the AIC technique does not appear in current airway guidelines, its use is simple, has a high success rate, and is widely reported.[26,27]

D. Reusable Design

The LMA Classic is reusable and designed to be used up to 40 times. An in vitro study suggested that the LMA Classic and ProSeal LMA may be reused up to an average of 130 and 80 times, respectively, before showing signs of failing the preuse tests recommended by the manufacturer, and in vivo work supports use up to 60 times.[28,29]

After use, the LMA Classic is cleaned (decontaminated) before sterilization by autoclave (up to 137° C for 3 minutes with the cuff fully deflated), and it is stored in sterile packaging thereafter. A 2001 bench-top study demonstrated that routine decontamination and sterilization failed to remove all proteinaceous material from airway devices and from the LMA Classic in particular.[30] At the same time, there was increasing public awareness about variant Creutzfeldt-Jakob disease (vCJD), especially in the United Kingdom. Concerns grew that residual prions, the infective, misfolded proteins responsible for vCJD, might remain and be passed from patient to patient. Several national bodies recommended using single-use devices "wherever possible,"[31] even though the estimated risk of such cross-contamination was 1 to 10 cases in 100,000 patients.[32] Brimacombe and coworkers described the rush toward single-use LMs as "driven by fears of the unknown and scientific misinformation."[33] Since then, the risk of vCJD has fallen dramatically, and the risk of transmission is likely to be vanishingly small.[34]

This risk must be balanced against other risks introduced by alternative equipment.[35] Blunt and Burchett found that even a small deterioration in safety as a result of using a single-use device of poorer quality in place of a reusable device increased the overall risk to patients and went against the recommendation of the Spongiform Encephalopathy Advisory Committee (SEAC).[32]

E. Absence of a Bite Block

The LMA Classic lacks a bite block and is prone to obstruction by biting in the agitated patient during emergence. Use of a bite block (e.g., rolled gauze placed between the molar teeth) is recommended until the LMA Classic is removed, and failure to adhere to this recommendation can lead to airway obstruction, hypoxia, and postobstructive pulmonary edema.[36] The LMA Flexible also has no bite block, but the intubating LMA (ILMA), ProSeal, and Supreme LMA do.

IV. EFFICACY, SAFETY, AND EVALUATION OF SUPRAGLOTTIC AIRWAY DEVICES

The market for SADs is extensive, and in the United Kingdom, which represents only a fraction of the global market, estimated sales are in excess of $10,000,000 per annum. The LMA has five variations (i.e., Classic, Flexible, ILMA, ProSeal, and Supreme) or eight if single-use variants are included. At least 10 other SADs of different design to the LMA are on the market. In the past decade, production has ceased for at least six SADs, and it is inevitable that in the next decade more new devices will arrive and some currently in use will depart.

About 30 distinct single-use and reusable LMs are marketed. They are somewhat different from one another in design and in manufacturing materials and processes. If all variants are included, more than 40 SADs are available for nonintubated adult patients.

A small survey of SAD manufacturers in 2003 examined several devices introduced around that time[35] and found that the number of patients in whom the device had been used before marketing was less than 150 all in cases but one. In most cases, no trials were published in peer-reviewed journals before launching the product. One device launched in 2001 and remained without published data 18 months later. Only two of seven devices were compared with the LMA Classic in randomized, controlled trials before marketing, and the largest of them enrolled only 60 patients. This situation has not changed, and many later devices have been introduced with little or no trial evidence of their efficacy.

How does an anesthesiologist start using a new airway device? Typically, a company representative supplies a few anesthesiologists with samples of the new device and provides education in its use. The anesthesiologists try the device on a few patients and form an opinion. Hundreds of anesthesiologists may go through this process, exposing perhaps thousands of patients to relatively untested devices before a consensus is reached. The quality of each evaluation varies with the individual's practice, experience, and diligence. Companies may use informal comments from one user to encourage other users. Individual uptake may be swayed considerably by limited personal experiences, and new devices can be introduced without adequate evaluation of clinical efficacy or safety, or the devices can be rejected without due cause. Some companies restrict the distribution of new devices to a few hospitals or to experts in the field. Others attempt to collect an informal assessment of the device's performance each time it is used. Some perform extensive laboratory, model, and clinical evaluations before marketing, but these practices are far from universal.

This raises a question about whether it is acceptable to evaluate new devices in such an ad hoc manner. This process should be contrasted with the introduction of a new drug, which must go through laboratory and preclinical studies even before clinical trials are considered. Results of the three phases of clinical trials are reviewed before release of the drug to the market, and postmarketing surveillance is mandatory and extensive.

What regulations govern the introduction of new medical devices, particularly airway devices? In the European Union, the use of medical devices is controlled by three European Directives as part of European law.[36] Some directives are specifically applicable to airway devices, and adherence is overseen by a regulatory body in each member country. The statutory body has responsibility for ensuring that medical devices do not threaten patients' health and safety. Statutory requirements are largely harmonized throughout Europe, and compliance with one country's requirements allows distribution and marketing of a device throughout the European Union. Although many countries have mechanisms that are designed to critically examine the efficacy of new technologies (e.g., National Institute of Clinical Excellence [NICE] in the United Kingdom), these bodies often have specific conditions (e.g., for NICE, new technology for new procedures) such that new (airway) equipment designed to do an old job tends to fall outside their areas of inspection and regulation.

The statutory requirements of safety and quality do include a statement to the effect that the device should function as intended by the manufacturer. However, in practice, the statutory assessments focus on production quality control and manufacturing standards. A mixture of self-assessment and external assessment is obtained, depending on the risk that the device may pose to patients. These assessments must be passed to allow continued marketing of a device. Airway devices are considered to be of low or intermediate risk and are primarily subject to manufacturers' self-assessment. Performance of the desired function, efficacy, and cost-effectiveness are not a focus of these assessments. Passing the statutory requirements and obtaining a Conformité Européenne (i.e., European Conformity [CE]) mark allows marketing of the device throughout Europe, and member countries are not allowed to impose other barriers to trade after a CE mark is applied. The CE mark implies that the device is fit for its intended purpose, but assessment of performance, efficacy, and cost-effectiveness are left to the manufacturers, distributors, and end users in the postmarketing phase.

After a device is marketed, clinical trials are not required to demonstrate efficacy or quality of performance. Manufacturers are legally bound to report serious or potentially serious adverse incidents.[37] The statutory body requires reporting of incidences in which "malfunction of or deterioration in the characteristics and performance of a device" leads to "actual or potential patient harm."[37] There is also a mechanism for voluntary reporting of incidents by users. Whether these mechanisms lead to reliable reporting of such incidents and whether these schemes identify devices that are poorly designed or underperform is not clear. Formal assessment of performance may come from postmarketing cohort or comparative studies. However, these studies are uncommon, and they usually are published at some interval after a device has been marketed.

Lack of timely reporting creates another problem. In light of clinical experience and customer feedback, new devices are often redesigned after their initial release onto the market. These "improved" devices go through a similar process to that described earlier, and they are again brought to market. Second-, third-, and fourth-iteration devices may then appear, often under the same name as the original. For example, one SAD was modified three times (the four versions were named identically) in the 18 months after it was initially marketed. Publication delay compounds the confusion, because the unsuspecting reader of journals may not realize that a recently published paper relates to a device that has subsequently been modified. Performance of the old version may be very different from that of the current version. In one review of the SAD with four versions, one half of the cited papers related to previous versions of the device. Although this does not make trials of the previous version of each device completely redundant, it does make interpretation of the limited data more difficult. It would arguably be better to determine the desirable features of a new airway device and use these to assess the design and function of it before and after it is marketed.

A. Desirable Features of Supraglottic Airway Devices

Certain issues influence the anesthesiologist's choice of an airway for an individual patient. Should the anesthesiologist choose a single-use device, a device that can be reused most often, the cheapest device, or the device that causes the least trauma? Do all devices maintain the airway reliably? To what extent do any of them protect the airway from regurgitation and pulmonary aspiration? Which devices enable safe and effective positive-pressure ventilation? Will the device enable access to the airway for intubation if required? Are there differences in ease of insertion and ability to ventilate patients' lungs between the various devices? How often are manipulations needed to maintain a clear airway during anesthesia? Which devices are tolerated best during emergence? What are the relative incidences of airway trauma and postoperative pharyngolaryngeal morbidity? Unfortunately, in most cases, remarkably few of these data are available. The manner in which new medical devices are regulated contributes to this situation.

The characteristics of an ideal SAD include efficacy, versatility, safety, reusability, and cost. The device should be made of good-quality, nontoxic materials and have a long shelf-life. Reusable devices should be robust enough to allow many uses and cleaning cycles without damage or deterioration of performance, and other desirable features may reflect the preferences of anesthesiologists and their patients.

The anesthesiologist wants a device that is inserted reliably on the first attempt, producing a clear airway for spontaneous and controlled ventilation. It should enable maintenance of hands-free anesthesia in a variety of patients in various head and neck positions. Device performance should be consistent and predictable, and it should allow emergence without complications. The incidence of airway trauma and postoperative sore throat should be acceptably low. Design features or clinical evidence for protection against aspiration is highly desirable, and the ability to reach the trachea through the device may also be a factor in choosing a SAD. It should function reliably as a rescue device and for difficult airway management. The ideal device should not cause intraoperative complications, trauma, or pharyngolaryngeal morbidity for the patient.

The anesthesiologist should be able to insert the SAD despite a limited mouth opening (most require 2 to 3 cm) and using a light depth of anesthesia (dose range for different airways varies approximately twofold). SADs requiring a muscle relaxant for insertion are of limited use.

All SADs may cause airway obstruction from epiglottic downfolding. This problem can be reduced by ensuring correct insertion technique and by using devices designed with a slim leading edge and a large airway orifice. The slim profile of the deflated Laryngeal Tube (LT, King Systems, Noblesville, IN) and LMA Classic and the deflation device and tip flattener that are provided with the PLMA are examples of designs that minimize the tip size. The epiglottis may cause obstruction by entering the orifice of the airway device. Several design features are aimed at avoiding this problem, including epiglottic bars (e.g., LMA Classic, LMA Flexible, some newer LMs), a large orifice that is too big to become obstructed (e.g., PLMA, i-gel), multiple airway holes (e.g., Combitube, LT), and an orifice with protective fins (e.g., Supreme LMA).

The first-time insertion success rate should be high, and initial insertion should require a minimum of manipulations. With current devices, the first-time insertion success rate ranges from less than 70% to more than 95%. The average number of manipulations required for insertion ranges from less than one manipulation in 25 cases to more than one per case.

The anesthesiologist requires an airway that does not require manipulations after insertion or repositioning during anesthesia, enabling hands-free anesthesia. The most functional devices require an intervention in less than 1 in 25 cases, but others require intervention in two thirds of cases.

The airway should be stable when the head and neck position varies, such as during rotation to improve surgical access or when the head and neck are repositioned for additional procedures. Limited evidence suggests that the stability of different SADs under these circumstances varies.

Intraoperative complications (e.g., airway obstruction, loss of airway, regurgitation, laryngospasm) should be uncommon. The published incidence of minor complications with existing devices ranges from less than 10% to 60%. Serious and minor repetitive complications or the need to perform repeated or continuous manipulations to maintain the airway may force early removal of the airway. This is the ultimate failure of the airway device, and it occurs with an incidence of less than 1 in 50 cases to more than 1 in 5 cases.

The ideal SAD should be reliable for spontaneous and controlled ventilation. Among the existing devices, several versions of one device function poorly during spontaneous ventilation, and another is designed specifically to facilitate controlled rather than spontaneous ventilation. Several devices that produce a low-pressure seal with the airway may be unsuitable during controlled ventilation because of the risk of gastric inflation and regurgitation. The role of second-generation SADs in protection of the airway is discussed later.

The ideal airway device causes no trauma to the airway. The incidence of trauma to the airway with the latest SADs, as evidenced by blood visible on the device, ranges from close to 0% to more than 50%. SADs commonly cause sore throat, dysphonia, and dysphagia, but these symptoms are usually minor, transient, and less common than after tracheal intubation. The possibility of nerve injuries is a greater concern. The ideal airway minimizes or eliminates both of these problems. However, the intra-cuff and mucosal pressures vary in intensity and location with different SADs. The overall incidence of sore throat varies from less than 10% to more than 40%. Clinically significant nerve injury is rare with all SADs, and the relative risks of individual devices are unknown.

In addition to maintaining the airway during anesthesia, a SAD may enable access to the airway. It is easy for this role to be overemphasized, because during routine anesthesia, it is rare that the SAD needs to be changed for an ETT, and when this exchange is required, the SAD usually can be removed before intubation is attempted conventionally. If the SAD is likely to be needed as a conduit for planned tracheal intubation or for management of a difficult airway, the device may be selected accordingly. The intubating LMA (ILMA) and Cookgas intubating laryngeal airway (ILA) are designed specifically for these roles, and several others (e.g., i-gel, PLMA) are likely to perform similarly well. Several techniques may be used, including blind use of an ETT or bougie and light-guided and fiberoptically guided techniques with an ETT or exchange catheter. Such techniques require the larynx to be visible from the airway orifice and the internal diameter of the SAD lumen and its orifice to be of adequate caliber. For various devices, the ability to view the laryngeal inlet from the airway orifice ranges from more than 90% to less than 40%. Variations in length and diameter limit the techniques that may be used with certain SADs. The proximal orifice of some SADs is too small to admit an ETT with an ID larger than 5.0 mm, whereas others accommodate ETTs with

an 8.0-mm ID. At their distal end, grills, bars, small orifices, and difficult angles may impede or prevent access to the trachea.

Although most devices are used by anesthesiologists, SADs may be used by individuals with less experience for anesthesia, out-of-hospital rescue, or resuscitation. The ideal airway should therefore be intuitive to use, have a high success rate for the naive user, and be easy to learn. The few available data suggest that insertion and airway maintenance by nonanesthesiologists and by naive users varies considerably among devices.

Many assume that reusable devices may be replaced by cheaper, single-use devices, and some think that single-use devices are intrinsically preferable. However, many single-use devices differ from the reusable devices they seek to replace in design and in the materials used. Some modifications appear to be minor, but the implications for performance have generally not been evaluated. The work on single-use laryngoscopes and intubation bougies provides evidence that changes in product material may alter performance considerably.[38,39] Data on the current versions of the single-use LM and comparisons between these and the LMA Classic remain largely unavailable.

No single device meets all the criteria for the ideal SAD. Some criteria are incompatible with others. For instance, a device that is large enough to accommodate a standard-sized ETT and that incorporates an adequate-caliber drain tube is unlikely to be as easily inserted as a smaller device. Epiglottic bars reduce airway obstruction but hinder instrumental access to the trachea. A single-use device is less likely than a more expensive reusable device to be made of the best materials to optimize handling characteristics and minimize pharyngolaryngeal trauma. It is likely that several different airways will always be needed for use in different clinical situations.

B. Efficacy Versus Safety

SADs may have several roles, and different designs and performance characteristics may be required for each role. The LMA Classic was originally used almost exclusively to provide anesthesia for brief, peripheral operations that were performed in slim patients, usually during spontaneous ventilation. The popularity of the LMA Classic has led to an evolution in practice such that SADs have become increasingly used for longer, more complex operations and for obese patients. SADs are increasingly used for laparoscopic and open intra-abdominal surgery, and their use during controlled ventilation has become commonplace.

Many of these expanded indications can benefit patients, but they also raise questions about efficacy and safety. During spontaneous ventilation, the LMA Classic provides a clear airway and enables hands-free anesthesia in more than 95% of cases. Efficacy of the LMA Classic for controlled ventilation diminishes rapidly as lung resistance increases (e.g., obesity, laparoscopy), and rates of hypoventilation and gastric distention increase, raising concerns about the safety of its use in these situations.

In the past decade, more than 40 SADs have been introduced. Most are attempts to mimic and compete with the LMA Classic to appeal to purchasers and managers. Anesthesiologists are more interested in SAD designs that improve performance (i.e., efficacy and safety) and thereby increase their clinical utility.

Many studies comparing SADs have been inadequately powered to determine efficacy, and none has addressed the issue of safety directly. Efficacy depends on several factors, including ease of insertion, manipulations required to maintain a clear airway throughout anesthesia, and tolerance during emergence. Efficacy during controlled ventilation requires the ventilation orifice of the SAD to be positioned over the larynx, and the SAD must seal well within the laryngopharynx (i.e., pharyngeal seal).

Safety encompasses avoidance of complications occurring at all stages of anesthesia and afterward. Prevention of aspiration requires a good-quality seal within the laryngopharynx and esophagus (i.e., esophageal seal) to prevent gas leaking into the esophagus and stomach and to prevent regurgitant matter passing from the esophagus into the airway. A functioning drain tube enables regurgitant matter to bypass the larynx and be vented outside, protecting the airway and giving an early indication of regurgitation to the anesthesiologist. Studies have shown that the extent of esophageal seal varies considerably among SADs. Those with a drain tube can effectively vent regurgitant fluid if the drain is not occluded.[12,40,41]

C. Structured Approaches to Evaluation of New Devices

New airway devices should undergo mandatory assessment of manufacturing quality and clinical performance before marketing. The characteristics of the ideal SAD outlined earlier provide a checklist against which function can be assessed. Several methods have been recommended.[35,42,43] Cook described a three-stage evaluation process[35]:

Stage 1. Bench evaluation using manikins or models designed to test function and basic safety
Stage 2. A rigorous cohort study to determine whether the device is effective and to further exclude major concerns about safety
Stage 3. A randomized, controlled trial against the current gold standard for the procedure for which the new device is expected to be used (e.g., LMA Classic, PLMA, ILMA)

In stage 1, the bench models include airway manikins and others, such as those specifically designed to test aspiration risk.[44] This stage is limited by lack of fidelity of available manikins.[45] With the increasing use of SADs during resuscitation, during out-of-hospital rescue, and by non-anesthesiologists, there is an urgent need to develop realistic manikins for testing and training. Data acquired from such studies require intelligent interpretation and knowledge of the relative performance of different manikins.[46-48] Results of manikins studies are considerably limited, and at best, they may be used to evaluate basic information on device performance and

durability and to identify major conceptual or design problems. Appropriate bench testing may lead to further development of a device before starting clinical studies.

In stage 2, a cohort study may be used for the first assessment of clinical performance in patients. This approach enables full clinical evaluation of the new device under routine clinical conditions. Functions that can be tested include ease of insertion, pharyngeal seal, airway resistance, stability of the device in different head and neck positions, ease of passage of a gastric tube, positioning of the airway over the larynx, and suitability for fiberscopic or catheter exchange techniques. Learning curves can be examined. A cohort study also enables assessment of function during spontaneous and controlled ventilation and determination of airway trauma or pharyngolaryngeal morbidity. The cohort must be large enough to enable identification of common problems, but unless it is very large, it cannot detect uncommon or rare problems. For instance, for an event that does not occur in a cohort study of n cases, the 95% confidence interval (CI) for frequency of that event is approximately 1 in $3/n$.[49] For example, if no nerve injuries occur in a cohort study of 100 cases, the upper limit of the 95% CI for risk of nerve injury is 1 in 33. A cohort of at least 100 patients is a reasonable compromise between being large enough to identify important uncommon events and remaining a practical size.

Stage 3 employs a randomized, controlled trial. After successful completion of bench and cohort evaluations, the need for further modifications of the device should be considered. Significant modifications necessitate repetition of the early evaluations. On successful completion of the early evaluations, the new device should be compared with its best existing competitor. In many cases, this is the LMA Classic. The randomized, controlled trial must be of adequate size to identify clinically important differences in function. Studies may be designed to test the hypothesis that the devices perform differently (i.e., superiority-inferiority trials) or that the test device does not perform significantly less well than the benchmark device (i.e., noninferiority trials).[50] Power calculations can be based on data acquired from phase 2, but trials of at least 100 patients provide more comprehensive and clinically useful comparisons. Economic evaluation of cost-effectiveness of the new device may take place at this stage. Data from the three phases of evaluation can be used to determine what role the new airway device has in the market.

In an ideal world, a license for only one aspect of airway care (e.g., spontaneous breathing only, controlled ventilation in patients with good pulmonary compliance, airway maintenance when tracheal access is likely to be necessary) would be offered based on the results of research. License extensions could be granted in light of further research. Current legislation designed to encourage market competition means that no such limits are imposed, as they are in drug development.

Implementation of the suggested methodology would still result in only 200 to 300 uses of the device in patients before release to market. Because this number is not enough to identify uncommon or unexpected problems, complications, and advantages, the proposed method of evaluation does not obviate the need for post-marketing surveillance or reporting of adverse incidents. A formal method of postmarketing evaluation could be developed. For instance, the first 5000 devices marketed could have evaluation cards attached, which would be returned after use. Some SAD manufacturers have used such a system in the past without making the resultant information available to the profession. Alternatively, the manufacturer could be required to seek reports of all adverse incidents for the first 2 years after release, similar to the Yellow Card system for new drugs that applies in the United Kingdom.

A second structured approach to evaluating and choosing new devices was made by Wilkes and colleagues.[43] In this proposal, a central body of experts would coordinate research to evaluate new devices, review available evidence and provide national recommendations on devices reaching standards of acceptability. Although potentially of value for a large population (e.g., a country), the barrier it may create to free trade and the likelihood of legal challenges are problems.

The UK Difficult Airway Society (DAS) has proposed a guideline whereby purchasers could adopt a minimum level of evidence before making a pragmatic decision about the purchase or use of an airway device.[42] This minimum level of evidence (i.e., level 3b: a case- or historical-controlled cohort study) would form the basis of a professional standard to guide those with responsibility for selecting airway devices.[51] Devices without this minimum level of evidence would not be purchased. The investigators argue that widespread adoption of this professional standard would lead to situations in which it was in the interests of manufacturers and purchasers to acquire such evidence and the DAS would support both parties in setting up research with this aim. The strength of this approach lies in purchasers driving the need to raise the evidence bar and manufacturers being encouraged to perform clinical trials at an early stage in device development. This approach is not anticompetitive because it creates no barriers to manufacturers bringing a device to market, but it does raise the level of expectation of the community of purchasers about what they wish to purchase.

Whether any of these methods of structured evaluation are officially adopted, each has potential advantages for the manufacturer, clinician, and patient. For successful devices, the manufacturer would have robust data to support performance claims and a clearer vision of the likely advantages and applications of the new device. This would enhance marketing and raise credibility. For devices that performed poorly, the manufacturer could avoid the expense of large-scale production and marketing of devices that would ultimately fail to achieve market share. The clinician would have better evidence on which to base medical decisions. Researchers would have clearer ideas about how a new device might be evaluated to define function further and investigate wider indications for use. The patient would be less likely to be exposed to unnecessary risk due to the use of an unevaluated device.

Anesthesiologists and patients expect equipment to be effective and safe during anesthesia. The relationship between manufacturer and clinician (acting for the patient) is symbiotic. Care of patients can improve only through a sustained effort by clinicians and manufacturers to improve the medical devices used during anesthesia. In this respect, much has been achieved in airway care in the past 20 years, and the practice of anesthesia has been transformed. Innovation is expensive, and much of the cost of advances or improvements accrues during research and development. This cost is borne entirely by the manufacturer. A more open relationship between interested parties and the early involvement of objective, structured evaluation of new airway equipment are recommended. This approach could prevent undertested or underdeveloped products from coming to market and thereby protect patients medically and manufacturers legally. An evaluation program should encourage and support equipment manufacturers to achieve these goals.

V. FIRST-GENERATION SUPRAGLOTTIC AIRWAY DEVICES

A. Generic Laryngeal Masks

Since 2005, many manufacturers have produced LMA-like devices designed to compete with LMAs. They included single-use (mostly polyvinyl chloride [PVC]) and reusable (PVC and silicone) devices. Because the term *laryngeal mask airway* (LMA) is registered, the newer devices are referred to as *laryngeal masks* (LMs). The manufacturers assert that the main driving force for the introduction of single-use devices has been the concerns about the sterility of cleaned, reusable devices. The financial opportunities of the SAD market are another reason for the increase in these devices.

For patent reasons, all LMs are different from the LMA Classic, and much variation exists between LMs. The patent on the basic design of the LMA Classic lapsed in 2005, but the patent for the epiglottic grills remained in place until 2008. All LMs designed before 2008, except those made by the original manufacturers of the LMA Classic, do not have the epiglottic bars at the distal end of the airway tube; some recent entrants into the market do. Some LMs have angulated stems, and others have enlarged masks. Some early LM designs featured more bulky masks and cuffs than the LMA Classic, and this design and the stiffer PVC material of which they were made impeded insertion. Particularly with the larger masks, there is a possibility of entrapping the tongue and drawing it backward during insertion (causing trauma) and downfolding the epiglottis after it is inserted (causing obstruction and trauma).

For cost reasons, most single-use LMs are made with a PVC cuff, which increases the rigidity of the device. PVC is cheaper than silicone and reduces the cost of these devices for the manufacturer and purchaser. PVC is less permeable to nitrous oxide than silicone, and during nitrous oxide administration, the increase in LM cuff pressure in the early phase of anesthesia is considerably less than when using a silicone device.[52,53]

PVC has two disadvantages. First, it is more rigid than silicone. Brain examined PVC as a material for LMA construction in the mid-1980s but rejected it because of its rigidity.[54] The increased rigidity of PVC LMs may cause problems, such as increased trauma to the airway during use and an increase in pharyngolaryngeal morbidity postoperatively. The rigidity, especially in masks with thicker cuffs, may lead to folds and wrinkles in the partially inflated cuff, which may affect the airway seal or create channels that enable regurgitant fluid to reach the larynx, altering efficacy and safety. The impact of these effects is not known for many devices because of the lack of published evidence. Some manufacturers use a softer form of siliconized PVC, which may obviate the problems described.

The second concern is the toxicity of phthalates, such as di-2-ethylhexyl phthalate (DEHP) or dioctyl phthalate (DOP), which are used in the manufacturing process to render the PVC softer. These chemicals are not linked to the plastic matrix and leach out slowly during use. They are considered potentially carcinogenic, mutagenic, and reprotoxic,[55] and there is particular concern about phthalates in products that may be placed in the mouth (e.g., children's toys, airway devices). The issue has been considered important enough by some for bills banning PVC in some products to be brought before the legislatures of some U.S. states and the European Parliament. Phthalates are banned from use in cosmetics in Europe, and in May 2005, the European Parliament voted to make permanent a temporary ban on six phthalates (including DEHP) in PVC used in children's toys and called for investigation into health care equipment.[55] It is easy to overstate the importance of phthalates in the safety of PVC LMs, but the unquantified low risk they pose bears comparison with the unquantified low risk of transmission of prion disease when using a reusable device. Alternative plasticizers, such as no-DOP formulas and di-isononyl-cyclohexane dicarboxylate (Hexamoll DINCH) are available for use in PVC applications, although at considerably increased cost. In the past few years, an increasing number of low-cost silicone LMs designed for single use and reuse have been introduced.

The greatest concern about the profusion of LMs on the market is the lack of rigorous evaluation. Typically, there is no robust evidence to inform whether the single-use or reusable LMs perform similarly to equivalent LMAs or to inform which LM performs best. The limited evidence does show that all LMs and LMAs are not equivalent. Of the approximately 30 devices available, only 2 have substantial publications that compare their efficacy with that of LMAs: the AuraOnce LM (Ambu Inc., Glen Burnie, MD) and the Portex Soft Seal LM (SSLM, Smiths Medical ASD, Keene, NH). For the other devices, there appears to be a void of published evidence. A publication from the National Health Service (NHS) Centre for Evidence-Based Purchasing illustrates the difficulty in determining the relative merits and demerits of these competitors to the LMA Classic. The document listed more than 25 alternative standard LMs and reported a total of 18 comparative trials for the devices. Some of these studies were of poor quality. This publication record contrasts with the more than 2500 publications on the LMA Classic.[56]

B. Features of Laryngeal Masks

1. Indications, Advantages, and Disadvantages

LMs are intended for use for the same indications as the LMA Classic—as an alternative to the face mask for achieving and maintaining control of the airway during routine anesthesia in fasted patients. They may be used for critical anesthesia procedures (e.g., airway rescue after failed mask ventilation, after failed intubation). LMs also may be used to establish a clear airway during resuscitation in the profoundly unconscious patient with absent glossopharyngeal and laryngeal reflexes who may need artificial ventilation. LMs are not intended to replace all functions of the ETT and are best suited for use in fasted patients undergoing surgical procedures in which tracheal intubation is not deemed necessary. However, in certain circumstances, procedures previously requiring intubation because face mask anesthesia was not suitable (e.g., airway access, hand position) may be suitably performed using a LM or LMA.

The disadvantages and advantages of LMs are extrapolated from the extensive evidence for the LMA Classic to LMs because of their design similarities. However, equality of performance for the LMA Classic and many LMs has not been confirmed. For most standard LMs, the airway seal is modest (16 to 24 cm H_2O). There are no specific design features to prevent aspiration, although good technique and insertion can minimize this risk by ensuring the mask encircles the larynx and the tip obturates the upper esophageal inlet. Standard LMs may be used during spontaneous ventilation or controlled ventilation. If used for controlled ventilation, peak airway pressure should be limited to less than 20 cm H_2O to avoid airway leak and gastric inflation. LMs therefore may not be appropriate for patients with reduced lung compliance or increased airway resistance. Airway resistance during ventilation increases dramatically if the LM is poorly positioned over the larynx or if laryngeal closure occurs due to an inadequate depth of anesthesia. The major disadvantage of LMs is that they do not protect against aspiration and do not secure the airway as effectively as an ETT. A LM cannot prevent or treat airway obstruction at or beyond the larynx.

2. Laryngeal Masks Compared with Face Mask Ventilation and Tracheal Intubation

LMs reduce dead space ventilation compared with face mask ventilation. If reasonable airway pressures are used and the mask is correctly positioned, gastric inflation is unlikely. Use of a LM or any SAD enables anesthesiologists to have their hands free for other tasks. Compression of the eyes and facial and infraorbital nerves is avoided, and operating room pollution from anesthetic gases is reduced.

Compared with ETTs, LMs are easier to place, do not require laryngoscopy and its associated problems, and are less invasive. Insertion does not require the use of muscle relaxants. Insertion causes negligible cardiovascular stimulation, and increases in intraocular pressure are minimal at insertion and removal. Removal of LMs can be delayed until the patient is fully awake with the return of protective airway reflexes. Coughing and hypoxia occur less frequently compared with removal of an ETT.

C. Single-Use Laryngeal Masks

Several single-use LMs and LMAs including flexible devices have been introduced in the past few years. Performance must be assumed because performance evaluations and comparative trials have not been performed.

In the United Kingdom, the Department of Health advises that all airway equipment used for tonsillectomy should be single use, and this recommendation is endorsed by the Royal College of Anaesthetists and other professional bodies. NICE did not consider LMAs when examining the risk of vCJD transmission. In this climate, the single-use LMA Flexible is likely to have a significant role. Two single-use LMs—the AuraOnce and the SSLM—have a significant body of published literature that allows a balanced analysis of their performance.

1. Ambu AuraOnce Laryngeal Mask

The Ambu AuraOnce LM was designed and produced between the fall of 2002 and February 2004, when it was launched by the Danish medical device manufacturer Ambu. Ambu offers a range of LMs. The Ambu Aura-Once is a single-use LM with a preformed curve. The Ambu Aura40 is a reusable version of the Ambu Aura-Once. The Ambu AuraSraight is a single-use device with a more conventional curve to the stem. The Ambu Aura-Flex is a single-use, reinforced, flexible LM, and the Ambu Aura-i is a modification of the AuraOnce that is designed to facilitate intubation in a fashion similar to that of the ILMA.

The Ambu AuraOnce is the most investigated model. It is a sterile, single-use product made of PVC with a preformed curve designed to replicate human anatomy (Fig. 23-2). This angled curve is designed to ensure that the patient's head remains in a natural position when the mask is in use and to facilitate insertion without exerting force on the upper jaw. A reinforced tip reduces the risk of the device folding back during insertion. Reinforcing internal ribs built into the curve of the airway tube provide a degree of flexibility and enable the airway tube to conform to individual anatomic variations and adapt to a wide range of head positions without loss of function.

The Ambu AuraOnce is molded in one piece with an integrated inflation line and no epiglottic bars at the airway orifice. The cuff is elliptical and is shaped to lie in the hypopharynx at the base of the tongue. The absence of epiglottic bars means there is no barrier to flexible fiberoptic devices. The product is sterile and latex free and is available in adult and pediatric sizes 1 through 5. The recommended size is based on the weight and height of the patient.

The Ambu Aura40 is the reusable, silicone version of the Ambu AuraOnce.[40] Its built-in curve is designed o replicate the natural human anatomy and offers the same features as the Ambu AuraOnce. It can be steam autoclaved up to 40 times.

The Ambu Aura-i (Fig. 23-3) is a modification of the Ambu AuraOnce that is designed to facilitate intubation in a fashion similar to that of the ILMA. It has a shorter, wider, and more rigid airway tube than the Ambu Aura-Once, and proximally, a rigid plastic sleeve acts as a handle for insertion and as a bite block. It is designed for use during routine airway maintenance and as a device for airway rescue and fiberoptic intubation. Sizes 3, 4, and 5 accommodate ETTs up to sizes 6.5-, 7.5-, and 8-mm ID, respectively. Ambu has released a single-use videoscope that may be used with the Ambu Aura-i.

a. APPLICATION

Familiarity with the manufacturer's warnings, precautions, indications, and contraindications is necessary before use, and the patient should be at an adequate depth of anesthesia (or unconsciousness) before attempting insertion. Before insertion, the following guidelines should be observed:

- The size of the Ambu AuraOnce must be appropriate for the patient. Use the manufacturer's guidelines combined with clinical judgment to select the correct size. Always have a spare Ambu AuraOnce ready for use.
- Resistance or swallowing may indicate inadequate anesthesia or inappropriate technique, or both.

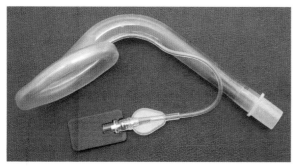

Figure 23-2 Ambu AuraOnce laryngeal mask as delivered. The red "tab" keeps the pilot balloon valve open so the cuff pressure is maintained at atmospheric pressure.

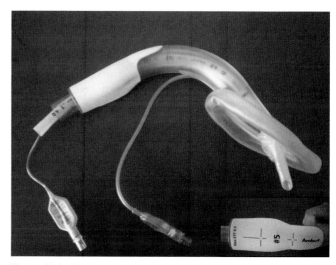

Figure 23-3 The Ambu Aura-i laryngeal mask with a tracheal tube passed through it illustrating its role as a conduit. Inset shows markings on posterior of stem.

Inexperienced users should choose a deeper level of anesthesia.

- The Ambu AuraOnce is inserted in a fashion similar to that described for the traditional LMAs in Chapter 22. Excess force must be avoided at all times. When the mask is fully inserted, resistance is felt. If the cuff fails to flatten or curls over as it is advanced, it is necessary to withdraw the mask and reinsert it. In case of tonsillar obstruction, a diagonal shift of the mask is often successful.

Intubation techniques through the Ambu AuraOnce are the same as those described earlier for the LMA Classic. The preformed curve may make this slightly less easy than in the more smoothly curved LMA Classic, but this difficulty is easily overcome with lubrication. The absence of bars at the end of the airway tube is an advantage over the LMA Classic.

The Ambu Aura-i is a single-use device that may be used in preference to the Ambu AuraOnce if intubation through the device is anticipated or planned.

b. INDICATIONS, ADVANTAGES, AND DISADVANTAGES

The Ambu AuraOnce has several features of potential advantage over some other LM designs. Its cuff is soft and flexible but has a reinforced tip; together with the preformed curve of the stem, these features facilitate insertion. Because it is molded in a single unit, it is free from ridges that may injure the airway during insertion, and component parts cannot separate during use.

Its disadvantages are those of all LMs. If used for controlled ventilation, the manufacturers recommend limiting peak airway pressure to 20 cm H_2O and the tidal volume to 8 mL/kg[2].

c. MEDICAL LITERATURE

Approximately 25 publications about the Ambu Aura-Once are listed on PubMed.

COHORT STUDIES. A multicenter study of the clinical performance of the Ambu AuraOnce was conducted by Hagberg and colleagues to evaluate ease of insertion, insertion success, airway seal, and ventilation.[57] Device placement was successful in all 118 nonparalyzed, anesthetized patients on the first or second attempt (92.4% and 7.6%, respectively). Adequate ventilation was achieved in all patients, and the vocal cords could be visualized by fiberoptic endoscopy in 91.5% of patients. Complications and patients' complaints were minor and were quickly resolved. The investigators reported that the curvature of the tube facilitated insertion and that the large, soft cuff allowed a higher oropharyngeal leak pressure than is commonly found in other LMs. The reinforced tip of the Ambu AuraOnce may avoid folding, which can lead to air leakage, a common problem with other LMs.

Genzwuerker and coworkers studied ventilation using the Ambu AuraOnce in different head positions in 30 patients.[58] Five different head positions were used: head on a standard pillow, head rotated 90 degrees to the left side, head rotated 90 degrees to the right side, head with chin lift on a standard pillow, and head flat on a table without a pillow. No changes in the performance of the device were observed in any position. The Ambu Aura-Once may be a useful SAD for cases in which head movement may be necessary during surgery.

RANDOMIZED, CONTROLLED STUDIES OF EFFICACY. Shariffuddin and Wang compared the Ambu AuraOnce with the LMA Classic during controlled ventilation in 40 patients in a randomized, crossover design.[59] The mean ± standard deviation oropharyngeal leak pressure was higher for the Ambu AuraOnce (19 ± 7.5 cm H_2O) than for the LMA Classic (15 ± 5.2 cm H_2O, P = 0.004). The Ambu AuraOnce also required fewer insertion attempts (P = 0.02) but more manipulations to achieve a patent airway (P = 0.045). Values for time to insert the device and intraoperative performance were similar.

Sudhir and associates performed a randomized, crossover study comparing the Ambu AuraOnce and LMA Classic in 50 patients.[60] Success rates for the first attempt success were similar (92% for the Ambu AuraOnce and 84% for the LMA Classic, P = 0.22). The volumes of air required to inflate the cuff to produce an effective airway seal were similar, but the cuff pressure was lower for the Ambu AuraOnce (median, 18 cm H_2O) compared with LMA Classic (27 cm H_2O, P = 0.007). Complications were similar in both groups.

Ng and coworkers compared the Ambu AuraOnce with the LMA Classic and reported the Ambu AuraOnce to be easier to insert, but they found no difference in time to insertion,[61] successful insertion on the first attempt, oropharyngeal leak pressure, hemodynamic response to insertion, or complications of placement.

Francksen and colleagues compared the performance of the Ambu AuraOnce and the LMA Unique in 80 patients undergoing minor routine gynecologic surgery.[62] They demonstrated that the time to insertion and failure rate were comparable and that oxygenation and ventilation variables were adequate with either device. Median airway leak pressures were slightly higher with the Ambu AuraOnce than with the LMA Unique (18 versus 16 cm H_2O, P < 0.013). No gastric inflation was observed with either device in this small study.

Francksen and coworkers also studied 120 patients scheduled for routine minor obstetric surgery who were randomly allocated to size 4 Ambu AuraOnce, LMA Unique, or SSLM.[63] The Ambu AuraOnce was fastest to insert by a few seconds. All three had high first-attempt insertion success rates (all >95%). Rates of subjectively rated excellent insertion were 75% for the LMA Unique, 70% for the Ambu AuraOnce, and 65% for the SSLM. All devices were judged acceptable.

Lopez and colleagues compared four single-use LMs (i.e., Ambu AuraOnce, Solus LM, LMA Unique, and SSLM) in 200 patients with ASA physical status class I, II, or III who were undergoing elective ambulatory surgery and for whom airway management was performed by inexperienced residents.[64] The Ambu AuraOnce (78%) and LMA Unique (80%) performed best in terms of ease of insertion, with the Solus requiring most reinsertions. Optimal ventilation was best with the LMA Unique (94%). Airway leak pressure was 27.3 mm Hg for the SSLM, 23.7 mm Hg for the Ambu AuraOnce, 22.1 mm Hg for the LMA Unique, and 20.9 mm Hg for the Solus. Blood staining occurred most frequently with the SSLM (38%).

OTHER STUDIES. Gernoth and colleagues compared the performance of the Ambu AuraOnce with the LMA Classic in 60 patients whose cervical spines were immobilized with an extrication collar before elective ambulatory interventions.[65] Insertion time, number of insertion attempts, and airway leak pressures were comparable (25.6 ± 5.3 cm H$_2$O for the Ambu AuraOnce and 26.5 ± 6.5 cm H$_2$O for the LMA Classic). The investigators concluded that both devices were suitable for rapid and reliable airway management in patients with cervical immobilization.

Using an in vitro test, Zaballos and coworkers examined the Ambu AuraOnce, LMA Classic, PLMA, LMA Unique, and i-gel using magnetic resonance imaging (MRI).[66] The Ambu AuraOnce and i-gel did not lead to artifacts, whereas each of the LMAs did.

Maino and associates examined the effect of nitrous oxide exposure on intracuff pressure of PVC and silicone LMs and the LMA Classic in vitro.[67] All cuffs were initially inflated with air to a pressure of 60 cm H$_2$O. The findings were not surprising given the physicochemical properties of PVC and silicone. When exposed to 66% nitrous oxide, the cuff pressure rose considerably more in the silicone cuffs than in the PVC devices. Among the PVC devices, the lowest increases in cuff pressure after 60 minutes of exposure were found in the Solus and LMA Unique (13 and 15 cm H$_2$O, respectively), and the increases in the cuffs of the Ambu AuraOnce and SSLM were notably higher (28 and 31 cm H$_2$O, respectively).

LITERATURE SUMMARY. Overall, the published literature shows that the Ambu AuraOnce performs similar to the LMA Unique and similar to or better than some other single-use LMs. Studies comparing it with the LMA Classic usually report almost equivalent performance. Only one study compared the Ambu AuraOnce with second-generation SADs. There are few reports of adverse events with the Ambu AuraOnce.

2. Soft Seal Laryngeal Mask

The SSLM is a disposable device made of PVC. Like the Ambu masks, it is one of few LMs with a body of published evidence on which its performance can be judged. Product development for this mask began in November 1998. Several prototypes were tried with features designed to improve insertion and performance. Evaluation included construction of a model oropharynx and testing in this replica and cadaver models. The final product was commercially launched in Australia in May 2002 and in the United States in January 2003, making it one of the earliest LMs to come to market.

The SSLM is a tubular oropharyngeal airway with a mask and an inflatable peripheral cuff attached to the distal end (Fig. 23-4). It is designed to produce an airtight seal around the laryngeal inlet to provide a secure airway suitable for spontaneous or controlled ventilation during general anesthesia.

The SSLM is available in sizes 1 through 5. The appropriate size is based on the weight and size of the patient. For adults, mask sizes 3, 4, and 5 are suitable for patients weighing 30 to 50 kg, 50 to 70 kg, and more than 70 kg, respectively. In broad terms, size 3 is suitable for small female patients, size 4 for many male and female patients, and size 5 for larger male patients.

Smiths Portex introduced a single-use silicone LM that includes epiglottic bars. It is available only outside North America.

a. APPLICATION

Insertion technique for the SSLM is similar to that recommended for LMAs in terms of patient position, device checking, preparation, and lubrication. Although many insertion techniques are used, insertion with the cuff partially inflated is recommended for the SSLM. If a muscle relaxant is administered before device insertion, use of a triple airway maneuver (i.e., mouth opening, head extension, and jaw thrust) should decrease the incidence of epiglottic downfolding.[68] The cuff should be inflated with air until a "just-seal" pressure is obtained. A maximum intracuff pressure of 60 cm H$_2$O is recommended.

The SSLM may be used as an intubation conduit. As with other LMs, this can be performed blindly (using an ETT or a bougie) or under fiberoptic guidance. Due to high failure rates for the blind technique, a fiberoptically guided technique is recommended, and use of an Aintree Intubation Catheter, as described previously, is a recognized and successful technique. The SSLM has a wider ventilation orifice than the LMA Classic; larger SSLM sizes can accommodate up to a 7.5-mm ETT. This and the absence of aperture bars facilitate intubation.

b. INDICATIONS, ADVANTAGES, AND DISADVANTAGES

Indications for the SSLM are the same as for the LMA Classic, which include routine anesthesia in fasted patients. The device can be used as a rescue airway in the "cannot intubate, cannot ventilate" (CICV) or the "cannot intubate, difficult to ventilate" (CIDV) situation, or it can be used as a primary airway for rescue of an unconscious patient whose airway is compromised or at risk. In all circumstances, the clinician must balance the risk of pulmonary aspiration against the benefits of obtaining an adequate airway or oxygenation of the patient.

The limitations of use of the SSLM are the same as for other LMs. The large bowl of the device and its PVC construction have been found by some to inhibit easy insertion. These limitations affect many PVC LMs.

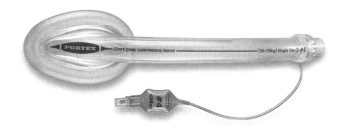

Figure 23-4 The Soft Seal laryngeal mask. (Courtesy of Smiths Medical ASD, Keene, NH.)

c. MEDICAL LITERATURE

There are approximately 27 publications about the SSLM in the medical literature.

RANDOMIZED, CONTROLLED STUDIES OF EFFICACY. Van Zundert and colleagues performed a randomized, controlled trial of the use of the size 4 SSLM and LMA Classic during spontaneously breathing anesthesia in 200 adult patients.[53] Insertion time, success, and fiberoptic position were equivalent. Further analysis of the cuff pressure change during nitrous oxide anesthesia, with the cuff pressure initially established at 45 mm Hg, showed that it increased in the LMA Classic to a mean of 100 mm Hg and that the mean final pressure in the SSLM was 47 mm Hg ($P < 0.001$).[69] There was a greater incidence of sore throat in the LMA Classic group at 2 hours postoperatively but not at 24 hours.

Similar to the low rates of trauma reported in the study by van Zundert's team, Hagberg and colleagues demonstrated that partial cuff inflation (30 mL of air) enhanced ease of insertion and minimized mucosal trauma.[70,71]

Shafik and associates performed a crossover comparison of the SSLM and LMA Classic in 60 patients.[72] The primary outcome measure was first-attempt insertion, for which success rates were equivalent (92% for the SSLM and 96% for the LMA Classic), as was ease of insertion.

Lopez and coworkers compared the SSLM with the LMA Classic in a randomized trial enrolling 60 patients.[73] Most performance characteristics were equivalent between devices, with the exception of a difference in airway seal (23 ±4 cm H_2O for the SSLM and 20 ±4 cm H_2O for the LMA Classic) and the fact that three patients in the SSLM group required the airway changed to an ETT.

Hanning and colleagues studied the SSLM and LMA Classic using a crossover design in a study of 35 healthy patients during paralyzed ventilation anesthesia.[74] The oropharyngeal leak pressure was higher with the SSLM than the LMA Classic (21 versus 16 cm H_2O).

In a crossover study, Brimacombe and colleagues compared the SSLM and LMA Unique in 90 healthy, paralyzed, anesthetized patients undergoing routine peripheral surgery.[75] The LMA Unique was superior to the SSLM in terms of ease of insertion, fiberoptic position, and mucosal trauma but similar in terms of oropharyngeal leak pressure and ease of ventilation.

In another randomized, crossover study, Paech and associates compared the SSLM and the LMA Unique in 168 anesthetized, spontaneously breathing patients.[52] The investigators reported that although both devices performed equivalently for first-time placement, the SSLM was subjectively rated more difficult to insert and more likely to cause mucosal trauma. However, the fiberoptic view of the larynx was better through the SSLM, and it more frequently provided a ventilation seal at 20 cm H_2O. In contrast to the LMA Unique, its cuff pressure did not increase during nitrous oxide anesthesia. In this study, there was a larger proportion of females, a smaller mask size was used for male and female patients, and the SSLM was inserted with a partially inflated cuff.

Cook and colleagues compared the SSLM with the LMA Unique in a randomized trial enrolling 100 patients.[76] The study was stopped early because of a high rate of airway trauma in the SSLM group. The investigators reported that the SSLM required more attempts for successful insertion ($P = 0.041$), more manipulations ($P < 0.0001$), failed more often ($P = 0.013$), and caused more complications ($P = 0.048$) than the LMA Unique. In 14% of SSLM uses, insertion or ventilation failed, and its use had to be abandoned. Leak pressure was higher with the SSLM (26.5 versus 20.5 cm H_2O, $P = 0.005$). Ventilation and fiberoptic view in those successfully inserted were not different for the two devices. The investigators also reported more complications during maintenance and sore throat postoperatively in recovery and at 24 hours for the SSLM. The SSLM was fully deflated before insertion in this study.

Francksen and coworkers studied 120 patients scheduled for routine minor obstetric surgery who were randomly allocated to the size 4 SSLM, Ambu AuraOnce, or LMA Unique.[63] The SSLM was slightly slower to insert than the Ambu AuraOnce and as fast as the LMA Unique. All three had high success rates (all >95%) for first-attempt insertions. Rates of subjectively designated excellent insertions were 75% for the LMA Unique, 70% for the Ambu AuraOnce, and 65% for the SSLM. All devices were judged acceptable.

Van Zundert and colleagues compared the SSLM with the LMA Unique and the CobraPLA in a study of 320 patients breathing spontaneously.[77] Insertion with the SSLM or LMA Unique was easier than with the CobraPLA ($P < 0.02$), but success rates and overall time to ventilation were similar. The SSLM and CobraPLA had higher airway seal than the LMA Unique ($P < 0.001$). Anatomic position was best with the CobraPLA, followed by the SSLM and LMA Unique. Blood staining occurred most frequently with the CobraPLA.

Hein and coworkers performed a crossover, randomized comparison of the SSLM and the SLIPA when inserted by trained medical students in 36 anesthetized patients.[78] Success rates for first-attempt insertions were similar (67% for the SSLM and 83% for the SLIPA), as were overall success rates (89% for the SSLM and 94% for the SLIPA). Time to ventilation with the SLIPA was faster, and there was an overall preference (67%) among participants for the SLIPA.

Tan and associates performed a randomized comparison of the SSLM, LMA Unique, and LMA Classic inserted by novice medical officers for anesthesia.[79] The novices had a total of five attempts with each mask. The SSLM was significantly slower to insert than the LMA Classic. The SSLM also had the lowest insertion success rate (80% for the LMA Classic, 77% for the LMA Unique, and 62% for the SSLM), although differences were not statistically significant. Although the SSLM achieved an airway seal of 4 to 5 cm H_2O higher than the other devices, blood on the airway was most common with the SSLM (32%) compared with the LMA Unique (9%) and the LMA Classic (6%), and sore throats were reported most frequently after use of the SSLM (42%) or LMA Classic (41%) compared with the LMA Unique (14%).

OTHER STUDIES. Boonmak and colleagues studied the use of the SSLM (sizes 3 and 4) for guiding fiberoptic intubation with a 6.0- or 6.5-mm ETT in 60 patients with normal airways.[80] The glottis was fully visible in 45% of patients after SSLM placement. Blind tracheal intubation succeeded in 5% of attempts, but with fiberoptic guidance, the success rate rose to 85%.

Danha and associates evaluated fiberoptically guided intubation through the SSLM and LMA Classic in 42 healthy patients with normal airways; a 6.0-mm, nasal, right-angle ETT was used for all evaluations.[81] Total intubation times and overall success rates were not different for the two devices. The success rate for first-attempt intubation through the SSLM was 76%.

Kuvaki and coworkers compared two insertion techniques for the SSLM in 100 patients randomized to different insertion techniques.[82] The SSLM was inserted in the two groups by a direct or a rotational technique, both without intraoral digital manipulation. The primary outcome measure was successful insertion at first attempt. The success rate for first-attempt insertion was higher with the direct technique (98%) than with the rotational technique (75%, $P = 0.002$), but insertion time was a few seconds faster with the latter method ($P = 0.035$). Final mask position over the larynx and airway morbidity were similar in both groups.

Keller and colleagues examined the pressure exerted in cadavers by the SSLM and LMA Unique on the larynx and pharyngeal wall during sequential inflation.[83] The SSLM had a lower elastance and lower intracuff pressure for a given inflation volume. Mucosal pressure increased with cuff inflation at most locations, and values were not different for the two devices at any site or cuff volume.

LITERATURE SUMMARY. A significant body of research has evaluated various aspects of the SSLM performance and compared it with other first-generation devices. Several studies comparing the SSLM with the LMA Classic and LMA Unique showed broadly equivalent performance, whereas others indicated the SSLM performed substantially less well. The airway seal of the SSLM is higher than that of the LMA Classic or LMA Unique. Insertion technique may be important. Some studies report the SSLM to be less easily inserted than the LMAs, and some report high rates of blood staining. Inflation with air before insertion appears to improve SSLM insertion and reduce trauma.

D. Intubating Laryngeal Airway

The Cookgas (St. Louis, MO) Intubating Laryngeal Airway (ILA) is distributed by Mercury Medical (Clearwater, FL). The ILA is a hypercurved intubating laryngeal airway invented by Daniel Cook. The ILA took more than 8 years to develop. In December 2004, it was introduced into clinical practice for airway management as a SAD or as a conduit for tracheal intubation. A single-use device has been launched.

The ILA is manufactured of medical-grade silicon and is latex free (Fig. 23-5). Ridges are located in the airway tube and the mask. The ridges below the airway connector were designed to improve the tube seal. They also allow easy removal of the connector during intubation through the device. The airway tube of the ILA is curved in a manner designed to mimic the anatomic curve of the upper airway; the design aims to eliminate the need to bend the tube further during use, which can lead to kinking.

The ILA tube accommodates large standard ETTs (≤8.5 mm for the larger ILA). The mask portion is large and cuffed, and it has a keyhole-shaped airway outlet designed to direct the ETT toward the laryngeal inlet. Three internal ridges located in the distal portion of the mask are designed to approximate the anatomic shape of the posterior pharynx and to create increased airway stability, smooth insertion, and improved airway alignment. When the ILA cuff is inflated, these ridges move against the posterior larynx and improve the anterior mask seal. The ILA was initially launched with three adult sizes available (2.5, 3.5, and 4.5), and two pediatric sizes were added (1.5 and 2). The increased range offers the possibility of use in small children and infants. The 2.5 is suitable for some children and adolescents 20 to 50 kg (smallest suitable ETT is 5.0 mm), the 3.5 is used in small adults (50 to 70 kg), and the 4.5 is used in large adults (70 to 100 kg). They are available in half-sizes to fit a broader range of patients.

After intubation, the ILA is removed using the Cookgas ILA Removal Stylet (Fig. 23-6), which is specifically designed for this use. The stylet stabilizes the previously inserted ETT and allows controlled removal of the ILA without dislodging the ETT from the trachea. The removal stylet consists of an adapter connected to a rod. The adapter is tapered from bottom to top and has horizontal ridges and vertical grooves. The ridges engage and grip the ETT, and the grooves create an airway passage for spontaneously breathing patients during removal of the ILA. The taper enables the stylet to accommodate standard ETTs in many sizes (5.0 to 8.5 mm). The stylet is manufactured from polypropylene and is reusable up to 10 times after washing in detergent, but cannot be autoclaved.

1. Application

After checking the patency of the device and integrity of the cuff by completely deflating and reinflating the cuff with the maximum recommended volume of air (Table 23-1), the device should be fully deflated before insertion. Performing this while pressing the anterior portion of the mask onto a sterile flat surface ensures an appropriately formed cuff for insertion. The posterior portion of the device should be prepared by applying a sterile, water-based lubricant just before insertion.

Insertion of the ILA is best performed with the patient's head and neck in the sniffing position, although other positions also may be used. The use of a jaw lift is recommended during insertion to lift the epiglottis off the posterior pharyngeal wall and increase pharyngeal space. The ILA is then inserted using a technique similar to that used for the LMA Classic, gently advancing the device while using the curvature of the ILA mask and airway tube as a guide. Some manipulation may be necessary to turn the corner into the upper pharynx. The

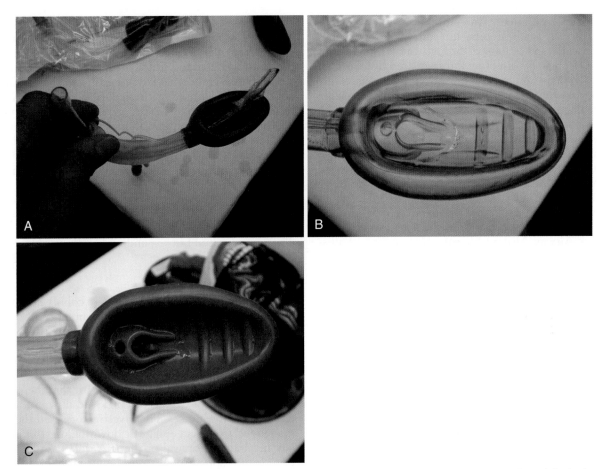

Figure 23-5   A to **C,** The Cookgas Intubating Laryngeal Airway. **A,** Reusable device with tracheal tube inserted. **B** and **C,** single-use and reusable devices showing "keyhole-like" airway orifice.

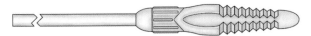

Figure 23-6   The Cookgas Removal Stylet is used with the Cookgas Intubating Laryngeal Airway.

TABLE 23-1
Intubating Laryngeal Airway Sizing

Mask Size	Patient Weight (kg)	Maximum Endotracheal Tube Internal Diameter (mm)
2.5	20-50	6.5
3.5	50-70	7.5
4.5	70-100	8.5

Courtesy of Tyco Healthcare, Schaffhausen, Switzerland.

device should be passed into the hypopharynx until resistance is met. The cuff should then be inflated with air (10 to 20 mL) until an effective seal is obtained or up to an intracuff pressure of 60 cm H$_2$O. Usually, cuff inflation with 10 mL of air is sufficient. The breathing system is then connected to the 15-mm connector, and adequacy of ventilation is assessed. If ventilation is inadequate, an up-down movement may be used to clear a downfolding

epiglottis. The ILA may then be used as a SAD for airway management. A bite block should be inserted alongside the tube and taped in place in the usual fashion.

If tracheal intubation is necessary or desired, ILA positioning should be assessed for optimal ventilation (e.g., easy airflow, higher tidal volumes). Before intubation, the risk of glottic closure should be minimized by administration of a muscle relaxant or topical local anesthesia. The patient should be fully preoxygenated. An appropriately sized ETT should be selected and prepared by fully deflating the cuff and lubricating the outer surface.

The ILA connector should be removed (but not discarded) and the ETT inserted through the ILA to a depth of approximately 12 to 15 cm, depending on the ILA size. This places the distal tip of the ETT at or just proximal to the opening of the ILA airway tube within the mask cavity. Several acceptable methods can then be used to advance the ETT into the trachea, although the literature supports a fiberoptically guided technique.

- Fiberoptic technique. A fiberoptic bronchoscope is passed through the ETT and into the trachea. When the carina is seen, the fiberscope can be left in place and the ETT advanced over it using the fiberscope as a guide (i.e., railroading). The ETT cuff can then be inflated, the scope removed, and the ETT connector replaced.

- Bougie technique. An intubation bougie (e.g., Eschmann tracheal tube introducer, Frova intubation catheter) is passed through the ETT and into the trachea. By directing the angulated distal end of the bougie anteriorly, the success rate is likely increased. By gently placing fingers over the cricoid cartilage, the stylet may be felt as it passes through the cricoid ring. When the bougie has been placed in the trachea, the ETT is passed over the bougie, through the laryngeal inlet, and into the trachea.
- Blind technique. The ETT is slowly advanced through the ILA. For spontaneously breathing patients, the anesthetic circuit can be attached to the ETT connector, and capnography may be used as a guide to successful tracheal placement. The Beck Airway Airflow Monitor (Great Plains Ballistics, Lubbock, TX) can also be used to facilitate blind tracheal intubation. If resistance to further advancement is encountered, the ILA should be repositioned.

After successful tracheal intubation has been achieved with any of these techniques, the ETT cuff should be inflated, and adequate ventilation should be assessed by observation of bilateral chest movement, auscultation, capnography, or spirometry, as appropriate.

When the appropriate position of the ETT is confirmed, the 15-mm connector of the ETT should be removed and the ILA Removal Stylet used to enable removal of the ILA. The removal stylet is placed, tapered end first, into the proximal end of the ETT until the adapter fits snugly and then rotated in a clockwise direction while applying firm inward pressure until the adapter firmly engages the ETT. The cuff of the ILA is deflated to enable easier removal of the device. While stabilizing the position of the removal stylet, the ILA is slowly withdrawn outward and out of the patient's mouth, leaving the ETT with attached removal stylet in place. The removal stylet is then unscrewed from the ETT in the counterclockwise direction while applying outward tension to disengage it from the ETT. The 15-mm connector can then be replaced on the ETT and the correct position of the ETT in the trachea reconfirmed.

2. Indications, Advantages, and Disadvantages

The ILA was designed for airway management as a SAD or as a conduit for blind, stylet-guided, or fiberoptically guided tracheal intubation. The ILA has a theoretical advantage over many other SADs because it is specifically designed to facilitate tracheal intubation. Its larger bowl and curved tube are designed to enhance entry into the mouth and passage along the oropharyngeal curve. The curve of its leading edge is designed to facilitate passage behind the epiglottis and arytenoid cartilages and into the upper esophageal inlet without the need for special deflation techniques or insertion devices. Each ILA accepts routinely used PVC ETTs (see Table 23-1).

The ILA does not necessarily require removal when it has been used as a conduit. It can remain in place and later be used during emergence as a bridge to extubation. The ILA Removal Stylet is designed with grooves that enable spontaneous ventilation through the ETT

during ILA removal, facilitating the performance of awake or asleep intubation during spontaneous ventilation.

The reusable ILA is nonsterile when delivered and requires cleaning and autoclaving before use. The non-sterile ILA Removal Stylet should be washed with soap and water and rinsed with alcohol before use. As with other first-generation SADs, the ILA does not provide protection against aspiration and should not be used in patients at risk of this complication. Due to the relatively low airway seal, the ILA is not suitable for patients with poor lung compliance, high airway resistance, or intraoral pathology.

3. Medical Literature

There is a limited but expanding literature on use of the ILA in adults.

a. COHORT STUDIES

Klein and Jones performed the first cohort study in 28 patients scheduled for gynecologic surgery; 22 of them were also intubated through the ILA.[84] The ILA was successfully placed (96.4%) on the first attempt in all but one patient. Leaks during manual ventilation were observed but were corrected with slight withdrawal of the device. The glottis was visible with the fiberscope in all patients, but a degree of epiglottic downfolding was observed in most cases. The investigators used the "Klein maneuver" to correct epiglottic downfolding: this involves jaw lift and withdrawal of the ILA, followed by reinsertion. Intubation through the ILA using fiberoptic guidance was 100% successful. The investigators reported that use of a flexible, reinforced ETT (Mallinckrodt) enhanced success during blind intubation.

Bakker and colleagues performed a cohort evaluation of controlled ventilation and tracheal intubation in 59 healthy patients undergoing elective surgery.[85] ILA insertion was successful in 100%, with a mean leak pressure of 19 ± 5 cm H_2O. Blind tracheal intubation was attempted in 19 patients. The first-attempt success rate was 58%, and the overall success rate for intubation was 74%. Postoperatively, 10% of patients had dysphagia, and one patient was diagnosed with bilateral lingual nerve injury, although this complication fully resolved after 4 weeks. The investigators concluded that the ILA was an adequate SAD for insertion and ventilation but that the proposed advantage of ease of tracheal intubation would require further investigation.

Joffe and associates reported a 70-patient cohort study of single-use and reusable ILAs.[86] The ILA insertion success rate was 100%, and in 57 patients, it was used as a primary airway only. The median airway leak pressures were 25 and 30 cm H_2O for the single-use and reusable devices, respectively. Fiberoptically guided intubation was successful in 12 (92%) of 13 attempts. Postoperatively, 26% of patients complained of mild sore throat.

Yang and coworkers studied 60 patients who were anticipated to be difficult to intubate and in whom the ILA was used for intubation; in one half, it was guided by a fiberscope and in one half by a Shikani Optical Stylet (SOS).[87] Insertion and ventilation through the ILA was successful in all patients. With the fiberscope, all but two were intubated on the first attempt, and they were successfully intubated on the second or third attempt. In the SOS group, 18 patients were intubated on the first attempt and 7 on the second attempt. The five failures in this group were all successfully intubated with the fiberscope. The fiberscope enabled faster intubation with a higher success rate. The hemodynamic changes recorded during intubation were minimal.

b. RANDOMIZED, CONTROLLED STUDIES OF EFFICACY

Using a noninferiority approach, Karim and colleagues compared the ILA and single-use ILMA during attempts at blind intubation in 154 healthy adults undergoing elective surgery.[88] The primary outcome measure was successful intubation within two attempts. This was achieved with the ILA in 77% (60 of 78) and with the ILMA in 99% (75 of 76) of patients (95% CI for the difference, 12% to 32%; $P < 0.0001$). After two failed blind attempts, fiberoptic guidance was used. In the ILA group, this enabled successful intubation of another 14 patients, but it failed in 4 patients. The overall intubation success rate using the ILA with three attempts (one with a fiberscope) was 95%. The investigators concluded that the single-use ILMA appears to be superior to the ILA as a conduit to facilitate blind tracheal intubation. A notable feature of this study was that one half of the patients had a body mass index (BMI) of 30 to 40 kg/m^2 including one fourth who had a BMI of more than 35 kg/m^2. BMI did not appear to influence the success rate of the ILA.

Erlacher and associates compared the ILA, ILMA, and CobraPLUS (Engineered Medical Systems, Indianapolis, IN) for ventilation and blind intubation in 180 healthy adults.[89] Ventilation was excellent with all devices, and minor repositioning was required in no more than 5% of patients in any group. Blind intubation was successful using the ILMA in 95% of cases, the ILA in 57%, and the CobraPLUS in 47%. Fiberoptic intubation was possible in all but one patient. Standard measures for predicting difficulty during routine intubation were not useful for predicting difficulty during blind intubation through these SADs.

c. OTHER STUDIES

Wong reported the use of an ILA combined with a lighted stylet to achieve intubation in a patient with a potentially difficult airway.[90] The patient had Hallermann-Streiff syndrome with oculomandibulofacial dystocia (i.e., bird-like appearance, mouth opening of 4 cm, receding chin, and Mallampati class III score). The lighted stylet (with the introducer removed) was placed inside the ETT, and transillumination was used to identify tracheal intubation.

d. LITERATURE SUMMARY

The available evidence suggests the ILA is an effective SAD that is usually easily inserted and enables ventilation. Blind tracheal intubation is successful at a higher rate than with most SADs but not as high as the ILMA. Use of a fiberscope increases the success rate, but several studies report some failures with this addition. Studies comparing the ILA with other SADs would be of value, as would determination of the role of the ILA in difficult airway management.

E. Laryngeal Tube

The VBM Laryngeal Tube (VBM Medizintechnik, Sulz, Germany) and King Laryngeal Tube (King Systems, Noblesville, IN) are SAD devices that were introduced to the European market in 1999 and to the United States in February 2003.[91] Between 1999 and 2002, several modifications were made to the original version of the laryngeal tube (LT), including a softer tip, a change from cuff inflation by separate pilot tubes to a single pilot tube, and alterations to the ventilation orifices and proximal cuff. Among the several distinct LTs, some are first-generation and others second-generation SADs.

There are five versions of the LT: the reusable LT, the disposable LT (LT-D), the reusable Laryngeal Tube Suction II (LTS-II), a disposable version of the LTS-II (LTS-D), and the Gastro-Laryngeal Tube (Gastro-LT). The LTS-II, LTS-D, and LT-G are considered later in "Second-Generation Supraglottic Airway Devices." The LT is designed for use during spontaneous breathing, controlled ventilation, and airway rescue.

The LT consists of an airway tube with two inflatable balloons or cuffs designed to lie above and below the laryngeal inlet (i.e., pharyngeal and esophageal, respectively), and both cuffs are inflated through a single pilot tube and balloon (Fig. 23-7).[91,92] When the device is inserted, it lies along the length of the tongue and extends distally into the proximal esophagus. Proximal and distal cuffs sit in the oropharynx and esophageal inlet, respectively. Inflation creates a seal, and ventilation occurs through orifices between the cuffs. Proximally, a 15-mm standard male adapter enables connection to the anesthetic circuit, and distally, several small airway orifices lie between the balloons (Fig. 23-8). Three black lines proximally indicate approximately correct depth of insertion.

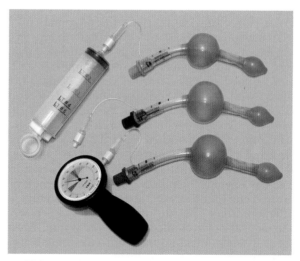

Figure 23-7 The VBM laryngeal tube (reusable versions, adult sizes shown). Also shown is a dedicated color-coded syringe (*top left*) for use with the LT and an inflation and cuff pressure monitor device (*bottom left*).

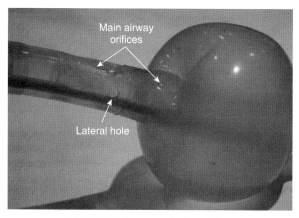

Figure 23-8 Laryngeal tube orifices.

TABLE 23-2

Characteristics of the Laryngeal Tube

Size	Patient Type	Sizing Selection Criteria	Color
0	Newborn	<5 kg	Transparent
1	Baby	5-12 kg	White
2	Child	12-25 kg	Green
2.5	Child	125-150 cm	Orange
3	Adult	<155 cm	Yellow
4	Adult	155-180 cm	Red
5	Adult	>180 cm	Purple

Courtesy of King Systems, Noblesville, IN.

The LT is made of silicon and is designed to be reused up to 50 times. The airway tube is slim, curved, and relatively short, with an average diameter of 11.5 mm and a blind tip. Seven sizes are available for use in neonates up to large adults (Table 23-2).[91,92] LT size selection should be based on the patient's weight for sizes 0 to 2 and on height for sizes 3 to 5. The disposable version (LT-D) is sold in sizes 2 to 5. Adult and child sizes (but not infant and newborn sizes) are supplied with a reusable, silicone bite block.

After correct device insertion, the proximal cuff lies in the hypopharynx and the distal cuff in the upper esophagus. Both cuffs have a high-volume, low-pressure design to avoid ischemic damage to mucosa and to achieve a good seal. The original version of the LT was designed with a single ventilation opening between the two cuffs in the ventral part of the tube. The current version has two main ventilation orifices.

The proximal cuff lies close to the proximal airway orifice, and there is a V-shaped dent in the pharyngeal cuff. As the cuff is inflated, soft tissue is deflected from the airway opening, helping to maintain a patent airway. The distal end of the airway tube slopes toward the distal ventilation orifice. The tip of the LT is a closed wedge shape, and it is surrounded by the distal cuff. Because there is a single inflation line, both cuffs inflate almost simultaneously.

In addition to the main ventilation orifices, there are two side eyelets, with one on either side of the main ventilation orifices. This design allows improved collateral ventilation if the epiglottis obstructs the main ventilation orifice. The latest version of the LT-D has three eyelets on each side. The efficacy of this design feature has not been formally tested. The LT-D is 1.0 cm longer than the LT to facilitate deeper placement of the device, aid correct positioning of the two main ventilation orifices, and improve the location of the proximal cuff beneath the tongue, so that the epiglottis is more likely to be raised with cuff inflation, in much the same manner as with a Macintosh laryngoscope blade.

1. Application

Before each use, the reusable LT must be cleaned and sterilized (by autoclaving) according to manufacturer's instructions. The device's general condition, tube patency, and integrity of both cuffs should be confirmed before use. Cuff integrity is tested by full deflation and inflation to check for leaks. The depth of anesthesia required before insertion is similar to that for other SADs: when the patient is unconscious, is apneic, and has no eyelash reflex or resistance to manipulation of the lower jaw. Muscle relaxants are unnecessary, but anesthesia should be deep enough to obtund airway reflexes. An appropriately sized LT should be chosen according to the selection criteria described previously. Before insertion, the cuffs must be fully deflated and lubricated. The LT may be inserted with a neutral head position or in the sniffing position; in the latter position, jaw lift may be needed to negotiate the angulation of the posterior pharynx.

The slim profile of the LT and easy insertion technique mean it can be inserted with either hand and with the anesthesiologist standing in a variety of positions. During routine use, the LT should be held in the dominant hand and inserted blindly along the midline of the tongue with the tip against the hard palate. It is passed smoothly along the palate into the hypopharynx until resistance is felt. If no resistance is felt, a thick, black line on the tube indicates the appropriate depth of insertion, and this line should lie at the incisors. After insertion, the cuffs should be inflated. As air is injected, the proximal cuff inflates first, stabilizing the device, followed by inflation of the distal cuff. A pressure gauge should be used to inflate the cuffs to a pressure of 60 cm H_2O. If a gauge is not available, a dedicated syringe can be used for cuff inflation. These 100-mL syringes have clear markings (in colors corresponding to the various LT color codes) indicating the approximate volumes of air needed for each size. The LT can then be connected to the breathing system. Indicators of correct LT placement are auscultation of bilateral lung sounds, bilateral chest excursion, absence of gastric insufflation, and an appropriate capnographic trace. When the LT is correctly positioned, the bite block, which is supplied with the device, can be attached to the tube.

After LT placement, manual, controlled, or spontaneous ventilation may be used. Initial use of positive-pressure ventilation may provide useful information about the correctness of LT placement. If ventilation is not ideal, the LT may be advanced or withdrawn slightly until ventilation is optimal. If controlled ventilation through the LT is problematic, spontaneous ventilation may also be difficult.

Correct placement of the LT may be verified using a test with a lightwand without the metallic stylet. The lightwand is inserted into the LT and advanced through it until a faint glow can be seen above the thyroid prominence. This indicates that the lightwand tip is just in front of the laryngeal inlet. When the LT is correctly positioned, the lightwand tip enters the glottic opening, and correct positioning is shown by a well-defined, circumscribed glow seen in the anterior neck slightly below the thyroid prominence. If transillumination shows a glow with a halo near the thyroid prominence, the test result is considered negative. This result may be caused by the lightwand tip lying against the epiglottis or the glossoepiglottic fold. A lateral glow indicates that the hole for ventilation is not in front of the laryngeal inlet, even if ventilation is effective.

At the end of anesthesia, the LT can be left in place until the return of the protective airway reflexes. Slight cuff deflation at this point improves tolerance of the oropharyngeal cuff. The device should be removed with the patient deeply anesthetized or totally awake; otherwise, laryngospasm, coughing, or gagging may occur. Before removal of the device, the cuffs should be completely deflated. Inadequate cuff deflation can make removal difficult, risking damage of the cuff and discomfort for the patient.

A well-lubricated ETT (up to 6.5 mm) can be inserted into the LT after the proximal connector has been removed. An attempt to intubate blindly through the LT is then possible, and success relies on alignment of the ventilation orifices and the glottis. The tip of the ETT is gently advanced until it passes through the glottic opening. Resistance may be caused by incorrect positioning of the LT, epiglottic obstruction of ETT passage, or inadequate lubrication of the ETT. A tube exchanger may be placed in this manner, and after removal of the LT, an appropriate ETT can be passed. Fiberoptic guidance is an alternative and likely a more successful technique. Alternative described methods include the use of a rigid video laryngoscope to view intubation from outside the LT during insertion and use of a Trachlight to guide and monitor intubation.

After intubation is achieved, the LT cuffs must be deflated before the device is removed. The shorter tube shaft of the LT compared with the LMA Classic allows the ETT to be inserted farther into the trachea and makes it possible to place the ETT cuff in the trachea without removing the LT. Unless indicated otherwise, there is an argument for leaving the LT in place with both cuffs deflated after tracheal intubation has been performed. It is possible to perform tracheal intubation through the LT with an Aintree intubation catheter (AIC, Cook Critical Care), but passage of the AIC through the ventilation holes is at the limit of what can fit.

There are disadvantages to using the LT as a conduit for intubation. The diameter of the ETT is limited by the LT size. The rather narrow LT airway orifice compared with many other SADs may cause problems because it does not lie opposite the glottis or because negotiating the fiberscope or tube into the glottis is difficult. The relatively narrow ventilation orifices of the LT, its narrow lumen, and the fact that axial rotation may lead to imperfect alignment of the airway and larynx mean that the LT is unlikely to be first choice if selecting a specific SAD for intubation.

2. Indications, Advantages, and Disadvantages

The LT is designed for use during spontaneous or controlled ventilation. Because the slim profile of the LT allows easy insertion through a narrow orifice, it can be considered for airway management in patients with restricted mouth opening. Insertion is relatively easy and provides a clear airway in most patients on the first attempt. Extensive training is unnecessary. Its insertion and performance characteristics have led to its being included as an airway device for use in the management of cardiac arrest in the 2010 guidelines of the International Liaison Committee on Resuscitation (ILCOR).[93]

Because of the design and length of the LT, inadvertent tracheal intubation is unlikely, although it has been reported with some versions of the device.[94] The LT is associated with a low incidence of minor traumatic sequelae, such as sore throat, hoarseness, or blood on the device after use. The slim design, soft materials used in construction, and high-volume, low-pressure cuffs offer advantages. These high-volume, low-pressure cuffs provide a good seal and reduce the risk of ischemic damage when used appropriately. Another advantage is the ability to insert the device from a variety of positions relative to the patient, making it useful in emergency situations.

The LT may be used to maintain ventilation during attempts at fiberoptic intubation. The fiberoptic bronchoscope and ETT can be advanced through the nose into the oral cavity without deflating the cuffs of the LT. After tracheal intubation has been accomplished, the cuffs of the LT can be deflated and the device removed.

Although the LT's distal cuff forms a good esophageal seal, the LT and LT-D do not have drain tubes, and the LT should not be used in anesthetized patients at increased risk of regurgitation or aspiration of gastric contents. As with other SADs, due to the relatively low-pressure airway seal, the LT may not be appropriate in patients with poor lung compliance, increased airway resistance, or lesions of the oropharynx or epiglottis.

As with any SAD, partial glottic closure or laryngospasm may lead to airway obstruction. This may occur if the LT is inserted at too light a depth of anesthesia or if there is excessive surgical stimulation without an appropriate depth of anesthesia. These changes may be identified by alterations in capnography, spirometry, or airway pressure during mechanical ventilation.

The slim LT can rotate within the airway along its longitudinal axis. When this happens, the airway orifices, which are smaller than those of some other SADs, become poorly aligned with the glottis, with the risk of increased airway resistance or airway obstruction. This risk is minimized by careful insertion and confirmation of correct positioning during initial placement and cuff inflation.

3. Medical Literature

There are more than 150 publications about the LT and its design variations. Because the LT was modified, studies reporting before 2003 are likely to have evaluated an LT device that is no longer in use.

a. COHORT STUDIES AND STUDIES OF GENERAL PERFORMANCE

Using earlier versions of the LT, Asai,[95] Doerges,[96] and their colleagues determined that after blind insertion, the device provided a patent airway in most patients at the first attempt. The LT can be inserted quickly without extensive training; it is considered a suitable airway management device with a high rate of successful insertion requiring a mouth opening as limited as 23 mm.[97,98] Acceptance of the ease of LT placement is high among physicians, nurses, and paramedics, although correct positioning may require more adjustments in patients with an increased BMI.[99-101] Insertion time is reported to be comparable to that for the LMA Classic.[96]

Several studies confirmed the efficacy of controlled ventilation with the LT and found that its airway seal was modestly better than that of the LMA Classic, with some patients achieving a seal above 30 cm H_2O.[96,102-105] Although numerous studies have shown the LT can be effective during mechanical ventilation, some studies, most notably that of Miller (inventor of the SLIPA), have found the LT to be unsatisfactory for spontaneous ventilation.[106] The findings of Miller and colleagues were based on a frequent failure rate (7 of 17 patients) caused by loss of airway control during surgery.[106] The investigators assessed use of a first-generation LT that did not feature a second, large ventilation aperture and two lateral ventilatory openings that are part of the newer version.

In another study by Hagberg and colleagues, the LT was demonstrated to provide a reliable airway during elective surgery with spontaneous ventilation.[105] In this study, the mean depth of insertion was greater than expected for each size of the LT, and as a result, the company now manufactures this device 1 cm longer in the silicon version and 2 cm larger in the disposable version. The success rate for first-time placement was 86%, consistent with the rates of 85% to 95% found in previous studies.[96,102-104]

The dose of propofol required for LT insertion is approximately the same as for the LMA Classic.[107] Nitrous oxide diffuses into the cuffs, and cuff pressures should be monitored during use. During 30 minutes of nitrous oxide anesthesia, Asai and coworkers demonstrated an increase of 15 cm H_2O in the intracuff pressure.[104,108]

Because of the ease of insertion and a good airtight seal, the LT has been studied for airway management during cardiopulmonary resuscitation. There is considerable data on its use by medical staff and paramedics for primary airway management out of hospitals and for airway management during cardiopulmonary resuscitation.[109-113] The LT is included in the 2010 ILCOR resuscitation guidelines.[93] Dengler and associates reported some cases of massive pulmonary aspiration and one of gastric overinflation during use of the LT in the emergency setting.[114] This followed ventilation with high peak airway pressures, and the investigators questioned whether the LTS-II or LTS-D would have been a more appropriate device.

Langlois and associates performed a cohort study of the LT-D in 50 anesthetized patients.[115] Insertion was successful in 94%, and the median insertion time was 38 seconds. Insertion difficulty occurred in 25%. Mean oropharyngeal leak pressure increased from 26 cm H_2O (range, 22 to 32.5 cm H_2O) to 34 cm H_2O (range, 29 to 40 cm H_2O) at the end of surgery. No cases of gastric inflation, regurgitation, or hypoxia were reported. The incidence of moderate sore throat was 6% in the recovery room and 0% at 24 hours.

b. RANDOMIZED, CONTROLLED STUDIES OF EFFICACY

Amini and colleagues performed a study comparing the LT with the LT-D in 100 anesthetized, paralyzed patients.[116] Both devices showed similar clinical performance in terms of insertion success (90% for the LT-D and 96% for the LT) and insertion time (28.4 and 23.6 seconds, respectively). There were no differences in airway leak pressure, fiberoptic position, or postoperative sore throat and dysphagia.

Yilidz and associates compared the LT with the LMA Classic in 132 patients.[117] Oxygenation and ventilation were possible in all patients. Insertion success rates after the first, second, and third attempts were 84.8% ($n = 56$), 12.1% ($n = 8$), and 3% ($n = 2$) for the LT compared with 56.1% ($n = 37$), 25.8% ($n = 17$), and 18.2% ($n = 12$) for the LMA Classic ($P = 0.001$). Blood on the cuff was seen at removal in one patient with the LT and in 10 patients with the LMA Classic. Six patients in the LMA Classic group complained of hoarseness ($P = 0.012$). The success rates for LMA Classic insertion are markedly lower in this study than in many others, which may influence many of the results.

Noor and coworkers compared the LT and LMA Classic for ventilation during manual in-line stabilization in 40 healthy, anesthetized, and paralyzed patients.[118] Three attempts were allowed. The success rates (100%), adequacy of ventilation, and hemodynamic changes were not different for the two devices. The LT has a higher first-attempt success rate (100% versus 85%) and was significantly faster to insert (25 versus 36 seconds, $P = 0.001$).

Kurola and colleagues studied insertion of the LT, ILMA, and CobraPLA by paramedical students in 96 anesthetized, paralyzed patients.[119] The success rates for first-attempt insertion were 75% for the ILMA, 44% for the LT, and 22% for the CobraPLA. Overall success rates were 97% for the ILMA and 79% for the LT and the CobraPLA. In this small study, the numeric differences were not statistically significant.

c. OTHER STUDIES

No studies have been published examining whether the lower cuff protects against aspiration. Khazin and associates studied hypopharyngeal pH changes as a marker of regurgitation during anesthesia with several SADs (e.g., LT, CobraPLA, LMA Classic, ILMA, and PLMA) and with ETTs in 180 patients.[120] One to five patients in each study group of 30 had regurgitation episodes, but the rates were not statistically different between groups. The clinical relevance of the study, particularly its relevance to aspiration protection, is questionable. Bercker and coworkers designed a study to compare the seal of seven SADs in a cadaver model of elevated esophageal pressure. SADs included the LMA Classic, PLMA, ILMA, LT,

LTS-II, Combitube, and EasyTube.[40] All were inserted into unfixed human cadavers with an exposed esophagus that had been connected to a 130-cm water column. Slow and fast increases of esophageal pressure were performed, and the water pressure at which leakage appeared was documented. The Combitube, EasyTube, and ILMA withstood the water pressure up to more than 120 cm H_2O. The PLMA, LT, and LTS-II blocked the esophagus despite 72 to 82 cm H_2O of pressure. The LMA Classic leaked at 48 cm H_2O, but only minor leakage was found in the trachea. Devices with an additional esophageal drain tube removed fluid sufficiently without pulmonary aspiration. The LTS-II and LTS-D are likely to provide better protection than the LT.

Ulrick-Pur and colleagues examined the mucosal pressures exerted by several SADs in fresh cadavers.[121] Using maximum cuff volumes according to the manufacturers' guidelines, the highest pharyngeal pressures were found with the ILMA. The LMA Classic, ILMA, and PLMA induced significantly higher pharyngeal pressures than the LT, EasyTube, or Combitube at maximum inflation. The maximum esophageal pressures were significantly higher using the EasyTube than with the Combitube. Tracheal mucosal pressures were significantly higher using the Combitube compared with the ETT and the EasyTube.

Asai and coworkers reported successful use of the LT in three patients in whom insertion of the LMA had failed, and they suggested the relative width of the devices was responsible for failure or success.[122] In these cases, the pharyngeal space was narrowed by swollen tonsils, goiter, and redundant oropharyngeal tissue, and the investigators recommended that when LMA insertion is difficult or impossible because of a narrowed pharynx, insertion of the LT should be attempted before considering tracheal intubation. Reported side effects with the LT are few but do include tongue engorgement.[123]

d. LITERATURE SUMMARY

The LT is an easily inserted SAD. Alterations over the years have improved performance. Insertion by anesthesiologists and less-experienced practitioners can be performed with success rates exceeding 90%. Controlled ventilation may be more reliable than spontaneous ventilation. Airway seal is better than the LMA Classic but not as good as the PLMA. Protection against aspiration is undefined, and there are better alternatives when this is a factor in choosing a device. The LT-D appears to perform similar to the LT. The LT has an important role in out-of-hospital use.

F. Cobra Perilaryngeal Airway

The Cobra perilaryngeal airway (CobraPLA, Engineered Medical Systems, Indianapolis, IN) (Fig. 23-9) was designed by David Alfery. It was based on a modification of the Guedel oral airway and was marketed in 1997. The initial idea was to modify the Guedel airway to accomplish mask ventilation in the most difficult airways encountered. It has since been adapted to create a SAD. The proximal portion of the airway was modified to enable attachment to an airway circuit, a circumferential

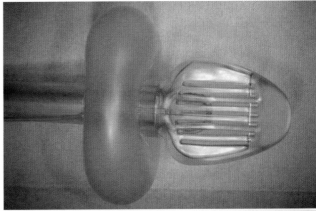
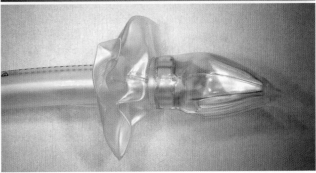

Figure 23-9 The Cobra perilaryngeal airway (CobraPLA) with cuff inflated *(top)* and deflated *(bottom)*.

cuff was added proximal to the distal breathing hole, and the distal end of the device was modified to form a cobra head shape. Later refinements included a distal flexible tip (tongue) and an internal ramp inside the cobra head to help guide an ETT toward the glottis. A modification of the CobraPLA, the CobraPLUS, incorporates an integrated temperature probe and a distal gas-sampling port.

The CobraPLA is made of PVC and polycarbonate. It consists of a breathing tube with a proximal, standard 15-mm adapter; a circumferential, inflatable cuff proximal to the ventilation orifice; and a distal, widened cobra-like head that surrounds the ventilation orifice. The anterior surface of the head consists of a grill of soft bars through which gas exchange takes place. The bars are soft enough to allow instrumentation of the larynx and upper airway if required. When in the proper position, the head lies in front of the laryngeal inlet and is designed to seal the hypopharynx. In this respect, it is different from many other SADs, because the distal tip lies proximal to the esophageal inlet. Internal to the head, there is a ramp to direct the breathing gas (or ETT) into the trachea. The head and anterior grill are designed to deflect the epiglottis off the head, preventing the epiglottis from obstructing the ventilation orifice. The cuff is circumferential and is designed to lie in the hypopharynx at the base of the tongue. When inflated, it raises the base of the tongue, exposing the laryngeal inlet, and it effects an airway seal, allowing positive-pressure ventilation to be carried out.

The device is named *Cobra* because of the shape of the distal part of the airway; when turned over and looked at on end, it appears similar to the head of a cobra snake.

This shape is designed to enable the device to pass more easily along the hard palate during insertion and to hold soft tissues widely away from the laryngeal inlet after the device is in place. *Perilaryngeal* describes its anatomic location and refers to the fact that the widened, distal Cobra end pushes soft tissues away from the laryngeal inlet.

The CobraPLA is available in eight sizes (1.5 through 6) designed to be used according to the weight and size of the patient. The recommended size is that which comfortably fits through the patient's mouth. Appropriate sizes are no. 3 for most female patients, no. 4 for most men, and no. 5 for larger men. When unsure about the appropriate size, especially when learning placement, use of the smaller of any two sizes under consideration is advisable. When a practitioner is comfortable with the insertion technique, especially when a muscle relaxant has been administered, use of a larger size may also be successful. The most important consideration is to choose a size that fits through the patient's mouth without undue difficulty, and the same device size may be appropriate for patients of considerably different weight, depending on their body habitus. The manufacturer suggests that two or more sizes may be acceptable for a particular height. Despite a relatively high weight, some patients may have a small mouth that necessitates a smaller CobraPLA.

Agro and colleagues suggested a modified method of size selection: no. 3 for less than 60 kg, no. 4 for 60 to 80 kg, and no. 5 for more than 80 kg.[100] In this study, relatively large CobraPLAs were used by skilled operators with techniques that included a combination of scissoring the mouth open and performing a jaw lift (i.e., Agro maneuver) in patients who had been given muscle relaxants. If using Agro's range or a relatively large CobraPLA, the cuff inflation volume can be reduced from the maximum recommended by the manufacturer. Use of the larger sizes achieves a higher degree of airway seal.

The CobraPLUS is a modified version of the CobraPLA which in its adult version has an integrated core temperature–measuring device and in its pediatric version also has a distal gas-sampling post within the device head. This is of particular interest in newborns and infants, in whom very rapid respiratory rates and low tidal volumes result in inaccurate gas-sampling values if using more proximal sampling sites.[124]

1. Application

The CobraPLA insertion technique is simple. After appropriate checks of integrity and patency, the cuff is fully deflated and folded back against the breathing tube. A lubricant is liberally applied to the front and the back of the Cobra head and to the cuff, with care taken to avoid obstructing the anterior grill. With the patient's head and neck in the sniffing position, the mouth is opened with a scissor maneuver using the nondominant hand and gently pulling the mandible upward. The CobraPLA tip should not be directed against the hard palate, as is often done when inserting an LMA Classic because this may increase the curve that the device tip must take at the back of the mouth and make insertion more difficult. The distal end of the CobraPLA is instead directed straight back between the tongue and hard palate. As the device is advanced into the mouth, an anterior jaw lift assists insertion. Pushing the jaw downward makes insertion more difficult. Modest neck extension (without a jaw lift) may aid passage of the device as it turns toward the glottis at the back of the mouth.

As the CobraPLA is advanced to the back of the mouth, it often turns caudally toward the larynx with minimal resistance as the flexible distal tip (tongue) guides the device downward. Sometimes, a gentle push past posterior resistance is needed. The CobraPLA is correctly seated when modest resistance to further distal passage is encountered as the device tip reaches the glottis. When the position is correct, the flexible tip lies under the arytenoids, the ramp-grill lifts the epiglottis, and the cuff lies in the hypopharynx at the base of the tongue.

After insertion, the cuff should be inflated initially with less than the maximum volume recommended until there is no leak with positive-pressure ventilation (i.e., minimal leakage technique). Providing an adequate depth of anesthesia is achieved, the cardiovascular response to CobraPLA insertion is similar to insertion of other SADs and therefore less than during laryngoscopy and tracheal intubation.

Manual ventilation assists the anesthesiologist in confirming correct placement and may determine the pressure at which an audible leak occurs. Indicators of correct placement are good lung ventilation, a normal capnographic trace, and no gastric insufflation.

Cuff inflation should be enough just to achieve a seal, and overinflation should be avoided. A cuff pressure gauge should be used to monitor intracuff pressure (approximately 60 cm H_2O). If adequate ventilation is not achieved, the CobraPLA may be inserted too far and should be withdrawn 1 to 2 cm. Spontaneous or mechanical ventilation can be used as indicated. Ventilation with an airway pressure above 25 cm H_2O should be avoided, even when testing for ventilation and cuff seal, because gastric insufflation may occur at pressures over this level. Low-pressure ventilation may be achieved by setting a low inspiratory flow rate and then adjusting the tidal volume. Pressure-controlled or pressure-limited modes of ventilation may also be useful to minimize peak airway pressure.

Some practical tips are worth considering. First, the patient should be at an adequate depth of anesthesia before insertion is attempted. Laryngospasm may occur during insertion if the patient is at too light a level of anesthesia. Second, if one CobraPLA is found to be unsuitable, an alternative size should be inserted before abandoning this technique. Third, if the CobraPLA is not inserted far enough, cuff inflation may cause tongue protrusion and a poor airway seal; the device should be advanced further or a smaller CobraPLA chosen. The cuff should not be visible at the base of the tongue when the mouth is opened. Fourth, if the CobraPLA is inserted too far, past the laryngeal inlet, ventilation is impossible. This may occur while learning the technique or if too small a CobraPLA is used. Pulling back the airway 1 to 2 cm usually resolves the situation. The CobraPLA is considered to have a steep learning curve, and the technique can be mastered in 5 to 10 insertions.[100]

Removal should be performed as the patient regains consciousness. When the patient is able to respond to simple commands (e.g., "open your mouth"), the Cobra-PLA cuff may be partially deflated and the device gently withdrawn from the patient. Partial deflation of the cuff enables it to squeeze secretions up and out of the mouth as the CobraPLA is removed.

The CobraPLA may be used as an intubation conduit. Its internal diameter is larger than the corresponding LMA Classic, and the largest CobraPLA has a 12.5-mm ID. This means that intubation through a CobraPLA with a relatively large ETT without an intubation guide or exchange catheter is feasible. Provided the proximal connector is removed, because the CobraPLA is shorter than many other SADS, a standard ETT may be passed through it far enough that the cuff lies below the vocal cords. This potentially makes the procedure technically easier than through an LMA Classic, and it does not require an extra-long ETT.

A standard ETT may be used for intubation through a CobraPLA, ideally guided by a fiberscope. As the fiberscope and ETT exit the ventilation orifice, the soft bars of the grill separate easily without impediment to advancement. The internal ramp directs the fiberoptic bronchoscope anteriorly, and if the larynx is anterior to the ventilation orifice, this approach should enable prompt intubation. The large diameter of the CobraPLA permits the passage of an adequately sized ETT (Table 23-3). The CobraPLA can be left in place with its cuff deflated if desired.

An alternative technique involves use of a lightwand to guide intubation, as has been described for other SADs.[99,125,126] The technique is described in the "Laryngeal Tube" section. Blind intubation through the CobraPLA by advancing an ETT through it or by using a bougie guide may be successful, but it has a significant failure rate, and the preceding techniques are far preferable when the equipment is available.

2. Indications, Advantages, and Disadvantages

The indications for use of the CobraPLA are similar to those for other first-generation SADs. This device cannot be relied on to protect the upper airway from aspiration in anesthetized patients. Unlike many other SADs, the tip of the device does not enter and obturate the

esophagus but is designed to lie above it. Elective use should be confined to patients not considered to be at risk for regurgitation of gastric contents.

The CobraPLA is designed for spontaneous and controlled ventilation. Like other SADs, the CobraPLA can be used as a rescue airway in CICV or CIDV scenarios, but it does not provide airway protection. If it is used to rescue the airway and regurgitation or aspiration is considered a risk, it is advisable to proceed to tracheal intubation if possible.

The relative ease of insertion is an advantage of the CobraPLA, which may make it suitable for use in airway emergencies even when it is used by personnel with little or no experience in the use of SADs. Some clinical evidence supports the efficacy of use by nonanesthesiologist physicians with minimal training in airway management.[127] Pediatric sizes of the CobraPLUS can monitor core body temperature and distal carbon dioxide levels.

As with many SADs, because airway pressures should be limited to no greater than 20 to 25 cm H_2O, the CobraPLA may not be appropriate for patients with reduced lung compliance or increased airway resistance. The major disadvantage of the device is that it does not protect against aspiration and does not secure the airway as effectively as the tracheal tube. Users should remember that the CobraPLA tip does not obturate the upper esophagus. Whether this increases the risk of aspiration compared with other SADs has not been determined definitively.

3. Medical Literature

Approximately 40 publications have described the CobraPLA or CobraPLUS. The CobraPLA was modified to aid insertion in 2006, as reported by the inventors, Alfery and Szmuk, in 2007.[128] The manufacturers modified the CobraPLA and the CobraPLUS by adding a distal bend in the breathing tube. It is likely that only publications after 2007 used the updated device, and this should be considered in interpreting these studies.

a. COHORT STUDIES

The first report of the use of the CobraPLA in a peer-reviewed journal was by Agro and coworkers in 2003; the study included 28 anesthetized and mechanically ventilated patients.[129] After mannequin training, the Cobra-PLA was inserted in patients within 10 ± 3 seconds with a 100% success rate. Immediate ventilation was achieved in 57% of patients, and 43% required a positioning maneuver (e.g., pulling back).

In a later study, Agro and colleagues studied 110 patients and reported 100% successful insertion in a mean time of 6.8 ± 2 seconds.[100] There were no adverse events or significant complications. Mean airway seal was 34 cm H_2O using very low cuff inflation volumes by choosing relatively large CobraPLAs.

In contrast, Cook and Lowe reported an aborted study with the CobraPLA.[130] During preparation for two studies, a total of 29 CobraPLAs were inserted, and two cases of significant aspiration were identified. The investigators raised concerns about the design of the Cobra-PLA and its safety in terms of aspiration protection. The manufacturers robustly rejected these assertions.[131-133]

TABLE 23-3

Sizing for Passage of an Endotracheal Tube in a CobraPLA

Cobra Size	ETT Size (mm)
½	3.0
1	4.5
1½	4.5
2	6.5
3	6.5
4	8.0
5	8.0
6	8.0

ETT, Endotracheal tube; *PLA*, perilaryngeal airway.

Park and associates studied the effect of changing head and neck positions on SAD performance, including the CobraPLA, in 139 patients.[134] Oropharyngeal leak pressure and cuff pressure were evaluated in four head and neck positions: neutral, 45 degrees of flexion, 45 degrees of extension, and 45 degrees of right rotation. Adverse events such as difficult ventilation or gastric insufflation were assessed. Airway leak pressures were well maintained with the CobraPLA, but "gastric insufflations occurred before the oropharyngeal leak in 37 of 45 patients."[134] The investigators concluded that caution is warranted when changing the position of the head and neck while using the Cobra-PLA because gastric insufflation may occur.

Nam and coworkers reported a case series of 50 uses of the CobraPLA in paralyzed patients undergoing elective surgery.[135] The success rate for first-attempt insertion was 82%, with a mean insertion time of approximately 16 seconds. Airway leak pressure (22.5 cm H_2O) was lower than other reports. The point of leakage was recorded as the neck (52%), abdomen (46%), or both sites (2%). The glottis was visible in 88% of patients through the CobraPLA. Postoperative blood staining was seen in 22%, mild dysphonia in 6%, mild dysphagia in 10%, and mild and moderate sore throat in 44% and 4%, respectively.

b. RANDOMIZED, CONTROLLED STUDIES OF EFFICACY

Akça and colleagues compared the CobraPLA with the LMA Unique in a randomized series of 81 patients, and the insertion times, airway adequacy, number of repositioning episodes, and minor complications were similar in both groups.[136] However, the cuff leak pressure of the CobraPLA was significantly greater than that of the LMA Unique (23 versus 18 cm H_2O). The investigators found lower airway leak pressures than Agro did, most likely because the Akça study used smaller CobraPLAs.

Gaitini and others, including the inventor, compared the CobraPLA with the LMA Unique during spontaneous ventilation in 80 anesthetized patients.[137] They reported no statistically significant difference between the devices regarding ventilatory variables, number and type of airway interventions required for placement, fiberoptic view, or incidence of adverse events. Reported benefits of the CobraPLA were a significantly higher airway leak pressure (27 versus 21 cm H_2O) and higher oxygen saturation (98% versus 97%) than for the LMA Unique. Conversely time for insertion was significantly shorter for the LMA Classic (24 versus 27 seconds), and insertion was slightly easier than with the CobraPLA.

In a crossover study between the CobraPLA and LMA Classic during controlled ventilation, Nam and associates reported a faster median insertion time for the CobraPLA (15 versus 25 seconds) and a higher median airway seal (23 versus 15 cm H_2O).[138] Other aspects of performance were not different.

Schebesta and coworkers compared the CobraPLA with the LMA Classic in 60 anesthetized patients.[139] The study focused on airway sealing and gas leakage, and despite confirming a higher airway leak pressure with the CobraPLA (24 versus 20 cm H_2O), use of the CobraPLA was associated with higher environmental nitrous oxide

(but not sevoflurane) levels during anesthesia. The study also reported the LMA Classic was associated with easier positioning and a lower peak airway pressure.

Galvin and colleagues studied the CobraPLA and LMA Classic for gynecologic laparoscopy.[140] Insertion characteristics, adverse events, and rates of throat morbidity were similar between devices. Peak airway pressures were higher with the LMA Classic than with the Cobra-PLA. Blood was observed on 40% of CobraPLAs after removal.

Turan and associates compared the CobraPLA with the LT and LMA Classic in 90 patients during short surgical procedures.[141] There were similar results for insertion times, number and type of airway interventions, and hemodynamic variables. Success rates for first-attempt insertion were highest in the CobraPLA group (95%) and lowest in the LMA Classic group (57%). However, blood staining was seen in 50% of cases using the CobraPLA and only 17% of cases using the LMA Classic or LT. The rate of sore throat was also higher in the CobraPLA group than with either of the other SADs.

c. OTHER STUDIES

Ben-Abraham and coworkers studied the ease of insertion of a CobraPLA in anaesthetized patients by residents in scrubs or in antichemical personal protective equipment (PPE).[127] Wearing PPE caused only a modest slowing of insertion time (i.e., median time increased 14 seconds) for anesthesia residents and nonanesthesia residents after training. After insertion, 42% of airway devices leaked, preventing adequate positive-pressure ventilation, and 13 devices (26% of the total) required replacement.

The CobraPLA has been used for difficult airway management in adults:

- For securing an obstructed airway and facilitating fiberoptically guided intubation after thyroidectomy[142]
- For rescuing the airway during cardiopulmonary resuscitation[143]
- For maintaining the airway during urgent percutaneous, dilatational cricothyroidotomy while enabling visualization of the procedure through a fiberscope[144]
- For a series of five percutaneous tracheostomies in a similar manner[145]
- For airway rescue followed by fiberoptically guided tracheal intubation in a "difficult to intubate, difficult to ventilate" patient undergoing rapid-sequence induction of anesthesia[146]

Complications reported during use of the CobraPLA include aspiration, hypoglossal nerve injury,[147] tube obstruction in a patient with a fixed flexed neck, and obstruction by incarceration of the epiglottis in the epiglottic bars.[148,149]

d. LITERATURE SUMMARY

The literature describes the positive and less positive aspects of the CobraPLA. The device usually is readily inserted and has a higher airway leak pressure than the LMA Classic and LMA Unique, although it is likely not higher than the PLMA and LMA Supreme. Some studies report issues with airway trauma and leakage, but interpretation is complicated by a change in design that occurred in 2006 and 2007. Intubation through the CobraPLA is possible but likely requires fiberoptic guidance to make it a reliable technique, like many SADs. Further studies comparing performance of the CobraPLA with second-generation SADs and further evaluation of the ability of the CobraPLA to protect the airway during regurgitation be welcome additions to the literature.

G. Tulip Airway Device

The Tulip airway device (Marshall Medical, Bath, United Kingdom) is a first-generation single-use SAD. It was designed by a British anesthetist Amer Shaikh and brought to market in 2010. It was designed for easy placement by anesthesiologists and others who are trained in its use. Its novel feature is that one size is intended to fit all adults.

Like the CobraPLA, the Tulip was named to reflect its overall shape and appearance. It is a simple airway tube with a distal airway orifice and surrounding distal cuff (Fig. 23-10). The device has a proximal, 15-mm standard connector. It is made of PVC and is designed for single use. The distal cuff is described as an inflatable polyhedral beveled cuff, which is designed to inflate below the soft palate, behind the tongue, above the epiglottis, and within the oropharynx.

The Tulip's design is similar to that of a cuffed oropharyngeal airway (COPA), but it has a larger, more distal, asymmetrical cuff and a shorter, softer, more smoothly curved stem. The stem of the Tulip is curved, and proximally, it has depth markings in three colors to indicate the correct depth of insertion for small (green), medium (orange), and large (red) adults.

1. Application

For insertion, the cuff is deflated and lubricated, except for the front, and the patient placed in the sniffing position. The device is held like a pen and advanced along the hard and soft palates and into the pharynx until the appropriate depth is achieved (according to scale on the tube and the patient size). The cuff is then inflated with the appropriate volume of air to achieve a low-pressure ventilating seal. The device is delivered with 30 mL in the cuff, and 20 to 30 mL can be added. The cuff volume should not exceed 80 mL. As the cuff is inflated, the breathing tube rises out of the mouth.

2. Indications, Advantages, and Disadvantages

Because the device is new and untested, its clinical characteristics are difficult to determine. The manufacturers

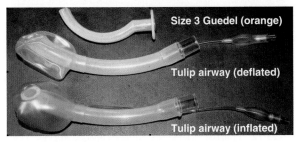

Figure 23-10 The Tulip airway device.

describe the device as suitable for operating rooms and emergency use because it bypasses the need for use of a Guedel oral airway and mask.

The main advantages of the Tulip are simplicity of size selection (i.e., one size fits all adults), a simple insertion technique, and low cost. The main disadvantage is the apparent lack of protection against aspiration. Because the device does not extend into the esophagus, it does not obturate the esophagus. In contrast to most other SADs, its design offers no protection against aspiration. If used for controlled ventilation at anything other than very low airway pressures, there is a risk of gastric inflation. Whether these concerns constitute a practical problem is unknown.

3. Medical Literature

The literature for the Tulip is limited to a single abstract, which describes very effective and swift deployment in a manikin with ventilation and positioning over the manikin's larynx as good as an i-gel and single-use LM.[150] The relevance of these provisional findings to clinical use are unknown. Early clinical experience confirmed its ease of use as a SAD, and clinical trials are being undertaken in the United Kingdom (Amer Shaikh, personal communication, 2009).

VI. SECOND-GENERATION SUPRAGLOTTIC AIRWAY DEVICES

When first introduced into anesthetic practice in 1988, the LMA Classic was greeted with a degree of skepticism. It was used almost exclusively for elective patients undergoing minor peripheral surgery while breathing spontaneously. The LMA Classic was avoided in all overweight patients and rarely used with controlled ventilation. Although this conservative approach was entirely appropriate, there has since been a gradual but inexorable widening of the applications and reduction in the contraindications to LMA Classic use. Whether the more laissez-faire approach to use of the device is appropriate is unknown, but the effect on routine anesthesia care that the LMA Classic has had is remarkable, as is its safety record. In 1993, a large study showed that 30% of all operations were performed with an LMA Classic. In 2009 in the United Kingdom, LMs were used for 56% of episodes of general anesthesia.[7]

First-generation devices that have appeared and disappeared from the market include the COPA, Airway Management Device (AMD), and the Pharyngeal Airway Xpress (PAXpress). Although several devices offered novel components of design, they had no clear advantages over other first-generation SADs, and some had several disadvantages. The main limiting factor to use of the LMA Classic and other-first generation SADs is a lack of protection against aspiration of gastric contents. A relatively low-pressure pharyngeal seal, leading to potential problems with efficacy and safety of controlled ventilation, is a secondary but important factor. In the past few years, newer SADs coming to market have offered the possibility of real technologic advances because they have design features intended to reduce the risk of aspiration, thereby increasing the safety of use. These

second-generation devices often create an increased pharyngeal seal, which ensures more effective and reliable
performance during controlled ventilation. Second-
generation devices overcome the main limitations of the
LMA Classic and other first-generation devices and offer
a genuine stride forward in the safety and effectiveness
of SADs (Fig. 23-11).

Seven SADs have design features that are intended to
reduce the risk of aspiration: the ProSeal LMA, LMA
Supreme, LTS-II, LTS-D, i-gel, SLIPA, and Baska mask.
The Combitube and EasyTube are crossover devices
between ETTs and SADs, and they have characteristics
of second-generation SADs, but they are rarely used for
anesthesia (see Chapter 27).

All second-generation SADs except the SLIPA have
drain tubes running from the tip of the device (correctly
positioned in the upper esophagus) to the proximal end
of the device (lying outside the mouth). If regurgitation
occurs, the correctly functioning drain tube has two
important functions. First, it enables the gastric contents
to bypass the larynx, pharynx, and mouth completely.
Second, even the smallest amount of gastric fluid visible
in the drain tube can alert the anesthesiologist that regurgitation has occurred and trigger an appropriate response.

SADs are increasingly used in more obese patients,
during laparoscopic surgery, during controlled ventilation, in the head-down position, and in those with minor
gastroesophageal reflux. Although all second-generation
SADs have features designed to lessen the likelihood of
gastric inflation, regurgitation, and aspiration, in several
cases, there is little or no evidence to support their performance (safety) benefits. Regurgitation and aspiration
are uncommon events, but the UK NAP4, a year-long
study of major airway complications in 2.9 million cases
of general anesthesia in 2008 through 2009, identified
aspiration as the most frequent cause of airway-related
death during anesthesia.[1] Review of the individual cases
identified numerous aspiration events when a first-
generation SAD was used in patients with clearly identifiable risk factors for aspiration.[151] These events were not
seen with second-generation SADs, although use of these
devices is considerably less common than first-generation
SADs in the United Kingdom, representing approximately 10% of SAD use.[7] Because harmful aspiration
events occur infrequently, evidence proving better safety
of one device compared with another can come only
from formal studies of several million patients, and these
studies are impractical. Instead, safety data must be

acquired by analyzing the design features, appropriate
bench models, surrogate measures of airway safety, and
clinical experience.

The PLMA and LMA Supreme are discussed in
Chapter 22, but it is worth noting that the PLMA is supported by a considerable body of data in terms of its
efficacy as a SAD and regarding its safety profile in separating the respiratory and gastrointestinal tracts and preventing aspiration.[23] No other second-generation SAD
has this body of evidence. The LMA Supreme is not a
single-use PLMA. It has numerous design differences, is
manufactured from a different material, and lacks the
body of evidence underpinning the PLMA. The PLMA is
therefore considered the benchmark against which other
second-generation SADs should be judged.

A. Laryngeal Tube Suction II, Disposable Laryngeal Tube Suction, and Gastro-Laryngeal Tube

In 2002, the Laryngeal Tube Suction (LTS) was introduced. It had a drain tube running posterior to the airway
tube to enable gastric tube placement and to prevent
gastric inflation during ventilation. Although the design
aimed to increase device safety (a similar design step to
that from the LMA Classic to the PLMA), the change in
design led to a much more bulky device, risking increased
insertion difficulty and possible trauma and thereby
losing two of the LT's major advantages. Several studies
found similar performances for the LTS and PLMA, but
one found marked differences in performance.[152-155]
Comparing the LTS and PLMA, Dahaba and colleagues
studied hemodynamic and catecholamine stress responses
to their insertion in 36 patients.[156] Mean arterial pressure,
heart rate, and epinephrine were significantly greater in
the LTS group than in the PLMA group.

In late 2005, the LTS was replaced by a considerably
modified LTS-II (Fig. 23-12). The LTS is no longer available. Like the PLMA, the LTS-II offers the potential for
expansion of the role of the LT. The scant literature suggests that the LTS-II is much easier to insert than the LTS
and that it provides a pharyngeal seal similar to that of
the PLMA. Like the LT, the LTS-II is reusable after

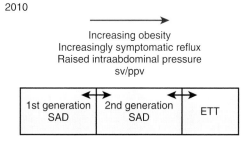

Figure 23-11 Second-generation supraglottic airway devices *(SADs)* available in 2010. *ETT,* Endotracheal tube. *ppv,* positive-pressure ventilation; *sv,* spontaneous ventilation.

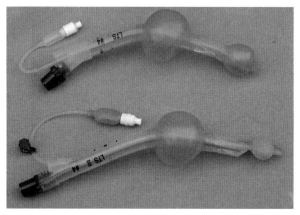

Figure 23-12 VMB Laryngeal Tube Suction devices. *Top,* LTS; *bottom,* LTS-II.

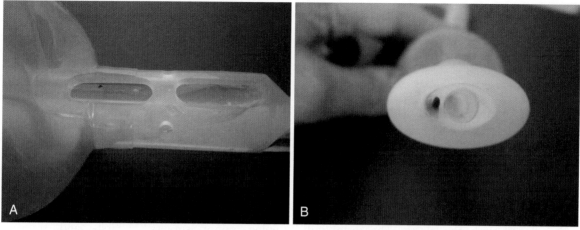

Figure 23-13 The Laryngeal Tube Suction II (LTS-II) airway orifices **(A)** and esophageal balloon **(B)**.

sterilization up to 50 times. Size selection and insertion technique for the LTS-II are identical to those for the LT. A single-use version of the LTS-II, called the LTS-D, is marketed. The latest LT is the Gastro-LT. It is designed specifically for use in upper gastrointestinal endoscopic procedures. It also can be considered a specialized second-generation SAD.

The LTS-II is designed for maintaining the patency of the airway during anesthesia and in emergency airway management. It consists of a translucent, double-lumen silicone tube with two inflatable cuffs with anterior ventilation orifices lying between the cuffs (Fig. 23-13). Both balloons are inflated through a single pilot tube and balloon, through which the cuff pressure can be monitored. When in position with the cuffs inflated, the larger, proximal balloon lies behind the tongue and lifts it forward while stabilizing the tube and isolating the ventilation orifice from the oral and nasopharynx above. The smaller, distal balloon obturates the esophageal inlet and is designed to isolate the ventilation orifice from the esophagus below. A drainage tube runs posterior to the airway tube and extends well beyond its tip. In the original version (LTS), the drain tube was only a little longer than the airway tube, and it ended in a rounded and somewhat bulky tip. The LTS-II has a smaller, considerably longer, and markedly modified tip and a redesigned distal balloon that is ovoid to mimic the shape of the upper esophagus and to provide axial stability for the SAD (see Figs. 23-12 and 23-13). The LTS-II also incorporates minor changes to the airway orifices and to the pilot balloon. The drain tube is designed for passage of a gastric tube up to size 16 F.

The Gastro-LT has a dramatically expanded drain tube and reduced-caliber airway tube (the opposite of the conventional LTS-II) (Fig. 23-14). The basic design principles remain the same as for the LTS-II, but all features of the airway tube are smaller. The drain tube is large enough to allow insertion of a gastrointestinal endoscope up to a diameter of 13.8 mm. The Gastro-LT is made of silicone, has an integrated bite block, and is reusable after decontamination and autoclaving. The device is designed to be used in adults 155 cm tall or taller.

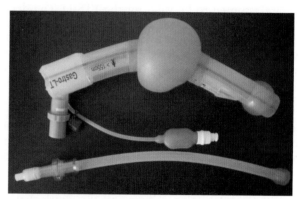

Figure 23-14 The Gastro-LT *(top)* and obturator *(bottom)*.

1. Application

The possibilities and limitations for intubation through the LTS-II are similar to those for intubation through the LT. Insertion and removal techniques for the LTS-II are those described earlier for the LT.

The LTS-II is designed for blind insertion without laryngoscopy. The airway tube has a 15-mm connector (color coded for different sizes) and has a dental line mark to indicate the correct depth of insertion. A bite block is supplied with both devices. The LTS-II is available in the full range of seven sizes from size 0 (newborn <5 kg) to size 5 (large adults >180 cm high), whereas the LTS-D is available only in adult sizes 3, 4, and 5.

2. Indications, Advantages, and Disadvantages

Indications for the LTS-II (and LTS-D) are anesthesia with spontaneous or controlled ventilation, emergency use as a rescue device during difficult airway management, and as a primary emergency airway, in settings such as during management of cardiac arrest outside the hospital.

LTS-II advantages similar to those of the LT include its simple insertion technique, a short learning curve, a relatively slim profile enabling insertion even with limited mouth opening, and the ability to insert the device with the patient's head and neck and the operator's body in a variety of positions. Compared with the LT, the LTS-II has a relatively large-caliber, noncompressible drain tube. This drain tube, which is semirigid and not prone to folding over or obstruction, enables access to the gastrointestinal tract (e.g., insertion of gastric tube) or egress of gastric contents (e.g., regurgitant gastric contents). It is large enough to accommodate small particles of food as well as liquids. Another advantage is that the asymmetrical distal balloon design anchors the device in the proximal esophagus, thereby reducing the likelihood of axial rotation, which has been observed with the LT.

The LTS-II forms a relatively high-pressure pharyngeal (airway) seal, enabling controlled ventilation in patients with reduced lung capacity, provided the airway orifice is correctly aligned with the glottis. The distal cuff forms an effective esophageal seal (approximately 72 to 82 cm H_2O).

Most attributes of the LTS-II described in the literature are assumed to be valid for the LTS-D. The design is identical, and materials are similar to those of the LTS-II. The cuffs of the LTS-D are made of thicker material. The Gastro-LT is designed to maintain the airway for upper gastrointestinal endoscopy during deep sedation or anesthesia with spontaneous or controlled ventilation.

Construction of the LTS-II is relatively rigid, and if used without due care, it can cause trauma to soft tissues. Adherence to manufacturer's guidance and well-practiced, careful technique should minimize this effect.

Despite the asymmetrical distal cuff, there is the possibility of axial rotation of the device leading to misalignment of the ventilation orifices and the glottis. Various rates have been reported for this complication. When it occurs, it may lead to airway obstruction during spontaneously ventilation, high airway pressures during controlled ventilation, and difficulty in accessing the trachea.

Because the airway orifice is a deficiency in the convex part of the curve of a semirigid device, poor insertion technique or undue force can flex the LTS-II at this point. Further advancement may lead to inadvertent tracheal intubation, which has been reported.[94] If inadvertent tracheal intubation occurs, the cuffs should not be inflated because the size of the distal cuff may damage the larynx.

3. Medical Literature

The medical literature should be interpreted with the knowledge that the LTS was replaced by the LTS-II in late 2005. Most studies before 2006 or 2007 studied the bulkier and less stable version of the device.

a. COHORT STUDIES

Mihai and coworkers reported an early cohort study of the LTS-II in 100 patients during controlled and spontaneous ventilation.[157] The success rates were 71% for first-attempt insertion and 100% for three attempts. Median insertion time was 15 seconds. Temporary airway obstruction occurred in six patients at insertion and in another eight during maintenance. Use of the device was abandoned once during insertion and once during maintenance. Median airway leak pressure was 29.5 cm H_2O. A gastric tube was passed through the drain tube in 97 of

99 patients. The glottis was visible during fiberoscopy in 51% of patients. Blood was visible on the device after removal in 12 patients. After the operation, 14 patients reported mild sore throat.

b. RANDOMIZED, CONTROLLED STUDIES OF EFFICACY

Genzwuerker and colleagues first compared the LTS-II and PLMA in 100 patients.[158] Overall performance was almost identical in terms of insertion success (96% for the LTS-II versus 98% for the PLMA), time to placement (25 versus 25.5 seconds), and airway seal (33 versus 32 cm H_2O). Similarly, rates of airway trauma and postoperative sequelae were equivalent in both groups.

Zand and associates randomized patients to the LTS-II or PLMA in a study of 100 anaesthetized patients undergoing minor surgery.[159] First- and second-attempt insertion success rates were comparable (86 versus. 88% and 96 versus 98%) in the LTS-II and PLMA groups, respectively); the two devices failed once after three attempts. The LTS-II was marginally favored over the PLMA in terms of insertion time (24.5 versus 28.8 seconds) and airway seal (20 versus 24.1 cm H_2O, $P = 0.04$). Of several postoperative pharyngeal morbidities, only hoarseness occurred more frequently in the LTS-II group.

Kikuchi and coworkers compared the LTS-II with the PLMA in 100 male patients.[94] Methods included assessing gas leakage with the cuff pressure reduced or when the device shaft was inclined and fluoroscopic examination of the position of the LTS-II. The LTS-II had a lower rate of successful placement than the PLMA (74% versus 96%), a lower tidal volume, and increased gas leakage. The airway seal lower in both groups compared with that reported elsewhere (16 cm H_2O for the LTS-II versus 21 cm H_2O for the PLMA). In 10% of uses, the LTS-II kinked and entered the trachea. Similar findings have not been published elsewhere.

Cavus and colleagues compared the LTS-II with the PLMA, EasyTube, and ETT in 88 patients.[160] Overall insertion success rates were 96% for the LTS-II and ETT, 91% for the PLMA, and 64% for the EasyTube. Time to first ventilation took significantly longer with the EasyTube. Airway leak pressure was highest with the LTS-II and lowest with the EasyTube (40 versus 19 cm H_2O). No major differences in objective or subjective performance were reported for the LTS-II, PLMA, and ETT.

Amini and associates compared the LTS-II and LTS-D in 60 healthy patients undergoing laparoscopic cholecystectomy.[161] First- and second-attempt success rates were similar (93% and 95% for the LTS-II and 86% and 93% for the LTS-D, respectively). After gas insufflation, tube replacement was required for one LTS-D and two LTS-II. Insertion times, success of gastric tube insertion, and postoperative complaints were similar for the two groups.

Thee and colleagues compared the LTS-II and ILMA with their respective disposable versions in 120 patients undergoing minor surgery.[162] Insertion success rates were 100%, except for one LTS-D failure. The LTS-D was faster to insert, had a higher airway leak pressure (40 cm H_2O), and was subjectively assessed to be easier to handle than the LTS-II.

c. OTHER STUDIES

A cadaver study of esophageal seal demonstrated a high-pressure seal (70 to 80 cm H_2O) for the LTS-II, similar to the PLMA seal and higher than the LMA Classic seal.[40]

Asai and colleagues demonstrated that the LT and LTS-II function less well with cricoid pressure applied before and during insertion.[163] Continuous cricoid pressure prolonged time to insertion, reduced the likelihood of successful ventilation, and decreased the airway seal.

Schalk and associates described modified insertion techniques for the LTS-D.[164,165] In the first variation, the LTS-D was inserted upside down (in the manner of a Guedel insertion) while a forced chin lift was performed with the other hand to create sufficient retropharyngeal space.[164] After insertion of one third of its length, the LTS-D was rotated by 180 degrees and pushed down the pharynx. The technique, performed by novices, almost halved insertion time and increased successful insertion within 45 seconds by threefold. When the LTS-D was inserted with the operator in front of the patient and by applying jaw thrust, insertion in patients with an immobilized neck was faster, and the success rate increased more than twofold.[165] Further evaluation suggested that a forceful jaw thrust was an important part of the success of the technique. In both studies, the baseline success rates for insertion were lower than in many other studies.

There is an emerging literature about use of the LTS-II and LTS-D in prehospital airway management, particularly in central Europe. Dengler and colleagues reported one case of massive pulmonary aspiration and one case of gastric overinflation during use of the LT.[114] In both cases, peak airway pressure had been high, and the investigators questioned whether the LTS-II or LTS-D would have been more appropriate. Shalk and colleagues reported 57 attempts with the LTS-D over a 40-month period by paramedics or medics, most of whom had limited prior experience.[166] The use was successful in all but one case, and most devices were inserted in less than 45 seconds. In a subsequent report, Shalk and coworkers described[167] use over 24 months with a 97% success rate; most users were relative novices with the LTS-D.[113] Its use was approximately equally spread between primary airway procedures and airway rescue after failed tracheal intubation. Three fourths of insertions took less than 45 seconds.

Park and colleagues studied the effect of changing the patient's head and neck position on SAD performance, including the LTS-II.[134] Leak pressure was well maintained with the LTS-II, but neck flexion led to ventilation difficulty in approximately 15% of patients.

The LTS-II has been used successfully in a patient with a cervical spine injury.[167] Scheller and associates reported emergency use of the LTS-II or LTS-D in eight patients with difficult airways.[168] In all cases, the device was successfully used as a bridge until a secure airway was established; in six, this was accomplished by cricothyroidotomy or surgical tracheotomy.

Reported complications of the LTS-II are few. In addition to the cases of inadvertent tracheal intubation, there are cases of pilot balloon obstruction by the bite block and a case of ulceration of the tongue and uvula after apparently uneventful use.[169,170]

A single publication described use of the Gastro-LT in 30 patients undergoing general anesthesia for endoscopic retrograde cholangiopancreatography.[171] The study reported 100% insertion success (90% at first attempt), and the mean time to achieve an effective airway was 26 seconds. Tidal volumes were well maintained, and the mean airway leak pressure was 34 cm H_2O.

d. LITERATURE SUMMARY

The LTS-II appears to be easy to insert, and it achieves a high airway seal. It has the advantages of a high-pressure esophageal seal and a drain tube. Ventilation is highly successful, and complications are few. Several studies suggest equivalence to the PLMA. The LTS-D appears to perform at least as well as the LTS-II. Neither device is ideally suited as a conduit for intubation. There is emerging literature on its role in prehospital care.

B. The i-gel

The i-gel (Intersurgical, Wokingham, United Kingdom) is a CE-marked, single-use device. Over several years, numerous prototypes of the i-gel were designed by Muhammed Nasir, a British anesthetist. It was marketed in 2007 and has not been modified since its introduction. In 2009, a full range of pediatric sizes was introduced.

The i-gel is a cuffless, single-use SAD made of a medical-grade thermoplastic elastomer gel (i.e., styrene-ethylene-butadene styrene) and designed for use during anesthesia and airway rescue. It is constructed with a stem and an anatomically designed mask portion; because of the absence of a cuff, inflation is not required after insertion (Fig. 23-15). To seal the airway, the i-gel relies on creating an anatomic seal with pharyngeal, laryngeal, and perilaryngeal structures.

Proximally, the device has a firm tube section that is rigid and noncompressible, acting as an integral bite block. The i-gel stem is elliptical and curved in cross section. Its large caliber lessens the likelihood of displacement or axial rotation after insertion. The mask portion is relatively large—similar to the size of an inflated cuffed SAD (e.g., LMA Classic, PLMA)—enabling the mask to occupy the whole hypopharynx and laryngopharynx. The mask has a relatively blunt tip. The airway tube has a wide bore and ends in a large ventilation orifice with no bars of grills. A ridge at the proximal end of the mask

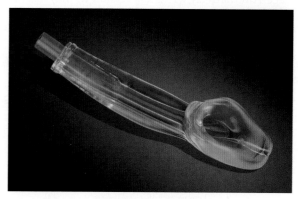

Figure 23-15   The i-gel.

bowl is designed to sit below the tongue base to prevent the i-gel from moving upward and out of position. A black line near the proximal end of the stem acts as a guide to the approximate correct depth.

The i-gel is included among the second-generation SADs because it incorporates throughout its length a drain tube running from the center of the mask tip to the proximal end of the stem. The drain tube is narrower than in some second-generation SADs (e.g., PLMA, LMA Supreme, LTS-II); the size 5 i-gel accommodates a 14-F gastric tube, and sizes 3 and 4 accommodate a 12-F gastric tube.

1. Application

The i-gel is supplied in a plastic cradle that maintains the stem's preformed curve and indicates the device size by its color. Seven sizes of i-gel are available (Table 23-4) and suitable for use in patients from neonates to large adults. Size selection is based on the patient's weight, but the manufacturers advise users to consider individual anatomic variations in selecting a size. For example, patients with long necks and wide thyroid and cricoid cartilages may require a larger size, and patients with central obesity may require the device size to be chosen on the basis of their ideal body weight.

The device should be inspected and checked for defects and obstructions before use. The back, sides, and front of the mask should be lubricated with a thin layer of water-soluble lubricant immediately before use. Excessive lubricant that may be aspirated, particularly from the anterior surface, should be avoided. The patient should be placed in the sniffing position and adequately anesthetized (i.e., to a level suitable for LMA Classic insertion). The patient's mouth should be opened and the i-gel advanced along the roof of the mouth and into the pharynx until resistance is met, indicating it is in position with the tip of the device sitting at the entrance to the esophagus.

Care should be taken to avoid catching the tongue in the bowl of the mask by ensuring the mouth is well open and that the mask tip is directed to the hard palate as it enters the mouth. If the tongue is caught, it may impede insertion and risk tearing the frenulum. Difficulty in negotiating the angle of the pharynx may be minimized by choosing the correct size of i-gel, lubricating as instructed, and extending the patient's head. A jaw lift or rotation of the device during insertion may also ease its passage. Alternatively, a rotatory technique may be chosen in which the device is inserted laterally and rotated into place as resistance is felt on reaching the posterior pharyngeal wall. If insertion is difficult or an adequate seal is not achieved, another device size should be tried.

After insertion, the i-gel should be held in place and secured with tape from "maxilla to maxilla." The anesthetic circuit should be attached to the 15-mm connector, and ease of ventilation should be confirmed with gentle manual ventilation. In most cases, the pharyngeal seal is approximately 20 to 30 cm H_2O. Although the manufacturers describe the use of muscle relaxants during controlled ventilation with the i-gel, many practitioners do not find this to be necessary if an adequate depth of anesthesia is maintained.

For most patients, the i-gel may be left in place after routine anesthesia until consciousness is regained and airway reflexes have returned. Gentle suction may be applied around the i-gel before removal, which should be performed when the patient is able to open his or her mouth in response to commands. The manufacturers describe removal under deep anesthesia and replacement with a Guedel airway for patients with a heightened gag reflex (e.g., smokers, asthmatics, patients with chronic obstructive pulmonary disease).

The i-gel has several features that make it suitable for use as a conduit for tracheal intubation, including a large-diameter lumen, relatively short airway tube, absence of bars or grills across the distal airway tube or airway orifice, and the large dimension of the mask bowl. The epiglottis is rarely folded over within the large mask bowl, and the glottis is usually easily visible. In this respect, the i-gel is similar to the PLMA. During endoscopy through the i-gel, the glottis usually is visible almost as soon as the endoscope exits the stem part of the airway tube, and the fiberscope can easily be negotiated to the glottis even if some manipulation is required. In some other SADs, such as the LMA Classic and LT family of devices, there is less space for manipulation. Table 23-5 shows the sizes of lubricated ETTs that can be passed through each size of i-gel.

Two high-quality studies compared the performance of the i-gel as a conduit for intubation with intubation through a single-use ILMA.[172,173] The first study found that the i-gel was a poor device for use with blind intubation (as are many SADs). The overall success rate for the first attempt was 15% through the i-gel and 69% through the ILMA ($P < 0.001$). In the second study, in which fiberoptic guidance was used, the i-gel performed very well and at least as well as the ILMA; the first-time success rate was 96% for the i-gel and 90% for the ILMA

TABLE 23-4

Sizing Guidelines for the i-gel Supraglottic Airway

i-gel Size	Patient Size	Guide Weight (kg)
1	Newborn	2-5
1.5	Infant	5-12
2	Small child	10-25
2.5	Large child	25-35
3	Small adult	30-60
4	Medium adult	50-90
5	Large adult	90+

TABLE 23-5

Sizing Guidelines for Inserting an ETT through an i-gel Supraglottic Airway

i-gel Size	Maximum ETT Size (mm)
1	3.0
1.5	4.0
2	5.0
2.5	5.0
3	6.0
e	7.0
5	8.0

ETT, Endotracheal tube.

($P = 0.21$). The findings support the use of the i-gel as a conduit for intubation as an elective technique and after airway rescue, but they strongly indicate that a fiberoptically guided technique should be used when possible.

2. Indications, Advantages, and Disadvantages

The i-gel is designed primarily for use during anesthesia and is suitable for spontaneous and controlled ventilation. The ease of insertion allied with a steep learning curve has led to recognition of its role in airway rescue. Its wide airway tube and large bowl reduce airway resistance and make it suitable for use as a conduit for intubation as an elective technique or after airway rescue. Because of its insertion and performance characteristics, it has been included as an airway device for use in management of cardiac arrest in ILCOR's 2010 guidelines.[93]

The i-gel has several design and performance advantages. Absence of a cuff may make insertion quicker and easier than many other SADs. Its remarkable slipperiness after lubrication and moderate rigidity increase ease of insertion. Its relatively large size and elliptical shape reduce the risk of displacement or rotation after insertion. The large, short, unobstructed airway lumen leads to low airway resistance during use and enables easy endoscopic access to the glottis if required. The drain tube and airway seal, which is usually a higher-pressure seal than that of the LMA Classic, indicate a degree of protection against aspiration and enable early identification of regurgitation (i.e., gastric contents seen in drain tube), although this advantage is largely unproven. Despite its size, it is well tolerated on emergence and may be removed with the patient fully awake. The incidence of sequelae after use of the i-gel (e.g., sore throat, dysphagia, dysphonia) appears to be low and perhaps as low as for any SAD.

The material the i-gel cuff is filled with is a thermoplastic gel. When warmed, its properties alter slightly, and several investigators have reported that the pharyngeal (airway) seal improves over time after insertion. Only limited evidence supports this effect, which has not been widely explored in other SADs. Alternative explanations include stress relaxation of pharyngeal muscles after distention, which may lead to improved airway seal sometime after insertion of the i-gel and other SADs. Although the clinical relevance of this feature remains undefined, the other features of the i-gel make it a useful and versatile device.

The i-gel is a suitable alternative to the LMA Classic and LMs during routine use, and it may have advantages over them. It is less well suited for some head and neck operations (suitable for the LMA Flexible) due to the bulky, rigid stem. Despite its soft feel, the relatively large size of the i-gel and its noncompressible design mean that care is required during insertion and removal to avoid injury, particularly to at-risk dentition and the frenulum of the tongue. There have been sporadic reports of congestion of the tongue, perhaps due to an incompletely inserted i-gel interfering with venous drainage. Good technique with full insertion and the device secured in place should minimize this risk.

In some series of i-gel uses, only a very-low-pressure airway seal can be achieved in a minority of patients. In about 2% to 5% of cases, manual ventilation may not be possible due to a gas leak. A change of size of device may resolve the problem.

One feature of the i-gel design may be an advantage and a disadvantage. The tip of the bowl of the i-gel is somewhat truncated. During the design phase, the inventor reduced the size of the tip to minimize disruption of the cricopharyngeus with the intention of reducing postoperative sore throat (Muhammed Nasir, personal communication, 2009 or 2010). Observational data suggest this modification has been successful in reducing postoperative sequelae, but a cadaver study has indicated that the esophageal seal of the i-gel is rather low (13 to 21 cm H_2O); this is less than one half of the equivalent seal of the LMA Classic (30 to 50 cm H_2O) or PLMA (50 to 80 cm H_2O) and less than one third of the seal achieved by the laryngeal tubes (70 to 80 cm H_2O).[12,40] The same studies demonstrate that regurgitant fluid is effectively vented by the i-gel drain tube, unless it is blocked. The drain tube may obviate the need for a high-pressure esophageal seal in protecting the pharynx from regurgitation, although the clinical importance of these findings remains uncertain. On the available evidence, it appears that an orogastric tube should not remain in the drain tube during use, because if the drain tube is occluded, the esophageal seal may not protect the airway; if inserted to drain the stomach, it should be used after suctioning. Cases of protection from aspiration with the i-gel are reported, as is one case of partial aspiration.

Overall, the increased protection against aspiration of the i-gel is supported by several design features but not formally proved by a clinical study. However, several million i-gel uses attest to the fact that the i-gel is a safe device.

3. Medical Literature

Despite the relatively new introduction of the i-gel, there are already more than 60 publications describing the device. This reflects the great interest in the device. Only the most important can be summarized here.

a. COHORT STUDIES

The first published i-gel study evaluated a series of 73 uses in 63 cadavers to determine its anatomic positioning after insertion using fiberscopic, radiologic, and dissection methods.[174] The full glottis was visible after 44 of 73 insertions, with only three epiglottis-only views. After eight reinsertions, more than half of the glottis was visible in all cadavers. In each of the 16 neck dissections and on eight radiographs, the bowl of the i-gel covered the laryngeal inlet.

Richez and colleagues reported use of the i-gel in 71 women.[175] Insertion success rate was 97%, and was rated easy in all cases. Mean airway leak pressure was 30 ± 7 cm H_2O, and peak airway pressure was 11 ± 3 cm H_2O. Gastric tube insertion was successful in 100% of cases. One case of coughing and one mild sore throat occurred.

Asai and Liu reported i-gel use in 20 patients breathing spontaneously.[176] In 19 patients, insertion was successful on the first attempt, and the mean insertion time was 12 seconds. The success rate for gastric tube insertion was 100%. No complications occurred during anesthesia, removal was uneventful, and no blood was detected on any device.

Kannaujia and colleagues performed a study of 50 i-gel uses, including assessment of stability during head and neck movement.[177] The success rate at first attempt was 90%, and 100% after two attempts, with a median insertion time of 11 seconds. Manipulations needed to achieve an effective airway were deeper insertion in 8% and jaw thrust or chin lift in 4%. Mean airway leak pressure was 20 cm H_2O. Gastric tube insertion was successful when attempted. There were no significant adverse events.

Gatward and coworkers evaluated 100 i-gels during controlled and spontaneous ventilation.[178] First-attempt insertion was successful in 86%, second-attempt in 11%, and third-attempt in 3% of patients. Fifty-three manipulations were required in 26 patients (median, 1) to achieve a clear airway. Median insertion time was 15 seconds. During ventilation, an expired tidal volume of $7 \text{ mL} \times \text{kg}^{-1}$ was achieved in 96% of patients. Median airway leak pressure was 24 cm H_2O. On fiberoptic examination, the vocal cords were visible in 87 patients (91%). There was one episode of regurgitation without aspiration. Other complications and side effects were mild and few.

In the largest cohort series of 1658 cases, insertion of the i-gel failed in 1.3% of cases, and 90% were judged to be an easy or very easy insertion.[179] Mean airway seal was 25 ± 8 cm H_2O, and 93% of cases were completed with the i-gel. Complications included laryngospasm or bronchospasm (0.8%), glossopharyngeal nerve injury (0.6%), glottic hematoma (0.6%), bilateral tip of the tongue paresthesia (0.6%), and bradycardia requiring cardiopulmonary resuscitation (0.6%).

Wharton and coworkers examined i-gel use by inexpert medical and paramedical users in 40 patients after manikin training.[180] The success rate was 82.5% (33 of 40) on the first attempt and 15% on the second attempt (6 of 40). After three attempts, there were no failures. Median insertion time was 17.5 seconds. Median airway seal was 20 cm H_2O (range, 13 to −40 cm H_2O). One case of regurgitation and partial aspiration occurred. Performance by these novices using the i-gel compared well with performance using other SADS, and it was remarkably similar to the performance by experienced anesthesiologists reported by the same group.[178]

b. RANDOMIZED, CONTROLLED STUDIES OF EFFICACY

In a small study, Uppall and associates compared leak volume (i.e., inspired volume − expired volume) during pressure-controlled ventilation (15, 20, and 25 cm H_2O) through the i-gel and cuffed ETT in 25 patients.[181] Leak volume did not vary at 15 or 20 cm H_2O, but at 25 cm H_2O, the i-gel leaked more than the ETT. No gastric inflation was detected.

Two studies compared the LMA Classic and i-gel and reported opposing findings. Janakiraman and colleagues compared the i-gel and LMA Classic in 50 healthy patients who were breathing spontaneously.[182] The investigators reported a much lower first-attempt insertion success rate (54%) for the i-gel than many other investigators and found this rate significantly lower than for the

LMA Classic (86%, $P = 0.001$). After two attempts and with a change in size, the insertion rates were similar (84% for the i-gel and 92% for the LMA Classic). Leak pressure was higher for the i-gel (median [IQR], 20 cm H_2O; 14 to 24 cm H_2O) than for the LMA Classic (17 H_2O; 12 to 22 cm H_2O; $P = 0.023$), and the fiberoptic view was statistically significantly better. The manufacturer suggested that the high failure correlated with a lack of lubrication of the front of the mask during this study.[183]

Helmy and coworkers also compared the i-gel and LMA Classic during spontaneous ventilation.[184] Neither device caused significant hemodynamic disturbance during insertion, and there was no difference in insertion attempts. The i-gel had a faster mean insertion time (15.6 ± 4.9 seconds versus 26.2 ± 17.7, $P < 0.1$), and it produced a higher leak pressure (25.6 ± 4.9 versus 21.2 ± 7.7 cm H_2O, $P = 0.016$). Gastric inflation was detected in 23% of LMA Classic uses and 5% of i-gel uses ($P = 0.016$).

Several studies have compared the i-gel with single-use LMs. Cattano and associates compared the i-gel and LMA Unique in 50 healthy patients.[185] There were no significant differences in the ease of insertion, leak pressures, or fiberoptic view. The i-gel was favored by faster insertion (21.0 ± 12.6 versus 30.0 ± 14.1 seconds, $P = 0.02$), but it required a second attempt at insertion more frequently, and in three patients, the i-gel was replaced by an LMA Unique. Patients weighing 80 to 90 kg were more likely to experience postoperative symptoms, such as sore throat and dysphagia. The investigators suggested the larger size might be restricted to patients who weighed more than 90 kg.

Uppal and colleagues conducted a study of 39 patients during controlled ventilation with the i-gel or LMA Unique. They reported similar insertion success, leak pressures (median, 25 cm H_2O for the i-gel versus 22 cm H_2O, for the LMA Unique) and leak volumes for both devices.[186] The i-gel was a few seconds faster to insert.

Francksen and coworkers compared the i-gel and LMA Unique in a study of 80 patients.[187] Overall performance measures were similar, but the i-gel had a higher leak pressure (29 versus 18 cm H_2O) and better fiberoptic view of the larynx. Postoperative symptoms were similar for the two devices.

Amini and Khoshfetrat compared the i-gel with the Solus LM (from the same manufacturers) in 120 patients.[188] The leak pressure was significantly higher in the Solus group (mean ± SD, 22.7 ± 7.7 versus 19.3 ± 7.1 cm H_2O, $P = 0.02$). The Solus provided a better fiberoptic view of the larynx and required less airway manipulation to maintain a clear airway. Both devices were considered to perform well.

Keijzer and associates studied postoperative symptoms in 218 patients whose airways were managed with the i-gel or La Premiere single-use LM.[189] The incidence of sore throat was significantly lower with the i-gel than with LM at three time points (1, 24, and 48 hours), with up to 40% of La Premiere uses leading to sore throat. The i-gel was also associated with less dysphagia and neck pain.

Heuer and colleagues compared the performance of the Ambu AuraOnce, LMA Classic, PLMA, and i-gel during ambulatory surgery; each group contained 40 patients.[190] The Ambu AuraOnce and LMA Classic were placed on the first attempt most often (both, 92.5%; PLMA, 85%; i-gel, 82.5%; $P < 0.05$).[190] Mean insertion times for the four devices were all within 2.5 seconds of each other. The investigators measured the proportion of cases in which the pharyngeal seal was above 15 and 20 cm H_2O; the respective rates were highest for the Ambu AuraOnce (97.5% and 67.5%), then for the PLMA (90% and 60%), the LMA Classic (85% and 62.5%), and the i-gel (72.5% and 50%); for both series, $P > 0.05$. More patients complained of a sore throat after using the LMA Classic ($P < 0.05$). The rather low airway leak pressures with the PLMA and i-gel and low insertion success rates with the i-gel are not consistent with the bulk of the literature.

Comparing the i-gel with the PLMA in 60 healthy patients, Singh and colleagues reported a somewhat higher first-time insertion success rate with the i-gel (29 of 30 versus 25 of 30 patients) and a lower leak pressure (25 versus 30 cm H_2O).[191] The i-gel group had fewer episodes of minor trauma, and the device was associated with more reliable gastric tube insertion.

Shin and associates compared the i-gel with the LMA Classic and the PLMA in a study of 167 healthy patients.[192] The airway leak pressures for the PLMA (30 cm H_2O) were higher than for the i-gel (27 cm H_2O) and LMA Classic (25 cm H_2O). Rates of insertion success and adverse events were similar, although there were more sore throats in the LMA Classic group.

Fernández Díez studied the i-gel and LMA Supreme in 85 patients.[193] First-attempt insertion success for the LMA Supreme (95%) was higher than for the i-gel (86%), and the time to insertion (27 versus 32 seconds) was not significantly different. The rate for passing a gastric tube on the first attempt was better for the i-gel (98%) than the LMA Supreme (86%). Leak pressure and compliance were similar in the two groups at the start of surgery and at 10, 30, and 60 minutes. Complications during surgery and at 90 minutes were not significantly different.

Theiler and colleagues compared the i-gel and LMA Supreme in a crossover study of 60 patients with simulated difficult airways through neck immobilization.[194] Insertion success was similar for the i-gel (93%) and LMA Supreme (95%, $P = 1.0$), as were tidal volumes and airway leak pressure (27 versus 26 cm H_2O, $P = 0.4$). The difference in success rates was 1.7% (95% CI, –11.3% to 7.6%). Insertion time was shorter for the LMA Supreme (34 versus 42 seconds, $P = 0.024$). The fiberoptic view through the i-gel showed less epiglottic downfolding. Two major studies comparing the i-gel with the single-use ILMA for intubation, blindly or with fiberoptic guidance, were described earlier.[172,173]

c. OTHER STUDIES

A U.K. national census of airway device use conducted from 2008 through 2009 recorded that 56.2% of all instances of general anesthesia are delivered with a SAD as the primary airway.[7] Most were LMs (including the LMA Classic, LMA Flexible, and other LMs). Only 10%

of SAD uses in this census were second-generation SADs, and the ratio of uses of i-gels to PLMAs was 2.5:1. The i-gels were used for 4% of all episodes of general anesthesia, and PLMAs were used for 1.7%.

Schmidbauers and coworkers' cadaver study showed the i-gel's esophageal seal to be lost at lower pressures than many others SADs.[12] During a slow increase in pressure, the i-gel lost its seal at 13 cm H_2O; 1 minute after maximum pressure had been applied, the device withstood a sustained pressure of 21 cm H_2O. Despite the lost seal, the i-gel drain tube vented liquids rapidly. The LMA Classic and PLMA created esophageal seals at considerably higher pressures (37 to 46 versus 58 to 59 cm H_2O). The clinical relevance of these findings is debated and requires further exploration.

Ismail and associates studied the changes in hemodynamics and intraocular pressure in 60 patients scheduled for nonophthalmic surgery with the i-gel, LMA Classic, or ETT.[195] Insertion of the i-gel did not increase intraocular pressure, whereas the ETT increased it 5 mm Hg, and the LMA Classic increased it marginally. Tracheal intubation led to a rise in all hemodynamic measures (i.e., heart rate, systolic blood pressure and diastolic blood pressure), but the increases were less with the LMA Classic. The i-gel led to significantly fewer changes. The perfusion index was decreased for 5 minutes by the ETT, 2 minutes by the LMA Classic, and not at all by the i-gel. Jindal and colleagues also examined the hemodynamics of insertion of the i-gel, LMA Classic, and SLIPA.[196] The i-gel produced the least hemodynamic changes. Zaballos and colleagues observed that the i-gel in vitro had no effect on MRI, whereas the LMA Classic, PLMA, and LMA Unique (but not the Ambu Aura-Once) did.[66] Novel applications of the i-gel include use for awake craniotomy with the head in a rotated position,[197] use in the prone position,[198] use for a patient with subglottic stenosis,[199] and use during placement of a bronchial blocker for single-lung ventilation in 25 patients without incident.[200]

The i-gel has been used in difficult airway management, including during rescue of an obstructed airway,[201,202] as an intermediate airway during difficult intubation,[203] as a conduit after failed intubation, and as a conduit for elective intubation in patients with predicted difficult airway.[204-206] All of these intubations use fiberoptic guidance.

Reported complications of i-gel use include tongue trauma,[207] severe laryngeal hemorrhage requiring intensive care unit admission,[208] regurgitation and aspiration,[178,209] and a variety of minor nerve injuries.[179,180,209-211]

d. LITERATURE SUMMARY

The i-gel is acquiring a reputation for ease of insertion, minimal stimulation, good performance during spontaneous or controlled ventilation, and excellent tolerance during emergence. Access to the glottis for intubation is reliable but requires fiberoptic guidance. Limitations are its occasional very poor seal and its moderate bulk. There is some uncertainty about the esophageal seal and drain tube capacity and therefore a degree of uncertainty about the additional protection against aspiration that the i-gel offers in the event of regurgitation.

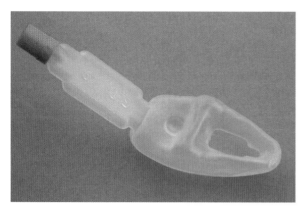

Figure 23-16 The Streamlined Liner of the Pharynx Airway (SLIPA).

TABLE 23-6			
SLIPA Size Selection			
SLIPA Size	Patient	Median Height (cm)	Height Range (cm)
47	Very small female	152	145-160
49	Small female	160	152-168
51	Medium female	168	160-175
53	Large female to small male	173	163-182
55	Medium male	180	173-193
57	Large male	190	180-200

SLIPA, Streamlined Liner of the Pharynx Airway.

C. SLIPA: Streamlined Liner of the Pharynx Airway

The SLIPA (Curveair, London, United Kingdom), which looks somewhat like a slipper, was developed by Donald Miller, a U.K.-based anesthetist.[212] The airway lines the pharynx and thereby controls it and provides an enlarged cavity (i.e., sump) for trapping regurgitated liquids and preventing pulmonary aspiration. The design does not require an inflatable cuff to achieve airway seal and such a cuff would also reduce storage capacity. A simpler device without a cuff makes manufacturing less expensive and the device suitable for single use. There were several iterations of the SLIPA before its commercial launch in Europe in June 2004.

The SLIPA is a cuffless single-use SAD made from firm plastic with a preformed shape designed to match the anatomy of the pharynx. Its hollow, blow-molded chamber is shaped like a pressurized pharynx and somewhat like a boot with a toe, a bridge that seals at the base of the tongue, and a heel that anchors the device in a stable position between the esophagus and nasopharynx (Fig. 23-16).[44] The anterior surface of the SLIPA has a series of bulges and indentations whose positions are designed to mimic human anatomy and enable close matching of the shape of the device and the patient's airway. For example, toward the toe side of two lateral bulges of the bridge are smaller, secondary lateral bulges that leave an indentation; the positions of the bulges were extrapolated from a study on cadavers to coincide with the tips of the hyoid bone. This design is intended to relive pressure at this vulnerable anatomic site and thereby reduces the risk of damage to the hypoglossal and recurrent laryngeal nerves.[213]

Because the device is hollow, a limited volume of pharyngeal secretions or regurgitated liquids can pass through the anterior airway orifice and be retained within the airway, potentially providing some protection from aspiration. The chamber has a considerably higher capacity than several other SADs (up to 70 mL for the SLIPA and less than 5 mL for a size 4 or 5 LMA Classic).[44] This design feature of the SLIPA is intended to reduce the risk of aspiration and is the reason it is classified as a second-generation device.

The SLIPA has six adult sizes (47, 49, 51, 53, 55, and 57) and no pediatric sizes. Many sizes are needed to closely match the SLIPA to the pharyngeal dimensions. Sizes 47, 49, and 51 are suitable for small, medium, and large female patients, and sizes 53, 55, and 57 are suitable for small, medium, and large male patients, respectively. The numbers refer to the widest transverse diameter (in millimeters) at the level of the bridge of the device. Matching this dimension to the distance between left and right cornu of the thyroid cartilage is one method of choosing the correct size. Guidance for sizing the device is shown in Table 23-6. Size selection is arguably more important for the SLIPA than other SADs because the lack of a cuff means that the airway seal and the ability to provide controlled ventilation depend on correct sizing. When there is doubt, the manufacturers recommend initially using the larger of two possible sizes.

1. Application

The insertion technique for the SLIPA is different from that of the LMA Classic, and it is not helpful to try pushing it against the hard palate. The device is lubricated, and the patient, who must be adequately anaesthetized, is positioned in the sniffing position. The device is advanced toward the esophagus until the heel of the device spontaneously locates itself in the nasopharynx. It usually passes the oropharyngeal curve with ease. The toe of the SLIPA may be used to lift the base of the tongue in a manner similar to a laryngoscope. As with most SADs, it is helpful if an assistant lifts the jaw forward during insertion. Alternatively, the anesthesiologist can lift the jaw forward with the thumb and finger. As the device moves into position, the angle between stem and shoe portion increases to be almost perpendicular. When it is in position, further pressure on the stem leads to clear resistance, indicating it is fully inserted. Because the heel enters the nasopharynx and anchors the device's position, the manufacturers indicate it is unnecessary to tie the device in place.

The SLIPA's plastic is relatively rigid at room temperature, and this may facilitate insertion. During use, the plastic softens as it warms, reducing the risk of airway trauma. After insertion, the toe of the device sits at the level of the cricopharyngeus (i.e., upper esophageal sphincter), the heal lies in the nasopharynx, and the stem lies over the tongue. The crescent shape of the toe is designed to lower the risk of obstructing the airway during insertion by folding the epiglottis down or causing laryngospasm. The bridge in the center of the chamber

TABLE 23-7

Fluid Retention by SLIPAs in Horizontal and 10-Degree Head-Down Positions

SLIPA Size (mm)	Horizontal Position (mL of Fluid)*	Head-Down Position (mL of Fluid)*
47	29 ± 0.3	45 ± 0.3
49	30 ± 1.0	48 ± 0.7
51	32 ± 1.3	54 ± 0.7
53	36 ± 1.0	62 ± 0.6
55	45 ± 1.2	68 ± 1.1
57	54 ± 0.8	72 ± 1.2

SLIPA, Streamlined Liner of the Pharynx Airway.
*Values are mean ± SD.
Courtesy of Donald Miller, MD.

with its two lateral bulges is designed to fit into the piriform fossa at the base of the tongue and displace it from the posterior pharyngeal wall, thereby preventing the epiglottis from closing on the glottis. The anterior opening in the SLIPA has a wider portion and a narrower, distal portion, which is designed to minimize the risk of obstruction by an elongated epiglottis. For patients with limited mouth opening (as little as 1 cm), the hollow chamber may be flattened to facilitate insertion.

The SLIPA can be removed while the patient is still anesthetized, in which case a bite block is not recommended for routine use. Removing the SLIPA requires dislodgement of the heel from its anchoring in the nasopharynx. The device should be gently pulled anterior and caudal at the same time as opening the mouth. If the intention is to remove the SLIPA after the return of airway reflexes, a bite block is recommended.

If regurgitation is suspected, the chamber can be emptied by passing a suction catheter into it. Directing the catheter laterally during insertion minimizes the risk of it passing through the ventilation orifice. Alternatively, the SLIPA can be removed and then the pharynx suctioned. The head-down position enlarges the capacity that a given SLIPA can accommodate (Table 23-7).

The SLIPA has not been evaluated as an intubation conduit. The instructions for use state that "the SLIPA is not recommended for pulmonary endoscopic procedures."

2. Indications, Advantages, and Disadvantages

The SLIPA is a simple, inexpensive, disposable SAD with design features intended to minimize the risk of aspiration during use. It can be used during anesthesia with spontaneous or controlled ventilation. Proposed advantages over first-generation SADs include simplicity of construction and use because of lack of a cuff, ease of insertion, ability to compress and insert when there is a reduced mouth opening, a shape designed to minimize pressure on at-risk nerves, no need to be secured, and the ability to capture regurgitant fluid. The limited amount of published literature on the SLIPA means that many of these proposed advantages remain unexamined and therefore unproven.

The SLIPA is recommended for patients who are fasted and is not recommended for use in patients with gastric volumes that are likely to exceed normal fasting

gastric volumes or in patients with gastroparesis. Because it relies on the chamber lying below the larynx, it is not recommended for use in positions such as prone or when the head and neck may be rotated. As with other SADs, use of the SLIPA does not require paralysis or laryngoscopy.

Because the SLIPA must be closely matched to the size of the pharynx to seal it effectively, many sizes are needed to ensure a correct fit for adult patients. Although patient height is an acceptable method for sizing the SLIPA, matching the width of the thyroid cartilage to the SLIPA's dimension aids in making the appropriate choice of device size. This range of sizes is not required for other SADs, and it may be considered an additional complexity, with an increased risk of selecting the wrong size.

The SLIPA is not designed to be used with the head rotated to the side, which may lead to loss of the seal. In the lateral or prone position, the utility of the SLIPA chamber to capture regurgitant fluid is reduced or lost.

3. Medical Literature

The literature on the SLIPA is complicated by several changes in its design over the years, which not all publications make clear. Many early studies were led or contributed to by the inventor. Later versions of the device have become more stable, and there have been more independent evaluations.

Fewer than 20 publications have described study of the SLIPA.

a. COHORT STUDIES

Miller and Lavelle reported an early cohort of 22 patients and a 91% success rate for use of the SLIPA.[212] Hein and colleagues performed a study of 60 insertions in patients undergoing minor surgical procedures.[214] Twenty SLIPAs were inserted by the experienced study lead and 40 by medical officers and anesthesiologists with various degrees of experience. Median time to ventilation was 20.4 seconds for the study lead and 24.8 seconds in the other group. The overall success rate for insertion was 100% for the study lead and 92.5% for the less-experienced group. Incidences of blood or sore throat score of more than 3 (scale of 0 to 10) were 23% and 7%, respectively. The less-experienced group reported the SLIPA to be easy to insert in 92% of cases.

Zimmermann and coworkers reported use of the SLIPA in 36 patients undergoing ophthalmic surgery.[215] Insertion was successful in 100% of patients, with 16% requiring manipulation to achieve a good seal. Four devices were replaced for other sizes. Ventilation was good, with no gastric inflation or regurgitation. In 17% of patients, blood was seen on removal of the device, and 22% reported slight pharyngeal discomfort.

b. RANDOMIZED, CONTROLLED STUDIES OF EFFICACY

In a study enrolling 120 patients, the inventor compared an early version of the SLIPA with the LMA Classic, with three sizes to choose from.[44] In overall performance (i.e., insertion success rate, airway seal, stress response to placement, postoperative trauma and sore throat), both devices were comparable. Insertion was successful for the

SLIPA and the LMA Classic in 59 of 60 patients. The airway leak pressure was higher with the LMA Classic, but the difference was not statistically significant.

Lange and associates compared the SLIPA with the LMA Classic in 124 patients undergoing ophthalmic surgery during general anesthesia.[216] SLIPA insertion failed in 2% and was easy in 88% of patients, and LMA Classic insertion failed in 0% and was easy in 90%. Airway leak pressure was not different between groups. Gastric inflation occurred in 19% of patients in the SLIPA group and 3% in the LMA Classic group ($P < 0.05$). No regurgitation was observed. Blood traces were more common in the SLIPA group (20% versus 11%, not statistically significant), as was postoperative sore throat (14% versus 2%).

In an early study by Miller and Camporota, the SLIPA was compared with the PLMA and ETT during 150 gynecologic laparoscopies.[217] The SLIPA and PLMA were comparable regarding ease of insertion, oropharyngeal leak (30 versus 31 cm H_2O), seal quality, systolic pressure in response to insertion, and time saved compared with tracheal intubation. There were fewer sore throats with the PLMA.

Woo and colleagues compared the SLIPA and PLMA in 101 patients undergoing gynecologic laparoscopy with controlled ventilation.[218] Insertion success rate, gastric insufflation, perilaryngeal leakage, anatomic fit, airway sealing pressure, respiratory mechanics, severity of sore throat, and incidence of blood and regurgitated fluid on the device were similar for the two groups. When the patient's head and neck position was changed, perilaryngeal leakage was less frequent with the SLIPA than with the PLMA (3 of 50 versus 11 of 51, $P = 0.026$). During peritoneal insufflation, perilaryngeal leakage did not occur with the SLIPA, but it occurred in four cases with the LMA ProSeal ($P = 0.045$).

Choi and coworkers reported a study of the SLIPA and PLMA in 60 patients.[219] Success rates for first-attempt intubation were 93% for the PLMA and 73% for the SLIPA, and the mean insertion times were 7.3 and 10.5 seconds, respectively. There was a greater hemodynamic response to SLIPA insertion than the PLMA. There was no statistically significant difference in the airway leak pressure, ventilation measures, postoperative sore throat, or other complication between the two groups. Blood stain on the device's surface was seen in 40% with the SLIPA and in 6.7% with the PLMA.

Puri and associates reported a high incidence of blood on the SLIPA at removal (40% versus 12% for the LMA Classic).[220]

c. OTHER STUDIES

Miller and Light used a lung model to study aspiration into the lungs, which could be quantitatively modeled in relation to regurgitation volumes during positive-pressure ventilation.[44] The model design had morphologic similarity to the SLIPA and was used to examine the SLIPA, LMA Classic, and PLMA. The SLIPA and PLMA compared favorably with the LMA Classic. Aspiration occurred after as little as 3.5 mL with the LMA Classic, whereas aspiration was prevented with the SLIPA until volumes of approximately 50 mL.

Hein and colleagues studied SLIPA and SSLM insertion in 36 anaesthetized patients by medical students trained on a manikin.[78] Rates of first-attempt insertion favored the SLIPA over the SSLM (83% versus 67%), as did the overall insertion success rate (94% versus 89%), but neither difference was significant. Median time to ventilation was shorter with the SLIPA (41 versus 67 seconds, $P = 0.004$) but only when it was used as the first device. Sixty-seven percent of the students expressed a preference for use of the SLIPA.

Fluid dynamic studies of various SADs revealed that there was less resistance to gas flow in the SLIPA than in other devices.[221] A surprising amount of the literature on the SLIPA examines hemodynamic changes in response to insertion. Xu and Zhong compared the SLIPA with the LMA Classic and ETT in 90 healthy patients scheduled for gynecologic laparoscopy.[222] Hemodynamic changes were greatest with the ETT. Puri and associates studied the hemodynamic response to insertion of the SLIPA and the LMA Classic in 100 patients.[220] Before SAD insertion, the Bispectral index was titrated to 40, a value indicating an appropriate level of general anesthesia. Both airway devices elicited hemodynamic changes, but they were greater and more prolonged in the SLIPA group. Both devices produced a similar increase in the Bispectral index after insertion. Similarly, Jindal and colleagues reported the SLIPA produced greater hemodynamic changes than the i-gel.[196] Choi and coworkers reported a greater hemodynamic response to the SLIPA than the PLMA.[219]

d. LITERATURE SUMMARY

There are too few studies to determine the efficacy of the SLIPA and whether the chamber does reduce the risk of aspiration. There is no substantial clinical evidence to support this claim. Although several studies have indicated adequate insertion and ventilation performance, including performance equivalent to the PLMA, several studies have indicated a high rate of airway trauma and sore throat. Clinical benefits of the SLIPA over other modern SADs require verification.

D. Baska Mask

The Baska mask is the newest entrant in the SAD market. It incorporates many features of the second-generation SADs with several novel features, which the inventor reports offer further advantages. It has been designed and developed over 11 years by Kanag Baska, an Australian anesthetist. The device came to market in Europe in 2011.

The Baska mask is a single-use, cuffless, silicone SAD. All parts that were deemed unnecessary were removed during design to minimize the bulk in the mask portion (Fig. 23-17). The stem, which has a 15-mm standard connector and an integrated, rigid bite block, has an oval cross section to provide axial stability. Two drain tubes run laterally on either side of the airway tube toward the mask portion. A soft, oval airway orifice at the distal end is surrounded by a soft, malleable mask portion. To either side of and posterior to the mask, the drain tubes open and extend to the mask tip (Fig. 23-18). The drainage system, incorporating one conventional drain tube and one active pharyngeal suction port, is intended to reduce the rate of aspiration. Proximally, an attachment enables suction to be attached to one of the ports to achieve continuous suction during insertion. Between the proximal anterior part of the mask and the distal stem is a strap designed to assist insertion.

The soft structure of the mask is compliant enough to change shape when pressure is applied. The manufacturers describe that as positive pressure is applied, the mask distends, increasing the pharyngeal seal, and as that pressure is released, the mask partially deflates, limiting any pressures applied to the pharyngeal tissues. Four sizes are available for small to large adults.

1. Application

The Baska mask is first sealed at both ends with fingers and compressed to assess its integrity. The posterior and sides of the mask should be lubricated with a water-soluble lubricant. The device may be inserted with the patient in several head and neck positions, but the neutral position is favored. The device is held in the dominant hand with the thumb, forefinger, and middle finger

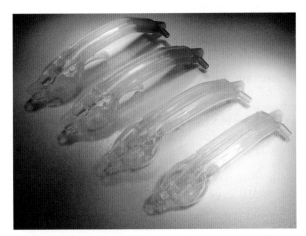

Figure 23-17 The Baska mask is a novel type of supraglottic airway device. Colors differentiate the different sizes of the device.

grasping the base of the mask and with the index and middle fingers exerting pressure on the mask in a posterior and downward direction. The device is inserted into the mouth and along the hard palate. On reaching the soft palate, the device is advanced into place by advancing the stem of the device. If difficulty is encountered in negotiating the pharyngeal corner, the anterior strap is pulled to flex the device tip and ease it around the corner. The device is fully inserted when resistance to advancement is felt. There is no cuff to deflate. Gentle manual ventilation is used to confirm the correct position of the device. Difficulties in ventilation may be resolved by minor advancement or withdrawal of the device. When this is not successful, a different size of Baska mask may be tried.

Continuous pharyngeal suction may be applied through one of the drain tubes during insertion to clear secretions in the pharynx. After insertion, the other drain tube may be used to insert a gastric tube and empty the stomach. At the end of surgery, the patient should be allowed to emerge until able to follow simple commands. At this point, the Baska mask may be removed by recovery staff or the patient.

The Baska mask has a wide lumen and a moderately large airway orifice without grills or impediments to the passage of tubes. Although it might be anticipated that the Baska mask performs similarly to other SADs as a conduit for fiberoptic-guided intubation (e.g., PLMA, i-gel), this depends on the ventilation orifice lying over the larynx and ease of passage of a fiberscope and tube. No reports or studies are available.

2. Indications, Advantages, and Disadvantages

The Baska mask can be used with spontaneous or controlled ventilation. It is new, and there are no publications reporting details of its routine use or defining the breadth or limits of its safe use. Specific disadvantages have not been determined due to a lack of experience.

3. Medical Literature

No published literature is available for this device, although at least two clinical studies are being conducted.

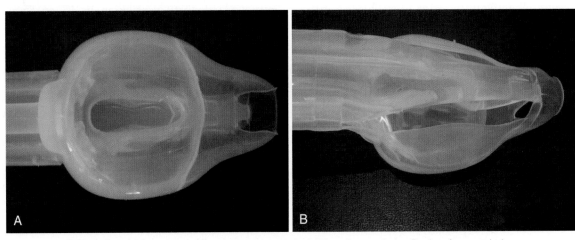

Figure 23-18 The mask portion of the Baska mask. **A,** View from anterior; **B,** view from posterior.

VII. PEDIATRIC SUPRAGLOTTIC AIRWAY DEVICES

SAD technology in pediatrics lags several years behind adult practice. In the past few years, some of the newer first-generation and second-generation SADs have become available in the full range of pediatric sizes. This represents an opportunity and a potential risk if not managed with care. There is an emerging selection of SADs for pediatric use and a supporting literature.

A. Ambu AuraOnce, Soft Seal Laryngeal Mask, and Other Laryngeal Masks

Monclus and associates studied the Ambu AuraOnce in 121 pediatric patients during MRI to look for a correlation between clinical measures such as insertion ease, leak pressure, and radiologic positioning.[223] Patients were between 4 months and 17 years old. Clinical data were collected, and saggital MRI cuts were reviewed to calculate neck flexion, LM position, and the device's relation to the trachea. The success rate for first-attempt insertion was 96%, and the rate for second-attempt insertion was 4%. Leak pressures ranged from 22.1 to 23.8 cm H_2O for different mask sizes, and values rose with patient age. Anomalous placement was seen on MRI for 23.5% of size 1.5, 10.9% of size 2, and 13.8% of size 2.5. No correlation was identified between anomalous LM position and leak pressure or ease of introduction.

Baker and coworkers studied several single-use LMs and the LMA Classic as conduits for pediatric flexible bronchoscopy in 100 patients.[224] Five devices (i.e., LMA Classic, Ambu AuraOnce, SSLM, LMA Unique, and Boss LM) were studied. Evaluation was based on subjective assessment of resistance to bronchoscopic manipulation within the SAD, laryngeal view, and measurement of time from starting insertion to visualizing the right upper lobe bronchus. Resistance to bronchoscopic manipulation was higher using PVC devices. The LMA Unique and Ambu AuraOnce were judged clinically inferior to the LMA Classic. The Boss Systems' single-use LM was as effective as the LMA Classic.

Glaisyer and Yule studied the use of the SSLM in 40 infants and children.[225] The SSLM was deemed a satisfactory airway in all patients. Insertion was achieved at the first attempt and was quick and easy. Repositioning during anesthesia was required in four cases.

B. Intubating Laryngeal Airway

Jagannathan and colleagues reported a 1-year, retrospective series of 34 uses of the ILA in children as a conduit for intubation.[226] Eight of these cases were emergencies. Patients were between 0.3 and 202 months old, and they weighed between 3.9 and 86 kg. Difficult airways (mostly craniofacial syndromes) were anticipated in 31 patients, and three difficult airways were unanticipated. The success rate for first-attempt intubation was 97% (33 patients), and the overall intubation rate was 100%; a fiberscope was used in 25, and a Shikani optical stylet in 7 patients. In two patients blind intubation succeeded

and in one it failed. The investigators suggest that visualized techniques offer a greater degree of success because of the potential for epiglottic downfolding when using the ILA in children.

In another prospective study, size 1.5 and 2.0 ILAs were studied in 100 healthy children with normal airways who were between 6 months and 8 years old.[227] ILA placement, fiberoptic tracheal intubation, and ILA removal were successful in all patients. The size 1.5 ILA cohort had a significantly higher rate of epiglottic downfolding compared with the size 2.0 ILA cohort ($P < 0.001$) despite adequate ventilation variables. A moderate negative correlation was found between weight and fiberoptic view ($r = -0.41$, $P < 0.001$), indicating that larger patients tended to have better fiberoptic grades. Compared with size 2.0, the size 1.5 ILA cohort took a significantly longer time for tracheal intubation, although this was of questionable clinical significance.

A few reports describe use of the ILA for management of difficult airways in children under anesthesia,[228-230] during extensive bleeding, and in an awake patient.[231,232] Several modifications of technique have been made for use in children. They include use of an airway exchange catheter or esophageal dilator to facilitate removal of the SAD after intubation.[233,234]

C. Laryngeal Tube and Laryngeal Tube Suction II

Genzwuerker and coworkers reported a comparative trial of the LT or LMA Classic with controlled ventilation in children between the ages of 2 and 8 years, who were scheduled for elective surgical interventions.[235] Insertion success was high for the LT group (30 of 30) and for the LMA Classic group (29 of 30). The LT was inserted slightly quicker than the LMA Classic (19 versus 23 seconds, $P < 0.05$) and achieved a higher airway leak pressure (19.2 versus 26.3 cm H_2O, $P < 0.001$). Peak airway pressure was slightly lower in the LMA Classic group.

Bortone and associates compared the LT and LMA Classic in 30 healthy children younger than 10 years.[236] Eleven children with an LMA Classic and two with an LT had adequate spontaneous or assisted ventilation after initial positioning ($P < 0.01$). Head positioning improved adequate ventilation in 15 of 15 with the LMA Classic and 11 of 15 with the LT ($P < 0.05$). Fiberoptic inspection revealed the vocal cords in 11 through the LMA Classic and none through the LT ($P < 0.001$).

Kaya and colleagues compared performance of the LT, LMA Classic, and CobraPLA in 90 healthy children undergoing short procedures with controlled ventilation.[237] Insertion times were similar for the LMA Classic (19 seconds), LT (21 seconds), and CobraPLA (18 seconds), as were the rates of successful insertion at first attempt for the LMA Classic (67%), LT (70.0%) and CobraPLA (73%). The number and type of airway interventions required and the hemodynamic, ventilation, and oxygenation variables throughout surgery were similar. Blood traces were seen on 20% of the LMA Classics, 20% of the CobraPLAs, and 10% of the LTs.

In a study of 24 children, Kim and associates reported that two methods of insertion—until resistance was felt and by inserting to a previously measured depth of the curved distance between the cricoid cartilage and the upper incisor—were more successful than the standard method of insertion (i.e., until the thick teeth mark on the tube was aligned with the upper incisors).[238] All children weighed between 12 and 25 kg, and a size 2 LT was used. Both alternative methods led to better ventilation and increased ability to identify the vocal cords with fiberoscopy (62.5% by the first method and 75% by the second) compared with standard method (12.5%).

Lee and colleagues compared complications of LT removal during anesthesia or after emergence in 70 healthy children between the ages of 1 and 12 years.[239] Anesthesia was induced and maintained with sevoflurane. In the anesthesia group, sevoflurane was maintained at 2%. Cough (37% versus 3%), hypersalivation (29% versus 6%), and desaturation (20% versus 0%) occurred more frequently in the awake group ($P < 0.05$), whereas airway obstruction (easily resolved by chin or jaw lifting) was more frequent in the anaesthetized group. The same group studied the optimal concentration of sevoflurane for removal of an LT (and LMA Classic) in children.[240] Forty unpremedicated children between the ages of 8 months and 12 years were studied during sevoflurane anesthesia. An up-down method was used to determine the optimal concentration for device removal (i.e., absence of coughing, teeth clenching, gross purposeful movement, breath-holding, laryngospasm, and desaturation). The end-tidal concentration of sevoflurane to achieve successful LT removal in 50% of children was 1.83%, and for a 95% success rate, it was 2%. For the LMA Classic, the concentrations were 1.9 %, and 2.15%. For both devices, this represents a minimum alveolar concentration (MAC) of 0.8 to 0.9.

The bulk of publications on the LTS-II in children describe its use in difficult airway management. Kim and associates reported on the effect of changes in head and neck position in LTS-II performance in 33 children scheduled for elective surgery.[241] The ventilation score (i.e., no leakage with an airway pressure of 15 cm H_2O, bilateral chest excursion, and a square wave capnogram, with each item scored 0 or 1 point) was measured in various positions. Leak pressure was reduced to 22 cm H_2O in the extended position, but ventilation was good without a leak at tidal volumes of 10 mL/kg.[99] In the neutral, extended, and rotated positions, the median ventilation scores were better (3 points each) than that with the head and neck flexed (1 point). Peak inspiratory pressure significantly increased in the flexed position. During fiberoptic examination, the vocal cords were more easily seen in extension and right rotation compared with the neutral position and flexion. The flexed position usually should be avoided.

Scheller and coworkers described the use of the LTS-II in 10 neonates and infants during difficult airway management, including failed mask ventilation, failed SAD ventilation, or failed intubation.[242] Use of the LTS-II was associated with a high level of success, securing the airway when other techniques had failed. The investigators support the use of the LTS-II over the LT in part because the drain tube enables gastric tube placement and can be used as an indirect indicator of correct placement. A modified insertion technique using an Esmarch maneuver was recommended. A single case report described use of the LTS-II to facilitate fiberoptic intubation in an infant.[243]

D. Cobra Perilaryngeal Airway

Passariello and coworkers studied the CobraPLA size 1.5 and 2 during controlled ventilation in 40 anesthetized children aged 1-10 years, weighing 10-35 kg.[244] The first-attempt insertion success rate was 90%, the median leak pressure was 20 cm H_2O, and the vocal cords were visible by fiberoscopy in 90% of patients. In 21% of patients, gastric inflation was observed at a peak inspiratory pressure of 20 cm H_2O or less.

Kaya and colleagues' study of the LT, LMA Classic, and CobraPLA in 90 healthy children undergoing short procedures with controlled ventilation was described earlier.[237]

Gaitini and coworkers compared the CobraPLA with the LMA Unique in 80 children undergoing elective general surgery of short duration during volume-controlled ventilation.[245] Time for and ease of insertion were similar. The CobraPLA needed more frequent jaw lifts, and the LMA Unique required more frequent head and neck adjustments. Fiberoptic scores were excellent with both devices. Respiratory variables were similar, except that plateau and peak pressures were higher in the CobraPLA group. Gas exchange was similar for both groups. Airway leak pressure was higher for the Cobra-PLA than the LMA Unique (27 versus 21 cm H_2O). There was a low rate of blood mucosal staining of the devices.

Szmuk and associates compared the CobraPLA with the LMA Unique in 200 children during positive-pressure ventilation.[246] The CobraPLA performed better in terms of airway seal, device stability, and gastric inflation. Capnography values (measured at the head of the Cobra-PLA) were higher than those of the Y piece of the circle circuit. This implies a greater accuracy, and the feature is incorporated in the CobraPLUS.

Szmuk and others have described the use of the CobraPLA as a conduit to facilitate tracheal intubation in two cases of known or predicted difficult airway.[247, 248] In a third case, a size 0.5 CobraPLA was used to maintain the airway of a neonate with airway difficulty (i.e., hypoplastic midfacies and subluxation of C5-C6) when intubation proved impossible.[249]

E. The i-gel

In the first published study of the i-gel in children the device was used in 50 healthy children weighing more than 30 kg who were undergoing short-duration surgery.[250] All devices were inserted on the first attempt. Mean airway leak pressure was 25 cm H_2O. There was no gastric inflation, and gastric tube insertion was achieved in all cases.

The i-gel was compared with the Ambu AuraOnce in 208 children up to 17 years old.[251] Insertion success was equivalent for the Ambu AuraOnce group (98%) and the i-gel group (93%), but i-gel insertion was slower (27 versus 24 seconds). Airway leak pressure was higher with the i-gel (23 versus 19 cm H_2O). Gastric tube placement was successful in 97% of the i-gel group. The fiberoptic view was good and equivalent between groups, and there were few side effects in either group. Almost one half of the i-gels needed taping to maintain the airway seal, especially in smaller children.

A study of 120 smaller children (<35 kg; median weight, 19 kg) reported insertion success on the first, second, or third attempt in 110, 8, and 1, respectively, with one failure.[252] Manual ventilation was possible in all cases, although excess leak precluded a tidal volume above 7 mL/kg in three children. Fiberoptic inspection through the i-gel showed a clear view of the vocal cords in 40 of 46 inspected cases. Median leak pressure was 20 cm H_2O. One child regurgitated without aspirating, and other complications and side effects were uncommon. The i-gel was inserted without complications, establishing a clear airway and enabling spontaneous and controlled ventilation in 113 (94%) children.

Initial findings suggest the pediatric i-gel requires careful insertion to avoid displacement: an inward force must be created by bimandibular taping. The stem of the device is unnecessarily long. The depth of insertion marker routinely lies some distance outside the mouth with the device correctly positioned, particularly for smaller size devices.

VIII. CONCLUSIONS

Since the introduction of the LMA into clinical practice, numerous alternative SADs have been developed. They have different sizes and shapes, and some are reusable, whereas others are designed only for single use. They have various intended uses. No single device meets all the criteria for the ideal SAD. Fortunately, use of these devices is easy to learn, and they can be used by experienced anesthesiologists and novice airway providers alike. Second-generation SADs are likely to provide better airway protection, and their use is increasing in clinical practice. Nonetheless, there are situations in which such devices should not be used (e.g., full-stomach patients) unless as a rescue device.

It is likely that several different airways will always be needed for use in different clinical situations. Airway providers should be skilled with several devices and techniques, including various SAD devices, to be considered competent in airway management. Clinical judgment born from experience is necessary to determine which of these devices is indicated in any situation.

IX. CLINICAL PEARLS

- Supraglottic airway devices (SADs) have several roles, including maintenance of the airway during spontaneously breathing or controlled-ventilation anesthesia, airway rescue after failed intubation or out of the hospital, use during cardiopulmonary resuscitation, and

use as a conduit to assist in the mangement of a difficult tracheal intubation.

- The risk of aspiration with SADs is considered to be relatively low in expert hands, which is achieved primarily by careful and appropriate case selection, expert insertion, and meticulous management of the airway after insertion.

- About 30 single-use and reusable laryngeal masks (LMs) are on the market. Each is different from other LMs in design and in manufacturing materials and processes.

- The greatest concern about the profusion of LMs on the market is the lack of rigorous evaluation. The limited evidence available shows that all LMs and LMAs are not equivalent.

- LMs are not intended to replace all functions of the ETT and are best suited for use in fasted patients undergoing surgical procedures when tracheal intubation is not deemed necessary.

- Airway devices are considered to be of low or intermediate risk and are primarily subject to manufacturers' self-assessment. Performance of the desired function, efficacy, and cost-effectiveness are not a focus of these assessments.

- The desirable features of an ideal SAD are efficacy, versatility, safety, reusability, and reasonable cost.

- Although most devices are used by anesthesiologists, SADs may be used by individuals with less experience in anesthesia, out-of-hospital rescue, or resuscitation.

- Familiarity with the manufacturer's warnings, precautions, indications, and contraindications is necessary before use, and the patient should be at an adequate depth of anesthesia or unconsciousness before attempting insertion.

- There is an emerging selection of SADs for pediatric use and a supporting literature.

SELECTED REFERENCES

All references can be found online at expertconsult.com.

6. Brimacombe JR, Berry A: The incidence of aspiration associated with the laryngeal mask airway: A meta-analysis of published literature. *J Clin Anesth* 7:297–305, 1995.
9. Graziotti PJ: Intermittent positive pressure ventilation through a laryngeal mask airway. Is a nasogastric tube useful? *Anaesthesia* 47:1088–1089, 1992.
20. Bernardini A, Natalini G: Risk of pulmonary aspiration with laryngeal mask airway and tracheal tube: Analysis on 65 712 procedures with positive pressure ventilation. *Anaesthesia* 64:1289–1294, 2009.
25. Atherton D, O'Sullivan E, Lowe D, Charters P: A ventilation-exchange bougie for fiberoptic intubations with the laryngeal mask airway. *Anaesthesia* 51:1123–1126, 1996.
42. Pandit JJ, Popat MT, Cook TM, et al: The Difficult Airway Society "ADEPT" Guidance on selecting airway devices: The basis of a strategy for equipment evaluation. *Anaesthesia* 66:726–772, 2011.
54. Brain AI: The development of the laryngeal mask—A brief history of the invention, early clinical studies and experimental work from which the laryngeal mask evolved. *Eur J Anaesthesiol Suppl* 4:5–17, 1991.

81. Danha RF, Thompson JL, Popat MT, Pandit JJ: Comparison of fiberoptic-guided orotracheal intubation through classic and single-use laryngeal mask airways. *Anaesthesia* 60:184–188, 2005.

109. Cook TM, Hommers C: New airways for resuscitation? *Resuscitation* 69:371–387, 2006.

173. Theiler L, Kleine-Brueggeney M, Urwyler N, et al: Randomized clinical trial of the i-gel and Magill tracheal tube or single-use ILMA and ILMA tracheal tube for blind intubation in anaesthetized patients with a predicted difficult airway. *Br J Anaesth* 10:243–250, 2011.

Chapter 24

Upper Airway Retraction: New and Old Laryngoscope Blades

RICHARD M. LEVITAN | CARIN A. HAGBERG

I. INTRODUCTION

Laryngoscopy performed for the purpose of tracheal intubation has historically involved a direct line-of-sight to the larynx. Newer fiberoptic and video imaging can visualize around the anatomic difficulties associated with difficult or impossible direct laryngoscopy. However, most intubations are still performed with direct laryngoscopy. Most direct laryngoscopy in adults is performed with a curved Macintosh blade, and less often, the narrow-lumen, straight Miller blade is used. Straight blades typically are used in pediatrics. This chapter reviews the evolution of the laryngoscope, some blades of historic interest and innovative designs, and subtleties of Macintosh and Miller blades. Major modifications have occurred in blade materials and illumination, and there has been a dramatic increase in the use of disposable laryngoscope blades for single cases.

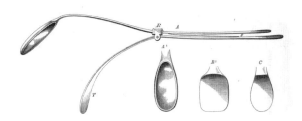

Figure 24-1 British physician Benjamin Babington combined a mirror and spatula. (From Mackenzie M: *Use of the laryngoscope in diseases of the throat*, ed 2, Philadelphia, 1869, Lindsay & Blakiston.)

II. HISTORY

Benjamin Babington first described mirror-based indirect laryngoscopy in 1829,[1] although it is often erroneously attributed to Manuel Garcia, a singer who described visualization of his own vocal cords in 1855.[2-8] Babington also hinged a tongue depressor to his initial mirror design, but he subsequently abandoned the depressor and focused on the mirror alone (Fig. 24-1). In 1844, John Avery combined a reflective speculum with an external light source to view the larynx (Fig. 24-2).[4] Mirror laryngoscopy for the investigation of laryngeal pathology was pioneered by

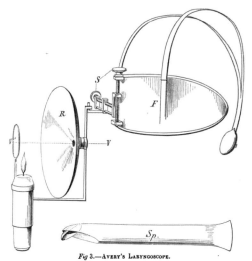

*Fig 3.—*AVERY'S LARYNGOSCOPE.

F. One side of the frontal-pad which supports the mirror. From it a double spring passes backward to a counter-pad which, when the instrument is worn, rests under the occipital protuberance. In the drawing, the occipital-pad is drawn forward by the unopposed strength of the spring.

S. Screws by which the reflector can be made to move laterally and perpendicularly.

R. Reflector.

VV¹, Line of vision.

Sp. The speculum.

Figure 24-2 Avery's reflective speculum. One side of the frontal pad *(F)* supports the mirror. From it, a spring passes backward to a counter-pad, which when the instrument is worn, rests under the occipital protuberance. As shown here, the occipital pad is drawn forward by the unopposed strength of the spring. The reflector *(R)* can be moved laterally and perpendicularly by screws *(S)*. *Sp,* Speculum; *V-V1,* line of vision. (From Mackenzie M: *Use of the laryngoscope in diseases of the throat*, ed 2, Philadelphia, 1869, Lindsay & Blakiston.)

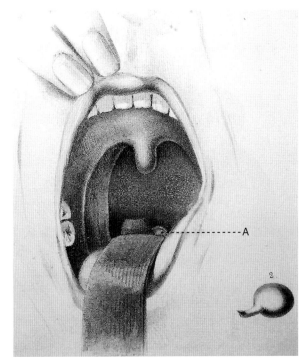

Figure 24-3 1845, Horace Green removed a laryngeal polyp *(2)* using a bent tongue spatula *(A)* to expose the larynx and polyp to direct vision. (From Green H: Morbid growths within the larynx. In Green H, editor: *On the surgical treatment of polypi of the larynx and oedema of the glottis*, New York, 1852, GP Putnam.)

Johann Czermak, who used instruments designed by Ludwig Turck in the late 1850s.[5-8] Czermak subsequently applied an external light source and a head-mounted mirror to improve visualization.[7]

Horace Green, widely considered to be America's first laryngologist, used tongue spatulas and probangs to examine and treat diseases of the larynx and trachea in the mid-1800s. In 1845, Green performed transoral removal of a laryngeal polyp in an 11-year-old girl using a bent tongue spatula to expose the larynx and polyp to direct vision (Fig. 24-3).[7,9] Green's technique[9] is remarkably similar to the indirect elevation of the epiglottis described almost 90 years later by Macintosh:

I drew forward and depressed the tongue, so as to enable me to see the condition of the epiglottis.... Whilst making this examination, and at the very moment the tongue was depressed, and the epiglottis in full view, the patient gave a sudden and rather violent cough, when a round white fibrous looking polypus appeared, momentarily, at the opening of the glottis, and then seemed as quickly to be drawn into the larynx.

Green goes on to describe the use of a hook and knife passed "nearly an inch into the glottis" to extract the polyp. Despite Green's accomplishments in direct laryngeal exposure, laryngeal surgery, and intubation, the first publication on direct laryngoscopy is credited to Alfred Kirstein in 1895, who called the new procedure *autoscopy* and devised techniques for use with the patient in sitting and supine positions.[10,11] Kirtsein's 1896 treatise on the procedure presages the development of laryngoscopy

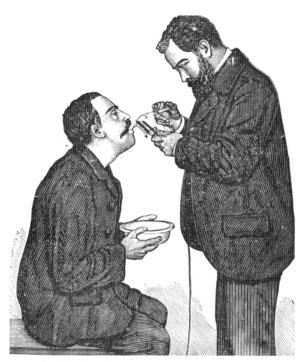

Figure 24-4 Alfred Kirstein performed autoscopy in the 1890s. (From Kirstein A, Thorner M: *Autoscopy of the larynx and the trachea (direct examination without mirror)*, Philadelphia, 1896, FA Davis.)

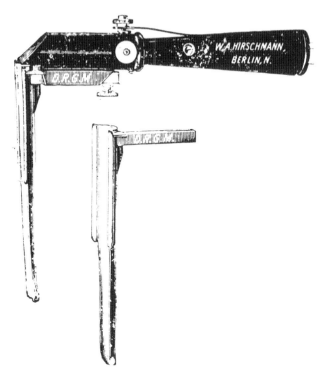

Figure 24-5 Kirstein's modified autoscope. A standard blade is attached to the handle, and an intralaryngeal blade is shown separately *(bottom)*. (From Hirsch NP, Smith GB, Hirsch PO: Alfred Kirstein—Pioneer of direct laryngoscopy. *Anaesthesia* 41:42, 1986.)

blades used in the modern era.[11] He observes that the tongue must be drawn forward and downward (with the patient sitting in front of the operator): "To get this position of the tongue, a tongue depressor is necessary (i.e., spatula)—which, however, unlike the ordinary spatula, must not be placed in front of the circumvallate papillae but must be applied behind the same to the root of the tongue" (Fig. 24-4). The epiglottis can be elevated *directly* by an instrument that projects over the epiglottis (e.g., the tip of the spatula introduced behind the epiglottis) or *indirectly* by a method described by Reichert in 1879 and promulgated by Kirstein[11]:

> *Pressure upon the base of the tongue and the median glosso-epiglottic ligament produces an elevation of the epiglottis on account of its close attachment to the tongue. As the first method requires previous cocainization, it should be reserved for exceptional cases; autoscopy must depend, in general, on the principle enunciated by Reichert—a principle which is already involved in the necessary instrumental depression of the base of the tongue.*

Kirstein developed two spatulas (Fig. 24-5). One had a distal, bent, bifid tip, which he called the *standard spatula*, that was designed for placement in the valleculae and pressed on the median glossoepiglottic ligament. Kirstein's intralaryngeal, perfectly straight spatula was designed to be introduced behind the epiglottis and press it against the root of the tongue. His descriptions of these instruments and intended uses portray exactly the functioning of modern curved- and straight-blade laryngoscopes.[11]

Chevalier Jackson, a professor of laryngology at Jefferson Medical College in Philadelphia (after Jacob de Silva Solis-Cohen, another Jefferson pioneer), refined laryngoscopy techniques in supine patients and established the principles of modern laryngoscopic exposure. Jackson created a tubed *glottiscope* in 1903 and was the first to apply enclosed distal lighting using a tungsten bulb that was connected to a large battery.[5-9,12] Subsequent versions of Jackson's tubular laryngoscope incorporated a removable, sliding floor that facilitated tube insertion, and he reported on the routine insertion of tracheal tubes using direct laryngoscopy in 1913 (Fig. 24-6).[12,13] In the same year, Henry Janeway, an anesthesiologist at Bellevue Hospital in New York City, described a smaller and more portable laryngoscope powered by batteries located in the handle (Fig. 24-7).[14] It featured a straight blade with a slight distal curve.[14] Janeway's blade did not achieve commercial success, but similar large, C-shaped, straight-blade designs created by Flagg, McGill, and Guedel became widely adopted.[15,16]

Laryngoscope blade design and laryngoscopy technique underwent little apparent evolution until Robert Miller's 1941 narrow-lumen, D-shaped, straight-blade design and Robert Macintosh's 1943 publication about a new curved-blade laryngoscope (Fig. 24-8, *A*).[17,18] The Macintosh and Miller blades have become universally adopted and the benchmarks against which all direct laryngoscope blades are compared. Although innumerable modifications of these standard designs have been described in the past 70 years, only a few alternative designs have achieved widespread use. In the 1970s, the

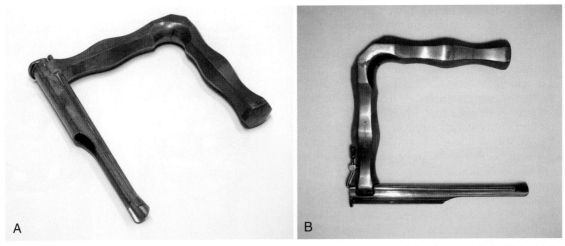

Figure 24-6 **A** and **B,** Chevalier Jackson's tubular laryngoscope incorporated a removable, sliding floor, which facilitated tube insertion.

flexible fiberoptic bronchoscope offered another option for use in difficult situations, and rigid fiberoptic devices such as the Bullard laryngoscope were first introduced in the late 1980s. The 1990s saw the introduction of additional rigid fiberoptic laryngoscopes and commercially available fiberoptic stylets. In the 21st century, video-assisted devices have been added to clinical practice.

III. DIRECT LARYNGOSCOPE DESIGN

A. Components of a Direct Laryngoscope

A laryngoscope consists of a handle, a blade, and a light source. There are marked variations in blade shape, tip design, and the mechanism and location of illumination systems (i.e., bulbs, or light-conducting fibers). The section of the blade that contacts the tongue is the *spatula*, and the left edge of the blade (from the operator's perspective) is the *flange*. (see Fig. 24-8, *B*). The proximal vertical flange is sometimes called the *vertical step*. At the base (or *heel*) of the blade is the *block*, which interacts with the top of the handle. The connection between the blade and handle causes the light to come on when the blade is opened. Blades are designed to

attach and detach from the handle with a standardized fitting (engaged at 45 degrees) that connects a *hook* on the blade to a small rod at the top of the handle.

Most laryngoscope blades are made from steel and most are chrome plated. Plastic blades have been produced by different manufacturers for approximately

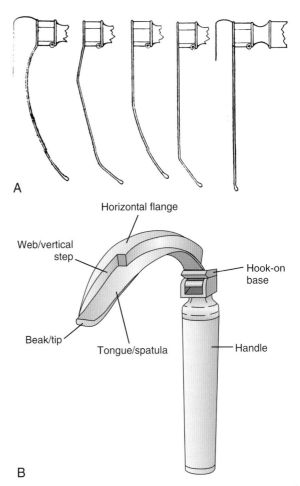

Figure 24-7 Henry Janeway produced a portable laryngoscope powered by batteries located in the handle.

Figure 24-8 **A,** Macintosh experimented with various blade shapes for the laryngoscope. **B,** The components of a direct laryngoscope with a Macintosh blade. (**A,** From Macintosh RR: Laryngoscope blades. *Lancet* 1:485, 1944; **B,** Courtesy of Anne Law.)

20 years. Plastic blades can be made very inexpensively, especially fiber-lit blades that use an acrylic rod for light conduction. The initial plastic blades had some flex and wobble; later designs have overcome these problems, and some are sturdy enough to be reusable.

The heel of a laryngoscope blade is a critical mechanical element. Many manufacturers decrease production costs using plastic heels on a metal blade, and some use metal fittings for the hook and base, even though the bulk of the heel is plastic. A potential problem with plastic-heeled blades is loosening of the paired ball bearings on either side of the heel. Some plastic blades have plastic flanges instead of bearings. A relatively new feature of some blades is a mechanism on the hook to prevent the blade from touching the handle when closed. This keeps a sterile blade from contacting the presumably dirty handle, although there is no requirement for laryngoscope blades to be supplied sterile.

B. Direct Laryngoscope Lighting

Visualization of the laryngeal inlet during direct laryngoscopy depends on adequate illumination of airway structures by the laryngoscope. Illumination is a function of the intensity and color of the supplied light and the area over which it falls. These factors depend on the nature of the laryngoscope blade's light source and the potential of the power source applied to it. Light can be measured in several ways: at its source (i.e., luminous flux, measured in lumens), at its receiving surface (i.e., illuminance, measured in lux), or by the amount of light re-emitted from a surface in a given direction (i.e., luminance, measured in candela per square meter [cd/m^2]).[19,20] During direct laryngoscopy, perception of the surface brightness of the larynx depends on light transmitted back to the laryngoscopist's eyes from the surface of the larynx; this is luminance.

A significant variable in the perception of adequate lighting during laryngoscopy is the operator. As clinicians age, they develop presbyopia (beginning in the fourth decade, regardless of visual acuity), and the amount of light needed for a given visual task increases. This is especially significant in performing direct laryngoscopy because the larynx is sighted with only one eye due to the severe visual restrictions of the procedure.[21] The procedure is visually analogous to looking down a 1-inch pipe at a target 12 to 18 inches away; visual restrictions include the mouth, teeth, tongue, blade, and epiglottis. Because the right and left eye are separated in the skull by 4 to 5 inches, the two views are disparate and cannot be merged into a stereoscopic view of the larynx. Subconsciously, we suppress the nondominant image through a phenomenon known as binocular suppression. It is not known what component of difficult laryngoscopy is related to inadequate lighting, but adequate illumination is especially important when landmarks are obscured by secretions, blood, and vomitus and when the epiglottis causes shadowing of the larynx.

Historically, there was no standard for laryngoscope light, but the International Organization for Standardization recently agreed on a standard of 500 lux after 10 minutes of operation.[22] The illuminance of a

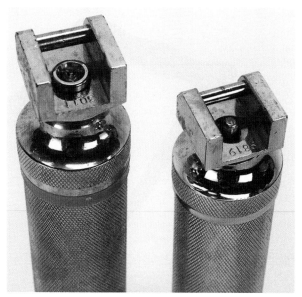

Figure 24-9 The conventional laryngoscope and fiber-lit laryngoscope use different, non-interchangeable fittings. In the United States, fiber-lit blades have a green dot on the base, and the handles have a green ring near the top *(left).*

laryngoscope light at the distal tip of the blade is a function of the distance from the light source to the tip of the blade, the type of bulb or fiberoptic-conducting system, and the battery type and charge status.[23] The light-to-tip distance is important because the amount of illuminance at a target is governed by the inverse square law (i.e., if the distance from the light source is doubled, one fourth of the amount of light lands on the target). Across different clinical settings, there may be dramatic differences in the illuminance of blade and handle pairs. Marked variation and poor light performance of laryngoscopes is widespread in anesthesia and emergency departments.[23,24] In a study of many emergency departments in Philadelphia, there was a 500-fold difference in the illuminance produced by different blade and handle pairs, ranging from 11 to more than 6000 lux.[24]

Bulb-on-blade laryngoscopes (called *conventional blades*) and fiber-lit laryngoscopes (in the United States, called *green-line scopes*) use different, non-interchangeable fittings (Fig. 24-9). Bulb-on-blade laryngoscopes have a simple electrical connection between the handle and blade. The electrical circuit is completed by opening the blade, providing power to the bulb, which is mounted on the distal aspect of the blade. Halogen and xenon bulbs are used by many manufacturers, but within the past 5 years, super-bright LED bulbs have become available. LED bulbs have tremendous advantages compared with other bulbs. They use a fraction of the energy of xenon or halogen bulbs, and they operate at much lower temperatures. The light they produce is much whiter, which may improve the discrimination of landmarks. The more yellow color of standard bulbs can be especially poor for distinguishing reddish yellow mucosal structures (e.g., epiglottis from the posterior pharyngeal wall). The primary reason LED lights will become standard on all instruments in the future is cost; as LEDs become much more commonly used on laryngoscopes and other

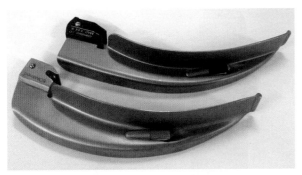

Figure 24-10 Examples of all-steel laryngoscope blades with LED bulbs on them. (Courtesy of SunMed, Largo, FL.)

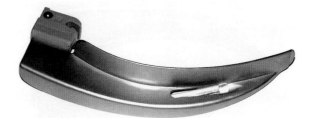

Figure 24-12 Disposable, fiber-lit blades are available in stainless steel with acrylic stems (SunMed Healthcare, Largo, FL).

portable medical instruments, the cost of the bulbs will continue to decrease. Some manufacturers already offer inexpensive, single-use, all-steel, LED-bulb blades (Fig. 24-10). Another advantage of LED bulb-on-blade designs is that they do not require expensive handle-battery systems because of their low energy requirements. This extends the operational and shelf life of the handle-battery pair dramatically, an important feature when stocking laryngoscopes in code carts and other settings.

An alternative illumination system uses light-conducting fibers in the blade with a bulb mounted in the top of the laryngoscope handle. In the United States, these blades have a green dot on the base, and the handles have a green ring on the top. Different types of fiber-lit blades and handles are not interchangeable. Fiber-lit systems depend on a good fit between the base of the blade and the top of the handle. A spring-loaded mechanism depresses the light at the top of the handle, making an electrical connection with the batteries. Problems with the spring may cause erratic performance, and a poor fit can allow light to escape between the bulb source in the handle and the fiberoptic bundle in the blade. The best light-conducting material is glass fiber, and the best designed of the glass fiber–lit blades use large arrays of fiber bundles (Fig. 24-11). There is significant variation in the size and quality of these glass fibers among manufacturers. Glass fiber is relatively expensive, and its light conduction deteriorates over time, depending on sterilization techniques.[25] Fast deterioration in light conduction, erosion of the bond between the glass and blade, and rusting of the blade occurs with lower-quality glass fiber blades.

Acrylic can be used for light conduction, and although it is not as effective a light conductor as glass, it is inexpensive and easy to integrate onto a laryngoscope blade (Fig. 24-12). Glass fibers must be wrapped in a steel rod and then attached to the blade or threaded through a channel that runs the length of the blade, but an acrylic rod can be easily attached as a separate component. Better acrylic fiber–lit blades enclose part or all of the acrylic rod to minimize light loss (Fig. 24-13). Acrylic fiber–lit blades usually are designed as single-use blades; they are inexpensive to produce, and their light conduction deteriorates significantly with sterilization. The inferior light-conducting performance of acrylic can

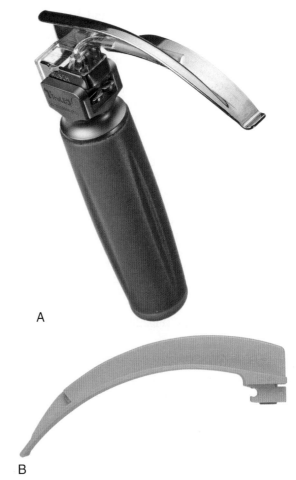

A

B

Figure 24-13 **A,** Wrapped acrylic rod (Truphatek International Ltd., Netanya, Israel). **B,** Heine XP disposable, fiber-lit blade (Heine Optotechnik, Herrsching, Germany).

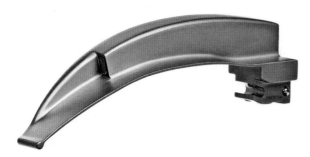

Figure 24-11 Large, glass-bundle blade (Emerald fiberoptic blade, Rüsch, Duluth, GA). Fiber-lit laryngoscopes use glass or acrylic fiber bundles to conduct light from the handle, along the blade, and to the distal tip.

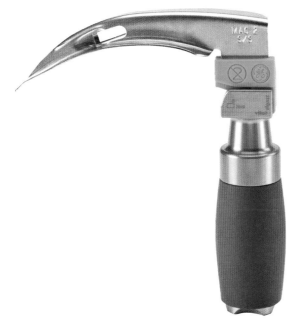

Figure 24-14 LED laryngoscope handle (General Electric, Fairfield, CT).

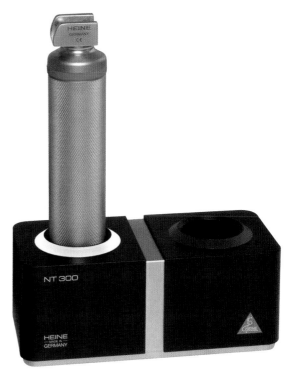

Figure 24-15 Rechargeable handle. (Courtesy of Heine Optotechnik, Herrsching, Germany)

be compensated by super-bright bulbs (LED is best) and powerful handles, but these features necessitate relatively expensive lamps, reflectors, and battery systems (Fig. 24-14).

A major variable in laryngoscope lighting involves the battery source. Standard handles use two C-sized batteries, and most pediatric handles or stubby handles use AA batteries. Several companies offer small handles that use a single, 3-volt, CR123 lithium battery (i.e., camera type). Compared with alkaline batteries, lithium batteries (regardless of size) have a flatter discharge curve, and they slowly diminish in power output over a long time. When lithium batteries start to fade, they die quickly; but during operation, they maintain a much more steady power output. Alkaline battery–powered handles continue to turn on even though light output has diminished dramatically. This phenomenon contributes to delayed battery replacement, because few clinical settings monitor blade and handle pairs using light meters. Many manufacturers offer rechargeable fiber-lit handles using nickel–metal hydride or nickel-cadmium batteries; combined with LED bulbs and special reflectors, these handles create brilliant white light that is far superior to older illumination technology (Fig. 24-15).

C. Direct Laryngoscope Blade Design

Laryngoscope blade design has evolved through trial and error and by sophisticated technical analysis. Macintosh published a series of blade design drawings with which he had experimented; models varied from the curved blade so widely accepted subsequently to entirely straight blades[18,26] (Fig. 24-16). Some investigators have made use of lateral head and neck fluoroscopy and radiography during laryngoscopy to help elucidate relationships of the tongue, hyoid bone, epiglottis, and laryngoscope blade during laryngoscopy.[27,28]

The scientific evaluation of laryngoscope blades has been impeded by the visual restrictions inherent to laryngoscopy; for example, the target is seen monocularly and therefore cannot be simultaneously viewed by two operators.[21] Although a head-mounted direct laryngoscopy video system was invented in 1998 that allowed routine recording of the procedure from the operator's perspective, few studies of laryngoscope blade design have used this objective tool.[29] Most studies have relied on subjectively reported laryngeal view (i.e., visualization of the larynx by the laryngoscopist for a few seconds). The standard reporting system of laryngeal view (i.e., Cormack-Lehane classification) has poor interobserver reliability and is not very sensitive because up to 99% of direct laryngoscopies involve Cormack-Lehane grade 1 or 2 views.[30] This grading system does not allow detection of differences between blade designs without a very large number of patients because of the relative scarcity of grade 3 and 4 views. The combination of restricted visualization, subjective reporting of the view, and lack of a sensitive means of reporting has historically retarded rigorous research on laryngoscopy blade design. As observed by McIntyre in a 1989 review article on blade design, "detailed evaluations of the performance of any particular laryngoscope blade are extremely rare and critical analysis virtually nonexistent." [31]

IV. DIRECT LARYNGOSCOPY BLADES

A. Macintosh and Related Curved Blades

1. Macintosh Laryngoscope Blade

Macintosh's 1943 publication of his curved-blade laryngoscope design defined a new blade and emphasized a

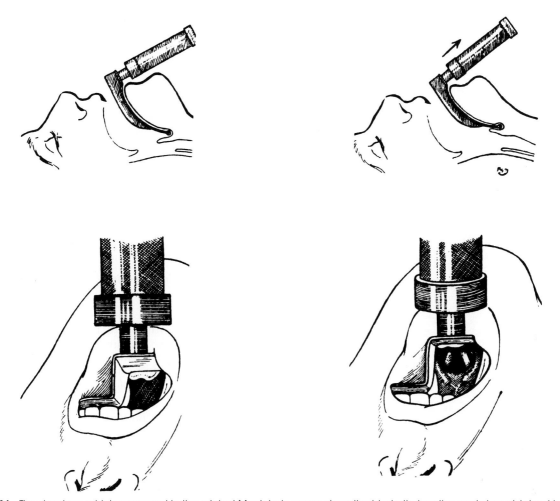

Figure 24-16   The drawings, which appeared in the original Macintosh paper, show the blade tip location and view obtained before *(left)* and after *(right)* lifting the laryngoscope. (From Macintosh RR: A new laryngoscope. *Lancet* 1:205, 1943.)

novel technique of laryngeal exposure for anesthesiologists (i.e., indirect elevation of the epiglottis) (see Figs. 24-8A and 24-16).[18] Although the pioneers of laryngology, including Green and Kirstein, were familiar with indirect elevation of the epiglottis, this technique was not widely appreciated in the new clinical discipline of anesthesiology. Macintosh stumbled into the design by accidentally exposing the larynx indirectly after inserting a Boyle-Davis mouth gag to keep the mouth open and depress the tongue during a tonsillectomy case: "Opening the mouth with the [Boyle-Davis] gag, I found the cords perfectly displayed.... Before the morning had finished, I had Richard Salt [senior technical assistant of his anesthesia department] ... [solder] the Davis blade onto a laryngoscope handle, and this functioned quite adequately as a laryngoscope."[32] The Crowe-Davis gag had been in use for several decades (Fig. 24-17); Boyle popularized the use of this mouth gag in England during World War II.[33]

Macintosh's classic article in *The Lancet* described using his shorter, curved blade by placing its tip in the vallecula between the epiglottis and the base of the tongue, with subsequent indirect elevation of the epiglottis.[18] Macintosh contended that he could use the blade at a lighter plane of anesthesia because of the predominant glossopharyngeal nerve innervation of the base of tongue

area rather than the superior laryngeal nerve innervation of the dorsal surface of the epiglottis. This was important before the widespread use of neuromuscular blockers. He also mentioned the need to insert the blade to the right of the tongue, with a sweep to the left to displace and control the tongue.[18] In this original communication,

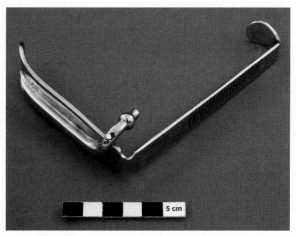

Figure 24-17   Davis blade. (Courtesy of the University of Melbourne Museum Image Archives, Melbourne, Australia.)

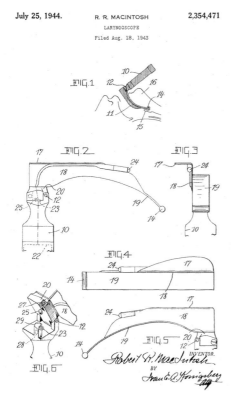

July 25, 1944.   R. R. MACINTOSH   2,354,471
LARYNGOSCOPE
Filed Aug. 18, 1943

Figure 24-18 Macintosh's patent images for the American version of the Macintosh blade were filed by the Foregger Company (with a misspelled MacIntosh signature).

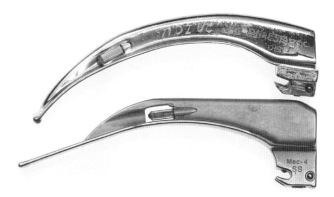

Figure 24-19 The English Macintosh blade *(top)* with its more accentuated curve and continued step and flange to distal blade is compared with the standard Macintosh blade *(bottom)*.

Macintosh stated and later reiterated that "the precise shape or curve of the blade does not seem to matter much provided that the tip does not go beyond the epiglottis."[18] However, numerous modifications of the Macintosh blade have been reported.

The specific design of the Macintosh blade has a circuitous history. Macintosh, a New Zealander, invented the blade while working in England. Richard Foregger, the son of Richard von Foregger, a manufacturer of early anesthesia devices, was stationed briefly in England during the Second World War. Macintosh gave his new blade to Foregger's son to bring to America, and he also gave blades to two English manufacturers (Medical Industrial Equipment and Longworth Scientific Instruments).[34] Macintosh did not pursue patents or royalties on his design. The U.S. patent application by the Foregger company shows Macintosh's name spelled incorrectly (with a capital I in the middle), and this incorrect spelling persists on many labels[34] (Fig. 24-18). The American and English Macintosh blade designs are descendants of the blades initially produced by the Foregger and Longworth companies, respectively.[34] Macintosh thought that one size would fit all adults, but the blade was initially used in obstetrics cases (i.e., only in women). Eventually, a larger size was devised, which evolved into the modern Macintosh 4, whereas the original design approximates what became the Macintosh 3. Although manufacturers have produced a Macintosh 2 and Macintosh 1, these sizes were not endorsed by Macintosh, and direct laryngoscopy in small children and infants usually is done with straight blades.

2. English Macintosh Blade

The English Macintosh laryngoscope, initially produced by Longworth in the United Kingdom, is continuously curved along the entire spatula, the flange runs to the tip of the blade, and the proximal flange is smaller[34-36] (Fig. 24-19). In contrast, many versions of the American Macintosh are straight in the distal portion, have a distal tip without a flange, and have a very large proximal flange. The bulb on an English Macintosh is closer to the distal tip, increasing illuminance measured at the tip. Although not standardized across all English-labeled Macintosh blades, most English designs use a clear bulb, whereas American Macintosh designs usually come with a frosted bulb. English blades and American Macintosh blades are also offered with fiber-lit illumination systems, which typically use smaller (2- to 3-mm), round bundles.

Asai and colleagues conducted a randomized crossover study of the English blade, comparing it with the standard Macintosh in 300 patients.[35] They found that the view with the English blade was better than the view with the standard blade in 34%, no different in 54%, and worse in 11% of patients. For the 42 patients with a Cormack-Lehane grade of 3 or worse with one blade, the view was rated better with the English blade than the standard blade in 60%, worse in 7%, and no different in 33% of patients.[35] Yardeni and colleagues, in performing an in vitro technical analysis of various blades, concluded that the English Macintosh 4 provided the best results, surpassing those delivered by the American size 4 and English Macintosh 3 blades, even at shallow insertion depths.[36] The flange heights on English Macintosh 4 and 3 blades are similar, but on the American Macintosh, the proximal flange on the 4 is much larger than the 3, and the larger size confers a significant risk of dental injury in some patients.

Levitan advocates the use of a narrow-flange-height Macintosh 4 German or English design on all adult emergency cases; if the full depth of the blade is not required, the flange height with these blades does not cause a problem (its height is the same as a Macintosh 3), but if more blade is needed, the depth can be increased without the need to switch the blade.[37] As stressed originally by Chevalier Jackson, epiglottoscopy must always be performed to find the epiglottis before making any effort to

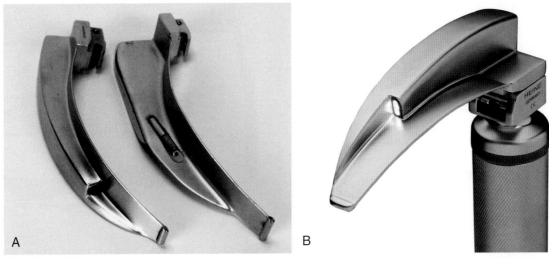

Figure 24-20 German Macintosh (i.e., German design) fiberoptic laryngoscope blades: Rüsch Emerald **(A)** and Heine **(B)**.

expose the larynx; otherwise, a large blade can be inserted too deeply and fail to identify landmarks.[38]

3. German Macintosh Blade

Heine, the German medical instrument company, pioneered incorporation of a rectangular, large (4.3-mm), glass-fiber bundle combined with a small flange height and full-length flange similar to that of an English Macintosh (Fig. 24-20). Like the English Macintosh, it has a small light-to-tip distance. When paired with rechargeable batteries and especially with an LED bulb, this large fiber bundle provides an extremely intense, white light. This design is easy to clean because it has no irregular surfaces. Other manufacturers have copied this design, with some labeling it a *German Macintosh*.

4. Improved-Vision Macintosh Blade

In Macintosh's original 1943 report of his curved-blade laryngoscope, the accompanying photograph of the blade showed a subtle flattening of the curve midblade. This disappeared early in the blade's history, probably because of manufacturing considerations.[32] In 1984, Gabor Racz described a modification in which the midportion of the Macintosh blade spatula was made concave (dorsally) in cross section, and the slight flattening of the midblade was reintroduced while the vertical step and flange were left intact (Fig. 24-21).[39] The combined modifications should help to reduce the crest-of-hill effect whereby the midblade convexity can encroach on the direct line of sight from eye to laryngeal inlet. Racz reported that the blade had been used successfully in several cases in which conventional laryngoscopy had failed.[39] The improved-view Macintosh is commercially available in multiple sizes from several manufacturers.

5. Bowen-Jackson Blade

Recognizing that curved and straight blades had advantages and disadvantages, Ronald Bowen and Ian Jackson attempted to create a blade that could be used in all difficult situations. The resulting blade is almost straight, but it has a fairly marked distal curve (Fig. 24-22). The distal

beak of the blade is bifid to allow straddling of the glossoepiglottic fold. The maximum depth of the vertical step is substantially less than that of the Macintosh blade, and it occurs midblade and tapers proximally to allow its use in patients with limited mouth opening or prominent teeth. When attached to the handle, the blade forms an angle of 100 degrees to help avoid contact with the chest.[40]

6. Left-Handed Laryngoscope

A mirror-image version of the Macintosh blade exists for use with the right hand. Inappropriately referred to as the left-handed laryngoscope, it is identical to the regular Macintosh blade except for the reversed configuration of the flange. Potential uses include laryngoscopy of patients in the right lateral decubitus position, procedures in those with right-sided facial or oropharyngeal abnormalities, and procedures in which the endotracheal tube (ETT) should be located on the left side of the mouth.[41,42]

7. Curved Blades with Exaggerated Distal Curvature

Several blades have been described with a more acute curvature of the distal spatula than that of the Macintosh. Of historical interest, the Gubuya-Orkin blade, described in 1959, was unique in having an S-shaped blade with a malleable distal 3 cm. The investigators described bending it through a range of 15 to 45 degrees, with an optimal position thought to be 35 degrees from the horizontal for indirect lifting of the epiglottis (Fig. 24-23).[43] Found to be effective in some cases in which Macintosh laryngoscopy had failed, the Gubuya-Orkin blade can be considered a forerunner of other blades with marked fixed or variable distal curvature.

Unlike the Macintosh blade, the Blechman blade has an accentuated curve at its distal tip. Its reverse-Z vertical step and flange begin distal to the block of the blade and extend only to within 5 cm of the blade tip. The curved Fink laryngoscope blade similarly has a sharper curve at the distal spatula and reduced vertical step proximally compared with the Macintosh. The ULX Macintosh

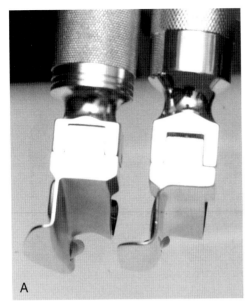

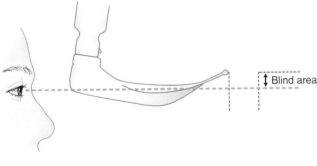

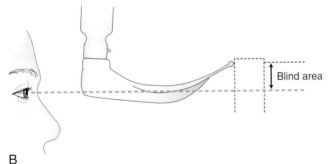

Figure 24-21 **A,** Cross section of the Improved Vision version of the Macintosh blade *(left)* compared with the standard blade *(right)*. Notice the concave, downward cross section of the midblade, potentially reducing the crest-of-hill obstruction to visualization that occurs with the standard Macintosh. **B,** The line of vision is improved and the blind area reduced by the redesigned blade *(top)* compared with the regular Macintosh blade *(bottom)*. (From Racz GB: Improved vision modification of the Macintosh laryngoscope (letter). *Anaesthesia* 39:1249–1250, 1984.)

(Upsher Laryngoscopy Systems, Mercury Medical, Clearwater, FL) blade has a more pronounced curve throughout the entire blade length than the standard Macintosh. The Wiemers or Freiburg blade, marketed in Europe, has less initial curvature than a Macintosh and has an acutely curved tip (Fig. 24-24).[44] As a group, these blades may have utility in patients with limitations of mouth opening, impaired head and neck mobility, or prominent upper incisors, in whom the tip of a Macintosh blade may fail

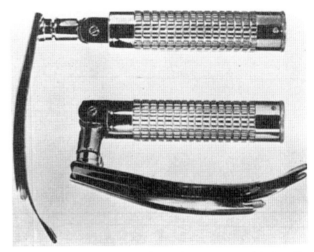

Figure 24-22 The Bowen-Jackson laryngoscope blade. (From Bowen RA, Jackson I: A new laryngoscope. *Anaesthesia* 7:254–256, 1952.)

to engage the glossoepiglottic fold at the appropriate angle. More specific indications for these blades await scientific evaluation.

B. Miller and Related Straight Blades

1. Miller Laryngoscope Blade

The use of straight blades, with entrapment and direct lifting of the epiglottis, was the common laryngoscopic technique when Miller introduced his modification of the straight laryngoscope blade in 1941. The blade he described was longer than the medium-sized blades available at the time, had a comparatively smaller flange height, was narrower at the tip, and featured a gradual curve starting 2 inches (5 cm) from the distal end (Fig. 24-25).[17] Miller contended that the smaller flange height would allow less mouth opening (permitting freer anterior movement of the mandible) and less potential for damage to the teeth. Although Miller's original design could accept a 38-F tube down the barrel, the flange height of modern Miller blades has become substantially smaller, and an adult-sized tracheal tube cannot fit down a Miller size 3 blade. Miller warned that the lumen should not be used for this purpose in his original description of the design.[17] With a smaller degree of mouth opening, Miller conceded that available room for tube manipulation would be less and that a stylet would be desirable.[17] In 1942, Cassels echoed Miller's contention that a greater distal curvature of the straight blade would facilitate exposure of the laryngeal inlet, accompanying his report with an elegant diagram to help illustrate his theory.[45] For a given position of the base of a straight blade between the teeth, especially when the mouth opening is limited, a curved distal tip can enable the laryngoscopist to visualize a more anterior aspect of the laryngeal inlet (Fig. 24-26). The Miller laryngoscope blade continues to be a commonly used straight blade.

2. Magill, Flagg, and Guedel Blades

Three older straight blades that warrant mention are the Magill, Flagg, and Guedel blades, which all predate the

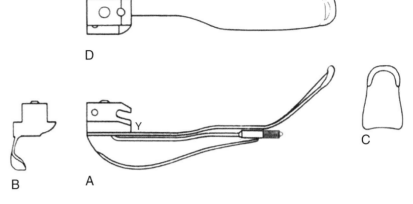

Figure 24-23 Schematic of the Gubuya-Orkin blade: side view **(A)**, fitting view **(B)**, end view of the tip section **(C)**, and top view **(D)**. (From Gabuya R, Orkin LR: Design and utility of a new curved laryngoscope blade. *Anesth Analg* 38:364–369, 1959.)

Miller. Miller developed his lower-profile, smaller-flanged straight blade partly in response to the perceived shortcomings of these relatively larger blades. Nonetheless, all three blades continue to be marketed in adult and pediatric sizes, attesting to their ongoing popularity.

The Magill blade, first marketed in 1921, is mainly straight, with a U-shaped step and flange concave to the right. The step and flange continue to within an inch of the end of the blade. The Flagg blade is straight with a very slight curve at the distal tip and was originally designed for use with Flagg catheters and tubes. With a light source placed quite distally, the C-shaped cross section tapers gradually from its proximal to distal end (Fig. 24-27).[46] The Guedel has an extremely large spatula and U-shape flange that is concave to the right. Its distal tip has slightly more curve than the Flagg, and the blade is angled on its base to result in a 72-degree angle with the handle to help promote a lifting action instead of using the teeth as a fulcrum.

3. Soper Blade

The straight Soper blade originally was described in 1947. When he was Wing Commander in the Royal Air Force Medical Division, Robert Soper developed the blade in response to the Macintosh's occasional failure to elevate a long, "flabby" epiglottis.[47] Although described as a modification of the Macintosh blade, it is largely straight except for a slight distal curvature. It retains the reverse-Z-shaped vertical step and flange of the Macintosh blade. A small, transverse slot cut into the blade a few millimeters from the tip is designed to help prevent the epiglottis from slipping off the blade (Fig. 24-28). The Soper blade is still commercially available in adult and pediatric lengths.

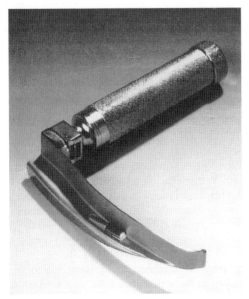

Figure 24-24 The Wiemers blade has a reduced initial curvature and sharply curved tip. (From Maleck WH, Koetter KP, Lentz M, et al: A randomized comparison of three laryngoscopes with the Macintosh. *Resuscitation* 42:241–245, 1999.)

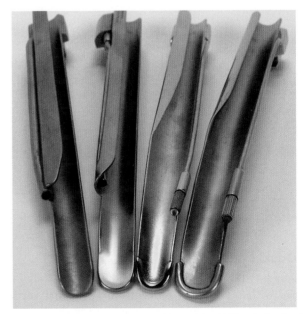

Figure 24-25 Original Miller blades. The original Miller design had a light on the right side of the flange when looking down the blade *(far right)*. Poorly designed Miller blades *(far left)* have the light on the leading edge of the left flange. The light embeds in the tongue and produces inadequate illumination.

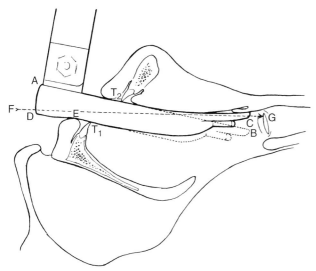

Figure 24-26 Cassels' 1942 diagram shows the advantages of a distal curve to an otherwise straight blade. With a compromised interincisor opening (T_1 to T_2), the limited upward angulation of a straight blade (A to B) may afford a view of only the posterior laryngeal inlet. Curving the distal blade (A to C) permits a more anterior view from point D looking along the line from F to G. (From Cassels WH: Advantages of a curved laryngoscope. *Anesthesiology* 3:580–581, 1942.)

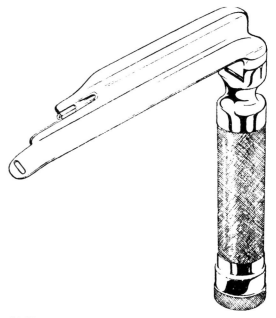

Figure 24-28 The Soper laryngoscope. (From Soper RL: A new laryngoscope for anaesthetists. *Br Med J* 1:265, 1947.)

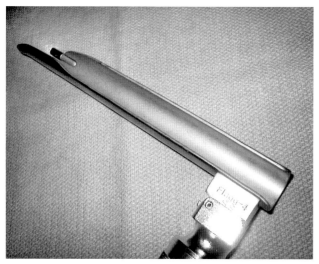

Figure 24-27 The Flagg blade.

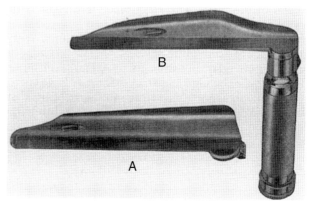

Figure 24-29 The Gould blade **(B)** is slightly longer, with a flattened vertical step proximally compared with the parent Soper blade **(A)**. (From Gould RB: Modified laryngoscope blade. *Anaesthesia* 9:125, 1954.)

4. Gould Blade

Gould, in 1954, modified a Soper blade by (1) lining the flange with rubber and reducing the proximal vertical step and (2) lengthening and blunting the distal end of the blade (Fig. 24-29). He made a similar modification to a Macintosh blade, although neither version attained widespread use.[48]

5. Wisconsin Blades

The Wisconsin blade is a large, straight blade with a circular flange. The original design had a slightly flared distal flange. The Whitehead modifications—the Wis-Foregger and Wis-Hipple blades—are variations of the original Wisconsin design with slightly modified flanges, bulb locations, and spatulas (Fig. 24-30).[46]

6. Snow Blade

In 1962, Snow recognized the advantages of a straight blade in certain difficult situations, but finding difficulty with epiglottic entrapment with the Wis-Foregger and problematic ETT passage with the Miller, he modified a straight blade by slightly curving the distal tip beginning

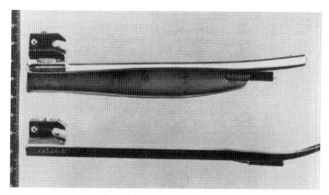

Figure 24-30   The Schapira blade *(bottom)* with minimal vertical component is compared with the Wis-Foregger blade *(top).* (From Schapira M: A modified straight laryngoscope blade designed to facilitate endotracheal intubation. *Anesth Analg* 52:553–554, 1973.)

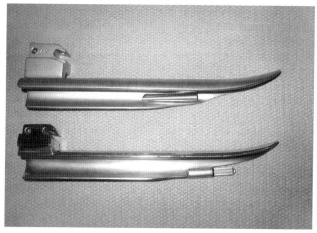

Figure 24-32   Two versions of the straight Phillips blade with a light tip that is protected *(top)* behind the vertical step and unprotected *(bottom).*

1 inch (2.5 cm) from its semirounded beak. He also increased the vertical step and flange combination to create a C-shaped groove that was concave to the right, which allowed a better view and easier tube passage (Fig. 24-31).[49]

7. Phillips Blade

Otto Phillips developed a blade similar to the Snow blade. In 1973, Phillips described it as a combination of the shaft of the Jackson blade and curved tip of the Miller blade. He thought that the Jackson shaft offered a good conduit for ETT passage and reasoned that the curved tip of the Miller would help to lift the hyoid bone and attached structures, affording good visualization of the glottis.[50] The light bulb is located on the left side of the blade, and in some versions of the blade, it may be unprotected from the tongue, although other versions use a fiberoptic carrier shielded by the vertical step (Fig. 24-32). The C-shaped vertical step and flange are less complete than a Wisconsin arc, are concave to the right, and extend to within 5 cm of the end of the blade. Phillips conducted an observational study of the use of the blade in the hands of experienced and inexperienced users in more

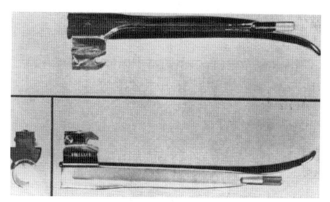

Figure 24-31   The Snow blade predates and is similar to the Phillips blade (see Fig. 24-32), with distal curve and C-shaped channel for endotracheal tube delivery. (From Snow JC: Modification of laryngoscope blade. *Anesthesiology* 23:294, 1962.)

than 1000 patients and found that successful intubation was achieved on the first attempt with the Phillips blade in 84% of cases.[50] The Phillips blade is produced in size 1 for pediatric patients and size 2 for adult patients. It is available commercially and has relatively widespread use.

8. Schapira Blade

Max Schapira described a blade that is straight with a slight distal anterior curvature but with a minimal vertical component and no horizontal flange (see Fig. 24-30).[51] The blade remains available commercially.

9. Henderson Laryngoscope

The Henderson laryngoscope blade (Karl Storz, Tuttlingen, Germany) is a modification of the straight blade. It was introduced by John Henderson of Glasgow, an enthusiastic proponent of straight-blade laryngoscopy in anesthesia practice.[52,53] The Henderson blade is straight over its entire length and has a semicircular vertical step and flange, resulting in a wide slot that permits easy ETT entry, passage, and exit. The step, flange, and light carrier continue to within 2.5 cm of the blade tip, which with the straight blade is designed to maximize light delivery. The fiberoptic light carrier is shielded from the tongue within the lumen of the blade (Fig. 24-33). The distal tip of the blade has a rounded, knurled edge, which can be seen when viewing down the barrel. Having a visible distal tip makes it easy to determine whether the blade has been advanced far enough to lift the epiglottis; when using a Miller blade or others with a distal upturned tip, repeated rounds of advancing and lifting are often required until the epiglottis is controlled.

The Henderson blade is available in small and large sizes. The 148- and 192-cm-long blades have lumens sufficiently large to accommodate passage of ETTs with 7- and 8-mm inner diameters (IDs), respectively. Henderson evaluated the blade in 300 patients and reported easy positioning of the blade in 91%, a grade 1 view in 93%, and successful direct ETT passage on the first attempt in 97% of patients.[53] He published a case series

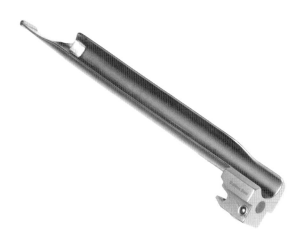

Figure 24-33 The Henderson blade features a completely straight spatula, protected light source, semicircular channel, and Macintosh-type beak. (Courtesy of John Henderson, MD, Glasgow, UK.)

documenting successful glottic exposure and intubation using paraglossal straight blade laryngoscopy in situations in which the Macintosh blade had failed.[52]

10. Dörges Universal Blade

The Dörges universal laryngoscope blade has been described as an effort to create a single blade with utility in many situations.[54] The blade is mainly straight with a slightly curved distal end, enabling its use by direct or indirect elevation of the epiglottis. It tapers gradually from the heel to 11 mm at its tip, corresponding to the width of a Macintosh 2 blade tip. The working length of 125 mm, however, is between those of Macintosh 3 and 4 blades. The angle of the blade tip with the handle is 76 degrees, as opposed to the usual 58 degrees of the Macintosh blade, potentially facilitating blade insertion into patients with a prominent sternal area. Similarly, the lower profile, 15-mm, reverse-Z-shaped vertical step and flange may facilitate the blade's insertion in patients with limited mouth opening. Two marks corresponding to a patient weight of 10 or 20 kg on the front and rear of the blade serve as a rough guide for insertion depth when using the blade in a pediatric patient (Fig. 24-34).

11. Grandview Blade

The Grandview laryngoscope blade (Hartwell Medical, Carlsbad, CA) was designed by a paramedic in the United

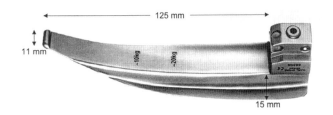

Figure 24-34 The Dörges universal laryngoscope blade has markings that indicate appropriate insertion depths for pediatric use. (From Gerlach K, Wenzel V, von Knobelsdorff G, et al: A new universal laryngoscope blade: A preliminary comparison with Macintosh laryngoscope blades. *Resuscitation* 57:63–67, 2003.)

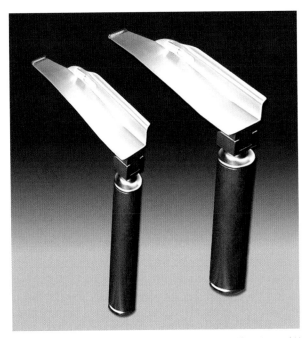

Figure 24-35 Two sizes of the Grandview blade. (Courtesy of Hartwell Medical, Carlsbad, CA.)

States, and it has achieved widespread use in U.S. Emergency Medical Systems.[55] It has a curvature somewhat similar to that of a Dörges blade, in that it is mostly straight but has a slightly bent distal tip. Its primary unique feature is its massive proximal spatula, and it is advertised as "the tongue tamer" (Fig. 24-35). Another feature of the Grandview is its use of a super-bright LED bulb. It comes in two sizes and in a reusable or single-use version. Its reusable version has a gold-colored tip to make tip visualization easier. There are no published clinical case series validating the Grandview blade as superior to a conventional Macintosh, although anecdotally, the manufacturer has received very positive feedback, and it has been successful commercially. Inadequate tongue control is a frequent error among novice intubators, and the larger spatula blade may be valued by those who intubate less frequently. Conversely, a larger blade volume may make it harder to reach the larynx in patients with a small displacement space (i.e., thyromental distance) and a large tongue-to-pharynx ratio.

C. Blades with Fixed and Various Degrees of Acute Angulation

1. Belscope

a. DESCRIPTION

The Bellhouse laryngoscope, or Belscope, is a straight blade bent 45 degrees at its midpoint.[56] The blade comes off the handle at a slightly offset angle and has a vertical step less than that of a Macintosh blade and no horizontal flange (Fig. 24-36). The Belscope is available in three lengths from tip to angle: 6.7, 8, and 9.3 cm. Because the blade typically is used to elevate the epiglottis directly, less compression and anterior displacement of the tongue may be needed to obtain a view of the larynx. The

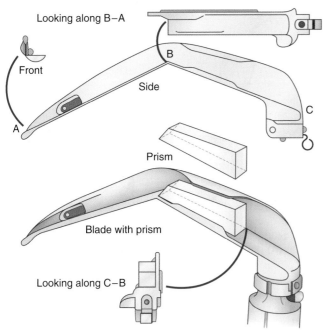

Figure 24-36   The Belscope angulated laryngoscope. The view *(top)* obtained from the blade angle along the distal blade *(line B-A)* is shown. Failing this, indirect visualization is possible with a prism *(line C-B)*. (From Bellhouse CP: An angulated laryngoscope for routine and difficult tracheal intubation. *Anesthesiology* 69:126–129, 1988.)

Belscope may be useful when poor atlanto-occipital extension, a large tongue, or a short mandible hinder optimal positioning of a Macintosh laryngoscope blade. If visualization remains suboptimal with the Belscope, a prism can be attached proximal to the angulation to provide an indirect view of the glottic opening.

b. BLADE USE

Without the prism, the Belscope can be used in a fashion similar to a straight blade. Displacing the tongue to the left, the blade may be inserted into the proximal esophagus and then withdrawn to expose the laryngeal inlet. Retraction of the upper lip may be advantageous. Because of the blade's 45-degree angulation, there may be less chance of the proximal blade applying pressure to the upper teeth. In the event that the larynx is not primarily visualized with the blade, use of the prism (suitably defogged) rotates the image of the larynx by 34 degrees (Fig. 24-37). Often, a styleted tracheal tube curved anteriorly is necessary for advancement through the glottis.[56]

c. CLINICAL EXPERIENCE

Bellhouse reported his experience of 3500 intubations in which he used the Belscope without failure.[56] The report included a subseries of 12 patients in whom the Belscope successfully exposed the glottis after the Macintosh had failed. Bellhouse emphasized the need for practice in the use of the blade because its feel was different from that of other blades.[56] Separately, Mayall reported a second series of 12 patients with Cormack-Lehane grade 3 laryngoscopies with the Macintosh blade, all of whom were converted to a "good view of the cords" with the Belscope without use of the prism.[57] In a crossover study by Sultana and colleagues comparing Macintosh and Belscope laryngoscopy, of 22 grade 3 views obtained, 19 were with the Macintosh blade. Tube passage using the Belscope required lip retraction by an assistant more frequently than with the Macintosh.[58]

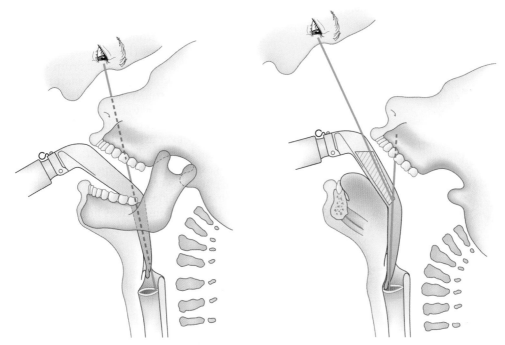

Figure 24-37   When using the Belscope by the right paraglossal route *(left)*, the view is assisted by retraction of the lip. Occasionally, use of the prism may be required for indirect visualization of the larynx *(right)*. (From Bellhouse CP: An angulated laryngoscope for routine and difficult tracheal intubation. *Anesthesiology* 69:126–129, 1988.)

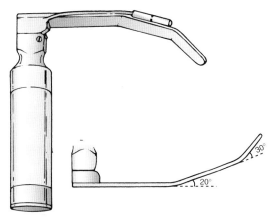

Figure 24-38 The Choi double-angle laryngoscope, with incremental 20-degree and 30-degree angles on its blade. (From Choi JJ: A new double-angle blade for direct laryngoscopy (letter). *Anesthesiology* 72:576, 1990.)

2. Choi Double-Angle Laryngoscope

In 1990, Choi described a double-angled blade with the spatula incorporating two incremental angles—the proximal (20 degrees) and the distal (30 degrees) (Fig. 24-38).[59] The spatula and beak are wide and flat for tongue or epiglottis control, and there is no vertical step or flange. The light source lies along the left edge of the blade between the two angles, with the bulb pointing toward the center of the glottis. The blade can be used with direct or indirect lifting of the epiglottis. It is commercially available in one adult and one pediatric size.[59]

3. Orr Laryngoscope

The Orr blade was developed to help eliminate contact with the upper teeth. Two right-angle bends (Fig. 24-39) are designed to enable the blade to sit down inside the mouth, shifting the fulcrum into the pharynx and away

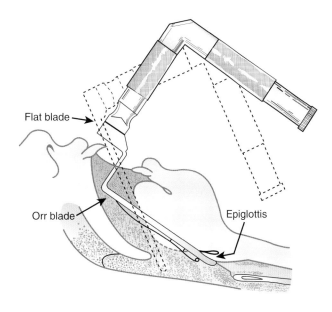

Figure 24-39 The Orr laryngoscope blade. (From Orr RB: A new laryngoscopy blade designed to facilitate difficult endotracheal intubation. *Anesthesiology* 31:377–378, 1969.)

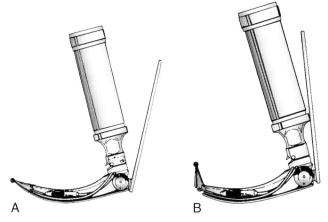

Figure 24-40 The Corazzelli-London-McCoy blade in the default position **(A)** and activated with the tip elevated **(B).** (From McCoy EP, Mirakhur RK: The levering laryngoscope. *Anaesthesia* 48:516–519, 1993.)

from the teeth. It typically is used to elevate the epiglottis directly, and the ETT is advanced from the right side of the mouth. Rarely used now, the Orr blade was available in two lengths.[60]

4. Levering Tip Laryngoscope

a. DESCRIPTION

The levering tip or articulating laryngoscope (Corazzelli-London-McCoy [CLM] blade, Mercury Medical, Clearwater, FL) is a modification of standard curved (and straight) laryngoscope blades. A curved blade first described in 1993 is marketed by several manufacturers (e.g., the Flipper, Rüsch, Duluth, GA; Heine Flex Tip, Heine Optotechnik, Herrsching, Germany). These laryngoscope blades have a hinged distal tip activated by a lever that lies adjacent to the handle of the laryngoscope. Depressing the lever toward the handle elevates the tip, located 25 mm from the end of the blade, by approximately 70 degrees (Fig. 24-40).[61] The lever acts on the tip through a spring-loaded drum on the proximal end of the blade, which pushes a shaft linking with the distal hinge. In the resting position, the blade looks and acts like a standard blade, with the vertical step of the distal adjustable tip locking with that of the rest of the blade. The blade-lever assembly can be used with any compatible standard handle. When activated, the levering tip laryngoscope may have the advantage of having a fulcrum at a point lower in the pharynx, helping to provide an optimal tip angle and contact with the hyoepiglottic ligament in situations such as limited mouth opening, a large tongue, or prominent or overriding upper teeth.

b. BLADE USE

The curved levering tip blade is most often used by placing the tip in the vallecula, although the tip can be placed beneath the epiglottis. If glottic visualization is poor, the lever can be depressed, activating the distal tip upward. This may help the blade tip make contact with the hyoepiglottic ligament, helping to lift the epiglottis and improve glottic visualization. Endotracheal intubation is then performed in a standard fashion. The lever is

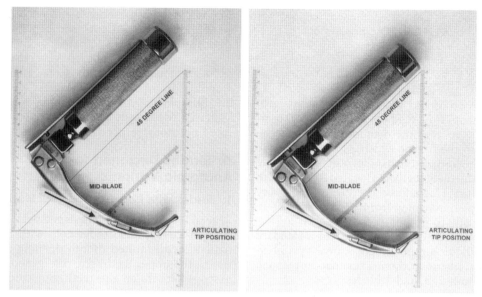

Figure 24-41   When the Corazzelli-London-McCoy blade improves the view *(left)*, the tip elevates the base of the tongue and the vallecula. However, if these structures are already maximally elevated, tip activation forces the blade posteriorly into the line of sight *(right)*, possibly worsening the view. (From Levitan RM, Ochroch EA: Explaining the variable effect on laryngeal view obtained with the McCoy laryngoscope (letter). *Anaesthesia* 54:599–601, 1999.)

released, and the blade is removed with the tip in the neutral position.

c. CLINICAL EXPERIENCE

Since the introduction of the CLM, several case reports have attested to its value in difficult situations.[62-69] Subsequent prospective series have confirmed the CLM's utility in some difficult situations and confirmed clinical suspicions that its use in otherwise easy situations may worsen the view. Studies have been consistent in their findings that without cervical spine precautions, improvement with the use of blade tip activation from Cormack-Lehane grade 3 views to grade 2 or better is significant, occurring in 44% to 91% of cases.[44,62-69] In most studies, the CLM blade has failed to meaningfully improve Cormack-Lehane grade 4 views.

The levering tip blade is less useful in otherwise easy laryngoscopies. Although one report documented a 66% improvement in 38 patients (arytenoids only) with Cormack-Lehane grade 2 laryngoscopic views, the same report revealed a 22% overall incidence of a worsening view obtained with tip activation, all in patients with Cormack-Lehane grades 1 and 2.[69] In easy laryngoscopic situations, the blade tip easily engages and can lift the hyoepiglottic ligament and hyoid bone at the appropriate angle. With no potential for further upward travel, blade tip activation instead forces the midportion of the blade downward and into the direct line of sight, potentially obscuring the view (Fig. 24-41).[70] The better the view before tip activation, the more likely this phenomenon appears to be.

Several studies have documented that the improvement in laryngoscopic view obtained with tip activation of the CLM is less than that obtained by external laryngeal pressure,[67,68,70] although application of external laryngeal pressure and tip activation has an additive effect.[67] McCoy and colleagues found that the force

incurred when using the levering tip blade was significantly less than that needed to visualize the larynx with the Macintosh blade.[62] There was no increase in heart rate, mean arterial pressure, or plasma norepinephrine levels with use of the levering tip blade,[62] possibly because there was less need to provide forward displacement of attached structures while elevating the epiglottis.

The CLM blade may be useful in patients requiring cervical spine precautions. In three studies simulating cervical spine precautions with use of manual in-line stabilization or application of a cervical collar, activation of the levering tip improved the Cormack-Lehane laryngeal view by at least one grade in 45% to 74% of patients, and in the patients with a grade 3 view, conversion to a grade 2 or better view occurred in 83% to 92% of cases.[71-73] In the 319 patients enrolled in these three studies, the view was worsened by use of the activated CLM blade in only one case. A separate study looking at head extension using external anatomic markers during CLM laryngoscopy demonstrated that 6 to 8 degrees less head extension was necessary for arytenoid-only and full-glottic exposure compared with Macintosh blade use.[74] MacIntyre and colleagues, using lateral radiographs to look at cervical spine movement with Macintosh and CLM blade use, could not demonstrate a significant difference in the degree of extension occurring between C0 and C3.[75] In a cadaver series with surgically induced lesions at C5-C6, Miller, Macintosh, and McCoy blade laryngoscopy use was assessed fluoroscopically. The Miller was superior to the Macintosh or the CLM blade at minimizing axial distraction, but no significant difference in anteroposterior displacement or angular rotation at the level of the lesion was demonstrated between blades.[76]

The CLM has been well studied since its introduction and appears to be useful in some difficult situations while not helping or worsening the view in easy cases of direct laryngoscopy. Published evidence suggests that it may be particularly useful when Cormack-Lehane grade 3 views have been induced by cervical spine precautions.

5. Flexiblade

a. DESCRIPTION

The Flexiblade (Arco Medic, Omer, Israel) incorporates a flexible component into a rigid blade. This direct laryngoscope is flexible in the intermediate portion of the blade. Activation of the trigger, which, unlike that in the CLM, lies along the front of the handle, results in variable flexion of six intermediate segments located 3.5 to 10 cm from the blade's tip. This adjusts the blade's curvature through a 20-degree arc, going from a shape similar to that of a Miller blade to that of a Macintosh blade (Fig. 24-42).[77] The Flexiblade can be attached to a standard laryngoscope handle or a remote light source by a fiberoptic cable. It is available in three sizes that correspond roughly to Macintosh 2, 3, and 4 blades.

b. MODIFIED HANDLES

Use of the Flexiblade is similar to the technique used with the CLM blade. With the tip of the blade located in the vallecula, activation of the trigger increases the amount of blade flexion, which may help with glottic visualization. ETT passage follows in the usual fashion.

c. ADAPTERS

Perera and coworkers evaluated the Flexiblade in 200 patients.[78] In patients with an initial Cormack-Lehane grade 3 view with the Flexiblade in the neutral position, blade activation converted the view to grade 2 or 1 in

84% of cases. In this series, blade activation worsened the view in only four patients, and as with the CLM blade, all of those patients had grade 1 or 2 views before blade flexion. Yardeni and colleagues[77] performed an in vitro technical analysis of the blade after the technique described by Marks and associates[28] and confirmed that the Flexiblade behaves in fashion similar to that of a Miller or Macintosh blade in the neutral and fully elevated positions, respectively.[78]

D. Blades Designed for Other Anatomic Variants

1. Blades with Reduced Vertical Step

Several blades have been designed with a reduced vertical step. In theory, this should help with blade insertion in patients with limited mouth opening and pose a lower risk to the upper teeth. The risk is increased if the laryngoscopist levers on the teeth, but studies have demonstrated that the horizontal flanges of well-used Macintosh blades show significant signs of wear at the level of the upper teeth, suggesting frequent contact with the blade, and other studies have demonstrated that even experienced clinicians generate significant axial force on the upper incisors.[79,80] Although these findings may suggest that one of the functions of the vertical step is to maintain mouth opening through contact with the upper teeth, most clinicians prefer to minimize contact with the upper teeth. To address the issue of step or flange contact with the upper teeth, several modifications to blades have been made.

a. BIZZARRI-GIUFFRIDA BLADE

The Bizzarri-Giuffrida blade was developed in response to the problem of the Macintosh blade's vertical step and flange proximally touching the upper teeth, causing difficulty in rotation of the blade into the hypopharynx and full insertion into the valleculae, particularly in patients with limited mandibular mobility. The blade is curved in fashion similar to that of the Macintosh blade and omits the vertical step, with the exception of a minimal amount at midblade, where it is needed to protect the light carrier (Fig. 24-43). The experience of several hundred patients was "complete satisfaction," particularly by those with buckteeth, a receding jaw, bull neck, or an anterior larynx. The investigators reported successful use of the blade during awake direct laryngoscopy.[81]

b. CALLANDER-THOMAS BLADE

In 1987, Callander and Thomas described a blade incorporating a reduction in the proximal portion of the vertical step and flange of the Macintosh blade (Fig. 24-44).[82] The reduction in the step height was postulated to improve the blade's utility in patients with limited mouth opening and to decrease the risk of dental damage.[82]

c. BUCX BLADE

A modification similar to the Callander-Thomas blade was made by Bucx and colleagues after technical analysis suggested it to be a good model.[83] This blade had a Macintosh-style curve and had the vertical step and flange reduced to a minimum from blade base to 8 cm

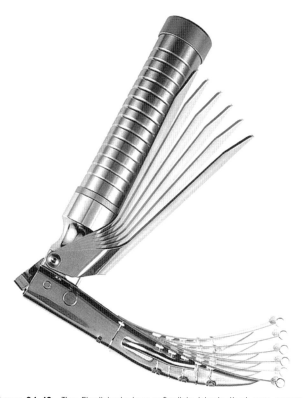

Figure 24-42 The Flexiblade has a flexible blade that can assume many positions. (Courtesy of Arco Medic, Omer, Israel.)

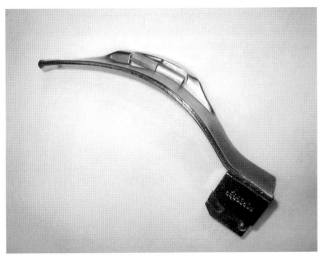

Figure 24-43   The Bizzarri blade has an almost no vertical step.

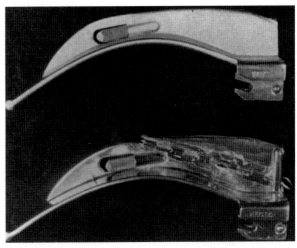

Figure 24-45   The Onkst blade *(bottom)* has a hinged vertical component compared with the standard Macintosh blade *(top)*. (From Onkst R: Modified laryngoscope blade. *Anesthesiology* 22:846, 1961.)

from the blade tip. Bucx and coworkers clinically evaluated the blade, randomly assigning 46 patients to two groups for laryngoscopy and intubation with a regular Macintosh or the modified blade.[84] Although the mean force exerted on the maxillary incisors was significantly reduced in the modified-blade group, there was a decided tendency toward anteflexion of the head during laryngoscopy with the modified blade and an increased need for the assistant to retract the upper lip to aid with intubation. Although the accepted purpose of the vertical step of laryngoscope blades is control of soft tissue, especially the tongue, this study suggests the possibility that the vertical step and flange at the level of the upper teeth may help to maintain mouth opening and counteract the tendency of the head to anteflex during laryngoscopy.

d. ONKST BLADE

In 1961, Onkst modified a Macintosh 3 blade to help avoid undue pressure on the upper incisors. The proximal portions of the blade's vertical step and flange are hinged and, although normally kept in the upright position by a

weak spring, allow the vertical step and flange to fold down in response to pressure on the teeth, theoretically avoiding dental damage (Fig. 24-45).[85]

e. RACZ-ALLEN HINGED-STEP BLADE

The Racz-Allen blade has a hinged step and flange.[86] The vertical step of this modified straight blade is maintained in position by a spring. During laryngoscopy, any pressure on the vertical step from the upper teeth causes an upward and lateral deflection of the hinged portion. The main blade is convex in cross section to a greater extent than the Miller blade to help maintain vision when the concave, hinged portion is displaced. A threaded shaft is removable, allowing disassembly of the two portions of the blade for cleaning (Fig. 24-46).[86] The blade length is intermediate between a Miller 2 and 3. Racz and Allen reported more than 2000 successful intubations at their institution with the blade.[86]

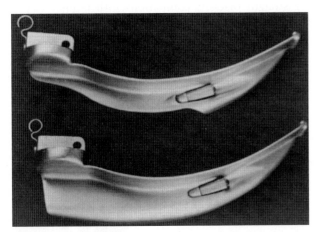

Figure 24-44   The Callander-Thomas blade *(top)* has a reduced vertical step proximally compared with the Macintosh blade *(bottom)*. (From Callander CC, Thomas J: Modification of Macintosh laryngoscope for difficult intubation (letter). *Anaesthesia* 42:671, 1987.)

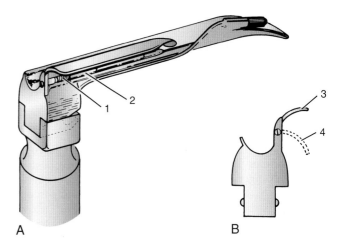

Figure 24-46   Side **(A)** and fitting **(B)** views of the Racz-Allen hinged blade. *1,* Spring; *2,* threaded screw; *3,* normal position; *4,* full displacement of the hinged component of the blade. (From Racz GB, Allen FB: A new pressure-sensitive laryngoscope. *Anesthesiology* 62:356–358, 1985.)

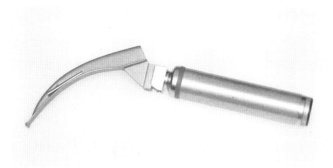

Figure 24-47 The Polio blade is a standard Macintosh blade that fits onto a standard handle at a very obtuse angle.

2. Blades and Devices That Avoid Chest Impingement

Several adaptations have been made to help avoid unwanted impingement of a laryngoscope's handle during laryngoscopy. This had been particularly important in morbidly obese patients, parturients with mammomegaly, and patients in an iron lung and during the application of cricoid pressure, when an assistant's hand is present. Equipment solutions have included shortened handles and making the angle between the laryngoscope handle and blade more obtuse by means of modifications to the blade or the handle or by insertion of adapters. However, appropriate positioning of the patient (e.g., ear-to-sternal notch horizontal alignment, head elevation relative to the chest) often renders these devices unnecessary.

a. MODIFIED BLADES

The Polio blade was introduced by Foregger in 1954 and designed for use during intubation of patients in iron lung respirators. It features a Macintosh-style blade that attaches to a battery handle at an obtuse angle of 170 degrees (Fig. 24-47).[87] It may still be used when a regular handle attachment setup encounters forward impingement (e.g., obesity, kyphosis with barrel chest deformity, mammary gland hypertrophy, a short neck),[87] although the extremely obtuse angle of the blade to the handle may make it difficult to generate an adequate lifting force. For obstetric cases, Kessell modified a Macintosh blade's block so that the blade comes off the handle at an angle of 110 degrees instead of the usual 90 degrees (Fig. 24-48).[88] Beaver described a straight blade with a handle set at 25 degrees to facilitate intubation of patients in "box" respirators.[89]

b. MODIFIED HANDLES

Handles with one half of the length of regular laryngoscope handles have been used to help avoid chest or breast impingement (Fig. 24-49). Patil and colleagues described a shortened, adjustable-angle laryngoscope handle incorporating a blade-lock device that allows blade positioning at 180, 135, 90, or 45 degrees to the handle (Fig. 24-50). When there is potential impingement of a laryngoscope handle on a patient's chest, the instrument can be inserted at 180 degrees; the angle of the blade to handle then can be reduced to 135 or 90 degrees, allowing laryngoscopy to be performed.[90]

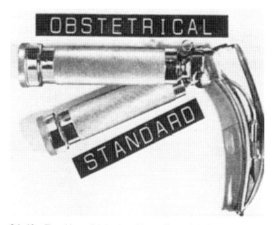

Figure 24-48 The Kessell blade. (From Kessell J: A laryngoscope for obstetrical use: An obstetrical laryngoscope. *Anaesth Intensive Care* 5:265, 1977.)

c. ADAPTERS

The Jellicoe adapter was described to overcome the true angle between the Macintosh blade tip and handle of 58 degrees. The adapter increases this angle to 90 degrees (Fig. 24-51), facilitating blade entry into patients' oral cavities in some situations.[91] In 1991, Dhara and Cheong described a multiple-angle laryngoscope adapter that fits between the handle and blade and that provides working angles of 65, 90, 110, 130, 150, and 180 degrees between blade and handle.[92] The Yentis adapter is a 2.5-cm cube block that fits between a standard handle and laryngoscope blade (Fig. 24-52). It allows insertion of the blade into the patient's mouth with the handle swung 90 degrees to the right. After the blade is inserted, the handle can be swung back to the normal position for laryngoscopy.[93]

3. Blades for a Small Infraoral Cavity

a. BAINTON BLADE

The Bainton blade is unique in this collection of blades because it is designed specifically for pathologic conditions that obliterate the hypopharynx. The very large and long straight blade is compatible with regular laryngoscope handles. The distal 7 cm of the blade has a squared,

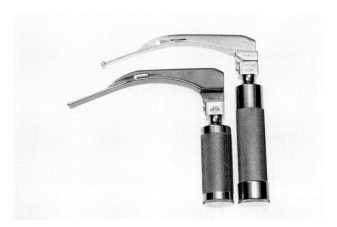

Figure 24-49 Shortened handles (*left*) help to avoid chest impingement during laryngoscopy.

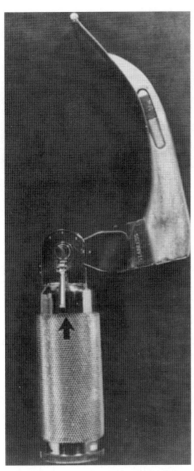

Figure 24-50 The shortened Patil handle allows positioning of the laryngoscope blade at an angle of 45, 90, 135, or 180 degrees. (From Patil VU, Stehling LC, Zauder HL: An adjustable laryngoscope handle for difficult intubations (letter). *Anesthesiology* 60:609, 1984.)

tubular design to help create a hypopharyngeal space where there may be none (Fig. 24-53). The lumen accepts an ETT up to size 8.0, and an intraluminal light source ensures that lighting is not compromised by tissues crowding the bulb. Bainton successfully tested his prototype in dogs with artificially induced hypopharyngeal swelling and in a small series of 12 patients with edematous conditions of the pharynx (one with a friable, bleeding tumor).[94]

b. DIAZ PEDIATRIC TUBULAR LARYNGOSCOPE

The Diaz pediatric tubular laryngoscope features a U-shaped handle and blade assembly. With a gradual distal curve, the blade is composed of two halves that are held together with a removable screw. A tubular scope with a straight blade design results when the two halves are attached (Fig. 24-54). The enclosed channel houses two light sources (one on each side) that are powered from an external fiberoptic light source. Endotracheal intubation is accomplished through the lumen of the scope, which must be disassembled by removal of the screw before the scope's removal from the patient.[95]

E. Pediatric Laryngoscopes

Macintosh and Miller blades are available in pediatric sizes. A size 1 in both blades is appropriate for an infant and a size 2 for a child. Additional Miller sizes 0 and 00 are available for the premature and small premature infant, respectively. Other pediatric blades are available commercially.

1. Oxford (Bryce-Smith) Blade

The Oxford, or Bryce-Smith, blade, was intended for neonates but is applicable for infants up to age 3 months. Primarily a straight blade, it tapers gradually from its proximal width of 1.8 cm to 1 cm distally. The step and flange are U-shaped, and although the distal 2.5 cm is open, a slight distal step remains for tongue control. The horizontal flange is quite broad proximally, helping to

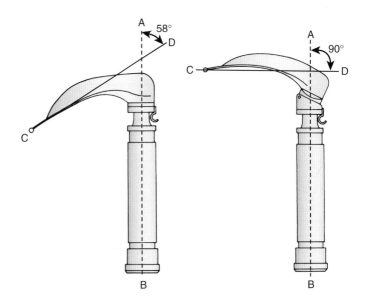

Figure 24-51 There is a 58-degree functional angle between the standard Macintosh blade tip and handle *(left)* and a 90-degree angle with the interposed Jellicoe adapter *(right)*. (From Jellicoe JA, Harris NR: A modification of a standard laryngoscope for difficult tracheal intubation in obstetric cases. *Anaesthesia* 39:800–802, 1984.)

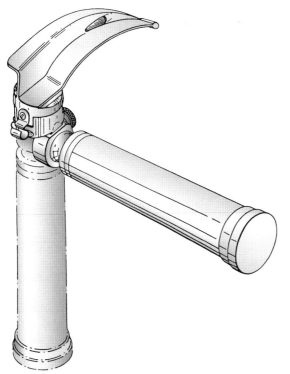

Figure 24-52 The Yentis adapter allows lateral pivoting of the laryngoscope handle to aid blade insertion. (From Yentis SM: A laryngoscope adaptor for difficult intubation. *Anaesthesia* 42:764–766, 1987.)

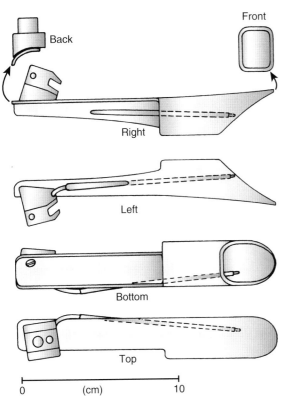

Figure 24-53 The Bainton laryngoscope blade is tubular distally to help overcome pharyngeal obstruction. (From Bainton CR: A new laryngoscope blade to overcome pharyngeal obstruction. *Anesthesiology* 67:767–770, 1987.)

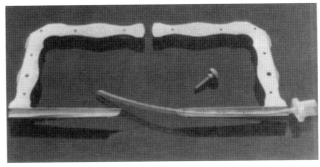

Figure 24-54 A tubular pediatric laryngoscope results when the two halves are attached by a removable screw. (From Diaz JH, Guarisco JL, LeJeune FE: A modified tubular pharyngolaryngoscope for difficult pediatric laryngoscopy. *Anesthesiology* 73:357–358, 1990.)

prevent the upper lip from obscuring the view and potentially helping in difficult cleft-palate situations (Fig. 24-55).[96]

2. Seward Blade

The Seward blade was created for use in the neonate, but additional sizes allow it to be used in children up to age 5 years. The primarily straight blade is 10.5 cm long, has a mild distal angulation and sharply tapering width, and ends in a thickened beak. The adult bulb is protected from the tongue on the inside of the reverse-Z-shaped step and flange (Fig. 24-56).[97]

3. Robertshaw Blade

Robertshaw originally modified a baby Soper straight blade by slightly curving the distal end while modifying the step and flange from the Soper's reverse-Z to a slight C shape. The light source was well protected from the tongue inside the vertical step. A subsequent modification exhibited additional leftward bending of the vertical step, creating a wider channel for visualization (Fig. 24-57).[98]

4. Other Blades

The Propper, or Heine, blade is straight with a slightly curved tip. The horizontal flange is in the reverse-Z configuration, curving away from the blade.[46] Other

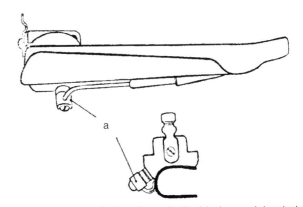

Figure 24-55 The Oxford, or Bryce-Smith, blade was intended for neonates but can be used for infants up to 3 months old. *a*, Light carrier. (From Bryce-Smith R: A laryngoscope blade for infants (letter). *Br Med J* 1:217, 1952.)

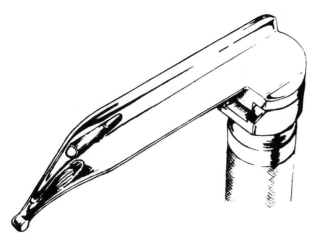

Figure 24-56 The Seward newborn laryngoscope blade. (From Seward EH: Laryngoscope for resuscitation of the newborn. *Lancet* 2:1041, 1957.)

modifications have been made for pediatric use. Matsuki described a widened, thin blade attached to the handle at a slightly obtuse angle to aid in control of the infant's tongue.[99] Rokowski and Gurmarnik described a modification of the standard Miller 0 blade in which the distal portion of the blade was widened to a triangular configuration for neonates or to a circular configuration for infants.[100] The width of the flange was reduced by 2 mm without modifying the height of the step to improve the area available for ETT manipulation and laryngeal visualization. Diaz combined several of the improvements in pediatric blades into one unit by modifying a Miller 1 blade to include an attached oxygen insufflation port, a corrugated lingual surface, and outward bending of the C-shaped flange to widen the cross-sectional area.[101] No formal evaluation has been published.

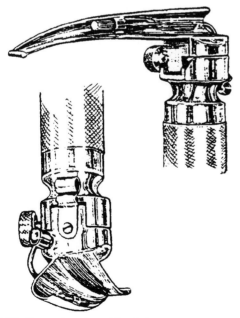

Figure 24-57 Second version of the Robertshaw blade. (From Robertshaw FL: A new laryngoscope for infants and children. *Lancet* 2:1034, 1962.)

F. Laryngoscope Blades with Accessory Devices

1. Blades with Integrated Oxygen Delivery Channels

Some blades, mainly in pediatric sizes, are available with integrated channels designed for the insufflation of oxygen during direct laryngoscopy. The concept has evolved from earlier reports of oxygen insufflation through feeding tubes taped to blades during laryngoscopy in neonates and infants.[102,103] Hencz described permanently affixing a wide-bore aspirating needle for the same purpose.[104] Todres and Crone formally described the Oxyscope laryngoscope, which incorporates a built-in oxygen insufflation channel.[105] It was originally made available in Miller 0 and 1 blades and subsequently in Macintosh blades. Studies during laryngoscopy in spontaneously breathing, anesthetized infants have demonstrated higher oxygen tensions with oxygen administration through these blades.[105,106] They continue to be marketed under various brand names, mainly in the Miller configuration.

2. Blades with Integrated Suction Channels

Some adult and pediatric blades have an integrated suction channel or blades that allow suction through an oxygen administration port.[107-109] The modified blades allow suctioning during ongoing laryngoscopy and may be useful in patients with copious secretions or emesis or in situations such as bleeding after tonsillectomy. The Khan blade has a 1.75-mm-ID tube welded to a straight blade with a proximal hub angled so that the laryngoscopist's thumb can occlude a port to control the amount of suction applied.[108] Tull suction blades, available in Miller and Macintosh versions, have a finger-controlled valve lying next to the laryngoscope handle to enable the laryngoscopist to apply suction at will.[46]

3. Blade with a Secondary Ultraviolet Light Source

In 2009, Intubrite introduced a new concept in laryngoscope blade illumination that combined a white LED light with a second ultraviolet (UV) or black light.[110] The UV light is a higher frequency (wavelength) than white light that lies in the invisible part of the electromagnetic spectrum. It overpowers the lower end of the white light spectrum, where reds and yellows cause a whitewash effect. According to Intubrite, the UV light reduces the scatter from standard white light and improves visualization of the airway. The ligamentous vocal cords contain high levels of phosphorus that, when struck by the black light (UV), phosphoresce (Fig. 24-58). The company claims that by varying the wavelength of UV light and adding a spectrally specific white LED light, this illumination system better outlines the texture and structure of the airway and diminishes the reflectivity from fluids within the passage.

The Intubrite blade requires 4.5 volts and is designed for use with unique, high-powered, ergonomic handles that have a conventional handle-blade connection. Intubrite blades cannot be used on the standard handles of conventional laryngoscopes because of their power

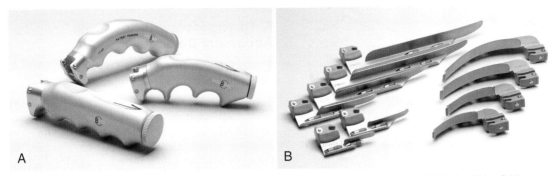

Figure 24-58 Intubrite handles **(A)** and laryngoscope blades **(B)**. (Courtesy of Intubrite, Vista, CA.)

requirements; traditional handles using 2 C batteries generate only 3.0 volts.

Intubrite blades come in sizes from neonatal to large adult, and they are offered in Macintosh and Miller designs. Blades are offered in single-use and reposable (i.e., limited multi-use) versions; the latter can be resterilized 20 times using a low-temperature sterilization process (e.g., Sterrad). No clinical studies have been published comparing the performance of these blades with that of standard illumination blades.

4. Ultra-lightweight Tactical Laryngoscope

The TruLite (Truphatek International Ltd., Netanya, Israel) is a single patient–use laryngoscope, which combines a low-profile Macintosh or Miller metal blade hinged to a small plastic handle (Fig. 24-59).[111] With two AA batteries, the laryngoscope blade and handle weighs only 120 g. The LED light provides a bright white light. The preconfigured and attached metal blade, extreme light weight, and small overall size and packaging make it ideal for tactical settings and use in aircraft medical operations. It is offered in three Miller sizes (1 to 3) and

four Macintosh sizes (1 to 4), all of which have small, narrow flange heights.

V. RIGID INDIRECT LARYNGOSCOPES WITH OPTICALLY ASSISTED VIEWS

Rigid indirect laryngoscopes enable a view of the laryngeal inlet indirectly through a fiberoptic bundle, video camera, or other optical aid. Examples of optically aided laryngoscopes include the Siker blade with its built-in mirror, blades using attachable prisms (e.g., Huffman, Belscope), and the Viewmax and EVO2 blades, which have integrated optical rods. Other indirect rigid laryngoscopes deliver an image endoscopically through a fiberoptic bundle or using video technology. The ensuing discussion is limited to mirrored blades and those that use prisms or optical rods. Fiberoptic instruments and video laryngoscopes are covered in Chapters 19 and 25, respectively.

A. Siker Laryngoscope

In 1956, Siker described an angled laryngoscope with an incorporated reflecting surface. The portion of the blade distal to the mirror is angulated at 135 degrees from the proximal section (Fig. 24-60). The stainless steel mirror is attached to the blade by means of a copper jacket to facilitate conduction of heat from the patient, thereby minimizing fogging of the mirror.[112] After blade insertion, if the laryngeal inlet cannot be directly visualized, the mirror can be used to indirectly identify the epiglottis and then the cords. Facility with the use of this blade takes some experience because the mirror inverts the reflected image. A styleted tube is essential; as the tube enters the larynx, it appears to move in a posteroinferior direction. In his original publication, Siker described the blade's use in 100 unselected patients. Laryngoscopy failed in just one patient because of excessive blade length. In three other patients with failed laryngoscopy and intubation with standard blades, the Siker succeeded. He emphasized the need for practice in the use of the blade.[112]

B. McMorrow-Mirakhur Mirrored Laryngoscope

McMorrow and Mirakhur described a modification of the levering tip laryngoscope that incorporates an adjustable

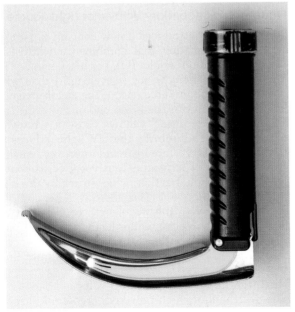

Figure 24-59 The Trulite (Truphatek International, Ltd., Netanya, Israel) is a disposable laryngoscope that combines handle and blade.

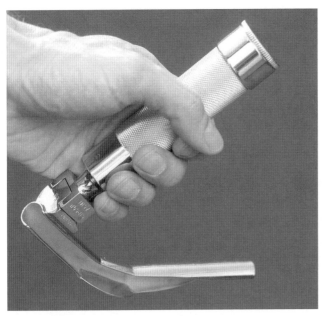

Figure 24-60 The Siker blade has a reflecting mirror located inferiorly at midblade.

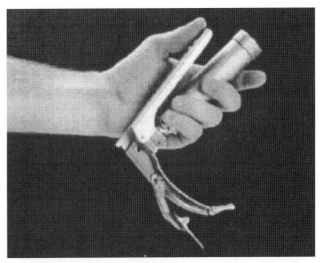

Figure 24-62 The McMorrow-Mirakhur laryngoscope is in the half-deployed position. The levering tip is activated, and the mirror is ignored. (From McMorrow RCN, Mirakhur RK: A new mirrored laryngoscope. *Anaesthesia* 58:998–1002, 2003.)

mirror.[113] Looking like a regular CLM (McCoy) laryngoscope in the resting position (Fig. 24-61), the McMorrow-Mirakhur laryngoscope can be operated as both a regular Macintosh blade or levering tip blade, as previously described. The difference is that it has a mirror lying posteriorly on the blade. As the levering tip is activated by moving the control lever toward the laryngoscope handle (Fig. 24-62), the mirror is deployed posteriorly and inferiorly with respect to the blade. If necessary, further depression of the control lever toward the handle changes the mirror pitch to a usable angle (Fig. 24-63), ultimately providing an additional 60-degree field of view compared with the Macintosh alone. If intubation is performed between the blade and the mirror, the scope has

to be removed in its activated state. The blade should be heated or the mirror defogged before each use.

McMorrow and Mirakhur tested the laryngoscope in 15 patients presenting for elective surgery and compared it with the Macintosh and McCoy blades. Manual in-line neck stabilization was used to create difficult conditions for laryngoscopy, and all patients had Cormack-Lehane grade 3 views with the Macintosh blade. Using the McMorrow-Mirakhur blade with mirror deployment, the view was improved from grade 3 to grade 1 in 50% of patients and to grade 2 in 21%. The view was considered worse in 7%, and no change was seen in 21% of patients.[113]

C. Huffman Prism

Although a prism had been described by Janeway in 1913, Huffman revisited the concept in 1968. He attached

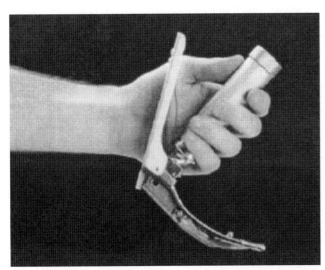

Figure 24-61 The McMorrow-Mirakhur laryngoscope in the resting position. (From McMorrow RCN, Mirakhur RK: A new mirrored laryngoscope. *Anaesthesia* 58:998–1002, 2003.)

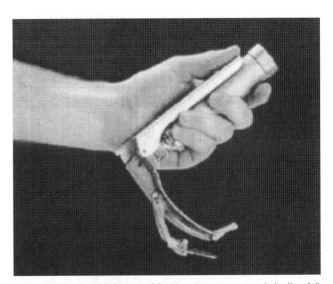

Figure 24-63 The McMorrow-Mirakhur laryngoscope is in the fully deployed position, with the distal mirror providing an additional 60 degrees of visual field. (From McMorrow RCN, Mirakhur RK: A new mirrored laryngoscope. *Anaesthesia* 58:998–1002, 2003.)

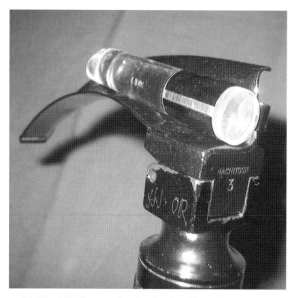

Figure 24-64 A Huffman prism is attached to a Macintosh 3 blade.

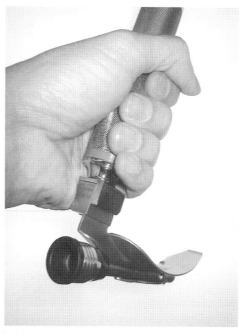

Figure 24-65 The lens system of the Rüsch Viewmax blade refracts the distal image by 20 degrees. (Courtesy of Rüsch, Duluth, GA.)

a Plexiglas prism to a Macintosh 3 blade by means of a steel clip. Because the image of the cords is deflected by approximately 30 degrees, Huffman theorized that less force on the tongue and hypopharynx would be needed to achieve laryngeal inlet visualization (Fig. 24-64).[114] Subsequently, he affixed a second prism distal to the first to achieve a total refraction of 80 degrees. He used the resulting instrument to inspect the larynx at light planes of anesthesia, but he speculated that it would be a useful tool for difficult laryngoscopy.[115] Huffman prisms continue to be available in various sizes for Macintosh blades.

D. Rüsch Viewmax Laryngoscope

1. Description

The Viewmax (Rüsch, Duluth, GA) laryngoscope blade is similar in shape to a Macintosh, but it incorporates a removable lens system (i.e., Viewscope) ending in a proximal eyepiece, which can refract the distal image 20 degrees from the horizontal (Fig. 24-65). This has the potential to improve laryngeal inlet visualization compared with that obtained by direct vision. The blade of the Viewmax is wider than that of a standard Macintosh,

and although the lens system provides some vertical component, the blade otherwise has little formal vertical step. With the resultant lessened ability to sweep the tongue to the left, the blade can be used midline in the patient's mouth. The Viewmax is available in an adult and a pediatric size, corresponding to Macintosh size 3½ and 2 blades, respectively. (The name *Viewmax* is also applied to another company's [Timesco, London, England] version of the improved-view Macintosh blade.) The Viewmax has received limited investigation in manikins and cadavers with mixed results compared to a standard Macintosh blade.[116-118]

2. Truview EVO2

The Truview EVO2 uses an optical rod similar to the Viewmax, but it has an angulated shape (Fig. 24-66). The EVO2 is made by Truphatek International, which also manufactures the Viewmax, a product distributed by Rüsch. The EVO2 has a 42-degree refraction angle to its

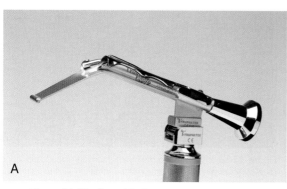

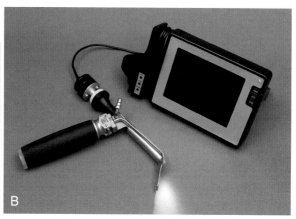

Figure 24-66 A and **B,** Truview EVO2 laryngoscope. (Courtesy of Truphatek International, Ltd., Netanya, Israel.)

optical system. Instead of a gently curved shape like the Viewmax, the EVO2 is an angulated blade; the proximal two thirds of the blade are straight, although it has a wide spatula, and the last third of the blade has a steep upward angle and a flat tip like a standard Macintosh blade. The optical lens system runs straight along the proximal two thirds of the blade.

A distinguishing feature of the EVO2 is an integrated oxygen port that allows delivery of up to 10 L/min of flow during laryngoscopy. The EVO2 is powered by a rechargeable fiber-lit handle (C or A battery sizes), and illumination is provided by a round, glass-fiber bundle. It comes in five sizes, from premature infant (0) to large adult (4). A 32-mm endoscopic coupler can be attached to the eyepiece, transforming the blade into a video laryngoscope system. The company offers a camera and monitor with the EVO2 (Truphatek PCD).

3. Clinical Experience

In pediatric and adult patients, the EVO2 has provided much improved laryngeal views compared with the standard Macintosh and Miller blades, although some studies have found slightly longer intubation times.[119-125] In adult patients with anticipated difficult laryngoscopy, the EVO2 has significantly improved the laryngeal view. In a small case series of cervical spine patients intubated while in a cervical collar, the EVO2 provided full glottic visualization, whereas the standard Macintosh blade provided very poor or nonexistent views.[120]

VI. CONCLUSIONS

Direct laryngoscopy for intubation confers the advantages of simplicity, direct glottic visualization, cost-effectiveness, equipment availability, and an overall success rate that is matched by few procedures in medicine. Although there is dramatically increased use of video laryngoscopes for many valid reasons, direct laryngoscopy is faster, and it is the most common means of rescuing failed video laryngoscopy. Direct laryngoscopy remains especially appropriate in emergency situations in which video or other imaging can be compromised by blood, vomitus, and secretions and in critical care scenarios in which there are very brief or nonexistent safe-apnea times. Clinicians should have redundant methods of intubation and ventilation immediately available to minimize the risk of failed intubation and to ensure patient safety.

VII. CLINICAL PEARLS

- Laryngoscope blades are not identical, and even within same designs (e.g., Macintosh and Miller), there is considerable variation among manufacturers. Depending on blade design, light source, battery type, and battery charge status, there can be a 500-fold difference in illuminance among blades in different clinical settings.

- With curved-blade laryngoscopes, design variables that are important to consider include the height of the proximal flange and the distance from the light source to the tip of the blade. Typically, a small flange is

advantageous, and a shorter light-to-tip distance creates more light at the target.

- Low-profile Macintosh 4 blades (German or English designs) can be used in all adults, by varying the depth of insertion. When using a blade with more length than may be needed, the practitioner should identify the epiglottis on insertion and avoid passing by this critical landmark. Starting with a longer blade eliminates the need for switching out to a larger blade in emergency situations. A smaller flange permits insertion even in small-mouthed persons.

- Whiter, brighter light is provided by LED and fiber-illuminated systems than with traditional bulb-on-blade devices. Battery status and battery type are important to ensure good light output. Lithium, nickel-hydride, and other battery types have better discharge profiles (i.e., more uniform output) for high-drain devices such as laryngoscopes than alkaline batteries, which have long run times but very diminished output over time.

- Fiber-lit laryngoscopes have light sources in the handle and use glass or acrylic rods to transmit light from the base to the tip of the blade. Conventional blades have an electrical connection at the top of the handle and base of the blade. There is wide variation in bulb types, and LED, xenon, and halogen bulbs are available in both systems.

- LED bulbs have several major advantages over other bulb types. They produce a very white light that may improve discrimination of the epiglottis edge against the mucosa of the hypopharynx, and they use markedly less energy than filament bulbs. They have become so inexpensive that many companies offer disposable conventional blades with an LED bulb on the blade.

- Considerations in straight-blade design include the flange height, spatula shape, and location of the light source. A light source on the left flange may embed in tissue and provide poor illumination. Large-flange and large-spatula designs provide easier tube delivery but have to displace more tissue to get to the larynx. The shape of the distal tip (e.g., slightly upturned distal tip of the Miller design) affects how the blade is advanced to lift the epiglottis directly.

SELECTED REFERENCES

All references can be found online at expertconsult.com.

5. Burkle CM, Zepeda FA, Bacon DR, Rose SH: A historical perspective on use of the laryngoscope as a tool in anesthesiology. *Anesthesiology* 100:1003–1006, 2004.

6. Cooper RM: Laryngoscopy—Its past and future. *Can J Anaesth* 51: R1–R5, 2004.

7. Zeitels SM: Universal modular glottiscope system: The evolution of a century of design and technique for direct laryngoscopy. *Ann Otol Rhinol Laryngol Suppl* 179:2–24, 1999.

18. Macintosh RR: A new laryngoscope. *Lancet* 1:205, 1943.

37. Levitan RM: *The airway cam guide to intubation and practical emergency airway management.* Wayne, PA, 2004, Airway Cam Technologies.

38. Jackson C: *Bronchoscopy and esophagoscopy: A manual of peroral endoscopy and laryngeal surgery.* Philadelphia, 1922, WB Saunders.

Chapter 25

Video Laryngoscopes

EROL CAVUS | VOLKER DÖRGES

I. INTRODUCTION

Although the use of video laryngoscopy for teaching the routine laryngoscopic technique of endotracheal intubation and for managing a difficult airway have been known for some years, anesthesiologists have been slow to recognize these advantages. Video-assisted techniques have been successfully used for decades in many surgical disciplines and have largely replaced open approaches in areas such as arthroscopy and laparoscopy (Box 25-1). The magnified and detailed view of the surgical site on a monitor makes it easier to coordinate the work of the surgical team and provides an effective teaching tool for novices. Anesthesiologists have observed this

development with interest but without realizing its potential for their own specialty. For years, anesthesiologists have applied video technology almost exclusively for imaging in bronchoscopy and fiberoptic intubation, but the past decade has witnessed some important innovations in the field of video-assisted airway management.

In 1996, Levitan introduced a video camera attached to a head ring (Airway Cam). With this technique, intubation performed with a standard laryngoscope is displayed on a video monitor so that it can be observed by other personnel in the room. The view of the glottis matches the visual field of the intubating physician and does not improve visualization of the glottic plane.

Airway pathology, difficult airway (e.g., trauma, tumor,
   previous surgery)
Immobilization of the cervical spine
Limited spatial conditions
Education, teaching
Documentation

Another principle forms the basis for development of
modern video laryngoscopes (VLs). By integrating optical
image guides and video cameras into standard laryngoscopes, a magnified and detailed view can be displayed
on an external monitor while conventional direct
laryngoscopy is performed. Various investigators made an
effort to advance this principle and integrated rigid or
flexible fiberoptics into laryngoscopes with different
shapes, such as the WuScope,[1] Bullard,[2] and Upsher-
Scope.[3] Henthorn and coworkers reported the combination of a flexible fiberoptic cable with a conventional
Miller laryngoscope blade,[4] which they used for student
education. Instructors and trainees found this forerunner
of modern VLs to be helpful in identifying the anatomy
of the upper airways and successfully performing the
intubation.

In 2001, Weiss and associates described a Macintosh
laryngoscope, the angulated video-intubation laryngoscope (AVIL), in which a thin fiberoptic cable can be
advanced through a guide channel in the laryngoscope
handle and blade to a point very close to the blade tip.[5]
Adapters can be used to connect the fiberoptic cable to
an external video unit, enabling a close-up view of the
larynx to be displayed on an external monitor. Another
option is to introduce the video scope into the endotracheal tube (ETT). However, there have been no other
publications on this device from other users, and it apparently has not found wide application.

The X-Lite (Rüsch, Duluth, GA) was introduced in
2001 in Vienna. This commercially available VL has an
image guide built into the blade and a video camera
installed in the handle. It was the first design to offer
interchangeable blade shapes and sizes that could be connected to the camera handle. Two fairly bulky and heavy
cables (i.e., light and image guides) emerge from the end
of the handle. These characteristics made the device more
cumbersome than a conventional laryngoscope, made the
device less rugged and more susceptible to technical
flaws, and hampered cleaning and disinfection.

In 2004, Kaplan and Berci introduced a further
improvement of a Macintosh VL, a direct coupled interface VL (DCI, Karl Storz, Tuttlingen, Germany), also
known as the VMS or V-MAC.[6] The DCI has an integrated camera and connectable blades equipped with a
fiberoptic light and image guide, and the handle and
blade are combined in a fixed unit.

Miniaturization of camera chip technology; improved,
rechargeable battery power and light output; and afford-
able, small liquid crystal display (LCD) monitors made
video laryngoscopy a booming technology, which led to
the introduction of different types of VLs. Because VLs
have different shapes, technical equipment, and applications, further classification of these devices is justified.[7]
The main difference in VLs arises from the type of blade
that is incorporated into the system. VLs that are based
on a conventional, established blade shape, such as the
Macintosh blade, have the option of visualizing the glottic
entrance by direct laryngoscopy. Users are familiar with
the handling of this blade type. Other VLs are designed
with highly curved or angled blades that pass around the
tongue and allow a "look around the corner" to the glottic
opening. These VLs allow the best visualization of the
glottis, although a direct view of the glottic entrance
usually is impossible (i.e., obligatory indirect visualization). Because of the high degree of blade angulation,
they must be used with a malleable or rigid styletted tube
in most cases.

A subcategory of obligatory indirect laryngoscopes has
a tube-guiding channel incorporated in the curved blade.
This design obviates the use of a tube stylet to guide the
tube to the glottic entrance, but it also does not allow
correction of the direction of the tube.

For hygienic purposes, all VL systems are available in
disposable forms. Compared with the reusable, stainless
steel designs that allow lower blade profiles, the disposable versions mainly use a plastic blade sheath, which
causes slightly larger blade profiles.

VL systems are available with an external or internal
monitor. The larger external monitor allows better orientation for the laryngoscopist and operating staff, who may
actively help with the intubation process (e.g., extralaryngeal maneuvers, suction). In systems with integrated
monitors, visual orientation is more difficult on the
smaller monitors. Others cannot easily follow the intubation process on the small monitor; this limitation may be
aggravated by adverse space or light conditions. Picture
or video documentation that can be obtained with external monitors usually is not available with the compact
design of the smaller monitor. The greatest advantages of
the systems with integrated monitors are their unrestricted mobility and minimal light and space requirements, which make them valuable for use in the
prehospital setting. Because all these devices are battery
operated, attention should be paid to the battery capacity
to prevent a system blackout during intubation.

II. VIDEO LARYNGOSCOPES USING MACINTOSH-BASED BLADES

A. A.P. Advance

1. Description

The A.P. Advance (Venner Medical, Kiel, Germany) is a
mobile VL that consists of a battery-containing handle, a
blade core, and a 3.5-inch LCD monitor that connects to
the handle magnetically. The size of the integrated
monitor is bigger than in competitive VLs; using National
Television System Committee (NTSC) video output, the
monitor signal can be exported to an external screen. The
monitor has an integrated, rechargeable battery, which
provides the monitor screen and handle with power. The
light source of the blade receives power from a battery

integrated in the handle, and the handle and blade may be used without a monitor attached (i.e., conventional direct laryngoscopy).

2. Instrument Use

The blade core can be used with three types of disposable blade sheaths. Two blades are adapted to the classic Macintosh shape (sizes 3 and 4), and one, the difficult airway blade (DAB), has been developed for use in the difficult airway. The DAB has a specific distal angulation and houses a tube-guiding channel in the distal one third of the blade, providing an obligatory indirect glottic view. For blade types with a guiding channel, the epiglottis should be lifted directly by the blade tip of the DAB, similar to the straight blade technique employed with a Miller blade.

3. Clinical Experience

No clinical experience has been published for the A.P. Advance, but in two mannequin studies, medical professionals used it in normal and difficult airway scenarios and reported good visualization and intubation success.[8,9] In another mannequin study, paramedics who had not previously used video laryngoscopy achieved earlier intubation and fewer unplanned advances of the tube compared with use of the GlideScope Ranger.[10]

B. Direct Coupled Interface (DCI) Video Laryngoscope System

1. Description

The DCI video laryngoscope was designed using a modified Macintosh blade with the same curvature as the original 1943 version and a laryngoscope handle. The batteries in the handle are replaced with a small video camera (i.e., DCI camera) and a combined image-light bundle that inserts into the Macintosh blade.[6] The DCI video laryngoscope system allows interchange of different devices, such as laryngoscopes (e.g., Macintosh, Dörges, Miller, D-Blade) and rigid (e.g., Bonfils intubation endoscope) and flexible fiberscopes (Fig. 25-1); however, mobility of the fiberoptic-based system is limited. The DCI system has been displaced by the mobile C-MAC video intubation system.

2. Instrument Use

Component of the DCI video laryngoscope system are assembled, and an antifog solution is applied to the tip of the image-light bundle. If a regular Macintosh blade is used, conventional direct laryngoscopy may be performed. On insertion of the scope into the patient's mouth, the image can be viewed on the video monitor. Even if the familiar Macintosh blade technique is used with this device, the distal viewing bundle may necessitate less anterior lift on the blade and may permit a view of part or all of the glottic opening in otherwise difficult laryngoscopies.

3. Clinical Experience

Kaplan and associates reported a series of 235 patients in whom they used the DCI video laryngoscope system.[6] Of these cases, 217 were predicted to be straightforward, and

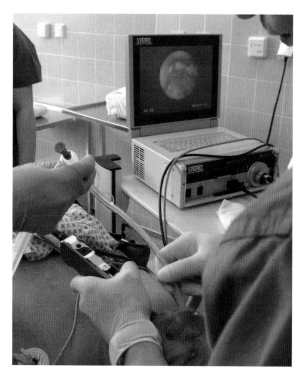

Figure 25-1 The DCI video laryngoscope system.

in all but one, the DCI video laryngoscope system was successfully used, with 10% requiring external laryngeal manipulation. A second group of 18 patients had anatomic predictors of difficult laryngoscopy; all in this group required external laryngeal manipulation but were successfully intubated with the DCI video laryngoscope system. In another study, Kaplan and colleagues compared the view obtained using DCI by direct vision with that obtained on the monitor and found that the image on the monitor was the same as or better than the direct line-of-sight view in most patients undergoing routine anesthesia.[11] Hagberg and colleagues describe the successful use in a patient who previously had an unexpected difficult laryngoscopy and impossible intubation and who was subsequently intubated with the DCI system after the first attempt.[12]

C. C-MAC Video Laryngoscope System

1. Description

The C-MAC (Karl Storz, Tuttlingen, Germany) video laryngoscope system is a modification of the Storz DCI system. The C-MAC VL can provide a useful alternative during routine induction of general anesthesia and in securing a difficult airway. The C-MAC is based on a modified Macintosh blade that has the same curvature as the original 1943 version,[13] but it is different from the original Macintosh blade in its thinner profile (maximum of 14 mm) and its beveled shoulder, which reduces the risk of oral and dental injury and facilitates insertion in patients with limited mouth opening. Optionally, the blade may be equipped with a guide channel for introducing a suction catheter to help maintain a clear visual field during laryngoscopy. The C-MAC system is compatible with various blades. The electronic module

(E-module) fits into the blade handle and allows a rapid exchange of Macintosh stainless steel blade sizes 2, 3, and 4, Miller sizes 0 and 1, and the D-Blade. A clip-on camera (C-CAM) can link the C-MAC system with rigid or flexible fiberoptics. The combined optical system of the C-MAC consists of a complementary metal-oxide semiconductor (CMOS) chip set (320 × 240 pixels), an optical lens with an aperture angle of 80 degrees, and a high-power, light-emitting diode (LED) at the distal third of the blade with effective antifogging properties. The blade handle with the E-module and the external, 7-inch LCD color monitor have push buttons that allow the operator to capture images from the screen and record video sequences, which are storable on standard SD memory cards, which have a 2-GB capacity. In the rare case that visualization of the glottic opening is still difficult, the D-Blade may be attached to the system within seconds. The higher curvature of the D-Blade allows a better look around the corner, and the low blade profile may permit use even in patients with limited mouth opening (e.g., 15 mm); however, direct laryngoscopy is not possible in most cases.

Other parts of the C-MAC system include the C-MAC pocket monitor (PM), which is a 2.4-inch LCD monitor combined with a lithium-ion battery–equipped E-module that fits in all available blades of the C-MAC system (e.g., Miller 0 and 1, Macintosh 2-4, D-Blade). The rechargeable battery supplies the monitor and the LED light source of the blades with 1 hour of energy without recharging, so that the VL is fully portable and can be used wireless. Power is turned on by a magnetic switch when lifting the monitor. Because this system is designed for mobile use, there are no other switches or connections for picture or video recording and exportation. To save battery capacity, the monitor turns off after 10 minutes automatically.

2. Instrument Use

For portable use, the monitor and blade handles can be packed separately in a rugged carrying bag, which permits use of all monitor buttons through the bag, even under difficult ambient conditions (e.g., prehospital settings). The C-MAC PM uses the identical blades, and the laryngoscopic technique is the same as with the conventional C-MAC system. However, successful handling of the device with the small monitor needs to be tested in clinical trials.

3. Clinical Experience

Several investigators showed superior visualization of the glottis with the C-MAC compared with conventional direct laryngoscopy.[14-17] Even if the application of a stylet cannot be eliminated completely, most intubations using a C-MAC VL can be performed without stylet use.[18,19] In a preliminary study by Cavus and associates of patients in whom conventional Macintosh laryngoscopy failed, use of the C-MAC D-Blade provided better glottic visualization and intubation success in all patients.[20] An observational study of 80 patients with the need for out-of-hospital emergency intubation (e.g. trauma, cardiopulmonary resuscitation) performed by physicians showed good handling and intubation success with the C-MAC

VL. In a few cases, video laryngoscopic intubation was impossible due to VL problems such as bright surrounding light, and only direct laryngoscopy with the same device resulted in fast, successful intubation.[17]

D. McGrath MAC Video Laryngoscope

1. Description

The McGrath MAC (Aircraft Medical, Edinburgh, United Kingdom) is a slim-profile, mobile VL that consists of a battery-containing handle, a steel blade core (CameraStick), and a 2.5-inch LCD monitor fixed to the handle. The proprietary lithium-ion battery pack provides approximately 250 minutes of power. The McGrath MAC is fully immersible for high-level disinfection. As in the McGrath Series 5 VL, there is no connection port to transfer the image to an external monitor.

2. Instrument Use

The McGrath MAC may be used with disposable Macintosh blades (sizes 3 and 4); there are no blades with higher angulation (as in the McGrath Series 5 VL) available for this VL. Because of the Macintosh blade shape, direct and indirect laryngoscopy can be performed.

3. Clinical Experience

The McGrath MAC has been used for double-lumen tube insertion and compared with conventional direct laryngoscopy. Glottic visualization and ease of double-lumen tube intubation were improved using the McGrath VL.[21]

E. GlideScope Direct

1. Description

The GlideScope Direct (Verathon Medical, Bothell, WA) is a stainless steel Macintosh blade that adds to the existing GlideScope system (see "Video Laryngoscopes Using Highly Curved Blades"). The purpose of this blade is to expand the system with the option to teach conventional laryngoscopy because the GlideScope Direct allows direct and indirect (video laryngoscopic) glottic visualization.

2. Instrument Use

The GlideScope Direct is primarily designed as an intubation trainer, but may also be used for clinical use. Due to the Macintosh shape, the GlideScope Direct provides both direct and indirect laryngoscopic view. It is available as a reusable and single-use device. In cases that need a more highly curved blade (e.g., GlideScope AVL, GVL), the whole blade including the cable has to be changed.

3. Clinical Experience

No clinical experiences have been published.

F. Truview Picture Capture Device

1. Description

The Truview picture capture device (PCD) VL (Truphatek International Limited, Netanya, Israel) has an integrated optical lens (optical view tube), a unique 42-degree blade tip angulation, and a view through a 15-mm eyepiece. The LED light source is stored in the handle, and the light is transmitted to the blade tip by fiberoptic strands. It is available in five blades sizes, and all of them allow direct laryngoscopy.

The blades are equipped with an integrated oxygen jet cleaning and insufflation system, which can connect to an external oxygen flow meter and provide oxygen at a rate of 4 to 6 L/min. The video properties of the optical Truview blade can be achieved by magnetic connection of the eyepiece to the camera of the Truview PCD screen.

2. Instrument Use

The Truview may be used like a conventional laryngoscope. Additional defogging maneuvers should be performed. The blade has an integrated channel that may allow apneic oxygenation of the patient during laryngoscopy.

3. Clinical Experience

The glottic view may be improved by use of the Truview compared with conventional laryngoscopy with a Macintosh blade, and this may result in a higher intubation success rate in difficult-to-manage airways.[22-25] Compared with conventional laryngoscopy with a Macintosh laryngoscope, intubation with the Truview may take more time, but intubation success rates may be comparable; however, rates of airway morbidity related to laryngoscopy may be lower.[23] In a study by Carlino and colleagues using the Truview as a teaching tool for anesthesiology residents, intubation success after the first attempt was almost doubled compared with that for conventional Macintosh laryngoscopy.[26] In patients with cervical spine immobilization, Malik and colleagues experienced inferior visualization and intubation compared with other VLs. The handling may be cumbersome, and fogging may impair visualization process.[22]

III. VIDEO LARYNGOSCOPES USING HIGHLY CURVED BLADES

Alignment of the oropharyngolaryngeal axis is not necessary using highly curved blades. With a look around the corner, optimal visualization of the glottis can be achieved without further manipulation (e.g., flexion or extension of the cervical spine). This may be important in patients with cervical immobilization, severe micrognathia, a fixed temporomandibular joint, or limited regional access.

High curvature of the blade typically makes it impossible to perform direct laryngoscopy; tracheal intubation requires indirect visualization. To follow the high curvature of the blade with an ETT, a tube guide or malleable stylet is necessary.[18,19] Although there is a tendency to focus on the video monitor, it is important to directly visualize the tube going into the mouth and advancing beyond the tongue before it becomes visible on the monitor. Perforations of the pharynx and hypopharynx have occurred with the GlideScope and the McGrath when operators have blindly inserted stylleted tubes while focusing only on the video monitor.[27,28] Highly curved, indirect VLs can be used with almost no forces applied to tongue and pharyngeal structures,

and these devices can be used in awake video laryngoscopic intubation as an alternative to awake fiberoptic intubation, assuming that attention is paid to possible contraindications for video laryngoscopy (e.g., mouth opening <15 mm, subglottic stenosis, tumor masses). Several case reports describe safe application of this technique.[29-35]

A. GlideScope

1. Description

The GlideScope is the prototype of modern, obligate indirect video laryngoscopes that display an image of the laryngeal inlet on an accompanying monitor. Made of medical-grade plastic, the laryngoscope is available in different sizes for fitting small children to morbidly obese patients. A high-power LED and miniature CMOS video camera are embedded posteriorly midway along the blade, resulting in a vertical profile up to 16 mm. Angulation of 60 degrees at midblade permits laryngeal inlet visualization with little tissue manipulation. An antifogging mechanism effectively maintains the view. The video image is transmitted to a 7-inch LCD monitor through a video cable; an integrated USB port allows recording of captured images and videos. A disposable version is available (GlideScope Cobalt AVL), which combines a nonsterile, reusable video baton and a sterile, single-use blade sheath. The monitor can be affixed to a mobile stand or be stored in a portable case. The GlideScope Ranger has been developed especially for mobile use in emergency situations (e.g., out of the hospital). The blade shape has been adapted to fit in the monitor box, and the size of the monitor screen has been reduced. A Macintosh-based steel blade (GlideScope Direct) has been added as an intubation trainer for educational purpose (see "Video Laryngoscopes Using Macintosh-Based Blades").

2. Instrument Use

Preparation for use of the GlideScope is limited to ensuring that the power is connected and turned on. After the instrument has been on for a few minutes, no additional defogging maneuver is needed. A stylleted ETT is needed with distal curvature of 60 to 90 degrees to aid access to the glottic opening (i.e., "hockey-stick" formation). The blade is inserted as done with a Macintosh blade, although in this indirect technique, the blade tip does not need to be advanced to the vallecula, and a lift does not need to be performed to the same extent as with a conventional Macintosh blade. When the best view of the glottis is achieved on the video monitor with or without external laryngeal manipulation, the ETT is advanced alongside and posterior to the blade. Because advancement of the styletted tube cannot directly be observed due to the blade curvature, caution is needed during advancement of the tube to avoid injury of pharyngeal structures.[27,36-38] Intubation can be achieved by positioning the ETT at the glottic opening and then advancing it off the stylet through the cords. If tube passage is difficult, relaxation of any upward tongue lift should be attempted; alternatively, backing away slightly from the laryngeal inlet with the scope may help. Good visualization of the process should be available throughout on the monitor.

3. Clinical Experience

The GlideScope is the prototype of modern obligate indirect VLs. Since its introduction in 2001, it has been studied in the operating room,[39-43] used in normal and difficult intubation scenarios,[38,44-49] and compared with other VLs.[16,18,22,50-55] In most patients, use of the Glide-Scope resulted in improved glottic visualization according to the Cormack-Lehane classification,[56] and it has provided successful intubation of difficult airways.[48,57] Aziz and colleagues analyzed 2004 GlideScope intubations and reported an overall intubation success rate of 97%. However, 3% could not be intubated with the GlideScope, and the investigators concluded that maintenance of competency with alternative methods of intubation was mandatory.[38] Intubation difficulties have changed from impaired visualization to difficult tube advancement. Despite optimal glottic visualization, the most difficult part of indirect video laryngoscopy is placing the curved tube in the glottic entrance and advancing it into the trachea.[58]

Use of the portable GlideScope Ranger has been studied predominantly in out-of-hospital settings and in emergency departments.[59-62] GlideScope Ranger use in an emergency setting improved glottic visualization and reduced the number of intubation attempts compared with conventional laryngoscopy.[57,63] However, Choi and colleagues reported some cases of unsuccessful intubation despite excellent visualization, which highlights the need for training on the device outside of emergency situations.[64]

B. McGrath Series 5

1. Description

One of the first fully portable and wireless devices with higher blade angulation and an integrated monitor is the McGrath Series 5 VL (Aircraft Medical Edinburgh, UK). It combines a steel blade with a length that may be adjusted according to the patient's body size and a single-size, disposable blade sheath. The low-profile blade has a disarticulating handle that can accommodate patients with limited mouth opening and severely limited neck mobility. There is no connection port for transferring the image to an external monitor. Two versions of the VL are available: a basic version with limited water protection and an improved version that is submersible in liquids, which may be essential for cleaning and disinfection purposes and for use in prehospital emergencies.

2. Instrument Use

The length of the blade can be adjusted before insertion into the patient's mouth. The McGrath Series 5 VL has three sizes, comparable in length to size 3, 4, and 5 Macintosh blades. After the instrument's power has been turned on for a few minutes, no additional defogging maneuver is needed. Similar to the GlideScope, a highly angulated, styletted ETT is needed to aid access to the glottic opening. Blade insertion is the same as for a Macintosh blade, although in this indirect technique, the

blade tip does not need to be advanced to the vallecula, and a lift need not be performed to the same extent as with the Macintosh blade.

3. Clinical Experience

Most clinical data show improved visualization and intubation success compared with conventional laryngoscopy with the Macintosh and Henderson straight blades.[65-68] Similar to the GlideScope, advancement of the styletted tube cannot directly be observed because of the blade's shape, and caution is needed during advancement of the tube to avoid injuries.[28]

C. A.P. Advance Difficult Airway Blade and the C-MAC D-Blade

The curved blades for use in difficult airways, the A.P. Advance DAB and C-MAC D-Blade, are additional components of the corresponding Macintosh-based video laryngoscopy systems.

IV. VIDEO LARYNGOSCOPES WITH TUBE-GUIDING CHANNELS

Some video laryngoscopes with high blade curvatures have integrated tube-guiding channels to improve tube passage without the use of a tube stylet. The VL and tube are directed together to the glottic entrance. Because of the surrounding channel, the tube cuff is reasonably protected from damage.

A. King Vision

1. Description

The King Vision (King Systems, Noblesville, IN) is a fully portable and wireless VL with high blade angulation. It has a reusable-battery–operated monitor and a disposable blade that also includes a CMOS video camera. The disposable blade is available with or without a tube-guiding channel, and one blade size is provided for adult use (tube sizes 6.0 to 8.0 mm). The King Vision's video output allows bystanders to view the images on an external medical monitor.

2. Instrument Use

The tube should be preloaded in the tube-guiding channel before insertion of the laryngoscope into the patient's mouth. The VL should be advanced toward the glottis, so that it barely lifts the epiglottis with the blade tip. With the channeled blade, better intubation conditions may be achieved if the VL is placed into the vallecula without uploading the epiglottis directly. When the glottic entrance is in the center of the screen, the tube can be advanced into the trachea under direct observation on the video screen. Because the monitor is attached to the blade without articulation, it may be necessary in obese or busty patients to connect the monitor first after introduction of the blade.

3. Clinical Experience

Clinical data for the use of the King Vision VL have not been published.

B. Pentax Airway Scope AWS-S100

1. Description

The Pentax Airway Scope (AWS-S100, Pentax Medical, distributed by AMBU, Inc., Glen Burnie, MD) is a fully portable, battery-operated, and wireless VL that is available in one size only. The AWS-S100 has a portable, transparent blade (PBlade) equipped with a port through which a suction catheter can be passed. It uses an LED light and flexible wire for a charge-coupled device (CCD) camera, rather than the CMOS camera chip used in other VLs.

2. Instrument Use

The AWS is the prototype of modern VLs that provide a blade-integrated channel for guiding a tube to the larynx. The standard technique for using the Pentax AWS involves direct elevation of the epiglottis for exposure of the vocal cords; however, it may also be used without elevating the epiglottis. A target symbol on the monitor assists in directing the tube to the glottic entrance. The AWS video output (NTSC composite) allows bystanders to view the images on an external medical monitor. According to the manufacturer, antifogging substances should be applied to the camera before use of the VL.

3. Clinical Experience

Because of the high angulation of the blade, the AWS has shown superior glottic visualization and intubation success compared with conventional laryngoscopy in patients with immobilization of the cervical spine.[22,69] In contrast, in a study of morbidly obese patients, Abdallah and colleagues showed faster intubation and higher first-pass success rates with a conventional Macintosh size 4 blade compared with the Pentax-AWS, despite inferior glottic visualization.[70] Several case reports describe the Pentax AWS VL for successful intubation of awake, spontaneously breathing patients.[31-33]

In morbidly obese patients, the relatively bulky design may cause difficulties during insertion in the mouth.[71] Problems with the guiding channel may arise if the cervical spine has a fixed rotation[72] or if otherwise the tube may not be redirected from the channel.[73] In principle, these problems may arise with all channeled-blade VLs.

C. Airtraq

1. Description

The Airtraq (Prodol Meditec, Guecho, Spain) is a single-use, indirect laryngoscope that incorporates two channels. One transfers the image to a proximal viewfinder through a series of prisms and lenses, and the other acts as a conduit for the ETT. A clip-on camera can transfer the image from the viewfinder to an external monitor. The Airtraq is available in different sizes for pediatric and adult patients. Nasal and double-lumen versions are available.

2. Instrument Use

Similar to the King Vision VL, the Airtraq tube should be preloaded in the tube-guiding channel before insertion of the laryngoscope into the patient's mouth. The laryngoscope should be advanced toward the glottis, so that it barely lifts the epiglottis with the tip of the blade.

3. Clinical Experience

Compared with conventional Macintosh laryngoscopy, the Airtraq has demonstrated promising results in patients at low or higher risk for difficult tracheal intubation and in patients with immobilization of the cervical spine.[74-76] McElwain and colleagues found that the Airtraq laryngoscope performed better than the C-MAC (with a Macintosh blade) and conventional Macintosh laryngoscopes in patients undergoing tracheal intubation with manual in-line stabilization of the cervical spine.[77] However, Trimmel and colleagues showed that the Airtraq laryngoscope had no benefit over conventional direct laryngoscopy in the prehospital setting if used by untrained physicians, and they could not recommend it in the prehospital setting without significant clinical experience obtained in the operation room.[78]

V. FIELDS OF APPLICATION

As more VLs are introduced into clinical practice and as airway managers become more skillful with the application of video laryngoscopy, it could become a standard part of management for patients with known or suspected difficult airway. However, because video laryngoscopic devices have different designs, technical issues, indications, and applications, it may take some time before a VL system is used for routine intubations.

VLs are available with external and integrated monitors. External monitors can provide optimal visualization of the intubation process to the entire team, who may anticipate actions such as extralaryngeal manipulations or suctioning. Captured images and videos can be recorded by external units. The smaller integrated monitors offer the greatest portability, which will be improved when wireless technology is implemented.

Video laryngoscopy has many nontraditional but useful applications in anesthesiology (Table 25-1). Suitable devices should be available when anesthesia is administered, and all airway practitioners should be skilled in their use. Although VLs can provide important savings in time and decreased patient morbidity, equipment cannot substitute for clinical proficiency, and traditional intubation skills should be maintained.

VI. DIFFICULT AIRWAY

At one time, the use of video laryngoscopy for managing the unexpected difficult airway was limited by restricted mobility and extended preparation time. This is no longer the case because current VLs are mobile and quick to set up. Serocki and colleagues found that video laryngoscopy was helpful in many clinical conditions with an expected difficult airway, including limited neck mobility, reduced thyromental distance, reduced inter-incisor distance, and retrognathia.[48] Their data confirmed that the DCI VL with a Macintosh blade and the GlideScope enhanced glottic visualization in patients with difficult conventional laryngoscopy.

TABLE 25-1

Overview of Video Laryngoscopes

Macintosh Type or Adapted Blades

Brand	C-MAC (Fig. 25-T1)	C-MAC PM (Fig. 25-T2)	McGrath MAC (Fig. 25-T3)	A.P. Advance (Fig. 25-T4)	Truview PCD (Fig. 25-T5)
Manufacturer	Karl Storz	Karl Storz	Aircraft Medical	Venner Medical/ distr. by LMA	Truphatek Intl.
Monitor size	7 inch	2.4 inch	2.5 inch	3.5 inch	5 inch
Resolution	800×400	320×240	NA	320×240	640×480
Camera chip	CMOS	CMOS	CMOS	CMOS	CCD (clip-on)
Illumination	LED	LED	LED	LED	LED
Multimedia	SD card for picture, video recording	—	—	Video output	USB-2, RCA video output
Accu	Lithium-Ion	Lithium-Ion	Lithium-Ion	Batteries $(1 \times AA)$	Batteries (rechargeable)
IP Prot. class	IP 54	IP X8	IP X7	IP 67/monitor 33	IP X0
Weight (g)	1500	180 (w/o blade)	200	435	NA

Highly Curved Blades (Obligatory Indirect)

Brand	GlideScope AVL, GVL (Fig. 25-T6)	GlideScope Ranger (Fig. 25-T7)	C-MAC D-Blade (Fig. 25-T8)	C-MAC PM with D-Blade (Fig. 25-T9)	McGrath Series 5 (Fig. 25-T10)	Pentax AWS (Fig. 25-T11)	King Vision (Fig. 25-T12)
Manufacturer	Verathon Medical	Verathon Medical	Karl Storz	Karl Storz	Aircraft Medical	Pentax/distr. by Ambu	King Systems
Monitor size	6.4 inch	3.4 inch	7 inch	2.4 inch	1.7 inch	2.4 inch	2.4 inch
Resolution	640×480	480×234	800×400	320×240	NA	NA	320×240
Camera chip	CMOS	CMOS	CMOS	CMOS	CMOS	CCD	CMOS
Illumination	LED	LED	LED	LED	LED	LED	LED
Multimedia	USB slot, NTSC video output	Recording (DVR optional)	SD card for picture, video recording	—	—	NTSC video output	Video output
Accu	Lithium-Ion	Lithium-Ion	Lithium-Ion	Lithium-Ion	Batteries $(1 \times AA)$	Batteries $(2 \times AA)$	Batteries $(3 \times AAA)$
IP Prot. class	NA	IP 68	IP 54	IP X8	IP 65	IP X7	NA
Weight (g)	1500	560	1500	180 (w/o blade)	325	375 (w/o batteries)	NA

Video Laryngoscopes with Tube-Guiding Channels

Brand	Pentax AWS (see Fig. 25-T11)	King Vision (see Fig. 25-T12)	Airtraq (Fig. 25-T13)	A.P. Advance DAB (Fig. 25-T14)
Manufacturer	Pentax/distr. by Ambu	King Systems	Prodol	Venner Medical/ distr. by LMA
Monitor size	2.4 inch	2.4 inch	—	3.5 inch
Resolution	NA	320×240	—	320×240
Camera chip	CCD	CMOS	None	CMOS
Illumination	LED	LED	LED	LED
Multimedia	NTSC video output	Video output	Clip-on camera	Video output
Accu	Batteries $(2 \times AA)$	Batteries $(3 \times AAA)$	Batteries $(3 \times AAA)$	Batteries $(1 \times AA)$
IP Prot. class	IP X7	NA	NA	IP 67/monitor 33
Weight (g)	375	NA	NA	435

CCD, Charge-coupled device; *CMOS,* complementary metal-oxide semiconductor; *DAB,* difficult airway blade; *distr.,* distributed; *LED,* light-emitting diode; *NA,* no data available; *NTSC,* National Television System Committee; *PCD,* picture capture device; *PM,* pocket monitor; *SD,* secure digital; *w/o,* without.

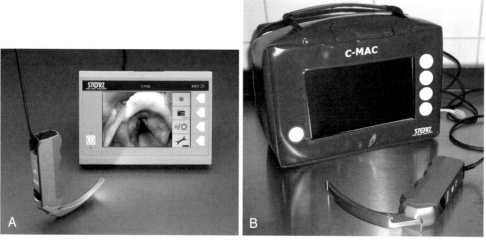

Figure 25-T1 C-MAC.

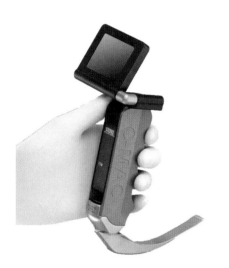

Figure 25-T2 C-MAC PM.

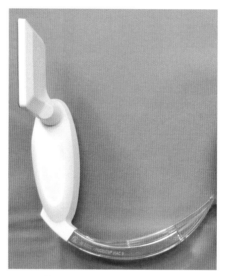

Figure 25-T3 McGrath MAC.

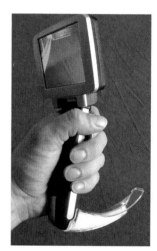

Figure 25-T4 A.P. Advance.

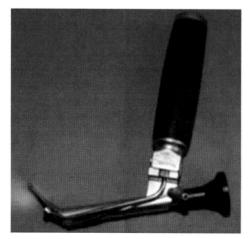

Figure 25-T5 Truview PCD.

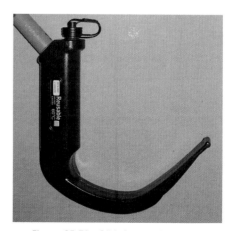

Figure 25-T6 GlideScope AVL/GVL.

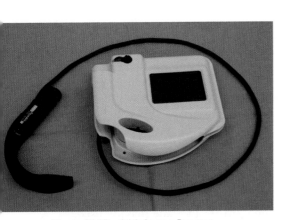

Figure 25-T7   GlideScope Ranger.

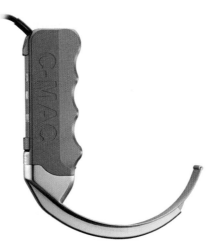

Figure 25-T8   C-MAC with D-blade.

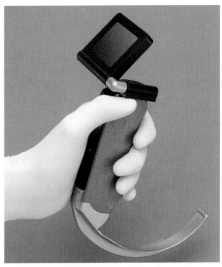

Figure 25-T9   C-MAC PM with D-blade.

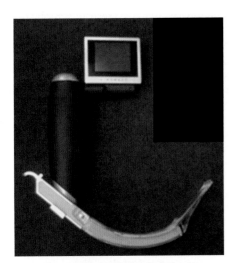

Figure 25-T10   McGrath Series 5.

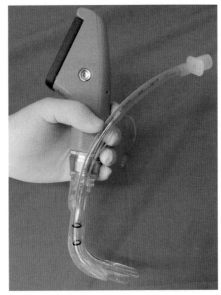

Figure 25-T11   Pentax AWS.

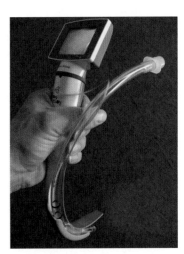

Figure 25-T12   King Vision.

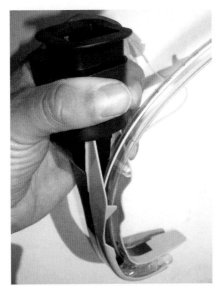

Figure 25-T13   Airtraq.

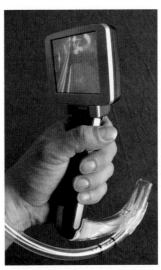

Figure 25-T14   A.P. Advance DAB.

Video laryngoscopy cannot replace awake fiberoptic intubation in many cases of predictable difficult airway. Nonetheless, in an expected difficult airway, video laryngoscopy may be a worthy addition as an awake intubation technique.[32,34,79] Although the American Society of Anesthesiologists (ASA) difficult airway guidelines highlight the approach of awake intubation as the preferred method to manage expected difficult airways, video laryngoscopy under general anesthesia should be considered for intubation if difficulty with intubation, but not mask ventilation, is expected.[80] Video laryngoscopy has successfully been applied for the management of the difficult airway in otonasolaryngologic and maxillofacial surgery,[48] neurosurgery,[81] obstetrics,[82] traumatology, pediatrics,[83] the intensive care unit,[84] the emergency department,[64] and in physician-based, out-of-hospital emergency medicine.[17]

VL systems may be advantageous over direct laryngoscopy for the exchange of one airway device for another. A case report demonstrated the use of video laryngoscopy to exchange a Combitube, which was placed by paramedics after failed direct vision intubation, for an ETT to establish a definitive airway.[12] It is not unusual for a supraglottic airway device, such as a Laryngeal Tube or Combitube, to be placed in the prehospital setting when direct laryngoscopy is unsuccessful and the patient's airway is difficult; exchanging this device for an ETT may be demanding. Anesthesiologists use VLs in routine cases without any suspicion of difficult airway management or before any attempt of direct laryngoscopy is performed, because VLs are simple to use and have a high rate of intubation success.

VLs have the advantage in the unanticipated situation because their rigidity facilitates rapid control of the position of the laryngoscope tip, and they can be ready for immediate use. These devices allow retraction of soft tissues so that there is a line of sight from the lens to the distal structures, without the necessity of aligning the oral and laryngotracheal axes with the naked eye. Even with a Macintosh VL that is used in the traditional Macintosh fashion (i.e., tip of blade in vallecula), the epiglottis may be directly elevated; the straight-blade technique offers improved viewing. This type of positioning is often performed for difficult airways. In a study of 60 patients by Cavus and associates,[15] a size 4 rather than a size 3 C-MAC blade was used in three patients with unexpected intubation difficulties. The Macintosh size 4 blade is more curved than the size 3, resulting in a higher angulation with a wider view of the glottis. In all three of these patients, the Cormack-Lehane score improved by two classes using this technique. Some practitioners position the tip over the dorsum of the tongue, proximal to the epiglottis, achieving indirect elevation of the epiglottis without conventional tensioning of the hyoepiglottic ligament.

Because of their optics, these devices allow the operator to visualize structures that may not be seen with the direct line-of-sight view available to the naked eye. When glottic visualization is difficult despite the use of a Macintosh-based VL, an obligate indirect VL such as the GlideScope or the C-MAC D-Blade may be used.[20,39] A direct view on the glottis is impossible with an obligate indirect VL in most patients. If secretions (e.g., blood, vomit), surrounding light, and battery failure impede the glottic view on the monitor, direct glottic visualization can be an important fall-back strategy.[17]

It may be advantageous to use a system in which different types of blades can be changed with minimal delay, such as C-MAC system or A.P. Advance.[9] In a stepwise approach, airway management can be changed from direct laryngoscopy by video laryngoscopy with a Macintosh blade to obligate indirect video laryngoscopy with a more highly curved blade (Fig. 25-2). Most VLs provide an output socket to an external monitor. Some offer video capture capabilities to record airway procedures for educational or documentation purposes (e.g., C-MAC, GlideScope). Control buttons are located on the handle or the monitor for recording videos and captured images.

The use of VLs has some restrictions. A training period outside an emergency situation is necessary to use the system correctly and obtain its full benefit. Additional training is also necessary for correct handling of the ETT while viewing the monitor instead of direct visualization of the larynx.

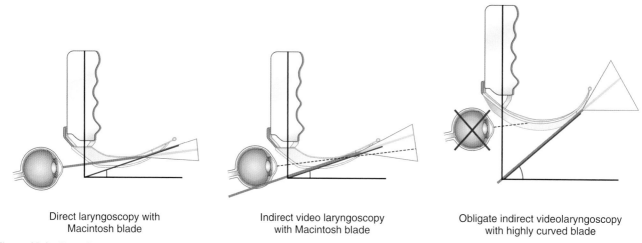

Direct laryngoscopy with Macintosh blade

Indirect video laryngoscopy with Macintosh blade

Obligate indirect videolaryngoscopy with highly curved blade

Figure 25-2 Stepwise approach to video laryngoscopy using interchangeable blades for conventional direct laryngoscopy, indirect video laryngoscopy, and obligate indirect video laryngoscopy.

VII. TEACHING

All VLs provide optimal visualization of the glottis on a video screen. The video presentation may be used to provide a "what to see during intubation" tutorial. Video laryngoscopy enables the supervising faculty member to directly observe the actions of the trainee, reducing the anxiety associated with allowing the trainee to perform the intubation. However, because the application of some devices varies significantly and only obligate indirect laryngoscopy may be possible, a limited number of VLs may be used in training for conventional laryngoscopy and intubation.

The demands for adequate clinical experience with airway management are increasing in training programs because providing acute airway management is often accomplished in high-stress settings. Allowing the trainee to manage the airway is a crucial decision by the faculty member, who must always consider the patient's level of acuity, the clinical circumstances, and the perceived confidence in the trainee who will be afforded the clinical experience.

VLs based on Macintosh blades offer the possibility for conventional direct laryngoscopy attempts by the trainee, and at the same time, the faculty member is able to analyze the airway on the monitor and make better-informed decisions about the prudence of allowing the trainee to continue. A study using video laryngoscopy to provide feedback for instructor showed that the student's success of intubation is increased and the rate of esophageal intubations was markedly decreased compared with instructor assistance based on standard cues.[85] In the absence of a VL system, the faculty member is more likely to take over the procedure earlier if a problem is encountered, reducing the experience afforded to the trainee.

VIII. DOCUMENTATION

VLs with external monitors can record and save video sequences and image captures from the screen. Video recordings of professional laryngoscopic attempts can be educational, and recordings of intubation attempts by students can be used as a teaching tool. Airway pathologies such as edema of the glottic opening and erythema after a burn injury can be documented. In newborns, the enlarged panoramic view and recordings of video laryngoscopy have assisted in correctly diagnosing vocal cord paralysis.[83]

Direct visualization of tube insertion with video recording can confirm correct tube placement and can detect esophageally misplaced ETTs quickly. Use of video laryngoscopy for routine intubations in the operating room, intensive care unit, emergency department, and prehospital emergency settings can increase intubation success rates and reduce the incidence of critical situations in airway management.[86]

IX. CONCLUSIONS

Direct laryngoscopy for intubation confers the advantages of familiarity, direct glottic visualization, cost-effectiveness, equipment availability, and a steep learning curve. However, the prevalence of Cormack-Lehane grade 3 views at direct laryngoscopy is stubbornly persistent. Adjunctive maneuvers such as external laryngeal manipulation and head lift, together with accessories such as ETT introducers (bougies), remain crucial to the success of unexpected difficult direct laryngoscopy. Alternative intubation techniques such as video laryngoscopy applied in a timely fashion are essential to achieving success in challenging situations. Because VLs are mobile and quick to set up, they play an important role in the management of an unexpected difficult airway. Use of a VL also may be considered in a predicted difficult airway if mask ventilation and oxygenation are warranted or in situations in which blind techniques are contraindicated (e.g., anatomic abnormalities of the airway) and video documentation is needed. However, the gold standard for management of predicted airway difficulties when oxygenation after induction of anesthesia cannot be ensured is the use of a flexible fiberoptic device in an awake, spontaneously breathing patient.

As more video-aided devices become available, clinicians must become familiar with some of them in elective cases to expect them to be useful in difficult situations. Teaching programs must ensure that excellent skills in direct laryngoscopy and flexible fiberoptics are taught and maintained and that anesthesiologists attain competence with different direct laryngoscopy blades.

X. CLINICAL PEARLS

- The main indication for video laryngoscopy is an unpredicted difficult intubation.

- If oxygenation of the patient can be ensured (e.g., by bag-mask ventilation), video laryngoscopy may be considered for some cases of predicted difficult intubation.

- Video laryngoscopes (VLs) have different technical requirements and handling conditions. Training with each device in elective situations is mandatory before use in airway emergencies.

- VLs with highly curved blades provide obligate indirect glottic visualization. In most cases, a tube stylet must be used. Despite optimal visualization of the glottic entrance, tube advancement into the trachea may be difficult due to the steep angle of the styletted, curved tube.

- VLs with Macintosh-type blades provide direct and indirect glottic views. The option of direct visualization may be particularly important in airway emergencies outside of the hospital.

- Ideally, VLs are available to cover a broad range of applications in patients of different ages and sizes (e.g., newborns, obese patients).

- Reusable, stainless steel blades have lower blade profiles, but disposable blades also should be available for hygienic reasons. Disposable blades are mandatory in some countries.

- Video laryngoscopy allows for image capture and video documentation that may be useful in a variety of settings (e.g., oropharyngeal pathologies, correct tube placement).

- Video laryngoscopy may be used for awake orotracheal intubation, but awake fiberoptic intubation remains the gold standard for patients with a predicted difficult airway, and skill in performing fiberoptic intubation must be maintained.

- Because VLs, especially those with interchangeable blades for direct laryngoscopy and obligate indirect laryngoscopy, aid education in conventional laryngoscopy and reduce patient morbidity, they may become the standard for routine intubation in the operating room, intensive care unit, emergency department, and prehospital emergency settings.

SELECTED REFERENCES

All references can be found online at expertconsult.com.

11. Kaplan MB, Hagberg CA, Ward DS, et al: Comparison of direct and video-assisted views of the larynx during routine intubation. *J Clin Anesth* 18:357–362, 2006.

15. Cavus E, Kieckhaefer J, Doerges V, et al: The C-MAC videolaryngoscope: First experiences with a new device for videolaryngoscopy-guided intubation. *Anesth Analg* 110:473–477, 2010.

18. Maassen R, Lee R, Hermans B, et al: A comparison of three videolaryngoscopes: The Macintosh laryngoscope blade reduces, but does not replace, routine stylet use for intubation in morbidly obese patients. *Anesth Analg* 109:1560–1565, 2009.

34. Doyle DJ: Awake intubation using the GlideScope video laryngoscope: Initial experience in four cases. *Can J Anaesth* 51:520–521, 2004.

38. Aziz MF, Healy D, Kheterpal S, et al: Routine clinical practice effectiveness of the GlideScope in difficult airway management: an analysis of 2,004 GlideScope intubations, complications, and failures from two institutions. *Anesthesiology* 114:34–41, 2011.

39. Cooper RM, Pacey JA, Bishop MJ, et al: Early clinical experience with a new videolaryngoscope (GlideScope) in 728 patients. *Can J Anaesth* 52:191–198, 2005.

58. Levitan RM, Heitz JW, Sweeney M, et al: The complexities of tracheal intubation with direct laryngoscopy and alternative intubation devices. *Ann Emerg Med* 57:240–247, 2011.

64. Choi HJ, Kang HG, Lim TH, et al: Endotracheal intubation using a GlideScope video laryngoscope by emergency physicians: A multicentre analysis of 345 attempts in adult patients. *Emerg Med J* 27:380–382, 2010.

73. Asai T, Liu EH, Matsumoto S, et al: Use of the Pentax-AWS in 293 patients with difficult airways. *Anesthesiology* 110:898–904, 2009.

85. Howard-Quijano KJ, Huang YM, Matevosian R, et al: Video-assisted instruction improves the success rate for tracheal intubation by novices. *Br J Anaesth* 101:568–572, 2008.

Separation of the Two Lungs: Double-Lumen Tubes, Endobronchial Blockers, and Endobronchial Single-Lumen Tubes

BRIAN L. MARASIGAN | ROY SHEINBAUM | GREGORY B. HAMMER | EDMOND COHEN

I. INTRODUCTION

The physiology, indications, and techniques of lung isolation and single-lung ventilation (SLV) are discussed in this chapter. Lung isolation is most commonly used during thoracic and cardiovascular procedures; however, it can often be useful and potentially life-saving in other situations. Newly designed double-lumen tubes (DLTs), single-lumen tubes (SLTs) with built-in endobronchial blockers (also called bronchial blockers), new bronchial devices, and enhanced fiberoptic technology are making lung isolation and SLV easier and safer to perform. Knowledge of these topics is requisite for a consultant anesthesiologist.

II. PHYSIOLOGY

The most common physiologic problem with SLV is the creation of a large intrapulmonary shunt. This shunt may result in hypoxia with severe irreversible end-organ damage. Most anesthesiologists aim to maintain arterial oxygen tension (PaO_2) at greater than 60 mm Hg as hemoglobin saturation drops sharply below this value.

In most surgical cases, patients are placed in lateral decubitus position with the ventilated lung dependent. The physiologic goal is to promote blood flow to the nonsurgical, dependent lung. By reducing the pulmonary vascular resistance (PVR) of the dependent lung to minimal levels, improved ventilation-perfusion ($\dot{V}/\dot{Q}$) matching may occur. Excess positive end-expiratory pressure (PEEP), airway pressures, hypoxia, hypercapnia, and hypovolemia may contribute to an increase in PVR of the dependent lung, thereby increasing the shunt fraction. Improvement of the shunt fraction can be accomplished by decreasing blood flow or supplying O_2 to the nondependent lung.

Hypoxic pulmonary vasoconstriction is a powerful reflex that increases the PVR of the hypoxic lung and the atelectatic lung, diverting blood to the well-oxygenated areas of lung. It is useful to limit agents that inhibit hypoxic pulmonary vasoconstriction, such as nitrates and high concentrations of volatile agents.

Supplementation of O_2 to the nondependent lung may also alleviate hypoxia. This can be accomplished by the application of an external continuous positive airway pressure (CPAP) circuit to the nondependent lung or simply by trapping partial inflations of the nondependent lung. The goal is to allow enough O_2 into the nondependent lung to reverse hypoxia while not obscuring the surgical field.

III. INDICATIONS FOR LUNG SEPARATION

A. Absolute Indications

Absolute indications for lung separation (Box 26-1) include protective isolation of the normal lung, establishment of adequate gas exchange when there is a change in pulmonary compliance or lung pathology, and unilateral bronchopulmonary lavage.

Accumulation of blood or any contaminant in the noninvolved lung can lead to severe atelectasis, pneumonia, sepsis, and death. Lung isolation may be life-saving by simply preventing immediate drowning of the ventilated lung or by preventing further deterioration of overall pulmonary function.

Several unilateral lung conditions lead to inadequate ventilation. A large bronchopleural or bronchocutaneous fistula can lead to little or no ventilation of the nonoperative, healthy lung. In this situation, the increased compliance of the diseased lung results in direction of most of the positive-pressure ventilation (PPV) toward the diseased lung, minimally ventilating the normal lung and producing inadequate gas exchange. Conversely, a relatively noncompliant transplanted lung cannot compete with the better compliance of the native lung, and as a result, the healthy transplanted lung can be severely underventilated. Another scenario involves a lung with bullous or cystic disease or a lung with tracheobronchial disruption.[1] Tension pneumothorax or tension mediastinum could result during these scenarios from elevated airway pressures that are often observed with SLV in the lateral decubitus position.

Patients with alveolar proteinosis may require unilateral bronchopulmonary lavage, which involves multiple instillations of large fluid volumes into the target lung with subsequent drainage of the effluent fluid.[2-4] Lung separation is mandatory to avoid lung cross-contamination and drowning caused by the large volume of fluid required to perform the lavage.

B. Relative Indications

Relative indications for lung isolation involve facilitating surgical exposure, avoiding lung trauma, and improving gas exchange. Operations such as repair of thoracic aneurysms, pneumonectomy, pulmonary lobectomies (especially of the upper lobe), video-assisted thoracoscopic surgery, esophageal surgery, and anterior spinal surgery all benefit from the optimized surgical exposure afforded by SLV (see Box 26-1). Lung isolation further improves recovery by minimizing lung instrumentation and trauma to the nonventilated, nondependent lung. In cases of unilateral lung trauma, oxygenation and recovery may be optimized with SLV by improving $\dot{V}/\dot{Q}$ matching.

Additional indications for SLV are bronchopleural and bronchocutaneous fistulas because they offer a low-resistance pathway for the delivered tidal volume during PPV. Another example is bronchopulmonary lavage for alveolar proteinosis or cystic fibrosis, because protection of the contralateral lung is necessary during separation. All other indications for SLV can be considered as the need for lung separation in which there is no risk of contamination of the dependent lung. This includes all relative indications that are necessary for surgical exposure, such as video-assisted thoracoscopy (VAT) for diagnostic and therapeutic procedures. Most procedures in which SLV is used are for lung separation; few require lung isolation. This distinction is important when selecting the method to provide SLV. In cases of lung isolation, DLTs are preferable to endobronchial blockers because they provide a superior protective seal to prevent contamination of the dependent lung.

Box 26-1 Indications for Separation of the Two Lungs or One-Lung Ventilation

Absolute Indications

Isolation of one lung from the other to avoid spillage or contamination
1. Infection
2. Massive hemorrhage

Control of the distribution of ventilation
1. Bronchopleural fistula
2. Bronchopleural cutaneous fistula
3. Surgical opening of a major conducting airway
4. Giant unilateral lung cyst or bulla
5. Life-threatening hypoxemia related to unilateral lung disease

Unilateral bronchopulmonary lavage
1. Pulmonary alveolar proteinosis

Relative Indications

Surgical exposure—high priority
1. Thoracic aortic aneurysm
2. Pneumonectomy
3. Thoracoscopy
4. Upper lobectomy
5. Mediastinal exposure

Surgical exposure—medium (lower) priority
1. Middle and lower lobectomies and subsegmental resections
2. Esophageal resection
3. Procedures on the thoracic spine

Pulmonary edema after cardiopulmonary bypass
Hemorrhage after removal of totally occluding, unilateral, chronic pulmonary emboli
Severe hypoxemia related to unilateral lung disease

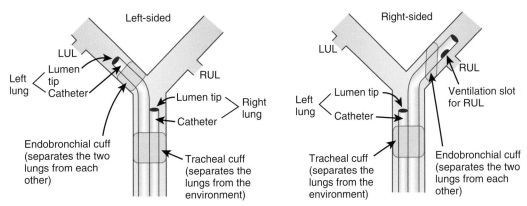

Figure 26-1 Essential features and parts of left-sided and right-sided double-lumen tubes. *RUL,* Right upper lobe; *LUL,* left upper lobe. (From Benumof JL: *Anesthesia for thoracic surgery,* Philadelphia, 1987, Saunders.)

IV. TECHNIQUES

A. Double-Lumen Tubes

1. Anatomy

DLTs are essentially two tubes bonded together with a design that allows each tube to ventilate a specified lung. DLTs are right-sided or left-sided devices. Left-sided DLTs have a bronchial port that extends into the left main stem bronchus and a tracheal port that is designed to sit above the carina. In right-sided DLTs, the bronchial port extends into the right main stem bronchus, and the tracheal port sits above the carina. The cuff of the right-sided DLT may be at an oblique angle to facilitate ventilation of the right upper lobe bronchus at the Murphy eye (Fig. 26-1).

The original DLTs were reusable, red rubber tubes with high-pressure cuffs that became stiff and brittle over time, making placement more difficult and traumatic. Newer DLTs are made of nontoxic plastic (the Z-79 marking) and are disposable. As the plastic warms up from the surrounding body temperature, the DLT conforms to the anatomy of the patient. This increased malleability, however, makes it more difficult to reposition the same tube. Current DLTs employ high-volume, low-pressure, color-coded cuffs. The bronchial cuff and its pilot balloon/connector are blue. The tracheal cuff and its pilot balloon/connector are clear or white. Cuff inflation pressure requires a balance between preserving an adequate seal and maintaining mucosal perfusion. Measured cuff pressures between 15 and 30 mm Hg achieve these goals.[5-8] In cases involving the use of nitrous oxide, the cuff pressures should be checked periodically.

DLTs come in various French (F) sizes: 28, 32, 35, 37, 39, and 41, and 1 F equals an approximately 0.33-mm measurement of the outer diameter (OD). In most adult men, a 39-F DLT fits well, having adequate length and appropriate diameter, while providing the capability of suctioning or fiberoptic bronchoscopy (FOB), and a 37-F DLT fits most adult women. A radiopaque line may be seen at the end of each lumen to allow for radiographic positioning. A Y-adapter for the proximal end allows ventilation of both lumens through a single circuit. The cross section of the DLT is designed as one round

bronchial lumen and one crescent-shaped tracheal lumen. Left- and right-sided DLTs are curved at the distal end to enable advancement into the respective main stem bronchus. DLTs from different manufacturers have their own characteristic feel and slight modifications to the basic design described. The depth required for insertion of the DLT correlates with the height of the patient. For any adult 170 to 180 cm tall, the average depth for a left-sided DLT is 29 cm. For every 10-cm increase or decrease in height, the DLT is advanced or withdrawn 1.0 cm.[9]

2. Advantages

The DLT has inherent advantages. When properly positioned, the DLT allows independent ventilation of each lung in unison or separately. This is a great advantage in cases in which each lung needs to be ventilated using different modalities. Treatment and prevention of desaturation is also easier with DLTs, because CPAP or partial lung inflation is easy to perform on the surgical lung while the opposite lung is ventilated normally. Suctioning and FOB are facilitated by the relatively large luminal accesses into each main stem bronchus. Access beyond each main stem bronchus also allows for egress of gases and lung deflation for surgical exposure. Other advantages include the solid structure and improved cuff seals of the DLTs, which prevent easy dislodgment after proper positioning.

3. Disadvantages

The most significant disadvantages of the DLT are related to its size. Intubation with a DLT is often more difficult than with an SLT.[6] Intubation is even more complex in patients with difficult airway anatomy.[10] In cases of a distorted or compressed tracheobronchial tree, placement of a DLT can be impossible due to its size and rigidity. DLT size can contribute to airway damage during placement and when the device is left in place for a long period. Because of some difficulty managing DLTs in the ICU with regard to weaning and pulmonary toilet, they are often exchanged for SLTs. The process of exchanging a DLT for an SLT can be dangerous, especially after procedures in which airway edema has occurred. Although DLT lumens are relatively large, FOB may be cumbersome due to the extended length of each tube and the

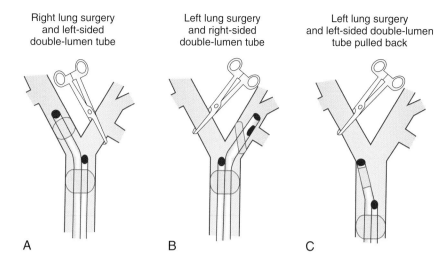

Right lung surgery
and left-sided
double-lumen tube

Left lung surgery
and right-sided
double-lumen tube

Left lung surgery
and left-sided double-lumen
tube pulled back

A　　　　　　　　　　　B　　　　　　　　　　　C

Figure 26-2 Use of left-sided and right-sided double-lumen tubes (DLTs) for left and right lung surgery is indicated by the clamp. When surgery is performed on the right lung, a left-sided DLT should be used **(A).** When surgery is performed on the left lung, a right-sided DLT may be used **(B).** However, because of uncertainty about the alignment of a right upper lobe ventilation slot to the right upper lobe orifice, a left-sided DLT can be used for left lung surgery **(C).** If left lung surgery requires a clamp to be placed high on the left main stem bronchus, the left endobronchial cuff should be deflated, the left-sided DLT pulled back into the trachea, and the right lung ventilated through both lumens (using the DLT as a single-lumen tube). (From Benumof JL: *Anesthesia for thoracic surgery,* Philadelphia, 1987, Saunders.)

narrowed crescent shape of the tracheal lumen. Multiple ports and connections further require a good working knowledge of the DLT anatomy to prevent errors in ventilation and management.

4. Selection

a. RIGHT-SIDED VERSUS LEFT-SIDED DOUBLE-LUMEN TUBES

To minimize tube displacement, it may be recommended that the nonoperated bronchus be intubated (i.e., using a left-sided DLT for a patient undergoing right lung surgery) (Fig. 26-2).[11] However, controversy exists in regard to left lung procedures because of the anatomic variability of the right upper lobe. The bronchial port of a right-sided tube may be difficult to position for adequate lung isolation and ventilation of the right upper lobe bronchus. This can result in difficulties during

surgery, including severe hypoxia during isolated right lung ventilation.[12]

Many anesthesiologists prefer to use left-sided DLTs for all lung surgeries (see Fig. 26-2); however, there are insufficient data to support actual increased safety, as opposed to the perception of safety when intraoperative hypoxia, hypercapnia, and high airway pressures are used as criteria.[13,14] If manipulation of the left main stem bronchus is required, the left-sided DLT is withdrawn and repositioned with the bronchial port above the carina. For operations on the left main stem, including sleeve resection, it may be preferable to use a right-sided DLT (Fig. 26-3).

Contraindications for use of a DLT include anatomic barriers that make positioning improbable or dangerous, such as carinal or bronchial lesions, strictures, vascular compression by aortic aneurysm, and aberrant

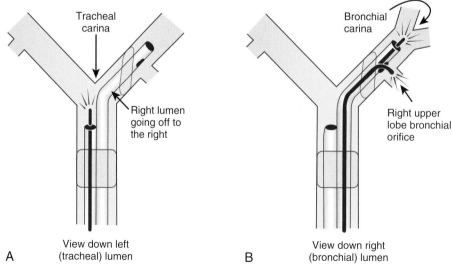

A　View down left (tracheal) lumen

B　View down right (bronchial) lumen

Figure 26-3 Schematic diagram portrays use of a flexible fiberoptic bronchoscope (FFB) to determine the precise position of a right-sided double-lumen tube. **A,** When the FFB is passed down the left (tracheal) lumen, the endoscopist should see a clear, straight-ahead view of the tracheal carina and right lumen going off into the right main stem bronchus. **B,** When the FFB is passed down the right (bronchial) lumen, the endoscopist should see the bronchial carina in the distance; when the FFB is flexed laterally and cephalad and passed through the ventilation slot of the right upper lobe, the bronchial orifice of the right upper lobe should be visible. (From Benumof JL: *Anesthesia for thoracic surgery,* Philadelphia, 1987, Saunders.)

Relation of Flexible Fiberoptic Bronchoscope Size to Double-Lumen Tube Size

FFB OD Size (mm)	DLT Size (F)	Fit of FFB inside DLT
5.6	All sizes	Does not fit
	41	Easy passage
	39	Moderately easy passage
4.9	37	Tight fit, needs lubricant,* hand push
	35	Does not fit
3.6-4.2	All sizes	Easy passage
Approximately 2.0	All sizes	Most operating rooms need special arrangements to obtain this size FFB

*Lubricant recommended is a silicon-based fluid made by the American Cystoscope Co.
DLT, Double-lumen tube; *FFB,* flexible fiberoptic bronchoscope; *OD,* outer diameter.

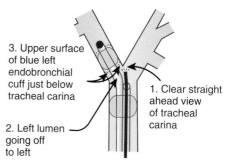

Figure 26-4 Use of a flexible fiberoptic bronchoscope down the right lumen to determine precise position of a left-sided double-lumen tube. The endoscopist should see a clear, straight-ahead view of the tracheal carina (1); the left lumen going off into the left main stem bronchus (2); and the upper surface of the blue left endobronchial cuff just below the tracheal carina (3). (From Benumof JL: *Anesthesia for thoracic surgery,* Philadelphia, 1987, Saunders.)

bronchus.[6,15,16] Right-sided DLTs may be indicated in cases with tortuosity and compression of the trachea or left main stem bronchus, which can make placement of a left-sided DLT impossible. Newly designed DLTs may be applicable for patients with special conditions including those with unusual anatomic variability.[17]

b. DOUBLE-LUMEN TUBE SIZE

The ideal size of a DLT is one that results in a near-complete seal of the bronchial lumen without inflation of the cuff. The high inflation pressures of a small tube can cause as much mucosal damage as forcing too large a tube into a small bronchus.[18] Even when height- and weight-based size estimates are used, it is impossible to choose the correct size of tube every time.[15,19] Commonly, a 39-F or 41-F DLT is selected for men and a 37-F or 39-F DLT for women of average height and build. The intentional use of smaller DLTs has not had significant clinical benefits.[20] A flexible fiberoptic bronchoscope (FFB) may be passed through the bronchial lumen to assess appropriate diameter and length of the DLT during placement (Table 26-1).

5. Positioning

Malposition of the DLT can lead to life-threatening consequences. Ventilation can be severely impaired, leading to hypoxia, gas trapping, tension pneumothorax, cross-contamination of lung contents, and interference with surgical procedures. Multiple studies have shown that DLTs are often malpositioned.[15,19] On the basis of these studies, indirect visualization with a FFB may be used routinely for confirmation of positioning. Various techniques using a FFB are discussed in the following sections.

a. PLACEMENT OF THE DOUBLE-LUMEN TUBE

DLTs are placed similar to SLTs but with some additional maneuvers and considerations. DLTs are larger in diameter and longer than SLTs, making them more difficult to place. It is important never to force a DLT into position. For laryngoscopy, the shoulder of a Macintosh blade provides better tongue displacement and more space through which to insert the tube. The use of a video laryngoscope has also been described as effective and potentially time-saving.[21] The bronchial tip of the DLT is placed through the cords, and the stylet is then removed to prevent trauma. After the bronchial portion has passed the cords, the DLT must be rotated 90 degrees toward the selected side of the bronchial lumen to sit properly. If resistance is encountered on rotating or advancing the tube, the use of a smaller tube needs to be considered. The average depth of insertion is 29 cm for a 170-cm individual. For each 10-cm increase or decrease in height, the tube depth is increased or decreased by 1 cm, respectively.[15] When the tube depth is reached, the tracheal cuff is inflated, and the patient is connected to the ventilator. Care must be taken not to tear or puncture the tracheal cuff during intubation. For example, covering the teeth with an unopened alcohol swab can minimize cuff damage.

After confirmation of CO_2 return and initiation of ventilation, an FFB is placed through the tracheal lumen (Fig. 26-4). The FFB is advanced, and the carina is identified. The bronchial lumen of the tube must be visualized entering the appropriate main stem bronchus (i.e., the bronchial lumen should be in the left main stem bronchus for a left-sided DLT). The balloon of the bronchial lumen should be inflated under direct vision and should lie just distal to the carina. The tube may have to be repositioned to visualize the balloon. Direct visualization of the balloon inflation helps to confirm tube position and size. Some DLTs have an indicator line just proximal to the bronchial cuff that should sit at the level of the carina. Direct visualization may be necessary to ensure that the bronchial balloon does not herniate over the carina or that the tracheal portion of the DLT does not encroach on the carina (Fig. 26-5).

Determination of right versus left main stem bronchus is done by visualization of the anterior and posterior aspects of the trachea. The anterior of the trachea is identified by the tracheal rings, which extend throughout the anterior two thirds of the trachea. Posteriorly, the trachea consists of the membranous component with longitudinal striations. After the anterior and posterior

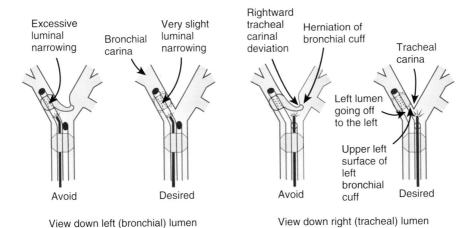

Figure 26-5 Desired views and views to be avoided when using a fiberoptic bronchoscope (FOB) to determine the position of a left-sided, double-lumen tube (DLT). *Left,* When an FOB is passed down the left lumen of a left-sided DLT, the endoscopist should see a slight, left luminal narrowing and a clear, straight-ahead view of the bronchial carina in the distance. Excessive left luminal narrowing should be avoided. *Right,* When the flexible FOB is passed down the right lumen of the left-sided DLT, the endoscopist should see a clear, straight-ahead view of the tracheal carina; the left lumen going off into the main stem bronchus; and the upper surface of the blue, left endotracheal cuff just below the tracheal carina. Excessive pressure in the endobronchial cuff, as manifested by tracheal carinal deviation to the right and herniation of endobronchial cuff over the carina, should be avoided. (From Benumof JL: *Anesthesia for thoracic surgery,* Philadelphia, 1987, Saunders.)

aspects of the trachea are identified, right and left orientation is obvious. It may be necessary to suction the DLT before insertion of the FFB. Lubrication and antifogging agents applied to the FFB can facilitate manipulation and visualization. The appropriate use of antisialagogues can also be useful in limiting secretions before DLT placement.

An alternative method of DLT placement is to use the FFB as an intubating stylet to guide the bronchial tip of the DLT directly into the correct main stem bronchus (Fig. 26-6). This is accomplished by inserting the FFB through the bronchial port of the DLT after the bronchial tip has passed the vocal cords. The FFB is then advanced down the trachea while identifying the anterior-posterior

and right-left orientation. The FFB is advanced further to identifying the carina and the right and left main stem bronchi, then advanced into the appropriate bronchus. The DLT is advanced over the FFB. It is then necessary to remove the FFB after confirming that the bronchial tip is not obstructed and is proximal to the secondary bronchial branches. The FFB is then placed in the tracheal lumen to confirm the position of the bronchial cuff and to ensure that the tracheal lumen is not encroaching on the carina. This technique allows for assessment of the carina and tracheal rings and allows placement in tortuous airways. However, it takes more time to perform, and in some patients with poor pulmonary reserve, this extra time can lead to desaturation.

Use of Fiberoptic Bronchoscope to Insert Left-Sided Double-Lumen Tube

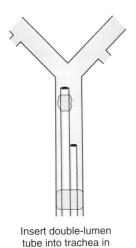

Insert double-lumen tube into trachea in conventional manner and ventilate both lungs

A

Pass fiberoptic bronchoscope down left lumen into left main stem bronchus

B

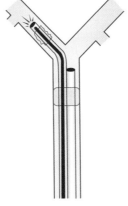

Push double-lumen tube in over fiberoptic bronchoscope until left lumen is in left main stem bronchus

C

Figure 26-6 A double-lumen tube (DLT) can be put into the trachea in a conventional manner, and both lungs can be ventilated by both lumens **(A).** A flexible fiberoptic bronchoscope (FFB) may be inserted into the left lumen of the DLT through a self-sealing diaphragm in the elbow connector to the left lumen; this allows continued positive-pressure ventilation of both lungs through the right lumen without creating a leak. After the FFB has been passed into the left main stem bronchus **(B),** it is used as a stylet for the left lumen **(C);** the FFB is then withdrawn. Final precise positioning of the DLT is performed with the FFB in the right lumen (see Figs. 26-19 and 26-20). (From Benumof JL: *Anesthesia for thoracic surgery,* Philadelphia, 1987, Saunders.)

b. CONFIRMATION OF PROPER PLACEMENT

Many maneuvers have been described to assess the proper position of a DLT,[22,23] including visualization of chest excursion while alternately clamping and unclamping the tracheal and bronchial ports, auscultation of lung fields while alternately clamping and unclamping the tracheal and bronchial ports (Fig. 26-7), and radiographic confirmation.[24,25]

The most important advance in checking for the proper position of a DLT is the FFB (Fig. 26-8). Smith and colleagues[26] demonstrated that when the disposable DLT was thought to be in the correct position by auscultation and physical examination, subsequent FOB showed that 48% of the tubes were malpositioned. Malpositions may not be clinically significant and may be missed by the clinician. When using a left-sided DLT, the bronchoscope is usually first introduced through the tracheal lumen to visualize the carina and to ensure that the bronchial cuff is not herniated. The upper surface of the blue endobronchial cuff should be just below the tracheal carina; the blue bronchial cuff of the disposable DLT is easily visualized. The bronchoscope is then passed through the bronchial lumen to identify the left upper lobe bronchial orifice. When a right-sided DLT is used, the carina should be visualized through the tracheal lumen, and the orifice of the right upper lobe bronchus should be identified when the bronchoscope is passed through the right upper lobe ventilating slot of the DLT.

Pediatric FOBs are available in several standard sizes: 5.6-, 4.9-, and 3.6-mm OD. The 4.9-mm OD bronchoscope can be passed through DLTs that are 37 F or larger. A 3.6-mm or smaller diameter bronchoscope is easily passed through all sizes of DLTs.[27-29]

DLT placement must be rechecked when the patient is repositioned, because movement of the tube is common. Training in the use of FFBs may be achieved during evaluation of any SLT-intubated patient and through the use of airway simulation and mannequins.[30]

6. Malpositioning and Complications

Use of a DLT is associated with a number of problems, the most important of which is malpositioning (see Fig. 26-7).[26,31] The tube can be malpositioned in several ways.

The DLT may be accidentally directed to the side opposite the desired main stem bronchus. In this case, the lung opposite the side of the connector clamp will collapse. Inadequate separation, increased airway pressures, and instability of the DLT usually occur. Because of the morphology of the DLT curvatures, tracheal or bronchial lacerations may result. If a left-sided DLT is inserted into the right main stem bronchus, it obstructs ventilation to the right upper lobe. It is essential to recognize and correct such a malposition as soon as possible.

The DLT may be passed too far down into the right or the left main stem bronchus. In this case, breath sounds are greatly diminished or not audible over the contralateral side. The tube should be withdrawn until the opening of the tracheal lumen is above the carina.

The DLT may not be inserted far enough, leaving the bronchial lumen opening above the carina. In this position, good breath sounds are heard bilaterally when ventilating through the bronchial lumen, but no breath sounds are audible when ventilating through the tracheal lumen because the inflated bronchial cuff obstructs gas flow from the tracheal lumen. The cuff should be deflated and the DLT rotated and advanced into the desired main stem bronchus.

A right-sided DLT may occlude the right upper lobe orifice. The mean distance from the carina to the right upper lobe orifice is 2.3 ± 0.7 cm in men and 2.1 ± 0.7 cm in women. With right-sided DLTs, the ventilatory slot in the side of the bronchial catheter must overlie the right upper lobe orifice to permit ventilation of this lobe. However, the margin of safety is extremely small and varies from 1 to 8 mm.[32] It is difficult to ensure proper ventilation to the right upper lobe and avoid dislocation of the DLT during surgical manipulation.

The left upper lobe orifice may be obstructed by a left-sided DLT. Traditionally, the take-off of the left upper lobe bronchus was thought to be at a safe distance from the carina and that it would not be obstructed by a left-sided DLT. However, the mean distance between the left upper lobe orifice and the carina is 5.4 ± 0.7 cm in men and 5.0 ± 0.7 cm in women.[33] The average distance between the openings of the right and left lumens on the left-sided disposable tubes is 6.9 cm. An obstruction of the left upper lobe bronchus is possible while the tracheal lumen is still above the carina. There is also a 20% variation in the location of the blue endobronchial cuff on the disposable tubes because this cuff is attached to the tube at the end of the manufacturing process.

Bronchial cuff herniation may occur and obstruct the bronchial lumen if excessive volumes are used to inflate the cuff. The bronchial cuff has also been known to herniate over the tracheal carina and, in the case of a left-sided DLT, to obstruct ventilation to the right main stem bronchus.

A rare complication with DLTs is tracheal laceration or rupture from the stiff tip of the bronchial lumen (Fig. 26-9). Overinflation of the bronchial cuff, inappropriate positioning, and trauma due to intraoperative dislocation that resulted in bronchial rupture have been associated with use of the Robertshaw tube and the disposable DLT.[34] The pressure in the bronchial cuff should be assessed and decreased if the cuff is overinflated. If lung isolation is unnecessary, the bronchial cuff should be deflated and then reinflated slowly to avoid excessive pressure on the bronchial walls. The bronchial cuff should also be deflated during any repositioning of the patient unless lung separation is absolutely required during this time.

In a prospective trial, 60 patients were randomly assigned to two groups. SLV was achieved with an endobronchial blocker or a DLT. Postoperative hoarseness and sore throat were assessed at 24, 48, and 72 hours after surgery. Bronchial injuries and vocal cord lesions were examined by bronchoscopy immediately after surgery. Postoperative hoarseness occurred significantly more frequently in the double-lumen group than the blocker group (44% versus 17%). Similar findings were observed for vocal cord lesions (44% versus 17%). The incidence of bronchial injuries was comparable between groups.[35]

Left Sided Double-Lumen Tube Malpositions

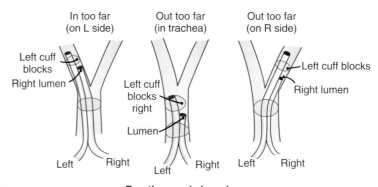

Procedure	Breath sounds heard		
	In too far (on L side)	Out too far (in trachea)	Out too far (on R side)
Clamp right lumen; both cuffs inflated	Left	Left and right	Right
Clamp left lumen; both cuffs inflated	None or faint right	None or very	None or faint left
Clamp left lumen; deflate left cuff	Left only or left and faint right	Left and right	Right only or right and faint left

Figure 26-7 Three major malpositions involving a whole lung are possible for a left-sided, double-lumen tube. The tube can be in too far on the left (i.e., both lumens are in the left main stem bronchus), out too far (i.e., both lumens are in the trachea), or down the right main stem bronchus (i.e., at least the left lumen is in the right main stem bronchus). In each of these malpositions, the left cuff, when fully inflated, can completely block the right lumen. Inflation and deflation of the left cuff while the left lumen is clamped creates a breath sound differential diagnosis of tube malposition. *L*, Left; *R*, right. (From Benumof JL: *Anesthesia for thoracic surgery*, Philadelphia, 1987, Saunders.)

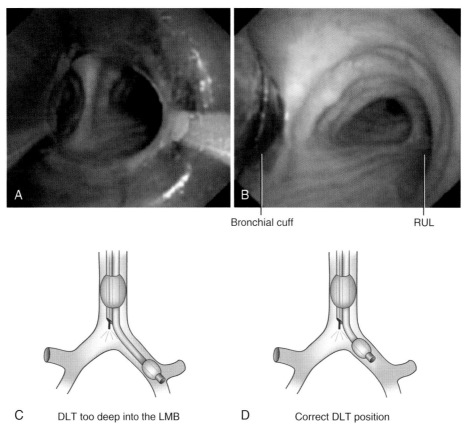

Figure 26-8 Fiberoptic bronchoscopy for a left-sided, double-lumen tube *(DLT)*. **A** and **C,** The DLT is too deep into the left main bronchus *(LMB)*. **B** and **D,** Correct DLT position. *RUL,* Right upper lobe.

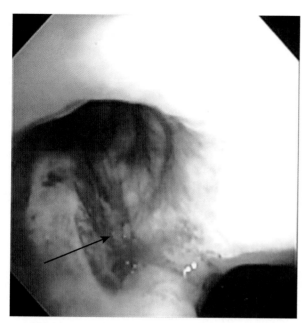

Figure 26-9 Injury (*arrow*) to the main left bronchus.

The most common minor complication is sore throat and temporary hoarseness. Other complications include laryngeal and bronchial injury, tracheobronchial tree disruption,[36] inadvertent suturing of the DLT to thoracic structures, and direct vocal cord injury.[37] Although most of the complications, except malpositioning, have been reported in the older-style DLTs (e.g., Carlens, Robertshaw), the newer designs can also pose risks.[38-40]

7. Exchanging the Double-Lumen Tube for a Single-Lumen Tube

a. PROCEDURE

It is often desirable to replace the DLT with an SLT at the end of the surgical procedure if the patient is to remain intubated postoperatively.

Replacement of a DLT with an SLT can be lifethreatening and must be performed with great caution. Before changing out a DLT, the anesthesiologist must ensure that the patient is prepared for reintubation, well preoxygenated and paralyzed. An SLT with stylet, face mask, and suction must be readily available. Individual bronchial suctioning may be considered, followed by bronchial cuff deflation and suctioning of the oropharynx.

Direct laryngoscopy is then performed, preferably with a Miller blade to allow control of the epiglottis. If the DLT and larynx are well visualized, the blade can be passed into the larynx just past the vocal cords. After the laryngoscope is positioned, an assistant deflates the tracheal cuff of the DLT on instruction, and the DLT is retracted under constant direct vision. When the DLT is removed, the assistant hands off the SLT, which is placed directly into the larynx. It is vital not to lose sight of the larynx and not to reposition the laryngoscope blade. Advancement of the Miller blade beyond the vocal cords may not be necessary, and the use of a Macintosh blade may also be adequate; however, the advantages of the techniques described here should be considered. When the SLT is beyond the cords, the cuff is inflated, the patient is ventilated, and CO_2 confirmation is obtained. If, on initial laryngoscopic inspection of the airway, the vocal cords are too edematous, bloody, or difficult to visualize, the tube exchange should be aborted.

b. AIRWAY EXCHANGE CATHETERS

Alternative techniques of tube exchange involve the use of airway exchange catheters (AECs). Of those available, the Cook AECs (CAECs; Cook Critical Care, Bloomington, IN) are easy to use and allow ventilation if the need arises. The technique involves placing an AEC through the existing DLT and then removing the DLT. The tracheal or bronchial port may be used. Although the bronchial port may provide more stability, it requires full extraction of the DLT to get hold of the AEC distally. Care must be taken to keep the AEC in place as the DLT is removed. After the DLT is removed, the SLT is guided over the AEC into the trachea. Then the AEC is removed while the SLT is kept in place. The cuff is inflated, and ventilation with confirmation of CO_2 is then obtained.

AECs are easy to dislodge at any point during the attempted exchange. The fit between the exchanger and the SLT is often such that the SLT becomes caught at the level of the vocal cords. Rotating the SLT with a corkscrew maneuver can overcome this obstruction, but it can also cause dislodgment of the endotracheal tube (ETT) and the AEC.

A combination technique using a tube exchanger under direct vision may be a safer approach. With this technique, the larynx and the DLT are visualized while an AEC is inserted through the DLT. The CAEC is seen passing into the distal airway; then, under direct vision, the DLT is withdrawn and the AEC position is confirmed. The SLT is advanced over the AEC while the larynx is visualized. The tube is guided under direct vision into the larynx, and the AEC is removed. Proper placement is determined by CO_2 detection and bilateral lung auscultation.

Several tube exchangers are commercially available from Cook Critical Care (Bloomington, IN) and Sheridan Catheter Corporation (Argyle, NY). On these tube exchangers, the depth is marked in centimeters. They are available in a wide range of ODs and easily adapted for oxygen insufflation or jet ventilation. The size of the tube exchanger and the size of the tube to be inserted should be tested before use in a patient. The 11-F tube changer can pass through a 35- to 41-F DLT, whereas the 14-F tube exchanger does not pass through a 35-F DLT.

To prevent lung laceration, the tube exchanger should never be inserted against resistance. Because the first generation of tube exchangers was very stiff, there was a risk for tracheal or bronchial laceration. A tube exchanger with a soft flexible tip was released by Cook Critical Care that is safer to use and is less likely to cause airway laceration. A laryngoscope should always be used to facilitate passage of a tube over the airway guide and past the supraglottic tissues.

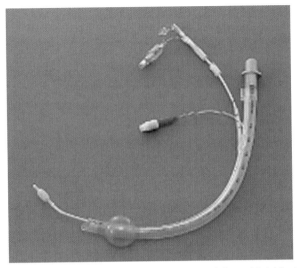

Figure 26-10 Univent single-lumen tube and bronchial blocker system. (Courtesy LMA North America, Inc., San Diego, CA.)

8. Contraindications

Not all patients requiring lung separation are candidates for a DLT. Contraindications to placement of a DLT can be separated into four categories: (1) known or anticipated technical difficulty in DLT placement, (2) dangerous anatomy, (3) difficult or small airways or small patient, and (4) unstable patient. For these patients, alternative means of lung separation are discussed later.

B. Single-Lumen Tubes

In some situations, lung isolation is required, but the use of a DLT is not practical. In these instances, the use of a modified SLT with integrated blockers (i.e., Univent tube [Fig. 26-10]) or the use of blockers in conjunction with a standard SLT is appropriate.

1. Indications

a. DIFFICULT AIRWAYS

Patients presenting with difficult airway anatomy can be a particular challenge for lung isolation, because the placement of a conventional DLT can be impossible in such patients.[41] Use of an SLT or a Univent tube (Fuji Systems, Tokyo, Japan) is advised, because these devices may be more easily placed than DLTs.[42]

For patients who have an SLT in place and have developed significant airway edema or are in the prone or lateral position and then require lung isolation, use of a bronchial blocker device is the safest technique to invoke lung isolation. Similarly, in patients who have an SLT and develop traumatized or bloodied airways, the insertion of a DLT is very difficult because of inability to visualize the airway anatomy properly through an FOB. The use of an SLT or Univent tube allows large-bore airway suctioning and improved safety for lung isolation.

Postoperative airway edema is inevitable in some cases, and the prospect of changing a DLT to an SLT postoperatively poses too great a risk to the patient. It is worth considering the use of an SLT with a bronchial blocker

or a Univent tube. The bronchial blockers can be withdrawn after they are no longer required, without removal of the ETT, and the patient may be transported to the ICU and weaned from the ventilator.

In patients with small airways anatomy, it is often not possible to place a DLT. The use of an SLT (with or without a bronchial blocker) or a Univent tube is the only method of isolating the lung without manual surgical compression of the lung. ETTs as small as 5.0 mm can accommodate blockers. With ETTs that are smaller than a 5.0-mm inner diameter (ID), it is not possible to pass the bronchial blocker and the FFB through the tube. In cases requiring a very small ETT (<5.0 mm), the technique of "main stemming" the ETT to achieve lung isolation can be used.

b. SEGMENTAL LOBE ISOLATION

Selective blockade of lung segments is sometimes desired. In these cases, a bronchial blocker device can be advanced into the desired lung segment.[43] For example, a patient with a left lung pneumonia and right lower lobe and right middle lobe bronchocutaneous fistulas would likely fail this method because of profound desaturation from inability to ventilate the healthy right upper lobe. Selective lobar blockade is considered an advantageous technique to avoid total lung collapse and improve oxygenation.[44] An SLT with a bronchial blocker isolating the right lower lobe and right middle lobe allows adequate saturation while the patient recovers from the pneumonia and the sealing of the bronchocutaneous fistula. It is very difficult to isolate lung segments with a DLT; combined use of a DLT and bronchial blocker devices would likely be required.

2. Disadvantages

a. LUNG DEFLATION

When bronchial blockers are used to isolate the lung, deflation of the blocked lung is slow because the gas trapped in the isolated lung cannot escape and must be reabsorbed. Deflation of the lung with the Univent tube is somewhat faster because of a small lumen extending through the blocker. It is also possible to administer suction to the blocker lumen of the Univent tube and facilitate lung deflation. To accelerate lung deflation, the patient should be ventilated with 100% O_2 for several minutes before bronchial cuff inflation. This accelerates deflation because O_2 is reabsorbed more rapidly than air. If the patient's pulmonary function permits, the patient can be temporarily disconnected from the ventilator circuit and both lungs allowed to deflate spontaneously. The bronchial blocker cuff is then inflated, and the patient is reconnected to the ventilator for SLV.

b. SECRETION REMOVAL

The relatively large lumens of DLTs allow passage of small suction catheters and good removal of blood or secretions. The same is not true of SLTs with bronchial blockers or Univent tubes; suctioning beyond the blockers is not possible during lung isolation. Suctioning of the nonblocked lung is possible, although care must be taken not to dislodge the bronchial blocker from its position.

c. BRONCHIAL MUCOSAL DAMAGE

Unlike DLTs, which use high-volume, low-pressure tracheal and bronchial cuffs, bronchial blockers and Univent tube blockers have low-volume, higher-pressure cuffs. Prolonged inflation of the bronchial balloons can result in mucosal ischemia and irreversible damage. For this reason, it is necessary to deflate the bronchial cuff at the earliest opportunity after lung isolation is no longer required.

Some practitioners advocate techniques of "just-seal" bronchial cuff inflation volumes to minimize mucosal ischemia and damage.[5,8] These techniques may be of little or no value, however, because most of those described are cumbersome and require specialized connectors between the ETT, the blocking device, and the circuit. The cuff pressure required for the bronchial blocker can change because of compliance changes of the ventilated lung.

d. TREATMENT OF DESATURATION

In all cases of SLV and desaturation, it is necessary to ensure that the patient is receiving 100% O_2, ensure adequate ventilation and perfusion, and verify tube and blocker placement. After these issues are resolved, the desaturation can be further treated.

With DLTs, desaturation with SLV can be treated by several maneuvers. The nondependent lung can have CPAP applied, the nondependent lung can be partially expanded, PEEP to the dependent lung can be altered, and if necessary, both lungs can be ventilated temporarily or throughout the procedure. Not all of these options are readily available for SLTs and Univent tubes. Because of the fully obstructive nature of the bronchial blockers, the nondependent lung cannot receive CPAP. Because of the lack of stability of the bronchial blocker line, deflation of the blocker results in shifting of its location, requiring FFB position confirmation each time. Intermittent partial or intermittent full inflation of the isolated lung may be cumbersome.

C. Univent Tubes

1. Anatomy

The Univent tube is a Silastic SLT with a built-in chamber that allows advancement of the integrated blocker (see Fig. 26-10).[41,45,46] The integrated blocker has a small lumen along its entire length that facilitates lung deflation and allows very limited suctioning. At the distal tip of the blocker is a small balloon, and the proximal end of the blocker section contains a lumen cap. This cap needs to be engaged when the blocker balloon is deflated during full lung ventilation. Failure to engage the cap when the blocker balloon is deflated results in a circuit leak. Univent tubes are available in many sizes (Table 26-2), all designated by internal lumen size. Because of the thickness of the tube wall and the integrated blocker chamber, the outer size of these devices is much larger than that of a similarly designated SLT. For example, a 7.5-mm Univent tube has an 11.2-mm OD, compared with the 10.2-mm OD of a 7.5-mm SLT. Despite the larger size, these tubes are very useful.

TABLE 26-2
Comparative Tube Sizes

Univent ID (mm)	Univent Gauge (F) of Single Main Lumen*	Univent OD (mm) Lateral/AP†	Equivalent SLT OD (mm)	Equivalent DLT (F)
7.5	31	11.0/12.0	9.6	35
8.0	33	11.5/13.0	10.9	37
8.5	35	12.0/13.5	11.6	39
9.0	37	12.5/14.0	12.2	41

*Marked on the tube.
†The AP diameter is greater than the lateral diameter because of the bronchial blocker lumen.
Data from MacGillivray RG: Evaluation of a new tracheal tube with a moveable bronchus blocker. *Anaesthesia* 43:687, 1988; and Slinger P: Con: The Univent tube is not the best method of providing one-lung ventilation. *J Cardiothorac Vasc Anesth* 7:108-112, 1993.
AP, Anteroposterior; *DLT,* double-lumen tube (Broncho-Cath); *F,* French measurement (1 F = OD in mm × 3); *ID,* internal diameter; *OD,* outer diameter; *SLT,* single-lumen tube (Shiley).

2. Positioning

Before the Univent tube is placed, it must be prepared. Preparation involves removal of the distal and proximal tension wires that help keep the Univent's shape during storage. The cuffs of the bronchial blocker and the main tube should be checked and deflated. After the tip of the bronchial blocker is bent to the shape of a hockey stick, it is retracted into the blocker chamber so that its distal tip is flush with the main tube. The tube is then inserted into the trachea with the tracheal balloon just distal to the cords. The main tube cuff is then inflated and secured at a distance of at least 2 to 3 cm between the distal tip of the main tube and the carina (Fig. 26-11) so that the curved shape of the blocker can be maintained and manipulated as it is advanced beyond the tip of the main tube. Failure to provide this adequate distance between the tip of the main tube and the carina makes directional control of the bronchial blocker very difficult.

Because the material of the Univent tube makes passage of a nonlubricated FFB difficult, the scope should be well lubricated before it is inserted into the main segment of the tube. It is often helpful to attach some type of self-sealing diaphragm device between the Univent tube and the elbow connection of the circuit. This allows continuous ventilation while the blocker is being positioned with the FFB. The FFB is advanced beyond the distal tip of the tube, and the anterior tracheal rings are identified, allowing proper orientation of the right and left main stem bronchi. The blocker portion of the tube is then visually advanced while the main tube position is maintained (see Fig. 26-11).

Placement of the blocker into the desired main stem bronchus is achieved by advancing the blocker with a clockwise or a counterclockwise rotation. If this maneuver is not sufficient to align the blocker into the desired bronchus, the entire Univent tube may be rotated in the desired direction to assist blocker orientation. The blocker is advanced into the correct location, and the locking cuff at the proximal end of the blocker is secured. It is useful

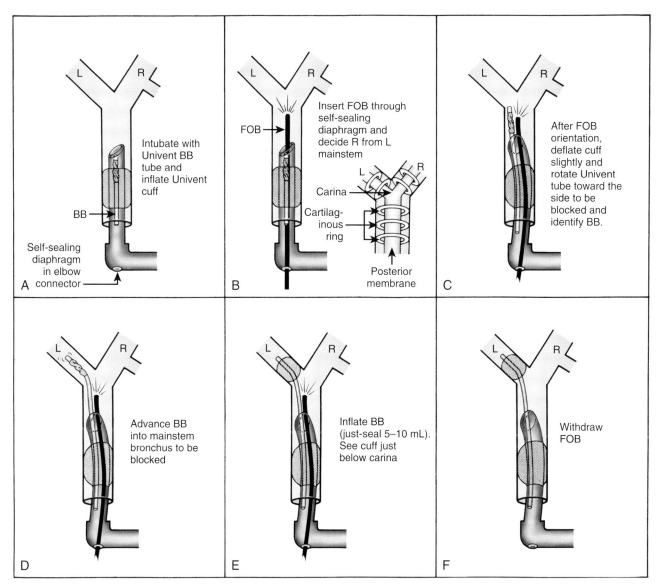

Figure 26-11 Sequential steps of the fiberoptically aided method of inserting and positioning the Univent bronchial blocker *(BB)* in the left main stem bronchus. Ventilation of one or two lungs is achieved by inflating or deflating, respectively, the bronchial blocker balloon. *FOB,* Fiberoptic bronchoscope; *L,* left; *R,* right. (From Benumof JL: *Anesthesia for thoracic surgery,* Philadelphia, 1987, Saunders.)

to note the distance marker on the blocker. If lung isolation is desired, the blocker cuff is inflated (best performed under direct FFB visualization), and the proximal cap of the blocker may be disengaged to enhance lung deflation (see Fig. 26-11). Blind placement of the blocker is often unsuccessful. Blind placement may result in trauma to the tracheobronchial tree, resulting in complications including bleeding or even tension pneumothorax. Limitations of the Univent tube shown in Table 26-3. The solutions related to Univent blocker issues may be applicable to other types of bronchial blockers.

D. Endobronchial Blockers

In modern thoracic anesthesia, lung separation can be achieved with a reusable bronchial blocker.[47] Inflation of the cuff at the distal end of the blocker blocks ventilation to that lung. All modern blockers have a lumen that permits suctioning of the airway distal to the catheter tip, and depending on the clinical circumstance, oxygen can be insufflated through the catheter lumen. The main advantage of these blockers is that they can be placed through a conventional SLT. When a blocker is placed in the right main bronchus, it usually is positioned close to the carina to block the right upper lobe. Because the blocker balloon requires a high distending pressure, it easily slips out of the bronchus into the trachea because of changes in position or surgical manipulation. That movement can result in obstructing ventilation and losing the seal between the two lungs. The loss of lung separation can be a life-threatening situation if it was performed to prevent spillage of pus, blood, or fluid from bronchopulmonary lavage. Bronchial blockers are rarely used for these types of cases in which lung isolation is required.

TABLE 26-3

Univent Bronchial Blocker Tube: Limitations and Solutions

Limitation	Solution
Slow inflation time	Deflate the bronchial blocker cuff, and administer a positive-pressure breath through the main single lumen. Then carefully administer one short, high-pressure (20-30 psi) jet ventilation.
Slow deflation time	Deflate the bronchial blocker cuff, and compress and evacuate the lung through the main single lumen. Then apply suction to the bronchial blocker lumen.
Blockage of bronchial blocker lumen by blood or pus	Suction, use a wire stylet, and then suction.
High-pressure cuff	Use a just-seal volume of air.
Intraoperative leak in bronchial blocker cuff	Ensure the bronchial blocker cuff is positioned below the carina. Increase the inflation volume, and rearrange the surgical field.

1. Indications

Indications for the use of a bronchial blocker are shown in Box 26-2. Because the blocker is placed through an SLT, it avoids the use of a DLT in a patient with a difficult airway. The use of a bronchial blocker also eliminates the need to change a DLT to an SLT at the conclusion of the procedure. This is important, because the airway at the conclusion of the procedure may be different from that in the initial period due to secretions and edema. In the past, Fogarty vascular embolectomy catheters were used for lung separation, but there is no indication for their use in the current practice of thoracic anesthesia. The balloon of the Fogarty is high pressure and low volume, and there is no lumen to allow egress of gas from the lung to facilitate deflation. The characteristics of bronchial blockers are summarized in Table 26-4.

2. Coaxial Stand-Alone Endotracheal Blockers

a. ARNDT ENDOBRONCHIAL BLOCKER

A snare-guided bronchial blocker, the Arndt Endobronchial Blocker (Cook Critical Care), was introduced to address the previously described problems. It is a wire-guided catheter with a loop snare (Fig. 26-12). A fiberscope is passed through the loop of the bronchial blocker and then guided into the desired bronchus. The

---

Box 26-2 Indications for the Use of Endobronchial Blockers

Lung isolation versus lung separation
Video-assisted thoracoscopy, increased number of patients who require one-lung ventilation
To avoid the need for tube exchange
Patients with difficult airways
  1. Patients after laryngeal or pharyngeal surgery
  2. Patients with a tracheotomy
  3. Patients with distorted bronchial anatomy (e.g., aneurysm compression, intraluminal tumor)
  4. Patients who require nasotracheal intubation
  5. Patients with an immobility or kyphoscoliosis
Surgical procedures not involving the lung
  1. Esophageal surgery
  2. Spinal surgery that requires a transthoracic approach
  3. Minimally invasive cardiac surgery
Special management circumstances
  1. Video-assisted thoracoscopy in which a quick look or wedge resection of the chest is planned
  2. Possible segmental blockade in a patient unable to tolerate one-lung ventilation
  3. Morbidly obese patients
  4. Small adult or pediatric patients
  5. Patients who require intraoperative lung isolation
  6. Patients who arrive in the operating room intubated from the intensive care unit

---

TABLE 26-4

Characteristics of Endobronchial Blockers

Characteristics	Arndt Blocker	Cohen Blocker	Uniblocker	EZ-Blocker
Size	9 F, 7 F, 5 F (pediatric)	9.0 F	9.0 F, 5.0 F (pediatric)	7.0 F
Guidance feature	Wire loop to snare the FB	Deflecting tip	Prefixed bend	Double-lumen bifurcated tip
Recommended ETT size (mm)	9-F 8.0 ETT 7-F 7.0 ETT 5-F 4.5 ETT	8.0 ETT	8.0 ETT	8.0 ETT
Central lumen	1.8 mm	1.8 mm	2.0 mm	1.4 mm (divided in half)
Murphy eye	Only in the 9-F device	Yes	No	No
Disadvantages	BB not visualized during insertion	Expensive	No steering mechanism; prefixed bend	Each lumen is too small; impossible to suction

BB, Bronchial blocker; *ETT,* endotracheal tube; *FFB,* flexible fiberoptic bronchoscope.

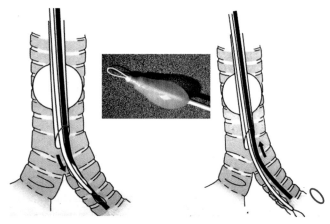

Figure 26-12 Arndt endobronchial blocker.

blocker is then slid distally over the fiberscope and into the selected bronchus. Bronchoscopic visualization confirms blocker placement and bronchial occlusion (Fig. 26-13).

This balloon-tipped catheter has a hollow lumen of 1.6 mm, which allows suction to facilitate the collapse of the lung and insufflation of oxygen to the nondependent lung. The balloon is available in a spherical or elliptic shape. The set contains a multiport adapter (Fig. 26-14) that allows uninterrupted ventilation during positioning of the blocker. The wire may then be removed, and a 1.6-mm lumen may be used as a suction port or for oxygen insufflation. In the first generation of this device, it was not possible to reinsert the string after it had been pulled out, losing the ability to redirect the bronchial blocker if necessary. External reinforcement of the wire allows its reintroduction through the lumen. The OD necessitates a large SLT (at least 8.0 mm) to accommodate the bronchial blocker. The Arndt blocker is available in a 7-F size for adults and in a 5-F pediatric size. A disadvantage of the Arndt blocker is that it is advanced blindly over the FFB into the desired main bronchus. In some cases, the tip of the blocker may get caught at the main carina or at the Murphy eye of the SLT.

b. COHEN FLEXITIP ENDOBRONCHIAL BLOCKER

The Cohen Flexitip Endobronchial Blocker (Cook Critical Care) is designed for use through an SLT with the aid of a small-diameter (4.0-mm) FOB (Fig. 26-15).[48] The blocker has a rotating wheel that deflects the soft tip by

Left-side blockade

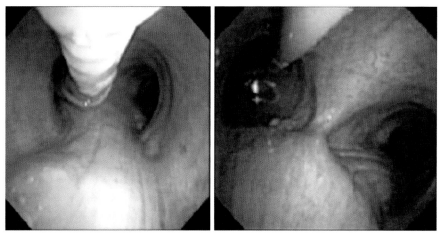

Right-side blockade

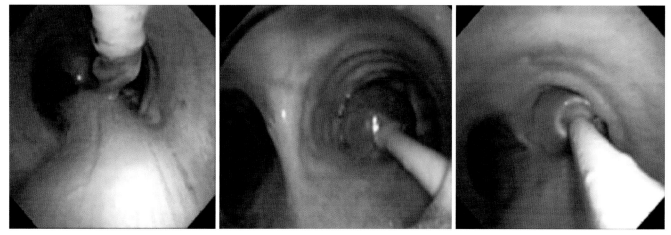

Figure 26-13 *Top,* Left main stem bronchus bronchial blocker in position before *(left)* and after *(right)* "just-seal" inflation. *Bottom left,* Right main stem bronchus bronchial blocker in the entering position. *Bottom center,* Bronchial blocker is too deep, occluding only the bronchus intermedius. *Bottom right,* Bronchial blocker in the right main stem bronchus with a just-seal inflation.

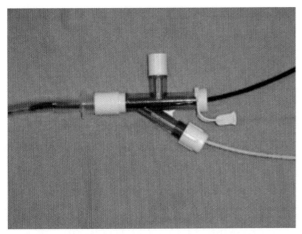

Figure 26-14 Multiport adapter for the Arndt endobronchial blocker.

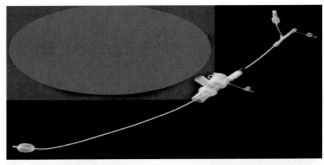

Figure 26-16 Uniblocker is a 9-F, balloon-tipped, angled blocker. (Courtesy of Fuji Systems Corp, Tokyo, Japan.)

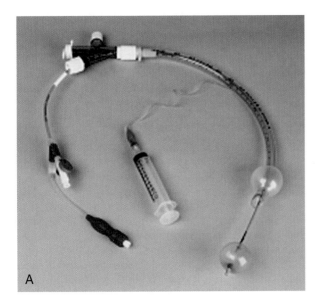

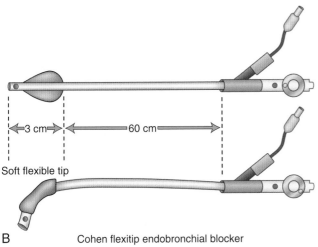

Soft flexible tip

Cohen flexitip endobronchial blocker

Figure 26-15 Cohen Flexitip endobronchial blocker. **A,** Equipment. **B,** Diagram.

more than 90 degrees and easily directs it into the desired bronchus. The blocker cuff is a high-volume, low-pressure balloon inflated through a 0.4-mm lumen inside the wall of the blocker. Its pear shape provides an adequate seal of the bronchus. It takes 6 to 8 mL of air to seal the bronchus with the cuff. The distinctive blue cuff is easily recognizable by FOB. It is best to inflate the cuff under direct vision by FOB, which is particularly important during right-sided blockade. In this case, the cuff is inflated near the carina, and proper position and cuff inflation are critical. The 9-F blocker has a central main lumen (1.6 mm) that allows limited suctioning of secretions and insufflation of oxygen to the collapsed lung.

c. UNIBLOCKER

Fuji Systems introduced a 9-F, balloon-tipped, angled blocker with a multiple-port adapter that is essentially the same design as the Univent tube blocker, but it can be used as an independent blocker passed by means of a special connector through a standard ETT (Fig. 26-16). It has a prefixed bend to facilitate insertion into the desired bronchus. This blocker is also available in a 5.0-F size for the pediatric population.

d. EZ-BLOCKER

The latest addition to the endobronchial blocker design is the EZ-Blocker (IQ Medical Ventures, Rotterdam, The Netherlands). It is a 7-F, four-lumen, 75-cm, disposable endobronchial blocker used to facilitate selective lung ventilation (Fig. 26-17). It has a symmetrical, Y-shaped bifurcation, and both branches have an inflatable cuff on each arm and a central lumen. The bifurcation resembles the bifurcation of the trachea. During insertion through a standard ETT, each of the two distal ends is placed into a main stem bronchus. The selected lung is isolated by inflating the blocker's balloon to the least volume necessary to occlude the main stem under bronchoscopic visualization. This device should offer an advantage during bilateral procedures, because each lung can be deflated without the need for repositioning the blocker. The clinical experience with this device is limited.

The effectiveness of lung isolation with three devices—the left-sided Broncho-Cath DLT, the Univent torque-control blocker, and the wire-guided Arndt—has been compared in a prospective, randomized trial. There was no significant difference in tube malpositions for the three devices, but it took longer to position the Arndt

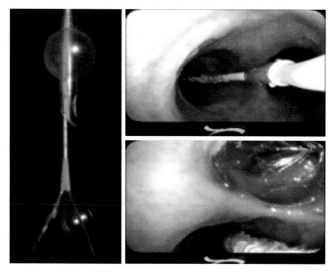

Figure 26-17 EZ-Blocker: device, insertion, and deployment.

blocker (86 versus 56 seconds) than the left-sided DLT and the Univent. Excluding the time for tube placement, the Arndt group also took longer for the lung to collapse (26 minutes), compared with the DLT group (18 minutes) or the Univent group (19.5 minutes). Unlike the other two groups, most of the Arndt patients required suction to achieve lung collapse. After lung isolation was achieved, overall surgical exposure was rated excellent for the three groups (Fig. 26-18). One minute longer to position a bronchial blocker or 6 minutes longer to collapse the lung with the bronchial blocker is insignificant considering the length of the thoracic procedure. The risk-benefit ratio and the patient safety profile for each patient and the clinical experience of the anesthesiologist should be considered when choosing the method for lung isolation.[49,50]

Another study evaluated the use of the Cohen blocker, the Arndt blocker, the Uniblocker, and a DLT in four groups of 26 patients in each group. The investigators found no differences among the groups in the time taken to insert these lung isolation devices or in the quality of the lung collapse.[51] The grading was done by the operating surgeons, who were blinded to which device was used. The number of cuff dislocations was higher among

the bronchial blocker groups, which was highest with the Arndt blocker, possibly because the study protocol used the elliptical cuff. Regardless of the type of bronchial blocker or DLT selected to provide SLV, the choice of technique depends on the clinical circumstances and the physician's experience and comfort with a particular device. However, the clinician should not limit his or her practice to the use of only one device but rather be versatile and comfortable in the use of several.

It is possible to perform lung isolation without the use of specialized tubes. In these cases, a bronchial blocking device is inserted through the lumen of an SLT (Fig. 26-19) or outside the SLT between the tracheal cuff and the trachea (Fig. 26-20). Placement is confirmed by FOB.

Any device that has a balloon-tipped catheter can be used as a bronchial blocker (see Fig. 26-19).[52] The most common devices used are Fogarty embolectomy catheters and the Cook bronchial blockers.[53]

a. FOGARTY CATHETERS

The Fogarty catheters come with a rigid wire stylet in place. This allows the creation of a hockey-stick curve at the distal end of the catheter, facilitating directional control of the blocker tip. After the catheter is positioned by FFB, the stylet is removed and a stopcock is placed over the balloon port. Under FFB visualization, the balloon is inflated until the desired lumen is occluded. The Fogarty is then secured to the ETT. The main disadvantage of this device is the inability to suction or insufflate distal to the high-pressure, low-volume cuff.

b. ARNDT AND COHEN BRONCHIAL BLOCKERS

Cook Critical Care has produced two specialized bronchial blockers, the Arndt and Cohen bronchial blockers. Each blocker uses a high-volume, low-pressure cuff and is introduced through a multiport airway adapter. This adapter has a sealing diaphragm that allows passage of blockers of different sizes and incorporates a separate port for introduction of the FFB. The multiport adapter can be used with any stand-alone bronchial blocker.

The Arndt bronchial blocker comes in various sizes and has a small central lumen to allow minimal insufflation and suctioning. It has a monofilament guide loop through which an FFB can be passed. On placement of the FFB in the desired tip position, release of the loop snare and advancement of the blocker to the tip of the FFB places the bronchial blocker in position while releasing the FFB from the loop. The Cohen bronchial blocker also comes in various sizes and employs a directional tip, which potentially makes placement of this device easier than placement of the Arndt bronchial blocker.

The main disadvantage of these commercial blockers is that their ODs are greater than those of the Fogarty catheters, making placement in ETTs with an ID smaller than 6.0 mm difficult to impossible. When a small ETT (<6.0-mm ID) is used, a Cook multiport adapter with a small Fogarty catheter may be preferred.

3. Para-axial Endotracheal Blockers

The advantage of placing the bronchial blocker device outside the SLT is that this method allows blocker placement with smaller ETTs because the blocker does not

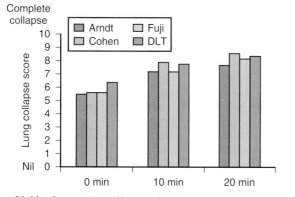

Figure 26-18 Comparison of lung collapse times for three bronchial blockers and a double-lumen tube.

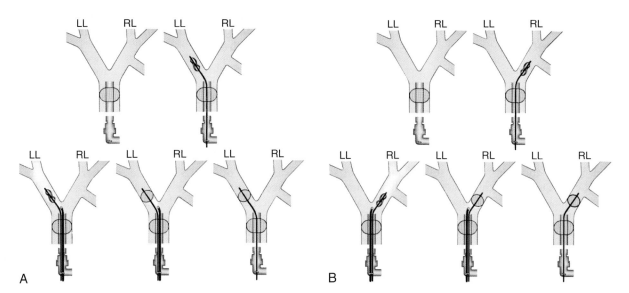

Figure 26-19   Sequence for lung separation with a single-lumen tube (SLT) and a bronchial blocker within the SLT. **A,** Left lung *(LL)* bronchial blocker. **B,** Right lung *(RL)* bronchial blocker. The bronchial blocker (Fogarty embolectomy catheter) is placed in the correct main stem bronchus under fiberoptic vision. (From Benumof JL: *Anesthesia for thoracic surgery,* Philadelphia, 1987, Saunders.)

share the ETT lumen (see Fig. 26-20). It is often easier to position the bronchial blocker with this method, because the blocker and the FFB do not become caught up with each other within the ETT lumen. Disadvantages of this para-tube technique include the need to perform laryngoscopy to place the bronchial blocker into the

trachea, the need to deflate the tracheal cuff while positioning the bronchial blocker, and the potential of rupturing the ETT cuff while manipulating the bronchial blocker. Because of these disadvantages, a coaxial placement may be advised, provided ETT lumen size is not an issue.

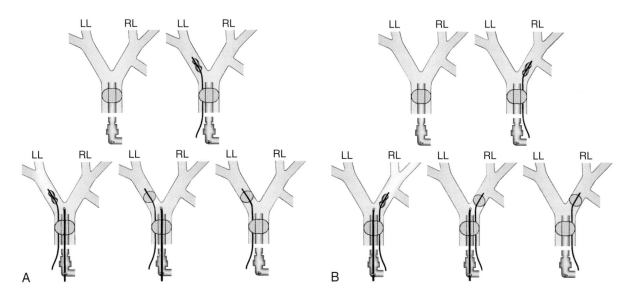

Figure 26-20   Separation of two lungs with a single-lumen tube (SLT), flexible fiberoptic bronchoscope (FFB), and a left lung **(A)** and a right lung **(B)** bronchial blocker that is outside the SLT. The SLT is inserted, and the patient is ventilated *(upper left diagrams).* The bronchial blocker is passed alongside the indwelling endotracheal tube *(upper right diagrams).* The FFB is passed through a self-sealing diaphragm in the elbow connector to the endotracheal tube and is used to place the bronchial blocker into the appropriate main stem bronchus under direct vision *(lower left diagrams).* The balloon on the bronchial blocker is inflated under direct vision and is positioned just below the tracheal carina *(lower middle diagrams).* During insertion and use of the FFB *(lower panels),* the self-sealing diaphragm allows the patient to continue to receive positive-pressure ventilation around the FFB but within the lumens of the ETT. *LL,* Left lung; *RL,* right lung. (From Benumof JL: *Anesthesia for thoracic surgery,* Philadelphia, 1987, Saunders.)

V. PEDIATRIC LUNG ISOLATION

A. Ventilation-Perfusion During Thoracic Surgery

Ventilation is normally distributed preferentially to dependent regions of the lung so that there is a gradient of increasing ventilation from the most nondependent to the most dependent lung segments. Because of gravitational effects, perfusion normally follows a similar distribution, with increased blood flow to dependent lung segments. Ventilation and perfusion are normally well matched. During thoracic surgery, several factors act to increase the $\dot{V}/\dot{Q}$ mismatch. General anesthesia, neuromuscular blockade, and mechanical ventilation cause a decrease in functional residual capacity (FRC) of both lungs. Compression of the dependent lung in the lateral decubitus position can cause atelectasis. Surgical retraction or SLV, or both, can result in collapse of the operative lung. Hypoxic pulmonary vasoconstriction, which acts to divert blood flow away from the underventilated lung, thereby minimizing the $\dot{V}/\dot{Q}$ mismatch, may be diminished by inhalational anesthetic agents and other vasodilating drugs. These factors apply to infants, children, and adults. The overall effect of the lateral decubitus position on $\dot{V}/\dot{Q}$ mismatching is different in infants than in older children and adults.

In adults with unilateral lung disease, oxygenation is optimal when the patient is placed in the lateral decubitus position with the healthy lung dependent and the diseased lung nondependent.[54] Presumably, this is related to an increase in blood flow to the dependent, healthy lung and a decrease in blood flow to the nondependent, diseased lung resulting from the hydrostatic pressure (or gravitational) gradient between the two lungs. This phenomenon promotes $\dot{V}/\dot{Q}$ matching in the adult patient who is undergoing thoracic surgery in the lateral decubitus position.

In infants with unilateral lung disease, on the other hand, oxygenation is improved when the healthy lung is nondependent.[55] Several factors account for this discrepancy between adults and infants. Infants have a soft, easily compressible rib cage that cannot fully protect the underlying lung. The FRC is closer to the residual volume, making airway closure likely to occur in the dependent lung even during tidal breathing.[56] When the adult is placed in the lateral decubitus position, the dependent diaphragm has a mechanical advantage because it is "loaded" by the abdominal hydrostatic pressure gradient. This pressure gradient is reduced in infants, reducing the functional advantage of the dependent diaphragm. The infant's small size also results in a reduced hydrostatic pressure gradient between the nondependent and dependent lungs. Consequently, the favorable increase in perfusion to the dependent, ventilated lung is reduced in infants.

The infant's increased O_2 requirement, coupled with a small FRC, predisposes to hypoxemia. Infants normally consume 6 to 8 mL of O_2/kg/min, compared with a normal O_2 consumption in adults of 2 to 3 mL/kg/min.[57] For these reasons, infants are at increased risk for significant O_2 desaturation during surgery in the lateral decubitus position.

B. Indications and Techniques for Single-Lung Ventilation in Infants and Children

Before 1995, almost all thoracic surgery in children was performed by thoracotomy. In most cases, anesthesiologists ventilated both lungs with a conventional ETT, and surgeons retracted the operative lung to gain exposure to the surgical field. During the past decade, the use of video-assisted thoracoscopic surgery (VATS) has dramatically increased in both adults and children. Reported advantages of VATS include smaller chest incisions, reduced postoperative pain, and more rapid postoperative recovery compared with thoracotomy.[58-60] Advances in surgical technique as well as technology, including high-resolution microchip cameras and smaller endoscopic instruments, have facilitated the application of VATS in smaller patients.

VATS is being used extensively for pleural débridement in patients with emphysema, lung biopsy, or wedge resections for interstitial lung disease; mediastinal masses; or metastatic lesions. More extensive pulmonary resections, including segmentectomy and lobectomy, have been performed for lung abscess, bullous disease, sequestrations, lobar emphysema, cystic adenomatoid malformation, and neoplasms. In selected centers, more advanced procedures have been reported, including closure of patent ductus arteriosus, repair of hiatal hernias, and anterior spinal fusion.

VATS can be performed while both lungs are being ventilated with the use of CO_2 insufflation and placement of a retractor to displace lung tissue in the operative field. However, SLV is extremely desirable during VATS because lung deflation improves visualization of thoracic contents and may reduce lung injury caused by the use of retractors.[11] There are several different techniques that can be used for SLV in children.

C. Single-Lumen Tube

The simplest means of providing SLV is to intubate the ipsilateral main stem bronchus with a conventional SLT.[61] When the left bronchus is to be intubated, the bevel of the ETT is rotated 180 degrees and the head is turned to the right.[62] The ETT is advanced into the bronchus until breath sounds on the operative side disappear. An FFB may be passed through, or alongside, the ETT to confirm or guide placement. When a cuffed ETT is used, the distance from the tip of the tube to the distal cuff must be shorter than the length of the bronchus, so that the cuff is not entirely in the bronchus.[63] This technique is simple and requires no special equipment other than an FFB. This may be the preferred technique of SLV in emergency situations such as airway hemorrhage or contralateral tension pneumothorax.

Problems can occur when using an SLT for SLV. If a smaller, uncuffed ETT is used, it may be difficult to provide an adequate seal of the intended bronchus. This may prevent the operative lung from adequately collapsing or fail to protect the healthy, ventilated lung from contamination by purulent material from the contralateral lung. One is unable to suction the operative lung using this technique. Hypoxemia may occur because of obstruction of the upper lobe bronchus, especially when the short right main stem bronchus is intubated.

Variations of this technique have been described, including intubation of both bronchi independently with small ETTs.[64-67] One main stem bronchus is initially intubated with an ETT, after which another ETT is advanced over an FFB into the opposite bronchus.

D. Balloon-Tipped Bronchial Blockers

A Fogarty embolectomy catheter or an end-hole, balloon wedge catheter may be used for bronchial blockade to provide SLV.[52,68-70] Placement of a Fogarty catheter is facilitated by bending the tip of its stylet toward the bronchus on the operative side. An FFB may be used to reposition the catheter and confirm appropriate placement. When an end-hole catheter is placed outside the ETT, the bronchus on the operative side is initially intubated with an ETT. A guidewire is then advanced into that bronchus through the ETT. The ETT is removed, and the bronchial blocker is advanced over the guidewire into the bronchus. An ETT is then reinserted into the trachea alongside the blocker catheter. The catheter balloon is positioned in the proximal main stem bronchus under fiberoptic visual guidance. With an inflated bronchial blocker balloon, the airway is completely sealed, providing more predictable lung collapse and better operating conditions than with an ETT in the bronchus.

A potential problem with this technique is dislodgment of the bronchial blocker balloon into the trachea. The inflated balloon blocks ventilation to both lungs and prevents collapse of the operated lung. The balloons of most catheters currently used for bronchial blockade have low-volume, high-pressure properties, and overdistention can damage or even rupture the airway.[71] One study, however, reported that bronchial blocker cuffs produced lower ratios of cuff to tracheal pressure than DLTs do.[72] When closed-tip bronchial blockers are used, the operative lung cannot be suctioned, and CPAP cannot be provided to the operative lung if needed.

Adapters have been used that facilitate ventilation during placement of a bronchial blocker through an indwelling ETT.[73,74] A 5-F endobronchial blocker that is suitable for use in children with a multiport adapter and FFB has been described (Cook Critical Care).[75] The risk of hypoxemia during blocker placement is diminished, and repositioning of the blocker may be performed with FFB guidance during surgery. Even with an FFB with a 2.2-mm OD, the indwelling ETT must have an ID of 5.0 mm or larger to allow passage of the catheter and FFB. This technique typically is limited to children older than 18 months to 2 years.

E. Univent Tube

The Univent tube is a conventional ETT with a second lumen containing a small tube that can be advanced into a bronchus.[45,76,77] A balloon located at the distal end of this small tube serves as a blocker. Univent tubes require an FFB for successful placement. Univent tubes are available in sizes as small as 3.5- and 4.5-mm ID for use in

children older than 6 years of age.[78] Because the blocker tube is firmly attached to the main ETT, displacement of the Univent blocker balloon is less likely than when other bronchial blocker techniques are used. The blocker tube has a small lumen, which allows egress of gas and can be used to insufflate O_2 or suction the operated lung.

A disadvantage of the Univent tube is the large amount of cross-sectional area occupied by the blocker channel, especially in the smaller tubes. Smaller Univent tubes have a disproportionately high resistance to gas flow.[79] The Univent tube's blocker balloon has low-volume, high-pressure characteristics, and mucosal injury can occur during normal inflation.[80,81]

F. Double-Lumen Tubes

All DLTs are essentially two tubes of unequal length molded together. The shorter tube ends in the trachea and the longer tube in the bronchus. Marraro described a DLT for infants that consists of two separate uncuffed ETTs of different length attached longitudinally.[82] This tube is not available in the United States. DLTs for older children and adults have cuffs located on the tracheal and bronchial lumens. The tracheal cuff, when inflated, allows PPV. The inflated bronchial cuff allows ventilation to be diverted to either or both lungs and protects each lung from contamination from the contralateral side.

Conventional plastic DLTs, previously available only in adult sizes (35, 37, 39, and 41 F), are now available in smaller sizes. The smallest cuffed DLT is 26 F (Rusch, Duluth, GA) and may be used in children as young as 8 years of age. DLTs are also available in sizes 28 and 32 F (Mallinckrodt Medical, St. Louis, MO), which are suitable for children 10 years of age or older.

DLTs are inserted in children by the same technique as is used in adults.[83] The tip of the tube is inserted just beyond the vocal cords, and the stylet is withdrawn. The DLT is rotated 90 degrees to the appropriate side and then advanced into the bronchus. In the adult population, the depth of insertion is directly related to the height of the patient.[84] No equivalent measurements are yet available in children. If FOB is to be used to confirm tube placement, an FFB with a small diameter and sufficient length must be available.[85]

A DLT offers the advantage of ease of insertion as well as the ability to suction and oxygenate the operative lung with CPAP. Left-sided DLTs are preferred to right-sided instruments because of the shorter length of the right main bronchus.[19] Right-sided DLTs are more difficult to position accurately because of the greater risk of right upper lobe obstruction.

DLTs are safe and easy to use. There have been very few reports of airway damage from DLTs in adults and none in children. Their high-volume, low-pressure cuffs should not damage the airway if they are not overinflated with air or distended with nitrous oxide while in place.

There is significant variability in overall size and airway dimensions in children, particularly in teenagers. For average-sized children 8 to 10 years of age, a 26-F DLT may be appropriate. However, in patients 11 to 14 years of age, appropriate DLT size may range from 26 to 32 F.

Estimation of the appropriate-sized cuffed-ETT may be used to correlate outer diameter measurements for proper DLT selection in these age groups. Difficulty in selection of DLT size contributes to use of other SLV techniques. Ultimately, proper evaluation of the patient with knowledge of anesthetic and surgical procedure requirements will determine proper modality selection and patient safety.

VI. CONCLUSIONS

The anesthesiologist caring for patients who require SLV and lung isolation faces many challenges. An understanding of the primary underlying lesion, as well as associated anomalies that may affect perioperative management, is paramount. A working knowledge of respiratory physiology and anatomy is required for the planning and execution of appropriate intraoperative care. Familiarity with a variety of techniques for SLV suited to the patient's needs allows maximal surgical exposure while minimizing trauma to the lungs and airways.

VII. CLINICAL PEARLS

- Lung isolation should be performed by well-trained and experienced practitioners who should understand the significant risks and benefits to such techniques.

- Absolute indications for lung separation include isolation of infection, contamination, or hemorrhage; control of ventilation distribution; and unilateral bronchopulmonary lavage.

- Relative indications for lung separation include surgical exposure and severe hypoxemia related to unilateral lung disease.

- Double-lumen tubes (DLTs) come in sizes 28, 32, 35, 37, 39, and 41 F, and the appropriate length is based on height, build, and airway examination. Positioning should be confirmed by flexible fiberoptic bronchoscopic (FFB) visualization, selective ventilation auscultation, or radiographic studies.

- DLTs are advantageous because they provide the capability of independent bilateral lung ventilation, bronchial suctioning, lung deflation, and stability, but they have the disadvantage of large size, rigidity, and difficulty in management for prolonged ventilation.

- For patients with difficult airways, anatomic anomalies, tracheal obstructions, tracheal-vascular distortions, or

need for segmental lung isolation, the use of single-lumen tube (SLT) isolation devices should be strongly considered.

- Disadvantages to SLT isolation techniques include difficulty with lung deflation, difficulty suctioning the isolated lung, difficulty with stability and positioning, and inability to independently ventilate the isolated lung portion.

- Univent tubes are SLTs with an external bronchial blocker attachment; they can be used as an effective device for lung isolation, including large segmental-lobar isolation.

- Bronchial blockers come as stand-alone devices and can be used with SLTs or DLTs that have a low-volume, high-pressure cuff system; they may be used para-axially or axially for whole or segmental lung isolation.

- Pediatric lung isolation techniques are similar, if not identical, to those used for adults, although SLT techniques are often used; however, pediatric anatomy and physiology differs from that of adults in regard to positioning and ventilation.

SELECTED REFERENCES

All references can be found online at expertconsult.com.

5. Brodsky JB, Adkins MO, Gaba DM: Bronchial cuff pressures of double-lumen tubes. *Anesth Analg* 69:608–610, 1989.
11. Benumof J: *Anesthesia for thoracic surgery*, ed 2, Philadelphia, 1995, Saunders.
14. Ehrenfeld JM, Walsh JL, Sandberg WS: Right- and left-sided Mallinckrodt double-lumen tubes have identical clinical performance. *Anesth Analg* 106:1847–1852, 2008.
19. Benumof JL, Partridge BL, Salvatierra C, et al: Margin of safety in positioning modern double-lumen endotracheal tubes. *Anesthesiology* 67:729–738, 1987.
22. Brodsky JB, Shulman MS, Mark JB: Malposition of left-sided double-lumen endobronchial tubes. *Anesthesiology* 62:667–669, 1985.
24. Benumof JL: The position of a double-lumen tube should be routinely determined by fiberoptic bronchoscopy. *J Cardiothorac Vasc Anesth* 7:513–514, 1993.
27. Hurford WE, Alfille PH: A quality improvement study of the placement and complications of double-lumen endobronchial tubes. *J Cardiothorac Vasc Anesth* 7:517–520, 1993.
45. Kamaya H, Krishna PR: New endotracheal tube (Univent tube) for selective blockade of one lung. *Anesthesiology* 63:342–343, 1985.
52. Ginsberg RJ: New technique for one-lung anesthesia using an endobronchial blocker. *J Thorac Cardiovasc Surg* 82:542–546, 1981.
68. Hammer GB, Manos SJ, Smith BM, et al: Single-lung ventilation in pediatric patients. *Anesthesiology* 84:1503–1506, 1996.

Chapter 27

Esophageal-Tracheal Double-Lumen Airways: The Combitube and EasyTube

MICHAEL FRASS | M. RAMEZ SALEM | SONIA VAIDA | CARIN A. HAGBERG

I. COMBITUBE

A. Use of the Endotracheal Tube for Intubation and Ventilation

Rapid establishment of a patent airway to facilitate adequate ventilation during cardiopulmonary resuscitation (CPR) is the primary task of the rescuer. Mouth-to-mouth ventilation carries the disadvantages of possible gastric insufflation and the danger of aspiration. Endotracheal intubation remains the gold standard in airway maintenance, but this skill is acquired only after intensive training and requires constant practice. The people performing resuscitation procedures often are untrained in intubation, which is sometimes difficult or impossible even for skilled personnel.[1] It requires good exposure of the patient's airway, a skilled endoscopist, and equipment or facilities for intubation. Because the main objectives of airway management are ventilation and oxygenation, the need arises for a simple and efficient alternative to endotracheal intubation.[2]

B. Use of the Esophageal Obturator Airway as an Alternative Airway Adjunct

The esophageal obturator airway was constructed by Don Michael and colleagues as an alternative to using the

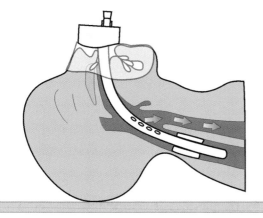

Figure 27-1 Esophageal obturator airway. Air is blown through the proximal port and travels through perforations into the hypopharynx *(arrows)* and trachea, because the mouth and nose are sealed by the mask and esophagus by the balloon.

endotracheal tube during emergency intubation.[3] The esophageal obturator airway is a 34-cm-long tube with a balloon at its distal tip (Fig. 27-1). The balloon should lie below the level of the tracheal bifurcation after insertion. The distal end is blocked. Proximal to the balloon, there are 16 holes that are positioned in the region of the hypopharynx after positioning the airway. At the proximal end, a face mask is connected to the airway, sealing the mouth and nose during ventilation.

The esophageal obturator airway is inserted by first grasping the back of the patient's tongue and the lower jaw with the thumb and index finger and then guiding the airway gently into the esophagus. The distal balloon is inflated to occlude the esophagus while the mask is pressed against the patient's face. Air enters the proximal end and then enters the hypopharynx through perforations because the distal end is blocked. From there, air is forced over the opened glottis into the trachea because the mouth and nose are sealed by the mask and the esophagus by the balloon (see Fig. 27-1).

1. Testing and Trials of the Esophageal Obturator Airway

Subsequent physiologic testing and field trials of the esophageal obturator airway have been performed. Schofferman and colleagues evaluated the airway in 18 patients suffering from cardiac arrest,[4] in whom resuscitation was performed by paramedics. Arterial blood gas analysis was obtained during ventilation with the esophageal obturator airway and subsequently with the endotracheal tube (ETT). There was little or no improvement in oxygenation after endotracheal intubation, implying that failure to oxygenate some patients did not result from the esophageal obturator airway.

Shea and associates compared two similar groups of patients during cardiopulmonary arrest with ventricular fibrillation[5]; 296 patients were intubated with an ETT or esophageal obturator airway. Survival rates and neurologic sequelae of survivors showed no statistically significant difference for the two groups. Hammargren and colleagues compared both devices after standardizing the method of oxygen delivery and ensuring true sampling

of arterial blood.[6] In 48 victims who had prehospital cardiac arrest, blood gases were sampled during ventilation with the esophageal obturator airway and subsequent ventilation with the ETT. There was no statistically significant difference between the two devices for the PaO_2 and $PaCO_2$ values. The investigators concluded that the esophageal obturator airway was an effective means of airway management, with the ventilation achieved equal to that of an ETT. Nevertheless, it soon became apparent from studies in the controlled environment of the operating room that considerable technical difficulties were associated with the esophageal obturator airway.[7]

2. Disadvantages of the Esophageal Obturator Airway

In the literature, the esophageal obturator airway remains controversial because of several possible complications:

1. There are significant difficulties in obtaining a tight face mask seal and maintaining the seal during transportation. Effective use requires at least two hands to seal the mask. Obtaining an adequate mask fit is particularly difficult in edentulous or bearded patients.[6,7]
2. Inadvertent or unrecognized tracheal intubation may occur.[8] The patient's airway is completely obstructed, and attempts at repositioning are usually unsuccessful.
3. Esophageal or gastric ruptures have been reported.[9-12] Ruptures of the esophagus or the stomach may be due to the length of the esophageal obturator airway. Because many cardiac arrest patients exhibit left atrial dilatation with subsequent lateral deviation of the lower half of the esophagus, the esophageal obturator airway may be forced in a left lateral direction in addition to the curved sagittal direction, which can lead to ruptures.

C. Development of the Combitube Esophageal-Tracheal Double-Lumen Airway

The previously described disadvantages and the idea that both tracheal and esophageal intubation allow ventilation and oxygenation led to the development of the Combitube. It was devised by Michael Frass in cooperation with Reinhard Frenzer and Jonas Zahler in Mödling and Vienna, Austria.[13-17]

The Combitube design was intended to deal effectively with the problem of managing the airway with the greatest success possible. Studies in large populations demonstrate that the Combitube provides a much better chance of ventilation and oxygenation than other devices[18-21] by isolating and protecting the airway from digestive regurgitation and aspiration.[22] The Combitube can be used when airway management is difficult independent of the cause, such as anatomic factors, the patient's position with respect to the operator, space and illumination restrictions, and presence of a full stomach. The Combitube does not need special equipment, energy, or complex techniques to be properly used. Because the Combitube is available in only two sizes (37 and 41 F),

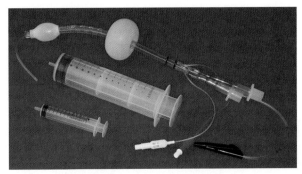

Figure 27-2 The Combitube has a large syringe for inflation of the oropharyngeal balloon and a small syringe for inflation of the distal cuff.

no time is lost in selecting the proper size among many alternatives.

D. Technical Description

The Esophageal Tracheal Combitube (Combitube; Tyco Healthcare, Mansfield, MA) is a device for emergency intubation that combines the functions of an esophageal obturator airway and a conventional ETT (Fig. 27-2). The Combitube is a double-cuff and double-lumen tube (Fig. 27-3). The oropharyngeal balloon is located at the middle portion of the tube and the tracheoesophageal cuff is located at the distal end.[23] The lumens are separated by a partition wall. Proximally, both lumens are opened and linked by short tubes with universal connectors. Distally, the pharyngeal lumen is blocked and has eight perforations at the level between the cuffs, and the tracheoesophageal lumen is open. This design allows ventilation when the Combitube is positioned in the esophagus through the perforations of the pharyngeal lumen and in the trachea through the opened distal end of the tracheoesophageal lumen. The pharyngeal balloon seals the oral and nasal cavities after inflation. Printed ring marks proximal to the oropharyngeal balloon indicate the limit of insertion.

The 37-F Small Adult (SA) Combitube may be used in patients 4 to 6.5 ft tall.[18,24,25] The 41-F model is used

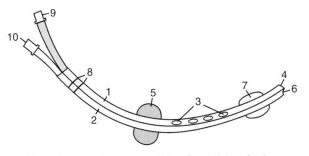

Figure 27-3 Cross-sectional view of the Combitube: *1,* pharyngeal lumen (i.e., longer tube with a blocked distal end); *2,* tracheoesophageal lumen (i.e., shorter tube with open distal end); *3,* perforations of esophageal lumen 1 in the pharyngeal section; *4,* blocked distal end of esophageal lumen 1; *5,* oropharyngeal balloon *(yellow); 6,* open distal end of tracheal lumen 2; *7,* distal cuff for obturating the esophagus or trachea; *8,* printed ring marks for indicating the depth of insertion between the teeth or alveolar ridges; *9,* connector for *(blue)* the tube leading to esophageal lumen 1; *10,* connector for *(transparent)* the tube leading to tracheal lumen 2.

in patients taller than 6 ft (with some overlap with the SA model). The 37-F SA Combitube usually is the preferred model because it works well in patients up to 6.5 ft tall.

E. Insertion Techniques

The Combitube can be successfully inserted independently of the patient's position with regard to the operator. The patient's head is preferably in the neutral position, or a small cushion may be used. The sniffing position may impede Combitube insertion.

1. Conventional Technique

With the operator behind the patient's head, the lower jaw and tongue are lifted by the thumb and index finger. The tongue is pressed forward by the thumb, and the tube is inserted in a curved downward movement until the printed ring marks lie between the teeth or the alveolar ridges in edentulous patients (Fig. 27-4A). The insertion should be performed along the tongue to avoid potential damage of the posterior pharyngeal mucosa. Sometimes, a rocking motion may alleviate problems encountered with insertion. Next, the oropharyngeal balloon is inflated with up to 85 mL of air for the 37-F SA Combitube (or up to 100 mL for the 41-F Combitube) through port no. 1 with the blue pilot balloon using the large syringe with the blue color code (see Fig. 27-4B). When the minimal-volume technique is used, enough air is added to inflate the balloon and obtain a seal (see "General Anesthesia"), or a cuff pressure gauge may be used to achieve a seal of 60 mm Hg. If sufficient sealing of the mouth and nose cannot be accomplished, the oropharyngeal balloon may be filled with an additional 50 mL of air, up to a total amount of 150 mL.[26]

During inflation, the tube may move slightly out of the patient's mouth because of the self-positioning properties of the balloon. A useful sign indicating malposition due to insufficient insertion is that the inflated pharyngeal balloon can be seen when looking into the patient's mouth (Fig. 27-5). If this occurs, the pharyngeal balloon should be deflated, and the tip's position should be reevaluated. The Combitube may become kinked during placement, and reinsertion may be necessary. The anatomic relationships of the oropharyngeal balloon have been demonstrated radiologically.[26] The balloon protrudes in an oral direction after overinflation so that it does not close the epiglottis. Figure 27-6 shows a cross-sectional magnetic resonance imaging (MRI) view of the Combitube in the esophageal position. It displays anterior movement of the larynx, a situation that can often be observed clinically. Knowledge of this may facilitate subsequent location of the larynx for endotracheal intubation.

The distal balloon is then inflated with 10 mL of air through port no. 2 with the white pilot balloon and using the small syringe.[27] With blind insertion, there is a high probability that the tube will be placed into the esophagus. Test ventilation is recommended through the longer, blue no. 1 tube leading to the esophageal lumen (see Fig. 27-4C). Air passes into the pharynx and then through the glottis into the trachea because the mouth, nose, and

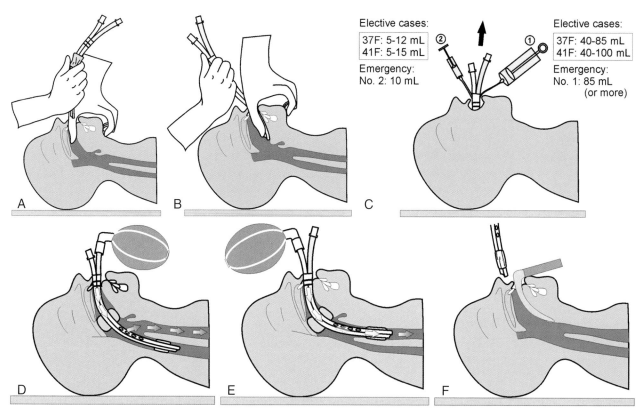

Elective cases:
| 37F: 5-12 mL |
| 41F: 5-15 mL |

Emergency:
No. 2: 10 mL

Elective cases:
| 37F: 40-85 mL |
| 41F: 40-100 mL |

Emergency:
No. 1: 85 mL
(or more)

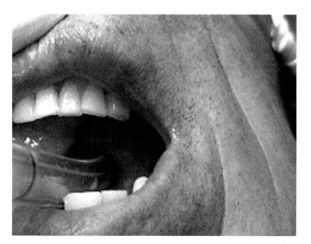

Figure 27-4 Guidelines for introduction of the Combitube. **A,** Insertion begins by lifting the chin and lower jaw. **B,** The Combitube is inserted in a downward, curved movement along the tongue. **C,** The oropharyngeal balloon is inflated with 85 mL of air, and the distal cuff is inflated with 5 to 10 mL of air. **D,** With the Combitube in the esophageal position, ventilation is performed through the longer no. 1 tube *(blue)*. Air flows through the holes into the pharynx and from there into the trachea *(arrows)*. **E,** With the Combitube in the tracheal position, ventilation is performed through the shorter no. 2 tube *(transparent)*. Air flows directly into the trachea *(arrows)*. **F,** The Combitube is inserted using a laryngoscope.

esophagus are blocked by the balloons. Auscultation of breath sounds in the absence of gastric insufflation confirms adequate ventilation when the Combitube is in the esophagus. Ventilation is then continued through this lumen. In this position, the Combitube allows closed suctioning and active decompression of the stomach.[28] Closed suctioning provides the advantage of reduced cross contamination between the bronchial system and gastric juices.[29] Gastric contents can be suctioned through

Figure 27-5 Seeing the inflated oropharyngeal balloon in the patient's mouth indicates malposition of the Combitube.

the unused tracheoesophageal lumen with the help of a small suction catheter (10 or 12 F) included in the kit.

The most common cause of failed ventilation through the blue connector is a tracheal position of the distal tip (see Fig. 27-4D). Without changing the position of the Combitube, ventilation is changed to the shorter, transparent no. 2 tube leading to the tracheoesophageal lumen, and the position is again confirmed by auscultation. Ventilation is then carried out through the tracheoesophageal lumen directly into the trachea. The oropharyngeal balloon may be deflated in case of regurgitation to allow suctioning with a conventional catheter. Otherwise, the balloon should remain inflated to stabilize the Combitube.

If no breath sounds are heard over the lungs or a capnographic curve is absent while ventilating through the blue connector, the second most common cause is that the Combitube has been inserted too deeply, and the oropharyngeal balloon lies just opposite the laryngeal aperture and occludes the airway.[30] In this situation, both balloons should be deflated and the Combitube pulled back about 2 to 3 cm out of the patient's mouth and then fixed in this position.

The third most common cause of failed ventilation is a phenomenon (e.g., laryngospasm, bronchospasm, pulmonary edema) leading to high airway pressure. In this situation, cause should be identified and treated. Unlike other airway devices, the Combitube allows ventilation

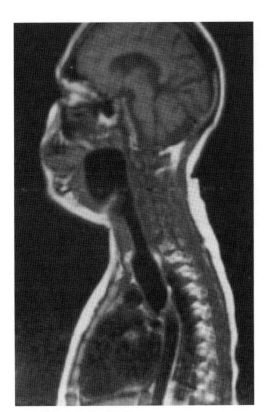

Figure 27-6 Cross-sectional MRI view of a patient intubated with Combitube in the esophageal position. (Courtesy of B. Panning, MD, Department of Anesthesiology, and C. Ehrenheim, MD, Department of Nuclear Medicine and Special Biophysics, Hannover School of Medicine, Hannover, Germany.)

against high airway pressure, and administration of inhaled bronchodilators[28,31] and proper treatment of the spastic phenomenon can be started immediately after full inflation of the balloon to ensure high-pressure ventilation.

An investigation by Wafai and coworkers was designed to test the reliability of the self-inflating bulb in identifying the location of the Combitube and facilitating its proper position in anesthetized patients.[32] In group 1 ($n = 26$), the Combitube was introduced blindly. In group 2 ($n = 20$), the tube was placed in the trachea (8 patients) or once in the trachea and once in the esophagus randomly (12 patients) under direct vision rigid laryngoscopy by the anesthesiologist performing the intubation. In both groups, the efficacy of the self-inflating bulb in identifying the location of the Combitube was tested by a second blinded anesthesiologist. In group 1, blind insertion of the Combitube resulted in esophageal placement in all patients, and in each case, it was correctly identified. The second anesthesiologist reported no reinflation when the compressed self-inflating bulb was connected to the distal lumen. When the compressed self-inflating bulb was connected to the proximal lumen, instantaneous reinflation was observed in 23 patients, delayed reinflation (2 to 4 seconds) in 2, and no reinflation (>4 seconds) in 1. Instantaneous reinflation occurred in these three patients after repositioning the Combitube. In group 2, the second anesthesiologist correctly identified the location of the Combitube in all cases. The results confirm previous findings that blind introduction of the

Combitube leads to esophageal placement and yields adequate ventilation. The self-inflating bulb can quickly identify the location of the Combitube and facilitate its positioning with the use of a simple algorithm. This can be important if the Combitube is used in a patient whose lungs cannot be ventilated by mask and whose trachea cannot be intubated.

2. Alternative Insertion Technique

Another way of inserting the Combitube has been described by Urtubia and colleagues.[33] This insertion technique (Fig. 27-7A and B) consists of grasping the upper teeth or the upper alveolar ridge with the index finger while pushing the chin with the middle finger. To avoid contact of the tip of the Combitube with the posterior oropharyngeal wall, Urtubia recommends keeping the Combitube bent as long as possible before blind insertion.[33] Similarly, Urtubia and associates describe a modification of the Lipp maneuver for blind insertion of the Combitube.[34]

For patients in sitting and prone positions or when the operator is facing the patient, a similar technique can be useful. The index finger grasps the lower teeth or alveolar ridge while the middle finger pushes the cheek (see Fig. 27-7C). The enlarged interincisor distance allows easier insertion of the Combitube, especially in partially edentulous patients and in patients with a limited oral opening (Fig. 27-8A and B). As with the original technique, it does not require any cervical movement, which makes it suitable for patients with cervical spine trauma.

The Combitube may be inserted blindly or with the aid of a laryngoscope. Use of a laryngoscope is recommended during the initial training period when endotracheal intubation using laryngoscopy fails (i.e., insert the Combitube with the laryngoscope still in place) and when blind insertion of the Combitube fails.[28]

F. Indications, Advantages, and Complications

1. Out-of-Hospital Emergency Intubation

The Combitube is especially suitable for emergency intubation in and out of the hospital when endotracheal intubation is not immediately possible. It may be used in the following three situations. First, in patients with difficult anatomy (e.g., bull neck, lockjaw, small mouth opening), the Combitube can be inserted in those with an interincisor distance (i.e., oral aperture) as small as 15 mm.[35] Second, the Combitube can be inserted in difficult spatial circumstances, such as limited access to a patient's head when the patient lies on the floor in a small room, when the patient is lying with his head close to the wall in the general ward or in the intensive care unit (ICU) with many lines at the side impeding quick access to the head, or when a patient is trapped in a car after an accident. Third, the Combitube can be inserted despite challenging illumination, such as bright light, massive bleeding, or regurgitation that can inhibit direct laryngoscopy. The Combitube prevents aspiration, which may occur with repeated suction maneuvers or vomiting.[22,24,36]

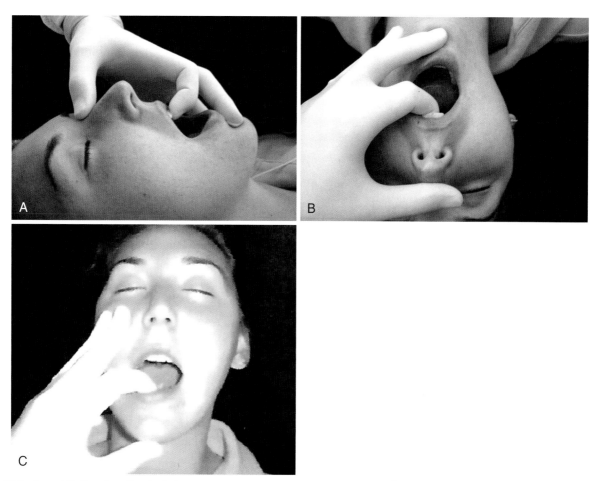

Figure 27-7 **A** and **B,** New insertion technique as described by Urtubia and coworkers.[33] **C,** Alternative insertion technique. (Courtesy of Carin Hagberg, MD, Houston, TX.)

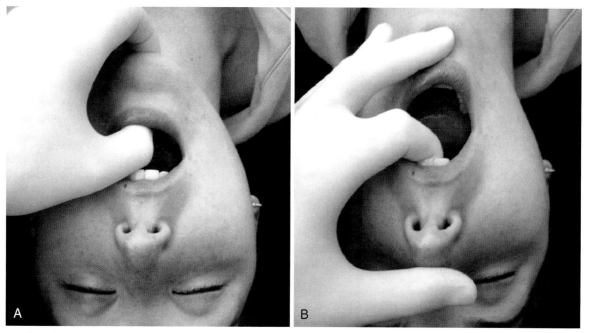

Figure 27-8 **A** and **B,** Comparison of the oral aperture in the two insertion techniques. Observe the larger interincisor distance in **B**. (Courtesy of Carin Hagberg, MD, Houston, TX.)

> **BOX 27-1** Suggested Indications for Use of the Combitube in Anesthesia and Emergencies
>
> I. Face abnormalities
>   A. Congenital (e.g., micrognathia, macroglossia)
>   B. Facial trauma[8,54,80]
>   C. Lockjaw[14,35,41]
>   D. Small interincisor distance[14,76]
> II. Cervical spine abnormalities
>   A. Bull neck[76]
>   B. Bechterew's disease
>   C. Klippel-Feil syndrome
>   D. Fractures and luxations[7,80,84,87]
>   E. Rheumatoid arthritis with subluxation of the atlantoaxial joint[36]
>   F. Morbidly obese patients[76,140]
> III. Further indications
>   A. Preoperative evaluation indications
>   1. Previous difficult intubation
>   2. Mallampati oropharyngeal classification class III or IV[93]
>   3. Cormack-Lehane laryngoscopic grade 3 or 4
>   B. Emergency situation
>   1. Accidental extubation in patients undergoing surgery in a prone or sitting position
>   2. Cervical hematoma after inadvertent puncture of the carotid artery[78]
>   3. Unexpected upper airway bleeding or continued vomiting[22,90]
>   4. Cesarean section[102-106]
>   5. Intubation in circumstances of limited space
>   6. Failed rapid sequence intubation[73,80]

2. Elective and Emergency Surgery

a. GENERAL ANESTHESIA

Use of the Combitube is indicated in routine surgery in patients for whom conventional intubation is not mandatory, such as singers and actors who may be afraid of damage to the vocal cords by endotracheal intubation, or in patients with rheumatoid arthritis with atlantoaxial subluxation. The main advantages of the Combitube in elective and emergency surgery are higher insertion and ventilation rates, reliable protection of the airway against regurgitation and aspiration of gastric contents (e.g., patients with a full stomach, gynecologic laparoscopy), and ventilation and oxygenation against high airway pressures (e.g., obesity, laryngospasm, bronchospasm). As with emergency intubation, it is especially suitable in patients with difficult anatomic conditions. When endotracheal intubation cannot be performed immediately, the Combitube should be considered (Box 27-1). The main advantage in the case of failed intubation or ventilation is immediate esophageal insertion of the Combitube under direct vision without removing the laryngoscope.

Some special considerations apply to the use of the Combitube by anesthesiologists who are expert in endotracheal intubation.

1. The patient's head does not have to be placed in the traditional sniffing position, as recommended for conventional endotracheal intubation. The patient's head should remain in a neutral position that allows free movement of the lower jaw. Depending on the situation, the chin may be pushed toward the patient's chest. Some clinicians prefer to extend the head or to use a small cushion. In patients with a cervical spine injury, the Combitube allows airway management while avoiding mobilization of the neck.

2. The position of the operator (Fig. 27-9) may be behind the patient, especially when a laryngoscope is used (see Fig. 27-9A); to the side of the patient's head (see Fig. 27-9B); or face to face, when the operator stands beside the patient's thorax and faces the patient (see Fig. 27-9C). In all three positions, it is necessary to insert the Combitube with a curved downward-caudal movement.

3. During elective surgery, it is always necessary to achieve an adequate depth of anesthesia, with or without additional relaxation. One half of the intubating dose of a neuromuscular blocking agent may be enough to ensure a smooth insertion.[18] Gaitini and colleagues have used the Combitube in patients with controlled mechanical ventilation and in spontaneously breathing patients without relaxation.[18] However, grasping and elevating the epiglottis with the fingers during insertion may reduce the need for relaxation.

4. Recommended induction agents are propofol or sevoflurane, with or without opioids.[37] In a study of 50 female patients undergoing gynecologic laparoscopy, Urtubia and associates successfully inserted the Combitube in 100% of cases using inhalational induction with sevoflurane as the sole agent,[38] without opioids or neuromuscular blockade. Use of a laryngoscope is recommended to avoid damage to the oral and pharyngeal mucosa. Nevertheless, with a well-performed blind insertion technique and an adequate level of anesthesia, the risk of damage is comparable to that with the laryngeal mask airway (LMA) or the ETT in terms of postoperative sore throat (16% to 25%).[18,24,27] With the laryngoscope, the Combitube is then intentionally introduced into the esophagus. When endotracheal intubation fails, a Combitube can be placed under direct visualization with the laryngoscope still in the patient's mouth.

5. Another method that may facilitate Combitube insertion and minimize insertion trauma is warming the Combitube in a bottle of warm saline or water, similar to the procedure performed with an ETT for nasal intubation. This technique also allows Combitube insertion without additional application of lubricant.

6. The minimal-volume technique should be applied in elective cases and in emergencies after stabilization of the patient. Studies have shown that adequate sealing of the oropharyngeal balloon can be achieved with 40 to 85 mL of air for the SA Combitube.[18,24,27,38-41] Gaitini and colleagues reported that the mean inflation volume of the oropharyngeal balloon at which an air leak was first observed was 45.5 ± 12.3 mL for the 37-F Combitube and

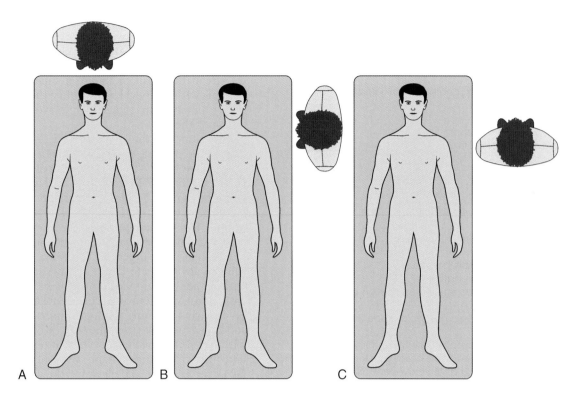

Figure 27-9 Position of the operator during insertion of the Combitube. **A,** The operator stands behind the patient, especially when using a laryngoscope. **B,** The operator stands to the side of the patient's head. **C,** The operator stands beside patient's thorax so that they are positioned face to face.

48.1 ± 12.1 mL for the 41-F Combitube.[40] The balloon should be initially filled with 40 mL of air only. If a tight seal can be achieved as evaluated by auscultation, comparable to inspiratory and expiratory tidal volumes and the flow-volume curve, the volume is not increased. If a leak is observed, additional increments of 10 mL of air each are added into the balloon until a tight seal is confirmed. The volumes of the oropharyngeal balloon also must be adjusted with the use of nitrous oxide and volatile anesthetics.

b. AWAKE INTUBATION

In an experiment on himself, Panning showed that the Combitube can be inserted easily with local pharyngeal anesthesia.[42] Keller and coworkers inserted the Combitube in four awake volunteers with topical anesthesia.[43] Nevertheless, unless an urgent insertion is required, the Combitube should always be inserted when gag reflexes are suppressed because of the risk of mucosal damage or vomiting.

c. REPLACEMENT OF THE COMBITUBE

The Combitube may be left in place for up to 8 hours.[44] Although emergency and routine surgical procedures may be successfully carried out during this period, the Combitube is not intended for long-term ventilation, because the pressure on the pharyngeal mucosa may be harmful. We recommend replacing the Combitube after a maximum duration of 8 hours. Replacement of the Combitube in the esophageal position by an ETT can be performed in several ways with no danger of aspiration:

1. While the distal cuff remains inflated, deflate the oropharyngeal balloon completely, with the Combitube remaining in the esophagus. Displace the Combitube to the left corner of the mouth, and insert an ETT by laryngoscopy or fiberoptic intubation.[45] After successful placement of the ETT, insert a suction catheter through the tracheoesophageal lumen into the esophagus, and during continuous suctioning, deflate the distal cuff, and remove the Combitube. If ETT insertion is impossible, push the Combitube back into its original midline position, reinflate the oropharyngeal balloon, and continue ventilating through the longer no. 1 lumen (blue) of the Combitube until the next endotracheal intubation attempt or until a surgical airway is established.

2. Gaitini and associates described another method.[46] The oropharyngeal balloon is partly deflated according to the minimal-volume technique so that the least amount of air allows adequate sealing of the oral and nasal cavities. During continued ventilation through the no. 1 lumen, a fiberoptic bronchoscope mounted with an ETT is introduced through the patient's mouth. Without a time limit, the bronchoscope may be advanced into the trachea. The unique feature of this method is that ventilation is not interrupted during the entire replacement procedure. All the patients in this study had Mallampati class III or IV oral cavity anatomy.

3. The Combitube may be replaced by surgical means, such as cricothyrotomy or tracheostomy.[47] These were the first surgical procedures performed with the Combitube. An advantage of this method is that the trachea is not occupied by an ETT, and ventilation can be continued while the surgical airway is established. A disadvantage is that the trachea is not protected against aspiration of blood generated during the surgical procedure.

4. If there is no danger of aspiration, the Combitube may be removed and replaced by conventional means (e.g., laryngoscopy, bronchoscopy). This approach may be advantageous because intubation around the Combitube can be difficult. In a cadaver study, the laryngeal view with and without the Combitube in place has been compared and the difficulty of intubation around the device evaluated.[48] Nine participants in an airway workshop placed 37-F Combitubes in eight non-embalmed cadavers. The pharyngeal balloon was deflated and laryngoscopy attempted with the Combitube in place. Each operator assessed the percentage of glottic opening (POGO) score and tried to pass a tracheal tube around the device. Difficulty of tube passage was rated by the operator. The Combitube was then removed and laryngoscopy (and POGO scoring) repeated without the device. POGO scores with and without the Combitube averaged 61% (95% confidence interval [CI], 49% to 73%) and 92% (CI, 89% to 95%), respectively. Fourteen (19%) of 72 intubation attempts with the Combitube failed. Major difficulty was reported for 22 (31%) of 72 attempts, and minor difficulty for 34 (47%) of 72. The investigators concluded that a previously placed Combitube significantly worsened the laryngeal view at laryngoscopy and prevented intubation in 19% of cases in this cadaver study. They suggest that removal of the Combitube is warranted if any difficulty with laryngoscopy is anticipated or encountered.

5. Harrison and colleagues described the successful replacement of the Combitube with an ETT by retrograde intubation.[49] The retrograde intubation was successfully performed without removing an in situ Combitube.

6. A Combitube in the tracheal position can be replaced by an ETT. After lubrication, a pediatric (8-F) tracheal tube exchanger (Cook Critical Care, Bloomington, IN) is introduced into the tracheo-esophageal lumen through the shorter no. 2 lumen (transparent) into the trachea, the Combitube is removed, and an ETT is advanced using the tube exchanger as a guide.[50,51] If not contraindicated, laryngoscopy should be performed, to facilitate advancement of the ETT through the glottis.

d. EXTUBATION

Extubation after surgery in the awake patient is possible, and the patient will not show signs of significant distress. It begins by deflating the oropharyngeal balloon, allowing communication with the patient. Deflation of the distal cuff and final extubation during continuous suctioning through the shorter no. 2 lumen should be performed only after recovery of protective reflexes.

After deflation of the oropharyngeal balloon, the pharyngeal structures may occlude the ventilating perforations of the Combitube. It is advisable to deflate the balloon up to the point at which breathing is normal. After spontaneous ventilation fully resumes, the Combitube can be withdrawn with a curved movement out of the patient's mouth in a fashion similar to insertion.

3. Advantages

The Combitube has a wide range of applications and advantages (Box 27-2). Those benefiting from its use include anesthesiologists and physicians in emergency departments,[18,19,23] paramedics and emergency medical technicians,[19,50,52-57] combat medics,[58] parkmedics,[59] and physicians in private practice (e.g., responding to anaphylactic reactions).[28,31] Cardiac arrests usually do not occur under ideal circumstances, and CPR often is performed in awkward locations, poorly lighted areas, and with limited access to the patient's head. Because the Combitube can be inserted without a laryngoscope, establishment of a patent airway is not hampered by adverse environmental factors or staff unskilled in endotracheal intubation.[27] It is safe against aspiration, and high ventilatory pressures may be applied.

There is no need for additional fixation of the Combitube after inflation of the oropharyngeal balloon,

---

> **BOX 27-2 Advantages of the Combitube and EasyTube**
>
> - Noninvasive compared with cricothyrotomy
> - Universal size (37-F Small Adult Combitube fits patients 4 to 6.5 ft)[18,23,104]
> - Universal model (one type only)
> - Easy to learn, even by untrained personnel[58,68,110,129,130]
> - No preparations necessary; tube and syringes are ready to use
> - Helpful under difficult conditions of space and illumination
> - Blind insertion technique
> - Neck extension unnecessary
> - Simultaneous fixation after inflation of the oropharyngeal balloon
> - Works in the tracheal or esophageal position
> - Active decompression of the esophagus and stomach
> - Minimized risk of aspiration[22,36,38,57,101,106]
> - Controlled mechanical ventilation possible at high ventilation pressures (≤50 cm H_2O)[19,24,27,36,51,93,101]
> - Independent of power supply (e.g., batteries of laryngoscope)
> - Well suited for obese patients[76,140]
> - May be used in paralyzed patients who cannot be intubated or mask ventilated
> - Only device for insertion in patients with trismus and limited mobility of cervical spine and those with combined pathologic conditions, such as trismus plus limited mobility of the spine and trismus plus tongue edema[129]
> - Fast, safe, and easy to use with successful skill retention[129,130]

because the anterior upper wall of the oropharyngeal balloon lies just behind the posterior end of the hard palate, thereby guaranteeing strong anchoring during ventilation and transportation. Providing a more secure airway is an attractive advantage of the Combitube compared with other devices used during transportation of emergency patients. Studies have shown that the Combitube is easy to learn and that the skills are retained over time.[57]

4. Disadvantages

A potential disadvantage of the Combitube is that suctioning tracheal secretions is impossible in the esophageal position. However, studies of use of the esophageal obturator airway in cardiac arrest patients have shown that the outcome of those cases is not statistically different compared with cases in which endotracheal intubation is used.[5,6] The Combitube is designed to bridge the short gap between the prehospital setting and admission of the patient to the emergency department. If prolonged ventilation is required, glycopyrronium bromide may be administered to suppress tracheal secretions (e.g., during surgery). Krafft and colleagues have described a redesigned Combitube in which two proximal anterior holes are replaced by one large hole, allowing a bronchoscope to pass for inspection and suctioning of the trachea and as a means for replacing the Combitube using a guidewire.[60]

5. Contraindications

The Combitube is contraindicated for use in patients with the following: intact gag reflexes (irrespective of the level of consciousness), height less than 6 ft (41-F Combitube) or less than 4 ft (37-F SA Combitube), central airway obstruction, ingestion of caustic substances, and known upper esophageal pathology (e.g., Zencker's diverticulum).

6. Complications

Ovassapian and coworkers observed livid discoloration of the tongue during ventilation with the Combitube in a few patients without further sequelae.[45] Tongue engorgement was described after 4 hours of Combitube use.[61] In an out-of-hospital study with paramedics as rescuers, two lacerations of the esophagus were found in autopsies of cardiac arrest patients ventilated with the Combitube.[62] However, the investigators found that the distal cuff was overfilled with 20 to 40 mL of air (instead of 10 ± 1 mL). As outlined in the instructions, the Combitube should not be advanced with use of force. Klein and associates reported an esophageal rupture after insertion of a Combitube, stiff suctioning catheter, LMA, laryngoscope, and ETT.[35] A traumatic procedure with one or more of these devices probably caused the complication.

Overinflation of the esophageal balloon was described in a case reporting airway obstruction secondary to tracheal compression. In this case, the esophageal balloon was inflated with 22.4 mL according to the computed tomography (CT) measurement.[63] Richards reported a case of piriform sinus perforation during the insertion of the Combitube.[64] This patient presented with cardiorespiratory arrest due to angioedema, probably caused by treatment with angiotensin-converting enzyme inhibitors. Another case of piriform sinus perforation during Combitube placement was reported by Moser.[65]

Oczenski and coworkers reported a very high number of complications for cases of elective surgery.[66] The total complication rate found by Oczenski's group[66] was fourfold that found in the studies led by Gaitini,[18] Hartmann,[27] and Urtubia.[24] This unexpectedly high rate of complications probably was caused by traumatic maneuvers during airway management, which is in accordance with an 8% rate of pharyngeal hematoma associated with the LMA. Vezina and colleagues retrospectively reviewed medical records of patients with cardiac or respiratory arrest.[67] The study was performed in the Quebec City Health Region, where paramedics use the Combitube as a primary airway device for patients with cardiorespiratory arrest. A high incidence of complications was reported.

The study of Oczenski and coworkers demonstrates that all precautions should be considered when there are obvious handling problems.[66] When facing difficulties during insertion, a laryngoscope should be used immediately to insert the Combitube intentionally into the esophagus under direct vision.

G. Medical Literature

1. Combitube in Cardiac Arrest Patients

a. IN-HOSPITAL STUDIES

Application of the Combitube during CPR has been investigated.[14-16,21] The first study consisted of two parts.[15] The first part considered the blood gas analyses of 19 patients after 15 minutes of ventilation with the Combitube. In the second part, the blood gas analyses of samples taken from 12 patients during ventilation with the Combitube were compared with those taken during subsequent ventilation with a conventional ETT. Blood gas analyses showed higher arterial oxygen pressures with the Combitube than with an ETT (124 ± 33 versus 103 ± 30 mm Hg; $P = 0.001$). Carbon dioxide pressure was not significantly different.

A second study reported the use of the Combitube during in-hospital CPR.[14] In a randomized sequence, the Combitube or a conventional ETT was used in 43 patients. After stabilization of the patients, each tube was replaced with the other type of tube. Blood gas analyses revealed increased oxygen tensions during Combitube ventilation, and the intubation time was significantly shorter with the Combitube.

Another study evaluated the safety and effectiveness of the 41-F Combitube as used by ICU nurses under medical supervision compared with an ETT established by ICU physicians during CPR.[68] The intubation time was shorter for the Combitube, and results of blood gas determinations for each device were comparable, although arterial oxygen tension was slightly higher during ventilation with the Combitube. The study suggests that the Combitube as used by ICU nurses is as effective as the ETT as used by ICU physicians during CPR.

b. OUT-OF-HOSPITAL STUDIES

Atherton and Johnson investigated the ability of paramedics in a nonurban emergency medical setting to use the 41-F Combitube.[52] Fifty-two cases of prehospital Combitube insertion by paramedics were examined, and 11 paramedics were evaluated for skill retention. Combitube insertion was attempted in 52 cardiac arrest patients in a prehospital setting, and 69% of them were intubated successfully. Paramedics recognized esophageal versus tracheal placement in 100% of cases. The Combitube was inserted successfully in 64% of patients who could not be tracheally intubated by direct visualization. The Combitube was inserted successfully in 71% of cases when used as a first-line airway adjunct. Fifteen months later, a follow-up study of 9 of 11 randomly selected paramedics demonstrated inadequate skill retention (e.g., improper insertion angle resulting in resistance and inability to insert the tube, inappropriate inflation of the balloons, insertion too deep or not deep enough). After this reevaluation and retraining, the success rate rose to almost 100%.[69] These results demonstrate that as with every device, there is a necessity for a reevaluation of skills after initial training. A study of emergency medicine residents suggests that they can learn and retain these airway skills.[70]

In a prehospital setting, three alternative airway devices and an oral airway were compared in a modified, randomized, crossover study by emergency medical assistants who were not trained in advanced life support (ALS) techniques.[20] The pharyngeal-tracheal lumen (PTL) airway, the LMA, and the 41-F Combitube were compared objectively for success of insertion, ventilation, and arterial blood gas and spirometry measurements performed on arrival at the hospital. Subjective assessment was carried out by emergency medical assistants and receiving physicians. Operating room training was performed only with the LMA. Autopsy findings and survival to hospital discharge were analyzed. The study took place in four non-ALS communities over 4.5 years and involved 470 patients in cardiac or respiratory arrest, or both. Emergency medical assistants had automatic external defibrillator training but no endotracheal intubation skills. Successful insertion and ventilation was highest for the Combitube (86% versus 82% with PTL airway and 73% with LMA, $P = 0.048$). Differences in subjective evaluation were significant. The Combitube was associated with the fewest problems with ventilation, and it was preferred by most emergency medical assistants. Unlike LMA use, no aspirations were found in autopsies after use of the Combitube.

A retrospective study was designed to determine the choice of airway devices used for nontraumatic,[21] out-of-hospital cardiac arrest patients and to evaluate the success and failure of insertion and airway control or ventilation by three airway adjuncts—the 41-F Combitube, the esophageal-gastric tube airway (EGTA), and the LMA—which were used in conjunction with the bag-valve-mask ventilation by emergency life-saving technicians in Japan. A survey of 1079 technicians was performed to identify the type of airway devices, the success rates of airway insertion, the effectiveness of airway control/ventilation, and associated complications in 12,020 cases of cardiac arrest. The choice of airway devices included bag-valve-mask ventilation for 7180 cases, EGTA for 545 cases, Combitube for 1594 cases, and LMA for 2701 cases. Successful insertion rates on the first attempt were 82.7% for EGTA, 82.4% for Combitube, and 72.5% for LMA ($P = 0.0001$). Rates of failed insertion were 8.2% for EGTA, 6.9% for Combitube, and 10.5% for LMA ($P = 0.0001$). Successful ventilation rates were 71.0% for EGTA, 78.9% for Combitube, and 71.5% for LMA ($P = 0.0004$). Six cases of aspiration were reported in the LMA group, whereas nine cases of soft tissue injuries, including one esophageal perforation, were reported in the 41-F Combitube group; 17.8% had vomited before or during airway placement. The Combitube appears to be the most appropriate choice among the airway devices examined.

The ability to train emergency medical technicians with defibrillation capabilities (EMT-Ds) to effectively use the 41-F Combitube for intubations in the prehospital environment was evaluated in a prospective field study lasting for 18 months.[71] Indications for use of the Combitube included unconsciousness without a purposeful response, absence of the gag reflex, apnea or a respiratory rate of less than 6 breaths/min, age older than 16 years, and height of at least 5 ft. Twenty-two EMT-D provider agencies involving approximately 500 EMT-Ds were included as study participants. Combitube insertions were attempted in 195 patients in cardiorespiratory arrest in a prehospital setting. An overall successful intubation rate of 79% was observed, with identical success rates for medical and trauma patients. The device was placed in the esophagus in 91% of cases. Resistance during insertion was the major reason for unsuccessful Combitube intubations. The overall hospital admission rate was 19%. No complications were reported. The study confirmed that EMT-Ds could be trained to use the Combitube as a means of establishing an airway in patients in the prehospital setting.

Rural EMTs were educated in selected advanced skills, and the safety and effectiveness of practice were evaluated.[55] After a minimum of 72 hours of training, EMTs employed three skills (i.e., Combitube insertion, glucometry, and automated external defibrillation) and seven medications (i.e., albuterol, nitroglycerin, naloxone, epinephrine, glucagon, activated charcoal, and aspirin). Congruence between prehospital assessment and emergency department diagnosis was assessed, along with correct use of airway skills (18 of 36 months). The Combitube functioned satisfactorily in 15 (79%) of 19 cases, and EMTs always correctly found the correct lumen to ventilate.

The purpose of another study was to assess the feasibility, safety, and effectiveness of the Combitube when used by EMT-Ds in cardiorespiratory arrest patients of all causes.[72] The EMTs had automatic external defibrillator training but no prior advanced airway technique skills. The prehospital intervention was reviewed using the EMTs cardiac arrest report, the automatic external defibrillator tape recording of the event, and the assessment of the receiving emergency physician. Hospital records and autopsy reports of 831 adult, cardiac arrest patients were reviewed in search of complications. Placement was successful in 725 (95.4%) of the 760 patients in whom

Combitube insertion was attempted, and ventilation was successful in 695 (91.4%) patients. An autopsy was performed in 133 patients, and no esophageal lesions or significant injuries to the airway structures were observed. Results suggest that EMT-Ds can use the Combitube for control of the airway and ventilation in cardiorespiratory arrest patients safely and effectively. In other field studies investigating the best time for postshock analysis after out-of-hospital defibrillation with automated external defibrillators, 86 (93.7%) of 96 patients were successfully intubated with the Combitube.[53,73] Similar results were found in a study by Cady and Pirrallo, who found a success rate of 89.4% for 860 Combitube insertions performed by paramedics experienced in endotracheal intubation.[74]

Mort reviewed an emergency intubation database to determine what airway devices were used as a backup to rescue the primary rescue device failures.[75] The bougie and the LMA have intrinsic failure rates. In each of the 18 patients, the Combitube was placed in the esophagus with no tracheal insertions identified. Carbon dioxide detection confirmed tracheal air exchange in each case. Minor adjustments were required to optimize the air exchange with the Combitube in nine cases and involved moving the Combitube distally (deeper) or proximally (shallower). Four of the 18 patients required a second attempt of Combitube placement when ventilation was obstructed despite repositioning (i.e., presumed epiglottic impingement by Combitube). After Combitube placement, effective ventilation and life-sustaining oxygen saturations (>92%) were established and maintained in each case until further steps were taken to secure the airway. Steps required to secure the airway (tracheal intubation) after successful placement of the Combitube varied. Eleven patients were tracheally intubated with the Combitube maintained in the esophageal position (i.e., direct laryngoscopy alone in four patients and direct laryngoscopy and bougie-assisted tracheal intubation in seven patients). Because of the poorly recognized periglottic anatomy with the Combitube in place, two patients had the Combitube exchanged to a Fastrach LMA as a successful intubation conduit. Five patients had unrecognizable periglottic anatomy due to excessive edema, significant secretions, and tissue trauma and therefore had a surgical airway created with the Combitube supporting ventilation and oxygenation (i.e., four cases in the emergency department and one general ward patient transported to the operating room for surgical airway procedure). The Combitube, commonly used in the emergency prehospital setting, appeared to be a useful secondary rescue device in the hospital setting when the bougie and LMA failed.

c. CASE REPORTS

Liao and Shalit reported a case of successful Combitube treatment of an acute respiratory arrest caused by an acute asthma exacerbation.[59] A level II EMT (National Park Service Parkmedic) used this device.[59] The female patient was successfully intubated and ventilated and was flown by helicopter for more than 2 hours. Despite repeated episodes of vomiting, no aspiration occurred in this patient. The Combitube was replaced by an ETT, and the patient was extubated 2 days later and discharged on day 3 after the initial event.

The Combitube was helpful in a bull-necked patient when movement of the neck and opening of the mouth were impossible and in the case of a rapidly enlarging cervical hematoma,[76,77] which caused upper airway obstruction and required immediate intubation after endotracheal intubation had failed because the epiglottis could not be visualized with a laryngoscope.[78]

In Chile, a 65-year-old woman with chronic renal insufficiency and atrial fibrillation experienced sudden respiratory arrest during the dialysis procedure at an out-of-hospital dialysis center. Ventilation with a face mask was impossible. As the patient's condition rapidly deteriorated, a nonskilled nurse reestablished her oxygenation by blind insertion of a Combitube.[79]

For a patient with acute respiratory failure,[22] attempts at endotracheal intubation failed due to continued vomiting that rendered fiberoptic visualization of the vocal cords impossible. Blind insertion of the Combitube led to successful ventilation, and replacement by an endotracheal airway was performed without danger of aspiration.

2. Combitube in Trauma Patients

a. STUDIES

Blostein and colleagues have prospectively studied use of the Combitube in trauma patients in whom orotracheal rapid-sequence intubation (RSI) failed.[80] Flight nurses were trained in the use of the Combitube by mannequin simulation, videotape review, and didactic sessions. Combitube insertion was attempted after failure of two or more attempts at orotracheal RSI. Over a 12-month period, 12 patients had successful Combitube insertion, and 10 cases qualified for review. Injuries, number of failed orotracheal RSI attempts, definitive airway control, initial arterial blood gas results, and outcome were recorded. Combitube insertion was successful in all 10 patients in whom placement was attempted. Definitive airway control was achieved by conversion to orotracheal intubation in seven patients, emergency department cricothyroidotomy in one patient, and operative room tracheostomy in two patients. No patient died because of failure to control the airway. Seven patients requiring Combitube had mandible fractures, four had traumatic brain injuries, two had facial fractures, and one had hemopneumothorax. Data suggest that Combitube insertion is an effective method of airway control in trauma patients who fail orotracheal RSI. It may be particularly useful in the patient with maxillofacial trauma and offers a practical alternative to surgical cricothyroidotomy in difficult airway situations.

The ability of paramedic RSI to facilitate intubation of patients with severe head injuries in an urban out-of-hospital system was evaluated by Davis and colleagues.[73] Adult patients with head injuries were prospectively enrolled over a 1-year period by using the following inclusion criteria: Glasgow Coma Scale score of 3 to 8, transport time greater than 10 minutes, and inability to intubate without RSI. Midazolam and succinylcholine were administered before laryngoscopy, and rocuronium was given after tube placement was confirmed by means of capnometry, syringe aspiration, and pulse oximetry. The Combitube was used as a salvage airway device. Outcome measures included intubation success rates, oxygen saturation values before and after intubation, arrival arterial blood gas values, and total out-of-hospital times for patients intubated en route versus on scene. Of 114 enrolled patients, 96 (84.2%) underwent successful endotracheal intubation, and 17 (14.9%) underwent Combitube intubation, with only 1 (0.9%) airway failure. There were no unrecognized esophageal intubations. On arrival at the trauma center, median oxygen saturation was 99%, mean arrival PaO_2 was 307 mm Hg, and mean arrival $PaCO_2$ was 35.8 mm Hg.[73,81]

Mercer and Gabbott considered the influence of neck position on ventilation with the Combitube, which was inserted in 40 patients undergoing general anesthesia.[77] A rigid cervical collar was then used to immobilize the neck of each patient. In all 40 subjects, adequate ventilation of the lungs was possible in this position as assessed by chest movement and auscultation, measurement of expired tidal volume, and maintenance of satisfactory arterial oxygen saturation. In 18 (45%) of 40 patients, small traces of blood were present on the Combitube after removal. Reducing the volume of air injected into the proximal balloon of the Combitube appeared to reduce the incidence of airway trauma during insertion.

In another study, a rigid cervical collar was used to immobilize the neck in 15 American Society of Anesthesiologists (ASA) physical class I or II patients under general anesthesia.[82] Insertion of the Combitube was then attempted. In 10 (66%) of 15 patients, blind insertion was impossible. In 5 (33%) of 15 successful blind insertions, the Combitube was in an esophageal position on each occasion. In 8 of 10 of the failures, reinsertion of the Combitube was attempted with the aid of a Macintosh laryngoscope. In 6 (75%) of 8 cases satisfactory placement was then possible, with the Combitube entering the esophagus on each occasion. Ventilation was satisfactory in all patients when insertion was successful. Blood staining of the Combitube was present in 7 (47%) of 15 patients. The investigators state that the Combitube cannot be recommended for use in patients whose necks are immobilized in rigid cervical collars. The alternative insertion technique may improve the rate of successful insertion in this group of patients, because it provides a larger oral aperture than the classic maneuver. However, in cases of suspected or evident cervical spine injury, manual in-line traction before intubation and application of a cervical collar is recommended.

In a 4-year, prospective study, Timmermann and colleagues followed the airway interventions performed by anesthesia-trained emergency physicians.[83] The Combitube or LMA was used in 2% of cases of failed intubation, with a success rate of 85% and 89%, respectively.

b. CASE REPORTS

A 14-year-old boy had been hit by a motorcycle while riding his bicycle. He suffered severe oronasal bleeding associated with craniofacial injury.[84] Computed tomography (CT) at admission indicated multiple craniofacial fractures (i.e., left frontal bone, maxilla, mandible, sphenoid bone, zygomatic bone, nasal bone, and ethmoid bone) with an epidural hematoma of the frontal lobe. His face was depressed about the nose. To keep the airway from oronasal bleeding, an emergency tracheostomy was performed after endotracheal intubation. Nasal and oral packing using Foley balloon catheters was performed but failed to control oronasal bleeding. Bradycardia appeared with ventricular fibrillation during the course because of marked hypovolemia. To get tighter packing, a Combitube was inserted. When the pharyngeal cuff of the Combitube was inflated, the blood pressure rose from 105/60 to 140/90 mm Hg, and the heart rate immediately decreased from 145 to 95 beats/min. Stable circulation was realized by this method during angiography. Embolization produced hemostasis. The Combitube was removed the next day. Surgery for facial fractures was conducted on the 16th hospital day, and the patient was discharged on the 70th hospital day. The Combitube was used in this case to effectively control severe oronasal bleeding before performing angiography. This method was easy to perform, and the investigators recommend the Combitube for oronasal bleeding before embolization.

In another case, an 18-year-old driver lost control of his car and crashed into a tree standing beside the street.[85] On arrival of the ambulance, the patient required immediate intubation, but he was trapped in the car. When the car struck the tree, the windshield was broken. Intubation was performed with the Combitube through the broken windshield with one hand only, and ventilation was performed successfully. The patient was then extracted and was intubated by an endotracheal airway. The patient survived and passed high school examinations soon after the accident.

A similar situation occurred for a 24-year-old man who was trapped in his jeep after a motor vehicle collision.[86] During his rescue, immediate intubation became mandatory. Because access to the patient's head was limited, a Combitube was inserted while standing in front of him, and ventilation was easily accomplished. The patient was admitted to the hospital and weaned from the ventilator 3 days later. After 4 weeks, he was discharged from the hospital without any neurologic sequelae. The Combitube appeared to be a valid alternative to endotracheal intubation in cases of difficult access to the patient's head.

Deroy and Ghoris described a case of elective anesthetic airway management in a patient with a cervical spine fracture.[87] In several unusual cases, the Combitube has proved superior to conventional endotracheal intubation. The Combitube proved to be useful in the case of neck impalement with a large, wooden splinter entering at the left angle of the mandible, traversing the pharynx and soft palate, and entering the right maxillary cavity below the floor of the orbit.[88]

Mercer reported a patient with a difficult airway who was in a halo frame for cervical immobilization.[89] The Combitube was successfully used after difficult bag-mask-valve ventilation and failed LMA ventilation.[89] Bhagwat and coworkers described the successful use of the Combitube to control oral cavity bleeding.[90] The patient had uncontrollable, torrential bleeding caused by the rupture of a right cheek and mandible arteriovenous malformation. The Combitube was used to ensure the airway and to control bleeding through the tamponade effect exercised by the pharyngeal balloon while performing external carotid artery ligation.

3. Anesthesiologic Studies

a. GENERAL ANESTHESIA

Function and effectiveness of the Combitube were first tested in animal experiments and subsequently in humans.[13,14] The effectiveness of ventilation with the Combitube was compared with ventilation with an ETT during routine surgery in a crossover study.[17] Twenty-three patients were ventilated first with the Combitube and then with an ETT (group 1). In group 2, application of the tubes was performed in a reversed order in eight patients. After 20 minutes of ventilation with each airway, arterial blood samples were analyzed. In all cases, patients were ventilated with the Combitube without problems, comparable to ventilation with an ETT. Arterial oxygen pressure was higher during ventilation with the Combitube (142 ± 43 mm Hg with the Combitube versus 119 ± 40 mm Hg with the ETT in group 1, $P = .001$; 117 ± 16 mm Hg with the endotracheal airway versus 146 ± 13 mm Hg with the Combitube in group 2, $P = .001$), whereas the differences in arterial carbon dioxide tension and pH were not significant.

The reasons for increased oxygen tension during ventilation with the Combitube were investigated in another study.[91] In 12 patients undergoing general anesthesia during routine surgery, a thin catheter was placed with its tip 10 cm below the vocal cords. Patients were then ventilated by mask, by the Combitube in the esophageal position, and by an ETT in a randomized sequence. Pressures were recorded in the trachea and at the airway openings. Blood gas analysis showed a higher arterial oxygen tension with the Combitube than with the ETT (151 ± 37 mm Hg versus 125 ± 32 mm Hg, $P < 0.05$) and a higher arterial carbon dioxide tension (36 ± 4 mm Hg versus 33 ± 4 mm Hg, $P < 0.05$). This slightly higher carbon dioxide tension with the Combitube may in part reflect integration of the hypopharynx into the physiologic dead space. Compared with mask ventilation, carbon dioxide tension was lower with the Combitube.

Several differences in intratracheal pressures were found. The rising pressure during inspiration was highest with the ETT (19 ± 6 mm Hg/sec with the ETT versus 14 ± 6 mm Hg/sec with the Combitube, $P < 0.05$). The smaller rising pressure with the Combitube may lead to a more favorable distribution of ventilation. Expiratory flow time was prolonged during ventilation with the Combitube (2.0 ± 1.0 seconds versus 1.3 ± 0.6 seconds with the ETT). This effect probably results from increased expiratory resistance because of the double-lumen design, and it may favor formation of a small, intrinsic, positive end-expiratory pressure (auto-PEEP). Auto-PEEP may also be caused by integration of the vocal cords into the airway with the Combitube, whereas they are bypassed by the ETT. The auto-PEEP does not exceed 2 mm Hg and therefore does not influence cerebral perfusion during CPR. The smaller rising pressure, prolonged expiratory-flow time, and auto-PEEP are responsible for the improved conditions for alveolar-arterial gas exchange.

Although peak pressures at the airway openings may be high due to the resistance of the double-lumen airway, intratracheal pressures were comparable for the two tubes. The peak endotracheal pressure was 10 ± 4 mm Hg with a Combitube and 12 ± 6 mm Hg with an ETT (P was not significant [ns]). The endotracheal-plateau pressure was 8 ± 2 mm Hg with the Combitube and 8 ± 4 mm Hg with the ETT (P = ns).[14] The Combitube may also be used for prolonged ventilation.[39] In seven patients in the ICU, the Combitube was used over a period of 2 to 8 hours during mechanical ventilation. Results showed adequate ventilation compared with subsequent endotracheal ventilation. Lipp and associates had an average time for insertion of the Combitube of 12 to 23 seconds.[92] In 3 of 50 patients, the Combitube had to be withdrawn 1 to 2 cm.

Urtubia and coworkers studied the proper use of the Combitube.[24] Although the manufacturer recommends that the SA Combitube be used in patients between 122 and 152 cm tall, the aim of this study was to evaluate whether ventilation was effective and reliable in patients taller than 152 cm with the Combitube in the esophageal position. They investigated whether airway protection was adequate and whether direct intubation of the trachea with the Combitube inserted in the esophagus was possible. Urtubia and colleagues studied 25 anesthetized, paralyzed, adult patients who were 150 to 180 cm tall.[24] Methylene blue was given orally to all patients before anesthesia induction. Under direct vision, an SA Combitube was inserted in the esophagus of all patients. The pharyngeal balloon inflation volume was titrated to air leak, and cuff pressures were measured. During surgery, a laryngoscope was inserted into the pharynx with the pharyngeal balloon deflated, and the laryngoscopic view was evaluated by using the Cormack-Lehane scale. The presence of methylene blue in the hypopharynx was investigated by direct laryngoscopy. Ventilation was effective and reliable in all 25 patients who were 150 to 180 cm tall (average, 169 ± 7 cm). A direct relationship between the pharyngeal balloon volume and patient height was established ($P < 0.05$) by using linear regression models, suggesting that the 37-F SA Combitube can be used in patients up to 6 feet (185 cm) tall and implying that the SA Combitube is the preferred size for most patients. The laryngoscopic view of the glottis was adequate to allow direct tracheal intubation. No trace of methylene blue was detected in the hypopharynx. The investigators concluded that the SA Combitube may be used in patients 122 to 185 cm tall. The trachea could be directly intubated with the Combitube in the esophageal position in patients with normal airways, and airway protection appeared to be adequate.

Gaitini and coworkers investigated the effectiveness of the Combitube in elective surgery during mechanical and spontaneous ventilation.[18] Two hundred ASA physical status I or II patients with normal airways who were scheduled for elective surgery were randomly allocated to two groups: nonparalyzed, spontaneously breathing

($n = 100$) or paralyzed, mechanically ventilated ($n = 100$). After induction of general anesthesia and insertion of the Combitube, SpO$_2$, EtcO$_2$, isoflurane concentration, systolic and diastolic blood pressure, heart rate, and breath-by-breath spirometry data were obtained every 5 minutes. In 97% of patients, it was possible to maintain oxygenation, ventilation, respiratory mechanics, and hemodynamic stability during mechanical or spontaneous ventilation for the duration of surgery, which was between 15 and 155 minutes. The results of this study suggest that the Combitube is an effective and safe airway device for continued management of the airway in 97% of elective surgery cases.

Walz and colleagues tested the smaller SA Combitube in patients exceeding 5 feet tall.[25] They studied 104 patients (66 men and 38 women between 3.93 [120 cm] and 6.5 ft [198 cm]) who received the SA Combitube during general anesthesia, most often during implantation of an automatic implantable cardioverter defibrillator. The duration of the procedures ranged from 45 to 360 minutes. In each case, the investigators were able to document with the use of pulse oximetry, capnometry, and ventilation parameters that the patients could be oxygenated and ventilated adequately. The oropharyngeal cuff volume of 85 mL, recommended by the manufacturer, was sufficient in 71 patients (68%). The remaining 33 patients required an additional insufflation volume of 25 to 50 mL in the oropharyngeal balloon to prevent air leakage. The group concluded that the SA Combitube could be used without restriction in patients exceeding 5 feet tall. Because of its smaller size, the SA Combitube is easier to use and seems to be less traumatic to soft tissues. Walz and colleagues preferred to use a laryngoscope during insertion of the SA Combitube, which resulted in less trauma and reduced the number of intubation failures.[25]

Evaluation of safety, efficacy, and maximum ventilatory pressures during routine surgery was investigated by Frass and coworkers.[93] Five hundred patients receiving general anesthesia were enrolled in the study. Type of surgery, duration of surgery, ease of airway insertion, and potential complications were recorded, along with maximum ventilatory pressures and leaks. The Combitube worked well in all but two patients. Duration of surgery varied between 30 and 360 minutes. The Combitube was placed in the esophagus in 97% of patients. More than 95% of the blind Combitube insertions were successful on the first attempt, with an average intubation time of less than 15 seconds. Efficacy of oxygenation and ventilation with the Combitube was evaluated by pulse oximetry and EtcO$_2$. An SpO$_2$ greater than 95% was documented in all cases, and the EtcO$_2$ was 35 to 45 mm Hg. Leak, expressed as a fraction of the inspired volume, did not increase more than 5%, up to a ventilation pressure of 50 cm H$_2$O. Data suggest that the Combitube is safe, easy to insert, and useful during routine surgery. The device may be used when ETT placement is not immediately possible.

Schreier and associates studied the 37-F SA Combitube in 20 children.[94] The average age was 9.3 ± 2.4 years, height was 137.3 ± 10.5 cm, and weight was 35 ± 10.8 kg. The Combitube worked well in all cases. This study shows that the 37-F SA Combitube can be used in "cannot intubate, cannot ventilate" (CICV) cases for children taller than 122 cm.

A 46-year-old, obese, white woman with a short neck was scheduled for excision of a thyroid goiter.[95] One hour after extubation, a hematoma was identified in the right anterior neck. Immediate intubation was mandatory. Fiberoptic intubation failed, but a blind attempt at inserting an ETT resulted in an esophageal intubation. An interincisor distance of 13 mm prevented insertion of a no. 3 LMA. An SA Combitube was then inserted blindly. Oxygen saturation rapidly improved and was maintained at 97% with an FiO$_2$ of 1.0. General anesthesia was completed, and after evacuation of the hematoma, ventilation improved as peak airway pressures declined. The Combitube was superior to the LMA in this case because of its slim design. The Combitube should be considered as an additional tool for managing patient airways in difficult circumstances.

Hagberg and colleagues reported successful use of the Combitube in a 50-year-old patient who had a severe contracture of the mouth and significant tracheal stenosis after prolonged intubation following a burn injury to the face.[96] His airway evaluation revealed a Mallampati class IV airway, one-finger-breadth mouth opening, and full range of neck mobility. Because of the patient's airway examination and concern about endotracheal intubation causing further subglottic tracheal stenosis, a Combitube was chosen for airway management. The otorhinolaryngology surgeons were present in the room when the patient's neck was prepared and draped and equipment was set up for a tracheostomy, if necessary. A fiberoptic bronchoscope was prepared for use. The investigators found the Combitube to be a very advantageous airway device in establishing an airway in this case and thought it should be considered for elective use in patients with limited mouth opening. They also recommended more extensive use of the Combitube in the operating room so that physicians are familiar with the device when it is needed emergently.[97,98]

The ease of learning to use the Combitube has been assessed. Enlund and associates reported a case in which conventional endotracheal intubation failed.[99] The patient was ventilated by a face mask in the sitting position while the Combitube was brought to the operating room. Although the surgeons were inexperienced in Combitube use, they read the manufacturer's instructions in the operating room and successfully inserted the Combitube. The device worked well throughout the entire surgical procedure.

Because tracheal suctioning is impossible with the Combitube placed in the esophageal position, the Combitube was redesigned.[60] The two anterior, proximal perforations of regular Combitubes were replaced by a larger, ellipsoid hole. Twenty patients with normal airways (Mallampati class I or II) were studied. During general anesthesia, patients were esophageally intubated with the Combitube. A flexible bronchoscope was inserted and guided through the modified hole and glottic opening down the trachea. For the replacement procedure, a J-tip guidewire was introduced through the bronchoscope. The bronchoscope and the Combitube were removed, and a standard ETT was advanced over a guide catheter. Bronchoscopic evaluation of the trachea and guided replacement of the Combitube by an ETT was successful in all 20 patients. The average time needed to perform airway exchange was 90 ± 20 seconds. Arterial oxygen saturation and $EtCO_2$ levels remained normal in all patients. No case of laryngeal trauma was observed during intubation or the airway exchange procedure. The redesigned Combitube enables fiberoptic bronchoscopy, finetuning of its position in the esophagus, and guided airway exchange in patients with normal airways. Further studies are warranted to demonstrate the value of this redesigned Combitube in patients with abnormal airways. This version is not commercially available.

b. LAPAROSCOPIC SURGERY

Airway management during laparoscopy is complicated by intraperitoneal carbon dioxide inflation, Trendelenburg position, increased airway pressures, and increased risk of pulmonary aspiration. The Combitube was used in 25 cases of laparoscopic cholecystectomy. Gastric insufflation could not be observed on the video film at the beginning or end of surgery.[100] Hartmann and coworkers investigated whether the SA Combitube was a suitable airway during gynecologic laparoscopy.[27] One hundred patients were randomly allocated to receive the SA Combitube ($n = 49$) or ETT ($n = 51$). Esophageal placement of the Combitube was successful at the first attempt (16 ± 3 seconds). Peak airway pressures were 25 ± 5 cm H_2O. An airtight seal was obtained using air volumes of 55 ± 13 mL (oropharyngeal balloon) and 10 ± 1 mL (esophageal cuff). Significant correlations were observed between the patient's height and weight and the volumes necessary to produce a seal. Similar findings were recorded for the control group; tracheal intubation was difficult in three patients. The SA Combitube provided a patent airway during laparoscopy. Nontraumatic insertion was possible, and an airtight seal was provided at airway pressures of up to 30 cm H_2O.

Exposure to sevoflurane and nitrous oxide (N_2O) during ventilation using an SA Combitube was compared with waste gas exposure using a conventional ETT.[101] Trace concentrations of sevoflurane and N_2O were assessed using a direct-reading spectrometer during 40 gynecologic laparoscopic procedures performed under general anesthesia. Measurements were made at the patients' mouths and in the anesthesiologists' breathing zones. Mean (±SD) concentrations of sevoflurane and N_2O measured at the patients' mouths were comparable in the SA Combitube group (0.6 ± 0.2 ppm of sevoflurane; 9.7 ± 8.5 ppm of N_2O) and ETT group (1.2 ± 0.8 ppm of sevoflurane; 17.2 ± 10.6 ppm of N_2O). These values caused comparable contamination of the anesthesiologists' breathing zones: 0.6 ± 0.2 ppm of sevoflurane and 4.3 ± 3.7 ppm of N_2O for the SA Combitube group, compared with 0.5 ± 0.2 ppm of sevoflurane and 4.1 ± 1.8 ppm of N_2O for the ETT group. Use of the SA Combitube during positive-pressure ventilation was not necessarily associated with increased waste gas exposure, especially when air conditioning and scavenging devices were available. The Combitube functioned satisfactorily in 22 patients scheduled for elective laparotomy.[91]

c. OBSTETRIC ANESTHESIA

Airway-related problems represent the most frequent cause of death among women who die of a complication of general anesthesia for cesarean delivery.[102] The Combitube has been included in algorithms for managing an unexpected difficult airway during general anesthesia for cesarean delivery.[102,103]

Urtubia and colleagues reported two cases of emergency cesarean delivery under general anesthesia in which an SA Combitube was used for first-line management of the airway.[104] Acute, severe fetal bradycardia in a 17-year-old, obese, pregnant girl did not allow time to perform spinal blockade. General anesthesia was induced, and the airway was maintained through a face mask while applying the Sellick maneuver. After delivery, an SA Combitube was blindly inserted into the esophagus while maintaining cricoid pressure. Ventilation and oxygenation were adequate. For a 27-year-old, deaf-mute, pregnant woman, emergent cesarean delivery was performed because of fetal distress under spinal anesthesia. Soon after surgery began, the patient demonstrated clear signs of pain, and general anesthesia was induced and ventilation performed through the SA Combitube inserted in the esophagus under laryngoscopic guidance. No postoperative pharyngeal symptoms and no respiratory complications were detected in both cases. The Combitube allowed adequate ventilation and airway protection for emergency cesarean delivery in these patients. The Combitube was quickly inserted blindly and with laryngoscopic guidance.

The Combitube was used as a rescue device in a CICV situation during induction of general anesthesia for a cesarean delivery. This case was followed by transient dysfunction of cranial nerves IX and XI, which was attributed to excessive pressure exerted on the pharyngeal mucosa.[105] This problem can be avoided by using the minimal inflation technique.[40]

Wissler used the Combitube in obstetric anesthesia.[106] He found that the Combitube was most easily and atraumatically inserted into the esophagus under direct vision using a laryngoscope. In his practice of obstetric anesthesia, the Combitube is his first choice for the anesthetized parturient who cannot be intubated or mask ventilated with cricoid pressure. He thinks it provides a better barrier against regurgitation and aspiration than the LMA.

In a pilot study performed by Hagberg and colleagues, the Combitube was determined to be comparable to the LMA regarding the incidence of gastroesophageal reflux (GER) and tracheal acid aspiration as detected by pH monitoring.[36] Fifty-seven patients were randomly assigned to receive an LMA or a Combitube for their elective surgical procedures. All patients were paralyzed and received positive-pressure ventilation. Two monocrystalline antimony catheters were used for pH monitoring of the trachea, oropharynx, and esophagus. One episode of GER occurred with the Combitube in place on extubation, but there were no pH changes reflected in the oropharyngeal or tracheal regions. Three patients in the LMA group met the pH criterion for aspiration (pH < 4.0 lasting at least 15 seconds), compared with only one patient in the Combitube group, but no patient

TABLE 27-1

Comparisons of Emergency Airway Equipment

Function	EasyTube or Combitube	Laryngeal Mask Airway or Laryngeal Tube	Esophageal Obturator Airway	Esophageal Gastric Tube Airway	Pharyngotracheal Lumen Airway
Provides barrier to minimize regurgitation of gastric contents	Yes	No	Yes	Yes	Yes
Allows buildup in esophagus of pressure and gastric contents during use	No	No	Yes	No	No
Functions when blindly passed into esophagus	Yes	NA	Yes	Yes	Yes
Functions when blindly passed into trachea	Yes	NA	No	No	Yes
Requires effective mask fit on face	No	No	Yes	Yes	No
Available in pediatric sizes	Yes/No	Yes	No	No	No
Needs taping	No	Yes	Yes	No	No
Safe against aspiration	Yes	No	No	No	No
Allows high ventilatory pressures	Yes	No	No	No	No

NA, Not applicable.
Modified from Wissler RN: The esophageal-tracheal Combitube. *Anesthsiol Rev* 20:147-152, 1993.

developed any clinical signs of aspiration. By providing reliable airway protection, the Combitube provides another alternative in managing a difficult airway.

Ideal insertion conditions for the LMA include lubrication and a special method of cuff deflation, whereas the Combitube is ready to use in its package. In an obstetric patient with increased oxygen consumption, decreased functional residual capacity, and airway obstruction, these differences in preparation time may be clinically important.

d. COMBITUBE COMPARED WITH ALTERNATIVE AIRWAY TECHNIQUES

The design of the Combitube has several advantages over other devices, including an open distal tip that allows decompression and suctioning of the esophagus and stomach in the esophageal position and ventilation in the tracheal position (Table 27-1).[106] Compared with other devices, the double-lumen design of the Combitube prevents lumen occlusion if the patient bites the tube, which avoids ventilation emergencies during the awakening period.

Compared with the LMA, the VBM Laryngeal Tube (LT; VBM Medizintechnik, Sulz, Germany), and other similar devices, the Combitube provides a decompression barrier (i.e., tracheoesophageal lumen) to minimize regurgitation of gastric contents and allows controlled mechanical ventilation with ventilation pressures higher than 20 cm H_2O.[91,107] Because the Combitube is safe against aspiration and avoids gastric insufflation during positive-pressure ventilation, use of the LMA is recommended only in elective cases without danger of aspiration. The LT is a device that simulates the design of the Combitube. Although the LT bears no lumen for active decompression, the VBM Laryngeal Tube Suction (LTS) does allow decompression of gastric contents. However, the device is very bulky and may be difficult to place in patients with a small interincisor distance. Another disadvantage is that analogous to the LMA, several sizes should be available to meet the needs of different sizes of patients.

In a training course for emergency care physicians, Winterhalter and associates compared emergency intubation with the Magill tube,[108] LMA, and Combitube in mannequins. The Combitube was rated highest with regard to effectiveness and ease of placement. In another comparative study involving nonanesthesia house officers, ventilation by face mask and LMA in a model led to gastric insufflation, but there was none with the Combitube.[109]

H. Recommendations for the Combitube

The Combitube has gained worldwide interest as an adjunct to standard airway equipment in many anesthesiology departments and ambulance services.[110-113] The Combitube has been recommended in the ASA practice guidelines for management of the difficult airway; the difficult airway algorithm calls for using the Combitube when an anesthetized patient can be neither intubated nor mask ventilated. Since 1992, it has been included in the guidelines for cardiopulmonary resuscitation and emergency cardiac care of the American Heart Association (AHA) as the first alternative airway, replacing the esophageal obturator as an alternative to the ETT.[114-117] The AHA has described the Combitube as a valuable tool for emergency intubation.[116]

In 2000, the Combitube was upgraded by the AHA to a class IIa device.[117] Recommendations for use of the Combitube have been included in the guidelines of the European Resuscitation Council, the Difficult Airway Society guidelines for management of unanticipated difficult intubations, and in many national guidelines.[118-121] The Combitube is included in the Street-Level Airway Management (SLAM) Emergency Airway Flowchart, a guideline created for advanced airway practitioners in anesthesiology, emergency medicine, and prehospital care.[113]

The Combitube is cited in many review articles as an alternative method for artificial ventilation, and it is recommended for patients with massive regurgitation or airway hemorrhage when visualization of the vocal cords may be impossible.[28,31,50,51,111,122,123] Gaitini and coworkers described the Combitube as an easily inserted, double-lumen/double-balloon supraglottic airway device.[18] The major indication for the Combitube is as a backup device for airway management. It is highly recommended for rescue ventilation in in-hospital and out-of-hospital environments and in situations of difficult ventilation and intubation, especially in patients with massive airway bleeding or limited access to the airway and those in whom neck movement is contraindicated.

Continued airway management with a Combitube that has been placed is a reasonable option in many cases. After securing the airway, it may not be necessary to abort the anesthetic or to continue with further airway management efforts. The Combitube is the perfect solution in places where a fiberoptic device is not available or when fiberoptic intubation fails.

Agró and colleagues emphasized that the Combitube is an easily inserted and highly efficacious device to be used as an alternative airway whenever conventional ventilation fails.[28] The Combitube allows ventilation and oxygenation whether the device is located in the esophagus (common) or the trachea (rare). Their review of the literature found the Combitube described as a valuable and effective airway in the emergency and prehospital settings, in cardiopulmonary resuscitation, in elective surgery, and in critically ill patients in the ICU. Some studies demonstrated the superiority of the Combitube over other supraglottic ventilatory devices in resuscitation as assessed by success rates for insertion and ventilation. Unlike the LMA, the Combitube may help in patients with limited mouth opening. It may especially benefit patients with massive bleeding or regurgitation, and it minimizes the risk of aspiration.

Because the Combitube is one of the three alternatives approved by the ASA for managing the CICV situation, its continued use is highly advisable, especially for trainees, to promote familiarity with it and allow its successful use during an emergency.

II. EASYTUBE

A. Development of the EasyTube Esophageal-Tracheal Double-Lumen Airway

The EasyTube (Rüsch EasyTube, Teleflex Medical, Research Triangle Park, NC) was developed to improve the standard of the Combitube. The outer appearance and handling are similar to those features of the Combitube.[124]

B. Technical Description and Insertion Technique

The EasyTube has a pharyngeal lumen that provides a supraglottic ventilation outlet ending just below the oropharyngeal balloon, which allows passage of a bronchoscope for inspection of the trachea, suctioning of tracheal secretions, or replacement, if necessary (Fig. 27-10). Because of this design, the longer tracheoesophageal lumen has a smaller outer tube diameter together and a

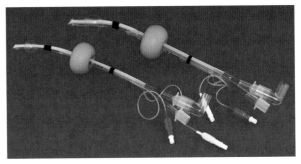

Figure 27-10 Two sizes of the EasyTube: 41 F (large) and 28 F (small).

larger inner diameter, and it ends like an ETT, decreasing the chance of injury to the pharyngeal and tracheal mucosa.

The distal end of the EasyTube is designed like that of a standard tracheal tube, with a tip diameter of 7.5 mm (41 F) or 5.5 mm (28 F). The device has kink-resistant outer tubes. It is a latex-free, sterile, single-use, double-lumen tube, and it is available in two sizes: 41 F for adult patients who are taller than 130 cm and 28 F for pediatric patients 90 to 130 cm tall. It provides sufficient ventilation when placed in the esophagus or the trachea.

The EasyTube may be positioned blindly or with the help of a laryngoscope. Laryngoscopic insertion is similar to that used for a standard tracheal tube. After placing the patient's head in a sniffing position and performing direct laryngoscopy, the trachea is intubated with the EasyTube. A black mark at the distal end of the tube indicates correct depth of insertion just below the vocal cords. Ventilation is performed through the transparent no. 2 lumen. In a CICV situation, the EasyTube can be inserted in the esophagus using a laryngoscope. Ventilation is then performed using the colored no. 1 lumen. The EasyTube also may be inserted blindly, as health care providers usually perform it, especially in the prehospital setting. While the patient's head is kept in a neutral position, the tube is inserted in a straightforward movement, parallel to the frontal axis of the patient, until the proximal black ring mark is positioned at the level of the upper incisor teeth. In the esophageal position, the no. 2 lumen may be used to drain gastric contents or allow insertion of a gastric tube. The pharyngeal and the distal cuffs are inflated with 80 and 10 mL of air, respectively, using the two prefilled syringes in the package (Fig. 27-11).

C. Indications, Advantages, and Complications

Indications for use of the EasyTube are the same as for the Combitube (see Box 27-1). It is designed for emergency intubation and for use in patients undergoing general anesthesia. It has been especially useful in various CICV situations. The 28-F pediatric size may be advantageous, because advanced airway management in children can be challenging, and the potential for morbidity is increased by failed attempts.[125] Nagler and Bachur posit that supraglottic rescue devices, including the LMA,

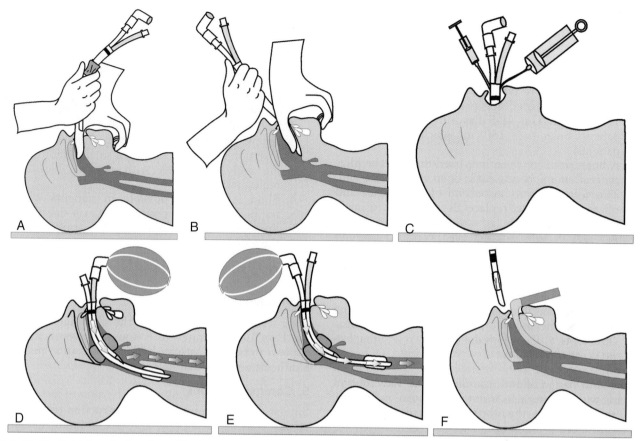

Figure 27-11 Guidelines for insertion of the EasyTube. **A,** Insertion begins by lifting the chin and lower jaw. **B,** The EasyTube is inserted in a downward, curved movement along the tongue. **C,** The oropharyngeal balloon is inflated with 80 mL of air and the distal cuff with 10 mL of air using the two prefilled syringes in the package. **D,** With the EasyTube in the esophageal position, ventilation is performed through the longer no. 1 tube *(blue)*. Air flows through the ventilation aperture into the pharynx and from there into the trachea *(arrows)*. **E,** With the EasyTube in the tracheal position, ventilation is performed through the shorter no. 2 tube *(transparent)*. Air flows directly into the trachea *(arrow)*. **F.** The EasyTube is inserted using a laryngoscope.

esophageal–tracheal double-lumen tube, and laryngeal tube, offer suitable ventilation strategies after failed intubation and in arrest scenarios.[125] They encourage pediatric providers to develop familiarity with emerging rescue ventilation devices and with advances in the practice of RSI and laryngoscopy.

1. Out-of-Hospital Emergency Intubation

Ease of use of the EasyTube makes it especially suitable for emergency intubation, which can be performed with the patient in almost any position. The dual lumens allow ventilation in the esophageal or tracheal position. Oral anchoring of the EasyTube is another feature that can be valuable during ventilation and transportation.

2. Elective and Emergency Surgery

a. GENERAL ANESTHESIA

The EasyTube was developed for use in general anesthesia cases. The dual system may be used to insert the EasyTube intentionally in the esophagus or the trachea. The ring mark below the distal cuffs enables correct positioning in relation to the vocal cords.

b. REPLACEMENT OF THE EASYTUBE

Analogous to the Combitube, the EasyTube can be replaced through a cricothyrotomy or tracheostomy or with the help of a video laryngoscope. Replacement also can be achieved with a bronchoscope and a guidewire inserted through the EasyTube working channel.

c. EXTUBATION

Similar to the Combitube, the oropharyngeal balloon of the EasyTube is deflated to allow communication with the patient. After recovery of protective reflexes, deflation of the distal cuff and final extubation during continuous suctioning through the shorter no. 2 lumen is performed. After full resumption of spontaneous ventilation, the EasyTube can be removed.

3. Advantages

The EasyTube provides several advantages over the Combitube:

1. The pharyngeal lumen of the EasyTube ends just below the oropharyngeal balloon. The tracheo-esophageal lumen is thinner than that of the

Combitube, which carries the two lumens down to the end. The thinner distal lumen of the EasyTube decreases the chance of injury to the pharyngeal and tracheal mucosa.

2. The oropharyngeal balloon is latex free.

3. The EasyTube is available in two sizes. The 28-F version is designed for pediatric patients 90 to 130 cm tall. The 41-F EasyTube is designed for patients taller than 130 cm, which includes most patients.

4. A fiberoptic scope can be passed through the pharyngeal lumen, because it is open at the distal end. This feature allows inspection of the trachea and offers one way to replace the EasyTube using a guidewire.

5. A larger suction catheter can be passed through both lumens (e.g., 16-F suction catheter in the 41-F EasyTube).

6. The eight small holes or ventilation apertures of the terminal oropharyngeal lumen of the Combitube may be responsible for a greater resistance, leading to larger differences in peak airway pressure measurements.[126] The EasyTube has only one supraglottic ventilation aperture.

The slim design allows insertion of the EasyTube in patients with an interincisor distance as small as 12 mm. As in the Combitube, the oropharyngeal cuff of the Easy-Tube prevents aspiration of blood or secretions from the oral or nasal cavity, and the distal cuff seals the esophagus preventing aspiration of esophageal or gastric secretions. This has been confirmed in a cadaver study.[107] Bercker and colleagues designed a study to compare the seal of seven supraglottic airway devices in a cadaver model of elevated esophageal pressure.[107] The Classic laryngeal mask airway (LMA-Classic), ProSeal laryngeal mask airway (PLMA), Fastrach intubating laryngeal mask airway (ILMA-Fastrach), Laryngeal Tube Suction (LTS), Laryngeal Tube Suction II (LTS II), Combitube, and Easy-Tube were inserted in unfixed human cadavers with an exposed esophagus that had been connected to a water column 130 cm high. Slow and fast increases of esophageal pressure were performed, and the water pressure at which leakage appeared was registered. The Combitube, EasyTube, and ILMA-Fastrach withstood water pressure up to more than 120 cm H_2O. The PLMA, LTS, and LTS II were able to block the esophagus until 72 to 82 cm H_2O. The LMA-Classic showed leakage at 48 cm H_2O, but only minor leakage was found in the trachea. Devices with an additional esophageal drainage tube drained fluid sufficiently without pulmonary aspiration. The investigators thought that the use of devices with an additional esophageal drainage lumen might be superior for use in patients with an increased risk of aspiration.[107] The Combitube, EasyTube, and ILMA-Fastrach showed the best capacity to withstand an increase of esophageal pressure.

Based on a review of the literature and his own experience as a paramedic and anesthesiologist, Bollig suggests that the Combitube and the EasyTube should be recommended in the Scandinavian guidelines for prehospital airway management.[127] He argues that the Combitube

has been recommended as an alternative airway device in the ALS guidelines of the European Resuscitation Council and in the ASA guidelines for CICV situations.[114,116] A review of the literature revealed the following advantages of the Combitube and EasyTube:

1. Insertion time is shorter for these devices than for endotracheal intubation.

2. The double-lumen airways offer better protection against aspiration than a laryngeal mask.

3. Insertion is possible despite a smaller mouth opening and in patients with massive bleeding or regurgitation.

4. Blind insertion is possible in patients who are trapped in a sitting position (e.g., car crash).

5. Epinephrine and lidocaine can be applied through the Combitube.

6. Mechanical ventilation in intensive care is possible for several hours using the Combitube.

4. Disadvantages

Long-term ventilation through the pharyngeal lumen of the EasyTube is limited to 8 hours. However, this time appears to be adequate for bridging the gap in managing a difficult airway situation.

5. Contraindications

Similar to the Combitube, any obstruction of the upper airways may be a relative or absolute contraindication for insertion of the EasyTube.

6. Complications

Possible complications comprise any damage, bleeding, or perforation of the oral, pharyngeal, or esophageal mucosa. However, because of the slimmer distal outer diameter of the tracheoesophageal lumen, the danger of injury is minimal. No major complications have been reported with the use of the EasyTube.

D. Medical Literature

1. Mannequin Studies

Based on the results from a mannequin study, the use of an impedance threshold valve for ventilation during CPR is possible in combination with the Combitube, Easy-Tube, or other supraglottic airway device.[128] Robak and coworkers reported the superiority of Combitube and EasyTube for controlling the airway in a mannequin under simulated pathologic airway conditions.[129] Fifty medical students assessed the success rate and insertion time for seven supraglottic airway devices: LMA Unique, LMA Fastrach single use, LMA Supreme, King LTS disposable (LTS-D), i-gel, Combitube, and EasyTube. All airways were inserted without problems, but only the Combitube and EasyTube were successfully inserted in simulated trismus, limited mobility of the cervical spine, and in cases of combined pathologic conditions such as trismus plus limited mobility of the spine and trismus plus tongue edema.

In another mannequin model, Ruetzler and colleagues studied the performance and skill retention of intubation by paramedics using seven airway devices: ETT, LMA

Unique, PLMA, LTS-D, i-gel, Combitube, and Easy-Tube.[130] After 3 months, 100% successful skill retention was reported for five of six supraglottic airway devices (i.e., LMA Unique, LTS-D, i-gel, Combitube, and Easy-Tube), and a rate of 58% was reported for endotracheal intubation.

2. In-Hospital Studies

Bollig and colleagues determined the difference in the rate of and time to successful airway placement and ventilation using tracheal intubation compared with use of the esophageal-tracheal Combitube or EasyTube. Twenty-six paramedics, who were trained in tracheal intubation, received additional training in the use of the Combitube and the EasyTube.[131] Each participant performed all three methods twice in a random order on a manikin. Time to successful ventilation (presented as the mean and standard deviation) and the success rate were recorded. Mean time to successful ventilation was significantly longer for tracheal intubation (45.2 ± 15.8 seconds) than for the Combitube (36.0 ± 8.6 seconds, $P = 0.002$) and the EasyTube (38.0 ± 15.3 seconds, $P = 0.023$), with no difference between the latter two methods ($P = 1.000$). The combined success rate for the Combitube and EasyTube (103 of 104 attempts) was significantly higher than for tracheal intubation (45 of 52 attempts) (odds ratio [OR] = 16.0; 95% confidence interval [CI], 1.9 to 134; $P = 0.002$). For the paramedics tested on manikins, the placement success rate was higher and less time was required for the Combitube and EasyTube than for tracheal intubation, with no differences identified between the Combitube and EasyTube.

In a study by Thierbach and Werner, 30 adult patients (ASA physical status I or II, Mallampati class I and II, and weight between 50 and 80 kg) undergoing minor surgery were randomly allocated to the esophageal EasyTube insertion group using a blind or laryngoscopically guided technique.[132] Data were collected for number of attempts, time taken to provide an effective airway, blood staining, and postoperative airway morbidity. The time to obtain an effective airway was measured from removal of the face mask to confirmation of normal ventilation and evaluated by bilateral chest movement and a normal capnography curve. There were no failures on inserting the device with either technique. First attempt and second attempt insertion rates were 86% and 14% for the blind insertion technique and 93% and 7% for the laryngoscopically guided technique, respectively. Time to achieve an effective airway was 31 ± 4 seconds for the blind technique and 33 ± 6 seconds for the laryngoscopically guided technique. After removal of the device, blood stains were observed in eight patients, with four patients in each group. The rate of sore throat in the postanesthesia care unit was 20% for both groups, and no patient required treatment. Data suggest that insertion of the EasyTube has the same success rate with or without using a laryngoscope. A study determined that pressures exerted on the oropharyngeal mucosa were lower than with laryngeal masks.[133]

Lorenz and associates studied the effectiveness, safety, and ease of placement of the EasyTube compared with an ETT in 200 patients randomized to one of these two groups.[134] Even though the number of insertions was equal in both groups, the insertion time was shorter with the EasyTube. (15.5 ± 3.6 seconds for the EasyTube versus 19.3 ± 4.6 seconds for the ETT, $P = 0.0001$). Ease of insertion was greater in the EasyTube group, and there was no difference in the incidence of sore throat, dysphagia, and hoarseness.

Gaitini and colleagues evaluated the ease of use of the EasyTube compared with the Combitube in 80 patients randomized to one of these two groups.[135] All patients were intubated blindly in the esophagus. Less time was required to achieve an effective airway using the Easy-Tube (19.4 ± 5.3 seconds) compared with the esophageal-tracheal Combitube (30.6 ± 4.1 seconds, $P < 0.001$). EasyTube insertion was rated significantly easier than Combitube insertion ($P = 0.008$) by anesthesiologists participating in the study. EasyTube insertion was rated easy in 36 cases and moderately difficult in 4 cases. Combitube insertion was rated easy in 26 cases and moderately difficult in 14 cases. No insertion in either group was rated difficult or impossible.

3. Out-of-Hospital Studies

In a prehospital setting, Chenaitia and coworkers evaluated the effectiveness and safety of use of the EasyTube in cases of difficult airway management by emergency physicians with minimal training with the device.[136] They performed a prospective, multicenter, observational study of patients requiring airway management conducted in a prehospital emergency setting in France by three mobile ICUs from October 2007 to October 2008. Data were available for 239 patients who needed airway management and were classified in two groups: the easy airway management group (225 patients [94%]) and the difficult airway management group (14 patients [6%]). All patients had a successful airway management. The EasyTube was used in eight men and six women; the mean age was 64 years. It was used for ventilation for a maximum of 150 minutes, and the mean time was 65 minutes. It was positioned successfully at first attempt, except for two patients; one needed an adjustment because of an air leak, and in the other patient, the EasyTube was replaced due to complete obstruction during bronchial suction. The investigators concluded that emergency physicians could use the EasyTube safely and effectively with minimal training in cases of difficult airway management. Because of its very high success rate for ventilation, the possibility of blind intubation, the low failure rate after a short training period, they thought it should be introduced in new guidelines for managing difficult airways in prehospital emergency settings.[133]

4. Study of the EasyTube in Emergencies

A preliminary study was undertaken by Thierbach and colleagues to assess early experiences with the EasyTube in prehospital and in-hospital emergency airway management procedures.[137] All airway management procedures with the EasyTube were recorded for a period of 18 months. The EasyTube was successfully used in 15 patients with unanticipated airway difficulties during anesthesia induction or prehospital airway management.

In all patients, the EasyTube was positioned successfully at the first attempt, with a median time of 31 seconds until start of ventilation. Effective supraglottic ventilation and oxygenation were achieved within 25 to 40 seconds. In three patients, the EasyTube needed one additional repositioning maneuver. On removal of the EasyTube, no blood was observed on the surface of the device, and no injuries were observed in the patients' mouth, pharynx, or esophagus. The investigators concluded that the device successfully established sufficient ventilation and oxygenation.[137]

5. Study Results and Applications

Studies demonstrate that the Combitube and EasyTube are effective alternatives to traditional intubation techniques. Both devices have been shown to be as effective as an endotracheal tube in emergency situations. The wide range of applications and ease of insertion make them valuable pieces of equipment in wards, operating rooms, and prehospital conditions, and the Combitube may be reused.[138] Operators involved in airway management should be familiar with the techniques described for these rescue devices to successfully manage an emergency and to avoid using the Combitube or EasyTube for the first time during a crisis.

Data suggest that the Combitube can be inserted successfully during microgravity (e.g., parabolic flights).[135,139] These results may aid in developing protocols for managing airway emergencies during space missions.

Studies show that double-lumen airways such as the Combitube and EasyTube are superior to other supraglottic devices in emergency situations.[20,21,75] Further study of these devices is recommended because they require less training than endotracheal intubation and are easier to insert than an endotracheal airway.[66]

III. CASE EXAMPLES OF AIRWAY MANAGEMENT WITH COMBITUBE, EASYTUBE, AND OTHER DEVICES

A 54-year-old, morbidly obese woman was admitted to the ICU because of respiratory failure.[140] Her neck was short and rigid, with thick, subcutaneous fat pads. Anatomic landmarks such as thyroid and cricoid cartilages were impossible to identify. Her tongue was very large, and the Mallampati score was class IV. Tracheal intubation by flexible fiberoptic bronchoscope (FOB) was performed under local anesthesia. Four days later, extubation was uneventful, and continuous positive airway pressure (CPAP) was initiated with the patient in the sitting position. Oxygen saturation ranged from 95% to 97%, but the patient was uncooperative and did not tolerate the CPAP mask. After removing the CPAP mask, supplemental oxygen (8 L/min) was given by an open face mask. Oxygen saturation decreased to 85%, she became rapidly cyanotic and dyspneic, and a severe bronchospasm was identified by direct thorax auscultation. Immediate tracheal intubation using the FOB was attempted under topical anesthesia, but respiratory parameters rapidly deteriorated. During intubation, the patient developed severe laryngeal spasm, which made passage of the FOB

through the vocal cords impossible. Oxygen saturation dropped to 60%, and the patient became unconscious and bradycardic. Three-handed mask ventilation was established with 100% supplemental oxygen and an oropharyngeal and two nasopharyngeal cannulas. Oxygen saturation increased to 80%. An expert anesthesiologist made one attempt at laryngoscopy, but only the tip of the epiglottis could be seen under direct vision. Laryngoscopy was immediately stopped because oxygen saturation dropped to 60% and the patient did not tolerate apnea. Cricothyrotomy was considered but excluded because it was impossible to identify the anatomic landmarks of the cricothyroid membrane. In view of the CICV situation, a 41-F Combitube was considered. Insertion was easy, and after checking the esophageal position by auscultation, ventilation was obtained using the device's pharyngeal tube. Inflation pressure appeared to be high, but oxygen saturation returned quickly to 95%. A 50-mg dose of atracurium was administered intravenously, and the patient was connected to a mechanical ventilator. Peak pressure was 45 cm H_2O. Residual bronchospasm was treated with 750 mg of aminophylline. The patient was transferred to the operating room for a tracheotomy while she was ventilated through the Combitube. The next day, the patient was fully awake and responsive, and she had no symptoms of neurologic damage. She was weaned from the ventilator 10 days after the tracheostomy and discharged from the ICU on day 22 after admission without neurologic sequelae.[140]

A female motor cyclist was hit by a truck and thrown onto the side of the street. On arrival of the ambulance, the patient was lying in a prone position. Because moving the body appeared to be dangerous, a 41-F EasyTube was inserted with the patient still in the prone position. Insertion and ventilation worked well.

A 45-year-old patient was scheduled for a neurosurgical procedure. Preoperative evaluation revealed a Mallampati score of class II. Endotracheal intubation was performed uneventfully, and the patient was moved into a prone position for surgery of the spine. Because of unintended movement of the ventilation tubes during surgery, extubation occurred. Immediate reintubation was mandatory, but insertion of a PLMA by an experienced anesthesiologist failed. An EasyTube was inserted without difficulty and remained in place during the 5-hour operation.

A 40-year-old man was scheduled for revision of scars caused by facial burns due to a gas explosion. The initial injury occurred 14 months before this procedure, and the patient had received a tracheostomy during his stay in the ICU. Preoperative evaluation revealed a reduced glottic opening and tracheal stenosis. Because of the existing airway pathology and the impossibility of using tapes, the EasyTube was elected for airway management. The EasyTube was inserted under direct vision with a laryngoscope into the esophagus and successfully used throughout the 130-minute surgical procedure.[141]

Paramedics failed to intubate a 51-year-old patient who was found unresponsive, but they successfully placed a Combitube. On arrival in the emergency department, it was decided to exchange the Combitube for an ETT. Three attempts to exchange the Combitube with an ETT using direct laryngoscopy failed. After deflation of the proximal cuff of the Combitube, an 8-mm ETT was advanced over a gum elastic bougie into the trachea under visualization of the oropharynx using a Direct Coupled Interface video intubating system.[142]

IV. CONCLUSIONS

The Combitube and EasyTube have proved to be valuable tools, especially in emergency and unexpected difficult airway situations. Compared with alternative supraglottic airways, these devices appear to be superior with respect to prevention of aspiration and application of high ventilatory pressures. Both airways can be inserted easily in patients with small interincisor distances.

The EasyTube has several advantages over the Combitube. First, the pharyngeal lumen of the EasyTube ends just below the oropharyngeal balloon. The tracheal-esophageal lumen is thinner than that of the Combitube, in which the two lumens continue to the distal end. Because the distal single lumen of the EasyTube is significantly thinner, the danger of mucosal damage is minimized. Second, the oropharyngeal balloon of the EasyTube is latex free. Third, the EasyTube is available in two sizes: 28 F for patients between 90 and 130 cm tall and 41 F for patients taller than 130 cm. Fourth, a fiberoptic scope can be passed through the pharyngeal lumen because it is open at the distal end. This feature allows inspection of the trachea and possible replacement of the EasyTube using a guidewire. Fifth, a larger suction catheter can be passed through both lumens of the EasyTube. Both airway devices can be considered for use in nonemergent or emergent situations, in patients with normal or difficult airways, and as a primary method of airway management or as a rescue device, as outlined in the ASA difficult airway algorithm.

V. CLINICAL PEARLS

- Train practitioners in alternate airways using manikins and intraoperatively
- Take care of aspiration risks
- Always have always a plan "B" available

SELECTED REFERENCES

All references can be found online at expertconsult.com.

1. Benumof JL: Management of the difficult adult airway. *Anesthesiology* 75:1087–1110, 1991.
18. Gaitini LA, Vaida SJ, Mostafa S, et al: The Combitube in elective surgery: A report of 200 cases. *Anesthesiology* 94:79–82, 2001.
20. Rumball CJ, MacDonald D: The PTL, Combitube, laryngeal mask, and oral airway: A randomized prehospital comparative study of ventilatory device effectiveness and cost-effectiveness in 470 cases of cardiorespiratory arrest. *Prehosp Emerg Care* 1:1–10, 1997.
24. Urtubia RM, Aguila CM, Cumsille MA: Combitube: A study for proper use. *Anesth Analg* 90:958–962, 2000.
27. Hartmann T, Krenn CG, Zoeggeler A, et al: The oesophageal-tracheal Combitube Small Adult. An alternative support during gynaecological laparoscopy. *Anaesthesia* 55:670–675, 2000.
32. Wafai Y, Salem MR, Baraka A, et al: Effectiveness of the self-inflating bulb for verification of proper placement of the Esophageal Tracheal Combitube. *Anesth Analg* 80:122–126, 1995.
72. Lefrancois DP, Dufour DG: Use of the esophageal tracheal Combitube by basic emergency medical technicians. *Resuscitation* 52:77–83, 2002.
73. Davis DP, Valentine C, Ochs M, et al: The Combitube as a salvage airway device for paramedic rapid sequence intubation. *Ann Emerg Med* 42:697–704, 2003.
130. Ruetzler K, Roessler B, Potura L, et al: Performance and skill retention of intubation by paramedics using seven different airway devices—A manikin study. *Resuscitation* 82:593–597, 2011.
139. Rabitsch W, Moser D, Inzunza MR, et al: Airway management with endotracheal tube versus Combitube during parabolic flights. *Anesthesiology* 105:696–702, 2006.

Percutaneous Translaryngeal Jet Ventilation

WILLIAM H. ROSENBLATT

I. INTRODUCTION

Invasive airway management is relegated to the category of rescue techniques that one must know but hopes never to use. Students may be able to witness a surgical crico-thyrotomy, and possibly to assist in the performance of an elective tracheostomy, but most anesthesiologists have successfully avoided incorporating these procedures into their practice. Although the modern airway armamentarium has made resorting to invasive procedures a rare event, the "cannot intubate, cannot ventilate" (CICV) scenario still occurs.[1] By equipping the clinician with an alternative to routine upper airway management, the potential for rescuing a failed airway and preventing devastating adverse outcomes is substantially increased.

Multiple studies have indicated that the incidence of the CICV scenario is between 0.01 and 2.0 cases per 10,000 anesthesias.[1-3] Although the root cause of this dire apneic or obstructive state may be fully or partially related to the patient's disease, it often has an iatrogenic component, being recognized at the time of anesthetic induction or as a result of other interventions. The American Society of Anesthesiologists (ASA), The Difficult Airway Society, and The Advanced Trauma Life Support guidelines, as well as the opinions of other expert organizations, concur that, although invasive airway access is rarely practiced or prepared for, this capability must be at the fingertips of any operator who is charged with airway management.[4-6] The conditions that commonly require the use of invasive airway access include facial fractures (32%), blood or vomit in the airway (32%), traumatic airway obstruction (7%), and failed intubation in the absence of other indications (11%).[7] A completely obstructed airway state does not have to exist for a patient to be at jeopardy. Any time the clinician cannot ensure adequate, life-sustaining gas exchange by virtue of a problem within the conveyance portions of the respiratory tract, further actions (noninvasive or invasive) are mandatory.

Although surgical cricothyrotomy has long been a standard of emergency invasive airway rescue, its use has declined, in part because of advances in noninvasive airway devices such as supralaryngeal airways (SLAs) and video laryngoscopes, the adoption of pharmacologic agents for rapid-sequence intubation in the emergency department, and increased requirements for trainee supervision.[8]

There is widespread agreement in the literature that percutaneous translaryngeal jet ventilation (PTJV),[5] using a small-bore catheter placed through the cricothyroid membrane (CTM), is a simple and effective treatment for the desperate CICV situation.[8,9] Compared with surgical cricothyrotomy and tracheostomy, the establishment of PTJV is ordinarily quicker, simpler, and therefore more efficacious for most anesthesiologists, who may not be practiced in more formal surgical techniques.[8,10] This may not hold true for the infant or small child, however. Although PTJV was faster to achieve than a surgical airway, it had an exceedingly high failure rate (83%) in a swine model of the juvenile population.[11] This is likely due to the lack of circumferential support offered by the immature cricoid cartilage.

The goal of this chapter is to present a clinically applicable discussion of the technique of PTJV. This will give the clinician the tools to perform PTJV rapidly and safely, but only if he or she is prepared. It is important that the clinician give advanced consideration to the technique—such as ensuring the immediate availability of appropriate cannulas, oxygen conveyance devices, and a high-pressure O_2 source—and to the situations that may call for its use.

A. A Note on Nomenclature

Although the acronym PTJV is used for this discussion, there are a number of names and acronyms in the literature that might be just as adequate but do not completely describe the current technique. Terms such as percutaneous (versus trans), tracheal (versus laryngeal), jet (versus insufflation), and oxygenation (versus ventilation) may all be appropriate, and at times one descriptor will fit better than another. The acronym PTJV is commonly used and describes most clinical situations in which it is likely to be used successfully.

The literature is replete with descriptions of PTJV techniques and of a number of devices, both commercial and "operating room [OR] rigged."[12-16] As discussed here, many of these OR-rigged PTJV setups have not undergone objective testing; although they are easy to construct, they may not be practical, robust, or life-sustaining.

Although the term "small-bore catheter" may be encountered in some texts and primary literature, authors use this term as a comparison to "surgical" options, which involve percutaneous cricothyrotomy and tracheostomy devices with an internal-bore diameter (ID) of 3 mm or greater. It should also be noted that the term "cannula-over-needle" is used in this text to refer to a device similar to the common intravenous catheter: a hollow, elongated plastic catheter with an inner coaxial sharp-beveled needle that is removed after in vivo positioning.

II. INCORPORATING PERCUTANEOUS TRANSLARYNGEAL JET VENTILATION INTO THE DIFFICULT AIRWAY PLAN

The 2003 ASA difficult airway (DA) algorithm lists three techniques that should be employed when circumstances are encountered in which one cannot intubate (i.e., via direct laryngoscopy) and cannot ventilate, either by bag-mask or with the use of a laryngeal mask airway (LMA; LMA North America, Inc., San Diego, CA). These techniques are insertion of an esophageal-tracheal Combitube (ETC; Ambu, Copenhagen, Denmark), use of PTJV, and provision of an emergency surgical airway. Because the LMA and ETC are familiar to most anesthesiologists, both of these noninvasive airways should be considered first in cases of supraglottic obstruction, unfavorable anatomy, or other CICV situations. Both have been demonstrated to be highly effective in this setting and are generally considered atraumatic.[4,17,18] Though other SLAs are likely to be as applicable, they are not mentioned in the 2003 practice guidelines. Whether or not future guideline revisions call for other devices or refer to generic SLAs, operator experience and comfort should guide choice. The preferred device should be immediately available whenever the possibility of a CICV situation might arise.[17]

If insertion of an SLA does not affect gas exchange quickly, the ASA DA algorithm recommends that the clinician move to an invasive airway access maneuver without hesitation or delay. Of the maneuvers suggested, PTJV may be the most familiar to the anesthesiologist. A distinct advantage of PTJV over surgical cricothyrotomy is that it can be practiced in nonemergency clinical care. The anesthesiologist who is practicing elective, awake intubation may choose to make the percutaneous transtracheal injection of lidocaine a routine technique, thereby practicing laryngeal catheter placement, and some have advocated the placement of prophylactic transtracheal catheters in high-risk airway situations or for elective laryngeal surgery.[19] It should be noted that severe subcutaneous emphysema is a rare complication of translaryngeal lidocaine injection, even in otherwise uncomplicated cases.[20]

III. INCIDENCE AND COMPLICATIONS

Barotrauma with resultant pneumothorax and hemodynamic changes has been reported with both emergent and elective use of PTJV.[8,19,21-31] In a retrospective chart review, Patel and associates described a 53-month experience with patients in acute respiratory failure in the intensive care unit.[21] Of the 352 patients requiring endotracheal intubation, 29 emergent PTJV attempts were made. The procedure was performed by house staff ($n = 5$) and attending physicians ($n = 24$). Successful cannulation of the airway was achieved in 79% of patients. Subcutaneous emphysema occurred in 2 of these patients. Orotracheal intubation was subsequently required in 22 patients, with 1 requiring a surgical tracheostomy. PTJV failed in 6 patients. These failures were attributed to recent thyroid surgery ($n = 1$), obesity ($n = 2$), kinking of the PTJV cannula ($n = 2$), and misplacement of the cannula ($n = 1$). Subcutaneous emphysema was seen in only 1 patient for whom PTJV failed. The other patient who suffered subcutaneous emphysema experienced severe pneumomediastinum treated with bilateral chest tubes. Of the 6 patients with failed PTJV, 2 were subsequently orally intubated with the aid of a bougie, and the remaining 4 died.

Smith and colleagues reported a 29% incidence of complications in 28 patients managed with PTJV to provide an emergency airway.[22] These complications included subcutaneous emphysema (7.1%), mediastinal emphysema (3.6%), exhalation difficulty (14.3%), and arterial perforation (3.6%), none of which were fatal.

Other complications, such as esophageal puncture, bleeding, hematoma, and hemoptysis, have been also reported after PTJV.[23]

In a review of 265 elective PTJV and other forms of jet oxygenation/ventilation for otolaryngologic surgery, Jaquet and colleagues wrote that PTJV was associated with hemodynamic instability (8 patients), subcutaneous emphysema of the neck (3 patients), posterior tracheal mucosa tear (1 patient), catheter kinking (3 patients), severe mediastinal/cervical subcutaneous emphysema (1 patient), unilateral pneumothorax (1 patient), and bilateral pneumothorax (1 patient).[19] The last 3 events were considered major complications, and all were associated with cough or laryngospasm during PTJV. Damage to the tracheal wall, witnessed by this group, was also demonstrated in a large-animal model of PTJV in which full-thickness erosion and hemorrhage of posterior tracheal mucosa was seen in all specimens.[29] Subcutaneous emphysema has been associated with cannula shaft lacerations in the absence of frank cannula misplacement.[30]

In another series of elective PTJV cases, there was an overall minor complication rate of 3%.[22] These complications (minor bleeding, subcutaneous emphysema) were typically seen when multiple attempts had to be made during cannula placement. The authors recommended that no more than two attempts should be made.

The site of PTJV access may also influence complications. In a swine tracheal model, Salah and coworkers studied trans-CTM versus transtracheal cannulation. With some percutaneous techniques, traumatic injury (including posterior wall tears or frank penetration and cartilaginous fractures) were more common when the PTJV cannula was inserted into the trachea.[31]

Complete or near-complete airway obstruction during PTJV may also contribute to hemodynamic instability.[24] In a controlled trial employing graded airway obstruction in dogs undergoing PTJV with 45 psi inflation pressures through a 13-G catheter, intratracheal pressures of 24 cm H_2O were associated with decreasing blood pressure and increased central venous pressure, even in the absence of pneumothorax. In complete upper airway obstruction simulated in dogs, intratracheal airway pressure rose precipitously as soon as the total lung capacity was exceeded. This was accompanied by a fall in systolic blood pressure and eventual rupture of the pulmonary system (pneumothoraces, pneumomediastinum, subcutaneous emphysema, cardiac fibrillation) when an intratracheal pressure of 250 cm H_2O was achieved.[25]

In one canine study, methylene blue instilled into the oral cavity was less readily aspirated into the trachea during PTJV, compared with controls.[26,27] The authors reasoned that the retrograde egress of gas from the larynx reduced oral content aspiration. A similar phenomenon has been noted in humans during O_2 insufflation through an endotracheal tube (ETT) exchange catheter.[28]

A. Mechanism of Barotrauma and Other Forms of Airway Trauma

Striving to verify the intraluminal position of a percutaneously placed cannula is mandatory during PTJV. Though cannula misadventures are responsible for many of the complications related to PTJV, complete upper airway obstruction during O_2 insufflation is likely responsible for most episodes of barotrauma. During involuntary obstruction of the upper airway (e.g., due to laryngospasm) intraluminal pressures, generally remaining in the safe range of 18 to 25 cm H_2O during PTJV, rise precipitously. In an artificial lung model, upper airway obstruction (airway resistance 200 cm H_2O/L/sec) resulted in an intratracheal pressure of 60 cm H_2O. Intraluminal pressures between insufflations did not rise above minimal levels (3 cm H_2O) until maximal airway resistance was produced, at which time there was an equilibration to maximal pressure.[32] In an adult sheep model, complete airway obstruction during constant tracheal insufflation of O_2 at 15 L/min resulted in a pressure of 96 cm H_2O in 12 seconds. When intermittent jet ventilation (JV) was used (inspiratory-to-expiratory [I:E] phase ratio, 3:5), a pressure of 108 cm H_2O was reached in 33 seconds.[25]

IV. CANNULA SIZE AND OXYGENATION

A wide variety of cannula-over-needle devices have been described in the PTJV literature in both in vivo and mechanical model trials and in case reports. Trials of cannulas smaller than 3 mm in diameter (equivalent to 8 G) have typically demonstrated the need for a high-flow regulator/conveyance apparatus. Although flow through cannulas of various diameters and lengths has been measured during simulated PTJV, actual flow varies with the clinical situation and is affected by factors such as airway resistance and pulmonary compliance. Table 28-1 lists experimental data on flow rates through cannulas of various sizes with the use of a 50 psi gas supply.[14,33,36]

TABLE 28-1

Flow Rates Through Cannulas in Various Models

Cannula Gauge	Internal Diameter (mm)	Flow (mL/sec)	Model	Reference
18*	1.4	50	Sheep (46-54 kg)	14
15*	2	150	Sheep (46-54 kg)	14
13*	2.5	250	Sheep (46-54 kg)	14
12*	3	340	Sheep (46-54 kg)	14
9*	4	800	Sheep (46-54 kg)	14
20	0.89*	400	Lung model	33
16	1.65*	500	Animal	
14	2.1*	1600	Lung model	33

*Approximate conversion.

Neff and colleagues insufflated gas through cannulas of various diameters in a sheep model.[25] Marginal oxygenation was achieved with a 1.4-mm-diameter (15-G) cannula using 15 L/min constant and 50-psi "pulsed" O_2 flow. Use of low-pressure systems, such as resuscitator bags and anesthesia machine circuits, which provide 1 to 2 psi, was futile for catheters smaller than 3 mm in diameter. However, Zornow and colleagues were able to produce "delayed" reoxygenation in a hypoxic swine model with a 14-G cannula and "vigorous" ventilation with an anesthesia machine circuit.[25,29] O_2 resuscitation was significantly faster when 50-psi supplies were used (15 versus 120 seconds).[25]

Some authors have speculated that entrainment of room air via a Venturi effect produced by the high velocity of the gas injected into the larynx during PTJV might add as much as 40% or 50% to the volume of inspired gas.[33-35] This hypothesis has been contradicted by the findings of arterial blood gas studies in both animals and healthy patients undergoing jet ventilation, which demonstrated O_2 tensions consistent with the insufflation of 100% O_2 (no entrainment of room air).[36-38]

Whereas complete upper airway obstruction has been associated with ineffective ventilation and barotrauma, partial obstruction may enhance both oxygenation and ventilation by driving gas flow toward the lower bronchial tree, facilitating tidal volume (V_T) and improving alveolar oxygen tension (PaO_2).[24]

In summary, cannulas smaller than 3 mm in diameter (8 G) are unreliable for oxygenation and ventilation unless high-pressure regulator systems are used and there is an egress for exhaled gas. Catheters smaller than 14 G are unreliable even with the use of high-flow regulators.

V. VENTILATION

Effective ventilation during PTJV requires a pathway for gas egress. Fortunately, most patients who present with life-threatening airway failure (e.g., laryngeal edema, epiglottitis, laryngeal tumor) have isolated inspiratory obstruction with no or partial expiratory obstruction.[39] This is true during spontaneous breathing as well as controlled ventilation through a face mask or SLA, and it is related both to the extrathoracic position of the upper airway and to the architecture of laryngeal and supralaryngeal structures. Complete obstruction to gas escape is a contraindication for PTJV and may be dependent on the devices used.

Because removal of CO_2 is dependent on sufficient volumes of gas entering and exiting the lung, low-pressure systems (e.g., resuscitation bags) are generally inadequate for ventilation, as they are for oxygenation. Zornow and colleagues, using a 14-G transtracheal cannula in a swine model, was able to effectively ventilate with a 50 psi O_2 source but could not reduce arterial CO_2 despite "vigorous" ventilation with an anesthesia machine circuit.[29] Whereas gas escaping from an in vivo ETT could be measured when PTJV was performed with the high-pressure source, no gas movement was appreciated with use of the low-pressure system.

Ward and coworkers examined no, partial, and complete upper airway obstruction during PTJV in dogs,

using 13-G catheters and a high-flow regulator delivering 45 psi of pressure.[40] With no or partial upper airway obstruction, CO_2 levels decreased during PTJV. Partial airway obstruction improved CO_2 removal, possibly by promoting improved alveolar expansion during the O_2 injection phase of PTJV.

A. Airway Rescue in Complete Upper Airway Obstruction

Although controversial and based on animal models, low-flow insufflation of O_2 into the pulmonary circuit has been proposed as a mechanism for maintaining oxygenation, although not effective ventilation, in the patient with a completely obstructed airway.[24,41,42] Several alternative techniques have been studied in the model of complete upper airway obstruction.

Frame and associates, using a canine model (20 to 29 kg), found that with complete airway obstruction, O_2 flows of 5 to 7 L/min through 10-G and 12-G catheters could maintain oxygenation with I:E phases of 1:4 seconds and provided reasonable ventilation ($PaCO_2$ <75 mm Hg).[41] When lower flow rates (3 L/min) were used, CO_2 tension increased rapidly after 5 to 20 minutes. Although this study demonstrated the successful use of low-pressure O_2 flow in complete airway obstruction (in an effort to avoid barotrauma), it must be cautioned that small animals and large insufflation catheters were used.

Low-flow translaryngeal rescue insufflation of oxygen (LF-TRIO) of as little as 2 L/min has been shown to maintain oxygenation in a large animal model (34-kg swine) for upwards of 60 minutes.[5] LF-TRIO recovered the animals from O_2 saturation nadirs of 50% in an average of 23 seconds. Cardiovascular parameters were stable in all animals for a minimum of 15 minutes. Although the animals experienced hypercapnia, the authors argued that this may be well tolerated if there are no specific comorbidities that may be aggravated by increasing CO_2 (e.g., head trauma). Although imaging in this study was limited to a small number of animals, there was no evidence of microatelectasis after 1 hour of LF-TRIO. LF-TRIO was considered by these authors to be a short-term rescue option when definitive surgical airway control is anticipated.

More recently, the concept of an active expiratory phase has been applied to PTJV (Fig. 28-1). In a series

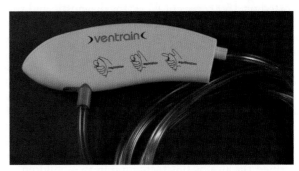

Figure 28-1 The Ventrain device uses a Venturi valve to apply negative pressure during the expiratory phase of percutaneous transtracheal jet ventilation. (Courtesy of Dolphys Medical BV, The Netherlands.)

of large-animal studies, Enk and Hamaekers described using the O_2 flow from a standard flowmeter to create a negative-pressure, transcatheter expiratory phase.[32] Bernoulli's principle, application of which is familiar to anesthesiologists in the functioning of the Venturi valve, states that when a fluid in a vessel passes through a constriction, dynamic energy (speed of flow) is increased, whereas static pressure (potential energy) exerted on the vessel side-wall is diminished. This setup can be manipulated to produce a subatmospheric pressure during an expiratory phase of PTJV. In an initial bench model, a prototype expiratory ventilation assistance (EVA) device reduced by half the time required for a 1000-mL injected V_T to be expired via a 2-mm ID cannula and also increased the effective minute ventilation by 33%.[32] In another large-animal study by the same group that included a complete obstruction of the upper airway, EVA restored oxygenation within 10 seconds and limited hypercarbia over 15 minutes.[42] However, EVA was less effective when the upper airway was unobstructed, possibly due to preferential entrainment of ambient air into the PTJV catheter via the lower-resistance upper airway path and, consequently, reduced removal of alveolar gases.[43]

B. Percutaneous Translaryngeal Jet Ventilation in Relief of Upper Airway Obstruction

The introduction of PTJV may encourage partial relief of upper airway obstruction. In a controlled study, Okazaki and colleagues demonstrated that induced airway obstruction (by simple neck flexion) was partially relieved by the insufflation of 10 L/min O_2, although not as well as by the chin lift–jaw thrust maneuver.[44] This finding implies a potential utility of transtracheal insufflation in patients who are at high risk for airway obstruction during post-anesthesia recovery.[44,45]

VI. ELECTIVE INDICATIONS

A. To Facilitate Operations of the Upper Airway

There have been several reports and various recommendations for the elective use of PTJV in surgical procedures to avoid tracheostomy, provide an unobstructed surgical field, or facilitate safe ETT. Singh and coworkers reported on 1500 cases of PTJV for diagnostic and surgical procedures of the upper airways, including bronchoscopy and esophagoscopy ($n = 1257$) and endolaryngeal surgery ($n = 135$).[46] PTJV support was continued for 24 to 48 hours into the postoperative period in 108 cases. Spoerel and Greenway, describing ventilation techniques during endolaryngeal surgery, similarly found adequate pulmonary ventilation with excellent conditions for microscopic surgery.[47] Smith and colleagues reported on elective transtracheal ventilation in children undergoing surgical procedures involving the head and neck.[48] They described the use of this technique in two children, one undergoing an operation for laryngeal stenosis and one who became obstructed and cyanotic in the recovery room. $PaCO_2$ measurement at the end of the procedures

indicated that the patients were moderately hyperventilated. Similarly, because PTJV leaves the entire airway from the vocal cords to the face accessible for surgical manipulation, it is not surprising that its elective use has been described for a large variety of procedures on these structures in adults.[49] In addition, Wagner and coauthors described a case in which high-frequency JV was used with success (thus avoiding tracheostomy) in a patient with a partial upper airway obstruction caused by a hypopharyngeal foreign body with sharp appendages.[50]

Dhara and colleagues reported on two cases in which a triple-lumen central venous catheter was placed through the CTM before induction of anesthesia.[51] Making use of all three lumens, this unique approach allowed the clinicians to measure tracheal CO_2 and intra-airway pressure, as well as providing jet oxygenation. In both cases, an upper airway egress for insufflated O_2 was maximized by use of a nasopharyngeal airway (NPA) or tongue retraction.

Depierraz and associates investigated the elective use of PTJV in pediatric patients (aged from less than 1 to 12 years) with significant upper airway obstruction.[52] They recited the major advantages of this technique: improved surgical exposure of the upper airway obstructive lesion, reduced manipulation of the lesion, reduced operative field movement during laser surgery, reduced danger of airway fire, and reduced risk of blowing particles into the distal airway.

B. To Permit Safe Intubation of the Trachea

In situations in which there is a significant risk of airway management failure, PTJV has been used electively to preclude the CICV situation. One report described the use of prophylactic PTJV to provide oxygenation in a patient who was known to be difficult to intubate.[53] PTJV enabled the patient to be anesthetized, muscle relaxed, and intubated in a safe, nonemergent manner. In another report of a 13-year-old girl with ankylosis of the temporomandibular joint resulting from a prior fracture, PTJV was electively instituted before the induction of anesthesia, and the trachea was subsequently intubated with the aid of fiberoptic bronchoscopy.[54] In a third report, PTJV was used to supplement spontaneous ventilation via the natural airway in a patient with a massive upper tumor so that the airway could be secured in a nonemergent manner.[55]

C. To Facilitate Training

Another benefit of the elective use of transtracheal techniques not to be ignored is training of students and anesthesiology residents as well as critical practice for attending physicians themselves. As discussed earlier, the 2003 ASA DA algorithm suggests four alternatives in the CICV situation: LMA, ETC, PTJV, and surgical airway.[4] The first two techniques can be practiced electively (the cost of the single-use ETC may be decreased by reprocessing).[56] Although a surgical airway can be electively practiced in appropriate patients, such as in a case of upper airway pathology when a tracheostomy is surgically planned and an otolaryngologist is available as a supervising physician, transtracheal catheter placement has definite clinical indications that can be employed for training purposes (e.g., awake intubation procedures, retrograde intubation). Many authors agree with this approach, especially because total airway obstruction may not be relieved by the SLA devices.[22,57,58] However, elective use of translaryngeal needle placement is not without its complications, as reviewed earlier.[20]

VII. EQUIPMENT

The literature is replete with manufactured and OR-rigged devices for delivering O_2 to a translaryngeal catheter. The great advantage of using a preassembled, commercially made PTJV system is the quality assurance that is built into a commercial product and the freedom from having to assemble the system. In addition, because low-pressure systems (e.g., anesthesia breathing circuit, self-inflating resuscitation bag) are typically ineffective when coupled with percutaneous catheters and because the anesthesia machine manufacturers limit the utility of the common gas outlet (CGO) for PTJV, commercial systems offer specifically designed components and joints for use with high pressure.[25] Many of the OR-rigged devices remain untested, and although they may resemble working systems, performance in a true clinical emergency is unknown.[59] In addition, a working system should be prepared or made available before the need for it arises. In the CICV situation, small delays contribute to devastating effects. Not only can it take many seconds to minutes to assemble a device, not all anesthetizing or resuscitative locations contain uniform equipment. Basic characteristics of a PTJV system are listed in Box 28-1.

A study testing four different OR-rigged devices arrived at the conclusion that only devices employing high pressure were capable of delivering adequate transcannula flows and maintaining oxygenation, although adequate ventilation was not consistently assured.[15]

Several of the described OR-rigged devices rely on intermittent occlusion of a port of a three-way stopcock with the intent of allowing diversion of the O_2 supply flow through the unoccluded port during the expiration phase (expired gas is meant to be removed via the upper airway, if it is unobstructed).[60-62] Hamaekers and colleagues showed that three-way stopcocks act as flow splitters.[63] Unoccluding the open limb of the stopcock does not halt all flow into the transtracheal catheter; this results in continuous O_2 flow into the trachea, possibly hindering CO_2 removal and contributing to hemodynamic instability. In the case of total upper airway occlusion, continued flow from these devices can contribute to barotrauma.[63]

By comparison, a relatively simple manufactured device is the Enk Flow Modulator (Fig. 28-2; Cook Critical Care, Bloomington, IN). Unlike many OR-rigged devices, forward gas flow in the PTJV catheter is minimal when the five 4-mm holes of the Enk Flow Modulator are released. This reduces positive end-expiratory pressure (PEEP) and other consequences of continued flow during the expiratory phase.[63,64] Some flow through the catheter during the expiratory phase may be desirable (when there is not complete upper airway occlusion). This flow may aid in elimination of CO_2 from the unoccluded airway, as well as enhancing oxygenation.[64]

In two studies, investigators surveyed their colleagues to determine what OR-rigged devices were preferred. In Morley and Thorpe's survey,[14] three different configurations were described, and the survey by Ryder and colleagues[15] described seven different configurations. In these studies, 5% and 10% of anesthesiologists, respectively, could not assemble any device, and only 5% and 40% of the devices, respectively, were considered adequate for PTJV. When clinicians were asked to assemble a device of their own choosing, they needed between 20 and 365 seconds (mean, 90 seconds) to produce a functional device, again raising doubts about the practicality of depending on unmanufactured systems.[15] Industrial-grade valves, which may mimic the function of the devices manufactured specifically for JV, typically contain lubricants and should not be used for medical indications.

The most critical element in the system employed for PTJV may be the availability of pressurized O_2, typically supplied at 45 to 60 psi. Central supply ("wall oxygen") is ubiquitous in ORs, intensive care units, and other areas of hospitals. Portable O_2 tanks are also fitted with regulators that are adjusted to deliver 50 psi. A variety of

---

BOX 28-1	**Characteristics of an Ideal Transtracheal Jet Ventilation Device**

Validated in clinical or laboratory studies
Minimum cannula size, 14 G
Low-compliance tubing, fixed component joints
Ability to connect to a high-pressure (50 psi) O_2 source
Ability to connect to anesthesia circuit, self-inflating bag (if ≥3 mm ID)
Kink resistant
Intratracheal pressure measurable
EtCO$_2$ measurable
Flow controllable
Pressure regulation provided
Available preassembled
Available sterile

EtCO$_2$, End-tidal carbon dioxide concentration; *ID*, internal diameter.

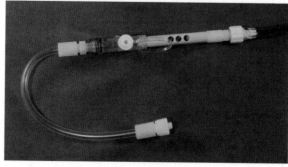

Figure 28-2 The Enk Flow Modulator uses a 15 L/min low-flow regulator/flowmeter to provide O_2 for percutaneous transtracheal jet ventilation. The operator manually covers the finger holes to direct flow to the patient. (Courtesy of Cook Critical Care, Bloomington, IN.)

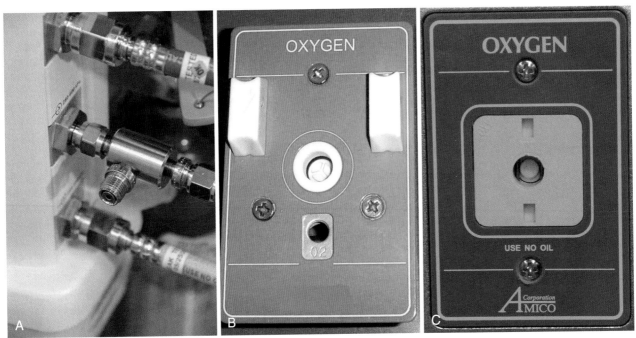

Figure 28-3 Indexed systems for central supply O_2 sources. **A,** Diameter-Index Safety System (DISS); **B,** Chemtron; **C,** Ohmeda.

indexed systems may be used to prevent mismatching of gas sources and clinical devices (Fig. 28-3). When purchasing new equipment for PTJV use, the specific indexing system, as well as the male versus female configuration, must be specified to the vendor. Many anesthesia machine manufacturers provide an outlet that is tied to the high-pressure gas supply and is accessible by Diameter-Index Safety System (DISS) fittings (see Fig. 28-3A). Although the anesthesia machine CGO was previously employed as a source of high-pressure O_2, its use is discouraged, and to this end, manufacturers have downregulated the available pressure when the machines' O_2 flush valve is activated (Fig. 28-4).[33]

All systems used to convey O_2 from high-pressure sources to the patient must have adjustable governors that limit static pressure or continuous flow in order to minimize barotrauma, and they must contain a

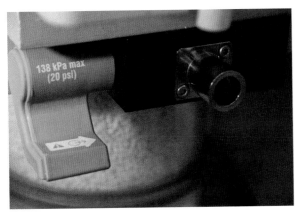

Figure 28-4 Accessory common gas outlet on an Asteva Anesthesia Machine from Datex-Ohmeda (Madison, WI). The maximum pressure from this outlet is downregulated by the manufacturer, who also supplies an accessory Diameter-Index Safety System (DISS) fitting on the rear of the machine.

mechanism for halting or diverting flow to produce an expiratory phase during PTJV. Two such systems are commonly used in PTJV: high-flow regulators (with manual triggers) and low-flow regulator-flowmeters (with flow diversion). High-flow regulator systems, such as the Manujet III (VBM Medizintechnik, Sulz, Germany) (Fig. 28-5), allow the user to preset the pressure delivered to the PTJV catheter (0 to 50 psi) during a no-flow state. Manual activation of a trigger starts the flow of O_2 to the translaryngeal catheter; release of the trigger halts gas flow. A disadvantage of this system is that it is closed—there is no path for gas escape during the expiratory phase. This may increase the risk of barotrauma or encourage more hypercapnia. Although these systems are capable of delivering 50 psi to the translaryngeal catheter, intratracheal pressures do not rise above 25 cm H_2O.

The second commonly studied system for O_2 conveyance is the low-flow regulator, which limits continuous flow from 0 to 15 L/min (Fig. 28-6). Low-flow regulators are commonly available on small (E-cylinder) O_2 transport tanks, on some anesthesia machines, and attached to central supply O_2.[34] Several studies have demonstrated the utility of these devices. When 15 L/min is delivered satisfactory V_T with 16- and 14-G PTJV catheters may be achieved within the first 0.5 seconds.[34] Low-flow regulators are ubiquitous in hospitals. Inexpensive systems have been developed to convey O_2 from low-flow regulators to the patient.

A study by Preussler and colleagues compared the two aforementioned conveyance systems.[65] This group compared a high-flow regulator (Manujet III) attached to a 50 psi O_2 source and low-flow, 15 L/min regulator-flowmeter fitted with an Enk Oxygen Flow Modulator.[66] Both systems were tested in anesthetized pigs using a specialized 15-G transtracheal cannula. The upper airway of the pigs was kept patent with an ETT and a 20-cm H_2O PEEP valve in order to simulate a clinical partially

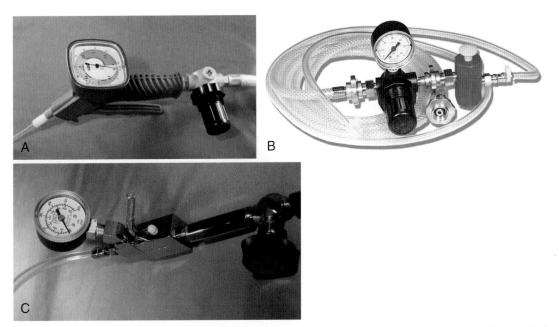

Figure 28-5   Three high-flow regulator-powered manual jet ventilators: **A,** Manujet III (VBM, Medizintechnik, Sulz, Germany); **B,** manual jet ventilator (Instrumentation Industries, Bethel Park, PA); **C,** jet ventilator (Anesthesia Associated, San Marco, CA). (**B,** Courtesy of Instrumentation Industries.)

obstructed airway. The investigators found that both device setups performed equally well, maintaining EtCO₂, PCO₂, and PaO₂ in acceptable ranges. The Enk Flow Modulator includes a Luer-Lok syringe port for administration of drugs into the trachea without interruption of ventilation or oxygenation. The Manujet III has a variable-pressure regulator and pressure gauge. Other bench models have shown that close-circuit gas injectors, such

as the Manujet III, achieve higher peak flows, greater V_T (650 mL), and higher intra-airway pressures, compared with the Enk Flow Modulator (240 mL).[64]

During total expiratory pathway occlusion in a bench model, intra-airway pressure rises precipitously with closed-circuit gas injectors (e.g., Manujet III) that have no facility for gas release during the expiratory phase via the transtracheal catheter. Lenfant and colleagues showed

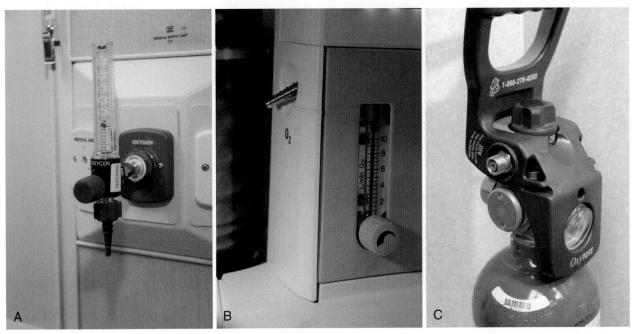

Figure 28-6   Three types of low-flow regulator-flowmeters: **A,** wall mounted; **B,** incorporated into an anesthesia machine (Datex-Ohmeda Avance model; Datex-Ohmeda, Madison, WI); **C,** incorporated into an E-cylinder tank regulator.

that when 3-bar pressure was applied via the Manujet in a completely occluded airway, intra-airway pressures of 136 cm H_2O were measured after two inspirations.[64] In contrast, systems that use flow diversion by allowing gas escape during the expiration phase (e.g., Enk Flow Modulator with 15 L/min gas flow) generated significantly lower intra-airway pressures after multiple breaths. In the completely occluded airway scenario, these systems may have an advantage, providing a pressure release pathway. The authors caution, however, that aggressive insufflation with any device can be dangerous in the completely occluded airway. The Enk Flow Modulator is not immune to producing high pressures in this situation.[64] In most cases of CICV, total airway occlusion does not occur. In situations in which high peak pressure is of concern, the driving pressure can be reduced. In the emergency clinical situation, close attention to chest rise (and fall, between insufflations) can guide adjustment.[64]

The last critical device in the PTJV setup is the translaryngeal cannula. Historically, a variety of intravenous catheter-over-needle devices have been employed.[22,55,67,68] Others have attempted to measure expired CO_2 and intratracheal pressure using alternative devices, such as triple-lumen central venous catheters.[51] Garry and colleagues used a needle-in-needle catheter assembly (a 14 G or 16 G catheter fitted within a 3-mm ID catheter).[69] O_2 was insufflated in the central needle while suction and CO_2 monitoring were applied to the annular space. Newer catheters constructed from kink-resistant materials have a preformed tip angulation, Luer-Lok connectors, 15-mm circuit adapters, or securing rings (Fig. 28-7).

VIII. TECHNIQUE OF PERCUTANEOUS TRANSLARYNGEAL JET VENTILATION

Emergent need for PTJV may be anticipated but is rarely expected. No clinician is likely to induce anesthesia when complete loss of airway control is a probable outcome. Conversely, most patient airways are managed without critical incident, and it is the job of the anesthesiologist to envisage the scenario in which invasive airway access could become necessary. Preparation for the use of PTJV may be the single most important aspect of its application. Table 28-2 lists the minimal materials and resources that must be available if PTJV is anticipated; my own opinion is that these should be accessible in any anesthetizing situation in a health care setting.

Willingness to use PTJV is the next step of preparation. Most anesthesiologists, by the nature of their training, prefer noninvasive methods. The tendency (and trend) is to reduce the use of even well-established invasive procedures (e.g., adoption of ultrasound guided nerve block versus nerve stimulation techniques). Given the proliferation of SLA devices and endotracheal intubation techniques during the last 20 years, it is unsurprising that surgical and percutaneous airway rescue procedures, even when performed adequately, are often applied too late in the lost-airway scenario to effect a change in outcome and prevent death or brain death.[70] Dogged perseverance with laryngoscopy and unsuccessful SLA ventilation must be avoided—evidence attests that this not only is futile but also contributes to a worsening outcome.[70,71]

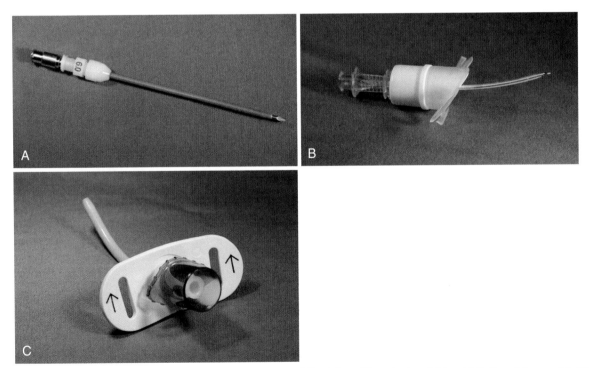

Figure 28-7 A, The Cook transtracheal jet ventilation catheter (Cook Critical Care, Bloomington, IN) is a 15-G, 5- or 7.5-cm, wire-reinforced, kink-resistant cannula. The proximal end has a female Luer-Lok type of adapter. **B,** The Ravusin 13- or 14-G jet cannula (VBM, Medizintechnik, Sulz, Germany) has rings for securing the cannula to the patient, both Luer-Lok and 15-mm proximal adapters, and a preformed curve. **C,** The Ardnt Emergency Cricothyrotomy Catheter (Cook Critical Care) is made of a precurved, kink-resistant material; unlike the other catheters, it is inserted with the use of an over-the-wire Seldinger technique.

TABLE 28-2

Equipment and Resources for Percutaneous Translaryngeal Jet Ventilation

	Description	Example
Minimal Resources		
Oxygen source	Wall or regulated tank, 50 psi	Indexed central supply or regulated tank O_2
	Low-flow O_2 flowmeter, 15 L/min minimal flow	Wall outlet or tank flowmeter
Needle catheter (specialized)	13-G ID or greater diameter	Cook Transtracheal Catheter*
		Ravusin catheter†
Conveyance device	Regulated and adjustable, hand-triggered valve with indexed O_2 source connection	Manujet III†
	O_2 flowmeter-powered, hand-regulated O_2 outlet	Enk Flow Modulator*
		Ventrain‡
Personal protective equipment	Protects operator from bloodborne acquired antigens	Gloves, face mask
Other	Syringe, Luer-Lok	5 or 10 mL
Preferred Accessories		
Skin-marking pen	To mark the location of the cricothyroid membrane	
Antiseptic solution, sterile drapes	For preparation of sterile field	
Scalpel	For small vertical skin incision	
Fluid	Helps to appreciate needle entrance into larynx	Saline, local anesthetic with epinephrine (1:200,000 dilution)
Fine-gauge needle	For local injection of anesthetic, epinephrine	22-25 G

*Cook Critical Care, Bloomington, IN.
†VBM, Medizintechnik, Sulz, Germany.
‡Dolphys Medical BV, The Netherlands.

A. Insertion of the Transtracheal Catheter

The right-hand–dominant operator stands on the left hand side of the patient. The CTM is palpated with the neck of the patient extended, unless an absolute contraindication exists (Fig. 28-8). The rate of misplacement of PTJV due to misidentification of the CTM is high, with one study showing that only 30% of clinicians were able to identify the overlying surface landmarks.[72] The literature is replete with methods of identifying the CTM (Box 28-2). When airway management difficulty is anticipated, it is not unreasonable (and is often encouraged) for the

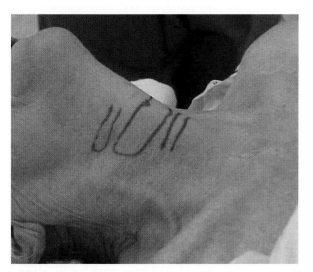

Figure 28-8 The location of the cricothyroid membrane is identified and marked. When difficulty is anticipated, this may be done in anticipation of percutaneous transtracheal jet ventilation.

clinician to identify the CTM before the start of any airway procedures such as anesthetic induction or preparation for awake management (see Fig. 28-8).[4] The DA Taskforce of the ASA encouraged assessing the feasibility of invasive airway use in any patient whose airway is to be controlled. Preanesthesia palpation and marking draws attention to the potential futility of attempting invasive management (e.g., in the patient with super-obesity) and may lead to an early change in the anesthesia plan.[1]

The CTM is the accepted entrance point for PTJV.[31] Insertion of a cannula-over-needle or surgical airway in the vicinity of the cricoid cartilage has several advantages. First, several landmarks have been described for CTM identification. Second, it is the only completely circumferential cartilage in the airway. The mature cricoid cartilage lends rigidity to the larynx, making it resilient to the anteroposterior pressure of an inserted cannula-over-needle, resulting in reduced trauma.[31] Third, the posterior wall of the cricoid cartilage extends from the trachea inferiorly to the inferior border of the thyroid cartilage. This provides a solid "backstop" for the probing PTJV cannula-over-needle placed through the CTM. Several reports have described intentional and unintentional tracheal PTJV cannula placement when the CTM was

BOX 28-2 Methods for Identifying the Cricothyroid Membrane

Operator's fingerbreadth below thyroid notch (adult)
Patient's fingerbreadth below thyroid notch
Second skin crease lies over cricoid cartilage
Four operator fingerbreadths above sternal notch (adult)
Two centimeters below thyroid notch (adult)

difficult to identify. Salah and colleagues, in a swine cadaveric airway study, noted increased trauma to the tracheal anatomy with some, but not all, percutaneous techniques, emphasizing the preference for CTM access.[9]

If time permits, a local anesthetic with epinephrine can be injected into the skin to reduce bleeding, thus improving visualization in the event that a surgical technique must be pursued. In the emergent situation, analgesia at the site of airway access is not an objective. Combined local anesthetic-epinephrine solutions are often used by surgeons for skin vasoconstriction because of their safe and reliable dilutions. An antiseptic solution can be rapidly applied, if time permits.

The previously identified translaryngeal cannula-over-needle is readied with a 5- to 10-mL syringe, with or without fluid. If it is not already preshaped by the manufacturer, a small-angle bend (15 degrees) can be placed 2.5 cm from the distal end.[73] This angulation helps prevent intratracheal cannula kinking or cephalad travel. The needle punctures the skin in the midline over the lower third of the surface landmarks of the CTM. The CTM is a relatively avascular structure, although blood is occasionally drawn into the syringe (this should not deter the intubator from completing this life-saving procedure). The cricothyroid artery and vein can be avoided by performing the puncture in the midline of the neck in the lower third of the CTM, just above the cricoid cartilage.[74,75] Initially, the axis of the cannula-over-needle is oriented at a 90-degree angle to the imagined location of the cervical spine. As downward pressure is exerted, constant negative pressure is applied to the syringe plunger. It is practically mandatory that the intralaryngeal position be identified by aspiration of gas. Except in the case of drowning or pulmonary hemorrhage, the larynx and trachea should be gas filled. Under no circumstance should the intubator assume that the larynx or trachea has been entered based on surface landmarks or tactile sense alone. Not only is the injection of pressurized O_2 into the subcutaneous tissue, the mediastinum, a large vessel, the pleural space, or other inappropriate location futile, but it may lead to rapid death and may obscure the anatomic planes needed to complete a surgical airway.

As bore diameter increases, passage of the cannula-over-needle through the skin becomes increasingly difficult. The requirement that large-gauge cannula be used for PTJV is counterbalanced by percutaneous insertion difficulty. If this is encountered, a small vertical incision through the skin can be made with a scalpel blade. Resistance to needle advancement may otherwise be caused by contact with the cricoid or thyroid cartilage, and the landmarks of the airway should be rapidly reassessed.

If a constant negative pressure is applied to the syringe, entrance into the larynx is heralded by air aspiration. The few bubbles that may be detected with needle exploration should not be construed to indicate airway entry. A 13-G or larger needle entering the airway will allow the effortless aspiration of voluminous air. Once air is aspirated from the larynx, the syringe is oriented 30 degrees cephalad, and the cannula is advanced off the needle and into the airway. When the hub of the cannula reaches the skin line, and the needle has been fully removed and safely discarded, air should once again be aspirated from

the in situ cannula to reconfirm the intralaryngeal location. From the moment the cannula is inserted into the trachea, a human hand should be dedicated to holding the transtracheal cannula in place until a definitive airway is established.

After reverification of the intra-airway cannula location, the available O_2 conveyance system is attached via its Luer-Lok connections. Initial insufflations of O_2 should be titrated to chest excursion. When a high-flow, hand-triggered regulator is used, a 1 second or less inspiratory time has been emphasized by several authors.[34,64] Though 50 psi may be needed to cause chest excursion, commencing PTJV with more modest pressures (25 to 30 psi) may be prudent to preclude the devastating complications of cannula misplacement. The ability to designate precise insufflation pressures may not be available on all high-flow regulators, underscoring the recommendation that equipment be prepared or adjusted before the need arises. The maximum and midrange output settings on the available high-flow regulator should be determined during equipment preparation.

A variety of I:E phase ratios have been suggested without absolute advantages being established, in part because of the wide variety of artificial and animal models that have been studied. In general, low respiratory rates (e.g., 4 breaths/min) result in improved ventilation, especially if partial airway obstruction exists. Respiratory rates as high as 12 breaths/min (e.g., a phase ratio of 1:4) have been studied.[64] Adhering to the principle of ensuring adequate chest wall recoil to guide the respiratory rate is of singular importance. Inadequate recoil may be caused by poor maintenance of upper airway patency, a shortened expiratory phase, or a fixed obstruction. Maneuvers to open the upper airway (e.g., oropharyngeal airways [OPAs], NPAs, SLAs, chin lift-jaw thrust) may be reassessed, and lengthening of the expiratory phase may be attempted. If the clinical history and course are consistent with a fixed upper airway obstruction, the strategies discussed earlier may be in order. As previously discussed, complete upper airway obstruction is a contraindication to the use of high-flow regulators.

When a low-flow regulator and conveyance system is in use (e.g., O_2 flow meter, Enk Flow Modulator), V_T will be reduced, yet the same oxygenation/ventilation strategies are applied.[64] The low-flow regulator should be set to 15 L/min; inspiratory time should be based on observation of chest wall excursion, although 1 second may be used as the initial standard. The phase ratio should be based on observations of chest fall but has been studied in ranges similar to those noted earlier for high-flow regulators. The use of active expiratory valves (e.g., EVA) should improve ventilation by allowing faster respiratory rates and by reducing, but not eliminating, the dangers of barotrauma and hypoventilation during complete upper airway obstruction.

IX. MAINTENANCE OF THE NATURAL AIRWAY

Unless an advanced EVA device such as the Ventrain (Dolphys Medical BV, The Netherlands) is in use, the driving pressure for the expiratory phase of PTJV is the elastic recoil of the chest wall and abdominal contents (10 to 20 cm H_2O). The hazards of an obstructed upper airway, apart from inadequate ventilation, have already been discussed. During PTJV, all efforts should be made to maintain a patent upper airway in order to avoid excessive intrathoracic pressure and to aid ventilation. Chin and jaw thrust maneuvers or use of an OPA, NPA, or SLA should be employed throughout the PTJV procedures.

X. CONCLUSIONS

The incidence of the CICV situation is 1 per 10,000 patients presenting to the OR, and it is higher in the emergency department. The degree to which SLA devices have reduced the occurrence of this critical circumstance, although dramatic, has yet to be defined. In most cases, the possibility of failed upper airway management can be anticipated and avoided. PTJV is a simple, easily mastered procedure that offers a remedy for this dire situation. The lungs of both healthy and critically ill patients have been successfully oxygenated and ventilated by this method, and it has a place in every anesthetizing situation. The systems of choice are dependent on the clinical situation, the physical plant in which the operator works, and the available conveyance devices. Translaryngeal ventilation systems using the anesthesia circle system (with reservoir bag), self-inflating resuscitation bags, and OR-rigged conveyance devices perform poorly in this dire clinical situation and may be helpful only if very large (>3 mm) cannulas are used.

Because there are a number of serious PTJV complications, this life-saving procedure should be undertaken only in desperate emergencies or in carefully thought-out elective situations. However, because desperate CICV emergencies continue to occur in association with the practice of anesthesia, I recommend that every anesthetizing location have PTJV equipment immediately available and that anesthesiologists become familiar with the technique.

XI. CLINICAL PEARLS

- Translaryngeal insufflation of O_2 requires a high-pressure O_2 source unless catheters 3 mm or larger in diameter are used. Anesthesia circuits and air-mask-bag units cannot provide adequate pressure.

- Before contemplating translaryngeal insufflation of O_2, the clinician should ensure that all materials and an O_2 source are available. This requires planning prior to the event.

- Only medical-grade devices should be used for these life-salvaging techniques. Jerry-rigged devices should not be used.

- Dedicated translaryngeal catheters, 14 G or larger, and not angiocatheters should be used.

- Translaryngeal insufflation of O_2 requires some degree of upper airway patency. If the airway is completely occluded, devices that allow exhalation of gas (passive or active) must be used. In any case, these patients demand a surgical airway as soon as possible.

- Whenever translaryngeal insufflation of O_2 is undertaken, an oropharyngeal device (e.g., supralaryngeal airway [SLA], oropharyngeal airway [OPA], nasopharyngeal airway [NPA]) should be in place to promote gas escape.

- Apart from and earlier than recovering O_2 saturation, chest recoil (not expansion) is the best monitor of well-performed translaryngeal insufflation.

SELECTED REFERENCES

All references can be found online at expertconsult.com.

8. Manoach S, Corinaldi C, Paladino L: Percutaneous transcricoid jet ventilation compared with surgical cricothyroidotomy in a sheep airway salvage model. *Resuscitation* 62:79–87, 2004.
9. Salah N, El Saigh I, Hayes N, et al: Comparison of four techniques of emergency transcricoid oxygenation in a manikin. *Anesth Analg* 110:1083–1085, 2010.
11. Johansen K, Holm-Knudsen RJ, Charabi B, et al: Cannot ventilate-cannot intubate an infant: Surgical tracheotomy or transtracheal cannula? *Paediatr Anaesth* 20:987–993, 2010.
19. Jaquet Y, Monnier P, Van Melle G, et al: Complications of different ventilation strategies in endoscopic laryngeal surgery: A 10 year review. *Anesthesiology* 104:52–59, 2006.
24. Carl ML, Rhee KJ, Schelegle ES, et al: Effects of graded upper-airway obstruction on pulmonary mechanics during transtracheal jet ventilation in dogs. *Ann Emerg Med* 24:1137–1143, 1994.
31. Salah N, El Saigh I, Hayes N, et al: Airway injury during emergency transcutaneous airway access: A comparison at cricothyroid and tracheal sites. *Anesth Analg* 109:1901–1907, 2009.
43. Hamaekers A, Theunissen M, Jansen J, et al: Emergency ventilation through a 2 mm ID transtracheal catheter in severe hypoxic pigs using expiratory ventilation assistance (EVA). Meeting Abstracts, September 2010, Society for Airway Management.
44. Okazaki J, Isono S, Atsuko T, et al: Usefulness of continuous oxygen insufflation into trachea for management of upper airway obstruction during anesthesia *Anesthesiology* 93:62–68, 2000.
66. Enk D, Busse H, Meissner A, et al: A new device for oxygenation and drug administration by transtracheal jet ventilation. *Anesth Analg* 86:S203, 1998.

Chapter 29

Performance of Rigid Bronchoscopy

SOHAM ROY | IRVING Z. BASAÑEZ | RONDA E. ALEXANDER

I. HISTORICAL BACKGROUND

Rigid bronchoscopy is an invasive surgical technique that is used to visualize the oropharynx, larynx, vocal cords, trachea, and proximal pulmonary branches. The origins of rigid bronchoscopy, like many aspects of modern medicine, can be traced back to Hippocrates (460-370 BC), who advised introducing a pipe into the larynx in a suffocating patient to assess the airways.[1] Because of limitations with lighting, the field was largely dormant until the 1800s, when incandescent light bulbs were invented. The development of local anesthesia in 1880 also made bronchoscopy more tolerable. In March of 1897, Gustave Killian passed an endoscope through the larynx and removed a piece of pork bone from the right main stem bronchus using cocaine anesthesia.[1] Chevalier Jackson further advanced the field of rigid endoscopy by developing improved lighting, auxiliary instrumentation for removal of foreign objects, and rigid bronchoscopy training programs.[2] He is recognized as the father of contemporary rigid endoscopy.[3] Since Jackson's time, many changes have been made to the bronchoscope, so that current rigid instrumentation and ventilation systems allow for more precise and accurate assessment of the aerodigestive tract.[3] H.H. Hopkins of England invented the first conventional lens system by using glass rods instead of small lenses, which produced a significantly brighter image, occupied less space, and allowed for greater visualization of an object in a single field.[1] This provided the basis for fiberoptic and modern rigid bronchoscopy.

II. INDICATIONS AND CONTRAINDICATIONS

The tracheobronchial tree can be directly observed with either rigid or flexible bronchoscopy. Although the advent of flexible bronchoscopy has given physicians improved access to more distal portions of the tracheobronchial tree with a more rapid learning curve and less patient discomfort compared with rigid bronchoscopy,[2] there are still several situations in which rigid bronchoscopy is more appropriate. The larger working port and rigid structure make rigid bronchoscopy useful for surgical interventions within the airway, such as the removal of foreign bodies or polyps (see "Foreign Body Removal").[4] At the same time, the bronchoscope can be used in establishing and maintaining airway control in patients with difficult ventilation, such as those with an acute airway obstruction or massive hemoptysis.[4] The major advantage of the rigid bronchoscope compared to the flexible one is that it has a ventilation port that can be directly connected to the anesthesia ventilator, allowing for maintenance of an airway and external ventilation while airway procedures are performed. In fact, the latest practice guidelines for the management of a difficult airway (DA) include the use of rigid bronchoscopy because it "reduces airway-related adverse outcomes."[5]

Other instances in which rigid bronchoscopy is indicated include deeper diagnostic biopsies when a fiberoptic specimen would be inadequate; dilatation of strictures; bronchial stenting; fracture reduction; application of laser therapy or cryotherapy; tumor removal; and diagnosis of vascular rings. Some of the indications for pediatric rigid bronchoscopy are listed in Box 29-1.

There are few contraindications to rigid bronchoscopy. In practice, most of the factors limiting rigid bronchoscopy are related to the general anesthesia used, such as an unstable cardiovascular or respiratory status.[6] One absolute contraindication to rigid bronchoscopy is an unstable cervical spine, because of the hyperextension of the head required during the procedure. In this instance, flexible bronchoscopy is indicated to avoid any further spinal injury during bronchoscopy. Other contraindications include laryngeal stenosis that prevents passage of the bronchoscope; limited range of motion of the mandible; severe kyphoscoliosis; uncontrolled coagulopathy; and extreme ventilatory/oxygenation demands.[7,8]

Stridor
Tracheostomy surveillance
Foreign body evaluation and management
Interval evaluation after laryngotracheal reconstruction
Chronic cough
Severe hemoptysis
Management of severe laryngotracheal infections
Airway trauma
Assessment of toxic inhalation or aspiration
Evaluation of laryngeal pathology
Management of mass lesions of the airway, including recurrent respiratory papillomatosis
Placement of stents
Assisting in laser therapy

Adapted from Hartnick CJ, Cotton RT: Stridor and airway obstruction. *In* Bluestone CD, Stool DE, Alper CM, et al (eds): *Pediatric otolaryngology*, ed 4, Philadelphia, 2003, Elsevier.

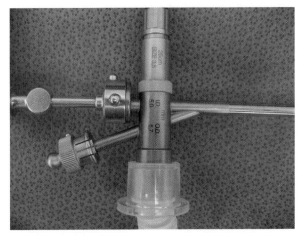

Figure 29-2 Close-up view of ventilating bronchoscope. The anesthesia circuit attaches inferiorly, the prismatic light source superiorly, and the suction port at an angle.

III. INSTRUMENTATION

The Storz endoscope with the Hopkins rod-lens optical system, introduced in 1966, is the most widely used rigid bronchoscope and has largely replaced the Jackson and Holinger endoscopes.[9] As described earlier, the rod-lens system provides better illumination, greater visualization, and angled views. The bronchoscope is a hollow, rigid metal tube that is tapered and beveled on the distal end and has a series of different-sized ports on the proximal end that serve different purposes. There are side holes at the end of the bronchoscope to allow for ventilation proximal to the tip.[10] The beveled edge of the tip is used to facilitate introduction of the bronchoscope into the airway and for resection of tumors. The inferior port is usually the ventilating port connected to the anesthesia circuit. The superior port connects to the prismatic light deflector and the light source (Figs. 29-1 and 29-2). The main port is the working channel for aspiration and for insertion of instruments such as telescopes, biopsy forceps, laser fibers, balloon devices, cryotherapy probes, and stents. The port can be left open to allow room air into the system or it can be closed to prevent leakage of air or anesthetic gases, depending on the ventilation and type of anesthesia being used.

Bronchoscopes vary in size, in length, and in internal and external diameter. Table 29-1 depicts the different sizes of Storz bronchoscopes used by patient age, although this choice needs to be tailored to the individual patient. The size chosen should maximize the surgeon's view while causing the least trauma to the airway.[9] Telescopes with different angles (0, 30, and 70 degrees), lengths, and diameters can be inserted through the main working port to visualize areas that are difficult to see with the rigid bronchoscope alone, namely the right and left upper bronchial orifices and the right middle bronchial orifice.[9] Illumination can be provided either through a light carrier rod that goes down a channel in older endoscopes, through the telescope, or by means of a port that attaches to a prismatic light deflector which subsequently attaches to a light source in newer endoscopes (Figs. 29-3 and 29-4). The last configuration has the advantage that it provides both proximal and distal illumination.

Rigid bronchoscopy should be performed either in an operating room (OR) or an endoscopy suite. As with all procedures that require general anesthesia, the room should be equipped with equipment for oxygen (O_2) saturation monitoring, carbon dioxide (CO_2) monitoring, blood pressure monitoring, and electrocardiography. A

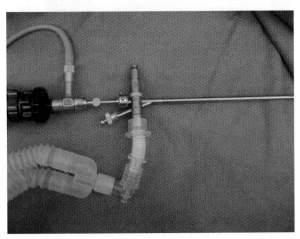

Figure 29-1 Bronchoscope with attachments to anesthesia circuit.

TABLE 29-1

Suggested Bronchoscope Sizes (Karo Storz Brand) According to Patient Age

Size	Length	ID (mm)	OD (mm)	Age
2.5	20	3.5	4.2	Premature
3.0	20, 26	4.3	5.0	Premature, newborn
3.5	20, 26, 30	5.0	5.7	Newborn–6 mo
3.7	26, 30	5.7	6.4	6 mo–1 yr
4.0	26, 30	6.0	6.7	1–2 yr
5.0	30	7.1	7.8	3–4 yr
6.0	30, 40	7.5	8.2	5–7 yr
6.5	43	8.5	9.2	Adult

ID, Internal diameter; *OD,* outer diameter.
Adapted from Tom LWC, Potsic WP, Handler SD: Methods of examination. *In* Bluestone CD, Stool DE, Alper CM, et al (eds): *Pediatric otolaryngology*, ed 4, Philadelphia, 2003, Elsevier.

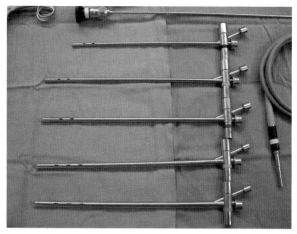

Figure 29-3 Bronchoscopes of varying sizes in example setup.

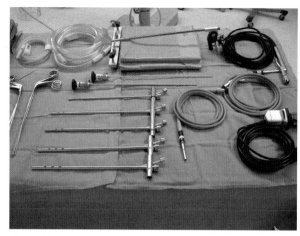

Figure 29-5 Additional setup including graspers and suction

full set of ventilating bronchoscopes (see Table 29-1 for sizes) and a backup light source should be available. The standard adult size rigid bronchoscopy is 8 mm in diameter and 40 cm long. Other instruments such as graspers, biopsy forceps, optical forceps, and suction devices should also be available to the surgeon (Fig. 29-5). Optional items include a flexible bronchoscope that can be passed through the rigid bronchoscope for further examination of the lower tracheobronchial tree. Video capability is also desirable but not required (Fig. 29-6).

IV. PREOPERATIVE CONSIDERATIONS

A thorough history should be taken to assess previous cardiac disease, such as a recent myocardial infarction or any documented dysrhythmias, or pulmonary disease (e.g., asthma) that may require bronchodilators before bronchoscopy.[4] To minimize the risk of bleeding, the patient should have a normal platelet count, prothrombin time, and partial thromboplastin time. Unless a bleeding history is known, a preoperative coagulation workup is not necessary. Because patients with uremia have qualitative platelet abnormalities that can predispose to excessive bleeding, creatinine and blood urea nitrogen values should be relatively normal.[4] Patients should also be

questioned about aspirin or anticoagulant use and timing of the last intravenous dose. Additional laboratory studies and tests may be ordered depending on the history.

A 12-lead electrocardiogram is required for patients with cardiac risk factors such as smoking, diabetes mellitus, arterial hypertension, or hypercholesterolemia and for those with a significant cardiac history. A chest radiograph may provide information regarding congestive heart failure, pulmonary consolidations, or the presence of chronic obstructive pulmonary disease (COPD). Arterial blood gas analysis can be performed to evaluate the patient's acid/base status in the setting of pulmonary disease.

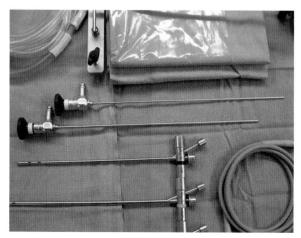

Figure 29-4 Optical telescopes for visualization through bronchoscopes.

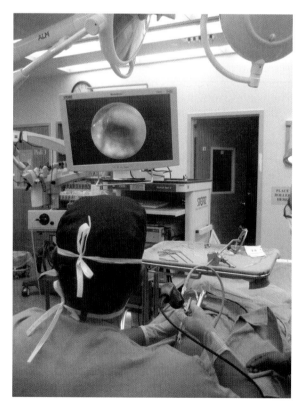

Figure 29-6 Bronchoscopist's view during a procedure. The monitor is shared so that it may be viewed simultaneously by the bronchoscopist and the anesthesiologist.

Pulmonary function tests are no longer indicated as routine preoperative assessment of respiratory disease but may be useful for determining the postoperative plan.[11] For example, patients with a forced vital capacity (FVC) of less than 20 mL/kg is at an increased risk for pulmonary complications postoperatively and may benefit from extended postoperative monitoring.[10] Also, patients with forced expiratory volumes of less than 50% are at risk for hypercarbia and hypoxia.[12] The clinical predictors of cardiac complications perioperatively or postoperatively with major risk are unstable or severe angina, decompensated congestive heart failure, significant dysrhythmias, and severe valvular disease.[13] Cardiac conditions should be evaluated and the medical therapies optimized before the surgery. Perhaps the simplest way to assess the patient's overall cardiopulmonary status is to inquire about exercise tolerance.

Often, rigid bronchoscopy is performed emergently with limited preoperative evaluation or testing in order to secure an airway, and knowledge and assessment of risk factors for cardiopulmonary mortality, difficult intubation (DI), and difficult mask ventilation (DMV) may be of importance for perioperative and postoperative management. DI may be predicted by weight, head and neck movement, jaw movement, receding mandible, "buck" teeth, Mallampati classification, thyromental distance, sternomental distance, and a history of DI.[5,14,15] There are five independent risk factors for DMV: age greater than 55 years, body mass index greater than 26 kg/m², presence of a beard, lack of teeth, and a history of snoring.[14] A careful evaluation of the patient's jaw and neck mobility should be made, because severe cervical spine disease is a contraindication to rigid bronchoscopy.

V. ANESTHESIA FOR BRONCHOSCOPY

Because of the nature of the procedure and sharing of the airway, the anesthesiologist and the surgeon must be in constant communication during a rigid bronchoscopy procedure. The goals for anesthesia during bronchoscopy are to provide anesthesia and analgesia, to provide sufficient relaxation, to diminish the reactivity and reflexes of the respiratory tract, to maintain adequate oxygenation, and to achieve prompt awakening at the conclusion of the procedure. General anesthesia is typically used to prevent unnecessary patient movement and possible unintentional damage to the airway. This can be accomplished with deep inhalational anesthesia, total intravenous anesthesia, or a combination of inhalational and intravenous anesthesia with or without neuromuscular blocking (NMB) agents depending on the specifics of the procedure and the preferences of the surgeon and anesthesiologist.

There are several different ventilation techniques that can be used with rigid bronchoscopy. The rigid bronchoscopes have ventilating ports that can be attached to the anesthesia circuit directly, allowing the anesthetic gases to flow concomitantly during the procedure. This is the most common and straightforward manner in which to keep a patient adequately ventilated during rigid bronchoscopy, although ventilation can also be achieved by the use of spontaneous ventilation, positive-pressure ventilation (PPV), apneic oxygenation, jet (Venturi) ventilation, or negative-pressure ventilation (NPV).

Traditionally in the pediatric population, inhalational anesthesia with spontaneous respiration has been used during rigid bronchoscopy, often with switching to a total intravenous anesthetic technique after induction. Disadvantages of inhalational anesthesia with spontaneous respiration include difficulty in maintaining an adequate plane of anesthetic depth and the anesthetic pollution of the surgical environment from a gas leak around the bronchoscope.[16] Malherbe and colleagues proposed total intravenous anesthesia with propofol and remifentanil and spontaneous respiration as a reasonable alternative to deep inhalational anesthesia that carries no major complications.[16] In the spontaneous respiration technique, the patient is not given an NMB agent and is allowed to breathe spontaneously. The ventilating port of the bronchoscope is attached to the anesthesia circuit with 100% O_2 flow (see Fig. 29-1). The advantage of spontaneous ventilation is that it allows for *continuous* ventilation during the procedure; the main disadvantage is that the depth of anesthesia required for the procedure itself may suppress both cardiac output and the respiratory drive, making spontaneous respirations difficult.[17] Another potential disadvantage is that the instrumentation required for the procedure itself provides increased airway resistance and may reduce the efficacy of spontaneous respirations.[18]

When PPV is used, it is typically achieved by first relaxing the patient with an NMB agent and subsequently connecting the ventilating port of the bronchoscope to the anesthesia circuit. Positive pressure is administered by squeezing the bag or by using the anesthesia ventilator, forcing gas pressure through the rigid bronchoscope.[19] Advantages include the prevention of atelectasis, improved oxygenation, and the ability to overcome the increased airway resistance caused by the instrumentation within the rigid bronchoscope.[18] A disadvantage to PPV is that a proximal eyepiece must be in place, which hinders the use of suction or other instrumentation during ventilation.[20] There is also usually some gas leak during PPV due to the absence of a tight seal, decreasing efficiency. Finally, the size of the bronchoscope and the presence of a telescope in the lumen increases resistance to airflow and increases dead space ventilation, making ventilation more difficult.

In apneic oxygenation, there are periods of time when the anesthesiologist withholds ventilation during which the surgeon works. The patient is first hyperventilated to produce a profound hypocarbia. Under direct visualization, a catheter is then passed to the carina, and the flow rate of O_2 is set. The period of time in which the surgeon can work is determined by the rise in CO_2, after which the patient is allowed an equivalent amount of time during the next ventilation cycle to return to baseline. The partial pressure of CO_2 (P_{CO_2}) is expected to rise continuously at a rate of 3 mm Hg per minute.[10] This technique is risky when it is used in patients who have a history of CO_2 retention (e.g., COPD), and intraprocedural awareness is also reported more frequently with this technique.

Jet ventilation is usually used during laser procedures, and it is provided by use of a jet-ventilator with a jet injection cannula (JIC), also known as a Saunders injector.[21] This technique is used to overcome the hypoventilation caused by air leaks during PPV.[22] The cannula has three lumens, two of which open proximally and deliver the jet ventilation; a distal lumen measures airway pressure.[21] The JIC is 3 mm in diameter, can have various lengths, and is made of stainless steel and therefore has a lower risk of endotracheal ignition.[21,22] The JIC is usually introduced distal to the lesion being accessed to provide optimal ventilation. High-pressure O_2 (50 psi) is delivered to the airway at high velocities, creating a negative pressure and causing a Venturi effect.[16] The negative pressure caused by the high velocity of air entering the airways induces a column of air from outside the injector to flow into the airways and expand the lungs. Exhalation is passive and relies on the collapse of the airway once the pressure is removed. Sufficient time must be allotted for air egress during this technique to prevent stacked breaths and progressive hyperinflation. This method is contraindicated during foreign body removal, because the high-flow air may dislodge the foreign body and cause a complete obstruction.[18] Of note, jet ventilation does not prevent acidemia or hypercarbia and may increase the risk of air embolism, pneumothorax, and particle dissemination into the lungs and distal airways.[20] Also, in patients with poor lung compliance, ventilation may be inadequate with this technique.[10]

NPV, compared with spontaneous assisted ventilation, reduces the administration of opioids, shortens recovery time from anesthesia, and prevents hypercarbia.[20] It can be accomplished by a poncho-wrap connected to a negative-pressure ventilator, with a 2-L/min O_2 flow, negative pressure of −25 hectopascals (hPa), a respiratory rate of 15 breaths/min, and an inspiration/expiration ratio of 1:1. NPV may be safer in patients with poor tolerance to hypercarbia, such as patients with myocardial ischemia.[20]

Intravenous and topical medications can be used provided the patient's history reveals no prior adverse reactions or if the potential benefit outweighs the expected risks. Opioids are often used for analgesia, for sedation, and to decrease the cough reflex. However, because they depress the respiratory drive, they should be withheld from patients who have signs of airway obstruction or a foreign body. A recent study by Yoon and colleagues comparing propofol sedation to a combination of both propofol and alfentanil showed that the propofol-only group had a higher average oxygen saturation as measured by pulse oximetry (SpO_2; 97.8 ± 1.6 versus 96.4 ± 1.1, $P < 0.01$). The degree of cough (measured using a 100 mm visual analogue scale), however, was not different between the groups (73.4 ± 22.7 versus 72.2 ± 18.5, respectively). This may be partially attributed to the intrinsic antitussive properties of propofol. Therefore, narcotics may not be required if the patient is being induced with propofol.[23]

Anticholinergics are often used to reduce airway secretions and have been shown to enhance the absorption and prolong the analgesic action of topical analgesics such as lidocaine which are administered to the airways to reduce reactivity, prevent bronchospasm, and dampen the systemic reaction to airway manipulation.[24] Intravenous anticholinergics are also commonly used to prevent the parasympathetic-mediated bradycardia and hypotension that can occur during rigid bronchoscopy.[11] Their routine use remains debated.[25] A steroid such as dexamethasone can be used to decrease intraoperative and postoperative edema that can result from airway instrumentation.

For emergence from anesthesia, all anesthetic gases are turned off, NMB agents are reversed, and the patient is ventilated until spontaneous respirations resume. Topical lidocaine may again be administered to prevent laryngospasm and diminish coughing.[12]

VI. SURGICAL TECHNIQUE

The surgeon should ensure that the necessary instrumentation is available before rigid bronchoscopy is initiated. In pediatric bronchoscopy, the size of the bronchoscope needed can be approximated by the patient's age, or by size of an appropriate endotracheal tube (see Table 29-1). In all patients, bronchoscopes one or two sizes smaller than the preselected one should be available in case the airway encountered is smaller than anticipated.[9] The surgeon should also select the appropriate size of instruments that will be used during the procedure, such as laryngoscopes, telescopes, endotracheal tubes, forceps, and suctions, and ensure that they are functioning properly. Teeth should be protected with rubber guards or with damp gauze, and the eyes should be protected with lubricant and tape.[4,12]

After informed consent for the procedure is obtained, the patient is taken to the OR or endoscopy suite. In pediatric bronchoscopy, the child should be positioned with the neck flexed on the body and the head extended at the neck.[9] This position is sometimes called the "sniffing" position, and is used to position the trachea anteriorly.[4] A shoulder roll to elevate the shoulders and a foam donut to stabilize the head are usually placed in older children; in younger children, a small donut for the head is sufficient. The goal is to align the oral, pharyngeal, and tracheal axes to facilitate insertion of the bronchoscope.

The anesthesiologist may induce anesthesia with either mask ventilation or intravenous agents, after which the surgeon begins the endoscopy by examining the oral cavity, oropharynx, and supraglottic larynx.[12] The vocal cords are identified and may at this point be sprayed with a topical agent such as lidocaine to diminish airway reactivity and laryngospasm. In pediatric bronchoscopy, especially in cases of airway obstruction due to a foreign object, a slotted laryngoscope can be used in combination with a telescope to examine the larynx and the airway before the rigid bronchoscope is inserted, because there is a possibility of dislodging the foreign object and causing a complete obstruction during the introduction of instruments.[12] O_2 can also be insufflated via a flexible large-bore catheter into the laryngeal inlet during the preliminary examination to allow the surgeon additional time to work in the airway (Fig. 29-7).[12]

Whereas in older children and adults the bronchoscope may be advanced directly into the trachea without laryngoscopic assistance, in younger children it is easiest

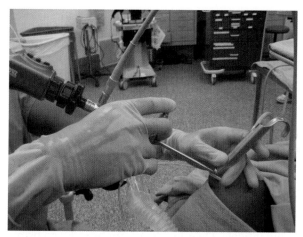

Figure 29-7 Bronchoscope in position for ventilation during a procedure.

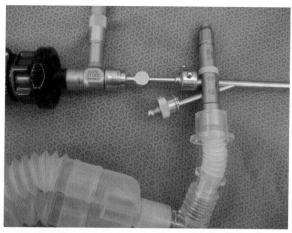

Figure 29-8 Rigid ventilating bronchoscope with telescope attached to camera posteriorly.

and safest to use a laryngoscope to guide the rigid bronchoscope.[9] The laryngoscope is introduced in the usual fashion into the vallecula until the glottis is in the field of vision. The rigid bronchoscope is then introduced within or adjacent to the lumen of the laryngoscope down to the level of the true vocal cords.[9] If the vocal cords are not open, then the patient is not sufficiently relaxed, and additional intravenous anesthetic or NMB agent should be given.[3] The rigid bronchoscope is then rotated 90 degrees to align the leading edge with the axis of the vocal cords as the bronchoscope passes through the glottic opening into the subglottis. This provides the path of least resistance and minimizes the risk of glottic damage.[7] A simple twisting motion may be required to advance the bronchoscope into the subglottic area.[9] Once it is distal to the glottis, it can be rotated back 90 degrees to its original orientation. Although the beveled tip of the rigid bronchoscope is conventionally directed anteriorly, some surgeons advocate placing the tip along the posterior wall of the trachea to prevent damage to the membranous trachea.[8]

In older children, adolescents, and adults, laryngoscopy is not always required. The patient's maxilla is grasped with the left hand while at the same time support is provided for the rigid bronchoscope, and the dentition is protected by the thumb of the surgeon's nondominant hand.[4,9] The bronchoscope is passed into the oral cavity in a plane perpendicular to that of the patient, and the posterior pharynx can be visualized. The bronchoscope is then rotated to a plane parallel with the airway axis. After visualization of the epiglottis, the tip of the bronchoscope is used to displace the epiglottis and tongue anteriorly. This maneuver requires gentle rocking of the bronchoscope on the thumb (*not on the teeth*) and brings the vocal cords into the field of vision.[4] Once the vocal cords are in view, the glottis can be approached and the subglottis may be entered, as previously described.[9]

For the intubated patient, the rigid bronchoscope may be advanced alongside the tube and then passed through the glottic opening as the tube is removed under direct visualization. If the patient has had the larynx surgically removed or closed, the rigid bronchoscope should be placed only through the laryngostoma.[8]

Once the bronchoscope has been successfully introduced into the trachea, the "sniffing" position can be converted to cervical hyperextension by removing the supporting pillow and donut from under the head and by lowering the headboard to extend the neck.[4,26] This maneuver is typically used in adults. The nondominant hand then holds the bronchoscope while the dominant hand is used for instrumentation of the airway for the duration of the procedure.[4] If any resistance is felt during the procedure, the surgeon should always reevaluate the patient's head and positioning, jaw opening, and bronchoscope size as well as ensuring that the patient's lips are not caught. At this point, the anesthesia circuit can be attached to the bronchoscope through the side port, and the catheter with O_2 flow can be removed (Fig. 29-8). Unless total intravenous anesthesia is being used, the lens cap to the main working port should be on to prevent leakage of anesthetic gas through the proximal end of the bronchoscope.

Before any intervention, an initial examination of the airway is performed. The subglottis and trachea are examined, and any masses or mucosal discolorations should be thoroughly investigated.[9] Even after premedication with an anticholinergic agent, secretions are frequently encountered during the bronchoscopy and can be suctioned by introducing a rigid or flexible suction cannula into the main working port. This or any other rigid instrumentation of the airway allows for escape of anesthetic gases into the OR environment and results in a loss of the closed anesthesia circuit. Flexible suction catheters can be used through a smaller side port to prevent the loss of the closed anesthesia circuit.[12]

Care must be taken not to suction the airways excessively, because this may lead to mucosal edema and inflammation and worsen the respiratory status of the patient. This effect can be mitigated by premedicating the patient with a steroid such as dexamethasone. The bronchoscope is then advanced to the level of the carina. The appearance and movement of the carina are noted during respirations. Decreased movement of the carina can be an indicator of hilar lymphadenopathy.[9] In order to advance the rigid bronchoscope to the main stem bronchus, the head should be slightly turned to the side opposite the intended bronchus. The distal airways may be evaluated by inserting different-angled telescopes to view the tracheobronchial tree. The 30- and 90-degree telescopes are especially useful to examine the segmental orifices of the upper lobes, in particular the right upper lobe, which is in a difficult location.[3,7] The distal tracheobronchial tree can also be examined by inserting the flexible bronchoscope through the rigid bronchoscope.[7]

After the preliminary evaluation of the airway is completed, the planned procedure is performed (see later discussion). For diagnostic bronchoscopy, the bronchial brushings, washings, and biopsies are performed, in that order.[3] If any bleeding is encountered, it can be controlled with electrocautery or local application of epinephrine, oxymetazoline, or phenylephrine.[3] Phenylephrine may result in pulmonary edema or cardiac depression and should be used very cautiously. This emphasizes the need for constant communication between the anesthesiologist and the surgeon during rigid bronchoscopy. The procedure must be paused periodically and the working port sealed to minimize leakage of anesthetic gases into the OR environment and to allow for adequate ventilation. After the procedure is completed, the secretions should be thoroughly suctioned to prevent atelectasis.[12] Once the anesthesiologist has prepared for postbronchoscopy ventilation, the bronchoscope can be removed under direct vision if O_2 saturation is greater than 90%.[3,12] Bronchospasm and temporary hypoxia are not uncommon after withdrawal of the bronchoscope, and the anesthesiologist must be ready to support ventilation via mask ventilation or endotracheal intubation until spontaneous ventilation resumes.[3,12]

VII. COMPLICATIONS

The complications that may occur during or after rigid bronchoscopy can often be avoided by a thorough preoperative evaluation and proper technique.[3] These include damage to dentition, arytenoid dislocation, respiratory depression, laryngospasm, bronchospasm, subglottic edema, hypoxia, dysrhythmias, mucosal or parenchymal bleeding, perforation, pneumothorax, pneumomediastinum, and death.[3,9,27] In pediatric rigid bronchoscopy, the complication rates range from 1.9% to 4%.[27] In adults, Lukomsky and associates reported a complication rate of 5%,[28] whereas Drummond and coworkers reported a rate of 13.4%.[29] Patients with an increased preoperative risk, neoplastic disease, presence of a foreign body, or carinal involvement should be monitored closely, because these conditions are particularly associated with an increased complication rate in adults.[29] The three risk factors identified by Hoeve and colleagues for an increased complication rate in children are a history of tetralogy of Fallot, need for biopsy or drainage of a lesion during bronchoscopy, and a history of foreign body aspiration.[27]

It is imperative that patients be evaluated preoperatively for poor dentition, because loose teeth are at risk for damage or dislodgement during the procedure. If cervical spine disease with a contracted neck is present, rigid bronchoscopy may not be safely performed; a limited range of cervical motion precludes safe advancement of the scope into the airway, resulting in

complications ranging from dental injury to perforation of the posterior pharynx, membranous trachea, or distal airway.[26] Such perforation of the airway may result in pneumomediastinum or pneumothorax but can be avoided by choosing an alternative method for examining the airway (e.g., flexible bronchoscopy) in susceptible patients.[16]

Hemorrhage can occur during bronchoscopy, especially during deep tissue biopsies. It may be controlled by use of the bronchoscope to apply pressure to the bleeding site, thorough suction, local application of epinephrine, or intravenous vasopressin. The patient's greatest danger when this occurs is aspiration rather than hemorrhagic shock.[27]

Bronchospasm and laryngospasm occasionally occur intraoperatively. Their incidence can be reduced by maintaining an adequate anesthetic plane and by the topical application of a local anesthetic, such as lidocaine. Other agents, including opioids and beta-blockers, can be used to blunt the hemodynamic response to airway stimulation.[16]

Late complications include airway edema, pneumothorax, and atelectasis.[12] Laryngeal edema is usually more serious in children, because their airway lumen is smaller and resistance increases exponentially with any airway swelling.[12] This condition can be improved with the administration of humidified O_2, racemic epinephrine, and steroids. If the patient does not respond to medical management, endotracheal intubation may be necessary. Laryngeal edema may be reduced by premedicating the patient with intravenous steroids.[16] In cases of Venturi ventilation or high ventilation pressures, pneumothorax may result from barotrauma.[10,12]

Rigid bronchoscopy requires excellent communication between the anesthesiologist and the surgeon. Failure to communicate may lead to inadequate control of the airway and can result in hypercarbia, hypoxemia, or death, especially in patients with impending complete airway obstruction.[26] This can be prevented by having all parties involved in the surgery familiarize themselves with the procedure before starting. A contingency plan must be in place in the event the airway is lost. This may entail preparation for tracheostomy or ventilatory bypass in an absolute emergency.

VIII. FOREIGN BODY REMOVAL

The removal of aspirated foreign bodies remains one of the main indications for rigid bronchoscopy, especially in children, in whom the use of flexible bronchoscopy is comparatively risky. In 2006, the total number of deaths caused by aspiration or ingestion of foreign objects, including food, totaled 3981.[30] Most deaths resulting from foreign body aspiration occur before hospital arrival.[31] The incidence of foreign body aspiration peaks in older infants and toddlers, with 74% of cases occurring in children younger than 3 years of age.[32] The male-to-female ratio is about 2:1 in children.[32] In adults, the peak incidence occurs in the sixth decade of life.[33]

The clinical progression of foreign body aspiration occurs in three stages. The initial stage is usually characterized by a choking episode followed by coughing, gagging, and even obstruction of the airway.[32] In a series of 100 cases published by Barrios and coworkers, the history of a choking crisis was the clinical parameter with the highest sensitivity (97%) and also had a fair specificity (63%).[34] Chest radiographs may appear normal, and symptoms can be minimal.[31,34] In cases of suspected foreign body aspiration, rigid bronchoscopy remains the gold standard for both diagnosis and treatment. Whereas atelectasis is more common in adults, air trapping is more common in children.[33] The location of the foreign object also differs between adults (right bronchial tree) and pediatric patients (central airway). The second stage is usually asymptomatic, because the initial symptoms resolve due to a fatigued cough reflex.[32] As many as 50% of initial presentations of foreign body aspiration go undiagnosed for longer than 7 days,[29] and this is more likely to occur in an adult.[33] The third stage indicates a complicated foreign body aspiration, which can be associated with pneumonia, hemoptysis, bronchiectasis, chronic cough, lung abscess, fever, or malaise.[32]

Radiographic evaluation includes anteroposterior and lateral views of the extended neck and chest. It is imperative that both inspiratory and expiratory views be obtained whenever possible to evaluate for unilateral air trapping.[32] The four main types of obstruction at a bronchial orifice are bypass valve obstruction, check valve obstruction, stop valve obstruction, and ball valve obstruction.[32] In bypass valve obstruction, the obstruction is incomplete and will result in a normal radiographic evaluation. In check valve obstruction, commonly seen acutely, the foreign body permits air flow into the lung segment but blocks the air flow out of the lung segment. This results in a mediastinal shift *away from* the obstruction on an expiratory film. Stop valve obstruction is seen when a foreign body has been present for an extended period; it is characterized by no airflow into, and subsequent collapse of, the affected lung segment. The rarest type of obstruction, the ball valve type, permits airflow out of the lung segment but not into it. This phenomenon results in atelectasis and a mediastinal shift *toward* the obstructed segment on an expiratory film. Other studies (e.g., fluoroscopy, videofluoroscopy) have been used when the diagnosis is uncertain.[31,32]

The management of an aspirated foreign body depends on the clinical picture. If an acute complete obstruction is suspected, rigid bronchoscopy must be performed promptly. More frequently, however, the patient presents in the second or third stage, when there is adequate time to plan a successful and safe bronchoscopy. If possible, the procedure should be scheduled when experienced personnel are available, the instruments have been appropriately selected, and the child is fasted appropriately to prevent aspiration of gastric contents.[19,32] Advanced planning for the procedure includes determining the nature of the foreign object to guide the selection of instruments for its retrieval.

Controversy remains regarding the anesthetic approach during bronchoscopy for foreign body aspiration. Those who advocate spontaneous ventilation argue that PPV may precipitate an acute obstruction with clinical deterioration,[18,32] whereas others advocate controlled ventilation with NMB to prevent the patient from moving and

decrease the probability of airway trauma. A retrospective series of 94 cases showed no difference in adverse events with either ventilatory management approach,[18] whereas a prospective study by Chen and colleagues consisting of 384 children found that patients managed with total intravenous anesthesia and spontaneous ventilation had increased intraoperative body movement, longer duration of emergence from anesthesia, lower percentage of successful foreign body removal, and more postoperative laryngospasm.[35] Chen's study also identified five risk factors for intraoperative hypoxemia (SpO_2 ≤ 90%): younger age, plant seed as the type of foreign body, longer operative time, presence of pneumonia before procedure, and spontaneous ventilation. Manual jet ventilation was found to decrease the risk of intraoperative hypoxemia. The factors associated with postoperative hypoxemia were plant seed as the foreign object and prolonged emergence from anesthesia. Patients with these characteristics should be closely monitored after the procedure.

If the foreign body is small enough, it can be removed through the lumen of the main working port. However, the objects are usually larger and need to be removed with the bronchoscope as a unit. Once the object is within the forceps, it is dislodged from the airway and the bronchoscope is advanced to cover the foreign object, preventing it being stripped off the forceps during withdrawal.[32] Removal of the bronchoscope may compromise the airway, so, again, communication during withdrawal is critical. Vegetable foreign bodies should be grasped lightly to avoid fragmentation of the foreign body into the distal airways.[32] After removal of the object, bronchoscopy should be repeated to ensure that no residual foreign body is left and to assess the patency of the airway distal to the previous obstruction. Bleeding is usually controlled with thorough suctioning and vasoactive agents. If residual granulation tissue is present and is the source of bleeding or residual obstruction, it may be resected at the repeat endoscopy.[32]

IX. CONCLUSIONS

Despite the advances that have expanded the applications for flexible bronchoscopy, rigid bronchoscopy remains a valuable tool in a surgeon's armamentarium. Rigid bronchoscopy is preferred when the airway is in peril and for procedures in which direct manipulation of the airway is needed. The two most common indications are foreign body aspiration or ingestion and massive hemoptysis, and rigid bronchoscopy is also often used to secure or assess an otherwise unstable airway. The wide lumen of the bronchoscope allows for instrumentation of the airway, which is required for endoscopic airway procedures such as biopsies and laser therapy. The procedure is performed with the patient under general anesthesia, although there are many different ventilation techniques.

The risk for complications increases significantly with inexperienced personnel, and the American College of Chest Physicians recommends that trainees perform at least 20 procedures under supervision to obtain basic competency and at least 10 procedures per year to maintain competency.[7] The importance of communication between the bronchoscopist and the anesthesiologist cannot be overstated. When applied appropriately, rigid bronchoscopy can be a life-saving intervention in airway management.

X. CLINICAL PEARLS

- Open communication between the surgeon and the anesthetist is of highest importance during rigid bronchoscopy.

- Inspect the equipment prior to the patient's arrival; ensure that the bronchoscopes, light sources, light carriers and connectors are all in working order.

- Check that instruments (suctions, graspers, telescopes) are appropriate length for the selected bronchoscope.

- Have a backup set that is a size smaller than what you plan to use.

- For pediatric patients, calculate the safe maximum dose of each topical medication (e.g., lidocaine), and restrict their presence in the operative field.

- Place dental/gingival protection, and never leave the bronchoscope on the teeth.

- Advance the scope only when there is an identifiable lumen.

SELECTED REFERENCES

All references can be found online at expertconsult.com.

5. Caplan RA, Benumof JL, Berry FA, et al: Practice guidelines for management of the difficult airway. *Anesthesiology* 98:1269–1277, 2003.
6. Beamis JF: Modern use of rigid bronchoscopy. In Bollinger CT, Mathur PN, editors: *Interventional bronchoscopy*, Basel, 2000, Karger, pp 22–30.
12. Pereira KD, Hessel AC: Performance of rigid bronchoscopy. In Haber CA, editor: *Benumof's airway management*, ed 2, Philadelphia, 2007, Mosby Elsevier, Chapter 27.
13. Eagle KA, Berger PB, Calkins H, et al: ACC/AHA guideline update for perioperative cardiovascular evaluation for noncardiac surgery: Executive summary. A report of the American College of Cardiology/American Heart Association Task Force on Practice Guidelines (Committee to Update the 1996 Guidelines on Perioperative Cardiovascular Evaluation for Noncardiac Surgery). *J Am Coll Cardiol* 39:542–553, 2002.
14. Langeron O, Masso E, Huraux C, et al: Prediction of difficult mask ventilation. *Anesthesiology* 92:1229–1236, 2000.
20. Natalini G, Cavaliere S, Vitacca M, et al: Negative pressure ventilation vs. spontaneous assisted ventilation during rigid bronchoscopy. *Acta Anaesthesiol Scand* 42:1063–1069, 1998.
27. Hoeve LJ, Rombout J, Meursing AE: Complications of rigid laryngobronchoscopy in children. *Int J Pediatr Otorhinolaryngol* 26:47–56, 1993.
31. Reilly J, Thompson J, MacArthur C, et al: Pediatric aerodigestive foreign body injuries are complications related to timeliness of diagnosis. *Laryngoscope* 107:17–20, 1997.
32. Darrow DH, Holinger LD: Foreign bodies of the larynx, trachea, and bronchi. In Bluestone CD, Stool SE, Alper CM, et al, editors: *Pediatric otolaryngology*, ed 4, Philadelphia, 2003, Saunders, pp 1543–1547.
33. Baharloo F, Veyckemans F, Francis C, et al: Tracheobronchial foreign bodies: Presentation and management in children and adults. *Chest* 115:1357–1362, 1999.

Chapter 30

Percutaneous Dilational Cricothyrotomy and Tracheostomy

DAVIDE CATTANO | LAURA F. CAVALLONE

I. DEFINITIONS AND CLASSIFICATIONS OF PERCUTANEOUS CRICOTHYROTOMY AND TRACHEOSTOMY

A. Cricothyrotomy and Percutaneous Dilational Cricothyrotomy

Cricothyrotomy is a technique for providing an opening in the space between the anterior inferior border of the thyroid cartilage and the anterior superior border of the cricoid cartilage for the purpose of gaining access to the airway. This area is considered to be the most accessible part of the respiratory tree below the glottis.[1-6]

Cricothyrotomy can be classified in several ways. Based on the urgency of the clinical situation, the procedure has been classified as emergent or elective. Emergent cricothyrotomy may be done in the prehospital setting, emergency room, intensive care unit (ICU), or operating room. Elective cricothyrotomy is usually done before surgery in the operating room. It also may be performed in critically ill patients in the ICU at the bedside.[7] Depending on the technique used, the procedure may also be classified as nonsurgical or surgical. The

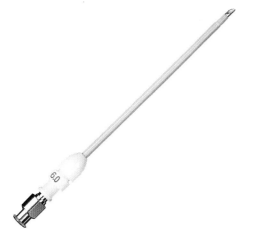

Figure 30-1 Cook cricothyrotomy catheter needle. (Courtesy of Cook Medical, Bloomington, IN.)

nonsurgical approach can be achieved by needle puncture or percutaneously over a guidewire, with or without a cricothyroid membrane (CTM) incision.[8]

A practical and clinical classification of cricothyrotomy techniques includes three categories. The first category includes techniques that use a needle or over-the-needle catheter placed directly into the cricothyroid space. The needle technique is used for transtracheal catheter ventilation or, more properly, transcricoid ventilation.[9] The cricothyrotomy needle (Fig. 30-1) and the Ravussin cannula (Fig. 30-2) are examples of these devices. Transtracheal catheter ventilation cannulas are also available, but they are inserted as described for the second category (Fig. 30-3).

The second category includes techniques requiring the introduction of a guidewire that is inserted through a needle or catheter and followed by dilation of the cricothyroid space. The needle or catheter placement can be preceded by an incision of the skin and of the CTM. An airway catheter is also introduced over the dilator threaded over the guidewire. These techniques allow

insertion of an airway considerably larger than the initial needle or catheter, often of sufficient internal diameter (ID) to allow ventilation with conventional ventilation devices, suctioning, and spontaneous ventilation. These techniques may properly be classified as percutaneous dilational cricothyrotomy (PDC).

The third category is surgical cricothyrotomy, which involves the use of a scalpel and other surgical instruments to create an opening between the skin and the cricothyroid space. It is discussed in Chapter 31.

B. Tracheostomy and Percutaneous Dilational Tracheostomy

1. Open Tracheostomy

Surgical tracheostomy, as described by Chevalier Jackson,[10] is a surgical procedure that provides an airway through the cervical trachea. It remains the standard against which all other procedures with the same aim must be compared in terms of success and complications rates. Classically, the procedure is performed in the operating room under general or local anesthesia, as dictated by the clinical situation. An open tracheostomy may be performed at the bedside in the ICU or in the emergency room in urgent situations. After an initial skin incision, sharp dissection is carried out to the thyroid isthmus, which is divided. The cervical trachea is then incised and a tracheostomy tube inserted.

2. Percutaneous Tracheostomy

Percutaneous tracheostomy is performed by means of a skin puncture into the trachea that is subsequently dilated to form a stoma, rather than creating a stoma by surgical incision.[11] Although there are many techniques for performing a percutaneous tracheostomy, the initial part of the procedure always involves a puncture through the skin into the trachea, which is then enlarged by dilation or with forceps to spread the puncture to a size that allows placement of an appropriate tracheostomy tube. These techniques are typically used in patients with an

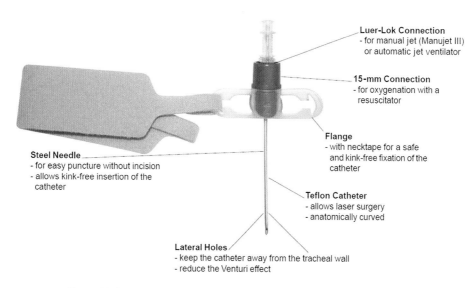

Figure 30-2 Ravussin cannula. (Courtesy of VBM Medical, Noblesville, IN.)

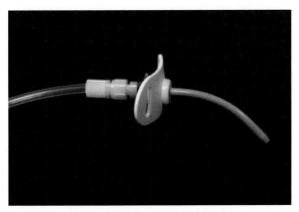

Figure 30-3 Arndt cannula for cricothyrotomy. (Courtesy of Cook Medical, Bloomington, IN.)

established airway (i.e., endotracheal tube [ETT] or laryngeal mask airway [LMA]) and are mostly used for intubated ICU patients.

Emergency situations were traditionally considered absolute contraindications to the use of this technique, but in the past few years, some reports have supported its safety and feasibility in selected emergent cases.[12,13] The Ciaglia technique, first described in 1985, is the original technique now described as percutaneous dilational tracheostomy (PDT). It involves making a very small skin incision, introducing a needle into the trachea, and dilating the opening with sequentially larger dilators to allow insertion of a tracheostomy tube of the selected size. As originally described, this procedure was performed blind, but it is increasingly performed under continuous endoscopic guidance.

Other modifications of the Ciaglia technique include the use of lower tracheal rings interspaces (originally performed in the interspace between the cricoid cartilage and the first tracheal ring) and the use of a single, curved dilator to replace the original multiple dilators. Of the percutaneous approaches described, the Ciaglia technique with continuous endoscopic visualization and use of a single dilator is considered by many to be the safest, and it is the most widely used in North America.

The Griggs guidewire dilating forceps technique involves placing a guidewire through an initial puncture site. The area is forcibly enlarged with the use of a dilating forceps (i.e., grooved Howard-Kelly forceps) to obtain a stoma of the desired size. One advantage of this technique is the reduced amount of compression on the airway by the forceps compared with other dilational methods. The procedure as originally described is performed blind and subject to complications such as false passage and subcutaneous emphysema. Concurrent endoscopic visualization reduces these risks, although bleeding may be a problem because of tearing of adjacent structures when inserting and opening the forceps.

The Fantoni technique is based on retrograde dilation of an initial tracheal puncture. During this procedure, a needle is inserted between the tracheal rings (i.e., first and second or second and third) and directed cranially. A guidewire is then passed through the needle and directed toward the oral cavity. Dilation is carried out by means of a conic cannula inserted over the guidewire through

the oral cavity. Ventilation at this stage is maintained by means of a special, small ETT that allows passage of the conic cannula alongside the ETT. The tracheostomy tube is ultimately brought out in a retrograde fashion through the cervical trachea and skin. This technique is used primarily in Italy, where it originated, but it has found little applicability in North America, because it is lengthy to perform and involves potential loss of the airway due to the many airway manipulations necessary to perform the procedure and secure the cannula in its final position.

3. Percutaneous Dilational Cricothyrotomy and Tracheostomy in Airway Control

a. THE PROBLEM OF AIRWAY CONTROL

Adverse outcomes related to respiratory events account for one of the two largest classes of injury in the American Society of Anesthesiologists (ASA) Closed Claims Project. As reported by Caplan and colleagues and Cheney and associates, the two major categories of anesthesia-related events or mechanisms causing death or brain damage between 1975 and 2000 were respiratory and cardiovascular difficulties, which together made up 68% of damaging events.[14,15] Three mechanisms of injury were responsible for most of the adverse respiratory events: difficult ETT placement (23%), inadequate ventilation (22%), and esophageal intubation (13%).

In an analysis of claims against the National Health System in England between 1995 and 2007,[16] airway and respiratory claims accounted for 12% of anesthesia-related claims, 53% of deaths, 27% of cost, and 10 of the 50 most expensive claims in the dataset. These claims most frequently described events at induction of anesthesia, involved airway management with a tracheal tube, and typically led to hypoxia and the patient's death or brain injury.

In the operating room, in the ICU (or in other hospital areas), and in the prehospital setting, three difficult scenarios have been repeatedly observed during attempts to control the airway: (1) the airway can be easily controlled by mask ventilation, but endotracheal intubation is not possible; (2) the airway cannot be mask ventilated but can be intubated; and (3) rarely, the airway cannot be mask ventilated or intubated. It is every anesthesiologist's nightmare to encounter a true difficult airway as depicted in the third scenario.[17] Five to 35 of 10,000 patients (0.05% to 0.35%) reportedly cannot be endotracheally intubated, and approximately 0.01 to 2.0 of 10,000 patients are difficult to mask ventilate and intubate.[18,19]

ASA guidelines provide a difficult airway algorithm and suggest strategies for evaluating, preparing for, and intubating the difficult airway. They also consider the relative merits and feasibility of alternative management choices, such as nonsurgical versus surgical techniques for the initial approach to ventilation, awake intubation versus intubation after induction of general anesthesia, and preservation versus ablation of spontaneous ventilation. The algorithm describes emergency and nonemergency pathways for managing the airway if intubation fails. The ASA guidelines also suggest that equipment suitable for "emergency surgical airway access" be among the contents of a portable storage unit readily available in the operating room. The algorithm suggests that emergency invasive airway procedures are "surgical or percutaneous tracheostomy or cricothyrotomy."

ASA guidelines offer a stepwise approach to the patient with a difficult airway, primarily focusing on difficulties encountered in the operating room, and offer strategies to anticipate and treat a difficult airway in this environment. However, the anesthesiologist is often called on to manage the airways of critically ill patients in other hospital environments, such as the emergency department, wards, diagnostic areas (e.g., radiology), or ICUs. In all settings, it is important that anesthesiologists are trained and prepared to recognize and manage situations in which cricothyrotomy or percutaneous tracheostomy, or both, are considered as preferred options.

b. ROLES OF THE ANESTHESIOLOGIST, OTOLARYNGOLOGIST, AND EMERGENCY MEDICINE PHYSICIAN

The anesthesiologist may be called immediately or after other physicians have attempted unsuccessfully to secure the airway or failed to recognize the futility of standard intubation techniques. In rare instances, the availability of a physician skilled in the technique of cricothyrotomy or percutaneous tracheostomy may be life-saving. This individual should be the anesthesiologist. Appropriate equipment for cricothyrotomy should be available throughout the hospital or as part of an emergency airway kit. No data exist regarding how frequently anesthesiologists are called to secure an airway outside the operating room, but in many hospitals, this responsibility seems to be handled more frequently by other physicians.[20-23]

Each institution should have a clear plan for alerting qualified individuals when emergency airway support is required in different areas of the hospital.[24] Many publications describe the use of various types of advanced airway equipment, report the availability of such devices, and explain the use of simulators to teach difficult airway management skills, and many articles identify the need to educate residents in advanced airway techniques.

Organizing resources and staff to manage a difficult airway and maintaining appropriate training are important for patient safety and clinical quality.[25,26] In 2000, Showan and Sestito proposed that the components of a successful airway management system include personnel, training, an emergency response system, an oversight process, standardized equipment, and patient education. As with any type of emergency, preparedness is the key when planning for response.[27-30]

In 1996, a comprehensive airway program was introduced at Johns Hopkins.[26] The core components of the comprehensive difficult airway program were communication and electronic medical record information (including airway documentation), equipment, personnel, and education. Investigators based their implementation on the causes that required a surgical airway and the inability of an anesthesiologist to intubate and ventilate. The causes were an inability to access the written medical record, resulting in a lack of preoperative information about the patient's airway; lack of immediate access to equipment and supplies necessary to manage a difficult airway; and lack of availability of trained personnel to help manage and secure the airway.

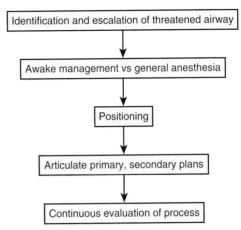

Figure 30-4 Progressive escalation sequence for a threatened airway.

Continuing medical education is essential to maintain skills in performing emergent cricothyrotomy, and standardized simulation alone may not be sufficient to warrant optimal training. Individual skills, availability of devices, and training in specific techniques may deviate from standard guidelines, making "at site, ad hoc" guidelines necessary.

A threatened airway protocol has been proposed for implementing an escalation-based model at The University of Texas Medical School at Houston.[31] The model is based on seven general principles to guide physicians in the identification and management of situations in which hospitalized patients may have rapid deterioration of a condition affecting the upper airway that requires immediate intervention to maintain or reestablish ventilation and oxygenation. These seven principles are concerned with appropriate communication among providers, maintenance of oxygenation, avoidance of sedation until the patient is in a safe environment, complete airway assessment, maintenance of spontaneous ventilation as long as possible, and avoidance of rapid-sequence induction (i.e., administration of a muscle relaxant without a prior attempt to ventilate), unless an easy airway and a full stomach are expected. Four main features constitute the cornerstones of management of a patient with a threatened airway: identification of the airway emergency and escalation of the approach to management, choice of appropriate sedation or anesthesia technique, positioning, and articulation of plans for intervention. A progressive algorithm (Fig. 30-4) that guides the progression of the necessary steps has been inspired by others' work.[31,32] The use of specific airway devices or tools is mandated in the primary and secondary plans by the success in securing the airway or depending on changes in airway viability (Fig. 30-5).

The otolaryngologist plays a critical role in airway management by contributing a skill set that is different from but complementary to that of the anesthesiologist. Circumstances may range from well-controlled elective situations to near-panic, last-ditch attempts to establish an airway when all else has failed.[33] The otolaryngologist possesses an excellent knowledge of the three-dimensional anatomy of the upper aerodigestive tract and the

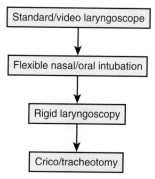

Figure 30-5 Airway approach algorithm for a threatened airway.

variations encountered in pathologic circumstances. This knowledge and expert endoscopy skills can assist the anesthesiologist in determining a difficult airway.

II. HISTORICAL PERSPECTIVE

Surgical manipulation of the trachea for emergent airway control is one of the oldest invasive procedures documented. It was performed in ancient Egypt and India more than 3000 years ago. Tracheostomy was mentioned in the writings and illustrations of the great Greek physician Galen (130 to 200 AD). He provided anatomic drawings of the airway and favored a vertical rather than horizontal incision in emergencies. He based his anatomic knowledge on dissections of animals and assumed that the structures were identical in the human body. Galen also stated that Asclepiades (124 to 56 BC), who practiced in Rome, recommended opening the trachea in its upper part to prevent suffocation. Antyllus (approximately 150 AD) described the indications for and technique of tracheostomy, advocating a transverse incision between two rings. Galenic teaching persisted for more than 1300 years, until Andreas Wesele Vesalius (1515 to 1564 AD) published *De Humani Corporis Fabrica*, detailing the first correct description of human anatomy. Vesalius secretly conducted extensive dissection of human cadavers and, at age 28, published his landmark work in seven volumes. Included was a detailed description of tracheostomy—control of the airway with the use of a cane or reed and assisted ventilation of the lung. He allegedly performed a tracheostomy and experimentally inflated the lungs of a dead Spanish nobleman, whose heart was reported to beat again. His action outraged the medical and clerical communities.

During the next 300 years, very few reports were published regarding the surgical control of the airway, and they were primarily limited to experimental control of breathing in laboratory animals. In *Respiratory Changes of Intrathoracic Pressure*, published in 1892, Samuel Meltzer described insertion of breathing tubes through a tracheostomy and successfully controlling ventilation in curarized animals. In France, Armand Trousseau recognized the importance of emergency tracheostomy in airways compromised by upper airway obstruction, diphtheria, and massive infection in the oropharynx and neck. In 1909, Chevalier Jackson,[10] a laryngologist at the Jefferson Medical School in Philadelphia, described the

technical details of surgical tracheostomy and standardized the procedure. Jackson's technique was for years considered the preferred method of surgical airway management. Jackson later published the results of 30 years' observation of his own tracheotomized patients and reported a very high incidence of laryngeal and subglottic stenosis in patients who underwent a procedure that he referred to as *high tracheostomy*, involving division of the cricoid or thyroid cartilage.[34] As a consequence, the high tracheostomy technique was abandoned for many decades.

In 1969, Toye and Weinstein described a technique for percutaneous tracheostomy based on the premise that a functional tracheal airway could be more rapidly and safely achieved percutaneously than with Jackson's method of surgical dissection.[35] The technique involved inserting a needle into the trachea and dilating the resultant needle tract to allow placement of a breathing catheter.

Cricothyrotomy, which differed from high tracheostomy because it involved opening of the CTM instead of dissection of the cricoid cartilage, was proposed again in 1976 by two Denver cardiothoracic surgeons, Brantigan and Grow. They published the results of 655 consecutive cricothyrotomies in which there were minimal complications and no reported incidence of subglottic stenosis. Subsequently, other clinical and experimental series have been reported, and cricothyrotomy has become generally accepted. The procedure was found to be faster, simpler, less invasive, and less likely to cause bleeding than tracheostomy. It is associated with lower morbidity and mortality rates than emergency tracheostomy, making it desirable as an emergency technique for gaining immediate airway control. Various modifications of the original technique have been developed. The use of the Seldinger technique for insertion, as described by Corke and Cranswick in 1988, enhances the safety of the procedure.[8]

Using a guidewire and passing a dilator to create a channel reduce the chance of incorrect placement and damage to surrounding blood vessels. Interest in cricothyrotomy as an alternative to endotracheal intubation is largely the result of the development of emergency medicine as a distinct specialty and the frequent treatment of patients with difficult airways in the prehospital and emergency department environments. Emergency physicians and prehospital providers often encounter patients with life-threatening injuries who cannot be intubated by conventional routes and who need immediate and definitive treatment. Most reports of the use of cricothyrotomy in emergent situations appear in the emergency medicine literature. For anesthesiologists, interest in PDT and PDC increased as part of a trend toward less invasive surgical procedures.

The Ciaglia technique, first described in 1985, is the original technique now described as PDT. In this technique, insertion of the guidewire is followed by serial dilations performed with multiple, progressively larger dilators.[36] The Rapitrach method, proposed in 1989 by Schachner and coworkers, entails the use of dilating forceps and a single-step dilating technique.[37]

In 1990, Griggs and colleagues presented the guidewire dilating forceps method, which was similar to the

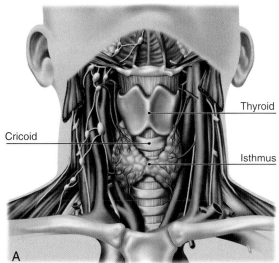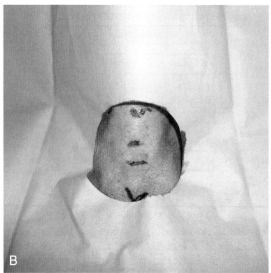

Figure 30-6 **A,** Dissection anatomy. **B,** External landmarks. (**A,** From De Leyn P, Bedert L, Delcroix M: Tracheotomy: Clinical review and guidelines. *Eur J Cardiothorac Surg* 32:412–421, 2007.)

Rapitrach method and based on a one-step dilating techinque[38] that used a modified forceps. In 1997, Fantoni proposed the translaryngeal tracheostomy technique based on retrograde dilation of an initial tracheal puncture by means of a conic cannula inserted through the oral cavity.[39]

The Ciaglia Blue Rhino, a modified version of the Ciaglia technique, was introduced by Cook Medical (Bloomington, IN) in 2000.[40] In this technique, the series of sequentially larger dilators of the original Ciaglia technique is replaced by a single, curved dilator with a hydrophilic coating, the Blue Rhino, that progressively dilates the stoma in one step.

In 2002, Frova and Quintel described the Percutwist tracheostomy technique. A "rotating dilation" is performed in a single step by means of a screwlike, rotating device.[41] In 2008, a further development of the Ciaglia technique was presented by Cook Medical: the Ciaglia Blue Dolphin balloon percutaneous tracheostomy introducer. This device combines balloon dilation and tracheal tube insertion into one step.

Many of the techniques proposed for PDC and PDT are performed over guidewires. Although anesthesiologists are familiar with the Seldinger technique for the insertion of vascular catheters, many are unacquainted with airway management techniques that use airway devices based on the same technology and concept.[27,42]

III. ANATOMY AND PHYSIOLOGY

Safe and rapid performance of cricothyrotomy requires a thorough knowledge of cricothyroid space anatomy (Fig. 30-6) and its relation to other structures in the neck.[1,6,43-47] The CTM ligament is 10 mm long and 22 mm wide and is composed mostly of yellow elastic tissue. It covers the cricothyroid space and is located in the anterior neck between the thyroid cartilage superiorly and the cricoid cartilage inferiorly. The cricothyroid space can be readily identified by palpating a slight dip or indentation in the skin immediately below the laryngeal prominence.

The CTM consists of a central anterior triangular portion (i.e., conus elasticus) and two lateral parts. The thicker and stronger conus elasticus narrows above and broadens below, connecting the thyroid to the cricoid cartilage. It lies subcutaneously in the midline and is often crossed horizontally in its upper third by the superior cricothyroid vessels. To minimize the possibility of bleeding, the CTM should be incised at its inferior-third portion. The two lateral parts are thinner, lie close to the laryngeal mucosa, and extend from the superior border of the cricoid cartilage to the inferior margin of the true vocal cords. On either side, the CTM is bordered by the cricothyroid muscle. Lateral to the membrane are venous tributaries from the inferior thyroid and anterior jugular veins. Because the vocal cords usually lie 1 cm above the cricothyroid space, they are not commonly injured, even during emergency cricothyrotomy.[48] The anterior jugular veins run vertically in the lateral aspect of the neck and are rarely injured, but tributaries may occasionally course over the cricothyroid space and be damaged during the procedure. Characteristically, the CTM does not calcify with age and lies immediately underneath the skin.

Variations in the anatomy and dimensions of the CTM are common. The anterior cricothyroid space is trapezoidal and has a cross-sectional area of approximately 2.9 cm². The mean distance between the anterior borders of the inferior thyroid cartilage and the superior cricoid cartilage is 9 mm (range, 5 to 12 mm), whereas the width of the anterior cricothyroid space ranges from 27 to 32 mm. The cricothyroid space is not much larger than 7 mm in its vertical dimension, and that space may be narrowed further by contraction of the cricothyroid muscle. The vertical distance between the undersurface of the true vocal cords and the lower anterior edge of the thyroid cartilage is between 5 and 11 mm. The vertical height of the CTM from the superior border of the cricoid cartilage to the inferior border of the thyroid cartilage in the midline varies from 8 to 19 mm (mean, 13.69 mm), a somewhat greater distance that can probably be explained by the fresh rather than fixed state of specimens.

The arterial and venous vessel patterns in the neck area surrounding the CTM vary considerably. Although the arteries always lie deep to the pretracheal fascia and are easily avoided during a skin incision, veins may be found in the pretracheal fascia and between the pretracheal and superficial cervical fascia. Vascular structures may cross vertically and anterior to the CTM, predisposing them to damage during cricothyrotomy. A small cricothyroid artery, which is a branch of the superior thyroid artery, commonly crosses the upper portion of the CTM, anastomosing with the artery on the other side. External visible and palpable anatomic landmarks are used to locate the CTM. The laryngeal prominence (i.e., thyroid cartilage or Adam's apple) and the hyoid bone above it are readily palpable. The CTM usually lies one to one and a half finger breadths below the laryngeal prominence. The cricoid cartilage is usually felt below the CTM. The importance of these landmarks is emphasized because it is disastrous to place the cricothyroid tube into the thyrohyoid space instead of the cricothyroid space.

Conscious effort to identify these landmarks reduces the possibility of committing this preventable error (see Fig. 30-6B). When the normal anatomy is distorted, identification of these landmarks is difficult. In these cases, the suprasternal notch may be used as an alternative marker. The small finger of the right hand should be placed in the patient's suprasternal notch, followed by placement of the ring, long, and index fingers adjacent to each other in a stepwise fashion up the neck, with each finger touching the one below it. When the head is in the neutral position, the index finger is usually on or near the CTM.

IV. INDICATIONS AND CONTRAINDICATIONS FOR PERCUTANEOUS DILATIONAL CRICOTHYROTOMY AND TRACHEOSTOMY

A. Cricothyrotomy

Cricothyrotomy is considered by many to be the standard approach to airway management when orotracheal or nasotracheal intubation and fiberoptic approaches have failed.[5,18,49] In the emergency room or prehospital setting,[50,51] cricothyrotomy is indicated for immediate airway control in patients with maxillofacial, cervical spine, head, neck, and multiple trauma and in patients in whom endotracheal intubation is impossible to perform or contraindicated. It is also used for the immediate relief of upper airway obstruction. In the operating room and in the ICU, the technique is indicated when conventional methods of intubation fail, such as in patients with traumatic facial injuries in whom other techniques of airway access are difficult or impossible to perform. Cricothyrotomy can also be used as an alternative to tracheostomy in patients with recent sternotomy who need airway access because the incision does not communicate with the mediastinal tissue planes. A needle-size cricothyrotomy with a Luer-Lok connection (for jet ventilation) or an anesthesia circuit–size connection is used for thoracic and other procedures involving the airways, especially the trachea, larynx, epiglottis, and base of the tongue.

Emergency cricothyrotomy has largely replaced emergency tracheostomy in the emergency department because of its simplicity, rapidity, and minimal morbidity, and percutaneous techniques are replacing surgical approaches.[52,53] Use of emergency tracheostomy is limited and indicated only when laryngeal trauma may be accompanied by local edema, hemorrhage, subcutaneous emphysema, and damage to the thyroid or cricothyroid cartilage, precluding the performance of cricothyrotomy.

Cricothyrotomy is difficult to perform in pediatric patients because the larynx is smaller and their airways contain less fibrous supporting tissue and have only loose mucous membrane attachments in the airway inlet. Absolute and relative contraindications to cricothyrotomy are rare. Patients who have been intubated translaryngeally for more than 3 days (7 days according to many investigators) should not undergo cricothyrotomy because of the propensity to develop subglottic stenosis. Those with preexisting laryngeal diseases, such as cancer, acute or chronic inflammation, or epiglottitis, have a higher morbidity rate when cricothyrotomy is performed. Distortion of the normal neck anatomy by disease or injury may render the technique impossible. Normal anatomic landmarks may be distorted, making identification of the CTM difficult. Bleeding diathesis and a history of coagulopathy predispose the patient to hemorrhage, making the procedure extremely dangerous.

Cricothyrotomy is technically problematic to perform in the pediatric population and should be performed with extreme caution in children younger than 10 years. It should not be performed at all in children younger than 6 years unless a wire can be placed in the cricothyroid space and placement within the trachea can be verified.[54] Emergency tracheostomy under controlled conditions is the preferred choice.[55] Physicians who are unfamiliar or inexperienced with the technique are discouraged from performing the procedure without adequate supervision from a more senior or knowledgeable member of the medical team. Inexperience has been implicated as the most important factor contributing to cricothyroid complications.[56-58] Accuracy in identifying anatomic landmarks significantly depends on the physician's experience but is poor overall, justifying the percutaneous technique in emergency conditions but supporting the use of ultrasound or video-enhanced visualization during elective procedures.

B. Percutaneous Dilational Tracheostomy

PDT is mainly indicated in adult intubated patients (Box 30-1). In this patient population, the main indications for performing a PDT are the same as those for surgical tracheostomy:

- Preventing upper airway damage due to prolonged intubation
- Facilitating pulmonary toilet

- Providing a stable airway in patients requiring long-term mechanical ventilation and oxygen support

Several benefits of performing a tracheostomy in patients who require prolonged ventilation have been postulated and are supported by different levels of evidence.[59] Shorter ICU and hospital stays and less need for sedation are the most widely recognized benefits, whereas improved patient comfort, decreased work of breathing, improved oral hygiene, better long-term laryngeal function, faster weaning from mechanical ventilation, lower risk of ventilator-associated pneumonia, and lower mortality rates have also been reported but are supported by a lower level of evidence.[59]

For the population of critically ill adult patients, PDT has been recommended as the procedure of choice for performing elective tracheostomy.[59,60] PDT is recommended on the basis of a lower risk of wound infection, being able to perform it at the bedside rather than transferring critically ill patients to the operating room, and better cost-effectiveness compared with surgical tracheostomy.[60]

Upper airway obstruction due to tumor, edema, infection, stenosis, or trauma represents the other major category of indications for tracheostomy. However, the overall safety of performing PDT in emergent situations and with unprotected airways is extremely controversial, and, in these conditions, the procedure should be reserved for selected patients and performed only by experienced providers.[13] Anatomic suitability for this procedure must be determined preoperatively with the patient's neck extended. Maximum neck extension increases the length of the cervical trachea and defines critical anatomic landmarks, such as the cricoid cartilage and sternal notch. A contraindication to the procedure is the inability to palpate the cricoid cartilage above the sternal notch. Similarly, the patient with a midline neck mass, high

innominate artery, or large thyroid gland should undergo open surgical tracheostomy in the operating room. Coagulopathies should be corrected preoperatively. Ideally, the functional platelet count should be 50,000 or greater, and the international normalized ratio (INR) should be corrected to 1.5 or less. However, there have been reports of PDT safely performed in patients with severe thrombocytopenia.[61]

Patients requiring a positive end-expiratory pressure (PEEP) of 15 cm H_2O or higher are at high risk for complications such as subcutaneous emphysema and pneumothorax, and when possible, the procedure should be postponed for these patients. PDT is relatively contraindicated in nonintubated patients with acute airway compromise and in the pediatric population. For airway compromise in nonintubated patients, the risks are related to the length of the procedure and the inability to perform the procedure under direct endoscopic visualization without an ETT. Reasons to avoid PDT in children include the different airway anatomy and dimensions and the technical difficulties of maintaining adequate ventilation with a bronchoscope within a small ETT. Selected cases may present an exception to these contraindications, depending on the experience of the providers.[13]

V. PERCUTANEOUS DILATIONAL CRICOTHYROTOMY

A. Principles and Planning

This chapter focuses on percutaneous dilational techniques. Surgical cricothyrotomy and transtracheal catheter ventilation are discussed elsewhere in Chapter 31.

PDC is fast and usually easy to perform, even on patients with short necks or with spinal injury. Cricothyrotomy may be performed for elective airway management in trauma patients with technically challenging neck anatomy in lieu of tracheostomy, because it does not require a surgeon's skill to gain airway access and has fewer operative and postoperative complications.[62-65] Several commercially available devices use this technology. These devices have in common the insertion of an airway catheter over a dilator, which is usually introduced over a guidewire. The guidewire is inserted through a needle or over-the-needle catheter (i.e., Seldinger technique) after making an initial skin incision. This technique, often used for the insertion of catheter introducer sheaths and central lines, is familiar to anesthesiologists. An airway over a dilator and guidewire is preferable because of the inherent safety of this technique and the ability to insert an airway of far greater diameter than the initial catheter.

The Nu-Trake device (Smiths Medical, Dublin, OH) introduces a housing that is similar to a dilator but made in two parts, with the needle loaded coaxially within it. After the needle is withdrawn, metal airways with obturators are serially introduced inside the housing until the desired diameter of tube is reached.

Several devices allow insertion of the dilator directly over a needle or directly into the skin incision. Although they lack the step of introducing a guidewire, they are included in this discussion because they require a skin incision and a dilator for insertion of the airway. PDC is gaining popularity in the emergency room, ICU, and operating room. It is similar to another popular ICU technique, PDT, which is an elective procedure.

Airways can be introduced rapidly by the Seldinger over-the-wire technique, which allows positive-pressure ventilation without modification of standard ventilation devices. Although the technique requires more time to perform than needle cricothyrotomy, it may be more effective in providing adequate ventilation and oxygenation.

Several cricothyrotomy sets (Melker Emergency Cricothyrotomy Catheter Set, Cook Critical Care, Bloomington, IN; Portex Mini-Trach II, Smiths Medical, Keene, NH; Pertrach, Pulmodyne, Inc., Indianapolis, IN) can be inserted by the PDC technique. The Melker device uses a skin incision, followed by insertion of a guidewire and insertion of a dilator and airway catheter (i.e., cricothyrotomy tube). The Melker set is available in 3.5-, 4.0-, and 6.0-mm-ID, uncuffed airway catheter sizes with lengths of 3.8, 4.2, and 7.5 cm, respectively. The Melker set also comes in a military version that is modified for direct insertion through an incision without the use of a guidewire (similarly, the Portex cricothyroidotomy kit [PCK] and Nu-Trake from Smiths Medical and the Quicktrach I and II from VBM are designed for single insertion without a guidewire). The 4.0-mm-ID airway catheter is 7.5 cm long. This allows use of a smaller-diameter tube of sufficient length for an adult neck. The military version is available with cuffed and uncuffed airway catheters. A cuffed, 5.0-mm-ID, 9-cm-long airway catheter also has been introduced into the market. These sets are available with adapters so that jet ventilators and conventional ventilators can be attached to the airway device. Pertrachs are available with 5.5- and 7.1-mm-ID cannulas.

The over-the-wire technique offers several advantages. Even if the over-the-needle or direct dilational technique, such as the Quicktrach, PCK, or the Melker military version, may be faster to perform, the reported difficulties and complications are greater. This is also true for the Nu-Trake device. Complications have included failure to gain airway access, multiple attempts at cannulation, mediastinal injury, pneumothorax, and severe bleeding. The wire-guided technique has the disadvantage of the wire kinking. Several clinical and cadaver-based studies have established the safety and efficacy of the percutaneous over-the-needle or -cannula, wire-guided technique.[42,66-71] For some of the devices, their use, diffusion, and success seem to have been influenced by local availability, original country of manufacturing, preliminary animal studies, and marketing, despite scarce clinical evidence of efficacy.

B. Insertion Techniques

1. Percutaneous Dilational Cricothyrotomy Device

The PDC device manufactured by Melker contains a scalpel blade; a syringe with an 18-G over-the-needle catheter or a thin-walled introducer needle, or both; a guidewire; a dilator of appropriate length and diameter; and a polyvinyl airway catheter with or without a cuff

(Fig. 30-7). A universal kit combines open cricothyrotomy and percutaneous tools in a single tray. (Although it defeats the concept of a percutaneous approach, it may be useful in remote or austere locations.) Detailed insertion instructions for this type of device are available from the manufacturer's Website, brochure, and CD. A description of the Melker insertion technique (Fig. 30-8) follows:

1. Position the patient supine, and if there is no contraindication, slightly extend the neck by using a roll under the neck or shoulders. If cervical spine injury is suspected, properly immobilize the head and neck, and maintain a neutral position.
2. Open the prepackaged cricothyrotomy set, and assemble the components. Whenever possible and appropriate, use aseptic technique and local anesthetic.
3. Identify the CTM between the cricoid and thyroid cartilages.
4. Carefully palpate the CTM, and while stabilizing the cartilage, make a vertical or horizontal skin incision using the scalpel blade (can also be performed after the Seldinger technique). Make a stab incision (vertical or horizontal) through the lower third of the CTM. An adequate incision eases introduction of the dilator and airway, but the incision can follow the placement of the guidewire.
5. Attach the supplied syringe to the 18-G introducer needle–plastic catheter (over the needle technique) system (same that you would use to place an angio-catheter), or alternatively attach the syringe to the introducer needle only (having removed the plastic catheter) if you prefer or are concerned the plastic catheter may kink. Insert the syringe-needle-catheter or syringe-needle only, and advance it through the incision into the airway at a 45-degree angle to the frontal plane in the midline in a caudad direction. When advancing the needle forward, entrance into the airway can be confirmed by aspiration with the syringe resulting in free air return or air bubbles in a saline-filled syringe.
6. Remove the syringe and needle, leaving the plastic catheter or introducer needle in place. Do not attempt to advance the plastic catheter completely into the airway, which may result in kinking of the catheter and an inability to pass the guidewire. Advance the soft, flexible end of the guidewire through the catheter or needle and several centimeters into the airway.
7. Remove the plastic catheter or needle, leaving the guidewire in place.
8. Advance the handled dilator inside the airway catheter (single dilation if a preincision was made), tapered end first, into the connector end of the airway catheter until the handle stops against the connector. With other sets, insert the dilator to the recommended depth, or insert the dilator over the guidewire for a preinsertion dilation (recommended if a preincision was not made). Use of lubrication on the surface of the dilator may enhance the fit and placement of the emergency airway catheter.

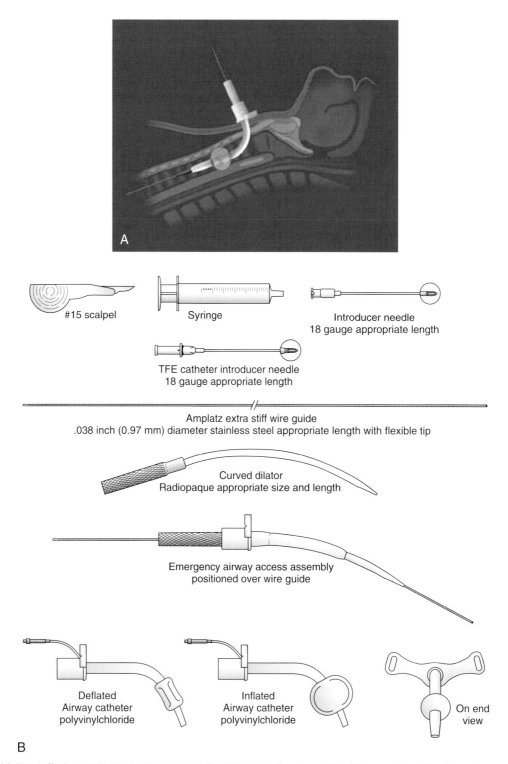

Figure 30-7 **A,** Melker cuffed cannula inserted in a model. **B,** Melker cricothyrotomy kit, which consists of the items shown and a tracheostomy cloth tape strip for fixation of an airway catheter. (Courtesy of Cook Medical, Bloomington, IN.)

9. Advance the emergency airway access assembly over the guidewire until the proximal stiff end of the guidewire is completely through and visible at the handle end of the dilator. Always visualize the proximal end of the guidewire during the airway insertion procedure to prevent its inadvertent loss into the trachea. Maintaining the guidewire position, advance the emergency airway access assembly over the guidewire with an in-and-out motion.

10. As the airway catheter is fully advanced into the trachea, remove the guidewire and dilator simultaneously.

11. If a cuffed tube is inserted, inflate it with 10 mL of air with the syringe provided.

12. Fix the emergency airway catheter in place with the cloth tracheostomy tape strip in a standard fashion.

13. Using its standard 15- to 22-mm adapter, connect the emergency airway catheter to an appropriate ventilatory device.

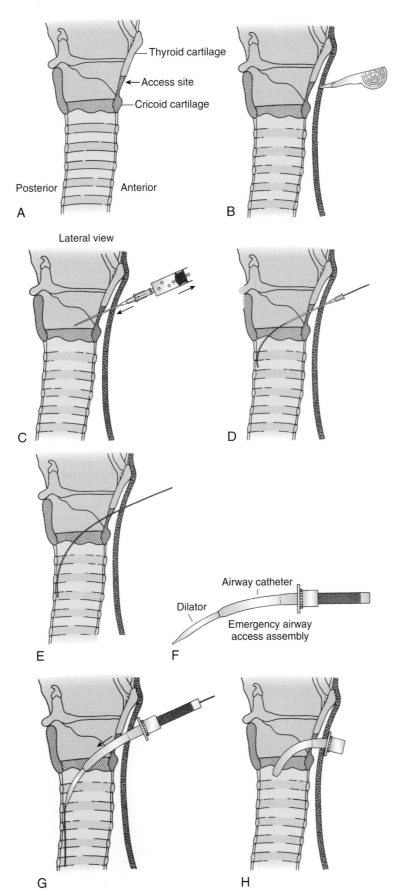

Figure 30-8 A to **H,** Melker insertion technique. (From Melker emergency cricothyrotomy sets: Suggested instructions for placement, instruction pamphlet. Cook Critical Care, Bloomington, IN, 1988.)

2. Skin Incision Before Needle Insertion

Few authors recommend an incision before introducing the catheter for two reasons. First, the catheter is more likely to kink when the needle is removed, making it difficult to pass the guidewire. Second, there have been reports of an inability to advance the dilator because the skin incision was not next to the guidewire. Extending the incision to the guidewire solved the problem. Anesthesiologists and critical care physicians usually make a skin incision after wire introduction. In that case, a firm incision next to the wire, which is carefully done to avoid cutting the wire, into the CTM is recommended. Predilation, which is done with the dilator only before inserting in the airway cannula, can help with placement, reducing the likelihood of the cannula grasping tissue (i.e., gap between the airway cannula and dilator).

3. Vertical Versus Horizontal Incision

It is unclear whether a horizontal or vertical skin incision is superior. The literature is evenly divided on this matter but usually refers to surgical cricothyrotomy. It can be argued that a vertical incision is better during emergency cricothyrotomy because it can be extended superiorly or inferiorly if the relationship of the skin and CTM changes (as frequently happens). A vertical stab through the CTM in the inferior third is recommended to ease placement of the dilator and avoid the cricothyroid arteries, which often anastomose in the midline superiorly.

4. Over-the-Needle Catheter Versus Introducer Needle

The guidewire through a needle tends to be superior when a skin incision is not used, but it has a similar success rate to that for an over-the-needle catheter if an incision is used initially. It appears that catheters kinked only when attempts were made to pass the total length of the catheter into the airway.

5. Percutaneous Dilational Cricothyrotomy

a. ARNDT

The Arndt cricothyrotomy cannula (Cook Medical) is technically a percutaneous dilational wire-guided cannula designed for transtracheal jet ventilation (Fig. 30-9; see Fig. 30-3).

b. PERTRACH

The Pertrach (Fig. 30-10) is similar to the previously described devices, except that the guidewire and dilator are a single unit. The introducer needle must be split after the distal end of the guidewire is advanced so that the dilator can be introduced (Fig. 30-11). This is cumbersome, especially in emergency situations, and requires the guidewire and dilator to be advanced far down the airway. A study in cadavers showed equal success for PDC with the Pertrach and surgical cricothyrotomy. Surgical cricothyrotomy was faster, but it was impossible to predict whether bleeding complications would have been higher with the surgical cricothyrotomies. The manufacturer and the users have reported problems with the needle, which is occasionally difficult or impossible to split.

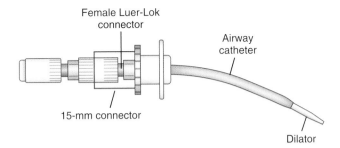

Figure 30-9 Arndt cricothyrotomy cannula components. (Courtesy of Cook Medical, Bloomington, IN.)

c. NU-TRAKE

The Nu-Trake device has a rigid airway and may be difficult to secure. The Nu-Trake requires far greater insertion forces than other devices, often resulting in the introducer-stylet embedding in the posterior wall of the trachea. The device has had frequent air leaks, and the lumen has a tendency to occlude on the posterior wall of the trachea. Subcutaneous emphysema, cricoid cartilage injury, cricotracheal ligament perforation, posterior wall perforation, and incidental submucosal airway hemorrhage have also been described.

d. QUICKTRACH AND PORTEX CRICOTHYROIDOTOMY KIT

The Quicktrach (Rüsch, VBM) (Fig. 30-12) and PCK (Portex) (Fig. 30-13) offer a single-step technique that is preceded by a skin incision, proceeds over a needle, and is not guided by a wire. The devices are technically faster to use but overall are less safe, carrying a higher complication rate (e.g., multiple attempts, inability to advance the cannula, false pas sage) than the Seldinger technique. The PCK (Fig. 30-14) has a Veress needle system, which is designed to detect pressure on the posterior wall of the

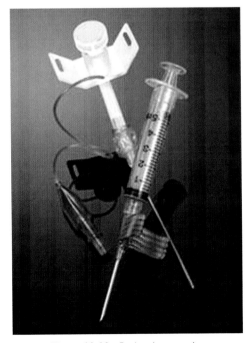

Figure 30-10 Pertrach cannula.

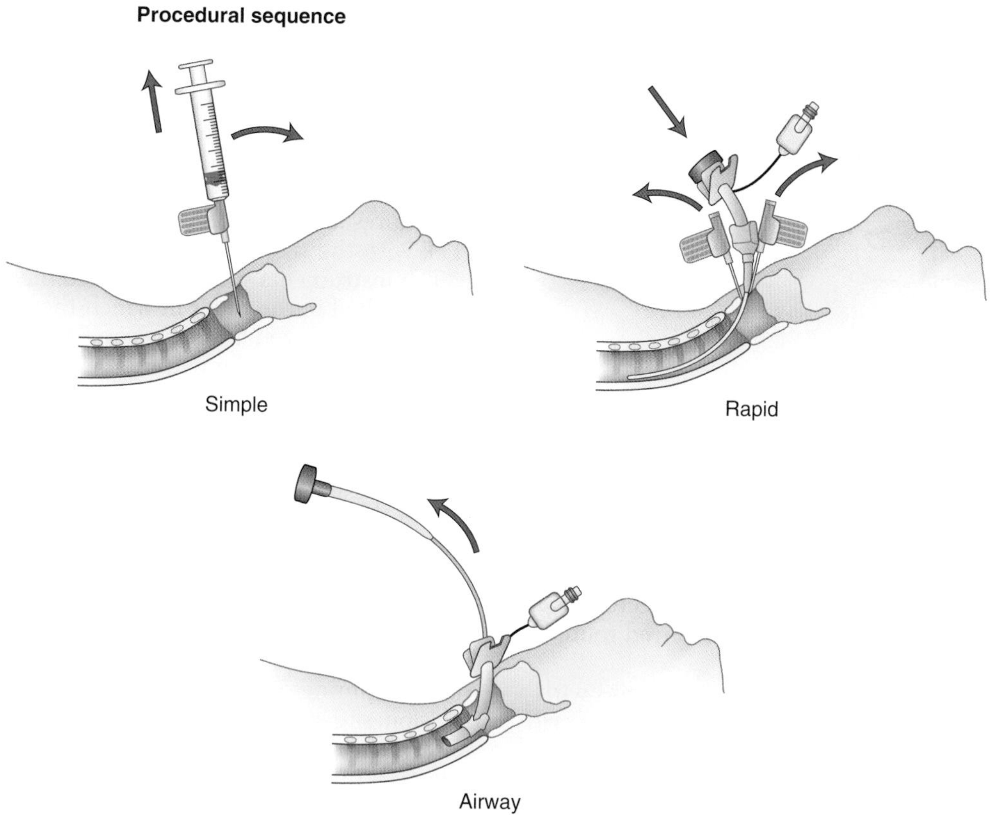

Procedural sequence

Simple

Rapid

Airway

Figure 30-11 Pertrach technique steps.

trachea. The PCK is inserted directly through the CTM after a skin incision (Fig. 30-15).

The fast access that these systems provide can be life-saving in remote locations and in treating a severely damaged airway, outweighing the potential complications. However, their use in less emergent situations may be questionable, especially by first-time users.

VI. PERCUTANEOUS DILATIONAL TRACHEOSTOMY

A. Principles and Planning

PDT is an accepted alternative to surgical tracheostomy, and it is gaining in popularity, particularly for patients in the ICU who have been intubated or are expected to

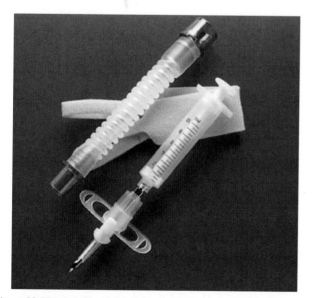

Figure 30-12 Quicktrach I standard set. (Courtesy of Teleflex Medical, Research Triangle Park, NC.)

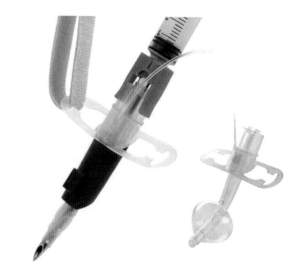

Figure 30-13 Quicktrach II cricothyrotomy set. (Courtesy of VBM Medical, Noblesville, IN.)

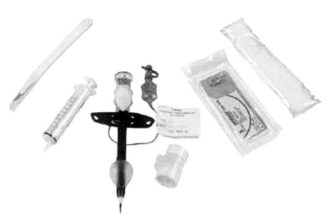

Figure 30-14 Portex cricothyroidotomy kit. (Courtesy of Smiths Medical, Dublin, OH.)

need endotracheal intubation for extended periods.[59,72-76] PDT is a mostly elective procedure, although there have been reports of PDT safely performed in selected emergent situations.[13] Cricothyrotomy is a preferred route for emergent airway access.

As with any procedure, proper planning begins with a history and physical examination, and palpation of critical landmarks, such as the cricoid cartilage and sternal notch, is mandatory. The neck must be inspected to exclude a high innominate artery or midline neck mass. Preoperative testing is minimal and includes a recent chest radiograph and serum determinations of hemoglobin, prothrombin time (PT), partial thromboplastin time, and platelets. The INR, which is calculated to reflect the PT, best reflects coagulation status. Although 1 is a normal value, an INR corrected to less than 1.5 is acceptable. Because bleeding is usually minimal, crossmatching of blood cell units is unnecessary, even in the presence of a low hemoglobin level.

A fully equipped difficult airway cart should be available nearby in the event of accidental extubation during the procedure. In patients with thick, large necks, consideration should be given to placement of an extra-long tracheostomy tube to prevent accidental decannulation or displacement into the pretracheal soft tissues. Ideally, four people are required for the procedure, including the operating physician, a resident or critical care colleague to perform the bronchoscopy, a respiratory technician or other qualified staff member to assist in adjusting ventilator settings and to hold the ETT firmly in position, and a nurse to administer medications, monitor vital signs, and assist in obtaining necessary materials and instruments. The surgeon and necessary instruments usually are positioned to the patient's right, the respiratory technician to the left, and the bronchoscopist at the head of the bed.

Many kits are commercially available for this procedure. The most widely used are those based on the original Ciaglia technique (Fig. 30-16A) and subsequent modifications that led to the single-dilator kits. Included in this category is the Ciaglia Blue Rhino G2 Advanced Percutaneous Tracheostomy Kit (Cook Medical), the Portex ULTRAperc Single-Stage Dilator (Smith Medical), and the Ciaglia Blue Dolphin balloon percutaneous tracheostomy kit (Cook Medical).

The Portex Griggs Percutaneous Dilation Tracheostomy Kit (Smiths Medical), based on the Griggs guidewire dilating forceps technique, is widely used. Detailed insertion instructions for these types of devices are available from the manufacturers' Web sites, brochures, and CDs. The following paragraphs offer a brief description of the general principles of appropriate planning for these procedures and detailed instructions on how to perform PDT with the single-dilator technique.

The instruments should be placed on a stand over the patient's bed in the order in which they will be used. An appropriately sized bronchoscope with a suction port must be chosen to fit within the ETT or nasotracheal tube while allowing adequate ventilation. A pediatric bronchoscope must be used when the ETT has an ID of less than 7.0 mm. A video monitor, if available, may be connected to the bronchoscope, allowing full visualization of the intratracheal portion of the procedure by the operating surgeon and staff. Any procedure involving manipulation of the trachea is highly stimulating to the patient and requires adequate local anesthesia supplemented by intravenous sedation. Local anesthesia, consisting of 1% or 2% lidocaine with a 1:100,000 solution of epinephrine, is used for generous infiltration of the incision site down to the level of the trachea. Topical anesthesia in the form of 2% to 4% lidocaine may be injected through the bronchoscope and is useful in decreasing the cough reflex during intratracheal instrumentation. Intravenous anesthesia is required, and the particular drug combination depends on the patient and the institution. Frequently used medications include midazolam, fentanyl, remifentanil, propofol, and dexmedetomidine. The presence of an anesthesiologist is recommended, but this depends on the hospital setting and availability. Care should be exercised in managing the ETT, performing the bronchoscopy, and administering drugs, particularly in elderly patients, because large fluctuations in blood pressure and heart rate may occur even with small doses. Muscle relaxation is recommended to facilitate procedures.

B. Insertion Techniques

1. Seldinger Guidewire and Single-Dilator Kit

1. The patient is positioned as for conventional tracheostomy with the head extended on the neck, and anatomic landmarks are marked (see Fig. 30-6, *B*). A standard preparation and drape are applied.
2. The skin and subcutaneous tissues are infiltrated with 2% lidocaine and a 1:100,000 solution of epinephrine one or two finger breadths below the previously palpated and marked cricoid cartilage (Fig. 30-17, *A*).
3. A 1.5-cm horizontal skin incision is made, and the subcutaneous tissues are bluntly separated with a curved hemostat. No attempt is made to manipulate the strap muscles or thyroid gland.
4. At this point, the fiberoptic bronchoscope (FOB) is advanced until its tip is aligned with the lower margin of the ETT (advance in a supraglottic device until the cricoid is visualized). External

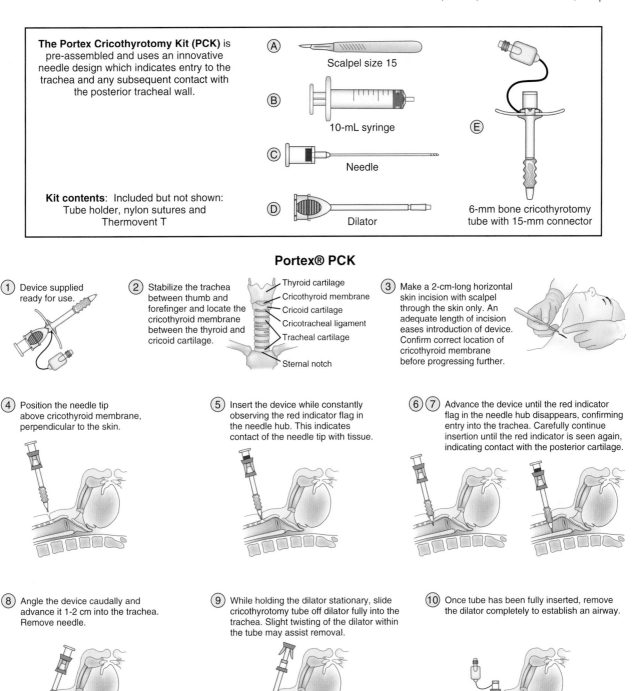

Figure 30-15 Portex cricothyroidotomy kit *(PCK)* insertion technique. (Modified from Smiths Medical, Dublin, OH.)

manipulation and transtracheal illumination can facilitate structure recognition.

5. Any ties securing the ETT are loosened, and the FOB and ETT are withdrawn slowly in unison until the incision is maximally transilluminated.

6. The FOB, which may be connected to a monitor, is maintained in this position throughout the procedure, allowing direct visualization of every step.

7. The 16- or 17-gauge introducer needle is inserted between the first and second or second and third tracheal rings (see Fig. 30-17, *B*).

8. A midline intercartilaginous placement is verified bronchoscopically.

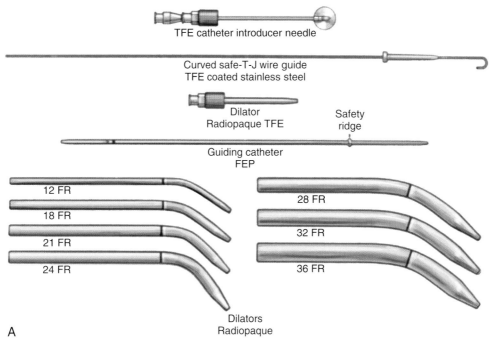

TFE catheter introducer needle

Curved safe-T-J wire guide
TFE coated stainless steel

Dilator
Radiopaque TFE

Safety
ridge

Guiding catheter
FEP

12 FR
18 FR
21 FR
24 FR

28 FR
32 FR
36 FR

Dilators
Radiopaque

A

Figure 30-16 **A,** Ciaglia kit. (Courtesy of Cook Critical Care, Bloomington, IN.)

9. The needle is withdrawn, leaving the overlying catheter sheath through which the guidewire can be inserted (see Fig. 30-17, C and D).
10. The sheath is removed and replaced by a 14-F introducer dilator, which is advanced over the guidewire (several times); this maneuver enlarges the tracheal aperture sufficiently to allow easy placement of the 12-F guiding catheter.
11. The guiding catheter and guidewire are left in place and form the backbone over which the single dilator is used.
12. The single dilator with the hydrophilic coating moistened is advanced over this unit (see Fig. 30-16, B), several times if necessary, until resistance is minimal. The chosen depth of dilation also depends on the size of the cannula to be inserted.
13. The dilator is replaced by the preloaded tracheostomy tube, which is advanced into the trachea. Some resistance may be encountered at the interface between the dilator and tracheostomy tube.
14. The guidewire, guiding catheter, and dilator are removed and replaced by the inner cannula.
15. The ventilatory apparatus is connected to the tracheostomy, which is secured with four corner sutures.
16. When ventilation is adequate, the ETT is removed while examining the vocal folds. A postoperative chest radiograph is obtained to rule out a pneumothorax. In a patient with a large, thick neck, a longer tracheostomy tube should be used to prevent accidental displacement of the tube into the pretracheal soft tissue. In the event of accidental decannulation within 5 days of the procedure, the ICU staff is advised to reintubate the patient orally rather than attempt to reinsert the tracheostomy tube.

Precautions in the performance of this technique include the following:

- Always confirm access into trachea by air bubble aspiration.
- Maintain safety positioning marks of the guidewire, guiding catheters, and dilator during the dilating procedure to prevent trauma to the posterior wall of the trachea.
- Tracheostomy tubes should fit snugly to the dilator for insertion. Generous lubrication of the surface of the dilator enhances fit and placement of the tracheostomy tube.

2. Ciaglia Blue Rhino G2 Advanced Percutaneous Tracheostomy Kit

The Ciaglia Blue Rhino G2 Advanced Percutaneous Tracheostomy Kit (Cook Medical) (Fig. 30-18, A) has a curved dilator that is advanced over a guiding catheter and creates a tracheostomy opening in one pass, obviating the need for multiple dilators as with previous kits (see Fig. 30-18, B). The softness of the dilator, the hydrophilic coating, and the one-passage technique are the main advantages of this widely used percutaneous tracheostomy system, which has been at least as safe as the PDT techniques in multiple trials.[40,77-81]

3. Ciaglia Blue Dolphin Balloon Percutaneous Tracheostomy Kit

The Ciaglia Blue Dolphin Balloon percutaneous tracheostomy kit (Cook Medical) offers an improvement on the single-dilator PDT technique. This system combines balloon dilation and tracheal tube insertion in a single step (Fig. 30-19). The underlying principle is that balloon dilation should minimize pressure on the anterior tracheal wall and deliver an even and controlled radial

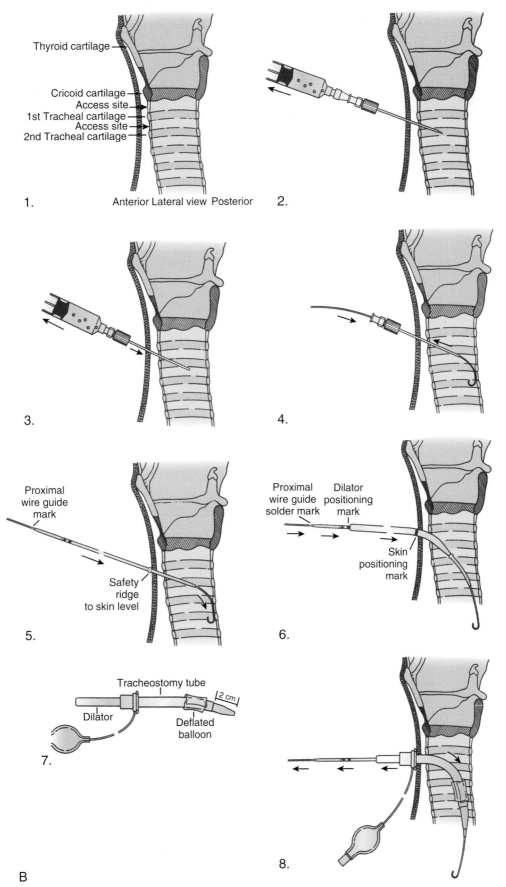

Figure 30-16, cont'd B, Detailed instructions (*1* to *8*) for insertion of the Ciaglia percutaneous tracheostomy set.

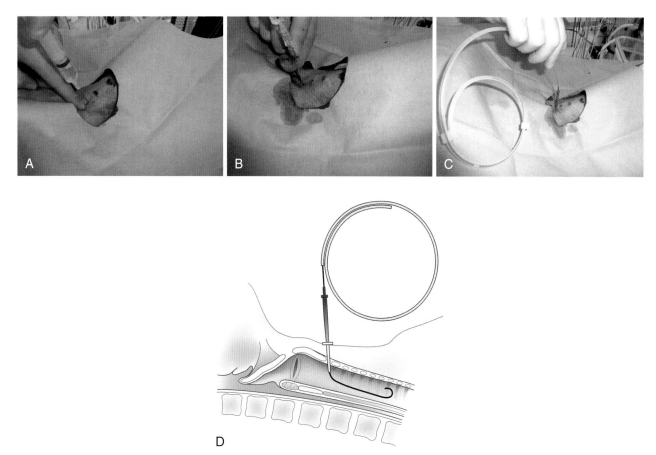

Figure 30-17 Use of a single dilator. **A,** Local anesthesia. **B,** Introducer needle, **C,** Guidewire insertion in a clinical case. **D,** Diagram of guidewire insertion.

dilation. Given the novelty of this device, data from the literature are insufficient to determine any advantage of this system compared with established methods and devices.

4. Portex ULTRAperc Single-Stage Dilator

The Portex ULTRAperc Single-Stage Percutaneous Dilation Tracheostomy Kit (Smiths Medical) is based on the widely accepted Seldinger guidewire technique. The kits are available with the Blue Line Ultra Suctionaid Tracheostomy Tube that features an integrated suction lumen for removal of pooled secretions (Fig. 30-20).

In a study comparing the ULTRAperc device with the Blue Rhino in mannequin and porcine models, dilation with the ULTRAperc set was subjectively easier and required less force, and the time for tracheostomy tube

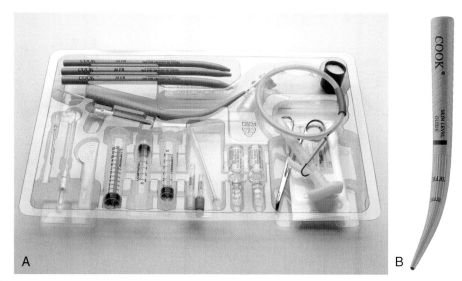

Figure 30-18 **A,** Ciaglia Blue Rhino G2 tray. **B,** Blue Rhino percutaneous tracheostomy dilator. (Courtesy of Cook Medical, Bloomington, IN.)

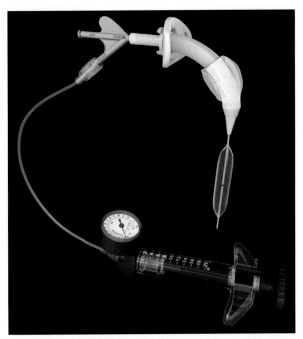

Figure 30-19   Ciaglia Blue Dolphin balloon percutaneous tracheostomy introducer. (Courtesy of Cook Medical, Bloomington, IN.)

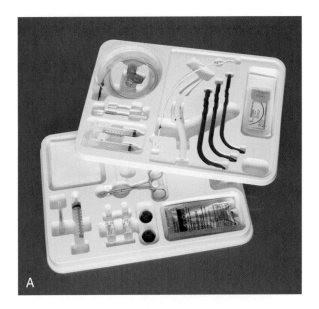

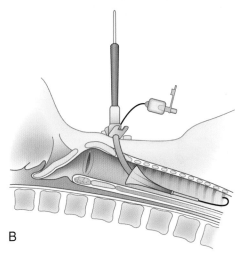

Figure 30-20   A, Portex ULTRAperc kit. **B,** Insertion of the ULTRAperc cannula with a handle introducer. (**A,** Courtesy of Smiths Medical, Dublin, OH.)

insertion was shorter.[82] The investigators suggest that the ULTRAperc set is subjectively easier to use, quicker, and causes less anterior-posterior tracheal compression during tracheostomy tube insertion compared with the Blue Rhino set in mannequin and porcine airway models. This advantage may be from the tracheostomy tube introducer in the ULTRAperc set that allows smooth passage of the tracheostomy tube through the dilated stoma.

5. Portex Griggs Percutaneous Dilation Tracheostomy Kit

The Portex Griggs Percutaneous Dilation Tracheostomy Kit (Smiths Medical) features guidewire dilating forceps that are central to the Griggs PDT technique (Fig. 30-21). Dilating forceps specially designed to slide along a prepositioned guidewire are used to open pretracheal tissue and the anterior tracheal wall in preparation for tube insertion. Use of the forceps causes less compression compared with the cone-shaped, single-stage dilators. In a prospective, randomized comparison of progressive-dilational versus forceps-dilational percutaneous tracheostomy,[83] the progressive-dilational tracheostomy took longer, caused more hypercapnia, and caused more minor and major difficulties than forceps-dilational tracheostomy. We agree that the guidewire dilating forceps technique is safe and easy to learn, and it may be quicker than the progressive-dilational technique. Sometimes, the forceps cannot be inserted to the full length due to thick subcutaneous tissue of the anterior neck. Switching from forceps to a progressive dilator allows completion of the procedure without complications.[31,84] The Portex Griggs Percutaneous Dilation Tracheostomy Kit also may be used in combination with Suctionaid tracheostomy tubes with an integral suction lumen to aid suctioning of secretions from above the cuff.

6. Percutwist

Increased control over the dilating maneuver from start to finish is one of the advantages of the Percutwist (Rüsch-Teleflex Medical) (see Fig. 46-19 in Chapter 46). Another is the possibility to lift the anterior tracheal wall, facilitating the endoscopic view of the dilation site during the procedure. Gradual application of the forces applied to produce dilation may increase the safety of this technique, although cases of posterior tracheal wall injury have been reported.[78,85]

7. Translaryngeal Tracheostomy Kit

The Translaryngeal Tracheostomy Kit (Mallinckrodt, Mirandola, Italy) is used mostly in European countries to perform translaryngeal tracheostomy according to the technique introduced by Fantoni in 1997. The critical steps of this procedure and use of this system are summarized in Figure 46-16 (see Chapter 46). Percutaneous tracheostomy has a learning curve and requires appropriate training. All studies comparing different methods

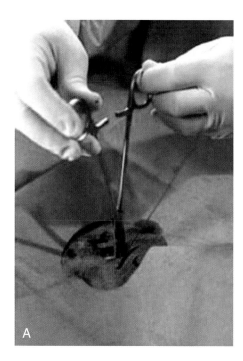

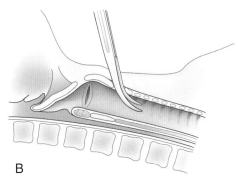

Figure 30-21 **A,** Portex Griggs forceps used for dilatation during surgery. **B,** Diagram of forceps dilatation. (**B,** Courtesy of Smiths Medical, Dublin, OH.)

should take into consideration potential differences in training of the personnel performing PDT with each proposed technique. Different environments and patient characteristics may dictate the choice of a specific technique or determine the preference for a specific system.

8. Controversies and Questions

a. USE OF BRONCHOSCOPY AND ULTRASOUND

The issue of bronchoscopy has been hotly debated in the literature over the past 2 decades. Those in favor argue that it is easy to perform and adds to the safety of the procedure by significantly decreasing or eliminating the risk of false passage, pneumomediastinum, pneumothorax, and subcutaneous emphysema. Bronchoscopy allows early detection and suctioning of intratracheal blood and secretions. The bronchoscope also allows proper midline needle placement between the second and third tracheal rings and prevents injury to the posterior tracheal wall.

Opponents argue that bronchoscopy increases the length and cost of the procedure and does not add to safety in experienced hands. Moreover, the presence of the bronchoscope within the ETT may result in CO_2 retention and difficulty ventilating the patient. The accumulated weight of evidence in the literature points to the advantages of bronchoscopy for safety reasons.[86,87] Nonetheless, a large meta-analysis was not able to demonstrate a clear advantage of bronchoscope-guided procedures in terms of decreasing overall mortality and major perioperative complications.[88]

Ultrasound has been proposed as a useful tool to identify the anatomy of airway, blood vessels, and other structures, such as the thyroid gland and isthmus. Ultrasound has in some cases replaced bronchoscopic guidance.[89] However, a combination of the two (depending on resource availability) may offer better results. Whether ultrasound can reduce the incidence of tracheal-innominate fistulas (a rare but deadly complication) needs further investigation.[90]

b. PATIENT'S HABITUS

Controversy exists regarding the suitability of percutaneous tracheostomy in obese patients. Obesity may preclude adequate palpation of critical landmarks and increase the risk of false passage or accidental decannulation into the soft tissues of the neck. Optimal positioning of the neck usually permits localization of the cricoid cartilage and sternal notch. Vigorous spreading of the subcutaneous tissues during the procedure facilitates palpation of the tracheal rings for precise needle placement. The risk of false passage may be addressed by always using a bronchoscope and ensuring step-by-step visualization.

Accidental decannulation in these patients is more likely to occur because of the displacement of the tube in the abundant soft tissues. Using proximally extended tracheostomy tubes dramatically reduces the risk of this complication. Ben Nun and colleagues presented a case series of 154 critically ill adult patients in whom percutaneous tracheostomy using the Griggs technique was performed at the bedside.[91] Eighteen of these patients had a short, fat neck as their only risk factor for PDT. Short, fat neck was defined as a neck circumference greater than 46 cm, with a distance between the cricoid cartilage and the sternal notch of less than 2.5 cm and distance between the cricoid cartilage and the pretracheal soft tissues of more than 2.5 cm. No complications were reported in this group. Heyrosa and coworkers reported their results for a series of 89 obese patients (body mass index [BMI] >35 kg/m²) undergoing PDT and 53 obese patients (same BMI) undergoing open tracheostomy, and they found the same complication rate (6.5%) for the two groups.[92]

Aldawood and colleagues performed PDT in 50 obese patients, mostly without bronchoscopic guidance.[93] They reported an increased rate of major complications compared with nonobese patients (12% versus 2%, $P = 0.04$) but a similar rate of minor complications for the two groups.[93] They defined obesity as a BMI of 30 kg/m² or higher. The most frequent major complication was "procedure aborted, not otherwise specified," but no surgical conversion, pneumothorax, or death occurred in either group. The investigators concluded that PDT could be performed safely in most obese patients.

In a prospective evaluation of endoscopic PDT in 500 consecutive intubated adults in the ICU, patients with a BMI of 30 kg/m^2 or greater had a significantly greater ($P < 0.06$) number of complications (15%) than the patients (8%) with a BMI less than 30 kg/m^2.[94] This risk was even more significant for patients with a BMI of 30 or more who were also in ASA physical status class 4 (11 of 56 [20%]) ($P < 0.02$). Byhahn and colleagues reported an extremely high complication rate (43.8%) for 73 obese patients and found that obese patients (BMI >27.5 kg/m^2) had a 2.7-fold increased risk for perioperative complications and a 4.9-fold increased risk for serious complications compared with nonobese patients.[95] The researchers concluded that percutaneous tracheostomy in obese patients was associated with a considerably increased risk for perioperative complications, especially for serious adverse events. Comparison of the results and conclusions from these studies is problematic because of the different criteria used in defining obesity, the dissimilar primary and secondary end points, and the use of different percutaneous techniques for PDT.

VII. POSTOPERATIVE CONSIDERATIONS

A. Cricothyrotomy

Cricothyrotomy is usually performed emergently to secure a difficult airway, but it can be performed electively.[7] When cricothyrotomy is performed under less than ideal circumstances, it should be considered a temporary measure, and when the patient is stabilized, endotracheal intubation with or without an FOB or a tracheostomy should be performed. The FOB affords an opportunity to evaluate the airway, especially at the site of the cricothyrotomy. The cricothyrotomy site should be examined frequently for signs of infection, and all patients should have a careful neurologic and airway evaluation before discharge from the hospital to ensure that there has been no damage to the vocal cords or other proximate structures. There is no consensus of opinion on what work-up is necessary after emergency cricothyrotomy, but any complaints by the patient of difficulty swallowing or phonating should be carefully evaluated. Complication rates from properly performed emergent cricothyrotomy are acceptably low.

B. Percutaneous Tracheostomy

With the termination of the intense stimulation produced by the procedure, the effects of the sedation may become more pronounced, and particular care must be taken in monitoring for changes in vital signs such as hypotension, tachycardia, or oxygen desaturation. In some cases, pharmacologic intervention may be required. Excess secretions or blood may compromise ventilation and result in an oxygen saturation drop, requiring suctioning. A postoperative chest radiograph is required to ensure the absence of pneumothorax and pneumomediastinum.

Many of these patients have copious secretions from the tracheostomy site because of their associated pulmonary condition. A tracheostomy tube with an inner cannula facilitates care and hygiene and ensures added safety by easy removal if obstruction from secretions occurs. The percutaneous technique is primarily dilational with minimal tissue dissection, resulting in a tighter tract and a very snug fit of the tracheostomy tube. The technique does not allow placement of traction sutures at the level of the trachea. Because of these factors, the patient should be reintubated orally in the event of accidental decannulation within the first 5 days of the procedure, while the tract is still relatively immature. Attempts at replacing the tracheostomy tube in an emergent situation may cause bleeding, the creation of a false passage, pneumomediastinum, hypoxia, or death.

1. Complications and Outcome Data

a. CRICOTHYROTOMY

The reported complication rate is 6% to 8% for elective cricothyrotomy and 10% to 40% for emergent procedures.[96,97] The morbidity and mortality rates for elective cricothyrotomy are similar to those for elective tracheostomy. Boyd and colleagues found 10 complications (6.8%) in 147 cricothyrotomies, but no differentiation was made between elective and emergency procedures. In 1976, Brantigan and Grow reported a 6.1% complication rate for 655 cases, most of which were correctable and self-limited, and this compared favorably with the complication rate associated with tracheostomy. The same investigators implicated the presence of acute laryngeal pathology (especially from prolonged intubation before cricothyrotomy) as the predisposing factor in the subsequent development of subglottic obstruction.[98]

Adverse effects of cricothyrotomy can be categorized as those that occur early and those that occur late in the postoperative period. Early complications include asphyxia related to failure to establish the airway, hemorrhage, improper or unsuccessful tube placement, subcutaneous and mediastinal emphysema, prolonged procedure time, pneumothorax, and airway obstruction. Esophageal or mediastinal perforation, vocal cord injury, aspiration, and laryngeal disruption may also occur.[99] Long-term complications include tracheal and subglottic stenosis (especially in the presence of preexisting laryngeal trauma or infection), aspiration, swallowing dysfunction, tube obstruction, tracheal-esophageal fistula, and voice changes.[100] Voice change is the most common complication, occurring in up to 50% of cases.[20] Voice problems include hoarseness, weak voice, or decreased pitch. The voice dysfunction may be caused by injury to the external branch of the superior laryngeal nerve, decreased cricothyroid muscle contractility, or mechanical obstruction related to narrowing of the anterior parts of the thyroid and cricoid cartilages.[101] Infection, late bleeding, persistent stoma, and tracheomalacia have also been reported. Although subglottic stenosis is the most frequently reported major complication after cricothyrotomy,[102] it is rare after tracheostomy. Pneumothorax and major blood vessel erosion are also associated with tracheostomy. Other complications associated with tracheostomy include mediastinal emphysema, accidental extubation, cardiac arrest, and death.

The complication rate for cricothyrotomy is higher in the pediatric population. Pneumothorax is the most common complication in children (5% to 7%) and is rarely seen in adults. Between 1% and 2% of adults develop subglottic stenosis after tracheostomy, compared with 2% to 8% of children. Children undergoing cricothyrotomy have a mortality rate up to 8.7%. Prehospital cricothyrotomy performed by emergency medical services (EMS) personnel carries a higher risk of morbidity than the in-hospital procedure. Spaite and Joseph reported an overall acute complication rate of 31% for 20 emergency patients. Failure to secure the airway accounted for the major complication rate (12%). Minor complications included right main stem intubation, infrahyoid placement, and thyroid cartilage fracture. Sixty surgical cricothyrotomies performed by trained aeromedical system personnel had a complication rate of 8.7%.[103] These complications included significant hemorrhage or soft tissue hematoma and incorrect placement. All the previous complications are from surgical or mixed surgical and percutaneous cricothyrotomy studies. Problems and complications associated specifically with percutaneous cricothyrotomy include difficulties with insertion, esophageal or mediastinal misplacement, and bleeding.[104] The overall reported complication rate is 5%. Complications included CTM calcification, blockage by secretions, dystrophic ossification, and heterotrophic bone formation. Displacement of the tube into the mediastinum may occur and can cause emphysema, respiratory distress, and pneumothorax.[105] Bleeding occurs in 2% of cases, but significant hemorrhage requiring surgical intervention is rare. The Seldinger technique appears to lessen the incidence of bleeding and promote a more precise technique of insertion.[106]

b. PERCUTANEOUS TRACHEOSTOMY

Most studies report excellent success and low complication rates with PDT.[90,107,108] Since PDT became common clinical practice, data on the utility of this procedure and its potential advantages over standard tracheostomy have been reported in many publications.[36,73,90,107,109,110]

Potential complications of tracheostomy, whether performed openly or percutaneously, can be described as intraoperative or postoperative and as early or late; they are listed in Box 30-2. The overall complication rate reported for PDT in large studies, systematic reviews, and meta-analyses ranges from about 6% to 15%.[85,111-114] It has been suggested that bronchoscopy-guided PDT might have a lower incidence of complications compared with PDT performed without bronchoscopy,[86,87,115] but the data on this issue are mixed, and other studies have not confirmed this hypothesis.[88] Among intraoperative complications, premature extubation and bleeding are most concerning and reported more frequently. Early postoperative complications include tube malpositioning, bleeding, subcutaneous emphysema, and pneumothorax. The most significant late complications are glottic and tracheal stenosis and stomal infection. A rare but deadly late complication is tracheal-innominate fistula.[90] Whether this complication is related to any specific technique or anatomic variants (e.g., tracheostomy performed too low, cannula not appropriately chosen, variant blood vessel anatomy) must be determined, as well as the possible contribution of ultrasound to reduce the incidence.

> **Box 30-2** Complications of Percutaneous Dilational Tracheostomy
>
> **Intraoperative Complications**
>
> Hemorrhage
> Loss of airway or premature extubation
> Pneumothorax
> Tracheal-esophageal fistula or posterior tracheal wall injury
> Hypoxia and ventilation problems
> Hypotension
> Cardiopulmonary arrest
> Recurrent laryngeal nerve injury
>
> **Postoperative Complications**
>
> *Early*
> Hemorrhage
> Stomal infection
> Pneumothorax and subcutaneous emphysema
> Tube obstruction
> *Late*
> Displaced tracheostomy tube or unplanned decannulation
> Granuloma
> Subglottic stenosis
> Stomal infection or infection of lower respiratory tract
> Tracheocutaneous fistula

However, because the incidence of this complication is low, a very large number of observations would be required to evaluate the value of an intervention to decrease it.

The differences between techniques used, operators' experience, patient selection criteria, and indications and timing of the procedures make it difficult to perform an accurate comparison of the data available from the literature on the overall safety of PDT with that for standard open tracheostomy. However, there seems to be a significant amount of evidence to support that PDT has a lower incidence of peristomal bleeding and wound infection compared with open tracheostomy.[73-76,88] For these reasons, it has been advocated that PDT should be considered the procedure of choice for performing elective tracheostomy in critically ill patients.[74,88] The decreased incidence of bleeding may be related to the lack of sharp dissection and the tamponade effect of the dilator. The much smaller wound created with the PDT technique reduces the surface area available for bacterial colonization and may explain the low rate of wound infection. Late outcome studies evaluating serious long-term complications associated with PDT indicate that the incidence of clinically significant tracheomalacia or stenosis requiring corrective intervention is low.[116]

After decannulation, 16 patients were evaluated by means of physical examination, standardized interviews, and fiberoptic laryngotracheoscopy. The subjective rating was good for all patients. Laryngotracheoscopy showed incidental tracheal changes in two patients consisting of soft tissue swelling and a membranous scar, respectively. Neither of these findings required treatment.[117] Histologic studies were conducted on 21 laryngotracheal specimens from patients who had undergone PDT or standard open tracheostomy. In the percutaneous group, cartilage fractures associated with a strong inflammatory response were found in one third of cases, compared with a more limited inflammatory response in the standard group. There was no clinical evidence of laryngotracheal stenosis in either group.

Carrer and associates, in a prospective observational study of 181 ICU patients receiving PDT over a 6-year period, reported a 0.7% rate of tracheal stenosis requiring tracheal stent placement and a 1.4% rate of recurrent granuloma of the stoma that was treated with laser resection. Late decannulation seemed the major risk factor for these infrequent but clinically significant late complications.[107]

2. Practical Applications of Cricothyrotomy

The superiority of the percutaneous technique over the surgical technique has turned attention toward the different cricothyrotomy kits available and their applications, success rates, and complications. An over-the-needle, wire-guided dilation technique is safer and adaptable to various practitioners (with different training time and specialties) and is still relatively fast. Over-the-needle techniques that do not use a guidewire, even if often reported to be faster and easier, can result in higher complication rates.

Another important issue is establishing indications based on patients' injuries and habitus and on clinical scenarios.[118,119] Percutaneous techniques are increasingly used in the prehospital setting and for major facial injuries, neck abnormalities, or challenging anatomy. Many patients can be assisted or ventilated with a bag-valve-mask if definitive cricothyrotomy is performed, and they can be jet ventilated or ventilated mechanically if a needle cannula has been placed.

Cricothyrotomy is an important tool for managing the impossible airway or the threatened airway, and it often is the last and only way to avoid anoxia. In the previous edition of this textbook, a simplified protocol was proposed for prehospital emergency trauma airway control (Fig. 30-22). The protocol can be expanded by including an in-hospital approach (see Fig. 30-23 and the Difficult Airway Society's "cannot ventilate, cannot intubate" scenario (http://www.das.uk.com/guidelines/cvci.html) or the ASA algorithm.[49] Both scenarios converge on an emergency pathway, in which the option of awake airway control or awakening the patient is not possible. In this emergency pathway, as interpreted by a modified ASA difficult airway algorithm (Fig. 30-24), cricothyrotomy performed surgically or percutaneously plays a fundamental role.

When dealing with difficult airways, planning includes ventilation and intubation. Regardless of the techniques and devices that may offer assistance with bag-mask ventilation or intubation, if one or the other fails, a supraglottic device is the first alternative to further attempts to intubate and bag-mask ventilate, and the last is an invasive airway approach (i.e., cricothyrotomy).

In the past few years, many changes in airway management occurred as a result of better airway equipment availability and implementation of airway protocols. As observed by Timmerman and colleagues and Combes and associates, cricothyrotomy is rare, even in emergency

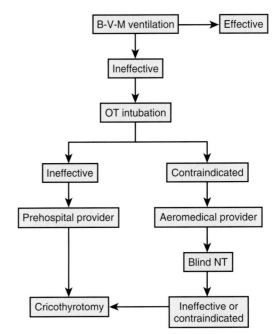

Figure 30-22 Emergency airway protocol for prehospital care. *B-V-M,* Bag-valve-mask; *NT,* nasotracheal; *OT,* orotracheal.

airway conditions, if an airway protocol is used (assuming no major neck trauma).[120,121] However, a careful reading of the literature shows a significant number of complications that may question the underuse of more invasive techniques and argue for the earlier use of these techniques, depending on the level of training, the setting, and clinical conditions. Appropriate training is fundamental to maintain proficiency in the technical skills required to perform these invasive procedures safely, rapidly, and effectively.

VIII. TRAINING MODELS

Because PDC is rarely performed, there is a need for quality teaching and training aids.[25,122] Although the technique closely mimics over-the-wire vascular insertion methods, it is sufficiently different that anesthesiologists ideally should practice on a regular basis.[27,57] Simple and inexpensive models can be made for training residents and inexperienced personnel, as well as maintaining the skills and proficiency of the trainees and experts.

Of the available animal models, dogs appear to be most similar to humans. The canine CTM, muscles, and cricothyroid area are similar to those in humans. The tracheal dimensions of the 25-kg dog are comparable to those of the adult human.[2] Cricothyrotomy has been performed on other animals, including pigs, sheep, and goats. The larynx is significantly smaller in these animal models, and 3.5- or 4.0-mm-ID sets must be used for teaching. In pigs, attempts to pass a needle or over-the-needle catheter into the cricothyroid space may result in hitting cartilage. The space can be entered only by directing the needle cephalad, not caudad. Dissection of the larynx revealed a projection on the inferior surface of the thyroid cartilage that articulated with the cricoid

Failed intubation, increasing hypoxemia and difficult
ventilation in the paralyzed anesthetised patient:
Rescue techniques for the "can't intubate, can't ventilate" situation

Failed intubation and difficult ventilation (other than laryngospasm)

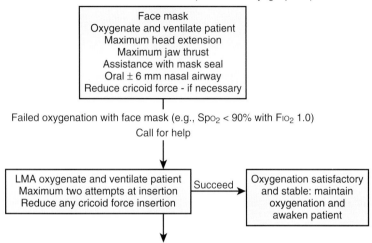

Figure 30-23 The Difficult Airway Society cannot intubate algorithm. (Courtesy of the Difficult Airway Society, London, United Kingdom.)

cartilage. This cornu had been previously described and had to be removed to perform cricothyrotomy studies.[101] The pig trachea model (professionally isolated and prepared) is used for airway training and is combined with manikin simulations for the education of residents and faculty in surgical and percutaneous cricothyrotomy in teaching institutions, workshops, and airway management courses (e.g., Society for Airway Management, Difficult Airway Workshop, American Society of Anesthesiologists Annual Meeting).

Fresh and embalmed cadaver specimens can be used.[67,123-125] The former are superior because the laryngeal structures of embalmed specimens are somewhat constricted because of muscle contraction, and it may be more difficult to discern the cricothyroid space. Mannequins can also be an acceptable model, and several products are available, but cheaper and simple models can also

be used for skill maintenance and simulation.[126] Simulation and practice-workshops are used in teaching programs or as part of dedicated airway management courses or meetings.[56,127-129]

IX. MISCELLANEOUS CONSIDERATIONS

A. Cuff Pressure

Tracheostomy tube cuffs are used to create a seal against the tracheal mucosa, thereby minimizing aspiration, and to facilitate positive-pressure ventilation by preventing leakage of air. Tracheal stenosis from low-volume, high-pressure, low-compliance cuffs was a major complication of tracheostomy during the 1960s. These cuffs may exert pressures as high as 180 to 250 mm Hg on the tracheal mucosa, far in excess of the normal capillary perfusion

1. One attempt for each.
2. Supraglottic method, laryngoscopy, or cricothyrotomy, either surgical or percutaneous.

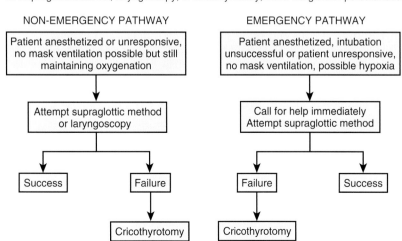

Figure 30-24 Modified American Society of Anesthesiologists cricothyrotomy airway algorithm. (Modified from the American Society of Anesthesiologists, Park Ridge, IL.)

pressures of 20 to 30 mm Hg. The result is a time-related, progressive ischemic injury ranging from inflammatory changes to chondronecrosis and tracheal stenosis or tracheomalacia. With the accumulated evidence attesting to the deleterious effects of low-volume, high-pressure cuffs, there has been a gradual shift in the past 3 decades toward the use of high-volume, low-pressure cuffs because they are safer.

The transition in the 1970s to high-volume, low-pressure cuffs decreased the incidence of cuff-related tracheal stenosis by 10-fold because of the ability of the cuff to seal the airway at pressures below the mucosal capillary perfusion pressure. These cuffs inflate symmetrically, adapt to the tracheal contour, and allow pressure distribution over a wide area. The risk of overinflation with resultant high intracuff pressures may be minimized by the following:

- Having a pressure-controlled cuff with a pressure pop-off valve, which prevents inflation beyond 20 mm Hg (although less than 20 mm Hg has been associated with increased risk of leakage of bacterial pathogens around the cuff into the lower respiratory tract)[130]
- Regular measurement of intracuff pressure with a manometer attached to a three- or four-way stopcock (the latter gives more accurate results)
- Cuff deflation for as long as safely possible in patients who do not require mechanical ventilation

B. Infections

1. Risk Factors

a. DISRUPTION OF HOST DEFENSES

Performing a tracheostomy requires a skin incision, thereby disrupting this highly effective natural barrier to infection. The resultant open surgical wound provides a wide surface area for colonization, which may occur from surrounding skin, preexisting infected pulmonary secretions, aspiration of oropharyngeal secretions, or instrumentation or handling of the tracheostomy tube.

The nose, paranasal sinuses, and pharynx, where filtration and humidification and local leukocyte antibacterial activity occur under normal circumstances, are all bypassed in the patient with a tracheostomy. Impaired vocal fold adduction in patients with tracheostomies and the presence of the tube prevent generation of an effective cough. Oropharyngeal secretions, often colonized with potentially pathogenic gram-negative organisms, are ineffectively cleared or swallowed, allowing some degree of aspiration and contamination of the tracheobronchial tree.

b. TRACHEOSTOMY TUBES

Most tracheostomy tubes, ETTs, and cuffs are made of polyvinyl chloride, a plastic to which bacteria readily adhere. Clumps of rod-shaped and coccoid bacteria have been identified on the surface of ETTs and, by extension, tracheostomy tubes. Cultures of this material have grown a variety of gram-negative and gram-positive bacteria, including *Pseudomonas aeruginosa*, *Proteus mirabilis*, *Staphylococcus aureus*, and *Staphylococcus epidermidis*.

These bacterial clumps may reach the tracheobronchial tree and lungs through detachment and aspiration or be dislodged during suction or bronchoscopy. Tracheostomy tubes that are made of polyvinyl chloride may serve as reservoirs for persistent contamination of the tracheobronchial tree.

2. Infection Sites

a. STOMAL INFECTION

Colonization of the surgical wound after tracheostomy occurs within 24 to 48 hours with primarily gram-negative organisms, including *Klebsiella*, *P. aeruginosa*, *Escherichia coli*, and occasionally *S. aureus*.[7,131] Wound edges may demonstrate mild erythema, and yellow or green secretions from the area may be copious, particularly in the first 7 to 10 days. These findings are more marked after standard open tracheostomy than PDT, probably because of the very small incision and tight tract in the latter procedure. Frequent and meticulous wound care with mechanical débridement, if necessary, is the best way to deal with this situation. Progressive cellulitis, despite aggressive local care, indicates infection, usually polymicrobial, and warrants systemic antibiotics. Rarely, necrotizing stomal infections may occur, with substantial loss of soft tissue down to and including the tracheal wall. This may create difficulties in maintaining adequate mechanical ventilation. Progression of the process may result in carotid artery exposure, with its attendant risks. Management involves replacing the tracheostomy tube with an ETT and aggressive wound débridement and cleaning with antiseptic dressings. Rarely, local flaps may be necessary to provide soft tissue coverage for vital structures.

b. TRACHEOSTOMY TUBES

Colonization of the wound, along with mechanical irritation from the tube, cuff, and tube tip, means that there is always some degree of localized, reversible tracheitis, which often manifests by increased secretions. Progression of this situation may lead to loss of tracheal support, resulting in tracheal stenosis or tracheomalacia. Full-thickness loss may result in life-threatening complications such as tracheal-esophageal or tracheal-innominate fistula. Selecting appropriate tube sizes, materials, and cuffs can minimize mechanical irritation. The cuff should be inflated only when necessary.

The known bacterial colonization of polyvinyl chloride devices makes a strong argument in favor of more frequent tube changes, perhaps weekly, in ventilator-dependent, critically ill patients.

c. HOSPITAL-ACQUIRED AND VENTILATOR-ASSOCIATED PNEUMONIA

Hospital-acquired pneumonia (HAP) accounts for up to 25% of all ICU infections and for more than 50% of the antibiotics prescribed.[132] Ventilator-associated pneumonia (VAP) occurs in 9% to 27% of all intubated patients.[133,134] In ICU patients, almost 90% of HAP episodes occur during mechanical ventilation. In mechanically ventilated patients, the incidence increases with duration of ventilation.[130] Important risk factors for HAP include exposure to invasive respiratory devices and aspiration of oropharyngeal pathogens or leakage of secretions containing bacteria around the ETT.[130]

Newly developed taper-shaped cuffs and suction above the cuff systems (Mallinckrodt TaperGuard Evac tube and Portex SACETT) seem to significantly reduce microaspiration compared with the Hi-Lo cuffs, reducing the incidence of VAP. The introduction of similar improvements for tracheostomy tubes may contribute to a reduction in the incidence of VAP in long-term mechanically ventilated patients.

d. CLEANING AND SUCTIONING

Under normal circumstances, the nose efficiently warms, humidifies, and filters inspired air; in the patient with a tracheostomy, these functions must be restored artificially. Dehydration of the respiratory tract results in impaired mucociliary function, causing inspissated secretions and atelectasis.[135] Providing adequate humidification is essential for all patients. Suctioning of secretions to maintain pulmonary toilet and patency of the tracheostomy tube constitutes an integral component of the care of the tracheostomy patient receiving mechanical ventilation and should be carried out according to the patient's needs.

Hypoxia, cardiac dysrhythmia, injury to the tracheobronchial tree, atelectasis, and infection have been associated with suctioning. These events can be minimized by close attention to technical details. Factors that may contribute to hypoxia include suctioning of oxygen-rich air for too long and the use of inappropriately large catheters. This can be prevented by applying suction for less than 2 seconds with a catheter less than one half of the size of the tracheostomy tube and ventilating the patient with 100% oxygen for at least 5 breaths before and after suctioning. A strictly aseptic technique using disposable catheters is mandatory to reduce the risk of cross-contamination.

Meticulous care of the tracheostomy tube and peristomal area is important for maintaining a patent airway and preventing infection and breakdown of the skin. Placement of a tracheostomy tube with an inner cannula is mandatory. This cannula should be removed and cleared several times daily in the early postoperative period. Complete occlusion of the lumen with blood, crusts, and secretions may occur, resulting in hypoxia or death; in this circumstance, rapid removal of the inner cannula is potentially life-saving.

Bacterial colonization of the peristomal area occurs and cannot be prevented with antibiotics. The wound should be cleaned of accumulated secretions and crusts with hydrogen peroxide to prevent breakdown of the skin and progression from wound colonization to infection. The skin under the tracheostomy neck plate should be kept dry with a thin, nonadherent dressing. Petroleum-based products should be avoided on open wounds because they may stimulate granulation tissue and result in myospherulosis.

e. SWALLOWING AND COMMUNICATION

In patients with tracheostomies in place who require mechanical ventilation, the incidence of swallowing dysfunction approaches 80%.[136,137] The cause in most cases is multifactorial and may include the following:

- Glottic injury from previous orotracheal or nasotracheal intubation, or both
- Limitation of normal laryngeal excursion by the tethering effect of the tracheostomy tube
- Compression of the esophagus, particularly in the presence of an inflated cuff
- Desensitization of the larynx and loss of protective reflexes related to chronic diversion of air through the tube
- Impaired vocal fold adduction
- The use of anxiolytics or neuromuscular blocking agents, or both
- Altered mental status or underlying neuromuscular illness

For patients on ventilators with minimal swallowing abnormalities and negligible aspiration, oral feedings may be possible, particularly with the help of the speech-language pathologist. Selection of appropriate food consistencies and emphasis on specific head positions may minimize or prevent aspiration. With mild or moderate aspiration, eligible patients on or off the ventilator may benefit from the use of a Passy-Muir valve. This device may reduce aspiration and improve deglutition by restoring subglottic air pressure.

Unfortunately, for most ventilator-dependent patients with a tracheostomy, the degree of swallowing dysfunction is such that oral intake is not an option. In these cases, enteral feeding is preferred when the gastrointestinal tract can be used safely. It is convenient, there are fewer metabolic and infectious complications, and the cost is lower than that of parenteral nutrition.

Placement of a cuffed, nonfenestrated tracheostomy tube necessarily results in aphonia. Every effort should be made to reestablish effective communication. Involving the speech-language pathologist and adequately assessing the patient's cognitive and linguistic skills are essential. Before establishing the best form of communication, the speech-language pathologist may seek the assistance of an otolaryngologist in confirming that the upper airway is patent and physiologically intact. When clinically possible, cuffed tracheostomy tubes may be exchanged for cuffless or fenestrated tubes, allowing speech by manual occlusion of the tube on expiration or by placement of a device, such as a Passy-Muir valve. This valve may also assist the patient in coughing and swallowing. Successful implementation of communication strategies or devices depends on detailed instruction, encouragement, and support by the speech-language pathologist of the nursing staff, patient, and family.

X. CONCLUSIONS

In the 1970s, after a 50-year hiatus, cricothyrotomy became recognized as an important procedure for emergency airway management. Despite considerable evidence that cricothyrotomy can be life-saving and has an acceptable low complication rate, controlled trials comparing various techniques have not been and are unlikely to be performed. This is largely the result of the infrequency with which physicians and other health care providers encounter patients requiring emergency cricothyrotomy. The lack of opportunity to perform cricothyrotomy or other emergency airway procedures is a problem for anesthesiologists, who are the recognized airway experts. Although the opportunity to perform a cricothyrotomy is rare, it must be performed expeditiously and correctly when required. We think that PDC should be easy for anesthesiologists to learn because it is similar to the Seldinger technique for insertion of catheters and sheaths, a technique used on a daily basis. The anesthesiologist should be well trained in emergency airway techniques and have appropriate equipment available at all times.

Although anesthesiologists practice primarily in the operating room, they are likely to be called on to perform emergency airway procedures in other settings. They are often asked by colleagues to lecture on difficult airways and emergency airways.

PDT is a safe and technically simple alternative to open surgical tracheostomy. It may be performed independently of operating room schedules and eliminates the need to move critically ill patients from one location to another, with all the associated risks. The simplicity of the procedure, however, does not alter the need for proper preoperative planning, meticulous preparation and execution of the procedure, and appropriate postoperative care.

XI. CLINICAL PEARLS

- Clinicians should quickly recognize a severe airway obstruction and a hypoxic condition to allow fast intervention.

- Proper airway anatomy recognition, even with an ultrasound-assisted evaluation, is the first step in successful management and avoidance of complications.

- The anesthesiologist should always consider the danger of piercing the posterior wall of the trachea and midline neck blood vessels.

- Cricothyrotomy is the technique of choice to secure the airway in emergencies and pending airway obstruction.

- Percutaneous dilational tracheostomy (PDT) is better performed under direct visualization (e.g., flexible fiberoptic bronchoscopy) below first tracheal ring.

- Training should be maintained by performing at least one procedure twice each year on live models and specialized mannequins.

- Percutaneous dilational techniques do not prevent complications. Disasters can be prevented by proper knowledge, preparation, anatomic identification, procedural indications, and skill acquisition and maintenance.

SELECTED REFERENCES

All references can be found online at expertconsult.com.

8. Corke C, Cranswick P: A Seldinger technique for minitracheostomy insertion. *Anaesth Intensive Care* 16:206–207, 1988.
11. Al-Ansari MA, Hijazi MH: Clinical review: Percutaneous dilational tracheostomy. *Crit Care* 10:202, 2006.
14. Caplan RA, Posner KL, Ward RJ, Cheney FW: Adverse respiratory events in anesthesia: A closed claims analysis. *Anesthesiology* 72:828–833, 1990.
16. Cook TM, Scott S, Mihai R: Litigation related to airway and respiratory complications of anaesthesia: An analysis of claims against the NHS in England 1995–2007. *Anaesthesia* 65:556–563, 2010.
18. Benumof JL: Management of the difficult airway: With special emphasis on the awake tracheal intubation. *Anesthesiology* 75:1087–1110, 1991.
20. Cole RR, Aguilar EA: Cricothyroidotomy versus tracheostomy: An otolaryngologist's perspective. *Laryngoscope* 98:131–135, 1988.
26. Berkow LC, Greenberg RS, Kan KH, et al: Need for emergency surgical airway reduced by a comprehensive difficult airway program. *Anesth Analg* 109:1860–1869, 2009.
36. Ciaglia P, Firsching R, Syniec C: Elective percutaneous dilatational tracheostomy: A new simple bedside procedure. Preliminary report. *Chest* 87:715–719, 1985.
91. Ben Nun A, Altman E, Best LA: Extended indications for percutaneous tracheostomy. *Ann Thorac Surg* 80:1276–1279, 2005.
123. Latif R, Chhabra N, Ziegler C, et al: Teaching the surgical airway using fresh cadavers and confirming placement nonsurgically. *J Clin Anesth* 22:598–602, 2010.

Chapter 31

Surgical Airway

MICHAEL A. GIBBS | NATHAN W. MICK

I. INTRODUCTION

A. General Principles

Emergency surgical airway management comprises four distinct but related techniques that gain access to the infraglottic airway. These are needle cricothyrotomy, percutaneous cricothyrotomy, surgical cricothyrotomy, and surgical tracheostomy. In emergency situations, cricothyrotomy is greatly preferred over tracheostomy because of its relative simplicity, speed, and lower complication rate. The airway is very superficial at the level of the cricothyroid membrane (CTM), separated from the skin only by the subcutaneous fat and anterior cervical fascia. The trachea moves progressively deeper in the neck as it travels caudally, making anterior access more difficult and introducing additional anatomic barriers (e.g., thyroid isthmus.) Needle cricothyrotomy with percutaneous transtracheal ventilation may provide temporary oxygenation in some patients, but the technique does not provide a secure (protected) airway and cannot support ventilation. Needle cricothyrotomy is reviewed elsewhere in this textbook (see Chapter 30). The emphasis in this chapter is on surgical and percutaneous cricothyrotomy; because the former, and in some cases the latter, places a cuffed endotracheal tube (ETT) in the trachea.

Any discussion of surgical airway management techniques must account for three important concepts:

1. Those Responsible for Surgical Airway Management Have Limited or No Experience

Most clinicians who are responsible for airway management have either limited or no experience with these procedures. Whether in the prehospital setting, the emergency department, the operating room, the inpatient unit, or the intensive care unit, surgical airway management is simply not required very often, largely because of high proficiency with direct laryngoscopy, increasing capability of identifying difficult airways (DAs) in advance, and the multitude of sophisticated alternative intubation devices that can be used when direct laryngoscopy is not possible or unsuccessful. The progressive diminution in use of emergency surgical airway procedures over the past two decades has many causes but is primarily the result of two evolutionary changes: (1) the shift in emphasis in trauma airway management from avoidance of oral laryngoscopy to widespread acceptance of gentle, controlled, oral laryngoscopy with in-line cervical spine immobilization and (2) the growing proficiency of clinicians from multiple specialties with rapid-sequence intubation (RSI).

Contemporary emergency department studies using RSI demonstrate high success rates (97% to 99%) and an infrequent need for surgical airway rescue (0.5% to 2.0%) even though the unselected nature of the patients and the large percentage with trauma result in a high proportion of DAs compared with those seen in elective surgery.[1-5] Despite increasing familiarity with alternative airway rescue devices (e.g., flexible and semirigid fiberoptic bronchoscopy, video laryngoscopy, retroglottic airways, supraglottic airways, retrograde intubation, lighted stylet) that further reduce the need for cricothyrotomy, the surgical airway remains the final pathway on all failed airway algorithms.[6] Therein lies the dilemma. As clinicians embrace new technologies and devices that make the need for surgical airway management increasingly rare, acquisition and maintenance of the skills necessary to perform surgical airway management, which in some cases is the only method capable of sustaining a patient's life, become increasingly elusive.

2. Surgical Airway Management Is Often Performed in Unstable Patients

Surgical airway management is infrequently, if ever, performed in stable patients and is often needed in a "cannot-intubate, cannot-ventilate" (CICV) situation, when failure to perform the technique properly and in a timely fashion may prove disastrous. The patient in need of emergency cricothyrotomy is typically one who has a significantly distorted airway anatomy or who has been subjected to multiple failed intubation attempts, or both. The operator is required to establish an airway in the presence of potentially overwhelming difficulty and with very little time.

3. If a Surgical Approach Fails, Few, If Any, Options Remain

Most would consider surgical cricothyrotomy to be the ultimate consideration among a series of airway management options. In addition, a failed surgical cricothyrotomy may result in bleeding, loss of airway integrity, or further airway distortion, making the success of subsequent rescue attempts highly unlikely.

In sum, emergency cricothyrotomy is a rarely performed procedure, done under duress by clinicians who may have limited experience, in patients in whom it is difficult to perform and who are likely to die if it fails. These challenges speak powerfully to those involved in airway management, counseling them to invest the time required to master this crucial technique. Fortunately, although it has been unfairly cloaked in mystique and represented as dramatic and difficult, cricothyrotomy is a relatively straightforward procedure that can be accomplished with a high success rate and a low rate of complications by providers with adequate but not extensive training. This training can be achieved by using various animal models (not whole animals) and through medical simulation.

B. Historical Perspective

The surgical airway as a life-saving procedure has been appreciated for thousands of years. The first depictions of surgical tracheostomy were found on Egyptian tablets dating from 3600 BC.[7] In the second century AD, Galen suggested tracheostomy, utilizing a vertical incision, as an emergency treatment for airway obstruction.[8-10] Vesalius later published the first detailed descriptions of tracheostomy in the 16th century, using a reed to ventilate the lungs. Ironically, his alleged resuscitation of a Spanish nobleman through tracheostomy and ventilation led to condemnation by the Spanish Inquisition and his ultimate death.[11] The first record of a successful tracheostomy performed in the United States was in 1852; the patient later died of airway stenosis, a common complication at that time. A paper from 1886 described a mortality rate of 50% for tracheostomy and a high incidence of stenosis, which accounted for many of the deaths.[12]

Chevalier Jackson published a landmark paper on tracheostomy in 1909, which enumerated principles still relevant today.[13] He described a surgical mortality rate of only 3%, which he attributed to several factors: optimal airway control before surgery, use of local anesthesia rather than sedation, use of a well-designed tube, and meticulous surgical and postoperative care. Jackson achieved international recognition; however, so did his condemnation of "high tracheostomy" as the cause of subglottic stenosis. The high tracheostomy he referred to was a cricothyrotomy, which at that time involved division of the cricoid or thyroid cartilage. Modern cricothyrotomy involves incision of the CTM only. In 1921, Jackson published a study of 200 patients referred to him for postcricothyrotomy stenosis. Aside from the obvious referral bias, the indication for a surgical airway at that time was primarily inflammatory lesions of the upper airway, which probably accounted for the high incidence of subglottic stenosis.[14]

Although in retrospect it was the technique and the underlying condition that were largely responsible for the high rate of stenosis, fear of this complication condemned the technique of cricothyrotomy for over half a century. In the interest of developing a technique that was safer and quicker than Jackson's open dissection, Toye and Weinstein described the first percutaneous tracheostomy in 1969.[15] However, cricothyrotomy was not widely reconsidered as a surgical airway option until 1976, when Brantigan and Grow published the results of cricothyrotomy for long-term airway management in 655 patients.[16] In their series, the rate of stenosis was 0.01%, no major complications were described, and the procedure was found to be faster, simpler, and less likely to cause bleeding than tracheostomy. Subsequent studies have supported their conclusion that cricothyrotomy is a safe and effective surgical airway procedure and should be the preferred technique when emergent surgical airway control is needed.[7,17,18] Contemporary case series have demonstrated that cricothyrotomy can be performed with a high success rate and a reasonably low complication rate by hospital-based physicians and other clinicians (i.e., nurses, paramedics) providing prehospital care.[13,19-25]

C. Definitions of the Surgical Airway

The definition of surgical airway can be so broad as to comprise all forms of airway management that require the creation of a new opening into the airway. *Cricothy-rotomy* is the establishment of a surgical opening in the airway through the CTM and placement of a cuffed tracheostomy tube or ETT. Cricothyrotomy has also been referred to as cricothyroidotomy, cricothyroidostomy, cricothyrostomy, laryngostomy, or laryngotomy; however, *cricothyrotomy* is presently the preferred term. *Tracheostomy* differs from cricothyrotomy in the anatomic location of entry into the airway. Tracheostomy is the establishment of a surgical opening in the airway at any level including at or caudal to the first tracheal ring.

Surgical airways may be further subclassified according to the technique used: (1) surgical (sometimes referred to as "open" or "full open" or "full surgical"); (2) percutaneous (more precisely described by the actual technique, such as Seldinger); (3) dilational (a distinct percutaneous approach); and (4) transtracheal catheter.

The terms *surgical cricothyrotomy* and *surgical tracheostomy* refer to the use of a scalpel and other surgical instruments to create an opening in the airway.[26,27] This technique allows the creation of a definitive, protected airway by the insertion of a cuffed tracheostomy tube with an internal diameter sufficient for ventilation, oxygenation, and suctioning.

The percutaneous dilational technique utilizes a kit or device that is intended to establish a surgical airway without requiring a formal surgical cricothyrotomy (see Chapter 30 for a detailed discussion). Following a small skin incision, the airway is accessed by a small needle through which a flexible guidewire is passed using the Seldinger technique. The airway device is then introduced over a dilator and passed over the guidewire and into the airway in a manner analogous to that of central line placement. An alternative percutaneous technique has been used that relies on placement of an airway device using a direct puncture into the airway; an example is the Nu-Trake Adult Emergency Cricothyroidotomy Device (Smiths Medical, Keene, NH). A large-bore metal needle or a sharp trocar within the catheter is used to puncture the airway directly, without the use of a guidewire. Direct puncture devices are more hazardous and have fallen out of favor because of a higher incidence of complications and a lower success rate compared with other percutaneous techniques.[28-32]

Transtracheal catheter ventilation, considered the least invasive surgical technique, involves the direct placement of a moderate-bore catheter through the CTM.[33] The small caliber of these devices does not allow adequate oxygenation without attachment to a high-pressure oxygen source or jet ventilator, except in small children, and does not support adequate ventilatory gas exchange. A 6-F reinforced fluorinated ethylene propylene, kink-resistant emergency transtracheal airway catheter (Cook Critical Care, Bloomington, IN) has been designed as a kink-resistant catheter for this purpose.

D. Role of the Surgical Airway

The relative merit of percutaneous dilational tracheostomy versus open surgical tracheostomy continues to be a subject of debate. Although formal open tracheostomies are primarily performed by surgeons, the percutaneous dilational tracheostomy is frequently performed by anesthesiologists and other nonsurgical intensivists, particularly in the intensive care setting. This technique was originally described by Toye and Weinstein in 1969, but it did not gain popularity until the results with a modified device were reported by Ciaglia and colleagues in 1985.[12,15] There have been no clinical studies to date demonstrating the superiority of any one approach over another or of any of these devices over formal surgical cricothyrotomy.

II. ANATOMY

An understanding of the anatomy of the upper airway and the neck is required for the successful and rapid performance of a surgical airway. Most emergent surgical techniques involve surgical fields that become rapidly obscured by blood and for this reason they are, essentially, "blind" procedures. The identification of anatomic landmarks is critical.

A. Bones and Cartilages

The horseshoe-shaped hyoid bone is the most cephalad rigid structure in the anterior neck, palpable approximately one finger breadth cephalad to the laryngeal prominence. It suspends the larynx during phonation and respiration by the thyrohyoid membrane and muscle.

The thyroid cartilage is the largest structure of the larynx and consists of two laminae fused in the midline to form the laryngeal prominence. The angle of this fusion is more acute in males, creating the more distinct prominence known as the Adam's apple. The separation of the laminae superiorly forms the palpable superior thyroid notch. The laryngeal prominence of the thyroid cartilage represents the most readily and consistently identified landmark in the neck when one is performing a surgical airway. The superior and inferior cornua of the thyroid cartilage are the posterior extensions of the upper and lower edges of the lamina. The thyrohyoid ligament attaches to the superior cornu, and the posterior cricoid cartilage articulates with the inferior cornu.

The cricoid cartilage, the only complete cartilaginous ring in the upper airway, defines the inferior aspect of the larynx (Fig. 31-1). It is shaped like a signet ring, with the wider lamina posterior. Superiorly, the lamina has synovial articulations with the arytenoids and thyroid cartilage. Anteriorly, the cricoid ring is attached to the inferior thyroid cartilage by the CTM.

B. Cricothyroid Membrane

The CTM is a fibroelastic tissue that covers the cricothyroid space, between the thyroid cartilage and the cricoid ring. It is trapezoidal in shape and in the average adult is 1 cm high and 2 to 3 cm wide. It is located in the midline, approximately 2 to 3 cm below the laryngeal prominence. The vocal cords are located 1 cm above the CTM and therefore are rarely injured during a cricothyrotomy.

Several anatomic characteristics make this membrane an ideal choice for emergency airway access. It is a subcutaneous structure located just beneath the skin, a small

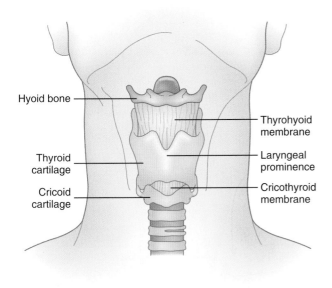

Figure 31-1 Surface anatomy of the larynx. (From Walls RM, Luten RC, Murphy MF, Schneider RE: *Manual of emergency airway management*, ed 2, Philadelphia, 2004, Lippincott Williams & Wilkins.)

Labels on figure: Hyoid bone; Thyroid cartilage; Cricoid cartilage; Thyrohyoid membrane; Laryngeal prominence; Cricothyroid membrane

amount of subcutaneous fat, and the anterior cervical fascia in most patients. Accordingly, it is easily palpated as a depression inferior to the thyroid cartilage, bounded on its inferior aspect by a hard ridge, the cricoid cartilage. The ligament does not calcify with age. It has no overlying muscles, major vessels, or nerves. It is supported by the anterior cervical fascia, which is not robust at this level.

C. Vascular Structures

The major arteries of the neck always lie deep to the pretracheal fascia and should not present a concern when incising the skin over the CTM. The paired superior thyroid arteries arise from the external carotid arteries, superior and lateral to the cricoid cartilage. The anterior branches of these arteries run along the upper thyroid isthmus to anastomose in the midline. The unpaired inferior thyroid artery also anastomoses with the superior thyroid artery at the isthmus. In 10% of the population, the potentially large thyroid ima artery ascends anterior to the trachea to join the anastomoses. A large venous plexus is found over the thyroid isthmus.

The right and left cricothyroid arteries are branches of the right and left superior thyroid arteries, respectively, and in most patients they cross the superior aspect of the CTM to anastomose in the midline.[34] Although they are at risk for injury during a cricothyrotomy, they do not appear to be clinically significant. Bleeding is often self-limited and is easily controlled with gauze packing. There is no venous plexus over the CTM.

D. Thyroid Gland

The isthmus of the thyroid gland lies anterior to the trachea, generally between the second and third tracheal rings, although it may extend to the first and fourth rings. Its size and location can be variable; however, its average height and thickness are 1.25 cm. A pyramidal lobe of the thyroid gland is present in one third of the population and extends superiorly from the isthmus, over the cricoid membrane and larynx to the left of the midline.

E. Anatomic Variations

In infants, the hyoid bone and cricoid cartilage are the most prominent structures in the neck. The laryngeal prominence does not develop until adolescence. The larynx also starts higher in the neck of the child; it descends from the level of the second cervical vertebra at birth to the level of the fifth or sixth in the adult.[35] The laryngeal prominence is more acute and therefore more prominent in adult males compared with females. This also results in longer vocal cords and accounts for the deeper voices of males.

The CTM varies in size among adults and can be as small as 5 mm in height. This space may narrow further with contraction of the cricothyroid muscle.[36] The CTM in the child is disproportionately smaller in area than that in the adult (Fig. 31-2). In an infant, the width of the membrane constitutes only one fourth of the anterior tracheal diameter, as opposed to three fourths in the adult. Because of this smaller area and the difficulty in identifying landmarks in children, emergency surgical cricothyrotomy is difficult and hazardous in small children and is not recommended in those younger than 10 years of age. In this age group, placement of a needle catheter with percutaneous transtracheal ventilation is the preferred method.

Identification of landmarks in the obese, edematous, or traumatized neck can be difficult. The CTM usually lies 1.5 finger breadths (using the patient's fingers) below the laryngeal prominence. Alternatively, its location may be estimated to be three to four finger breadths above the suprasternal notch when the neck is in a neutral position.

There can be significant variation in the arterial and venous pattern in the anterior vessels of the neck, which can result in a major artery's crossing the midline. This is rarely a problem for cricothyrotomy, because most anomalous vessels are present lower in the neck.

III. SURGICAL CRICOTHYROTOMY
A. Indications and Contraindictions

The primary indication for an emergent surgical airway (Box 31-1) is the failure of endotracheal intubation or alternative noninvasive airway techniques in a patient who requires immediate airway control. The American Society of Anesthesiologists (ASA) DA algorithm advocates a surgical airway as the final end point for the unsuccessful arm of the emergency pathway.[37,38] There are a number of other DA algorithms in the literature, as well as numerous modifications of the ASA guidelines; however, all comprehensive pathways include the surgical airway as the technique of choice when others have failed.[38-40] Despite the introduction of numerous

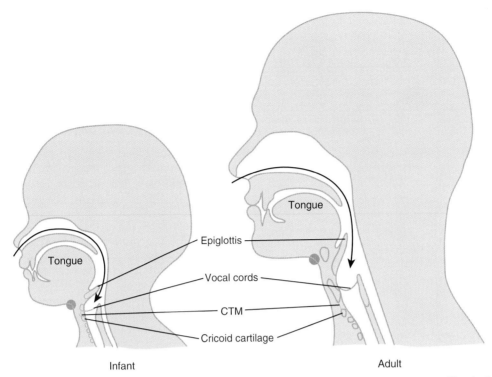

Figure 31-2 Anatomic differences in the pediatric compared with the adult airway: (1) higher, more anterior position for the glottic opening; (2) relatively larger tongue in the infant, which lies between the mouth and glottic opening; (3) relatively larger and more floppy epiglottis in the child; (4) the cricoid ring is the narrowest portion of the pediatric airway (in the adult, the narrowest portion is the vocal cords); (5) different position and size of the cricothyroid membrane *(CTM)* in the infant; (6) sharper, more difficult angle for nasotracheal intubation; (7) larger relative size of the occiput in the infant. See text for details. (From Walls RM, Luten RC, Murphy MF, Schneider RE: *Manual of emergency airway management,* ed 2, Philadelphia, 2004, Lippincott Williams & Wilkins.)

alternative rescue devices, the most common error in the management of the DA is persistent attempts at laryngoscopy in a failed airway situation.[41-43] This behavior has been associated with increased morbidity and mortality.[41] Identification of the CICV scenario should result in immediate consideration of surgical airway access. If alternative methods are tried despite inability to oxygenate and ventilate the patient by bag and mask, precious time may be lost in what are ultimately futile attempts, and by the time cricothyrotomy is undertaken and

accomplished, delays in achieving airway control and oxygenation will have led to hypoxic brain injury.

In most circumstances, cricothyrotomy is regarded as an emergency rescue technique when other noninvasive rescue techniques, such as the laryngeal mask airway, have failed, are predicted to fail, or are unavailable.[1] There are occasions, however, when a cricothyrotomy is the primary airway of choice. An example is the patient who has such severe facial trauma that nasal or oral approaches to the airway are deemed impossible. There also has been a renewed interest in the role of elective cricothyrotomy in the operative setting. Some cardiothoracic surgeons prefer cricothyrotomy to a tracheostomy in their patients with a median sternotomy, believing that the higher location of the airway wound reduces the potential for contamination of the sternal wound.[11] A study described the use of elective cricothyrotomy instead of tracheostomy in the intensive care unit for trauma patients with technically challenging neck anatomy. The procedure was described as simpler with no difference in short- or long-term complications.[44]

Cricothyrotomy is considered safe in trauma patients with unstable cervical spine injuries provided that cervical spine immobilization is maintained.[45,46] Although coagulopathy has been described as a relative contraindication, there are reports of successful cricothyrotomy after systemic fibrinolytic therapy for acute myocardial infarction.[47]

Often, the main hurdle to performing cricothyrotomy is simply making the initial decision to forego further

---

Box 31-1   Indications for Cricothyrotomy

Inability to Secure the Airway Using a Less Invasive Technique

1. Massive upper airway hemorrhage
2. Massive regurgitation
3. Maxillofacial trauma
4. Structural abnormalities of the airway (congenital or acquired)

Airway Obstruction

1. Traumatic
   a. Airway edema (includes thermal/inhalation injury)
   b. Foreign body
   c. Airway stenosis or disruption
2. Nontraumatic
   a. Airway edema
   b. Mass effect (e.g., tumor, hematoma, abscess)
   c. Upper airway infection (supraglottitis)

attempts at laryngoscopy or with other rescue devices and to proceed with a surgical airway. Noninvasive airway management methods are used so successfully that cricothyrotomy is often viewed as a procedure that will never be required. However, the single-minded pursuit of multiple noninvasive airways with resultant delay in the initiation of a surgical airway can result in hypoxic disaster, particularly if the patient is not able to be oxygenated and ventilated adequately with a bag and mask between attempts.

The decision to proceed to a surgical airway must also take into account some other important variables. The airway provider must appreciate whether the surgical airway will bypass the airway problem anatomically. For example, if the obstructing lesion is infraglottic, performing a cricothyrotomy may be a critical waste of time. The patient's anatomy and pathology must be considered when weighing the difficulty of performing a cricothyrotomy. Placement of the initial skin incision is based on palpation of the pertinent anatomy. Adiposity, burns, trauma, or infection may make palpation difficult; they do not represent absolute contraindications, but the strategy may need to be adjusted. The operator must also consider the type of invasive technique (i.e., open surgical or percutaneous). This consideration takes into account provider preference based on experience, the patient's presentation, and equipment availability.

Contraindications for surgical airway management are few and, with one exception, are relative. That one exception is young age. Children have a small, pliable, mobile larynx and cricoid cartilage, making cricothyrotomy extremely difficult. For children younger than 10 years, unless the larynx and cricoid cartilage are teenage or adult sized, percutaneous transtracheal ventilation should be used as the surgical airway management technique of choice. Two other situations have been proposed as absolute contraindications: tracheal transection and laryngeal fracture.[48] In either situation, tracheostomy has been recommended as the preferred method. Although anatomically and philosophically appealing, this assertion is clinically impractical. First, these injuries may not be readily apparent at the bedside. Second, there may be no other means of securing the airway in a dying patient. Third, expert surgical backup may not be readily available, and tracheostomy is a much more complicated procedure than cricothyrotomy. Therefore, these, too, should be considered relative contraindications; cricothyrotomy should be recognized as carrying significant risk in these situations and used when there is thought to be no other method to secure the airway. Relative contraindications also include preexisting laryngeal or tracheal pathology such as tumor, infections, or abscess in the area in which the procedure will be performed; hematoma or other anatomic destruction of the landmarks that would render the procedure difficult or impossible; coagulopathy; and lack of operator expertise.

The presence of an anatomic barrier in particular should prompt consideration of alternative techniques that might result in a successful airway. However, in cases in which no alternative method of airway management is likely to be successful or timely enough,

cricothyrotomy should be performed without hesitation. The same principles apply for both the cricothyrotomy and percutaneous transtracheal ventilation. Percutaneous transtracheal ventilation is the surgical airway method of choice for children younger than 10 years of age. The cricothyrotomes have not been demonstrated to improve success rates or time or to decrease complication rates when compared with surgical cricothyrotomy. As with formal cricothyrotomy, experience, skill, knowledge of anatomy, and adherence to proper technique are essential for success when a cricothyrotome is used. The large size and cutting characteristics of the insertion part of the cricothyrotome are likely to cause more damage in the neck than either an open cricothyrotomy or a Seldinger-based technique.

B. Procedure

1. Equipment

Tracheostomy tubes are made in a variety of designs and materials.[15] They may have a single lumen, but many have an inner cannula that can easily be removed to allow routine cleaning and prevention of mucous obstruction. Most tubes also come with a blunt-tipped obturator that is used to facilitate insertion and reduce trauma. The tubes may be rigid or flexible and kink resistant, and they may have variable curves, angles, and sizes, depending on the anatomic needs of the patient. Tracheostomy tubes are secured with twill or with a padded fastener that goes around the neck and attaches to the neck plate of the tube. Tubes may be cuffed or uncuffed. Cuffs should be kept at inflation pressures of 20 to 25 mm Hg, but over the short term, inflation can be judged by palpation of the reservoir balloon.[49] Underinflation can increase aspiration, whereas high cuff pressures can cause mucosal ischemia and subsequent tracheal stenosis or tissue necrosis.

It is critical that whatever surgical technique is chosen, the instrument and its location are familiar to the airway providers. The kit needs to be easily accessible, compact, and ideally located in a DA cart that is positioned in the room or otherwise readily accessible (Fig. 31-3). The operating room tracheostomy surgical trays are not appropriate for this purpose because of their size and complexity. It is recommended that a custom

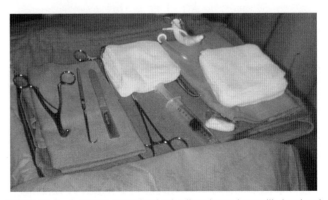

Figure 31-3 A simply organized cricothyrotomy tray with tracheal hook, Trousseau dilator, scalpel, and tracheostomy tube. (Photograph courtesy of R. M. Walls, Boston, MA)

cricothyrotomy kit be assembled with the components listed in Box 31-2 or that a commercial kit designed for this purpose be utilized. A commercial kit has become available that offers both the Seldinger technique and the necessary instruments for a surgical cricothyrotomy with a cuffed tracheostomy tube all in one system (Fig. 31-4).

2. Landmarks

The CTM is the anatomic site of access in the emergent surgical airway, regardless of the technique used. The CTM is identified by first locating the laryngeal prominence of the thyroid cartilage. This may be easier to appreciate in males because of their more prominent thyroid notch. Approximately 1 to 1.5 patient finger breadths below the laryngeal prominence, the membrane may be palpated in the midline of the anterior neck as a soft depression between the inferior aspect of the thyroid cartilage above and the rigid cricoid ring below. The thyrohyoid space, which lies superior to the laryngeal prominence and inferior to the hyoid bone, should also be identified. This space should be distinguished from the CTM to avoid misplacement of the tracheostomy tube above the vocal cords. In children, the CTM is disproportionately smaller because of a greater overlap of the thyroid cartilage over the cricoid cartilage. For this reason,

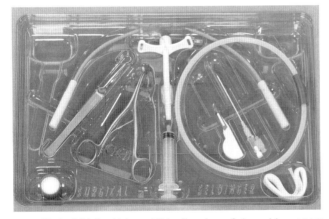

Figure 31-4 A Melker Universal Cricothyrotomy Set combines capability for a percutaneous, Seldinger-based cricothyrotomy *(right side)* with a simple instrument set for a full surgical cricothyrotomy *(left side)*. The same cuffed tracheostomy tube is used for either technique, but a blunt introducing cannula is substituted when surgical insertion is desired. (Photograph courtesy of Cook Critical Care, Bloomington, IN. Copyright by Cook Critical Care.)

cricothyrotomy is not recommended in children younger than 10 years of age.

The same anatomic or physiologic abnormalities (i.e., trauma, morbid obesity, congenital anomalies) that precipitated the surgical airway may also hinder easy palpation of landmarks. The location of the CTM can be estimated by placing four fingers on the neck, vertically, with the small finger in the sternal notch. The membrane is approximately located under the index finger, and this can serve as a point at which the initial incision is made. A vertical skin incision is preferred in the emergent situation because of the location of major blood vessels as well as ease in locating the membrane. Palpation through the vertical incision can then confirm the location. Identification may be assisted by using a locator needle attached to a syringe containing saline or lidocaine. Aspiration of air bubbles suggests entry into the airway, but this does not distinguish between the CTM and an intertracheal space.

Although palpation of the CTM is easily performed on most patients, the particular condition creating the airway difficulty may obscure traditional landmarks. The urgency and anxiety associated with a failed airway may further compound this difficulty. Therefore, it is the practice of some anesthesiologists to mark the skin overlying the approximate location of the CTM before the procedure begins if a possible DA is anticipated. Routinely palpating the CTM on patients is also recommended to become familiar with the landmarks.

C. Surgical Cricothyrotomy Techniques

1. Traditional Surgical Cricothyrotomy: The "No-Drop" Technique

a. PREPARATION OF THE NECK

Appropriate antiseptic solution should be applied and sterile technique observed as much as possible. The procedure should not be delayed if time does not allow ideal preparation. Suction, a bag-valve-mask, and oxygen should be immediately available. The tracheostomy tube should be opened and prepared for insertion at this time. There may be circumstances (e.g., conscious patient) in which it is desirable to infiltrate the skin and subcutaneous tissues with 1% lidocaine. The operator may wish to localize the membrane at this time using a 20-G needle. On aspiration of air into syringe, lidocaine can be injected into the airway. The injection precipitates a cough in the patient with intact airway reflexes; however, this serves to disperse the lidocaine and diminish further stimulation in the conscious patient. Caution is advised in patients with potentially unstable cervical spine injuries.

b. LANDMARK IDENTIFICATION

An emergent cricothyrotomy is best thought of as a procedure that is done by touch rather than by visualization. The identification of the external landmarks before initiating the incision and the use of a method to maintain knowledge of the anatomic relationships (see later discussion) are keys to success. The operator should be positioned on the same side of the patient as the operator's dominant hand (i.e., the hand that will be used to make

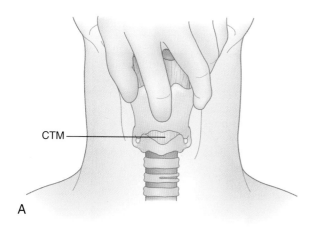

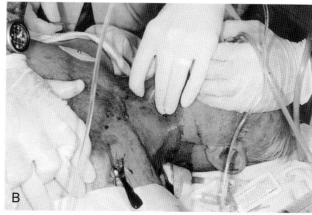

Figure 31-5   A and **B,** With the superior cornua of the larynx firmly immobilized by the thumb and long finger of the nondominant hand, the index finger is free to palpate and locate the cricothyroid membrane *(CTM)*. (**A** adapted from and **B** from Walls RM, Luten RC, Murphy MF, Schneider RE: *Manual of emergency airway management,* ed 2, Philadelphia, 2004, Lippincott Williams & Wilkins.)

the incisions); for example, a right-handed operator stands to the patient's right. After identification of the laryngeal prominence, the superior horns of the thyroid cartilage are firmly grasped between the thumb and long finger of the nondominant hand. This leaves the index finger ideally positioned to localize the CTM and re-identify its location at any time during the procedure by capitalizing on the constancy of the relationship as long as the thyroid cartilage is not released. Therefore, it is critical that control of the larynx with this hand be maintained until the placement of the tracheal hook (Fig. 31-5).

c. VERTICAL SKIN INCISION

The operator uses the dominant hand to make a generous vertical incision in the midline, with its center over the CTM. The incision should be at least 2 cm in length and may need to be extended in patients with significant obesity or if identification is difficult. The incision should go through subcutaneous tissues down to, but not into, the thyroid and cricoid cartilages (Fig. 31-6).

d. CONFIRMATION OF MEMBRANE LOCATION

With the thumb and long finger maintaining control of the thyroid cartilage, the index finger may now be inserted into the incision. Without interposed skin and tissues, it is much easier to appreciate the structures of the anterior neck and to confirm the location of the CTM. The index finger can be left in the wound, resting on the inferior aspect of the anterior larynx, indicating the superior limit of the CTM (Fig. 31-7).

e. HORIZONTAL INCISION OF THE CRICOTHYROID MEMBRANE

The index finger may be withdrawn just prior to incision or left in the wound to serve as a guide. The CTM should be incised horizontally for a distance of 1 to 2 cm (Fig. 31-8). It is recommended that an attempt be made to incise the lower half of the membrane to avoid the superiorly placed cricothyroid artery and vein. This can be difficult to achieve, and inadvertent injury to these vessels is rarely clinically significant. Despite the exposure obtained with the skin incision, bleeding from the skin and various vascular structures eliminates a clear view of

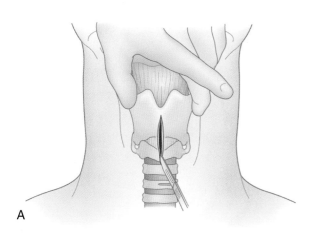

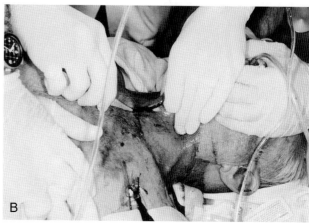

Figure 31-6   A and **B,** A vertical skin incision is made down to, but not through, the airway. (**A** adapted from and **B** from Walls RM, Luten RC, Murphy MF, Schneider RE: *Manual of emergency airway management,* ed 2, Philadelphia, 2004, Lippincott Williams & Wilkins.)

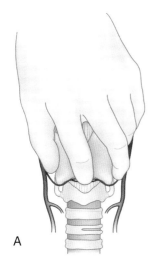
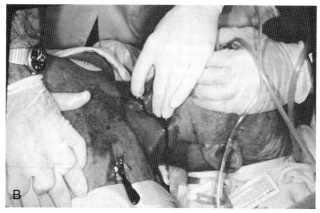

Figure 31-7 **A** and **B,** The index finger can now directly palpate and relocate the cricothyroid membrane. (**A** adapted from and **B** from Walls RM, Luten RC, Murphy MF, Schneider RE: *Manual of emergency airway management,* ed 2, Philadelphia, 2004, Lippincott Williams & Wilkins.)

the field in most cases. Time does not permit the operator to attempt to deal with bleeding so as to achieve a bloodless field. Maintenance of the anatomic relationships outlined previously allows the procedure to be completed expeditiously without the need for direct visualization of the structures of interest. If significant bleeding occurs, it can be dealt with (usually by simple wound packing) after the airway has been secured.

Attempts at ventilation (which have to be discontinued at this point) may result in the presence of air bubbles appearing in the wound and tissues of the neck in synchrony with respirations. The index finger may also be reinserted into the opening to confirm the proper location of the incision in the membrane.

f. INSERTION OF THE TRACHEAL HOOK

Laryngeal control should be maintained with the thumb and long finger of the nondominant hand. The hook is held in the dominant hand, turned so that it is oriented transversely, and then inserted into the trachea through the surgical opening (Fig. 31-9). The index finger of the nondominant hand can serve as a guide to help place the hook into the incision. Once through the CTM, the device hook is rotated so that the hook is oriented in the cephalad direction. The hook is firmly applied to the inferior border of the thyroid cartilage, and gentle upward and anterior traction with the hook handle at a 45-degree angle to the anterior neck skin can be used to bring the airway up to the skin (Fig. 31-10). The hook is then passed to an assistant to maintain immobilization and control of the larynx. The assistant will not release the hook under any circumstance until a definitive airway has been successfully inserted and placement is confirmed; thus the term "no drop technique." The operator's nondominant hand may then be released for completion of the procedure, with the proviso that the tracheal hook is maintaining control and should not be removed until confirmation of tube placement has been obtained.

g. DILATION OF THE OPENING WITH DILATOR

The Trousseau dilator is then inserted using the dominant hand. It is our preference to insert the dilator so that the

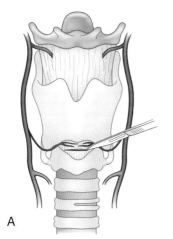
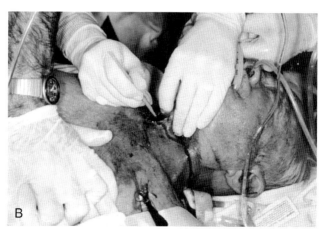

Figure 31-8 **A** and **B,** A transverse incision is made in the cricothyroid membrane staying low to attempt to avoid the cricothyroid artery and vein. (**A** adapted from and **B** from Walls RM, Luten RC, Murphy MF, Schneider RE: *Manual of emergency airway management,* ed 2, Philadelphia, 2004, Lippincott Williams & Wilkins.)

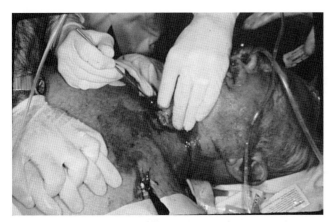

Figure 31-9 The tracheal hook is inserted into the wound, oriented transversely, and then rotated to pick up the inferior edge of the thyroid cartilage. (From Walls RM, Luten RC, Murphy MF, Schneider RE: *Manual of emergency airway management*, ed 2, Philadelphia, 2004, Lippincott Williams & Wilkins.)

prongs are oriented to dilate the opening in the rostral-caudal direction rather than transversely (Fig. 31-11). Although the dilator appears to be designed to insert directly into the airway and dilate transversely, it is the rostral-caudal dimension of the CTM that provides the most resistance to cannulation, so it is desirable to dilate in this plane. The Trousseau dilator is inserted only a couple of millimeters into the airway and then opened to dilate the airway. With the airway thus opened, the dilator, in situ, is transferred from the operator's dominant hand to the nondominant hand, where it can be held from underneath (see Fig. 31-11). This frees the dominant hand to insert the tracheostomy tube.

h. INSERTION OF THE TRACHEOSTOMY TUBE

The tracheostomy tube is then inserted with the obturator in place (Fig. 31-12). To avoid unnecessary delays at this juncture, the tube should have been removed from its packaging before initiation of the procedure and the blunt-tipped obturator should already have been inserted. The tube is oriented along the handle of the dilator (i.e.,

at a 90-degree angle to the patient) and inserted between the dilator blades, following their natural curve. As the tracheostomy tube gains the airway and is passing between the prongs of the Trousseau dilator, it is helpful to rotate the dilator handle counterclockwise 90 degrees (see Fig. 31-12) so that the dilation occurs in the transverse rather than the rostral-caudal dimension. The reason is that when the tracheostomy tube has gained access into the airway, the prongs of the Trousseau dilator may themselves inhibit successful passage of the tip of the tracheostomy tube down the trachea. Through rotation of the Trousseau dilator, the prongs are moved out of the way to either side of the tube, but dilation is continued to assist in placing the tracheostomy tube until it is firmly seated against the anterior neck. The dilator is gently removed as the tube is being advanced, just before it is seated in its final position (Fig. 31-13).

i. CUFF INFLATION AND SECURING THE TRACHEOSTOMY TUBE

The cuff should be inflated. The obturator is then removed, and the inner cannula, if one is present, is inserted to allow the attachment of the ventilation bag. Care must be taken during the initial assembly of the tracheostomy tube not to lose track of the inner cannula, which is needed for the attachment of ventilation devices. The tracheostomy tube can be secured with twill or with a padded fastener that goes around the neck and attaches to the neck plate of the tube.

j. CONFIRMATION OF TUBE POSITION

The tracheostomy tube position can be confirmed using the same methods as those used to confirm ETT position. Carbon dioxide detection can be used to confirm correct placement in the airway. If there is concern that the tube is placed outside the trachea, a nasogastric tube may be gently inserted. In the airway the tube advances easily, but resistance is met if the tube is in a false passage. Auscultation of both lungs and the epigastric area is also recommended, although esophageal placement of the tube is highly unlikely. A chest radiograph can be helpful in the identification of barotrauma. Only after the position of the tube is certain should the tracheal hook be

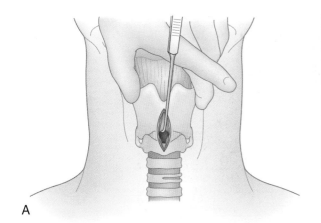

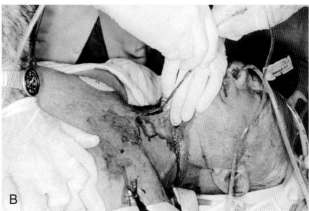

A   B

Figure 31-10 **A** and **B,** The tracheal hook exerts light traction on the inferior aspect of the thyroid cartilage. (**A** adapted from and **B** from Walls RM, Luten RC, Murphy MF, Schneider RE: *Manual of emergency airway management*, ed 2, Philadelphia, 2004, Lippincott Williams & Wilkins.)

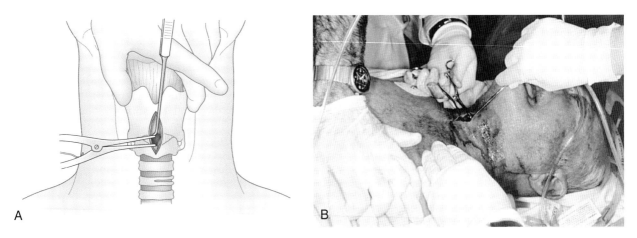

Figure 31-11 A and **B,** The Trousseau dilator is used to enlarge the vertical dimension of the membrane, the aspect providing the most resistance to insertion of the tube. (**A** adapted from and **B** from Walls RM, Luten RC, Murphy MF, Schneider RE: *Manual of emergency airway management,* ed 2, Philadelphia, 2004, Lippincott Williams & Wilkins.)

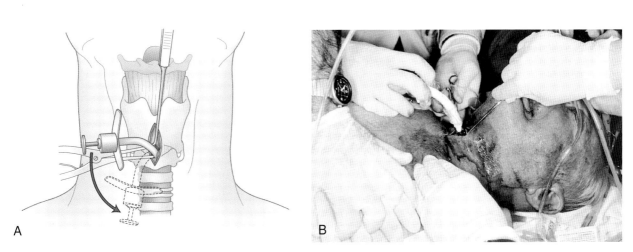

Figure 31-12 A and **B,** The tracheostomy tube is inserted, and the dilator can then be rotated counterclockwise 90 degrees to facilitate passage of the tube. (**A** adapted from and **B** from Walls RM, Luten RC, Murphy MF, Schneider RE: *Manual of emergency airway management,* ed 2, Philadelphia, 2004, Lippincott Williams & Wilkins.)

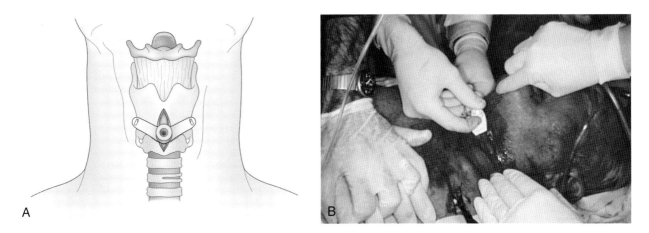

Figure 31-13 A and **B,** The tube is firmly seated, and the dilator can be removed. It is best to leave the hook in situ until placement is confirmed and the cuff has been inflated. (**A** adapted from and **B** from Walls RM, Luten RC, Murphy MF, Schneider RE: *Manual of emergency airway management,* ed 2, Philadelphia, 2004, Lippincott Williams & Wilkins.)

removed. This should be done with great care to avoid hooking a part of the tracheostomy tube and inadvertently extubating the patient. If the tube was inadvertently placed in a false passage, correction is greatly facilitated with the hook still in place.

2. Rapid Four-Step Technique

The rapid four-step technique (RFST) is an attempt to simplify the cricothyrotomy procedure by using a horizontal stab incision through the skin and membrane simultaneously, followed by tracheal hook traction applied caudad at the cricoid ring.[16] Cadaveric studies have shown RFST to be simple to learn and faster in obtaining a surgical airway than the open technique just described.[50-52] Other advantages include the following: (1) less equipment is necessary (it is performed with a scalpel, hook, and tracheostomy tube); (2) it may be performed independently; and (3) the operator is positioned at the head of the bed, similar to the stance for performance of orotracheal intubation.

Acute complications from RFST may be more common than with the traditional "no-drop" method. The stab technique may increase the incidence of trauma to the posterior trachea and anterior aspect of the esophagus. In cadaveric models, an increase in damage to the cricoid ring due to direct traction on the ring with the tracheal hook was found.[1,50-52] This may be remedied through the use of a double-hook device that disperses the forces across the cricoid ring.[1,51]

RFST may not be as desirable in patients in whom landmark identification is difficult. In this circumstance, we recommend beginning with a vertical incision, similar to the traditional technique described previously.[16] There are no clinical studies that report the success rates and associated acute and delayed complications of RFST compared with traditional methods in live patients. The choice between the RFST and the traditional technique is an individual one, because there is no clear evidence that either method is superior or more likely to bring success than the other.

As with other techniques, attempts should be made to oxygenate and ventilate the patient maximally before and during the procedure. The anterior neck should be prepared as described earlier for the "no-drop" technique. From a position at the head of the bed, RFST is performed in the following manner.

a. LANDMARK IDENTIFICATION

As in traditional cricothyrotomy, the airway is accessed through the CTM. Therefore, the identification of landmarks is exactly the same as described previously (Fig. 31-14; see Fig. 31-5). Because of the horizontal stab incision, however, it is even more critical to be confident of the location of the membrane. If there is uncertainty, it is recommended to begin with a vertical incision first, as described earlier.

b. HORIZONTAL STAB INCISION

A single horizontal stab incision using a no. 20 scalpel is made directly through the skin, subcutaneous tissues, and CTM. The incision should be approximately 1.5 cm wide, and because of the size of the no. 20 blade,

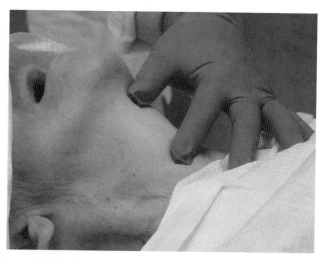

Figure 31-14 The landmarks are palpated as for the "no-drop" technique, but the horizontal skin incision leaves little room for error, so extra care is needed. (From Walls RM, Luten RC, Murphy MF, Schneider RE: *Manual of emergency airway management*, ed 2, Philadelphia, 2004, Lippincott Williams & Wilkins.)

widening of the opening is rarely required (Fig. 31-15). If the anatomy is not readily palpable through the skin, an initial vertical incision should be created to allow subsequent palpation of the anatomy and identification of the CTM. Once the CTM has been incised, the no. 20 blade is maintained in the airway until the tracheal hook is secured.

c. STABILIZATION OF THE LARYNX WITH THE TRACHEAL HOOK

A tracheal hook is placed parallel to the scalpel on the caudal side of the blade (Fig. 31-16). The hook is rotated to secure and control the cricoid ring, and the scalpel is then removed from the airway. The tracheal hook is used to apply gentle traction on the cricoid ring to lift the airway up toward the surface of the skin and to provide modest stoma dilation (Fig. 31-17). The direction of force on the hook is reminiscent of the "up and away" direction

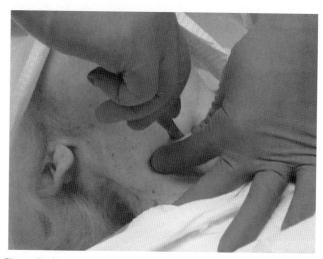

Figure 31-15 A single, horizontal, stab incision is made through skin and membrane. (From Walls RM, Luten RC, Murphy MF, Schneider RE: *Manual of emergency airway management*, ed 2, Philadelphia, 2004, Lippincott Williams & Wilkins.)

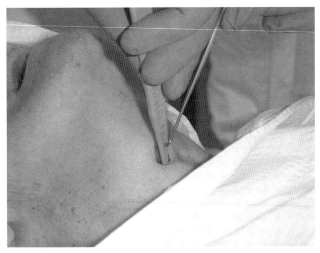

Figure 31-16 The hook is oriented transversely and inserted alongside the scalpel before the scalpel is removed. (From Walls RM, Luten RC, Murphy MF, Schneider RE: *Manual of emergency airway management*, ed 2, Philadelphia, 2004, Lippincott Williams & Wilkins.)

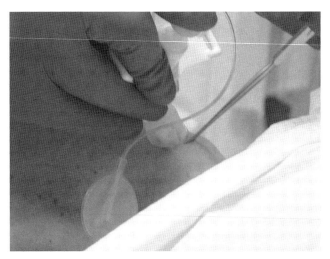

Figure 31-18 The tracheostomy tube is inserted and then verified and secured in the usual fashion. (From Walls RM, Luten RC, Murphy MF, Schneider RE: *Manual of emergency airway management*, ed 2, Philadelphia, 2004, Lippincott Williams & Wilkins.)

employed with laryngoscopy. The amount of traction force required for easy intubation (18 newtons) is significantly lower than the force that is associated with breakage of the cricoid ring (54 newtons); however, the chance of trauma may be further reduced by using a double-tined hook.[1] Use of the hook in this direction usually provides sufficient widening of the incision to obviate the need for further dilation (i.e., Trousseau dilator). Placement of the hook on the cricoid ring may also reduce the possibility of intubating the pretracheal potential space, which is essentially eliminated due to the apposition of the airway and the subcutaneous fat by the traction on the hook.

d. INSERTION OF THE TRACHEOSTOMY TUBE

With adequate control of the airway using the hook placed on the cricoid ring, a tracheostomy tube is gently

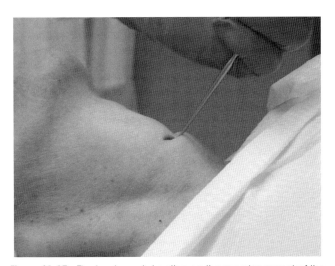

Figure 31-17 The hook exerts traction on the superior aspect of the cricoid cartilage and skin, pulling the airway up into the field. (From Walls RM, Luten RC, Murphy MF, Schneider RE: *Manual of emergency airway management*, ed 2, Philadelphia, 2004, Lippincott Williams & Wilkins.)

inserted through the cricothyroid space into the trachea (Fig. 31-18). The cuff is then inflated, the tube is secured, and its location is confirmed by the same methods described earlier.

3. Percutaneous Cricothyrotomy Techniques

Numerous commercial cricothyrotomy devices are available, many of which use a modified Seldinger technique to assist in the placement of a tracheal airway (see Fig. 31-4). There are aspects of this technique that may make it appealing to the anesthesiologist. This method is similar to the one commonly used for placement of central venous catheters and offers some familiarity to the operator who is uncomfortable or inexperienced with the surgical cricothyrotomy technique described earlier. This technique can be learned quickly. By the fifth practice attempt on a mannequin model, 96% of anesthesiologists achieved success within 40 seconds.[6] However, the technique still requires knowledge of the anatomy and the ability to localize the membrane and has several steps, so it approaches the open technique in complexity. When compared with the standard open technique in cadavers and dog models, there were no differences in performance times or complications.[53-55] It is estimated that the procedure may be accomplished in 40 to 100 seconds.[6,27,53-55] Also, the percutaneous cricothyrotomy kits are preassembled and commercially available, whereas at present the surgical tools used in the traditional approach are not (except in the combination kit shown in Fig. 31-4). It seems intuitive that the percutaneous technique should result in less bleeding, but no studies have been performed to assess the significance of any difference. One of the limitations is the relatively smaller lumen, which is of no real concern in an emergency, and in some models the absence of a cuff, which could be an issue if airway protection from emesis or hemorrhage is needed. It is suggested that a device with a cuff be selected, because many of these procedures are performed on patients who have not been fasted or are actively hemorrhaging and require further airway protection. The Melker

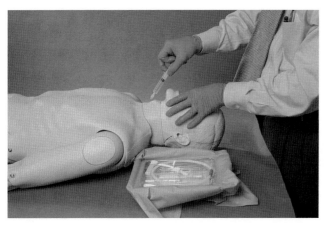

Figure 31-19 The finder needle is inserted through the cricothyroid membrane. A small, vertical skin incision may be made before insertion of the needle or later, just before insertion of the airway and dilator. (Photograph from STRATUS Center for Medical Simulation, Brigham and Women's Hospital, Boston, MA, used with permission.)

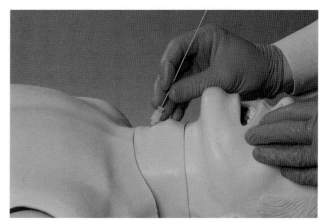

Figure 31-20 The wire is fed through in a caudad direction; then the needle is removed. (Photograph from STRATUS Center for Medical Simulation, Brigham and Women's Hospital, Boston, MA, used with permission.)

Cuffed Emergency Cricothyrotomy Catheter Set and the Melker Universal Cricothyrotomy Set are available with a cuffed airway catheter (Cook Critical Care).

As with other techniques, attempts should be made to preoxygenate and ventilate the patient maximally before and during the procedure. The anterior neck should be prepared as described earlier. Although the kits may vary, most of the percutaneous cricothyrotomy kits use the Seldinger technique and share the following steps.

a. LANDMARK IDENTIFICATION

The CTM is identified using the same methods described previously. The nondominant hand is then used to control the larynx and maintain identification of the landmarks.

b. INSERTION OF LOCATOR NEEDLE

The introducer needle is then inserted through the skin and the CTM in a slightly caudal direction. The needle is attached to a syringe and advanced with the dominant hand while negative pressure is maintained on the syringe. The sudden aspiration of air indicates placement of the needle into the tracheal lumen (Fig. 31-19).

c. INSERTION OF THE GUIDEWIRE

The syringe is then removed from the needle, and a soft-tipped guidewire is inserted through the needle into the trachea in a caudal direction. The needle is then removed, leaving the wire in place. As with most Seldinger techniques, control of the wire must be maintained at all times (Fig. 31-20).

d. SKIN INCISION

A small skin incision is then made adjacent to the wire. This facilitates passage of the airway device through the skin. Alternatively, the skin incision may be made vertically over the membrane before insertion of the needle and guidewire.

e. INSERTION OF THE AIRWAY

The airway catheter provided in the kit (3 to 6 mm internal diameter), with an introducing dilator in place, is then inserted over the wire into the trachea. If resistance is met, the skin incision should be deepened and a gentle twisting motion applied to the airway device (Fig. 31-21). After the airway device is firmly seated against the skin, the wire and obturator are removed together, leaving the tracheostomy tube in place. Tube location should then be confirmed, as described previously, and secured properly. The devices are radiopaque.

IV. TRAINING ISSUES

A survey published in 1995 found that although 80% of anesthesiology programs taught cricothyrotomy as part of their curriculum, most of them did so through lectures only, with no practical experience.[21] In a survey published in 2003, only 21% of anesthesiologists claimed skills to perform cricothyrotomy.[56] Most anesthesiology graduates have never performed a cricothyrotomy during their training.[6]

The merits of a procedure are irrelevant if hesitancy on the part of the provider leads to a significant delay in establishing a definitive airway. Discomfort with a procedure is usually overcome with technical proficiency obtained through stepwise practice; however, this procedure is performed so rarely that proficiency must be obtained through scheduled, simulated learning. Invasive airway methods, like any other invasive procedures, must be learned and practiced at regular intervals to maintain proficiency.

The advent of emergency medicine as a specialty with its own airway expertise has resulted in a significant decrease in exposure to emergency airways for anesthesiology trainees. The success of RSI in the emergency setting, as well as advances in airway management techniques in anesthesiology, have prompted editorials concerned with the problem of gaining and maintaining competence in invasive airway management.[57-59] Studies suggest a current cricothyrotomy rate of approximately 1% of all emergency airways and a dramatically lower rate in the operating suite. Regardless of the setting, this incidence is too low to ensure adequate training, but it

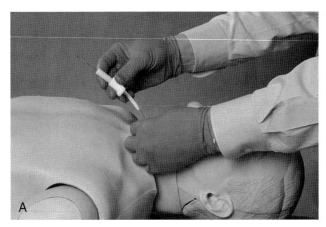
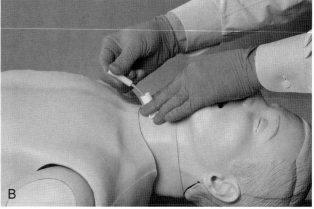

Figure 31-21 A, The airway is inserted over the guidewire with the dilator in place. **B,** The dilator and wire are then removed together. (Photograph from STRATUS Center for Medical Simulation, Brigham and Women's Hospital, Boston, MA, used with permission.)

highlights the probability that most airway managers will be called on to perform an invasive airway at some point in their career.

The practice required to obtain familiarity with the equipment and technique must take place outside the clinical setting. Of anesthesiology programs that instruct their residents on cricothyrotomy, 60% use lectures only, which is a poor teaching technique for developing proficiency in manual skills.[21] One study using a mannequin model determined that five cricothyrotomies were necessary to reach a steady performance state in which the procedure could be completed in 40 seconds.[25]

No studies have identified the optimal interval between training episodes for retention, although one small report suggested increased retention when training was repeated monthly versus every 3 months.[38] Studies in cadavers performed primarily to compare different surgical airway techniques incidentally identified a similar rapid learning curve.[60,61] There are no studies examining the clinical correlation of these training techniques, but the high success rate of emergency cricothyrotomy suggests that retention and competence have occurred.

On the basis of the limited available literature, some recommendations regarding the learning and retention of invasive airway techniques can be made: (1) identify a preferred method of invasive airway management that is immediately available; (2) become trained in the procedure by performing a sufficient number of repetitions under the supervision of a qualified instructor, using an animal or simulator model, or both; and (3) practice the technique in one to two refresher sessions per year on animal or simulator models, with five repetitions per session.

Animal tracheas may be obtained from a slaughterhouse at relatively low cost, and the technique may be attempted multiple times on each specimen (pigs and sheep are most commonly used). Simulators represent a significant capital investment, but newer simulators are much less expensive and much simpler to operate than older models. Models specifically for cricothyrotomy training are also available. Formal training under expert guidance is available through some difficult airway continuing medical education (CME) courses.

V. CHOOSING THE RIGHT TECHNIQUE

As described in the introduction, the typical clinical milieu in which an emergency surgical airway is performed will inevitably be impacted by four simultaneous challenges: (1) the patient will be compromised; (2) there will be very little time to establish the airway; (3) few, if any, other options will remain if the procedure is unsuccessful; and (4) the operator will have limited experience with the technique. It therefore becomes imperative to select a method with the highest likelihood of success and the lowest complication rate.

Guidance from the literature on choosing the best technique is limited and difficult to translate into clinical practice. There are no human studies comparing the various surgical airway techniques. The available comparative evidence is based almost entirely on studies using animal, cadaveric, or mannequin models.

Acknowledging this limitation, several generalizations can be made:

- Dilational techniques that rely on direct puncture into the airway are associated with an unacceptably high rate of complications, including injury to airway structures and catheter misplacement.[28-31] These techniques cannot be recommended unless other options are unavailable.
- The success rates of open surgical and percutaneous guidewire (Seldinger) cricothyrotomy are roughly comparable.[62]
- The complications associated with open surgical and Seldinger cricothyrotomy are distinctly different. When complications arise with open surgical cricothyrotomy, bleeding or injury to airway structures is the predominant problem. With Seldinger cricothyrotomy, the most common complication is misplacement of the airway into the pretracheal or paratracheal spaces.[62]

Equipment availability, experience, and backup resources play a significant role in technique selection. In weighing the priorities at hand when performing an emergent surgical airway, the prime directive must always be successful placement of the airway. Based on the third generalization, confidence with the identification of surgical airway landmarks becomes a critical question in the decision-making process.

If surgical airway landmarks are easily identifiable, the clinician can confidently employ whichever technique he or she feels most comfortable performing. Conversely, if airway landmarks are difficult or impossible to palpate (e.g., in a patient with morbid obesity), the Seldinger technique has a predictably high rate of airway misplacement. If a definitive airway is urgently needed in this situation, the open technique is preferred. Another option is to perform a hybrid technique during which a formal vertical skin incision is made to better palpate the CTM, and the technique is then continued using the Seldinger method.

VI. COMPLICATIONS

The rate of complications associated with emergency cricothyrotomy is difficult to quantify with precision. A critical review of the literature reveals that many of apparent complications are the result of the patient's underlying illness or occur as a consequence of the unsuccessful attempts at airway management preceding cricothyrotomy. In addition, the definition of complications, variations in technique, and the skill of the operators vary widely from study to study.

With these limitations in mind, the complication rate after surgical cricothyrotomy is highly variable, ranging from 14% to 50% depending on the technique, clinical setting, definition of complications, and experience of the operator.[2,9,18,52,63-67]

A. Hemorrhage

When surgical cricothyrotomy is performed, venous hemorrhage is the rule rather than the exception. This seldom interferes with successful completion of the procedure, and bleeding can usually be controlled with direct pressure or postprocedure suture closure of the incision. Major arterial hemorrhage can result from inadvertent laceration of the thyroid ima artery located near the isthmus of the thyroid, but this would require considerable misplacement of the skin incision from that described here. If the dissection strays far from the midline, the carotid artery or jugular vein can be injured. Arterial bleeding is distinctly unusual if the procedure is performed as described previously. Although it may seem intuitive that bleeding would be less likely after percutaneous cricothyrotomy, this has never been assessed in randomized human trials.

B. Tube Misplacement

Tracheostomy tube misplacement is the most important potential complication of both surgical and percutaneous cricothyrotomy. Whether it is considered a complication or a failure of the procedure, inadvertent placement of the tube in either the pretracheal or paratracheal soft tissues can be a lethal error. If ventilation is attempted before misplacement is recognized, massive subcutaneous emphysema and distortion of the neck can ensue, making subsequent efforts to gain the airway extremely difficult. This is perhaps the strongest argument for the use of surgical (rather than percutaneous) cricothyrotomy; in the former, the entry into the airway is confirmed by palpation and by direct insertion of the hook, dilator, and tracheostomy tube through an open incision.

C. Accidental Extubation

Replacing a decannulated tube into a recently performed tracheostomy can be extremely difficult, and great care must be taken to ensure that decannulation does not occur. Tracheostomy ties should be applied immediately after tracheal entry has been confirmed by capnography and under the direct supervision of the operator. Additional care should be taken to prevent excessive neck movement or entanglement by monitor lines or intravenous tubing if the patient is being transported. Violent coughing or exaggerated neck movement may also cause the tube to dislodge, and the patient should be appropriately sedated. Finally, self-extubation can occur if the patient is not unconscious or sedated.

D. Other Complications

Injury to the posterior laryngeal wall or esophagus can occur if an excessively deep incision is made when entering the airway. This is easily avoidable, provided careful technique is used. Insertion of a cricothyrotome adjacent to or through the airway can result in significant local tissue damage, including vascular injury and esophageal injury.

VII. CONCLUSIONS

Surgical cricothyrotomy is a rare procedure that is often performed by clinicians with little or no experience in situations in which a patient cannot be intubated via the orotracheal route and rescue ventilation has not been successful. Several different techniques are described in the literature, including open surgical or percutaneous (Seldinger or dilational percutaneous) technique. Each technique is a viable option. Which technique is chosen is based on provider comfort and the equipment available. Children younger than 10 years of age are a unique patient population in which the anatomy precludes traditional surgical or percutaneous cricothyrotomy and a transtracheal catheter-based procedure should be considered the method of choice. It is critical that any clinician who manages the airway in a patient have the knowledge and ability to perform a surgical cricothyrotomy or catheter-based procedure.

VIII. CLINICAL PEARLS

- New technology and improved skill in performing direct laryngoscopy have reduced the need for emergent surgical cricothyrotomy, and this has implications for skill retention among physicians managing airways in the emergency setting.

- Surgical cricothyrotomy is indicated in the "cannot intubate, cannot ventilate" (CICV) situation, in which direct laryngoscopy and rescue techniques have failed.

- Surgical cricothyrotomy can be performed via a percutaneous Seldinger technique or an open technique, and there is few data on which method is optimal.

- The presence or absence of adequate anatomic landmarks can help guide the clinician with technique selection. If the cricothyroid membrane is easily identifiable, either method can be used. If landmarks are difficult to identify (e.g., in obese patients), the open technique is more likely to be successful.

- Needle cricothyrotomy is preferred in children younger than 10 years of age because of the unique anatomic differences (i.e., small cricothyroid membrane) in this patient population.

SELECTED REFERENCES

All references can be found online at expertconsult.com.
1. Bair AE, Filbin MR, Kulkarni RG, et al: The failed intubation attempt in the emergency department: Analysis of prevalence, rescue techniques, and personnel. *J Emerg Med* 23:131–140, 2002.
35. Davis DP, Bramwell KJ, Hamilton RS, et al: Safety and efficacy of the rapid four-step technique for cricothyrotomy using a Bair Claw. *J Emerg Med* 19:125–129, 2000.
52. Holmes JF, Panacek EA, Sackles JC, Brofeldt BT: Comparison of 2 cricothyrotomy techniques: Standard method versus rapid 4-step technique. *Ann Emerg Med* 32:442–447, 1998.
57. Chang RS, Hamilton RJ, Carter WA: Declining rate of cricothyrotomy in trauma patients with an emergency medicine residency: Implications for skills training. *Acad Emerg Med* 5:247–251, 1998.
61. Eisenberger P, Laczika K, List M, et al: Comparison of conventional surgical versus Seldinger technique emergency cricothyrotomy performed by inexperienced clinicians. *Anesthesiology* 92:687–690, 2000.

Chapter 32

Confirmation of Endotracheal Intubation

M. RAMEZ SALEM | ANIS S. BARAKA

I. OVERVIEW

A. American Society of Anesthesiologists Closed Claims Studies

For the past several decades, the Committee on Professional Liability of the American Society of Anesthesiologists (ASA) has studied adverse anesthetic outcomes based on closed claims files of nationwide insurance carriers.[1] From the beginning, it was evident that adverse outcomes involving the respiratory system constitute the single largest class of injury, representing one third of the overall claims. Generally involving healthy adults undergoing nonemergency surgery with general anesthesia, three mechanisms of injury accounted for approximately three quarters of the adverse respiratory events in the 1970s and early 1980s: inadequate ventilation (38%), esophageal intubation (18%), and difficult endotracheal intubation (DI; 17%). The remaining adverse respiratory events were produced by a variety of low-frequency (≤2%) mechanisms, including airway obstruction, bronchospasm, aspiration, premature and unintentional extubation, inadequate inspired oxygen delivery, and endobronchial intubation.[1]

Care was judged to be substandard in more than 80% of the cases of inadequate ventilation and esophageal intubation. Almost all (>90%) of the claims for inadequate ventilation and esophageal intubation were considered preventable with better monitoring, compared with only 36% of claims for DI. Death and permanent brain damage were more frequent in claims for inadequate ventilation and esophageal intubation (>90%) than in claims for DI (56%). Median payments were $240,000 for inadequate ventilation, $217,000 for esophageal intubation, and $76,000 for DI.[1]

In 23% of the claims for esophageal intubation, there was documentation of DI; in 73%, there was sufficient information to reconstruct the time to detection of esophageal intubation. Within this latter subset, 3% of esophageal intubations were detected within 5 minutes, 61% in 5 to 10 minutes, and 36% after 10 minutes. Auscultation of breath sounds (presumed) was documented in 63% of the claims for esophageal intubation. In 48% of cases, auscultation led to the erroneous conclusion that the tube was in the trachea. This diagnostic error was eventually recognized in a variety of ways, including reexamination with direct laryngoscopy, absence of the endotracheal tube (ETT) in the trachea at the time of an emergency tracheostomy, resolution of cyanosis after reintubation, and discovery of esophageal intubation at autopsy. Cyanosis was documented in 52% of the claims and preceded the recognition of esophageal intubation in only 34% of the cases.[1]

Because pulse oximetry and capnography have been used since the mid-1980s, data from the closed claims project were analyzed in 1999 to determine whether these monitoring modalities correlated with improvement in patients' safety. After monitoring was instituted, respiratory events decreased, primarily in claims for injuries caused by inadequate ventilation and, to a lesser extent, esophageal intubation (Fig. 32-1).[2]

1. Pediatric Versus Adult Anesthesia Closed Malpractice Claims

Outcome studies in pediatric patients revealed that adverse respiratory events constitute a leading cause of morbidity and mortality.[3-5] The ASA closed claims study provided a database to compare pediatric and adult cases in which an adverse outcome occurred.[5] The pediatric claims presented a different distribution of damaging events compared with claims of adults (Tables 32-1 and 32-2). Respiratory events and mortality rate were greater in pediatric claims.[5] Anesthetic care was more often judged "less than appropriate," and the complications more frequently were considered preventable with better monitoring. The median payment to the plaintiff was greater for pediatric claims than for adult claims. Cyanosis (49%), bradycardia (64%), or both often preceded cardiac arrest, resulting in death (50%) or brain damage (30%) in previously healthy children.[5]

B. The Magnitude of the Problem of Endotracheal Tube Misplacement

Outcome studies have repeatedly identified adverse respiratory events including unrecognized esophageal intubation as a leading and recurring cause of injury in anesthetic practice.[6-10] The report on confidential enquiries into maternal deaths in England and Wales in 1979-1981 revealed that 8 of 22 deaths attributable to anesthesia were related to difficulty in endotracheal

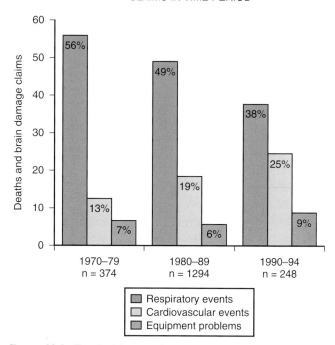

PERCENT OF DEATHS AND BRAIN DAMAGE CLAIMS IN TIME PERIOD

Figure 32-1 The incidence of respiratory, cardiovascular, and equipment-related damaging events as a percentage of total claims for death and brain damage in each time period ($P \le 0.5$, Z test). (Modified from Cheney FW: The American Society of Anesthesiologists Closed Claims Project: What have we learned, how has it affected practice, and how will it affect practice in the future? *Anesthesiology* 91:552–556, 1999.)

intubation.[9] In 4 patients, the ETT proved to be misplaced in the esophagus.[9] An investigation of anesthesia deaths in Australia revealed that 69% were related to airway management, with esophageal intubation once again identified as an important contributing factor.[8]

All anesthesiologists experience esophageal intubations sometime in their career, especially during training and when difficulty in visualizing the larynx is encountered. Most esophageal intubations are immediately and easily recognized. What is intriguing is the rare situation in which misplacement of the ETT in the esophagus is

TABLE 32-1

Comparison of Pediatric and Adult Damaging Events with Special Reference to the Respiratory System

Damaging Event	Pediatric Cases (*n* = 238) (%)	*P*	Adult Cases (*n* = 1953) (%)
Respiratory system	43	≤0.01	30
Inadequate ventilation	20	≤0.01	9
Esophageal intubation	5	NS	6
Airway obstruction	5	NS	2
Difficult intubation	4	NS	6
Inadvertent extubation	3	NS	1
Premature extubation	3	NS	1
Aspiration	2	NS	2
Endobronchial intubation	1	NS	1
Bronchospasm	0	NS	2
Inadequate FIO_2	0	NS	<0.5

FIO_2, Fraction of inspired oxygen; *NS*, not significant.
Data from Morray JP, Geiduschek JM, Caplan RA, et al: A comparison of pediatric and adult anesthesia closed malpractice claims. *Anesthesiology* 78:461, 1993.

TABLE 32-2

Comparison of Pediatric and Adult Demographic, Injury, and Payment Data

	Pediatric Cases (n = 238) (%)	P	Adult Cases (n = 1953) (%)
Age			
0-14	28	—	—
Sex			
Male	65	≤0.01	38
Female	32	≤0.01	62
Unknown	3	≤0.05	<0.5
ASA Physical Status			
1	35	≤0.01	22
2	14	≤0.01	22
3	6	≤0.01	13
4	4	NS	3
5	<0.5	NS	1
Unknown	40	NS	40
Poor medical condition and/or obesity	6	≤0.01	41
Death	50	≤0.01	35
Brain damage	30	≤0.01	11
Less than appropriate anesthetic care	54	≤0.01	44
Preventable with better monitoring	45	≤0.01	30
Median payment	$111,234	≤0.05	$90,000

ASA, American Society of Anesthesiologists; NS, not significant.
Data from Morray JP, Geiduschek JM, Caplan RA, et al: A comparison of pediatric and adult anesthesia closed malpractice claims. *Anesthesiology* 78:461, 1993.

not recognized, resulting in grave consequences. Failure to recognize esophageal intubation is not limited to junior residents or inexperienced personnel; it has occurred with experienced anesthesiologists. A case was reported in which three "consultant anaesthetists" failed to recognize esophageal intubation.[6] There are also many case reports describing anesthetic catastrophes and near-disasters in patients whose esophagus had been unintentionally intubated and in whom some or many of the common signs indicative of proper ETT placement were misleading.[8,11-17]

Unintentional esophageal intubation occurs more frequently in emergency airway management, in critically ill patients, and in patients who suffer cardiac arrest during out-of-hospital paramedic intubation.[18-20] In one report, esophageal intubation occurred in 8% of emergency intubation attempts in critically ill patients.[20] In a study of paramedics trained in direct laryngoscopic endotracheal intubation, there were 14 esophageal intubations in 779 patients, an incidence of 1.8%.[18] Esophageal tube placement was recognized and corrected in 11 of the 14 patients; three esophageal intubations (0.4% of the total) were not recognized and remained uncorrected. In another study, 25% of tracheas intubated in the prehospital setting had improperly placed ETTs detected on arrival at the hospital.[21] Contributing factors to this high incidence of esophageal intubation include intubation under less than optimal conditions; unavailability of monitoring equipment, protocols, or algorithms; violation of

the standard technique of auscultation of lung fields and the epigastrium; and intubation attempts by nonexpert personnel.[18-22]

It is obvious that grave consequences can occur if the ETT is misplaced in the esophagus or in a main stem bronchus or if inadvertent extubation occurs. Therefore, whenever endotracheal intubation is performed, clinicians should verify that the ETT is placed in the trachea and that the tube is positioned at an appropriate depth inside the trachea.

II. CONFIRMATION OF ENDOTRACHEAL TUBE PLACEMENT

A. Is There an Ideal Test for Confirmation of Endotracheal Tube Placement?

Over the years, the search has continued for an ideal test for confirmation of ETT placement. Such a test should be simple, quick, reliable, safe, inexpensive, and repeatable and should require minimal training. It should function in patients of different age groups, in various locations, and during DI. It should not yield false results, even in patients with cardiac arrest.

Unfortunately, such a perfect test does not yet exist. Many clinical signs and technical aids have been described to confirm endotracheal intubation. A number of these reports relied on the placement of two ETTs, one in the trachea and the other in the esophagus.[23-25] This scenario makes the observer's decision as to which tube is in the trachea or esophagus much easier and helps in the recognition of esophageal intubation. However, the clinician does not have the luxury of choice between two ETTs in a given clinical situation.[24,25]

In the assessment of these tests, the reader must understand what is meant by false-negative and false-positive results. Although not all reports are in agreement, most use the term *false-negative* when the ETT is in the trachea but the test fails and *false-positive* when the ETT is in the esophagus but the result mimics that of endotracheal intubation.[24,25] For capnography, a false-negative result occurs when the ETT is in the trachea but the waveform is absent, and a false-positive when the ETT is in the esophagus but the waveform is present.[24,25] To avoid confusion and to maintain conformity, these definitions are retained throughout the discussion that follows.

B. Methods of Verification of Endotracheal Tube Placement

Methods of verification of ETT placement (or detection of esophageal intubation) can be classified into non-failsafe, almost failsafe, and failsafe types, depending on their reported reliability and specificity.

1. Non-Failsafe Methods

a. OBSERVATION AND PALPATION OF CHEST MOVEMENTS

Commonly used maneuvers to confirm endotracheal intubation are observation of symmetrical bilateral chest movements and palpation of upper chest excursions during compression of the reservoir bag. These signs can easily distinguish tracheal from esophageal intubation in most patients. However, in obese patients, women with large breasts, and patients with a rigid chest wall, barrel chest, or less compliant lungs, these signs can be misinterpreted to indicate that the ETT is in the esophagus.[26] More important, upper chest wall movements simulating ventilation of the lungs can be seen and felt with an esophageally placed ETT. This phenomenon has been described in many instances of what ultimately proved to be esophageal intubation, and it has been reported in patients with intrathoracic hiatal hernia and after gastric pull-up operations.[11-17,26]

Pollard and Junius studied chest movements during esophageal ventilation in a male cadaver after a cuffed ETT was placed into the esophagus and attached to an inflating bag.[16] As they reported, "Chest and epigastric movements observed when the bag was compressed were indistinguishable from those normally seen in ventilation of the lungs even in the upper chest area." When the body was dissected starting with the epigastrium, it was noted that "the stomach was being inflated and was spontaneously deflating via the esophagus, the feel of the inflating bag being indistinguishable from normal pulmonary ventilation." Even when the lower end of the esophagus was occluded, "chest movements still appeared identical to those seen when the lungs are inflated." After the chest was entered, it was observed that "chest movements were caused by the flat esophagus distending into a firm tube that lifted the heart and upper mediastinal structures forward, elevating the sternum and ribs." The lifting of the chest wall by the distended esophagus is the most plausible explanation for the presumed chest movements seen during esophageal ventilation. Another possible mechanism is that gastric insufflation causes upward displacement of the diaphragm and outward movement of the lower chest. With release of bag compression, gas escapes from the stomach up the esophagus, allowing the diaphragm to move downward and the lower chest to move inward.[16]

b. AUSCULTATION OF BREATH SOUNDS

Auscultation of bilateral breath sounds is the most common method used to ensure proper ETT placement. It can be done repeatedly anywhere endotracheal intubation is performed and whenever change in the position of the tube is suspected. In almost all cases, breath sounds heard near the midaxillary lines leave very little doubt regarding the position of the ETT. However, in numerous anecdotal reports, deceptive breath sounds were heard in cases that proved to be esophageal intubation.

There are several reasons why sounds heard with esophageal intubation may mimic breath sounds from the lungs. The combination of esophageal wall oscillations with gas movement and acoustic filtering can produce inspiratory or expiratory wheezes indistinguishable from sounds arising from gas movement in the airway.[13,27,28] The high flow rate, distribution, and volume of gas delivered through the esophagus may lead to auscultation of predominantly bronchial breath sounds.[13] In infants and children, esophageal sounds can be easily transmitted to wide areas of the chest wall.[29] The quality of breath sounds may also differ depending on whether the chest is auscultated near the middle line or laterally near the axilla and may vary with the presence of pulmonary disease and from patient to patient.

Sounds retrieved by an esophageal stethoscope are different from those heard with a precordial stethoscope and should not be used to differentiate endotracheal from esophageal intuation.[16,25] In patients with a thoracic stomach or hiatal hernia, many of the clinical signs of esophageal intubation may be obscured. Because of the intrathoracic location of a large distensible viscus, bilateral breath sounds may be heard during manual ventilation.[12] For these reasons, whenever abnormal breath sounds are heard, they should not be relied on to confirm endotracheal intubations.[30]

Proper verification of ETT placement by auscultation is dependent on the clinician's experience.[31] In one study in the critical care setting, experienced clinicians identified ETT location correctly, whereas inexperienced examiners were correct in only 68% of cases.[31]

c. ENDOBRONCHIAL INTUBATION

Intentional endobronchial intubation has been used to discriminate between endotracheal and esophageal intubation when doubt exists.[32] The ETT is advanced until breath sounds are lost on one side and unilateral breath sounds are heard on the other side. That should not happen if the tube is in the esophagus. The ETT is then gradually withdrawn 1 to 2 cm beyond the point at which bilateral breath sounds are heard. This technique has been used in infants and children, particularly in infants with tracheoesophageal fistulas.[33] However, it is not recommended for routine use because it can precipitate carinal irritation and bronchospasm.[34]

d. EPIGASTRIC AUSCULTATION AND OBSERVATION FOR ABDOMINAL DISTENTION

Auscultation of the epigastric area to elicit air movement in the stomach has been suggested as a routine maneuver after endotracheal intubation, even before auscultation of the chest.[14,15,25,26] However, normal vesicular breath sounds from the lungs can be transmitted to the epigastric area in tracheally intubated patients who are thin or small.[26] On rare occasions, esophageal intubation may not be easily distinguishable from endotracheal intubation if epigastric auscultation alone is used. Furthermore, there are circumstances, such as obstetric emergencies, in which prepping of the abdomen before induction of anesthesia precludes epigastric auscultation after intubation.[25]

Abdominal distention caused by gastric insufflation after compression of the breathing bag in cases of esophageal intubation can be readily observed in most patients. Occasionally, this sign may not be a reliable indicator of esophageal intubation for the following reasons[16,26,35]:

1. Gastric insufflation and abdominal distention might have occurred during prior mask ventilation.
2. Gastric distention may not be apparent in obese patients.
3. A previously placed nasogastric tube (NGT) can cause intermittent decompression of the stomach.

4. Gradual gastric filling can be difficult to distinguish from normal abdominal movements because of the esophageal reflux of gases.

Conversely, gastric distention can occur in patients with congenital or acquired tracheoesophageal fistula despite placement of the tube in the trachea.[33]

e. COMBINED AUSCULTATION OF EPIGASTRIUM AND BOTH AXILLAE

In a study of 40 adult patients intubated in both the trachea and the esophagus, "blinded" observers auscultating both axillae failed to diagnose esophageal intubation in 15% of cases.[36] When movement of the abdominal wall alone was used to assess ETT position, false results were obtained in 90% of cases. In contrast, the combined auscultation of the epigastrium and both axillae was found to be totally reliable in diagnosing esophageal intubation.[36] These findings emphasize the importance of combining tests to achieve a high degree of reliability in assessing ETT placement.

Detection of misplaced ETTs by auscultation of the chest and epigastrium is probably more difficult in infants than in adults. Uejima reported on two children,[29] aged 7 months and 5 years, in whom esophageal intubation occurred. In both, bilateral chest movements and breath sounds were heard over four areas of the chest and over the epigastrium. However, these "breath sounds" were not vesicular in nature. The ease of transmission of sounds from the esophagus to the chest and epigastrium may mimic breath sounds, especially in infants, emphasizing again that whenever any but normal vesicular breath sounds are heard, they should not be relied on to confirm endotracheal intubation.[25]

Attempts have been made to quantify and assess breath sound characteristics using electronic stethoscopes placed over each hemithorax and the epigastrium. With the use of computerized analysis, researchers digitized and filtered breath sounds to remove selected frequencies. Preliminary results suggested that this technique, when incorporated into a three-component, electronic stethoscope-type device, provides an accurate, portable mechanism to reliably detect ETT position in adults.[37] However, before this method gains wide acceptance, further evaluation is necessary in a broader population of patients with a variety of pathologic states and with different conditions and environments.

f. RESERVOIR BAG COMPLIANCE AND REFILLING

Manual compression of the reservoir bag after endotracheal intubation and cuff inflation yields a characteristic feel of compliance of the lungs and chest wall, whereas passive exhalation on release of bag compression is accompanied by rapid bag refilling. In almost all esophageal intubations, compressing the reservoir bag does not inflate the chest and is not followed by appreciable refilling. However, exceptions to this rule do occur, as has been shown in reports of accidental esophageal intubations. In these cases, repeated filling and emptying of the stomach resulted in concomitant emptying and refilling of the reservoir bag, leading to the erroneous conclusion that the ETT was in the trachea.[13,14,16,17,35]

It is possible that high fresh gas flow might have contributed to reservoir bag refilling in these cases. To enhance the reliability of this test, it has been suggested that the fresh gas flow should be shut off temporarily.[38] If this is done, chest inflation and rapid bag refilling can be repeatedly done (three to five times) in tracheally intubated patients but not in esophageally intubated patients. Because changes in lung or chest wall compliance can be misinterpreted by the clinician compressing the reservoir bag and high airway resistance can lead to slow refilling, this test, used alone, should not be relied on to distinguish esophageal from endotracheal intubation.[26]

g. RESERVOIR BAG MOVEMENTS WITH SPONTANEOUS BREATHING

Movement of the reservoir bag during spontaneous breathing has been considered one of the signs indicative of endotracheal intubation. However, it has been demonstrated that this sign can be unreliable. In a group of anesthetized patients, the trachea and esophagus were intubated and the patients were allowed to breathe spontaneously.[39] With the ETT intentionally occluded, the high negative intrapleural pressures generated with spontaneous breathing efforts were transmitted to the esophagus, resulting in reservoir bag movements and measurable tidal volumes (V_T) up to 180 mL. Therefore, slight reservoir bag movements or measurements of small V_T during spontaneous breathing are not reliable indicators of endotracheal intubation.[39]

h. CUFF MANEUVERS AND NECK PALPATION

The higher-pitched sound produced by leakage around a tube placed in the trachea with the cuff deflated during compression of the reservoir bag, compared with the "flatus-like" sound of leakage around a tube placed in the esophagus, has been used as a distinguishing test.[26] As has been shown in case reports, when the cuff of an esophageally placed ETT is inflated close to the cricoid cartilage, the characteristic guttural sound may be absent or may become higher pitched, resembling leakage around a tracheally placed ETT.[16]

Palpation of the cuff on each side of the trachea between the cricoid cartilage and the suprasternal notch while moving the tube has been proposed to confirm endotracheal intubation.[26] After intubation and cuff inflation, 2 or 3 fingers are placed above the suprasternal notch. Several rapid inflations of the cuff are performed (up to 10 mL of air). An outward force is felt by the palpating fingers if the ETT is in correct position. Intermittent squeezing of the pilot balloon of a slightly overinflated cuff with the thumb and index finger while sensing the transmitted pulsations in the neck has also been suggested as a sign for confirming ETT placement.[40] Likewise, a maneuver using the pilot balloon as a sensor has been proposed.[34] A high-volume, low-pressure, prestretched cuff may not be palpable despite correct placement.[34] Conversely, an inflated cuff can be palpated in the neck in cases of esophageal intubations.[17] Therefore, these maneuvers should not be relied on in verifying endotracheal intubation.[25,26,30]

If an assistant gently palpates the trachea in the suprasternal notch or applies cricoid compression during endotracheal intubation, an "old washboard-like" vibration is appreciated as the ETT rubs against the tracheal rings.[41] It has been suggested that there should be no false-positive results of this sign if the ETT is misplaced in the esophagus, because the esophagus is soft and lies posterior to the trachea. Thus far, there have been no controlled studies to confirm the validity of this sign.

i. SOUND OF EXPELLED GASES DURING STERNAL COMPRESSION

Pressing sharply on the sternum while listening over the proximal end of the ETT to detect a characteristic feel and sound of expelled gases from the airway is occasionally used to distinguish esophageal from endotracheal intubation.[16] This test is mistrusted by many because of (1) inability to distinguish gases expelled passing through the ETT from gases passing through or around a tube misplaced in the esophagus, (2) inability to distinguish gases being expelled through the nose, and (3) inability to distinguish esophageal and stomach gases present from prior mask ventilation.[16]

j. TUBE CONDENSATION OF WATER VAPOR

The basic principle of tube condensation as a sign of ETT placement is that water vapor seen in clear plastic ETTs is more likely to be present with gases exhaled through a tracheally placed tube than with gases emanating from the stomach through a tube in the esophagus (Fig. 32-2). Two studies have demonstrated water condensation in all cases in which ETTs were placed in the trachea.[36,42] However, water condensation can and does occur when ETTs are placed in the esophagus. The fact that condensation was noticed in 85% of esophageal intubations in one study and in 28% in another study should strongly discourage its presence from being interpreted as a reliable indicator of a successful intubation.[36,42]

k. NASOGASTRIC TUBES, GASTRIC ASPIRATES, INTRODUCERS, AND OTHER DEVICES

A test devised to distinguish between tracheal and esophageal placement of an ETT involves threading a lubricated NGT through the tube in question, applying continuous suction, and attempting to withdraw the NGT.[43] This test exploits the distinguishing feature that the esophagus will collapse around the NGT when suction is applied, whereas free suction applied in the trachea will continue.

In a study of 20 patients in whom both trachea and esophagus were intubated, the ability to maintain suction and the ease of withdrawal during continuous suction clearly distinguished between the two positions.[43] When the NGT was in the trachea, suction applied to it could be maintained easily because the trachea remained patent and air was entrained through the open end of the tube. This allowed the NGT to be withdrawn easily despite suctioning. In contrast, when suction was applied to the NGT in the esophagus, the esophageal wall collapsed around it, thereby obstructing suction and interfering with easy withdrawal of the NGT. Although the length of the NGT that could be easily inserted before an impediment or resistance was felt (5 to 15 cm distal to the tip of the tube) identified correct tracheal placement, it was less useful in identifying esophageal intubation. Similarly, the nature of the aspirate (mucus versus bile or gastric juice) was found to be of limited value in most patients. Because the total time spent to make these observations was 20 to 30 seconds, the authors concluded that the test is reliable.[43] Despite their enthusiasm, this test is very rarely used because of the availability of better methods.

The Eschmann introducer is a 60-cm-long device (10 cm shorter than other similar devices) composed of two layers: a core of tube woven from Dacron polyester threads and an outer resin layer to provide stiffness, flexibility, and a slippery, water-impervious surface. Frequently, the device is referred to as a "gum elastic bougie"—despite the fact that it is not gum, not elastic, and not a bougie.[44] The introducer has a 35-degree kink located 2.5 cm from its distal end. Because its outer diameter (OD) is 5 mm, it can be used with ETTs with an inner diameter (ID) of 6 mm or greater. The device has been used for many years to facilitate intubation and has been introduced to differentiate tracheal from esophageal intubation in emergencies when there is doubt about the ETT location.[26] When inserted through the lumen of the ETT, the curved tip of the lubricated introducer may be felt rubbing over the tracheal rings, and resistance is encountered as the tip of the introducer meets the carina or a main stem bronchus at approximately 28 to 32 cm in the adult. If the ETT is in the esophagus, the introducer passes without resistance to the distal end of the esophagus or stomach.[26] Forceful insertion of an excessive length of the introducer could conceivably result in bronchial rupture or other injuries. This has led the manufacturer to discourage its use as an ETT changer, because other devices specifically designed for this purpose are now available.[45]

l. TRANSTRACHEAL ILLUMINATION

The success of transillumination of the soft tissues of the neck anterior to the trachea in accomplishing guided oral or nasal intubation has culminated in the development of improved lighted stylets and introducers (see

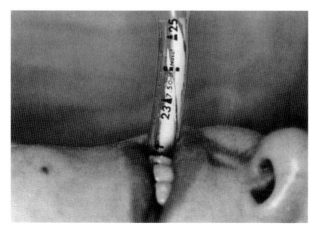

Figure 32-2 Condensation of water vapor seen in an endotracheal tube after endotracheal intubation during exhalation.

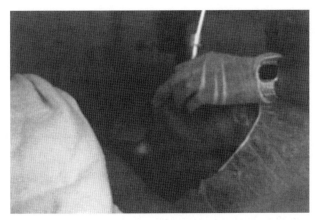

Figure 32-3 When the lighted stylet (or introducer) enters the larynx, an intense, circumscribed, midline glow seen in the region of the laryngeal prominence is suggestive of endotracheal intubation.

Chapter 21).[46-48] It has also prompted investigators to use transtracheal illumination to differentiate esophageal from tracheal ETT placement and to position the ETT accurately inside the trachea. Transmission of light through tissues depends on thickness, compactness, color, density, and light absorption characteristics of the tissue; wavelength, quality, and intensity of the light; proximity of the tissue to the light source; and the ambient lighting conditions in the room.[49] Typically, endotracheal intubation with the lighted stylet or introducer inside the ETT or placement of the stylet in the lumen of the ETT after intubation gives off an intense, circumscribed, midline glow in the region of the laryngeal prominence and sternal notch (Fig. 32-3). The illumination is mostly seen opposite the thyrohyoid, cricothyroid, and cricotracheal membranes. In the event of esophageal intubation, the light is either absent or perceived as dull and diffuse.

To enhance transillumination, darkening the room, dimming the overhead lights, and applying cricoid pressure (to approximate the tracheal wall to the light source and stretch the soft tissues anterior to the light source) have been recommended.[46-49] Newer lighted stylets or introducers, battery operated or incorporating a fiberoptic light source, have brighter lights than earlier prototypes. Consequently, dimming of the overhead lights or application of cricoid pressure may not be necessary. The reliability of transtracheal illumination in distinguishing esophageal from endotracheal intubation in adults has been demonstrated.[49,50] In one study conducted on five cadavers, only 1 of 56 intratracheal placements was misidentified as esophageal, whereas of 112 extratracheal placements (esophageal or pyriform fossa), 1 was misidentified as intratracheal.[50] In another study of 420 adult patients, tracheal transillumination was graded as excellent in 81% of patients and as good in the remaining 19%.[49] In contrast, transesophageal illumination could not be demonstrated in any patient. Despite these reports, false-negative results (ETT in trachea but no transillumination) with the use of the newer lighted stylets and introducers in patients with neck swelling or dark skin and in obese patients have been noticed.[31] Similarly, occasional false-positive results have been observed in thin patients. Nonetheless, the use of transillumination could

reduce unrecognized esophageal intubations, especially outside the operating room where other technical aids are not available.[49,50]

Reports have delineated several complications with these transillumination devices.[51-53] Loss of the bulb into the lung necessitating bronchoscopic removal has been reported.[51] A change in design involving encasement of the bulb in a plastic retaining cover has virtually eliminated the possibility of this complication in future.[47] Other reports have described arytenoid subluxation.[52,53] However, this complication can occur after conventional intubation, and there is no evidence of an increased incidence with the use of lighted stylets.

m. PULSE OXIMETRY AND DETECTION OF CYANOSIS

Although unrecognized esophageal intubation ultimately leads to a severe fall in O_2 saturation (and detectable cyanosis), minutes may elapse before this happens. A disturbing finding that emerged from the ASA closed claims study is that detection of esophageal intubation required longer than 5 minutes in 97% of cases.[1] Furthermore, detectable cyanosis preceded the recognition of esophageal intubation in only one third of cases. Several factors contribute to the delay in diagnosing esophageal intubation by pulse oximetry or in detecting cyanosis, or both.

Reliance on the appearance of cyanosis as a clue to esophageal intubation can contribute to such a delay. Recognition of cyanosis usually necessitates the presence of more than 5 g/dL of reduced hemoglobin, which corresponds to 75% to 85% O_2 saturation.[54] The detection may also depend on the concentration and type of hemoglobin. With severe anemia, cyanosis may not be apparent until the arterial oxygen saturation (Sao_2) falls to 60%. An infant with a high proportion of fetal hemoglobin may still look "pink" at an arterial partial pressure of oxygen (Pao_2) near 40 mm Hg because of the increased blood affinity of O_2 and leftward shifting of the fetal oxyhemoglobin dissociation curve; for this reason, a serious reduction in Pao_2 may develop before cyanosis is apparent.[55] Recognition of cyanosis is influenced by the limited exposure of the patient's body and the insensitivity of the human eye to changes in skin color or even the color of the blood during arterial desaturation. It could also be affected by variations in room lighting and the color of the surgical drapes.

Noninvasive monitoring of oxygen saturation by pulse oximetry (SpO_2) has proved to be a reliable indicator of Sao_2.[56,57] It is undoubtedly quicker to detect changes in SpO_2 than to rely on clinical detection of cyanosis. The main limitation of pulse oximetry is that it does not measure Pao_2, which may fall long before SpO_2 is affected.

Preoxygenation of the patient's lungs before anesthetic induction extends the period of time before a decrease in Sao_2 occurs in case of esophageal intubation.[58,59] In general, O_2 deprivation or apnea after air breathing results in a substantial fall in Pao_2 within 90 seconds, whereas Pao_2, after O_2 breathing, remains higher than 100 mm Hg for at least 3 minutes of apnea, and Sao_2 does not change during this period.[54,58] Consequently, pulse oximetry after preoxygenation does not immediately indicate that the esophagus has been intubated.[59] Because of this prolonged interval with normal SpO_2 being recorded initially after the intubation attempt, misplacement of the ETT may not be suspected later when SpO_2 begins to decrease.[1,59] Furthermore, the risk of misinterpretation of clinical findings suggestive of esophageal intubation may be greater when other clues such as decrease in SpO_2 or cyanosis are not yet manifest.[1] This "hazard" of preoxygenation has led a few clinicians to abandon such a practice so that esophageal intubation can be more readily appreciated.[60] One does not need to go to such extremes as to abandon a practice that has definite merits. However, the presence of normal pulse oximetry readings after intubation should not be taken as evidence of successful endotracheal intubation, and after preoxygenation, oxyhemoglobin desaturation, as indicated by pulse oximetry, is a relatively late manifestation of esophageal intubation.[1,13,59,61-63]

Both O_2 consumption and cardiac output can influence the Sao_2 through their effects on mixed venous oxygen tension ($P\bar{v}O_2$) and mixed venous oxygen content ($C\bar{v}O_2$).[54] A decrease in O_2 consumption associated with anesthetic induction or an increase in cardiac output or both can lead to an increase in $P\bar{v}O_2$ and $C\bar{v}O_2$. The high $P\bar{v}O_2$ retards the decrease in PaO_2 in the event of O_2 deprivation resulting from esophageal intubation and consequently may delay its recognition. Conversely, in patients with low Sao_2 and in those who have high O_2 consumption (e.g., children, women in labor, morbidly obese patients) or decreased functional residual capacity (FRC), oxyhemoglobin desaturation may occur faster.

With the vocal cords open, manual ventilation into the esophagus can result in alveolar gas exchange. In 18 of 20 patients studied after intentional intubation of both the esophagus and the trachea, ventilation into the esophagus caused cyclic compression of the lungs by the distending stomach and esophagus, leading to some gas exchange evidenced by recording of carbon dioxide at the proximal end of the ETT.[35] Although in this situation esophageal ventilation causes ventilation of the lungs with room air, it considerably delays the onset of cyanosis and oxyhemoglobin desaturation. Similarly, respiratory efforts by a spontaneously breathing patient through the unintubated trachea may delay the recognition of esophageal intubation. Esophageal ventilation may also be effective in yielding apneic oxygenation if the cords are open and there is a leak around the cuff of the misplaced esophageal tube.

n. THE BECK AIRWAY AIRFLOW MONITOR

The Beck Airway Airflow Monitor (BAAM; Great Plains Ballistics, Lubbock, TX) consists of a cylindrical plastic whistle with a 2-mm-diameter aperture (Fig. 32-4). When connected to the proximal end of an ETT in a spontaneously breathing patient, the airflow is forced through the small lumen, producing a loud whistle.[64] The pitch during inspiration and exhalation differs because of varying airflow velocities. The BAAM has been used to assist blind intubation and guide the ETT into the trachea. The loudness of the whistle indicates proximity to the tracheal air column, whereas cessation of the sound implies esophageal intubation, obstruction of the ETT, or excessive leak around the ETT. In patients who are not breathing spontaneously, a gentle squeeze of the chest

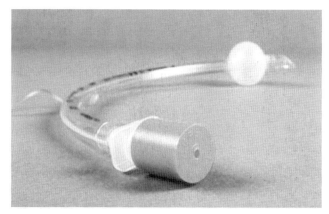

Figure 32-4 The Beck Airway Airflow Monitor (BAAM) attaches to a standard 15-mm endotracheal tube connector and magnifies airway-airflow sounds. (Courtesy of Life-Assist, Inc., Rancho Cordova, CA.)

produces whistling if the ETT is in the trachea. Because the whistle is produced by the airflow, an ETT in the pharynx can produce a whistle. Reports on this device have been limited to case reports and one study in neonates.[64] More research is needed to determine its validity.

o. CHEST RADIOGRAPHY

A chest radiograph can diagnose esophageal intubation if the ETT is located in the lower esophagus distal to the carina (Fig. 32-5).[65] Because a tube in the esophagus is

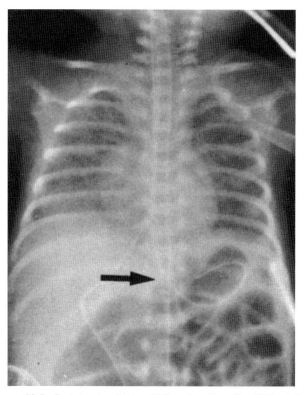

Figure 32-5 Endotracheal tube (ETT) malposition. The ETT is at the gastroesophageal junction (*arrow*). Moderate intestinal dilation is seen. (From Mandel GA: Neonatal intensive care radiology. In Goodman LR, Putman CE, editors: *Intensive care radiology: Imaging of the critically ill*, Philadelphia, 1983, WB Saunders, p 290.)

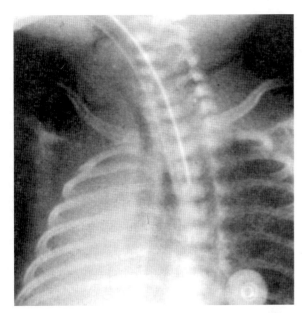

Figure 32-6 Right posterior oblique portable chest radiograph with patient's head turned to the right shows air-filled trachea projecting to right of endotracheal tube (ETT). The ETT aligns with the air-filled distal esophagus. This is the best position for diagnosis of esophageal intubation. (From Smith GM, Reed JC, Choplin RH: Radiographic detection of esophageal malpositioning of ETTs. *AJR Am J Roentgenol* 154:23, 1990.)

often projected over the tracheal air column on anteroposterior chest radiographs, the radiologic features of esophageal intubation are usually difficult to assess.[63] However, it should be suspected in the following situations[63,65]:

- If any part of the border of the ETT is seen outside or lateral to the air column of the tracheobronchial tree (in the absence of a pneumomediastinum)
- In the presence of esophageal air and gastric distention, particularly if an NGT is in place
- If there is a noticeable deviation of the trachea caused by an overinflated cuff.

Although a lateral view of the chest could precisely reveal esophageal intubation, such views are often difficult to obtain. However, in one study, ETT location was identified correctly in 92% of the films taken with the patient in a 25-degree right posterior oblique position with the head turned to the right side.[63] Because the esophagus is located slightly to the left as well as behind the trachea, this projection presents the relationship *en face* with respect to the radiologic beam, resulting in avoidance of superimposition of the trachea over the esophagus (Fig. 32-6). Because radiography is time-consuming and not failsafe, it should never be relied on for diagnosis of esophageal intubation, even in the critical care setting.

p. IMPEDANCE RESPIROMETRY

Impedance respirometry, which measures electrical conductivity of the thorax, has been used to monitor respiratory rate in the critical care setting and to monitor apnea in infants. The ability of impedance respirometry to distinguish esophageal from endotracheal intubation has

been explored.[66,67] A high-frequency alternating current is passed between two electrodes placed on the anterior chest wall. With the increase in lung volume during inspiration, there is an associated decrease in lung electrical conductivity and therefore increased impedance.[66,67] These changes can be measured and displayed as a waveform. If the esophagus is intubated, such an effect on thoracic impedance should be absent. Although assessment by thoracic impedance plethysmography was found to have 100% sensitivity in the detection of esophageal ETT placement in a study in adult patients,[66] it correctly identified only 76 of 80 ETTs in children.[67] Of those incorrectly identified, one was in the trachea and three were in the esophagus. Obviously, more studies are needed before any conclusions can be made. Although it is not a perfect test, use of impedance respirometry could decrease the time taken to identify incorrect placement when combined with other methods of ETT verification.[67]

2. Almost Failsafe Methods

a. IDENTIFICATION OF CARBON DIOXIDE IN EXHALED GAS

The availability of capnometry (measurement of CO_2 in expired gas) and capnography (instantaneous display of the CO_2 waveform during the respiratory cycle) for intraoperative monitoring has prompted clinicians to extend their use to facilitate detection of esophageal intubation.[35,68-71] The principle of use stems from the fact that exhaled CO_2 can be reliably detected during controlled or spontaneous ventilation in patients with adequate pulmonary flow whose trachea is intubated, whereas no CO_2 can be detected in gases emanating from an ETT in the esophagus.

Studies have revealed that the combined use of capnography and pulse oximetry could avert more than 80% of mishaps considered preventable.[72] In an amendment to its original basic intraoperative monitoring standards, the ASA stated the following: "When an ETT is inserted, its correct positioning in the trachea must be verified by clinical assessment and by identification of CO_2 in the expired gas. End-tidal CO_2 ($Etco_2$) analysis, in use from the time of ETT placement, is strongly encouraged." (Standards for Basic Anesthetic Monitoring, 2003 Directory of Members, American Society of Anesthesiologists, Park Ridge, IL, p 493.) Identification of CO_2 in the exhaled gas has emerged as the standard for verification of proper ETT placement. Furthermore, interruption of CO_2 sampling in the exhaled gas due to disconnection, obstruction, accidental tracheal extubation, or total loss of ventilation is immediately detected. Two main methods are currently used: capnography and colorimetric detection of CO_2.

CAPNOGRAPHY. Currently available CO_2 analyzers use various principles to measure CO_2 in the inspired and exhaled gases on a breath-to-breath basis and display the CO_2 waveform by mass spectrometry, infrared absorption spectrometry, or Raman scattering. A normal capnographic waveform in relation to the respiratory cycle is shown in Figure 32-7.[73] A mass spectrometric tracing showing CO_2 waveforms after esophageal intubation and

NORMAL CAPNOGRAM

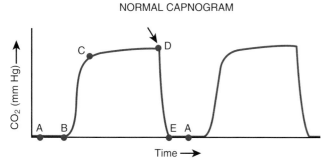

Figure 32-7 The CO_2 waveform. *A,* Expiratory pause begins. *A–B,* Clearance of anatomic dead space. *B–C,* Dead space air mixed with alveolar air. *C–D,* Alveolar plateau. *D,* End-tidal partial pressure of CO_2 registered by capnograph *(arrow)* and beginning of inspiratory phase. *D–E,* Clearance of dead space air. *E–A,* Inspiratory gas devoid of CO_2. (Modified from May WS, Heavner JE, McWorther D, Racz G: *Capnography in the operating room: An introductory directory,* New York, 1985, Raven Press, p 1.)

after correct placement of the ETT in the trachea is shown in Figure 32-8. Although capnography typically distinguishes tracheal from esophageal intubation, false-negative results (i.e., ETT in trachea, absent waveform) and false-positive results (i.e., ETT in esophagus or pharynx, present waveform) have been reported.

Since the advent of capnography to confirm ETT placement, there have been reports of markedly different problems yielding unexpected false-negative results. For

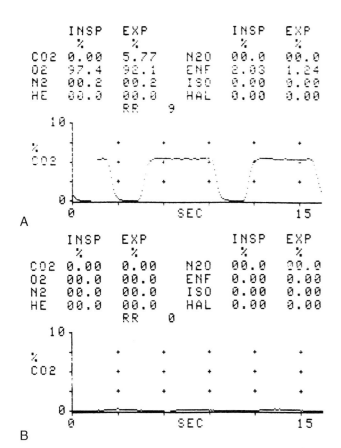

Figure 32-8 A, Normal capnograph, endotracheal tube (ETT) in trachea. **B,** Absent capnograph, ETT in esophagus.

example, disconnection of the ETT from the breathing apparatus, apnea, and equipment failure may be misinterpreted as absent waveform caused by esophageal intubation.[74] A kinked or obstructed ETT interferes with sampling of exhaled gas and may lead to an absent or distorted waveform. Lack of a CO_2 waveform caused by severe bronchospasm has also been reported.[74] Unintentional application of positive end-expiratory pressure (PEEP) to a loosely fitted or uncuffed ETT can cause exhaled gases to escape around the distal lumen of the tube and may result in a sampling error and absent waveform.[75] In addition, dilution of exhaled gases by high fresh gas flow in a Mapleson D system when proximal sidestream sampling is used in infants weighing less than 10 kg leads to erroneous sampling.[76,77] This problem can be corrected by distal sampling from the ETT, up to the 12 cm mark; by use of a mainstream sampling device; or by use of special ventilators.[77] Lower sampling flow rates and gas sampling line leaks can result in artifactually low exhaled CO_2 values and an abnormal waveform.[78,79]

Marked diminution of pulmonary blood flow increases the alveolar component of the dead space.[54,70] Low cardiac output, hypotension, pulmonary embolism, pulmonary stenosis, tetralogy of Fallot, and kinking or clamping of the pulmonary artery during pulmonary surgery all cause a decrease in end-tidal carbon dioxide partial pressure (P_{ETCO_2}), reflecting an increase in alveolar dead space.[54,80,81] Other factors contributing to the increased alveolar dead space during anesthesia include patient age, large V_T, use of negative phase during exhalation, short inspiratory phase, and presence of pulmonary disease.[54,81] As a result of the widespread destruction of alveolar capillaries in patients with chronic obstructive pulmonary disease, an increased alveolar dead space ensues. An increase in alveolar dead space is manifested as a decrease in P_{ETCO_2} and an increase in the Pa_{CO_2} to P_{ETCO_2} difference (normally 0 to 5 mm Hg).[54,81] If capnography alone is relied on to confirm ETT placement in patients who have a very large alveolar dead space, the low P_{ETCO_2} values might mislead the clinician into thinking that the ETT was not placed in the trachea.

An abrupt reduction in cardiac output reduces P_{ETCO_2} by two mechanisms: First, a reduction in venous return causes a decrease in CO_2 delivered to the lungs, and second, the increase in alveolar dead space dilutes the CO_2 from normally perfused alveoli, thus decreasing P_{ETCO_2}.[82-84] When cardiac arrest ensues, CO_2 is no longer delivered to or eliminated through the lungs even if ventilation is adequate, and consequentially P_{ETCO_2} values exponentially decrease to remarkably low values (<0.5%). Ninety seconds after experimentally induced ventricular fibrillation, P_{ETCO_2} is usually decreased by 90%.[85] Accordingly, a decision regarding the location of the ETT based on capnographic findings alone during cardiac arrest may lead to a misdiagnosis.

Experimental cardiac arrest demonstrated a remarkably high correlation between P_{ETCO_2}, cardiac output, and coronary perfusion pressure during closed-chest precordial compression, during open-chest cardiac massage, and after resuscitation.[86,87] Similar observations were reported during episodes of cardiac arrest in critically ill patients.[86,87] The restoration of spontaneous circulation is

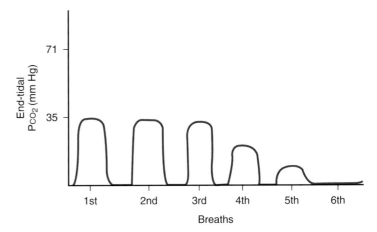

Figure 32-9 CO_2 waveforms obtained in a 10-year-old boy with an esophageal intubation. The waveform looks normal during the first three breaths but becomes flat very quickly. (From Sum Ping ST: Esophageal intubation. *Anesth Analg* 66:483, 1987.)

heralded by a rapid increase in P_{ETCO_2} within 30 seconds. This overshoot in P_{ETCO_2}, which is characteristic of successful resuscitation, may exceed the prearrest value and reflects washout of CO_2 that has accumulated in venous blood and in tissues during circulatory arrest.[86,88] In patients in whom resuscitative efforts fail to restore spontaneous circulation, P_{ETCO_2} remains low or even declines, whereas in those who eventually regain spontaneous circulation, P_{ETCO_2} reaches 19 mm Hg or higher. These observations suggest that capnography can be used for monitoring the adequacy of blood flow generated by precordial compression during cardiopulmonary resuscitation and can serve as a prognostic indicator of successful resuscitation.[86,88]

False-positive results can occur when the ETT is misplaced in the esophagus after exhaled gases are forced into the stomach during bag-mask ventilation preceding intubation attempts.[85,89] If enough alveolar gas reaches the stomach, a CO_2 concentration greater than 2% may be initially detected, and the CO_2 waveform may be indistinguishable from that observed with endotracheal intubation.[35,89,90] In fact, CO_2 waveforms have been observed in one third of esophageal intubations,[90] but repeated ventilation results in rapidly diminishing CO_2 levels while the waveform becomes rather flat and irregular (Fig. 32-9).[35,89] As a result of the dilution with successive ventilation, it is very unlikely that any CO_2 would be detected after the sixth breath or after 1 minute in cases of esophageal intubation, making it easy to distinguish esophageal from endotracheal intubation.[35] It has also been observed that compression of the chest caused clear, peaked CO_2 elevation in 18 of 20 tracheally intubated patients but no changes in esophageal intubation.[35] This simple, quick maneuver together with other signs can confirm proper ETT placement.

False-positive results can potentially occur in cases of esophageal intubation after ingestion of carbonated beverages or antacids.[91-93] High CO_2 levels (20%) are present in all carbonated beverages.[92] Sodium bicarbonate, an ingredient found in most antacids (except sodium citrate), reacts with hydrochloric acid in the stomach, releasing CO_2 levels comparable to those found in alveolar gas. With carbonated beverages, CO_2 levels as high as 5.3% can be measured initially with esophageal ventilation, rendering correct assessment of ETT placement rather difficult.[92] However, rapid decline in CO_2 levels occurs with successive ventilations (Fig. 32-10). The abnormal CO_2 waveform may give an important clue in the early detection of esophageal intubation.[92] Because a normal-looking CO_2 waveform during the first few ventilations is no guarantee of correct ETT placement, the waveform must be watched closely for at least 1 minute after placement of the tube.

It should be emphasized that a normal waveform is not synonymous with presence of the tube in the trachea.[89] A normal waveform may be observed without a tube present in the trachea during spontaneous or controlled ventilation in cases of face mask anesthesia, use of a laryngeal mask airway, and use of the esophageal-tracheal Combitube (ETC) (Tyco-Healthcare-Kendall-Sheridan Corporation, Mansfield, MA), with which ventilation is carried out through the pharyngeal perforations.[94,95] A normal waveform may also be present and sustained if the distal end of the ETT is in the pharynx but not necessarily in the trachea.[94] This situation should be suspected by the unusual volume of cuff air required to stop the leak and an increased peak inspiratory pressure.

Although capnography has been widely used in operating rooms, its use in emergency rooms, intensive care units, and hospital floors has been rather limited because of the need for warm-up and careful calibration time; the requirement for an external power source, which limits use in emergency situations; and the fact that the technology is not easily transferable to the patient's side. Portable apnea monitors that use infrared spectrometry for sensing CO_2 have been used for confirmation of ETT placement.[96] Although they do not accurately quantify CO_2 concentration, a moving-bar indicator with seven light-emitting diodes does provide an estimate of 1.5 percentage points per illuminated diode. Gas is aspirated through plastic tubing attached to the elbow connector proximal to the ETT, allowing the monitor to sense CO_2 in the first exhalation after intubation. The device is cheap and portable, operates for 90 minutes on batteries, and requires neither warm-up time nor calibration. This electronic instrument can also function as a breathing circuit disconnection alarm.[96]

COLORIMETRIC END-TIDAL CARBON DIOXIDE DETECTION. Early studies attempted to quantitate the amount

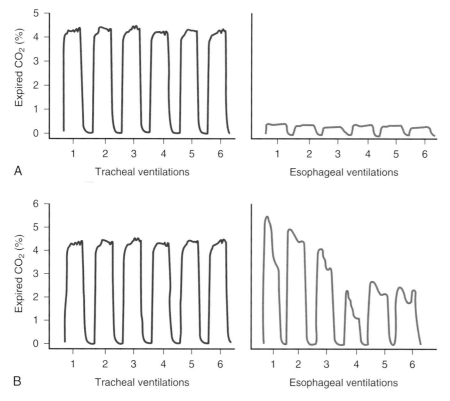

A Tracheal ventilations   Esophageal ventilations

B Tracheal ventilations   Esophageal ventilations

Figure 32-10 Expired CO_2 waveform during tracheal and esophageal ventilations before **(A)** and after **(B)** addition of a carbonated beverage in the stomach. (From Sum Ping ST, Mehta MP, Symreng T: Reliability of capnography in identifying esophageal intubation with carbonated beverage or antacid in the stomach. *Anesth Analg* 73:333–337, 1991.)

of CO_2 in exhaled gas and relied on the reaction of CO_2 with another substance such as barium hydroxide to produce a color change.[97] Thereafter, chemical indicators that change colors in the presence of increased hydrogen ion concentrations were used. The Einstein CO_2 detector was constructed by attaching a 15-mm adapter to one end of a DeLee mucus trap containing a mixture of 3 mL of phenolphthalein and 3 mL of cresol. When the exhaled gas is bubbled through the chamber, carbonic acid formation causes a dramatic color change from red to yellow within seconds. Failure of the solution to change from red to yellow should suggest esophageal intubation.[98]

Several disposable colorimetric CO_2 detectors are currently available. The Easy Cap II CO_2 Detector (Nellcor Puritan Bennett, New York, NY; Fig. 32-11) can be connected between an ETT and a breathing circuit or bag-mask assembly.[99-104] The detector contains filter paper impregnated with a colorless liquid base and a pH-sensitive indicator (metacresol purple) that reversibly changes from purple to yellow as a result of pH change when exposed to CO_2 and reverts to purple when CO_2 is no longer present. The color changes are made visible through a transparent dome in the plastic housing of the device. In general, a purple color (A range) indicates a CO_2 level of 0.5% or less. The B range is a dusty tan color, reflecting levels of 0.5% to 2%. When the detector is exposed to CO_2 levels greater than 2%, the color brightens to a yellow-tan color, the C range.

Studies have shown that colorimetric $PETCO_2$ monitoring is reliable in verifying proper ETT placement in nonarrested patients.[99-104] In one study,[103] the mean minimum CO_2 concentration required for detection of the perceivable color change was 0.54% (4.1 mm Hg) and ranged from 0.25% to 0.60% (1.9 to 4.6 mm Hg). When an ETT is correctly placed in a patient with adequate pulmonary blood flow, the detector should register C. The color change occurs immediately with the first breath in almost all patients. In the nonarrested patient when the device registers low or absent CO_2 (A reading), esophageal

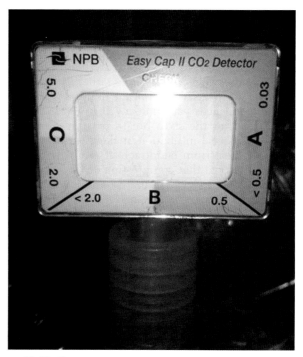

Figure 32-11 The colorimetric carbon dioxide detector. (Easy Cap II CO_2 Detector, Nellcor Puritan Bennett, New York, NY).

intubation should be strongly suspected. If a C reading is obtained in an arrested patient, proper ETT placement is confirmed. In contrast, an A reading (absence of color change) during manual ventilation in a patient with cardiac arrest is consistent with either an esophageal or an endotracheal intubation in patients with profound low-flow state resulting from prolonged arrest or inadequate resuscitation. In another study, for 28 of 106 endotracheal intubations in "pulseless" patients the detector did not show any color change, indicating a $PaCO_2$ of less than 4 mm Hg.[104] A multicenter trial of a colorimetric CO_2 detection device found that all cardiac arrest patients who survived to admission had a value of C registered on the monitor.[105] No patient in whom the detector failed to register color change survived. Therefore, the device may be useful as a prognostic indicator of successful resuscitation.[104]

Although the availability of such a device is considered a great leap forward, it has its own pitfalls and is not a substitute for assessment skills. Because the device has a dead space of 38 mL, the manufacturer does not recommend its use in children weighing less than 15 kg, although its efficacy in verifying endotracheal intubation has been confirmed in infants as young as 6 months.[106] The color change may be difficult to discern under low-light conditions and may be misinterpreted by color-blind individuals. The detector is not sensitive to temperature, but it is eventually affected by humidity. Water vapor interferes with the chemical reaction and inactivates the device; it can be rendered ineffective within 15 minutes if the patient is receiving humidified gases. It has been suggested that trapping the humidity with a passive moisture exchanger may extend the useful life of the device.[106] The manufacturer cautions against use of the device in conjunction with a heated humidifier or nebulizer and emphasizes that it is not intended to be used for longer than 10 minutes after intubation. Because the indicator permanently changes color if exposed for a prolonged period to low CO_2 or other acids in the air, the device is packaged in a gas-impermeable metallic foil and is marketed as a single-use item. The packaged detector has a shelf life of 15 months if left unopened but may not function properly if the package is accidentally opened and the device is exposed to room air for several hours. For this reason, it is essential to verify that the indicator color is purple before use. Clinicians should familiarize themselves with the $EtCO_2$ detectors in their institutions and the appropriate color changes before use of these detectors.

Widespread use of colorimetric CO_2 detectors has been hampered by limitations in their performance characteristics. Newer colorimetric CO_2 indicators seem to have overcome some of these limitations.[107] With this improved technology, it is expected that detectors will be more durable during prolonged exposure to heat, humidity, and CO_2. Furthermore, they will be cheaper and will have a longer shelf life. However, there are potential sources of rare errors with the use of colorimetric CO_2 monitoring, even in the nonarrested patient. After manual bag-mask ventilation before intubation, CO_2 from the exhaled air may be blown into the stomach and may result in detectable CO_2 levels, yielding a false-positive

yellow color if the ETT is misplaced in the esophagus. Ventilating the patient with six breaths results in a washout of CO_2 to near-zero if the ETT is misplaced in the esophagus. Close observation of the color of the detector is essential during and after the delivery of six quick breaths so that false-positive results are avoided.

Concerns about inadvertent detection of gastric CO_2 from ingested beverages after esophageal intubation, which can potentially vitiate colorimetric CO_2 detection, have been raised.[101] In a study of carbonated beverage ingestion and esophageal intubation in the cardiac arrest porcine model, the amount of CO_2 released did not result in spurious color change of the detector in the four animals studied and did not cause difficulty in interpretation of the readings.[108] Therefore, concern that false-positive results might be caused by esophageal placement in a patient who has recently ingested carbonated beverages appears to be unwarranted.[104,108]

Colorimetric CO_2 is a simple, safe, highly sensitive, reliable, and quick method for confirming ETT placement in the nonarrested patient. Unlike capnography, it is portable (pocket sized) and does not require calibration or a power source. It is useful in places where capnography is unavailable, such as hospital floors, emergency departments, and prehospital settings. As with capnography, false-negative results (i.e., ETT in trachea, no color change) may occur. Very rarely, false-positive results (i.e., ETT in esophagus, with color change) can occur with the first few breaths. In the arrested patient, interpretation of "no color change" requires caution because it may indicate circulatory arrest, inadequate resuscitation, or esophageal intubation.

b. ESOPHAGEAL DETECTOR DEVICE/SELF-INFLATING BULB

Use of the esophageal detector device (EDD) is based on anatomic differences between the trachea and the esophagus.[109] The trachea in the adult is 10 to 12 cm long, and its diameter can vary from 13 to 22 mm. The trachea remains constantly patent because of C-shaped rigid, cartilaginous rings that are joined vertically by fibroelastic tissue and closed posteriorly by unstriped trachealis muscle. The esophagus is a fibromuscular tube, 25 cm long in adults, which extends from the cricopharyngeal sphincter to the gastroesophageal junction; there is no intrinsic structure to maintain its patency.

Wee and O'Leary and their colleagues introduced a new method using a simple device to distinguish esophageal from endotracheal intubation.[109,110] The principle underlying use of the EDD is that the esophagus collapses when a negative pressure is applied to its lumen, whereas the trachea does not. The device consists of a 60-mL syringe fitted by an adapter that can be attached to an ETT connector. When the syringe is attached to an ETT placed in the trachea, withdrawal of the plunger of the syringe aspirates gas freely from the patient's lungs without any resistance apart from that inherent in the device (Fig. 32-12). If the ETT is in the esophagus, withdrawal of the plunger causes apposition of the walls of the esophagus, occluding its lumen around the ETT, and a negative pressure or resistance is felt when the plunger is pulled back. Wee conducted a study in 100 patients in whom placement of ETTs and esophageal tubes was

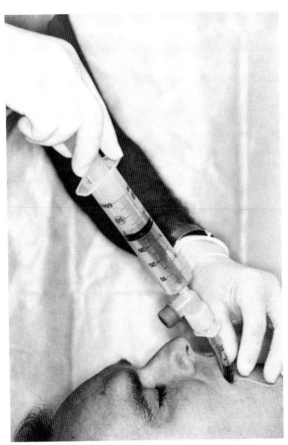

Figure 32-12 The esophageal detector device consists of a 60-mL syringe fitted by an adapter to an endotracheal tube connector.

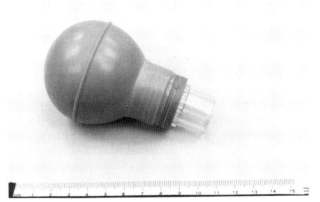

Figure 32-13 The self-inflating bulb is fitted with a standard 15-mm adapter. (From Salem MR, Wafai Y, Joseph NJ, et al: Efficacy of the self-inflating bulb in detecting esophageal intubation: Does the presence of a nasogastric tube or cuff deflation make a difference? *Anesthesiology* 80:42–48, 1994.)

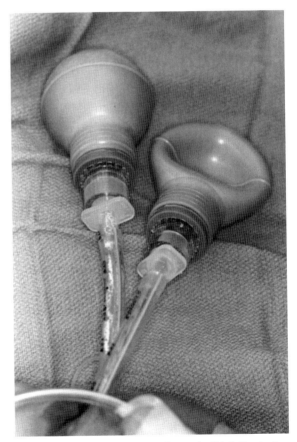

Figure 32-14 In a demonstration, collapsed self-inflating bulbs were connected simultaneously to tracheally and esophageally placed endotracheal tubes (ETTs) in the presence of a nasogastric tube. The bulb connected to the ETT in the trachea instantaneously reinflated, whereas that connected to the ETT in the esophagus remained collapsed. (From Salem MR, Wafai Y, Joseph NJ, et al: Efficacy of the self-inflating bulb in detecting esophageal intubation: Does the presence of a nasogastric tube or cuff deflation make a difference? *Anesthesiology* 80:42–48, 1994.)

assessed using the EDD.[109] There were 99 first-time correct identifications of ETT placement, and the mean time required to diagnose tube placement was 6.9 seconds. Application of constant but slow aspiration has been recommended to avoid the suction effect and prevent mucosal damage. Endotracheal intubation is confirmed if 30 to 40 mL of gas is aspirated without resistance in adults or 5 to 10 mL in children older than 2 years of age.[109-111]

Nunn simplified the EDD by replacing the syringe with an Ellik evacuator, which is a self-inflating bulb (SIB) with a capacity of 75 to 90 mL.[112] After intubation, the device is connected to the ETT, and the bulb is compressed. Compression is silent, and refill is instantaneous if the ETT is in the trachea. In contrast, if the ETT is in the esophagus, compression of the SIB is accompanied by a characteristic flatus-like noise, and the SIB remains collapsed on release. The test can be accomplished easily within 3 seconds, and the outcome is unmistakable.[113] This technique has been further modified by compressing the SIB before, rather than after, connection to the ETT connector.[114] Investigations that used the latter technique confirmed earlier studies and demonstrated that the sensitivity, specificity, and predictive value of the SIB are 100% (Figs. 32-13 and 32-14).[115-118]

Despite the efficacy of both the EDD and the SIB in differentiating esophageal from endotracheal intubation in essentially healthy patients, there have been reports of false-negative results (i.e., the ETT is in the trachea, but gas cannot be aspirated by the EDD or the SIB does not reinflate). The EDD or the SIB may fail to confirm ETT placement in infants, in whom the tracheal wall is not held open by rigid cartilaginous rings; if the ETT is obstructed by kinking or by the presence of material in the ETT; and in patients with severe bronchospasm.[119-122] Slow or no reinflation of the SIB may be encountered if the tube bevel is at the carina or in the right main stem bronchus.[24] In such cases, slight retraction or rotation of the ETT usually corrects the position of the tube and orientation of the bevel, resulting in instantaneous reinflation of the SIB.[121,123] The SIB may also fail to reinflate or may reinflate slowly when connected to a properly placed ETT in patients with morbid obesity (MO)[123,124] and in patients who have a marked reduction in expiratory reserve volume, such as in those with pulmonary edema or adult respiratory distress syndrome, parturients undergoing cesarean section, and patients undergoing chest compression during resuscitation. The presence of secretions causing airway obstruction may also lead to a false-negative result.[123,125]

In a study involving 2140 consecutive anesthetized adult patients,[123] the overall incidence of false-negative results with the SIB (i.e., no reinflation or reinflation delayed for longer than 4 seconds) was 3.6%. It was apparent that the choice of technique used can contribute to false-negative results. When the SIB was fully compressed before connection to the ETT in 1117 patients, the incidence was 4.6%, whereas false-negatives were reduced to 2.4% in 1023 patients when the SIB was compressed after connection to the ETT. Most of the patients (85.5%) in whom false-negative results were obtained had MO (body mass index >35 kg/m²) (Table 32-3). We surmise that this phenomenon seen in patients with MO and in pregnant women is related to marked

TABLE 32-3

Demographics of False-Negative Results in Determining Correct ETT Placement with the Self-Inflating Bulb

Patient Condition	T1	T2
Morbid obesity	45	20
Severe bronchospasm	2	2
Elderly with chronic obstructive pulmonary disease	2	2
Main stem intubation	1	0
Pulmonary secretions	1	0
Pulmonary edema	0	1
Total	51	25

In T1, the self-inflating bulb (SIB) is compressed before it is connected to the endotracheal tube (ETT). In T2, the SIB is first connected to the ETT and is then compressed. See text for details.
From Wafai Y, Salem MR, Joseph NJ, Baraka A: The self-inflating bulb for confirmation of endotracheal intubation: Incidence and demography of false negatives. *Anesthesiology* 81:A1303, 1994.

reduction in FRC after anesthetic induction and muscular paralysis in the supine position leading to reduced caliber of intrathoracic airways and collapsibility of the trachea on application of subatmospheric pressure by the SIB.[123-125] It is also possible that the negative pressure generated (greater than –50 cm H_2O) may cause collapse and invagination of the posterior tracheal wall. Further compression can occur as a result of mediastinal compression.[124,125] The chain of events that may lead to failure of the SIB to confirm endotracheal intubation is presented in Figure 32-15. If the SIB is compressed after connection to the ETT rather than before, a volume of gas is first introduced into the airway before subatmospheric pressure is generated by the SIB; this would limit the collapse of the SIB that is observed when it is compressed before connection to the ETT.[123-125]

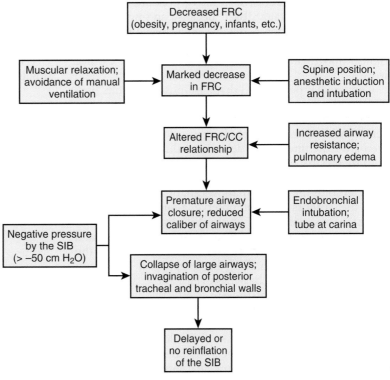

Figure 32-15 Chain of events leading to false-negative results when using the self-inflating bulb *(SIB)* to confirm endotracheal intubation in patients with decreased functional residual capacity. *CC,* Closing capacity; *FRC,* functional residual capacity. (From Lang DJ, Wafai Y, Salem MR, et al: Efficacy of the self-inflating bulb in confirming endotracheal intubation in the morbidly obese. *Anesthesiology* 85:246–253, 1996.)

Advantages of the SIB include low cost, unlimited shelf life, no power source, usability with one hand, and usability in areas of low light. It is quick to use (<10 seconds) and is unaffected by ingested carbonated beverages, antacids, or exhaled CO_2 in the event of esophageal intubation. Unlike capnography, it can confirm endotracheal intubation before manual ventilation is initiated, thus avoiding the undesirable effects of esophageal ventilation.[116,118] The performance of the SIB should not be affected by a cardiac arrest, the presence of an NGT, or cuff deflation.[118] Studies found the EDD/SIB to be more accurate in verifying proper ETT placement in patients with out-of-hospital cardiac arrest and during emergency intubations than CO_2 detection methods.[126,128] Indeed, it has been the method preferred by emergency medical personnel.[126-128] Verification of ETT placement with the SIB enables physicians and emergency personnel to proceed with other resuscitation duties. Other studies found the SIB to be complementary to CO_2 detection.[31,129,130]

Some studies have found a high incidence of false-negative results with the use of the SIB in patients with out-of-hospital cardiac arrest.[130,131] Although the SIB correctly identified all esophageal intubations, it identified only 72% of ETTs placed in the trachea, whereas 60% of the latter were identified by CO_2 detection. Combining the SIB with CO_2 detection enhanced the sensitivity to 90.8%.[130] Possible reasons for incomplete or no reinflation of the SIB were similar to those presented in Table 32-3.

Based on the findings in a porcine cardiac arrest model, it has been suggested that the decreased muscle tone of the posterior tracheal wall that occurs during cardiac arrest could result in mucosal aspiration, airway blockage, and increased false-negative results associated with the use of EDDs.[132] These findings, however, could be explained by the excessive negative pressure generated with the use of certain SIBs.[133] Because no single test for verifying ETT position is reliable, all available modalities should be tested and used in conjunction with proper clinical judgment in cases of out-of-hospital cardiac arrest.[130,131]

Concern has been raised that false-positive results (i.e., ETT in esophagus, but SIB reinflates) may occur as a result of gastric insufflation after bag-mask ventilation before intubation. In one study, it was demonstrated that even after the intentional delivery of three small breaths (300 to 350 mL each), the SIB was effective in detecting esophageal intubation in all 72 patients.[116] In another study, despite the use of mask ventilation before intubation, the authors did not observe a single instance of instantaneous reinflation of the SIB from the esophagus.[113] In a study of one pig, Foutch and associates[134] used a syringe similar to that of Wee[109] and found that the device was effective in detecting esophageal intubation even after 1 minute of bag-mask ventilation.[132] Although these studies imply that the SIB is effective in detecting esophageal intubation after mask ventilation (and modest gastric insufflation), it may fail occasionally in cases of massive gastric insufflation or if the lower esophageal tone is decreased.[125,135] It is recommended that, when the SIB is used to confirm endotracheal intubation, the test

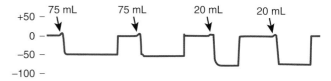

Figure 32-16 Representative tracing of negative pressure (mm Hg) generated by large (75 mL) and small (20 mL) self-inflating bulbs (SIBs) when the SIB is compressed before it is connected to the endotracheal tube placed in the esophagus. The small SIB generates greater negative pressure than the large SIB. See text for details.

should be undertaken before ventilation is initiated through the ETT.

It is essential that the SIB be of an appropriate size.[118,119] Although a smaller SIB (capacity 20 mL) has a smaller radius and therefore generates a higher negative pressure (Fig. 32-16), it is unreliable in detecting esophageal intubation if the SIB is compressed after connection to the ETT.[136] The larger SIB (capacity 75 mL) is recommended because it does not yield false-positive results when either technique is used.[137] Although SIBs can be constructed by fitting a bulb with a standard 15-mm adapter, they are commercially available for single use. The devices are checked before use by connecting the compressed SIB to a clamped ETT; absence of reinflation is an indication of airtightness (Fig. 32-17). We have found that proper function of the device is not affected when a bacterial or viral filter is placed between the device and the ETT connector.

An SIB that incorporates a colorimetric CO_2 detector is now available (Fig. 32-18). This new device (Salem SIB; Mercury Medical, Clearwater, FL) should enable clinicians to assess reinflation of the SIB after connection to the ETT and simultaneously to observe the color change indicative of the presence or absence of CO_2 in the expired gas during reinflation of the SIB. The use of this device should eliminate most of the false results and lead to accurate verification of the location of the ETT before manual ventilation is initiated.

Use of the SIB has been extended to identify the location of the ETC and facilitate its proper positioning using

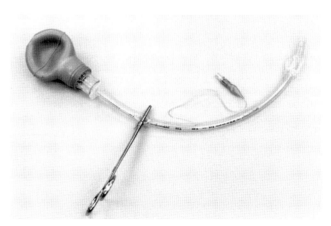

Figure 32-17 Testing the self-inflating bulb for leakage. The compressed bulb is connected to a clamped endotracheal tube. Absence of reinflation is indicative of airtightness. This test reveals any leakage from the bulb or the connector (such as a cracked connector or loose fitting).

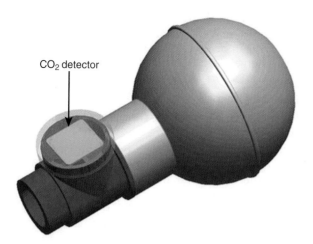

Figure 32-18 Salem self-inflating bulb. See text for details. (Courtesy of Mercury Medical, Clearwater, FL.)

a simple algorithm (Figs. 32-19 and 32-20).[95] This may be of importance if the ETC is used in patients whose lungs cannot be ventilated by mask and whose trachea cannot be intubated. After blind placement, the compressed SIB is connected to the distal lumen. Instantaneous reinflation implies that the ETC is in the trachea and ventilation is carried out through the distal lumen; absence of reinflation is indicative of esophageal placement, which is very common. In this position, the pharyngeal balloon and the distal cuff are inflated and the compressed SIB is connected to the proximal lumen; instantaneous reinflation is expected to occur because the compressed SIB aspirates gas from the lungs through the

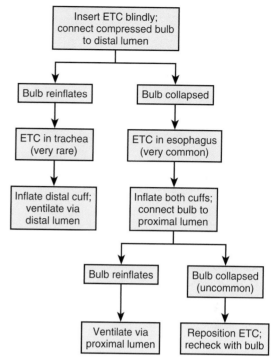

Figure 32-20 Algorithm for identifying the position and facilitating proper placement of the esophageal-tracheal Combitube *(ETC)* after blind placement. (From Wafai Y, Salem MR, Baraka A, et al: Effectiveness of the self-inflating bulb for verification of proper placement of the esophageal-tracheal Combitube. *Anesth Analg* 80:122–126, 1995.)

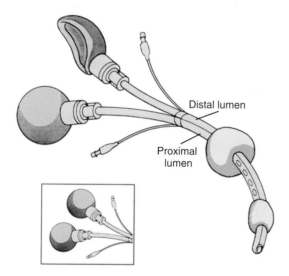

Figure 32-19 Schematic diagram depicting outcome when the compressed self-inflating bulb is connected to the distal and proximal lumens of an esophageal-tracheal Combitube in the esophageal position. Notice that the bulb connected to the distal lumen remains collapsed, whereas that connected to the proximal lumen instantaneously reinflates. The insert depicts the outcome when the Combitube is in the trachea: Both bulbs instantaneously reinflate. (From Wafai Y, Salem MR, Baraka A, et al: Effectiveness of the self-inflating bulb for verification of proper placement of the esophageal-tracheal Combitube. *Anesth Analg* 80:122–126, 1995.)

pharyngeal perforations. If slow or no reinflation of the SIB occurs, repositioning the ETC (pulling it back 1 to 2 cm) may be indicated, and rechecking with the SIB confirms proper placement. Controlled ventilation is then carried out through the proximal lumen. Proper positioning and adequacy of ventilation can be further confirmed by the presence of breath sounds, absence of gastric insufflation, capnography or colorimetric CO_2 detection, and pulse oximetry.[95]

c. ACOUSTIC DEVICES AND REFLECTOMETRY

Devices that use sonic techniques as the basis for distinguishing tracheal from esophageal intubation have been developed. The mechanism of action of the Sonomatic Confirmation of Tracheal Intubation (SCOTI) device (Penlon; Abingdon, Oxfordshire, UK) is recognition of the resonating frequencies, which vary according to whether the tube is in an open structure (trachea) or a closed structure (esophagus).[138] Although the concept is intriguing, the inability to configure the device correctly with all types and lengths of ETTs has limited its usefulness as an indicator of endotracheal intubation.[139-142] Disappointing sales led to withdrawal of the device from the market in 1996.[143]

Another approach employs the principle of acoustic reflectometry by projecting a series of sonic impulses into the airway and placing a miniature microphone in the ETT wall to monitor sound pressure.[144] The presence of deflection at the ETT tip allows discrimination between esophageal and endotracheal intubation. With acoustic

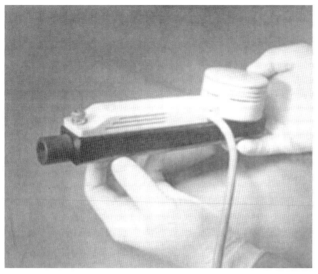

Figure 32-21 A Hood Labs (Pembroke, MA) two-microphone acoustic reflectometer. (From Raphael DT, Benbassat M, Arnaudov D, et al: Validation study of two-microphone acoustic reflectometry for determination of breathing tube placement in 200 adult patients. *Anesthesiology* 97:1371–1377, 2002.)

reflectometry, one-dimensional image of a cavity, such as the airway or the esophagus, is constructed. The reflectometric area-distance profile consists of a constant cross-sectional area segment (length of the ETT), followed either by a rapid increase in the area beyond the tube in case of endotracheal intubation or by an immediate decrease in the area in case of esophageal intubation.[145] In a study of 200 endotracheal intubations confirmed by capnography, acoustic reflectometry correctly identified 198 (Figs. 32-21 through 32-23). In 2 patients, endotracheal intubations were interpreted as an esophageal intubation. However, all 14 esophageal intubations were correctly identified.[146] Because it is noninvasive and rapid (<3 seconds), acoustic imaging may become popular in future in the determination of the location of ETT placement in patients with cardiac arrest, particularly when visualization of the glottis is not possible. With technical improvement in the computer-based system, acoustic reflectometry may have value as an imaging adjunct device that can be used in the diagnosis and treatment of airway emergencies.[146]

3. Failsafe Methods

a. DIRECT VISUALIZATION OF THE ENDOTRACHEAL TUBE BETWEEN THE CORDS

Sighting of the ETT passing through the larynx during intubation or confirmation of the presence of the ETT between the cords after intubation is one of the most reliable methods to ensure correct ETT placement. Two maneuvers can be helpful to assist direct visual confirmation of endotracheal intubation, one during and the other after intubation.

If the ETT is introduced directly posterior to the laryngoscope blade, as shown in Figure 32-24A, the laryngoscopist's view of the cords may be obscured and the ETT may inadvertently enter the esophagus. This can be avoided by directing the ETT from the right corner of the mouth toward the larynx. As seen in Figure 32-24B, this maneuver can allow visualization of the ETT entering the larynx, thus confirming endotracheal intubation. The other maneuver that can be performed after intubation but before removing the laryngoscope from the mouth involves gentle posterior displacement of the ETT toward the palate (Fig. 32-25).[147] The backward push on the tube against the forward traction of the laryngoscope blade exposes the cords by altering the direction of the ETT as it enters the larynx.[147] This maneuver can be helpful in cases in which the cords are obscured by the ETT as it enters the larynx.

Viewing the ETT entering the larynx cannot be accomplished in all cases of direct laryngoscopy, especially if intubation is difficult and during blind nasal intubation. Even after visualization of the ETT entering the larynx, the tube may slip out of the larynx while the laryngoscope is being removed, during taping of the tube, while the patient is being positioned, or during transportation. This tends to occur more frequently if

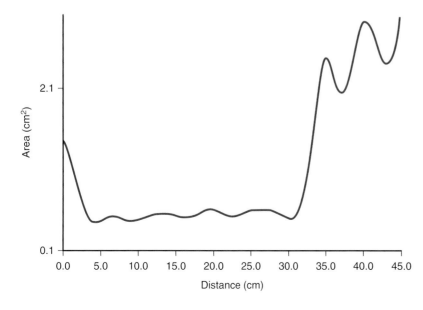

Figure 32-22 An acoustic reflectometry area-distance profile consists of a plot of the total cross-sectional area of the cavity versus axial length down into the cavity. If the endotracheal tube (ETT) is placed in the trachea, the reflectometric profile consists of a constant cross-sectional area segment (length of ETT), followed by a rapid increase in the area beyond the carina. (From Raphael DT, Benbassat M, Arnaudov D, et al: Validation study of two-microphone acoustic reflectometry for determination of breathing tube placement in 200 adult patients. *Anesthesiology* 97:1371–1377, 2002.)

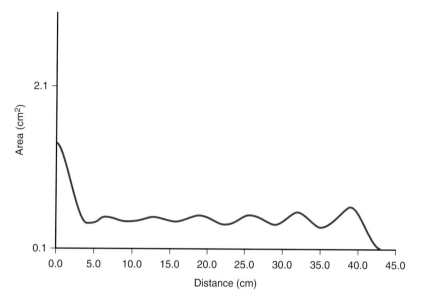

Figure 32-23   If the endotracheal tube (ETT) is placed in the esophagus, the reflectometric profile consists of a constant cross-sectional area segment (length of ETT), followed by an immediate decrease in the area distal to the tube. (From Raphael DT, Benbassat M, Arnaudov D, et al: Validation study of two-microphone acoustic reflectometry for determination of breathing tube placement in 200 adult patients. *Anesthesiology* 97:1371–1377, 2002.)

the distal end of the ETT lies just below the cords or high in the trachea.

b. FLEXIBLE FIBEROPTIC BRONCHOSCOPY

A sure method for confirmation of endotracheal intubation is visualization of the tracheal rings and carina with a flexible fiberoptic bronchoscope (FFB) after intubation.[147-149] This is convenient only when an FFB is readily available or when the instrument is used to aid intubation (see Chapter 19). It should be emphasized that visualization of the vocal cords and tracheal rings through the FFB before the ETT is threaded over it does not guarantee endotracheal intubation. There are three reasons why the ETT may not follow the path of the FFB into the trachea.[148,150-152] First, a stiff, large ETT may carry a relatively thin FFB into the esophagus even if the tip of the scope was originally placed in the larynx and trachea.[148,150] Second, the tip of the tube and its Murphy eye are at 90 degrees to the right when the concavity of the ETT is facing anteriorly.[148,152] Consequently, the tip

of the tube may be blocked from entering the larynx by the right arytenoid cartilage, the vocal cord, or both. If excessive force is used, the tube may slip into the esophagus. This problem can be corrected by a 90-degree counterclockwise rotation.[148,152] Third, if the scope is inserted through a tube placed nasally, the FFB may exit the tube through the Murphy eye and may actually enter the trachea, but in this case it will be impossible to thread the tube over the scope.[148,151] To ensure that endotracheal intubation has been accomplished, the FFB should be withdrawn after placement of the tube and then reintroduced to visualize the tracheal rings and carina and to determine the distance from the distal end of the tube to the carina.[148]

III. VERIFICATION OF ENDOTRACHEAL TUBE INSERTION DEPTH

According to the ASA closed claims analysis, the combination of inadvertent extubation and main stem

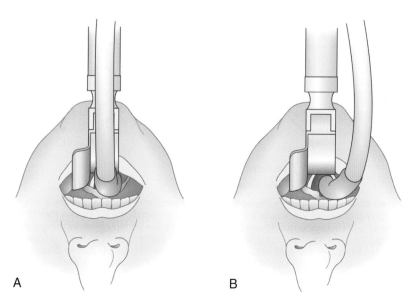

Figure 32-24   **A,** When the endotracheal tube (ETT) is introduced directly posterior to the blade, the view of the cords may be obscured and the tube may enter the esophagus instead of the trachea. **B,** Directing the ETT from the right corner of the mouth toward the larynx can allow better visualization of the tube entering the larynx.

A   B

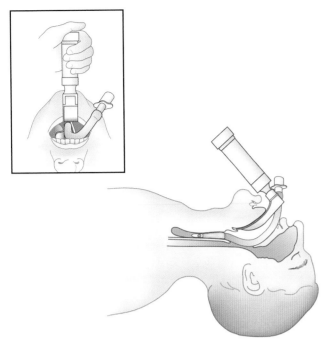

Figure 32-25 Posterior displacement of endotracheal tube restores the view of the larynx. (From Ford RW: Confirming endotracheal intubation: A simple manoeuvre. *Can Anaesth Soc J* 30:191–193, 1983.)

intubation, is 4%.[20] Applying a strict definition of "acceptable ETT placement" as more than 2 cm but no more than 6 cm above the carina (with the head in a neutral position) in adult patients after emergent intubation, Schwartz and colleagues found an incidence of 15.5% of inappropriately placed ETTs according to radiologic assessment, with a higher incidence in women than in men.[154]

Fortunately, endobronchial intubation is not a common cause of death, but if it remains unrecognized, it can lead to hypoxemia secondary to collapse of the contralateral lung and hyperinflation of the intubated lung with resultant tension pneumothorax. The ensuing hypoxemia depends on the degree of venous admixture ($\dot{V}/\dot{Q} > 0$), the magnitude of intrapulmonary shunting where $\dot{V}/\dot{Q} = 0$, the fraction of inspired oxygen (FIO_2), the degree of inhibition of hypoxic pulmonary vasoconstriction, and the level of $S\bar{v}O_2$. Unintentional main stem intubation can result in one of several scenarios depending on the location of the distal end of the tube (Fig. 32-26).[155] Placement of the ETT high in the right main bronchus (or even at the carina) may result in preferential ventilation of the right lung. Retrograde gas flow may lead to partial ventilation of the left lung if the ETT cuff does not provide a tight seal (see Fig. 32-26A).[153] A biphasic CO_2 waveform may be noticed (when the two lungs have different time constants).[156] Ventilation with high flow rates through an ETT whose tip is placed just proximal to the orifice of the right upper lobe bronchus promotes negative pressure (Bernoulli effect) and atelectasis of the right upper lobe (see Fig. 32-26B). Placement of the ETT further down the right main bronchus prevents ventilation of the left lung and occludes the right upper lobe bronchus (see Fig. 32-26C). An ETT placed in the lower portion of the trachea may obstruct a congenital tracheal bronchus, causing upper right lobe atelectasis (Fig. 32-27; see Fig. 32-26D).[157,158] In this rare anomaly, the bronchus to the right apical lung segment or the bronchus to the right upper lobe arises directly from the trachea, usually less than 2 cm from the carina.

intubation accounts for 2% of all adverse respiratory events in adults and 4% in pediatric patients.[1,5] Analysis of the Australian Incident Monitoring Study (AIMS) found that "accidental" bronchial intubation accounted for 3.7% of the total incidents reported. Most of the bronchial intubations were detected in the operating room (93.5%), during maintenance of anesthesia (77.9%), and by unexplained O_2 desaturation alone (63.6%). Capnography remained normal or unremarkable during 88.5% of episodes.[153] The incidence of main stem intubation in the critical care setting, not detected by clinical examination but discovered on chest radiography after

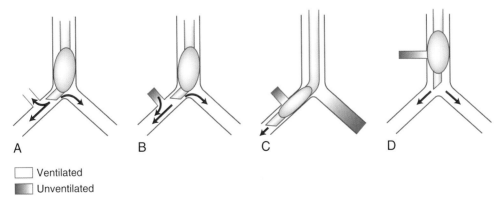

☐ Ventilated
▨ Unventilated

Figure 32-26 Unintentional intubation of the main stem bronchus can result in one of several scenarios, depending on the location of the distal end of the endotracheal tube (ETT). **A,** Placement of the ETT high in the right main bronchus may result in preferential ventilation of the right lung. Retrograde gas flow may lead to partial ventilation of the left lung if the ETT cuff does not provide a tight seal. **B,** Ventilation with a high flow rate through an ETT whose tip is placed just proximal to the orifice of the right upper lobe bronchus promotes negative pressure and atelectasis of the right upper lobe. **C,** Placement of the ETT further down the right main bronchus prevents ventilation of the left lung and occludes the right upper lobe bronchus. **D,** A tube placed in the lower portion of the trachea may obstruct a congenital tracheal bronchus, causing upper right lobe atelectasis. (Modified from Mecca RS: Management of the difficult airway. In Kirby RR, Gravenstein N, editors: *Clinical anesthesia practice*, ed 2, Philadelphia, 2007, Saunders, pp 921–954.)

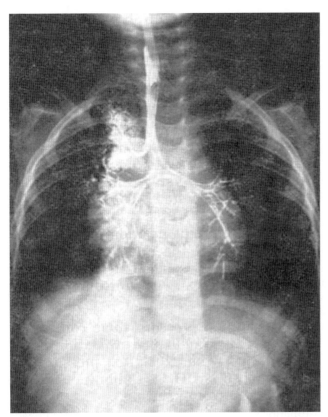

Figure 32-27 Bronchographic study revealing the presence of an apically displaced right tracheal bronchus. The left tracheal shadow at the level of the first rib is suggestive of a vascular ring, although this was not verified by cardiac catheterization or esophagograms. The potential for inadvertent intubation or occlusion of this lower airway anomaly is apparent. (From Venkateswarlu T, Turner CJ, Carter JD, Morrow DH: The tracheal bronchus: An unusual airway problem. *Anesth Analg* 55:746, 1976.)

A. Methods of Verification of Endotracheal Tube Insertion Depth

To decrease the likelihood of main stem intubation and unintentional extubation, clinicians should aim at positioning the distal end of the ETT in the middle third of the trachea. Various methods can be used before, during, or after intubation to locate the ETT at an appropriate depth in the trachea.

1. Referencing the Marks on the Tube Before and After Intubation

In one method, the ETT is placed alongside the patient's face and neck with the tip of the tube lying at the suprasternal notch and the tube aligned to conform externally to the position of the nasal or oral ETT. The centimeter marking at which the tube intersects with the teeth or gums for oral intubation, or the naris for nasal intubation, is noted so that the ETT can be secured in that position after intubation. In another method, the orally placed ETT is secured at the upper incisor teeth (or gums) at the 23-cm mark in men and the 21-cm mark in women of average adult size.[159] This method was found to be reliable in anesthetized patients but not in critically ill patients.[20,159] We have observed that in tall men and in patients in whom excessive head extension is needed, the

ETT may need to be secured at the 24- or 25-cm mark; in some shorter women, it may need to be secured at the 19-cm mark for optimal placement of the distal end of the ETT in the middle of the trachea. Formulas regarding the appropriate length of the ETT are available for infants and children. The reader is referred to pediatric anesthesia texts for this information.

2. Direct Visualization of the Tube and Its Cuff

Positioning of the distal end of the ETT in the middle of the trachea is a relatively easy maneuver when the ETT can be seen entering the larynx during direct laryngoscopy. Because the length of the trachea is 10 to 13 cm in an average adult, placing the upper end of the cuff of an ETT (7 or 8 mm ID in size) 2 cm below the vocal cords positions the distal end of the tube approximately 4 cm from the carina. In a simple study based on measurements, it was found that, except in cases of short tracheas, placing the upper end of the cuff 2 cm below the cords predictably positioned the distal end of the ETT in the middle of the trachea.[160] This maneuver should be used whenever orotracheal intubation is performed under direct laryngoscopy.

3. Prevention of Endotracheal Tube Displacement After Intubation

Despite initial proper positioning, the ETT can still slip out of the larynx (or move closer to the carina) while the laryngoscope blade is being removed, during taping of the tube, after the position of the head is changed, during positioning of the patient, or during transportation. Several precautions should be undertaken to prevent ETT displacement (Box 32-1).

4. Influence of Positioning on Endotracheal Tube Insertion Depth

Excessive movement of the ETT can occur during extension and flexion of the head.[161,162] In a radiologic study in adults, Conrardy and coworkers demonstrated an average 3.8-cm movement of the ETT toward the carina when the head was moved from full extension to full flexion (Fig. 32-28).[161] In some patients, this movement reached as much as 6.4 cm. With lateral head rotation, the ETT moved an average of 0.7 cm away from the carina. Because the average movement of the ETT when the head is moved from the neutral position to full extension or full flexion is 1.9 cm in the adult, it is unlikely that

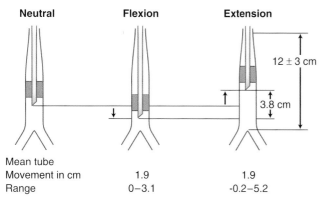

	Neutral	Flexion	Extension
Mean tube Movement in cm		1.9	1.9
Range		0–3.1	-0.2–5.2

Figure 32-28 Mean movement of an endotracheal tube (ETT) with flexion and extension of the neck from the neutral position. The mean ETT movement between flexion and extension is about one third to one fourth of the length of an adult trachea (12 ± 3 cm). (From Conrardy PA, Goodman LR, Lainge F, et al: Alteration of ETT position: Flexion and extension of the neck. *Crit Care Med* 4:8–12, 1976.)

extubation or main stem intubation would occur during this movement if the distal end of the tube is in the middle of the trachea, but it could occur if it is too high or too low in the trachea.

Malpositioning of the ETT can occur with changes in patient positioning,[163] with displacement of the diaphragm, and during surgical manipulation of the trachea or esophagus, especially if the ETT is not initially placed in the middle of the trachea. A high incidence of main stem intubation has been reported after institution of the Trendelenburg position. The weight of the abdominal organs results in cephalad shift of the diaphragm and the carina, which may cause a taped ETT to relocate into a main stem bronchus. The opposite can happen when the reverse Trendelenburg position is used.

Many reports have confirmed tracheal tube migration on creation of a pneumoperitoneum during laparoscopic procedures, increasing the risk for endobronchial intubation.[164-169] Although the Trendelenburg tilt can lead to further migration, movement can also occur during upper abdominal laparoscopic procedures performed in the reverse Trendelenburg position.[165] The mechanism is similar to that for the Trendelenburg position, but the diaphragm is displaced cephalad by the insufflated gas rather than the weight of the abdominal contents. After positioning of the tip of the ETT at 30 to 40 mm from the carina, it was found that the distance significantly decreased to 26 mm (range, 17 to 35 mm) in patients undergoing laparoscopic cholecystectomy. The maximum distance of tube migration was 8 mm (range, 0 to 15 mm). One fifth of the patients would have been at risk of bronchial intubation if the ETT had not been carefully positioned.[167] ETT migration occurs more often in obese patients undergoing laparoscopic procedures compared with open abdominal surgery. In 17% of obese patients, the tube advances into the right bronchus.[168] ETT displacement also occurs in children undergoing laparoscopic procedures. In one study,[169] maximal displacement was 0.5 + (0.05 × age in years) for 20-degree head-down tilt, 0.6 + (0.09 × age) after insufflations, and 1.2 + (0.11 × age) for 20-degree head-down

tilt and insufflations. However, in no patient did endobronchial intubation occur when the ETT was placed according to the intubation depth marking as recommended by the manufacturer.

Obviously, the tip of the ETT should be placed in the middle of the trachea, or 3 to 4 cm above the carina in adults. If the ETT moves toward the carina, then carinal stimulation may cause tachycardia, hypertension, or bronchospasm and increase the risk of bronchial intubation.[163] If the ETT moves outward, the cuff may cause injury to the vocal cords and increase the risk of accidental extubation. If the ETT is placed appropriately in the middle of the trachea, it is very unlikely (except in infants) that endobronchial intubation or extubation will ensue.

Because the trachea and the esophagus are invested in the same cervical fascia, pulling on either structure during surgery can misplace an ETT. This can occur during repair of esophageal atresia in infants and during esophagoscopy. Excessive movement of the head and neck of intubated patients must be avoided; however, if such movements are necessary, they should be done carefully. The position of the ETT should be rechecked when the patient's position is altered; when the head is moved; after surgical manipulation of the trachea or esophagus; whenever displacement of the diaphragm is suspected (e.g., changes in FRC, changes in position, abdominal insufflation); and when an unexplained decrease in SaO_2, increased airway pressure, cuff leak, or biphasic CO_2 waveform is noticed.

The ease with which main stem intubation can occur with head flexion and unintentional extubation with head extension is of particular concern in the infant, especially in the neonate, whose trachea is only 4.7 to 5.7 cm long (Fig. 32-29).[170,171] When endotracheal intubation is performed in infants, precautions should be taken to ensure that the ETT is placed far enough in the trachea but not in a main stem bronchus. One precaution is to use an ETT that has circumferential marks at 2.2 cm from the distal end and to introduce the marker on the ETT as far as the cords in term infants, slightly above the cords in preterm infants, and slightly below the cords in older infants. Another alternative that has been recommended is to use ETTs with diameters of 2.5, 3.0, and 3.5 mm and marks at 2.2, 2.4, and 2.6 cm, respectively, from the distal end. The reader is referred to pediatric anesthesia texts for more details.

5. Observation and Palpation of Chest Movements and Auscultation of Breath Sounds

Observation or palpation of an asymmetrical chest movement and detection of unequal bilateral breath sounds should alert the clinician to the possibility of a main stem intubation (usually on the right side). In addition, absence of right apical movement or breath sounds, or both, implies that the ETT and its cuff are obstructing the right upper lobe bronchus. Gradual withdrawal of the tube should correct the problem. Although auscultation of bilateral breath sounds is the most common method used in detecting main stem intubation, investigations revealed that this may not be a reliable diagnostic modality.[153,172,173] Brune and colleagues observed that

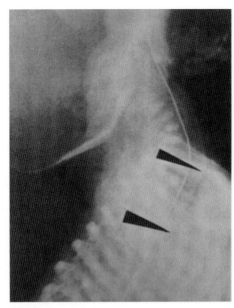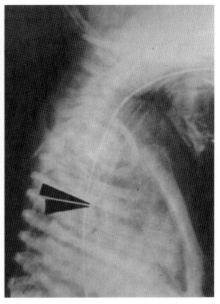

Figure 32-29   Radiographs illustrate the effect of head position on placement of the endotracheal tube (ETT) in newborn infants. The upper arrow indicates the tip of the ETT; the lower arrow indicates the tip of the carina. Notice the marked excursion of the tip of the tube with head flexion *(right)*. (From Todres ID, deBros F, Kramer SS: Endotracheal tube displacement in the newborn infant. *J Pediatr* 89:126–127, 1976.)

60% of endobronchial intubations occurred despite the presence of equal breath sounds on auscultation.[172]

The inaccuracy of the auscultation method may be related to the structure of the tip of the ETT when it is placed near the carina.[174] The Murphy eye, which is present in most ETTs, is a 1.0-cm elliptical port located 0.8 cm from the tip on the right side of the tube, opposite the bevel. The eye was originally designed to allow ventilation of the lungs if the bevel becomes occluded and also to allow ventilation of the right upper lobe if the ETT is accidentally advanced into the right main stem bronchus.[144] Studies confirmed that the Murphy eye can maintain gas flow through the space between the ETT cuff and the right main stem bronchus and that it permits ventilation (albeit inadequate) of the left lung, thus allowing breath sounds to be heard bilaterally, until the tip is inserted 2 cm beyond the carina. Unilateral breath sounds may not be heard until the tube tip is further advanced to 3.2 cm beyond the carina.[174] Accordingly, the Murphy eye reduces the reliability of chest auscultation in detecting endobronchial intubation.[174]

Despite the limitations of auscultation of bilateral breath sounds, continuous or repeated auscultation to detect intraoperative complications such as bronchial intubation and obstructed airway has been emphasized.[175] The limitations and difficulties encountered in continuously and simultaneously auscultating right and left breath sounds have led investigators to explore other methods to amplify breath sounds.[37,176] In one method, already discussed, breath sounds are quantified using electronic stethoscopes placed over each hemithorax and epigastrium.[37] In another, a system that makes it possible to "visualize" breath sounds is used. The visual stethoscope allows real-time fast transformation of the sound signal and three-dimensional color rendering of the results on a computer with simultaneous processing of two individual sound signals.[176] With continuous bilateral

breath sounds displayed, the clinician can monitor left and right breath sounds simultaneously and can rapidly detect any changes.[176] This system has potential advantages in assessing breath sounds throughout the surgical procedure, not just to verify ETT placement. Furthermore, more than one individual can monitor breath sounds.

Preliminary studies of both the electronic and the visual stethoscope showed precise accuracy for detecting endobronchial intubation.[37,176] During advancement of the ETT, alterations of the shape of the visualized breath sounds appeared before changes in breath sounds were detected by auscultation. However, these studies were conducted in nonobese patients without lung pathology in a quiet operating room. Further evaluation is needed in patients with a variety of pathologic conditions and under different ambient conditions.[37,176]

6. Cuff Maneuvers and Neck Palpation

Various maneuvers involving palpation of the ETT cuff on each side of the trachea above the suprasternal notch (e.g., rapid cuff inflations, intermittent squeezing of the pilot balloon of a slightly overinflated cuff, use of the pilot balloon as a sensor while palpating the cuff in the neck) have been proposed to ensure that the ETT is not in a main bronchus.[177,178] Suprasternal palpation of the cuff provides a high degree of confidence that the distal tip of the tube is more than 2 cm from the carina, whereas if the cuff is not palpable, the tip is probably close to the carina.[178]

7. Use of Fiberoptic Bronchoscopes

During fiberoptic intubation, the distance from the distal end of the ETT to the carina should be determined and the position of the ETT can be easily corrected, if necessary.[148,149] The distal end of the tube is usually positioned approximately 4 cm from the carina in adult patients.

The use of FFB to evaluate the position of the ETT has been extended to the critical care setting to obviate the necessity of frequent chest radiographs.

8. Transtracheal Illumination

Transillumination techniques can help position the ETT tip at a reliable distance above the carina. Two methods have been suggested. In one, the flexible lighted stylet is placed inside the ETT so that the stylet bulb is positioned at the tube's distal opening before intubation.[49,50] By observing maximal illumination at the sternal notch (a consistent anatomic landmark) during intubation, the tip of the tube can be placed consistently 5.0 ± 1.0 cm from the carina.[50] In the other method, the tip of the lighted stylet is placed inside the ETT, just proximal to the cuff, before intubation. Visualization of transillumination distal to the cricoid cartilage is indicative of proper cuff positioning. In this position, the distance between the tip of the ETT and the carina varies from 3.7 to 4 cm in adults. Use of either method can reduce the need for radiographic confirmation of ETT positioning.

9. Capnography

In cases of main stem intubation, the capnographic waveform usually shows a normal pattern. If a biphasic waveform is noticed, main stem intubation or impingement of the tube on the carina should be suspected.[156] Other causes of biphasic waveforms should be excluded, such as lateral decubitus position, kyphoscoliosis causing compression of the lung, pulmonary disease, spontaneous breathing efforts, hiccups, and sampling line leak.[30,79,156]

10. Use of the Esophageal Detector Device/Self-Inflating Bulb

The EDD with SIB is of no value in diagnosing main stem intubation. However, main stem intubation should be suspected if there is slow reinflation of the SIB.[137] Rotation or gradual pullback of the ETT, or both, may lead to instantaneous reinflation of the SIB.

11. Chest Radiography

In critically ill patients, a portable chest radiograph can easily detect main stem intubation and can determine the location of the distal end of the tube in relation to the carina (Fig. 32-30).[20,65,154] Because malpositioned ETTs may not be detected by routine clinical assessment, some investigators are recommending that chest radiographs should remain the standard practice in the critical care setting.[65,154]

IV. CONCLUSIONS

The goals of endotracheal intubation are to place the ETT in the trachea and to position the tube at an appropriate depth inside the trachea. Unrecognized esophageal intubation and ETT malposition are a leading cause of injury involving the respiratory system in anesthetic practice and in the prehospital setting. Although they are rare events, the outcome is so devastating that awareness of their occurrence is essential whenever endotracheal intubation is performed.

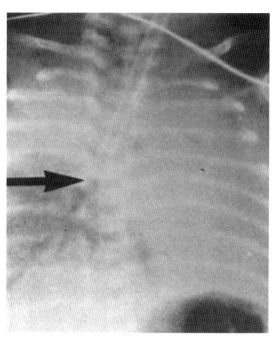

Figure 32-30 Malposition of the endotracheal tube (ETT). The ETT is in the bronchus intermedius *(arrow)*. Notice the airless left lung and right upper lobe. (From Mandel GA: Neonatal intensive care radiology. In Goodman LR, Putman CE, editors: *Intensive care radiology: Imaging of the critically ill,* Philadelphia, 1983, WB Saunders, p 290.)

A vast array of methods has been described to verify ETT placement. In most patients, these methods (alone or in combination) can successfully and quickly differentiate esophageal from endotracheal intubation. Nevertheless, almost all of these methods have been documented to fail under certain circumstances. It is crucial that clinicians involved in endotracheal intubation have the necessary airway management skills, perform these tests accurately, and interpret their results correctly. Obviously, not all of these tests can be applied in every situation, but the clinician should be familiar with and use as many tests as possible. Prioritization of these tests depends on many factors, including experience, availability of devices, condition of the patient, and the setting in which endotracheal intubation is performed.

Viewing the ETT passing between the cords during direct laryngoscopy and visualization of the tracheal rings and carina with an FFB after intubation are the only foolproof methods of confirming endotracheal intubation. In the nonarrested patient, CO_2 monitoring can quickly differentiate tracheal from esophageal intubation. In the arrested patient, CO_2 monitoring can be unreliable, although it can be useful as a prognostic indicator of the efficacy of resuscitation. Devices such as the EDD/SIB may be more useful in patients with cardiac arrest, but they can also yield false results.

Placing the distal tip of the ETT in the middle of the trachea can be accomplished by positioning the upper end of the cuffed ETT 2 cm below the vocal cords during direct laryngoscopy or by placing the distal tip of the tube 4 cm above the carina with the aid of an FFB in adults. The position of the ETT should always be verified by clinical assessment (auscultation of both axillae and the epigastrium). If direct visualization cannot be done,

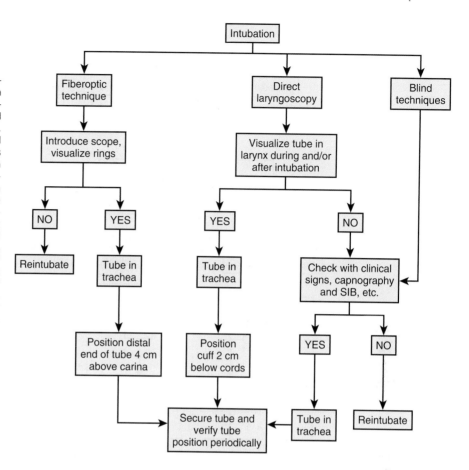

Figure 32-31 *Proposed algorithm for verification of endotracheal tube (ETT) position and insertion depth during elective endotracheal intubation. Intubation is performed using an ETT of appropriate size and length. Blind techniques include blind nasal or oral intubation and intubation with introducers or intubating stylets. Verify tube position periodically, especially in the following situations: changes in ETT position, changes in head or body position, suspected decrease in functional residual capacity or displacement of the diaphragm, traction on trachea or esophagus, unexpected fall in arterial oxygen saturation (Sao₂), biphasic CO_2 waveform, and unexpected cuff leak. Cuff leak after adequate cuff inflation can be a result of leakage around the cuff or loss of air from the cuff; causes include cuff protruding above cords, ETT too small, extremely compliant airway, tracheomalacia, tracheoesophageal fistula (very rare), defective cuff or damage to cuff during intubation, defective pilot-balloon system, and kinking of connecting tubing. SIB, Self-inflating bulb.* (From Salem MR: Verification of ETT position. *Anesthesiol Clin North Am* 19:813–839, 2001.)

referencing the marks on the ETT, use of transillumination techniques, or cuff maneuvers can be helpful. In emergency and critical care settings, a chest radiograph can easily detect malpositioned ETTs that may not be detected by routine clinical assessment. Other techniques (use of an FFB, cuff maneuvers, transillumination) can obviate the necessity for frequent chest radiographs.

On the basis of available information, two algorithms are proposed: one for verification of ETT position in elective intubation (Fig. 32-31) and the other for emergency intubation (Fig. 32-32). These algorithms are designed to assist the clinician and should not be a substitute for clinical judgment. Under no circumstances should clinical signs be ignored in the presence of conflicting information from monitors and technical aids.

V. CLINICAL PEARLS

- The ideal test for confirmation of endotracheal tube (ETT) placement should be simple, quick, and repeatable; it should function in patients of different age groups, in various locations, and during difficult intubation (DI); and it should not yield false results even in patients with cardiac arrest.

- Contributing factors to the high incidence of esophageal intubation in patients who experience cardiac arrest during out-of-hospital paramedic intubation include intubation under less than optimal conditions; unavailability of monitoring equipment, protocols, or algorithms; violation of the standard technique of auscultation; and intubation attempts by nonexpert personnel.

- Whenever "abnormal" breath sounds are heard by auscultation, they should not be relied on to confirm endotracheal intubation.

- Tube condensation of water can and does occur when an ETT is placed in the esophagus, and its presence should not be interpreted as a reliable indicator of a successful intubation.

- Oxyhemoglobin desaturation is a relatively late manifestation of esophageal intubation.

- CO_2 levels as high as 5% can be detected initially in cases of esophageal intubation after the ingestion of carbonated beverages or antacids. However, rapid decline in CO_2 levels occurs with successive ventilation.

- Capnography and use of colorimetric end-tidal CO_2 detectors can provide a prognostic indicator of successful resuscitation.

- Visualization of the tracheal rings through a flexible fiberoptic bronchoscope (FFB) before the ETT is threaded over it does not guarantee successful endotracheal intubation.

- Common causes of false-negative results with the use of the self-inflating bulb (SIB) include decreased FRC (e.g., obesity, pregnancy, infants), ETT at the carina or main stem bronchus intubation, bronchospasm, and secretions.

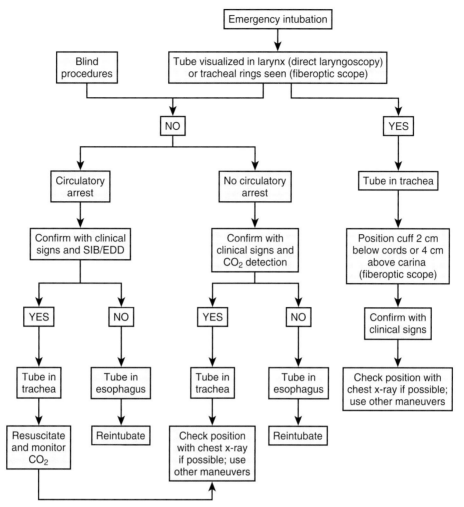

Figure 32-32 Proposed algorithm for verification of endotracheal tube (ETT) position and insertion depth during emergency intubation. In the emergency and critical care settings, chest radiographs (frequently obtained) can easily detect malpositioning of a tracheally placed ETT. Other techniques (e.g., flexible fiberoptic bronchoscopy, cuff maneuvers, transillumination) can decrease the need for frequent chest radiographs. In patients with circulatory arrest, CO_2 monitoring can be unreliable. In these patients, devices such as the self-inflating bulb/ esophageal detector device *(SIB/EDD)* are more helpful. During cardiopulmonary resuscitation, monitoring of CO_2 can serve as a prognostic indicator of the efficacy of resuscitation. (From Salem MR: Verification of ETT position. *Anesthesiol Clin North Am* 19:813–839, 2001.)

- The Murphy eye reduces the reliability of chest auscultation in detecting endobronchial intubation.

SELECTED REFERENCES

All references can be found online at expertconsult.com.

1. Caplan RA, Posner KL, Ward RJ, et al: Adverse respiratory events in anesthesia: a closed claims analysis. *Anesthesiology* 73:828–833, 1990.
20. Schwartz DE, Matthay MA, Cohen NH: Death and other complications of emergency airway management in critically ill adults. *Anesthesiology* 82:367–376, 1995.
63. Smith GM, Reed JC, Choplin RH: Radiographic detection of esophageal malpositioning of endotracheal tubes. *AJR Am J Roentgenol* 154:23–26, 1990.
86. Falk JL, Rackow EC, Weil MH: End-tidal carbon dioxide concentration during cardiopulmonary resuscitation. *N Engl J Med* 318:607–611, 1988.
116. Salem MR, Wafai Y, Baraka A, et al: Use of self-inflating bulb for detecting esophageal intubation after "esophageal ventilation." *Anesth Analg* 77:1227–1231, 1993.
124. Lang DJ, Wafai Y, Salem MR, et al: Efficacy of the self-inflating bulb in confirming tracheal intubation in the morbidly obese. *Anesthesiology* 85:246–253, 1996.
146. Raphael DT, Benbassat M, Arnaudov D, et al: Validation study of two-microphone acoustic reflectometry for determination of breathing tube placement in 200 adult patients. *Anesthesiology* 97:1371–1377, 2002.
167. Inada T, Uesugi S, Kawachi S, Takubo K: Changes in tracheal tube position during laparoscopic cholecystectomy. *Anaesthesia* 51:823–826, 1996.
174. Sugiyama K, Yokoyama K, Satch K, et al: Does the Murphy eye reduce the reliability of chest auscultation in detecting endobronchial intubation? *Anesth Analg* 88:1380–1383, 1999.
178. Pollard R, Lobato E: Endotracheal tube location verified reliably by cuff palpation. *Anesth Analg* 81:135–138, 1995.

PART 5

Difficult Airway Situations

Chapter 33

Prehospital Airway Management

EDWARD R. STAPLETON | MICHAEL F. MURPHY

I. INTRODUCTION

Prehospital airway management ranges from the use of basic airway maneuvers in the management of the unresponsive patient to the need for a surgical airway (i.e., cricothyrotomy) in the "cannot intubate, cannot ventilate" (CICV) situation. Because transport time from the scene of an emergency is often delayed by distance, traffic conditions, and victim extrication, skilled providers can be assets to the most seriously ill or injured patients. However, the scope of practice for emergency medical services (EMS) providers throughout North America varies broadly. In some systems, airway management is provided exclusively by basic emergency medical technicians (EMTs) who are not trained in endotracheal intubation, cricothyrotomy, or extraglottic airway devices, leaving the airway uncontrolled and susceptible to gastric inflation and aspiration induced by bag-mask ventilation, which produces a difficult airway or complete airway obstruction that may be impossible to resolve. Other systems use highly trained paramedics and allow the use of medication-assisted intubation and a variety of airway devices, which opens the door to potential clinical errors and complications such as airway trauma, misplaced tubes, and unrecognized esophageal intubation.

The variability in EMS systems throughout North America is dictated by several factors, including historical system design, state laws, system size, volunteer versus paid provider status, physicians' preferences, and economic issues. For example, in large urban systems, a lack of high-quality medical direction and monitoring may make medication-assisted intubation difficult to successfully implement and sustain. In rural systems, the frequency of intubation may be low, making it difficult to acquire and maintain the necessary skill levels.

Prehospital intubation can be challenging compared with the in-hospital environment. EMS providers work in a variety of conditions that complicate the task of airway management, ventilation, and oxygenation. Extreme weather, enclosed working spaces (e.g., cars, small rooms, hallways), bystander distractions, and a variety of other challenging situations face the EMT and paramedic.[1]

Some aspects of an EMS system design are essential for maximizing provider competency. The frequency with which any provider performs advanced airway management is critical for maintaining skill competency.[2,3] Some systems have reported very low rates of intubation, especially for pediatric patients.[4-6] How can competency be maintained when providers intubate three or four times per year?[2,7-9] Should they intubate when the frequency is so low? System medical directors must answer these questions when designing, evaluating, or refining an EMS system. Physicians must be artful in selecting airway strategies, training providers, monitoring interventions, and maintaining quality.[7]

II. HISTORY OF AIRWAY MANAGEMENT BY EMERGENCY MEDICAL SERVICES

Before the 1950s, prehospital airway management was provided by relatively unskilled providers in most EMS systems throughout the United States. Progressive systems of the time provided bag-mask ventilation with an oropharyngeal or nasopharyngeal airway. In some cases, training was limited to basic first aid without training in airway adjuncts.[10-12]

In the 1960s, the quality of prehospital care came into focus with publication of *Accidental Death and Disability: The Neglected Disease of Modern Society* by the National Research Council and development of a national standards curriculum for EMTs that defined minimal training and equipment.[13] Standards included training in the use of basic equipment such as bag-mask ventilation, oropharyngeal and nasopharyngeal airways, and suction.

In the late 1960s, the concept of advanced-level care was introduced first in Northern Ireland under the leadership of Dr. Frank Pantridge and subsequently implemented in several cities in the United States, including New York, Miami, Seattle, and Pittsburgh. In these systems, paramedics were trained to provide endotracheal intubation in the field along with other advanced life support interventions. Most programs included training in the operating room under the supervision of an anesthesiologist. This innovation was helpful for victims of respiratory and cardiac arrest who were unresponsive. However, there were still challenges for patients with respiratory failure, shock, or other premorbid conditions who were responsive but in need of definitive airway management. In the absence of sedation and rapid-sequence intubation (RSI) protocols, intubation for these conditions was often performed by employing *brutane*— the use of force to assist in performing a medical procedure, such as intubating the trachea.

In the 1970s, some paramedic systems began to use neuromuscular blocking drugs to manage patients' airways with great success. These programs provided significant medical oversight that included monitoring successful outcomes and complications associated with endotracheal intubations.[14] System medical directors had concerns about the use of medication-assisted intubation, including the issue of increased time at the scene by paramedics and complications such as unrecognized esophageal intubation.[15-17]

Drug-assisted intubation is a relatively new idea that is used on a limited basis in EMS systems in North America. Because success rates for drug-assisted endotracheal intubation vary greatly among EMS groups, it is not routinely recommended.[8,9] However, the National Association of EMS Physicians has developed guidelines for implementing drug-assisted intubation programs that include provider training, patient selection, use of standardized protocols and resources for storage and delivery of medications, training in verification and monitoring of end-tidal carbon dioxide, a continuous quality improvement program, and research on a system level to verify effectiveness of the program.[18]

Alternative airway devices have been used in prehospital care since the advent of prehospital advanced life support. Devices include the esophageal obturator, gastric tube airway, esophageal-tracheal Combitube, and King laryngeal tube (LT) airway. Many studies have demonstrated their relative effectiveness compared with bag-mask ventilation and endotracheal intubation (ETI) ventilation.[19-21]

III. PREHOSPITAL CARE OF AIRWAY PATIENTS

Prehospital care of airway patients addresses the spectrum of clinical conditions faced in emergency departments, critical care units, and operating rooms. In the ideal world, providers would be prepared to deal with airway management and ventilation for all possible conditions, but the scope of practice and provider skill levels vary in North America. In other parts of the world, where physicians staff EMS vehicles, skill levels may be more uniform. At the entry level of emergency medical response (EMT-Basic), forced positive pressure with bag-mask ventilation and rapid transport may be the only options available. ETI has been considered the gold standard for definitive airway management, but the diverse skill levels found in prehospital care and the use of extraglottic airway devices in EMS have challenged this idea. High rates of unrecognized esophageal or hypopharyngeal placement or dislodgement have raised concerns about ETI as a default strategy for EMS providers.[16,17]

A. Basic Airway Management

Most EMS providers are equipped to manage the patient who is unresponsive or in respiratory or cardiac arrest. Since the late 1960s, EMT-Basic training has included the use of oropharyngeal and nasopharyngeal airways, bag-mask ventilation, and suctioning. Training has emphasized appropriate mask seal, controlled volumes and inspiratory times, and the avoidance of hyperventilation in cardiac arrest and shock states.[11,22-24]

Complete airway obstruction by acute epiglottitis, foreign bodies, laryngeal-tracheal trauma, airway hematomas, and numerous other conditions is a challenge in hospitals staffed by highly skilled airway managers and particularly in the prehospital environment, where the necessary tools and skills may not be available. In these unfavorable settings, rapid transport to surgical intervention may be the only practical option. In rural environments where transport times are prolonged, upper airway obstruction is more likely to be a fatal condition.

B. Extraglottic Airway Devices

Use of the King LT as a primary and alternative airway device has been an effective prehospital airway strategy.[17,25,26] Because alternative airway devices do not provide definitive protection against aspiration, they typically are used temporarily until ETI can be achieved in the field or in the emergency department. In one case report, the King LT resulted in tongue engorgement when left in place for approximately 3 hours.[27]

The double-lumen esophageal-tracheal Combitube is an alternative airway device commonly used in EMS. It has been used by Basic and Advanced EMTs as a primary airway device and by paramedics as a rescue device. Effectiveness of the Combitube has varied among studies in prehospital care. Cady and colleagues found it had no effect on patient outcomes compared with ETI.[28] In a study of prehospital physicians, the Combitube was superior to ETI in the management of cardiopulmonary arrest.[29] When the King LT and Combitube were compared in a study of EMS providers, nurses, and physicians, the King LT was inserted faster and preferred by 96% of the participants.[30]

For patients with acute respiratory distress and acute pulmonary edema, continuous positive airway pressure

(CPAP) has significantly improved outcomes and reduced the need for intubation in prehospital care.[31] CPAP has also proved to be cost-effective in the prehospital environment.[32]

Some studies have shown increased morbidity rates with prehospital intubation. Others have demonstrated no increase in mortality rates despite significant errors such as esophageal intubation, dislodgement, or failed ETI.[33] A study of patients with acute respiratory distress showed a decrease in mortality rates when advanced interventions such as ETI were used in the prehospital environment.[33]

Some investigators think that ETI should not be standard operating procedure for EMS systems. Variables cited as key factors in determining whether a given EMS system should use ETI include low case exposure and inadequate operating room training for paramedics and paramedic students. However, it has been shown that if a minimum number of intubations is used as the criterion to permit ETI in the field, the overall numbers of ETI performed in the field decrease because fewer providers meet the minimum number needed to permit continued performance of the skill.[2] Additionally, supraglottic devices have demonstrated equivalency to ETI in many studies, and many advocate using alternative strategies for ensuring the success rates for intubations, such as simulation and cadaver training.[21,34,35] When time in the operating room is made available to paramedics, it can be a significant training adjunct for clinical practice.

The U.S. National Highway Traffic Safety Administration (NHTSA) requires only five intubations to be eligible for paramedic certification.[22-24] This level is well below the recommended level of 35 ETIs for emergency medicine residents. Anesthesiology residents must perform between 45 and 60 ETIs to achieve at least a 90% success rate in the controlled setting of the operating room.[36] Wang and colleagues calculated the learning curves for paramedic students performing ETI and found that at 20 to 25 ETIs in live subjects must be performed to achieve success rates of at least 90%.[2] This finding argues that paramedics with only five ETIs during training may have little skill in performing intubations.

Medical oversight is a critical part of any EMS airway program. Direction by physicians has enhanced the cognitive (though not the technical) skills of paramedics and improved patient selection.[7]

IV. SYSTEM STRUCTURE AND TYPES OF PROVIDERS

The foundation for any EMS program is provided by system-wide protocols. Almost every system in North America has protocols that delineate the specific steps of care, types and dosages of medications, and other special considerations needed to rescue patients. Protocols usually are designed by a group of physicians, an EMS medical advisory committee, or an EMS medical director. In the case of advanced airway management in the United States, protocols relating respiratory failure, cardiac arrest, and airway obstruction are derived from the National EMS Education Standards and from guidelines for CPR and emergency cardiac care by the American Heart Association (AHA), International Liaison Committee on Resuscitation (ILCOR), and other reputable bodies.[37-39]

The guidelines for airway management have significantly changed over the past decade. The most striking modification is incorporation of waveform capnography as the gold standard for endotracheal tube confirmation and continuous verification of intratracheal positioning. In some EMS jurisdictions, waveform capnography has become a requirement for all intubations. The value of this strategy was established by Silvestri and colleagues, who demonstrated no unrecognized esophageal intubations when capnography was used in their EMS system.[16]

A. Emergency Medical Technicians

Typically, EMTs are trained in the use of basic airway methods that include, use of oral and nasal airways, and administration of oxygen and suction. Some EMT programs permit the use of extraglottic devices.

B. Advanced Emergency Medical Technicians

Advanced training includes skills such as electrocardiogram interpretation, advanced or alternative airway management (e.g., ETI, use of dual-lumen airway devices), intravenous fluid therapy, and intravenous administration of certain medications. Advanced EMT training is shorter and more focused than paramedic training. Advanced EMT programs are more commonly used in rural, volunteer EMS systems because the ability to attend longer training programs may not be feasible and the call volume is less than in larger markets.

C. Paramedics

Paramedics have the highest level of EMT training in the United States and Canada. A paramedic completes a course that follows the standardized national curriculum (e.g., as prescribed by NHTSA) or meets the standards of some other educational paradigm. A paramedic performs advanced tasks, such as electrocardiogram interpretation, drug therapy administration, invasive airway techniques, and manual defibrillation. Paramedics also may be involved in critical care transport operations. For these services, EMS providers are involved primarily in the transfer of acutely ill and injured patients from one care center to another. EMS providers who function in this role often have additional training in specialized devices, such as intravenous infusion pumps, ventilators, and counterpulsation aortic balloon pumps. Paramedics and critical care nurses are commonly employed in medical evacuation (Medevac) programs that use helicopters for transport (also referred to as Helicopter EMS or HEMS). These programs are designed to transport a critically ill patient from the scene of an emergency or a local community hospital to a specialized care facility.

V. PHYSICIAN OVERSIGHT AND CONTINUOUS QUALITY ASSURANCE

Physician oversight of prehospital care has been an essential component since the earliest EMS advance life support programs.[10] It has included training and evaluation, protocol development, radio communications with providers in the field, review and observation of patient care delivery, and continuous quality assurance programs. Airway management has been a central issue in advanced EMT and paramedic training since the early 1970s.

A. Training

High-quality training is the most important part of any EMS system. EMS airway management and ventilation training has ranged from basic skill instruction on a manikin to supervised clinical application in the operating room, emergency department, and prehospital environments. Innovative strategies have included cadaver practice and manikin practice in a simulation environment.

B. Continuous Quality Improvement

The most important role for a physician in prehospital care is continuous quality improvement. Poor airway management in prehospital care can result in brain injury and death. Every case of airway management and ventilation should be reviewed by the medical director's staff. At a minimum, this includes tracking success rates for intubation and alternative airway devices and documenting end-tidal carbon dioxide values at the scene, during transport, and on arrival at the hospital. The receiving emergency department should be routinely contacted by the medical director's staff for confirmation of airway device placement on arrival. Figure 33-1 is a review form that might be used for this purpose. Figure 33-2 is a more comprehensive form used by a hospital-based program using RSI.

VI. CONCLUSIONS

Depending on the level of training, EMTs can offer emergency care that includes many airway management techniques. ETI performed by personnel other than physicians is under intense scrutiny to ascertain its benefit. In the meantime, medical oversight as part of a comprehensive quality program is essential for successful airway management. For a physician planning an EMS system, the training strategy should be appropriately matched to the level of provider, protocols, system issues (e.g., response times, hospital transport times, environmental factors), and scope of practice. Factors that can limit the introduction of advanced skills such as use of supraglottic devices, ETI, and medication-assisted intubation include volunteer EMTs with limited training time, an inability to closely monitor providers, and failure to employ a comprehensive airway management quality program.

VII. CLINICAL PEARLS

- Emergency medical services (EMS) provide a variety of prehospital care, including airway management.

- Emergency medical technicians (EMTs) work in many environments that complicate the task of airway management, including extreme weather, small, enclosed working spaces, and bystander distractions.

- EMS programs and EMT training are based on established protocols that delineate the specific steps of care, types and dosages of medications, and other special considerations needed to rescue patients. Protocols usually are designed by a group of physicians, an EMS medical advisory committee, or an EMS medical director and are based on national standards and curricula.

- EMTs are trained to assess a patient's condition and to perform the procedures needed to maintain a patent airway with adequate breathing and cardiovascular circulation until the patient can be transported to a hospital for definitive medical care.

- EMTs can mange the patient who is unresponsive or in cardiorespiratory arrest. Depending on the level of training and local protocols, they can use bag-mask ventilation, suctioning, drug-assisted intubation, oropharyngeal and nasopharyngeal airways, and alternative devices such as the Combitube and King laryngeal tube (LT) airway.

- The most important role for a physician in prehospital care is continuous quality improvement, because poor airway management can result in brain injury and death.

Medical Control
Follow-up Runsheet

EMS Provider Details:

ET/EGD placement confirmed by (check all that apply):

Auscultation   Direct visualization   Disposable Colormetric etCO$_2$ Electronic Capnography

Esophageal Detection Device   Other _____

ET/EGD secured by (check all that apply):

Commercial tube holder   Tape   Tie   Head immobilization

ET/EGD placement at hospital confirmed as:

Tracheal   Esophageal   Oropharyngeal   None

Tube size_____   **Patient height** ___' _____"

If Combitube used, ventilation through:

Blue tube   White tube

Person at ED confirming placement_____ **Title** _____

NYS ETI QI form completed by tech   QI form faxed by Medical Control

Emergency Department follow-up details:

ET/EGD placement at ED confirmed as:

Tracheal   Esophageal   Oropharyngeal   No device in place

ET/EGD placement confirmed by (check all that apply):

Auscultation   Direct visualization   Disposable colormetric etCO$_2$ Electronic Capnography

Esophageal Detection Device   Chest X-Ray   Ultrasound

Complications (check all that apply):

Dental trauma   Oropharyngeal trauma   Right mainstem intubated

Emesis aspiration   Accidental extubation   Other _____

etCO$_2$ at scene _____ mm Hg   etCO$_2$ at hospital arrival _____ mm Hg

Figure 33-1   The medical control follow-up runsheet is completed by a paramedic based at County Medical Control who collects information from the field provider after the call. Through voice and fax communications, additional data are collected from the emergency department staff, who confirm proper placement of the airway device. Regional hospitals cooperate in this county-wide initiative to ensure quality airway management. *ED,* Emergency department; *EGD,* extraglottic airway device. *EMS,* Emergency medical services; *ET,* endotracheal tube; *ETI,* endotracheal intubation; *NYS,* New York State; *QI,* quality improvement.

ETI/RSI
Decision and Confirmation CQI Form

MRN: _____ Date: ____/____/____ Time: _____:_____

This form should be completed by the scene Paramedic and Emergency Department Physician and reviewed by the Medical Control Physician.

Predictors of Difficult Bag-Mask Ventilation or Intubation Present with Patient

Check all positive findings:

☐ **M** – poor **M**ask seal predicted
☐ **O** – **O**bese habitus
☐ **A** – **A**dvanced age
☐ **N** – **N**o teeth
☐ **S** – **S**tiff lungs (COPD, hemo/pneumothorax, burns, etc)

☐ **L** – **L**ook externally (short-bull neck, micrognathia, etc.)
☐ **E** – **E**valuate distances. "3,3,2" <3 fingerbreadths for incisor distance
        <3 fingerbreadths for hyoid/mental distance, <2 fingerbreadths for thyroid to mouth distance
☐ **M** – **M**allampati class 3 or 4 airway
☐ **O** – **O**bstruction of airway
☐ **N** – **N**eck mobility limited (e.g., suspected cervical injury)

Backup Devices Prepared

☐ BVM   ☐ Bougie   ☐ King LT
☐ Glide Scope   ☐ Combitube   ☐ Other

Indication For RSI

☐ **Head trauma or ICH with:**
  • ↓ LOC - GCS_____
  • Hypoxia – SpO$_2$ <90%
  • Combativeness
  • Failure to maintain airway
    - Secretions
    - Sonorous breathing
    - Emesis

  * Lidocaine 1 mg/kg: _____ mg

☐ **Respiratory Failure**
  • Hypoxia – SpO$_2$ <90% **with** assist
  • etCO$_2$ – >60 mm Hg
☐ **Loss of Airway Reflexes**
  • Depressed level of consciousness
  • Active seizure
☐ **Anticipated Deterioration**
  • Severe multi-trauma
  • Major OD
  • Other_____

RSI Medications		**Patient Characteristics**
Etomidate (0.3 mg/kg)	_____ mg	
Succinylcholine (1.5 mg/kg)	_____ mg	Age: _____ years
Rocuronium (0.6 mg/kg)	_____ mg	
Vecuronium (0.1 mg/kg)	_____ mg	Weight: _____ kilograms
Paralysis and Sedation		
Rocuronium (0.6 mg/kg)	_____ mg	Height: _____ feet, inches
Ativan (1-2 mg)	_____ mg	

Figure 33-2 The decision and confirmation continuous quality improvement form is used at a hospital-based emergency medical service. It is completed by the field paramedic who treated the patient and then by the emergency department physician. *BVM,* Bag-mask ventilation; *CQI,* continuous quality improvement; *ETI,* endotracheal intubation; *GCS,* Glasgow Coma Scale score; *ICH,* intracerebral hemorrhage; *LOC,* level of consciousness; *LT,* laryngeal tube; *MRN,* medical record number; *OD,* overdose; *RSI,* rapid-sequence intubation. (Courtesy of Stony Brook University Medical Center, Department of Emergency Medicine, Stony Brook, NY.)

Difficulty	Alternate Techniques
☐ Low ☐ High ☐ Failed ☐ # Attempts _____	☐ Tomahawk ☐ Bougie ☐ Other_____

ETT Diameter: _____
ETT Depth: _____
Secured with: _____

Glottic Visualization

☐ Cormack-Lehane Grade (I–IV) _____

Paramedic (Check all that apply)	**ED Physician** (Check all that apply)
☐ Waveform Capnography • _____mm Hg ☐ Direct visualization of tube passing the vocal cords ☐ Equal breath sounds ☐ Absent epigastric sounds ☐ O_2 Saturation <u>sustained</u> >95% ☐ Secured after confirmation ☐ Backup device used_____ ☐ Adjuncts used _____ Name: _____ Signed: _____	☐ Waveform Capnography • _____mm Hg ☐ Direct visualization of tube placement between vocal cords ☐ Equal breath sounds ☐ Absent epigastric sounds ☐ O_2 Saturation <u>sustained</u> >95% ☐ Re-intubation necessary Name: _____ Signed: _____

Please affix a strip showing pre-hospital pulse, SpO_2 and $etCO_2$ waveform below:

Figure 33-2, cont'd

SELECTED REFERENCES

All references can be found online at expertconsult.com.

2. Wang HE, Abo BN, Lave JR, et al: How would minimum experience standards affect the distribution of out-of-hospital endotracheal intubations? *Ann Emerg Med* 50:246–252, 2007.

4. Gausche M, Lewis RJ, Stratton SJ, et al: Effect of out-of-hospital pediatric endotracheal intubation on survival and neurological outcome: A controlled clinical trial. *JAMA* 283:783–790, 2000.

7. Cushman JT, Zachary Hettinger A, Farney A, Shah MN: Effect of intensive physician oversight on a prehospital rapid-sequence intubation program. *Prehosp Emerg Care* 14:310–316, 2010.

16. Silvestri S, Ralls GA, Krauss B, et al: The effectiveness of out-of-hospital use of continuous end-tidal carbon dioxide monitoring on the rate of unrecognized misplaced intubation within a regional emergency medical services system. *Ann Emerg Med* 45:497–503, 2005.

18. National Association of EMS Physicians (NAEMSP): Drug-assisted intubation in the prehospital setting: Position statement of the National Association of Emergency Physicians. *Prehosp Emerg Care* 10:260, 2006.

23. National Highway Traffic Safety Administration (NHTSA): National emergency medical services education standards, 2010. Available at http://www.ems.gov/education/overview.html (accessed March 2012).

33. Wang HE, Cook LJ, Chang CC, et al: Outcomes after out-of-hospital endotracheal intubation errors. *Resuscitation* 80:50–55, 2009.

37. Hinchey PR, Myers JB, Lewis R, et al: Improved out-of-hospital cardiac arrest survival after the sequential implementation of 2005 AHA guidelines for compressions, ventilations, and induced hypothermia: The Wake County experience. *Ann Emerg Med* 56:348–357, 2010.

38. Brain Trauma Foundation: Prehospital severe traumatic brain injury guidelines. Available at http://tbiguidelines.org/glHome.aspx (accessed March 2012).

39. Walls R, Murphy M: *Manual of emergency airway management*, ed 3, Philadelphia, 2008, Lippincott, Williams & Wilkins, pp 303–325.

Chapter 34

Disaster Preparedness, Cardiopulmonary Resuscitation, and Airway Management

JOSEPH H. MCISAAC III | LAUREN C. BERKOW

I. INTRODUCTION

Disasters happen. They happen frequently, but they are not uniformly distributed in time and geography. Any particular place tends to experience them infrequently. Although there are many definitions of disaster, the most common medical definition of a disaster is an "event that results in casualties that overwhelm the health care system in which the event occurs."[1] Typically, disasters degrade the fundamental infrastructure necessary for a viable economy and civil society. This disruption magnifies the impact of the event by widening the gap between needed and available resources (Fig. 34-1).

In most parts of the world, natural disasters, such as floods, major storms, earthquakes, wildfires, tsunamis, and epidemics, occur at higher frequencies than man-made disasters, such as wars or technologic events. Catastrophic events can be viewed by scale (local versus regional), proximity (happens locally versus somewhere else), time scale (discrete versus continuous), degree and type of infrastructure degradation (minimal versus total, physical

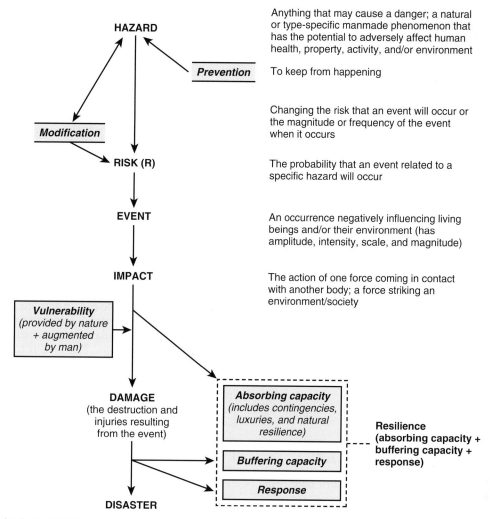

Figure 34-1 Standardized definitions of terms used to communicate by the various disciplines involved in disasters. (Modified from Task Force for Quality Control of Disaster Medicine (TFQCDM)/World Association for Disaster and Emergency Medicine (WADEM): *Health disaster management: guidelines for evaluation and research in the Utstein style,* vol 1. Available at http://www.wadem.org/guidelines/chapter_3.pdf [accessed March 2012].)

destruction versus loss of personnel), and casualty spectrum.

II. DISASTER TRIAGE

Triage is the act of sorting casualties. It implies that numbers of casualties exceed available medical resources. During routine circumstances in modern hospitals, the sickest patients receive the highest priority. During mass casualty events, patients are sorted into several levels based on the ability to help the greatest number while conserving scarce resources. Several systems are in use, and all are based loosely on military systems but have not been scientifically validated.[2] Patients who require intense resources with little likelihood of salvage are called *expectant*. They are expected to die and are given comfort measures only. Those with severe but treatable conditions are marked as *immediate*. Wounded who can wait are referred to as *delayed* or *minimal* (Fig. 34-2). Because triage depends on resources, repeat triage should occur

when there is a change in patient status, available care, and transfer to another facility.

III. SURGE CAPACITY

The concept of *surge capacity* is important beyond the emergency department. As the number of arriving patients peaks, the ability to expand services and number of beds is critical. Although temporarily increased capacity can result from cancellation or delay of routine patient load, there ultimately must be an expansion of overall facility capacity or introduction of new facilities into the system.[3] This can be done by adding portable facilities, recruiting administrative space within the institution, or using municipal buildings (e.g., schools) for treatment space. Unless providers and supplies can be augmented from outside the disaster zone, creative allocation of resources is the only option. The Agency for Healthcare Research and Quality (AHRQ) has developed an online, disaster-specific hospital surge model that can be used for planning.[4]

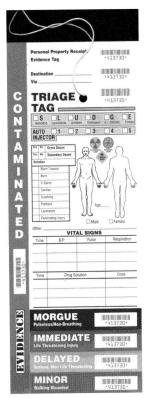

Figure 34-2 Example of a triage tag. (Courtesy of Disaster Management Systems, Inc., Pomona, CA.)

IV. ALTERED STANDARDS OF CARE

In large-scale disasters, an altered standard of care must be implemented. Chronic diseases such as diabetes, hypertension, and hypothyroidism become uncontrolled as the medication supply is depleted. Life-threatening conditions such as coronary ischemia and dialysis-dependent renal failure can no longer be treated adequately. Scarce resources are more appropriately directed to others. Loss of sanitation and hygiene increase the frequency of wound infection, respiratory diseases and gastrointestinal diseases. Acute shortages of antibiotics can become a major limitation, and determination of the standard of care can be set regionally (e.g., in pandemic influenza) or done on an ad hoc basis.[5]

V. HOSPITAL INCIDENT COMMAND SYSTEM

All U.S. hospitals are required by The Joint Commission (TJC), formerly the Joint Commission on Accreditation of Healthcare Organizations (JCAHO), and by governmental policies to have disaster plans prepared and tested twice per year. The most accepted standard for hospital disaster response is the Hospital Incident Response System (HICS) (http://www.hicscenter.org/index.php [accessed March 2012]). HICS consists of a command and control framework headed by the incident commander and prioritized task lists for each designated subordinate. Modeled on military combat systems and perfected by the California Fire Service, HICS is a time-tested system.

VI. OPERATING ROOM PREPARATION

On notification of a disaster situation, the local institution's operating room disaster standard operating procedure should be used.[6] HICS does not delineate how a surgical service should organize the operating room. The HICS model should be used with a single chief of the operating room, preferably a senior anesthesiologist who is in communication with the emergency department, intensive care units, postanesthesia care unit, the chief of perioperative nursing, and the hospital's surgical chief.

VII. ANESTHETIC AND RESUSCITATION TECHNIQUES

A. Emergency Airway Management and Ventilation

Emergency airway management strategies during disasters are closely coupled with triage plans and available resources. Resources are not expended on casualties that are designated as expectant. In a mass casualty situation, patients requiring ventilator support may be beyond the capabilities of the system. The goal is to have all patients breathe spontaneously. Placing patients in a lateral (rescue) position may be the most reasonable approach in some situations. Oral airways, nasal airways, supraglottic devices, and surgical airways are relatively low-technology options. Anecdotal reports from World War I describe using a midline tongue retraction suture or piercing the tongue with a piece of wood, but these methods are of questionable value.

Tracheal intubation, except when performed blindly, requires a light source and a laryngoscope. Typically, the intubated patient requires controlled ventilation. Use of a surgical airway is rarely indicated, but it remains an option in selected cases. The expenditure of effort and resources for such a patient may not be consistent with the most good for the greatest number, but care should not be denied to a salvageable casualty when time and resources are available. Advanced techniques are only as good as their availability and the skill of the practitioner. Several types of portable ventilators can be used during a respiratory disease pandemic if normal infrastructure (i.e., electrical power and compressed gas) is available. Figure 34-3 shows a portable ventilator.

B. Anesthetic Techniques

Trauma often is regarded as the predominant source of surgical disease among mass casualties in a disaster. Although that is usually the case at the outset, routine surgical disease evolves to become a major concern over time because of delays in caring for victims. Some maladies (e.g., strangulation of an incarcerated hernia) progress to the acute stage, whereas others (e.g., lacerations, fractures) progress to infection and gangrene because of deferred care and difficulty with hygiene and sanitation. Babies continue to be born, and the complications of childbirth must be addressed.

Choice of anesthetic technique depends on the resources available and the skill of the practitioner. Total

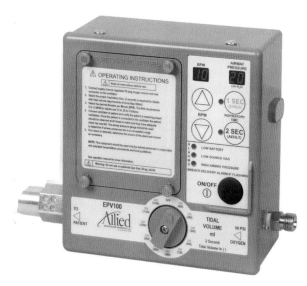

Figure 34-3 Example of portable ventilator used for treating mass casualties. (Courtesy of Allied Healthcare Products, Inc., St. Louis, MO.)

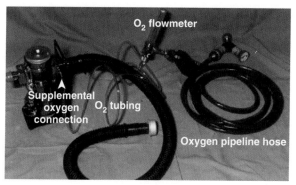

Figure 34-4 Omeda Universal Portable Anesthesia Complete (U-PAC) drawover anesthesia system. (Courtesy of GE Healthcare, Fairfield, CT.)

intravenous anesthesia (TIVA) with local anesthetic infiltration has been the default option when resources are constrained. Needed quantities of parenteral agents such as ketamine, narcotics, benzodiazepines, propofol, and barbiturates are compact, easy to transport, and easy to store. Judicious infiltration of local anesthetics can provide acceptable conditions for short procedures when used alone. Baker and colleagues[7] described three levels of military anesthesia care on the battlefield: sevoflurane inhalation using standard anesthesia machines at the highest level, drawover vaporizers at the intermediate level, and TIVA at the lowest level. Regional anesthesia, particularly nerve blocks placed with a nerve stimulator or ultrasound if available, has enjoyed popularity in war zones and during the 2010 Haiti earthquake.[8]

The Omeda Universal Portable Anesthesia Complete (U-PAC) drawover anesthesia system (GE Healthcare, Fairfield, CT) has been deployed with the U.S. military. Drawover features include durability, compactness,

portability, low capital investment, low operating expense, and no requirement for compressed gas or electricity.[9] Components of a drawover system include a vaporizer powered by patient respiration or a self-inflating bag with a one-way valve (Fig. 34-4).

VIII. PLANNING AND PREPARATION

The key to successful management during a disaster is good preparation and planning, which starts with a realistic understanding of the situation. When preparing to meet the needs of a distant event, the response should be tailored to the acute and endemic disease spectrum, climate, degree of infrastructure impairment, and cultural particulars of the affected area. An area with inadequate transportation; total loss of power, water, and sanitation; and tenuous security after a major earthquake has significantly different needs from an area experiencing pandemic influenza (Fig. 34-5). Logistics are always the major limiting factor. Resupply may be uncertain or nonexistent. Local manufacture of substitutes (e.g., boiled linen for sterile dressings) may be the only option. Compressed gas and intravenous fluids are heavy, bulky, and in short supply. Lack of refrigeration limits use of certain pharmaceuticals. Modern sterilization methods may not be available, requiring improvisation. Boiling metal

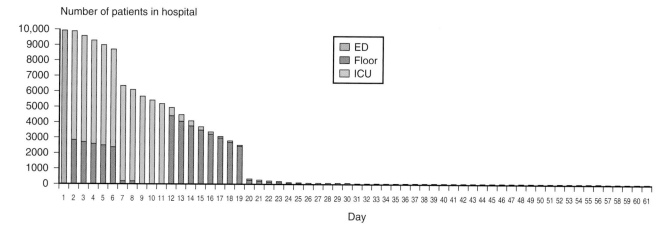

Figure 34-5 Time course of hospitalized patients after a 10-kT nuclear detonation. *ED,* Emergency department; *ICU,* intensive care unit. (From U.S. Department of Health and Human Services: Hospital surge model. Available at http://www.hospitalsurgemodel.org (accessed March 2012).)

instruments for 15 to 30 minutes renders a high degree of asepsis. After thorough cleaning with soap or detergent, soaking heat-intolerant equipment in common household bleach (i.e., sodium hypochlorite solution) is an excellent means of sterilization, but it tends to degrade many materials after repeated application.

A. The U.S. National Disaster System

The National Incident Management System (NIMS) provides a systematic,[10] proactive approach to guide all levels of governmental departments and agencies, nongovernmental organizations, and the private sector to work seamlessly to prevent, protect against, respond to, recover from, and mitigate the effects of incidents, regardless of cause, size, location, or complexity, to reduce the loss of life and property and harm to the environment. NIMS works hand in hand with the National Response Framework (NRF).[11] NIMS provides the template for the management of incidents, and the NRF provides the structure and mechanisms for national-level policy for incident management.

The National Disaster Medical System (NDMS) is a nationwide partnership designed to deliver quality medical care to the victims of and the responders to a domestic disaster.[12] NDMS provides state-of-the-art medical care under any conditions at the disaster site, in transit from the impacted area, and in participating definitive care facilities.

B. National Disaster Medical System Teams

The NDMS consists of several teams: Disaster Medical Assistance Team (DMAT), Disaster Mortuary Operational Response Team (DMORT), Veterinary Medical Assistance Team (VMAT), and National Medical Response Team (NMRT).

DMATs provide primary and acute care, triage of mass casualties, initial resuscitation and stabilization, advanced life support, and preparation of sick or injured for evacuation. The basic deployment configuration of a DMAT consists of 35 persons, including physicians, nurses, medical technicians, and ancillary support personnel. They can be mobile within 6 hours of notification and are capable of arriving at a disaster site within 48 hours. They can sustain operations for 72 hours without external support. DMATs are responsible for establishing an initial (electronic) medical record for each patient, including assigning patient-unique identifiers to facilitate tracking throughout the NDMS.

NMRTs provide medical care after a nuclear, biologic, or chemical incident. This team can provide mass casualty decontamination, medical triage, and primary and secondary medical care to stabilize victims for transportation to tertiary care facilities in a hazardous material environment. The basic deployment configuration of an NMRT consists of 50 persons.

C. Strategic National Stockpile

The Strategic National Stockpile is a national repository of antibiotics, chemical antidotes, antitoxins, life-support medications, intravenous administration and airway maintenance supplies, and medical and surgical items. The Strategic National Stockpile is designed to supplement and resupply state and local public health agencies in the event of a national emergency anywhere and at anytime within the United States or its territories.

D. Surgical Specialty Teams

Besides military medical assets controlled by the federal government, the NDMS has several International Medical Surgical Response Teams (IMSuRT) for rapid deployment of surgical expertise to disaster zones. The NDMS is organizing a prototype Multispecialty Surgical Enhancement Team (MSET) consisting of anesthesiologists, trauma surgeons, neurosurgeons, and orthopedic surgeons. No specific doctrine has been announced. It can be anticipated that multiple teams will be formed.

E. Infrastructure Resiliency

Disaster preparedness must consider infrastructure resilience. This can be accomplished through hardening of existing infrastructure such as utilities and communications or through the acquisition of alternatives. Examples are alternative power sources such as solar-, mechanical-, and steam-powered engines; amateur radio as a substitute for standard communications; and food prepared for long-term storage.

F. Anticipating Surprise

Expect the unexpected. Failure to predict surprise can result in panic, paralysis, and a sense of defeat. Developing a psychology to anticipate unexpected occurrences and then training for such contingencies creates an atmosphere of resilience. Attitude is probably the most important characteristic that determines outcome. In retrospect, most surprises can be seen as having indicators that were overlooked or recognized but rejected as unbelievable. Typically, they are high-impact, low-probability events.[13]

G. Decontamination, Personal Protective Equipment, and Isolation for Chemical, Biologic, and Radiologic Events

Personal protective equipment (PPE) is used by medical personnel to prevent occupational exposure to infectious, radiologic, or chemical agents. Gloves, gowns, and masks are a normal part of responders' daily lives under universal precautions. High-risk infections such as tuberculosis require the use of high-efficiency particulate air (HEPA) filtration masks, most commonly the N95 mask, a filter found to remove at least 95% of airborne particles during worse-case testing. Negative-pressure isolation rooms and wards are used to keep airborne infection risks contained.

It is important to distinguish between decontamination and isolation. Infectious patients cannot be decontaminated because the infection is internal. Patients with external chemical and radiologic contamination should be decontaminated to minimize the patient's exposure to the agent and the exposure of the treating staff. Removal of clothing and washing with copious amounts of water (with or without soap) constitute the best universal decontamination strategy. This can be accomplished for mass casualties through a formal decontamination system or by any improvised method that accomplishes the goal. Employing a method for assessing the effectiveness of decontamination (e.g., testing patients after decontamination with a Geiger counter, chemical meter, or using a surrogate tracer) can increase confidence in the system, but studies have consistently shown several orders of magnitude of contamination reduction using only clothing removal and shower. The main exception to this rule is a gross level of contamination by persistent chemicals used by the military, such as thickened nerve agents and some vesicants. These scenarios are more likely to occur in large-scale chemical warfare, which is unlikely to occur because most armies have eliminated their inventories. First responders at the hospital level typically wear level C PPE, whereas first responders at a site of high agent concentration often wear level A or B PPE.[14]

Use of PPE imposes a burden on the caregiver. Besides the psychological impact and heat stress, there are measurable impediments to vision, hearing, communications, and manual dexterity. Suyama and colleagues found that for a non–PPE-wearing operator,[15] needle-to-skin time favored intravenous placement over intraosseous but that an intraosseous approach provided faster vascular access when wearing PPE. The affect of PPE on airway management seems less clear. Although Greenland and coworkers found that PPE affected bronchoscopy but not intubation,[16] Castle and colleagues found that chemical-biologic-radiologic-nuclear (CBRN) PPE significantly impaired intubation but not laryngeal mask airway placement while kneeling,[17] sitting, or lying on the floor.

IX. BASIC LIFE SUPPORT AND CARDIOPULMONARY RESUSCITATION GUIDELINES

The 2005 American Heart Association (AHA) guidelines for basic life support (BLS) and cardiopulmonary resuscitation (CPR) recommended the sequence of airway, breathing, and circulation (A-B-C).[18] The first steps in the 2005 BLS were opening the airway, checking for breathing, and providing two rescue breaths if adequate breathing is not detected. The third step was to initiate chest compressions (Fig. 34-6). To check for breathing, lay rescuers and health care providers were advised to "look, listen, and feel." Health care providers were then advised to check for a pulse after delivery of the initial rescue breaths to a nonresponsive, nonbreathing individual.

The 2005 CPR guidelines recommended two rescue breaths, each given over 1 second, with sufficient tidal volume to produce visual chest rise. If an advanced airway was in place, the guidelines recommended 8 to 10 breaths per minute without synchronizing breaths between chest compressions.

Updated BLS and CPR guidelines were released by the AHA in 2010.[19-21] Table 34-1 summarizes these guidelines. The recommended sequence was changed to circulation, airway, and breathing (C-A-B). In conditions of low blood flow (e.g., cardiac arrest), oxygen delivery to the brain and heart is limited primarily by blood flow instead of arterial oxygen content.[22] Using cardiac-only resuscitation and minimizing delays or interruptions in chest compressions can improve survival.[23] Evidence does not show any difference in survival rates between chest compressions delivered alone and chest compressions combined with positive-pressure ventilation.[23-25] The AHA currently recommends that chest compressions be initiated before rescue breaths or advanced airway placement. Rescue breaths are provided after the first cycle of chest compressions (Fig. 34-7). "Look, listen, and feel" has been removed from the 2010 algorithm.

Although the optimal oxygen concentration to be delivered during CPR has not been defined, current AHA guidelines recommend initial delivery of 100% oxygen during resuscitation. After return of spontaneous circulation, the 2010 guidelines recommend titration of oxygen administration to maintain an oxygen saturation level of 94% or greater to avoid hyperoxia when appropriate monitoring is available. Box 34-1 summarizes the changes pertaining to airway management during CPR that were introduced in the 2010 AHA guidelines.

X. INITIAL AIRWAY MANAGEMENT DURING CARDIOPULMONARY RESUSCITATION

A. Rescue Breathing

Initial rescue breathing during CPR should be provided through a mouth-to-mouth method, mouth-to-barrier device, or bag-mask ventilation (if available). Each rescue breath should be given over 1 second with a sufficient tidal volume to produce a visible chest rise. Two ventilations should be provided after every 30 compressions (30:2 compression-to-ventilation ratio). Trained lay rescuers or health care providers should initiate rescue breathing. An *untrained* lay rescuer should provide chest compressions only and not initiate rescue breathing. If a pulse is present, one rescue breath should be given every 6 seconds and the pulse rechecked every 2 minutes.

The airway should be opened by a head tilt–chin lift maneuver, unless a cervical spine injury is suspected. If a cervical spine injury is suspected, a jaw thrust should be performed with the head maintained in a midline position.

B. Airway Adjuncts

Oropharyngeal airways can be used to assist bag-mask ventilation by displacement of the tongue, which can occlude the airway. Oropharyngeal airways are recommended for unconscious patients and should be placed by rescuers trained in their use.

Nasopharyngeal airways are better tolerated in conscious patients than are oral airway adjuncts, and they can assist ventilation by relieving nasopharyngeal obstruction.

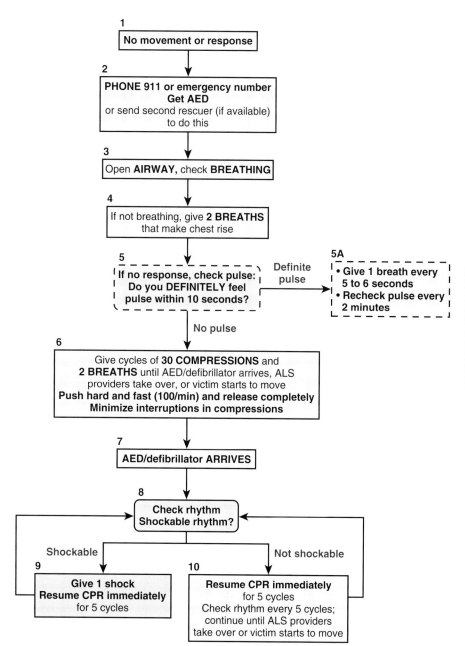

1
No movement or response

2
PHONE 911 or emergency number
Get AED
or send second rescuer (if available)
to do this

3
Open **AIRWAY**, check **BREATHING**

4
If not breathing, give **2 BREATHS**
that make chest rise

5
If no response, check pulse:
**Do you DEFINITELY feel
pulse within 10 seconds?**

Definite
pulse →

5A
• **Give 1 breath every
5 to 6 seconds**
• **Recheck pulse every
2 minutes**

No pulse

6
Give cycles of **30 COMPRESSIONS** and
2 BREATHS until AED/defibrillator arrives, ALS
providers take over, or victim starts to move
**Push hard and fast (100/min) and release completely
Minimize interruptions in compressions**

7
AED/defibrillator **ARRIVES**

8
**Check rhythm
Shockable rhythm?**

Shockable   Not shockable

9
**Give 1 shock
Resume CPR immediately**
for 5 cycles

10
Resume CPR immediately
for 5 cycles
Check rhythm every 5 cycles;
continue until ALS providers
take over or victim starts to move

Figure 34-6 The 2005 adult basic life support health care provider algorithm. *AED,* Automatic external defibrillator; *ALS,* advanced life support; *CPR,* cardiopulmonary resuscitation. (From Emergency Cardiovascular Care (ECC) Committee, Subcommittees, and Task Forces of the American Heart Association: 2005 American Heart Association Guidelines for Cardiopulmonary Resuscitation and Emergency Cardiovascular Care. *Circulation* 112(Suppl):IV1–IV203, 2005.)

Nasal airway adjuncts should be placed by a rescuer trained in their use, and they should be used with caution if a basilar skull fracture or coagulopathy is suspected.

XI. ADVANCED AIRWAY MANAGEMENT DURING CARDIOPULMONARY RESUSCITATION

Endotracheal intubation during CPR should be performed by trained health care providers, and interruptions of chest compressions should be minimized. Endotracheal intubation through direct laryngoscopy may be more difficult if performed during chest compressions. Prolonged attempts at tracheal intubation should be avoided, especially if chest compressions are halted during attempts. Placement of an endotracheal tube or other advanced airway device has not been associated with any improvement in return of spontaneous circulation. Endotracheal intubation attempts by inexperienced providers may result in complications such as failed intubation or esophageal intubation.[26]

After endotracheal tube placement, ventilations are delivered without interruption of chest compressions at a rate of one breath every 6 to 8 seconds. Certain resuscitation medications (Box 34-2) can be delivered through the endotracheal tube. Secretions can be removed from the airway through the endotracheal tube, and the endotracheal tube cuff may provide a barrier against aspiration.

A. Confirmation of Endotracheal Tube Placement During Cardiopulmonary Resuscitation

The 2005 CPR guidelines recommended the use of exhaled carbon dioxide (CO_2) detectors or esophageal

TABLE 34-1

Basic Life Support Components for Adults, Children, and Infants

Component	RECOMMENDATION		
	Adults	*Children*	*Infants*
Initial response	Unresponsive	Unresponsive	Unresponsive
	No breathing or no normal breathing (i.e., only gasping)	No breathing or only gasping	No breathing or only gasping
	No pulse palpitated within 10 sec for all ages (HCP only)		
CPR sequence	C-A-B	C-A-B	C-A-B
Compression rate	At least 100/min	At least 100/min	At least 100/min
Compression depth	At least 2 inches (5 cm)	At least one-half AP diameter About 2 inches (5 cm)	At least one-half AP diameter About 1.5 inches (4 cm)
Chest wall recoil	Allow complete recoil between compressions	Allow complete recoil between compressions	Allow complete recoil between compressions
	HCPs rotate compressors every 2 min	HCPs rotate compressors every 2 min	HCPs rotate compressors every 2 min
Compression interruptions	Minimize interruptions in chest compressions	Minimize interruptions in chest compressions	Minimize interruptions in chest compressions
	Try to limit interruptions to < 10 sec	Try to limit interruptions to < 10 sec	Try to limit interruptions to < 10 sec
Airway	Head tilt and chin lift (HCP suspects trauma: jaw thrust)	Head tilt and chin lift (HCP suspects trauma: jaw thrust)	Head tilt and chin lift (HCP suspects trauma: jaw thrust)
Compression-to-ventilation ratio (until advanced airway placed)	30:2—one or two rescuers	30:2—one rescuer 15:2—two HCP rescuers	30:2—one rescuer 15:2—two HCP rescuers
Ventilations when rescuer untrained or trained and not proficient	Compressions only	Compressions only	Compressions only
Ventilations with advanced airway (HCP)	1 breath every 6 to 8 sec (8 to 10 breaths/min)	1 breath every 6 to 8 sec (8 to 10 breaths/min)	1 breath every 6 to 8 sec (8 to 10 breaths/min)
	Asynchronous with chest compressions	Asynchronous with chest compressions	Asynchronous with chest compressions
	About 1 sec per breath	About 1 sec per breath	About 1 sec per breath
	Visible chest rise	Visible chest rise	Visible chest rise
Defibrillation	Attach and use AED as soon as available	Attach and use AED as soon as available	Attach and use AED as soon as available
	Minimize interruptions in chest compressions before and after shock	Minimize interruptions in chest compressions before and after shock	Minimize interruptions in chest compressions before and after shock
	Resume CPR beginning with compressions immediately after each shock	Resume CPR beginning with compressions immediately after each shock	Resume CPR beginning with compressions immediately after each shock

*Excluding the newly born, in whom the cause of arrest usually is asphyxia.

A, Airway; *AED,* automated external defibrillator; *AP,* anterior-posterior; *B,* breathing; *C,* circulation; *CPR,* cardiopulmonary resuscitation; *HCP,* health care provider.

Modified from American Heart Association: Highlights of the 2010 American Heart Association guidelines for CPR and ECC. Available at http://static.heart.org/eccguidelines/pdf/90-1043_ECC_2010_Guidelines_Highlights _noRecycle.pdf (accessed March 2012).

Box 34-1   2010 Advanced Cardiac Life Support Guidelines: Changes in Airway Management

1. The basic life support sequence has changed from A-B-C to C-A-B for adults, children, and infants. Initiate chest compressions *before* ventilations.
2. Use of cricoid pressure during ventilations is not recommended.
3. Instruction to "look, listen, and feel for breathing" has been removed from the algorithm.
4. Excessive ventilation should be avoided.
5. Continuous quantitative capnography is recommended to confirm endotracheal tube placement.
6. Oxygen concentration is weaned after return of spontaneous circulation to maintain oxygen saturation at 94% or greater.

A, Airway; *B,* breathing; *C,* circulation.

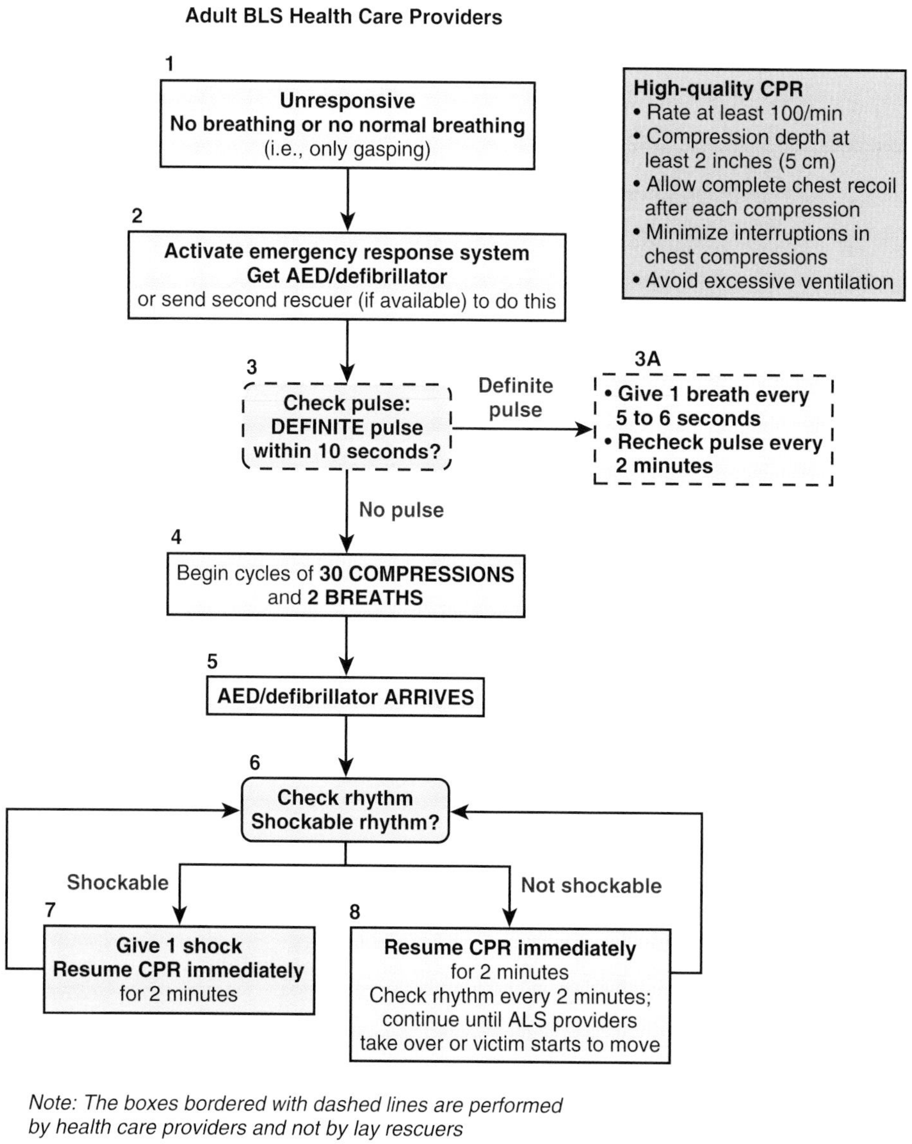

Adult BLS Health Care Providers

Figure 34-7 The 2010 adult basic life support (*BLS*) health care provider algorithm. *AED,* Automatic external defibrillator; *ALS,* advanced life support; *CPR,* cardiopulmonary resuscitation. (From Berg RA, Hemphill R, Abella BS, et al: Part 5: Adult basic life support: 2010 American Heart Association Guidelines for Cardiopulmonary Resuscitation and Emergency Cardiovascular Care. *Circulation* 122:S685–S705, 2010.)

Box 34-2	**Resuscitation Medications That Can Be Delivered Through an Endotracheal Tube**

Administer two to three times the intravenous dosage, followed by 10 mL of normal saline:

Lidocaine
Epinephrine
Atropine
Vasopressin
Naloxone

---

detectors for confirmation of endotracheal tube placement in addition to clinical assessment by auscultation and direct visualization. Exhaled CO_2 detectors may produce a false-negative result due to decreased blood flow and CO_2 delivery to the lungs, pulmonary embolus, pulmonary edema, or severe airway obstruction.[27] False-positive readings have been detected when the stomach contains large amounts of carbonated liquids.[28]

The 2010 CPR guidelines recommend the use of continuous waveform capnography for confirmation of endotracheal tube placement during CPR, although the use of exhaled CO_2 detectors or esophageal detectors is considered acceptable if waveform capnography is not available. Continuous waveform capnography may have decreased specificity and sensitivity during prolonged resuscitation and decreased perfusion.

Thoracic impedance measurement may aid in detection of esophageal intubation, but evidence is insufficient to recommend its use for confirmation of endotracheal tube placement. Thoracic impedance is significantly higher during inspiration than during expiration, and changes in impedance, which can be measured by defibrillation pads, occur only if the endotracheal tube is correctly placed.[29]

B. Use of Cricoid Pressure During Cardiopulmonary Resuscitation

The 2005 CPR guidelines recommended the use of cricoid pressure by a third rescuer if the victim is deeply unconscious. Evidence suggests that applying cricoid pressure may impede ventilation and interfere with the placement of advanced airway devices or intubation.[30,31] The 2010 guidelines recommend *against* the routine use of cricoid pressure as part of airway management during CPR.

C. Supraglottic Airway Devices

The 2005 and 2010 AHA CPR guidelines support the use of a supraglottic airway device as an alternative to endotracheal intubation. Box 34-3 lists the supraglottic devices that have been studied for use in cardiac arrest and acknowledged by the AHA. Because intubation through a supraglottic airway does not require glottic visualization, placement may be faster than endotracheal intubation, and it may result in shorter no-flow times (i.e., period when chest compressions are halted for other interventions).[32,33] Supraglottic airway placement should be considered as an option if endotracheal intubation fails. Ventilations are delivered through a supraglottic airway device in the same ratio as through an endotracheal tube (i.e., one breath every 6 to 8 seconds without interruption of chest compressions).

If available, newer supraglottic airway devices that provide a conduit for intubation can be considered. Preliminary evidence supports their use in the prehospital environment, especially if difficulty with intubation is encountered.[34,35]

D. Role of Advanced Airway Devices

Advanced airway management techniques such as fiberoptic intubation and video laryngoscopy have not been widely studied as intubation techniques for airway management during CPR. Preliminary evidence suggests that video laryngoscopy may be an acceptable alternative to conventional laryngoscopy, especially for difficult intubations.[36,37] Advanced airway devices may not be easily accessible in the prehospital environment. Inadequate light conditions and the lack of electricity may limit the usefulness of video laryngoscopy outside the hospital setting.

Box 34-3 Supraglottic Airways Approved by American Heart Association for Use in Cardiopulmonary Resuscitation

Esophageal-tracheal tube (Combitube)
Laryngeal mask airway (LMA)
Laryngeal tube (LT)

XII. ALTERNATIVE METHODS OF OXYGEN DELIVERY DURING CARDIOPULMONARY RESUSCITATION

A. Oxylator

The Oxylator (CPR Medical Devices, Ontario, Canada) is a fixed-flow automatic resuscitation management system with an adjustable pressure limit. Several models exist, including the Oxylator EMX, which is recommended for prehospital use (Fig. 34-8). The Oxylator delivers oxygen flow at 30 L/min until an adjustable maximum pressure (up to 45 cm H_2O) is reached, at which point passive exhalation occurs to an airway pressure of 2 to 4 cm H_2O. The device allows manual (rescuer initiated) and automatic inhalation modes. The Oxylator works with medical oxygen or hospital air supply, tank, or compressor; it does not require electricity; and it can be connected to a face mask, supraglottic airway, or endotracheal tube.

Potential advantages of the Oxylator over bag-mask ventilation include consistent ventilation and oxygenation to a set pressure; possible avoidance of hyperventilation, excessive ventilation, or gastric insufflation; and early detection of airway obstruction.[38] Use of the Oxylator in the automatic mode can free the CPR provider to focus on other resuscitation tasks. The Oxylator may be useful in austere environments in which access to the patient's head and airway may be limited.

B. ResQPOD

The ResQPOD (Advanced Circulatory Systems, Roseville, MN), designated an AHA class 2A recommendation for patients in cardiac arrest, is an impedance threshold device. By regulating thoracic pressure during ventilation, the device increases blood flow to the heart and brain, increases systolic blood pressure, and increases the success rate of defibrillation. By preventing excess air from entering the thorax during ventilation, the device increases thoracic negative pressure and increases blood flow to the heart. It is placed proximal to a face mask, supraglottic

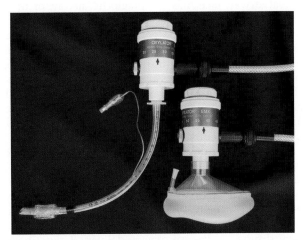

Figure 34-8 The Oxylator EMX is a positive-pressure resuscitation and inhalation system. (Courtesy of Lifesaving Systems, Inc., Roswell, GA.)

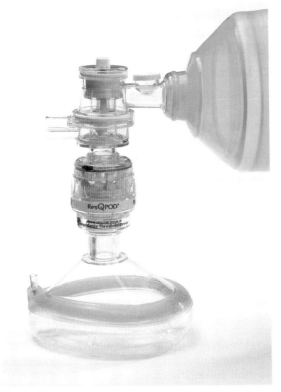

Figure 34-9 The ResQPOD is an impedance threshold device that provides perfusion on demand (POD) by regulating pressures in the thorax during states of hypotension. (Courtesy of Vygon, Ecouen, France.)

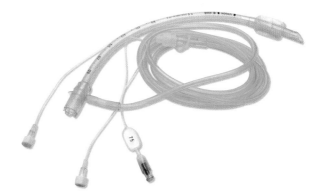

Figure 34-10 The Boussignac endotracheal tube contains capillaries through which oxygen is delivered by continuous insufflation, generating a constant positive alveolar pressure. (Courtesy of Vygon, Ecouen, France.)

airway, or endotracheal tube and connects to the source of ventilation (Fig. 34-9). The ResQPOD also contains timing-assist lights to guide proper ventilation rates and prevent hyperventilation. Use of this device during CPR has improved survival rates.[39]

C. Passive Oxygen Insufflation

Oxygen can be delivered passively through an oropharyngeal airway, face mask, supraglottic airway, or modified endotracheal tube (Boussignac endotracheal tube, Vygon Corporation, Montgomeryville, PA). The Boussignac tube contains capillaries through which oxygen is delivered by continuous insufflation, generating a constant positive alveolar pressure. The proximal end of the tube remains open to allow exhalation (Fig. 34-10). The changes in intrathoracic pressure that occur during chest compressions trigger passive inhalation and active exhalation, allowing adequate gas exchange.

Passive oxygen delivery does not require the use of a rescuer to deliver ventilations, minimizes interruptions in chest compressions, and may reduce the risk of barotrauma caused by excessive ventilation. Evidence shows passive oxygen delivery to be as effective as bag-mask ventilation or mechanical ventilation through an endotracheal tube.[40,41] Passive oxygen delivery is described as an alternative but not a replacement for ventilation during CPR in the 2010 AHA guidelines.

XIII. CHALLENGES OF AIRWAY MANAGEMENT DURING CARDIOPULMONARY RESUSCITATION

When a patient requires CPR in an emergency situation, immediate airway management is required. In the prehospital setting, no general medical history or intubation history is available to guide airway management decisions. Within the hospital setting, patient information may or may not be accessible. Even if it is available, adequate time may not exist to review the information. Knowledge of previous difficulty with ventilation or intubation is often unknown.

A. Access to the Airway

Access to the airway during CPR may be limited in the prehospital and hospital settings. Outside of the hospital, CPR may be required in whatever location or situation the victim presents, and access may be limited by the outside environment or accident scene. Airway access may also be challenging inside an ambulance or helicopter. Other equipment required to resuscitate the patient and treat life-threatening injuries may also limit access to the patient. Within the hospital setting, access to the patient's airway may be limited by equipment, invasive lines or monitors, or the small size of many hospital rooms and intensive care suites. During mass casualty disasters, PPE or chemical protection gear may make airway management more difficult.

B. Cervical Spine Injury

Cervical spine injury has been diagnosed in 2% to 5% of patients after traumatic injury.[42] If the anterior and posterior columns of the cervical spine are injured, the injury is considered unstable.[43] Most trauma patients are placed in a cervical collar until cervical injury is ruled out; some of these patients may require CPR and emergent airway management before a radiologic examination can be obtained. Significant head injury is associated with traumatic cervical spine injury; patients with a Glasgow

> **Box 34-4** **Airway Management Recommendations for Patients with Suspected Cervical Spine Injury**
>
> Rapid-sequence intubation is most often recommended.
> Manual in-line stabilization of the cervical spine minimizes movement during intubation.
> No safe amount of cervical spine movement has been defined.
> A selection of laryngoscope blades and sizes should be available.
> Supraglottic airway devices can be used as airway adjuncts.
> No specific intubation method is recommended.
>
> Modified from Ollerton JE, Parr MJA, Harrison K, et al: Potential cervical spine injury and difficult airway management for emergency intubation of trauma adults in the emergency department—a systematic review. *Emerg Med J* 23:3–11, 2006.

Coma Scale score of 8 or less often require emergent airway management.[44]

Manual in-line stabilization of the cervical spine is recommended for airway management in patients with a suspected or known cervical spine injury to reduce the potential for neck movement. Neck traction is not recommended. The presence of a cervical collar increases the difficulty of intubation. If necessary, the collar may be removed for airway management, provided that manual in-line stabilization is maintained.

No one method of intubation has been proved to be safest, and rapid-sequence intubation by direct laryngoscopy is the most commonly reported technique. Evidence shows that some degree of cervical spine motion occurs with all methods of intubation,[45,46] but data are lacking about whether the small amount of movement that occurs during airway management is clinically significant. A higher incidence of cervical spine limitation and difficult intubation may exist among elderly patients.[47] Box 34-4 describes recommendations for airway management in the patient with a suspected or known cervical spine injury.

C. Equipment Challenges

In the prehospital environment, airway management must be provided with the equipment that is available. Depending on the resources, a full complement of airway equipment, including oxygen supplies, may or may not be available. Equipment also may be unavailable within the hospital if airway management is required in a location remote from the operating room or intensive care setting. The type of airway management provided may be dictated by the available supplies and equipment, and adjunct airway devices for difficult airway management may not be quickly accessible. In the emergent setting, bag-mask ventilation should be initiated and maintained until additional airway equipment becomes available.

XIV. CONTROVERSIES

A. Role of Hyperventilation

Evidence suggests that hyperventilation may decrease overall survival and should be avoided.[48] Excessive ventilation should also be avoided because of the risk of gastric insufflation, regurgitation, or aspiration. Hyperventilation increases intrathoracic pressure and results in reduced coronary perfusion pressures.[49]

B. When to Secure the Airway

Existing information is inadequate to guide the ideal timing of advanced airway device placement. Evidence supports the practice of initiating chest compressions early, before the start of airway management. Airway management strategies should minimize interruptions in resuscitation. Newer, advanced airway devices that can be placed quickly and that do not require direct visualization of the vocal cords may achieve this goal.

XV. CONCLUSIONS

Disasters occur frequently but rarely in any one place. Triage, surge capacity, and altered standards of care are ways to ration scarce resources when demand outstrips supply. Planning and preparing for disasters can help to mitigate their impact. The HICS is used in U.S. hospitals for management during major incidents. The NDMS, operating under the National Incident Command System, is responsible for addressing major disasters within the United States.

The updated CPR guidelines stress initiation of chest compressions before airway management. Advanced airway devices such as supraglottic airways can be considered if access to the patient is limited or endotracheal intubation fails. Airway management during CPR or disaster situations is often guided by the resources available to the provider, which may be limited.

XVI. CLINICAL PEARLS

- Disaster management should start with a bottom-to-top approach, followed by a multiple-scale approach.

- Communication, preservation of infrastructure, and mitigation techniques are essential during a disaster response.

- The 2010 AHA CPR guidelines recommend beginning chest compressions before initial airway management (i.e., circulation, airway, and breathing).

- Hyperventilation during CPR should be avoided, and it may reduce overall survival.

- Limited access to the patient may make airway management and resuscitation during disasters more challenging.

SELECTED REFERENCES

All references can be found online at expertconsult.com.

19. Berg RA, Hemphill R, Abella BS, et al: Part 5: Adult basic life support: 2010 American Heart Association Guidelines for Cardiopulmonary Resuscitation and Emergency Cardiovascular Care. *Circulation* 122(Suppl 3):S685–S705, 2010.

20. Neumar RW, Otto CW, Link MS, et al: Part 8: Adult advanced cardiovascular life support: 2010 American Heart Association Guidelines for Cardiopulmonary resuscitation and Emergency Cardiovascular Care. *Circulation* 122(Suppl 3):S729–S767, 2010.

23. SOS-KANTO study group: Cardiopulmonary resuscitation by bystanders with chest compression only (SOS-KANTO): An observational study. *Lancet* 369:920–926, 2007.

43. Crosby ET: Airway management in adults after cervical spine trauma. *Anesthesiology* 104:1293–1318, 2006.

Chapter 35

The Patient with a Full Stomach

ASHUTOSH WALI | UMA MUNNUR

I. INTRODUCTION

Anesthetic administration in a patient with a full stomach poses three challenges to the anesthesia provider: prevention of gastric regurgitation, prevention of pulmonary aspiration, and institution of appropriate airway management. The accepted safe anesthesia management plan for reducing pulmonary aspiration of gastric contents in these patients involves identifying those at risk for gastric regurgitation and pulmonary aspiration by using practice guidelines for preoperative fasting, implementing prophylactic pharmacologic therapies, and applying appropriate airway management techniques that may reduce the risk of pulmonary aspiration. A review of the relevant literature suggests that the incidence of perioperative pulmonary aspiration is declining.[1] Mortality rates for this dreaded complication have dramatically decreased over the past few decades.[1]

II. DEFINITION OF PULMONARY ASPIRATION

Perioperative *pulmonary aspiration* of regurgitant gastric contents is defined as the presence of bilious secretions or particulate matter in the tracheobronchial tree. The term *bronchoaspiration* has been used to describe the same phenomenon, but the previous nomenclature for pulmonary aspiration is used in this chapter.[2] Pulmonary aspiration can occur at any time preoperatively until 2 hours after terminating anesthesia. Diagnosis is made by direct examination of the airway, bronchoscopic assessment of the tracheobronchial tree, or postoperative imaging that demonstrates lung infiltrates not previously identified on the preoperative radiograph.[3] The incidence, morbidity, and mortality from pulmonary aspiration are considered in Chapter 12.

III. TIMING OF PULMONARY ASPIRATION

Patients with a full stomach are considered to be at high risk for pulmonary aspiration, which may occur before or during induction of anesthesia or at emergence from anesthesia. Most adult cases of pulmonary aspiration occur during induction of anesthesia (i.e., before laryngoscopy and tracheal intubation) (50%), during laryngoscopy (29%), or during and after emergence from anesthesia.[1,4] In the pediatric population, most cases of pulmonary aspiration occur during induction with an inhalation anesthetic or tracheal intubation without a muscle relaxant, and more than 30% take place during emergence and extubation.[3]

Although most instances of pulmonary aspiration coincide with anesthetic induction, laryngoscopy, or surgery, they can also occur postoperatively.[5] Patients who are at risk before surgery are also at risk during the postoperative period because the residual effects of anesthetic agents, muscle relaxants, and narcotic analgesics decrease protective airway reflexes.

IV. PHYSIOLOGIC RISK FACTORS IN THE PERIOPERATIVE PATIENT

Several physiologic risk factors predispose to aspiration pneumonitis (Table 35-1):

1. Increased gastric fluid volume (GFV) with acidic pH, increased bacterial count, or solid material

2. Delayed gastric emptying
3. Impaired protective physiologic mechanisms, which include reduction in lower esophageal sphincter (LES) and upper esophageal sphincter (UES) pressure
4. Loss of protective airway (laryngeal-pharyngeal) reflexes

A. Gastric Volume and pH

The widely cited criteria for aspiration pneumonitis (GFV = 0.4 mL/kg and pH < 2.5), which were generated from the study of a single Rhesus monkey and extrapolated to humans, have been refuted.[6] Current evidence supports a dose-response relationship for gastric volume instilled directly into the lung and gastric acidity. The lethal dose for acid pulmonary aspiration has been studied in numerous animal models.[5,7,8] James and colleagues demonstrated that hydrochloric (HCl) acid instilled directly into rat tracheas resulted in a high mortality rate.[9] Late mortality rates were 90% with a volume of 0.3 mL/kg at a pH of 1.0 and 14% with a volume of 1 to 2 mL/kg at a pH less than 1.8. An investigation involving primates demonstrated that aspiration of large volumes (0.8 to 1.0 mL/kg) of acid at a pH of 1 was associated with severe pneumonitis. Instillation of smaller volumes (0.4 to 0.6 mL/kg) produced mild radiologic and clinical changes but no deaths. The median lethal dose for acid aspiration into the lungs was 1.0 mL/kg. Extrapolation of these data to humans provides a critical volume of approximately 50 mL for severe pulmonary aspiration in adults.[10]

The effect of aspiration of milky products into the lungs has also been studied in animals.[11] Acidification of human milk to a pH of 1.8 with HCl acid increased the severity of aspiration pneumonitis compared with 5%

TABLE 35-1

Physiologic Risk Factors for Regurgitation and Aspiration of Gastric Contents

Physiologic Effect	Risk Factors
Increased gastric volume, pressure, and acidity	Less than 6 hours of NPO (e.g., recent meal, drink, alcohol)
	Gastric insufflation (e.g., mask ventilation)
	Acid hypersecretion (e.g., hypoglycemia, alcohol, increased gastrin secretion)
Delayed gastric emptying	Intestinal obstruction (e.g., opioids, anticholinergics)
	Drugs
	Pregnancy
	Obesity
	Diabetes, peptic ulcer disease, trauma
	Sympathetic stimulation (e.g., acute pain, anxiety, stress)
Impaired protective physiologic mechanism	Autonomic neuropathy (e.g., diabetic gastroparesis)
Decreased LES tone	Pregnancy
	Gastroesophageal reflux
	Hiatal hernia
	Laryngoscopy
	Cricoid pressure application
Decreased UES tone	General anesthesia and sedation
Loss of protective airway (laryngeal-pharyngeal)	Altered mental state or head injury reflexes
	CNS-depressant drugs
	Cerebral hemorrhage or infarct
	Neurologic diseases (e.g., multiple sclerosis, Guillain-Barré, cerebral palsy, Parkinson's disease)
	Neuromuscular diseases (e.g., muscular dystrophies, myasthenia gravis)

CNS, Central nervous system; *LES*, lower esophageal sphincter; *NPO*, nil per os (no oral intake); *UES*, upper esophageal sphincter.

dextrose acidified to a pH of 1.8 with HCl acid. Acidification of human breast milk with gastric juice instead of HCl acid did not increase the severity of lung injury. Instillation of soy-based formula or other dairy milk formula into the lungs caused a less severe form of acute injury.[12] Human milk is particularly noxious when aspirated compared with other types of milk.

In normal, healthy children, the range of residual gastric volume at the time of anesthetic induction is broad. Cote and coauthors reported values of 0.11 to 4.72 mL/kg, which were higher than the values (0.01 to 4.08 mL/kg) reported by Splinter and associates.[13,14] Children in clinical studies typically have average gastric volumes greater than 0.4 mL/kg and acidic pH levels,[14-22] but they rarely have (1 in 10,000 anesthetics) aspiration pneumonia associated with anesthesia.[23] Instead of focusing on GFV at induction, the emphasis to prevent pulmonary aspiration should be on patients' comorbidities, their risk factors, type of anesthesia, and characteristics of the aspirate.

B. Delayed Gastric Emptying

Patients who have delayed gastric emptying are considered to have a full stomach and to be at risk for pulmonary aspiration. Patients' conditions that delay gastric emptying include obesity, pregnancy, diabetes, peptic ulcer disease, trauma, stress, and acute pain.

C. Impaired Protective Physiologic Mechanisms

1. Lower Esophageal Sphincter Tone

The LES forms a border between the stomach and the esophagus, with the lower esophagus creating a sling around the abdominal esophagus.[24] Barrier pressure is the difference between LES pressure and gastric pressure. Intragastric pressure is normally less than 7 mm Hg. Normal resting LES pressure in conscious individuals is 15 to 25 mm Hg higher than intragastric pressure. An incompetent LES reduces barrier pressure and increases the risk of regurgitation of gastric contents.

LES tone reduction is the major problem in patients with gastroesophageal reflux (GER) during anesthesia and in disease states. In patients presenting with hiatal hernia, the maximum pressure at the gastroesophageal junction was lower (17.1 mm Hg) than the pressure in healthy volunteers (28 mm Hg).[25] Intragastric pressure increases to 35 mm Hg when the stomach is distended.[26] Gastric distention with increased intragastric pressure and reflex relaxation of the LES causes spontaneous GER. When esophageal pressure equals gastric pressure, the development of a common cavity leads to spontaneous GER.[27]

Patients with coexisting gastroesophageal pathology presenting for anesthesia are susceptible to GER. The mechanism for reflux is a transient relaxation of the LES.[27,28] Anesthetic agents and techniques relax the LES, reduce barrier pressure, and predispose the patient to GER.[29] Cricoid pressure application and laryngoscopy during anesthesia also lower LES tone.[30] Drugs that lower LES tone include anticholinergics, benzodiazepines,

dopamine, sodium nitroprusside, ganglion blockers, thiopental, tricyclic antidepressants, β-adrenergic stimulants, halothane, enflurane, opioids, and propofol.[29] Inhalation agents can reduce the LES pressure below the intragastric pressure, depending on the degree of relaxation.[29,31] Propofol has no effect on barrier pressure except for a transient decrease in LES tone and gastric pressure at 1 minute, which return to baseline values later.[32] Drugs that increase LES pressure include antiemetics, cholinergic drugs, succinylcholine, pancuronium, metoclopramide, domperidone, edrophonium, neostigmine, metoprolol, metoprolol, α-adrenergic stimulants, and antacids.[29,32]

2. Upper Esophageal Sphincter Tone

The cricopharyngeus muscle acts as the functional UES. It is one of the two inferior constrictor muscles of the pharynx. It extends around the pharynx from one end of the cricoid arch to the other and is continuous with the circular, muscular coat of the esophagus.[24] In the conscious, healthy patient, the UES helps to prevent pulmonary aspiration by sealing off the upper esophagus from the hypopharynx.[33]

Various anesthetic techniques and agents (except ketamine) reduce the UES tone and predispose the patient to regurgitation of material from the esophagus into the hypopharynx. Residual neuromuscular blockade (even with train-of-four ratio of 0.7) puts the patient at risk for pulmonary aspiration because of a reduction in UES tone and impaired swallowing.[34-38]

D. Loss of Protective Laryngeal-Pharyngeal Airway Reflexes

Four well-defined reflexes in the upper airway protect the lungs from aspiration. They are apnea with laryngospasm, coughing, expiration, and spasmodic panting that involves the glottic area and the true or false vocal cords.[39] Impaired laryngeal-pharyngeal function usually results from an altered consciousness level. Patients with central nervous system disorders, cerebrovascular injuries, head trauma, alcohol intoxication, and neuromuscular disorders (particularly myotonia dystrophica and scleroderma) have an increased pulmonary aspiration risk due to diminished pharyngeal sensation and diminished protective airway reflexes.[40]

Anesthetic agents that result in the loss of UES tone impair protective reflexes.[41] Prevention of protective laryngeal closure permits entry of this foreign matter into the tracheobronchial passages, causing regurgitation of gastroesophageal contents into the pharynx.

V. PATIENTS AT RISK FOR PULMONARY ASPIRATION

Recognition of patients who have any of the aforementioned risk factors for pulmonary aspiration is the first step toward minimizing the incidence of perioperative pulmonary aspiration. These patients can be categorized in two groups: those with a full stomach (i.e., history of ingestion of a meal with less than 6 hours fasting time)[42] and those designated as having a full stomach despite a prolonged preoperative fast.

Patients who are at high risk for pulmonary aspiration are at the extremes of age, have altered consciousness, have ingested solids or liquids despite orders to take nothing by mouth (*nil per os* [NPO]), are pregnant (particularly those in labor), or have sustained trauma. Trauma, even if not abdominal, delays gastric emptying.[43,44] Trauma patients, especially those in acute pain who are scheduled for emergency surgery, have decreased gastrointestinal motility and increased gastrointestinal secretion despite fasting preoperatively.[45] The incidence of pulmonary aspiration increases markedly after trauma because of recent ingestion of food, depressed consciousness, diminished or absent airway reflexes, or gastric stasis induced by raised sympathoadrenal influx of catecholamines. In 53 adults with Glasgow Coma Scale scores less than 8 who were intubated by the London Helicopter Emergency Medical Service, the incidence the of gross pulmonary aspiration was 38%.[46,47]

Other factors increase the risk of pulmonary aspiration. Medications that delay gastric emptying affect the protective physiologic mechanisms. Patients receiving narcotics are expected to have delayed gastric emptying,[48,49] but it has also been demonstrated that administration of opioids in a single dose to healthy patients did not delay gastric emptying or affect acidity.[50-52]

Long-standing diabetes and gastroparesis are risk factors. Diabetic gastroparesis impairs gastric emptying and may compromise LES function.[1,53-55] Patients who are morbidly obese can have delayed gastric emptying, increased abdominal pressure, and a difficult airway, all of which are potential risks for pulmonary aspiration. The gastric volumes in 71% of these patients are in the at-risk range compared with the levels found in normal subjects.[56] The risk of aspiration also is increased for patients with stress and acute pain, raised intracranial pressure, and neuromuscular disorders.

Certain types of surgery are associated with pulmonary aspiration. The incidence of silent gastric regurgitation is higher in esophageal,[1,4] upper abdominal,[57] and emergency laparoscopic operations.[58,59] Comorbidities are more likely in patients with American Society of Anesthesiologists (ASA) IV or V physical status. Emergency surgery, especially when performed at night, is a risk factor for aspiration.

Failed tracheal intubation of a patient with a difficult airway can lead to hypoxia associated with gastric regurgitation and pulmonary aspiration. General anesthesia administration in patients with a full stomach necessitates tracheal intubation to protect the airway from pulmonary aspiration. If tracheal intubation that is undertaken to isolate the airway and avoid pulmonary aspiration proves to be difficult, the procedure itself can lead to pulmonary aspiration. A difficult intubation can be predicted in only two thirds of cases. Problematic anesthetic inductions compounded by difficult tracheal intubation, difficult mask ventilation, inadequate anesthesia with coughing or straining, difficult emergence, or difficult extubation constitute prime conditions for gastric regurgitation and pulmonary aspiration, and they have been reported in up to 77% of these cases.[60-63]

Regional anesthesia may be followed by complications. Regional anesthesia is usually considered safe in patients at risk for pulmonary aspiration because they are awake and have intact protective airway reflexes.[64] However, after administration of spinal anesthesia, some patients develop extensive sympathetic block followed by hypotension, vomiting, difficulty swallowing, or impaired cough reflex.[1] The risk of pulmonary aspiration is exacerbated by difficulty in swallowing because of a high level of sympathetic block. Concomitant administration of narcotics or sedatives can obtund the protective airway reflexes, leading to gastric regurgitation and pulmonary aspiration.[39,65,66] Vomiting associated with sympathetic blockade–induced hypotension requires turning the patient's head to the lateral position and placing the patient in the Trendelenburg position to avoid pulmonary aspiration of gastric contents.

VI. PERIOPERATIVE ANESTHESIA CONSIDERATIONS IN FULL-STOMACH PATIENTS

Anesthetic management in patients with a full stomach involves preemptive methods to minimize pulmonary aspiration and its morbidity. Goals are to minimize the volume of gastric contents, reduce GER, and prevent perioperative pulmonary aspiration. Preemptive measures to accomplish these goals include preoperative fasting, pharmacologic therapies to decrease gastric acidity, facilitation of gastric emptying or drainage, and competent LES tone maintenance. Full-stomach precautions dictate the anesthetic induction technique. Appropriate airway management techniques include effective cricoid pressure (CP) application, tracheal intubation, or the use of other airway devices.

A. Preoperative Fasting

Historically, adult patients have fasted 8 to 12 hours before surgery to reduce the volume of gastric contents and the aspiration pneumonitis risk. The National Confidential Enquiry into Perioperative Deaths highlighted the issue of preoperative starvation.[67] NPO after midnight is an accepted preoperative order. Long fasting before an elective operation is uncomfortable and creates detrimental effects by causing thirst, hunger, irritability, noncompliance, and resentment in adult patients.[57] Prolonged fasting is especially deleterious in children because it produces dehydration or hypoglycemia.[21,68] During the past 20 years, several scientific papers have challenged the traditional practice of preoperative fasting for more than 8 hours. The current understanding of gastric emptying physiology has generated revised preoperative fasting policies.[3,21,50,69-77]

Despite the knowledge that the stomach handles emptying solids and liquids differently, physicians traditionally lumped consideration of them together in the standard preoperative order: NPO after midnight the day before surgery. After an extensive review, the ASA task force revised policies and published specific practice guidelines for preoperative fasting.[42,78]

The Fourth National Audit Project (NAP4) was conducted by the Royal College of Anaesthetists and the Difficult Airway Society. The large-scale review of airway-related complications was published in 2011 after analyzing the events included in NAP4 from September 1, 2008, to August 31, 2009.[63] The NAP4 examined records for major complications among the 2.9 million general anesthetics in the operating rooms, airway management procedures in intensive care units (ICUs), and airway management techniques in the emergency departments across the United Kingdom.[63] The data revealed 184 serious airway-related complications that led to death, brain damage, emergency invasive airway access through the neck, unanticipated admission to the ICU, or prolonged ICU stay.[63] The most frequent fatal complication from general anesthesia was pulmonary aspiration of regurgitated gastric contents, which was implicated in 50% of the deaths.[63] Cook and colleagues thought that pulmonary aspiration was a well-recognized problem for patients under general anesthesia and that it should be preventable in most cases. However, in some cases reported in the study, proper precautions were not taken.[63] The incidence in NAP4 was three to five times higher than that found in the analysis of the ASA Closed Claims Project database reported from the United States.[79]

1. Liquids

Residual gastric volume is directly related to regurgitation and pulmonary aspiration. However, the ASA Task Force on Preoperative Fasting, despite extensive scrutiny of the existing data, has been unable to establish a link between residual gastric volume and pulmonary aspiration.[78,80]

a. CLEAR LIQUIDS

Clear liquids in healthy patients empty exponentially. The gastric emptying half-life ($t_{1/2}$) of clear liquids is 12 minutes, which is considerably faster than for solids. Theoretically, for a patient who consumes 500 mL of clear liquid, almost 97% of the liquid is eliminated from the stomach after five half-lives (i.e., 60 minutes).[81-83] The rate of gastric emptying after a liquid meal has been well studied in adults.[74,76,80] The studies demonstrated that after drinking 750 mL of pulp-free orange drink, the mean $t_{1/2}$ ranged from 10 ± 7 to 20 ± 11 minutes. The fastest $t_{1/2}$ for an individual subject was 2.9 minutes, and the slowest $t_{1/2}$ was 41.6 minutes, indicating that almost complete gastric emptying could be accomplished in 2 hours (approximately five half-lives) after a clear liquid drink was consumed. Even in individuals with the slowest emptying rates, only 10% or less of the original liquid was retained in the stomach after 2 hours.[72,75,84-86]

The ASA Committee on Standards and Practice Parameters supports a fasting period of 2 hours after the ingestion of clear liquids for all patients.[78] Clear liquids include water, fruit juices without pulp, carbonated beverages, clear tea, and black coffee. The clear liquid category does not include alcohol. The volume of liquid ingested is less important than the type of liquid.

b. MILK

In term and preterm infants, breast milk leaves the stomach more rapidly than formula milk. The gastric emptying $t_{1/2}$ for breast milk is approximately 25 minutes; for formula milk, it is twice as long.[87,88] Consultants and the ASA Committee on Standards and Practice Parameters recommend fasting 4 hours after breast milk and 6 hours after infant formula.[78]

2. Solids and Nonhuman Milk

Gastric emptying for solids occurs in a linear pattern with time, and 10% to 30% of ingested solids may remain in a patient's stomach after 6 hours.[89] Gastric emptying is inhibited when the duodenum is distended; when the chyme contains a high concentration of acid, proteins, or fats; or when the osmolarity is not iso-osmolar. Gastric emptying after solid ingestion also depends on body posture after intake, exercise, meal weight, size of food particles, amount of food, and the type of food.[90,91] Lack of readily available, appropriate methodology makes the assessment of stomach contents in the perioperative period difficult.

Miller and coworkers investigated patients who ate a light breakfast of a slice of buttered toast and a cup of tea or coffee with milk 2 to 4 hours before surgery.[92] Gastric contents were measured by inserting a gastric tube after anesthetic induction. There was no significant difference in gastric volume or pH between the control group (fasting) and the study group. Soreide and associates investigated a group of healthy, female volunteers who ingested a standard hospital breakfast of one slice of white bread with butter or jam, one cup (150 mL) of coffee without milk or sugar, and one glass (150 mL) of pulp-free orange juice.[93] Gastric contents were measured by repeated ultrasonography and paracetamol absorption techniques. No solid food was detected in any volunteer 240 minutes after breakfast. The latter test determined that at least 4 hours between eating and surgery are needed for solid foods to empty from the stomach.

It is appropriate to fast at least 6 hours after intake of a light meal or nonhuman milk before elective procedures. The ASA Committee on Standards and Practice Parameters revised the guidelines because the members found that intake of fried or fatty foods or meat could prolong gastric emptying time. In these situations, 8 hours or more may be needed for preoperative fasting.[78]

3. Patients with Diabetes

Radioisotopic techniques and electrical impedance tomography have been used to show that type 1 diabetic patients have delayed gastric emptying.[55] After ingestion of a semisolid meal, the mean $t_{1/2}$ of gastric emptying was 54.8 ± 26.6 minutes in diabetic patients compared with 40.4 ± 8.6 minutes in nondiabetic control subjects. Diabetic patients require a longer fasting period (8 hours) than nondiabetic patients.

4. Ambulatory Patients and Anxiety

Anxiety delays gastric emptying and increases acid secretion.[94,95] Ambulatory surgery increases anxiety. A background study showed that the mean gastric volume was 69 mL in outpatients and 33 mL in inpatients, with an average pH of less than 2.5 in both groups.[96]

To test the hypothesis that preoperative stress affects residual GFV and pH in pediatric patients, children between the ages of 3 and 17 years were randomly assigned to three groups: outpatients, inpatients, and patients who had multiple operations.[13] There were no differences in the residual GFV between the three groups and no differences in gastric contents between inpatients and outpatients. The relationships among oral premedication, preoperative anxiety, and gastric contents showed that premedication reduces anxiety. However, there were no correlations among the type of premedication, level of anxiety, gastric volume, and gastric pH.[97]

B. Fasting Guidelines Summary

Almost 80% of elective operations are scheduled for ambulatory patients or those with same-day admittance. The ASA Task Force on Preoperative Fasting recommends avoiding anesthetizing a patient with a full stomach to reduce the risk of pulmonary aspiration.[80] The ASA practice guidelines about minimum fasting period for ingested material include the following recommendations: clear liquids, 2 hours; breast milk, 4 hours; infant formula, nonhuman milk, and a light meal, 6 hours. A fast should precede elective procedures requiring general anesthesia, regional anesthesia, or sedation or analgesia (i.e., monitored anesthesia care). The guidelines also recommend a fasting period for a meal that includes fried foods, fatty foods, or meat of 8 hours or more before elective procedures. Diabetic patients need 8 hours or more for gastric emptying after ingesting semisolid material.

Most anesthesiologists practicing outpatient anesthesia in the United States have conformed to the recommendation of the ASA practice guidelines for preoperative fasting time.[77] Similar opinions from associations linked to the World Federation of Societies of Anesthesiologists and from the current literature have led to changes in preoperative fasting guidelines worldwide.[69-71,98,99]

C. Role of Preoperative Ultrasonography

Ultrasonography has been proposed as a useful, noninvasive, bedside tool to determine gastric content and volume in the perioperative period based on studies in parturients,[100] a pilot phase study enrolling 18 healthy adult volunteers,[101] and a follow-up phase II study enrolling 36 adult volunteers that suggested the gastric antral cross-sectional area was a reliable indicator of the quantitative assessment of gastric volume in the right lateral decubitus position.[101] Another prospective trial performed an ultrasonographic qualitative and quantitative analysis of the gastric antrum in 200 fasted patients undergoing elective surgery by assigning a grade to each patient on a 3-point grading scale. Eighty-six patients were categorized as grade 0, suggesting an empty antrum (0 mL); 107 patients as grade 1, suggesting minimal fluid volume (16 ± 36 mL) detected only in the right lateral decubitus position; and 7 patients as grade 2, suggesting a distended gastric antrum with fluid 180 ± 83 mL visible in supine and right lateral decubitus positions.[102] Results of this study of elective surgical patients indicates that preoperative ultrasonography may be able to help identify patients who are at higher risk of pulmonary aspiration. Because certain patient populations, such as trauma patients undergoing surgery, are known to be at high risk for pulmonary aspiration with associated morbidity and mortality,[46] it seems prudent to use ultrasonography as a screening tool preoperatively for these patients.

D. Pharmacotherapy

The ASA practice guidelines do not recommend the routine preoperative use of gastrointestinal stimulants, medications that block gastric acid secretion, antacids, prokinetics, antiemetics, or anticholinergics to reduce the risk of pulmonary aspiration in patients who have no apparent increased risk.[78,80]

Proton pump inhibitors (PPIs) reduce intragastric acidity and gastric juice volume, and they have been advocated for preanesthetic use to prevent pulmonary aspiration.[103] Peptic ulcer bleeding is common, and recurrent bleeding is an independent risk factor for mortality. A PPI infusion prevents recurrent upper gastrointestinal bleeding after endoscopic therapy.[104] A study from Japan showed that rabeprazole may be a suitable alternative to standard H_2-blocker prophylaxis against acid aspiration pneumonia.[105]

Surveys on pulmonary aspiration prophylaxis in the full-stomach, nonobstetric population are rare. The accepted pharmacologic regimens include an attempt to manipulate the gastric pH, volume, and barrier pressure.[106-114] Other surveys of antacid prophylaxis are limited to obstetric anesthesia.[115-120] Most studies suggest improved safety from reduced gastric volume or an increase in gastric pH, or both.[1,121-131] However, no data show evidence of improved outcome after the use of antacids, H_2-receptor blockers, PPIs, or prokinetics. Because of the paucity of data and a lack of evidence to prove the value of pharmacologic therapies for preventing pulmonary aspiration, it is not possible to provide a cost-benefit ratio.[78,80]

E. Preoperative Gastric Emptying

Preoperative stomach emptying through a gastric tube is beneficial for patients at risk for pulmonary aspiration (e.g., small bowel obstruction). Any contents emptied from the stomach make anesthesia induction safer for the patient.

Preoperative gastric emptying concerns include the effect of routine gastric tube insertion before emergency surgery for at-risk patients, the effect of an in situ gastric tube on the efficacy of CP application during induction of anesthesia, and the effect of the gastric tube on GER and pulmonary aspiration in mechanically ventilated patients.

1. Preoperative Gastric Tube Insertion Before Emergency Surgery

Preoperative gastric emptying is not without hazards. Preoperative insertion of a gastric tube and subsequent gastric emptying in an awake, unsedated patient elicits a profound sympathetic response and oxygen desaturation.[132] This response, which is similar to the cardiovascular response after tracheal intubation without analgesia,[133,134] puts the patient with cardiac problems at risk for cardiac ischemia and dysrhythmias. Routine preoperative nasogastric tube placement is not recommended except in selected patients with small bowel or gastric outlet obstruction. Although the gastric tube helps to reduce intragastric volume and pressure, it does not guarantee that the stomach is completely empty. Preoperative nasogastric tube insertion and stomach decompression are recommended only in patients with a distended stomach (e.g., bowel obstruction).

2. In Situ Gastric Tube During Induction

The disposition of an existing gastric tube during induction of general anesthesia is a debatable issue. After the stomach is decompressed, the gastric tube can be removed or left in situ during a rapid-sequence induction (RSI). Although the presence of the gastric tube may impair the function of the UES and LES,[135] studies with cadavers have shown that the efficacy of CP application during induction of anesthesia is not impaired.[136,137] If the patient has a nasogastric tube, it need not be withdrawn before induction of anesthesia because it acts as an overflow valve and prevents pressure buildup in the stomach; it also allows drainage during anesthesia induction.[138]

3. Effects of Gastric Tube Placement in Mechanically Ventilated Patients

The third concern was tested in mechanically ventilated ICU patients to determine the effect of the nasogastric tube size on the incidence of GER.[139] The concern about GER is that it can result in pulmonary aspiration and bacterial pneumonitis. Investigators found no significant difference in GER and pulmonary aspiration with the use of small-gauge and large-gauge nasogastric tubes.

4. Sealing the Esophagus by Inflatable Cuffs

Inflating a cuff at the gastroesophageal junction to prevent gastric reflux is considered to be unsafe. A newly designed, but similar nasogastric device with an inflatable balloon to occlude the gastric cardia (Aspisafe, Braun, Melsungen, Germany) was first studied in pigs (Fig. 35-1).[140] After gastric filling with large volumes, despite maneuvers and drugs used to promote regurgitation, the new nasogastric device did not produce GER.[140] The same experiment was duplicated in healthy volunteers and surgical patients considered to be at risk for pulmonary aspiration, and findings were similar.[140] Use of this device is considered safe because there was no test evidence of GER after RSI.[39]

The device was subsequently studied in conjunction with the use of a laryngeal mask airway (LMA). A dye indicator injected into the stomach revealed that the balloon tube prevented GER.[141] Future clinical studies should decidedly prove balloon tube safety and usefulness in preventing regurgitation during induction and emergence.

VII. GENERAL ANESTHESIA MANAGEMENT

The goals of general anesthesia in full-stomach patients include skillful airway management and prevention of pulmonary aspiration of gastric contents. Airway

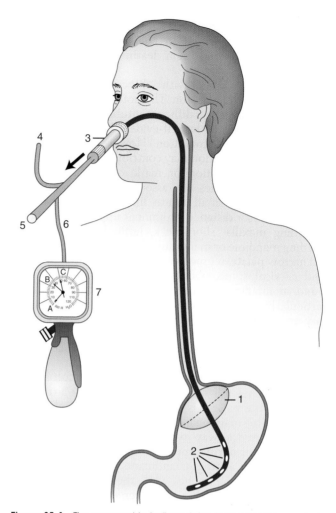

Figure 35-1 The nasogastric balloon tube that is used to occlude the cardia in a patient has several components: *1*, inflatable balloon; *2*, lateral openings to aspirate stomach contents and equilibrate pressure between the stomach and the outside air; *3*, pliable nose stopper with a foam ring and locking device (enlarged drawing to illustrate); *4*, separate lumen ("slurp lumen"); *5*, main lumen with an aspiration connection; *6*, branch tube with the subsidiary lumen leading into the inside of the balloon; *7*, pressure monitoring device (*A*, pressure level in the deflated state of the balloon; *B*, pressure level in the inflated state of the balloon; *C*, pressure level when the aspiration tube is pulled tight, resulting in close appositional contact of the balloon with the cardia). (From Roewer N: Can pulmonary aspiration of gastric contents be prevented by balloon occlusion of the cardia? A study with a new nasogastric tube. *Anesth Analg* 80:378–383, 1995.)

management techniques used to isolate the trachea from the gastrointestinal tract with a cuffed tracheal tube include intubation of the trachea in an awake patient using a flexible fiberoptic bronchoscope (FOB), optical stylet, or a video laryngoscope and use of RSI and tracheal intubation technique after preoxygenation and effective CP application.

A. Awake Tracheal Intubation in Patients at High Risk for Pulmonary Aspiration

The advantages of securing the airway with the patient awake compared with RSI and intubation in patients with a full stomach and a difficult airway are the avoidance of loss of protective reflexes, failure of CP to prevent pulmonary aspiration, failed tracheal intubation leading to hypoxia and brain death, and cardiovascular collapse.

A full-stomach patient with a difficult airway warrants an awake tracheal intubation. The potential for managing a difficult airway (i.e., difficult intubation or difficult mask ventilation) may be self-evident because of a pre-existing or acquired condition. However, normal individual anatomic variation may contribute to the difficulty with tracheal intubation or mask ventilation. Various physical characteristics are associated with a difficult airway, including a small mouth, limited mouth opening, short interincisor distance, prominent upper incisors with overriding maxilla, short neck, limited neck mobility, receding mandible or mandibular hypoplasia, high-arched and narrow palate, temporomandibular joint dysfunction, rigid cervical spine, obesity, and congenital anomalies found in infancy. Morbidly obese patients and infants particularly are at risk for a difficult airway and pulmonary aspiration. No single feature on physical examination accurately predicts a difficult intubation, but a variety of simple diagnostic tests have been suggested to identify patients with difficult airways.[142-154]

A priority in managing patients with a difficult airway and a full stomach is securing the airway with a tracheal tube while the patient is awake. This has several advantages, including maintenance of protective airway reflexes, uncompromised airway exchange and oxygenation, and maintenance of normal muscle tone, which helps in the identification of anatomic landmarks.

Intubation of the trachea while the patient is awake is a useful technique with a high degree of acceptance by patients, and it is considered a fail-safe method of choice when gastric regurgitation and pulmonary aspiration are likely.[155] Awake intubation is useful in situations of anticipated difficulties in tracheal intubation and in patients with intestinal obstruction, gastrointestinal hemorrhage, or upper airway obstruction; in seriously ill or moribund patients; and in those with respiratory failure.[156]

In patients with intestinal obstruction, paralytic ileus with abdominal distention, or upper gastrointestinal hemorrhage, the timing of regurgitation of gastric contents into the pharynx, particularly between the loss of consciousness and tracheal intubation, is greatly increased. Intubation of the trachea while the patient is awake is therefore a sound practice that affords protection against inhalation of gastric contents, loss of the airway, hypoxia, and cardiovascular collapse. Successful accomplishment of awake intubation in patients at risk for pulmonary aspiration depends on several factors, including adequate psychological preparation, use of an intravenous antisialagogue to dry up the oropharyngeal secretions, judicious intravenous sedation, topicalization of the airway, skills and experience of the endoscopist, and the nature and urgency of the surgery.

Before topicalization of the airway, the administration of anticholinergic drugs minimizes secretions, allowing adequate penetration of local anesthetic through the mucosa, enhancing the local anesthetic effects, and enabling better visualization through the bronchoscope. The drawback of using anticholinergic drugs in patients with a full stomach is that it can reduce LES tone and barrier pressure, creating a potential risk for pulmonary aspiration.

Efficacy and safety of awake intubation in full-stomach patients can be accomplished with the use of minimal sedation, administration of oxygen by nasal cannula during intubation, and application of local anesthetic to the pharynx, larynx, and trachea. The premise of conscious sedation is to balance the comfort of the patient and tolerance of the procedure and still have a patient responsive to commands. Judicious sedation with small amounts of short-acting benzodiazepines and narcotics helps allay anxiety and helps the patient who is awake tolerate any discomfort that occurs during tracheal intubation. Ovassapian and colleagues presented the concept of awake fiberoptic intubation using judicious sedation and topicalization of upper and lower airways in patients at high risk for pulmonary aspiration.[157] An accompanying editorial stated that this study of 121 patients was too small to accept the safety of the technique of awake intubation, sedation, and topicalization of the airway.

Topicalization of the lower airway (i.e., below the vocal cords) in an awake patient at risk for pulmonary aspiration is controversial. However, topicalization of the airway adds to the patient's comfort and enhances the chances of successful awake tracheal intubation. There are several ways to anesthetize the upper and lower airway, including administering local anesthetic spray to the mucosa, administering lidocaine jelly to the base of the tongue, bilateral blockade of the internal branch of the superior laryngeal nerve (i.e., sensory to the base of the tongue, vallecula, epiglottis, and larynx up to the level of the cords), bilateral glossopharyngeal nerve blocks (i.e., eliminates gag reflex), and transtracheal injection of local anesthetic through the cricothyroid membrane (i.e., anesthetizes the airway below the vocal cords).

After judicious sedation and topicalization of the airway, several techniques can be used to accomplish awake intubation, including blind nasal intubation, FOB intubation, use of optical stylets, use of video laryngoscopy, intubating laryngeal mask airways (ILMAs), lightwand-guided intubation, and retrograde intubation. There are advantages and drawbacks with each of these techniques.

B. Rapid-Sequence Induction

RSI of anesthesia to protect the airway from pulmonary aspiration of gastric contents has evolved since the introduction of succinylcholine in 1951 and the first description of CP by Sellick in 1961.[135] The primary objective of RSI is to minimize the time interval between loss of consciousness and tracheal intubation. The essential features of RSI include preoxygenation with 100% oxygen, administration of a predetermined induction dose, application of effective CP, and avoidance of positive-pressure ventilation until the airway is secured with a cuffed tracheal tube.[158,159] Many emergency physicians use RSI of anesthesia as their technique of choice to facilitate orotracheal intubation in patients presenting to the emergency room.[160-165] Having specialized equipment for management of failed tracheal intubation is an integral part of RSI.[42,166-168]

RSI plays a major role in emergency anesthesia and is used almost universally for obstetric general anesthesia in the United Kingdom and United States[158]; however, it is practiced less widely in mainland Europe.[169] A survey of French anesthetists showed that only 23% used a full complement of measures to prevent pulmonary aspiration, and CP was rarely used,[1,170] but the incidence of fatal aspiration in France is lower than in other countries (1.4 per 10,000 versus 4.7 per 10,000 episodes of anesthesia).[1,170]

No prospective studies identify the efficacy of RSI in preventing morbidity or its safety. In the past decade, changes in available induction agents, muscle relaxants, airway adjuncts, and increased research in airway management have led to opportunities for RSI in general anesthesia practice to evolve further.

Preoxygenation is a standard component of RSI.[159] Preoxygenation with fresh gas flows of 100% oxygen through a mask with a good fit for 3 to 5 minutes is recommended. Alternatively, a series of four vital capacity breaths of 100% may be used in an emergency.[159] Thiopental remains the most popular induction agent for RSI,[159] although propofol also is used extensively. Other intravenous induction agents include ketamine and etomidate.[171,172]

Succinylcholine remains the muscle relaxant of choice for use in RSI.[159] Certain conditions may preclude the use of succinylcholine, as in burns and spinal cord injuries, because administration of succinylcholine can result in adverse effects such as hyperkalemia and dysrhythmias. Several studies have demonstrated that rocuronium in adequate doses (0.8 to 1.2 mg/kg) produces intubation conditions rapidly comparable to those with succinylcholine 1 mg/kg.[173,174] However, this large dose leads to prolonged duration of action of up to 1 hour.[175] In a patient with a difficult airway, this drug may allow less margin for error than succinylcholine.[176] Fifty percent of cases of difficult intubation occur without preoperative predictive signs and can increase the risks of gastric regurgitation and pulmonary aspiration in full-stomach patients.[177]

1. Modified Rapid-Sequence Induction

RSI is a well-established technique in anesthesia practice. During standard RSI, patients are made apneic and unconscious without establishing the ability to ventilate the lungs. Positive pressure usually is avoided to prevent gaseous distention of the stomach and subsequent pulmonary aspiration in RSI. However, avoidance of ventilation of the lungs during RSI precludes the ability to test the airway and verify that a patient's lungs can be ventilated by mask before the administration of a muscle relaxant. The technique of RSI therefore involves inherent risks to the patient, including the possible inability to secure an airway or to ventilate the lungs and oxygenate the patient who is unconscious and apneic. During RSI, failure to secure the airway can lead to many attempts at tracheal intubation with subsequent trauma to the airway, and failure to ventilate the lungs can lead to hypoxia, hypercarbia, and alterations in heart rate and blood

pressure, resulting in significant morbidity. These risks may not be warranted or appropriate, particularly in patients who are at risk for gastric regurgitation and pulmonary aspiration. For them, appropriate management can include modification of the standard RSI technique consisting of preoxygenation, laryngoscopy using an elevated-head position,[178] induction of anesthesia, application of CP, apneic diffusion oxygenation,[179] and the added step of gentle positive-pressure ventilation of the lungs before tracheal intubation.[135,180]

A modified RSI technique allows the anesthesia provider to confirm that the patient's lungs can be ventilated and the patient can be oxygenated by mask before insertion of a cuffed tracheal tube. Positive pressure is provided by a face mask before and after the administration of the muscle relaxant. However, the risks and benefits of modified RSI have to be considered in a patient with a full stomach and a potentially difficult airway. The risks of being unable to intubate the trachea and ventilate the lungs have to be weighed against the risk of pulmonary aspiration; the results of both complications can be disastrous if they are not managed appropriately. However, the risk of cerebral hypoxia due to inadequate oxygenation must outweigh the risk of pulmonary aspiration. Cerebral hypoxia is not treatable and can result in devastating morbidity and mortality, whereas pulmonary aspiration is treatable and has a good outcome in current clinical practice.

2. Cricoid Pressure

CP is an integral component of RSI and is an accepted standard of care during anesthesia and to a lesser extent during resuscitation in patients with a full stomach.[159,181-183] As early as the 1770s, CP was recognized as an important method to occlude the esophagus and prevent gastric distention during lung ventilation of drowning victims.[184] However, it was almost 200 years later that Sellick introduced CP into clinical anesthesia practice.[135] Although studies cite increasing concerns regarding the safety and efficacy of CP, it is still widely practiced.[185-187]

The cricoid cartilage is a complete circle shaped like a signet ring. It is attached superiorly to the thyroid cartilage by the cricothyroid ligament and inferiorly to the first tracheal ring by the cricotracheal membrane. The esophagus begins at the lower border of the cricoid cartilage, and the cricopharyngeus muscle guards the esophageal opening. The cricoid cartilage is different sizes and has different locations in adults and children.

The CP, a force measured in newtons (N), must be of sufficient amount applied during induction of general anesthesia to prevent regurgitation from the esophagus and stomach. Regurgitation of stomach contents depends on esophageal pressure, gastrointestinal pathology, intragastric pressure, UES and LES pressures, and the effectiveness of occluding the esophageal lumen. On the basis of several studies,[136,188-192] a force (CP) of 44 N (9.8 N = 1 kg = 2.2 lb) was accepted as the gold standard for prevention of gastric regurgitation in adults when applied in the standard or tonsillectomy position.[192] CP greater than 44 N prevents gastric regurgitation. When appropriate force is applied, the upper end of the esophagus is occluded and compressed against the C6 vertebra. In paralyzed intubated patients, lowering the CP to 40 N increased esophageal pressure to more than 38 mm Hg.[193] In a study using the double-lumen Salem sump tube in 20 women undergoing emergency cesarean delivery under general anesthesia,[194] the mean gastric pressure was 11 mm Hg (range, 4 to 19 mm Hg). It was predicted that 99% of women undergoing emergency cesarean delivery having a gastric pressure of 25 mm Hg were unlikely to have regurgitation of fluid. Evidence from a cadaver study showed that a CP of 30 N prevents regurgitation of esophageal fluid even with gastric pressure at 42 mm Hg. Anatomic studies suggest that a CP of 30 N is adequate and should reduce the risk of esophageal rupture.[137,193]

The CP necessary to provide an adequate occlusive effect in children of different age groups is debatable. No data are available to clarify this issue. An observational study using the bench model indicated that the mean cricoid force applied clinically to a 5-year-old child should be 22.4 to 25.1 N.[195]

a. HEAD AND NECK POSITION

Sellick made the original recommendation to use the tonsillectomy position, without a pillow, with CP applied at the C5 vertebra.[135] The rationale for the tonsillar position is that it increases the concavity of the cervical spine, stretches the esophagus, and prevents lateral displacement of the esophagus. Unfortunately, this mode of CP application often worsens the view at laryngoscopy.[196] The head position must be ideal for intubating with head extension on the neck, neck flexion, and a pillow beneath the occiput.[197]

b. TIMING OF CRICOID PRESSURE APPLICATION

The timing and amount of CP applied during induction of general anesthesia are important. The original recommendation was synchronous CP application; moderate pressure in an awake, conscious individual; and a gradual increase to a full force of 44 N immediately on loss of consciousness. Applying a full force of 44 N before induction in a conscious individual is detrimental; it produces significant discomfort, complete airway obstruction,[198] retching, and vomiting.[181] Vomiting with continued CP application can cause death from pulmonary aspiration or a ruptured esophagus.[199,200]

A cricoid yoke has been used to apply pressure in awake volunteers without considerable pain or coughing.[189] The accepted practice is to apply a lower CP (20 N) before induction of anesthesia and increase it to 30 N as the patient loses consciousness.[201]

Reluctance to use CP stems from faulty technique of its application and its effect on airway management, reported cases of pulmonary aspiration, and esophageal rupture. CP application causes anatomic distortion of the upper airway, making airway management more difficult. Most data were collected with a CP of 40 N. Studies show that a CP of 30 N applied in an upward and backward manner improves the laryngoscopic view during intubation.[201] Similarly, Randell and colleagues showed that CP,[202] modified to backward, upward, rightward pressure (BURP) on the thyroid cartilage, improved the view in 57 of 68 cases. The thyroid cartilage is the surface

marking for the glottic opening, and application of BURP on the thyroid cartilage therefore improves the glottic view at laryngoscopy.[203]

c. SINGLE-HANDED CRICOID PRESSURE

For single-handed CP, the thumb and middle finger are placed on either side of the cricoid cartilage, and the index finger is placed above to prevent lateral movement of the cricoid.[135] The laryngoscopic view is better with the head in the Magill position and better with single-handed CP than with double-handed CP.[204]

Another single-handed method is to place the palm of the hand on the sternum, applying pressure with only the index and middle fingers.[205] This technique improved the laryngoscopic view of the glottis. In infants and children, the single-handed technique compressing the cricoid cartilage is performed with the little or middle finger while the same hand holds the face mask.[206]

CP should be applied with the left hand from the left side of the patient. This prevents interference with laryngoscopy, specifically when the laryngoscope blade is inserted from the right corner of the mouth.

d. DOUBLE-HANDED CRICOID PRESSURE

The bimanual or two-handed CP technique uses the single-handed technique in addition to using the assistant's right hand to provide counterpressure beneath the cervical vertebra for neck support. This maneuver provides support to the hyperextended arch of the vertebral column to maintain the efficacy of CP and to optimize the laryngoscopic view. Variations of this technique include placing the left hand behind the head and holding the extended head to maintain the Magill intubating position.[207]

e. CRICOID PRESSURE IN CLINICAL PRACTICE

In clinical practice, application of a predetermined CP can be sustained by the assistant for only a short period. Application of CP with a flexed arm can be sustained only for a mean time of 3.7 minutes at 40 N, with considerable onset of pain at 2.3 minutes. This limitation has important clinical implications in cases of failed tracheal intubation in full-stomach patients. Application of CP in clinical practice may interfere with airway management (i.e., tracheal intubation, face mask ventilation, and LMA placement), and failure to manage the airway appropriately is a more frequent cause of morbidity and mortality than pulmonary aspiration.[208]

VIII. MANAGEMENT OF THE DIFFICULT AIRWAY IN THE FULL-STOMACH PATIENT

Management of difficult RSIs in full-stomach patients is little studied. Airway catastrophes occur predominantly when airway difficulty is not recognized before anesthesia is administered.[209,210] Although airway difficulty should be anticipated in 90% of cases, a prospective study showed that only approximately 51% of difficult intubations were recognized and expected.[211] Difficult and failed tracheal intubations occur more frequently during an emergency than during elective surgery, during nights than during days, and during weekends than during weekdays.[97,212,213] Unanticipated difficult intubations in full-stomach patients undergoing emergency surgery poses additional problems. There is no option for anesthesiologists to postpone surgery, and the risk of pulmonary aspiration of gastric contents is much greater.

In full-stomach patients, repeated attempts to intubate the trachea increase the risk of airway trauma, bleeding, and laryngeal edema, and failure to secure the airway can increase the incidence of pulmonary aspiration.[214] Hypoxia and death can result from failure to oxygenate the patient and ventilate the patient's lungs or from unrecognized intubation of the esophagus, neither of which is caused solely by failed tracheal intubation.[142]

Significant advances in airway management have been made in the past 2 decades. New airway devices and adjuncts to assist in the tracheal intubation of difficult airways are available. In most cases of difficult intubation, a partial view of the glottis is possible (i.e., grade III laryngoscopic view).[97,167,212] Of the many airway devices available to physicians in the United Kingdom and Canada, the Eschmann stylet (gum elastic bougie) is used to facilitate tracheal intubation in more than 95% of grade III laryngoscopic views.[215] Another commonly used device is the McCoy laryngoscope (CLM, Mercury Medical, Clearwater, FL), which can improve visualization of the larynx in up to 50% of cases with difficult laryngoscopic views.[216,217]

Additional levering laryngoscopes include the Flipper (Rusch, Research Triangle Park, NC) and the Heine Flex Tip (Heine USA, Dover, NH). These laryngoscopes were designed to provide greater flexibility and improved visualization of the larynx in patients with a difficult airway, smaller mouth opening, or restricted head and neck movement.[218]

A practical classification proposes subdividing the grade 3 Cormack-Lehane laryngoscopic view into two grades: grade 3A, in which the epiglottis is visible and can be elevated with the laryngoscope blade, and grade 3B, in which the epiglottis is visible but cannot be elevated.[219] This new classification is as sensitive and more specific than the Cormack-Lehane classification in predicting difficult tracheal intubation, but it is more sensitive and more specific in predicting easy tracheal intubation.[219]

A manikin-simulated difficult airway study showed that the Eschmann stylet and a fiberoptic stylet were effective in facilitating tracheal intubation in a simulated grade 3A Cormack-Lehane view, with success rates of 100% and 98%, respectively.[220] The mean times to successful intubation were similar between groups: 31 seconds for the Eschmann stylet and 29.2 seconds for the fiberoptic stylet.[220] However, in the simulated grade 3B Cormack-Lehane view, use of the fiberoptic stylet significantly improved the success rate (98% for the fiberoptic stylet and 9% for the Eschmann stylet) and reduced the mean time to successful tracheal intubation (31 seconds for the fiberoptic stylet and 45.6 seconds for the Eschmann stylet).[220]

A. Difficult Airway Management Using the Laryngeal Mask Airway

Before 1990, the choice of airway devices was limited to the face mask or the tracheal tube. The LMA (LMA North America, San Diego, CA) is one of the most significant and important airway devices introduced for airway management. Several supraglottic airway devices have been developed since then, including the Air-Q (Mercury Medical, Clearwater, FL); i-gel (Intersurgical Ltd., Berkshire, United Kingdom); Streamlined Liner of the Pharynx Airway (SLIPA, Curve Air Ltd., London, United Kingdom); and Ambu Aura Laryngeal Mask (Ballerup, Denmark). Second-generation supraglottic devices include the esophageal-tracheal Combitube (Tyco Healthcare, Mansfield, MA) and the King Laryngeal Tube Suction (LTS) and the King LTS disposable (LTS-D) (King Systems, Noblesville, IN).

Archie Brain, the inventor of the LMA, has continued to develop variations of the original device. These modifications include eight sizes of the original Classic Laryngeal Mask Airway (LMA Classic, LMA North America, Inc., San Diego, CA), the LMA Classic with a disposable connector to facilitate tracheal intubation (LMA Classic Excel), a single-use LMA (LMA Unique), a reinforced but flexible LMA (LMA Flexible), an LMA specifically designed for blind tracheal intubation (ILMA-Fastrach), an LMA fitted with an integral gastric access or venting port (LMA ProSeal), and its disposable version (LMA Supreme). The LMA is a recognized part of the ASA difficult airway algorithm. As a ventilatory device or intubating conduit, or both, the LMA fits into the difficult airway algorithm in several places.

1. Classic Laryngeal Mask Airway

The use of the LMA Classic is contraindicated in full-stomach patients and patients at high risk for pulmonary aspiration because of gastrointestinal pathology, obesity, GER, or emergency surgery. The main disadvantage of using the LMA Classic in patients with a full stomach or obstetric patients is an increased risk of gastric regurgitation and pulmonary aspiration. The LMA Classic design is such that even when correctly placed, its tip lies against the UES, and the device does not isolate the respiratory tract from the gastrointestinal tract. Because the esophagus is included in the rim of the LMA Classic, it does not protect the lungs from regurgitated gastric contents. Full-stomach and pregnant patients may be vulnerable to gastric regurgitation and pulmonary aspiration with the use of this device.[221]

Studies of gastric regurgitation and pulmonary aspiration rates associated with using these supraglottic devices have mainly focused on the LMA Classic. A meta-analysis of 547 publications suggested that the overall incidence of pulmonary aspiration associated with the LMA Classic is about 2 cases per 10,000 patients,[222] a figure corroborated by a large number of studies. This rate is comparable to that of outpatient anesthesia administered with a face mask and tracheal tube (Table 35-2).[53] Studies also have demonstrated that the use of the LMA Classic is associated with a reduction in barrier pressure at the LES.[223] In comparing the cuffed tracheal tube with the

TABLE 35-2

Incidence of Aspiration with the Laryngeal Mask Airway

Study	Cases per Patient Population
Haden, et al, 1994[309]	1:3500
Wainwright, 1995[310]	0:1877
Verghese and Brimacombe, 1996[228]	1:11910
Brimacombe, 1996[311]	0:1500
Lopez-Gil, et al, 1996[312]	0:2000

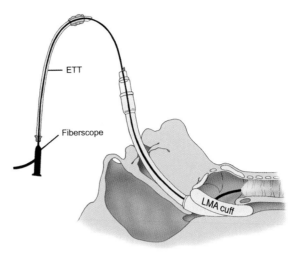

Figure 35-2 Fiberoptic-guided intubation. The laryngeal mask airway (LMA) is inserted and the cuff is inflated. The fiberscope is inserted through the LMA, through the vocal cords, and into the trachea. The endotracheal tube (ETT) is mounted on the fiberscope. The ETT is threaded over the flexible fiberoptic bronchoscope into the LMA shaft with the bevel pointed 90 degrees to the left; as it enters through the maximum aperture bars, it is rotated anteriorly. After it is located in the trachea, placement is confirmed by detection of end-tidal carbon dioxide. (Courtesy of Publications and Creative Services, Baylor College of Medicine, Houston, TX.)

LMA Classic during general anesthesia with positive-pressure ventilation, Valentine and colleagues (using a pH electrode placed in the midesophageal zone) determined that there were significantly more episodes of reflux among the LMA Classic patients.[224] In contrast, Agro and associates found no episodes of reflux with the use of LMA Classic in patients undergoing elective orthopedic surgery.[225] The association between GER and the LMA Classic is not clear. However, there is insufficient evidence to support the hypothesis that the reduction in lower esophageal pH is influenced directly by the pressure or the volume in the cuff of the LMA Classic.[226] Application of CP reduces LES pressure[30]; a similar reflux may occur because of the increased pharyngeal pressure exerted by the LMA Classic. There is controversy about the effect of the LMA Classic on LES tone, with some studies reporting a reduction in tone and others reporting no change.[223,227] However, it is accepted that UES function is relatively unimpaired by the LMA Classic. Some anesthesiologists believe that the LMA Classic is contraindicated in patients with a full stomach and in obstetric patients.

Despite the pulmonary aspiration risks with an LMA Classic (with or without CP) being the same as those encountered with a face mask,[222,228] particularly in patients with a full stomach, there are several case reports documenting the use of the LMA Classic after failed tracheal intubation attempts during emergency cesarean section. In these cases, the LMA Classic device provided a clear airway and was useful in rapidly providing oxygenation and relieving hypoxia. There were no reports of pulmonary aspiration.[222,229-233] In 1346 elective cesarean sections, the LMA Classic was used as an alternative to tracheal intubation to ventilate lungs. The tracheal tube was blindly inserted with minimal cardiovascular responses, and there was no incidence of pulmonary aspiration in 98% of cases.[234] In another study, the LMA Classic was used in 1067 patients undergoing elective cesarean sections.[98] After RSI with CP, the LMA Classic was inserted, and an effective airway was obtained in 1060 patients (99%). There were no episodes of pulmonary aspiration, hypoxia, laryngospasm, or gastric insufflation.[235]

The major benefit of using the LMA Classic after failed tracheal intubation attempts in a patient with a full stomach is that it serves as a rescue device and provides oxygenation.[236] However, because of the potential for gastric regurgitation and the risk of pulmonary aspiration, a choice must be made about whether to use the LMA Classic as a definitive airway or as a conduit for tracheal intubation. Technical problems associated with the LMA Classic include the less than ideal position of the device in relation to the glottic opening and downfolding of epiglottis in the LMA Classic aperture bars. The blind passage of a tracheal tube through the LMA Classic has an unacceptably low degree of success. Difficulties include catching the tracheal tube tip on the aperture bars or the anterior commissure because of the natural bend in a standard polyvinyl chloride tracheal tube and the natural bend where the tube exits the LMA. When CP was not applied, Heath and Allagain could intubate the trachea blindly through the LMA Classic in 72% of patients at first attempt and in most patients when time was not limited.[237] However, the blind technique of tracheal intubation through the LMA Classic often requires significant manipulation of the head and neck to accomplish the intubation. An Eschmann stylet can be used to aid tracheal intubation. A high success rate was obtained for patients in whom difficult intubation was not anticipated by inserting the Eschmann stylet with its angulated end pointing anteriorly until it passed through the grille of the LMA Classic and then rotating the Eschmann stylet by 180 degrees.[238] Failures, however, have been reported with this visually unassisted guided technique of endotracheal intubation through the LMA Classic.[239] Because of the potential problems, in an urgent situation, blind tracheal intubation through the LMA Classic may not be advisable. Fiberoptic-guided tracheal intubation through the LMA Classic has been shown to be the most reliable technique, which has a much higher success rate than other approaches (Fig. 35-2).[213-237]

If the LMA Classic is used as a definitive airway without the passage of a tracheal tube, timing of the removal of the device in a patient with a full stomach becomes crucial. A randomized, controlled trial demonstrated that the pH in the lower esophagus was significantly higher in patients in whom the LMA Classic remained in situ until the end of the case, at which point the patient was able to follow commands. It is suggested that the LMA Classic should be removed only when the patient has fully regained consciousness at the end of the anesthetic.[240]

2. Fastrach Intubating Laryngeal Mask Airway

After attempts to intubate the trachea of patients with a full stomach have failed, an alternative to using the LMA is to use the Fastrach intubating laryngeal mask airway (ILMA-Fastrach). The ILMA-Fastrach is designed specifically to overcome the problems associated with blind tracheal intubation using the LMA Classic. The ILMA-Fastrach consists of a rigid, anatomically curved airway tube made of stainless steel with a standard 15-mm connector. The tube is wide enough to accommodate an 8.0-mm tracheal tube and short enough to ensure passage of the tracheal tube beyond the vocal cords.

The highest degree of success in intubating the trachea blindly through the ILMA-Fastrach can be achieved by using the special tracheal tube (Euromedical ILM Tracheal Tube, Euromedical, Sungai Petani, Kedah, Malaysia) supplied with the device. This silicon tube is soft tipped, straight, wire reinforced, and cuffed. Ferson and colleagues reported their clinical experience with the ILMA in 254 patients with difficult airways,[241] including patients with Cormack-Lehane grade 4 views; patients with immobilized cervical spines; those with airways distorted by tumors, surgery, or radiation therapy; and those wearing stereotactic frames. The device was particularly useful in patients undergoing emergency or elective surgery for whom tracheal intubation with a rigid laryngoscope had failed.[242-244] Similar multicenter trials and reports have described the use of an ILMA-Fastrach in patients with difficult airways and failed tracheal intubation (including emergency cases at risk for aspiration).[245-251] The ILMA-Fastrach has been used as a rescue device by emergency room physicians after failed RSI.[252] Our institution has reported cases in which the device proved to be a lifesaving rescue device after failed tracheal intubation during emergency cesarean section.[253,254]

3. ProSeal Laryngeal Mask Airway

The ProSeal laryngeal mask airway (PLMA) is a complex and potentially useful device for patients particularly at risk for gastric regurgitation and pulmonary aspiration. Some anesthesiologists refuse to use the LMA Classic because of concerns regarding gastric distention with positive-pressure ventilation and the potential for pulmonary aspiration. To address these issues, the primary goal of designing the PLMA was to construct a device with improved ventilatory characteristics that also offered protection against gastric insufflation and regurgitation. The principal feature of the PLMA is a double mask forming two end-to-end junctions: one with the respiratory tract and the other with the gastrointestinal tract. In contrast, the original LMA Classic forms a single end-to-end junction with the respiratory tract. The PLMA has a modified posterior cuff that provides high seal pressure—up to 30

cm H_2O—providing a tighter seal against the glottic opening with no increase in mucosal pressure. The PLMA also offers a better airway seal at a given pressure than the LMA Classic.[255] When properly positioned, the distal orifice of the PLMA lies against the UES and separates the esophagus and stomach from the glottic area. It has an integral gastric access and venting port that allows passage of a 14-F gastric tube, allowing suctioning of gastric contents.

In awake volunteers, neither the PLMA nor the LMA Classic appeared to interfere with UES or LES tone.[256] No manometric studies have been performed to assess LES function in anesthetized patients, but FOB inspection of the PLMA drainage tube showed that the UES was completely open in 3% to 7% of paralyzed patients and in 9% of nonparalyzed patients.[257,258] This effect, which may have implications for the frequency of regurgitation into the drainage tube, may be mechanical, a local reflex, or result from direct exposure to atmosphere through the drainage tube.

The PLMA is easy to insert and is a more effective ventilatory device when using positive-pressure ventilation. A meta-analysis using Fisher's method has shown that the PLMA forms a more effective seal with the respiratory tract than the LMA Classic.[259] The efficacy of the seal with the gastrointestinal tract has been determined by measuring the airway pressure at which air leaks into the drainage tube in anesthetized adults. Depending on cuff volume,[260] the efficacy of the seal for air is at least 27 to 29 cm H_2O,[255,261] and for fluid, the efficacy is 19 to 73 cm H_2O, with a similar seal mechanism for the respiratory tract.

The drainage tube provides a conduit to the gastrointestinal tract. It is also possible to insert a gastric balloon tube to further reduce the risk of pulmonary aspiration.[141] The success rate for gastric tube insertion is 88% to 100%.[258,261] Inserting a gastric tube has several advantages. The tube allows removal of gas or fluid from the stomach, the process of insertion provides information about the position or patency of the drainage tube, and the tube can function as a guide for PLMA reinsertion if accidental displacement occurs.[262]

The incidence of gastric insufflation seems to be low, even at high airway pressures.[255,263] Gastric insufflation has been detected in only 1 of 572 patients (data from seven studies).[255,257,258,261,263-265] Gastric insufflation is less common with the PLMA than with the LMA Classic when high positive-pressure ventilation is used.[255]

There are at least two reports of the PLMA being used in the difficult airway scenario. Keller and colleagues,[263] in a prospective study of morbidly obese patients (i.e., patients at risk for gastric regurgitation and pulmonary aspiration), found that the PLMA was successful in 11 of 11 patients who were difficult or impossible to intubate with a laryngoscope. However, there are two case reports of pulmonary aspiration of gastric contents using the PLMA. In the first patient, brownish fluid was seen ejecting from the drainage tube of PLMA after administration of reversal agents at the end of surgery. There were clinical signs of pulmonary aspiration without any radiologic changes.[266] In the second patient, foldover malposition of the distal cuff against the posterior oropharyngeal wall

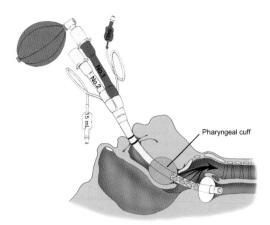

Figure 35-3 Esophageal-tracheal Combitube (ETC) in the esophagus. The ETC tube is advanced until the black rings are at the level of the teeth or alveolar ridges. The distal cuff is inflated with 15 mL of air to seal the esophagus, and the proximal cuff is inflated with 85 mL (37-F ETC) to 100 mL (41-F ETC) of air; this secures the tube in the correct position and occludes the nasal and oral passages. Ventilation is attempted through lumen no. 1. (Courtesy of Publications and Creative Services, Baylor College of Medicine, Houston, TX.)

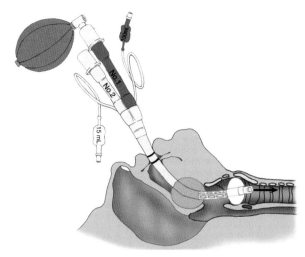

Figure 35-4 Esophageal-tracheal Combitube (ETC) in the trachea. The ETC is placed in the trachea, and the ventilation is shifted to lumen no. 2. (Courtesy of Publications and Creative Services, Baylor College of Medicine, Houston, TX.)

(confirmed later by FOB) during insertion was cited as the reason for pulmonary aspiration.[267]

In two reports, the PLMA was used successfully in obstetric patients after failed tracheal intubation.[268] Keller and colleagues showed that the PLMA was a rescue device after failed tracheal intubation in an obstetric patient with hemolysis, elevated liver enzymes, and low platelet count (HELLP syndrome) and proved to be useful for postoperative respiratory support for 8 hours until the platelet count had increased and the patient was hemodynamically stable.[268]

Emergence characteristics for the PLMA seem to be similar to those for the LMA Classic.[257] Practical considerations include suctioning the gastric tube and reversing any residual neuromuscular blockade before beginning of emergence. As with the LMA Classic, the patient should not be disturbed, and the PLMA should be removed only when the patient is conscious and obeys commands. When the patient is fully awake and responsive to verbal commands, the device is removed with the cuff inflated along with the gastric tube on continuous suction to prevent any oropharyngeal secretions from entering the laryngopharynx.

B. Esophageal-Tracheal Combitube in the Full-Stomach Patient

The Combitube, developed by Frass and colleagues, is a disposable, polyvinyl chloride, double-lumen airway device that combines the features of an esophageal obturator airway and a tracheal tube.[269] It functions well in both the esophageal and tracheal positions.[270] Using the Lipp maneuver,[271] the Combitube is inserted blindly. Insertion usually results in esophageal placement (Fig. 35-3), and ventilation is initiated through the gastric lumen.[272] With both cuffs inflated, ventilation through the proximal lumen allows airflow through eight oval fenestrations from the hypopharynx into the trachea. An effective seal of the latex oropharyngeal cuff prevents the

escape of air from the mouth and nose. Instead, air is forced into the trachea and lungs. If the Combitube is placed in the esophagus, gastric fluids can be aspirated through the gastric lumen. If breath sounds are not heard, the Combitube has more than likely been placed in the trachea (Fig. 35-4). Without removing the Combitube, ventilation is switched to the tracheoesophageal lumen and confirmed with auscultation and capnography.

Unsatisfactory ventilation through either lumen indicates that the Combitube is too far advanced into the esophagus to produce airway obstruction by the oropharyngeal cuff (Fig. 35-5A). In this situation, the distal esophageal cuff and the oropharyngeal cuff are deflated, and the Combitube is withdrawn approximately 2 to 3 cm (see Fig. 35-5B). The esophageal cuff and the oropharyngeal cuff are then reinflated, and pulmonary ventilation is resumed.[119]

The Combitube serves as a rescue device for establishing an airway in the "cannot intubate, can ventilate" and "cannot intubate, cannot ventilate" situations, and it is particularly useful in the full-stomach patient. It is inserted blindly or under direct laryngoscopy,[273] can secure the airway easily and rapidly, and requires minimal preparation (i.e., can be properly used with relatively little formal training).[60] Combitube placement by inexperienced personnel (e.g., ICU nurses) under medical supervision was found to be as safe and successful in providing effective oxygenation and ventilation of the lungs as tracheal intubation performed by ICU physicians during cardiopulmonary resuscitation.[274] As a rescue device, it is helpful in securing the airway if vocal cord visualization is compromised or if oropharyngeal bleeding has occurred.

The Combitube prevents pulmonary aspiration during cardiopulmonary resuscitation,[270] especially when protective airway reflexes are absent, protecting the airway from pulmonary aspiration of gastric contents.[275] Frass and coworkers found that the tracheoesophageal lumen served as a conduit for decompression of gastric contents

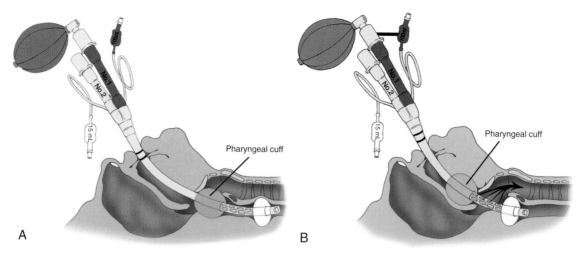

A

B

Figure 35-5 Placement of the esophageal-tracheal Combitube (ETC). **A,** Excessive insertion depth of the ETC causes obstruction of the glottic opening, and ventilation is impossible. **B,** Correct positioning is achieved by readjustment of the ETC, which is pulled back 2 to 3 cm (indicated by the two black rings), and ventilation through lumen no. 1 allows the passage of gas from the side orifices into the trachea (*arrow*). (Courtesy of Publications and Creative Services, Baylor College of Medicine, Houston, TX.)

and allowed gastric suctioning.[270] Urtubia and associates administered methylene blue orally to 25 patients before induction of anesthesia and found no evidence of methylene blue in the hypopharynx during laryngoscopy before Combitube placement or after its removal.[275] Hagberg and colleagues determined that the incidence of pulmonary aspiration is comparable for the Combitube and the LMA.[276]

C. Esophageal-Tracheal Combitube for Prevention of Pulmonary Aspiration

Many case reports attest to the safety of the Combitube and the use of the tracheoesophageal lumen as an effective decompression channel for regurgitated gastric contents, which prevents pulmonary aspiration during cardiopulmonary resuscitation or during anesthesia.[276-278] The 10-F orogastric tube, available in the prepackaged Combitube kit, can be readily used for esophageal and gastric suctioning. The Combitube has been used successfully as a primary airway device in seven obstetric patients (R.M. Urtubia, personal communication, 2001), two of whom were reported.[279] They did not have a history of difficult tracheal intubation, and they underwent general anesthesia for emergency cesarean section. The Combitube was used as the initial airway device, and it allowed adequate oxygenation, ventilation, and protection from pulmonary aspiration of gastric contents.[279] Wissler reported the use of the Combitube under direct laryngoscopy during obstetric anesthesia.[280] The Combitube has become his primary choice for managing an anesthetized parturient whose trachea cannot be intubated or whose lungs cannot be mask ventilated while applying CP.[280]

If tracheal intubation becomes necessary, it can be achieved using the FOB with the Combitube in place. The fiberscope is passed alongside the Combitube, the oropharyngeal balloon is partially deflated, and tracheal intubation is achieved visually and is followed by removal of the Combitube without interruption of airway control,

oxygenation, or ventilation (Fig. 35-6). This technique has been used for spontaneously breathing and mechanically ventilated patients.[44,281] One of the authors (AW) managed a morbidly obese, 550-pound woman with obstructive sleep apnea, who had been in the medical intensive care unit (MICU) with a Combitube in situ. Tracheal intubation was requested by the MICU team to help with weaning the patient from the ventilator. Using the hybrid technique of direct laryngoscopy and fiberoptic bronchoscopy, tracheal intubation was successfully accomplished, and was followed by Combitube removal.

Video film recordings of 25 patients undergoing laparoscopic cholecystectomy under general anesthesia and mechanical ventilation using the Combitube revealed no gastric insufflation at the beginning or end of surgery.[282]

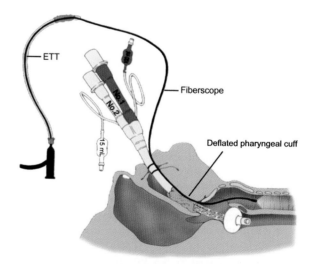

Figure 35-6 Tracheal intubation using a fiberscope can be achieved with the esophageal-tracheal Combitube (ETC) in place. The fiberscope is passed alongside the ETC with the pharyngeal cuff partially deflated. After tracheal intubation is established, the ETC is removed without interruption of airway control, oxygenation, or ventilation. *ETT,* Endotracheal tube. (Courtesy of Publications and Creative Services, Baylor College of Medicine, Houston, TX.)

A large, retrospective survey of 12,020 cases of nontraumatic cardiac arrest in Japan revealed 1594 instances of Combitube use without any evidence of pulmonary aspiration of gastric contents.[277]

The Combitube has several advantages compared with the LMA:

1. Preparation time is minimal.
2. The device is ideal for full-stomach patients and pregnant patients (especially after failed tracheal intubation), for whom oxygenation, avoidance of arterial desaturation, and pulmonary aspiration are important factors.
3. Lubrication is not required.
4. No special method is required for cuff inflation or deflation.

The few case reports of complications related to the use of the Combitube primarily involve the original version (41 F) of the device and are attributed to its stiffer, rather large, and potentially traumatic design.[283] These complications have included esophageal rupture, subcutaneous emphysema, piriform sinus rupture, pneumomediastinum, and pneumoperitoneum.[284,285] Common factors in these cases included difficult ambient conditions in the field or prehospital environment, multiple attempts to insert the device, resistance with insertion, and the use of excessive force.[286]

Several recommendations help to minimize the complications and to enhance the rate of successful placement of the Combitube:

1. Use the smaller Combitube SA universally for patients between 4 and 6 ft tall.
2. Briefly dip the device in warm saline before use.
3. Use the Lipp maneuver (i.e., holding the two ends of the Combitube together to bend it into a semicircle for a few seconds before insertion) during placement of the device.
4. Place the device under direct laryngoscopy.[273]
5. Use a gentle technique to reduce the hemodynamic response from stimulation of the proprioceptors at the base of the tongue.[283]
6. Inflate the oropharyngeal balloon slowly to the minimum volume necessary for an airtight seal to reduce soft tissue injury.[283]
7. Employ a reliable technique, using direct laryngoscopy as an aid to Combitube placement if necessary.[273]

Although there are no large, randomized studies that indicate the relative safety of the Combitube in preventing pulmonary aspiration of gastric contents, these recommendations are useful and appealing to health care personnel managing patients who have a full stomach, with or without a difficult airway.

D. King Laryngeal Tube Suction Airways in the Full-Stomach Patient

The King LTS and its disposable version, the King LTS-D, are second-generation supraglottic airways that are modifications of the Combitube. They are slightly shorter, softer, and smaller than the Combitube and may have a lower complication profile.[287] These devices are placed using gentle, blind insertion along the surface of the tongue from the mouth into the upper esophagus (see Fig. 37-7A in Chapter 37) . They have twin lumens, one for ventilation and the other for gastric suctioning with an 18-F orogastric tube and passive venting, thereby isolating the trachea from the esophagus (see Fig. 37-7B in Chapter 37). In contrast to the Combitube, they have a single pilot balloon for the proximal oropharyngeal nonlatex cuff and the distal esophageal cuff, preventing confusion regarding the choice of pilot balloon required for a particular cuff. They are easily placed,[288] use low-pressure cuffs,[289] allow exchange for a tracheal tube by passing an FOB preloaded with an Aintree airway exchange catheter[290] (see Fig. 37-7C in Chapter 37), and have been used during controlled ventilation and during spontaneous respiration.[288,291] Based on the literature, The device has potential for successful use in the full-stomach patient. A study comparing the LMA Classic and the King LT in 22 patients showed that the mean leak pressure was significantly higher for the King LT and that gastric insufflation was not observed with King LT.[289] A second study enrolling 30 patients showed that a ventilatory seal of 40 cm H_2O was easily obtained without gastric insufflation.[287] A case report of an obstetric patient demonstrated the successful use of King LTS in providing access for oxygenation and ventilation after failed tracheal intubation during an emergency cesarean section.[292]

IX. EXTUBATION

When an awake intubation or RSI is indicated to prevent pulmonary aspiration, an awake tracheal extubation should be considered to prevent airway complications and to enhance patient safety during emergence from general anesthesia, at extubation, and in the postanesthesia care unit.[293] The patient should be awake, conscious, and appropriately responding to commands before extubation. Daley and colleagues performed a survey of tracheal extubation of adult surgical patients who were still deeply anesthetized.[294] Most respondents in the survey, who otherwise used the technique for extubation, considered the risk of pulmonary aspiration a contraindication to deep tracheal extubation.

X. MANAGEMENT OF PULMONARY ASPIRATION

When a fully conscious person aspirates foreign substances into the tracheobronchial tree, a brief but effective bout of coughing can clear the aspirate. Patients with observed pulmonary aspiration under sedation should have the mouth and pharynx suctioned immediately so that the patency of the upper airway is restored. Suctioning solid or liquid material allows recovery of the aspirated material so that it is not absorbed by the lungs, and it stimulates coughing to further expel the aspirate. After asphyxiation has been averted, bronchoscopy can be performed to clear the obstructing material from the lower airways. Bronchoscopy should not be routinely performed; it should be reserved for patients who have aspirated sufficient solid material to cause significant airway obstruction.[293] Damage to the mucosa of the tracheobronchial tree occurs within seconds, but the bronchial secretions neutralize the aspirated acid within minutes.[295] Attempts to neutralize the acid aspirate with saline or bicarbonate lavage have proved to be futile and may increase the damage.[296]

The treatment of pulmonary aspiration of gastric contents is aimed at restoring pulmonary function to normal as soon as possible. If the patient is awake and able to maintain a reasonable arterial oxygen tension (PaO_2), a conservative approach is to provide supplemental oxygen through a nasal cannula or a face mask. The inspired oxygen concentration (FIO_2) can be increased to maintain PaO_2 at approximately 60 to 70 mm Hg. This may suffice in a patient with a mild condition, but more aggressive therapy is indicated if aspiration is more severe. Severe bronchospasm may be treated by aminophylline infusion or the inhalation of a β-adrenergic bronchodilator.[296,297]

When severe pulmonary aspiration is suspected, early ventilatory support is the mainstay of treatment. Early continuous positive airway pressure (CPAP) is indicated in awake and alert patients who do not respond to a face mask. CPAP up to 12 to 14 mm Hg can be administered through a tight-fitting mask. If higher levels are required, mechanical ventilation should be considered. The level of CPAP can be reduced as the patient improves, but it should not be completely withdrawn before the alveoli can maintain stability. A high FIO_2 level can be used initially but should be decreased as soon as possible.[298]

If the patient is obtunded, a tracheal tube should be placed and mechanical ventilation initiated. Positive end-expiratory pressure (PEEP) should be applied, and FIO_2 should be decreased as soon as possible while adequate oxygenation is maintained. PEEP is commonly used to elevate functional residual capacity and prevent atelectasis resulting from poor ventilatory efforts.[297] It also improves the ventilation-perfusion ($\dot{V}/\dot{Q}$) ratio and allows the use of less toxic levels of oxygen to be administered, giving the lungs a chance to recover.[295] Caution should be exercised when using PEEP because high levels can worsen pulmonary damage by causing increased transudation of fluid through injured capillary beds.[299] Cereda and coworkers investigated the effect of PEEP in patients with acute lung injury and found that a PEEP of at least 15 cm H_2O was needed to prevent a decay in the respiratory system compliance.[300]

Despite these measures, if hypoxemia persists along with bilateral lung infiltrates and poor lung compliance, management should be similar to that for the acute respiratory distress syndrome (ARDS). A large, multicenter, randomized trial sponsored by the National Institutes of Health compared ventilation with lower versus traditional tidal volumes in patients with ARDS.[301] Smaller tidal volumes (6 mL/kg predicted body weight) and hypoventilation with permissive hypercapnia were associated with a 10% reduction in mortality, along with a shorter period using mechanical ventilation. The lower tidal volume ventilation approach protected the lungs from excessive stretch, improving several important clinical indicators of outcome in patients with ARDS.[301] An alveolar recruitment maneuver using a CPAP of 40 cm H_2O for 40 seconds improved oxygenation in patients with early ARDS who did not have impairment of the chest wall.[302] A recruitment maneuver with a smaller tidal volume was associated with a survival rate of 62%, compared with a rate of 29% when using conventional ventilation without the recruitment maneuver.[303]

Use of prophylactic antibiotics is not recommended.[304] Antibiotics alter the normal flora of the respiratory tract, which predisposes the susceptible patient to secondary infection with resistant organisms. Mitsushima and colleagues demonstrated that acid aspiration–induced epithelial injury led to subsequent bacterial infection in mice.[305] Approximately 20% to 30% of patients who manifest initial gastric content aspiration eventually develop a secondary infection.[202] Antibiotics should be reserved for patients who show signs of clinical infection and for patients who have aspirated grossly contaminated material into their lungs.

Wolfe and coworkers found that pneumonia resulting from gram-negative bacteria was more common after pulmonary aspiration among patients treated with corticosteroids than those who were not treated.[306] Corticosteroids interfered with the healing of granulomatous lesions in rabbit models.[307] The consensus appears to be that corticosteroids play no role in the treatment of aspiration pneumonitis.[308]

XI. CONCLUSIONS

Anesthetic intervention in patients with a full stomach presents the anesthesiologist with three challenges: prevention of gastric regurgitation, prevention of pulmonary aspiration, and appropriate airway management. Large surveys of pulmonary aspiration in general surgical patients found a low incidence of pulmonary aspiration of gastric contents and only a slightly greater risk among obstetric and pediatric patients. The resulting morbidity is also low, and death is rare. Changes in anesthetic practice and training probably have contributed to the decline in this dreaded complication. Preoperative fasting was introduced to reduce the risk and severity of aspiration pneumonitis. Adequate time (6 hours) must be allowed before surgery for solid foods to be emptied, but the evidence supports a reduction in the preoperative fluid fast for pediatric patients and allowance of unlimited clear fluids until 2 hours before any scheduled surgery. The routine preoperative use of multiple pharmacologic agents in patients who have no apparent risk for pulmonary aspiration is not recommended. Meticulous attention to airway management of patients at risk for pulmonary aspiration is crucial. RSI and CP, although accepted in routine practice, have never had scientific validation. Many patients at risk for pulmonary aspiration because of pregnancy, obesity, extremes of age, or comorbidities are likely to desaturate more rapidly during prolonged periods of apnea associated with difficult tracheal intubation during RSI. Awake tracheal intubation and being prepared to deal with difficult or failed tracheal intubation in patients with a full stomach are essential to the successful management of these patients.

XII. CLINICAL PEARLS

- The incidence of pulmonary aspiration in the general surgical population is low, but it is slightly increased among obstetric, pediatric, and trauma patients.

- Recommendations for preoperative fasting times are 2 hours for clear liquids and 6 hours for solids.

- Preoperative ultrasonography of the gastric antrum may be used to screen patients at risk for perioperative pulmonary aspiration of regurgitant gastric contents.

- Routine preoperative use of gastrointestinal stimulants, H_2-receptor antagonists, and proton pump inhibitors (PPIs) is not recommended in patients with no increased risk of pulmonary aspiration.

- Meticulous attention to airway management during induction, through emergence, and after extubation is crucial for patients at risk for pulmonary aspiration.

- Awake tracheal intubation and dealing with a difficult or failed airway in a patient with a full stomach requires expertise in advanced airway management.

- Airway management skills should be advanced by participating in workshops and by frequently using them in routine clinical practice.

SELECTED REFERENCES

All references can be found online at expertconsult.com.

2. Beck-Schimmer B, Bonvini JM: Bronchoaspiration: Incidence, consequences and management. *Eur J Anaesthesiol* 28:78–84, 2011.
62. Mhyre JM, Riesner MN, Polley LS, Naughton NN: A series of anesthesia-related maternal deaths in Michigan, 1985-2003. *Anesthesiology* 106:1096–1104, 2007.
63. Cook TM, Woodall N, Frerk C, for the Fourth National Audit Project: Major complications of airway management in the UK: Results of the Fourth National Audit Project of the Royal College of Anaesthetists and the Difficult Airway Society. Part 1: Anesthesia. *Br J Anaesth* 106:617–631, 2011.
78. American Society of Anesthesiologists Committee: Practice guidelines for preoperative fasting and the use of pharmacologic agents to reduce the risk of pulmonary aspiration: Application to healthy patients undergoing elective procedures: An updated report by the American Society of Anesthesiologists Committee on Standards and Practice Parameters. *Anesthesiology* 114:495–511, 2011.
102. Perlas A, Davis L, Khan M, et al: Gastric sonography in the fasted surgical patient: A prospective descriptive study. *Anesth Analg* 113:93–97, 2011.
110. Nishina K, Mikawa K, Maekawa N, et al: A comparison of lansoprazole, omeprazole, and ranitidine for reducing preoperative gastric secretion in adult patients undergoing elective surgery. *Anesth Analg* 82:832–836, 1996.
135. Sellick BA: Cricoid pressure to prevent regurgitation of stomach contents during induction of anaesthesia. *Lancet* 2:404–406, 1961.
203. Roth JV: Cricoid pressure is for full stomachs, thyroid pressure is for assisting intubations [letter]. *Anesth Analg* 104:219, 2007.
214. Mort TC: Emergency tracheal intubation: Complications associated with repeated laryngoscopic attempts. *Anesth Analg* 99:607–613, 2004.
301. Acute Respiratory Distress Syndrome Network: Ventilation with lower tidal volumes as compared with traditional tidal volumes for acute lung injury and the acute respiratory distress syndrome. The Acute Respiratory Distress Syndrome Network. *N Engl J Med* 342:1301–1308, 2000.

Chapter 36

The Difficult Pediatric Airway

RANU R. JAIN | MARY F. RABB

I. INTRODUCTION

One of the most challenging aspects facing anesthesiologists is maintaining the technical skills that are necessary for the management of the difficult airway (DA). The American Society of Anesthesiologists (ASA) guidelines define a *difficult airway* as the clinical situation in which a conventionally trained anesthesiologist experiences difficulty with face mask ventilation of the upper airway, difficulty with endotracheal intubation, or both.[1] Recent reports demonstrate how important skilled airway management is to the practice of pediatric anesthesia. Data from the ASA Pediatric Closed Claims Data Base demonstrate a greater frequency of adverse respiratory events in the pediatric population.[2] In the pediatric closed claims analysis, respiratory events accounted for 43% of all adverse events, most frequently related to inadequate ventilation (20%). Esophageal intubation, airway obstruction, and *difficult intubation* (DI) combined accounted for 14% of the remaining adverse respiratory events. In the Pediatric Perioperative Cardiac Arrest (POCA) registry, 20% of all cardiac arrests were attributed to the respiratory system.[3] Airway obstruction and DI were responsible for 27% and 13% of these events, respectively. Incidence of difficult mask ventilation in nonobese children is 2.1%. Most of the patients who experience arrests from airway obstruction or DI have an underlying disease or syndrome.

In addition, infants and small children display anatomic differences compared with adults. Knowledge of these differences, as well as congenital syndromes and different disease states, is required for management of the DA. Airway management in the pediatric patient may require general anesthesia before intubation attempts, which might not be a primary approach in a cooperative adult patient.

II. ANATOMY OF THE PEDIATRIC AIRWAY

The pediatric airway, particularly in infants, is different from the adult airway. Understanding these differences is important when managing the pediatric airway. Following is a brief review of the anatomy of the normal pediatric airway.[4-7]

A. Larynx

The larynx is situated more cephalad at the third and fourth cervical vertebrae (C3-C4) level in the infant and migrates to the adult C5 level by 6 years.[6] Because the infant's larynx is more rostral (higher), the tongue is located closer to the palate and more easily apposes the palate. As a result, airway obstruction may occur during induction or emergence from anesthesia. A common misnomer is that the infant's larynx is more "anterior" when it is really more "rostral" or "superior" in the neck, compared with the adult larynx. In syndromes associated with mandibular hypoplasia, such as Pierre Robin, the larynx is actually positioned more posteriorly than normal. This results in a greater acute angulation between the laryngeal inlet and the base of the tongue. In this circumstance,

direct visualization of the glottis may be difficult or impossible. Because of the cephalad position of the larynx and the large occiput, the "sniffing" position does not assist in visualization of the pediatric larynx.[4,7] Elevating the head only moves the larynx into a more anterior position. Infants should be positioned with the head and shoulders on a flat surface with the head in a neutral position and the neck neither flexed nor extended.[5]

B. Epiglottis

The infant epiglottis is long, stiff, and often described as Ω or U shaped.[6] It projects posteriorly above the glottis at a 45-degree angle. Because the epiglottis is more obliquely angled, visualization of the vocal cords may be difficult during direct laryngoscopy. It may be necessary to lift the tip of the epiglottis with a laryngoscope blade to visualize the vocal cords. Straight laryngoscope blades are often preferred for this reason. If the patient is not paralyzed, use of a Macintosh blade is less stimulating because it is not necessary to lift the epiglottis.

C. Subglottis

The cricoid cartilage is the narrowest portion of the infant's airway, about 5 mm in diameter, compared with the vocal cords of the adult airway.[6] The infant's larynx is funnel shaped with a narrow cricoid cartilage, whereas the adult airway is cylindrical. Tight-fitting endotracheal tubes that compress the mucosa at this level may cause edema and increase resistance to flow. Resistance to flow is inversely proportional to the radius of the lumen to the fourth power (r^4). One millimeter (1 mm) of edema can reduce the cross-sectional area of the infant trachea by 75%, versus 44% in the adult trachea.

III. EVALUATION OF THE PEDIATRIC AIRWAY

No completed studies have evaluated the predictors of DI in children. Physical examination to predict the potentially difficult airway should be guided from the knowledge of normal anatomy and the syndromes associated with the DA.

The evaluation of the pediatric airway should begin with a history and physical examination of the head and neck. The examinations mostly involve subjective experience, and consistent evaluation criteria should improve the ability to predict the DA. Clues to a potentially difficult airway include snoring, noisy breathing, difficulty breathing with feeding or an upper respiratory tract infection, and recurrent croup. Review of previous anesthesia records should be performed if available. If a DA is encountered, documentation of events and the ability to mask-ventilate is helpful for future caregivers. A prior uneventful anesthesia does not guarantee success the next time.[4,7]

Knowledge of syndromes that may adversely affect the airway is crucial to the management of the difficult pediatric airway. The presence of one anomaly mandates a search for others. A common feature in patients with many of these syndromes is *micrognathia*. Micrognathia creates more difficulty with displacement of the tongue during direct laryngoscopy, thus increasing the chance that the glottis will be difficult to visualize.[4,7] The ability to intubate often changes as the child grows. Intubation often becomes easier with syndromes associated with micrognathia (e.g., Pierre Robin) as the patient ages. In mucopolysaccharide disorders or abnormalities involving the cervical spine (e.g., Klippel-Feil syndrome), intubation may become more difficult as the child ages.[5]

Abnormalities of the ear or the presence of ear tags has been suggested as an indicator of DI.[5] In one study, *bilateral microtia* was associated with an increased incidence of DI (42%, vs. 2% in unilateral microtia). Mandibular hypoplasia was associated with bilateral microtia 10 times more than with unilateral microtia (50% vs. 5%), thus allowing bilateral microtia to be used as an indirect predictor of DI.[8]

Physical examination must focus on the head, neck, and cervical spine. Many evaluations used to predict DA in adults have not been extrapolated to the pediatric population. Cooperation of the patient is necessary for precise evaluation. In the young or uncooperative child, appropriate evaluation is limited. Preliminary data indicate that the Mallampati classification may be an insensitive predictor of DI in the pediatric population.[9] Pediatric anesthesiologists are at a disadvantage because they are anesthetizing patients with less objective airway information available. This underscores the need for a skilled approach to the difficult pediatric airway.

Evaluations should focus on the size and shape of the mandible, size of the mouth and tongue, absence or prominence of teeth, presence of loose teeth, and the neck length and range of motion. Berry[10] suggests that the appropriate thyromental distance in infants is one finger breadth (1.5 cm). Lateral examinations of the head and neck may provide clues to the presence of micrognathia. Mandibular enlargement has also been identified as a risk factor for DI.

Cherubism is a childhood disease consisting of painless mandibular enlargement with or without maxillary involvement that progresses rapidly in early childhood and then regresses during puberty. In cherubism, the potential displacement space is encroached on by mandibular enlargement.[11] Palpation of the soft tissue of the potential displacement area may reveal the problem.

A. Diagnostic Evaluation

Magnetic resonance imaging (MRI) and computed tomography (CT) may be extremely helpful in the evaluation of airway pathology. Flexible fiberoptic endoscopy may be of benefit before intubation when visualization of vocal cords is thought to be difficult or when airway pathology is suspected. In patients with unilateral hemifacial microsomia, radiographic classification of the mandibular anatomy can help predict ease of intubation.[12]

Radiographic evaluation of patients with airway obstruction may be obtained in patients who present to the emergency room only if they are not in respiratory distress. Radiographs should be obtained in the upright position because obstruction may worsen in the supine position.[13] In this situation, it is mandatory that a clinician skilled in airway management and capable of managing a difficult pediatric airway accompany the patient along with the appropriate equipment.

Radiographs have high sensitivity (>86%) for the diagnosis of airway foreign body, exudative tracheitis, and innominate artery compression. For laryngomalacia and tracheomalacia, radiography has much lower sensitivity (5% and 62%, respectively).[13] Radiologic evaluation should not take precedence over airway control in patients with a compromised airway. Other physicians, especially the otolaryngologist, may be consulted and may support a DI.

IV. CLASSIFICATION OF THE DIFFICULT PEDIATRIC AIRWAY

Difficulty with ventilation, intubation, or both is the definition of a difficult airway according to the ASA DA management guidelines.[1] Recognition of the DA along with the circumstances that predispose to airway problems is crucial to the safe management of the pediatric airway. Classification of the difficult pediatric airway may be made according to the anatomic location affected. Major anomalies of the head, face, mouth and tongue, nasopharynx, larynx, trachea, and neck are listed.

V. PEDIATRIC AIRWAY EQUIPMENT

To manage a DA successfully, the appropriate equipment should be immediately available. We recommend the creation of a difficult pediatric airway cart stocked with equipment for patients ranging from premature infants to small adults. In addition, the American Academy of Pediatrics Section on Anesthesiology recommends the creation of a DA cart for all locations anesthetizing children.[14] This cart should be dedicated only for use in a DA or a "cannot intubate, cannot ventilate" scenario (Box 36-1).

Box 36-1   *Pediatric Difficult Airway Cart*
Assortment of laryngoscope handles or blades
Oxyscope
Endotracheal tubes (ETTs): 2.0-7.0 mm
Oral/nasopharyngeal airways
Bite blocks
Masks
Stylets
Endotracheal tube exchangers
Laryngeal mask airways (LMAs): all sizes
Fiberoptic intubation (FOI) equipment
Bronchoscopic swivel connector
Retrograde intubation kit
Percutaneous cricothyrotomy kit
Laryngoscope
McGill forceps
Albuterol adapters (for metered doses)
Intravenous (IV) catheters
Defogger
Yankauer: pediatric and adult sizes
Suction catheters
Lidocaine solution/jelly

A. Face Mask

When managing the DA, the ability to ventilate with a mask is more important than endotracheal intubation. When dealing with the pediatric airway, and especially the difficult pediatric airway, it is important to have a selection of masks readily available. Disposable clear-plastic masks with an inflatable rim are typically used. These masks should extend from the chin to the bridge of the nose. A leak-free seal should be obtained with minimal pressure applied to the face or mandible. Transparent masks allow visualization of secretions or vomitus during induction. These masks can be purchased in different flavors or scented before induction to make them less intimidating.

Face masks have been modified for fiberoptic intubation (FOI) in a variety of ways.[15-18] Frei and colleagues[16,17] described modifying a commercially available mask (Vital Signs) by drilling a hole into the lateral aspect of the mask and attaching a corrugated silicon tube. The center of the mask is fitted with a plastic ring covered by a silicon membrane. A hole 1 to 2 mm smaller than the outer diameter (OD) of the bronchoscope is punched into the membrane. This airway endoscopy mask has been used to facilitate fiberoptic bronchoscopy (FOB) in patients ranging in age from 3 days to 12 months with spontaneous ventilation and propofol sedation.[15] A commercially available face mask with a ventilation side port (MERA, Senko Ika Kogyo, Tokyo) was modified and used successfully to intubate fiberoptically nine patients age 3 months to 11 years under inhalational anesthesia with continuous manual ventilation.[18]

B. Oropharyngeal Airway

Upper airway obstruction may occur during induction of anesthesia because the infant's tongue is large in relation to the oropharynx. Appropriately sized oropharyngeal airways are necessary for air exchange. Guedel and Berman airways are the most common airways available. By holding the airway next to the child's face, the correct size can be estimated. If the airway is too short, obstruction may be worsened. If the airway is too long, the epiglottis or uvula may be damaged. Use of a tongue depressor to insert the oropharyngeal airway is recommended to avoid impaired lymphatic drainage of the tongue.[4]

C. Nasopharyngeal Airway

Nasopharyngeal airways are available in sizes 12 to 36 French (F) and are used with caution in pediatric patients with hypertrophied adenoids. The *modified nasal trumpet* was first described by Beattie, followed by its use in pediatric airway management as described by Holm-Knudsen in 2005 (Fig. 36-1).

D. Endotracheal Tube

Endotracheal tubes (ETTs) in a variety of sizes (2.5-7.0 mm) should be available for the pediatric patient. Laser-resistant, nasal/oral Ring-Adair-Elywn (RAE), and

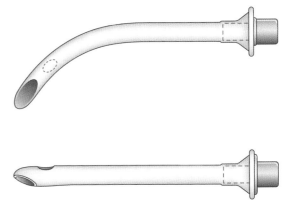

Figure 36-1 Modified nasal trumpet airway by Beattie is a nasal airway with an endotracheal tube connector wedged into the flared end. The patient can be ventilated through this modified nasal trumpet. The mouth, lips, and the other naris should be closed.

wire-reinforced ETTs are available for use depending on the surgical requirement. Determination of correct ETT size is based on the patient's age and weight. ETTs one-half size larger and smaller than the calculated size should be available (Fig. 36-2). Traditional teaching advocates the use of *uncuffed* ETTs in patients younger than 8 years. Pediatric ETTs with low-pressure high-volume cuffs are available for use in patients with low lung compliance or those at risk for aspiration. For *cuffed* ETTs, a half-size smaller tube should be used because the OD of the tube is larger with the cuff.[19]

Maintenance of air leak pressure at less than 25 cm H_2O with or without a cuff is recommended to minimize the occurrence of *postintubation croup*. Use of a manometer is recommended to avoid overinflation of the cuff. Koka and associates[20] cite the incidence of postintubation croup as 1%. In a prospective study of more than 5000 children, however, Litman and Keon[21] found that seven patients developed croup, defined as inspiratory stridor at least 30 minutes in duration, for an incidence of 0.1%. In that study, ETTs with air leak pressures greater than 40 cm H_2O were replaced with the next smaller size.[21] The presence or absence of a leak depends on the level of anesthesia and the use of muscle relaxants. Many clinicians use the degree of difficulty in passing the ETT below the vocal cords as the indicator of proper fit.

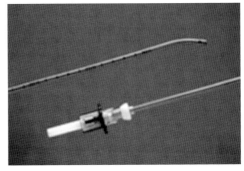

Figure 36-2 Frova Intubating Introducer (Cook Critical Care, Bloomington, IN) catheter is available in a pediatric size (8 F) that allows placement of a 3.0-mm endotracheal tube. It is hollow with two side ports, is blunt tipped, and has a Rapi-Fit adapter.

TABLE 36-1

Suggested Endotracheal Tube Size for Infants

Age	Size (mm ID)
Preterm (>1000 g)	2.5
Preterm (1000-2500 g)	3.0
Newborn to 6 months	3.0-3.5
1-2 years	4.0-4.5
>2 years	(Age +16)/4 = ID

ID, Internal diameter.

In general, there are many formulas to calculate the appropriate size of ETT. Formulas for selecting an uncuffed ETT in children older than 2 years include (age + 16)/4 or (age/4) + 4. The use of cuffed ETTs in newborns and children under 8 years has been studied. In a group of 488 patients, patients were randomly allocated to receive a cuffed or an uncuffed ETT.[22] The formula for the cuffed tube was (age/4) + 3. This formula was appropriate for 99% of patients. In that study, three patients in each group were treated for croup symptoms. Formulas for length of insertion of an oral ETT include length (cm) + 3 times internal diameter (mm) or length (cm) = age (years)/2 + 12.[19] In the premature or newborn infant, the rule is tip-to-lip distance in cm = 6 + weight (kg).[23] Whatever method is chosen, correct ETT position should be confirmed by auscultation of bilateral breath sounds (Tables 36-1 and 36-2). Also, leak should be checked to a permissible pressure.

Double-lumen tubes are not available for use in pediatric patients younger than 6 to 8 years. The Arndt Endobronchial Blocker (Cook Critical Care, Bloomington, Ind) has been used to provide one-lung ventilation in infants.[24] The 5.0-F blocker is available; the recommended ETT size is 4.5 mm. The Univent tube (Fuji Systems, Tokyo) is a single-lumen tube with an incorporated movable bronchial blocker inside.[25] Pediatric sizes of the Univent tube are available: 3.5-mm internal diameter (ID) and 4.5-mm ID. The 3.5-mm Univent tube does not have a lumen for suctioning or administration of oxygen to the blocked lung. FOB is needed for placement. Further detail regarding one-lung ventilation is provided in Chapter 26.

E. Endotracheal Tube Exchangers

Endotracheal tube (ETT) exchangers have multiple uses; they can be used to exchange damaged ETs and provide

TABLE 36-2

Formula for Endotracheal Tube (ETT) Size and Depth of Insertion

Type/Insertion	Formula
Uncuffed ETT	(Age + 16)/4 or ETT >2 years, Age/4 + 4
Cuffed ETT	Age/4 + 3
Length of insertion (oral)	Age (years)/2 + 12 or 3 × ID (mm)
Length of insertion (nasal)	3 × ID (mm) + 2

ID, Internal diameter.

a conduit for reintubation, if necessary. Many different types of exchangers are available for use in adult patients. These tube exchangers are long, semirigid catheters that fit inside ETTs. The Frova Intubating Introducer (Cook Critical Care) is available in a pediatric size (8 F) that allows placement of a 3.0-mm ETT. It is 33 cm in length with a hollow lumen and a blunt curved tip that is shaped like the gum elastic bougie. The blunt curved tip can be passed "blindly" into the trachea when visualization of the glottis is inadequate. The Frova catheter has a hollow lumen and two side ports and is packaged with removable Rapi-Fit adapters that allow ventilation and a stiffening cannula[26] (Fig. 36-2).

Cook also manufactures airway exchange catheters (AECs) in four sizes. These catheters are blunt tipped and hollow, with distal side ports and a Rapi-Fit adapter. The 8-F size is 45 cm in length and can be used in 3.0-mm ETTs.[26]

F. Laryngoscopes

1. Straight vs. Curved Blades

Laryngoscope blades in different sizes and shapes should be available before induction of anesthesia. Laryngoscope blades fall into two categories: straight and curved. Because the epiglottis is angled posteriorly, visualization of the glottis may be difficult. *Straight* laryngoscope blades are often recommended for use in neonates and infants to lift the epiglottis. The most common straight blades include the Miller, Wisconsin, Wis-Hipple, and Wis-Foregger blades. *Curved* blades are more suitable for older children.

2. Oxyscope

The Oxyscope is a fiberoptic Miller no. 1 blade with a port for insufflation of oxygen during intubation. Oxygen insufflation during laryngoscopy in spontaneously breathing, anesthetized infants has been shown to minimize the decrease in transcutaneous oxygen tension, thus making airway instrumentation safer.[27]

3. Anterior Commissure Laryngoscope

The anterior commissure laryngoscope is frequently used by otolaryngologists for visualization of the glottis. It is a rigid, tubular, straight-blade laryngoscope with a distally located, recessed light source. This design permits enhanced visualization by preventing the tongue from obscuring the field of view.[28]

4. Bullard Laryngoscope

The Bullard laryngoscope (Circon ACMI, Stanford, Conn), developed by Dr. Roger Bullard at the Medical College of Georgia, is an indirect laryngoscope that utilizes fiberoptic and mirror technology to visualize the larynx.[29] Use of fiberoptics and a curved blade enable visualization of the larynx "around the corner" of the blade, thus eliminating the need to align the oral, pharyngeal, and tracheal axes. A standard laryngoscope handle or a flexible fiberoptic cable connected to a light source powers the fiberoptic light source. This laryngoscope is manufactured in three sizes: adult, pediatric, and pediatric long.[30] The adult size, with a blade that is

2.5 cm wide, is suitable for children older than 10 years. The *pediatric* version (newborn to age 2 years) has a blade 1.3 cm wide that extends 0.6 cm beyond the fiberoptics. This blade is recommended for use in neonates, infants, and smaller children. The *pediatric long* version is available for use in infants and small children up to age 10; it has a longer blade (1.4 cm) and a wider flange (1.6 cm). In the pediatric long version, a multifunctional stylet is attached to the fiberoptic bundle between the eyepiece and handle and aligns the tip of the ETT beneath the flange of the blade. The smallest ETT that passes over the stylet in the pediatric long version is 4.5 mm.[30]

The Bullard laryngoscope requires minimal mouth opening for its insertion (0.64 cm in cephalad-caudad axis). It has been used to intubate patients with unstable cervical spine or with Pierre Robin, Treacher Collins, Noonan's, or Klippel-Feil syndrome, among others.[29] The adult Bullard laryngoscope has been used successfully to intubate patients older than 12 months with normal airways.[31] Contact with the right aryepiglottic fold and, in children, contact with the anterior vocal cord occurred.[31,32] Compared with the Wis-Hipple 11/2, the adult Bullard laryngoscope provided a similar view and required a slightly longer time for intubation in children 1 to 5 years of age.[32]

5. Angulated Video-Intubation Laryngoscope

The angulated video-intubation laryngoscope (AVIL), invented by Dr. Marcus Weiss of Zurich, is an endoscopic intubation device. The AVIL consists of a cast-plastic Macintosh 4 laryngoscope, with the blade angulated distally, and an integrated fiberoptic endoscope (1.8 m long, OD 2.8 mm, VOLPI, Schlieren, Switzerland). The distal blade tip is angulated about 25 degrees to provide increased viewing for the fiberoptic lens. With the angulated tip, the AVIL resembles an activated McCoy blade. Flattening of the blade's vertical flange enables the device to be used in children. The fiberoptic endoscope runs from the handle to the tip of the blade. The AVIL uses conventional laryngoscopy techniques coupled with video monitoring from the blade tip. Styletted ETTs, in a "hockey stick" configuration, are passed along the vertical flange of the blade under video control.[33]

The AVIL has been used in patients ranging in age from 3 months to 17 years with manual in-line neck stabilization. In infants and small children, care should be taken with insertion of the blade; initial insertion of the blade was too deep in these patients.[34] Several reports document the use of this device in pediatric patients with a DA. The video laryngoscope has been used successfully to intubate children with Morquio's syndrome as well as a 3-day-old neonate with Pierre Robin syndrome.[33,35]

6. Truview Laryngoscope

The Truview (Truphatek International, Netanya, Israel) is a recently introduced rigid laryngoscope that has an angulated tip and an optical assembly that provides an illuminated and magnified view of the larynx. The optical system consists of a lens and a prism, which extends the view beyond the tip of the blade. The tip of the device is narrow to accommodate small mouth openings and angulated 46 degrees anteriorly to provide a wider view of the larynx using light refraction. This laryngoscope also has a side port that allows for oxygen insufflation and can be attached to video monitoring to assist with training. The height of the laryngoscope blade is 8 mm. Compared with traditional laryngoscopes, the Truview EVO2 laryngoscope offers various advantages and improves laryngoscopic view. A study by Singh and colleagues[35a] of 60 neonates and infants comparing the Truview EVO2 with the Miller blade demonstrated an improved laryngoscopic view with the Truview blade, with an increased time to intubation that was statistically but not clinically significant.

7. GlideScope Video Laryngoscope

The GlideScope Video Laryngoscope (Cobalt, Verahon) has a reusable video baton and single-use laryngoscopy blades in two sizes. The laryngoscope comes with a monitor screen, and a video recording unit is also available. The GlideScope Cobalt model features a 10-mm laryngoscope blade. The blade is inserted in the midline without displacing the tongue.[36] Two studies have been reported using the GlideScope in children with normal airways. Both studies found it suitable for intubation in pediatric patients.[37,38] In one of the studies, the time required for intubation was longer.

8. Airtraq Optical Laryngoscope

The Airtraq Optical Laryngoscope (AOL; Prodol, Vizcaya, Spain) is a single-use indirect laryngoscope for tracheal intubation. The Airtraq comes in two pediatric sizes: infant (size 0) for ETT 2.5 to 3.5 and pediatric (size 1) for ETT sizes 3.5 to 5.5. Both sizes require a mouth opening of 12 to 13 mm. The rubber eyepiece may be used or a camera may be attached and used with a wireless monitor. Images from the distal tip of the blade are projected to the proximal eyepiece. The Airtraq is inserted midline, and the tip may be placed in the vallecula or used to lift the epiglottis. Once the glottis is visualized, the ETT is slowly advanced. For intubation, it is important to lubricate the ETT so that the tube advances easily. Problems with advancement of the ETT may be caused by too large diameter of the ETT, the guide channel, or incorrect angle of the ETT.[36] Two case reports documented the use of the Airtraq in pediatric patients with difficult airways: a 9-year-old child with Treacher Collins syndrome who weighed 23 kg[37] and a 4.8-kg infant with Pierre Robin syndrome.[38] Other case reports have documented difficulty with advancement of the ETT into the trachea despite a good view of the larynx.[39]

G. Stylets

There are various types of stylets available as adjuncts to endotracheal intubation, including the traditional malleable stylet, lighted stylets, and optical stylets. Stylets should be available for the DA. The stylet is inserted into the ETT until the distal end of the stylet is just short of the ETT tip. The ETT and stylet are bent into the desired shape, usually a hockey stick configuration. Complications associated with use of stylets include tracheal trauma, ETT obstruction, and shearing of the stylet.

When removal of a stylet becomes difficult, the tip should be examined.[40]

1. Lighted Stylets

Several different types of lighted stylets, or *lightwands*, are currently commercially available, including the Vital Signs Light Wand Illuminating Stylet (Vital Signs, Totawa, NJ) and the Tube Stat Lighted Stylet (Xomed, Jacksonville, Fla). Pediatric versions are available for use with ETTs as small as 2.0 to 4.0 mm. The use of the lighted stylet to guide blind endotracheal intubation relies on the principle of *transillumination*. The presence of a well-defined glow in the neck indicates tracheal placement. Esophageal placement is indicated by the absence of a glow in the neck. Several different reports describe successful intubation of pediatric patients with the lightwand.[41,42] Successful technique includes the following principles:

1. A small shoulder roll should be used to keep the head in a neutral to slightly extended position. This is extremely important in a small infant, whose neck naturally flexes when lying on a flat surface because of the large occiput.
2. The lightwand should be advanced in the midline; if the light deviates to one side, the lightwand should be withdrawn and repositioned.
3. The epiglottis is elevated by lifting the jaw with the nondominant hand.
4. Transillumination should be assessed before advancing the lightwand too far.
5. Blind nasal intubation in children is often easier with the rigid stylet left in place.
6. The wand is bent less sharply than for an oral intubation.

Benefits of light-guided tracheal intubation include use in obstructed conditions, low acquisition costs, and disposable components that eliminate the need for disinfection of equipment. As with any new technique, experience in patients with normal anatomy should be obtained before attempts in patients with a DA.

2. Optical Stylets

The first optical stylet, described in 1979, was a Hopkins telescope with a fiberoptic external light source (Karl Storz, Tuttlingen, Germany).[43] The Seeing Optical Stylet (SOS) system (Clarus Medical, Minneapolis) is a new, reusable, high-resolution fiberoptic endoscope with a malleable stainless steel stylet.[36] It combines the features of an FOB and a lightwand. The Shikani Seeing Stylet is portable, lightweight, and available in pediatric and adult versions. The pediatric version is compatible with ETTs 3.0 to 5.0 mm in size. The SOS can be inserted directly into an ETT, allowing intubation to be performed under direct vision. Illumination is provided by a standard green line fiberoptic laryngoscope handle or the included SITElite halogen handle. An adjustable tube stop with an oxygen port, which goes over the shaft of the stylet, allows supplemental oxygen to be delivered. Many factors do not affect the SOS, including cervical spine injury, small mouth, large tongue, and reduced jaw mobility.[36]

Pfitzner and colleagues[44] described the use of the Shikani SOS on eight occasions in seven patients with DA. There were seven successful intubations; one patient, who had previous surgery and radiotherapy for a retropharyngeal rhabdomyosarcoma, could not be intubated by any method. Two patients with limited mouth opening and one patient with a C1-C2 subluxation were intubated on the first attempt. A patient with Hunter's syndrome was intubated on the second attempt. A potential difficulty mentioned with the SOS is loss of the visual field, which occurs when the lens is next to a mucosal surface. Maneuvers to increase the operating space available are use of a laryngoscope to retract the base of the tongue, lifting the mandible, and pulling the tongue forward.[45]

The Shikani Stylet is inserted into the ETT after lubrication with silicon spray. The fiberoptic cable can be connected to a video monitor. The mandible is lifted with the left hand and displaced anteriorly until the lower teeth are anterior to the upper teeth.[45] The stylet with the loaded ETT is advanced into the trachea under direct vision. Laryngoscopy may be useful in cases of DI (Fig. 36-3). The Shikani Optical Stylet (Clarus Medical) is a portable video stylet.

3. Video-Optical Intubation Stylet

Another video-optical intubating stylet (Acutronic Medical Systems, Hirzel, Switzerland) consists of a flexible fiberoptic endoscope (developed by Dr. Weiss of Zurich). A sliding connector locks the video stylet onto the ETT adapter; it does not require neck extension but does require mouth opening. One report documents successful use of the video-optical intubating stylet in patients age 6 to 16 years, with a simulated grade III laryngoscopic view; 46 of 50 patients were intubated on the first attempt; four attempts were considered failures because of prolonged intubation time (>60 seconds).[46]

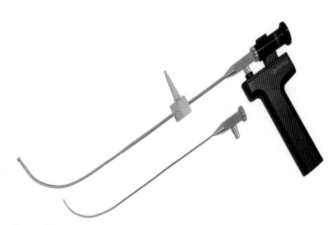

Figure 36-3 Shikani Seeing Optical Stylet (Clarus Medical, Minneapolis) is a reusable, high-resolution fiberoptic endoscope. The pediatric version is compatible with endotracheal tubes in the range of 3.0 to 5.0 mm. Supplemental oxygen can be delivered through the oxygen port. It can be used with the SITElite halogen handle (as shown) or a standard green line fiberoptic laryngoscope handle.

TABLE 36-3

LMA Classic Mask Size with Corresponding Cuff Volumes, ETT, and FOB

Mask Size	Weight (kg)	Maximum Cuff Volume (mL)	Maximum ETT Size	Maximum FOB (mm)
1	Infants up to 5	Up to 4	3.5 uncuffed	2.7
1.5	5-10	Up to 7	4.0 uncuffed	3.0
2	10-20	Up to 10	4.5 uncuffed	3.5
2.5	20-30	Up to 14	5.0 uncuffed	4.0
3	30-50	Up to 20	6.0 cuffed	5.0
4	50-70	Up to 30	6.0 cuffed	5.0
5	70-100	Up to 40	7.0 cuffed	5.0
6	>100	Up to 50	7.0 cuffed	5.0

LMA, Laryngeal mask airway; *ETT*, endotracheal tube; *FOB*, fiberoptic bronchoscope.

H. Laryngeal Mask Airways

1. LMA Family

The laryngeal mask airway (LMA North America, San Diego), introduced in 1983 and approved for use in 1991 by the U.S. Food and Drug Administration (FDA), is a standard part of the ASA DA algorithm.[1,47] Pediatric versions of the LMA Classic, as well as the disposable LMA, are available for use and are part of the pediatric DA algorithm, as described by Steward and Lerman.[48] Application of the LMA requires minimum training and can be useful in neonatal resuscitation.[49] The LMA Flexible is available in sizes 2 and 2.5, and the LMA ProSeal is available in a size 2. The size of the LMA in children is determined by the patient's weight, although a new method has been suggested. With the hand extended and palm side facing up, the thumb and little finger are extended. The second, third, and fourth fingers are placed together. The fully inflated LMA is placed against the palmar side of the patient's fingers, keeping the widest part of the LMA in line with the widest part of the three fingers. In a study of 163 children at birth to 14 years old, this method was correct in 78%. In the remaining patients, a difference of only one size was observed.[50]

The LMA has been described as a conduit for blind intubation as well as a conduit for fiberoptic intubation.[51-55] Awake placement of the LMA has been described in an infant with Pierre Robin syndrome.[56] Anterograde intubation through the LMA with a guidewire was also described in an infant with micrognathia who could not be intubated with conventional methods. A soft-tipped guidewire was advanced through the LMA and the position confirmed by fluoroscopy. An ETT was inserted over the guidewire, followed by removal of the LMA.[57] A review of the literature demonstrates different insertion techniques.

The standard technique described with the cuff *deflated* for adults has also been advocated for children. In addition, a rotational or reverse technique has been described. The LMA is inserted with the cuff facing the hard palate and then rotated and advanced simultaneously. An alternative technique involves inserting the LMA with the cuff partially inflated. Reports on placement of the LMA with the different techniques are conflicting. In children, one study compared two insertion techniques. The partially inflated cuff insertion technique does not increase the incidence of downfolding of the epiglottis and is an acceptable alternative to the standard technique.[58] In another study, insertion of the partially inflated LMA required less time and was associated with a higher success rate on first attempts compared with the standard (deflated) technique.[59] Results from a study detailing the fiberoptic positioning of the LMA in children with a DA show that 29.5% of patients had a grade I (full) view of the glottis, 29.5% had a grade II (partial) view, and 41% a grade III (epiglottis only) view. Children with a mucopolysaccharide disorder had a grade III view 54% and a grade I view 14% of the time.[60]

The ProSeal LMA is now available in pediatric sizes. This LMA has a second mask to isolate the upper esophagus with a second dorsal cuff to increase the seal against the glottis. Lopez-Gill and coworkers[61] found that it was easily inserted, and oropharyngeal leak pressure was greater than 40 cm H_2O (Table 36-3).

2. Air-Q Intubating Laryngeal Airway

The Air-Q Intubating Laryngeal Airway (ILA) (Cookgas, Mercury Medical, Clearwater, Fla) is a supraglottic device used both for airway maintenance during routine anesthesia and as a conduit for tracheal intubation for patients with a DA. Unlike the LMA, the ILA was designed primarily to allow for the passage of conventional cuffed tracheal tubes when used for blind tracheal intubation, and it has the option for subsequent removal. The ILA also shares some structural features with the intubating laryngeal mask airway (ILMA). Compared with the LMA, the ILA allows for straightforward passage of a cuffed tracheal tube when used as a conduit for tracheal intubation because of three design differences. First, the airway tube of the ILA is wider, more rigid, and curved. Second, removal of the detachable 15-mm proximal connector increases the ID of the airway tube. Third, the ILA's shorter length allows for easier removal after successful tracheal intubation. The Air-Q ILA is available in six sizes (1, 1.5, 2, 2.5, 3.5, and 4.5) for single use and in four sizes (2.0, 2.5, 3.5, and 4.5) for reuse. Sizing of the pediatric Air-Q ILA is similar to the LMA, in that it is weight based (size 1 for patients <5 kg; size 1.5 for 5-10 kg; size 2 for 10-20 kg).

The self-pressurized Air-Q ILA (ILA-SP) is a new first-generation supraglottic airway for children with a self-adjusting cuff and lack of a pilot balloon. A newer version of the ILA-SP was recently introduced into our practice for routine airway maintenance in children. The ILA is currently the only supraglottic device available in pediatric patients designed to act as a conduit for tracheal intubation with cuffed tracheal tubes.

I. Rigid Ventilating Bronchoscope

The rigid ventilating bronchoscope is extremely useful for ventilating patients with a DA and is included in the most recent version of the ASA DA algorithm as an alternative device in the "cannot ventilate, cannot intubate" situation. In any situation of potential airway collapse, the otolaryngologist and the rigid ventilating bronchoscope should be immediately available (see Chapter 29).

VI. INDUCTION TECHNIQUE

The principles outlined in the ASA guidelines for DA management apply to the pediatric patient. Evaluation, recognition, and preparation are key elements.[1] Preoxygenation of pediatric patients, although difficult, should be attempted before any DA intervention, if possible. Studies have demonstrated that the optimal time for preoxygenation in pediatric patients is different from that in adults. Values ranging from 80 to 100 seconds have been reported for adequate preoxygenation in healthy children.[62,63] Summoning help early, using *awake intubation*, and preserving spontaneous ventilation during intubation attempts are also important when managing the DA. The awake or awake sedated approach is preferred in most circumstances when managing the DA. However, in pediatric patients, the patient's cooperation may limit the usefulness of awake intubation. One well-tolerated technique is placement of a lubricated LMA in awake infants, which provides an airway for inhalational induction.[56]

The traditional approach to the difficult pediatric airway has been maintenance of spontaneous ventilation under inhalational anesthesia. Premedication with oral or intravenous atropine (0.01-0.02 mg/kg) is indicated for vagolytic and antimuscarinic effects. Inhalation induction may be performed with sevoflurane in 100% oxygen. Sevoflurane has been used in the management of the DA with success.[64,65] The low blood gas solubility of sevoflurane and consequent rapid induction and emergence are advantageous when managing the DA. When the ability to ventilate the patient by mask is demonstrated, a small dose of muscle relaxant or propofol may be given to facilitate intubation.

For patients who can tolerate an *awake sedated* intubation technique, a variety of drugs can be used. One must always keep in mind the risk/benefit ratio when sedating a patient with a DA. Sedatives may further compromise an airway. Sedatives should not be given to any patient in acute distress or with the potential for acute obstruction. Use of sedatives should be based on careful physical examination, anesthesiologist experience with agents involved, and overall patient condition. If no other options are available, slow titration of pharmacologic agents to effect, without loss of spontaneous ventilation, should be performed. Use of pharmacologic agents that are easily antagonized is recommended. For older children and adolescents, a combination of midazolam and fentanyl may be used. Remifentanil can also be used. Dexmedetomidine has been used successfully to perform an awake fiberoptic intubation in a morbidly obese patient with facial, cervical, and upper thoracic edema.[66] In extreme circumstances, parental presence at induction may be allowed. Careful preparation of the parent must be performed prior to induction. As soon as the patient separates or begins to lose consciousness, a designated member of the operating room (OR) staff should immediately escort the parent out of the OR.

Another important aspect for successful airway management is *topicalization* of the airway with local anesthesia. In pediatric patients, this may be obtained by nebulizing, spraying, or swabbing local anesthetic solution or by applying viscous gel to a gloved finger. FOB with suction ports can be used to spray local anesthesia on the vocal cords under direct vision. The maximum dose of local anesthetic allowed should be calculated before topicalization. The drug of choice is *lidocaine* because it has the best safety profile. Maximum doses of lidocaine are 5 mg/kg. Agents containing benzocaine (e.g., Cetacaine spray; Americaine ointment; Hurricane ointment, gel, or spray) should be avoided in infants and young children because of the risk of methemoglobinemia.[7]

VII. AIRWAY MANAGEMENT TECHNIQUES

A. Techniques for Ventilation

Obstruction of the upper airway is a common occurrence in pediatric patients undergoing an inhalation induction. Techniques for overcoming this type of obstruction include insertion of an appropriate-size oropharyngeal airway or a nasopharyngeal airway, or both. Another common mistake is occlusion of the submandibular space with incorrect placement of the anesthesiologist's hand. Care should be taken to position the hand on the tip of the mandible and not on the submandibular space. Chin lift or jaw thrust combined with continuous positive airway pressure (CPAP) at 10 cm H_2O has been shown to improve upper airway patency.[67]

Additional techniques are available for mask ventilation. The two-person technique involves either one person holding the mask with both hands while an assistant compresses the reservoir bag or a second person assisting in jaw lift while the first person continues to compress the reservoir bag. Another option is using the anesthesia ventilator to provide ventilation so that one person can hold the face mask with both hands.[68]

B. Techniques for Intubation

1. Direct Laryngoscopy

Tips for successful visualization of the larynx include proper use of external laryngeal pressure and positioning. Direct laryngoscopy involves alignment of the oral, pharyngeal, and laryngeal axes in order to visualize the glottis. Because the larynx is situated in a more cephalad position and the occiput is large, the sniffing position in infants does not assist in visualization of the larynx.[4,7] The infant should be positioned with the head in a neutral position with the neck neither flexed nor extended.[69] A small shoulder or neck roll may be beneficial. Optimum external laryngeal manipulation (OELM) should also be used with a poor laryngoscopic view to improve visualization. OELM may improve the laryngoscopic view by at least one whole grade in adults. This is not cricoid pressure but rather pressing posteriorly and cephalad over the thyroid, hyoid, and cricoid cartilages. Benumof and Cooper[70] suggest that OELM should be an instinctive and reflex response to a poor laryngoscopic view. This maneuver has also proved effective in pediatric patients.[71] The main mechanism seems to be shortening of the incisor-to-glottis distance.

The two-anesthesiologist technique involves manipulating the larynx under direct vision by the laryngoscopist and intubation by a second anesthesiologist. This technique has been used successfully to intubate a 6-month-old infant with Pierre Robin syndrome and concomitant tongue-tie (ankyloglossia).[72]

The *retromolar* or *paraglossal* technique has been advocated as useful in cases of DI related to a small mandible.[73] A straight laryngoscope blade is introduced into the extreme right corner of the mouth overlying the molars, thus reducing the distance to the vocal cords. It is advanced in the space between the tongue and lateral pharyngeal wall until the epiglottis or glottis is visualized. The head is rotated to the left to improve visualization while applying external laryngeal pressure displacing the larynx to the right. Advancement of the ETT is facilitated by retracting the corner of the mouth to allow placement of the ETT. The styletted ETT should be shaped into the classic hockey stick configuration. An alternative approach involves placement of the ETT from the left side of the mouth.[74] Lateral placement of the laryngoscope blade reduces the soft tissue compression because the tongue is essentially bypassed. The maxillary structures are also bypassed by the lateral blade placement, thus improving the view.[4] Because there is a reduced space for displacement of the tongue in syndromes with micrognathia, this approach may be useful. The retromolar technique has been described as an alternative method for intubation of patients with Pierre Robin syndrome.[75] A pediatric version of the Bonfils Retromolar Intubation Fiberscope is the Brambrink Intubation Scope (Karl Storz). It is an optical stylet that allows a retromolar approach to the DA.[26]

In adults the *left molar* approach with a Macintosh blade and OELM has been reported to improve the glottic view in cases of difficult laryngoscopy.[76] Suspension laryngoscopy is often employed by otolaryngologists as an alternative technique for visualization of the difficult larynx. Intubation of an infant with Goldenhar's syndrome was accomplished by *suspension laryngoscopy*.[77] This method is similar to standard laryngoscopy by the retromolar technique.

With any direct laryngoscopy technique, limiting the number of attempts is recommended. Edema can rapidly occur and create a "cannot ventilate, cannot intubate" scenario.

2. Blind Intubation Technique

a. BLIND NASOTRACHEAL INTUBATION

Blind nasotracheal intubation requires preservation of spontaneous ventilation either under general anesthesia or with adequate vasoconstriction and topicalization of the nasal mucosa. The tip of the ETT is directed toward the larynx by listening to the intensity of the breath sounds or by the capnograph tracing. This technique requires extensive practice before use. Tips for this technique include external pressure on the neck, which may direct the glottis toward the ETT; placement of a stylet through the ETT after passage through the nasopharynx to direct the tip to the glottis; inflating the ETT cuff with air to center it at the glottis and then deflating it for actual passage; and repositioning of the head (flexion/extension) if the initial intubation attempt fails.[48] Pediatric patients with enlarged adenoids may be at risk for bleeding and trauma with this technique. Blind nasotracheal intubation of a neonate with Pierre Robin syndrome has been described.[78]

b. DIGITAL ENDOTRACHEAL INTUBATION

Digital intubation is a blind technique that is relatively easy to learn. Intubation of an 8-day-old, 3.3-kg neonate with Pierre Robin syndrome has been reported.[79] The left index finger is passed midline along the surface of the tongue until it passes the epiglottis. The left thumb may apply cricoid pressure to steady the larynx. The ETT, using the left index finger as a guide, is advanced into the trachea. This technique has been used as the primary method of intubating neonates in some neonatal centers.[80] As with any new technique, practice is required.

c. LIGHTWAND INTUBATION

Intubation with a lightwand is a blind technique that has found success in management of the difficult pediatric airway.[41,42] The success rate increases with experience; practice is thus required. As with any new technique, experience with patients who have normal anatomy should be gained first. Contraindications to the use of the lightwand include tumors, infections, trauma, and foreign bodies of the upper airway.[37] Causes of failed intubation include entrapment in the vallecula or the aryepiglottic folds. A shoulder roll helps to extend the head and neck and increase the exposure of the anterior neck. After preparation of the lightwand, the jaw is lifted with the nondominant hand or a laryngoscope blade. The lightwand is inserted in the midline into the patient's mouth, rotated around the patient's tongue, then gently rocked back and forth. If the ETT wand is in the trachea, a well-defined bright light (size of a quarter) is visible at the level of the subglottis on the anterior surface of the neck.

3. Fiberoptic Laryngoscopy

Aids for fiberoptic intubation (FOI) include face masks, oropharyngeal airways, guidewires, and the LMA.[81] The Frei mask previously described or variations of commercially available masks have been used with success.[15,16,82] The Patil-Syracuse mask is available in a size 2, but it is difficult to achieve a good seal with this mask. An endoscopy mask can be made by attaching a swivel fiberoptic bronchoscope (FOB) adapter to a pediatric face mask in one of two ways[81]: a commercially available swivel adapter (Instrumentation Industries, Bethel Park, Pa) can be attached directly to the mask, or an adapter designed for attachment to the ETT (e.g., Portex bronchoscope adapter) can be connected to the face mask with a 15-mm to 22-mm adapter.

Oropharyngeal airways may also be modified for use in pediatric FOI. A strip may be cut from the convex surface of a Guedel-style airway to produce an aid for oral fiberoptic laryngoscopy, creating a channel. The fiberscope is placed in the channel, which helps maintain a midline position. The use of a smaller airway than predicted is suggested so that one may visualize the base of the tongue and epiglottis. Modified oropharyngeal airways are not effective as bite blocks, and one must be careful.[81] Also, a nipple from a baby bottle has been modified to act as a conduit for FOI in an infant with an unstable cervical spine. In this case, a hole was cut obliquely into the end of the nipple. After topicalization of the airway with 2% lidocaine, FOI was performed with a 4.0-mm uncuffed ETT.[83]

Flexible fiberoptic laryngoscopy is one of the cornerstones of DA management. Preparation for fiberoptic laryngoscopy should include preparation of the patient (antisialogue) and checking of the FOB, light source, and suction as well as standard airway equipment. An assistant is necessary for monitoring of the patient and providing a jaw lift, which is useful because it elevates the tongue from the posterior pharynx.[7] For older children and adolescents who will be sedated for the procedure, explanation and reassurance in a calm manner are helpful. A method of delivering oxygen is necessary as well. This can be accomplished in a variety of ways, either blowby from the anesthesia circuit or by nasal cannula. For patients who are anesthetized, an LMA or an endoscopy mask may be used to ventilate the patient while the intubation is being performed. Tips for successful oral intubation include midline placement of the FOB, advancement of the FOB only when recognizable structures are visualized, and retraction of the tongue with gauze or clamps if needed.[7] If the view from the fiberscope is pink mucosa, the FOB is slowly pulled back until a recognizable structure is seen. If the nasal route is chosen, a topical vasoconstrictor may be used to reduce the chance of bleeding. In a series of 46 patients with DA, fiberoptic nasal intubation was successful on the first attempt in 37 patients (80.4%) and on the second or third attempt in 7 patients (15.2%). Two failures occurred: one related to bleeding and the other to inability to introduce the scope nasally.[84]

Flexible fiberoptic laryngoscopy may be performed in a variety of ways. The standard technique involves passage of the ETT over the FOB. The ultrathin fiberoptic laryngoscope with a directable tip allows FOI to be performed with ETTs as small as 2.5 mm. Intubation of a 3-month-old infant with the Pierre Robin syndrome has been successfully performed with an ultrathin fiberscope.[85] A new 2.5-mm ultrathin flexible FOB with a 1.2-mm suction channel has been used to intubate a newborn with a DA.[86] This FOB has a 2.5-mm OD, 1.2-mm working suction channel, angle of deflection of 160 degrees up and 130 degrees down, and a working length of 450 mm.

In scenarios where the available bronchoscope is too large for the required ETT, a staged technique may be employed.[87] A FOB with a working channel, a cardiac catheter, and a guidewire are required. The guidewire is passed into the working channel of the fiberscope before intubation. The FOB guidewire assembly is then introduced into the mouth and positioned above the larynx. The guidewire is advanced into the trachea under direct visualization, followed by removal of the FOB. A cardiac catheter (used to stiffen the wire) is threaded over the guidewire. Finally, an ETT is advanced into the trachea over the guidewire-catheter assembly, which is then removed. A modification of this technique involves passage of the ETT over the guidewire without the reinforcing cardiac catheter. This has been used to intubate nasotracheally a 3-day-old infant with Pierre Robin syndrome.[88]

The fiberoptic bronchoscope may also be used as an aid for nasal intubation either under direct vision or with a guide. In these cases, FOB is introduced into one of the nares while the ETT is advanced into the trachea through the other naris.[38] Alternatively, if the ETT cannot be manipulated into the glottis, a guide may be placed in the opposite naris and directed into the trachea. The ETT is then removed and threaded over the guide. A urethral catheter has been used in this manner to assist in the intubation of a 2-week-old neonate with Klippel-Feil syndrome, occipital meningocele, and microretrognathia.[89] Another variation of the staged technique involves placement of a larger ETT into the larynx under fiberoptic visualization, followed by removal of the FOB, leaving the larger ETT in the larynx. A bougie is placed through the larger ETT into the trachea, and the ETT is removed. An appropriate-size ETT is then advanced over the bougie into the trachea.[90]

Flexible FOB intubation through the LMA has been successful.[52,53,91] Staged intubation techniques involving the LMA, FOB, guidewires, and catheters (dilators) have been reported, including the use of LMA-assisted wire-guided fiberoptic endotracheal intubation. In a series of 15 cases, Heard and colleagues[92] demonstrated that this technique was safe, successful, and easy to learn. After the FOB is placed through the LMA and the vocal cords are visualized, the guidewire is passed through the suction port of the bronchoscope and into the trachea. The LMA and FOB are carefully removed, and the ETT is advanced over the wire. A variation of this theme involves fiberoptic visualization of the glottis through the LMA followed by passage of a guidewire through the suction port of a FOB into the trachea as before. The fiberscope is then removed and an airway catheter or a ureteral dilator passed over the wire into the trachea through the LMA. The LMA is then removed and an ETT advanced over the catheter into the trachea.[93] This technique has been used successfully to manage the airway in children with mucopolysaccharidoses. The use of an LMA, an airway exchange catheter (AEC), and a 2.2-mm–OD FOB has also been described.[94] After placement of the LMA and visualization of the vocal cords, the fiberscope is removed. The fiberscope is placed into the lumen of a size 11 AEC, which had been cut to 25 cm. This combination was advanced through the LMA into the trachea by a connector. The LMA and FOB are removed, and an ETT is advanced over the Cook AEC.

Przybylo and coauthors[95] reported the performance of a retrograde FOI through a tracheocutaneous fistula in a child with Nager's syndrome. The ultrathin FOB was passed through the fistula in a cephalad direction past the vocal cords and exiting the nares. The ETT was then advanced over the FOB into the trachea.

4. Bullard Laryngoscope

The pediatric Bullard laryngoscope is placed into the oropharynx in the horizontal plane. After passing the tongue, the handle is rotated to a vertical position. One must be careful to stay in the midline as the blade slides around the tongue. The handle then is lifted to visualize the glottis.[29] Once the glottis is visualized, a styletted ETT is advanced under direct vision into the trachea.

5. Dental Mirror–Assisted Laryngoscopy

The dental mirror can be used as an adjunct to direct laryngoscopy in order to view an anterior larynx. After direct laryngoscopy is performed, the dental mirror is inserted on the right side of the mouth and angled so that the vocal cords are seen. The handle of the mirror is moved to the left and held by the left hand. An appropriately shaped, styletted ETT then is advanced into the trachea while looking at the dental mirror. Practice is required to develop the necessary coordination. A Stortz no. 3 dental mirror and a Macintosh no. 1 laryngoscope have been used to intubate a 3.9-kg, 2.5-month-old infant.[96]

6. Retrograde Intubation

The classic retrograde technique involves percutaneous placement of an intravenous catheter through the cricothyroid membrane into the trachea followed by placement of a guidewire. The guidewire exits the mouth or nose and the ETT is then exchanged over the guidewire. If resistance to ETT passage occurs, counterclockwise rotation of the ETT may facilitate placement. This technique has been used for intubation of an infant with Goldenhar's syndrome.[97] A 14-F retrograde intubation set is commercially available from Cook for use with ETTs of ID 5.0 mm or greater.

A combined technique using the FOB and retrograde intubation has been used successfully in management of the difficult pediatric airway as well, as previously mentioned.[98]

A fiberoptic bronchoscope with a working channel is necessary for the combined technique. The guidewire is threaded into the suction port of an intubating FOB that has a preloaded softened ETT on it. The FOB is passed along the guidewire until it is past the vocal cords. When the scope is past the vocal cords, the wire is withdrawn and the ETT correctly positioned. This technique allows passage without obstruction from the arytenoid cartilage or epiglottis. Oxygen insufflation can be performed through the suction port as well, even with the wire in place. Care must be taken to limit flow to avoid tracheobronchial injury from excessive gas velocity. Audenaert

and colleagues[99] used this technique in 20 patients with DA age 1 day to 17 years and reported no major complications. Retrograde wire-guided direct laryngoscopy has also been reported for airway management in a 1-month-old infant.[100] In that patient, attempts to pass a 2.5-mm ETT over the wire itself were unsuccessful, but endotracheal intubation was achieved over the wire with direct laryngoscopy.

7. Emergency Access

Emergency access is divided into the emergency surgical and the emergency nonsurgical airway.[1] Emergency *surgical airway* access is often difficult and requires the presence of a skilled anesthesiologist. It is the last resort in the "cannot ventilate, cannot intubate" arm of the ASA DA algorithm.[101] Three procedures are referred to in this category: emergency tracheostomy, emergency cricothyroidotomy, and percutaneous needle cricothyroidotomy. In children younger than 6 years, emergency tracheostomy is usually the procedure of choice because the cricothyroid membrane is too small for cannulation.[99] In older children, percutaneous needle cricothyroidotomy is often preferred over a surgical approach because most anesthesiologists can perform this technique rapidly. Also, there is less risk of injury to surrounding structures.[4] Emergency cricothyroidotomy kits are available from Cook with 3.5-, 4-, and 6-mm–ID airway catheters.

The emergency *nonsurgical airway* access includes use of the LMA, esophageal-tracheal Combitube, and transtracheal jet ventilation (TTJV).[1] The Combitube is available in a small-adult size and is contraindicated in patients less than 4 feet tall.[7] The LMA is useful in the management of the difficult pediatric airway, as stated previously, as an supraglottic airway device or as a conduit for intubation. However, in the presence of glottic or subglottic obstruction, the LMA is ineffective; TTJV is considered the technique of choice in this situation, as reported in two cases for laser endoscopic surgery.[102] Caution with TTJV is urged because serious complications may result from its use.[103] TTJV below a glottic or subglottic obstruction may result in barotrauma because the pathway for egress of air and oxygen is limited. Tension pneumothorax has been reported with jet ventilation through an AEC in an adult.[104]

VIII. COMPLICATIONS OF AIRWAY MANAGEMENT

Complications that result from intubation in adults can occur in the pediatric population as well. Airway injury accounted for 6% of claims in the ASA closed-claims database.[105] Four percent of the airway injury claims involved pediatric patients younger than 16 years. The most frequent sites of injury reported were the larynx (33%), pharynx (19%), and esophagus (18%). Injuries to the esophagus and trachea were more frequently associated with DI. Laryngeal injuries included vocal cord paralysis, granuloma, arytenoid dislocation, and hematoma. Pharyngeal injuries included lacerations, perforation, infection, sore throat, and miscellaneous injuries (foreign body, burn, hematoma, and diminished taste).

An oropharyngeal burn related to the laryngoscope lamp occurred in a term baby weighing 3.6 kg who was easily intubated at birth.[106] The laryngoscope was switched on before intubation. Lightbulb laryngoscopes, in contrast to fiberoptic laryngoscopes, can reach temperatures that would result in burns to the oropharynx. Filaments may overlap with use, and it is common for two or more coils to touch.[106] The resistance of the lamp decreases and the current increases, thus increasing the temperature. Koh and Coleman[106] recommend that all lightbulb laryngoscopes be switched on for less than 1 minute; if left on, the temperature of the bulb should be manually checked before intubation.

Difficult intubation accounted for 62% of all esophageal injuries, with most involving esophageal perforation (90%). Esophageal perforation following DI has been reported in a neonate.[107]

Laryngotracheal stenosis may be classified as glottic, subglottic, or tracheal. Prolonged intubation seems to be the major etiology. The mechanism responsible seems to be ischemic necrosis caused by pressure from the ETT against the glottic and subglottic mucosa. This results in an inflammatory reaction with a secondary bacterial infection and scar formation. Risk factors include too large an ETT, prolonged intubation, repeated intubation, laryngeal trauma, sepsis, and chronic inflammatory disease.[108]

The incidence of postintubation croup varies from 0.1% to 1%.[20,21] Risk factors include age under 4 years, tight-fitting ETT, repeated intubation attempts, duration of surgery exceeding 1 hour, patient's position other than supine, and previous history of croup. Reports are conflicting concerning the risk from a concurrent upper respiratory tract infection. Classic treatment consists of humidified air, nebulized racemic epinephrine, and dexamethasone. In pediatric trauma patients, absence of an air leak at extubation was the strongest predictor of postextubation stridor requiring treatment.[109]

IX. AIRWAY DISEASES AND IMPLICATIONS

A. Head Anomalies

Airway management can be adversely affected by conditions that involve enlargement of the head. Mass lesions and macrocephaly can interfere with mask ventilation or direct laryngoscopy, or both.

1. Airway Implications

Airway management in children with macrocephaly requires proper head and neck positioning and care of the associated airway anomalies that are a frequent finding in patients with mucopolysaccharidosis. If preoperative evaluation suggests presence of a DA, awake methods of endotracheal intubation should be initially attempted.

In children, awake intubation may require careful use of sedatives in addition to topical anesthesia to the oropharynx, larynx, and nasopharynx (for nasotracheal intubation). A limited number of attempts at direct laryngoscopy may be made. If these are not successful, one of the various techniques of nonvisual or indirect laryngoscopy as detailed earlier may be used to secure the airway. If the patient does not comply with awake endotracheal intubation without the use of an amount of sedative that risks respiratory compromise, general anesthesia may be induced as long as mask ventilation is possible. The patient may breathe a potent vapor anesthetic until a level of anesthesia is achieved that allows endotracheal intubation. Other options include fiberoptic laryngoscopy in a patient breathing spontaneously through a mask or an LMA, use of a lighted stylet, use of a Bullard laryngoscope, and the retrograde technique. When mask ventilation is known to be easy in children, muscle relaxants may be used if their use notably improves the chance of endotracheal intubation.

The pathologic conditions that involve enlargement of the head and affect the airway are encephalocele, hydrocephalus, and mucopolysaccharidosis, along with other, less common conditions, such as phakomatoses, cranioskeletal dysplasias, or conjoint twins with face-to-face encroachment of the heads or proximity of the chests (thoracopagus).

2. Specific Anomalies

a. ENCEPHALOCELE

Patients with encephalocele may have other diseases that complicate airway management. The only two syndromes associated with encephalocele in which survival past infancy is likely are Roberts-SC phocomelia syndrome (includes pseudothalidomide syndrome, hypomelia-hypertrichosis–facial hemangioma syndrome) and facio-auriculovertebral spectrum (includes first and second brachial arch syndrome, oculoauricular vertebral dysplasia, hemifacial microsomia, Goldenhar's syndrome). Encephaloceles, or neural tube defects of the head, usually occur in the occipital area, although they may involve the frontal and nasal regions. When large, they affect airway management by interfering with mask fit or laryngoscopy.[110]

b. HYDROCEPHALUS

Hydrocephalus is associated with more than 30 malformation syndromes. Some craniosynostosis syndromes are associated with hydrocephalus and result from bone compression that prevents free flow of cerebrospinal fluid; examples include achondroplasia, Apert's syndrome, and Pfeiffer's syndrome. Some of these diseases may affect the airway by more than one mechanism (e.g., children with hydrocephalus who also have Arnold-Chiari malformation). Difficulties with airway management are usually associated with the underlying pathology and interference with face mask ventilation.

c. MUCOPOLYSACCHARIDOSES

The mucopolysaccharidoses are a group of seven inherited lysosomal storage disorders caused by the deficiency of specific lysosomal enzymes required for the degradation of glycosaminoglycans (GAGs), which are complex macromolecules. The inability to degrade GAGs leads to their lysosomal accumulation and the subsequent clinical features of the disorders, which can include facial coarsening, corneal clouding, valvular heart disease, hepatosplenomegaly, and dysostosis multiplex accompanied by short stature.

Mucopolysaccharidosis (MPS) type I, which results from the deficiency of L-iduronidase activity, can manifest as one of three different clinical phenotypes: Hurler's syndrome (i.e., MPS type IH), Scheie's syndrome (i.e., MPS type IS), or Hurler-Scheie syndrome (i.e., MPS type I H/S). Of these, Scheie's syndrome is the mildest form of the metabolic defect. The other mucopolysaccharidoses are Hunter's syndrome (type II), Sanfilippo's syndrome (type III), Morquio's syndrome (type IV), Maroteaux-Lamy syndrome (type VI), and Sly's syndrome (type VII).

The anesthetic morbidity of the mucopolysaccharidoses is 20% to 30%.[111] Morbidity is almost always related to respiratory difficulties. Intubation and maintenance of the airway might be difficult because of a variety of upper airway abnormalities, including micrognathia, macroglossia, patulous lips, restricted motion of the temporomandibular joints, friable tissues, and the presence of copious viscous secretions. Semenza and Pyeritz,[112] in a retrospective study on 21 patients with the diagnosis of MPS, found that the anatomic factors affecting respiratory status included (1) upper airway narrowing by hypertrophied tongue, tonsils, adenoids, and mucous membranes; (2) lower airway narrowing by GAG deposition within the tracheobronchial mucosa; (3) decreased thoracic dimensions related to scoliosis and thoracic hyperkyphosis; and (4) decreased abdominal dimensions because of lumbar hyperlordosis, gibbus formation, and hepatosplenomegaly. In addition, a short neck and an anterior and narrowed larynx may lead to an increased incidence of difficult or failed intubations.[113] In particular, patients with Hunter's, Hurler's, or Maroteaux-Lamy syndrome have significantly more airway difficulties as they grow older than MPS patients with other syndromes.[114]

The incidence of difficult intubation is high. In one review of 34 patients who underwent 89 anesthesias, the overall incidence of DI was 25% and failed intubation, 8%.[113] In children with Hurler's syndrome, incidence of DI was 54% and failed intubation, 23%. Herrick and Rhine[115] administered 38 anesthetics to nine patients with MPS (Hunter's, Hurler's, Sanfilippo's, and Morquio's syndromes) and found an overall incidence of airway-related problems of 26%, with a 53% incidence in patients with the Hurler's or Hunter's syndrome.

Belani and associates[116] reported their experience with 141 anesthetics in 30 patients with MPS. Visualization of the vocal cords during laryngoscopy was easier in children with Hurler's syndrome when they were younger (23 vs. 41 months; $P \leq 2.01$) and smaller (12 vs. 15 kg; $P \leq 2.05$). Also, children with preoperative obstructive breathing had a significantly higher incidence of postextubation obstruction. A total of 28 children underwent bone marrow transplantation; this reversed upper airway obstruction and also reversed intracranial hypertension.

Failure to insert an LMA or nasopharyngeal airway and fatal outcomes have been reported.[93,117,118] Consequently, nasotracheal intubation is not recommended, because of difficulties with the anatomy of nasal passages and potential hemorrhage from soft tissue trauma. Accumulation of mucopolysaccharides in the trachea may require a much smaller ETT than usual.[117] Tracheostomy can also be difficult technically in these patients and in one case was impossible even postmortem.[119]

Cervical instability, potential spinal cord damage, and severe thoracic and lumbar skeletal abnormalities make positioning and intubation difficult. In their series, in children with Hurler's syndrome, Belani and associates[116] found a 94% incidence of odontoid dysplasia, whereas 38% demonstrated anterior C1-C2 subluxation. To avoid cervical cord damage in patients with cervical instability, Walker and colleagues[113] described manual in-line stabilization during intubation and concluded that a pediatric FOB should be available for all known difficult intubations.[113] Tzanova and coworkers[120] reported successful anesthesia in a 23-month-old girl with Morquio's syndrome and unstable neck. The Truview laryngoscope has been used successfully in patients with unstable neck and those with cervical collars. Fiberoptic nasal intubation with spontaneous ventilation has been suggested as the method of choice.

A number of other skeletal deformities should also be considered in MPS patients. Chest cage dysfunction related to kyphoscoliosis leads to reduced vital capacity and restrictive pulmonary disorder.[69] Cardiac diseases are common in these patients. Both clinical and histologic studies of the cardiovascular system show progressive involvement of the coronary arteries, heart valves, and myocardium. The lumen of the coronary arteries is narrowed as a result of deposition of collagen and mucopolysaccharides in the intima. Coronary artery involvement and valvular involvement in patients with Hurler's syndrome have been reported.[114,121,122] Complications with 141 anesthetics in 30 patients with MPS included one child with intraoperative stroke and another with pulmonary edema; severe and extensive coronary obstruction was responsible for two intraoperative deaths, and coronary angiography underestimated coronary artery disease.[116]

Considering the high rate of DI in MPS patients, regional anesthesia seems a good alternative in older children. Failed epidural anesthesia was reported in one patient.[117] The deposition of mucopolysaccharides in either the general epidural space or the sheath of the nerve fibers, preventing direct access of the local anesthetic to the nerve, was suspected.

B. Facial Anomalies: Maxillary and Mandibular Disease

The pediatric airway may be complicated by a large number of syndromes involving the head, neck, and cervical spine. The airway and associated structures are deviated from the branchial arches. The first arch develops into the maxilla, mandible, incus, malleus, zygoma, and a portion of the temporal bone. The second arch develops into stapes, the styloid process of the temporal bone, and a portion of the hyoid. The third arch develops into the reminder of the hyoid. The fourth and six arches fuse to form the laryngeal structures, including the thyroid, cricoid, and arytenoid cartilages. The pharyngeal muscle develops from the fourth arch, whereas the sixth arch gives rise to the laryngeal musculature. Failure of any of these to develop properly may lead to characteristic anomalies.

1. Tumors

a. CYSTIC HYGROMA

Cystic hygromas are multiloculated cystic structures that are benign in nature. They form as the result of budding lymphatics and thus may occur anywhere in the body, although most frequently in the neck (75%) and axilla (20%). As the tumor grows, it may cause symptoms from pressure on the trachea, pharynx, blood vessels, tongue, and nerves and eventually may severely compromise the airway. The tongue often protrudes outside the mouth and prevents its closure, making maintenance of the airway difficult if not impossible. Airway obstruction is the most critical complication of the cystic hygroma in the neck. The safest approach in these children seems to be nasal intubation,[123] either blind or with fiberoptic assistance with the patient awake. In extreme cases, tracheostomy may be necessary.

b. NECK TERATOMA

Teratomas of the head and neck are interesting because of their obscure origin, bizarre microscopic appearance, unpredictable behavior, and often dramatic clinical presentation. The reported incidence of cervical teratomas ranges from 2.3% to 9.3% of all teratomas. A teratoma is a true neoplasm, which includes four groups: dermoid cysts, teratoid cysts, true teratomas, and epignathi (pharyngeal teratomas).

Teratomas of the head and neck frequently arise with respiratory distress or even asphyxia at delivery, and a well-established plan for early airway management should be prepared. If they are untreated, the mortality of patients with these masses is 80% to 100%.[124] Fetal ultrasonography has been used since the 1970s to aid in the prenatal diagnosis. Antenatal diagnosis is important for two reasons. First, elective cesarean section should be planned to avoid dystocia and fetal trauma. Second, because immediate establishment of a patent airway is essential for survival, a team of pediatric airway experts must be available.

The ex utero intrapartum technique (EXIT) allows the continuance of fetoplacental circulation during cesarean section. Initially, only the infant's head and shoulders (but not the placenta) are delivered, thus maintaining uteroplacental blood flow. Intramuscular fentanyl and vecuronium are given, the infant's airway is secured, and then the umbilical cord is clamped and delivery of the infant completed. The EXIT has proved useful in cases of anticipated DA instrumentation of the neonate (e.g., large fetal neck masses causing airway obstruction).[125] Once the head of the neonate is delivered, a multitude of choices are available for airway management: direct laryngoscopy, FOI, pediatric Bullard laryngoscopy,[124] or tracheostomy. The EXIT procedure has proved to be safe and efficacious, allowing establishment of an airway in a controlled manner because the placenta allows continued gas exchange during airway manipulation.[126,127] Early identification of these masses allows controlled delivery of the neonate in a setting where pediatric anesthesiologists, surgeons, and neonatologists can develop strategies to minimize the risk of a postnatal respiratory death.

c. CHERUBISM

Cherubism is a familial disease of childhood in which patients acquire mandibular and sometimes maxillary enlargement. The mandibular rami hypertrophy, limiting the submandibular space for displacement of the tongue and making visualization of the glottis during direct laryngoscopy difficult.[11]

2. Congenital Hypoplasia

a. ACROCEPHALOSYNDACTYLY

Maxillary hypoplasia results from premature synostosis of facial and cranial sutures and usually manifests as one of multiple abnormal features in a group of rare but complex syndromes called *acrocephalosyndactylies*. Acrocephalosyndactyly encompasses a number of dysostoses, not all of which can be distinguished clearly. The midface retrusion gives the appearance of prognathia, although in reality the mandible is smaller than normal. In addition, there may be associated anomalies of the central nervous system (CNS; increased intracranial pressure, absent corpus callosum), the extremities, and in a small percentage of patients the heart.[128] Both the upper and the lower airway may be compromised in these patients.[129]

Multiple pathologic conditions may be seen; maxillary regression may be associated with choanal stenosis or atresia, reduction in nasopharyngeal space,[130] and palate deformity (narrow, high arched, or cleft). These features may cause respiratory compromise or obstructive apnea early in life, although as the child grows, obstruction can worsen because of continued restriction in growth of the maxillary region.[131-134] In one series, upper airway obstruction arose more frequently in Crouzon's disease and Pfeiffer's syndrome than in Apert's syndrome.

The incidence of airway obstruction has been addressed.[135] Of a total 40 patients with severe "syndromic" craniosynostosis (13 had Apert's syndrome and 27 had Crouzon's disease), 40% presented with airway obstruction (12.5% severe and 27.5% mild obstruction). There was no significant difference in the distribution of airway status between patients with Apert's syndrome and Crouzon's disease. The severe obstruction in the five patients resulted from midface hypoplasia, lower airway obstruction, tonsillar and adenoid hypertrophy, and choanal atresia.

Lower airway disease in the acrocephalosyndactylies occurs in the form of tracheomalacia, bronchomalacia, solid cartilaginous trachea lacking tracheal rings, and tracheal stenosis. Patients with tubular cartilaginous trachea have displayed a propensity for easy tracheal injury, edema, and stenosis and a potential for lower airway infection (tracheitis and bronchitis) and mucous plugging, because tracheal ciliary activity may be deficient. Sleep apnea was described in association with tracheal cartilaginous sleeve in a patient with Pfeiffer's syndrome.[136]

Airway problems can be divided into those arising from the nasal passages, nasopharynx, palate, or trachea.

Nasal septal deviation is a common feature of craniosynostosis patients and is considered a principal finding in Saethre-Chotzen syndrome. Narrowing of the nasal passages arises from maxillary hypoplasia. Although choanal atresia can occur, the usual picture is generalized narrowing. The nasopharynx is shallow because of hypoplasia of the maxilla and the altered angulation of the skull base. Palatal abnormalities further impinge on the nasopharynx. These deformities may consist of arched or ridged palates or increased thickness of the soft tissue. The degree of airway obstruction varies among these patients, being among the worst in those with Apert's syndrome. Complications have included cor pulmonale and even death from airway obstruction. Lower airway obstruction may result from a number of abnormalities, including subglottic stenosis and vertically fused tracheal cartilage. Subglottic stenosis is especially common in Crouzon's patients. Vertically fused tracheal cartilage has been reported in patients with Apert's, Crouzon's, and Pfeiffer's syndromes; the entire trachea is encased in a tube of nonsegmented cartilage. These children can be difficult to manage and usually present with episodes of recurrent lower respiratory tract infections, reactive airways disease, and chronically retained secretions.

Acrocephalosyndactyly disorders include Apert's syndrome (type I) and Apert-Crouzon (Crouzon's) disease. Acrocephalosyndactyly also occurs with other diseases, including Chotzen's (Saethre-Chotzen) syndrome and Pfeiffer-type acrocephalosyndactyly.

i. **APERT'S SYNDROME.** Apert's syndrome is characterized by agenesis or premature closure of the cranial sutures, midface hypoplasia, and syndactyly of the hands and feet that is symmetrical and involves at least the second, third, and fourth digits. Prevalence is estimated at 1 in 65,000 live births (~15.5 per 1 million population). Apert's syndrome accounts for 4.5% of all cases of craniostenosis. Concerning CNS abnormalities, intelligence varies from normal to mental deficiency, although a significant number of patients are mentally retarded. Malformations of the CNS may be responsible for most cases. Papilledema and optic atrophy with loss of vision may be present in cases of subtle increased intracranial pressure. Other abnormalities include cervical spine fusion, which is common and almost always involves C5-C6; osseous fusions may also be evident in other joints of the extremities and in the spine, tracheal cartilage anomalies, and diaphragmatic hernia.[137]

Airway Anomalies. These result from facial abnormalities, which include small nasopharynx and hypoplastic and retropositioned maxilla. DI in Apert's syndrome has been reported. One of the suggested mechanisms is trismus related to temporalis muscle fibrosis.[138] Both upper and lower airway can be compromised by complete or partial cartilage sleeve abnormalities of the trachea and obstructive sleep apnea.[129]

ii. **CROUZON'S SYNDROME.** Crouzon's syndrome (Crouzon's disease, craniofacial dysostosis) is closely related to Apert's syndrome. In 1912, Crouzon described the triad of skull deformities, facial anomalies, and exophthalmos.[139] Crouzon's syndrome is an autosomal dominant disorder with complete penetrance and variable expressivity.[140,141] About 50% of cases represent sporadic mutations, and 40% are familial. In the United States, prevalence is 1 per 60,000 live births (~16.5 per 1 million population). Crouzon's syndrome makes up approximately 4.8% of all cases of craniosynostosis at birth.[142] Crouzon's disease is associated with acanthosis nigricans (5%) and CNS defects such as chronic tonsillar herniation (73%), progressive hydrocephalus (30%), and syringomyelia.[143] Multiple sutural synostoses frequently involve premature fusion of the skull base sutures, causing midfacial hypoplasia, shallow orbits, a foreshortened nasal dorsum, maxillary hypoplasia, and occasional upper airway obstruction.[144]

Airway Anomalies. Crouzon's syndrome is characterized by premature closure of calvarial and cranial base sutures as well as those of the orbit and maxillary complex (craniosynostosis). Other features include beaked nose; short upper lip; mandibular prognathism; overcrowding of upper teeth; malocclusions; V-shaped maxillary dental arch; narrow, high, or cleft palate and bifid uvula; hypoplastic maxilla; and relative mandibular prognathism. Cervical fusion of C2-C3 and C5-C6 is present in 18% of cases.

iii. **SAETHRE-CHOTZEN SYNDROME.** Chotzen's syndrome is an autosomal dominant acrocephalosyndactyly that affects between 1 and 2 of every 50,000 people. Craniosynostosis, facial asymmetry, low frontal hairline, ptosis, brachydactyly, and cutaneous syndactyly of the fingers and of the second and third toes are characteristic features.[145]

b. **ACROCEPHALOPOLYSYNDACTYLY**

Acrocephalopolysyndactyly includes the following four types of syndromes:

- Noack's syndrome: similar to acrocephalosyndactyly type V (Pfeiffer type)
- Carpenter's syndrome: mental retardation, bradydactyly
- Sakati-Nyhan syndrome: hypoplastic tibias; deformed, displaced fibulas
- Goodman's syndrome: congenital heart defect, clinodactyly, camptodactyly, ulnar deviation, intact intelligence

i. **PFEIFFER'S SYNDROME (TYPE I).** Pfeiffer's (Noack's) syndrome (type I) is also a close relative of Apert's syndrome, although it is less severe. Pfeiffer's syndrome has three clinical subtypes and is manifested by craniosynostosis, broad thumbs and toes, variable maxillary retrusion, and partial soft tissue syndactyly. *Type I* is classic Pfeiffer's syndrome; affected patients have normal intelligence and a good prognosis. *Type II* is associated with cloverleaf skull, severe proptosis, and ankylosis of the elbows (Fig. 36-4). *Type III* is manifested by the absence of cloverleaf skull but the presence of elbow ankylosis and high morbidity in infancy. Other abnormalities are severe exorbitism that puts patients at risk for corneal exposure and damage, high-arched palate, crowded teeth, hydrocephalus, and seizures.[146]

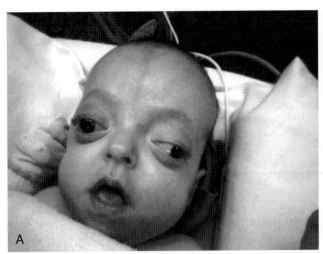
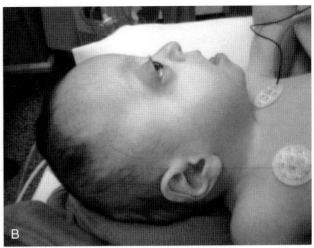

Figure 36-4 Pfeiffer's syndrome. Craniosynostosis, marked proptosis, and maxillary retrusion are present. Upper and lower airway obstruction may be present as well.

Airway Implications. As with Apert's syndrome, Pfeiffer's syndrome can arise with upper and lower airway obstruction. Congenital tracheal stenosis,[147] tracheal obstruction related to congenital tracheomalacia,[148] and obstructive sleep apnea have been reported.[149] In addition to a high incidence of vertebral fusion (73%), other radiologic abnormalities include hypoplasia of the neural arches, hemivertebrae, and a "butterfly" vertebra.[150] The C2-C3 level was most often involved, although fusion was noted at all levels of the cervical spine.

ii. **CARPENTER'S SYNDROME (TYPE II).** Carpenter's syndrome (type II) is typically evident at or shortly after birth. Because of craniosynostosis, the top of the head may appear unusually conical (acrocephaly) or the head may seem short and broad (brachycephaly). In addition, the cranial sutures often fuse unevenly, causing the head and face to appear dissimilar from one side to the other (craniofacial asymmetry). Other malformations of the skull and facial (craniofacial) region may include downslanting eyelid folds (palpebral fissures), a flat nasal bridge, malformed (dysplastic), low-set ears, small dental malformations,[151] and underdeveloped (hypoplastic) upper or lower jaw (maxilla or mandible), or both.

Additional abnormalities may include short stature, structural heart malformations (congenital heart defects), mild to moderate obesity, protrusion of portions of the intestine through an abnormal opening in the abdominal wall near the navel (umbilical hernia), or failure of the testes to descend into the scrotum (cryptorchidism) in affected males. Both normal intellect and mild mental retardation have been reported in patients with Carpenter's syndrome.[152,153]

Airway Implications. Difficult intubation might be expected in Carpenter's patients with hypoplastic upper or lower jaw, oral malformations, and obesity.

c. MANDIBULAR HYPOPLASIA

Mandibular hypoplasia is one of the main anomalies of the mandible, with a profound effect on airway management. Micrognathia results in posterior regression of the tongue and a small hyomental space. The mandible develops from the first branchial arch and is a feature in many rare syndromes (e.g., Pierre Robin, Treacher Collins, Goldenhar's, Nager's).[154] Although micrognathia is a feature typically shared by these syndromes, they often present additional specific features with adverse effects on the airway.

The finding of periauricular skin tags or abnormally developed external ears, which also develop from the first branchial arch, may be used as a marker for a potentially difficult airway.

Micrognathia may affect the airway in three ways: (1) the tongue may not be easily moved during laryngoscopy; (2) if the tongue is not pulled forward in the normal developmental manner, the laryngeal inlet appears more anterior and difficult to visualize; and (3) the oral aperture is not opened as easily or as widely.[155] Glossoptosis may further complicate the airway in micrognathic children. Glossoptosis makes displacement of the tongue to the left difficult, so the airway is difficult to visualize.

i. **PIERRE ROBIN SYNDROME.** Pierre Robin sequence, which affects 1 in 8500 newborns,[156] was described in 1923 by Pierre Robin as airway obstruction associated with glossoptosis and hypoplasia of the mandible. At present, this syndrome is characterized by retrognathia or micrognathia, glossoptosis, and airway obstruction. An incomplete cleft of the palate is associated with the syndrome in approximately 50% of these patients (Fig. 36-5). Pierre Robin sequence results from failure of mandibular growth during the first several weeks of embryogenesis. This causes posterior displacement of the tongue, which prevents normal growth and closure of the palate.

The Pierre Robin sequence represents a spectrum of anatomic anomalies whose common features include mandibular hypoplasia, glossoptosis, and cleft palate. Four types of airway obstruction have been described in patients with Pierre Robin sequence; in only 50% is the obstruction totally related to posterior positioning of the tongue.[157] Therefore, glossopexy fails to relieve airway

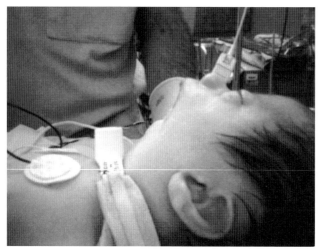

Figure 36-5 Pierre Robin syndrome. Marked micrognathia, glossoptosis, and cleft palate are evident. The micrognathia causes posterior displacement of the tongue, preventing normal development of the palate. Because of the upper airway obstruction present, an elective tracheostomy was performed.

obstruction in approximately half of all symptomatic patients with the Pierre Robin sequence. This may explain why the use of an oral or nasopharyngeal airway alone may not improve an already-difficult mask airway. Patients who fail to improve after glossopexy or nasopharyngeal airway placement, or both, usually require tracheostomy.[56]

Airway Implications. A large body of literature details airway management of patients with Pierre Robin sequence. Preoperative or postoperative airway obstruction and mask ventilation difficulties have been a frequent problem in these patients. In a 10-year retrospective study of 26 infants with Pierre Robin syndrome, Benjamin and Walker[158] found that awake intubation without general anesthesia proved to be safer and less difficult when a special-purpose slotted laryngoscope was used. Li and colleagues[159] reviewed the airway management in 110 children with Robin sequence. Prone posturing was effective in the treatment of mild airway obstruction in 82 patients (90.2%) who had noisy breathing sounds. Only 30% of the patients required endotracheal intubation and 6.6% required tracheostomy (all were eventually decannulated).

Alternative intubation techniques used successfully in patients with Pierre Robin syndrome include LMA,[56,160-162] FOB intubation,[88,163,164] FOI through an LMA,[52] rigid nasoendoscope with video camera or video intubation laryngoscope,[35] Trachlight with a homemade lighted stylet,[165-167] and retrograde intubation.[168] Digitally assisted endotracheal intubation and elective endotracheal intubation in prone position have also been reported.[78,79]

ii. TREACHER COLLINS SYNDROME. Treacher Collins syndrome (mandibulofacial dysostosis, Franceschetti's syndrome) results from a deficient vascular supply to the first visceral arch during the initial 3 to 4 weeks of gestation and is believed to be caused by a change in the gene on chromosome 5 that affects facial development and leads

to hypoplasia of the facial bones, especially the zygoma and the mandible. There is a 50% chance that the child will pass the trait on to future generations. It is often associated with DI and airway obstruction, mainly related to micrognathia.

Facial clefting causes a hypoplastic facial appearance, with deformities of the ear, orbital, midface, and lower jaw regions. The clinical appearance is a result of the zygoma (malar bone) failing to fuse with the maxilla, frontal, and temporal bones. Highly variant degrees of involvement (complete, incomplete, abortive) can be seen, but common facial features include hypoplastic cheeks, zygomatic arches, and mandible; microtia with possible hearing loss; high-arched or cleft palate; antimongoloid slant to the eyes; colobomas; increased anterior facial height; malocclusion (anterior open bite); small oral cavity and airway with a normal-sized tongue; and pointed nasal prominence.

Most children with Treacher Collins syndrome have normal development and intelligence. However, additional physical findings have included a 40% hearing loss, dry eyes, cleft palate, and breathing problems. Both acute and obstructive sleep apneas have been described.[169,170]

An extensive array of complications can affect management. Because of the small jaw and airway, combined with the normal size of the tongue, breathing problems can occur at birth and during sleep when the base of the tongue obstructs the small hypopharynx. This can also cause serious problems during the induction of general anesthesia. Consequently, a tracheostomy may be required to control the airway adequately.

Airway Implications. The airway of children with Treacher Collins syndrome had been successfully managed with an LMA,[171-173] the Bullard intubating laryngoscope,[30] Augustine stylet,[174] and FOB. Rasch and coauthors[175] recommend that children with obstructive symptoms have laryngoscopy before anesthetic induction. If the glottic opening is visualized, inhalational induction can proceed. If the glottic structures cannot be visualized, the anesthetist must choose between awake oral or nasal intubation, elective tracheostomy, or FOI.

iii. GOLDENHAR'S SYNDROME/HEMIFACIAL MICROSOMIA. Synonyms of Goldenhar's syndrome (hemifacial microsomia) are first and second branchial arch syndrome, facioauricular vertebral spectrum, oculoauricular vertebral dysplasia, and oculoauriculovertebral spectrum disorder. The main feature of this condition is unilateral underdevelopment of one ear (which may not even be present) associated with underdevelopment of the jaw and cheek on the same side of the face. When this is the only problem, it is normally referred to as *hemifacial microsomia*, but when associated with other abnormalities, particularly of the vertebrae (hemivertebrae or underdeveloped vertebrae, usually in neck), it is referred to as *Goldenhar's syndrome*. However, these are likely two ends of the spectrum of the same condition.

The muscles of the affected side of the face are underdeveloped. There are often skin tags or pits in front of the ear or in a line between the ear and the corner of the mouth.

Children with the Goldenhar end of the spectrum may have congenital heart diseases in 5% to 58% of cases (ventricular septal defect, patent ductus arteriosus, tetralogy of Fallot, coarctation of aorta). A variety of kidney abnormalities may also be present (e.g., ectopic kidneys, renal agenesis, hydronephrosis).

Airway Implications. Difficulties in airway management result from mandibular hypoplasia, cleft or high-arched palate, cervical vertebral anomalies, and scoliosis.[176] Suggested airway management approaches include using a lighted stylet,[177] suspension laryngoscopy,[77] or LMA under anesthesia or using awake FOI through a laryngeal mask.[178,179]

iv. NAGER'S SYNDROME.

Nager's syndrome (mandibulofacial dysostosis) is a rare craniofacial disorder with fewer than 100 cases reported in the medical literature. The morphologic features of Nager's syndrome include downslanted palpebral fissures, malar hypoplasia, a high nasal bridge, atretic external auditory canals, and micrognathia (severe underdevelopment of the lower jaw). Proximal limb malformations include absent or hypoplastic thumbs, hypoplasia of the radius, and shortened humeral bones.[180] Many of the characteristic facial features may be similar to those of Treacher Collins syndrome. However, patients with Treacher Collins syndrome have more severe maxillary and zygomatic hypoplasia, downslanting palpebral fissures, and lower lid coloboma.

Among the additional problems of children with Nager's syndrome are stomach and kidney reflux and hearing loss. Cardiac and spine defects have been also reported.[181] Danziger and coworkers[181] reported four patients with a cardiac defect (type unspecified), and tetralogy of Fallot was reported in another patient.[154]

Airway Implications. Difficulties with airway management and postoperative airway obstruction may occur secondary to mandibular hypoplasia with micrognathia, restricted jaw mobility, and microstomia. Associated cleft lip or cleft palate, or both, and maxillary hypoplasia with midface deformities may further complicate airway management and appropriate mask fit during mask ventilation. The airway has been successfully managed with LMA,[182] retrograde intubation,[95] and FOI.[183]

d. SMITH-LEMLI-OPITZ SYNDROME

Smith-Lemli-Opitz syndrome (SLOS) is an autosomal recessive syndrome characterized by congenital anomalies affecting the airway; cardiorespiratory, gastrointestinal, and genitourinary systems; and CNS. SLOS has an incidence between 1 in 26,500 pregnancies in Canada and 1 in 50,000 pregnancies in the United States.[184,185] The syndrome results from an inborn error of cholesterol biosynthesis involving a deficiency of 3β-hydroxysterol δ7-reductase, the enzyme that catalyzes the reduction of 7-dehydrocholesterol to cholesterol.[186] Patients with SLOS can have severe growth failure, congenital anomalies affecting most organ systems, early death, developmental delay, and self-injurious and ritualistic behavior.[187-189]

Airway Implications. Patients with SLOS can be a challenge for airway management because of the typical dysmorphic facial features, including micrognathia, prominent incisors, cleft palate, and a small and abnormally hard tongue. There are several reports of DI and abnormal laryngoscopic views in patients with SLOS.[190-192] An LMA was used successfully in managing the airway in a newborn infant with SLOS.[193]

Quezado and associates[194] presented experience from a series of 20 anesthesias in 14 SLOS patients, prospectively deciding to use fiberoptic laryngoscopy as the initial technique of intubation in spite of the possible gastroesophageal reflux,[184] muscle rigidity,[192] and behavioral abnormalities in these patients.[189] In all patients, adequate spontaneous ventilation was maintained throughout the airway management. One patient had laryngospasm during induction, and one was intubated by an otolaryngologist.

e. CORNELIA DE LANGE (CRYPTOPHTHALMOS) SYNDROME

Cornelia de Lange syndrome (CDLS) is a syndrome of multiple congenital anomalies transmitted in an autosomal dominant pattern, characterized by a distinctive facial appearance, prenatal and postnatal growth deficiency, feeding difficulties, psychomotor delay, behavioral problems, and associated malformations mainly involving the upper extremities. The incidence is 1 per 30,000 to 50,000 live births.[195] A most important feature is a striking delay in the maturation of structure and function of most organ systems, including the CNS.[196] CDLS patients are short in stature (the syndrome is also called Amsterdam dwarfism),[197] have microcephaly (98%), and the facial features are perhaps the most diagnostic of all the physical signs. Cardiac defects occur in 15% of patients.[198]

Airway Implications. Intubation may be difficult because of a short (86%), often webbed neck; a high-arched (66%), sometimes cleft palate; and a small mouth with micrognathia (84%). There is also a high incidence of gastroesophageal reflux (58%) and hiatal hernia. There are a number of case reports of DI in CDLS; the airway was successfully managed by blind nasal intubation in one case.[199] Lumb and Carli[200] reported respiratory arrest in a 3-year-old child after caudal injection of bupivacaine and hypothesized that changes in intracranial pressure secondary to caudal injection might be the cause of the cardiac arrest.

f. HALLERMANN-STREIFF SYNDROME

Hallermann-Streiff syndrome (oculomandibulodyscephaly with hypotrichosis or oculomandibulofacial syndrome) is rare, with approximately 150 cases reported.[201] Cardinal features are dyscephaly with bird facies; frontal or parietal bossing; dehiscence of sutures with open fontanelles; hypotrichosis of scalp, eyebrows, and eyelashes; cutaneous atrophy of scalp and nose; mandibular hypoplasia; forward displacement of temporomandibular joints; high-arched palate; small mouth; multiple dental anomalies; and proportionate small stature.[202,203] Children with Hallermann-Streiff syndrome can have a multitude of cardiorespiratory problems. The incidence of cardiac anomalies is 4.8% and includes septal defects, patent ductus arteriosus, and tetralogy of Fallot. Upper airway obstruction may result from small nares and glossoptosis secondary to micrognathia, which may lead to cor pulmonale.[201]

Airway Implications. The patients have natal teeth, which are brittle and may be easily broken or avulsed during laryngoscopy. The temporomandibular joint (TMJ) may be easily dislocated. At times, the TMJ is absent, making placement of the ETT by the oral route impossible. Small nostrils, deviated nasal septum, high-arched palate, and anterior larynx preclude blind nasotracheal intubation. The ascending ramus of the mandible is either underdeveloped or absent, resulting in a small mouth cavity. Intubation was achieved with difficulty in two cases with the patient under inhaled anesthesia. In both cases, mask ventilation was impossible.[203,204] Most patients with Hallermann-Streiff syndrome may require elective tracheostomy because of respiratory difficulty.[202]

g. TURNER'S SYNDROME

Turner's syndrome (gonadal dysgenesis) is caused by the absence of a second X chromosome. Manifestations of the syndrome include primary amenorrhea, genital immaturity, and short stature; intelligence is usually normal. Additional associated features that may influence the management of anesthesia include hypertension, short neck, high palate, micrognathia, the occasional presence of aortic stenosis or coarctation of aorta, and an absent kidney.

Airway Implications. Despite the micrognathia and the short neck, only one case of DI has been published.[205] Because of the small stature, unexpected unilateral endobronchial intubation was reported.[206]

3. Inflammatory Disease

a. JUVENILE RHEUMATOID ARTHRITIS (STILL'S DISEASE)

Juvenile rheumatoid arthritis (JRA) is a systemic disease of mesenchymal tissues, which may affect collagen and connective tissue of any organ and in which arthritis is one manifestation. Although it is beyond the scope of this review to describe this complex disease, the possible involvement of the heart (36% pericarditis confirmed by echocardiography) should be mentioned.

Abnormalities predisposing to DA management include temporomandibular ankylosis, mandibular hypoplasia, and cricoarytenoid arthritis. Atlantoaxial or low cervical subluxation may occur. The vertebrae may fail to grow, and ankylosis of the apophyseal joints may result.

Difficulty in maintaining the airway patency and inability to intubate the trachea are the most serious anesthetic problems in these children. Severe respiratory distress requiring endotracheal intubation has been reported in children with JRA.[207-210] Vetter[210] reported an acute exacerbation of JRA, manifesting as acute arytenoiditis and resulting in marked upper airway obstruction. Symmetrical swelling of the arytenoids and moderate swelling of the epiglottis were noted at laryngoscopy. In another case, direct laryngoscopy demonstrated immobile vocal cords, which were approximated to each other in the midline secondary to arthritis of the cricoarytenoid joints.[209] In both patients, intubation was achieved with some difficulty during direct laryngoscopy, and both recovered after large doses of steroids. Nevertheless, a fiberoptic bronchocope should always be available in case of failure.

C. Mouth and Tongue Anomalies

1. Microstomia

Microstomia (a small mouth opening) is uncommon and may be congenital or acquired. Pediatric microstomia may be congenital (in Freeman-Sheldon [whistling face], Hallermann-Streiff, and otopalatodigital syndromes) but is more often acquired after accidental thermal injuries, such as biting an electrical extension cord or ingesting household lye.[98]

a. CONGENITAL MICROSTOMIA

i. FREEMAN-SHELDON SYNDROME. Freeman-Sheldon syndrome (whistling face syndrome, windmill-vane-hand syndrome, craniocarpotarsal dysplasia, distal arthrogryposis type 2) is a rare congenital disorder defined by facial and skeletal abnormalities. The three basic abnormalities are microstomia with pouting lips, camptodactyly with ulnar deviation of the fingers, and talipes equinovarus.

Airway Implications. Anesthetic challenges include DA management, intravenous cannulation, and regional technique. Patients may be at increased risk for malignant hyperthermia and postoperative pulmonary complications. Oral FOI is considered the preferred airway management technique; the nasal route cannot be used because of small nostrils.[211] An LMA was used successfully in one patient after direct laryngoscopy proved to be impossible.[212,213]

ii. HALLERMANN-STREIFF SYNDROME. As discussed earlier, Hallermann-Streiff syndrome is a rare congenital disorder in which the presence of mandibular hypoplasia and microstomia makes intubation difficult.

Airway Implications. Again, these patients have brittle natal teeth that may be easily broken or avulsed during laryngoscopy. The TMJ may be easily dislocated[214] and at times is absent, making oral intubation impossible. The small nostrils, deviated nasal septum, high-arched palate, and anterior larynx preclude blind nasotracheal intubation. The ascending ramus of the mandible may either be underdeveloped or absent, resulting in a small mouth cavity. The options available to circumvent these problems are awake intubation, intubation over a fiberoptic bronchoscope, retrograde intubation,[214] and intubation under inhalational anesthesia. Even tracheostomy proved to be difficult in these cases; thus an experienced pediatric otolaryngologist should be available.[215]

b. ACQUIRED MICROSTOMIA

i. EPIDERMOLYSIS BULLOSA HEREDITARIA DYSTROPHICA. See "Pharyngeal Bullae or Scarring" under "Nasal and Palatal Anomalies."

Postburn contractures of the neck following a burn injury may hamper cervical hyperextension and lifting of the mandible. Direct laryngoscopy may also be difficult because of rigid scar tissue, which obscures the mandibular and laryngeal anatomy, or microstomia after retraction of scar tissue in facial burns.[216] Fiberoptic intubation is the method of choice for securing the airway,[217] but LMA can also be used successfully. Kreulen and colleagues[216] described a quick surgical neck release of contractures to facilitate endotracheal intubation in postburn patients. Bilateral commissurotomy to allow insertion of the laryngoscope into the mouth is also reported.[98]

ii. BURNS FROM LYE INGESTION. Microstomia from lye ingestion may be associated not only with limited mouth opening but also with such severe intraoral scarring that common landmarks guiding either rigid or flexible fiberoptic laryngoscopy are obscured, rendering oral and nasal intubation difficult or impossible.[98,218]

2. Diseases of the Tongue

Increase in tongue size is known as *macroglossia*, defined as a resting tongue that extends beyond the teeth or alveolar ridge.[219]

a. CONGENITAL DISEASE

i. HEMANGIOMA Hemangiomas are the most common tumor seen during infancy and affect 10% to 12% of white children.[220] Most hemangiomas (70%) are seen during the first weeks of life as an erythematous macula or a telangiectasia. All hemangiomas proliferate during the first year of life. Complications include ulceration, high-output cardiac failure, airway obstruction, and the *Kasabach-Merritt syndrome*, which results from platelet sequestration and destruction within the hemangioma as well as consumptive coagulopathy. It is fatal in 60% of children.

ii. LYMPHANGIOMA. Lymphangioma is a rare congenital disease of unknown etiology.[221] Cystic hygroma of the head and neck, with large lymphatic endothelium-lined cysts, is amenable to surgical excision. Cavernous or microcystic lymphangioma, however, is composed of small lymphatic spaces and poses a therapeutic dilemma by its propensity to cause airway and feeding difficulties and by its tendency to recur despite extensive surgery. All lymphangiomas are present at birth, even though they may not become apparent until the first or second year of life. Although the lymphatic malformation affects preferentially the submandibular space and the neck, it may extend cephalad and invade the tongue and surrounding structures.[221]

Airway Implications. Lymphangiomatous involvement of the tongue is generally diffuse and may result in dramatic macroglossia, extending the tongue outside the mouth beyond the lip margins. It is associated with airway obstruction as well as dysphagia and speech, orthodontic, and aesthetic problems. Acute enlargement of the tongue has been reported following trauma or upper respiratory tract infections. Of the multiple therapeutic methods

advocated, surgical laser resection is the mainstay. Repeat laser resection may be necessary because of the tendency for recurrence. Spontaneous resolution is uncommon. In many patients, if lymphangioma is left untreated for extended periods, pulmonary hypertension and cor pulmonale may develop.

In one series, 9 of 18 patients (50%) reviewed required tracheostomy because of the size of the lymphoma and the tendency for recurrence.[222] Nasal fiberoptic intubation was used successfully in these patients.[223]

b. TRAUMATIC INJURY

Burns of the face and mouth can affect the tongue and pharynx. Aspiration of hot liquid can occur in conjunction with upper-body scald burns, leading to acute compromise of the airway, "thermal epiglottitis." Clinical features and radiologic findings are similar to those seen in patients with acute infectious epiglottitis.[224] Thermal epiglottitis can be an extremely difficult problem if subtle signs of impending airway compromise are not appreciated. The treatment should be approached with the same caution and preparedness for emergency airway management as in acute infectious epiglottitis. Immediate endotracheal intubation should be performed in those with acute respiratory distress, and prompt investigation by direct laryngoscopy in the OR is appropriate in those who have not yet developed overt respiratory distress.[225] Surprisingly, only 9.2% of 1092 burn patients admitted to the Shriners Burns Institute in Galveston, Texas, over a 5-year period needed endotracheal intubation or tracheostomy for more than 24 hours.[226] A similar incidence of endotracheal intubation (10%) was found after accidental inhalation of caustic substances.[227]

i. LYMPHATIC OR VENOUS OBSTRUCTION. Tongue swelling may result from prolonged surgical traction and local mechanical pressure. This may be caused by transesophageal echocardiography probe or by dentures in adults.[228,229] Angioneurotic edema or other reactions to drugs can cause marked swelling of the tongue, leading to life-threatening airway emergencies.[230-232]

c. METABOLIC DISORDERS

The *Beckwith-Wiedemann syndrome* (BWS) comprises a constellation of clinical features including the presence of omphalocele, macroglossia, hypoglycemia (related to hyperinsulinism), inguinal hernia with gigantism, organomegaly, renal medullary dysplasia, cardiac defects, and embryonic tumors occurring less frequently.[233]

Airway Implications. The anesthetic management of children with BWS may be complicated by a potentially difficult airway related to macroglossia.[234-236] Because of the high rate of omphalocele in this syndrome, anesthetic care is frequently required during the neonatal period. The LMA was used successfully in children with BWS.[233] Even though endotracheal intubation was possible in most case reports,[234,236,237] airway obstruction presented a major concern, especially after extubation. Swelling, secretions, and blood may precipitate complete airway obstruction. Because of the size of the tongue, additional pathology (tongue hematoma and bleeding) can increase the difficulty of airway management and cause postoperative obstruction.[235]

i. GLYCOGEN STORAGE DISEASES. Glycogen storage diseases (GSDs) are a heterogeneous group of inherited disorders involving one of the several steps of glycogen synthesis or degradation. They occur in approximately 1 in 20,000 live births. Isolated deficiencies of virtually all the enzymes involved in glycogen processing have been described. The glycogen present in patients with GSD is abnormal in structure, amount, or both. Of the 10 Cori-type GSDs, only Cori's type II (*Pompe's disease*, also known as generalized glycogenosis or [lysosomal] acid maltase deficiency) is associated with glycogen infiltration of the skeletal muscle of the tongue, which can lead to macroglossia and potential airway issues.[238]

Airway Implications. Severe macroglossia may lead to airway obstruction during anesthetic induction, emergence from anesthesia, or the postoperative period. Associated cardiomyopathy, myopathy, nervous system involvement (especially the motor neurons in the brainstem and spinal cord), and alterations in the regulation of serum glucose concentrations are part of the clinical presentation. Only a few reports address airway problems related to macroglossia in patients with GSD.[239,240]

ii. LIPID STORAGE DISEASES. Lipid storage diseases are characterized by abnormal sphingolecithin metabolism, which results in an abnormal amount of lipid products being stored in the cells of the reticuloendothelial system. The lipids include cholesterol (xanthomatosis), cerebroside (Gaucher's disease), and sphingomyelin (Niemann-Pick disease). In *Gaucher's disease*, accumulation of the substrate leads to multiorgan dysfunction involving the brain, spleen, liver, lymph node, and bone marrow. Airway difficulties may arise because of trismus, limited neck extension, and upper airway infiltration with glucocerebroside. Kita and colleagues[241] found it was impossible to insert an LMA in a 9-year-old child with Gaucher's disease because of trismus and a narrowed oral cavity. Subsequently, FOI was performed successfully.

iii. NEUROFIBROMATOSIS. Neurofibromatoses are a group of hereditary diseases transmitted in an autosomal dominant manner and characterized by a tendency to form tumors of ectodermal and mesodermal tissues. Two distinct forms recognized on clinical and genetic grounds are designated neurofibromatosis type 1 (NF1) and neurofibromatosis type 2 (NF2).[242] *Von Recklinghausen's neurofibromatosis* (NF1) is one of the most common genetic disorders related to an autosomal dominant mutation and occurs at a frequency of 1 in 3000 to 4000 live births.[243] The clinical features of NF1 include café au lait spots; neurofibromas involving the skin, deeper peripheral nerves, nerve roots, and blood vessels; intracranial and spinal cord tumors; kyphoscoliosis; short stature; and learning disability. One feature common to all patients is disease progression over time. NF1 also is associated with a higher incidence of malignant disease than NF2.

Airway Implications. Possible problems in airway management of the patient with NF1 include the presence of intraoral lesions, tumors compromising the airway, and the presence of thoracic deformities or neurologic lesions. Although their presence in the upper airway is rare, neurofibromas may pose a serious problem in airway management. An estimated 5% of NF1 patients have intraoral manifestations of the disease.[244] Discrete neurofibromas may involve the tongue or the larynx.[245,246] This may cause obstruction, as well as symptoms of dyspnea, stridor, loss or change of voice, or dysphagia, and should warn the anesthetist of potential airway problems.[247] Airway obstruction after induction of anesthesia has been reported in patients with a tongue neurofibroma and a neurofibroma involving the laryngeal inlet.[244,247] Both patients required emergency tracheostomy. Even if intraoral pathology is recognized preoperatively, elective awake fiberoptic endotracheal intubation may fail because of a grossly distorted anatomy. In addition, the presence of macroglossia, macrocephaly, mandibular abnormalities, and cervical spine involvement may contribute to difficulties of airway management.[242]

d. TONGUE TUMORS

i. LINGUAL TONSIL HYPERTROPHY. The lingual tonsil, a normal component of Waldeyer's ring, consists of lymphoid tissue located at the base of the tongue. Acute inflammation and hypertrophy of lingual tonsils can occur and has been reported as one of the unusual causes of unexpected difficulty with both mask ventilation and endotracheal intubation.[248,249] Lingual tonsil hypertrophy (LTH), or lingual tonsillar hyperplasia, has occasionally been reported in children but more often occurs in adults, particularly in atopic individuals.[250,251] The etiology is unclear. However, LTH is thought to be a compensatory mechanism following removal of the palatine tonsils or secondary to a chronic, low-grade infection of the tonsils.[251,252]

Airway Implications. Clinically, LTH is not detectable on routine preoperative physical examination.[253] Although many patients are asymptomatic, others may complain of a globus sensation, alteration of voice, chronic cough, choking, or dyspnea.[254] Jones and Cohle[253] were the first to report a death secondary to failed airway management in a patient with unrecognized LTH. Asai and colleagues[248] reported a case of suboptimal ventilation and failed endotracheal intubation using various intubation strategies, including the intubating LMA and FOB.

Enlarged lingual tonsils can impinge against the epiglottis, displacing it posteriorly. This can make mobilization of the epiglottis difficult during direct laryngoscopy. Similarly, FOI is often equally difficult because the posterior displacement of the epiglottis causes interference with the insertion of the tip of the endoscope under it. These difficulties may be compounded by the presence of redundant pharyngeal tissue interfering with fiberoptic exposure and the use of muscle relaxants.[253] With the onset of neuromuscular blockade, the pharyngeal musculature relaxes, causing further posterior movement of the tongue and epiglottis.[255]

In a retrospective study of unexpected DI in 33 patients, Ovassapian and coworkers[256] reported that the only finding common to all patients was LTH observed on fiberoptic pharyngoscopy. Most of the patients had normal airway measurements (Mallampati class of I or II), and 36% of patients were difficult to ventilate.

The LMA has been used in "cannot intubate, cannot ventilate" situations caused by LTH with both success and partial success.[257-260] Asai and colleagues[248] highlighted that the LMA cannot always solve a truly glottic or subglottic problem; rather, the ventilatory mechanism must get below the lesion. If an airway cannot be established with an LMA, TTJV and cricothyrotomy are other options. Crosby and Skene[258] recommended the Bullard laryngoscope (which can be fitted with a camera) as the airway device of choice for LTH patients because its robust construction permits gentle manipulation of airway tissues, allowing it to create the necessary endoscopic airspace.

Other masses situated at the base of the tongue may displace the epiglottis and may distort the airway anatomy. Such masses include thyroglossal duct cysts and thyroid tumors.

D. Nasal and Palatal Anomalies

Nasal obstruction in pediatric patients may result from choanal atresia or stenosis, nasal masses, foreign body, trauma, or adenoidal hypertrophy, as well as choanal stenosis combined with nasal mucosal edema.[261,262] These lesions may become evident at birth or later in childhood. Nasopalatal anomalies can result in airway obstruction and feeding difficulty and can complicate airway management.

1. Choanal Atresia

Choanal atresia is a congenital anomaly of the nasal choana that results in lack of continuity between the nasal cavity and the pharynx. This entity is rare and results from failure of resorption of the nasobuccal membrane at the sixth to seventh week of gestation. Congenital choanal atresia is usually bony and unilateral, versus membranous and bilateral. Complete nasal obstruction in a newborn may cause death from asphyxia. During attempted inspiration, the tongue is pulled to the palate, obstructing the oral airway. Vigorous respiratory efforts produce marked chest retraction. Death may occur if appropriate treatments are not available; however, if the infant cries and takes a breath through the mouth, the airway obstruction is momentarily relieved. The crying then stops, the mouth closes, and the cycle of obstruction is repeated.

Many patients have associated narrowed nasopharynx, widened vomer, medialized lateral nasal wall, or arched hard palate. Associated malformations occur in 47% of infants without chromosomal anomalies. Such malformations include cleft palate, cleft lip, and Treacher Collins syndrome. The upper airway abnormalities are present in 56% of patients with choanal atresia.[263] Nonrandom association of malformations can be demonstrated using the CHARGE association, which appears to be overused in clinical practice. The components of the CHARGE association are coloboma, 80%; heart disease, 58%; atresia choanae, 100%; retarded growth, 87%; development, or CNS anomalies, 97%; genital hypoplasia, 75%; and ear anomalies or deafness, 88%. Other airway abnormalities, as part of the CHARGE association, may be present.[264]

A high level of suspicion is required to diagnose bilateral choanal atresia. Symptoms of severe airway obstruction and cyclic cyanosis are the classic signs of neonatal bilateral atresia. If bilateral, choanal atresia is a medical emergency that becomes evident after birth with severe respiratory distress and cyanosis. These signs resolve with crying and recur when crying stops or the infant attempts to feed. In unilateral disease, the signs and symptoms are less evident and thus may result in delayed diagnosis. These patients come to medical attention with unilateral nasal discharge and mouth breathing. Respiratory distress occurs when the second nostril becomes obstructed, as during an upper respiratory tract infection. Older children display nasal discharge, inability to blow the nose on the affected side, nasal speech, and mouth breathing.

The diagnosis is based on history and physical examination, inability to pass a nasal catheter into the nasopharynx, flexible fiberoptic examination, and radiologic studies. CT scan is useful in demonstrating the atretic area.

Airway Implications. Treatment of the choanal atresia is directed at providing the patient with a patent airway. Infants may benefit from the placement of an oral airway. Feeding may take place in the form of gavage. Endotracheal intubation is usually not needed unless there are associated congenital anomalies, and tracheostomy is not necessary. Surgical correction is not an emergency and uses an endonasal or a transpalatal approach, to remove the bony or membranous obstruction and part of the vomer and stent the newly created path. In infants, the transpalatal approach is used less often because of the risk of injury to the palatal growth center.

Roger and associates[265] evaluated the need for a tracheostomy and its timing in 45 patients during the evolution of CHARGE association. They found a high percentage of associated airway abnormalities: pharyngolaryngeal anomalies leading to dyspnea (58%; discoordinate pharyngolaryngomalacia, glossoptosis, retrognathia, laryngeal paralysis, DI) and tracheobronchial anomalies (40%; tracheoesophageal fistula, esophageal atresia, tracheomalacia). Tracheostomy was necessary in 13 patients (29%) despite that the posterior nasal choanae were patent in 10 patients. The authors concluded that often a tracheostomy could not be avoided in these patients, regardless of choanal patency, and that tracheostomy needs to be performed early to avoid hypoxic events.

Asher and coworkers[266] studied the association between catastrophic airway events and developmental delay in patients with CHARGE association. They found that children with CHARGE association have a propensity for airway instability, and that cerebral hypoxia contributed to the developmental delay in some of the patients. They recommended early tracheostomy rather than early choanal atresia repair in these patients to protect the CNS.

If micrognathia or subglottic stenosis is present, a difficult endotracheal intubation should be anticipated. Awake endotracheal intubation, direct laryngoscopy, indirect visual techniques, or nonvisual intubation techniques may be tried. If the patient with choanal atresia has tracheal stenosis, a smaller-than-usual ETT must be available.

2. Nasal Masses

Nasal mass lesions are rare disorders in the pediatric population, with an incidence of 1 in 20,000 to 40,000 live births.[267,268] Nasal mass lesions are a diverse group of lesions that include anomalies of embryogenesis, such as encephaloceles, dermal and nasolacrimal duct cysts, tumors, and inflammatory processes.[267] *Encephaloceles* represent herniation of CNS tissue at the level of the cranium. Although most encephaloceles are located in the occipital area, some occur anteriorly and may contain various quantities of brain tissue. Encephaloceles may be associated with midline defects. *Dermal cysts* become evident as hard intranasal masses that result from herniation of dura and subsequent contact with the skin. These midline defects may manifest as a nasal obstruction without a facial mass. There is a risk of local abscess formation and intracranial infection.

Tumors located in the nasal area in children are rare and include hemangiomas, neurofibromas, angiofibromas, hamartomas, lipomas, and rhabdomyosarcomas. Radiologic studies (CT, MRI, angiography) can elucidate the size and position of the mass and display coexistence of any cranial bone defect. The mainstay of treatment is surgery.

A foreign body in the nostril is a finding in small children, usually a toy part or food substance. This typically manifests as nasal discharge, which may be purulent, foul smelling, or bloody, and obstruction of the affected side. Diagnosis is made by history, examination of the nares, and occasionally, radiologic evaluation.

Airway Implications. Nasal masses can affect the management of the airway by interfering with mask ventilation or with direct laryngoscopy and endotracheal intubation. Nasotracheal intubation in these patients should be avoided. Extension of a cephalocele through a palatal defect interfered with endotracheal intubation in one patient.[269] All the airway implications previously discussed under choanal atresia with unilateral (or even bilateral) obstruction are valid in patients with nasal airway obstruction.

3. Palatal Anomalies

Cleft lip and cleft palate are the most common of the craniofacial anomalies, with an incidence of approximately 1 in 800 live births; 25% of cleft lip cases are bilateral, 85% of which are associated with cleft palate. There has been a move toward earlier surgical repair of both cleft lip and palate, with cleft lip repair being performed in the neonatal period in some centers.

Anomalies of the palate include cleft and high-arched deformities and hypertrophy of the alveolar ridge area. In two studies of children undergoing palate repair, the incidence of difficult laryngoscopy (Cormack and Lehane grades III and IV) was 6.5% and 7.4%.[263,270] Of the 59 patients with difficult laryngoscopy in Gunawardana's study,[263] 2.95% had unilateral cleft lip, 45.76% had bilateral cleft lip, and 34.61% had retrognathia. Interestingly, endotracheal intubation was successful in 99% of patients in whom laryngoscopy was difficult (failed intubation was 1%). There was a significant association between age and laryngoscopic view: 66.1% of patients with difficult laryngoscopies were younger than 6 months, 20.3% were 6 to 12 months, and 13.6% were 1 to 5 years old.

The presence of other associated congenital anomalies, including cardiac and renal anomalies, should always be remembered, particularly in children with isolated cleft palate. More than 150 syndromes have been described in association with cleft lip or palate, but fortunately all are rare. Some, however, have considerable anesthetic implications, and many involve potential airway problems, including the well-known Pierre Robin, Treacher Collins, and Goldenhar syndromes. Other, such as Klippel-Feil syndrome, may include abnormalities of the cervical spine.[271]

Henriksson and Skoog[272] reviewed the records of 154 patients who underwent closure of the palate and found that 84% had isolated cleft palate, 12% had Pierre Robin syndrome, and the rest had other identified syndromes. The risk of anesthetic complications was four times greater with surgery in children less than 1 year of age, with a sixfold increase when a more elaborate velopharyngoplasty technique was used.

The postoperative airway complications ranged between 5.6% and 8% in two surveys.[273,274] As a rule, patients with cleft palate with the Pierre Robin sequence or other additional congenital anomalies had an increased risk for airway problems after palatoplasty.

Palatal edema or hematoma may also develop. Swelling limited to the soft palate or uvula can cause posture-dependent airway obstruction in children.[275] Edema may result from instrumentation of the airway, burn injury, allergy, or infectious agents.

Many methods of management of DA in patients with cleft palate have been described. The use of firm pressure over the larynx (cricoid pressure) to aid laryngoscopy, with a bougie as a guide to endotracheal intubation, is relatively simple to perform by any competent anesthetist and is usually successful.[263] Other techniques (e.g., LMA, FOB) have been described,[271] especially when cleft palate is associated with different syndromes.

4. Adenotonsillar Disease

Together, the lingual tonsils anteriorly, the palatine tonsils laterally, and the pharyngeal tonsils (adenoids) posterosuperiorly form a ring of lymphoid or adenoid tissue at the upper end of the pharynx known as Waldeyer's tonsillar ring. All the structures of Waldeyer's ring have similar histology and function, and regarding airway management, they produce similar symptoms and require treatment. In response to recurrent infections, adenoids and tonsils can hypertrophy and lead to airway obstruction.[276]

Adenoidal hypertrophy peaks at 4 to 6 years of age and disappears by adolescence. Although a disease of the older child, hypertrophy can occur in the infant. One of the major complications of adenoidal hyperplasia is *obstructive sleep apnea* (OSA). Signs and symptoms of airway obstruction include snoring and restless sleep, somnolence during the day, noisy breathing, mouth breathing, hyponasal speech, persistent nasal secretions, apnea, choking during feeding, respiratory distress, and behavioral disturbances.[163] If the condition is left untreated, failure to thrive; a characteristic, long adenoid facies with open mouth, palate, and dental malformations; and cardiovascular changes (cor pulmonale) reflective of chronic hypoxemia and hypercapnia may develop.[277]

Airway obstruction resulting from adenoid tissue is determined not by the absolute size of the adenoids but rather by their size relative to the volume of the pharynx.[249] Patients with preexisting diseases that reduce nasopharyngeal size or alter its integrity may have airway obstruction with only mild degrees of adenoidal hyperplasia. Examples are children with craniofacial anomalies (in whom the nasopharynx may be reduced in size) and those with nasal polyps, septal or turbinate malformations, MPS, or deficient pharyngeal support (Down syndrome).

Tonsillar hyperplasia is a physiologic phenomenon of childhood that peaks at about 7 years of age. It can cause OSA with restless sleep and an irregular breathing pattern, snoring, and intermittent periods of apnea as well as daytime somnolence, irritability, and poor school performance.[278] Long-standing partial obstruction of the airway can be associated with repeated hypoxic episodes and may result in pulmonary hypertension, cor pulmonale, and right-sided heart failure. Acute exacerbation of adenotonsillar hypertrophy may necessitate an emergency securing of the airway.[279,280]

The treatment of adenoidal and tonsillar hyperplasia is adenoidectomy and tonsillectomy. These are among the most common surgical procedures in children. There are multiple indications for excision of tonsils and adenoids.[276] Upper airway obstruction is of most concern for the anesthesiologist because these patients may have airway obstruction both during induction of anesthesia and in the postoperative period.

Airway Implications. Upper airway obstruction may occur after premedication, during induction of anesthesia, or following tracheal extubation. Visualization of the glottis during direct laryngoscopy may be difficult with tonsillar hypertrophy. Resection of tonsils and adenoids may not result in immediate relief of airway obstruction. Bleeding and edema can make the child susceptible to postoperative airway obstruction. Although it usually causes chronic upper airway obstruction, adenotonsillar hypertrophy can result in acute airway obstruction.[279-281] Airway assessment and management of patients with OSA caused by adenotonsillar hypertrophy are detailed in the next section.

Peritonsillar abscess in children manifests as a purulent mass surrounded by the tonsillar capsule. It occurs more frequently in untreated children with chronic tonsillitis or those who have been inadequately treated.[276] Signs and symptoms include fever, sore throat, tonsillar mass, dysphagia, drooling (caused by odynophagia and

dysphagia), muffled voice, trismus (caused by irritation of pterygoid muscle by pus and inflammation), and variable degrees of toxic state. Peritonsillar abscess requires intravenous antibiotic therapy. If symptoms of airway obstruction develop or the patient fails to respond to medical therapy, needle aspiration, incision, and drainage with tonsillectomy are recommended.[276] In a prospective study of 50 adult patients with peritonsillar abscess, the Mallampati score did not correlate with the Cormack and Lehane glottic view during laryngoscopy because of palatopharyngeal arch distortion. There were no DIs in this study group.[282]

Peritonsillar abscess affects the airway in a manner similar to tonsillar hypertrophy, except that the patients may have trismus. There may be associated edema of the supraglottic area, uvula, and soft palate that exacerbates airway obstruction. Patients are susceptible to airway obstruction during either spontaneous breathing or manual mask ventilation. During direct laryngoscopy, care should be taken not to rupture the abscess. When large, the abscess may interfere with visualization of the vocal cords.

5. Obstructive Sleep Apnea

a. DEFINITION

Obstructive sleep apnea syndrome (OSAS) in children is a disorder of breathing during sleep characterized by prolonged partial upper airway obstruction or intermittent complete obstruction (obstructive apnea) that disrupts normal ventilation during sleep and normal sleep patterns.[283]

b. PREVALENCE OF SNORING

The prevalence of primary snoring ranges from 3.2% to 12.1%,[39] whereas the prevalence of OSAS ranges from 0.7% to 10.3%.[39,284,285] The ability to maintain upper airway patency during the normal respiratory circle is the result of a delicate equilibrium between various forces that promote airway closure and dilatation. This "balance of pressure" concept was first proposed independently by Remmers and colleagues[286] in 1978 and Brouillette and Thach[287] in 1979 and represents the current thought regarding the pathophysiologic mechanisms of OSAS.

The four major predisposing factors for upper airway obstruction are as follows:

- *Anatomic narrowing.* The upper airway behaves as predicted by the Sterling resistor model; the maximal inspiratory flow is determined by the pressure changes upstream (nasal) to a collapsible site of the upper airway, and flow is independent of downstream (tracheal) pressure generated by the diaphragm.
- Children with OSAS close their airways at the level of enlarged adenoids and tonsils at low positive pressures, whereas healthy children require subatmospheric pressures to induce upper airway closure.[288]
- *Abnormal mechanical linkage between airway dilating muscles and airway walls.* Control of the upper airway size and stiffness depends on the relative and rhythmic contraction of a host of paired muscles, which include palatal, pterygoid, tensor palatini, genioglossus,

TABLE 36-4

Adult vs. Childhood Obstructive Sleep Apnea Syndrome (OSAS)

Features	Adult OSAS	Childhood OSAS
Snoring	Intermittent	Continuous
Mouth breathing	Uncommon	Continuous
Obesity	Common	Uncommon
Failure to thrive	—	Common
Daytime hypersomnolence	Common	Uncommon
Gender predilection	Male	None
Most common obstructive event	Apnea	Hypopnea
Arousal	Common	Uncommon treatment
Nonsurgical	CPAP in majority	CPAP in minority
Surgery	Selected cases in majority	T&A

CPAP, Continuous positive airway pressure; *T&A*, tonsillectomy and adenoidectomy.

geniohyoid, and sternohyoid. With contraction, these muscles promote motion of the soft palate, mandible, tongue, and hyoid bone. The activity of these muscles is dependent in particular on the brainstem respiratory network. Wakefulness conveys a supervisory function that ensures airway patency, and sedative agents that compromise genioglossal muscle activity may result in significant upper airway compromise. Roberts and others[289] demonstrated that mechanoreceptor- and chemoreceptor-mediated genioglossal activity is critical for maintenance of upper airway patency in both normal and micrognathic infants.

- *Muscle weakness.* There is little evidence to suggest that intrinsic muscle weakness is a major contributor to upper airway dysfunction. Nevertheless, in patients with neuromuscular disorders, airway obstruction is frequently observed during sleep.[290]
- *Abnormal neural regulation.* Subtle alterations in central chemoreceptor activity were found by different researchers. Gozal and others[291] reported that arousal to hypercapnia was blunted, whereas Onal and coworkers[292] found that upper airway musculature is more stimulated than the diaphragm.

c. PATHOPHYSIOLOGY AND CLINICAL PICTURE

The etiology and pathophysiology of obstructive sleep apnea in children are multifactorial, with anatomic and neuromuscular abnormalities playing a major role in the disorder.[293-297] Others, however, downplay the role of neuromuscular factors because the vast majority of children with OSAS can be cured by correcting anatomic obstructions. The narrowing of the airway lumen by hypertrophied lymphoid tissue, compliance, elasticity of the pharyngeal soft tissue, facial morphology, and the physiologic changes that occur in the pharyngeal dilators during sleep determine the severity of airway collapse.

Patients with dysmorphic constricted craniofacial development, such as those with Pierre Robin sequence; Treacher Collins, Apert's, or Crouzon's syndrome; or neuromuscular abnormalities, as in cerebral palsy and anoxic encephalopathy, have a much higher incidence of severe OSAS.

Adenotonsillar hypertrophy plays a major role in the pathogenesis of OSAS in children. The volume of lymphoid tissue in the upper airway increases from about 6 months of age up to puberty, with the maximum proliferation occurring in the preschool years, which coincides with the peak incidence of OSAS in children. Despite this narrowing of the upper airway by lymphoid tissue, most children do not develop OSAS. A normal child's airway is less likely to collapse in sleep than the adult airway.

One of the hallmarks of sleep-disordered breathing is fragmentation and disruption of normal sleep architecture. By definition, deeper levels of sleep, especially rapid eye movement (REM) sleep, are less susceptible to arousal from various stimuli, including adverse ventilatory events.[298] Oxyhemoglobin desaturation therefore tends to be more frequent and more severe during REM sleep. The hypercapnia and hypoxemia and resulting arousals associated with OSAS, at least in part, often result in a reduction in REM sleep.[298,299]

Although OSAS and hypertension are often associated in adults, children with OSAS also tend to have higher diastolic blood pressure. The cardiovascular changes appear to be the result of an increase in sympathetic tone that results from the sleep arousals, which in turn are related to the obstructive respiratory events.[300] The clinical presentation of OSAS in children has many similarities and important differences compared with the disorder in adults[245,299,301] (Table 36-4).

Unlike findings in adults, obesity is not a common factor in pediatric OSAS, although its role increases with the age of the child.[302] Abnormal sleep positions with preference for an upright position and hyperextension of the neck have been noted in children with sleep-related breathing disorders.[303]

Prolonged exposure to hypoxia and hypercarbia results in compensatory changes in the pulmonary vasculature. Pulmonary vascular resistance increases, causing increased right ventricular strain.[304] Severe cases may progress to pulmonary hypertension, dysrhythmias, and cor pulmonale.[305]

d. LABORATORY EVALUATION

Polysomnography (PSG) remains the gold standard for the diagnosis of OSAS in adults and children. In 1995 the American Thoracic Society adopted guidelines for performing PSG in children.[306] Use of PSG was recommended to differentiate primary snoring, which does not require any form of treatment, from OSAS, which can lead to cardiopulmonary dysfunction and functional

TABLE 36-5

Normal Sleep Study Measurements in Children

Measurement	Normal Values
Sleep latency (minutes)	>10
TST (hours)	>5.5
REM sleep (%)	>15% TST
Stage 3 and 4 non-REM sleep (%)	>25% TST
Respiratory arousal index (no./hr TST)	>5
Periodic leg movements (no./hr TST)	>1
Apnea index (no./hr TST)	>1
Hypopnea index (nasal/esophageal pressure catheter; no./hr TST)	<3
Respiratory disturbance index (RDI) (Apnea/hypopnea index)	<1
Nadir oxygen saturation (%)	<92
Mean oxygen saturation (%)	<95
Desaturation index (<4% for 5 sec; no./hr TST)	<5
Highest CO_2 (mm Hg)	52
CO_2 < 45 mm Hg	>20% TST

TST, Total sleep time; *REM,* rapid eye movement.

impairment if left untreated.[307] In general, studies show that history alone does not have sufficiently high diagnostic sensitivity or specificity to be the basis for recommending therapy.[308]

In a study of 50 healthy children, Marcus and colleagues[309] reported normal PSG values for the various respiratory events. The apnea indices (number of apneas per hours of total sleep time, TST) were 0.1 ± 0.5, with the minimum oxygen saturation being 96%, maximal drop in saturation 4%, and CO_2 over 55 mm Hg no more than 0.5% of TST. An abnormal study includes an apnea index greater than 1, oxygen desaturation greater than 4% more than three times an hour or associated with a greater than 25% change in heart rate, oxygen desaturation less than 92%, and elevation of end-tidal CO_2 to more than 52 mm Hg for more than 8% of TST, or 45 mm Hg for more than 60% of TST (Table 36-5).

e. AIRWAY IMPLICATIONS

Medical therapy of pediatric OSA is not considered to be consistently effective. Systemic or topical *steroids* may shrink lymphoid tissue, but the long-term effectiveness is not known, and a short course of systemic corticosteroids appears to be ineffective. Topical intranasal steroids appear to reduce the severity of OSAS.[310]

Adenotonsillectomy remains the mainstay of treatment for pediatric OSA.[311] The optimal age for adenotonsillectomy is 4 to 7 years, although a young age, even under 1 year, is not a contraindication for surgery for airway obstruction or OSA. Children with Down syndrome deserve further comment because they frequently have severe OSA.[312] Although data are conflicting on the usefulness of adenotonsillectomy in this group, it appears worthwhile if the tonsils or adenoids are obstructing the airway. If an adenotonsillectomy fails or is not considered appropriate therapy, uvulopalatopharyngoplasty may be effective.[39]

Several studies demonstrated the relative safety of adenotonsillectomy performed on an outpatient basis with a suitable period of postoperative observation and

hydration. It appears that if children meet standard discharge criteria (normal respiratory parameters, no bleeding, adequate oral intake and pain control, normal mental status) at 4 to 6 hours after surgery, they can be safely discharged home regardless of age or preoperative diagnoses.

Minimal specific evidence exists for or against the use of *opiates and sedatives* in the perioperative period in children with OSAS. To date, there are only anecdotal reports of respiratory depression in children in response to sedatives such as chloral hydrate and in the postoperative period,[313,314] including hypoxia.[315-317] Children with OSAS appear to have increased sensitivity to opioids.

Waters and associates[318] found that children with OSAS develop more pronounced *respiratory depression* than with aged-matched control subjects when breathing spontaneously under anesthetic with the upper airway secured.[318] Addition of a small dose of opioids increased the respiratory depression in children with OSAS. The low dose of fentanyl used (0.5 µg/kg) precipitated central apnea in 46% of the OSAS group. In this study, the best predictor of opioid-induced central apnea was an increase in end-tidal CO_2 to levels greater than 50 mm Hg during spontaneous breathing after anesthetic induction. In contrast to the previous studies,[316,318-320] Wilson and coauthors[321] found no correlation between the preoperative cardiorespiratory sleep study (PSG and home sleep studies) parameters and opioid administration and postoperative outcome.

Few studies provide data pertaining to complications of surgery in children undergoing adenotonsillectomy for upper airway obstruction. All specifically address the risk of postoperative *respiratory obstruction*[315-317,319-324] (Table 36-6). The authors define "respiratory compromise" in various ways but generally consider the need for supplemental oxygen as a minimum criterion. The papers report a wide range for the incidence of postoperative respiratory complications (0-27%), primarily because their populations include different proportions of children with neuromuscular, chromosomal, and craniofacial disorders.

Young age (<3 years) and associated medical problems were found in most studies to define the highest-risk groups. A high preoperative respiratory disturbance index (apnea/hypopnea index) also seems to be a risk factor for postoperative complications.[316,317] Time to onset of respiratory compromise after adenotonsillectomy appears to be brief, although McColley and others[316] reported that one patient required 14 hours to manifest respiratory symptoms. Postobstructive *pulmonary edema* may develop in some children undergoing adenotonsillectomy for relief of upper airway obstruction. The incidence of this complication is unknown, and pulmonary edema often manifests immediately after endotracheal intubation.

The patient's position, especially after extubation, seems to be important for the development of airway obstruction. Ishikawa and colleagues[325] found that prone position increases upper airway collapsibility in anesthetized infants. Isono and associates,[326] in a study of adult patients, reported that lateral position structurally improves maintenance of the passive pharyngeal airway in OSA patients. These findings are in concordance with

TABLE 36-6

Respiratory Compromise After Adenotonsillectomy in Children with Obstructive Sleep Apnea Syndrome (OSAS)

Author	Year	Methodology and Rating	Inclusion Criteria	No.	Rate of Respiratory Compromise	Comments
McGowan et al.[324]	1992	Case series, level IV	Clinical upper airway obstruction	53	25%	Risk factors for complications were prematurity, adenoidal facies, preoperative respiratory distress.
McColley et al.[317]	1992	Case series, level IV	Abnormal PSG	69	23%	Onset up to 14 hours postop. Main risk factors were age and preop RDI.
Price et al.[318]	1993	Case series, level IV	Clinical upper airway obstruction, nap PSG	160	19%	Associations with risk factors (age, preop PSG) asserted but not quantitated.
Rosen et al.[319]	1994	Case series, level IV	Abnormal PSG	37	27%	Postop obstruction occurred within hours of surgery. All patients with complications were complex and had a higher mean RDI preop.
Helfaer et al.[320]	1996	Case series, level IV	Mild OSAS by PSG (no severe cases)	15	0%	No postop desaturation or obstruction in children with mild OSAS.
Geber et al.[321]	1996	Case series, level IV	Questionnaire	292	15% (38% if age <3 yr)	Included complex patients. Respiratory compromise developed only in patients who snored preop.
Rottschild et al.[325]	1994	Case series, level IV	Clinical diagnosis	69	7%	Specific diagnostic criteria for OSAS not specified.
Bivati et al.[320]	1997	Case series, level IV	Clinical diagnosis	3552 3 with PSG	25% (36% with abnormal PSG)	Included complex patients. No patient with normal PSA has postop respiratory complications.
Wilson et al.[322]	2002	Case series, retrospective	Abnormal PSG	163	21%	96% were managed in recovery room or ward setting.

PSG, Polysomnography; *postop,* postoperative/ly; *preop,* preoperative/ly; *RDI,* respiratory disturbance index.

the current practice of extubating and transporting children in the lateral position.

In a retrospective study of 163 OSAS children, Wilson and coworkers[321] found a 21% incidence of respiratory compromise requiring medical interventions after adenotonsillectomy. Ninety-six percent of the children with OSAS were managed in a recovery room or ward setting. Six children required postoperative admission to the intensive care unit (ICU).

Most of the polysomnographic studies done weeks after adenotonsillectomy in children with OSAS reported a cure rate between 85% and 100%.[327,328] A major concern in the immediate postoperative period is the effect of residual anesthesia, pain, sedative and analgesic medication, and edema of the pharyngeal tissues on the complication rate in this category of patients. Helfaer and coauthors[315] tried to respond to this question by comparing preoperative and first-night postoperative polysomnograms in children with mild OSAS.[315] Surprisingly, most of the children had improvements in their sleep studies on the night of surgery. These findings were not affected by the choice of intraoperative anesthetic. Specifically, intraoperative administration of narcotics was not associated with postoperative respiratory impairment. Even though this study was performed on a relatively small number of patients with mild disease, it was concluded that children with mild OSAS can be safely discharged home on the day of surgery (see Table 36-6).

In our institution, the criteria for postoperative admission are severe OSAS; age less than 3 years; associated craniofacial anomalies (including Down syndrome); associated neuromotor, cardiac, or pulmonary diseases; upper airway burn; hypotonia; morbid obesity; or children with recent upper respiratory tract infection.

In conclusion, the anesthetic management of OSAS should be directed toward assessing and managing the coexisting cardiac or pulmonary diseases; managing the airway, especially in syndromic children; minimizing the amount of opiates used intraoperatively; using capnography in postoperative period; and preventing and managing the possible postoperative complications. Preoperative sleep studies are necessary for a positive diagnosis and for decisions regarding postoperative monitoring. Therefore, anesthesiologists need to be familiar with reading a sleep study and interpreting PSG results.

6. Retropharyngeal and Parapharyngeal Abscesses

The various cavities and virtual spaces in the pharynx and neck are in anatomic continuity with one another. The retropharyngeal, parapharyngeal, peritonsillar, and submandibular spaces intercommunicate, and infection in one can extend to the others. The superior limit of the retropharyngeal space is the base of the skull; inferiorly, it extends into the mediastinum to the level of the tracheal bifurcation.

Retropharyngeal abscess is a rare but potentially fatal infection of the pharyngeal wall. It occurs primarily in pediatric patients; in one study more than half of the patients were younger than 12 months.[329] In children, it usually results from suppurative involvement of lymph nodes located in the retropharyngeal space. These nodes drain lymph from the pharynx, nasopharynx, paranasal sinuses, and middle ear. The most common pathogens are *Staphylococcus aureus* (25%), *Klebsiella* species (13%), group A streptococci (8%), and a mixture of gram-negative and anaerobic organisms (38%).[329,330] Other causes of retropharyngeal abscess include spread of infection from pharyngitis or peritonsillar abscess, penetrating trauma, and foreign body ingestion.

Clinical presentation of retropharyngeal abscess varies with the patient's age. Most children have fever, some degree of toxic appearance, a hyperextended or stiff neck, dysphagia, drooling, trismus, muffled voice, and respiratory distress. Infants and young children may have stridor. Older children with mediastinal involvement may, in addition, complain of chest pain. Physical examination may reveal cervical lymphadenopathy and pharyngeal swelling. A lateral radiograph of the neck typically shows widening of the retropharyngeal prevertebral soft tissue. CT is helpful in the diagnosis of retropharyngeal abscess but has difficulty differentiating cellulites and abscess. Lateral neck radiography was found to be very specific when the air sign was present.[331] Ultrasound imaging can also distinguish between suppurative and presuppurative stage.[332] Chest radiographs may show mediastinal involvement and tracheal deviation.[333]

Complications of retropharyngeal abscess include airway obstruction, abscess rupture, pneumonia, sepsis, and extension of the disease into the mediastinum and the carotid sheath, causing mediastinitis, jugular vein thrombosis, or penetration into the carotid artery. Treatment consists of airway support, antibiotic therapy, and early incision and drainage.

Airway Implications. The danger of retropharyngeal abscess is related to the potential for rapid progression to airway obstruction. In one report, 5 of 65 patients required tracheostomy.[334] There is also an ever-present risk of abscess rupture and aspiration of pus into the airway. The clinical presentation of children with retropharyngeal abscess can mimic that of children with epiglottitis and croup. The mortality rate is high; exact incidence is not known. In a retrospective study, Ameh[335] reported two deaths among 10 children surveyed; one child died before the abscess was drained, and the other died in the postoperative period because of laryngospasm. Coulthard and Isaacs[329] reported two deaths in 31 children with retropharyngeal abscess.

All patients with the diagnosis of retropharyngeal abscess must be considered to have a DA. The management depends on the severity of airway distress and degree of patient's cooperation. In most children, general anesthesia is required for airway management because few patients, if any, accept an awake technique. General anesthesia may be induced by inhalation of sevoflurane and oxygen with emergency plans for securing the airway should airway obstruction develops. If not in place, an intravenous line should be secured and atropine administered. It is advantageous to maintain spontaneous ventilation because neuromuscular blockade may relax the pharyngeal musculature and potentiate airway obstruction with an already-reduced pharyngeal space.

After adequate anesthetic depth is achieved, gentle direct laryngoscopy should be attempted, taking care not to rupture the abscess. If endotracheal intubation is not possible after limited attempts at direct laryngoscopy, a surgical airway should be considered for those with large lesions. In children with minimal respiratory distress and adequate mask air exchange, other intubation techniques (indirect visual or nonvisual) may be tried first. It is important to take special precautions not to traumatize the abscess during endotracheal intubation. Blind attempts at intubation, insertion of an LMA or oral airway, or overzealous direct laryngoscopy may result in rupture of the abscess.

7. Pharyngeal Bullae or Scarring

Epidermolysis bullosa (EB) describes a group of genetically determined mechanobullous disorders that vary in course and severity, ranging from relatively minor disability to death in early infancy.[336,337] They are characterized by an excessive susceptibility of the skin and mucosa to separate from the underlying tissues and form bullae following minimal mechanical trauma. The affected areas can be considerable in size as the bullae enlarge by expanding and tracking along the natural tissue planes. As with all blisters, they can be extremely painful. More than 20 types of EB are described,[338] with three major subtypes: *dystrophic, simplex,* and *junctional,* with each broad category of EB containing several subtypes.

a. DYSTROPHIC EPIDERMOLYSIS BULLOSA

Dystophic epidermolysis bullosa (DEB), which was first described by Fox in 1879, is probably the most frequent type of EB to have surgical treatment.[339,340] The prevalence of DEB is approximately 2 in 100,000 children.[341] The majority of DEB patients have wounds that are present at birth or shortly after, with a variety of blister sizes, some even exceeding 10 cm in diameter. The blisters of DEB are usually flaccid and filled with either a clear or a blood-stained fluid. New blisters tend to develop less frequently as the child ages. Scarring is unusual after a single episode of blistering, but blistering is much more easily provoked in previously blistered areas; it is this recurrence that causes atrophic scars to form. As a result of repeated skin infection, injury, and healing, patients with the dystrophic form develop *contractures,* which may involve the skin of the neck and mouth.

Oral, pharyngeal, and esophageal blistering is common in DEB. The recurrent blistering leads to progressive contraction of the mouth (causing limited opening) and fixation of the tongue. The associated pain and resulting dysphagia lead to a reduction of nutritional intake because eating is a painful, slow, and exhausting experience. Gastroesophageal reflux (GER) is common in patients with DEB. Esophageal scarring leads to dysmotility and the formation of strictures or webs, which contributes to the dysphagia by exacerbating oral, pharyngeal, and esophageal ulceration and also by increasing dental decay.

b. EPIDERMOLYSIS BULLOSA SIMPLEX

Almost all cases of epidermolysis bullosa simplex (EBS) are inherited in an autosomal dominant manner.[339] Although the exact prevalence of EBS is not known, it is thought to be approximately 1 or 2 in 100,000 children.[336] There are three major subtypes: Dowling-Meara, Weber-Cockayne, and Koebner.

Only the *Dowling-Meara* type (EBS herpetiformis) has airway implications. The onset of this type of EBS is usually in early infancy. There is a great range in the severity of Dowling-Meara, from relatively mild to exceptionally severe with death during the neonatal period. Oral involvement is usually not prominent, but a number of severely affected neonates exhibit extreme oropharyngeal involvement, which interferes with feeding. Patients may also have a tendency for GER and aspiration. Laryngeal involvement, causing a hoarse cry, is also regularly seen in Dowling-Meara EBS.

c. JUNCTIONAL EPIDERMOLYSIS BULLOSA

There are three major subtypes of junctional epidermolysis bullosa (JEB): Herlitz, non-Herlitz, and JEB with pyloric atresia. *Herlitz* JEB is the most common form. Formerly known as "lethal" JEB, it affects the larynx, producing a characteristic hoarse cry in infancy. This hoarseness is usually followed by recurrent bouts of stridor (caused by granulation tissue and not usually fresh blisters), each with the potential risk of fatal asphyxiation. The mouth and pharynx are often severely affected, causing substantial pain and feeding difficulties, which in turn lead to a profound failure to thrive. Death in the first 2 years of life is usual in Herlitz JEB, either from acute respiratory obstruction or from overwhelming sepsis related to a poor nutritional state.

d. AIRWAY IMPLICATIONS

Children with EB, especially DEB, are more likely to have airway management problems, with the risk of DI secondary to contracture formation. In addition to oral, pharyngeal, and laryngeal problems, head and neck skin involvement and contractures may make positioning for laryngoscopy difficult.[342] A DI should always be suspected and contingency plans made before embarking on anesthesia. To avoid prolonged facial manipulation during the procedure, airway maintenance by intubation is often preferred.[343] To reduce the risk of new laryngeal bullae formation, an ETT a half to one size smaller than predicted may be necessary. If a cuffed tube is required, the cuff should be slightly inflated. The risk of bullae formation after intubation is low because the larynx and trachea are lined with ciliated columnar epithelium rather than the squamous epithelium that lines the oropharynx and esophagus.[344]

Although securing the ETT by wiring it to a tooth has been advocated,[345] a more conservative approach is to tie the tube in place with either ribbon gauze or Vaseline gauze and a collar of adhesive tape around the ETT to prevent the ties from slipping. Nasal intubation can be performed, preferably with a fiberoptic scope, but blind nasal intubation should be avoided. Blind techniques (e.g., blind oral intubation or lighted stylet) have been

used successfully but may result in trauma to the laryngeal structures if multiple unsuccessful attempts are required and probably should be avoided.[346]

The lips are lined with lubricated gauze at the place they touch the ET and also underneath the tie to prevent chafing. An intravenous cannula should be secured with a nonadhesive dressing. Central venous and arterial cannulas, if required, should be sutured in place.

In caring for patients with EB, it is important to take general precautions to protect the integrity of the skin from trauma, friction injury, and adhesive products. Areas susceptible to pressure (e.g., below face mask) should be generously lubricated. Patients receiving systemic corticosteroid therapy may need perioperative supplementation.

E. Laryngeal Anomalies

1. Laryngomalacia

Laryngomalacia is the most common congenital abnormality of the larynx and is characterized by a long, narrow epiglottis and floppy aryepiglottic folds.[341] It is the most common cause of noninfective *stridor* in children.[341] Stridor, usually present at birth, may appear after weeks or months. It may appear only with crying or in the presence of an acute upper respiratory infection. The stridor is inspiratory, high pitched, and more obvious in the supine position.[197] In the mild form, stridor peaks at 9 months and then levels off, declines, and disappears by 2 years of age.[347] Severe laryngomalacia may cause upper airway obstruction, cyanosis, failure to thrive, and cor pulmonale. GER has been reported as well, and antireflux therapy is recommended.[348]

Diagnosis of laryngomalacia is by endoscopy, particularly laryngoscopy. Indirect laryngoscopy is not practical for infants and children. Flexible endoscopy or rigid endoscopy may be necessary. General anesthesia is required.

Airway Implications. Patients with laryngomalacia are at risk for airway obstruction, and preparations for management of the difficult pediatric airway must be made. A gradual inhalation induction with 100% oxygen is performed, maintaining spontaneous ventilation. CPAP with 10 cm H_2O may be necessary to overcome obstruction, along with an oral airway and jaw lift. The time required for an adequate depth of anesthesia may be delayed in cases of airway obstruction. When deep levels of anesthesia are achieved, direct laryngoscopy may be performed. Topicalization of the vocal cords prior to laryngoscopy decreases the incidence of coughing. As stated previously, one should calculate the maximum dose before topicalization so that toxic doses are avoided.

Surgical treatment consists of either aryepiglottoplasty or laser excision of redundant supraglottic tissue.[349] Endoscopic division of the aryepiglottic folds has been suggested as the first-line therapy for severe laryngomalacia.[350]

2. Epiglottitis

Epiglottitis, more appropriately called *supraglottitis*, is a life-threatening infection of the epiglottis, aryepiglottic folds, and arytenoids. It is a true airway emergency because supraglottitis may progress rapidly to complete airway obstruction. Supraglottitis is classically described as occurring between 2 and 8 years of age, although it can occur in infants, older children, and adults.[351] *Haemophilus influenzae* type B (Hib) is the most common causative agent, although other organisms have been reported. *Pseudomonas*, group A β-hemolytic *Streptococcus*, and *Candida* have been reported in the literature as etiologies of epiglottitis as well.[351-353] The introduction of the *H. influenzae* conjugate vaccine has dramatically reduced the incidence of supraglottitis, but vaccine failure does occur.[353] A high index of suspicion for the diagnosis of supraglottitis should be maintained because the disease has not been completely eliminated.

Children with epiglottitis often present with the four Ds of supraglottitis: drooling, dyspnea, dysphagia, and dysphonia. These children are described as "toxic appearing" and anxious, preferring to rest in the tripod position (upright sitting position, leaning forward with the mouth open).[352] High fevers and signs of respiratory distress evolve over a few hours. Stridor, if present, is usually inspiratory.[354]

Diagnosis is usually based on clinical findings. Radiographs are indicated only if the child has no respiratory distress and a physician capable of controlling the DA is in attendance. A lateral neck radiograph obtained with hyperextension during inspiration is the single best exposure. Classic findings include round, thick epiglottis (thumb sign), loss of the vallecular airspace, and thickening of the aryepiglottic folds.[351] Definitive diagnosis is made at laryngoscopy in the OR. No one should attempt to visualize the posterior pharynx in the emergency room. Dynamic airway collapse may occur, and complete obstruction ensues.

Airway Implications. The mainstay of therapy for supraglottitis is to obtain an airway, usually with a multidisciplinary approach in an organized and controlled manner. An otolaryngologist capable of performing an emergency tracheostomy is present at the induction. The difficult pediatric airway cart, a rigid bronchoscope, and tracheostomy set must be in the OR. When dealing with the child with epiglottitis, it is vital that the child remain calm. If separation from the parents is too stressful, parental presence at induction, after proper preparation, should be considered. Sedation is not advised in this situation. After placement of a precordial stethoscope and pulse oximeter, a gradual inhalation induction with 100% oxygen is performed with the child in the sitting position. Maintenance of spontaneous ventilation is crucial; CPAP at 10 cm H_2O may be beneficial in maintaining a patent airway. Once anesthesia is induced, an intravenous line is placed and a volume bolus of 10 to 30 mL/kg of lactated Ringer's solution is given. The rest of the monitors are applied, and atropine or glycopyrrolate is given intravenously before laryngoscopy for its antimuscarinic effect. After an adequate depth of anesthesia is obtained, direct laryngoscopy is performed and an oral ETT is placed. Identification of a cherry-red edematous epiglottis is diagnostic. A tip for successful intubation is that gentle pressure applied to the chest may reveal expiratory gas

bubbles. A styletted ETT, one or two sizes smaller than predicted, is placed into the trachea.[354] If the patient cannot be intubated, the DA algorithm is followed. Rigid FOB may be attempted if the condition permits, or a surgical airway is obtained.

After the appropriate cultures are obtained, antibiotic therapy is initiated. Some advocate changing the oral ETT to a nasotracheal tube because of the greater stability of the nasotracheal tube. The mean duration of intubation ranges from 30 to 72 hours. Extubation is performed when the patient demonstrates clinical improvement and there is evidence of an air leak around the ETT. Some clinicians advocate the use of dexamethasone before extubation to reduce the incidence of postextubation stridor.[351]

3. Congenital Glottic Lesions

Congenital laryngeal anomalies include laryngomalacia, vocal cord paralysis, laryngeal web, and atresia. *Vocal cord paralysis* is the second most common cause of congenital laryngeal malformations.[355] Bilateral vocal cord paralysis is often associated with CNS abnormalities such as Arnold-Chiari malformation. Birth trauma may also induce vocal cord paralysis. The presentation of bilateral vocal cord paralysis is high-pitched inspiratory stridor and a normal or mildly hoarse cry. Severe airway obstruction may develop that requires emergency intubation or tracheostomy.[355] Occasionally, vocal cord paralysis resolves spontaneously or after a ventriculoperitoneal shunt is placed.[356] In unilateral paralysis, the left side is more frequently affected. Cardiovascular and mediastinal problems are often associated with unilateral paralysis.[355] Unilateral paralysis arises with a weak cry.[276] It seldom requires surgery.[356]

Laryngeal webs occur when there is failure of recanalization of the larynx during embryologic development. In general, webs occur at the level of the glottis, causing respiratory distress at birth. They may be thin and limited to the glottis, with minimal airway obstruction. Significant airway obstruction is usually the result of more extensive webs. These webs are thick, extending into the subglottis. Surgical treatment is endoscopic division of the web for smaller webs. Laryngotracheal reconstruction may be needed for extensive webs.

Laryngeal atresia is a rare and often fatal anomaly. Survival depends on the presence of an associated tracheoesophageal fistula or immediate tracheostomy at birth.[355]

Airway Implications. The degree of obstruction determines the method used for airway management. Severe forms require a surgical airway; milder cases may be managed with intubation. Intubation may be performed either awake or after inhalation induction, depending on the patient and the situation. Preparations for a failed intubation should be made.

4. Recurrent Respiratory Papillomatosis

Laryngeal papillomatosis, or recurrent respiratory papillomatosis (RRP), is the most frequent benign tumor of the larynx, with an incidence in the United States of 4.3 per 100,000 children. It is caused by the human papillomavirus (HPV) types 6 and 11. It is also the second most common cause of hoarseness in children.[357] Laryngeal papillomas are located primarily in the larynx on the vocal cord margins and epiglottis; however, any part of the respiratory tract may be affected.[358] RRP may affect children and adults. The juvenile form is often more aggressive than the adult form of the disease. Pediatric patients with RRP often wheeze and the diagnosis may be delayed. The primary symptom of RRP is hoarseness or a weak cry. Stridor is often the second symptom to develop, usually starting as inspiratory and progressing to biphasic with advancing disease.[357] Other symptoms may include chronic cough, paroxysms of choking, failure to thrive, and respiratory fatigue.[358] Diagnosis is made with a flexible fiberoptic nasopharyngoscope. If patient's cooperation limits the examination, general anesthesia may be needed. Treatment consists of CO_2 laser microlaryngoscopy, which vaporizes the lesions and causes minimal bleeding. Frequent surgical procedures may be required to control the disease. Medical management includes the use of acyclovir, interferon-α, cidofovir, and indole 3-carbinol.[358]

Airway Implications. Airway obstruction has been reported with induction of anesthesia in patients with RRP.[359] Anesthetic evaluation should include careful preoperative assessment of the airway and the emotional status of the child.[360] Sedation is necessary because these patients require frequent surgeries, but it should be avoided in patients with respiratory compromise. In appropriate cases, parental presence in the OR may be beneficial. Anesthesia should be induced with an inhalational induction in 100% oxygen while maintaining spontaneous respirations. Patients may be apprehensive about the mask, and an alternative technique, such as cupping the hands around the circuit to increase the concentration of the inhalational agent, may be useful.[360] This is a recognized DA, and appropriate equipment and personnel should be in the OR before induction.

5. Laryngeal Granulomas

Laryngeal granulomas are frequently the result of prolonged endotracheal intubation.[108] However, granuloma formation has been reported after short-term intubation as well. Other factors contributing to granuloma formation include female gender, size of the ETT, position of the ETT, traumatic intubation, and excessive cuff pressure.[82] The incidence in adults has been described as 1 in 800 to 1 in 20,000.[361] Typically, granulomas form in the posterior glottis on the medial aspect of the arytenoids.[106] Hoarseness is a common feature. Treatment consists of inhaled steroids, antireflux measures, antibiotics, and surgical removal under direct visualization.[82]

Airway Implications. If the granulomas are large or pedunculated, airway obstruction may be seen. Awake intubation may be indicated in the adult population, or rarely, inhalation induction with intubation in the pediatric population. ETTs smaller than predicted should be immediately available.

6. Congenital and Acquired Subglottic Disease

a. SUBGLOTTIC STENOSIS

Subglottic stenosis may be classified as congenital or acquired. It is defined as the presence of an abnormally small subglottic lumen (<3.5 mm in diameter in newborn).[355] *Congenital subglottic stenosis* is the third most common congenital anomaly.[356] Patients may present with mild or severe airway obstruction. Another common presentation is recurrent croup.[355] Patients who develop recurrent croup with upper respiratory tract infections during the first years of life should be evaluated for congenital subglottic stenosis. Acquired subglottic stenosis is usually the result of endotracheal intubation. Definitive diagnosis is made with rigid endoscopy. Treatment consists of anterior or multiple cricoid splitting with cartilage graft interpositioning (mitomycin). The success rate for these procedures is approximately 90%.[356]

b. CROUP

Croup, or *laryngotracheobronchitis*, is the most common cause of infectious airway obstruction in children. The incidence of croup in the United States is 18 per 1000 children annually. The peak incidence is 60 per 1000 among children 1 to 2 years of age.[351] Croup affects children between the ages of 6 months and 4 years, with peak incidence in early fall and winter. Parainfluenza type I is the most common etiologic agent responsible for croup. This is a viral infection that affects the subglottic region of the larynx, causing edema. The disease has a gradual onset, usually arising after an upper respiratory tract infection. Symptoms include inspiratory stridor; suprasternal, intercostal, and subcostal retractions; and a croupy or barking cough. Anteroposterior films of the neck show the classic church steeple sign (symmetrical narrowing of the subglottic air).[351]

For mild cases, treatment consists of breathing humidified air or oxygen.[351] In severe cases, treatment with nebulized racemic epinephrine (0.25-0.5 mL in 2 mL of saline) is indicated. Repeated treatments, every 1 to 2 hours, may be necessary. Because the duration of action is brief (<2 hours), rebound respiratory distress may develop after treatment, and observation is necessary. Studies suggest that patients may be discharged from the emergency room after a 3-hour observation period provided that the parents are reliable and easy access to the ER is available. Racemic epinephrine should be used with caution in patients with tachycardia or underlying cardiac abnormalities, such as tetralogy of Fallot or idiopathic hypertrophic subaortic stenosis.[362]

After years of debate, the use of *steroids* in the treatment of mild to moderate viral croup has gained acceptance.[363-365] Treatment with steroids has been associated with a reduction in admissions and length of stay.[365] Dexamethasone, 0.6 mg/kg (maximum dose, 10 mg) intravenously, is the standard dose. Dexamethasone (0.6 mg/kg) given orally was associated with more rapid resolution of symptoms than nebulized dexamethasone.[363] *Heliox*, a mixture of helium and oxygen, has also been used in the treatment of viral croup. Helium is an inert, nontoxic gas that has low specific gravity, low viscosity, and low density. Because of these properties, helium reduces airway resistance by decreasing turbulent flow in the airway.[366] If the preceding measures fail, intubation is necessary.

Airway Implications. As with all cases of upper airway obstruction, preparations for management of a difficult pediatric airway must be made. The appropriate equipment and personnel must be in the OR at induction. A gradual inhalation induction is performed with 100% oxygen maintaining spontaneous respirations. Intubation is performed with an ETT one or two sizes smaller than predicted, to decrease the risk of subglottic stenosis. Extubation is performed after an adequate air leak around the ETT is demonstrated.

F. Tracheobronchial Anomalies

1. Tracheomalacia

Tracheomalacia is characterized by weakness of the tracheal wall related to softness of the cartilaginous support. This allows the affected portion to collapse under conditions where the extraluminal pressure exceeds the intraluminal pressure.[367] Tracheomalacia may be classified into either congenital (primary) or acquired (secondary). *Congenital tracheomalacia* may be further subdivided into idiopathic or syndromic conditions. Tracheoesophageal fistula, CHARGE syndrome, and DiGeorge's syndrome are associated with congenital tracheomalacia. *Acquired tracheomalacia* is typically caused by extrinsic compression of great vessels or is secondary to bronchopulmonary dysplasia. Symptoms include episodic respiratory distress, persistent dry cough, wheezing, dysphagia, and recurrent respiratory infections. Failure to wean from the ventilator or failure of extubation may also be indicative of tracheomalacia.[367]

Airway Implications. Airway obstruction has been reported in patients with tracheomalacia during general anesthesia, even in asymptomatic patients.[368,369] Collapse of the affected segment occurs during expiration and with particularly forceful expiration or coughing. CPAP with or without intermittent positive-pressure ventilation (PPV) can alleviate the obstruction.[370] Noninvasive PPV through a face mask has been used successfully to prevent reintubation in an infant with tracheomalacia postoperatively.[371]

2. Croup

See previous discussion.

3. Bacterial Tracheitis

Bacterial tracheitis, formerly called *pseudomembranous tracheitis* or *membranous laryngotracheobronchitis*, is a potentially life-threatening disease. It is an infection of the subglottic region, and progression to full airway obstruction is possible. Bacterial tracheitis is believed to result from a bacterial superinfection preceded by a viral upper respiratory tract infection.[372] The peak incidence is in the fall and winter, affecting children from age 6 months to 8 years. *S. aureus, H. influenzae,* α-hemolytic *Streptococcus,* and group A *Streptococcus* are the usual causative agents. Patients usually present with a several

day history of viral upper respiratory symptoms followed by rapid deterioration. The patient develops high fever, respiratory distress, and a toxic appearance. In contrast to those with supraglottitis, these patients have a substantial cough, appear comfortable when supine, and tend not to drool.[351]

In contrast to those with laryngotracheobronchitis, patients with bacterial tracheitis do not respond to racemic epinephrine or corticosteroids. Radiographs of the airway often show irregular tracheal densities and subglottic narrowing.[372] Patients with severe respiratory distress should be taken to the OR for rigid endoscopy and intubation.

Airway Implications. Patients with bacterial tracheitis have the potential for airway obstruction. Preparations for management of the difficult pediatric airway must be made, including a rigid bronchoscope. Inhalation induction with maintenance of spontaneous respirations is preferred. Endoscopy is performed with removal of the sloughed mucosa. Intubation is performed, and specimens for culture and Gram stain are taken. Broad-spectrum antibiotics are started and continued for 10 to 14 days. Intubation is usually required for 3 to 7 days.[351]

4. Mediastinal Masses

Anesthesia for patients with mediastinal masses, usually *anterior* mediastinal masses, is associated with a high risk of airway obstruction, hemodynamic instability, or even death from extrinsic compression of three structures: the heart, great vessels (primarily superior vena cava), and the trachea and bronchi.[373] Induction of anesthesia and PPV may exacerbate the airway compression in a variety of ways. Loss of intrinsic muscle tone, reduced lung volumes, and a reduced transpleural pressure gradient combine to increase the effects of extrinsic compression. Cardiac arrest, superior vena cava syndrome, and airway occlusion are problems that can occur during induction of anesthesia.[374-376] Airway compression during induction of anesthesia can occur even in asymptomatic patients.[375] These complications may be unresponsive to position changes or open cardiac massage.

Mediastinal masses may be divided into anterosuperior, visceral, and posterior. The anatomic location of the mediastinal mass varies with age. In children, mediastinal masses are predominantly found in the *posterior* mediastinum. *Neurogenic tumors,* especially neuroblastomas, are the most common mediastinal tumor in young children. *Germ cell tumors* are the second most common anterior mediastinal mass in children. In adolescents, *lymphomas* are the most common anterior mediastinal mass.[373]

Symptoms such as orthopnea, stridor, and wheezing are ominous signs of airway obstruction.[377] Positional dyspnea, tachyarrhythmia, and syncope suggest right-sided heart and pulmonary vascular compression. Syncope during a Valsalva maneuver suggests significant vascular encroachment.[373] Children usually display symptoms earlier than adults. Small decreases in airway diameter result in increased resistance. Preoperative evaluation should focus on symptoms of respiratory compromise in the supine and standing positions. Intolerance of the supine position indicates compression by the mass on the trachea, heart, pulmonary artery, or superior vena cava. Preoperative CT scan should be obtained. Minimum criteria for safe administration of general anesthesia should be a tracheal cross-sectional area at least 50% of predicted and a peak expiratory flow rate at least 50% of predicted value.[378]

Airway Implications. Patients with a mediastinal mass are considered difficult to ventilate. Avoidance of general anesthesia, muscle relaxants, and PPV are the mainstay of anesthetic management for patients presenting for biopsy before irradiation or chemotherapy. Biopsies should be performed, if at all possible, under local anesthesia.[379] Ketamine, local anesthesia, and a 50:50 mixture of O_2 and nitrous oxide (N_2O) while maintaining spontaneous ventilation have been used successfully for a diagnostic biopsy in a 13-year-old patient.[380] Placing the patient in reverse Trendelenburg position may help.

With pediatric patients, general anesthesia may be needed for biopsy. Recommendations have been made for a rigid pediatric bronchoscopy and femoral-to-femoral bypass standby.[375,381] If possible, irradiation of the mass before general anesthesia may reduce the risk associated with anesthesia. Peripheral shielding of the mediastinum may allow subsequent tissue biopsy.[382] For older children, an awake fiberoptic intubation or FOB should be performed to assess the degree of obstruction after topicalization of the airway. In small infants and children, an awake intubation is not practical. In these patients, an inhalation induction with maintenance of spontaneous ventilation is recommended. Intravenous access must be obtained in a lower extremity before induction.[381] Induction of anesthesia in the lateral semi-Fowler position has been recommended.[376] Maintenance of spontaneous ventilation is vital; however, this is not foolproof.[383] Heliox (80% helium, 20% O_2) has been used for induction with sevoflurane and an LMA for successful airway management in a 3-year-old patient with severe respiratory distress related to a massive mediastinal mass.[384]

If airway obstruction or hemodynamic collapse occurs with induction, the following steps are suggested. First, one attempts to pass the ETT down the least obstructed bronchus. If passage of the ETT is not possible, rigid bronchoscopy to bypass the obstruction is attempted. Position changes to the lateral or prone position may alleviate the obstruction by changing the weight distribution of the tumor. Finally, cardiopulmonary bypass has been recommended.[375] Airway obstruction may occur during emergence as well. Extubation should be performed with the patient awake. These patients should be monitored postoperatively in the ICU.

5. Vascular Malformations

Vascular malformations result from abnormal development of the arterial component of the branchial arch system, resulting in complete or incomplete encirclement of the trachea or esophagus, or both.[385] In 1945, Gross[386] introduced the term *vascular ring* to describe this anomaly. Patients with vascular rings may present with symptoms of respiratory distress or dysphagia because of

tracheoesophageal compression. Patients may present with respiratory distress after birth or may be asymptomatic for life. Most children with vascular rings present with nonspecific symptoms such as stridor, dyspnea, cough, or recurrent respiratory tract infection.[387] Dysphagia is often the primary symptom in adults with vascular ring.[385] In a retrospective review of vascular rings, 74% of the malformations were symptomatic, with inspiratory stridor and wheezing as the main complaints.[387]

Various types of vascular rings have been described, including double aortic arch and right aortic arch with aberrant left subclavian artery. The *double aortic arch* usually arises earlier than other varieties requiring surgical correction.[385] Associated cardiac anomalies are often present with the vascular ring. Diagnosis is confirmed by radiologic studies. A chest radiograph may indicate the site of the ascending and descending aorta. A barium esophagogram may disclose extrinsic compression of the esophagus. Angiography has been considered the gold standard for identifying vascular rings. CT and MRI scans are able to assist in the diagnosis of vascular ring and determine the anatomy. The diagnosis of vascular ring may be delayed because of the nonspecific symptoms.[387] Patients who are symptomatic should undergo surgery. Surgical correction is by a left thoracotomy, right thoracotomy, or median sternotomy.[385]

Airway Implications. Patients with a vascular ring are at risk of airway obstruction from compression of the trachea. Tracheomalacia may be present as well. Maintenance of spontaneous ventilation until the trachea is intubated with a reinforced ETT may be beneficial. A rigid bronchoscope should be available to serve as an airway stent in the event of airway collapse.

6. Foreign Body Aspiration

Foreign body aspiration is a cause of significant morbidity and mortality in the pediatric population. Young children are at increased risk for foreign body aspiration, with children less than 2 years old most often affected.[388] A second peak of aspiration occurs between ages 10 and 11 years.[389] Most of the deaths occur in children younger than 1 year. The objects most frequently aspirated are food products. There is only a slight propensity for the object to lodge on the right side because of symmetrical bronchial angles in children under 15 years old. The left main stem bronchus is displaced by the aortic knob by age 15, creating a more obtuse angle at the carina.[390]

Witnessed events are easier to diagnose. A history of choking, gagging, or coughing is usually given. Patients may be asymptomatic at the time or may develop symptoms of acute distress. A persistent cough, wheezing, or recurrent pneumonia may be the initial sign if the aspiration occurred in the past. The American Academy of Pediatrics has developed guidelines for the management of choking episodes. For children under 1 year, back blows and abdominal thrusts with the child in a head-down position are recommended. The Heimlich maneuver is reserved for older children and adults.[391]

Classically, peanuts should be removed promptly because of the inflammatory reaction to the peanut oil.

Emergency removal is indicated if the patient is in distress or if the foreign body is in a precarious location. If the patient is stable, radiographs may be taken to assist in localizing and identifying the foreign body. If the foreign body is radiopaque, it is easily identified. Radiolucent foreign bodies may demonstrate soft tissue density in or narrowing of the airway.[13] Indirect signs of air trapping, mediastinal shift, or atelectasis may be present. Lateral decubitus films are helpful in infants and younger children because they cannot cooperate with expiratory films.[390] The downside lung should be deflated unless it is obstructed with a foreign body.[389]

Airway Implications. In general, inhalation induction *without* cricoid pressure is the favored technique for removal of foreign bodies in the airway, regardless of the type of object, according to a postal survey of members of the Society for Pediatric Anesthesia.[388] (For foreign bodies in the upper esophagus, a rapid-sequence induction without cricoid pressure was the preferred technique, whereas for objects in the lower esophagus and stomach, a rapid-sequence induction *with* cricoid pressure was chosen.) Cricoid pressure may cause harm if the foreign body is sharp or positioned in the larynx. If the case is not an emergency, one can wait until the appropriate nothing-by-mouth time has passed. In a retrospective review of anesthetic management for tracheobronchial foreign body removal, neither spontaneous nor controlled ventilation was associated with an increased incidence of adverse events.[392]

With an inhalation induction, a prolonged induction may occur because of airway obstruction. CPAP at 5 to 10 cm H$_2$O and assisted ventilation may be needed at times to maintain a patent airway. After an adequate level of anesthesia is obtained, topicalization of the airway may decrease the incidence of coughing or laryngospasm. Use of a ventilating rigid bronchoscope allows ventilation during the procedure. High oxygen flow rates may be needed to overcome the presence of an air leak around the FOB. Communication between the anesthesiologist and the endoscopist is crucial because this is a shared airway. The patient may require intermittent ventilation if desaturation occurs during the FOB. When the foreign body is grasped, the glottis should be relaxed for removal. Short-acting muscle relaxants, propofol, or deeper inhalational anesthesia may be used. The forceps and the bronchoscope are removed from the trachea as a single unit.[354] Dislodgement of foreign bodies at the glottic or subglottic area has been reported.[393] If a foreign body is dislodged and obstructs the trachea, the bronchoscope must be used to push the foreign body into a main stem bronchus to enable ventilation of one lung. FOB with tracheotomy removal of a bronchial foreign body has been used successfully to remove an object that was too large to pass through the subglottis.[394]

When the foreign body is removed, the patient is usually intubated with an appropriate-size ETT. Depending on the amount of edema from the procedure, the patient should be able to be extubated. Postoperatively, racemic epinephrine (0.5 mL of 2.25% solution in 3 mL of saline) may be used for stridor. Dexamethasone is often given for edema.

7. Other Tracheal Disease

Tracheal stenosis is congenital or acquired. *Congenital* stenosis may be associated with congenital airway malformations such as tracheoesophageal fistula, hypoplastic lungs, and tracheomalacia. Congenital complete *tracheal rings* are also a cause of tracheal stenosis. In this condition, the rings are fused posteriorly and there is no posterior membranous wall. *Acquired* stenosis is usually attributed to prolonged intubation, inhalational injuries, trauma, or tumors. Symptoms include stridor, wheezing, croup, tachypnea, and cough. For mild lesions, conservative therapy is warranted. Surgical treatment involves tracheal resection with primary reanastomosis for short-segment lesions. Anterotracheal split procedures may be used for longer segmental lesions. Laser excision of granulation tissue at the repair site may be needed.[276]

Airway Implications. Tracheal stenosis may cause difficulty with ventilation or ETT advancement. Minimal trauma to the airway can lead to acute airway obstruction.[276] Use of an LMA has been described in two patients with subglottic stenosis in whom the stenotic areas were 2 mm or less.[395,396] Passage of the rigid bronchoscope should be performed only at definitive repair.

G. Cervical Spine Anomalies

1. Limited Cervical Spine Mobility

Limited cervical spine mobility may be caused by congenital or acquired disorders. The two congenital disorders that limit the mobility of the cervical spine are Klippel-Feil syndrome and Goldenhar's syndrome.

a. KLIPPEL-FEIL SYNDROME

Klippel-Feil syndrome is characterized by fusion of two or more cervical vertebrae. Other features include short neck, a low posterior hairline, scoliosis, and congenital heart disease.[397] Difficulty with airway management usually arises in the latter half of the first decade of life. The degree of difficulty with airway management depends on the severity of neck fixation.

b. GOLDENHAR'S SYNDROME

See under "Mandibular Hypoplasia."

c. JUVENILE RHEUMATOID ARTHRITIS

Juvenile rheumatoid arthritis is a chronic arthritis with variable manifestations. Several different subgroups of disease have been identified: systemic onset (Still's disease), polyarticular, and oligoarticular (see under "Facial Anomalies: Maxillary and Mandibular Disease").

d. AIRWAY IMPLICATIONS

Careful preoperative evaluation of patients with limited cervical mobility must be done before anesthetic induction. Previous anesthetic records, if available, should be reviewed for any relevant information. Because a DA is presumed to exist, preparation for management of the difficult pediatric airway must be made. In cases of limited cervical mobility, the ability to align the oral, pharyngeal, and laryngeal axes for visualization of the glottis is impaired. The presence of TMJ involvement may limit mouth opening as well. Awake endotracheal intubation is recommended in this scenario. Many techniques are available for use, including FOB, Bullard laryngoscope, retrograde wire technique, and lightwand. This may not be suitable in younger patients. For patients who will not cooperate with an awake technique, a mask induction with 100% O_2 and spontaneous ventilation is indicated. Retrograde intubation, suspension laryngoscopy, and fiberoptic intubation through the LMA have all been reported in pediatric patients with Goldenhar's syndrome.[77, 97, 398] The lightwand was used to intubate an 18-day-old infant with right hemifacial microsomia.[42]

2. Congenital Cervical Spine Instability

Cervical spine instability, if unrecognized, is a potential cause of serious morbidity and even mortality during airway management. Cervical spine instability or subluxation most often involves the atlanto-occipital joint. Congenital syndromes such as trisomy 21, Hurler's syndrome, Hunter's syndrome, and Morquio's syndrome are associated with cervical spine instability.[399] Of these, trisomy 21 is the syndrome most often encountered by anesthesiologists.

a. DOWN SYNDROME

Trisomy 21 (Down syndrome) occurs in approximately 1 of every 660 live births. Mental retardation, congenital heart disease, OSA, and congenital subglottic stenosis may be present. Approximately 20% of patients have ligamentous laxity of the atlantoaxial joint, which may allow atlantoaxial instability. This may predispose them to cervical spinal cord compression. Children are at risk for injury during hyperextension, hyperflexion, or increased rotation of the neck.[275,400] Signs of cervical spinal cord compression include loss of ambulatory function, spasticity, hyperreflexia of the lower extremities, extensor plantar reflexes, and loss of bowel and bladder control. Other signs may include increased fatigue with walking and torticollis.[400] Preoperative evaluation of the patient with Down syndrome must attempt to discover any preexisting signs or symptoms of spinal cord compression. The issue of screening for atlantoaxial instability in patients with Down syndrome is controversial. The American Academy of Pediatrics Committee on Sports Medicine and Fitness decided that the value of cervical spine radiographs is uncertain in screening for possible catastrophic neck injury in athletes with Down syndrome.[400] However, Pueschel[401] argued that patients should be screened for atlantoaxial instability. A survey of the Society of Pediatric Anesthesia found that members obtain preoperative radiographs (18%) or subspecialty consultation (8%), or both, for asymptomatic patients. For symptomatic patients, radiographs and preoperative consultations are obtained 64% and 74% of the time, respectively. The majority of respondents attempt to maintain the head in a neutral position for both symptomatic and asymptomatic patients.[402]

Airway Implications. Airway management for patients with Down syndrome should consider the possibility of cervical spine instability with cord compression. In addition, the large tongue and potential for OSA can lead to upper airway obstruction. Patients who have symptoms of cord compression should have radiographic evaluation before any elective surgical procedure. Lateral extension and flexion radiographs of the upper cervical spine can reveal atlantoaxial subluxation. An odontoid process (axis) to anterior arch (atlas) distance greater than 4.5 mm indicates abnormal instability.[400]

For emergency surgery, cervical spine precautions should be used in patients who are symptomatic. In-line stabilization of the cervical spine for direct laryngoscopy should be used. Techniques for airway management that require minimal neck movement may be useful (e.g., Truview or Bullard laryngoscope, lightwand, angulated video laryngoscope, SOS).

3. Acquired Cervical Spine Instability

Acquired cervical spine instability in pediatric patients can result from multiple trauma or head and neck trauma. Any pediatric patient with a severe head injury should be treated as though a cervical spine injury is present.[403] An estimated 1% to 2% of pediatric patients with multiple trauma have a cervical injury.[391] Pediatric patients with underlying medical conditions such as Down syndrome may be more susceptible to cervical cord injury.[391] Pediatric patients less than 8 years old are at increased risk for injury to the upper cervical spine and craniovertebral junction. Only 30% of cervical injuries occur below C3 in children younger than 8. They also have a higher incidence of *spinal cord injury without radiographic abnormality* (SCIWORA).[404] Immobilization of a patient with suspected cervical injury is crucial so that further damage to the cord is prevented. A hard collar, spine board, and soft spacing devices between the head and securing straps are needed. The occiput is large, and a blanket under the torso allows the neck to rest in a neutral position.

Airway Implications. The choice of airway management depends on the degree of urgency associated with the intubation. Techniques that minimize head extension and cervical flexion are mandatory. Trauma patients are considered at risk for aspiration, and appropriate measures need to be taken.

For an urgent airway in a patient with a DA or facial fractures, a surgical airway may be the best option. If time allows, a limited number of attempts at direct laryngoscopy may be performed. The Truview or Bullard laryngoscope may be useful in this situation. In an emergency, the LMA may be used to ventilate or oxygenate the patient until a formal airway is established. This does not provide protection against aspiration.

For a nonurgent intubation, further evaluation of the cervical spine is warranted. When the cervical spine has been "cleared" by the neurosurgeon or trauma surgeon, a rapid-sequence induction with cricoid pressure may be performed after adequate preoxygenation if the airway appears reasonable. If the cervical spine is unstable, a rapid-sequence induction with cricoid pressure may be performed with in-line stabilization. Fluoroscopy was used to assist the intubation of an 11-year-old patient with an unstable subluxation of C1-C2 after a motor vehicle crash.[405] Awake techniques such as flexible fiberoptic laryngoscopy, Bullard laryngoscope, lightwand, SOS, or retrograde intubation may be indicated if the patient has an unstable cervical spine and a DA.

X. PEDIATRIC TRAUMA

All pediatric trauma patients are considered to have a cervical spine injury until proved otherwise. In addition, these patients are at risk for aspiration. Oxygen should be administered and ventilation assisted if needed as soon as possible. Trauma patients should be immobilized on a spine board with a rigid collar as previously described. After an evaluation of the airway, one should decide on the method of intubation. If the airway is judged to be adequate, a rapid-sequence induction with cricoid pressure and manual in-line stabilization should be employed. If the airway cannot be secured, the ASA DA algorithm should be followed. In a DA scenario, one of the previously described awake techniques may be used. In certain cases, awake tracheostomy or surgical cricothyrotomy may be indicated. A multidisciplinary approach to the management of the difficult pediatric trauma airway is necessary.

XI. EXTUBATION OF THE DIFFICULT AIRWAY

The management of the difficult pediatric airway does not end until the plan for extubation has been established. Choices include extubation over an airway catheter or guidewire or extubation when an air leak develops, as with epiglottitis. Preparations for the difficult pediatric airway must be made because an extubation may lead to a reintubation. If airway edema is suspected at the end of the surgery, because of either the intubation process or the surgery, dexamethasone may be of benefit. Postoperative ventilation may be indicated as well until the edema resolves. Extubation has been successfully performed over an airway exchange catheter in an adolescent with a DA.[406] Alternatively, a 0.018-inch guidewire has been used to maintain airway access in a 2-year-old child with severe micrognathia and tetralogy of Fallot.[407]

XII. CONCLUSIONS

Unexpected difficulties with airway management in otherwise healthy children are rare after exclusion of predictors of difficult intubation, such as mandibular hypoplasia, limited mouth opening, and facial asymmetry, including abnormalities of the ear, syndromes, obstructive sleep apnea syndrome, and stridor. Difficulties that occur are probably a result of inexperience or inadequate supervision and lack of pediatric airway training. Thorough preoperative assessment and anticipation of airway difficulties, as well as education, continuous training, and regular practice in basic airway management, are necessary to reduce the incidence of pediatric airway difficulties. Besides inexperience with the pediatric airway, most morbidity and mortality in pediatric airway management is attributed to a failure to recognize and overcome functional airway problems because of insufficient depth of anesthesia or muscle paralysis, and not to a failure to intubate.

XIII. CLINICAL PEARLS

- The pediatric airway anatomy is different in children. Their larynx is located higher in the neck with a relatively larger tongue; they have a differently shaped epiglottis; and the vocal cords are angled.

- The newborn rib cage is oriented parallel, and the intercostal muscles are not as effective at increasing intrathoracic volume with inspiration.

- The work of breathing for each kilogram of body weight is similar in infants and adults.

- The oxygen consumption of a full-term newborn (6 mL/kg/min) is twice that of an adult (3 mL/kg/min), which results in increased respiratory rate.

- The infant's tidal volume is relatively fixed.

- Minute alveolar ventilation is more dependent on increased respiratory rate than on tidal volume.

- Functional residual capacity of an infant is similar to FRC of an adult when normalized to body weight, because the ratio of alveolar minute ventilation to FRC is doubled (with hypoxia or apnea or under anesthesia), the infant's FRC is diminished, and desaturation occurs more precipitously.

- In infants, most airflow resistance occurs in the bronchial and small airways.

- Resistance to airflow is inversely proportional to the radius of the lumen to the fourth power for laminar flow, and to the radius of the fifth power (r^5) for turbulent flow.

- Radiographic evaluation may be extremely helpful to diagnose a difficult airway.

- Radiographs of the upper airway (AP and lateral films, fluoroscopy) may show site and cause of airway obstruction.

- When necessary, MRI and CT provide more detailed information if time permits.

SELECTED REFERENCES

All references can be found online at expertconsult.com.

3. Morray JP, Geiduschel JM, Ramamoorthy C, et al: Anesthesia-related cardiac arrest in children. *Anesthesiology* 93:6–14, 2000.
4. Coté CJ, Todres ID: The pediatric airway. In Coté CJ, Todres ID, Goudsouzian NG, Ryan JF, editors: *A practice of anesthesia for infants and children*, ed 3, Philadelphia, 2001, Saunders.
9. Kopp VJ, Bailey A, Valley RD, et al: Utility of the Mallampati classification for predicting difficult intubation in pediatric patients. *Anesthesiology* 83:A1147, 1995.
14. American Academy of Pediatrics, Section on Anesthesiology: Guidelines for the pediatric perioperative anesthesia environment. *Pediatrics* 103:512–515, 1999.
16. Frei FJ, aWengen D, Rutishauser GE, et al: The airway endoscopy mask: useful device for fiberoptic evaluation and intubation of the paediatric airway. *Paediatr Anaesth* 5:319–324, 1995.

22. Khine HH, Corddry DH, Kettrick RG, et al: Comparison of cuffed and uncuffed endotracheal tubes in young children during general anesthesia. *Anesthesiology* 86:627–631, 1997.

52. Ellis DS, Potluri PK, O'Flaherty JE, et al: Difficult airway management in the neonate: a simple method of intubating through a laryngeal mask airway. *Paediatr Anaesth* 9:460–462, 1999.

76. Bonfils P: Schwierge Intubation bei Pierre Robin–Kindern, eine neue Methode: Der retromolare Weg. *Anaesthesist* 32:363–367, 1983.

256. Crosby ET, Cooper RM, Douglas MJ, et al: The unanticipated difficult airway with recommendations for management. *Can J Anaesth* 45:757–776, 1998.

273. Henriksson TG, Skoog VT: Identification of children at high anaesthetic risk at the time of primary palatoplasty. *Scand J Plast Reconstr Surg Hand Surg* 35:177–182, 2001.

Chapter 37

The Difficult Airway in Obstetric Anesthesia

MAYA S. SURESH | ASHUTOSH WALI

I. INTRODUCTION

Difficult laryngoscopy, failed intubation, and inability to ventilate or oxygenate after induction of general anesthesia (GA) for cesarean delivery (C/D) are major contributory factors leading to maternal morbidity and mortality. In Western countries, the recognition of adverse maternal and neonatal outcomes associated with difficult airway (DA) management has led to a dramatic decline in the use of GA for both elective and emergency C/D.[1-3]

The overall general anesthesiology practice in industrialized countries in the last 2 decades has undergone a dramatic change. Management of the DA has emerged as one of the most important patient safety issues. Guidelines and strategies for management of the DA have been published by the American Society of Anesthesiologists (ASA),[4] the Difficult Airway Society (DAS) in the United Kingdom,[5] and the Canadian,[6] French[7] and Italian[8] national societies' work groups on difficult airway management. These guidelines are applicable to the general surgical population. However, none of the guidelines address management of the DA in an obstetric situation, especially in the context of urgency in delivering the baby.

There are differences among these standards, guidelines, algorithms, recommendations, and protocols, but in practice and in medicolegal cases, the distinction between terminologies can be blurred (Table 37-1).[9] Published literature shows that the guidelines from the ASA Task Force on Management of the Difficult Airway have been discussed in 18% of nonobstetric medicolegal cases and were useful both in defending care (defense, 8%) and in criticizing care (plaintiff, 3%).[10] Expert witnesses also have used these guidelines in litigated obstetric DA management cases.

II. DEFINITIONS

There is no consensus on a standard definition of the DA in the literature. The ASA Task Force defined DA as a clinical situation in which a conventionally trained anesthesiologist experiences difficulty with face mask ventilation, difficulty with intubation, or both. The original ASA description of difficult intubation (DI) included a limit of 10 minutes or multiple attempts. The wisdom of this definition must be questioned in obstetrics especially, given the fact that GA is generally reserved for emergency C/D in which delivery of the baby is of the utmost urgency. The common practice in obstetric anesthesia is to use a single dose of succinylcholine when anesthetizing for C/D under GA. In the obstetric situation, *difficult intubation* is the inability of an experienced anesthesiologist to intubate within one dose of succinylcholine.[11] A more apt definition of *failed intubation* in obstetric patients is inability to secure the airway with two attempts using a conventional laryngoscope or an alternative airway device to assist with tracheal intubation.

III. ANESTHESIA-RELATED MATERNAL MORTALITY

Although the total number of maternal deaths has been decreasing steadily in the last few decades both in the United States and United Kingdom (Table 37-2),[12,13] anesthesia-related complications rank seventh among the leading causes of maternal death, in both countries (Fig. 37-1).[14,15] Even in the developing countries, anesthesia is emerging as an additional risk for maternal mortality and remains largely under-reported.[16,17] Failures in airway management are a primary cause of anesthesia-related maternal deaths in the underdeveloped countries.[18]

The first national study of anesthesia-related maternal mortality in the United States between 1979 and 1990 was published in 1997.[19] Most of these deaths (82%) took place during C/D. Death rates for GA during C/D increased from 20 per million in 1979-1984 to 32.3 per million in 1985-1990. Conversely, the death rate for regional anesthesia (RA) during the same periods declined from 8.6 to 1.9 per million, respectively. The relative risk for GA increased to 16.7 from 1985 to 1990. The case fatality risk ratio for GA was. 2.3 times that of RA from 1979 to 1984 and increased to 16.7 times from 1985 to 1990.[19] The majority of maternal deaths were related to difficult or failed intubation, pulmonary aspiration, or respiratory complications.

A follow-up study examined 12 years of anesthesia-related maternal deaths between 1991 and 2002 and

TABLE 37-1

Definition of Terms and Degree of Obligation

Terms	Definitions	Degree of Obligation
Standards	Generally accepted principles for patient management; exceptions are rare, and failure to follow is often difficult to justify	Mandatory
Strategy	A well-planned series of steps for achieving a goal	Voluntary
Guidelines	Systematically developed statements to assist practitioners for specific clinical circumstances; incorporates the best scientific evidence with expert opinion	Voluntary
Practice policies	Describe present recommendations issued to influence practitioners in reaching decisions about interventions	Voluntary
Recommendations	Suitable and useful strategy; not as strict as standards or guidelines	Voluntary
Options	Different possibilities are available; neutral assessment	Voluntary
Protocols and algorithms	Stepwise procedures or decision trees to guide practitioners through diagnosis and treatment of various clinical problems	Voluntary

From Henderson JJ, Popat MT, Latto IP, Pearce AC: Difficult Airway Society guidelines for management of the unanticipated difficult intubation. *Anaesthesia* 59:675–694, 2004.

Anesthesia-Related Maternal Deaths in the United States and United Kingdom, 1979-2001

Year of Death	United States*	United Kingdom†
1979-1981	4.3	8.7
1982-1984	3.3	7.2
1985-1987	2.3	1.9
1988-1990	1.7	1.7
1991-1993	1.4	3.5
1994-1996	1.1	0.5
1997-1999	1.2	1.4
2000-2002	1.0	3.0

*Maternal deaths per million live births.
†Maternal deaths per million maternities (live births, stillbirths, pregnancy terminations, ectopic pregnancies, and abortions).
(From Hawkins JL, Chang J, Palmer SK, et al: Anesthesia-related maternal mortality in the United States: 1979-2002. *Obstet Gynecol* 117:71, 2011.)

compared them with data from 1979 to 1990 to estimate trends over time and to compare the risks of GA and RA during cesarean delivery.[13] Results showed that 86 pregnancy-related deaths were associated with complications of anesthesia, accounting for 1.6% of the total. Case-fatality rates for GA declined from 16.8 per million in 1991-1996 to 6.5 per million in 1997-2002 (Table 37-3).

Complications related to anesthesia still occur, despite the decrease of almost 60% in anesthesia-related maternal mortality between 1979-1990 and 1991-2002. Although deaths from GA during C/D declined, about two thirds of the anesthesia-related deaths were caused by intubation failure or induction problems.[13] The decline in GA-related case fatalities was explained by improvements in management of the DA and failed intubation and by increased expertise of anesthesiologists with the laryngeal mask airway (LMA) and other airway devices.[13]

A review of maternal mortality in Michigan from 1985 to 2003 identified eight anesthesia-related deaths.[20] Seven of these deaths were due to anesthesia-related factors. Interestingly, there were no deaths during induction of GA. The deaths were caused by airway obstruction or hypoventilation during emergence, lapses in monitoring, or lack of supervision in the postoperative period. Other risk factors included African-American race and obesity. This study highlighted the importance of airway-related problems during emergence, particularly in obese patients and in the African-American population, as well as the importance of vigilance in monitoring and management in the postoperative period for prevention of airway-related complications.

In the United Kingdom, despite the decline in the total number of maternal deaths, anesthesia-related causes consistently accounted for approximately 10% of the total direct deaths. During the period 1982-1984, anesthesia was the third leading cause of maternal death, resulting in 19 of 243 deaths, of which 15 were due to airway-related difficulties.[21] The confidential enquiry spanning 1994-1996 showed that anesthesia was responsible for only 1 of 268 maternal deaths. In the Confidential Enquiry into Maternal and Child Health (CEMACH) 2000-2002 study, there were six direct deaths, all related to GA.[15] Maternal deaths from complications of GA included a risk of 1 maternal death in 20,000. These

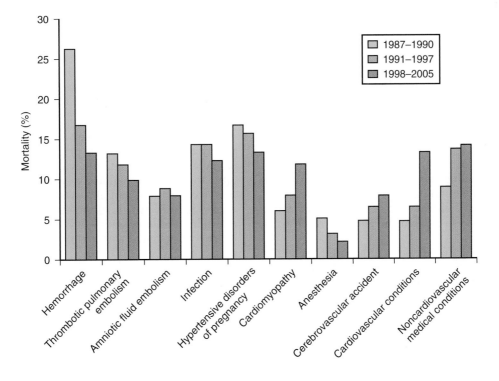

Figure 37-1 Maternal mortality in the United States. (From Berg CJ, Callaghan WM, Syverson C, Henderson Z: Pregnancy-related mortality in the United States, 1998 to 2005. *Obstet Gynecol* 116:1302–1309, 2010.)

TABLE 37-3

Case-Fatality Rates and Rate Ratios of Anesthesia-Related Deaths during Cesarean Delivery by Type of Anesthesia, United States, 1979-2002

Year of Death	CASE-FATALITY RATES*		Rate Ratio (95% Confidence Interval)
	General Anesthesia	Regional Anesthesia	
1979-1984	20.0	8.6	2.3 (1.9-2.9)
1985-1990	32.3	1.9	16.7 (12.9-21.8)
1991-1996	16.8	2.5	6.7 (3.0-14.9)
1997-2002	6.5	3.8	1.7 (0.6-4.6)

*Deaths per million general or regional anesthesias.
From Hawkins JL, Chang J, Palmer SK, et al: Anesthesia-related maternal mortality in the United States: 1979-2002. *Obstet Gynecol* 117:71, Table 3, 2011.

cardiopulmonary arrests and deaths were related to difficult or failed intubation, difficult pulmonary ventilation resulting in failure to oxygenate, pulmonary aspiration, or acute respiratory distress syndrome (ARDS). In all of these cases, the anesthesia care was considered substandard.[15]

IV. OBSTETRIC ANESTHESIA CLOSED CLAIMS STUDIES

The 2009 closed claims study published in the United States revealed that obstetric anesthesia claims for injuries from 1990 to 2003 had declined compared with claims for injuries before 1990.[1] In the period 1990-2003, the proportion of maternal death or brain damage and that of newborn death or brain damage decreased. Respiratory causes of injuries also decreased, from 24% to 4% in claims from 1990 or later. Claims related to inadequate oxygenation or ventilation and those related to aspiration also decreased.

Despite the decrease in claims, one of the most common anesthesia-related causes of maternal death or damage associated with GA was difficult tracheal intubation. Airway-related claims involved multiple attempts at tracheal intubation leading to progressive difficulty with ventilation. In two of the claims, tracheal intubation was assessed to be difficult preoperatively with a backup plan to awaken the patient and perform fiberoptic intubation. However, progressive airway difficulties occurred while attempts were made to awaken the patients, resulting in adverse outcomes.

The number of claims related to difficult tracheal intubation after 1990, compared with pre-1990 claims, was unchanged.[1] However, the overall improvement in closed claims statistics and the decline in anesthesia-related maternal mortality in more recent years were probably attributable to implementation of a minimum standard of care requiring the use of respiratory system monitors (pulse oximetry and capnography) during anesthesia in modern practice, enhanced awareness of the risk of pulmonary aspiration of gastric contents in the obstetric patient, decreased use of GA in obstetric practice, and use of advanced airway management techniques.

V. WHY IS ADVANCED AIRWAY MANAGEMENT IMPORTANT?

There have been tremendous advances in airway management in recent years, including an explosion in the use of airway devices as adjuncts to airway management. There has been a vast increase in the body of knowledge and in publications worldwide in this field. Improvements in advanced airway management have led to a documented decline in the incidence of airway-related perioperative morbidity in the surgical population.[22] Similarly, in the last 2 decades, anesthesiologists' focus on improving management of the DA and of failed intubation, experience with the LMA, application of the ASA difficult airway algorithm (DAA), and advanced airway management strategies have helped decrease GA-related case fatalities in obstetric cases.[13]

Because GA for cesarean delivery is frequently reserved for true emergencies, these high-level stress situations may lead to inadequate airway assessment or preparation, which can contribute to the risk of difficult or failed tracheal intubation, leading to the possibility of morbidity and mortality in both mother and baby.

Because the medical-legal liability associated with airway-related adverse maternal outcomes is high,[1] it is essential that all those practicing obstetric anesthesia as part of airway management should do the following:

1. Assess risk factors that predispose to airway-related complications
2. Be cognizant of predictors of the DA
3. Have appropriate algorithms and airway devices and equipment immediately available in the labor and delivery suite and in the operating room to manage the DA
4. Have an airway rescue plan, within the framework of the ASA DAA, for managing the DA
5. Be cognizant of the twin goals of urgently delivering the baby and preventing pulmonary aspiration, which can be hard to balance
6. Acquire and maintain advanced airway management skills.

A heightened awareness of the difficult obstetric airway among all anesthesia practitioners and use of video laryngoscopes, alternative devices to assist with tracheal intubation, and supraglottic devices as a bridge to ventilation, oxygenation, and airway management may further minimize or even help eliminate airway-related maternal morbidity and mortality. Unfortunately, there is a learning curve associated with acquiring these advanced airway skills.

VI. RISK ASSESSMENT

Anatomic and physiologic factors alter the airway during pregnancy, placing the parturient at risk for difficult laryngoscopy, difficult tracheal intubation, and difficult mask ventilation (DMV). There is no single factor that explains the high incidence of failed tracheal intubation and respiratory-related injury in obstetrics. Difficult laryngoscopy or DMV may be related to excessive weight gain and upper airway edema during pregnancy, compounded by breast enlargement and by additional changes in preeclampsia. Rapid onset of hypoxemia associated with DA may be caused by respiratory changes, cardiovascular impairment from aortocaval compression, gastrointestinal changes placing the parturient at risk for pulmonary aspiration, and acute respiratory distress syndrome secondary to respiratory-related complications.

A. Airway

Airway changes occur during pregnancy, labor, and delivery.[23] Further, the incidence of Mallampati (MP) class III and class IV scores increases during labor compared with the prelabor period, and these changes are not reversed by 48 hours after delivery. Therefore, it is absolutely necessary to examine the airway of a parturient in labor before administering anesthesia for a cesarean delivery.[24]

An increase in the ground substance of the airway connective tissue, caused by elevated levels of estrogen during pregnancy, an increase in total body water, and an increase in interstitial fluid and blood volume, results in hypervascularity and edema of oropharynx, nasopharynx, and respiratory tract. Excessive weight gain during pregnancy, preeclampsia, iatrogenic fluid overload, excessive bearing-down efforts during labor, and increase in venous pressure all lead to increased upper airway mucosal edema. Additional upper airway changes include tongue engorgement during pregnancy, which leads to decreased mobility of the floor of the mouth and changes in the MP score.[25] Several published reports have described development of airway edema during labor and delivery, in preeclampsia, and after massive fluid and blood transfusion resuscitation following postpartum hemorrhage.[26-30] In some of these reports, the associated difficulties in tracheal intubation were secondary to changes in the MP score.

Because of the increased vascularity and engorgement of the mucosa, the parturient is at increased risk for epistaxis after manipulation of the nasopharynx with nasotracheal intubation and for swelling of the airway and is vulnerable to increased trauma with repeated attempts at intubation.[31] Avoidance of manipulation of the nasopharynx, use of smaller-sized tracheal tubes, and strict adherence to no more than two attempts at tracheal intubation[32] are vital measures to avoid airway-related trauma, complications, and catastrophes.

B. Respiratory Changes

The enlargement of the uterus during the course of pregnancy causes a 25% decrease in expiratory reserve volume and a 15% decrease in residual volume, resulting in an overall 20% decrease in functional residual capacity (FRC). In the supine position, the FRC is 70% of its normal capacity measured in the upright position. The supine position, particularly in an obese parturient, can result in airway closure and an increase in the alveolar-arterial gradient during normal tidal respiration, predisposing the parturient to lower partial pressure of oxygen. At the same time, oxygen consumption is increased by 20% secondary to the metabolic needs of the growing fetus, uterus, and placenta. The increase in oxygen consumption, along with decreased FRC, places the parturient at increased risk for hypoxemia and its consequent adverse neurologic effects (brain death), especially during DI, failed intubation, and DMV.

C. Cardiovascular Changes

The gravid uterus compresses the inferior vena cava in the supine position, resulting in a decrease in venous return and cardiac output. The reduction in cardiac output, together with elevated oxygen consumption, can further decrease oxygen saturation. The decrease in cardiac output and the ensuing hypoxemia during a "cannot intubate, cannot ventilate" (CICV) situation predisposes the mother to myocardial hypoxemia, cardiovascular arrest, and compromised uteroplacental perfusion, which can also place the fetus' well-being at risk. Maintaining left uterine tilt, establishing an airway with adequate ventilation and oxygenation in a timely manner, maintaining adequate perfusion in mother and baby, and ensuring cardiovascular stability become extremely important to ensure a safe outcome for both mother and bady.

D. Gastrointestinal Changes

Other risk factors include pregnancy-related hormonal, anatomic, and physiologic gastrointestinal changes that place the parturient at risk for gastric regurgitation and pulmonary aspiration during GA. The gravid uterus shifts the stomach cephalad and changes the angle of the gastroesophageal junction, resulting in incompetence of the gastroesophageal pinchcock mechanism. The lower esophageal tone is decreased, leading to increased gastric reflux. There is a progesterone-mediated smooth muscle relaxant effect on the gastrointestinal mucosa. Furthermore, gastric emptying is prolonged during labor. Therefore, the parturient is at risk for gastric regurgitation, active vomiting, and pulmonary aspiration during GA, in case of a DA, or during failed intubation. Aspiration-related deaths during pregnancy occur from complications associated with induction problems such as DI, esophageal intubation, and inadequate attempts at ventilation.[12]

E. Obesity

Weight gain during pregnancy results from the increasing size of the uterus and fetus, increased blood and interstitial fluid volumes, and deposition of new fat. There is a correlation between weight gain and an increase in the MP score.[30] Pregnancy also results in a significant increase in breast size and engorgement. In the supine position, the enlarged breasts can encroach into the neck area, impeding effective application of cricoid pressure and leading to difficulty with laryngoscope blade insertion.

Obesity has reached epidemic proportions in the United States, and the incidence of obesity in pregnancy has doubled in the last 10 years. A body mass index (BMI) greater than 25 kg/m^2 is considered overweight, and a BMI greater than 30 kg/m^2 is considered obese.[33] In the nonobstetric population, a BMI greater than

26 kg/m^2 results in a threefold increased incidence of DMV and a 10-fold increased incidence of difficult tracheal intubation.[34,35] Both prepregnancy obesity and excessive weight gain during pregnancy are associated with comorbidities such as hypertension or preeclampsia with intrauterine growth retardation, diabetes and macrosomia, and dysfunctional labor, thus increasing the incidence of operative cesarean delivery. The incidence of postpartum hemorrhage is higher in these patients, leading to increased likelihood of a GA intervention.

Because weight gain and obesity are associated with an increase in the MP score, the incidence of a partially obliterated oropharyngeal space in an obese parturient is doubled compared with that in nonpregnant patients. The aforementioned changes, the breast engorgement, and anthropometric differences between patients create a risk for difficult laryngoscopy, DI, and DMV.[30,36,37] DI is encountered more frequently in morbidly obese parturients weighing more than 130 kg.[38] Mask ventilation tends to be difficult because of low chest wall compliance and increased intra-abdominal pressure. In obesity, the respiratory-related changes of pregnancy are even more significant, with a marked decrease in FRC such that the closing capacity exceeds the FRC during tidal breathing, leading to a decrease in arterial oxygen tension and predisposing the parturient to a much higher risk of hypoxemia during a DI or DMV encounter. Obesity compounds all the risk factors associated with normal pregnancy, including DA, difficult laryngoscopy, DI, DMV, and aspiration-related complications.

In the obese parturient, a thorough preoperative assessment, a review of comorbidities, and a previous anesthetic history for difficulty with tracheal intubation are essential to allow for proper preparation and appropriate interventions. Placing the obese parturient in the so-called ramped position before induction of GA is critical to facilitate ventilation and improve laryngoscopic visualization of the glottis for intubation. The aim is to achieve the best alignment of the three axes (oral, pharyngeal, and laryngeal) in obese patients, thereby enhancing the success rate of intubation at the first attempt.

VII. INCIDENCE OF DIFFICULT OR FAILED INTUBATION IN OBSTETRICS

In 1998, the incidence of difficult laryngoscopy or tracheal intubation in the nonobstetric population was 0.1% to 13%.[39] In the obstetric population, the incidence of difficult tracheal intubation was found to be 1/250[40] to 1/280,[41] 1/300,[42] and 1/750.[36]

A review of GA for cesarean deliveries from 1990 to 1995 showed the incidence of difficult tracheal intubation to range from a high of 16.3% to a low of 1.3%.[2] There was a sentinel CICV incidence of 1 in 536 cases; in this patient, multiple attempts at intubation, unsuccessful mask ventilation, failed Combitube placement, and unsuccessful cricothyroidotomy resulted in cardiopulmonary arrest followed by surgical tracheostomy. Resuscitation was accomplished, but the mother remained in a coma until death, and the baby suffered significant neurologic injury.

In a review of GA for cesarean deliveries from 2000 to 2005, the incidence of CICV was 1 in 98. The single case of CICV occurred after failed tracheal intubation, unsuccessful LMA placement, and hypoxemia; successful cricothyroidotomy resulted in a good outcome for both mother and baby.[43]

VIII. PREDICTION OF DIFFICULT AIRWAY MANAGEMENT

The ASA DAA recommended an airway-related history to detect medical, surgical, and anesthetic factors that might indicate the presence of a DA. The guidelines also recommended an airway physical examination using assessment of multiple airway features before initiation of anesthetic care and airway management in all patients.[4] The ASA closed claims analysis (2005) showed that 8% of patients did not have a preoperative history or airway physical examination.[10]

A retrospective audit was performed of all obstetric GAs, a total of 3430 cases over an 8-year period.[44] None of the patients had a failed or esophageal intubation. There were 23 DIs, an incidence of 1:156. Anticipated difficult tracheal intubation occurred in 9 patients, 3 of whom underwent awake fiberoptic intubation; in the remaining 6 patients, who were morbidly obese, the DI was managed by senior trainees or consultants. Unanticipated difficulties occurred in 14 patients (61%). The preoperative assessment was found to be inadequate in these cases, being either not recorded (6 cases) or poorly documented (8 cases).

The first step in management of the high-risk airway is recognition of its presence. Research involving the best practices in promoting patient safety in airway management with rapid-sequence induction (RSI) suggests performing an adequate preoperative evaluation and examining the airway so as to be able to better predict difficult laryngoscopy, DI, and DMV. Similarly, because of the airway-related changes that occur during pregnancy, the obstetric airway should be considered a high-risk airway and therefore a thorough preoperative airway assessment and documentation should be required.

A. Preoperative Assessment

1. History and Evaluation

According to the ASA Task Force, an airway history and a focused review of medical records must be conducted when feasible.[4] Obviously, airway evaluation and prediction of DA in an obstetric patient starts with a thorough, focused airway-related history and evaluation of specific airway-related examination findings.[45] A thorough history addresses any difficulty with previous GAs, obstructive sleep apnea (OSA) or snoring, head and neck abnormalities, and diseases that might impair the airway and result in difficult tracheal intubation. A history of DA management should be considered a strong predictor of problems unless the history was related to a specific reversible disease process such as a dental abscess. The history may be available from verbal recollections by the patient, previous anesthetic records, hospital notes, a letter describing DA management, or a

Medic-Alert bracelet. The introduction of anesthesia information management systems and mandatory electronic medical records should be extremely useful in the future as "airway alerts" are built in to notify future practitioners of the specific details encountered with DA management in a particular patient.

Preexisting conditions that can lead to difficulties in managing the airway include bull neck (neck circumference >16 cm in women), large breasts, large tongue, limited cervical movement, limited mouth opening, prominent upper incisors, and receding jaw.

The physical examination should include assessment of facial and neck masses, quality of dentition, buck teeth, small or large chin, maxillary and mandibular position, pharyngeal structures and high arched palate, and any deformity resulting from trauma, tumor, or inflammation.

2. Predictors of Difficult Airway

Numerous investigators have attempted to predict DA by using a simple bedside physical examination. There are numerous publications describing univariate or multivariate predictors of DI in nonobstetric patients and a handful relating the use of multivariate predictors of the DA, such as MP classification.

Yentis described the problems with many studies examining the prediction of DA.[46] It is appropriate here to delineate the terms used to describe the accuracy and predictive power of these tests. A test to predict DI should have high *sensitivity*, so that it will identify most of the patients in whom intubation will be truly difficult. It should also have a high *positive predictive value* (PPV), so that only a few patients with airways actually easy to intubate will be subjected to the protocol for DA management. The test should also have a high specificity, so that it will identify most patients in whom tracheal intubation will be truly easy (Table 37-4).[46] Excellent interobserver reliability is essential for any test to have high specificity, sensitivity, and PPV in predicting a DA.

B. Quantitative Evaluation of Difficult Intubation

Multiple external features are associated with difficult laryngoscopy and intubation. In an urgent or emergent

---

BOX 37-1   LEMON Airway Assessment Method

L—Look externally for anatomic features that may make intubation difficult
E—Evaluate the 3-3-2 Rule
　　Mouth opening (3 finger breadths)
　　Hyoid-chin distance (3 finger breadths)
　　Thyroid cartilage-floor of mouth distance
　　　(2 finger breadths)
M—Mallampati score
　　Class I: soft palate, uvula, pillars visible
　　Class II: soft palate, uvula visible
　　Class III: soft palate, base of uvular visible
　　Class IV: hard palate visible
O—Obstruction: Examine for partial or complete upper airway obstruction
N—Neck mobility

From Reed MJ, Dunn MJ, McKeown DW: Can an airway assessment score predict difficulty at intubation in the emergency department? *Emerg Med J* 22:99–102, 2005.

---

obstetric situation, a practical, systematic, and rapid evaluation of the airway is necessary and important to predict a potentially difficult laryngoscopic view and DMV before initiation of RSI for GA in a cesarean delivery. The evaluation should dictate the management plan and the availability of airway rescue devices.

The LEMON mnemonic represents one such assessment that is simple and quick, can be performed on any emergency patient, and has proved to have high PPV.[47] The LEMON mnemonic represents the following five elements for preanesthetic assessment (Box 37-1):

L: Look externally—The initial impression of potential airway difficulty is based on assessment for any obvious anatomic distortions or external features that may make intubation difficult, such as facial and periorbital edema in a preeclamptic patient.
E: Evaluate the 3-3-2 Rule—Measuring the geometry of the airway can predict the anesthesia practitioner's ability to align the oral, pharyngeal, and tracheal axes.
  • Mouth opening—The interincisor distance between the patient's incisor teeth or the mandibular opening in an adult should be at least 4 cm or 3 finger-breadths

---

TABLE 37-4

Statistical Terminology and Calculation*

Term	Calculation
True positive (TP)	Difficult intubation that had been predicted to be difficult
False positive (FP)	Easy intubation that had been predicted to be difficult
True negative (TN)	Easy intubation that had been predicted to be easy
False negative (FN)	Difficult intubation that had been predicted to be easy
Sensitivity	Percentage of correctly predicted difficult intubations as a proportion of all intubations that were truly difficult—that is, TP/(TP+FN)
Specificity	Percentage of correctly predicted easy intubations as a proportion of all intubations that were truly easy—that is, TN/(TN+FP)
Positive predictive value	Percentage of correctly predicted difficult intubations as a proportion of all predicted difficult intubations—that is, TP/(TP+FP)
Negative predicted value	Percentage of correctly predicted easy intubations as a proportion of all predicted easy intubations—that is, TN/(TN+FN)

*The sensitivity, specificity, and positive predictive value of each test are calculated using the Cormack-Lehane score as the constant variable.
Adapted from Yentis SM: Predicting difficult intubation: Worthwhile exercise or pointless ritual? *Anaesthesia* 57:105–109, 2002.

- The distance from the hyoid cartilage to the chin should be at least 3 cm or 2 finger breadths (under the chin). The ability of the mandible to accommodate the tongue can be estimated between the mentum and the hyoid bone. A smaller mandible is less likely to accommodate the tongue, which can impair visualization during laryngoscopy. An unusually large mandible can elongate the oral axis.
- The distance between the thyroid notch and the floor of the mandible (top of the neck) should be at least 2 finger breadths.

M: Mallampati score—The degree to which the tongue obstructs the visualization of the posterior pharynx has some correlation with the ability to visualize the glottis. The MP score can be estimated by having the patient, in a sitting position, open the mouth fully and protrude the tongue as far as possible without phonation. The relationship of the base of the tongue to the oropharyngeal structures—uvula and tonsillar pillars and fauces—is assessed as follows:

- Class I : Soft palate, uvula, faucial, and tonsillar pillars visible (easy intubation)
- Class II: Soft palate, uvula visible
- Class III: Soft palate, base of uvula visible
- Class IV: Hard palate only visible (DI)

O: Obstruction—Pathologic conditions such as edema, glottic tumor, lingular tonsil, hyperplasia, and trauma can cause obstruction and can make laryngoscopy and ventilation difficult.

N: Neck mobility—This is a vital requirement for successful intubation. The sniffing position is the optimal, classic position of the head and neck for facilitating intubation. The extension of the atlanto-occipital (A-O) joint on the cervical spine so as to be able to align the three axes (oral, pharyngeal, and laryngeal) during laryngoscopy enhances the ease of laryngoscopy and tracheal intubation. Normal A-O joint extension of the head over the neck is 35 degrees. It can be assessed easily by getting the patient to place the chin down on the chest and tilt the head backward as far as possible. A reduction in A-O joint extension of 12 degrees (33%) or more correlates with intubation difficulty; complete joint immobility significantly compromises the laryngeal view. Limited A-O joint extension is present in certain pathologic states such as spondylosis, rheumatoid arthritis, and cervical spine stenosis, resulting in symptoms of nerve compression with cervical extension. Complete A-O joint immobility (e.g., hard-collar neck immobilization) can compromise the view of the glottis during laryngoscopy.

C. Additional Tests

Difficult laryngoscopy was defined by the ASA Task Force as the inability to visualize any part of the vocal cords despite multiple attempts at conventional laryngoscopy.[4] The original Cormack and Lehane classification of laryngoscopic views was used to describe the visibility of the glottis during laryngoscopy with a conventional laryngoscope and to predict the ease of intubation.[48] The view at laryngoscopy was divided into four grades on the basis of a study in obstetric patients.[49] The entire glottis is visible in a grade 1 view, whereas in a grade 2 view only the posterior portion of the glottis is visible; in a grade 3 view, only the epiglottis is seen, and in grade 4 view not even the epiglottis is seen. Grades 3 and 4 are considered to indicate DI.

1. Thyromental Distance

The thyromental distance (TMD) is defined as the distance from the chin (mentum) to the top of the notch of the thyroid cartilage with the head fully extended; it must be measured with a ruler for accuracy. The TMD gives an estimate of the mandibular space and helps in determining how readily the laryngeal axis will fall in line with the pharyngeal axis when the A-O joint is extended[50]:

- A TMD measurement of 6.5 cm or greater with no other abnormalities indicates the likelihood of easy intubation.
- A TMD measurement of 6.0 to 6.5 cm indicates that alignment of the pharyngeal and laryngeal axes will be challenging and that difficulty with laryngoscopy may result. However, intubation is possible with the use of adjuncts such as an Eschmann introducer or an optical stylet.
- A TMD measurement of less than 6 cm indicates difficult laryngoscopy; specifically, intubation may be impossible.

TMD, in conjunction with other parameters such as the MP classification, has been used to predict DI.

2. Sternomental Distance

The sternomental distance (SMD) is measured from the sternum to the tip of the mandible with the head fully extended and the mouth closed. The normal measurement is 13.5 cm. The SMD and the corresponding laryngoscopic view were documented in 523 parturients undergoing elective or emergency C/D under GA.[51] An SMD of 13.5 cm or less had a sensitivity of 66.7%, a specificity of 71%, and a PPV of only 7.6%. Eighteen patients (3.5%) had a Cormack-Lehane grade 3 or 4 laryngoscopic view and were classified as having potentially difficult tracheal intubations. The SMD on its own as a sole indicator of DI was not useful, and the suggestion was to incorporate it with other tests in the preoperative airway examination.

3. Jaw Protrusion

Jaw protrusion (also termed *prognathism* or *subluxation*) is assessed by the mandibular protrusion test, which demonstrates the extent to which the lower incisors can be slid in front of the upper ones[52]:

- Class A: The lower incisors can be protruded anterior to the upper incisors.
- Class B: The lower incisors can be brought edge-to-edge with the upper incisors.
- Class C: The lower incisors cannot reach the top incisors.

Class C protrusion was associated with difficult laryngoscopy and DMV, whereas class A protrusion rarely produced any difficulty.

4. Studies Assessing Predictors of Difficult Airway in Obstetrics

a. MALLAMPATI CLASSIFICATION

A number of studies in both general surgical and obstetric patients have indicated that the MP classification is a simple, reproducible, reliable, and important parameter in evaluating and assessing the airway. It has been used as a single predictor and as a part of multivariate analysis to predict difficult tracheal intubation. However, studies have shown that the MP classification by itself has limited discriminative power in accurately predicting difficult tracheal intubation.

In obstetric patients, the MP score has been used as a single parameter to illustrate the dramatic airway changes that occur in pregnancy and to highlight the importance of preoperative assessment of the airway. Pilkington and coworkers (1995) evaluated the MP class at 12 weeks' and 38 weeks' gestation[30]; photographs taken at the two time periods demonstrated the increase in MP class in the same patient as gestation advanced. The MP score correlated with the increase in body weight, implying that oropharyngeal edema was responsible for the increase in the MP score.

b. MULTIVARIATE PREDICTORS

Rocke and colleagues (1992) were the first to use multivariate predictors to predict difficult tracheal intubation.[36] They evaluated the MP classification as modified by Samsoon and Young, referring to it as the Modified Mallampati Test (MMT), along with other predictors in 3440 patients undergoing elective or emergency C/D under GA. Data were collected on 1606 patients, representing 46.7% of the obstetric surgical patients. Of the patients studied 1500 underwent general anesthesia. Other risk parameters for DA that they assessed included short neck, which equates with decreased A-O joint extension; receding mandible or decreased TMD (<3 finger breadths); and protruding maxillary incisors indicating significant overbite, which would equate to the current class C jaw protrusion or class III upper lip bite test.[53]

Rocke's group made subjective assessments of the ease or difficulty of tracheal intubation according to the following scale (Table 37-5)[36]:

- Grade 1: Easy—intubation at first attempt with no difficulty

- Grade 2: Some difficulty—insertion of tracheal tube not achieved at first attempt; no difficulty but successful intubation after adjustment of laryngoscope blade and/or adjustment of head position, not requiring additional equipment, removal and reinsertion of the laryngoscope, or senior assistance
- Grade 3: Very difficult—requiring removal of the laryngoscope, further oxygenation by mask ventilation, and subsequent intubation with or without the use of airway adjuncts (e.g., Eschmann introducer, alternative laryngoscope blade) or intubation by a senior colleague
- Grade 4: Failed intubation—several attempts at intubation or unrecognized esophageal intubation by resident, followed by subsequent tracheal intubation by senior anesthesiologist

Based on these various parameters, the relative risk of experiencing difficult tracheal intubation (compared with an uncomplicated MMT class I airway) was determined as follows: 3.23 for MMT class II, 7.58 for MMT class III, 11.3 for MMT class IV, 5.01 for short neck, 9.71 for receding mandible, and 8.0 for protruding incisors. The investigators analyzed the univariate individual risk factor (i.e., MMT class) and combinations of the various risk factors and showed that a patient with an MMT III or IV classification plus protruding incisors, a short neck, and a receding mandible would have a probability of difficult laryngoscopy greater than 90% (Fig. 37-2). This study highlighted the importance of preoperative airway assessment to determine the best anesthetic intervention and the importance of prospectively preparing for airway interventions in the true obstetric emergency C/D under GA.

Gupta and colleagues evaluated the obstetric airway,[54] using the MMT and the Wilson risk sum, to assess the potential for DA in 372 patients undergoing elective or emergency C/D under GA. The Wilson risk sum score was ascertained by adding scores for five factors (weight, head and neck movement, jaw movement/jaw protrusion, receding mandible, and buck teeth). The investigators also compared the sensitivity, specificity, and PPV of the MMT score (60%, 97.6%, and 65%, respectively) with the data published by Rocke and coworkers[36] for laryngoscopy (59.2%, 74.1%, and 4.0%, respectively). The MMT was reproducible and was more sensitive than the Wilson risk sum score. As a screening test for prediction of DI, the Wilson risk sum score was less sensitive

TABLE 37-5

Association between Oropharyngeal Structures Visualized Preoperatively and Subsequent Difficulty at Tracheal Intubation*

Difficulty at Intubation	OROPHARYNGEAL STRUCTURES VISUALIZED (NO. PATIENTS (%))				
	Class I	Class II	Class III	Class IV	Total
Grade 1: Easy	461 (96.4)	566 (90.6)	264 (82.2)	58 (76.3)	1349 (89.9)
Grade 2: Some difficulty	15 (3.1)	48 (7.7)	43 (13.4)	13 (17.1)	119 (7.9)
Grade 3: Very difficult	2 (0.42)	10 (1.6)	13 (4.0)	5 (6.6)	30 (2.0)
Grade 4: Failed	0 (0)	1 (0.2)	1 (0.3)	0 (0)	2 (0.1)

*Values are significant at P < 0.001. See text for details.
From Rocke DA, Murray WB, Rout CC, Gouws E: Relative risk analysis of factors associated with difficult intubation in obstetric anesthesia. *Anesthesiology* 77:69, 1992.

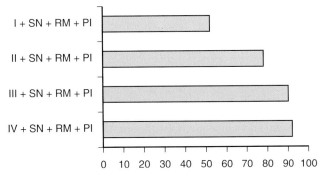

Figure 37-2 Probability of experiencing difficult intubation for varying combinations of risk factors. Roman numerals refer to Modified Mallampati Test (MMT) class. *PI*, Protruding incisors; *RM*, receding mandible; *SN*, short neck. See text for details. (From Rocke DA, Murray WB, Rout CC, Gouws E: Relative risk analysis of factors associated with difficult intubation in obstetric anesthesia. *Anesthesiology* 77:67, 1992.)

(36%) but had almost the same specificity (98.5%) and PPV (64%) as the MMT. When both tests were combined as predictors, the sensitivity was improved to 100%, the specificity was marginally decreased to 96.2%, and the PPV (64.8%) remained almost the same, compared with the MMT score alone. Gupta and colleagues concluded that, in obstetric patients, use of the Wilson risk sum score along with the MMT score resulted in high sensitivity, high specificity, and a high PPV.[54] This study highlighted the importance of incorporating multiple predictors rather than using single (univariate) predictors of difficult laryngoscopy and intubation. There was a significant relationship between increased weight and external laryngeal manipulation.

Merah and associates studied the potential of five airway measurements to predict a difficult direct laryngoscopy in 80 West African obstetric patients during C/D under GA.[37] The five bedside tests that were evaluated were MMT, TMD, SMD, horizontal length of mandible, and interincisor gap. Eight patients (10%) had difficult laryngoscopy. The MMT as a sole predictor had a sensitivity, specificity, and PPV of 87.1%, 99.6%, and 70%, respectively. In light of the current state of knowledge with respect to airway evaluation, the investigators concluded that this prediction tool would behave similarly in Caucasians as in West Africans. Weight contributed to the prediction of difficult laryngoscopy. The difference between the mean weights of difficult-to-intubate patients (109 ± 12.4 kg) and easy-to-intubate patients (81 ± 12.0 kg) was statistically significant. The combination of MMT and TMD yielded values of 100%, 93.1%, and 61.5% for sensitivity, specificity, and PPV, respectively. The researchers concluded that MMT can be used as the sole predictor of difficult tracheal intubation.

Kodali and colleagues performed a two-part study to evaluate airway changes during labor and delivery.[23] In part I, they used the conventional Samsoon modification of the MP airway classification. The airway was photographed at the onset of labor ("prelabor") and at the end of labor ("postlabor"). Pregnant women with MP class IV airways were excluded from this initial part of the study. In part II, prelabor and postlabor upper airway volumes were measured by acoustic reflectometry. In part I

($n = 61$), there was a significant increase in MP class between prelabor and postlabor measurements ($P < 0.0001$). The airway increased by one class in 20 parturients (33%) and by two classes in 3 parturients (5%). At the end of labor, there were 8 parturients with MP class IV ($P < 0.01$) and 30 with MP class III or IV ($P < 0.0001$). In Part II ($n = 21$), there were significant decreases in oral volume ($P < 0.05$) and in pharyngeal area ($P < 0.05$) and volume ($P < 0.001$) after labor and delivery.

Boutonnet and associates methodically evaluated the changes in MP class at four time intervals in 87 pregnant patients: during the eighth month of pregnancy (T_1), at placement of the epidural catheter (T_2), at 20 minutes after delivery (T_3), and at 48 hours after delivery (T_4).[24] MP class did not change for 37% of the patients. The proportion of patients falling into MP class III or IV at the various times of assessment were as follows: T_1, 10.3%; T_2, 36.8%; T_3, 51%; and T_4, 20.7%. The differences in the percentages were all significant ($P < 0.01$). The incidence of MP classes III or IV increased during labor compared with prelabor period, and these changes were not reversed by 48 hours after delivery.

The studies by Kodali and Boutonnet and their colleagues confirmed the frequent increase in MP score during pregnancy and particularly during the course of labor.[23,24] These findings suggest that it is imperative to evaluate the airway in early labor and to reevaluate it before anesthetic management for operative delivery.

c. META-ANALYSIS OF BEDSIDE SCREENING TEST PERFORMANCE

Shiga and colleagues systematically determined the diagnostic accuracy of bedside tests for predicting difficult tracheal intubation in patients with no airway pathology.[55] Thirty-five studies comprising 50,760 patients, including both surgical and obstetric patients, were selected from electronic databases (Table 37-6).

The overall incidence of difficult tracheal intubation was 5.8% (95% confidence interval [CI], 4.5% to 7.5%). Screening tests included the MP oropharyngeal classification, TMD, SMD, mouth opening, and Wilson risk score. Each test yielded poor to moderate sensitivity (20% to 62%) and moderate to fair specificity (2% to 97%). The meta-analysis found that the most useful bedside test for prediction was a combination of the MP classification and TMD (positive likelihood ratio, 9.9; 95% CI, 3.1 to 31.9). The study concluded that in surgical patients, this combination of tests added some incremental diagnostic value compared with the value of each test alone.[55]

The meta-analysis showed that in the obstetric population (2155 patients), the prevalence of difficult tracheal intubation was 3.1% (95 % CI, 1.7 to 5.5). The diagnostic performance of the MP classification in obstetric and obese populations was similar to that in the overall surgical population. The diagnostic odds ratios in these populations were similar, and the trend toward poor sensitivity and fair specificity remained. In the obstetric patients, the MP classification yielded a sensitivity of 56%, a specificity of 81%, and a likelihood ratio of 0.6%. The meta-analysis data in the obstetric patients remained inconclusive because of the small number of studies and heterogeneity.

TABLE 37-6

Pooled Estimates of Bayesian Statistics from Six Bedside Tests for Difficult Intubation (DI)*

Diagnostic Test	No. Studies	No. Patients	Prevalence of DI (95% CI), %	Pooled Sensitivity (95% CI), %	Pooled Specificity (95% CI), %	POOLED LIKELIHOOD RATIO (95% CI) Positive	POOLED LIKELIHOOD RATIO (95% CI) Negative	Pooled Log Diagnostic Odds Ratio (95% CI)
Overall Population								
MP class	31	41,193	5.7 (4.4-7.3)	49 (41-57)	86 (81-90)	3.7 (3.0-4.6)	0.5 (0.5-0.6)	2.0 (1.7-2.3)
TMD	17	29,132	6.5 (4.6-9.1)	20 (11-29)	94 (89-99)	3.4 (2.3-4.9)	0.8 (0.8-0.9)	1.7 (1.2-2.1)
SMD	3	1,085	5.4 (3.1-9.2)	62 (37-86)	82 (67-97)	5.7 (2.1-15.1)	0.5 (0.3-0.8)[†]	2.7 (1.4-3.9)
Mouth opening	3	20,614	5.6 (2.2-14.5)	22 (9-35)	97 (93-100)	4.0 (2.0-8.2)	0.8 (0.7-1.0)	1.7 (1.2-2.3)
Wilson risk score	5	6,076	4.0 (1.8-9.0)	46 (36-56)[†]	89 (85-92)[†]	5.8 (3.9-8.6)	0.6 (0.5-0.9)	2.3 (1.8-2.8)
MP class + TMD	5	1,498	6.6 (2.8-15.6)	36 (14-59)	87 (74-100)	9.9 (3.1-31.9)	0.6 (0.5-0.9)	3.3 (1.5-5.0)
Obstetric Subgroup								
MP class	3	2,155	3.1 (1.7-5.5)	56 (41-72)[†]	81 (67-95)	6.4 (1.1-36.5)	0.6 (0.4-0.8)[†]	2.5 (0.6-4.4)
Obese Subgroup (BMI > 30)								
MP class	4	378	15.8 (14.3-17.5)[†]	64 (51-97)	74 (62-87)	2.9 (1.6-5.3)	0.4 (0.2-0.8)[†]	2.1 (0.8-3.3)

BMI, Body mass index (kg/m²); *CI*, 95% confidence interval; *MP class*, Mallampati classification; *OR*, odds ratio; *SMD*, sternomental distance; *TMD*, thyromental distance.

*Post-test probability = ((pretest odds) • likelihood ratio)/(1 + (pretest odds) • likelihood ratio); where pretest odds = pretest probability/(1 − pretest probability). The DerSimonian-Laird random-effects model was used throughout. Significant heterogeneity (*P* < 0.1) was found except where indicated.

[†]Difference not significant.

From Shiga T, Wajima Z, Inoue T, Sakamoto A: Predicting difficult intubation in apparently normal patients. *Anesthesiology* 103:429–437, 2005.

Whereas in the obese patients (BMI > 30 kg/m²), the incidence of difficult tracheal intubation was 15.8 % or three times higher than in the overall population. Obese patients with a 15% pretest probability of DI had a 34% risk of difficult tracheal intubation after a positive MP class result, which is twice the risk of the overall population with a 5% pretest probability. Similarly, obese pregnant patients also had a higher incidence of difficult tracheal intubation. Because of the higher incidence of difficult tracheal intubation, the MP classification may yield higher post-test probability of difficult tracheal intubation in obese patients than in the overall population.[55]

5. Trends in Anesthesia in Obstetrics

Cesarean delivery is the commonest major surgical procedure carried out in the United States (U.S. Centers for Disease Control and Prevention National Center for Health Statistics Report 2010) and the incidence is increasing worldwide.[56] The increased incidence of maternal morbidity and mortality associated with GA in obstetric patients and the heightened awareness among anesthesia practitioners of the risk for DA and failed intubation in obstetrics has led to an increased use of RA techniques. A 2009 closed claims analysis found that use of RA was 65% before 1990 and increased to more than 80% since then, whereas the use of GA declined from 33% before 1990 to 17% after 1990.[1] National Health Service maternity statistics show that the number of obstetric GAs for C/D administered in the United Kingdom fell from over 50% in 1989-90, to as low as 5%

in 2004-2005.[57] Johnson and colleagues similarly found a marked decline in GA for C/D, from 79% to less than 10% over the same period.[58]

The current trend in the United States and the United Kingdom is to use GA mainly for the true emergency C/D, if there is insufficient time for a regional technique, or in cases in which there is a contraindication to RA. Despite the decline in the use of GA for C/D, the incidence of difficult tracheal intubation was not found to be significantly different (5% before 1990 versus 3% after 1990).[1] Encountering a DA in the obstetric population is not uncommon; therefore, the emerging problem of declining airway skills is important, as evidenced by a rise in the rate of failed tracheal intubation, from 1:300 between 1978 and 1983 to 1:250 in 1994.[40,59,60] It is uncertain whether these concurrent trends are interrelated. The risk of failed tracheal intubation is considerably higher for emergency than for elective C/D, with 80% of airway-related fatalities occurring during emergency C/D (nights and weekends) and usually involving trainees.[40] A review of GA for C/D at a tertiary hospital during the period 1990-1995 showed a decline in the use of GA, from 7.2% to 3.6%.[2] A further review of GA for C/D from 2000 to 2005 in the same institution showed that GA use had further declined to a low incidence of about 1%.[43]

Because of the decreased use of GA for C/D, anesthesia trainees' experience of GA in obstetric patients is also on the decline. The lack of opportunities for training and maintenance of airway skills is an emerging concern.[58,61,62]

IX. RECOMMENDATIONS FOR MANAGEMENT OF THE DIFFICULT AIRWAY

Guidelines for the management of anticipated and unanticipated DA have been published by various national societies. The guidelines of the ASA Task Force were originally developed as a consequence of the high number of perioperative respiratory adverse events during airway management.[63,64] The updated version of the DAA was published in 2003 (Fig. 37-3).[4] The ASA DAA guidelines include evaluation of the airway, physical examination (as described earlier), basic preparation for the DA, and follow-up care. Although these points are applicable to the obstetric patients as well, some elements of the ASA DAA and their adaptability to the obstetric DA cannot be assessed due to the lack of strong evidence. The available evidence on management of the DA in the obstetric patient is mainly in the form of case reports. The ASA DAA provides a framework for management of the DA and should be modified and adapted to the obstetric patient where applicable.

A key point of the ASA DAA and its strength is the recommendation of a clear strategy for management of both the anticipated and the unanticipated DA. This strategy, however, depends on the skills and preferences of the anesthesia practitioner. The ASA Task Force strongly recommended the use of strategies to maintain oxygenation throughout the process of airway management. It is the cornerstone of airway management in situations including the nonemergency pathway, the emergency pathway, and increasing hypoxemia during the CICV critical airway situation. Crucial elements of the ASA DAA include an early attempt at insertion of the LMA if face mask ventilation is not adequate (strengthened in the updated version), the possibility of awakening the patient, and simple "call for help" at an early stage. These are all applicable in the obstetric DA scenario and add to the strength of the algorithm. As mentioned earlier, the ASA DAA offers many options; however, it is not specific for an urgent obstetric situation.

X. EQUIPMENT (DIFFICULT AIRWAY CART)

The ASA DAA recommended that anesthesia personnel familiarize themselves with the patients and the airway equipment in advance. Likewise, the ASA Practice Guidelines for Obstetric Anesthesia recommended that airway equipment should be readily available in the labor and delivery area.[45] Based on our own experience, we believe that equipment and anesthesia personnel should actually be *immediately* available in the labor and delivery area, throughout the 24-hour shift, on a daily basis. Our current practice is to have a designated DA cart immediately available inside our obstetric operating rooms for use in airway emergencies, and this policy has proved to be invaluable on many occasions.[65-67]

The fiberscope is located in a predesignated slot on the side of our DA cart. The top shelf has all the equipment and local anesthetics required for an awake tracheal intubation as well as an optical stylet for optimizing the glottic view during a DI under GA. The next three drawers are organized to follow the sequence of clinical scenarios that one might encounter during an unanticipated DA:

- Drawer A: Supraglottic airways of sizes 3 and 4 (LMA Excel, Fastrach LMA, ProSeal LMA) for use in the nonemergency pathway
- Drawer B: Specialized supraglottic airways (Combitube 37 F, King LTS-D sizes 3 and 4) for use in the emergency pathway
- Drawer C: Equipment available for invasive airway access (cricothyroidotomy kit, transtracheal jet cannula with adapter) for use in the emergency pathway, critical airway situation

XI. ANTICIPATED DIFFICULT INTUBATION

Because the incidence of difficult tracheal intubation is significantly higher in the obstetric population, especially during emergency C/D and on nights and weekends,[40] it is only prudent to avoid GA for C/D if other safe anesthetic choices are available. In modern obstetric anesthesia practice, neuraxial anesthesia is administered to some patients who would have received GA in the past, such as patients with severe preeclampsia with lower platelet count, placenta previa without active bleeding, or umbilical cord prolapse in a parturient with a functioning epidural catheter.

The use of neuraxial anesthesia is based on current evidence in the literature, which includes the following:

1. An increased use of epidural anesthesia during labor in high-risk parturients
2. A heightened awareness that an in situ functioning epidural catheter may decrease the necessity for GA in an urgent situation
3. Understanding that the presence of a functioning epidural catheter allows analgesia to be converted to epidural anesthesia, if necessary for a C/D
4. Appreciation of the risks of airway complications associated with GA for C/D
5. Improvement in the quality of intraoperative and postoperative pain management, with the addition of opioids to the local anesthetic, during spinal and epidural blocks
6. Keeping parturients awake and allowing for bonding with the baby during C/D

The current practice of placing epidural catheters prophylactically, early in labor, in high-risk parturients who have clinical conditions such as morbid obesity, DA, or obstetric comorbidities or complications has reduced the risk of an unanticipated GA. This is considered best practice and is in keeping with the most recent ASA guidelines for obstetric anesthesia.[45] The practice guidelines advocate this concept of using a prophylactic epidural in high-risk parturients, which basically involves the placement of a catheter and the confirmation of functionality with small amounts of local anesthetic, early in labor, and possibly before a request for analgesia. This provides a readily available neuraxial route of anesthesia, should an

DIFFICULT AIRWAY ALGORITHM

1. Assess the likelihood and clinical impact of basic management problems:
   A. Difficult ventilation
   B. Difficult intubation
   C. Difficulty with patient cooperation or consent
   D. Difficult tracheostomy
2. Actively pursue opportunities to deliver supplemental oxygen throughout the process of difficult airway management
3. Consider the relative merits and feasibility of basic management choices:

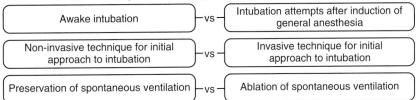

4. Develop primary and alternative strategies:

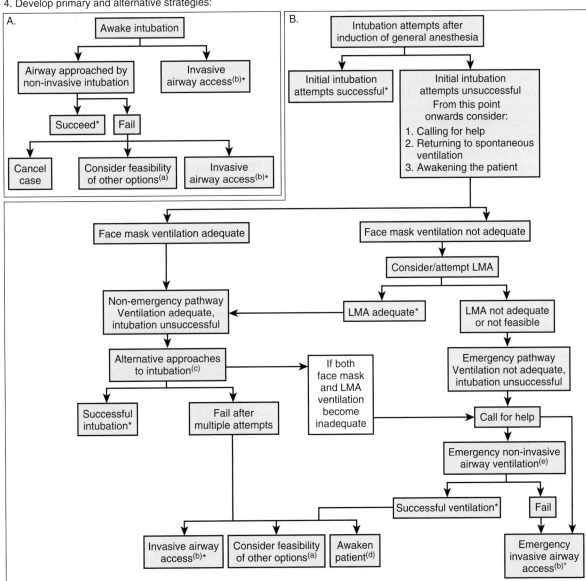

*Confirm ventilation, tracheal intubation, or LMA placement with CO_2.

a. Other options include (but are not limited to): surgery utilizing face mask or LMA anesthesia, local anesthesia infiltration or regional nerve blockade. Pursuit of these options usually implies that mask ventilation will not be problematic. Therefore, these options may be of limited value if this step in the algorithm has been reached via Emergency Pathway.

b. Invasive airway access includes surgical or percutaneous tracheostomy or cricothyrotomy.

c. Alternative non-invasive approaches to difficult intubation include (but are not limited to): use of different laryngoscope blades, LMA as an intubation conduit (with or without fiberoptic guidance), fiberoptic intubation, intubating stylet or tube changer, light wand, retrograde intubation, and blind oral or nasal intubation.

d. Consider re-preparation of the patient for awake intubation or canceling surgery.

e. Options for emergency non-invasive airway ventilation include (but are not limited to): rigid branchoscope, esophageal-tracheal Combitube ventilation or transtracheal jet ventilation.

Figure 37-3 Difficult airway algorithm (DAA). *LMA,* Laryngeal mask airway. (From American Society of Anesthesiologists Task Force on Management of the Difficult Airway: Practice guidelines for management of the difficult airway: An updated report by the American Society of Anesthesiologists Task Force on Management of the Difficult Airway. *Anesthesiology* 98:1269–1277, 2003.)

emergent operative delivery be necessary. If the epidural catheter is not functioning well, it should be replaced with either a functioning continuous epidural catheter or a continuous spinal catheter.

Current evidence confirms the efficacy of dosing in situ epidural catheters in achieving decision-to-delivery intervals (DDI) for C/D and is comparable to that achieved with GA.[68,69] Evidence suggests that it is necessary to allow the shortest DDI for the true fetal distress situation; additionally, the recommended 30-minute DDI for emergency cesarean deliveries is appropriate[18] and allows the administration of a spinal anesthetic. Holcroft and colleagues showed the outcomes classified by type of anesthesia.[70] DDI for GA was almost 15 minutes shorter than for spinal anesthesia and 13 minutes shorter than for epidural anesthesia ($P = 0.0002$). The epidural group had functioning labor epidurals that were converted to surgical anesthesia for C/D, whereas the spinal anesthesias were performed after the decision for C/D was made. There were no differences in the incidence of 1-minute Apgar scores lower than 7 based on anesthesia type, but there was a significant increase in 5-minute APGAR scores lower than 7 in the GA group. There was no difference in the umbilical arterial pH between the groups, but the base excess was significantly worse in the GA group. The investigators concluded that although GA is considerably faster than either spinal or epidural anesthesia, it is well established that GA poses greater maternal risk.[13,71] Therefore, the benefits of obtaining anesthesia sooner versus the risk of a maternal complication must be weighed and determined by the obstetrician and anesthesiologist working in consultation together in each individual case. The American Congress of Obstetricians and Gynecologists (ACOG) Committee Opinion entitled, "Anesthesia for Emergency Deliveries" endorsed the following stance: "Cesarean deliveries that are performed for a nonreassuring fetal heart rate pattern do not necessarily preclude the use of regional anesthesia."[72] These guidelines require both familiarity and knowledge for application in an urgent C/D situation.

Another option for neuraxial techniques for C/D is deliberate continuous spinal analgesia using the Tuohy needle and an epidural catheter. A recent study by Palanisamy and colleagues confirmed that (1) the rate of use of GA for cesarean delivery between 2000 and 2005 was low, approximately 1%; (2) 85% of GAs were administered for emergent deliveries; (3) most were performed because of a perceived lack of time, particularly for the emergency deliveries; (4) very few GA cases resulted from failure of neuraxial anesthesia techniques; and (5) there was a very low incidence of GA-related morbidity with no cases of mortality.[43] This study confirmed first, that the policy of placing epidural catheters prophylactically in high-risk parturients, particularly obese parturients with potential DA, has reduced the risk of unanticipated GA. Second, the adoption of a more aggressive approach toward management of inadequate neuraxial block (by replacing epidural catheters for suboptimal analgesia during labor) may have reduced the incidence of intraoperative conversion to GA. Third, the willingness to perform emergent spinal anesthesia,

including intentional continuous spinal techniques, especially in patients with certain comorbid conditions (e.g., severe preeclampsia)[73,74] or morbid obesity,[75] may have been partly responsible for the reduction in GAs.

The use of a combined spinal/epidural technique for labor analgesia in a high-risk parturient may not be the most prudent choice. Even though several studies have found a lower incidence of failed epidural analgesia after initiation of analgesia with a combined spinal/epidural technique,[76,77] there is a disadvantage in that the correct placement of the epidural catheter in the epidural space cannot be verified until the spinal anesthesia wanes. Therefore, if a functioning epidural is important, so as to be able to convert to surgical anesthesia for emergency C/D, especially in a parturient who has a high probability of a DA or a nonreassuring fetal status, then a combined spinal/epidural technique is not the preferred technique for labor analgesia.

If neuraxial anesthesia is contraindicated due to maternal hemorrhage, coagulopathy, or umbilical cord prolapse, one may have to resort to GA. The DA cart should be immediately available in the operating room and should include other advanced airway devices such as a cricothyroidotomy kit and transtracheal jet ventilation (TTJV) equipment. It is prudent to inform the ear, nose, and throat surgeon or the general surgeon to remain readily available in these situations.

XII. AIRWAY MANAGEMENT STRATEGIES

A. Cesarean Delivery

The anesthesia practitioner must have a clear and effective plan for managing a patient with DA, a difficult or failed intubation, or a CICV in a parturient undergoing C/D under GA. The ASA DAA is a beginning for an organized approach to DA problems.[4] All anesthesia practitioners must be familiar with the ASA DAA. Although this algorithm is commendable in providing a logical, well-organized overview of the DA, it is not easily memorized and is not easy to implement in emergency situations, especially when two lives (mother and baby) are at risk. The United Kingdom DAS basic guidelines[5] are more linear and emphasize a four-point approach with each plan consequent on failure of the previous plan (Fig. 37-4):

- Plan A: Initial intubation attempt
- Plan B: Secondary intubation attempt
- Plan C: Maintain oxygenation and ventilation using rescue techniques with supraglottic devices and bail out
- Plan D: Invasive techniques for the CICV situation

Two principles are emphasized in these guidelines: (1) maintenance of oxygenation during the execution of each plan and (2) seeking the best assistance available as soon as difficulty with laryngoscopy is experienced.

For purposes of this discussion, we have adapted our recommendations for airway management strategies in the obstetric patient with due consideration to both the ASA DAA guidelines and the U.K. DAS guidelines.

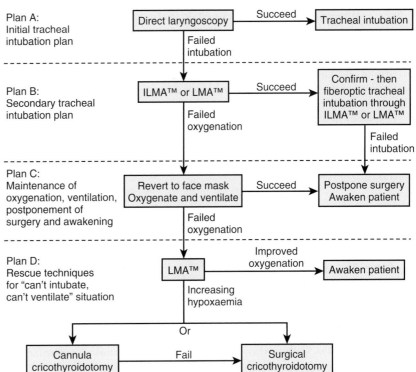

Figure 37-4 Airway management strategies for patients undergoing cesarean delivery. *ILMA*, Intubating laryngeal mask airway; *LMA*, laryngeal mask airway. (Adapted from Henderson JJ, Popat MT, Latto IP, Pearce AC: Difficult Airway Society guidelines for management of the unanticipated difficult intubation. *Anaesthesia* 59:675–694, 2004.)

B. Awake Fiberoptic Intubation

In a parturient who has a known history of DA, an anticipated DA, morbid obesity, certain anatomic features indicating that tracheal intubation by conventional means is likely to be difficult or impossible, or contraindications to RA and is undergoing C/D, a safe option is to secure the airway with the tracheal tube while the patient remains awake. If RA is not an option and time is not an issue, an awake tracheal intubation can be performed safely with the use of either a flexible fiberscope or a video laryngoscope.[78,79] The following paragraphs describe the logical approach to awake tracheal intubation.

Adequate preparation is crucial to the success of an awake tracheal intubation and has several aspects:

- Psychological preparation of the patient.
- Administration of an antisialagogue such as glycopyrrolate, 0.2 to 0.3 mg intravenously, 10 to 15 minutes before the application of topical anesthesia to dry the oropharyngeal secretions. Excessive secretions interfere with the effects of local anesthetics. Glycopyrrolate, being a quaternary ammonium compound, does not cross the placenta.
- Judicious sedation with midazolam (1 mg) and fentanyl (50 to 100 μg) intravenously, so that the patient is calm and cooperative, without risking respiratory depression in the mother or neonate. Opioids produce analgesia and depress the airway reflexes to facilitate smooth oropharyngeal and laryngeal instrumentation.
- Adequate topicalization of the airway with local anesthetic to make it nonreactive to physical

stimulation. Topical anesthesia of the oropharynx is achieved with 4 or 5 short sprays of 4% lidocaine to the palate, base of the tongue, and lateral and posterior pharyngeal walls. Two minutes after the spray of local anesthetic, 2% lidocaine gel is spread on the base of the tongue with a tongue blade, to supplement the topical anesthesia and to prevent gagging. Use of a good topical anesthetic before endoscopy prevents coughing, gagging, and laryngeal spasm and contributes to the success of the technique. Depressed gag and airway reflexes can make the parturient more susceptible to pulmonary aspiration of gastric contents. Ovassapian and colleagues[80] presented the concept of topicalization of the lower airway and awake fiberoptic tracheal intubation in patients at high risk for pulmonary aspiration and have helped diffuse that controversy.
- The "Spray as you go" technique with local anesthetic spray of 2% lidocaine. This is used for application of the topical anesthetic and for anesthetizing the upper airway from the tip of the tongue to the trachea.
- The advanced airway management skills of the operator. The skill of the anesthetist is equally important for success of the technique.

Research has documented the successful use of awake fiberoptic tracheal intubation in 60 parturients with DAs undergoing C/D.[81] These parturients received judicious sedation and underwent full topicalization, including transtracheal injection of lidocaine (except that those parturients with coagulopathy received nebulized lidocaine), and there were no cases of pulmonary aspiration.

Lower esophageal tone is maintained in patients who are not oversedated and prevents pulmonary aspiration regardless of the extent of topicalization. In our own institution, we are occasionally faced with similar clinical situations and have successfully used awake, oral fiberoptic intubation to secure the airway before administration of GA for cesarean delivery.[82]

The nasal route for awake, fiberoptic tracheal intubation has been used occasionally in pregnant women. However, it should be used with caution because of the hyperemic nasal mucosa and the potential for inducing epistaxis.

XIII. UNANTICIPATED DIFFICULT TRACHEAL INTUBATION

A. Step 1: Initial Tracheal Intubation Attempt

We propose a five-step flow chart for unanticipated difficult tracheal intubation after induction of GA in the obstetric patient (Fig. 37-5). It is based on the ASA DAA and the U.K. DAS algorithm and is modified for the obstetric patient. Each step should not take longer than 30 to 45 seconds, so no more than 5 minutes should elapse before the decision is made to use invasive airway access in the emergency pathway—critical airway scenario.

If the decision is made to proceed with GA, and before induction of anesthesia and intubation, one must strictly adhere to certain basic principles: use of gastrointestinal prophylaxis to prevent aspiration; optimal positioning, including the placement of a wedge under the right hip to offset any aortocaval compression; and use of the ramped-up position in obese parturients to facilitate laryngoscopy, tracheal intubation, and ventilation.

Induction of anesthesia is preceded by preoxygenation to effectively denitrogenate the lungs; effective use of a preoxygenation technique that maximizes oxygen stores (preoxygenation for 3 to 5 minutes or 4 deep breaths over 30 seconds)[83]; and the first attempt at direct laryngoscopy should always be performed in optimal conditions. After succinylcholine administration and confirmation of adequate muscle relaxation, appropriate head and neck position, and use of effective cricoid pressure, proceed with RSI and tracheal intubation. The application of optimal external laryngeal manipulation to optimize the laryngoscopic view may be critical. All these elements are important in managing the DI scenario (see Fig. 37-5, Step 1) and are discussed in detail in the following sections.

1. Aspiration Prophylaxis

Because of the risk for gastric regurgitation and pulmonary aspiration, all pregnant patents are considered to have a "full stomach" regardless of their preoperative fasting status. Aspiration risk can be mitigated by oral administration of triple pharmacologic prophylaxis that includes sodium citrate to neutralize the acidic contents of the stomach; intravenous (IV) administration of a histamine (H_2) receptor antagonist to reduce gastric acid secretion; and IV administration of a gastrokinetic drug, such as metoclopramide, to speed up gastric emptying and increase the tone of the lower esophageal sphincter.

2. Positioning

Proper positioning of the patient is an often missed critical step in facilitating laryngoscopy, tracheal intubation, and mask ventilation, if needed. The optimal sniff position (slight flexion of the neck and extension of the head on the neck), which aligns the oral, pharyngeal, and laryngeal axes into a straight line, is mandatory to facilitate tracheal intubation.[52] The neck should be flexed on a pillow and the A-O joint extended to achieve the optimal sniffing position. However, in morbidly obese patients including parturients, one should utilize the head-elevated laryngoscopy (HELP) position and create a ramp, using folded towels or blankets under the shoulders and head to ensure that the head and shoulders are higher than the chest.[84] The HELP position is determined by drawing an imaginary horizontal line that connects the patient's sternal notch with the external auditory meatus, so that the head and neck are at a slightly higher elevation than the chest. The Troop Elevation Pillow (Mercury Medical, Clearwater, FL) is shaped like a ramp and is designed to optimize the HELP and sniffing positions.

3. Cricoid Pressure

Cricoid pressure has played an important role in prevention of pulmonary aspiration since its introduction by Sellick.[85] It is an integral part of the flow chart for the patient having RSI for cesarean delivery. Sellick first described a neck maneuver to compress the esophagus between the cricoid cartilages anteriorly and the body of the sixth cervical vertebra posteriorly in order to prevent regurgitated gastric contents from entering the hypopharynx during induction of GA.[85] Typically, a cephalad and posteriorly pointing force of 10 newtons (N), applied by the thumb and index finger of the assistant, is required in the awake patient; this force increases up to 30 N in the unconscious patient.[86,87] On the other hand, as important as cricoid pressure is to prevent regurgitation of gastric contents into the oropharynx,[88] excessive cricoid pressure may obscure the glottic view by displacing the vocal cords anteriorly or laterally.[89] The assistant may be asked to transiently reduce or release cricoid pressure, with suction at hand, so that the glottic area and vocal cords can be visualized, despite the possible risk of pulmonary aspiration in the event of gastric regurgitation.[90,91] Aspiration is treatable, whereas irreversible hypoxia is not.

4. External Laryngeal Manipulation

Various steps taken to optimize the laryngoscopic view with external laryngeal manipulation, referred to as the BURP maneuver (i.e., backward, upward, rightward pressure on the thyroid cartilage) and the use of an Eschmann introducer can maximize the success of tracheal intubation. The use of optimal external manipulation (i.e., the BURP maneuver) involves pressure on the thyroid cartilage and displacement of the larynx in three specific directions—posteriorly against the cervical vertebrae, as far superiorly as possible, and slightly laterally to the right.[92] Because the thyroid cartilage is the surface

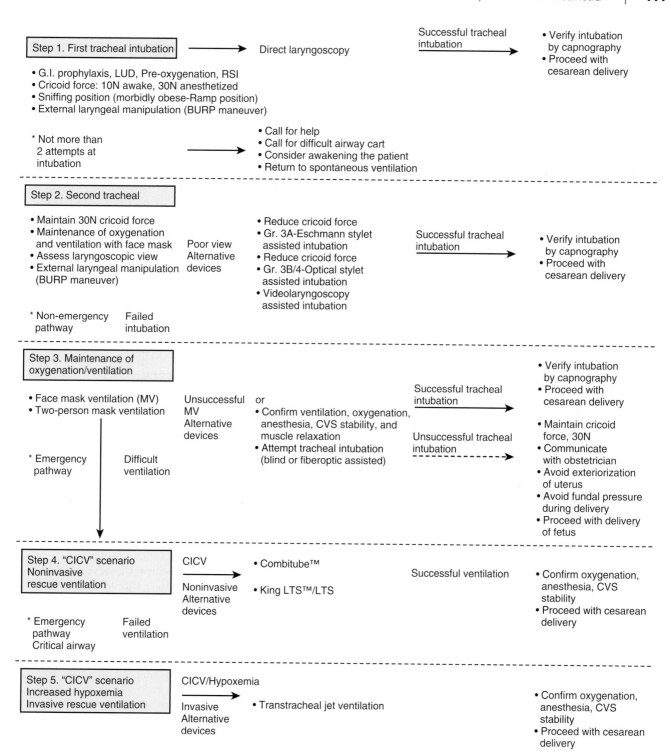

Figure 37-5 Five-step approach to unanticipated difficult tracheal intubation during rapid-sequence induction (*RSI*) of anesthesia in the obstetric patient. The BURP maneuver consists of backward, upward, and rightward pressure on the thyroid cartilage. *CICV,* "Cannot intubate, cannot ventilate"; *CVS,* cardiovascular system; *G.I.,* gastrointestinal; *Gr.,* Cormack-Lehane grade (laryngoscopic view); *LUD,* left uterine displacement; *N,* newtons (unit of force).

marking for the laryngeal aperture, proper application of the BURP maneuver improves the laryngoscopic view. In a study comparing glottic views with and without use of the BURP maneuver, it was shown that the BURP maneuver improved the glottic view by at least one whole grade and reduced the incidence of failure to view any portion of the glottis from approximately 9.2% to 1.6%.[92]

B. Step 2: Second Tracheal Intubation Attempt

1. Consider Calling for Help, Returning to Spontaneous Ventilation, and Awakening the Patient

In all but the most urgent situations, one can consider awakening the mother and reassessing the fetus before proceeding with an alternative plan. However, in urgent and emergent C/D situations under GA, the goal should be to balance maternal oxygenation, prevention of pulmonary aspiration, and expeditious delivery of the fetus. Such a situation dictates addressing management of the DA after a failed tracheal intubation attempt. Appropriate initial management and procedures after failed attempts at tracheal intubation can influence and even ensure the final optimal and best outcome for both mother and baby. Calling for help is critical; it should be done sooner rather than later. Immediate access to the DA cart is critical as well.

Despite use of optimal positioning and the BURP maneuver, if the first attempt at intubation fails because of a poor view, particularly a grade 3 laryngoscope view, other alternative intubation devices (i.e., Eschmann introducer, optical stylet, video laryngoscope) should be considered to assist in the second attempt at intubation (see Fig. 37-5, Step 2). There should be no more than two attempts at tracheal intubation in an obstetric patient. The second attempt at laryngoscopy should be considered the "best attempt at tracheal intubation." To increase the success rate, it should be performed by a reasonably experienced anesthesiologist, the optimal sniff or ramped position should be used, and external laryngeal manipulation should be applied. Additionally, the laryngoscope blade type and handle may need to be changed. If necessary, cricoid pressure may be transiently released to optimize the glottic view.

Persistent attempts during emergency tracheal intubation have shown that there was a significant increase in the rate of airway-related complications as the number of laryngoscopic attempts increased (comparing ≤2 with >2 attempts), resulting in hypoxemia (11.8% versus 70%), regurgitation of gastric contents (1.9% versus 22%), aspiration of gastric contents (0.8% versus 13%), bradycardia (1.6% versus 21%), and cardiac arrest (0.7% versus 11%) ($P < 0.001$).[32] We also recommend limiting the intubation attempts to two in an emergent obstetric case.[93-95]

2. Role of Eschmann Introducer (Gum Elastic Bougie)—Grade 3A Laryngoscopic View

The Eschmann introducer, commonly referred to as the gum elastic bougie, is used universally to facilitate difficult tracheal intubation.[96] The original Cormack and Lehane classification of laryngoscopic view[50] was recently modified by Cook,[97] who proposed subdividing grade 3 into grades 3A and 3B (Fig. 37-6). In grade 3A, the glottic aperture cannot be seen but the epiglottis can be visualized and elevated; hence, a role for indirect methods, such as the Eschmann introducer, is indicated. Success rates have been shown to be similar between the Eschmann introducer and optical stylets in the grade 3A airway (31 versus 29.2 seconds).[98]

3. Role of Optical Stylets—Grade 3B/4 Laryngoscopic View

In grade 3B, when the glottic aperture cannot be seen and the epiglottis is visualized but cannot be elevated, other alternative methods may be used (see Fig. 37-6).[99] Optical stylets have been used successfully to facilitate rapid tracheal intubation in the grade 3B laryngoscopic view and to help confirm tracheal tube placement.[98] The success rate has been shown to be higher with optical stylets than with the Eschmann introducer, and the time required is shorter with optical stylets in the grade 3B view (31 versus 45.6 seconds).[98]

4. Role of Video Laryngoscopy

Video technology has become widespread across medical/surgical disciplines and allows improved visualization of anatomic detail. Besides allowing management of the DA, video laryngoscopy can be a useful teaching tool during both direct and indirect laryngoscopy.[100] The portability of video laryngoscopes should facilitate their use in the operating room and also in managing airway calls in emergency departments, intensive care units, endoscopy suites, and radiology suites. It seems only natural that video laryngoscopy will become the norm in managing and teaching the DA in the near future.

Perhaps, in situations in which traditional laryngoscopy fails during the first attempt, the next attempt (best attempt at tracheal intubation) should be the use of a video laryngoscope with which the operator is familiar. Some of the devices available include the Berci Kaplan DCI, Glidescope, McGrath Scope, and CMAC Storz. The Glidescope has been successfully used in large studies and case series.[78,101] Potential difficulty can be overcome by using a rigid stylet and shaping the tracheal tube before attempting insertion.

Channeled video laryngoscopes include the AirTraq, Pentax, and KingVision. These scopes are designed to provide an easy glottic view without aligning the oral, pharyngeal, and tracheal axes and have a channel for holding the tracheal tube. There has been one report of two cases of rapid tracheal intubation using Airtraq in morbidly obese parturients undergoing emergency cesarean delivery after failed tracheal intubation.[102]

Some centers have already implemented the practice of video laryngoscopy as the "first-look" airway device for immediate C/D under GA, and for the anticipated difficult tracheal intubation. The use of alternative devices such as the Eschmann introducer, optical stylets, and video laryngoscopes can enhance the intubation success rate during the second tracheal intubation attempt.

Cook's modification of Cormack and Lehane's Laryngeal Grades of the Airway

	Visualized oral opening	Potential intubation implications
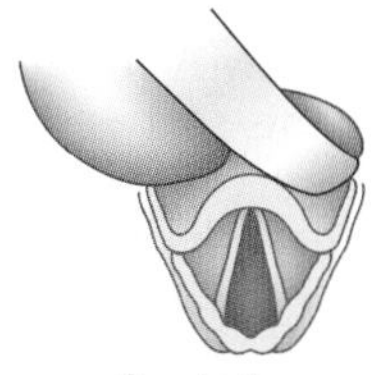 Grade 1	Entire glottic opening from the anterior to posterior commissure	Should facilitate an easy intubation
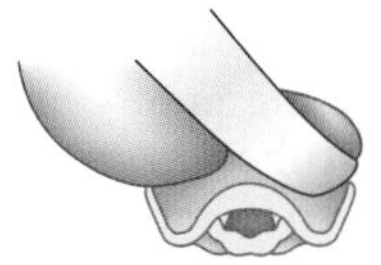 Grade 2	Just the posterior portion of glottis	Normally not difficult to pass a styletted otracheal tube through the laryngeal aperture
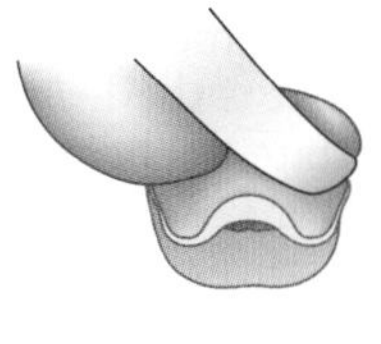 Grade 3a*	Epiglottis only (epiglottis can be lifted using a laryngoscope blade)	Intubation is difficult but possible using a bougie introducer or flexible fiberoptic scope
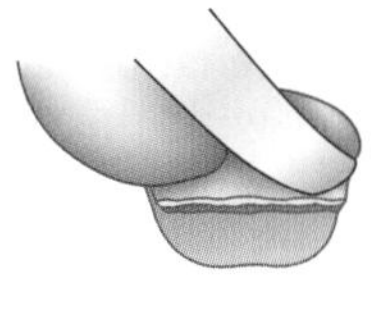 Grade 3b*	Epiglottis only (but epiglottis cannot be lifted from the posterior pharynx using a laryngoscope blade)	Intubation can be difficult because insertion of a bougie introducer (e.g., gum elastic bougie) may be impeded, which can directly affect the successful use of a bougie introducer or a flexible fiberoptic scope
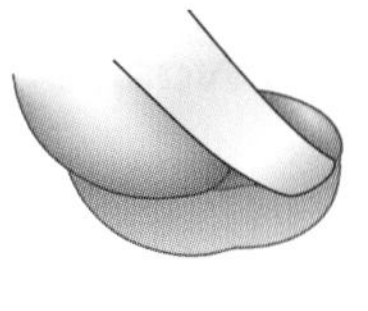 Grade 4*	Only soft tissue, with no identifiable airway anatomy	Difficult intubation, requiring advanced techniques to intubate the trachea

*Tracheal intubation normally requires an advanced airway technique beyond direct laryngoscopy

Figure 37-6 Cormack and Lehane's laryngeal grades of the airway, as modified by Cook. (Adapted from Cook TM: A new practical classification of laryngeal view. *Anaesthesia* 55:274–279, 2000.)

C. Step 3: Maintenance of Oxygenation and Ventilation

The goals and priorities in airway management strategies after a failed second tracheal intubation should include (1) maintenance of maternal oxygenation, (2) prevention of gastric regurgitation, (3) airway protection, and (4) expeditious delivery of the fetus (see Fig. 37-5, Step 3).

Maintaining oxygenation in the parturient is of paramount importance. Pregnancy-related changes can result in rapid development of hypoxemia and acidosis.[103] Because adequate oxygenation is critical, mask ventilation in the presence of cricoid pressure is attempted. If mask ventilation is difficult, an optimal or best attempt at ventilation (i.e., two-person mask ventilation via a conventional face mask) is initiated while cricoid pressure (30 N) is maintained.[95]

The algorithm then divides into two pathways, determined by the presence or absence of adequate face mask ventilation.

After a failed second attempt at tracheal intubation, if oxygen saturation is maintained, the patient is considered to be on the *nonemergency pathway* (cannot intubate, but can ventilate), and use of the classic LMA, the intubating laryngeal mask airway (ILMA), or the ProSeal laryngeal mask airway (PLMA) as a rescue device must be considered. The revised ASA DAA, based on evidence in the literature, supports the role of the LMA in airway management.[104,105] The LMA not only is useful to provide maternal oxygenation, ventilation, and anesthesia but also serves as a conduit for intubation. Cricoid pressure may have to be reduced or released transiently to allow proper placement of the LMA.[91] The LMA or ILMA may be used as a conduit for tracheal intubation, either blind or fiberoptically assisted (see Fig. 37-5, Step 3).

1. The Classic Laryngeal Mask Airway

The classic LMA has been widely used for the difficult obstetric airway without any episodes of gastric regurgitation or pulmonary aspiration.[40,106-109] Han and colleagues successfully used the classic LMA as a ventilatory device in 1060 of 1067 parturients undergoing elective cesarean delivery.[110] No episodes of hypoxia, regurgitation, or aspiration were reported. Multiple case reports in the literature have described successful use of the classic LMA after failed tracheal intubation in obstetric patients.[107,111-114] In patients requiring tracheal intubation, fiberoptic-guided tracheal intubation through the classic LMA is reliable.[115] However, a longer tracheal tube (e.g., Endotrol, Microlaryngeal, or Nasal Ring-Adair-Elwyn) is needed. The Aintree exchange catheter (Cook Medical, Bloomington, IL) may also be used to facilitate intubation through the classic LMA.

The fiberscope/Aintree catheter exchange technique is extremely useful in switching from an LMA to a tracheal tube.[116] The Aintree catheter is 56 cm long and, once preloaded on the fiberscope, allows the distal 3 to 4 cm of the fiberscope to be available for manipulation and passage via the LMA into the trachea. The inner diameter of the Aintree catheter is 4.8 mm, allowing it to be preloaded on no larger than a 4.0-mm pediatric fiberscope. Its removable Rapi-fit connector allows for oxygen insufflation, if necessary, during the airway exchange. Its external diameter is 6.5 mm, allowing it to be used as an airway exchange catheter (AEC) for tracheal tubes that have an internal diameter of 7 mm or more. This airway exchange technique involves the following steps (see Fig. 35-2 in Chapter 35):

1. Insertion of LMA and cuff inflation
2. Confirmation for easy ventilation and oxygenation
3. Passage of fiberscope, preloaded with Aintree catheter, via the LMA into the trachea under vision
4. Removal of fiberscope, leaving the Aintree catheter in the trachea, with the LMA in situ
5. Deflation of LMA cuff, followed by removal of LMA
6. Passage of tracheal tube of at least 7 mm internal diameter over the Aintree catheter into the trachea

2. The Intubating Laryngeal Mask Airway

The LMA Fastrach or ILMA is designed to specifically overcome the problems associated with blind tracheal intubation through the classic LMA.[117] The ILMA is particularly useful during failed intubation in an emergency C/D because it provides oxygenation and a conduit for blind tracheal intubation and prevents pulmonary aspiration. Several studies have shown successful use of the ILMA to help visually unassisted tracheal intubation in patients with a DA.[115,117,118] The ILMA was used successfully after failed tracheal intubation during an emergency C/D in a patient who was morbidly obese and eclamptic and in a second case in which RA had failed and was followed by GA resulting in failed tracheal intubation.[66,67] The ILMA proved to be a life-saving device in both parturients.

3. The ProSeal Laryngeal Mask Airway

The PLMA is a unique device that represents a substantial change in LMA design. The PLMA offers several advantages over the classic LMA for failed tracheal intubation in obstetrics: (1) the seal is 10 cm H_2O higher, giving it greater ventilatory capability[119]; (2) it enables correct positioning in which the glottis is isolated from the esophagus and therefore may provide airway protection and protection against pulmonary aspiration[120,121]; (3) it facilitates gastric tube insertion to empty the stomach of fluid and air insufflated during difficult face mask ventilation. The PLMA has been used successfully after failed intubation during emergency C/D.[120,122-124]

After failed tracheal intubation, and once the anesthesia practitioner is able to successfully achieve pulmonary ventilation and oxygenation through the LMA, caution must be used in selecting a nonirritating inhalation anesthetic and in providing an adequate depth of anesthesia. Sevoflurane provides rapid, smooth induction and adequate depth of anesthesia; it is the least irritating volatile agent,[125] and it helps facilitate tracheal intubation through the LMA in patients with a DA.[126]

If tracheal intubation is difficult via the LMA and the fetal or maternal condition warrants immediate surgery, the obstetrician should be asked to proceed with cesarean delivery while the anesthesia care team maintains cricoid pressure and provides oxygenation and anesthesia via the LMA. Communication with the obstetrician should include the need to avoid both exteriorization of the uterus and fundal pressure during cesarean delivery, because of the unprotected airway and the risk of regurgitation and aspiration (see Fig. 37-5, Step 3).

D. Step 4: CICV—Noninvasive Rescue Ventilation

1. Emergency Pathway

If face mask ventilation was not adequate and the LMA was ineffective in providing oxygenation and ventilation, the patient is considered to be on the *emergency pathway* (CICV) and will require rescue ventilation with other noninvasive devices[4] such as the Combitube. King LTS/LTS-D may be a suitable alternative to the Combitube (see Fig. 37-5, Step 4).

2. Combitube

The Combitube should be considered in emergency airway situations, especially when patients are at risk for pulmonary aspiration, tracheal intubation has failed, and LMA is not effective.[127,128] The ASA DAA suggests use of the Combitube after failed pulmonary ventilation with conventional face mask and LMA.[4] The successful use of the Combitube has been described after failed tracheal intubation in an emergency C/D.[127]

Even though the Combitube is losing its popularity in Canada and the United Kingdom, it is still a part of the ASA DAA, the American Heart Association guidelines, and the European Resuscitation Council guidelines. The ASA DAA incorporated use of the Combitube in the emergency pathway (i.e., the life-threatening CICV situation) in which establishing ventilation and oxygenation is critical. It may also be particularly useful for difficult or failed tracheal intubations in obstetric patients, who are at increased risk for gastric regurgitation and pulmonary aspiration.

When properly positioned, the Combitube allows ventilation with a higher seal pressure than the classic LMA, protects against regurgitation, and allows a subsequent attempt at fiberoptic intubation while the inflated esophageal cuff maintains airway protection.[127,129] Although there have been failures,[130] the Combitube has been used successfully in cases of difficult tracheal intubation[127,131] and CICV,[132,133] including failure with the LMA.[134] The Combitube may offer significant advantages over the LMA in parturients. These advantages include isolation of the stomach from the glottic area and minimal need for preparation. Oxygenation and pulmonary ventilation can be achieved rapidly, especially because the parturient is prone to rapid arterial oxygen desaturation. The Combitube has been shown to prevent pulmonary aspiration during cardiopulmonary resuscitation and to protect the airway from pulmonary aspiration of gastric contents during obstetric anesthesia.[129,135]

The Combitube is a disposable double-lumen tube with two cuffs and two pilot balloons that is designed for blind insertion. If blind insertion is difficult or unsuccessful, the Combitube may be placed in the upper esophagus under direct vision with the use of a laryngoscope. Ventilation is initially attempted through lumen 1, which forces air into the trachea (see Fig. 35-3 in Chapter 35). Causes of failed ventilation with the Combitube include inadvertent tracheal placement (5%), deep insertion laryngospasm, and bronchospasm. The steps in troubleshooting Combitube use are important to understand, especially when one is confronted with a critical airway. The Combitube is designed to enter the esophagus after blind insertion. If ventilation is difficult through the blue lumen 1, the Combitube could be in the trachea, and ventilation must be switched to the clear lumen 2, allowing air to enter the trachea directly through the open end. If the Combitube is inserted too deep (see Fig. 35-5A in Chapter 35), ventilation is impossible and the pharyngeal balloon must be deflated, the Combitube pulled back 1 to 2 cm, and ventilation switched back to the blue lumen 2 (see Fig. 35-5B in Chapter 35). The original Combitube is a large, bulky device and can cause esophageal damage; therefore, the small adult (SA) size is recommended.[136]

3. Other Alternative Airway Devices

The King LT (known as the laryngeal tube in Europe) differs from the Combitube by being smaller, shorter, and softer and having a non-latex oropharyngeal cuff. The design of the King LT allows easy insertion, provides vertical positioning latitude, uses low-pressure cuffs,[119,137] and allows passage of an AEC while simultaneously providing an esophageal barrier (Fig. 37-7A).[138] It is a versatile airway device that can be used in elective or emergent conditions or DA, and ventilation can be spontaneous or controlled.[139]

The King LTS/LTS-D is the double-lumen version. It has dedicated ventilation and gastric access lumens and allows passage of an 18-F orogastric tube via the gastric drainage lumen (see Fig. 37-7B). Ventilatory seal with the King LT and airway pressure of 40 cm H_2O was found to be possible without gastric inflation in 30 patients.[140] The LMA was compared with King LT in 22 patients, and the mean leak pressure was significantly greater for the King LT[141]; gastric insufflation did not occur with the King LT. The King LTS/LTS-D may be useful in situations in which the patient is at risk for aspiration. In a case report, the King LTS was used successfully to establish ventilation and oxygenation after failed intubation in an emergency C/D.[142]

Exchange of the King LT for a tracheal tube can be accomplished with a fiberscope and an AEC (see Fig. 37-7C).[138] The incidence of complications and adverse airway events is minimal with the use of this device.[119]

If oxygenation and ventilation are not established with either the LMA, the Combitube, or the King LT and the patient develops increasing hypoxemia (associated with bradycardia), the patient is considered to be in the *emergency pathway—critical airway* situation, which is a life-threatening emergency requiring immediate invasive intervention and rescue ventilation with either percutaneous cricothyroidotomy, TTJV, or surgical tracheostomy (see Fig. 37-5, Step 5).[4,5]

E. Step 5: CICV with Increasing Hypoxemia—Invasive Rescue Ventilation

1. Emergency Pathway—Critical Airway

All current airway guidelines[4-6] recommend management of the CICV situation using either cannula cricothyroidotomy with percutaneous TTJV or surgical cricothyroidotomy.

The scenario of failed intubation, increasing hypoxemia, and difficult ventilation often occurs secondary to repeated unsuccessful attempts when a "can ventilate" situation rapidly develops into a CICV situation, resulting in significant maternal morbidity, including hypoxic brain damage, and maternal mortality. The fetus is also at risk for severe neurologic injury. Rapid development of severe hypoxemia, particularly if associated with bradycardia, is an indication for imminent intervention with an invasive airway rescue technique.

Once the decision is made to perform an invasive procedure, it is essential to use an effective technique. Rapid reoxygenation is critical and is best achieved with a combination of an invasive airway device and a ventilation technique that is capable of delivering effective ventilation and high minute ventilation with a fraction of inspired oxygen (FIO_2) of 1.0.

2. Cricothyroidotomy and Transtracheal Jet Ventilation

The risks of invasive rescue techniques must be constantly weighed against the risks of hypoxic brain damage or maternal death.[143] In Palanisamy's study,[3] among the 98 parturients who received GA for C/D, there was a sentinel case of DI, resulting in a critical airway incident (CICV) that necessitated a surgical cricothyroidotomy.

Correct Position of the King LTS-D in the Esophagus

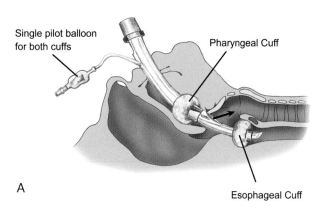

Single pilot balloon for both cuffs

Pharyngeal Cuff

A

Esophageal Cuff

Correct Position of the King LTS-D in the Esophagus with OGT *in-situ*

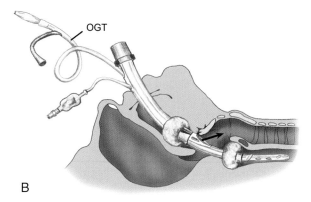

OGT

B

Tracheal Intubation via King LTS-D Using Aintree Catheter and Fiberscope

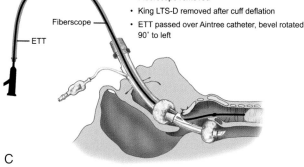

Fiberscope

ETT

- King LTS-D inserted, cuff inflated
- Fiberscope, with preloaded Aintree catheter, inserted into trachea via King LTS-D
- Aintree catheter passed into trachea
- Fiberscope removed
- King LTS-D removed after cuff deflation
- ETT passed over Aintree catheter, bevel rotated 90° to left

C

Figure 37-7 King LTS-D supraglottic airway. **A,** Correct position in the esophagus. **B,** Correct position with orogastric tube *(OGT)* in situ. **C,** Tracheal intubation using Aintree catheter and fiberscope. *ETT,* Endotracheal tube. (Courtesy of Baylor College of Medicine, Houston, TX.)

The investigators reported that the total time taken from RSI of anesthesia to surgical cricothyroidotomy was less than 5 minutes.[3]

The anesthesia practitioner must be prepared to use invasive techniques to secure the airway via the cricothyroid membrane. Success depends on understanding the anatomy of the cricothyroid membrane and factors that determine efficacy of ventilation airway devices.[144,145]

a. CANNULA CRICOTHYROIDOTOMY WITH PERCUTANEOUS TTJV

This technique involves the combination of insertion of a cannula or catheter through the cricothyroid membrane and use of a high-pressure source for ventilation. TTJV can provide effective ventilation[146,147]; however, it is fraught with barotrauma hazards and is associated with a low success rate.[148-150] It is important to keep the upper airway patent and open to allow for deflation of the lungs and exhalation through the upper airway. If an LMA has been used, it can be left in place to allow for exhalation.

The needle cricothyroidotomy entails insertion of a catheter (usually an intravenous catheter) through the cricothyroid membrane; the needle through the catheter

is then removed, and the anesthetist advances the guidewire through the catheter using the Seldinger technique. Next, a dilator is advanced over the guidewire, then removed, and a tracheostomy tube is inserted.

b. SURGICAL CRICOTHYROIDOTOMY

A simplified cricothyroidotomy technique can be performed in 30 seconds.[151] This technique consists of the following four steps:

Step 1—Identification of the cricothyroid membrane
Step 2—Horizontal stab incision (no. 20 scalpel) through skin and membrane
Step 3—Caudal traction on the cricoid membrane with a tracheal hook
Step 4—Intubation of the trachea

Cricothyroidotomy can be particularly difficult in the obese patient. Insertion of the tube can be facilitated by passage of an introducer (bougie) through the incision or by the use of a tracheal retractor.[152]

Guidewire techniques of cricothyroidotomy can be successful. The Melker guidewire intubation set is now available with a cuffed tube. It has been shown that the technique can be performed in 40 seconds after practice in a mannequin.[153]

3. Extubation

The ASA Task Force regarded the concept of an extubation strategy as a logical extension of the extubation process.[4] The closed claims analysis for DA management in surgical patients concluded that development of management strategies covering emergence and the recovery phase after extubation may improve patient safety.[10]

An emerging problem in obstetric patients is respiratory-related complications after emergence and maternal mortality after extubation.[20] The data from the Confidential Enquiries into Maternal Death from the United Kingdom and a study from the United States on anesthesia-related deaths in Michigan indicated that airway management of the obstetric patient during induction of GA,[20,154] including intubation, was without complications; however, critical airway and ventilation incidents including hypoventilation or airway obstruction occurred during emergence, extubation, or recovery.

Current literature does not provide a sufficient basis for evaluating the merits of an extubation strategy.[4] The focus has been mainly on addressing strategies, safety concerns, and techniques for intubating the trachea after induction of anesthesia, with relatively little attention paid to extubation strategies. The U.K. data specifically mentioned lack of training as partly responsible for the undesirable outcomes after extubation. The review from Michigan identified eight anesthesia-related deaths between 1985 and 2003. All of these deaths occurred as a result of airway obstruction or hypoventilation during emergence and recovery. Lapses in standard postoperative monitoring and inadequate supervision by an anesthesiologist were identified. Obesity and African-American race also seemed to be important risk factors for anesthesia-related maternal mortality.

Proposals to improve patient safety in obstetrics must require identification of preexisting comorbidities that can lead to postoperative respiratory complications. Standard monitoring in the postoperative period that includes pulse oximetry must be mandatory. As perioperative physicians, anesthesiologists are uniquely qualified to supervise the anesthesia care team; to manage and minimize anesthesia-related maternal risk; to provide peripartum medical diagnosis and treatment; to facilitate life-saving airway management interventions; and to lead prompt, coordinated, and effective resuscitation efforts to prevent airway catastrophes in obstetric patients.

Further attention is required for high-risk extubation patients, such as obese parturients and patients with an edematous airway, obstructive sleep apnea, or known or suspected airway management difficulties. Development of a strategy to maintain continuous access to the airway, so as to facilitate potential rescue of the airway, must be considered. Postextubation hypoventilation, airway compromise, ventilation-perfusion inequalities, and airway obstruction due to respiratory fatigue or apneic episodes may affect the patient in the operating room during emergence or in the immediate postoperative recovery period. Maintenance of continuous access to the airway

after extubation with an AEC can be an important component of an extubation strategy in these selected patients.[155] The AEC is well tolerated by most patients (90%) and therefore is a valuable option.[155] Currently, there are no evidence-based guidelines regarding the optimal period of time for which to maintain airway access after extubation via an indwelling AEC. Experts have suggested at least 30 to 60 minutes or until the likelihood of reintubation is minimized.[156-159] Patients with the potential for periglottic edema may benefit from extending the duration of the in-dwelling AEC to 60 to 120 minutes.[155]

The presence of an AEC to assist in reintubating and resecuring the airway is another major step toward improving patient safety and must be considered for obstetric patients who are potentially at high risk for airway-related catastrophes during emergence and after extubation.

XIV. COMMUNICATION AND DOCUMENTATION

After a failed tracheal intubation and successful airway management in a patient undergoing C/D, the following measures need to be adopted at the conclusion of the procedure:

1. Comprehensive documentation in the patient's chart outlining the problem and measures taken to manage the airway
2. Communication with the patient and the family
3. A detailed letter for the patient to carry describing the events that took place and their subsequent management
4. An airway alert in the electronic medical record
5. Application for a Medic-Alert band for the patient
6. Notification to the DA registry

XV. CONCLUSIONS

Difficult laryngoscopy, failed tracheal intubation, and inability to ventilate or oxygenate after induction of GA for C/D are major contributory factors leading to maternal morbidity and mortality. Management of the DA has emerged as one of the most important safety issues. The necessity of a focused history, physical examination, and airway evaluation for predictors of DI and difficult ventilation allows the anesthesia practitioner to develop appropriate strategies of management for the obstetric patient. Heightened awareness of GA-related maternal mortality has led to a dramatic increase in the use of neuraxial anesthesia techniques in obstetric patients, with a consequent decrease in anesthesia-related maternal mortality. Despite the decrease in maternal mortality, however, DI continues to be a high-liability issue.

Emergency airway management after failed intubation in obstetrics presents a challenge for the anesthesia practitioner. The dictum of having preformulated strategies for airway management in place before induction is important. Working within the framework of the ASA DAA; seeking help sooner rather than later; deciding to restrict the number of attempts to no more than two after failed tracheal intubation; using alternative devices to assist tracheal intubation; using supraglottic airways; maintaining oxygenation throughout the execution of the plan; and using invasive techniques such as cricothyroidotomy in a CICV situation are keys to successful outcome for both mother and baby.

The declining use of GA in obstetrics is concerning because of the diminished airway management skills of anesthesia trainees in obstetrics. Solutions to the problem include a dedicated and structured advanced airway management (AAM) rotation for anesthesia trainees, formal curriculum and teaching of the DAA, and systematic practice and repetition of AAM clinical skills in the operating room in surgical patients. High-fidelity simulation training with formal instruction in management of failed tracheal intubation, difficult ventilation, and cricothyroidotomy skills in obstetric emergency situations should be taught and practiced. Simulator training and protocols to deal with airway management issues may enhance the skills of the anesthesia trainee for future management of airway issues in obstetric patients.

XVI. CLINICAL PEARLS

- Cesarean delivery is the most common major surgical operation carried out in the United States (U.S. Centers for Disease Control and Prevention's National Center for Health Statistics report) and is increasing in incidence throughout the world.

- Anesthesia-related maternal complications rank seventh in the United States and the United Kingdom as a cause of maternal mortality; airway-related causes feature as a predominant category and are preventable.

- Pregnancy-related anatomic and physiologic changes predispose parturients to difficulty with intubation, ventilation, and extubation.

- Early preoperative assessment for patients undergoing labor and delivery must include a thorough airway history and examination and a rescue plan for potential failed tracheal intubation. Appropriate airway equipment and personnel must be immediately available in labor and delivery sites to manage the difficult airway (DA).

- Regional anesthesia (RA) is safe in most parturients undergoing cesarean delivery; in certain exceptional situations, an awake tracheal intubation is considered the safest choice in cases of anticipated or known DA in a parturient undergoing cesarean delivery.

- Adequate preoxygenation, left uterine displacement, head-elevated positioning, and use of supplementary high-flow oxygen via nasal cannula enhances oxygenation.

- Alternative airway devices such as optical stylets or video laryngoscopy should be used after a failed second attempt at tracheal intubation in the unanticipated DA (cannot intubate, can ventilate) scenario.

- First generation supraglottic airways such as the laryngeal mask airway (LMA) and second-generation supraglottic airways such as the King LTS-D should be considered as ventilatory devices in the unanticipated DA ("cannot intubate, cannot ventilate" [CICV]) scenario.

- Invasive airway access with a percutaneous/surgical cricothyrotomy or transtracheal jet ventilation (TTJV) may be necessary in the situation of critical airway with hypoxemia.

- Problems related to emergence and extubation have emerged as the most common cause of airway-related maternal mortality in recent reports from United States and the United Kingdom.

- Documentation should be provided in the patient's record if difficulty is encountered with laryngoscopy, tracheal intubation, ventilation, or tracheal extubation.

SELECTED REFERENCES

All references can be found online at expertconsult.com.
1. Davies JM, Posner KL, Lee LA, et al: Liability associated with obstetric anesthesia: A closed claims analysis. *Anesthesiology* 110:131–139, 2009.
3. Palanisamy A, Mitani AA, Tsen LC: General anesthesia for cesarean delivery at a tertiary care hospital from 2000 to 2005: A retrospective analysis and 10-year update. *Int J Obstet Anesth* 20:10–16, 2010.
4. American Society of Anesthesiologists Task Force on Management of the Difficult Airway: Practice guidelines for management of the difficult airway: An updated report by the American Society of Anesthesiologists Task Force on Management of the Difficult Airway. *Anesthesiology* 98:1269–1277, 2003.
5. Henderson JJ, Popat MT, Latto IP, Pearce AC: Difficult Airway Society guidelines for management of the unanticipated difficult intubation. *Anaesthesia* 59:675–694, 2004.
10. Peterson GN, Domino KB, Caplan RA, et al: Management of the difficult airway: A closed claims analysis. *Anesthesiology* 103:33–39, 2995.
12. Hawkins JL: Anesthesia-related maternal mortality. *Clin Obstet Gynecol* 46:679–687, 2003.
20. Mhyre JM, Riesner MN, Polley LS, Naughton NN: A series of anesthesia-related maternal deaths in Michigan, 1985-2003. *Anesthesiology* 106:1096–1104, 2007.
24. Boutonnet M, Faitot V, Katz A, et al: Mallampati class changes during pregnancy, labour, and after delivery: Can these be predicted? *Br J Anaesth* 104:67–70, 2010.
93. Wali A, Suresh MS: Maternal morbidity, mortality, and risk assessment. *Anesthesiol Clin* 26:197–230, ix, 2008.
97. Cook TM: Classification of laryngoscopic view. *Anaesthesia* 55:1029–1030, 2000.
98. Kovacs G, Law JA, McCrossin C, et al: A comparison of a fiberoptic stylet and a bougie as adjuncts to direct laryngoscopy in a manikin-simulated difficult airway. *Ann Emerg Med* 50:676–685, 2007.
101. Cooper RM, Pacey JA, Bishop MJ, McCluskey SA: Early clinical experience with a new videolaryngoscope (GlideScope) in 728 patients. *Can J Anaesth* 52:191–198, 2005.
153. Wong DT, Prabhu AJ, Coloma M, et al: What is the minimum training required for successful cricothyroidotomy?: A study in mannequins. *Anesthesiology* 98:349–353, 2003.
155. Mort TC: Continuous airway access for the difficult extubation: The efficacy of the airway exchange catheter. *Anesth Analg* 105:1357–1362, 2007.

Chapter 38

Anesthetic and Airway Management of Microlaryngeal Surgery and Upper Airway Endoscopy

VLADIMIR NEKHENDZY | MICHAEL SELTZ KRISTENSEN | REBECCA E. CLAURE

I. GENERAL CONSIDERATIONS

The range and precision of laryngologic surgical procedures have dramatically expanded over the past decade. Patient outcomes have improved due to technologic advances such as the introduction of high-magnification operating microscopes and video endoscopes, instrument miniaturization, new injection materials, and the use of powered instrumentation and optical fiber–based lasers.[1-5]

Advances and demands of the new surgical techniques and an expanding patient population that was previously considered unsuitable for surgery have created novel challenges for the anesthesiologist. State-of-the-art anesthesia and airway management for laryngeal surgery require the anesthesiologist to be adept with various methods of managing the difficult airway and performing airway exchange, to competently execute intraoperative ventilation strategies, to be proficient with inhalational and total intravenous anesthesia, and to quickly tailor

785

anesthetic techniques to the various durations of the surgical cases. New challenges have developed with the widespread introduction of minimally invasive laryngeal robotic surgery, which demands a fully open surgical field for three-dimensional visualization and superior motor control.[4,6,7]

Successful anesthetic management of microlaryngeal cases requires a high degree of cooperation with the surgeon, a reciprocal understanding of the potential problems, and adequate preparation on both sides to meet the anticipated challenges that may arise.[1,3,8,9] Thorough appreciation by the anesthesiologist of the complexity of the upper airway anatomy, the pathologic process involved, and all steps of the surgical procedure is necessary for devising a rational anesthetic plan and maintaining a good working relationship with the surgeon.[1,8,10] The expert ability to safely share the patient's airway with the surgeon, in conjunction with an intimate knowledge of possible immediate intraoperative and early postoperative complications of laryngeal surgery, greatly contributes to safe patient management in the perioperative period.[8]

Microlaryngeal surgery encompasses a wide range of laryngeal procedures that can be organized in two broad categories: phonomicrosurgery (i.e., benign and malignant vocal cord lesions, laser laryngeal surgery, and vocal cord augmentation) and laryngeal framework surgery (i.e., vocal cord paralysis and motion disorders, scarring, stenosis of the glottic, subglottic, and tracheal areas, and laryngeal trauma).[1] For practical purposes, these may be further categorized as involving endoscopy alone, surgical excision, injection, dilation, or a combination of these approaches.

This chapter focuses on airway management and anesthesia for microlaryngeal surgery, diagnostic direct laryngoscopy, and endoscopy (i.e., bronchoscopy and esophagoscopy). A combination of these three interventions, called *panendoscopy*, is typically performed as part of the diagnostic work-up for patients with head and neck cancer, and is accompanied by surgical biopsies of the base of the tongue, piriform sinuses, nasopharynx, and other diseased or suspicious areas.[11-13] Additional surgical indications for bronchoscopy and esophagoscopy are discussed in the corresponding sections of this chapter, and management of pediatric patients is discussed separately from approaches to adults.

II. PATIENT PREOPERATIVE EVALUATION AND PREPARATION

Patients presenting for phonomicrosurgery may have a variety of comorbidities contributing to their voice symptoms and affecting anesthetic management. Changes in voice quality can be exaggerated by inadequate airflow production (e.g., chronic obstructive pulmonary disease [COPD]) or vocal fatigue caused by neuromuscular disorders (e.g., myasthenia gravis, muscular dystrophy, Parkinson's disease).[1] Various rheumatologic and musculoskeletal ailments can alter posture, impairing voice quality, and endocrine disorders, such as hypothyroidism, can cause dysphonia as a result of swelling in the Reinke's

space (i.e., superficial lamina propria) of the vocal cords.[1]

Almost one half of the patients presenting with laryngeal and voice disorders have silent laryngopharyngeal reflux as the primary cause or as a significant etiologic factor.[1,14] Coexistent significant glottic insufficiency (e.g., vocal cord paralysis) may place these patients at increased risk for aspiration of gastric contents,[13,15] and it can usually be diagnosed during a routine preoperative flexible fiberoptic laryngoscopy or laryngostroboscopy performed by the surgeon. Those presenting for esophagoscopy for evaluation and treatment of esophageal obstructing lesions, achalasia, Zenker's diverticulum, active gastrointestinal bleeding, or esophageal foreign body removal constitute another category of patients at high risk for aspiration. Even when gastroesophageal reflux is not clinically significant, adequate preoperative pharmacologic control of the symptoms is warranted: the combination of acid exposure and direct trauma from the operating procedure and the endotracheal intubation can lead to laryngeal mucosal injury.[16]

Many patients presenting for laryngeal surgery and panendoscopy have a long history of heavy smoking and drinking,[17] which are directly linked to the development of squamous cell carcinoma of the larynx, the second most common malignancy of the head and neck.[18] It is not uncommon for these patients to present with anemia.[18] Appropriate laboratory studies should be obtained, and the electrolyte and fluid status of these patients should be optimized preoperatively.

Chronic cigarette smoking and alcohol use can cause induction of the cytochrome P450 multi-enzyme system, leading to increased perioperative requirements for opioids and neuromuscular blockers and generation of higher levels of potentially toxic metabolites of volatile halogenated anesthetic agents.[19-22] Patients with chronic alcohol consumption require preoperative evaluation of liver function and coagulation status. For those with advanced liver disease, controlled hypotensive techniques should be avoided, and intraoperative hypotension should be treated aggressively to prevent adverse outcomes associated with prolonged decrease in hepatic circulation and further deterioration of liver function.[23]

Many patients who present for laryngeal surgery are elderly and have cardiovascular disease. Appropriate diagnostic tests are indicated for them as part of the preoperative work-up. The pulmonary status of COPD patients should be optimized to decrease airway reactivity and the possibility of postoperative pulmonary complications. Patients with significant lung disease and ventilation-perfusion ($\dot{V}/\dot{Q}$) mismatch may not be suitable candidates for intraoperative ventilation techniques, such as spontaneous ventilation, apneic intermittent ventilation (AIV), or jet ventilation (JV),[22-24] which may be required for microlaryngeal surgery (see "Intraoperative Ventilation Techniques and Strategies for Microlaryngeal Surgery").

The rate of difficult endotracheal intubation may reach almost 16% among patients presenting for ear, nose, or throat cancer surgery,[25] which is on average six times higher than among the general surgical patient population.[25-29] Comprehensive preoperative airway

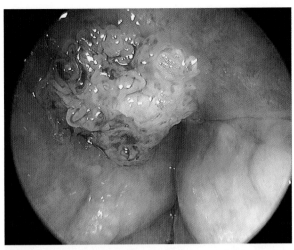

Figure 38-1   Epiglottic carcinoma. (Courtesy of Edward Damrose, MD, Stanford University Medical Center, Stanford, CA.)

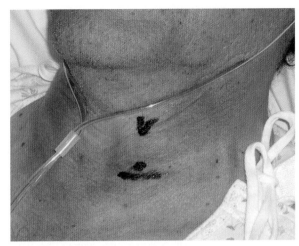

Figure 38-3   Patient with a laryngeal carcinoma, fixed hemilarynx, and severe inspiratory stridor presented for panendoscopy and subsequent tracheostomy. The *black check mark* indicates a thyroid notch, a *horizontal black line* corresponds to the top of the cricoid cartilage, and a *black dot* represents the location of the cricothyroid membrane. Notice the inflammatory skin changes. The vocal cords were visible during preoperative nasal endoscopy. Endotracheal intubation was successfully accomplished by video laryngoscopy after inhalational induction.

assessment is paramount (see Chapter 8); however, standard anesthesia airway assessment tests fail to account for aspiration risk, lower airway problems, and base of the tongue pathology (e.g., epiglottic cancer, epiglottic and vallecula cysts, lingual tonsillar hypertrophy). Pathology of the base of the tongue may be encountered with increased frequency in patients presenting for panendoscopy and microlaryngeal surgery (Fig. 38-1).

Postradiation changes in the neck and decreased mandibular protrusion are important factors predicting the risk of impossible mask ventilation, difficult mask ventilation, and difficult intubation in patients at risk for these conditions (see Chapter 8),[30,31] and these risk factors may occur with increased frequency among patients presenting for microlaryngeal surgery or panendoscopy.[12] The pharyngeal space may also be reduced by limited submandibular compliance of the soft tissues (e.g., cancerous involvement, masses, inflammation, previous radiation therapy) (Fig. 38-2), which may result in difficult intubation or failed intubation due to the restriction of the space that accommodates the tongue during direct laryngoscopy.[32]

Pharyngeal restriction can be further accentuated by a large tongue or intraoral masses that can be exophytic and mobile.[32] Drooling, dysphagia, and expiratory snoring are the signs of marked pharyngeal restriction,[17,32] but inspiratory stridor at rest represents the most worrisome sign, suggesting a reduction in airway diameter at the supraglottic, periglottic, or glottic level of at least 50%.[15,31-33]

Airway compromise in these patients may also involve the lower airways. Airway narrowing at the tracheal or tracheobronchial level is typically characterized by expiratory stridor, whereas biphasic inspiratory-expiratory stridor usually points to obstructive subglottic lesions.[8] In some cases, preoperative examination of the flow-volume loops may be helpful.[34]

It is prudent to assess the laryngeal mobility, the degree of tracheal deviation, and the location of the cricothyroid membrane (CTM).[18] Significant tracheal deviation, especially in combination with the fixed hemilarynx (Fig. 38-3) and poor or absent visualization of the vocal cords during preoperative nasal endoscopy, can be an ominous sign,[33,35] warranting performance of an awake tracheostomy, if technically feasible. Usually, the extent of disease in elective cases has been comprehensively evaluated preoperatively by routine chest radiography, computed tomography (CT), magnetic resonance imaging (MRI), and flexible fiberoptic laryngoscopy, providing the anesthesiologist with valuable information regarding the location, size, spread, and vascularity of the obstructive lesions; the degree of obstruction; the mobility of the vocal cords; and the extent of laryngeal and tracheal deviation or compression.[8,18,36] Preoperative discussion of these findings with the surgeon helps to devise safe and rational airway management and anesthetic plans for the patient.[18]

Other airway considerations for patients presenting for microlaryngeal surgery or panendoscopy include

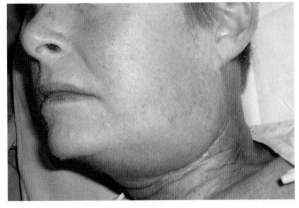

Figure 38-2   Postradiation neck changes and decreased submandibular compliance in a patient presenting for panendoscopy. Notice the postincisional neck scar, and Postradiation changes that have resulted in fibrotic changes in the skin and subcutaneous tissues of the neck and induration of the submandibular space.

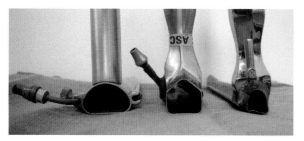

Figure 38-4 Commonly used operating laryngoscopes. The posterior apertures of the Kleinsasser *(left)*, Dedo *(center)*, and Holinger *(right)* operating laryngoscopes are shown. The bigger size and wider channel of the Kleinsasser and Dedo laryngoscopes allows passage of the surgical instruments and binocular microlaryngeal surgery. Notice the metal cannula inserted into the left side port of the Kleinsasser laryngoscope for supraglottic jet ventilation (JV). In the Dedo scope, the JV port is integrated with the lumen, and it can be used for smog evacuation during laser surgery. The Holinger laryngoscope is monocular but has greater maneuverability. It is widely used for diagnostic laryngoscopy and visualization of the anterior commissure. The left side channel of the Holinger laryngoscope is occupied by a light guide. Supraglottic JV through the Holinger laryngoscope requires insertion of a metal cannula inside its lumen (see Fig. 38-15).

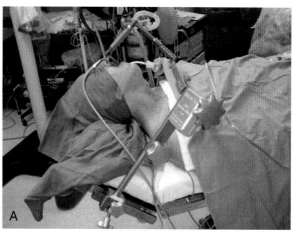

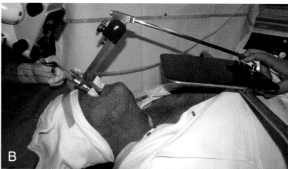

Figure 38-5 Types of suspension laryngoscopy. **A,** Gallows-type suspension device. **B,** Fulcrum-type suspension device (Storz apparatus). Notice the patients' neck flexion and head extension, which are required for suspension laryngoscopy. (**A,** From Rosen CA, Simpson CB, editors: *Operative techniques in laryngology,* Berlin, 2008, Springer-Verlag, p 68.)

anticipation of the presence of supraglottic and glottic edema due to inflammation, infection, tumors, previous radiation therapy or repeated endoscopies,[37] and careful dental assessment. Gentle airway manipulation during direct laryngoscopy is essential. The use of a smaller-diameter endotracheal tube (ETT) is frequently warranted, and the absence of dental trauma should be documented before surgical instrumentation of the patient's airway commences.

III. OPERATIVE LARYNGOSCOPY AND MICROLARYNGEAL SURGERY

A. Special Considerations and Anesthesia Objectives

In contrast to direct laryngoscopes used by the anesthesiologists, which are designed only to identify the glottic opening, operating laryngoscopes can provide excellent and wide laryngeal exposure and allow diagnostic examination, biopsy, and operation on structures in the larynx and pharynx, with minimal distortion of the areas of surgical interest.[16,38] The handles of these laryngoscopes are integrated with the blades and have a wide proximal aperture that facilitates the passage of instruments during suspension laryngoscopy.[38,39] Many types of laryngoscopes exist (Fig. 38-4), each offering certain advantages for its intended application, such as the ability to better expose supraglottic, glottic, or subglottic areas.[38] Many laryngoscopes are multipurpose, and selection is frequently dictated by individual or institutional preference.[38]

With the use of these laryngoscopes, systematic endoscopy of the larynx and pharynx frequently proceeds in three stages, progressing from handheld examination to suspension laryngoscopy (for more detailed evaluation with the straight and angled telescopes) and then to microlaryngoscopy using the operating microscope for image magnification, biopsy, microsurgery, or laser surgery.[38] Suspension laryngoscopy (Fig. 38-5) frees the surgeon's hands for precision bimanual surgery and facilitates maintenance of a stable plane of anesthesia.[38,40] The use of a video monitor by the surgeon permits the anesthesiologist to observe the surgical procedure and monitor the patient's airway.

The essential requirements for precision microlaryngeal surgery and optimal preservation of function include a clear and still surgical field, absence of patient movement, and allocation of sufficient time to carefully complete the procedure in an unhurried manner.[9,38,39,41] The patient's airway must be protected from blood, debris, and irrigation fluid, and ventilation must be adequately controlled.[3,8,41] The anesthesiologist must safely share the patient's airway with the surgeon, and must be prepared to skillfully and confidently switch from one ventilation technique to another during the case if needed or dictated by surgery.

In most surgical procedures, the patient's airway is shared with the surgeon, and immediate access to the airway is difficult or impossible because the operating room (OR) table is turned 90 or 180 degrees away from the anesthesiologist. The ETT must be secured diligently to prevent accidental extubation under the surgical drapes or withdrawal of the ETT into the larynx, resulting in a sudden air leak or possible compression of the anterior branch of the recurrent laryngeal nerve by the ETT cuff.[42,43]

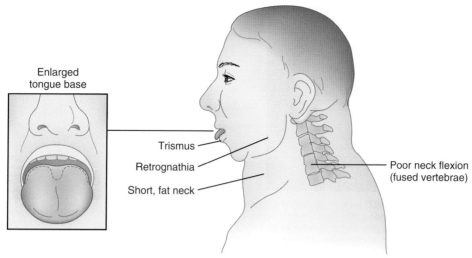

Figure 38-6   Anatomic features associated with a difficult airway exposure. Difficult laryngeal exposure during direct or suspension laryngoscopy may be encountered in patients with retrognathia; lingual hypertrophy or poor palatal visualization; trismus or reduced interincisor opening; short, thick neck; and limited neck extension. (From In Rosen CA, Simpson CB, editors: *Operative techniques in laryngology*, Berlin, 2008, Springer-Verlag, p 56.)

Performance of conventional and operative direct laryngoscopy, supraglottic tissue distention, and laryngeal stimulation elicit intense cardiovascular responses, resulting in tachycardia, arterial and pulmonary hypertension, and arrhythmias.[44-46] Although these responses are usually short lived, myocardial ischemia and compromise of cerebral circulation may occur in high-risk patients, resulting in adverse outcomes.[47-49] Anesthetic technique should ensure a stable plane of anesthesia, nonstimulating emergence from anesthesia, a rapid return of consciousness, and protective airway reflexes, and it should facilitate quick discharge of patients, because most of these surgical procedures are done on an outpatient basis.[3,8]

Special attention should be directed to adequately protecting the patient's eyes and arms to prevent accidental injury or compression by heavy surgical instrumentation.[9] When rigid endoscopy is planned, a tooth guard should be used routinely.[34] It may be prudent to warn the patients in advance of the potential for dental trauma, and any previous dental damage should be carefully documented.[34,43]

Patients who are vocal performers or use the voice in some professional capacity present unique challenges.[16] The anesthesiologist must frequently think outside the box and exercise different advanced airway management options to avert trauma to the patient's vocal cords and cricoarytenoid joints.

B. Airway Management for Microlaryngeal Surgery

1. Conventional and Advanced Airway Management

Patients presenting for diagnostic direct laryngoscopy and microlaryngeal surgery frequently have a difficult airway. The chosen approach to this airway depends on the pathology and the patient's symptoms. In situations with critical airway compromise, an awake tracheostomy may be warranted from the outset, but it may prove to be technically challenging or impossible and may require

general anesthesia. Even if an awake tracheostomy is chosen as a primary approach, full backup preparation for alternative airway management is necessary.

Video laryngoscopy reliably improves laryngeal exposure by at least one grade,[50-54] allows continuous observation of the entire intubation procedure by the entire team, and may therefore be a near-ideal technique for managing difficult airways in patients presenting for microlaryngeal surgery. Choosing the video laryngoscopic device depends on the operator's preference and must consider the nature and location of the lesions. For example, it may be safer to navigate around tumors at the base of the tongue with the Pentax Airway Scope, whose blade engages under the epiglottis, unlike other devices that typically require the tip of the blade to be placed in the vallecula. Video laryngoscopes that use the steering technique (i.e., styleted ETT), such as the Glidescope video laryngoscope, offer better control of intubation and may facilitate ETT maneuvering around the intraoral masses.[55] Although the use of the Glidescope may be less traumatic compared with the Airtraq in patients presenting for microlaryngeal surgery,[56] in the largest published series of Glidescope-assisted intubations in more than 2000 patients with difficult airways,[57] the strongest predictor of the steering technique failure was altered neck anatomy with presence of a surgical scar, radiation changes, or a mass. These conditions are frequently encountered in patients presenting for diagnostic direct laryngoscopy and microlaryngeal surgery.

Although advanced airway management techniques can be highly successful when direct laryngoscopy fails, the patient's unfavorable anatomy (Fig. 38-6) may not be modifiable for the surgical exposure, which requires the use of the largest operating laryngoscope and placement of the patient's head in the Boyce-Jackson position using a combination of cervical flexion and atlantooccipital extension (see Fig. 38-5).[1,38,58,59] If suspension laryngoscopy fails or if the location of the lesion is not easily accessible, it can be performed, to the extent microlaryngeal surgery permits, with the help of the flexible

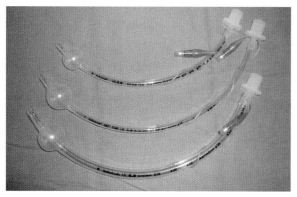

Figure 38-7 Microlaryngeal tracheal (MLT) tube. A standard endotracheal tube (ETT) with an inner diameter (ID) of 5.0 mm *(top)* is compared with a 5.0-mm ID MLT tube *(center)* and 8.0-mm ID ETT *(bottom)*. A greater length and bigger cuff diameter of the MLT tube (equivalent to a standard 8.0-mm ID ETT) allows a sufficient depth of tracheal placement, a connection to the anesthesia circuit, and an adequate seal of the trachea.

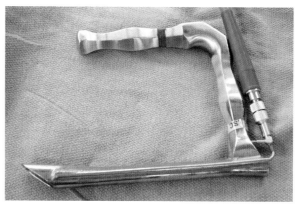

Figure 38-8 Holinger anterior commissure laryngoscope. The pointed tip and the leverage capability of the laryngoscope facilitate visualization of at least part of the glottis. An anterior flare at the tip of the laryngoscope allows it to serve as a guide to endotracheal intubation.

fiberoptic bronchoscope (FFB) inserted through the laryngeal mask airway (LMA).[60-62] The intubating laryngeal mask airway (iLMA) offers certain advantages, such as a rigid, wide metal tube that can accommodate a large-diameter FFB,[61] optimal alignment of the iLMA aperture with the glottic opening,[63] diminished hemodynamic responses compared with suspension laryngoscopy,[61] and superior ventilation capabilities.[63-66]

The iLMA is associated with an outstanding success rate for blind endotracheal intubation in patients with difficult airways.[63,65] Unfortunately, the manufacturer-supplied iLMA ETTs are too big for most microlaryngoscopic surgery. An ETT with a smaller inner diameter (ID) (e.g., 5.0-mm ID microlaryngeal tracheal [MLT] tube) is typically required to maximize the surgical view (Fig. 38-7). Placement of MLT tubes through the iLMA can be achieved with the help of a small-diameter FFB; however, passage of the ETT through the laryngeal inlet into the trachea is blind. Blind advancement of the ETT may cause inadvertent laryngeal trauma and core out pedunculated supraglottic or glottic tumors, nodules, or cysts.[56,67] When the FFB route (with or without the use of a supralaryngeal airway device) is chosen for endotracheal intubation, it is advantageous to closely match the outer diameter (OD) of the scope with the ID of the ETT to minimize the risk of complications associated with blind ETT advancement. Use of optical stylets (e.g., Bonfils, Shikani, Clarus Video System) may also be beneficial in that regard, because the ETT will follow the trajectory of the stylet navigated under direct vision through the vocal cords. However, most of the available adult-size stylets require the use of an ETT with a minimum ID of 5.5 to 6.0 mm.

The decision to proceed with an awake or asleep approach to an anticipated difficult airway should follow the American Society of Anesthesiologists (ASA) difficult airway algorithm,[68] with special attention directed to predictors of difficult mask ventilation, impossible mask ventilation, and their association with difficult intubation (see Chapter 8). The anesthesiologist also should review the pertinent preoperative findings identified on flexible fiberoptic laryngoscopy, chest radiography, CT, and MRI and should discuss these findings with the surgeon.

If an asleep approach to the difficult airway is chosen, several preformulated alternative airway management plans must be in place before induction of anesthesia. If the airway is marginal, the patient's neck should be prepped, and the surgical team should be present on induction, ready to perform an emergent cricothyrotomy or tracheostomy, or to employ rescue techniques such as the use of the surgical anterior commissure scope or a rigid bronchoscope.[11,18,69,70] The anterior commissure scopes (e.g., Holinger, Ossoff-Pilling, Benjamin Slimline/Super-Slimline, Jackson) (Fig. 38-8; see Fig. 38-4) have great leverage capabilities, incorporate the recessed lighting and concurrent rigid microsuction, and can be very effective in handling poor laryngeal exposure or glottic obstruction.[1,13,38,69] The anterior flare at the distal oval end allows these scopes to be used as a conduit for orotracheal intubation when the bougie introducer or the ETT is passed directly down the lumen (Fig. 38-9).[69]

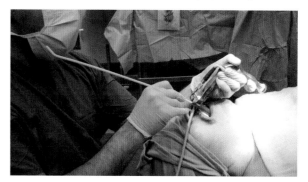

Figure 38-9 Airway rescue is achieved with a bougie introducer and a Holinger laryngoscope in a patient with difficult laryngeal exposure. The endotracheal tube (ETT) cannot be directly advanced down the narrow barrel of the Holinger laryngoscope due to impaired visualization during tube advancement. The bougie introducer is used first, followed by removal of the laryngoscope and railroading the ETT over the bougie into the patient's trachea. The ETT can be directly advanced through the wider lumen of other laryngoscopes, such as the Lindholm or Dedo (see Fig. 38-14).

In experienced hands, rigid bronchoscopy may be used to rescue failed direct laryngoscopy and failed intubation and to manage a "cannot intubate, cannot ventilate" (CICV) situation.[68] It also serves as an indispensable tool for managing acute airway obstruction resulting from foreign bodies, hemoptysis, or tumors.[71] After the bronchoscope is placed into the patient's trachea by the surgeon, manual (Fig. 38-10) or JV can commence in a safe manner through the lumen of the bronchoscope. Subsequent airway exchange to the ETT can be performed using a bougie introducer (Fig. 38-11).[72,73] This exchange technique can also be conducted when the rigid bronchoscope is employed first as part of a panendoscopy procedure in patients with abnormal airway.

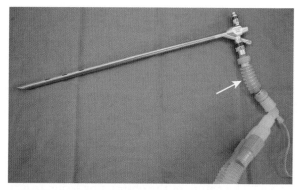

Figure 38-10 A rigid bronchoscope is connected to the anesthesia circuit by a Racine adapter *(arrow)*. A flexible diaphragm of the Racine universal adapter (SunMed, Largo, FL) connects a side arm of a rigid bronchoscope to the anesthesia breathing circuit.

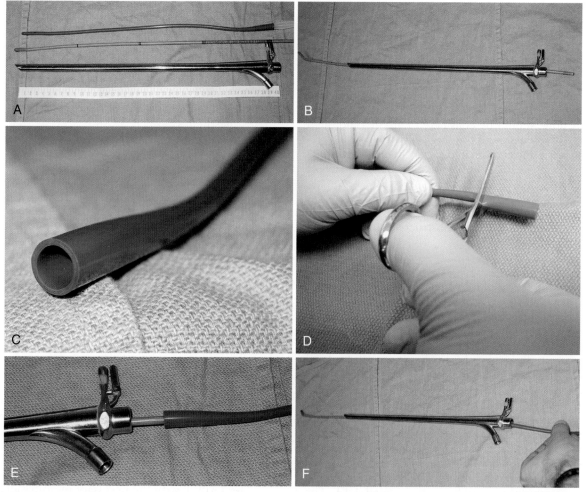

Figure 38-11 Airway exchange can be achieved with a rigid bronchoscope and a bougie introducer. **A,** The 9-F, 40-cm-long, rigid bronchoscope (CL Jackson Fiberoptic Bronchoscope, Pilling Inc., Fort Washington, PA); 15-F, 60-cm-long, multiple-use gum elastic bougie (GEB) (Eschmann Tracheal Tube Introducer, SIMS Portex Inc., Keene, NH); and 16-F, 41-cm-long, rounded, closed-tip suction catheter (Robi-Nel catheter, Kendall Dover, Mansfield, MA) are used to facilitate an airway exchange. The exchange technique involves several steps: deliberately passing the curved tip of the GEB **(B)** through the lumen of the bronchoscope into a bronchus (eliciting a distal hold up sign); stabilizing and extending a proximal straight tip of the GEB with a precut, distal, funnel-shaped end of the Robi-Nel suction catheter **(C-E);** safe removal of the bronchoscope over the extended GEB-catheter assembly **(F);** and removal of the catheter and railroading the endotracheal tube over the GEB into the patient's trachea. Anchoring a round, atraumatic tip of the GEB in a large-caliber bronchus maintains a stable position of the intubation guide and prevents its distal end from accidentally springing backward out of the trachea during bronchoscope withdrawal. This approach is superior to the use of the airway exchange catheter (AEC), whose placement below the carina is not recommended because of the recognized risk of lung perforation by the straight tip of the device. Reliably maintaining proximal positioning of the AEC tip during the airway exchange is difficult, because the AEC centimeter markings mapping the distance to the carina will become embedded inside the bronchoscope during its withdrawal. (**A, B,** and **E,** From Nekhendzy V, Simmonds PK: Rigid bronchoscope-assisted tracheal intubation: Yet another use of the gum elastic bougie. *Anesth Analg* 98:545–547, 2004.)

Patients with an advanced airway obstruction and inspiratory stridor at rest comprise some of the most feared and complicated cases for the anesthesiologist.[33] The incidence of difficult mask ventilation and impossible mask ventilation among patients with severe stridor and upper airway obstruction of more than 75% of the lumen reaches 40% and 6%, respectively,[74] compared with 1.4% and 0.15% for the general surgical population.[30,31,75] These patients frequently present for panendoscopy and microlaryngeal surgery on an emergent or semi-emergent basis, yet they require a systematic and thoughtful approach by the anesthesiologist and the surgeon.[38] The nature of the obstructing lesion (e.g., vascular, submucosal, pedunculated, inflammatory) and its location (e.g., supraglottic, glottic, subglottic, midtracheal, lower tracheal, and bronchial [mediastinal]) may require completely different intubation considerations and approaches.[17,33,34,36,38,69,71]

In the context of laryngeal surgery, the optimal technique of airway management of the stridorous patient with an advanced proximal airway obstruction (i.e., supraglottic, glottic, and subglottic levels) remains a subject of controversy. An awake flexible fiberoptic intubation, inhalational induction, and intravenous induction with muscle relaxants[17,33,74,76] have been used successfully, but none should be considered fail-safe. Thorough preoperative discussion of the surgical pathology and formulation of closely coordinated airway management plan with the surgeon are essential for safe management of these patients.

Based on our experience and review of the pertinent literature,[17,33,35,38,69,71,74,76-80] current recommendations for management of the critically obstructed airway can be outlined as follows:

1. For patients with severe stridor (e.g., symptoms exaggerated at night, hypoxemia-induced agitation or panic attacks, use of accessory muscles on inspiration, a large tumor, fixed hemilarynx, gross anatomic distortion, a larynx not visible on preoperative nasal endoscopy or flexible fiberoptic laryngoscopy), strongly consider tracheostomy under local anesthesia without sedation.

2. Patients with moderate stridor and a significant lesion seen on nasal endoscopy or flexible fiberoptic laryngoscopy, but who are considered possible to intubate, are best managed with an inhalational induction or an awake fiberoptic intubation. All airway instrumentation should proceed in a careful and gentle manner. Endotracheal intubation should be accomplished rapidly, with a small ETT. The number of attempts should not exceed two, because critical airway obstruction can quickly progress to complete as a result of manipulation of the airway.

3. If an inhalational induction is chosen, a sufficiently deep and stable plane of anesthesia is essential to avoid loss of the airway (e.g., avoidance of cough, laryngospasm). Endotracheal intubation should be performed under direct vision (e.g., direct laryngoscopy, video laryngoscopy, flexible fiberoptic bronchoscopy). Muscle relaxants should be avoided until after the intubation is completed to prevent

sudden, complete airway obstruction, especially when the tumor is subglottic. The patient's neck should be prepared, and the surgical team should be present and ready to attempt an airway rescue with an anterior commissure scope or a ventilating rigid bronchoscope or by emergent cricothyrotomy or tracheostomy.

4. If endotracheal intubation under direct vision (e.g., direct laryngoscopy, video laryngoscopy, flexible fiberoptic bronchoscopy) fails in an anesthetized or awake patient or is deemed problematic, tracheostomy should be performed expeditiously, with the patient breathing spontaneously.

5. An awake fiberoptic intubation should be used with caution, because sudden loss of the airway can be precipitated by one or more of the following factors:
   - Bleeding from a friable tumor on impaction with the FFB or seeding parts of the broken tumor into the trachea
   - "Cork in the bottle" effect, when the scope is introduced into the critically narrowed airway
   - Inhibitory effect of local anesthetics on the tongue and upper airway musculature, laryngeal muscles, and function
   - Central nervous system depressant effect of local anesthetics
   - Local anesthetic-precipitated laryngospasm
   - Patient's apprehension and agitation during the procedure, resulting in hyperventilation and "sucking in" mobile, pedunculated tumors

6. Additional fallback strategies may include the following:
   - Placement of a transtracheal jet ventilation (TTJV) catheter before induction of anesthesia in an attempt to provide apneic oxygenation or high-frequency TTJV (see "Intraoperative Ventilation Techniques and Strategies for Microlaryngeal Surgery")
   - High-frequency jet ventilation (HFJV) through the supralaryngeal airway device (e.g., LMA)
   - JV approaches require caution, especially in the presence of subglottic lesions, to avoid air trapping and barotrauma

7. Patients with inspiratory obstruction due to bilateral vocal cord paralysis or fixation of cricoarytenoid joints typically do not present ventilation or intubation problems.

8. If tracheostomy is avoided, an extubation strategy must be decided on with the surgeon. Extubation should be performed over an airway exchange catheter (AEC), with the necessary reintubation equipment immediately available. Some patients should remain intubated until the airway inflammation and edema subside, and the patient's airway is then reevaluated.

2. Intraoperative Ventilation Techniques and Strategies for Microlaryngeal Surgery

Surgery can be conducted in an awake patient, frequently under conscious sedation, or with the patient anesthetized (Box 38-1). The ventilation options under general anesthesia consist of "tube" (i.e., endotracheal intubation)

> **Box 38-1   Ventilation Techniques and Strategies for Microlaryngoscopic Surgery**
>
> I. Awake airway surgery (conscious sedation)
> II. Asleep airway surgery (general anesthesia)
>   II.1. Endotracheal intubation (cuffed microlaryngeal tracheal (MLT) tube)
>   II.2. Tubeless techniques
>   a. Spontaneous ventilation
>   Inhalational anesthesia (insufflation)
>   Total intravenous anesthesia
>   b. Apneic intermittent ventilation
>   c. Jet ventilation
>   Supraglottic
>   Subglottic
>   Low frequency
>   High frequency
>   Superimposed high frequency

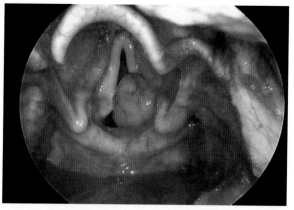

Figure 38-12 A right vocal process granuloma is located in the posterior glottis. The location and the nature of the pathology preclude the use of the microlaryngeal tracheal (MLT) tube and require the use of jet ventilation. (Courtesy of Edward Damrose, MD, Stanford University Medical Center, Stanford, CA.)

and "tubeless" techniques, with the latter represented by the techniques of spontaneous ventilation, AIV, and JV.[8,13,38,81,82]

a. AWAKE AIRWAY SURGERY WITH CONSCIOUS SEDATION

For selected patients, many laryngoscopic procedures can be safely and effectively performed in an office-based setting, including diagnostic endoscopy, laser surgery, panendoscopy for cancer screening and biopsies, and therapeutic vocal cord injections.[2-5,16] The key to success for office-based surgery remains adequate topical and regional anesthesia of the patient's airway, which is usually performed by the surgeon and typically follows preparation of the patient for awake oral and nasal flexible fiberoptic intubation (see Chapter 19). Although highly motivated patients can undergo office-based laryngoscopic surgery strictly under local anesthesia, most desire sedation and amnesia.[3]

If presence of the anesthesiologist is requested, the main objectives are to monitor for possible local anesthetic toxicity (see Chapter 19), to supplement local anesthesia with a rapidly titratable and reversible state of sedation, and to treat acute hyperdynamic responses that can occur in up to 20% to 30% of patients, despite seemingly adequate topical anesthesia of the airway.[3,83] Judicious use of intravenous opioids or sedatives/hypnotics, or both, is paramount, because a loss of patient cooperation may result in intraoperative injury.[3,16,34] Sedation of the patients with obstructive sleep apnea and morbid obesity should be performed with extreme caution.[84,85]

b. ASLEEP AIRWAY SURGERY WITH GENERAL ANESTHESIA

General anesthesia for microlaryngeal surgery represents a unique example of some of the conflicting intraoperative goals that exist between the surgeon and the anesthesiologist with regard to the patient's airway control and maintenance. For the surgeon, ideal operating conditions would be completely unobstructed surgical visualization, unimpeded surgical manipulation, and absence of movement in the surgical field. From the anesthesiologist's perspective, the ideal anesthetic technique would allow adequate protection of the patient's lower airway from aspiration and the use of stable, controlled mechanical

ventilation with the ability to measure the concentration of anesthetic gases, peak inspiratory pressure (PIP), inspired oxygen concentration (FIO_2), and end-tidal carbon dioxide level ($EtCO_2$).[81] In most cases, these objectives can be balanced by the use of a small MLT tube, maximizing the patient's safety and the success of surgery.

ENDOTRACHEAL INTUBATION WITH MICROLARYNGEAL TRACHEAL TUBES. The use of a small (5.0-mm ID) MLT tube with positive-pressure ventilation remains the standard for airway management in most nonlaser microlaryngeal surgery, and it is associated with minimal or no intraoperative complications.[86,87] (For anesthetic management of the laser airway surgery see Chapter 40.) Adequate gas exchange can be maintained through small-ID ETTs in most adult patients,[88,89] unless the duration of surgery approaches 2 hours (which happens rarely).[88] Even then, despite a consistent trend toward progressive hypercapnia and respiratory acidosis, the pH and $EtCO_2$ values remain within physiologic range.[89]

With most glottic pathology originating in the anterior two thirds of the larynx,[90] consistent positioning of a small MLT tube between the arytenoid cartilages in the posterior part of the glottis leaves most of the surgical field unobstructed to the surgical view and manipulations.[4,13,16,38,91] Even with many posterior glottic disorders, it may be possible for the surgeon to gently displace the MLT tube anteriorly with the microsurgical cupped forceps or to perform the surgery using the specially designed posterior glottic laryngoscopes.[90,92]

However, if the posterior glottis is occupied by a significant surgical pathology (e.g., posterior glottic or subglottic stenosis, transglottic tumor) (Fig. 38-12), use of alternative, tubeless ventilation techniques becomes necessary.[38] Because of the surgeon's preference, tubeless ventilation can also be requested as a primary ventilation mode from the outset of the procedure.

TUBELESS TECHNIQUES

Spontaneous Ventilation. Spontaneous ventilation is rarely used in adult microlaryngeal surgery,[93-95] but it is commonly employed in the pediatric patient population,

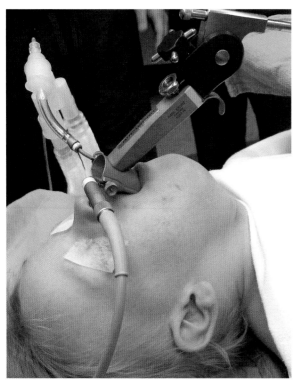

Figure 38-13 A child in suspension laryngoscopy using the spontaneous ventilation (insufflation) technique. Notice the precut endotracheal tube connecting the anesthesia circuit to a metal cannula inserted into a side port of the suspension laryngoscope. (Courtesy of Peter Koltai, MD, Stanford University Medical Center, Stanford, CA.)

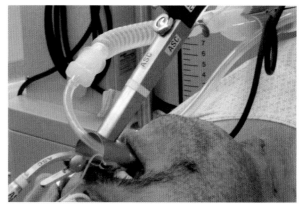

Figure 38-14 Apneic, intermittent ventilation during microlaryngeal surgery. The endotracheal tube is intermittently placed through the lumen of a suspension (Lindholm) laryngoscope by the surgeon and connected to the anesthesia breathing circuit for positive-pressure ventilation.

for whom it offers the additional ability to evaluate dynamic airway function and the level of obstruction (see "Anesthesia for Pediatric Airway Endoscopy and Microlaryngeal Surgery"). Anesthetic gases can be delivered (insufflated) through a nasal trumpet connected through an ETT adapter to the anesthesia circuit,[96-99] an ETT positioned in the nasopharynx,[82,100,101] a metal cannula, a side port of the rigid bronchoscope or operating laryngoscope (Fig. 38-13; see Fig. 38-10),[38] or a catheter placed through the vocal cords into the patient's trachea.[9,102,103] Scavenging of anesthetic gases can be facilitated with an open suction tube at the corner of the patient's mouth.

Although this technique offers free access to the larynx, it does not provide a still surgical field for precision surgery, it affords no protection of the lower airway, and it contaminates the OR environment.[34,87,103] Deep planes of anesthesia are usually required to blunt the laryngeal responses and to prevent patient movement, which tends to provoke cardiovascular instability and ventilatory compromise (i.e., hypoxemia, hypercarbia, and short periods of apnea).[8,39,104] With careful technique, inhalational agents can be substituted for total intravenous anesthesia (TIVA).[82,96,105] However, control of the patient's movement and a stable plane of anesthesia frequently remains problematic.[104] Monitoring an adequate hypnotic state (e.g., processed electroencephalographic activity) may be advisable for these patients.

The protagonists of spontaneous ventilation technique may wish to routinely supplement general anesthesia with topical or local anesthesia of the airway (usually

done by the surgeon after deployment of suspension laryngoscopy), which facilitates maintenance of a more stable and lighter plane of anesthesia, promotes hemodynamic and respiratory stability, and decreases the incidence of intraoperative laryngospasm.[39,82,96,103,105,106]

Apneic Intermittent Ventilation. AIV remains a relatively popular technique for microlaryngeal surgical procedures of short duration in some surgical centers.[87] Compared with spontaneous ventilation, it affords more stable and controlled anesthetic conditions, as well as full muscle relaxation. After induction of anesthesia, the patient's lungs are ventilated by a face mask or an LMA, which is followed by a period of apnea to allow deployment of a suspension laryngoscope by the surgeon. The patient's trachea is subsequently intubated by the surgeon with a small-diameter, preferably uncuffed ETT that is placed through the lumen of the laryngoscope,[87] and the patient's lungs are hyperventilated with an FiO_2 of 1.0 (Fig. 38-14). The ETT is then removed to provide a fully unobstructed and still surgical view of the larynx. The ETT is withdrawn and reinserted as frequently as necessary to maintain an oxygen saturation by pulse oximetry (SpO_2) of 90% or greater and $EtCO_2$ between 40 and 60 mm Hg,[18,87,107] allowing periods of apnea up to 5 to 10 minutes in healthy adult patients.[87,108] Apneic oxygenation through the hypopharyngeal catheter, preceded by an adequate period (10 minutes) of preoxygenation and denitrogenation of the patient's lungs, can be tried in anesthetized and paralyzed patients.[108]

TIVA is typically used for maintenance. Monitoring the hypnotic state of anesthesia is advisable during AIV, because the incidence of awareness and recall may reach 4% (30 times higher than in the general surgical population), especially when the inhalational agents are used to supplement intravenous anesthesia.[109,110]

The disadvantages of AIV include slowing the pace of surgery, disruption of the surgical field, possible trauma to the vocal cords and lower airway due to repeated endotracheal intubation, and a propensity for laryngospasm.[87] In a study of more than 350 patients,[87] the incidence of intraoperative laryngospasm with AIV was

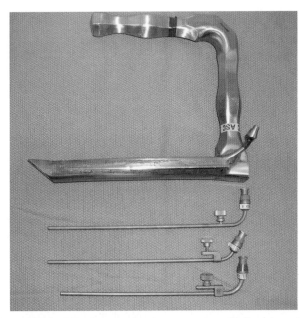

Figure 38-15   A Dedo operating laryngoscope with the integrated side port *(top)* can be used for supraglottic jet ventilation, and different jetting metal cannulas *(bottom)* can be inserted through the side ports of the operating laryngoscopes or directly through their lumen (see Fig. 38-4).

1.4%. The AIV may not be suitable for patients with significant lung or cardiovascular disease,[107] and it leaves the patient's lower airway unprotected to aspiration.[18]

Appropriate and successful phonomicrosurgery can rarely be performed using AIV, because the apnea periods are too short to permit unhurried precision surgery.[1,111] This technique may be better reserved for short, uncomplicated cases.

Jet Ventilation. Supraglottic JV (i.e., jet nozzle above the glottic opening) for microlaryngeal surgery can be performed through the side port of a suspension operating laryngoscope, with the jet cannula attached to the lumen of the laryngoscope (Fig. 38-15; see Fig. 38-4)[1,24,59,112] or through a specialized jet laryngoscope.[113,114]

Subglottic JV (i.e., jet nozzle below the glottic opening) is established by bypassing the larynx from above (i.e., translaryngeal or transglottal approach) or below (i.e., percutaneous approach) through the CTM or the upper TTJV rings.[74,86,87,111] Transglottal JV typically employs specialized, laser-safe, small-diameter, orally placed, double-lumen catheters (Fig. 38-16),[24,81,115,116] in which the large port is used for jetting and the smaller lumen

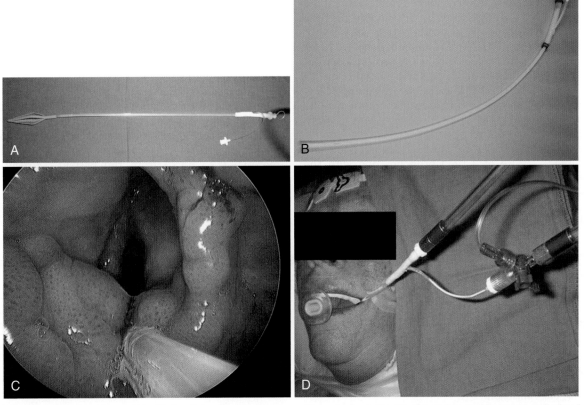

Figure 38-16   The Hunsaker Mon-Jet Ventilation Tube (Medtronic Xomed Inc., Jacksonville, FL) **(A)** and a double-lumen catheter (LaserJet, Acutronic medical systems AG, Hirzel, Switzerland) **(B)** are laser-resistant, come with the metal stylet to facilitate tracheal placement, and have a large port that is used for jet ventilation (JV) and a smaller port that is used for monitoring the distal airway pressure and respiratory gases. The green, basket-shaped distal end of the Hunsaker Mon-Jet tube **(A)** facilitates self-centering of the tube within the trachea, preventing the catheter "whip" that may lead to submucosal gas injection and possible occlusion of the distal end of the jet tube by tracheal mucosa. **C,** The small-diameter Hunsaker Mon-Jet tube is placed through the glottis to facilitate a clear surgical view and surgical access. **D,** The Hunsaker Mon-Jet tube is taped in place during JV, with the monitoring port connected to the ventilator through a three-way stopcock. The jet ventilator tubing is suspended to prevent kinking, and an oral airway is inserted to facilitate full egress of air during JV. (**B,** Courtesy of Acutronic medical systems AG, Hirzel, Switzerland; **C** and **D,** from Davies JM, Hillel AD, Maronian NC, et al: The Hunsaker Mon-Jet tube with jet ventilation is effective for microlaryngeal surgery. *Can J Anaesth* 56:284–290, 2009.).

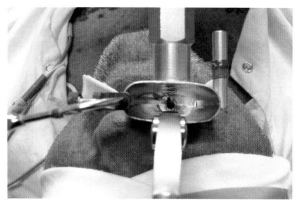

Figure 38-17 Subglottic high-frequency jet ventilation (JV) through a movable metal jet nozzle. Transglottal JV is provided through the metal jet nozzle (Brock & Mechelsen A/S, Birkerod, Denmark) and is secured on the suspension laryngoscope for the operation for vocal cord carcinoma.

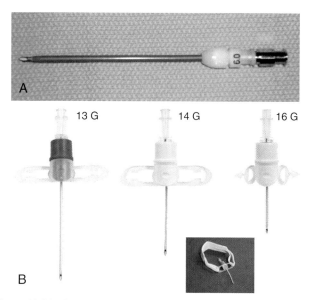

Figure 38-18 Devices for transtracheal jet ventilation (TTJV). **A,** The 7.5-cm long, 2-mm inner diameter TTJV catheter (Cook Medical Inc., Bloomington, IN) is mounted on a 14-gauge (G) needle. The catheter is wire reinforced to prevent kinking. **B,** Different sizes of the Ravussin-type cricothyrotomy catheter (VBM Medizintechnik GmbH, Sulz, Germany) for TTJV. The 13-gauge, 1.3-mm outer diameter catheter with the fixation flange and foam Velcro neck tape is most frequently used in adults. (Courtesy of Acutronic Medical Systems, GmbH, Salzburg, Austria.)

for monitoring the distal airway pressure and respiratory gases. Long, single-lumen catheters (typically 1.5- to 3-mm ID), some of which are laser resistant, may be used and can be placed through the oral or nasal route[24,34,87,102,117-119]; however, they lack concurrent monitoring capability. Alternatively, a small-diameter, movable, metal jet cannula can be passed through the glottis by the surgeon after the suspension laryngoscope is in position (Fig. 38-17).[87,120] For transglottal JV, midtracheal placement of the catheter or cannula is usually preferred. TTJV is typically administered through a long catheter or Ravussin-type cannula (Fig. 38-18).[74,86,121] For TTJV catheter or cannula placement, the use of an FFB or a rigid bronchoscope may be advocated to monitor the procedure[87,111,122] and to minimize the risk of unnoticed posterior tracheal wall laceration, which may lead to submucosal gas injection and barotrauma.[87,111] Use of a rigid bronchoscope with the bevel turned posteriorly may be especially efficacious, because the posterior tracheal wall is protected by the bronchoscope from the needle entry.[87] For transglottal JV and TTJV, endoscopic control also allows adjustment of

the position of the distal end of the catheter or cannula to optimize HFJV.[24,86,87,122]

Compared with endotracheal intubation, supraglottic and subglottic JV techniques have distinct advantages of providing the surgeon with an enlarged, clear or minimally impeded, and undistorted view of the endolarynx, facilitating surgical access and eliminating flammable material (i.e., ETT) from the patient's airway during laser surgery.[24,115] Although supraglottic and subglottic ventilation techniques can use low-frequency jet ventilation (LFJV), HFJV, or superimposed high-frequency jet ventilation (SHFJV) modes,[34,86,111,123-125] the

TABLE 38-1

Preferred Use of Jet Ventilation Techniques for Microlaryngeal Surgery

Method of Ventilation	Low-Frequency Jet Ventilation	High-Frequency Jet Ventilation	Superimposed High-Frequency Jet Ventilation
Supraglottic Jet Ventilation			
Suspension laryngoscope	± a	± b	−
Jet laryngoscope	± a	± b	+
Subglottic Jet Ventilation			
Catheter	± c	+	−
Metal cannula	± c	+	−
Transtracheal jet ventilation	± c, d	+	−
Rigid bronchoscope	+ e	+ e	+ e

a, Probably best reserved for uncomplicated, relatively short procedures; b, may not be able to provide adequate gas exchange in patients with severe pulmonary disease or advanced laryngotracheal stenosis; c, should be used with caution; manual low-frequency jet ventilation is best avoided; d, also can be used as a rescue mode in "cannot ventilate, cannot intubate" situation; e, Used to bypass tracheal obstruction, and in central/distal airway surgery. A specially designed multilumen rigid bronchoscopes, or multilumen adapters for conventional rigid bronchoscopes, are required for high-frequency jet ventilation and superimposed high-frequency jet ventilation.

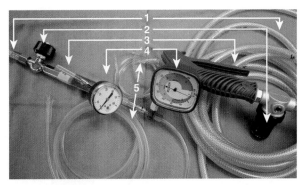

Figure 38-19 A simple Sanders-type injector (AA Jet Ventilator, Anesthesia Associates, San Marcos, CA) *(left)* and a manual jet ventilator (QuickJet, Rusch-Teleflex Medical, Durham, NC) *(right)* are used for manual (Venturi) low-frequency jet ventilation. Both devices contain a pressure hose *(1)*, an adjustable pressure-regulating valve *(2)*, a manual lever for delivering the pressurized gas *(3)*, an easily readable pressure gauge *(4)*, and noncompliant jet ventilation tubing *(5)*. QuickJet allows presetting a desired level of driving pressure, indicated by the colored scale on the pressure gauge.

use of these modes in clinical practice is usually more restrictive (Table 38-1).

The use of manual supraglottic LFJV (i.e., Venturi jet ventilation) at a rate of less than 60 breaths/min continues to predominate in clinical practice,[111] probably because of the low cost and easy accessibility of manual JV devices (Fig. 38-19) (a manual mode also can be preset on commercially available jet ventilators, where available).[59,111,126,127] Although an overall incidence of complications with manual supraglottic LFJV may be low (0.42%),[120] a survey of 229 U.K. centers revealed that it was responsible for most major complications (e.g., significant hypoxemia, barotrauma, unplanned admission to the intensive care unit) and for all deaths, especially when applied subglottically.[111] This suggests that LFJV should be reserved for uncomplicated, elective procedures of short duration and that it may not be regarded as a standard of practice for microlaryngeal surgery.[24] For increased safety, LFJV should be started with a low driving pressure ($\leq$10 psi), which is gradually increased until visible chest excursions are observed, and adequate oxygen saturation is maintained.[24,59,111]

The subglottic HFJV mode (respiratory rate of 100 to 300 breaths/min; tidal volumes [V_T] of 1 to 3 mL/kg), delivered through specialized automated jet ventilators, is typically used.[24,34] Compared with supraglottic LFJV, in which intermittent apnea is frequently required due to significant vocal cord movement, subglottic HFJV significantly reduces laryngeal motion and affords a quiet surgical field without the need for interrupting ventilation.[125] If vocal cord movement becomes a problem, HFJV driving pressure can be decreased, and the respiratory frequency can be increased to provide a smoother gas flow, or the ventilator can be turned off during particularly delicate parts of the procedure.[24,125]

Despite very small V_T values, CO_2 elimination during subglottic HFJV is facilitated by the upstream turbulent convective flow of CO_2 along the decreasing gradient from the alveoli to the conducting airways.[34] The alveolar-arterial CO_2 gradient in patients with normal lung function is largely maintained within normal range.[34,128]

Monitoring $EtCO_2$ during HFJV can be accomplished by briefly switching to LFJV mode on the ventilator to get a reliable signal or by using transcutaneous Pco_2 monitoring.[24] Administration of subglottic HFJV also results in a higher inspired O_2 concentration, because entrainment of air is reduced deep inside the airway.[24,86] Improved oxygenation is further enhanced by generation of continuous positive end-expiratory pressure in small airways (auto-PEEP), leading to alveolar recruitment and increased functional residual capacity (FRC).[24,34,119] Nevertheless, patients with severely restricted lung compliance, $\dot{V}/\dot{Q}$ mismatch or shunting, and reduced FRC (e.g., morbid obesity) remain at increased risk for hypoxemia.[86]

In contrast to supraglottic LFJV, with which contamination of the lower airway due to air entrainment is possible,[34,81] a continuous, upward-directed flow of gas during subglottic HFJV creates a positive-pressure build-up, preventing blood and surgical debris from being directed down an unprotected airway.[111,119,129] However, increased airway pressure creates concern about air trapping and barotrauma, mandating maintenance of adequate gas outflow at all times.[130]

Before the suspension laryngoscope is secured, with the patient anesthetized and a subglottic JV catheter or cannula in place, strategies for minimizing the risk of barotrauma on initiation of subglottic HFJV may include starting ventilation with low driving pressures (<15 to 30 psi), allowing sufficient exhalation time by avoiding high-frequency ventilation (i.e., starting with LFJV first), and maintaining the patient's airway patency with the assistance of an oral airway or providing a jaw lift, if needed.[74,86,87,125,131] Alternatively, initiation of the subglottic HFJV can be held off until the suspension laryngoscope is deployed, and ventilation is supported conventionally through a face mask or the LMA. It may be prudent to confirm absence of the subglottic catheter or cannula obstruction by the $EtCO_2$ return and to check the catheter or cannula position endoscopically before subglottic HFJV commences.[86,125]

On emergence from anesthesia, small V_T values and low peak and mean airway pressures associated with subglottic HFJV enable the patient to breathe spontaneously, facilitating a transition to adequate spontaneous ventilation.[24,34,86,132,133] This transition can be further assisted at the end of surgery by increasing the frequency of ventilation to 300 breaths/min, increasing FIO_2 to 1.0, and setting a ventilator driving pressure at about 10 psi (0.8 bar), which enables almost continuous flow of O_2 and apneic oxygenation, as well as a rise in the carbon dioxide (CO_2) level.[24] If the conversion to spontaneous ventilation through a small subglottic catheter proves difficult, the patient's airway can be supported through a face mask, LMA, or ETT, as required; these conventional bridge airway strategies equally apply to transitioning from supraglottic JV. If obstructive airway lesions exist, subglottic HFJV must be used with extreme caution. If upper airway obstruction is greater than 50%, the position of the jet nozzle should be proximal to the site of the obstruction to prevent barotrauma, or the obstruction must be bypassed by a rigid bronchoscope first.[24,79]

Total outflow obstruction with resultant barotrauma during subglottic HFJV can be quickly precipitated by surgical instrumentation, glottic edema, laryngospasm, or closure of the vocal cords due to inadequate depth of anesthesia or inadequate muscle relaxation.[81,86,130] Modern automated jet ventilators (e.g., Monsoon III Universal Jet Ventilator [Acutronic Medical Systems AG, Hirzel, Switzerland], Twin Stream [Carl Rainer GmbH, Vienna, Austria]) incorporate multiple safety features, including automatic ventilator shutdown, if the user-preset pressure limits are exceeded.[24,74] This design has enabled some experienced providers to successfully use high-frequency TTJV in patients with massive supraglottic lesions and severe airway compromise,[74] for which the use of supraglottic or subglottic JV was not possible or surgically feasible. The presence of a second anesthesiologist to facilitate monitoring and maintenance of an upper airway was required and deemed an important safety factor in preventing intraoperative pressure-related complications in all cases.[74] Although no major complications were observed in this series of 50 patients,[74] the incidence of minor complications reached 20%, a more than threefold increase compared with the instances when high-frequency TTJV has been used in patients with less severe airway compromise.[87] Study results hold some promise that a simple,[134,135] portable expiratory ventilation assistance (EVA) device may be able to facilitate egress of gas through the jet catheter during TTJV, thereby increasing the safety of this technique; however EVA suitability for microlaryngeal surgery remains to be established.

Compared with the transglottal approach, high-frequency TTJV is associated with a significantly higher combined major and minor (e.g., transient hypoxemia) complication rate (see "Intraoperative Complications"),[86,87] and it represents an independent risk factor for complications during JV for microlaryngeal surgery.[87] Modern automated JV may not be able to remediate all possible causes of barotrauma associated with high-frequency TTJV; complications may be related to the TTJV catheter insertion problems, laryngospasm, and high-pressure episodes (e.g., coughing, active expiration) during the recovery period.[80,86] Notwithstanding the attractive features of high-frequency TTJV, such as a motionless surgical field and a particularly easy transition to spontaneous respiration,[86] it may be advisable to reserve the elective use of this technique (especially in cases of severe supraglottic airway obstruction) for the most complicated patients[74] and to designate operators with significant clinical experience and expertise.[74,80,86,111]

SHFJV, which combines high-frequency and low-frequency ventilation modes, has been used effectively in surgical treatment of high-grade laryngeal and tracheal stenosis, even with a remaining glottic opening as small as 2 to 3 mm.[136] SHFJV is delivered supraglottically through a specialized jet laryngoscope, which incorporates welded low-frequency and high-frequency jet nozzles (Fig. 38-20).[113,136,137] As the streams (LFJV of 12 to 20 breaths/min; HFJV of 100 to 900 breaths/min) get simultaneously directed from the ventilator toward the center of the distal end of the jet laryngoscope, LFJV entrains air (Fig. 38-21) and produces cyclic changes in V_T (similar to supraglottic LFJV), facilitating maintenance of $PaCO_2$ at near-normal limits and allowing HFJV to be adjusted as needed.[136,137] HFJV builds up a

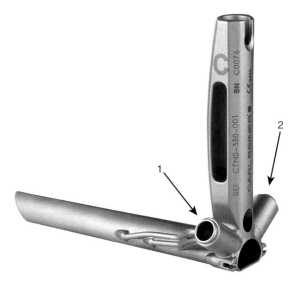

Figure 38-20 Jet laryngoscope for superimposed high-frequency jet ventilation. The jet laryngoscope (Carl Reiner GmbH, Vienna, Austria) incorporates a port for jet ventilation (1) with two welded jet nozzles for high-frequency and low-frequency ventilation and a port for pressure and gas monitoring (2). (Courtesy of Carl Reiner GmbH, Vienna, Austria.)

continuous PEEP and promotes alveolar recruitment, maintaining $PaCO_2$ even in the presence of the low FIO_2 required for laser surgery.[136-139] Safety of SHFJV is enhanced by an integrated port for continuous pressure (PIP and PEEP) and gas (FIO_2 and $EtCO_2$) monitoring at the end of the jet laryngoscope (see Fig. 38-21)[137] and of an automatic pressure-triggered ventilator shutdown feature, similar to an isolated HFJV mode.

To achieve adequate SHFJV, it appears to be sufficient to generate a PIP of 15 to 30 cm H_2O, as measured

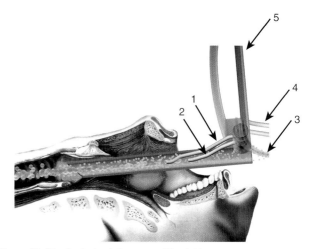

Figure 38-21 Technical diagram of the jet laryngoscope and superimposed high-frequency jet ventilation. High-frequency and low-frequency jet ventilation are simultaneously delivered to the patient from the ventilator through the high-frequency (1) and low-frequency (2) jet nozzles connected to the ventilator input tubing (3). The gas flow to the patient is augmented by air entrainment (blue circles). The pressure monitoring system (4) and jet laryngoscope handle (5) are indicated. (Modified image courtesy of Carl Reiner GmbH, Vienna, Austria.)

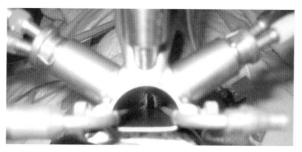

Figure 38-22   Superimposed high-frequency jet ventilation allows a completely unobstructed surgical view through the jet laryngoscope. Notice the ventilator input tubing *(green, left)* and the pressure or gas monitoring system *(red and yellow, right)* connected to the jet laryngoscope. (Courtesy of Lise Nørrekjær, MD, Department of Anaesthesia, Køge Sygehus, Køge, Denmark.)

at the end of the jet laryngoscope, which closely correlates with the PIP at the glottic and tracheal levels (i.e., no further increase in pressure occurs in the distal airway).[136,138] The PEEP values may not exceed 2.5 to 5 cm H_2O.[137,138] As a result, no adverse hemodynamic effects and barotrauma were observed in more than 1500 adult and pediatric patients who had undergone supraglottic SHFJV for laryngotracheal surgery, and endotracheal intubation was required in only 3 patients (0.2%), with concomitant significant restrictive or obstructive pulmonary disease.[136] Due to the HFJV component, vocal cord movement is greatly attenuated during SHFJV; if a perfectly still surgical field is requested by the surgeon, HFJV can be further increased, LFJV decreased or stopped, or a short period of full apnea instituted.[24,136,137]

SHFJV is a completely tubeless, laser-safe, open breathing system that allows a fully unobstructed surgical field (Fig. 38-22). It enables an easy switch between different JV modes and parameters, and it offers greater versatility and ventilation capabilities over the single-frequency JV techniques, especially in patients with preexisting compromised gas exchange. However, its effective use requires

optimal laryngoscope alignment and adjustability in relation to the glottic opening.

Despite the increased safety profile of SHFJV, clinical monitoring of the patient to prevent barotrauma should remain the standard of care for all JV techniques (Fig. 38-23).[86,87] Close cooperation between the surgeon and the anesthesiologist is essential; if the operating laryngoscope moves or is removed and obstructs the airway without a warning to the anesthesia team, major barotrauma may result.[16] Ensuring an adequate level of anesthesia, analgesia, and muscle relaxation; painstaking attention to maintaining unobstructed exhalation; and close monitoring of vital signs and chest excursions are essential for the patient's safety.[59,86,87,138] The main advantages and disadvantages of the ventilation techniques used for microlaryngeal surgery are compared in Table 38-2.

C. General Anesthesia Management for Panendoscopy and Microlaryngeal Surgery

1. Premedication and Monitoring

The main anesthesia objectives and special considerations for microlaryngeal surgery are discussed in "Special Considerations and Anesthesia Objectives." Premedication can frequently be omitted. Administration of an antisialogogue (e.g., 0.2 mg of glycopyrrolate given intravenously) may be desired by the surgeon to facilitate the surgical field, especially in patients with copious secretions,[3,10] but it does not constitute the standard of care.[43] Mucosal intake of drying agents may result in increased vocal cord viscosity and impaired vibration, markedly changing the patient's voice postoperatively and contributing to postoperative dysphonia.[140] Steroids (e.g., 8 to 12 mg of dexamethasone given intravenously) are frequently used to prevent or minimize excessive postoperative swelling,[16,34] although controlled studies documenting this beneficial effect appear to be lacking.[34]

Standard OR monitors are used. Invasive arterial blood pressure monitoring is rarely indicated, and its use should

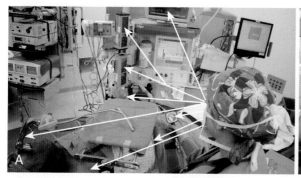
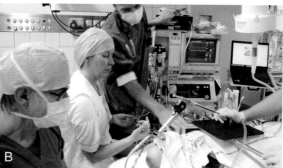

Figure 38-23   Challenges of intraoperative jet ventilation (JV). **A,** Manual, supraglottic low-frequency JV using QuickJet, connected *(red arrow)* to the suspension laryngoscope. The position and attentiveness of the anesthesiologist are required for multitasking and the challenging situations that exist. The anesthesiologist's attention *(white arrows)* must be simultaneously directed at maintaining close communication with the surgeon, observing the chest excursions, looking at the epigastric area for possible gastric distention, controlling driving pressure of the jet ventilator, maintaining adequate neuromuscular blockade (evaluated in this case at the ulnar nerve), ensuring a stable level of anesthesia delivered intravenously through the programmable infusion pumps, and observing the patient's vital signs. **B,** Automated, subglottic high-frequency JV in an 11-month-old child with recurrent respiratory papillomatosis. The JV is accomplished transglottally through a movable metal jet nozzle that is closely controlled by the anesthesiologist. Notice a different operating room setup compared with that in **A** and presence of two anesthesiologists, which increases the patient's safety.

TABLE 38-2

Advantages and Disadvantages of Ventilation Techniques Used for Microlaryngeal Surgery

Technique	Advantages	Disadvantages
Awake airway surgery	Avoidance of general anesthesia Unobstructed surgical field and free surgical access to the larynx Increased patient cooperation Ability to evaluate dynamic airway function Ability to monitor voice quality throughout the surgery Possible improvement in surgical outcomes Convenience for the surgeon and the patient Cost savings	Success depends on adequate topical and regional anesthesia of the airway Local anesthetic–induced side effects Lack of powered magnification Lack of precision afforded by a still surgical field May require conscious sedation Loss of patient cooperation may result in injury Limited ability to handle major intraoperative complications, such as bleeding and edema Limited amount of tissue biopsied or excised May not be suitable for patients with significant PD or CVD or for young pediatric patients
Endotracheal intubation (microlaryngeal tracheal tube)	Adequate surgical field and surgical access to the larynx in most cases Still surgical field Adequate airway protection Control of patient immobility and vocal cord movement with adequate NMB Stable and controlled ventilation technique Ability to continuously and reliably monitor FIO_2, $EtCO_2$, PIP, and anesthetic gases Suitable for prolonged procedures	Largely unsuitable for surgery of the posterior glottic pathology (e.g., posterior glottic or subglottic stenosis, transglottic tumor) Unsuitable for laser if the need arises May not be used according to the surgeon's preference
Spontaneous ventilation (insufflation and total intravenous anesthesia)	Unobstructed surgical field and free surgical access to the larynx Ability to evaluate dynamic airway function and obstruction Suitable for laser surgery	Unprotected lower airway Precision surgery difficult or impossible in the moving surgical field Contamination of operating room environment with anesthetic gases, if insufflation technique is used Difficulty controlling adequate depth of anesthesia and absence of patient movement Inability to continuously and reliably monitor FIO_2, $EtCO_2$, and anesthetic gases May not be suitable for patients with significant PD or CVD or for very young pediatric patients Best reserved for short, uncomplicated cases
Apneic intermittent ventilation	Unobstructed surgical field and free access to the larynx Still surgical field Control of patient immobility and vocal cord movement with adequate NMB Ability to intermittently control gas exchange Suitable for laser surgery	Unprotected lower airway Possible airway trauma and disruption of the surgical field due to repeated passage of the endotracheal tube Possible propensity for intraoperative laryngospasm Inability to continuously and reliably monitor FIO_2, $EtCO_2$, and anesthetic gases May not be suitable for patients with significant PD or CVD or for very young pediatric patients Slows the pace of surgery Best reserved for short, uncomplicated cases
Jet ventilation (JV)	Unobstructed or minimally impeded surgical field and surgical access to the larynx Still surgical field Control of patient immobility and vocal cord movement with adequate NMB Ability to monitor and control FIO_2, $EtCO_2$, driving pressure, PIP, and PEEP with automated jet ventilators Suitable for prolonged procedures	Sole dependence on total intravenous anesthesia Association with most major (e.g., barotrauma) and minor intraoperative anesthesia-related complications Dependence on sophisticated automated jet ventilators for safe use Limitations of manual JV and transtracheal JV Significant experience and presence of two operators often required May not be suitable for patients with significant PD or CVD

CVD, Cardiovascular disease; *EtCO₂*, end-tidal carbon dioxide; *FIO₂*, fraction of inspired oxygen; *JV*, jet ventilation; *NMB*, neuromuscular blockade; *PD*, pulmonary disease; *PEEP*, positive end-expiratory pressure; *PIP*, peak inspiratory pressure.

be dictated by the patient's medical history, physical examination results, and special considerations such as prolonged JV or intraoperative problems (see "Jet Ventilation Problems"), for which intermittent sampling of arterial blood gases may become necessary. Monitoring the degree of neuromuscular blockade (NMB) with a conventional nerve stimulator should constitute the standard of care during panendoscopy and microlaryngeal surgery (see "Neuromuscular Blockade").

2. Anesthesia Induction and Maintenance

Conventional and advanced airway management is discussed in "Conventional and Advanced Airway Management." In most patients, standard intravenous induction can be safely performed. Difficulty in maintaining the airway during inhalational induction in patients with large, pedunculated tumors, granulomas and cysts should be anticipated, even if preoperative symptoms of airway obstruction are mild,[38] and early application of continuous positive airway pressure (CPAP) can help to stent the airway open. Another useful strategy involves preparing the patient's nares with a mixture of a vasoconstrictor and a topical anesthetic before induction, which will allow early passage of a nasal airway if the airway obstructs.[17,33]

Sevoflurane is most commonly used for inhalational induction in adult and pediatric patients.[34,141] The minimum alveolar concentration (MAC) of sevoflurane required to provide adequate endotracheal intubating (EI) conditions in 50% of unpremedicated adult patients (MAC_{EI50}) is 4.5% (95% confidence interval [CI], 3.9% to 5.2%), and the 95% effective dose (ED_{95}) for endotracheal intubation is 8%.[142] Although the ED_{95} time for achieving this target concentration in patients with normal airway is approximately 7 minutes,[143] up to 20 minutes may be required in patients with partial airway obstruction due to preexisting increase in minute ventilation and $\dot{V}/\dot{Q}$ mismatch.[17,34] This time can be shortened with the addition of small intravenous doses of midazolam or fentanyl,[141,144] although at the expense of an increased risk of apnea and loss of the airway.

If the patient's airway is reassuring, TIVA with propofol and an opioid is most commonly used during induction and maintenance of anesthesia for panendoscopy and microlaryngeal surgery.[34,74,86,87,111] TIVA offers many practical advantages, such as delivering a stable, consistent level of anesthesia in cases of JV and other settings in which the delivery of inhalational anesthetics is compromised. TIVA facilitates maintenance of induced hypotension, resulting in improved surgical visibility; ensures rapid return of protective airway reflexes; promotes rapid awakening and early postanesthesia recovery; and decreases the incidence of postoperative nausea and vomiting.[70,145-150] A propofol-based anesthetic results in profound depression of pharyngeal and laryngeal musculature and reflexes, and it effectively blocks the catecholamine release and hyperdynamic cardiovascular responses.[145,151-153] Full synergistic effect of propofol with rapidly acting opioids (e.g., remifentanil, alfentanil) allows rapid titration of anesthetic to the desired clinical effect.[154-156]

Remifentanil and alfentanil are widely used because of their favorable pharmacokinetic profile. Remifentanil is superior to fentanyl and alfentanil in promoting intraoperative hemodynamic stability, improving respiratory and general recovery, and facilitating patients' discharge after outpatient surgery.[157-162] The recommended induction doses are an intravenous bolus of 0.5 to 2 μg/kg of remifentanil and intravenous bolus dose of 1 to 2 mg/kg of propofol, followed by continuous maintenance infusions of 0.1 to 0.5 μg/kg/min of remifentanil and 80 to 180 μg/kg/min of propofol.[48,156-158,160,163] For alfentanil, an intravenous bolus of 20 to 30 μg/kg is commonly used for induction, followed by a continuous maintenance infusion of 0.25 to 1 μg/kg/min.[159,160,164,165]

Compared with conventional weight-based manual infusions, target-controlled infusions allow easier and more rapid titration of analgesia to the individual patient's responses, avoiding overshoot, improving the time course of the drug effect, and facilitating perioperative hemodynamic control.[166-168] Targeting propofol concentrations of 3 to 3.5 μg/mL and remifentanil concentrations of 2 to 5 ng/mL should be sufficient for most otherwise young (18 to 65 years old) and healthy (ASA physical class I or II) patients during the maintenance stage of anesthesia if adequate NMB is maintained.[166,169-171]

Severe bradycardic response to remifentanil should be treated promptly: activation of afferent parasympathetic fibers during direct and suspension laryngoscopy and endotracheal intubation or instrumentation may result in severe cardiac arrhythmias and asystole.[172,173] Pediatric patients and adults with high vagal tone may be at highest risk for these grave complications,[172] and pretreatment with anticholinergic agents may prevent or attenuate vagus-mediated cardiac arrhythmias. Treatment of reflex bradycardia and asystole during direct or suspension laryngoscopy must include immediate cessation of the offending stimulus, prompt administration of anticholinergics (e.g., atropine), and cardiopulmonary resuscitation, if necessary; infusion of isoproterenol or cardiac pacing may be required.[172]

Sevoflurane can be effectively combined with remifentanil and alfentanil for microlaryngeal surgery, producing good operating conditions, cardiovascular stability, and rapid emergence from anesthesia.[162] Compared with other inhalational anesthetics, sevoflurane may be preferred for outpatient microlaryngeal surgery. It improves the quality of postoperative patient recovery and shortens the discharge time, is associated with a reduced incidence of coughing compared with desflurane,[174] and produces less somnolence and postoperative nausea and vomiting compared with isoflurane.[175] Compared with TIVA, sevoflurane decreases salivary gland excretion, potentially promoting better visibility for the surgeon,[176] although clinical significance of this effect is unknown.

3. Neuromuscular Blockade

Maintenance of adequate NMB for microlaryngeal surgery is recommended,[1,34,38,86,111] but this advice is not universally followed.[111,177] Lack of appreciation for the benefits of adequate muscle relaxation constitutes a significant area for improvement in anesthesia care in general[177] and microlaryngeal surgery in particular.

Full muscle relaxation facilitates smooth endotracheal intubation, which should be accomplished in patients presenting for microlaryngeal surgery without the use of an ETT stylet when possible.[1] Maintenance of adequate NMB can prevent disastrous consequences of sudden patient movement, such as bucking or coughing while in suspension or during bronchoscopy or esophagoscopy,[43] and it can facilitate respiratory compliance during JV.[34] For some short surgical interventions, for which adequate muscle relaxation is only transiently required, combined administration of 2 µg/kg of remifentanil, 2 mg/kg of propofol, 1.5 mg/kg of lidocaine, and only one half of an intubating dose of rocuronium (0.3 mg/kg) can be administered, producing intubating conditions similar to intravenous administration of 1.5 mg/kg of succinylcholine.[178] For very short diagnostic procedures, for which muscle relaxants can be completely avoided, a bolus dose of 3 to 4 µg/kg of remifentanil (or intravenous bolus of 40 to 60 µg/kg of alfentanil), administered over 90 seconds and followed by an intravenous bolus of 2 to 2.5 mg/kg of propofol should provide excellent conditions for endotracheal intubation[179-181] or a quick "surgical look."

For most adult microlaryngeal surgical and panendoscopy procedures, maintenance of a high degree of NMB is strongly preferred and is most commonly achieved by administration of intermittent intravenous bolus doses of intermediate-acting, non-depolarizing neuromuscular blockers or succinylcholine infusion.[86] In the absence of contraindications to succinylcholine, the choice may be largely influenced by the duration of the procedure, the anesthesiologist's preference, and special surgical requirements. If rapid or intermittent return of spontaneous ventilation is required intraoperatively, an intravenous bolus of succinylcholine followed by an infusion may be preferred.[34] A succinylcholine infusion at a rate of 0.1 mg/kg/min (95% CI, 0.06 to 0.14 mg/kg/min) provides 100% twitch depression to the train-of-four (TOF) stimulation of the ulnar nerve (adductor pollicis muscle) and can be easily titrated to effect due to its linear kinetics.[182] The infusion should be started after the intubating dose of succinylcholine has dissipated and a twitch response has reappeared.[182,183] For practical purposes, it should be titrated to a barely visible single twitch during TOF stimulation of the ulnar nerve, which corresponds to 95% to 98% of twitch depression.[182] The observed increased succinylcholine requirements (i.e., tachyphylaxis) should alert the anesthesiologist to a rapidly developing transition from phase 1 to phase 2 NMB.[183,184] Similar phenomena are observed in children.[185]

In the absence of a phase 2 block, succinylcholine infusions may avoid postoperative residual curarization (PORC). The incidence of PORC with the use of the intermediate-acting, non-depolarizing muscle relaxants reaches 20% to 30% in the general surgical population.[186,187] PORC is associated with delayed discharge from the recovery room, even in the absence of respiratory compromise.[186] The use of mivacurium, despite its short duration of action, is associated with an almost 10% incidence of residual block, unless its action is pharmacologically reversed.[188] This highlights the need for vigilant intraoperative monitoring of NMB and routine

reversal of NMB after microlaryngeal surgery to ensure adequate TOF recovery to a level of more than 0.9.[189-192] Even small degrees of residual paralysis (TOF of 0.7 to 0.9) are associated with impaired pharyngeal function and increased risk of aspiration, significant attenuation of the hypoxic ventilatory response, unpleasant symptoms of muscle weakness, and weakness of the laryngeal and upper airway muscles, which may contribute to the possibility of acute upper airway obstruction postoperatively (see "Postoperative Complications").[192]

During microlaryngeal surgery, access to the patient's arms is frequently difficult or impossible, and the anesthesiologist is faced with an alternative choice of monitoring NMB at the temporal branch of the facial nerve (i.e., orbicularis oculi muscle) or posterior tibial nerve (i.e., flexor hallucis brevis muscle). Monitoring TOF at the orbicularis oculi correlates best with NMB at the laryngeal adductor muscles, which are responsible for vocal cord movement and glottic closure[193] and may constitute the surgeon's preference.[43] For adequate orbicularis oculi monitoring, the following guidelines should be followed[194,195]:

1. The electrodes should be positioned just lateral to the eye or with one electrode lateral to the eye and one in front of the ear.
2. Small currents (20 to 30 mA) and small electrodes should be used to avoid stimulation of other facial muscles.
3. The responses to stimulation should be observed in the middle of the eyebrow.

The onset of and the recovery from non-depolarizing NMB at the larynx and orbicularis oculi are similar and faster than at the ulnar nerve.[191,193-196] Significantly quicker recovery of NMB is observed in adults at the flexor hallucis brevis muscle (i.e., great toe) compared with the hand muscles.[191] Assessment of the residual block at the end of the surgery must still be guided by a twitch recovery at the ulnar nerve, because the adductor pollicis muscle recovers last.[191,194,196]

The anesthesiologist must maintain constant communication with the surgeon to match the maintenance of adequate NMB with the duration of surgery. If additional muscle relaxation is requested at the end of the procedure to abolish vocal cord movement, administration of non-depolarizing muscle relaxants should be avoided, and deepening the level of anesthesia and/or administration of additional analgesia (e.g., intravenous bolus of remifentanil) should be performed instead.[43] Pharmacologic reversal of non-depolarizing NMB should be routinely done at the end of microlaryngeal surgery.

Sugammadex, a selective relaxant binding drug, can antagonize any level of NMB, including the profound blockade induced by rocuronium, adding flexibility to the use of non-depolarizing relaxants.[197] The recommended dose is 2 to 16 mg/kg, depending on the level of the block.[188,197] Profound NMB induced by rocuronium can be reversed in less than 3 minutes.[198] Sugammadex, however, has no affinity for atracurium, cisatracurium, or succinylcholine; is not widely available; and is very expensive.[197]

4. Conventional and Operative Direct Laryngoscopy

The intense sympathoadrenal response observed during direct laryngoscopy and endotracheal intubation (see "Special Considerations and Anesthesia Objectives") may be further accentuated by continuous deployment of the suspension laryngoscope and intralaryngeal or intratracheal surgical manipulations, resulting in a 10% to 17% incidence of transient intraoperative myocardial ischemia.[199] The administration of 1.5 to 2 mg/kg of esmolol by intravenous bolus, followed by continuous intravenous infusion at a rate of 100 to 300 µg/kg/min, may be particularly effective in promoting hemodynamic stability and preventing intraoperative myocardial ischemia.[200-202] Potentiation of the action of opioids and anesthetic agents by esmolol further results in decreased postoperative opioid analgesic requirements,[203-206] facilitates emergence from anesthesia, and shortens a discharge time after outpatient surgical procedures.[207-210]

5. Jet Ventilation Problems[24,34]

a. INSUFFICIENT OXYGENATION

A sudden drop in SpO_2 may be the result of acute barotrauma and pneumothorax, which should be promptly treated. A gradual decline in SpO_2 usually results from insufficient alveolar ventilation or limited lung diffusion capacity, and it is most commonly associated with preexisting restrictive or obstructive pulmonary disease. The steps of therapeutic intervention include increasing FiO_2 in the jet gas, gradually increasing the driving pressure, increasing the ratio of the duration of inspiration to the duration of expiration (I:E ratio), reducing the ambient air entrainment by adding an O_2 bias flow, and switching from supraglottic to the more efficient subglottic JV until the problem is corrected. Increasing the respiratory frequency or PEEP level should be avoided, because this may lead to lung overexpansion and reduced venous return. If these measures are exhausted without achieving adequate oxygenation, the anesthesiologist should switch to AIV or endotracheal intubation with an MLT tube.

b. INSUFFICIENT CARBON DIOXIDE ELIMINATION

Intraoperative hypercapnia can be observed in patients with severe COPD and reduced lung compliance. Slightly increasing the driving pressure is recommended until the problem is corrected. If $EtcO_2$ or $Paco_2$ levels continue to rise despite maximal driving pressure, permissive hypercapnia can be allowed in selected patients. Studies indicate that $Paco_2$ values as high as 100 mm Hg may be well tolerated intraoperatively.[211] A switch to conventional endotracheal intubation and intermittent positive-pressure ventilation always remains an option.

The higher ASA physical status correlates with the higher incidence of complications with transglottal and TTJV techniques,[87] and these patients should be given special attention if JV is planned. Patients with previous neck radiation therapy are at higher risk for multiple attempts at TTJV catheter placement and subsequent risk of developing intraoperative barotrauma.[86]

6. Bronchoscopy and Esophagoscopy

Diagnostic and therapeutic forms of endoscopy (i.e., bronchoscopy and esophagoscopy) are typically performed as part of the panendoscopy procedure. The use of operating flexible and rigid bronchoscopy in central and distal airway surgery, including tracheal and endobronchial stent placement, is beyond the scope of this discussion, and JV is most commonly employed for these surgical procedures. Operating esophagoscopy is commonly used for endoscopic resection of Zenker's diverticulum.

If rigid bronchoscopy is planned first, general anesthesia is induced in a standard manner, and the patient's lungs are hyperventilated through the face mask with an FiO_2 of 1.0. With the onset of complete muscle relaxation, the patient is immediately turned over to the surgeon without securing an airway.[43] Quick and gentle direct laryngoscopy for the purpose of applying topical laryngotracheal anesthesia (3 to 4 mL of 4% lidocaine) before rigid bronchoscopy can be tried to help blunt hemodynamic responses to subsequent surgical manipulation; however, the risk of residual laryngeal anesthesia should be kept in mind if the procedure is short.[212]

After the rigid bronchoscope is introduced into the patient's trachea, JV can be instituted, or ventilation can commence manually through the OR anesthesia circuit by using the Racine universal adapter connected to the side arm of the bronchoscope (see Fig. 38-10). A rigid telescope and many accessory instruments such as forceps, suction catheters, laser fibers, or silicone stent delivery systems can be placed by the surgeon through the central lumen of the bronchoscope.[213] Although balanced inhalational anesthesia has been used successfully in this setting,[34] TIVA can provide a more stable plane of anesthesia. With manual ventilation, high gas flows are usually required because of the variable leak around the end of the bronchoscope. Close communication with the surgeon is essential for decreasing the manual inflating pressures when the bronchoscope is introduced into a main stem bronchus and to ensure complete exhalation.[43]

After rigid bronchoscopy is completed, if endotracheal intubation is planned, a resumption of adequate mask or LMA ventilation with an FiO_2 of 1.0 is advisable before direct laryngoscopy. If necessary, the airway can be exchanged with the ETT through the in situ rigid bronchoscope (see Fig. 38-11).[72,73]

If endotracheal intubation is chosen, a small-diameter (e.g., 6.0 mm ID), wire-reinforced ETT may be preferred for rigid esophagoscopy to avoid possible compression of the ETT lumen; however, if suspension laryngoscopy with endotracheal intubation is planned next, a 5.0 mm ID MLT tube should be used instead. The ETT should be moved over to the left side of the patient's mouth to facilitate introduction of the surgical instruments and securely taped to the lower jaw, facilitating full opening of the patient's mouth by the surgeon.[43]

Intraoperative flexible fiberoptic bronchoscopy can be performed by the surgeon through an appropriately sized ETT, alongside the small ETT with its cuff deflated; through the LMA; or through Patil-Syracuse endoscopy mask (Ambu Inc., Glen Burnie, MD) (Fig. 38-24). If

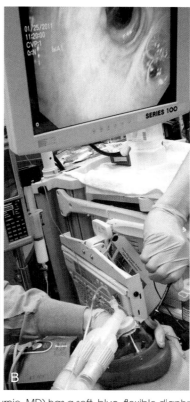

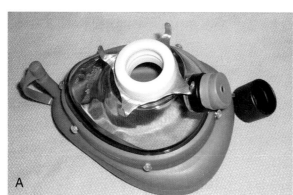

Figure 38-24 A, The reusable, clear-view Patil-Syracuse mask (Ambu Inc., Glen Burnie, MD) has a soft, blue, flexible diaphragm that facilitates passage of flexible endoscopes and endotracheal tubes. A black cap seals off the diaphragm and allows positive-pressure ventilation (PPV) through the anesthesia circuit when endoscopy is not in use. **B,** Flexible fiberoptic bronchoscopy is performed through the Patil-Syracuse mask. Placement and manipulation of the flexible fiberoptic bronchoscope by the surgeon is aided by a concomitant use of a pink Williams oral airway intubator, which facilitates central positioning and maneuvering of the fiberoptic bronchoscope. Maintenance of a good seal through the flexible diaphragm allows adequate PPV by the anesthesiologist.

flexible fiberoptic bronchoscopy is performed through the ETT (7.5 to 8.0 mm ID) using a swivel bronchoscopy adapter, ventilation is better controlled manually because of increased resistance to the gas flow and high PIP. Gentle, manual ventilation with small tidal volumes and an FIO_2 of 1.0 is usually well tolerated by the patient over the short course of the procedure. The efficacy of ventilation through the Patil-Syracuse mask during flexible fiberoptic bronchoscopy is greater than through the Classic LMA or iLMA,[214] and the Patil-Syracuse mask can be used to facilitate flexible esophagoscopy.

After endoscopy through the Patil-Syracuse mask is completed, an appropriate ventilation strategy can be instituted for the performance of operative direct laryngoscopy and suspension microlaryngeal surgery. If no further surgery is planned, the patient can be allowed to emerge from anesthesia, breathing spontaneously through the Patil-Syracuse mask or the LMA.

7. Emergence from General Anesthesia

Although highly stimulating intraoperatively, panendoscopy and microlaryngoscopic surgical procedures are typically characterized by low postoperative pain scores, even when the operation is prolonged.[43] Use of remifentanil infusions frequently allows reduction of the total dose of supplemental intravenous fentanyl to 1 to 2 μg/kg or avoidance of intraoperative use of fentanyl completely. In the recovery room, intermittent intravenous

bolus doses of fentanyl in combination with oral analgesics are usually sufficient for pain control.[43] Remifentanil-induced hyperalgesia has not been an issue in our experience, possibly because of the short duration of most cases and the relatively low infusion rates that are typically required intraoperatively (0.1 to 0.3 μg/kg/min). If increased pain occurs postoperatively, it should raise an alert about possible surgical complications, such as esophageal perforation (see "Intraoperative and Immediately Postoperative Complications").

Antiemetic prophylaxis should be routine,[43] and it is most commonly achieved by intravenous administration of a serotonin $5HT_3$ receptor antagonist (e.g., ondansetron). Multimodal antiemetic prophylaxis should be employed for patients at high risk for postoperative nausea and vomiting.

If endotracheal intubation was performed, smooth, nonstimulating emergence from anesthesia constitutes one of the most challenging tasks.[1,43] Patient's straining, bucking, or coughing with the ETT in situ results in an attempted forceful glottic closure, which may provoke additional trauma to and ulceration of the mucosal surface of the vocal cords, leading to wound formation.[140,215,216] Emergence phenomena such as a patient's agitation and uncontrolled head movements and postextubation laryngospasm may exacerbate the surgically compromised vocal cords further.[140] Subsequent vocal cord wound healing leads to remodeling of the superficial layer of the vocal cord lamina propria and the epithelium, which may result in formation of vocal cord nodules, polyps, and cysts.[215]

Three strategies can facilitate smooth tracheal extubation. First, the patient's trachea can be extubated at a deep plane of anesthesia, and the airway supported by a mask until the patient resumes spontaneous ventilation and emerges from anesthesia. Although this may be a viable approach, it is time and labor consuming, carries an increased risk of post-extubation laryngospasm, and leaves the patient's airway unprotected. It should be undertaken only if airway management on induction was uncomplicated. The second approach (i.e., Bailey maneuver), with the patient still anesthetized, involves insertion of a supralaryngeal airway (usually an LMA) behind the existing ETT, removal of the ETT, and administration of the supraglottic ventilatory support until the patient resumes spontaneous ventilation and awakens from anesthesia.[217] With the third, pharmacologic approach, the anesthesiologist relies on a low-dose remifentanil infusion to blunt the tracheal responses and to promote smooth extubation and awakening at the end of surgery.

Remifentanil is ideally suited for the control of tracheal extubation, because the return of consciousness and the cough reflex occur almost simultaneously.[17] Although the optimal dose of remifentanil required to blunt tracheal responses to extubation remains to be determined, current data indicate that a remifentanil infusion of 0.05 to 0.06 µg/kg/min (target concentration of 1.5 ng/mL) during emergence is likely sufficient; it reliably and effectively suppresses the cough reflex in awake intubated patients while promoting hemodynamic stability.[218,219]

IV. INTRAOPERATIVE AND IMMEDIATELY POSTOPERATIVE COMPLICATIONS

Most common, clinically relevant major and minor complications of panendoscopy and microlaryngeal surgery are summarized in Table 38-3. The incidence of complications is small and is largely related to the experience of the anesthesiologist and the surgeon, as well as their cohesive team work, the characteristics of the patient population treated, and the status of the treating institution (e.g., academic, tertiary care, private practice).[2,40,220-222]

A. Intraoperative Complications

Panendoscopy and microlaryngeal surgery remain very safe procedures. The mortality rate is exceedingly low (0.02% to 0.6%).[221,223] In a large, single-institution, retrospective review of 1093 endoscopic laryngeal surgery cases, Jaquet and colleagues[87] reported no intraoperative deaths, an incidence of major complications of 0.37% (all related to barotrauma during subglottic JV), and no major complications for 281 pediatric patients between the ages of less than 1 year and 16 years.

Loss of the airway on induction, requiring emergent cricothyrotomy or tracheostomy, can be sudden, especially in patients with critical airway obstruction. Proper preparation of the OR team is the key to promptly and efficiently dealing with intraoperative airway

TABLE 38-3

Complications of Panendoscopy and Microlaryngeal Surgery

Major Complications	Minor Complications
Intraoperative	**Intraoperative**
Death	Oropharyngeal mucosal
Loss of the airway	trauma
Major barotrauma	Dental trauma
complications	Minor barotrauma
Hypoxemia and hypercarbia	complications
Major hemodynamic	(subcutaneous
instability (e.g., myocardial	emphysema, gastric
ischemia, stroke)	distention)
Intraoperative awareness	Minor hemodynamic
Massive bleeding	instability (e.g., transient
Tracheobronchial tree	arrhythmias, vasovagal
perforation	events)
Esophageal perforation	Laryngospasm
Pulmonary aspiration	Corneal abrasion
Postoperative	**Postoperative**
Airway obstruction	Sore throat
Laryngospasm	Cranial nerve dysfunction
Negative pressure	(e.g., lingual,
pulmonary edema	glossopharyngeal,
Pulmonary aspiration	hypoglossal)
	Respiratory compromise
	Hemoptysis
	Temporomandibular joint
	disorder aggravation

Data from references 1, 2, 13, 33, 38, 40, 43, 213, 220-222.

emergencies.[38] An overall incidence of major barotrauma complications (e.g., cervicomediastinal emphysema, pneumothorax, tension pneumothorax) is small (0.2% to 0.5%),[87,111,120] and these complications are most frequently observed during TTJV (1.1%).[87] Intraoperative bronchial or transbronchial biopsy represents an independent risk factor for intraoperative pneumothorax (about 10%).[221] These patients also carry a higher risk of developing pulmonary edema after transbronchial biopsy.[221] Although the overall incidence of cardiovascular compromise may reach 20% to 50%,[2,83,142] major cardiac and cerebrovascular complications are rarely observed (0% to 2.2%).[86,87,111,221] Massive bleeding is rare and may be encountered in patients while coring out friable vascular tumors or during inadvertent perforation of the tracheal or bronchial wall with the laser or rigid bronchoscope.[71,213] Ensuing respiratory failure with an inability to wean the patient from the ventilator has been described.[71] The rigid bronchoscope should be used by experienced operators, because improper technique frequently results in dental or oropharyngeal trauma.[213] Particular care must be exercised when introducing a rigid bronchoscope into the airway of patients considered at high risk for cervical spine (C-spine) dislocation during neck extension (e.g., elderly, patients with rheumatoid arthritis, those with congenital C-spine abnormalities).[71] Prospective trials identify the incidence of dental trauma after suspension laryngoscopy at 0% to 6.5%,[40,224] depending on the operator's experience, methodology of the study, dental injury criteria, preexisting dentition status of the patient, and suspension technique used.[40]

Esophageal perforation is a rare event if flexible esophagoscopy is used.[2] A significantly higher complication rate (2.6%) was reported for rigid esophagoscopy, in which case patients with a history of head and neck cancer present a particular risk.[220] Pulmonary aspiration remains a particular concern when the patient's airway is left unprotected (e.g., JV), especially in patients at increased risk for aspiration of gastric contents. Intraoperative airway soiling may occur from aspiration of blood, secretions, surgical debris, or tumor cell contamination of the lower airway.[38]

Minor intraoperative anesthesia-related complications happen infrequently (2.6%).[87] The incidence of minor intraoperative laryngospasm during microlaryngeal surgery has been reported by Jaquet and colleagues as 3.1%[87]; it was exclusively related to the use of AIV and was associated with a light plane of anesthesia. In contrast, prospectively recorded, surgery-related minor complications are common (37.5% to 73%).[40,222] Minor surgical complications, such as sore throat, mucosal injury (e.g., cuts, edema, hematoma), and cranial nerve dysfunction (e.g., lingual, glossopharyngeal, hypoglossal), are most commonly observed.[1,40,221,222] The latter are likely caused by direct pressure or stretch injury associated with laryngoscopy or suspension of the laryngoscope,[40] and they are related to the size of the operating laryngoscope used and the duration of suspension.[1,40] Presenting symptoms in the recovery room may include dysesthesia and taste alteration, swallowing problems, and deviation of the tip of the tongue.[40,222]

B. Postoperative Complications

The risk of postoperative airway compromise is significantly greater among the patients who underwent diagnostic laryngoscopy and panendoscopy than those in the general surgical population.[225] The residual effects of anesthetics, analgesics, and inadequately reversed NMB may further contribute to the development of hypoventilation, atelectases, and poor mobilization of secretions in the early postoperative period.[34] Airway surgery invariably produces a certain degree of traumatic edema, which may precipitate acute airway obstruction postoperatively in an already compromised airway.[13] Development of airway obstruction should be suspected if the patient has symptoms such as dyspnea, respiratory distress, and particularly inspiratory stridor.[34] Aggressive early treatment with humidified oxygen and nebulized racemic epinephrine constitutes the first reasonable therapeutic intervention.[13,34] Postoperative laryngospasm may precede or accompany airway obstruction[226,227] and quickly lead to development of acute negative-pressure pulmonary edema.[34,226] Although the incidence of these complications in the general surgical population is small (0.3% and 0.09%, respectively),[226,228] negative-pressure pulmonary edema is preceded by laryngospasm in more than 50% of cases.[227] Treatment is supportive and consists of reestablishment of airway patency, O_2 supplementation, ventilatory support (i.e., CPAP or endotracheal intubation with positive-pressure ventilation and PEEP), management of

fluid shifts, and maintenance of normal intravascular volume.[34,226-228] Postoperative hemoptysis is usually associated with interventional bronchoscopy, for which the incidence may reach as high as 41%.[221] It is common for the suspension laryngoscopy to aggravate preexisting temporomandibular joint disease, and these patients should be advised accordingly before surgery.[1]

V. ANESTHESIA FOR PEDIATRIC UPPER AIRWAY ENDOSCOPY AND MICROLARYNGEAL SURGERY

A. General Considerations

The general principles of adult airway endoscopy can be applied to infants and children, although important anatomic, physiologic, and pathologic differences in the airway exist (see Chapter 36). Some of the most common indications for flexible and rigid airway endoscopy in pediatric patients and neonates are listed in Table 38-4. Usually, examination of the entire airway, including the nasopharynx, larynx, the subglottic region, and the remaining tracheobronchial tree is indicated, because abnormalities at more than one site are found in 10% to 20% of patients.[229-231]

TABLE 38-4

Indications for Flexible and Rigid Airway Endoscopy in Pediatric Patients

Flexible Endoscopy	Rigid Endoscopy
Airway obstruction	Airway obstruction
Stridor or noisy breathing	Stridor or noisy breathing
History of laryngomalacia	History of laryngomalacia or tracheomalacia
Persistent or recurrent wheezing	
Chronic cough	Persistent or recurrent wheezing
Hoarseness or weak cry	
Pulmonary abnormalities	Cyanosis or apnea
Atelectasis	Hoarseness or weak cry
Recurrent or persistent consolidations	Foreign body evaluation or management
Atypical or diffuse infiltrates	Evaluation and treatment of laryngeal pathology
Removal of mucous plugs	Evaluation and treatment of lesions of the airway
Evaluation of the artificial airway	Evaluation after laryngotracheal reconstruction
Assessment before extubation	
Confirmation of endotracheal tube position	Aspiration or gastroesophageal reflux
Tracheotomy surveillance	Toxic inhalation or aspiration
Foreign body evaluation	Airway trauma
Toxic inhalation or aspiration	
Tracheoesophageal fistula	
Special procedures	
Bronchoalveolar lavage	
Bronchial or endobronchial biopsy	

Data from references 232, 233, and 269.

B. Patient Preoperative Evaluation and Preparation

Preoperative assessment of the pediatric patient should consider the likely diagnosis,[232,233] the extent of airway compromise, and the degree of urgency of the procedure. A complete history, including a history of prematurity, any concurrent diseases, and an overview of the child's progress since birth, should be obtained.

Preterm infants, infants whose gestational age at birth is less than 37 weeks, are at higher risk for postoperative respiratory depression and apnea when exposed to anesthesia.[234-238] The postconceptual age (PCA; i.e., gestational age plus postnatal age) is inversely related to the risk of postoperative apnea,[234,235,237] with infants younger than 44 weeks' PCA at the greatest risk.[238,239] The former preterm infant with a PCA of more than 60 weeks can be sent home safely using standard discharge criteria.[238,239] Infants with a PCA of less than 60 weeks should be admitted for monitoring at least 12 hours postoperatively or overnight.[239] Comorbidities to consider when assessing increased risk of postoperative apnea include apnea at baseline, anemia, neurologic disease, and chronic lung disease.[235,237,238,240,241] Elective procedures in preterm infants should be postponed until more than 60 weeks' PCA.[238,239] Apnea after anesthesia has also been reported in term infants,[242-244] and elective procedures should be postponed until the infant is more than 44 weeks' PCA.[239]

The physical examination should focus on the airway, respiratory system, and cardiovascular system. The patient should be examined carefully for indicators of a potentially difficult airway, such as craniofacial abnormalities, micrognathia, retrognathia, limited mouth opening, or C-spine abnormalities. Abnormal airway noises (stridor is the most common) should be evaluated carefully.

Routine laboratory studies are not indicated for most children. Preoperative hemoglobin levels should be considered for procedures with the potential for blood loss for children with hemoglobinopathies, former preterm infants, and those younger than 6 months old.[239] Preoperative fasting guidelines should be followed unless the procedure is deemed emergent.

C. Operative Pediatric Airway Endoscopy and Microlaryngeal Surgery

1. Special Considerations and Anesthesia Objectives

Some of the most commonly used general purpose (diagnostic or intubating) operating laryngoscopes are the Storz and Parsons laryngoscopes (Storz, Tuttlingen, Germany), which are available in different sizes.[245] The Parsons laryngoscope (Fig. 38-25) can also be used for bronchoscopy, and after suspension, for some types of microlaryngeal surgery.[245] The Benjamin-Lindholm laryngoscope (Storz) provides a more panoramic view of the larynx and facilitates access for microlaryngeal surgery.[246] The Parsons and Benjamin-Lindholm laryngoscopes allow continuous insufflation of O_2 or anesthetic gases through a channel on the left side of the device (see Fig. 38-13). The pediatric rigid bronchoscopes manufactured by Storz are used almost universally.[229] The OD of the

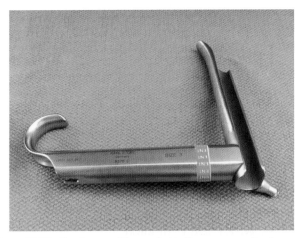

Figure 38-25 The flange of the pediatric Parsons operating laryngoscope (Storz, Tuttlingen, Germany) is open on the right side, allowing the passage of a rigid bronchoscope, if desired.

bronchoscope typically is larger than an ETT with the same ID, and careful attention to choosing a bronchoscope with the appropriate OD is important to avoid damage to laryngeal structures.[247]

The anesthesia objectives in pediatric patients are similar to those in adults (see "Special Considerations and Anesthesia Objectives"). Because of the shared airway, communication between the surgeon and the anesthesiologist before and during the procedure is critical, and it is probably the most important factor in avoiding complications.[248]

2. Intraoperative Ventilation Techniques and Strategies

Pediatric patients undergoing upper airway endoscopy and microlaryngeal surgery frequently present with difficult airway problems. Alternative techniques for pediatric difficult airway management are addressed in Chapter 36. The approach to ventilation of the pediatric patient usually follows the one used for adults (see "Intraoperative Ventilation Techniques and Strategies for Microlaryngeal Surgery").

a. AWAKE APPROACH

In pediatric patients, the awake approach is typically limited to a diagnostic evaluation of the upper airway and its dynamic function with a nasopharyngolaryngoscope or a FFB.[249] It can be safely performed in an office setting under topical anesthesia without sedation in children of all ages, even neonates,[249-251] but it may also be performed in the OR as part of a more complete examination. The limitation of performing this procedure in an office setting without sedation is the inability to pass the scope below the vocal cords.[249,251]

b. SPONTANEOUS VENTILATION

Under general anesthesia, spontaneous ventilation is generally preferred over controlled ventilation for endoscopy of the pediatric airway.[229,247,252] However, the multiple techniques in use indicate that no single method is universally accepted.[229,247]

Spontaneous breathing techniques in neonates and infants should be limited to shorter examinations. Under anesthesia, a combination of reduced FRC, high compliance of the pediatric airways and chest wall, increased O_2 consumption, and further airflow limitations imposed by the surgical instrumentation inside and around the airway can lead to a rapid hypoxemia if spontaneous ventilation is maintained.[229,253-255] Nevertheless, successful intraoperative spontaneous ventilation has been reported in neonates as young as 2 weeks,[256-258] and it is more easily maintained during the entire procedure in older infants and children. If spontaneous ventilation fails due to apnea or hypoventilation, institution of alternative ventilation techniques must be promptly implemented.

c. APNEIC INTERMITTENT VENTILATION

For the physiologic reasons outlined previously, AIV in young pediatric patients is suitable for only very short procedures, such as a diagnostic bronchoscopy.

d. LASER-SAFE ENDOTRACHEAL TUBE

Small, laser-safe ETTs are not commercially available for infants and small children.[255] Regular pediatric ETTs can be wrapped with a fire-resistant foil for laser surgery.[254] Preparation of these wrapped ETTs is becoming less common because it is time consuming and cumbersome. Potentially dangerous gaps in the wrapping may allow ignition of the ETT, and fragments of wrapping material can serve as foreign bodies.

e. JET VENTILATION

In children, supraglottic JV is probably most commonly used.[255,259,260] Subglottic JV is used less frequently,[87] because the smaller, compliant airways of infants and small children may not allow adequate exhalation, potentially leading to a higher incidence of barotrauma.[254] In infants, even a small cannula can obstruct the surgical field. The use of TTJV in infants and small children is uncommon.[87]

3. General Anesthesia Management for Pediatric Airway Endoscopy and Microlaryngeal Surgery

a. PREMEDICATION AND MONITORING

Routine, noninvasive monitoring usually is sufficient. If quantitative assessment of CO_2 is not available due to the method of airway management, the anesthesiologist should visually monitor chest excursions and auscultate breath sounds using a precordial stethoscope.[261]

The goals of premedication in children include alleviation of anxiety, a smooth separation from parents, and facilitation of the induction of anesthesia. If the child is symptomatic and there is a possibility of airway obstruction or respiratory compromise, premedication using a smaller amount than customary should be considered. Premedication can decrease the likelihood of crying and struggling on induction and thereby prevent worsening of the airway symptoms. Infants 9 to 10 months old typically benefit from premedication.[262] Recommended dosages for midazolam are 0.25 to 0.5 mg/kg taken orally or 0.05 to 0.1 mg/kg administered intravenously.[263]

If intravenous access has already been established, an antisialagogue can be given to decrease secretions. Glycopyrrolate is preferred in children because it has no central effects, and it causes less tachycardia than atropine.[264,265] Intramuscular injections of any medication are painful and should be avoided if possible.[266] Administration of 0.5 mg/kg of dexamethasone, with a maximum dose of 10 to 20 mg, is recommended to minimize postoperative airway edema.[247]

b. ANESTHESIA INDUCTION AND MAINTENANCE

For children without intravenous access, gentle inhalational induction with sevoflurane is recommended, and the intravenous access is secured after sufficient depth of anesthesia is reached. Preserving spontaneous respiration initially is critical to allow dynamic assessment of the vocal cords, larynx, and tracheobronchial tree,[229,261,267] and it is strongly preferred when a high-grade obstruction of the upper airway is suspected or a difficult airway is anticipated.[261,268] If only a short endoscopic examination is planned, the nasopharyngolaryngoscope or FFB is passed through the nose into the pharynx by way of a bronchoscopic swivel adapter attached to a standard anesthesia mask.[269] Alternatively, the anesthesia mask can be removed to facilitate the examination. The FFB can also be passed through a laryngeal mask or an ETT if visualization of the upper airway is not required.[269]

When the depth of anesthesia is sufficient to tolerate laryngoscopy, the surgeon performs direct laryngoscopy and topicalizes the airway with lidocaine, which typically is applied to the vocal cords by atomizer or sprayed with a 3-mL Luer-Lok syringe fitted with a plastic or metal cannula.[247] The usual concentration of lidocaine is 2% for children (1% for small infants), and the maximum dose is 3 to 5 mg/kg[229,270]; toxicity is possible with excessive doses, and seizures have been reported.[271] When appropriately applied, the lidocaine provides surface analgesia to the glottis, subglottis, and proximal trachea, decreasing the chance of laryngospasm or coughing when the bronchoscope is inserted and reducing the general anesthetic requirements. After the airway has been successfully topicalized, the surgeon performs a second laryngoscopy to evaluate the larynx and the vocal cords more completely.

Depending on the pathology, the surgeon may choose to pass the telescope for a rapid assessment. This has the advantage of producing less airway trauma than by the larger bronchoscope. If there is significant narrowing, the telescope may pass beyond the narrowing more easily. The surgeon may choose to place the child in suspension at this point. A rigid bronchoscope is then passed through the vocal cords. A thinner telescope with an optical eyepiece is subsequently placed through the bronchoscope, allowing the subglottis and trachea to be examined. After the bronchoscope is introduced past the vocal cords, the anesthesia circuit is connected to the side arm of the bronchoscope, allowing gas exchange and continued ventilation, similar to the technique used in adults (see Fig. 38-10). With the optical telescope in place, gas exchange occurs in the space between the telescope and the bronchoscope sheath. Partial occlusion of the bronchoscope lumen by the optical telescope increases resistance to ventilation, especially when the 2.5-, 3.0-, and 3.5-mm ID bronchoscopes are used.[247] The smallest optical telescope should be used to prevent increased airflow resistance.[259]

After an appropriate diagnosis has been established, the surgeon may choose to immediately initiate treatment of the pathology. Endoscopic surgery can include the use of microdebriders, dilating balloons, stents, or lasers.[272,273] Many pediatric airway centers are using laser less frequently, because alternatives such as microdebriders and balloon dilation become preferred.[272,273]

TIVA with propofol and remifentanil is used most frequently for maintenance of anesthesia, even during spontaneous ventilation. Infusions of 150 to 500 µg/kg/min of propofol and 0.05 to 0.2 µg/kg/min of remifentanil have been reported.[258,267] A bolus dose of propofol (1 to 5 mg/kg) may be administered to achieve steady-state conditions rapidly.[258,274] Remifentanil infusion may require a more dilute solution in neonates and infants to provide sufficient delivery volume.[275] Infusions must be carefully titrated to effect to avoid apnea, and they should be delivered as close to the intravenous catheter as possible to minimize delays in response to changes in infusion rates.[275]

Dexmedetomidine may be a particularly useful adjunct to TIVA when the spontaneous ventilation technique is used, because its administration is characterized by lack of respiratory depression and stable hemodynamic profile, even at high doses.[276-278] MRI of the upper airway in spontaneously breathing children with a high-dose intravenous infusion of dexmedetomidine (3 µg/kg/hr) showed only small reductions in upper airway diameter and no clinical evidence of upper airway obstruction.[279] For the preservation of spontaneous ventilation, a combination of an intravenous bolus (0.25 to 1 µg/kg) and intravenous infusion (2 to 2.5 µg/kg/hr) of dexmedetomidine with an intravenous infusion (200 to 300 µg/kg/min) of propofol appears to be well tolerated.[277,278]

Several manual infusion schemes exist for TIVA in children. Devices that allow target-controlled intravenous infusions of anesthetics in children are not widely available,[274,280] and the target concentrations for neonates and infants or for critically ill children have not been fully investigated.[281] Significantly higher propofol doses per unit of body weight are necessary in healthy children for induction and maintenance of anesthesia.[274] Compared with adults, to achieve blood concentration of propofol of 3 µg/mL, the bolus dose should be increased by more than 50%, and the infusion rate should be almost doubled (19 mg/kg/hr for 10 minutes, followed by 15 mg/kg/hr for 10 minutes and 12 mg/kg/hr thereafter).[274] Similarly, the reported target concentration of remifentanil necessary to block the response to a skin incision under target-controlled propofol anesthetic in pediatric patients between the ages of 3 and 11 years is almost twice that needed in adults (0.15 µg/kg/min, 95% CI, 0.13 to 0.17 versus 0.08 µg/kg/min, 95% CI, 0.06 to 0.12).[282]

c. EMERGENCE FROM ANESTHESIA IN THE PEDIATRIC PATIENT

After airway endoscopy is completed, an ETT can be placed in the trachea to control the airway, or more commonly, the child can be allowed to emerge breathing 100% O_2 by mask.[247,267] If the child is intubated, the usual criteria for extubation should be applied. In the recovery room, these patients should be carefully monitored for signs of airway edema or respiratory distress.

4. Complications of Pediatric Airway Endoscopy

Major and minor complications of pediatric airway endoscopy largely replicate those observed in adult patients (see "Intraoperative and Immediately Postoperative Complications").[249,267,283] No major complications were recorded with different intraoperative ventilatory techniques in more than 280 pediatric patients.[87] Intraoperatively, adverse airway events are most likely to occur with an inadequate depth of anesthesia.[267] Interventions that seem to decrease complications are careful and effective topicalization of the airway, close observation of the child for any movement or response to initial stimulation, and immediate withdrawal of the laryngoscope or bronchoscope with patient response until an adequate depth of anesthesia is reestablished.[267] In two large series of pediatric patients undergoing rigid bronchoscopy, the complication rate was 2% to 3%.[232,284] Stridor due to airway edema is the most commonly seen complication in the immediate postoperative period, and it should be treated with nebulized racemic epinephrine.

5. Recurrent Respiratory Papillomatosis

Recurrent respiratory papillomatosis (RRP) (Fig. 38-26) is the most common benign neoplasm of the respiratory tract in children, and it is characterized by the proliferation of exophytic squamous papillomas within the respiratory tract.[285-287] Because of the recurrent nature of the disease, most children return frequently for treatment. The average enrollee in the National Registry for Juvenile-Onset Recurrent Respiratory Papillomatosis underwent a mean of 5.1 operations annually.[288] Repeated surgical treatment may lead to laryngeal web formation and irreversible damage to the vocal cords.[287,288]

The most common symptoms of RRP are related to laryngeal obstruction and include hoarseness, abnormal cry or voice change, and stridor.[187,289] The larynx and glottis are affected in almost all cases, followed by supraglottic involvement and subglottic involvement. Distal spread to the trachea, bronchi, and lungs has been

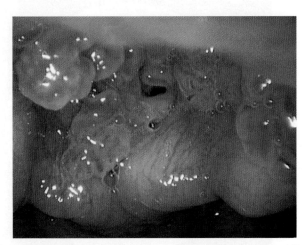

Figure 38-26 Recurrent respiratory papillomatosis. (Courtesy of Alan Cheng, MD, Stanford University Medical Center, Stanford, CA.)

reported.[286,287] Pulmonary lesions can cause bronchiectasis, pneumonia, and declining pulmonary status.[286]

Anesthesia and airway management for patients with RRP can employ tubeless spontaneous ventilation,[290] AIV, and JV[247,267,291]; the advantages and disadvantages of each technique have been discussed (see "Intraoperative Ventilation Techniques and Strategies for Microlaryngeal Surgery"). A 2002 survey of members of the American Society of Pediatric Otolaryngology showed a preference for spontaneous ventilation or AIV (63.5%), followed by JV (24.3%) and laser-safe ETTs (9.6%),[285] although a theoretical risk of carrying the human papillomavirus (HPV) particles into the distal airways with AIV or JV exists.[267,291] A higher incidence of apnea and laryngospasm may be observed during spontaneous ventilation in RRP patients under TIVA compared with positive-pressure ventilation through an ETT.[292]

Current surgical preference for debulking RRP lesions appears to favor the use of the microdebrider over the CO_2 laser,[285,286] because it shortens the operating time, eliminates the risk of a laser fire, and is associated with decreased postoperative pain.[293] With microdebrider surgery, the ETT can be used for the entire procedure, although it limits the surgeon's access to the posterior glottis.

D. Foreign Bodies in the Airway and Esophagus

1. Foreign Body Aspiration

Foreign body aspiration in the airway is most common in children 1 to 3 years old[289,294] and is a leading cause of accidental death in children younger than 5 years.[295] Food products (especially nuts and seeds) are the most commonly aspirated airway foreign bodies (77% to 86%).[296] Nuts with oils on the surface can be particularly problematic because they may stimulate a significant inflammatory response.[297]

Foreign body aspiration is suspected when a child has an acute choking event or severe coughing with respiratory distress, but in many instances, the diagnosis is delayed.[297-299] Foreign bodies in children with a delayed diagnosis may be more difficult to extract,[300] and these children are also at higher risk for complications.[300,301] Symptoms and signs associated with bronchial aspiration include coughing, wheezing, dyspnea, and decreased breath sounds on the affected side, whereas coughing, stridor, dyspnea, and cyanosis are more common with laryngeal or tracheal foreign bodies.[302]

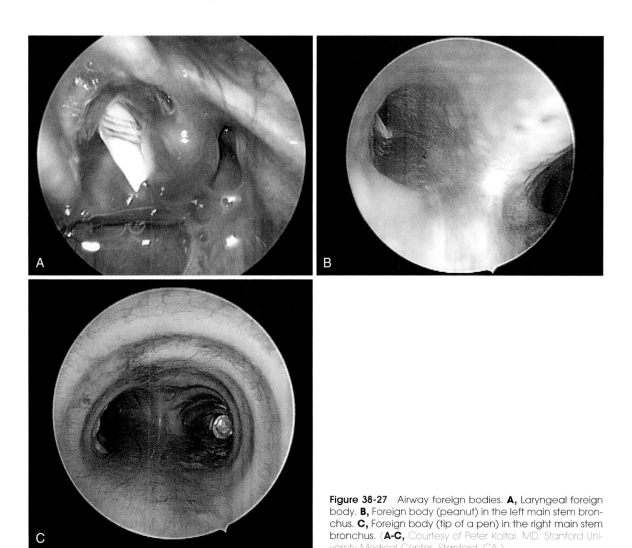

Figure 38-27 Airway foreign bodies. **A,** Laryngeal foreign body. **B,** Foreign body (peanut) in the left main stem bronchus. **C,** Foreign body (tip of a pen) in the right main stem bronchus. (**A-C,** Courtesy of Peter Koltai, MD, Stanford University Medical Center, Stanford, CA.)

Most airway foreign bodies lodge in the bronchial tree (85% to 91%), preferentially on the right side, with the remainder catching in the larynx or trachea[233,296] (Fig. 38-27). A foreign body in the bronchus can cause a ball-valve obstruction with hyperinflation of the distal lung, and if the obstruction is complete, the distal lung collapses.[229]

Preoperative assessment should consider the likely position of the foreign body, the extent of airway compromise, and the urgency of the procedure. Physical examination may reveal diminished breath sounds and rhonchi on the affected side. A chest radiograph should be obtained just before surgery to confirm that the coin, for example, has not already passed into the stomach. Because many objects are radiolucent, the chest radiograph should also be reviewed for evidence of secondary changes, such as distal air trapping, infiltrates, or atelectasis.

The treatment of choice for airway foreign bodies is prompt endoscopic removal under conditions of maximal safety and minimal trauma.[297,301] Following preoperative fasting guidelines is recommended if the procedure is not an emergency.[299] An intravenous catheter should be inserted in most cases. In an emergency situation or with a distressed infant, establishing intravenous access immediately after inhalation induction is acceptable.[299] As with most pediatric endoscopy cases, glycopyrrolate should be administered to decrease secretions, and intravenous dexamethasone is recommended to minimize postoperative airway edema.[247]

Before induction of anesthesia, the possibility of complete airway obstruction should be anticipated. Distal airway foreign bodies are more difficult to remove, whereas proximal foreign bodies are more likely to obstruct the airway.[299] A backup plan should include emergency rigid bronchoscopy, deliberate advancement of the foreign body into a main stem bronchus, tracheotomy, and thoracotomy in selected cases.

Induction and maintenance of anesthesia are similar to anesthesia described earlier for direct laryngoscopy and rigid bronchoscopy. The choice between maintaining spontaneous respiration and controlling ventilation remains controversial, with both techniques producing equally good results.[289,299,303] For airway foreign bodies, pediatric anesthesiologists seem to prefer maintenance of spontaneous ventilation,[304] because positive pressure can force the foreign body deeper into the smaller airways.[299,303] For the esophageal foreign bodies, controlled ventilation with an ETT is the preferred technique.[304]

When the airway foreign body is too large to withdraw through the lumen of the bronchoscope, the bronchoscope, forceps, and foreign body are removed as a single unit.[289,294] If the foreign body is dropped in the proximal airway and cannot be immediately retrieved, it should be pushed distally into the bronchus. If the foreign body is pushed into the contralateral bronchus, there is a potential for complete obstruction from edema in the original bronchus.[305] The FFB can be preferentially used when the foreign body is lodged far into the periphery of the lung.[297]

Esophageal foreign bodies (usually coins) are considered less serious than airway foreign bodies, and most pass through the gastrointestinal tract harmlessly.[306-308] For asymptomatic esophageal coins, an observation period of 8 to 16 hours is considered appropriate[309]; batteries and magnets are exceptions and should be removed expeditiously.[310,311] Esophageal foreign bodies most commonly lodge at the level of the cricopharyngeal muscle,[294] and foreign body impaction is most frequently associated with vomiting, gagging, odynophagia, dysphagia, poor feeding, and excessive salivation.[308] A large esophageal foreign body may cause symptoms of airway obstruction by compression or irritation of the upper airway, necessitating emergent intervention.[301]

2. Complications of Endoscopy for Foreign Body Removal

a. INTRAOPERATIVE COMPLICATIONS

Intraoperative complications during foreign body removal are usually minor, and include laryngospasm, bronchospasm, and O_2 desaturations. In a large review of almost 13,000 tracheobronchial foreign bodies in children, major complications, such as tracheal or bronchial laceration requiring repair, pneumothorax or pneumomediastinum, failed bronchoscopy requiring tracheostomy or thoracotomy, cardiac arrest, and hypoxic brain damage, occurred in about 1% of cases.[296] Fatal complications have been reported, but they are rare (0.4%).[297,298]

b. POSTOPERATIVE COMPLICATIONS

The most common immediate postoperative complications include laryngeal edema and traumatic laryngitis.[297] Long-term complications, such as granulation tissue and stricture formation, can occur at the site of the foreign body.[301] Persistent pneumonia and atelectasis may be seen after removal of long-standing foreign bodies.[294,297] After esophagoscopy, the most common complications are vomiting, aspiration, fever, and a second, missed foreign body.[301]

VI. CONCLUSIONS

The field of laryngeal surgery is complex and continues to expand rapidly. It is likely that the mounting complexity of microlaryngoscopic procedures will benefit from perioperative involvement of a dedicated anesthesia team. Lack of collaboration and planning between the surgeon and the anesthesiologist can turn even a simple microlaryngoscopic case into a chaotic, life-threatening airway crisis.[1] As anesthetic challenges continue to grow, so will the demand for a wide range of unique skills and expertise from the anesthesiologist to ensure patient safety and favorable surgical outcomes.

VII. CLINICAL PEARLS

- Close communication between the anesthesiologist and the surgeon throughout the perioperative period is critical for the success of the operation and for patient safety.

- A structured and stepwise approach to a tenuous and partially obstructed airway is necessary for successful management.

- Core surgical and anesthesia objectives include an anesthetic plan suitable for variable or unpredictable duration of surgery, an immobile and clear surgical field, absence of the patient's movement, maintenance of a stable plane of anesthesia, competent execution of different intraoperative ventilation techniques and strategies, full return of the patient's protective airway reflexes, smooth and rapid emergence from anesthesia, and fast-tracking patients for discharge.

- The principles and practice of jet ventilation must be well understood and adhered to by the anesthesiologist and the surgeon.

- Total intravenous anesthesia (TIVA) is preferred, especially when delivery of inhalational anesthetics is compromised.

- Neuromuscular blockade (NMB) should be adequately maintained.

- In pediatric patients, spontaneous ventilation technique typically is preferred over controlled ventilation.

- The possibility of post-extubation airway edema, laryngospasm, and postoperative airway obstruction should be anticipated and treated appropriately.

SELECTED REFERENCES

All references can be found online at expertconsult.com.

1. Rosen CA, Simpson CB: *Operative techniques in laryngology,* Berlin, 2008, Springer-Verlag.
18. Xiao P, Zhang XS: Adult laryngotracheal surgery. *Anesthesiol Clin* 28:529–540, 2010.
24. Biro P: Jet ventilation for surgical interventions in the upper airway. *Anesthesiol Clin* 28:397–409, 2010.
33. Mason RA, Fielder CP: The obstructed airway in head and neck surgery. *Anaesthesia* 54:625–628, 1999.
86. Bourgain JL, Desruennes E, Fischler M, et al: Transtracheal high frequency jet ventilation for endoscopic airway surgery: A multicentre study. *Br J Anaesth* 87:870–875, 2001.
87. Jaquet Y, Monnier P, Van Melle G, et al: Complications of different ventilation strategies in endoscopic laryngeal surgery: A 10-year review. *Anesthesiology* 104:52–59, 2006.
111. Cook TM, Alexander R: Major complications during anaesthesia for elective laryngeal surgery in the UK: A national survey of the use of high-pressure source ventilation. *Br J Anaesth* 101:266–272, 2008.
229. Benjamin B: Anesthesia for pediatric airway endoscopy. *Otolaryngol Clin North Am* 33:29–47, 2000.
232. Hoeve LJ, Rombout J: Pediatric laryngobronchoscopy: 1332 procedures stored in a data base. *Int J Pediatr Otorhinolaryngol* 24:73–82, 1992.
267. Collins CE: Anesthesia for pediatric airway surgery: Recommendations and review from a pediatric referral center. *Anesthesiol Clin* 28:505–517, 2010.
296. Fidkowski CW, Zheng H, Firth PG: The anesthetic considerations of tracheobronchial foreign bodies in children: A literature review of 12,979 cases. *Anesth Analg* 111:1016–1025, 2010.

Chapter 39

The Difficult Airway in Conventional Head and Neck Surgery

ALEXANDER T. HILLEL | DAVID A. DIAZ VOSS VARELA | NASIR I. BHATTI

I. INTRODUCTION

Airway management in head and neck surgery is unique because the operative field is the upper airway itself or the adjacent structures and the anesthesiologist must share access to the airway throughout all phases of the procedure. The head and neck surgeon is uniquely qualified to help diagnose and manage the compromised airway, and a collegial relationship and ongoing communication between the surgeon and the anesthesiology team are essential.

Acute airway situations in head and neck surgery should be approached in a systematic manner. The simplest adequate form of control should be selected, and the lowest level (i.e., supraglottis, glottis, subglottis, or trachea) of airway obstruction should be ascertained; control should be established by securing an airway below that level. Acute airway problems often evolve in association with other medical problems. Obvious and potential difficult mask ventilation or difficult intubation should

be discussed with the head and neck surgeon, and thoughtful discussion about sequential steps of airway management should take place before anesthetic induction and especially before attempting intubation. Ideally, if time allows, an action plan addressing airway management, including the initial strategy and two backup measures, should be communicated to all team members in the room. Maintaining lines of communication during the intubation procedure can reduce morbidity and mortality associated with difficult airway management.[1]

The spectrum of head and neck surgery is broad, including simpler procedures such as tonsillectomy, major ablative oncologic resections in the head and neck, and extensive reconstructive procedures. The risk of a difficult airway is relatively high for patients undergoing head and neck surgery. Bag-bask ventilation (BMV) and endotracheal intubation may be potentially or obviously difficult because of the nature of the patient's underlying condition.

The severity or completeness of airway obstruction is categorized as follows:

1. Complete obstruction: no detectable airflow in or out of lungs
2. Partial obstruction: patient with stridor or dyspnea from narrowing of the major airway
3. Potential or impending obstruction: concern that a patient will develop airway compromise because of a known anatomic or physical condition if the respiratory physiology or the consciousness level is altered

This chapter addresses current principles and techniques for securing and safely managing the airway of patients undergoing conventional head and neck surgery. The discussion emphasizes prevention of difficult airway events associated with common and uncommon procedures in otolaryngology and in head and neck surgery, ranging from a tonsillectomy to a resection of oral and oropharyngeal cancer.

II. AERODIGESTIVE ONCOLOGIC SURGERY

A. Preoperative Airway Assessment

The preoperative airway assessment must include a comprehensive general medical history, focused history related to upper airway symptoms, general and head and neck physical examination, a thorough assessment of previous anesthetic records, details of surgical steps and alternative plans, and when indicated, laboratory and imaging studies. Patients with an upper aerodigestive tract malignancy may have limited cardiopulmonary reserve because of the disease process, dysphagia, and toxic effects of the chemotherapeutic agents. The risk of regurgitation and aspiration should be considered at the time of induction of general anesthesia.

1. History

Tobacco and alcohol use are associated with most cases of head and neck cancer and predispose these patients to chronic obstructive pulmonary disease, pneumonia, hypertension, coronary artery disease, and alcohol withdrawal. Information about previous surgical and anesthetic procedures with an emphasis on a history of anesthetic difficulties or difficult intubations, or both, must be obtained and communicated. Previous difficult airway management is considered to be one of the most important predictors of subsequent airway management difficulties.[2,3] Patients with a history of obstructive sleep apnea (OSA), especially those without an obvious anatomic abnormality, need careful assessment because their redundant pharyngeal mucosa and soft palate anatomy may hinder BMV and the ability to intubate. Common presenting symptoms of airway obstruction include dyspnea at rest or on exertion, voice changes, dysphagia, stridor, and cough. Physical findings may include hoarseness; agitation; and intercostal, suprasternal, and supraclavicular retraction. Voice changes provide an early suggestion of the anatomic level and severity and progression of the lesion. A muffled voice may indicate

TABLE 39-1	
Evaluation of Stridor	
Factor	Features
Definition	Harsh, high-pitched sound from partial obstruction of upper airway
Typical characteristics	Inspiratory Monophonic High pitched
Airway obstruction Inspiratory versus expiratory	Inspiratory stridor suggests that the lesion is extrathoracic. Expiratory stridor suggests that the lesion is intrathoracic.
Awake versus asleep	Obstruction that is worse when awake or with exertion suggests a laryngeal, tracheal, or bronchial origin. Obstruction that is worse when asleep suggests a pharyngeal origin.

supraglottic disease, whereas glottic lesions often result in a coarse, scratchy voice. If there is suspicion of an anterior mediastinal, pharyngeal, or neck mass resulting in partial airway obstruction, initiating anesthesia in the patient in the supine position without first securing the airway may lead to complete airway obstruction and therefore deserves special preoperative evaluation.

2. Physical Examination

A systematic and comprehensive evaluation of the patient's upper airway is mandatory. The condition of dentition, facial hair (beard), size and mobility of the tongue, thyromental distance, Mallampati score, and limitations in neck flexion and extension must be evaluated. A thyrocervical distance of less than 6 cm in a fully extended adult neck is a good indicator of difficult laryngoscopy and an inability to visualize the vocal cords. The presence and character of stridor should be appreciated, because it may suggest the location of airway narrowing (Table 39-1). Postirradiation changes, neck masses, and previous neck surgery may result in reduced neck mobility, causing difficult mask ventilation and difficult intubation. Findings of morbid obesity, evidence of any oropharyngeal or lip edema, and signs of upper aerodigestive tract bleeding may direct the preferred method of airway management. Lower cranial nerve dysfunction from tumor or previous surgery may also result in airway difficulty related to aspiration or obstruction.

3. Laboratory and Imaging Studies

Laboratory and imaging studies can provide additional information before definitive airway management, depending on the urgency or emergency of the situation. In nonurgent cases, assessment of pulmonary function in patients with chronic pulmonary diseases may be helpful, along with arterial blood gas and pulmonary function tests. Similarly, computed tomography (CT) and magnetic resonance imaging (MRI) may help in determining the size, location, and nature of the obstruction. Even in airway urgencies, flexible laryngoscopy or indirect laryngoscopy performed by an otolaryngologist (i.e., head and neck surgeon) may help with anticipation and planning for a difficult airway.

B. Securing the Airway

There are many approaches to securing the airway of patients undergoing head and neck surgery in a safe manner. Determining the optimal approach may depend on the surgery being performed, location of a lesion or infectious mass, or tolerance of the patient. For example, in a patient undergoing maxillomandibular fixation to repair a fractured mandible, nasotracheal intubation is ideal to keep the endotracheal tube (ETT) out of the oral cavity. In a patient with severe supraglottic angioedema, flexible fiberoptic intubation through the nose with the patient upright is preferred to enable identification of the airway with fiberoptic visualization and to avoid pharyngeal collapse in the supine position. Establishing a sequential airway plan with backup options and open communication between the anesthesiology and surgical teams facilitate preparedness and patient safety. An analysis of anesthesia-related cardiopulmonary arrests revealed that up to one third of severe complications result from an inability to establish an optimal airway after the induction of general anesthesia.[4]

1. Examination of the Airway in the Awake Patient

For a potentially difficult airway, the anesthesiologist may elect to evaluate the airway in an awake patient with the help of judicious intravenous sedation and topical anesthesia. This assessment helps to determine the optimal approach to securing the airway without compromising the patient's spontaneous breathing. The successful execution of this technique requires constant meaningful contact with the patient and adequate use of topical agents, such as 4% lidocaine spray, with the ultimate goal of not compromising the ability of the patient to breathe spontaneously and to protect the airway. Percutaneous blocks of the superior laryngeal nerves or translaryngeal instillation of lidocaine is best avoided in patients with a head or neck tumor. After the patient is adequately prepared, careful direct laryngoscopy is performed to assess whether to proceed with an awake intubation or to induce general anesthesia for subsequent intubation. A reasonable airway in an awake patient may change to a compromised airway immediately after induction of general anesthesia, with loss of tone of the pharyngeal wall and anterior displacement of the larynx.[5] If direct laryngoscopy with sedation is too risky to perform, consideration should be given to awake, flexible fiberoptic laryngoscopy to assess the airway and the possibility of awake, nasotracheal, flexible fiberoptic intubation.

2. Choice of Endotracheal Intubation Technique

a. ENDOTRACHEAL INTUBATION AFTER INDUCTION OF GENERAL ANESTHESIA

In patients with no obvious or expected airway compromise, the ETT can be placed during direct laryngoscopy after induction with a short-acting paralyzing agent, such as succinylcholine. Because it is difficult or impossible to empty the stomach with a nasogastric tube in the case of a large pharyngeal or esophageal tumor, the patient is assumed to have a full stomach.[6] Risk of aspiration is reduced by preinduction administration of ranitidine, metoclopramide, and oral sodium citrate–citric acid buffer (Bicitra, Willen Drug Co., Baltimore, MD). The Hollinger anterior commissure laryngoscope is a valuable tool in difficult airway management, and it should be considered when other techniques have failed. This scope may accommodate a 5.0-mm or smaller cuffed ETT, but the insufflation port may become lodged in the barrel of the scope. To avoid this issue, a trial passage of the ETT through the laryngoscope should be attempted before the performance of direct laryngoscopy.[7]

b. NASOTRACHEAL INTUBATION IN THE AWAKE PATIENT

If a difficult airway or difficult intubation is anticipated from the preoperative examination or awake assessment of the airway has mandated an awake intubation, nasotracheal or orotracheal intubation of an awake patient may be performed. The choice of route is directed by the surgical requirement and by the physical condition of the patient. Continuous administration of supplemental oxygen (O_2) during the entire process is mandatory.

The nasotracheal route is useful in cases of small mouth opening, severe trismus, large tongue, receding lower jaw, large oral cavity tumor, planned maxillomandibular fixation, or tracheal dilatation. Operator and equipment positioning relative to the patient is depicted in Figure 39-1. For nasal intubation, the nose is prepared with a nasal decongestant spray, such as pseudoephedrine (Afrin) and topical 4% cocaine. Cocaine is more advantageous than lidocaine because it is a vasoconstrictor in addition to being a very effective surface anesthetic. The potential for abuse by the personnel is occasionally a deterrent for its routine use. In placing the ETT through the nose, it is necessary to remember that the nasal floor usually runs in a horizontal plane perpendicular to an

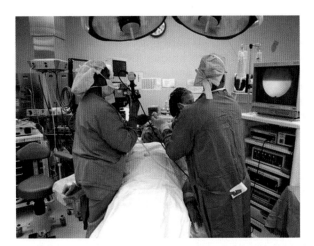

Figure 39-1 The optimal setup for fiberoptic intubation includes elevation of the patient's head to minimize airway collapse. The intubator should be facing the patient, allowing the entire team to observe the procedure on the video monitor. (From Bhatti NI: Surgical management of the difficult adult airway. In Flint PW, editor: *Cummings otolaryngology–head and neck surgery*, ed 5, Philadelphia, 2010, Elsevier, pp 121–129.)

imaginary vertical line connecting the glabella and the pogonion. The ETT is advanced to approximately the 15-cm mark, and the connector is removed. The flexible fiberoptic bronchoscope (FFB) is then used to visualize the glottic opening and to introduce the tube into the trachea.

c. FIBEROPTIC-GUIDED OROTRACHEAL INTUBATION

Orotracheal intubation is facilitated with an oropharyngeal airway (OPA), such as a Williams or Ovassapian OPA. Similar to nasotracheal intubation, optimal topical anesthesia of the oral cavity and oropharynx is warranted to overcome the patient's gag reflex. The lubricated ETT, with its connector removed, is loaded onto the proximal end of the FFB. The tip of the scope is then introduced through the OPA and passed behind the epiglottis into the glottic opening leading into the trachea. When the scope is past the vocal folds, the tracheal rings should be identified before advancing the ETT. The ETT is then eased into the trachea over the scope, and placement is confirmed with a combination of bilateral chest auscultation and end-tidal carbon dioxide (EtCO$_2$) measurement. After confirmation of the placement, general anesthesia is induced.

d. RIGID BRONCHOSCOPY

The rigid bronchoscope, a hollow stainless steel tube through which a rigid telescope is placed, provides excellent access to the airways. The distal end of the rigid bronchoscope is usually beveled to facilitate intubation and lifting of the epiglottis. The updated American Society of Anesthesiologists (ASA) protocol states that in the "cannot intubate, cannot ventilate" (CICV) scenario, "a rigid bronchoscope for difficult airway management reduces airway-related adverse outcomes."[8] This modality is recommended as a technique for cases of difficult mask ventilation. Other indications for rigid bronchoscopy include massive airway hemoptysis, foreign body retrieval, laser or photodynamic therapy, and placement of airway stents.[9]

e. RETROGRADE INTUBATION

Though rarely used, retrograde intubation represents another alternative technique for intubation of the difficult airway in head and neck patients. This technique can also be used in patients with trismus, trauma to the cervical spine, temporomandibular joint ankylosis, upper airway masses, or failed intubation. This technique begins with puncture of the cricothyroid membrane (CTM) or cricotracheal membrane with a small needle angled superiorly to pass a guidewire through the larynx, and it is then guided through the nose or mouth. The ETT is then advanced over the guidewire with a Seldinger technique into position in the trachea.[10]

Retrograde intubation may also be used to facilitate other approaches. For example, a combination of conventional, fiberoptic, and retrograde techniques can be used to intubate successfully.[11] An FFB with a suction port can be used as an anterograde guide over a retrograde wire. A direct laryngoscopic view can facilitate placement of the tip of a fiberoptic scope into or near the glottic aperture. After the FFB is past the vocal folds and tracheal

rings have been identified, the preloaded ETT may be passed over the FFB into the trachea.

f. TRACHEOSTOMY WITH LOCAL ANESTHESIA

If a patient is in acute respiratory distress because of upper airway obstruction and the patient is considered unable to be safely intubated under general anesthesia after evaluation (including FFB), the best choice is to perform a planned but urgent awake tracheostomy.[12] This should be performed under local anesthesia with minimal intravenous sedation to avoid loss of spontaneous breathing. Tracheostomy under local anesthesia in an awake patient is also an excellent method to secure the airway in the following situations: upper airway abscess that may be in the way of or distorting the pathway for endotracheal intubation; bulky, friable supraglottic or glottic mass; and glottic stenosis with presumed bilateral cricoarytenoid joint fixation. In these situations, attempts at direct laryngoscopy and intubation may result in abscess rupture or aspiration of purulent material, blood, or material from a friable tumor, or in the case of cricoarytenoid joint fixation, the fixed, medialized vocal folds do not allow passage of the ETT without severe damage to the membranous vocal folds.

3. Difficult or Failed Intubation

An unanticipated difficult intubation or failed intubation is not an uncommon occurrence in head and neck surgery. When this situation is encountered after induction of general anesthesia, a very systematic, well-designed plan should be followed. Maintenance of oxygenation is paramount, and BMV should be continued between each intubation attempt. Repeated attempts at intubation carry the risk of traumatizing the larynx and should be minimized. Trying different neck positions and different laryngoscope blades should be limited to three or four attempts, because the time and ability to think clearly are limited under these circumstances, and each anesthesiology team should have an algorithm to follow routinely. The subsequent course of action depends on the team's ability to achieve satisfactory BMV.

a. ADEQUATE BAG-MASK VENTILATION

If BMV is adequate, a potent inhalational agent is used to continue general anesthesia. The Hollinger anterior commissure laryngoscope may be used to visualize the vocal cords. This laryngoscope has a flared superior flange that can lift the epiglottis to visualize anteriorly placed vocal cords. An Eschmann stylet is passed through the glottic opening, and an ETT is then passed over it after withdrawing the laryngoscope. The anesthesiology team can practice visualizing the larynx with this tubed anterior commissure laryngoscope, which is available on the otolaryngologist's laryngoscopy cart.

As an alternative, in a patient who is adequately BMV, the ETT may be passed with oral fiberoptic-guided laryngoscopy.[13] An OPA bite block is placed in the patient's mouth, and the regular mask is replaced with an endoscopy port (i.e., Patil-Syracuse endoscopy mask).[14] The lubricated FFB is passed through the mask's diaphragm into the OPA and into the trachea through the glottis.

The ETT is then threaded over the FFB into the patient's trachea. As described earlier, a scope can also be used to pass an ETT through the nose. The nose is decongested with topical Afrin, and topical 4% cocaine is used to anesthetize the nose. The appropriately sized, well-lubricated ETT is then placed along the floor of the nose, and an FFB is passed through the tube. An assistant occludes the other nostril and the mouth, and a triple connector is used so that the scope and O_2 delivery can be simultaneously introduced.

Despite multiple attempts and use of the preceding techniques, intubation attempts may continue to be unsuccessful. If BMV is still possible, anesthesia should be discontinued and the patient allowed to awaken. The anesthesiologist should then proceed with an awake intubation.

b. FAILED BAG-MASK VENTILATION

In situations of inadequate BMV of an anesthetized patient, after unsuccessful attempts at chin thrust and placement of a nasopharyngeal airway or OPA, the ASA algorithm should be followed.[8] The laryngeal mask airway (LMA) was integrated into the ASA difficult airway algorithm in different locations in 1996,[15] as a supralaryngeal airway or ventilation device or as an intubation conduit. If LMA ventilation is not adequate or feasible, the emergency pathway should be followed, and if the patient cannot be ventilated with a bag-mask or awakened safely, emergency surgical airway remains the next option (see Chapters 10 and 31). Use of LMAs is increasing in many situations of inadequate BMV,[16,17] but they should be used with extreme caution in conventional head and neck surgery, even by those with adequate experience with these devices. If ventilation with the LMA is the only option, we recommend definitive endotracheal intubation before initiation of surgery by advancing an ETT through the LMA or advancing an Aintree intubation catheter (Cook Critical Care, Bloomington, IN) over an FFB passed through the LMA into the trachea. In the latter case, the LMA is then removed, and an ETT is passed over the Aintree catheter and into the trachea. It should be kept in mind that only ETTs 7.0 mm or larger can be used with this technique.

4. Cricothyrotomy

Cricothyrotomy (i.e., coniotomy) is a procedure for establishing an emergency airway when other methods are unsuitable or impossible. Emergency cricothyrotomy is performed in approximately 1% of all emergency airway cases in the emergency department.[18] The access site is the CTM. This procedure is especially suited for gaining control of the airway when severe hemorrhage or massive facial trauma, foreign bodies, or emesis does not permit visualized intubation. Other cases arise when teeth are clenched, when intubation repeatedly fails, and when there is a possibility of cervical spine injury. In these cases, cricothyrotomy represents the safest and quickest way to obtain an airway because minimal soft tissue dissection is required between the skin and the CTM.[19] If a patient has sustained a respiratory insult associated with burns or smoke inhalation, an elective prophylactic cricothyrotomy may be performed early to prevent fatal respiratory obstruction occurring during transport.[20]

a. SURGICAL TECHNIQUE

The CTM is identified by palpating a slight indentation in the skin superior to the prominence of the cricoid cartilage. The CTM is immediately subcutaneous with no overlying large veins, muscles, or fascial layers, allowing easy access. A vertical skin incision and a horizontal entrance into the CTM are advised. For an incision into the CTM itself, a low horizontal stab is made to avoid laterally placed vessels.[21] A small tracheostomy tube or a small standard ETT can be used in a cricothyrotomy. If an ETT is placed through the cricothyrotomy, it should be minimally advanced so it does not enter a bronchus because of the short distance between the CTM and carina. Tube size is important in ensuring successful cannulation without excessive trauma. After the patient is stabilized, the cricothyrotomy should be converted to a formal tracheotomy for adequate ventilation and to minimize risk of injury to the vocal folds, which attach into the thyroid cartilage just superior to the CTM (Fig. 39-2). This technique is contraindicated in patients who are at increased risk for subglottic stenosis, preexisting laryngeal disease, malignancy, nearby inflammatory processes, epiglottitis, severe distortion of normal anatomy, or bleeding diathesis and contraindicated in infants and children.[22]

b. NEEDLE TECHNIQUE

Needle cricothyrotomy is performed in dire emergencies when the appropriate equipment or knowledge to perform a formal emergency cricothyrotomy or intubation is unavailable or in children younger than 2 years with airway obstruction and an inability to be intubated. A large-gauge needle and cannula with a syringe attached are introduced through the CTM until air can be aspirated (Fig. 39-3). The cannula is then advanced off the needle down the airway (Fig. 39-3). The cannula is connected to an oxygen supply. The patient can then be oxygenated, but ventilation to remove carbon dioxide (CO_2) is not achieved, and respiratory acidosis may ensue rapidly. A needle cricothyrotomy ensures a supply of O_2 for a short time only, and it must be converted to a surgical cricothyrotomy or tracheotomy in a timely fashion to allow adequate ventilation.[23]

The transtracheal needle ventilation technique can be used to great advantage in the emergency setting. This technique requires access to 100% O_2 at 50 psi and a Luer-Lok connector. Adequate ventilation through the catheter is not possible with a conventional ventilator or a handheld anesthesia bag.[24] The airway is controlled by puncturing the trachea or CTM with a 16-gauge, plastic-sheathed needle. The needle is withdrawn, leaving the sheath in the trachea; the sheath is then attached to the high-pressure line through a pressure regulator control, and ventilation is accomplished using a manual interrupter switch. The patient can be fully ventilated with this technique for only 45 minutes. The only way the gas or O_2 inspired through transtracheal jet ventilation (TTJV) can escape is through the patient's own airway, and attempts at securing the airway must continue. The equipment to perform adequate TTJV should be

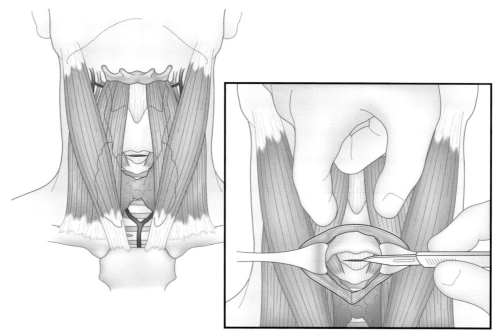

Figure 39-2 Cricothyrotomy. The cricothyroid membrane is palpated through the skin by using the thyroid notch and cricoid cartilage as reference points.

available in the operating room, and the anesthesiology team should familiarize themselves with its assembly.

5. Percutaneous Dilatational Tracheostomy

Percutaneous dilatational tracheostomy (PDT) is placement of a tracheostomy tube without direct surgical visualization of the trachea. The general consensus is that PDT should be performed only on intubated patients.[25]

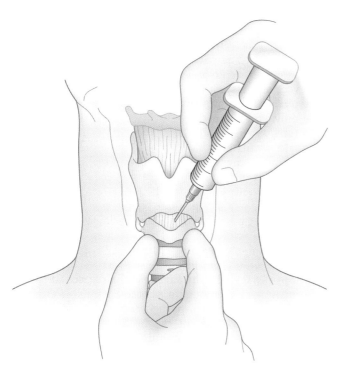

Figure 39-3 Needle cricothyrotomy. A large-gauge needle and cannula with a syringe attached are introduced through the cricothyroid membrane until air can be aspirated.

It is considered to be a minimally invasive bedside procedure that is easily performed in the intensive care unit (ICU) or ward, with continuous monitoring of the patient's vital signs.[7] The criteria for PDT are more stringent than those for open surgical tracheostomy.[26] A PDT should be performed on patients whose cervical anatomy can be clearly defined by palpation through the skin. Moreover, two preoperative criteria must be met: the ability to hyperextend the neck and ensuring that the patient can be reintubated in case of accidental extubation. Obese patients, children, and those with severe coagulopathies should not be considered candidates for this procedure (Table 39-2).[26]

Several systems and approaches for performing a percutaneous tracheostomy have been marketed since the inception of the idea, and many comprehensive accounts of the evolution of this approach are available in the literature. Controversy surrounding this procedure lingers, but there have been many large series with acceptable rates of complications as long as proper selection of

TABLE 39-2

Contraindications to Percutaneous Dilatational Tracheostomy

Absolute Contraindications	Relative Contraindications
Emergent airway access	Anatomic abnormalities
Infants	(e.g., deviated trachea,
Infection at insertion site	enlarged superficial veins)
High positive end-expiratory	Enlarged thyroid or other
pressure (PEEP) or	neck mass
oxygenation requirements	Coagulopathy
	Previous neck surgery
	Obesity

patients and adherence to a procedural protocol are ensured.[27]

Ciaglia and colleagues described a technique in which there is no sharp dissection beyond the skin incision.[28] The procedure is done with the patient under general anesthesia, and all steps are performed under bronchoscopic vision. The patient is positioned and prepared in the same fashion as for a standard surgical tracheostomy. A skin incision is made, and the pretracheal tissue is cleared with the help of blunt dissection. The ETT is withdrawn enough to place the cuff at the level of the glottis. The endoscopist places the tip of the bronchoscope such that the light from the tip shines through the surgical wound. The operator then enters the tracheal lumen below the second tracheal ring with an introducer needle. The track between the skin and the tracheal lumen is serially dilated over a guidewire and stylet. A tracheostomy tube is placed under direct bronchoscopic vision over a dilator. Placement of the tube is confirmed again by visualizing the tracheobronchial tree through the tube. The tube is then secured to the skin with sutures and tracheostomy tape.

In another technique for percutaneous tracheostomy, Schachner and colleagues made a small skin incision and passed a dilator tracheotome (Rapitrac) over a guidewire into the trachea to dilate the tract fully in one step.[29] The tracheotome has a beveled metal core with a hole through its center that accommodates a guidewire. Inside the trachea, the tracheotome is dilated, and a conventional tracheotomy cannula fitted with a special obturator is passed through the tracheal opening. The dilator and obturator are then removed.

A novel method called translaryngeal tracheostomy (i.e., Fantoni's technique) is different from other techniques. For Fantoni's tracheostomy, the initial puncture of the trachea is carried out with the needle directed cranially and the tracheal cannula inserted with a pull-through technique along the orotracheal route in a retrograde fashion. The cannula is then rotated downward using a plastic obturator. The main advantage of Fantoni's tracheostomy is that a minimal skin incision is required, and almost no bleeding is observed.[30,31] The procedure can be carried out only under endoscopic guidance, and rotating the tracheal cannula downward may pose a problem, demanding more experience.

The routine use of bronchoscopy during PDT, other than Fantoni's tracheostomy, is controversial.[32,33] There are reports of lower rates of acute complications under endoscopic guidance.[33] For critically ill patients or those with head injuries, it is important to consider the resultant hypercarbia when choosing to perform an endoscopically guided PDT. However, endoscopic guidance plays a critical role in the training of physicians, during percutaneous tracheostomy in patients with complex anatomy, and in removing aspirated blood. Another consideration that supports the use of bronchoscopy is the ability to better define the exact location of the tracheal puncture.[34] A cadaver study in autopsies of patients who had undergone PDT found that the tracheal puncture site varied greatly.[35] It seems logical that bronchoscopic guidance during PDT can confirm the initial airway puncture site, although a controlled study is necessary to settle this issue.[34]

The technique of PDT is relatively easy to learn, but it has been repeatedly reported that a learning curve exists, which may be overcome by performing a number of supervised procedures. The time required for performing a bedside PDT is considerably shorter than that required for performing an open tracheostomy.[36] In ICU patients, one of the major advantages of PDT is elimination of the scheduling difficulty associated with the operating room and anesthesiology teams. Bedside PDT also precludes the necessity to schedule the surgery and to transport critically ill patients who require intensive monitoring to and from the operating room.[37] PDT expedites the performance of the procedure in most cases. The cost of performing a PDT is roughly one half that of an open surgical tracheostomy. The major savings are operating room charges and anesthesia fees.[38]

C. Intraoperative Airway Management

1. Positioning of the Endotracheal Tube

Otolaryngology procedures require specific positioning of the ETT, because the operative field is shared by the anesthesiology and surgical teams. Procedures such as oropharyngeal tumor resection with reconstruction and cases requiring maxillomandibular fixation mandate the nasal placement of the ETT. The ala of the nose must be well protected from the risk of necrosis by pressure from the ETT. An alternative is placement of a tracheostomy tube at the beginning of the case. For operations with a tracheostomy, the tracheostomy tube can be exchanged for a reinforced tube (anode tube) rather than an ETT, which avoids kinking of the tube. If positive-pressure ventilation is necessary for the surgical procedure, an uncuffed tracheostomy tube should be replaced by a cuffed tracheostomy tube. A tracheostomy tube exchanger, such as the Weinmann Tracheostomy Exchange Set (Cook Critical Care) should be used to facilitate the exchange when the tracheostomy tube has been in place for 7 days or less.

2. Surgical Field Requirements

Head and neck surgery often requires the operative team to be on both sides of the table, and the operating table has to be positioned to accommodate this need. Bulky anesthetic equipment must be kept clear of the surgical field. The ETT and the connectors should be nonkinking, have a low profile, and be secured to the head so that head movement does not compromise the anesthetic circuit. Exact positioning of the ETT should be planned with the head and neck surgeon. The ETT should be taped to the oral commissure or around the nose to prevent downward pressure leading to the risk of accidental extubation or pressure necrosis of the nasal ala or the tip. The position of entry of the ETT into the airway has to be switched during certain head and neck procedures such as during a tracheostomy. Correct positioning of the second tube must be ensured before removing the first tube.

3. Considerations During a Tracheostomy

When a tracheostomy is being performed, there are important considerations that require clear communication between the anesthesiology and otolaryngology teams. Administration of 100% O_2 is advised before tracheal opening so that, in case of loss of airway at the time of placement of a tracheostomy tube, there is sufficient reserve in the lungs to prevent hypoxemia. Most procedures on the neck and around the upper airway involve routine use of Bovie cautery. As the dissection approaches the trachea, it is advisable to avoid the use of Bovie cautery directly over the airway to avoid an airway fire. If Bovie cautery is necessary, it is mandatory to reduce the fraction of inspired O_2 to the lowest possible level compatible with optimal O_2 saturation.

As the tracheal incision is about to be made, the surgical team should communicate with the anesthesiology team to deflate the ETT cuff to prevent cutting the cuff. After the trachea is entered and the surgeon is able to visualize the ETT, the anesthesiologist should loosen the tape and should be able to withdraw the ETT so that the distal tip is just above the opening into the trachea. An adapter and a short, flexible tube (e.g., Jolly tube) are placed onto the cuffed tracheostomy tube to avoid pull on the trachea. A successful operating room tracheotomy requires excellent planning on the part of the anesthesiology and surgical teams to avoid mishaps.

Correct placement of the tracheostomy tube is confirmed by the appearance of an $EtCO_2$ waveform and by the presence of bilateral breath sounds on auscultation. To prevent contamination of the tracheobronchial tree with blood and secretions above the tracheostomy site, this area should be meticulously suctioned at the time of changing to a more permanent tracheostomy tube. When the tracheostomy is performed as part of a head and neck resection and reconstructive procedure and when a reinforced tube is placed, it is mandatory to secure it to the chest wall with sutures. This prevents accidental slipping of the tube into a main stem bronchus, which can result in oxygenation problems or bronchospasm if the anesthesia is light at that point. At the completion of the case, the anode tube is replaced with a tracheostomy tube.

III. EXTUBATION IN HEAD AND NECK SURGERY

Accidental extubation is a risk in head and neck surgery because the surgical team is frequently operating around the oral and nasal cavities. The anesthesiologist should be attentive to this possibility and remain in constant communication with the surgical team to avoid inadvertent extubation. The preparations and plans to reintubate should be in place before extubation in case the situation arises. In head and neck procedures in which the patient does not have a tracheostomy, there is risk of supraglottic and glottic edema because of the presence of an ETT and intraoperative manipulation. Intraoperative measures, such as administration of short-acting intravenous steroids (e.g., dexamethasone [Decadron]), minimizing the movement of the ETT, and keeping the head of the patient slightly elevated, can help reduce this risk. Excessive intravenous fluid administration should be avoided. Patients undergoing lengthy ablative and reconstructive procedures may benefit from remaining intubated and lightly sedated overnight in the ICU.

Extubation can then be planned for the next day in the presence of experienced anesthesiology and surgical personnel with equipment available for securing the airway. Planning for extubation should include instruments to enable a bedside cricothyrotomy or a tracheostomy, if necessary.

A. Planned Extubation of the Endotracheal Tube

In most situations, extubation proceeds smoothly after patients meet extubation criteria, including spontaneous ventilation and the ability to follow commands. In others, it may be more challenging than the intubation. It may not be possible to use BMV because of postsurgical edema and changes related to the reconstruction. The use of OPA and nasopharyngeal airway devices may not be feasible because of concern about disrupting delicate surgical repair in the oropharynx or nasopharynx.

To ensure a safe extubation, the anesthesiology team should consider the following questions. First, is there an air leak around the tube after deflating the cuff? Second, if the patient develops acute airway obstruction on extubation, are the equipment and personnel available to secure an airway to prevent hypoxia? This may include options for an emergency cricothyrotomy, TTJV, or a tracheostomy. If the answer is an affirmative, extubation should proceed. If the preceding criteria cannot be met, extubation should be delayed for another 24 hours, or the anesthesiologist should consider extubating over an airway exchange catheter (AEC) or a jet stylet.[39] A hollow AEC with a small internal diameter is inserted through the ETT into the patient's trachea. The ETT is then withdrawn over the catheter; the AEC can be used as a means of jet ventilation or a reintubation guide, or both.[11] This approach is especially useful when an ETT needs to be exchanged or replaced.

B. Managing Accidental Decannulation of a Fresh Tracheostomy

Accidental decannulation of a fresh tracheostomy may be life-threatening because of the rapid closure of the tracheostomy tract in the immediate postoperative period. Options to reestablish an airway are challenging in obese patients, patients with a short thick neck, small retrognathic jaw, intermaxillary fixation, or a deep and posterior airway. Initially, an attempt should be made to immediately place a tracheostomy tube or an ETT through the tracheostomy opening. If this is unsuccessful, BMV should be applied immediately and a call for help initiated. The patient should be placed supine with the neck extended and a shoulder roll in place. A tracheal dilator or cricoid hook, or both, and ample light can enable replacement of a one-size-smaller tracheostomy tube or an ETT. No more than one or two attempts should be made, especially if the BMV is optimal. An experienced anesthesiologist should place an orotracheal tube with direct laryngoscopy. In experienced hands, a Hollinger anterior commissure laryngoscope and Eschmann stylet can be a lifesaving combination in this situation. When the airway is secured from above, the patient can be taken back to the operating room for replacement of the tracheostomy tube.

IV. TONSILLECTOMY AND OTHER OROPHARYNGEAL PROCEDURES

A. Preoperative Considerations

Tonsillectomy is one of the most frequent procedures performed by the otolaryngologist, with about 737,000 performed in 2006.[40] Most of these operations are performed on healthy adults and children. Current indications include history of recurrent tonsillitis, tonsillar hypertrophy, OSA, asymmetrical tonsils, recurrent peritonsillar abscess, and tonsillar malignancy.[41] Performance of these procedures in patients with coagulation disorders is uncommon but can be challenging if the diagnostic workup fails to alert the surgical and anesthesiology teams about the presence, nature, and extent of the problem.

B. Obstructive Sleep Apnea

OSA can lead to serious and potentially life-threatening conditions if left untreated. They include hypertension, pulmonary hypertension, coronary artery disease, cor pulmonale, and congestive heart failure.[42] Nonsurgical options are available for patients with mild to moderate sleep apnea, but many patients with severe sleep apnea, tonsillar hypertrophy, and soft palate redundancy can benefit from tonsillectomy, uvulectomy, and uvulopalatopharyngectomy. Adults with this disorder must have a preoperative assessment of the severity of the problem with an overnight polysomnogram. The severity of OSA, the extent of desaturation, and the number and duration of apneic episodes have significant implications, especially for postoperative monitoring of these patients. Induction of general anesthesia relaxes the pharyngeal muscles in a manner similar to the effect of rapid-eye-movement (REM) sleep.[39] This makes BMV difficult to maintain, and the OPAs and nasopharyngeal airways do not always significantly improve the airway. Excessive pharyngeal tissue exacerbates the obstruction caused by the redundant soft palate and base of the tongue, hindering a good view of the cords during laryngoscopy. Patients with OSA are more sensitive to sedative and narcotic analgesics. This necessitates extreme caution and a need for slow titration in using these agents. Awake fiberoptic intubation may be considered before induction of general anesthesia.

C. Peritonsillar and Parapharyngeal Abscess

Anesthetic management of patients with peritonsillar abscess is a challenging task in head and neck surgery. These patients have severe odynophagia, upper airway edema, and distortion of the normal anatomy. The limited mouth opening resulting from local pain and inflammation increases the degree of difficulty when securing the airway. The anesthesiologist should expect a difficult airway on induction of general anesthesia and make alternative plans to be able to achieve a secure airway. Spontaneous or traumatic rupture of the abscess is a real risk, and the consequential aspiration of pus into an unprotected airway remains a possibility. The head and neck surgeon may attempt needle aspiration for decompression of the abscess under local anesthetic.[43] Awake intubation or direct laryngoscopy is a safe option only if the abscess is relatively small and does not distort the route of intubation. A possible alternative is nasal, awake fiberoptic intubation using topical anesthesia. Topical anesthesia can be accomplished using the "spray-as-you-go" technique or translaryngeal injection of 3 to 4 mL of 4% lidocaine.[13] For a sizable abscess or airway distortion, a tracheostomy done under local anesthesia with minimal or no sedation is the safest approach.

D. Airway Management During Routine Tonsillectomy and Oral Procedures

The surgeon places a mouth gag (e.g., Crowe-Davis) into the mouth to increase exposure of the oropharynx. The ETT is held in a groove under the blade of this gag. There is a small but real danger of extubation during placement, adjustment, and removal of this blade. The ETT should always be secured with a tape to the lower lip. To monitor for kinking or obstruction of the ETT, the anesthesiologist must pay close attention to $EtCO_2$, bilateral chest auscultation, and peak airway pressures. The oral cavity and oropharynx should be gently but meticulously suctioned at the end of the procedure to prevent aspiration of blood, causing laryngospasm. The patient's head should be turned to the side at the end of the procedure to minimize blood in the endolarynx and resultant laryngospasm.[29]

E. Postoperative Airway Problems After Tonsillectomy

Monitoring patients for OSA after tonsillectomy has been a controversial issue. Children with severe and mixed (obstructive and central) sleep apnea should be monitored overnight in a postanesthesia care unit (PACU).[44] Relief of airway obstruction increases the risk of postoperative pulmonary edema and does not address central apneic episodes, which may be unmasked and result in O_2 desaturation and loss of respiratory drive.[44] The postoperative care of adults with OSA after tonsillectomy and similar procedures should be individualized. Care should be based on the severity of sleep apnea preoperatively and performance in the PACU in the immediate postoperative period.

F. Management of Bleeding After Tonsillectomy

Post-tonsillectomy bleeding may take place in the immediate postoperative period (i.e., reactionary bleeding) or 7 to 10 days after the surgery (i.e., secondary bleeding, often from infection). Preventive measures, such as meticulous hemostasis for reactionary bleeding and hydration and administration of oral antibiotics for secondary bleeding, are routinely recommended by surgeons.

Obstruction of the airway by a combination of bleeding and postoperative airway edema is the most frequent cause of post-tonsillectomy morbidity.[45] Post-tonsillectomy bleeding occurs usually at a slow rate, allowing a large volume of blood to be swallowed by the patient without awareness. Postoperative nausea and vomiting and loss of blood may result in severe hypovolemia before a fall in the hemoglobin level is detected. Reduced hemoglobin level and aspiration of blood may result in hypoxemia in the patient, especially in a young child. Careful serial monitoring of hemoglobin levels and judicious use of packed red cell transfusions are important considerations, particularly in children.

If surgical treatment is required for post-tonsillectomy hemorrhage, the patient should be assumed to have a full stomach with blood in the airway.[39] Awake intubation under direct laryngoscopy in adults or rapid-sequence induction of anesthesia with etomidate or ketamine is the preferred choice in this situation. A work-up for coagulation disorders should take place in case of recurrent hemorrhage. An angiogram or a CT scan to rule out a pseudoaneurysm of the carotid may be needed in rare cases of recurrent and severe post-tonsillectomy hemorrhage.

V. SURGERY ON THE ANTERIOR SKULL BASE

The scope of head and neck surgery has expanded to include craniofacial, maxillofacial, and anterior skull base surgery. Indications may include trauma, syndromic skeletal abnormalities, sleep apnea, orthognathic deformities, and tumor removal. The anesthetic team must discuss and understand the approach, nature, and extent of the proposed surgical procedure to be able to anticipate airway problems.[46] Most patients undergoing these procedures are previously healthy adults or children, but a few have anatomic abnormalities that predispose them to challenging airway problems, including limited mouth opening, retrognathia, protruded maxilla, and presence of orthodontic appliances.[47]

A. Airway Management

Anesthesiologists should be prepared for fiberoptic intubation if a difficult airway is anticipated during the preoperative work-up. The nasal route is preferred because access for most of these procedures involves intraoral incisions. The possibility of maxillomandibular fixation at the end of the case is another reason for considering nasotracheal intubation. Nasotracheal intubation is achieved using the technique previously described. The regular adapter of the ETT is replaced with a curved adapter with a flexible extension, which is connected to the ventilator. The extension is then padded and taped over the patient's forehead so as to come off the top of the head and not interfere with the surgical approach.

B. Extubation in Skull Base Surgery

In maxillomandibular fixation, an attempt at extubation should be considered only if the patient is fully awake, is following commands, and has intact airway reflexes. Appropriate wire-cutting instruments should always be at hand for patients with such an impediment to access to the airway. After endoscopic resection of skull base tumors or repair of cerebrospinal fluid leaks, deep extubation is recommended to keep intracranial pressures low and ensure the integrity of the repair.

VII. CONCLUSIONS

The risk of a difficult airway is relatively high in the otolaryngology patient population undergoing operative management of glottic and subglottic stenosis and among head and neck cancer patients. The anesthesiology and otolaryngology teams should consider many options to secure the airway and should communicate the airway plan of action before intubation. Applying these principles can optimize airway management in head and neck surgical patients.

VIII. CLINICAL PEARLS

- The risk of a difficult airway is relatively high for patients undergoing head and neck surgery.

- Communication during the intubation procedure reduces the morbidity and mortality associated with difficult airway management.

- The optimal approach to securing the airway of patients undergoing head and neck surgery depends on the operation being performed, location of the lesion or infectious mass, tolerance of the patient, and comfort level of the anesthesiology and otolaryngology team.

- Establishing a sequential airway plan with backup options optimizes patient safety.

- The Hollinger anterior commissure laryngoscope is one of the most useful tools for difficult airway management, and it should be considered when other techniques for orotracheal intubation have failed.

- Nasotracheal fiberoptic intubation is useful in cases of a small mouth opening, severe trismus, large tongue, receding lower jaw, large oral cavity tumor, planned maxillomandibular fixation, or tracheal dilatation.

- If a patient is in acute respiratory distress because of upper airway obstruction and is unable to be safely intubated under general anesthesia, the best choice is to perform a planned but urgent awake tracheostomy.

- Cricothyrotomy is a procedure for establishing an emergency airway when other methods are unsuitable or impossible.

SELECTED REFERENCES

All references can be found online at expertconsult.com.

1. Arriaga AF, Elbardissi AW, Regenbogen SE, et al: A policy-based intervention for the reduction of communication breakdowns in inpatient surgical care: Results From a Harvard Surgical Safety Collaborative. *Ann Surg* 253:849–854, 2011.
4. Keenan RL, Boyan CP: Cardiac arrest due to anesthesia. A study of incidence and causes. *JAMA* 253:2373–2377, 1985.

7. Bhatti NI: Surgical management of the difficult adult airway. In Flint PW, editor: *Cummings otolaryngology–head and neck surgery*, ed 5, Philadelphia, 2010, Elsevier, pp 121–129.

8. Practice guidelines for management of the difficult airway: An updated report by the American Society of Anesthesiologists Task Force on Management of the Difficult Airway. *Anesthesiology* 98:1269–1277, 2003.

11. Benumof JL: Management of the difficult adult airway. With special emphasis on awake tracheal intubation. *Anesthesiology* 75:1087–1110, 1991.

15. Benumof JL: Laryngeal mask airway and the ASA difficult airway algorithm. *Anesthesiology* 84:686–699, 1996.

20. Milner SM, Bennett JD: Emergency cricothyrotomy. *J Laryngol Otol* 105:883–885, 1991.

37. Freeman BD, Isabella K, Cobb JP, et al: A prospective, randomized study comparing percutaneous with surgical tracheostomy in critically ill patients. *Crit Care Med* 29:926–930, 2001.

39. Kirk GA: Anesthesia for ear, nose, and throat surgery. In Rogers MC, Tinker JH, Covino BG, Longnecker DE, editors: *Principles and practice of anesthesia*, vol 2, St. Louis, 1993, Mosby, pp 2257–2274.

43. Donlon JV, Jr: Anesthesia for eye, ear, nose, and throat surgery. In Miller RD, editor: *Anesthesia*, vol 2, New York, 1990, Churchill Livingstone, pp 2001–2023.

Chapter 40

Anesthesia for Laser Airway Surgery

ANIL PATEL

I. INTRODUCTION

The use of laser technology in medicine and surgery has expanded greatly since its development in the 1960s, and lasers are found in some form throughout most hospitals in the world. Laser technology has been incorporated into most aspects of modern life, from computers to supermarket bar code readers, and lasers have been used increasingly in a wide variety of clinical applications, from diagnostic medicine to laser airway surgery.

In medical practice, the type of laser used depends on the procedure to be undertaken, the type of surgery, the location, and the requirements of the physician. They are used in superficial or cutaneous procedures, such as those

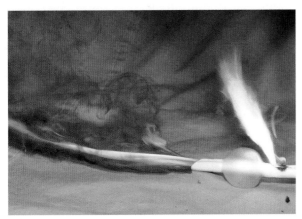

Figure 40-1 Catastrophic laser-induced blowtorch fire of a polyvinyl chloride endotracheal tube (ETT). The ETT had 100% O_2 flowing through it and had a sustained CO_2 laser strike proximal to the cuff on the outer surface, from which a second flame is emerging.

involving dermatologic, dental, opthalmic, and plastic surgery, and those involving introduction of lasers into the body, such as interventional or diagnostic cardiovascular procedures and thoracic, neurologic, urologic, gynecologic, and general surgery.

Airway surgery is unique in that it involves the anesthesiologist and surgeon working in the same anatomic field. Even without the use of a laser in a shared airway, procedures are challenging when the airway is compromised. The addition of a laser beam (i.e., ignition source) into a shared airway can cause a catastrophic fire, and to avoid these disasters, all operating room staff must recognize that a team approach is essential (Fig. 40-1).[1-39] If a high-risk situation exists, all team members must proactively agree on how a fire will be prevented and managed.[1] The importance of a team approach cannot be overstated.

For safe laser airway surgery, the surgeon and anesthesiologist should be familiar with the principles of a laser, types of laser available, hazards of laser use, and management approach for an airway fire. They should understand the advantages and disadvantages of the various anesthesia techniques available.

II. PRINCIPLES OF LASER TECHNOLOGY

A. History

Laser is an acronym for light amplification by the stimulated emission of radiation. Photons are released in a very narrow, intense, high-energy beam as a result of a stimulated emission.

The history and development of lasers parallels our understanding of electromagnetic radiation, ions, molecules, and atoms. In 1900, Max Planck revised his earlier work on radiation and the absorption of light and heat by a black body (i.e., a perfect absorber).[40] He proposed that electromagnetic energy could be emitted only in quantized form. In this process, called the *photoelectric effect*, electrons are emitted from matter as a consequence of their absorption of energy from short-wavelength electromagnetic radiation, such as visible or ultraviolet light.

In 1905, Albert Einstein described how the photoelectric effect was caused by absorption of quanta of light (i.e., photons) and explained that the energy of these quanta was directly related to the frequency of the radiation absorbed. From these observations, Einstein developed his ideas on quantum mechanics, and in 1917, he developed the quantum theory of radiation,[41,42] in which he discussed the interactions of atoms, ions, molecules, photons, and electromagnetic radiation. According to the quantum theory of radiation, electrons, atoms, molecules, and photons interact with electromagnetic radiation of quantum units by absorption, spontaneous emission, and stimulated emission.[43]

In 1954, Charles Townes described the first amplification and generation of electromagnetic waves by stimulated emission by using microwaves, which he called microwave amplification by the stimulated emission of radiation (MASER). In 1960, Theodore Maiman produced light amplification by the stimulated emission of radiation (LASER) using a ruby crystal and red light. Throughout the 1960s and 1970s, many substrates and ions were tried as the laser medium. Some, such as the carbon dioxide (CO_2) laser, were successfully developed, found to be useful in medical practice, and are still used.[44]

B. Physics

An atom consists of a nucleus around which electrons orbit in discreet shells. These shells, or orbits, have specific energy levels associated with them. Electrons in the stable ground state occupy the lowest orbit, which is closest to the nucleus and has the lowest energy level. Electrons can move from one orbit to a higher-level orbit by absorbing energy, or they can move from a higher-level orbit to a lower level by emitting energy. The energy absorbed or emitted is exactly equal to the difference between the orbital energy levels, and it can take the form of a photon, which is the elementary particle of light and a quantum of electromagnetic energy.

In *absorption*, an electron is boosted to a higher energy level by absorption of the energy of a colliding photon. The natural state for matter is to be at the lowest energy level. An electron in a higher orbit will spontaneously drop back to the lowest-energy orbit possible and emit energy as a photon, which is exactly equal to the photon required to take the electron to the higher orbit. This process, known as *spontaneous emission*, occurs in a random manner that results in incoherent light.

In 1917, Einstein postulated that if a photon released from an excited atom collided with another atom already in the excited state, the second atom would release two photons with the same wavelength, phase, and direction (i.e., identical photons). If these two photons stimulated more excited atoms, more identical photons would be released. Einstein called this process *stimulated emission of radiation*, and it is the basic principle of laser physics (Fig. 40-2).[45]

The energy of a photon is proportional to the frequency of light and is described by the following equation:

$$e = h\lambda$$

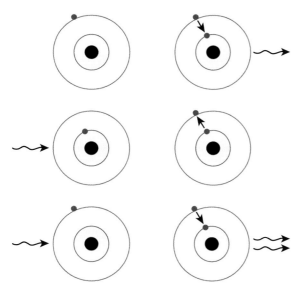

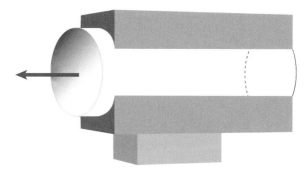

Figure 40-3 Laser apparatus. A power source (yellow box) stimulates the lasing medium (inside the cylinder within the gray box). The spontaneous emission of photons from electrons in the excited state stimulates the emission of more photons. The parallel mirrors (circles at the ends of the gray box) reflect the photons traveling along the axis of the laser, amplifying the intensity of the radiation. This results in a coherent monochromatic laser beam emerging from the partially reflective mirror (*red arrow*).

Figure 40-2 The processes of absorption, spontaneous emission, and stimulated emission are necessary for a laser to operate. *Top*: In an excited state (i.e., electron in a higher-energy orbit), the electron is unstable and reemits this energy (i.e., spontaneous emission). *Middle*: A photon or light packet with energy (*hv*) or another power source can provide the energy necessary to raise the energy level of electrons from the ground state to an excited state (i.e., absorption). *Bottom*: A photon of the appropriate energy impinging on an electron in the excited state causes the release of a second photon of the same energy (i.e., stimulated emission). The latter photon travels in the same direction and is in phase with the first photon.

where
e = quantum energy
h = Planck's constant
λ = wavelength

All lasers consist of a *laser medium* (e.g., CO_2, argon) contained in an *optical cavity* between *two mirrors,* one totally reflecting and one partially reflecting mirror. An *external energy source* continuously excites or pumps the laser medium, causing many of the atoms to reach a higher energy level (Fig. 40-3). When more than one half of the atoms are in an excited state, a population inversion has taken place. In this state, spontaneous emission occurs in every direction, but photons emitted in the direction of the optical cavity strike the mirror and are reflected back, striking excited atoms, and resulting in stimulated emission. This process repeats itself at an increasing rate with each passage of the photons reflected off the mirrors through the laser medium, generating a huge number of identical photons that all have the same wavelength, phase, and direction. The partially reflecting mirror lets a small amount of this energy escape through the aperture, creating the laser beam.

Laser light may be in the invisible infrared, visible, or ultraviolet part of the electromagnetic radiation spectrum. It is monochromatic, with all the photons having the same wavelength, and collimated, allowing the beam to be intense and unidirectional, with no divergence, preventing spread as the light moves farther away. The laser light is coherent spatially and temporally, with all the photons in phase, and it has high energy density.

C. Laser Parameters

The operator can select three parameters to alter the effectiveness of the laser on tissue by adjusting the exposure time, spot size, and power.

1. Exposure Time

Exposure time is the time that the tissues are exposed to the laser light. The exposure time is influenced by the pulse structure of the laser, which is influenced by the type and configuration of laser and which may be fixed. The pulse structure can be in a continuous mode, with the laser emitting continuous laser light when switched on. The pulse structure can also be in a pulsed mode in which a single, brief (0.5 microseconds to 100 milliseconds) pulse of laser light is emitted. Early versions of these pulsed-mode lasers showed that the pulse was a series of irregular spikes. Q-switching produces a very short laser pulse, reducing the interval of the pulse and increasing high peak power. By using the pulsed mode with high intensity and short pulse duration, the laser beam can ablate tissues quickly and before thermal energy spreads damaging adjacent tissues.

2. Spot Size

After the laser light has emerged from the optical cavity of a laser system, it may pass through a lens that focuses the beam to a very small diameter, or spot size, ranging from 0.1 to 2.0 mm. The optical properties of each focusing lens determine the focal length, or distance from the lens to the intended target tissue.[46]

3. Power

When using lasers in clinical practice, power often is measured in watts (W), although a more useful term is the *power density*. For a given power, the effects vary according to the spot size and the time of exposure. The relationship between power and depth of tissue injury becomes logarithmic when the power and exposure time are kept constant and the spot size is varied.[47] Power density describes the amount of power (W) arriving at a surface area (W/cm^2).

$$\text{Power density } (W \cdot cm^{-2}) = \text{Power output of laser } (W) / \\ \text{Area of focal spot } (cm^{-2})$$

D. Laser-Tissue Interaction

When a laser interacts with tissues, the energy can be reflected, absorbed, conducted as heat, or scattered. The extent to which these processes occur depends on the type of laser used and the tissue with which it interacts. Laser wavelengths depend on the medium, and the degree of absorption depends on the target tissue components. The CO_2 laser (10,600-nm wavelength) is particularly well absorbed by water, whereas the neodymium:yttrium-aluminum-garnet (Nd:YAG) laser (1064-nm wavelength) is absorbed less by water and creates more energy scatter. The argon laser (488- and 514-nm wavelengths) and potassium titanyl phosphate (KTP) laser (532-nm wavelength) are in the visible spectrum, and their energies are absorbed well by pigments such as melanin and hemoglobin. For the most commonly used lasers in medicine, absorption of laser energy excites the atoms within tissues, which produces heat (Fig. 40-4).

The CO_2 laser heats the water within cells, and as the temperature rises to about 65° C, proteins denature and thermal necrosis occurs. As the heating continues and the temperature reaches 100° C, the water within the cell boils and produces water vapor; this leads to an explosive vaporization, and the cell explodes. The tissue surface in contact with the CO_2 laser disintegrates and undergoes charring, with carbon debris deposited at about 350° C. There is little damage to the underlying structures. Surrounding the charred area is a zone of thermal necrosis, and around this is an area of thermal conductivity and repair.[48]

E. Laser Classification

The American National Standards Institute (ANSI Z136 report on safe use of lasers) and the International Standard International Electrotechnical Commission (IEC 60825 report on the safety of laser products) define four classes of laser according to their power and wavelength:

Class 1. These lasers are considered safe, with no risk when viewed by the naked eye. Class 1M denotes that the beam is potentially hazardous if it is viewed with an optical instrument, such as a microscope.

Class 2. These lasers emit low-power visible radiation in the range of 400 to 700 nm. An aversion reaction or blink reflex limits exposure to less than 0.25 seconds and provides protection from equipment such as a laser pointer. Class 2M devices are the same as class 2, but they may be hazardous if viewed with an optical instrument.

Class 3. A class 3R laser is considered safe with restricted beam viewing, and if the maximum permissible exposure is exceeded, the risk of injury is low. Class 3B lasers are hazardous if the eye is exposed directly, and protective eyewear is required if direct viewing of a laser beam may occur. A key switch and safety interlock must be present on all class 3B lasers.

Class 4. Most medical lasers belong in this class and pose dangers to the eye, skin, and combustible material. They are a fire risk and produce air contaminants and plumes. All class 3B and class 4 lasers must be operated by trained, authorized personnel and be equipped with a key switch and a safety interlock.

F. Types of Laser

Lasers are named according to their medium, which can be a gas, solid, liquid, or semiconductor. Many types of lasers exist, and their clinical application depends on their wavelength, tissue absorptive characteristics, cost, ease of use, and safety. Lasers have differences in their emitted wavelength, output power, mode of operation (i.e., pulsed or continuous mode), and application (i.e., contact or noncontact). For laser airway surgery, the CO_2, argon, Nd:YAG, KTP, and diode lasers are the most commonly used (Table 40-1).

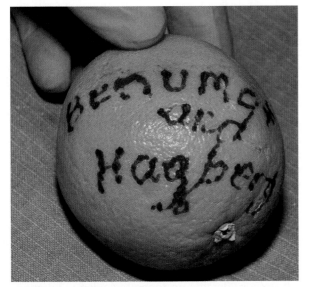

Figure 40-4   The surface of an orange after a CO_2 laser strike shows charring and carbon debris deposited at around 350° C. The words *Benumof and Hagberg* can be seen.

TABLE 40-1

Characteristics of Commonly Used Medical Lasers

Type of Laser	Laser Wavelength (nm)	Color	Fiberoptic Transmission
Gas			
Helium-neon	633	Red	Yes
Argon	500	Blue-green	Yes
Carbon dioxide	10,600	Invisible	No
Solid			
Ruby	695	Red	Yes
Nd:YAG	1,060	Invisible	Yes
KTP	532	Green	Yes

KTP, Potassium titanyl phosphate; *Nd:YAG*, neodymium:yttrium-aluminum-garnet.
Adapted from Sosis MB: *Probl Anesth* 7:160, 1993.

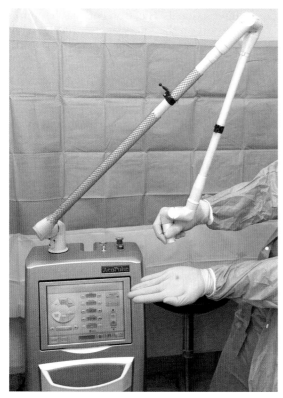

Figure 40-5 The CO_2 laser (AcuPulse, Lumenis, Yokneam, Israel) has an articulating arm for attachment to a surgical microscope or handheld device. The coaxial helium-neon, low-intensity laser can be seen as a continuous, visible red light.

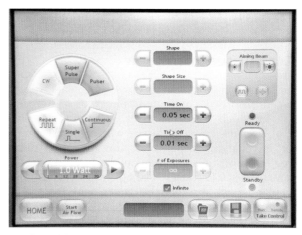

Figure 40-6 CO_2 laser parameters include continuous, pulsed, and superpulsed modes.

1. Carbon Dioxide Laser

The CO_2 laser has been used for many otolaryngology and head and neck surgical procedures and in gynecologic surgery for the treatment of intraepithelial neoplasms, condylomata acuminata, and other lesions. It is the most commonly used laser for airway surgery and is particularly suited to laryngeal and head and neck surgical procedures (Fig. 40-5).

This laser uses CO_2 mixed with nitrogen and helium as its medium. The nitrogen is used to aid in energy transfer to the upper excitation level of the CO_2 molecule. The CO_2 laser emits invisible infrared light at a wavelength of 10,600 nm in the infrared range of the electromagnetic spectrum, and the light cannot be seen by the human eye. To allow the CO_2 laser to be seen, a second, coaxial helium-neon (He-Ne) laser is incorporated into the CO_2 laser and acts as a pointer. The low-intensity (0.8-mW) He-Ne laser has a wavelength of 6328 nm, which is within the visible part of the electromagnetic spectrum, and the light is red. As soon as the CO_2 laser is switched on, this visible red light is seen continuously and independently of the status of the CO_2 laser. The He-Ne laser must be aligned with the CO_2 laser in the coaxial arrangement, and the alignment must be checked before use. If the coaxial arrangement is not aligned, the CO_2 laser and the He-Ne beam will strike different areas, resulting in destruction of healthy tissue or increasing the risk of an airway fire.

The CO_2 laser is preferred for laryngeal lesions. It is used for the treatment of benign laryngeal pathology, such as nodules, polyps, papillomas, granulomas, Reinke's edema, webs, hemangiomas, subglottic stenosis, and arytenoidectomy, and for phonosurgical procedures. CO_2 lasers allow precise cutting and shallow penetration of tissues. These qualities are imperative for removal of lesions situated in the supraglottic or immediate subglottic regions. It can be used for leukoplakia on the vocal cord and within the oral cavity. Transoral laser procedures use a CO_2 laser to excise and debulk tumors within the oral cavity and from the vocal cord itself. Many early vocal cord tumors are treated with excision by a CO_2 laser.

The CO_2 laser can be used in a continuous, pulsed, or superpulsed mode. The superpulsed mode reduces the exposure time to a few nanoseconds while delivering high energies of 400 to 500 W with each peak (Fig. 40-6). The rest time between each peak allows the tissues to cool and reduces thermal injury to adjacent tissues.

The CO_2 laser can be attached to an operating microscope or a handheld device so it can be used for intraoral procedures such as palatal surgery. CO_2 laser energy is highly absorbed by water, and because water is the primary component of most biologic tissue, CO_2 laser energy is highly absorbed by most tissues. It is readily absorbed by the first 200 µm of biologic materials, independent of tissue pigmentation.

The CO_2 laser has advantages that make it an effective surgical tool. Its use with an operating microscope allows the surgeon to precisely destroy targets approximately 2 mm in diameter under binocular vision. This degree of precision may be impossible to achieve with conventional cautery. During CO_2 laser surgery, the surgical field is usually bloodless because of the laser's considerable hemostatic action. Vessels up to 0.5 mm in diameter usually can be sectioned without bleeding.[49] The CO_2 laser has been used successfully to excise vascular lesions, even in patients with a bleeding diathesis.[50] The use of more traditional surgical tools, such as cautery, usually results in considerable postoperative edema. Edema does not usually occur after using the CO_2 laser because of the sharp line of tissue destruction, with virtually no injury to surrounding tissue. Ninety percent of the laser's energy is absorbed within 0.03 mm.[51] There is no manipulation of tissues because laser treatment is usually a noncontact technique. Microscopic examination of tissue after CO_2 laser surgery reveals a discrete line of destruction, with preservation of capillaries and normal features of adjacent tissues. The preservation of adjacent tissues is thought to account for the rapid healing, minimal scarring, and reduced pain often observed after CO_2 laser surgery.[49]

The CO_2 laser is a safe and extremely useful surgical modality in the airways and the digestive tract.[52] It is best suited for widening benign tracheal stenoses and for removal of granulation tissues.[53]

2. Flexible-Fiber Carbon Dioxide Laser

A drawback of CO_2 lasers is that they are fixed to a line-of-site delivery mechanism and cannot be transmitted through ordinary fiberoptic bundles, which limits their use to areas accessible by a straight approach. Flexible-fiber CO_2 lasers (Omniguide, Cambridge, MA; Fiberlase CO_2 Fiber, Lumenis, CA) have been developed for use in airway procedures, including base of tongue tumors, laryngeal tumors, tracheal tumors, laryngeal papillomas, tracheal stenosis, and laryngeal lesions.[54-59]

Flexible-fiber CO_2 lasers have a photonic band gap mirror lining, which guides light through a hollow core. The mirror lining reflects the CO_2 laser energy along the hollow core to the distal tip. The hollow core also delivers a cooling flow of inert gas, usually helium, that helps to prevent the fiber from overheating, clears the surgical field of blood, minimizes tissue heating, and ensures the hollow core is clear. The flexible laser fiber can be passed through a rigid bronchoscope or flexible bronchoscope or can be used with a handpiece.

The anesthesiologist should be aware of the risk of a gas emboli, and this possibility should be monitored. Pressurized gas exiting the fiber tip during the laser procedure may cause gas emboli, and the fiber tip should not be brought into direct contact with blood vessels or vascular tissues. Pressurized gas exiting the fiber tip during the laser procedure may cause separation of submucosal flaps or mild emphysema under superficial layers of tissue, and the CO_2 fibers should not be used for lesions below the carina. The flexible CO_2 laser allows access to areas inaccessible by traditional line-of-sight CO_2 lasers, including the nasal cavity, oral cavity, tongue base, larynx, subglottis, and trachea up to the carina.

3. Potassium Titanyl Phosphate Laser

The KTP laser is strongly absorbed by hemoglobin and melanin, and it is used for otolaryngologic lesions, vascular diseases, and hemorrhages.[60] The KTP laser has been used to treat several skin conditions, including port wine stains, hemangioma, telangiectasia, spider nevi, and red scars of the skin (Fig. 40-7).

The KTP laser is generated by passing the light of a rapidly pulsed Nd:YAG laser through a potassium titanyl phosphate crystal, which doubles the frequency and halves the wavelength to 532 nm, producing a beam in the bright green visible spectrum that has a tissue penetration of 0.5 to 2 mm.[60] The radiation is able to pass

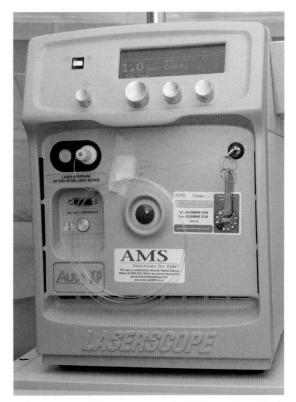

Figure 40-7   Potassium titanyl phosphate (KTP) laser (AuraXP, American Medical Systems, Minnetonka, MN). The flexible fiber is coiled in front of the laser.

through a flexible fiberoptic bundle and is used in a pulsed mode. It is used in vascular lesions within the airway, and because it can be transmitted through clear substances and can pass through a flexible fiberoptic fiber, it can be used in areas where a direct line-of-site laser cannot. The KTP laser has been used for laryngotracheal stenosis, laryngeal paralysis, and choanal atresia. The convenience of fiber delivery, concomitant telescopic control, and low-grade edematous reaction were the main advantages over the CO_2 laser. Healing time was longer for the KTP laser than for the CO_2 laser.

4. Argon Laser

The argon laser contains argon gas and produces a visible blue-green beam with wavelengths of 488 nm and 514 nm, which are absorbed selectively by hemoglobin, melanin, and other pigments that lie under the retina. The beam is readily transmitted down a fiberoptic bundle, allowing endobronchial surgery (Fig. 40-8).

Applications of the argon laser include ophthalmologic surgery, especially for retinal and anterior chamber procedures. Because the laser passes readily through fluid inside the eye without damage, it is used in the treatment of retinal vascular lesions, including diabetic retinopathy, retinal detachment, glaucoma, and macular degeneration. Its applications in dermatologic and plastic surgery include the removal of port wine stains, hemangiomas, and tattoos because of the laser's absorption by hemoglobin and other pigments. Because the tissue penetration is 0.5 to 2 mm, it is useful for superficial coagulation of capillary vessels. Port wine stains are lightened without

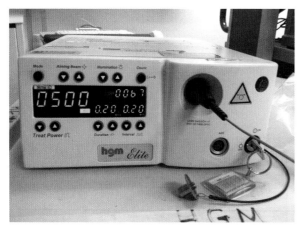

Figure 40-8 HGM Elite argon laser (HGM Medical Laser Systems, Salt Lake City, UT) has a flexible fiberoptic bundle protected by a red lead.

scarring after treatment with the argon laser.[50] To vaporize tissues, the power density is increased to produce a small focal spot; this allows argon laser stapedotomy. The argon laser has been used in infants to remove obstructive endobronchial lesions due to traumatic suction catheter injuries by passing argon laser fibers through the suction port of the fiberoptic bronchoscope (FOB) and targeting the obstructive endobronchial lesion with the argon laser beam.

5. Neodymium: Yttrium-Aluminum-Garnet Laser

The Nd:YAG laser has been used for photocoagulation and deep thermal necrosis in the treatment of gastrointestinal bleeding and obstructing bronchial lesions. The Nd:YAG laser uses a clear, solid, crystalline medium that emits radiation in the infrared region of the electromagnetic spectrum; the radiation has a wavelength of 1060 nm and is invisible (see Table 40-1). Conventional fiberoptic bundles readily transmit Nd:YAG laser radiation at high power, which is applied in a continuous or pulsed mode. The radiation is more readily absorbed by dark tissue. Blue or black pigmentation enhances Nd:YAG absorption, whereas pale colors enhance its penetration.[61,62] Nd:YAG radiation penetrates tissues to a depth of 2 to 6 mm and provides good homeostasis for blood vessels up to 0.5 cm in diameter. However, the depth of penetration is less predictable than that of the CO_2 laser. The power density below the tissue surface depends on the color of the surface, which makes laser penetration more difficult with the Nd:YAG laser than with the CO_2 laser.

The Nd:YAG laser is recommended for lesions distal to the larynx and for bulky, vascular endobronchial neoplasms. The advantage of the Nd:YAG laser is that the radiation can be transmitted through fiberoptic bundles. Excision of lesions that are located distal to the larynx is complicated because it is difficult to reach the tumor with the laser beam. In these situations, the Nd:YAG laser is preferred because it can be used with a rigid bronchoscope or an FOB.[62] Nd:YAG lasers are less precise in cutting, penetrate the tissue deeper, and have improved photocoagulation and superior hemostasis compared with other lasers.

Dumon and coworkers,[63] reporting a large series of cases, recommended the use of rigid rather than flexible bronchoscopy for treating obstructive pulmonary lesions by means of endoscopic Nd:YAG laser surgery. Brutinel and associates reported difficulty ventilating and oxygenating patients' lungs through an endotracheal tube (ETT) during Nd:YAG surgery with an indwelling FOB in place.[64] Casey and colleagues reported combustion of the FOB and ETT in a patient undergoing Nd:YAG laser airway surgery.[65] The use of a rigid bronchoscope for the treatment of obstructing pulmonary lesions facilitates the removal of tissue and the treatment of complications.[66] Power levels less than 50 W given in short pulsations decrease the chances of impingement on vital underlying structures.[66] McDougall and Cortese reported two patients who died during Nd:YAG laser endoscopic treatment of airway obstructions using very high power.[67] At high power, the penetration of tissues by the Nd:YAG laser cannot be readily controlled, and perforation of a large blood vessel is possible.

6. Ruby Laser

The ruby laser uses a solid medium of a crystal aluminum oxide (i.e., sapphire) containing chromium ions. It emits visible red radiation at a wavelength of 695 nm (see Table 40-1). The ruby laser is used only in the pulse mode. The radiation is not readily absorbed by water but is significantly absorbed by pigments such as melanin and hemoglobin. The ruby laser can easily penetrate the anterior structures of the eye. It is used to photocoagulate vascular and pigmented retinal lesions. Use of this laser has decreased with the availability of newer types, and the ruby laser is not commonly used for laser airway surgery.

7. Diode Laser

The diode laser is another addition to a growing array of tools for laser surgery. This laser is effective for treatment of hyperplastic inferior nasal turbinates and provides good hemostasis and a sufficient reduction of tumors in otolaryngology practice.[60] The continuous-wave, semiconductor diode laser emits radiation at wavelengths of 810 and 940 nm in the near-infrared spectrum. The radiation is delivered by a flexible fiber coupled with an aiming beam. The diode laser penetrates tissue to a depth of 1 to 3 mm, and it is suitable for vascular lesions. It is used to remove and debulk airway pathology, including tumors throughout the airway.

8. Other Lasers

Other lasers may have krypton, gold, copper, xenon, erbium:YAG, or holmium:YAG as their medium, but none is used for laser airway surgery.

III. LASER HAZARDS

General laser hazards exist for any type of surgery being done with a laser. Hazards include eye, skin, and drape damage; laser plumes; gas embolism; and misdirected laser beams.

Airway laser hazards exist when a surgeon is using a laser within the airway. The greatest danger is an airway

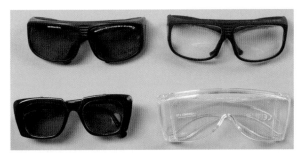

Figure 40-9 In the selection of laser glasses, notice the protection offered by the sides of the glasses, which wrap around the eye.

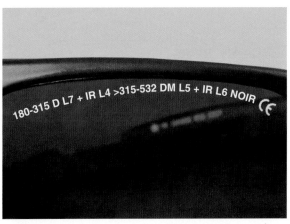

Figure 40-11 The correct protective eye glasses must be used with any given laser. The optical density value, the wavelengths against which protection is afforded, and maximum radiant exposure or irradiance to which eyewear is exposed are part of the design of laser glasses.

fire. Fires require three components known as the *fire triad*: a fuel source, an oxidant source, and an ignition source.

A. General Laser Hazards

1. Eye Damage

Lasers can easily damage the eyes by direct or indirect exposure, causing serious corneal and retinal injuries that may be irreversible. Eye protection is essential for anyone within the operating room, including the patient, auxiliary staff, nursing staff, surgeon, and anesthesiologist (Fig. 40-9). General precautions for the patient include taping the eyes closed and avoiding the use of petroleum-based eye lubricants. Further protection includes saline-soaked eye pads, protective eye glasses, or metal eye goggles, depending on the wavelength and type of laser used.

All laser glasses should be labeled clearly with the optical density value, the wavelengths against which protection is afforded, and maximum radiant exposure, or irradiance, to which the eyewear can be exposed (Figs. 40-10 and 40-11).[68] The correct protective eye glasses must be used for the type of laser used for the procedure; failure to do so provides no protection for the eyes. In hospitals where only one type of laser is in use, this is less of a problem, but care must be taken in hospitals with many types of lasers and protective eye goggles.

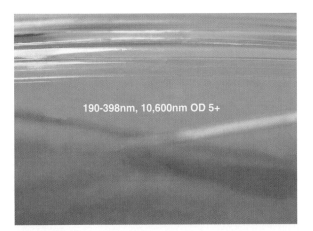

190-398nm, 10,600nm OD 5+

Figure 40-10 Eyes must be protected from laser energy. Laser glasses are labeled with the optical density value, the wavelengths against which protection is afforded, and maximum radiant exposure or irradiance to which eyewear is exposed.

For CO_2 lasers, the damage to the eye is limited to the cornea because its radiation is largely absorbed by water, and the cornea is more than 75% water.[61,69] There is no risk to the retina. For airway use, the patient's eyes should be taped, protective saline-soaked eye pads placed, and surgical drapes applied and covered with another layer of saline-soaked swabs placed over the drapes. For the operating room staff, CO_2 laser–protective eyeglasses should be worn. Contact lenses protect only the area covered and provide inadequate protection. Regular conventional eyeglasses can protect against the CO_2 laser beam if the beam has been directed or reflected straight onto the eyeglass; however, if the beam is reflected accidentally into the side of the eyeglasses, damage to the eye can occur. When working with CO_2 lasers, all operating room staff should use eyeglasses that wrap around the eye, protecting from CO_2 laser entry from the side. The surgeon does not need to use CO_2 laser protective eyeglasses when working with the operating microscope because the optics of the microscope provide protection[70]; however, if the surgeon uses the CO_2 laser with a handpiece, the surgeon must also wear protective eyeglasses.

For Nd:YAG lasers, unprotected eyes may absorb and focus laser light at the ocular fundus, resulting in irreparable damage. Radiation from the KTP and other lasers such as the Nd:YAG can penetrate the cornea and lens of the eye, resulting in severe retinal damage. The endoscopist is at greatest risk because of the Nd:YAG laser's potential for backscatter.[62] The patient and all operating room staff should wear protective eyeglasses. Filters that absorb the Nd:YAG wavelength of 1.06 μm can be placed into rigid and flexible bronchoscopes. If the fibers break during laser surgery, the beam may be deflected to anywhere in the operating room.

For KTP and argon lasers, all operating room personnel require protective amber-colored eyeglasses, and for laser procedures on the face, metal goggles are used (Fig. 40-12). For rigid and flexible endoscopes and operating microscopes, filters that absorb the KTP wavelength can be introduced.

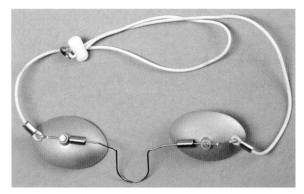

Figure 40-12 Metallic goggles are used during laser procedures on surface skin.

2. Skin and Drape Damage

Laser burns to the skin can occur, and the face or exposed areas should be protected with wet towels and drapes. For laser airway procedures involving a suspension laryngoscope, all of the area around the surgical laryngoscope and face should be completely covered with wet towels, which must be kept wet throughout the procedure. Care should be taken, particularly around the draping of the proximal portion of the surgical laryngoscope, to ensure that the lips and nose are fully protected because this region is more likely to be struck by a reflected laser beam from the proximal rim of the surgical laryngoscope (Fig. 40-13).

Preparation solution should not contain alcohol. Oxygen saturation monitors are a standard of care and should be used because detection of cyanosis is difficult with the patient's face covered. Disposable surgical drapes are a potential fire hazard. They are treated with flame-retardant chemicals and are water resistant, but all types of surgical drapes are potentially flammable. Many cases of drapes catching fire have been reported. When the drapes catch fire, it is difficult to extinguish because the drapes are water resistant, and the water rolls off them. A CO_2 fire extinguisher should be available. Drapes,

once ignited, go up in flames immediately, causing the operating room to be inundated with smoke and making it difficult for everyone to see and breathe.[71-73] It is important to keep the towels moist, or they can become flammable.

3. Laser Plume

The plume of smoke produced by vaporization of tissues in electrocautery or laser surgery may be hazardous. The smoke contains fine particles (mean size, 0.31 µm; range, 0.1 to 0.8 µm) that can be efficiently transported and deposited in the alveoli.[74] In rat lungs, the deposition of laser plume particles could produce interstitial pneumonia, bronchiolitis, a reduction in mucociliary clearance, inflammation, and emphysema.[75,76] The laser's smoke plume acting as a vector for viruses is a controversial idea. Viral DNA has been detected in plumes from condylomas and skin warts but not from laryngeal papillomas.[77-80] CO_2 lasers seem to produce the most smoke from vaporization of tissue. Operating room personnel can be protected by using an efficient smoke evacuator at the surgical site (Fig. 40-14).[81,82] Ordinary operating room masks can filter particles no smaller than 3.0 µm. Laser masks that are more efficient should be used to protect the operating room personnel from plume particles.

4. Gas Embolism

Gas embolism has been reported with Nd:YAG laser resection of tracheal and bronchial tumors, and it may be a risk factor for flexible-fiber CO_2 lasers introduced into the bronchial tree.[83,84] Gas embolism has been reported in laparoscopic surgery that used Nd:YAG laser probes that required a gas cooling system.[85,86]

5. Misdirected Laser and Laser Protocol

A misdirected laser may result from equipment failure or an inadequate knowledge of that equipment. Safety protocols should be in place to prevent this problem. Burn (discussed earlier) can occur even with an unfocused laser.

The intensity of the laser and the potential for tissue damage and combustion with a misdirected beam necessitates that strict safety precautions are followed.

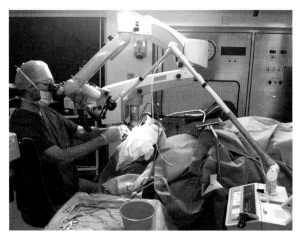

Figure 40-13 Care should be taken to ensure complete coverage of the face and area around the surgical laryngoscope with wet towels. A CO_2 laser is attached to the operating microscope by an articulating arm.

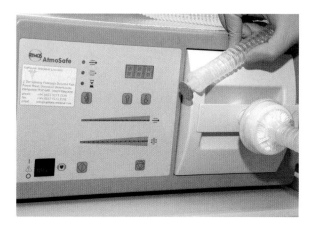

Figure 40-14 The AtmoSafe smoke evacuator (Atmos Medical Limited, Hampshire, United Kingdom) holds a metal coin by its suction.

Hospitals should have a laser safety officer or advisor, access to laser technicians, a laser register, and adequate staff training.

Lasers should always be set to the standby mode, except when they are ready to fire, to prevent inadvertent actuation. They should be used in the pulsed (shuttered) mode rather than the continuous mode whenever possible to limit the energy delivered by the laser and to allow the area being lasered to cool between firings. The laser radiation should never be allowed to strike highly polished or mirror-like surfaces. Most instrumentation for use with lasers has a dull or matte finish, and blackened instruments are widely used. This is important because reflection of the coherent laser beam may not disperse it, and injury to the patient or operating room personnel is possible, even from a reflected laser beam. Any instruments that become hot as a result of laser radiation may cause burns.[68,87] Tracheal laceration, tooth damage, injury to soft tissue, and cutaneous burns to operating room personnel have been described during laser surgery.[88]

The Nd:YAG and argon lasers can penetrate glass, and any windows in the operating room should have an opaque covering to prevent penetration by laser radiation. A warning sign should be placed on the operating room door so that anyone entering is informed that the laser is in use (Figs. 40-15 and 40-16). To prevent personnel inadvertently entering the operating room during laser surgery, the doors may be automatically locked when the operating room is in laser mode (Fig. 40-17). Extra goggles should be available for personnel entering the operating room.

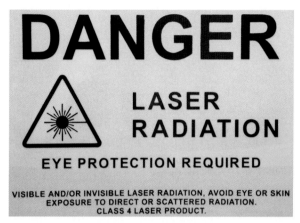

Figure 40-16 A warning sign should be placed on the operating room door to prevent personnel from inadvertently entering during laser surgery.

B. Airway Laser Hazards

The high energy of the laser and its potential for combustion can cause an airway fire when the surgical field is near to the airway (Fig. 40-18). When a laser strikes the unprotected external surface of a tracheal tube during laser airway surgery, the surface starts to disintegrate and can catch fire. If the fire is not recognized and the laser continues to be applied, it can produce a hole in the tracheal tube and expose the burning surface to the oxidant-rich gas within the anesthesia system. At this stage, an explosive blowtorch-like fire may occur and

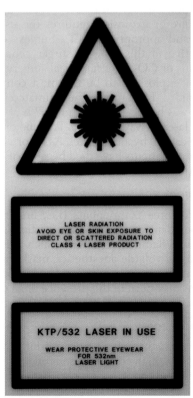

Figure 40-15 The sign warns personnel entering the operating room that a KTP laser is being used.

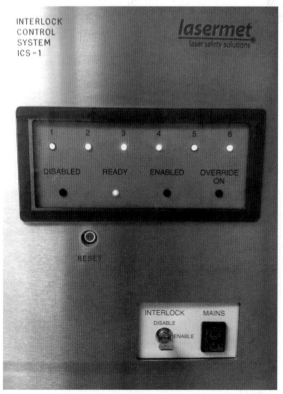

Figure 40-17 Interlock control system in the operating room prevents entry during laser use. When these systems are engaged, operating room doors are locked automatically.

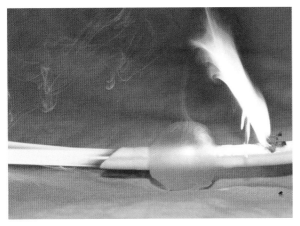

Figure 40-18 An airway fire results when a laser strikes the polyvinyl chloride endotracheal tube.

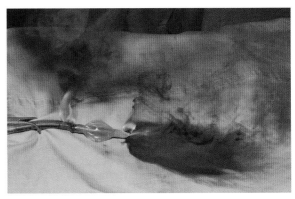

Figure 40-20 Smoke, molten material, and other particulate material spread out after an airway fire.

rapidly spread in a distal and proximal manner. Any airway fire is a life-threatening complication, but the blowtorch fire is especially feared (Fig. 40-19).

If the cuff of an ETT is punctured, the oxidant-rich gas within the circuit becomes exposed to the external surface of the ETT, and the risk of an airway fire, including a blowtorch fire, is increased significantly. Examination of an ETT after a blowtorch laser fire reveals total or near-total destruction of the ETT, with molten material, smoke, and other particulate material spreading out from the distal end of the tube (Figs. 40-20 and 40-21).

It is thought that operating room fires are underreported and that there are probably 100 to 200 operating room fires in the United States per year. Of the reported fires, 20% result in serious injury to the patient. One or two deaths per year are caused by airway fires.[89]

Many options are available for anesthesia management during airway laser surgery. Selection of the ventilation method and type of laser depends on the nature and location of the lesion, the condition of the patient, and the availability of equipment and expertise. Different anesthesia management techniques have been described in the treatment of recurrent respiratory papillomatosis using the CO_2 laser.[90] In a 1995 survey, 92% of otolaryngologists preferred using a CO_2 laser for removal of recurrent

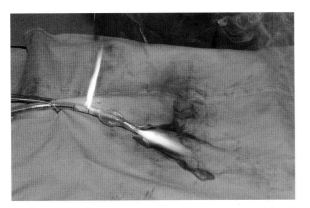

Figure 40-19 Continued laser application can produce a hole in the tracheal tube and expose the burning surface to the oxidant-rich gas within the anesthesia system, producing a blowtorch airway fire.

respiratory papillomas. However, there is no consensus with respect to anesthesia management. About 46% preferred using a laser-safe ETT, 26% favored using jet ventilation, 16% preferred an apneic technique, and 12% preferred spontaneous ventilation.[91] Other options include awake with topical anesthesia, general anesthesia through an ETT, rigid bronchoscopy with general anesthesia, and general anesthesia by a laryngeal mask airway (LMA). The possibility of complete airway collapse or an inability to ventilate must be taken into consideration when deciding on spontaneous or positive-pressure ventilation.

When general anesthesia for laser airway surgery is conducted without an ETT, special techniques are used. They include Venturi jet ventilation, intermittent apneic technique, LMA, and insufflation, which are discussed later in this chapter.

If ventilation through an ETT is proposed, prevention of an ETT fire or explosion requires the use of special techniques and appropriate ETTs. Surveys of otolaryngologists active in this type of surgery concerning the complications of CO_2 laser laryngeal surgery have found ETT fires or explosions to be the most common major complication.[52,92] Historically, the estimated incidence of airway fires was between 0.4% and 0.57% of the patients undergoing laser airway surgery.[39] The one or two deaths per year are caused by airway fires. As reported by Cozine and colleagues, patients have died because of combustion of an ETT during CO_2 laser surgery.[93]

1. Fuel Source

Fires require three components (i.e., fire triad): a fuel source, an oxidant source, and an ignition source. Fuel source includes flammable material, such as ETTs, gauze, sponges, drapes, volatile anesthetics, masks, nasal cannulas, suction catheters, gloves, gowns, endoscopes, and any material that may burn in the presence of an oxidant-rich atmosphere. The only exception is stainless steel.

2. Oxidant Source

An oxidant-rich atmosphere exists within closed breathing circuits when high concentrations of oxygen or nitrous oxide are present, and this increases the chances of an airway fire. An oxidant-rich atmosphere also can occur under drapes or masks and can increase the likelihood of a fire.

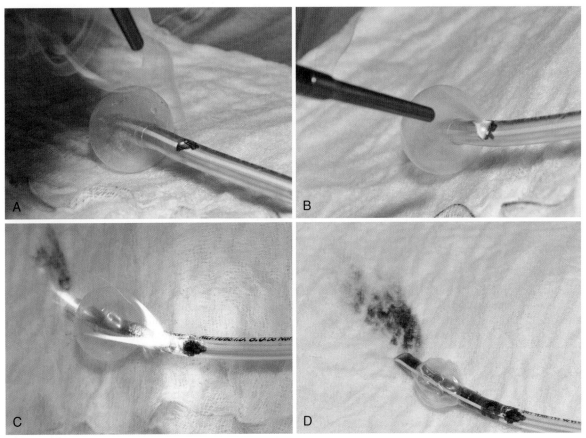

Figure 40-21   A laser striking the polyvinyl chloride endotracheal tube (ETT) created an airway fire. **A,** Smoke emerges from the outer shaft of the ETT after a continuous laser strike. **B,** The outer surface glows orange. **C,** After perforation into the inner aspect of the ETT in the presence of 100% oxygen flow, flames emerge from the puncture site and distal ETT. **D,** After the fire is extinguished, damage to ETT and material spreading out from its distal end can be seen.

3. Ignition Source

Any high-energy source has the potential to ignite a fire. During laser airway surgery, the laser is the ignition source. Other ignition sources include electrocautery devices, fiberoptic cables, light cables, defibrillator pads, heated probes, and drills. The influence of special equipment and anesthesia on airway fires is discussed later in this chapter.

IV. PREVENTING AIRWAY FIRES

The risk of an airway fire during laser airway surgery depends on the many factors that affect the three components of the fire triad. The first component is the fuel source, and the most common fuel source is the ETT. Attempts have been made to reduce the risks of a fire by protecting the tube shaft by covering it with metal foil, protecting the tube shaft by covering it with laser-protective coatings, adding saline to the tube cuff, and developing specially manufactured laser tubes suitable for laser airway surgery.

The second component is the oxidant source. An understanding of the effect of anesthetic gases on tracheal tube flammability is required, as well as an appreciation of the flammability limits of potent inhaled anesthetics.

The third component is the ignition source. The different types of lasers, power settings, modes of operation, exposure times, and spot sizes have been discussed. Most of these parameters depend on the type and site of surgery undertaken, but the anesthesiologist should understand the factors that increase the risk of an airway fire.

A. Fuel Source Considerations

1. Use of Metallic Foil Tapes to Protect Endotracheal Tubes

Metal foil tape wrapped around a standard ETT that is used during laser surgery in adults is of historical interest, but it is not commonly used for laser airway surgery. Foil tapes were first suggested as a simple, inexpensive means of protecting the shafts of combustible ETTs from laser beams by Strong and Jako in 1972.[49] Their use during laser surgery was described during the 1970s and 1980s,[94-97] when specially manufactured laser-resistant ETTs were not available or performed poorly.

Metallic foil tapes provide protection only from the direct impact of the laser beam. Indirect combustion caused by sparks or heat from gaseous or tube combustion is still possible because the ETTs used typically were combustible and usually had an enriched concentration of oxygen flowing through them. Problems with the use of metallic foil tape have included obstruction of the airway when the tape came loose from a wrapped ETT[98,99]

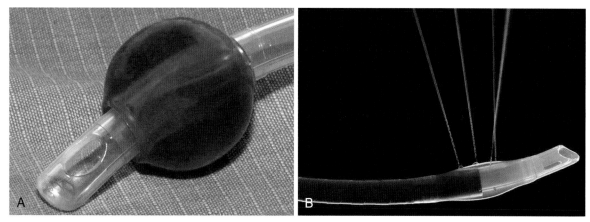

Figure 40-22 **A,** The endotracheal tube cuff is filled with saline and methylene blue dye. **B,** Perforation of the saline-filled cuff results in jets of water.

and aluminum foil tape becoming trapped in the trachea after laser airway supraglottoplasty.[100]

No metallic foil tapes are manufactured for medical applications, and the U.S. Food and Drug Administration has not sanctioned their use. The physician who wraps an ETT with metal foil tape incurs some product liability risk as a noncertified "manufacturer" if injury occurs.[101] One manufacturer, when questioned, cautioned against the use of its aluminum tape for medical purposes.[102]

Wrapping the metal foil tape in a spiral, overlapping manner should cover the shaft from the cuff to the most proximal region possible and should include the pilot tube. Poor wrapping may cause some areas of the shaft to be unprotected, and bending of the tube may expose unprotected areas. Foil-wrapped tubes may loose flexibility, and their foil edge surface may traumatize. The type of metallic tape used to protect combustible ETTs is important.[102]

The possibility of changes in the composition of any metallic foil tape requires every batch of tape to be evaluated for its incendiary characteristics before use.[95] Metal foil tape wrapped around a standard ETT is not recommended for laser airway surgery.

2. Laser-Guard Protective Coating

The Merocel Laser-Guard (Medtronic Xomed Corp, Mystic, CT) ETT protective coating is no longer available in many parts of the world and is largely of historical interest. It can be regarded as an advance from the use of metallic foil tape to cover a combustible tracheal tube, but its use has been replaced by specially manufactured tracheal tubes for laser airway surgery. The Merocel Laser-Guard consisted of a rectangular sheet of embossed silver foil covered with a thin, absorbent Merocel sponge layer on one side and adhesive on the other.

3. Prevention of Endotracheal Tube Cuff Fires with Saline

During laser airway surgery, the ETT cuff is particularly vulnerable to a laser strike. The high-volume, low-pressure cuff is thin and relatively large because the tube size chosen is undersized to provide the best exposure of the larynx for the surgeon.

The laser beam is aligned along the axis of an operating laryngoscope, which is along the same axis as the ETT but is almost perpendicular to the cuff, which expands away from the tracheal tube until it reaches the tracheal wall. Because undersized ETTs are used, the cuff size is large, and the area exposed to a laser strike is greater than for a larger ETT. A laser strike of the cuff can result in an airway fire at the cuff or lead to a leak of anesthetic gases from within the circuit and expose the outer part of the tracheal tube to an oxidant-rich environment, increasing the chance of a shaft- or cuff-related airway fire or blowtorch fire.

During the 1970s and 1980s, attempts were made to improve the laser-resistant properties of the shaft of combustible ETTs. In 1982, LeJeune and colleagues suggested that filling ETT cuffs with saline could protect them from the CO_2 laser, because a laser strike on the cuff results in a jet of water that acts as a "built-in fire extinguisher" (Fig. 40-22).[103] The saline also can act as a heat sink. Sosis and Dillon compared air-filled and saline-filled cuffs, and they found the saline-filled cuffs,[104] although perforated by the laser beam as rapidly as air-filled cuffs, were significantly slower to deflate, allowing more time before reaching the point at which airway pressure could no longer be maintained. Saline-filled cuffs prevented ETT ignition by the CO_2 laser set to 40 W (Table 40-2) in a statistically significant number of cases compared with the control group of air-filled cuffs, and saline filling of ETT cuffs was recommended for laser airway surgery. A small amount of dye, such as methylene blue, should be added to the saline so that laser-induced ETT cuff perforation becomes

TABLE 40-2

Incidence of Endotracheal Tube Combustion with Air- and Saline-Filled Cuffs with the Carbon Dioxide Laser Set to 40 W

Cuff Type	Number of Cases	Combustion (%)
Air	5	100*
Saline	5	20*

*$P < 0.05$, Mann-Whitney U test.

From Sosis MB, Dillon FX: Saline-filled cuffs help prevent laser-induced polyvinylchloride endotracheal tube fires. *Anesth Analg* 72:187, 1991.

obvious to the surgeon, who can immediately terminate operation of the laser. Further protection of the ETT cuffs can be obtained by placing moistened pledgets above them and keeping the pledgets moist throughout the procedure.[105]

4. Special Endotracheal Tubes for Laser Airway Surgery

Beginning in the 1970s, laser surgery of the airway became increasingly popular, and as the dangers of an airway fire became clearer, many attempts were made to reduce this risk. Two strategies were used to reduce the risk. The first involved the anesthesiologist using a standard combustible ETT and covering it in some form of protective coating. Early attempts involved protection of the shaft by metal foil and then specially designed protective coatings. The second approach involved manufacturers producing tracheal tubes that had laser-resistant properties. Some of the early manufactured laser tubes were not particularly effective, but they were thought to allow any type of laser use, and subsequently, a number of airway fires were reported. It is useful to discriminate between laser-proof and laser-resistant devices.

Laser proof implies that irrespective of the oxidant environment and the power of the laser, the ETT cannot catch fire. With a laser-proof ETT, a continuous laser strike with extremely high power in a 100% oxygen environment does not produce a fire of the tube. Only one laser-proof tracheal tube (Norton) has been designed, and it is discussed later.[106]

All other manufactured ETTs for laser airway surgery are only laser resistant. Laser-resistant tubes provide some degree of protection against a laser strike, but these tubes vary in their materials, protective coating, relative size, and number of cuffs used. Any laser-resistant tube can result in an airway fire or blowtorch fire (Fig. 40-23) if it is used outside of its limits, such as a laser strike on an unprotected area between the tube shaft distal and the cuff, at the unprotected proximal part of the shaft, or at the cuff itself. The anesthesiologist should appreciate the maximum power settings for which a laser-resistant tube has been tested, the range within which ignition does not occur, and the effect the oxidant environment has on the laser resistance characteristics. All laser-resistant tubes are

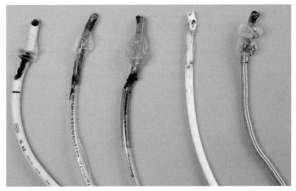

Figure 40-23 Laser-induced fire damage to endotracheal tubes (ETTs). Left to right, the first three are standard nonlaser polyvinyl chloride ETTs, and all three have been damaged by an airway fire. The two ETTs on the right are designed for laser use. Both tubes have sustained fire damage in their unprotected areas distal to the cuff by high-energy, sustained CO_2 laser strikes to the ETTs with 100% oxygen passing through them.

not laser proof, and they must not be used outside of their limits.

a. NORTON LASER ENDOTRACHEAL TUBE

The Norton ETT (V. Mueller, Baxter Healthcare Corp., Niles, IL), first described in 1978 by Norton and De Vos, was the only laser-proof tracheal tube produced (Fig. 40-24).[106] It was constructed from interlocking, spiral-wound, stainless steel parts. It is no longer manufactured. Because it was made of steel, it was extremely resistant to multiple uses and autoclaving, and it may still exist in some hospitals.

The Norton ETT had a matte or sand-blasted finish, rather thick walls, and a ribbed exterior. It came in three sizes: 4.0-, 4.8-, and 6.4-mm internal diameter (ID) (Table 40-3).[107] The matte finish diffused reflected laser beams.[106] A 4.8-mm-ID Norton ETT has a wall thickness of 1.4 mm. The thick wall of this ETT is considered a disadvantage because the tube can obscure the surgeon's view more than an ETT with the same ID but with thinner walls—an important consideration during laser airway surgery. This ETT's large size and stiffness may make surgical exposure and laryngoscope positioning

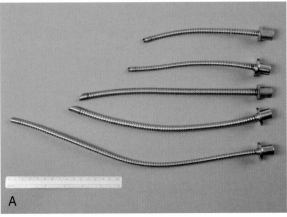
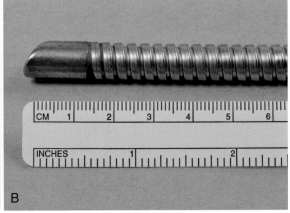

Figure 40-24 A and **B,** In the selection of Norton laser tubes, notice the absence of a cuff and ribbed exterior.

TABLE 40-3

Internal Diameter, External Diameter, and Wall Thickness for the Norton Laser Endotracheal Tube

Endotracheal Tube Size (F)	Internal Diameter (mm)	External Diameter (mm)	Wall Thickness* (mm)
24	4.0	6.6	1.3
26	4.8	7.4	1.3
28	6.4	9.3	1.45

*Calculated.
Courtesy of V. Mueller, Niles, IL.

difficult, and it can make passage through the glottis traumatic. It is usually necessary to use a stylet to introduce the Norton ETT.

The Norton tube had no cuff, but a separate latex cuff was available and could be attached to it. If an external cuff was added to the device, it was no longer laser proof because the cuff and pilot tube could act as a fuel source for an airway fire. The separate latex cuff is no longer manufactured, and because they degraded over time, they are not commonly found.

Alternatively, the pharynx may be packed with wet gauze, sponges, or packs to seal the system to allow positive-pressure ventilation of the lungs, but this introduces a potential fuel source and can cause an airway fire, particularly if they are allowed to dry out. Even if ventilation of the patient's lungs is not compromised by leakage, the presence of anesthetic gases in the oropharynx increases the possibility of combustion in the surgical field and increases operating room pollution.

The relatively small diameter and ridged internal surface produce turbulent airflow and an increased resistance to airflow. Woo and Strong suggested Venturi ventilation through the Norton tube in an attempt to overcome the ventilation issues of increased resistance,[108] airflow, and air leaks.

b. XOMED LASER-SHIELD I ENDOTRACHEAL TUBE

The Xomed Laser-Shield I ETT (Xomed-Treace, Jacksonville, FL) is no longer manufactured and is of historical interest only. The silicon rubber tube was coated with a silicon elastomer to which metallic particles had been added, and it was designed to be used only with a CO_2 laser. Several airway fires were reported with its use.[109-112] It is a useful reminder of the limitations of a laser-resistant ETT and the dangers of using a device outside of its intended range.

c. BIVONA LASER ENDOTRACHEAL TUBE

The Bivona (Gary, IN) laser ETT is no longer available in many parts of the world and is mainly of historical interest. It was designed to limit the effect of cuff perforation by a laser strike, because the polyurethane foam cuff with its silicone envelope maintained the cuff seal even when penetrated. The Bivona laser ETT was designed to be used only with a CO_2 laser. Blowtorch airway fires were reported with this tube.[112]

d. XOMED LASER-SHIELD II ENDOTRACHEAL TUBE

The Xomed Laser-Shield II ETT (Xomed Surgical Products, Jacksonville, FL) has a laser-resistant overwrap of aluminum foil tape and a Teflon cover. The proximal and distal ends of the silicon elastomer shaft and cuff are not protected and therefore are not laser resistant (Fig. 40-25). The metallic tape provides protection against laser impact. The Teflon tape gives the tube a smooth surface to minimize mucosal injury from tube manipulation. No adhesives are used because adhesives with metallic tape increase the risk of an ETT fire.[98] Dry methylene blue dye has been placed in the cuff inflation valve to enable detection of a cuff rupture. The Xomed Laser-Shield II comes packaged with neurosurgical cottonoid, which is used wet to protect the distal shaft and cuff for an added margin of safety.

Dillon and associates evaluated the combustibility of the Xomed Laser-Shield II ETT and compared it with 3M's no. 425 aluminum foil–wrapped, combustible, polyvinyl chloride (PVC) ETTs used with a CO_2 laser and an Nd:YAG laser.[113] Exposure of the bare silicon rubber shaft of the Laser Shield-II ETT to CO_2 laser radiation resulted in combustion in 2.1 ± 0.7 seconds; Nd:YAG laser radiation–induced combustion occurred at 3.3 ± 4.5 seconds ($P = 0.05$). The silicon rubber burned with a bright flame and disintegrated. It was difficult to extinguish. Dillon and colleagues concluded that the foil-wrapped shaft of the Laser Shield-II ETT provided adequate protection against high-power, continuous-mode Nd:YAG and CO_2 laser radiation.[113]

Ossoff and colleagues also studied the Laser-Shield II for combustibility with CO_2 and KTP lasers. They evaluated the Laser-Shield II dry, with blood, with a blood/K-Y jelly mixture, and with K-Y jelly alone on the ETT. Each tube was clamped, and 100% oxygen was delivered at 3 L/min through it. All trials were performed with 3 minutes of continuous output. The maximum power output was 40 W for the CO_2 laser and 15 W for the KTP laser. These settings far exceed the clinical settings used. With the KTP laser (13.5 to 15 W), no fires were observed, regardless of surface penetration. For the CO_2 laser, no fires were observed at 40 W for 3 minutes on continuous mode with the dry ETT. Blood or KY-jelly, or both, decreased the resistance of the ETT to CO_2 laser radiation. For the tube with blood alone, 25 W was the highest power that the tubes withstood without ignition. For the K-Y jelly/blood mixture, the maximum power was reduced to 19 W. With K-Y jelly alone, no fire occurred at the maximum power setting of 40 W.[114]

The Xomed Laser-Shield II ETT offers the potential advantage of an adhesive-free foil wrapping for ETT protection. Silicon, however, disintegrates during combustion, whereas rubber and PVC tend to retain their integrity. The Teflon overwrap around the foil raises questions because pyrolysis of Teflon may liberate toxic fumes that can cause polymer fume fever.

Medtronic Xomed recommends only the Xomed Laser-Shield II for all surgical procedures involving the use of CO_2 or KTP lasers in a normal-pulsed or continuous mode of noncontact delivery. It is contraindicated for use with any Nd:YAG laser, argon laser, or any laser other

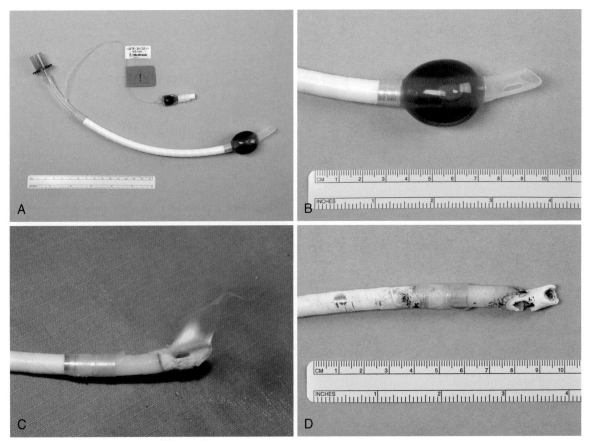

Figure 40-25 Xomed Laser-Shield II endotracheal tube (Xomed Surgical Products, Jacksonville, FL). **A,** The proximal and distal ends of the silicon elastomer shaft and cuff are not protected. **B,** The laser-resistant aluminum foil tape can be seen proximal to the cuff. **C** and **D,** An airway fire occurred in the distal, unprotected area after a sustained, high-power CO_2 laser strike in 100% oxygen.

than the CO_2 or KTP. When the laser beam hits the Laser-Shield II Teflon, the reflective aluminum wrapping may be exposed, and it is possible for the beam to be reflected into the patient's tissue. The sizes of Xomed Laser-Shield II ETTs are given in Table 40-4.

e. MALLINCKRODT LASER-FLEX ENDOTRACHEAL TUBE

Mallinckrodt (Glens Falls, NY) Laser-Flex ETTs have corrugated stainless steel shafts. They are designed as a

TABLE 40-4

Internal Diameter, External Diameter, and Wall Thickness for the Xomed Laser-Shield II Endotracheal Tube

Internal Diameter (mm)	External Diameter (mm)	Wall Thickness (mm)*
4.0	6.6	1.3
4.5	7.3	1.4
5.0	8.0	1.5
5.5	8.6	1.55
6.0	9.0	1.5
6.5	10.0	1.75
7.0	10.5	1.75
7.5	11.0	1.75
8.0	11.5	1.75

*Calculated.
Courtesy of Xomed-Surgical Products, Jacksonville, FL.

single-use item, and the manufacturer states that this type of ETT should be used only with the CO_2 and KTP lasers. The adult version of this ETT incorporates two PVC cuffs. The manufacturer suggests that the distal cuff can be used if the laser damages the proximal one. The adult tube's distal end, including its Murphy eye and the proximal 15-mm connector, is constructed from combustible PVC (Fig. 40-26). The Laser-Flex cuffs are inflated by means of two 1-mm-diameter PVC pilot tubes that are located on the inside of the ETT. An Nd:YAG or other laser fiber should never be inserted through this tube. Heyman and colleagues found that prolonged laser impingement on the shaft of a Mallinckrodt Laser-Flex ETT could prevent cuff deflation, and they stressed the importance of aspirating the saline from the cuff in a slow, gentle manner.[115]

The adult sizes of Mallinckrodt Laser-Flex ETTs available with the double-cuff system are 4.5-, 5.0-, 5.5-, and 6.0-mm ID. Three pediatric sizes (3.0-, 3.5-, and 4.0-mm ID) of uncuffed Mallinckrodt Laser-Flex ETTs are also available. They are all stainless steel, except for a PVC 15-mm adapter. They are not equipped with Murphy eyes (Table 40-5).

Unlike the all-stainless-steel Norton ETT, the Mallinckrodt Laser-Flex ETT has an airtight shaft. However, the walls of both types of tubes are somewhat rough. In their product information for the uncuffed pediatric tubes, Mallinckrodt states, "Due to the spiral design of the tube,

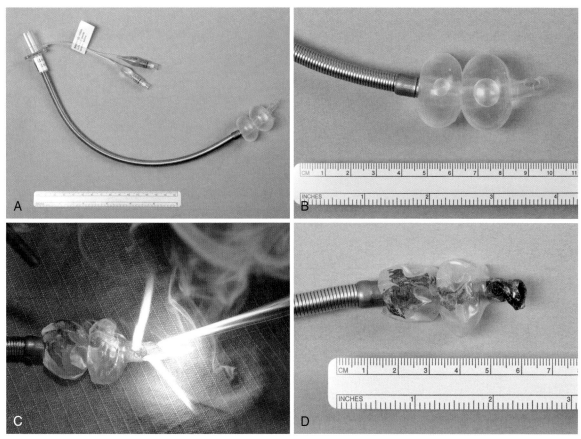

Figure 40-26 **A** and **B,** The Mallinckrodt Laser-Flex endotracheal tube (Covidien, Hazelwood, MO) has a corrugated stainless steel shaft and double cuff filled with saline. **C** and **D,** An airway fire occurred in the distal, unprotected area after a sustained, high-power CO_2 laser strike in 100% oxygen.

the airflow resistance for a given size will be approximately equal to a PVC tube, which is 0.5 mm smaller." They add, "Due to the bore size of the tube, patients should be monitored closely to guard against overinflation of the respiratory system and a build-up of expiratory gases."[116]

Sosis and coworkers studied the resistance to CO_2 laser radiation of size 4.5-mm-ID Mallinckrodt Laser-Flex ETTs.[117] The tubes were positioned horizontally on

TABLE 40-5

Internal Diameter, External Diameter, and Wall Thickness for the Mallinckrodt Laser-Flex Endotracheal Tube

Type of Endotracheal Tube	Internal Diameter (mm)	External Diameter (mm)	Wall Thickness* (mm)
Cuffed	4.5	7.0	1.25
	5.0	7.5	1.25
	5.5	7.9	1.20
	6.0	8.5	1.25
Uncuffed	3.0	5.2	1.10
	3.5	5.7	1.10
	4.0	6.1	1.05

*Calculated.
Courtesy of Mallinckrodt Medical, Inc., St. Louis, MO.

a stainless steel tabletop covered with a wet towel. An oxygen flow of 5 L/min passed through the tubes as a Sharplan (Tel Aviv, Israel) model 734 CO_2 laser was aimed at an ETT's shaft. A laser power setting of 35 W was used with a beam diameter of 0.6 mm. This resulted in a power density of 13,400 W/cm^2. The laser, set to the continuous mode of operation, was activated for 90 seconds or until combustion occurred. Blowtorch combustion occurred in one of five Laser-Flex ETTs studied. However, when human blood was applied to the shafts of four 4.5-mm-ID Mallinckrodt Laser-Flex ETTs, blowtorch combustion occurred in all cases.

In another study, Sosis and Dillon noted that there is less danger of a reflected laser beam causing damage when the Mallinckrodt Laser-Flex ETT is used compared with foil-wrapped ETTs.[118] In an evaluation of the Laser-Flex ETT with the Nd:YAG laser, Sosis found that the shaft of the Laser-Flex ETT could be ignited in all cases by the Nd:YAG laser when operated at high power.[97] Clinical Laser Monthly reported the occurrence of an airway fire during a case in which a Mallinckrodt Laser-Flex ETT was used during a laser excision of vocal cord polyps.[119] They stated that the patient had minor burns. They reported that, at the time of the fire, the cuffs of the ETT were not inflated with saline as recommended by the manufacturer.

f. SHERIDAN LASER-TRACH ENDOTRACHEAL TUBE

The Sheridan (Argyle, NY) Laser-Trach ETT is a single-use, red rubber tube that has a spiral-wrapped, nonflammable, embossed copper foil from cuff to the proximal end of the tube. The copper foil is covered by an outer, absorbent fabric. The company recommends saturating the outer layer with sterilized isotonic saline before use, and it must remain saturated during the procedure, because a laser strike on a dry outer coating of fabric will produce a fire.

The outer covering reduces heat buildup and must be vaporized before the copper foil is reached. The Sheridan Laser-Trach is recommended only for use with CO_2 and KTP lasers. The outer fabric coating adds additional size to any given internal diameter and these tubes are therefore relatively large compared to other laser-resistant tracheal tubes.

Sosis and associates compared 6.0-mm-ID Sheridan Laser-Trach ETTs with plain (bare) Rüsch red rubber ETTs of the same internal diameter.[120] Five liters per minute of oxygen flowed through the tubes being studied. The tubes were subjected to continuous radiation at 40 W from a Sharplan CO_2 laser or 40 W of continuous output from a Laserphotonics (Orlando, FL) Nd:YAG laser. The Nd:YAG laser radiation was propagated by a 600-μm fiber bundle. Each type of laser was directed perpendicular to the ETT being studied. The laser's output was continued until a blowtorch fire occurred or 50 seconds elapsed. No ignition occurred after 60 seconds of CO_2 laser fire to the shafts of eight Sheridan Laser-Trach ETTs tested. However, blowtorch ignition of all eight bare rubber ETTs tested occurred after 0.87 ± 21 (mean $\pm$ SD) seconds of CO_2 laser fire. Nd:YAG laser contact with the Sheridan copper and fabric-covered rubber ETTs resulted in perforation and blowtorch ignition in all tubes tested after 18.79 ± 7.83 seconds. This was significantly ($P < 0.05$) longer than the 5.45 ± 4.75 seconds required for blowtorch ignition of all eight plain red rubber ETTs tested with the Nd:YAG laser.

It was concluded that under the conditions of the study, the Sheridan Laser-Trach ETT was resistant to CO_2 laser radiation. It is not recommended for use with the Nd:YAG laser. Table 40-6 lists the sizes of the Sheridan Laser-Trach ETTs available.

g. LASERTUBUS ENDOTRACHEAL TUBES

Lasertubus (Rüsch, Duluth, GA) is a laser-resistant ETT with a shaft made of soft white rubber and a laser guard

---

TABLE 40-6

Internal Diameter, External Diameter, and Wall Thickness for the Sheridan Laser-Trach Endotracheal Tube

Internal Diameter (mm)	External Diameter (mm)	Wall Thickness*
4.0	8.2	2.10
5.0	9.5	2.25
6.0	10.6	2.30

*Calculated.
Courtesy of Sheridan Catheters, Argyle, NY.

---

approximately 17 cm long, consisting of a Merocel sponge and silver foil with a double cuff. A cuff within a cuff arrangement exists and the sponge surface should be soaked to reduce the risk of an airway fire in a manner similar to that for the Sheridan Laser-Trach. According to the manufacturer, the Lasertubus offers resistance to all types of medical lasers, such as argon, Nd:YAG, and CO_2, with wavelengths ranging from 488 to 1060 nm. Sosis and colleagues evaluated the Rüsch Lasertubus in vitro.[121]

Jacobs and colleagues reported crimping of the Lasertubus, resulting in hypoxemia in a patient.[122] After placement of the Lasertubus, the surgeon extended the patient's head and neck and within 30 seconds, peak inspiratory pressures increased, oxygen saturation decreased, and no end-tidal CO_2 was evident. Immediate direct laryngoscopy confirmed that the ETT was correctly placed. On inspection, no kinks or obvious obstruction was seen. Ultimately, the laser tube was removed and the patient reintubated with a PVC ETT. The patient's oxygen saturations returned to 100%. On inspection of the Lasertubus, the tube had crimped under the tape. Although this was a small defect not obvious to cursory inspection, it resulted in complete obstruction to airflow. The investigators then experimented by bending unused laser tubes and found that a weakness within the wall of the tube remained, predisposing to crimping with minimal force and producing complete obstruction to airflow.[122]

B. Oxidant Source Considerations

1. Effect of Anesthetic Gases on Endotracheal Tube Flammability

The anesthetic gases used during airway laser surgery can profoundly influence combustibility. Nitrous oxide should never be considered an inert gas during laser airway surgery. Although nitrous oxide cannot support life, it can readily decompose into oxygen, nitrogen, and energy according to the following equation:

$$N_2O = N_2 + \tfrac{1}{2} O_2 + energy$$

In an experiment analogous to one with oxygen, a glowing match thrust into a vessel containing nitrous oxide bursts into flames. Nitrous oxide supports combustion to approximately the same extent as oxygen, and the addition of nitrous oxide in an attempt to dilute oxygen makes no difference to the flammability.[123]

Chilcoat and coworkers stressed that the reduction in oxygen concentration on dilution with nitrous oxide did not provide any additional safety when performing laryngeal laser surgery.[124] They recommended the use of either nitrogen, air, or helium when it was desired to reduce the oxygen concentration in anesthetic gas mixtures to levels of 30% or less for laser surgery.[124] Wolf and Simpson showed that nitrous oxide and oxygen are linearly additive in their ability to sustain combustion.[125] Nitrous oxide should not be considered safe, and careful consideration is required before using it with laser surgery.

Helium and nitrogen are inert gases, and when added to oxygen, they can delay ETT flammability (Table 40-7). Pashayan and Gravenstein and Osoff found that helium was more protective than nitrogen in retarding

TABLE 40-7
Physical Properties of Helium and Nitrogen at 26° C

Physical Properties	Helium	Nitrogen
Thermal conductivity (cal (sec•cm^2 °C•cm^{-1}•10^{-6})$^{-1}$)	360.36	62.40
Thermal capacity (cal•g^{-1}•K^{-1})	1.24	0.249
Density (g•L^{-1})	0.179	1.25
Thermal diffusivity (cm^2•sec^{-1})	1.621	0.199

From Pashayan AG, Gravenstein JS: Helium retards endotracheal tube fires from carbon dioxide lasers. *Anesthesiology* 62:274, 1985.

laser-ignited ETT fires.[110,126] The protective effect of helium is probably due to its high thermal diffusivity (i.e., quantity of heat passing through 1 cm^2 of cross-sectional area per unit of time) or thermal conductivity (i.e., time rate of transfer of heat by conduction). Presumably, helium diffusivity prevents a rise in temperature around the site of laser exposure, preventing the laser-irradiated ETT from reaching its temperature of spontaneous ignition.

Pashayan and Gravenstein studied the CO_2 laser–induced combustibility of 2-cm segments of PVC ETTs in various oxygen, helium, and nitrogen environments.[126] At oxygen concentrations of 30% and 40%, the mean time to ignition with nitrogen was significantly shorter than the time for the same concentration of oxygen in helium. Pashayan and Gravenstein concluded that helium in concentrations of 60% or greater delayed CO_2 laser–induced combustion of PVC ETTs if the laser power output was 10 W or less.[126] They also concluded that the radiopaque barium stripe on the PVC ETT was more combustible than the clear portions of the ETT and that they should be positioned away from the laser. Reflected beams may reach a stripe that appears to be out of the direct line of sight, and using an ETT without such stripes is preferred.

Ossoff compared the incendiary characteristics of three ETTs in various oxygen concentrations diluted with either helium or nitrogen using a CO_2 laser. They found that helium was better than nitrogen as an inert mixture with use of the CO_2 laser to decrease flammability. They also showed that the safest anesthetic gas mixture was 30% oxygen in helium.[110]

Al Haddad and Brenner studied the combustion of 1- to 2-inch PVC ETT segments with the KTP laser and CO_2 laser in helium-oxygen and nitrogen-oxygen atmospheres.[127] They compared these two lasers because of their different wavelengths and penetration characteristics that are commonly used in airway laser surgery. The CO_2 laser mean ignition time in helium was prolonged compared with nitrogen ($P < 0.001$), whereas increasing the oxygen concentration reduced the ignition time for both nitrogen and helium. With KTP, there was no significant difference for ignition among the five groups of oxygen concentrations or between nitrogen and helium. Al Haddad and Brenner reconfirmed that helium, as part of the mixture with 30% oxygen, is safest for the CO_2 laser but concluded that the use of helium instead of

nitrogen conferred no added safety during KTP laser surgery.

Simpson and colleagues determined the flammability of four types of ETTs in mixtures of helium and oxygen or nitrous oxide compared with mixtures of nitrogen and oxygen or nitrous oxide.[128] The ETTs were initially ignited in oxygen and nitrogen, and the nitrogen was quickly discontinued and replaced with helium. The helium concentration was increased until the candle-like flame on the ETT was extinguished. The oxygen concentrations just before the flame's extinction with helium were defined as the *oxygen/helium index of flammability* by the researchers. A similar experimental design was used with mixtures of nitrogen and oxygen until the propane torch–induced combustion of the four types of ETTs was extinguished. This was defined as the *oxygen/nitrogen index of flammability*. Next, the oxygen was replaced by nitrous oxide, and the procedure was repeated to determine the *nitrous oxide/helium* and *nitrous oxide/nitrogen indices of flammability*. The indices of flammability of each type of ETT studied were averaged, and the results were compared using Bonferroni corrected *t*-tests. These results show that the PVC ETT is flammable in 27.4% oxygen with the remainder consisting of helium and in 25.4% oxygen with the remainder nitrogen. In all cases, the oxidant oxygen/helium values were statistically significantly higher than the oxygen/nitrogen values for the same type of ETT ($P < 0.05$). The oxidant nitrous oxide/helium indices were statistically higher than the nitrous oxide/nitrogen indices for all except the Xomed ETT.

Simpson and colleagues observed that the differences between helium and nitrogen indices determined in this study were not clinically significant. For example, for a PVC ETT, the difference between 27.4% oxygen in helium and 25.4% oxygen in helium needed for combustion is very small. Their study also showed that the PVC ETTs were less flammable than the red rubber, silicon, and Xomed ETTs.

In summary, oxygen and nitrous oxide support combustion very well; dilution of oxygen by nitrous oxide makes no difference to the flammability and should be avoided; helium and nitrogen are inert gases, and their use can reduce the risk of an airway fire; and helium was better than nitrogen as an inert mixture with the CO_2 laser, but this difference was not clinically significant. Moreover, in clinical practice, administration of air and oxygen is most frequently used during laser airway surgery because most anesthesia machines do not allow the delivery of helium. The oxygen concentration should be kept as low as clinically feasible while the laser is in proximity to the tube.

2. Flammability Limits of Potent Inhaled Anesthetics

In 1850 in Boston, Massachusetts, the first recorded fire occurring in the operating theater was reported during facial surgery. With the use of ether, acetylene, ethylene, and cyclopropane, many more reports followed.[129] The range of flammability of potent inhaled anesthetics used in modern practice is well above the alveolar concentrations that would be applied to patients in clinical practice.

TABLE 40-8

Minimum Flammable Concentrations of Halothane, Enflurane, and Isoflurane

Anesthetic Agent	MFC of Agent in 20% O_2/Remainder N_2O (%)*	MFC of Agent in 30% O_2/Remainder N_2O (%)*
Halothane	3.25	4.75
Enflurane	4.25	5.75
Isoflurane	5.75	7.0

*The minimum flammable concentration (MFC) was determined by igniting each anesthetic in a mixture of 20% or 30% oxygen (O_2), with the remainder composed of nitrous oxide (N_2O).
Adapted from Leonard PF: The lower limits of flammability of halothane, enflurane, and isoflurane. *Anesth Analg* 54:238, 1975.

Leonard,[130] in investigating the lower limits of flammability of halothane, enflurane, and isoflurane, observed that halogenation rendered these compounds less flammable but might not prevent their combustion under all circumstances. He found that it was possible to ignite a mixture of 4.75% halothane in 30% oxygen with the remainder composed of nitrous oxide (Table 40-8). In 20% oxygen with the remainder nitrous oxide, halothane concentrations greater than 3.25% were combustible. In oxygen–nitrous oxide mixtures of 20% and 30% oxygen, enflurane could be ignited at concentrations greater than 4.25% and 5.75%, whereas isoflurane required 5.25% and 7.0%, respectively. These values were obtained under laboratory conditions designed to encourage flammability. A closed combustion vessel was used that contained no water vapor, CO_2, or nitrogen. Ignition was initiated with a 15-kV transformer that delivered a 60-mA current across a 0.25-inch gap. However, because the spark duration was not specified, the total energy delivered could not be calculated. The ignition power used (900 W) was, however, higher than the maximum power output delivered by most electrosurgical equipment. Leonard observed that the energy used in this experiment was much greater than that of a static discharge in the operating room. He concluded that even if the fraction of nitrous oxide administered to the patient exceeds 70%, the lowest flammable concentration of each of the three volatile halogenated anesthetic agents is above that which would be used clinically, except perhaps at the beginning of an inhalation induction.

A study by Pashayan and Gravenstein showed that the addition of 2% halothane to a mixture of 40% oxygen and 60% helium significantly decreased the mean time to combustion of PVC ETT segments that were subjected to CO_2 laser radiation.[126] Ossoff and colleagues found that the addition of 2% halothane significantly retarded the ignition of Rüsch red rubber ETTs in atmospheres of 30%, 40%, and 50% oxygen–balance helium at power settings of 10, 15, and 20 W.[95]

The ratio (3.3) of the percentage of desflurane at the lower limits of flammability in 70% nitrous oxide to the minimum alveolar concentration (6%) is not markedly different from what Leonard reported with enflurane (3.4), halothane (6.3), or isoflurane (6.1).[96,110] Sevoflurane is considered to be nonflammable over the entire anesthetizing concentration range in the presence of air, oxygen, and nitrous oxide.[96,131]

C. American Society of Anesthesiologists Practice Advisory for the Prevention and Management of Operating Room Fires

In 2008, a report by the American Society of Anesthesiologists (ASA) Task Force on operating room fires published a practice advisory for the prevention and management of operating room fires.[1] Practice advisories are systematically developed reports that are intended to assist decision making in areas of patient care.[1] They are based on scientific literature, expert opinion, clinical feasibility data, open forum commentary, and consensus surveys. They are not intended as standards, guidelines, or absolute requirements and can be adopted, modified, or rejected according to clinical needs and constraints.[1] This practice advisory looked at operating room fires, surgical fires, airway fires, and high-risk procedures.

The practice advisory defined an operating room fire as a fire that occurred on or near patients who are under anesthesia care and included surgical fires, airway fires, and fires within the airway circuit. A surgical fire was defined as a fire that occurred on or in a patient. An airway fire was a special type of surgical fire that occurred in a patient's airway and that may or may not include fire in the attached breathing circuit.[1] A procedure was designated as high risk when an ignition source came close to an oxidizer-enriched atmosphere (e.g., tracheostomy, laryngeal surgery).

The task force developed the advisory by a seven-step process that involved consensus on the criteria for evidence; systematic review of originally published, peer-reviewed studies; expert opinions of consultants asked to participate in surveys on the effectiveness of various strategies for fire prevention, detection, and management and comment on a draft of the advisory; comments of active members of the ASA on the advisory; open forum discussions at a major national meeting; survey of consultants on the feasibility of implementing the advisory; and all available information that was used to build consensus within the task force to formulate the advisory statements

The ASA Task Force's primary findings commented on education, operating room fire drills, preparation for every case, and prevention and management of operating room fires. The anesthesiologist should collaborate with all members of the procedure team throughout the procedure to minimize the presence of an oxidizer-enriched atmosphere in proximity to an ignition source.[1]

For all procedures, surgical drapes should be configured to minimize the accumulation of oxidizers (i.e., oxygen and nitrous oxide) under the drapes and to keep them from flowing into the surgical site. Flammable skin prepping solutions should be dry before draping. Gauze and sponges should be moistened before use near an ignition source.[1]

For high-risk procedures, the anesthesiologist should notify the surgeon whenever there is a potential for an ignition source to be in proximity to an oxidizer-enriched atmosphere or when there is an increase in oxidizer concentration at the surgical site. Any reduction in supplied oxygen to the patient should be assessed by monitoring pulse oximetry and, if feasible, inspired, exhaled, and delivered oxygen concentrations.[1]

For laser procedures, a laser-resistant ETT should be used. The laser-resistant ETT used should be chosen to be resistant to the laser used for the procedure (e.g., CO_2, Nd:YAG, argon, erbium:YAG, KTP). The ETT cuff of the laser tube should be filled with saline and colored with an indicator dye such as methylene blue.[1]

Before activating a laser, the surgeon should give the anesthesiologist adequate notice that the laser is about to be activated.[1] The anesthesiologist should reduce the delivered oxygen concentration to the minimum required to avoid hypoxia, stop the use of nitrous oxide, and wait a few minutes after reducing the oxidizer-enriched atmosphere before approving activation of the laser.[1]

For cases involving an ignition source and surgery inside the airway, cuffed tracheal tubes should be used when clinically appropriate.[1] The anesthesiologist should advise the surgeon against entering the trachea with an ignition source (e.g., electrosurgery unit).

Before activating an ignition source inside the airway, the surgeon should give the anesthesiologist adequate notice that the ignition source is about to be activated. The anesthesiologist should reduce the delivered oxygen concentration to the minimum required to avoid hypoxia, stop the use of nitrous oxide, and wait a few minutes after reducing the oxidizer-enriched atmosphere before approving the activation of the ignition source.[1] In some cases (e.g., surgery in the oropharynx), scavenging with suction may be used to reduce oxidizer enrichment in the operative field.[1]

For a fire in the airway or breathing circuit, remove the ETT as fast as possible, stop the flow of all airway gases, remove all flammable and burning materials from the airway, and pour saline or water into the patient's airway.[1] If the airway or breathing circuit fire is extinguished, reestablish ventilation by mask, avoiding supplemental oxygen and nitrous oxide, if possible. Extinguish and examine the ETT to assess whether fragments were left in the airway. Consider bronchoscopy (preferably rigid) to look for ETT fragments, assess the injury, and remove residual debris. Assess the patient's status and devise a plan for ongoing care.[1]

D. Management of an Airway Fire

Many factors must be considered when an airway fire occurs. All operating room personnel must be prepared for the possibility of an airway fire during laser endoscopic surgery. If an airway fire occurs, sterile isotonic saline or water should be immediately available in a 30- or 60-mL syringe. Another laser and PVC ETT should be available. A plan of action should be rehearsed by operating room personnel so that rapid action can be taken if a fire occurs.

Schramm and colleagues discussed immediate management of an airway fire.[132] The management protocol calls for immediate removal of the ETT.[132] Sosis wrote a laser airway fire protocol in which certain steps should be taken simultaneously by the anesthesiologist and

Box 40-1 Laser Airway Fire Protocol
• Cease ventilation and turn off all anesthetic gases, including oxygen.*
• Extinguish flames with a saline solution.*
• Remove endotracheal tube (ETT) after deflating cuff,* and ensure the whole ETT has been removed.
• Ventilate the patient's lungs by mask after all burning material has been removed and extinguished.
• Examine the airway for burns and foreign bodies such as fragments of the ETT or packing materials.

*These steps should be taken simultaneously by the anesthesiologist and surgeon.
Adapted from Sosis MB: *Probl Anesth* 7:160, 1993.

surgeon (Box 40-1).[133] In the event of an airway fire, the protocol calls for immediate cessation of ventilation and turning off of all anesthetic gases, especially oxygen, by disconnecting the hose from the common gas outlet, detaching the ETT from the anesthetic circuit, or clamping the ETT or turning off the flow meters. At the same time, the flames should be extinguished with a sterile saline or water solution. Presuming an easy airway, the protocol calls for the ETT to be removed immediately because it no longer provides an airway and may be on fire. After the ETT has been removed and the fire completely extinguished, the patient's lungs should be ventilated with 100% oxygen by bag and mask.

Chee and Benumof described "a patient scheduled for an elective tracheostomy whose airway evaluation revealed an in situ 8-mm-ID PVC ETT, swollen lips, an edematous tongue protruding out of the mouth and an oropharynx filled with secretions."[134] General anesthesia was induced with 300 mg of intravenous propofol and maintained with 0.4% inspired isoflurane (Forane) and a 35% oxygen-air mixture. The vital signs remained stable. Electrocautery was used for coagulation by the surgeons. The patient was administered 100% oxygen immediately before insertion of the tracheostomy tube. Suddenly, the surgeons reported a blue flame shooting up vertically from the patient's neck. The breathing circuit was disconnected immediately from the ETT, and 20 mL of 0.9% saline was flushed in the ETT. The fire was extinguished promptly. The ETT was not removed because the ability to reintubate was uncertain. Despite a leak around the perforated cuff, the seal was sufficient to generate a peak inspiratory pressure of 20 cm H_2O. Meanwhile, the surgeons were able to insert a tracheostomy tube into the trachea. Fiberoptic bronchoscopy was performed in the operating room and postoperatively revealed generalized upper airway edema consistent with prolonged intubation, no distal airway burn injury, and minimal burn injury to the proximal aspect of the tracheostomy site. The patient experienced no sequelae from the airway fire.

Each patient before laser surgery must be evaluated for risk of possible difficult intubation. If the patient is difficult to intubate or potentially a high risk for difficult intubation and an airway fire occurs, the patient will still be difficult to intubate. In these circumstances, the risk of removing the ETT and not being able to reestablish an airway outweighs the risk of leaving the tube in after the airway fire is extinguished. Van Der Spek and coworkers suggested that if the patient is not easy to intubate,[135] a long stylet can be passed through the existing tube before removing it to facilitate the passage of a new one. Chee and Benomuf also suggested that the ETT can serve as a conduit for a tube exchanger.[134] For reintubation, an airway exchange catheter is placed through the ETT with the assistance of a laryngoscope, if possible, to facilitate the passage of a new ETT over the airway exchange catheter. To minimize the risk of failing to pass an ETT over the airway exchange catheter, the operator can use a relatively small ETT over a relatively large airway exchange catheter. The airway exchange catheter allows ventilation, which allows time for an alternative reintubation strategy, such as a surgical airway or FOB.[136]

After the airway is reestablished, the extent of the airway damage should be assessed. Foreign bodies (e.g., pieces of tube, metal foil, pledgets) should be removed. This may entail fiberoptic bronchoscopy through an ETT or rigid bronchoscopy. Careful clinical judgment must be used to decide whether to extubate. Extensive burns should be managed with controlled ventilation of the lungs through an ETT or tracheostomy. The use of antibiotic and steroids should be considered if burns are severe. All inhaled gasses should be humidified.

V. AIRWAY PATHOLOGY

Patients presenting for laser airway surgery range from young, otherwise fit, and healthy individuals with minor vocal cord lesions with no anticipated airway problems to elderly patients with advanced glottic carcinoma, stridor, and significant airway compromise. An understanding of the different types of pathology seen and the use of lasers for their resection and removal is useful.

1. Nodules are benign lesions of the vocal fold (Fig. 40-27). They can be bilateral and are usually caused by vocal abuse. They can be resected by fine surgical instruments augmented by a laser.
2. Polyps are benign lesions of the vocal fold (Fig. 40-28). They are common in adults, are usually unilateral, and can be resected surgically augmented by a laser.

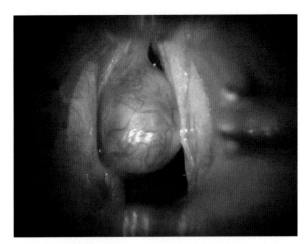

Figure 40-28   Large vocal fold polyp.

3. Cysts are benign lesions of the vocal folds (Fig. 40-29). They are commonly seen in professional voice users. They are caused by obstruction of a glandular duct, resulting in a mucous retention cyst. Surgery involves careful resection and may involve a laser.
4. Granulomas are benign lesions induced by healing granulomatous tissue that develops after microtrauma. They are usually found on the posterior third of the vocal process after trauma during intubation or extubation. Removal involves surgical instruments augmented by a laser.
5. Papillomas of the vocal folds are caused by human papillomavirus infection (Fig. 40-30). Most are benign lesions, but they rarely can undergo malignant transformation. In adults, hoarseness is usually the main symptom, although in severe cases, significant airway compromise with stridor can occur. In children, any airway obstruction has a significant effect on airflow, and near-total airway obstruction can occur. Laser resection usually involves a CO_2 laser, and after surgery, the airway obstruction and airflow are improved. Papillomas can recur, and some patients require repeated laser surgery at 1- to 12-month intervals.

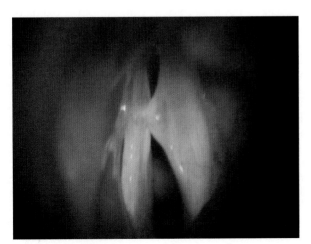

Figure 40-27   Nodule of right vocal fold.

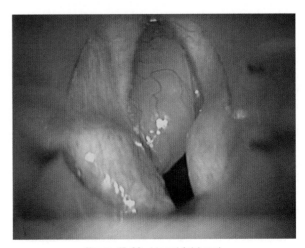

Figure 40-29   Vocal fold cyst.

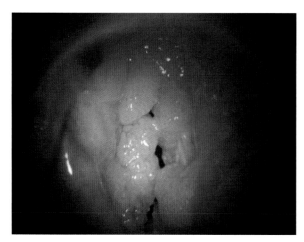

Figure 40-30 Extensive vocal fold papilloma.

6. Malignant tumors of the vocal cord are usually unilateral and occur mainly in the middle third of the vocal fold. Eighty percent are found in men 45 to 65 years old. More than 90% of patients are smokers with a high alcohol intake. Treatment depends on tumor staging and involves local resection, radiotherapy, transoral laser resection, hemilaryngectomy, or laryngectomy.

7. Other lesions on the vocal cord are caused by hemangiomas, submucous hemorrhage, Reinke's edema, chronic laryngitis, amyloidosis, sarcoidosis, tuberculosis, and rheumatoid arthritis. These lesions can be resected by a laser and any subsequent bleeding controlled with a laser.

VI. ANESTHETIC TECHNIQUES FOR LASER AIRWAY SURGERY

A. Laryngeal Mask Airway

The LMA was first described in 1983.[137] It is used in routine anesthetic practice and for management of the difficult airway.[119] The LMA and reinforced flexible laryngeal mask airway (fLMA) have been used for awake and anesthetized patients undergoing fiberoptic bronchoscopy for diagnostic and airway evaluation.[138,139] It has also been used for laser pharyngoplasty.[140] Carinal obstruction was managed using a combination of Nd:YAG laser therapy through a FOB inserted through an LMA and subsequent Nd:YAG through an FOB with a rigid bronchoscope.[141] Other reports described the use of a LMA and high-frequency jet ventilation for resection in tracheal surgery.[142]

The LMA and fLMA are constructed from silicon rubber that contains silica filler, which provides high-temperature resistance and some flame-retardation ability. The same material has been used to manufacture laser-resistant ETTs.[137] Pennant and colleagues did a limited study of the incendiary characteristics of the LMA and fLMA, suggesting that they are resistant to CO_2 lasers at power densities below 1.25 to 2.35 × 10^3 W/cm^2, but 1.2 × 10^4 W/cm^2 produced immediate ignition.[143] Brimacombe looked at the incendiary characteristics of the LMA and fLMA with the CO_2 laser and compared them with two standard PVC ETTs: Mallinckrodt reinforced armored tube and Mallinckrodt RAE tube. Continuous firing led to light smoke production and penetration of the tube in 20 to 30 seconds. Both PVC tubes were penetrated in 0.5 to 2 seconds, and ignition occurred at 2 to 6 seconds with 100% O_2 and 2 to 8 seconds with an O_2-N_2O mixture.[144]

At intermediate power density (4.7 × 10^3 W/cm^2), LMA and fLMA were penetrated at 0.5 to 2 seconds and ignited in 2 to 5 seconds with 100% O_2 and an O_2-N_2O mixture. At the highest power setting (9.8 ×10^3 W/cm^2), all four (i.e., LMA, fLMA, and two PVC ETTs) ignited in 0.05 to 0.1 seconds with 100% O_2. The LMA and fLMA are more resistant to CO_2 laser fire than standard PVC tubing. The CO_2 laser at power densities below 2.35 × 10^3 W/cm^2 appears to be safe with use of the LMA and fLMA.

Pandit and colleagues showed that at laser outputs and distances of the KTP fiber tip from the fLMA normally encountered in clinical practice, the fLMA was not penetrated or ignited.[145] Keller and associates looked at the standard LMA (silicon based) and fLMA (silicon based with metal wire) and at a disposable LMA (PVC based) and intubating LMA (silicon and steel based) and PVC-based ETTs using KTP and Nd:YAG lasers at two power densities used commonly in airway surgery (570 and 1140 W/cm^2).[146] Each airway device was fixed to a table in room air and attached to a closed-circuit breathing system with 30% oxygen in air delivered at 3 L/min. The laser was fired at the same distance of 3 mm. They also evaluated the marked and unmarked parts of the airway device and the unmarked device after application of 0.1 mL of unclotted fresh human blood. They evaluated the cuff with air or undiluted methylene blue dye.

There was no ignition of any airway device. The impact sites of the silicon-based LMA for both lasers revealed a layer of silica ash just like that found by Pandit and colleagues. The silicon-based tubes were less easily penetrated than the PVC-based tubes, except for the intubating LMA, which flared sooner than with the KTP laser at both densities. The disposable LMA cuff was more resistant to penetration than the silicon LMA cuff or PVC ETT. The cuffs filled with air were penetrated more rapidly than those with methylene blue.[99]

Pandit and Keller and their colleagues showed that the cuff was more vulnerable to a laser strike with the CO_2 and KTP lasers, especially when filled with air. Pandit filled the cuff with saline, and Keller filled the cuff with nondilute methylene blue, and both found increased resistance to the laser strike. The disadvantage of using saline in the cuff is that the manufacturers recommend filling the cuff only with air. It has been reported that if not all the saline is withdrawn from the cuff after use in the standard reusable LMA, the cuff may rupture during autoclaving.[147,148] Coorey and colleagues reported a technique in which they were able to empty the saline-inflated LMA reliably by a syringe without the plunger with the cuff held above the syringe to facilitate gravitational drainage. The cuff was then manually squeezed. The LMA with the syringe barrel attached was placed in a warming cupboard at 60° C for 12 hours. They found that filling the LMA cuff with saline was a viable option for laser airway surgery.[149]

The other option is the disposable LMA, for which filling the cuff with saline is not a concern because it is used only one time. The only concern is that the disposable LMA shaft is more easily penetrated than the silicon-based LMA, but the disposable LMA cuff was more resistant to penetration than the silicon-based LMA or PVC ETT cuffs. When filled with methylene blue dye and with the Nd:YAG laser power density at 570 W/cm^2, none of the cuffs was affected after 30 seconds.[146]

B. Management of Anesthesia

Operations on the airway are unique in that the surgeon and anesthesiologist are working in the same area. This can be challenging, and the anesthesiologist has to allow the surgeon adequate exposure to any lesions within the airway and at the same time oxygenate the patient, remove CO_2, maintain anesthesia, prevent soiling of the tracheobronchial tree, and maintain safe conditions and prevent an airway fire.

An ideal laser airway technique would be simple to use; provide complete control of the airway with no risk of aspiration; control ventilation with adequate oxygenation and CO_2 removal; provide smooth induction and maintenance of anesthesia, provide a clear and motionless surgical field that is free of secretions; not impose time restrictions on the surgeon; not be associated with the risk of airway fire or cardiovascular instability; allow safe emergence with no coughing, bucking, breath holding or laryngospasm; produce a pain-free, comfortable, alert patient at the end of the operation; and be laser proof.

The ideal technique does not exist, and some of these ideal conditions conflict. The presence of a cuffed ETT provides control of the airway and prevents aspiration but may obscure a glottic lesion and is not laser safe. A cuffed laser tube provides some protection against laser-induced airway fires but has a greater external-to-internal diameter ratio and may obscure laryngeal lesions. Jet ventilation techniques require specialist equipment and knowledge and an understanding of their limitations, and they do not protect the airway from soiling.

Safe laser airway surgery requires an understanding of the airway pathology, its location within the airway, the type of laser used, the surgical requirements, and the patient's comorbidities. It is essential that careful communication and cooperation between anesthesiologist and surgeon takes place before, during, and after any procedure.

During laser airway surgery, Rontal and colleagues used a video monitor during all laser endoscopic procedures so that the entire operating room team could observe the procedure.[150] The use of a video monitor to observe the impact of the laser beam on tissues in shared airway procedures is used by many surgical units and allows the operating room nurses to anticipate the surgeons' needs and the anesthesiologist to communicate better, adjust the anesthesia accordingly, and act quickly if there is an airway fire (Fig. 40-31). Without a video monitor, only the surgeon can see the surgical site and the impact of the laser beam; vital seconds may be lost

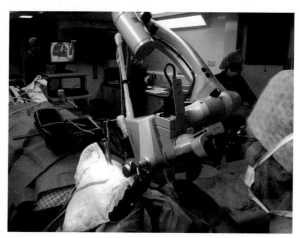

Figure 40-31 Video monitor allows all operating room staff to observe the procedure.

before the team recognizes an airway fire is happening, but it would have been obvious on a monitor screen. The presence of a video monitor has no disadvantage, but its absence may be detrimental, and some units regard it as a standard requirement for shared laser airway surgery.

1. Preoperative Evaluation

The preoperative evaluation attempts to identify factors that may cause difficulty during the perioperative course and involves assessment with a thorough medical evaluation for all patients coming to surgery. Laser airway surgery is carried out on a wide spectrum of patients and airway pathologies. Some patients are young, fit, and healthy with no airway compromise and require laser removal of minor airway lesions. At the other end of the spectrum, some patients have significant tobacco and alcohol intake, cardiovascular and respiratory dysfunction, and large obstructing tumors of the airway. Laser airway surgery for cancer patients is often palliative and can be a high-risk procedure when patients present in a suboptimal state with nutritional and metabolic derangements and limited time for correction before the airway deteriorates. Optimizing nutritional, metabolic, cardiovascular, and respiratory parameters is the aim before any surgery, but in cases of critical airway obstruction, this may not be possible, and the anesthesiologist, surgeon, patient, and relatives need to be aware of and accept the increased risks.

At the end of the preoperative assessment, the anesthesiologist should have some idea of the size, mobility, and location of the lesion. Standard airway assessments to predict the ease of ventilation, visualization of the laryngeal inlet, and tracheal intubation should be performed. Airway pathology and its impact on airway management should be assessed. The severity and size of lesions at the glottic level are assessed by direct or indirect laryngoscopy, undertaken by surgeons in an outpatient setting, and a photograph or image of the findings is often added to the record. Information about subglottic and tracheal lesions is provided by chest radiography, computed tomography (CT), and magnetic resonance imaging (MRI). The size of the lesion gives an indication of potential airflow obstruction. Stridor indicates a

1. History of endoscopic procedures, previous difficulties, medical record, and chosen technique
2. Hoarse voice: occurs with minor vocal fold lesions and significant pathology
3. Voice changes: nonspecific symptom
4. Dysphagia: significant
5. Altered breathing position: significant
6. Inability to lie flat: significant
7. Difficulty breathing during sleep: significant
8. Stridor: significant
9. Stridor on exertion: suggests obstruction becoming critical
10. Stridor at rest: indicates critical airway obstruction
11. Inspiratory stridor: suggests extrathoracic airway obstruction
12. Expiratory stridor: suggests intrathoracic airway obstruction

significantly narrowed airway. In the adult, stridor implies an airway diameter of less than 4 to 5 mm, but the absence of stridor does not exclude a significantly narrowed airway (Box 40-2).

Very mobile lesions (e.g., multiple, large vocal cord polyps, papillomas) may cause partial airway obstruction after induction of anesthesia, but total airway obstruction is extremely uncommon. Airway obstruction is worse with a spontaneously breathing patient after induction of anesthesia because of the loss of supporting tone in the oropharynx and hypopharynx.

Supraglottic lesions, if mobile, can obstruct the airway or make visualization of the laryngeal inlet difficult. Subglottic lesions may allow a good view of the laryngeal inlet but cause difficulty during the passage of an ETT.

The recognition of a compromised or anatomically distorted upper airway is paramount in the preoperative assessment of these patients. For elective procedures, a detailed history, examination, and other investigations should be undertaken, but for more urgent procedures with severe airway compromise, investigations may not be possible. Patients' old anesthesia records should be available to obtain the history of prior intubations. The major concerns are as follows:

1. Airway or head and neck problems: The anesthesiologist should know the underlying pathology of the lesion, anatomic characteristics, and severity of obstruction. An extensive evaluation of the degree of airway obstruction should be undertaken. A history should be obtained of signs of airway obstruction possibly related to edema or tumor, such as obstructive sleep apnea, difficulty breathing, difficulty swallowing, shortness of breath, snoring, stridor, wheezing, or difficulty clearing secretions. The airway should be examined for the Mallampati classification, mouth opening, prognathia, size of the tongue, neck range of motion, prominent teeth, and tracheal deviation from external compression. The precise location and extent of the tumor should be defined by chest radiography, CT, and MRI.[151] However, the patient's general condition may preclude obtaining imaging. The test results should be reviewed for the luminal size of the trachea and tracheobronchial obstruction. These studies should include chest radiography (i.e., anteroposterior and lateral for possible pulmonary collapse and consolidation, presence of air-filled lung bullae, or pneumothorax), CT or MRI, flow-volume loops, and barium swallow.

2. Respiratory problems: The concerns are upper airway obstruction and coexisting pulmonary problems, such as a history of chronic obstructive pulmonary disease, emphysema, or newly diagnosed asthma; wheezing; and decreased exercise tolerance. Whether the patient requires home oxygen should be determined. Physical examination includes auscultation of the lungs for wheezing or decreased breath sounds and looking for clubbing or cyanosis. The examiner should review the chest radiograph, percent of oxygen saturation, baseline arterial blood gas determination, flow-volume loop, and pulmonary function tests to determine the amount of pulmonary reserve and involvement of the extrabronchial structures.

3. Cardiovascular problems: The concerns are related to potential cardioarterial disease. History of chest pain, shortness of breath with exertion, decreased exercise tolerance, and previous myocardial infarction or congestive heart failure are of interest. Examination includes auscultation of the heart for rate, rhythm, and heart murmurs and assessment of the lungs for rales. The examiner should look for jugular venous distention, for congestive heart failure, and for possible subclavian venous occlusion due to the tumor. Tests that may be needed are a 12-lead electrocardiogram, cardiac echocardiogram, dipyridamole (Persantine) thallium, and exercise stress test.

4. Other system problems: The gastrointestinal system should be assessed for aspiration potentials, such as hiatal hernia, acid reflux, nighttime cough, and obesity. Routine blood work should be done unless otherwise indicated.

The patient's physical status should be optimized before surgery. Many airway procedures can cause sustained hypertension and tachycardia, both of which stress the cardiovascular system. Patients should receive nothing by mouth according to the ASA recommendation or hospital policy.

2. Premedication

Premedication to reduce secretions and anxiety may be useful in patients with minor airway lesions but should be avoided in patients with severe airway compromise. An antisialagogue to minimize oral and tracheobronchial secretions may be given: 0.2 mg of glycopyrrolate intravenously or 0.4 mg intramuscularly or 0.4 to 0.5 mg of atropine subcutaneously or intramuscularly. Caution should be taken if the patient has difficulty mobilizing secretions because the antisialagogue thickens pulmonary secretions. Thick secretions may block narrowed airways further, may be difficult to cough out by the patient, and may in extreme circumstances totally obstruct critically narrowed airways.

Any premedications given to patients should be given in the holding area of the operating room, where they can be monitored. During the preoperative visit, the anesthesiologist should attempt to allay the patient's fears. For patients with moderate obstruction, decreasing anxiety may be beneficial because quieter breathing results in decreased airway resistance. For patients with severely narrowed airways, respiratory depression must be avoided. Careful deliberation is needed before giving any anxiolytic or opioids or combination thereof, which can act synergistically in producing respiratory depression. Midazolam (0.5 to 1 mg intravenously, with repeated doses) may be given for anxiolysis but not for critically obstructed airways because a significant risk of total airway obstruction exists.

Patients should be monitored with a three- or five-lead electrocardiogram, depending on the cardiac history, pulse oximetry, capnography, oxygen analyzer, precordial stethoscope, peripheral nerve stimulator, and noninvasive blood pressure cuff. An invasive arterial blood pressure line should be considered for patients with cardiovascular instability to monitor closely hemodynamic changes and arterial blood gases intraoperatively.[152]

A difficult airway cart should be in the room that contains a complement of airway equipment and local anesthetics for topicalization. Airway equipment that should be available includes different laryngoscopes, oral and nasal airways, LMA, intubating LMA, fiberoptic scope, retrograde and cricothyrotomy kits, and jet ventilation. A rigid bronchoscopy and tracheostomy tray should also be in the room.

3. Induction and Maintenance of Anesthesia

a. GENERAL ANESTHESIA

The technique for induction and maintenance of general anesthesia for laser airway surgery is determined by the general condition of the patient, the location and size of the lesion, the planned surgical procedure, and most importantly, the degree of airway compromise. All patients with airway compromise should be considered as a possible difficult intubation, whereas not all patients with a difficult intubation have airway compromise.

When airway compromise is not an issue, most procedures are routine and uneventful with the use of most standard induction techniques. An intravenous induction technique is suitable for most benign and early malignant glottic lesions when airway obstruction is not present or anticipated. After intravenous induction of anesthesia and administration of neuromuscular blockade appropriate to the length of surgery, laryngoscopy is undertaken to visualize the larynx, establish laryngoscopy grade, and administer a local anesthetic. Confirmation of pathology is important because the disease may have progressed and the anesthesia plan may have to change.

When airway compromise is an issue, traditional teaching suggests any technique that uses inhalational induction and maintains spontaneous ventilation is safest in the presence of airway obstruction.[111,114] Spontaneous breathing has traditionally been thought of as critical with

intrathoracic obstructive lesions of the large airways. During spontaneous breathing, large airways are stented open during inspiration by the negative intrathoracic pressure that is generated. This permits some inspired tidal volume to get past the obstruction. When the chest wall expands during inspiration, the negative pressure generated is beneficial in preventing collapse of the tumor mass onto the large airways and vessels. These two safeguards are removed when spontaneous ventilation ceases.

Traditional teaching for inhalational induction and maintenance of spontaneous ventilation in obstructed airways has been questioned. Inhalational induction for advanced laryngeal tumors with airway obstruction is difficult and challenging. Physiologic problems include a reduction in airflow with spontaneous ventilation, an increased collapsibility of the airway, increased work of breathing, critical instability at points of narrowing leading to further airway collapse, and a reduction in functional residual capacity.[113] Induction is slow with apneic periods, and episodes of obstruction are common. Controversy exists about the suitability of "taking over" the patient's own spontaneous ventilation with bag-mask ventilation. The advantage of retaining spontaneous ventilation throughout is the theoretical inherent advantage of this technique. However, taking over ventilation allows a suitable depth of anesthesia for laryngoscopy to be achieved quicker. This avoids the long periods of spontaenous ventilation while waiting for an adequate depth of anesthesia, during which the patient may become unstable.

Traditional teaching advices caution if muscle relaxants are used. The airway can collapse with loss of muscle tone, and this may not be overcome by positive-pressure ventilation, resulting in total loss of the airway. Traditional teaching advises that before abolishing the ability to breathe spontaneously by administering a muscle relaxant or inducing a deep plane of anesthesia, it is prudent to establish that patients can be ventilated with positive pressure by face mask.

The administration of a muscle relaxant provides optimal ventilation and intubating conditions. Calder and Yentis commented on the perceived safe practice of not giving muscle relaxants until face mask ventilation has been documented and argued the theoretical advantage is not fulfilled in practice.[153] They considered two studies and looked at the incidence and prediction of difficult and impossible mask ventilation in which no patient was awakened and suggested that when a patient has an obstructed airway,[154,155] it was not feasible to await awakening and something had to be done to ventilate the lungs before catastrophic desaturation occurred.[153]

General anesthesia is used in pediatric patients. In small children with airway obstruction, attempting bronchoscopic procedures with sedation alone is not recommended. General anesthesia using inhalation agents allows better airway control and permits the operator to concentrate on the procedure.[156] In a retrospective review of pediatric patients undergoing diagnostic bronchoscopic procedures in the intensive care unit with sedation, ketamine was associated with a 20% rate of adverse reactions. Complications were mostly in children younger than 3 years with severe underlying disease.[157]

A tubeless spontaneous respiration technique has been used for pediatric microlaryngeal surgery. It allows an unrestricted view and surgical access to the larynx. This can be accomplished by delivering inhalation agents proximal to the larynx or by using propofol. Halothane (0% to 5% at 4 to 10 L/min) is delivered by the suction channel of the microlaryngoscope. Propofol (2 mg/kg) as a bolus is followed by an infusion of 100 µg/kg/min. In pediatric microsurgery, satisfactory results were obtained in two groups of children using halothane or propofol.[158]

General anesthesia is preferred in most adults to the same extent. Airway control that is possible with general anesthesia is fundamental in situations of airway obstruction and severe respiratory distress. There is better control of the airway and easier clearance of blood and mucus with use of a rigid bronchoscope.[159] For the insertion of a rigid bronchoscope, general anesthesia is necessary.

Rigid bronchoscopy can be performed in a spontaneously breathing patient using an inhalation technique. This technique requires experience, particularly in the presence of significant airway obstruction. A deep plane of anesthesia is needed to prevent coughing. Laryngospasm or bronchospasm can complicate induction if the instrumentation is attempted too hastily. This can disastrously worsen the situation, causing total airway obstruction resulting in hypoxemia, hypotension, and trauma to the trachea. Because the uptake of any inhalation agent is delayed by airway obstruction, induction times are always longer than usual. Sufficient time must be spent making sure that the patient is "deep enough" for intubation. Judging the appropriate depth of anesthesia is often difficult. Excess anesthesia may result in hypoventilation in a spontaneously breathing patient.[160] Caution should be exercised in monitoring the patient when using inhalation agents at such critical periods. The concentration required for an adequate depth of anesthesia to permit instrumentation of the trachea may not be tolerated by the cardiovascular system, causing hypotension and hemodynamic instability. Consequently, the margin of safety for inhalation agents may be very narrow. This is especially true in infants and in elderly patients. In children, sevoflurane seems to cause fewer complications, such as dysrhythmias and laryngospasm, than halothane.

Patients with significant tracheal obstruction benefit from sitting up and receiving supplementary humidified oxygen. A coughing spell may critically exacerbate the obstruction and should be avoided. In the operating room glycopyrrolate (0.2 to 0.3 mg) may be helpful in controlling secretions, and midazolam (2 to 4 mg intravenously) may be used for sedation. If an inhalation induction is chosen, the patient is preoxygenated with 100% oxygen, gradually induced with sevoflurane, and allowed to breathe spontaneously. For total intravenous anesthesia, the patient is induced with a sleep bolus of 2 mg/kg of propofol followed by a propofol infusion of 100 to 150 µg/kg/min. Before administering a muscle relaxant, it has traditionally been thought prudent to establish the ability to ventilate the patient by positive pressure through a face mask, although this approach has been questioned.[153] Positive-pressure ventilation may become impossible in the presence of certain large lesions in the airway. Urgent measures are necessary when the situation deteriorates to acute central airway obstruction. An ETT may be inserted to bypass the obstruction. Positive-pressure ventilation and suctioning may not be enough in certain situations. Rigid bronchoscopy may be required urgently to force the tube and establish an airway under direct vision.[161]

Muscle relaxation is often necessary to hold a quiescent surgical field for laser excisions. Medium- or short-acting muscle relaxants are preferred. Mivacurium (0.2 to 0.25 mg/kg intubating dose, 3 to 15 µg/kg/min infusion), rocuronium (0.6 mg/kg), and cisatracurium (0.15 to 0.25 mg/kg) have been used. Anesthesia can be supplemented with fentanyl (bolus dose of 2 to 15 µg/kg, maintained at an infusion rate of 0.03 to 0.1 µg/kg/min) or remifentanil (bolus dose of 0.5 to 1 µg/kg, maintained at an infusion rate of 0.1 to 0.4 µg/kg/min).

b. SEDATION AND TOPICAL ANESTHESIA

Selected adult populations undergoing flexible fiberoptic laser excision can be managed by experienced individuals with sedation and topical anesthesia. Topical anesthesia with sedation is suitable for adults who are cooperative and for a short endoscopy period with a flexible bronchoscope. This is a favored method for lesions in the middle or lower third of the trachea. Complications are rare. Bleeding seems the most life-threatening complication.[162]

Sedative drugs can decrease ventilation and should be used judiciously in small children and elderly patients. Two distinct mechanisms are accountable for this reduction: decreased respiratory drive and upper airway obstruction. Sedatives alter normal respiratory responses to hypercarbia and hypoxia, thereby decreasing the respiratory drive. Brief hypercarbia and acidosis that may develop under these circumstances are ordinarily inconsequential. However, airway obstruction is a real and more dangerous outcome of sedation because it can quickly lead to oxygen desaturation. Hypoxemia from airway obstruction can have devastating consequences.[163] The exact mechanism of upper airway obstruction during sedation or anesthesia is not clear. It may be caused by decreased muscular tone and increased collapsibility of the upper airway. Midazolam induces upper airway obstruction during deep sedation. Flumazenil relieves this obstruction in addition to reversing the sedative effects of midazolam.[71]

Introduction of additional obstruction to a patient with an airway that is already narrowed by a fixed lesion is fraught with danger. A perilous scenario can ensue, with progressively increasing obstruction resulting in total loss of the airway. Prompt measures must be undertaken to relieve the obstruction. They include asking the patient to take deep breaths, jaw thrust, chin lift, and insertion of an oral or a nasal airway. Chin lift or jaw thrust may not always relieve the obstruction. However, when these two maneuvers are combined with positive airway pressure, the pharyngeal airway is widened, counteracting airway narrowing.[164] If a procedure being performed under sedation becomes prolonged, additional, unplanned drugs have to be administered, increasing the risk of excessive intraoperative sedation and of postoperative somnolence.

VII. ANESTHESIA MANAGEMENT FOR LARYNGEAL LASER SURGERY

Many laryngeal lesions are resected and removed with the aid of a laser, including papillomas, vocal cord cysts, vocal cord polyps, Reinke's edema, vocal cord granulomas, vocal cord microwebs, and scar tissue after intubation. For most of these lesions, airway obstruction is not significant, and several anesthesia techniques are appropriate. It is important that the preoperative assessment identifies the type and size of laryngeal lesion to establish the extent of airway compromise and establishes the general medical status of the patient. The exact anesthesia technique chosen is determined by the experience of the anesthesiologist, surgical preference and access, equipment available, type of laser used, duration of the procedure, type and vascularity of the lesion, and protection against airway soiling from blood and secretions. Two approaches are used: closed systems, in which a cuffed laser tracheal tube is used, and open systems, in which a cuffed laser tracheal tube is absent. Open systems use spontaneous ventilation or jet ventilation techniques.

The technique chosen for a procedure is not absolute and may have to change as surgical and anesthesia requirements change. For example, an open system using jet ventilation on a lesion thought to be relatively avascular may change to a closed system employing a cuffed laser tube if the lesion is bleeding and there is a risk of soiling the tracheobronchial tree. Conversely, a system employing a cuffed laser tube may have to change during surgery to an open system if the laser tube overlies a lesion, making surgery very difficult or impossible.

A. Laser Tube

Closed systems are familiar to all anesthesiologists and involve the placement of a laser tube. The different types of laser tubes and their relative laser-resistant properties have been discussed. Placement of laser tubes is routine, although care should be taken to prevent traumatizing the laryngeal lesion as the laser tube is passed through the glottis and into the trachea. After the laser tube is in position and the cuff inflated, there is protection of the lower airway from blood and secretions. Routine control of the airway and ventilation are established, and because the system is closed, there is little danger of pollution of oxygen or volatile agents unless the cuff is compromised. It is important to appreciate immediately any cuff compromise due to a laser strike because it causes oxygen and volatile agent leaks around the laser tube, increasing the fire risk. All laser tubes have a greater outer diameter for any given internal diameter because of their laser-resistant coverings, and this may limit surgical access and visualization of laryngeal lesions. Because the surgeon requires adequate exposure, small laser tubes usually are placed, which can lead to higher inflation pressures.

B. Spontaneous Ventilation and Insufflation Techniques

Open systems can be used during anesthesia for laser procedures on the vocal cords, and spontaneous ventilation techniques have been used in adults and in children. Spontaneous ventilation techniques with insufflation are particularly suitable for infants and children in whom it is not possible to pass a tube past a lesion or when a laser tube obscures the lesion.

Spontaneous ventilation and insufflation techniques are useful in the removal of foreign bodies, evaluation of airway dynamics (e.g., tracheomalacia), and laser airway surgery. The technique requires a spontaneously breathing patient and provides a clear view of an unobstructed glottis. Insufflation of anesthetic gases and agents can be achieved by several routes: a small catheter introduced into the nasopharynx and placed immediately above the laryngeal opening; a tracheal tube cut short and placed through the nasopharynx, emerging just beyond the soft palate; a nasopharyngeal airway; and the side arm or channel of a laryngoscope or bronchoscope.

The absence of any fuel source (e.g., tube) within the airway makes this a laser-safe procedure for laryngeal lesions. However, great care must be taken to prevent the catheter or nasopharyngeal airway from getting very close to or entering the larynx. This would provide a fuel source that could easily cause an airway fire if struck by a laser beam. If the catheter is inadvertently inserted too far, it may enter the esophagus, causing marked gastric distention and possible regurgitation.

Inhalational induction may be commenced with sevoflurane in 100% oxygen. At a suitable depth of anesthesia, as assessed by clinical observations of the rate and depth of respiration, pupil size, eye reflexes, blood pressure, and heart rate changes, laryngoscopy is undertaken and topical lidocaine administered above, below, and at the level of the vocal cords. One hundred percent oxygen is administered by face mask with spontaneous ventilation and anesthesia continued with inhalational (insufflation) or an intravenous route (propofol infusion). At a suitable depth of anesthesia assessed by clinical observations, the surgeon undertakes rigid laryngoscopy or bronchoscopy.

Movements of the vocal cords are usually minimal with a spontaneously breathing technique, provided an adequate level of anesthesia is maintained. If the depth of anesthesia is too light, the vocal cords may move, the patient may cough, or laryngospasm may occur. If the depth of anesthesia is too great, the patient may become apneic with cardiovascular instability. Careful observation throughout the procedure, observing movements, respiratory rate and depth, cardiovascular stability, and unobstructed breathing, is vital, with the concentration of the volatile anesthetic adjusted accordingly. The insufflation technique requires close cooperation between the anesthesiologist and the surgeon.

The limitations of spontaneous ventilation or insufflation techniques include the lack of control over ventilation and the potential for airway soiling. Operating room pollution due to insufflation of volatile agents is also an issue and requires high-intensity suction catheters near the mouth (see Fig. 40-14). Insufflation techniques may not be suitable for large, soft, floppy lesions, particularly in the supraglottis or glottis, which may obstruct the airway after the onset of general anesthesia with spontaneous ventilation.

Rita and associates used the CO_2 laser successfully to excise subglottic stenosis in infants,[165] avoiding a tracheostomy, and reported that ETTs of any size in this group make surgery in infants difficult or impossible because the operative field is obstructed. They reported that in some infants with subglottic stenosis, even a 2.5-mm-ID ETT, was difficult to pass through the stenotic area. Rita and associates concluded that although the insufflation technique is potentially hazardous,[165] if it is done correctly, it provides an appropriate anesthetic technique for surgery on the larynx of infants.[166] They reported good results with this technique over the course of many years.

C. Intermittent Apneic Technique

Weisberger and Miner described the use of an intermittent apneic technique for laser laryngeal surgery in the resection of juvenile papillomatosis of the larynx without the use of an ETT.[167] The investigators stated that a clear, unobstructed view of the airway and complete immobility of the surgical field were essential for the surgeon during these cases (see Fig. 40-30). During a 2-year period, 51 procedures were performed by the investigators on nine patients who had juvenile laryngeal papillomatosis. Their average age was 10.5 years (range, 3.5 to 37 years). After induction of general anesthesia, the patients were paralyzed with atracurium or vecuronium and anesthesia maintained with halothane or enflurane in 100% oxygen. The patients' tracheas were intubated with small-caliber ETTs wrapped with foil tape. In cases of extensive papillomatosis, resection was started with the ETT in situ while the patients' lungs were ventilated with 40% oxygen. Otherwise, the ETTs were removed and the surgery started. The surgery was interrupted when the oxygen saturation decreased. The patients' tracheas were then reintubated, and they were hyperventilated with 100% oxygen. This resulted in a rapid rise in the oxygen saturation so that repeated extubations and surgery could continue. The median number of apneic episodes required for each procedure was two, with a range of one to five. The duration of apneic episodes was 2.6 minutes, with a range of 1 to 4.5 minutes. A suspension laryngoscope and microscope, which provided excellent visualization of the larynx, were used in these cases so that endotracheal intubation could be readily accomplished without moving the laryngoscope. The apneic technique removes all the flammable material from the larynx during laser actuation and is thought to decrease greatly the possibility of an airway fire. Weisberger and Miner stated that the apneic period should be shortened for small children because of their decreased functional residual capacity.[167] The technique is contraindicated in patients in whom visualization of the larynx is difficult.

D. Jet Ventilation Techniques

Jet ventilation techniques are suitable for ventilation during laser surgery of most adult vocal cord lesions. The main limitation for their use is the experience of the anesthesiologist and the absence of suitable equipment. Jet ventilation techniques involve the intermittent administration of high-pressure jets of air, oxygen, or oxygen-air mixtures that entrain room air and lower the delivered pressures. The risk of life-threatening barotrauma is the most serious complication, and it occurs when entrainment of room air is absent. This results in the delivery of very high driving pressures, leading to pneumomediastinum, pneumothorax, and surgical emphysema.[168-170]

In 1967, Sanders first described a jet ventilation technique using a 16-gauge, high-pressure source (jet) placed down the side arm of a rigid open bronchoscope.[171] Sanders used intermittent manual ventilation with a rate of 8 L/min and a driving pressure of 700 torr to entrain room air and showed the technique could maintain supranormal oxygen pressure and prevent a rise in the CO_2 partial pressure. Since 1967, modifications to Sanders' original jet ventilation technique have been made for endoscopic airway surgery. These modifications include frequency of ventilation (i.e., low-frequency, high-frequency, or superimposed frequency jet ventilation) and the site at which the jet emerges in the airway (i.e., supraglottic, subglottic, or transtracheal).

The frequency of ventilation and the location of the jet cannula should be selected according to the degree of airway obstruction and the location of the lesion. Specially designed catheters, laryngoscopes, bronchoscopes, and ventilators are available for the clinician to choose from. Many techniques have been described, claiming different advantages over the other methods.

There is no clear consensus about the ideal ventilation modes or the laser techniques. Selection must be done on the basis of a thorough understanding of the pathophysiology of airway obstruction and individual experience with use of these devices. Hunsaker introduced a laser-safe subglottic monojet ventilation tube.[109,172]

High jet pressure increases the risk of subcutaneous emphysema related to facial plane dissection in the neck, especially when there is disruption of the mucous membrane during surgery. If mucosal disruption is noticed, the jetting catheter should be positioned away from the mucosal opening because pressure drops rapidly with the distance from the jetting orifice. Because there is no ETT to protect the airway, vomitus, blood, smoke, or debris and seeding of papillomas down the tracheobronchial tree can occur. There is a possibility of polluting the operating room with infectious agents or the anesthetic gases. Mucosal dehydration and inspissated secretions can result from dry jetting gases. End-tidal CO_2 cannot be easily measured. Volatile agents cannot be used, and scavenging of gases is required.

1. Site of Jet Delivery

a. SUPRAGLOTTIC JET VENTILATION

Supraglottic jet ventilation describes a technique in which the jet of gas emerges in the supraglottis by attachment of a jetting needle to the rigid surgical suspension laryngoscope. High- or low-frequency ventilation can be used. Supraglottic jet ventilation techniques allow a clear, unobstructed view for the surgeon with no risk of a laser

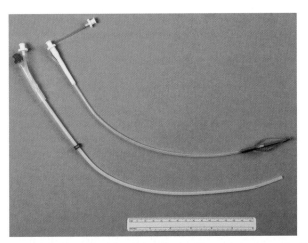

Figure 40-32   Hunsaker Mon-Jet catheter (Xomed, Jacksonville, FL) and Acutronic subglottic catheter for jet ventilation (Acutronic Medical Systems, Hirzel, Switzerland). The green basket of the Hunsaker catheter reduces catheter tip movement within the trachea.

airway fire. However, if the surgeon places surgical swabs into the operating field, there is a risk of an airway fire with the swab acting as a fuel source.

Supraglottic techniques have limitations: misalignment of the suspension laryngoscope to the glottic inlet, which results in poor ventilation and the risk of gastric distention with entrained air; blood, smoke, and debris blown into the distal trachea; considerable vibration and movement of the vocal cords, which may require ventilation to be stopped whilst operating; inability to monitor end-tidal CO_2 concentration; and risk of barotrauma with pneumomediastinum, pneumothorax, and subcutaneous emphysema.

b. SUBGLOTTIC JET VENTILATION

Subglottic jet ventilation involves placing a small (2 to 3 mm external diameter) catheter or specifically designed tubes (e.g., Benjet, Hunsaker, Acutronic, Carl Reiner) through the glottis and into the trachea, which allows delivery of a jet of gas directly into the trachea (Fig. 40-32). This means a fuel source is present within the airway, and care must be taken during laser airway surgery. Many of the subglottic catheters that are commercially

available have some laser-resistant properties, but if their tolerance is exceeded, the catheters can degrade and fracture. If after a fracture of the catheter and after a laser strike, jet ventilation is resumed, the distal fragment may be forced into the distal airways. Some catheters (e.g., Hunsaker) have metal wires within the catheter to reduce the chances of this distal fragmentation.

Subglottic jet ventilation is more efficient than supraglottic jet ventilation and results in reduced driving pressures, minimal vocal cord movements, a good surgical field, and no time constraints for the surgeon in the placement of the rigid laryngoscope. The main disadvantage is the potential for a laser-induced airway fire due to the presence of a potential fuel source within the airway and a greater risk of barotrauma than in supraglottic jet techniques (Fig. 40-33).

c. TRANSTRACHEAL JET VENTILATION

Elective transtracheal catheter placement under local anesthesia in individuals with significant airway pathology or under general anesthesia for elective laryngeal surgery has been described.[173] Transtracheal jet techniques carry the greatest risks of barotrauma. Other potential problems include blockage, kinking, infection, bleeding, and failure to site the catheter. None of the commercially available transtracheal catheters is specifically designed for laser use, and transtracheal jet ventilation techniques for endoscopic laser surgery of the larynx require a careful evaluation of the potential risks and benefits.

2. Jet Ventilation Frequency

a. LOW-FREQUENCY JET VENTILATION

Low-frequency ventilation typically describes ventilatory rates of less than 60 breaths/min (1 Hz), and in practice, most low-frequency ventilation is accomplished by a manual Sanders-type device at rates of 15 to 25 breaths/min. With sufficient driving pressures, this leads to near-normal tidal volumes, visible chest inflation, and passive chest deflation. A metal jet needle or cannula is positioned inside a laryngoscope or a rigid bronchoscope and is connected to a source of oxygen. To prevent barotrauma, a reducing valve and a pressure regulator should

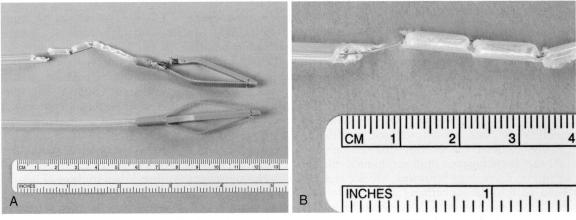

Figure 40-33   **A,** Hunsaker Mon-Jet catheter after it sustained a high-power CO_2 laser strike in 100% oxygen. **B,** The internal stainless steel wire prevented fragmentation.

be in line so that the oxygen pressure is limited to 50 psi for adults. In children, extreme caution should be used. The anesthesiologist should start with much lower values and gradually increase the pressure while observing the chest movements. Holding down the handheld lever controls the duration and frequency of the jet of oxygen. The actual delivered tidal volume, concentration of oxygen, and inspiratory pressures depend on the amount of air entrainment by the jet, length of the cannula and its alignment to the trachea, size of the laryngoscope, and lung compliance. These factors are hard to measure in a clinical situation with any great precision and at best are estimates. Adequate ventilation is accomplished in most patients who are anesthetized and given muscle relaxants.

The minimal possible pressure that can provide adequate ventilation should be used. The Venturi jet must be kept in perfect alignment with the trachea to achieve streaming of the flow into the lungs. Anesthesiologists should be watchful after any readjustment of the operating laryngoscope to which the jet is clamped, which may impair ventilation of the lungs. Oxygen saturation must be constantly monitored and chest movement continually observed.

During supraglottic jet ventilation, there is considerable movement of the laryngeal structures, and the timing of each breath can be coordinated with the surgeon operating the laser. Even small movements are magnified under the operating microscope. This movement is much less of an issue with subglottic jet ventilation. Intravenous agents, such as propofol infusions, are used to maintain anesthesia. Short-acting muscle relaxants are used to prevent movements of the patient that can be dangerous during a laser operation. Gastric distention with possible regurgitation may occur with a misaligned cannula,[174] and a nasogastric tube may be required. Adequate fluids are given intraoperatively, and gases may be humidified in the postoperative period to prevent mucosal drying.

Jet ventilation is helpful in many situations in which a laser is not used. Intermittent jet ventilation has been applied through the instrument channel of the flexible FOB to expand atelectatic lungs and through the Hunsaker jet ventilation tube for one-lung ventilation for lobectomy.[175] However, extreme care should be taken to avoid pulmonary barotrauma.

b. HIGH-FREQUENCY JET VENTILATION

During high-frequency jet ventilation (HFJV), small tidal volumes are delivered at a rate of 60 to 150 cycles per minute from a high-pressure source (5 to 50 psi), with inspiration taking 20% to 40% of each cycle. This is an effective ventilation method that provides adequate gas exchange. This method has been used in rigid bronchoscopy. Hautmann and colleagues described a technique of delivering HFJV through a noncompliant insufflation catheter.[176] The catheter can be threaded through the sidearm of the bronchoscope and positioned in the trachea or in the main stem bronchus. Medici and coworkers used an insufflation catheter with a side hole in the contralateral main stem to deliver high-frequency positive-pressure ventilation during endobronchial surgery using an Nd:YAG laser.[177] HFJV catheters can be placed transtracheally; however, in a prospective multicenter study, the rate of subcutaneous emphysema was 8.4%.[178]

An advantage of HFJV is that it provides excellent views and access to the surgical site. Catheters are small and obstruct the surgical field less than larger conventional ETTs. To-and-fro movements of the major airways that are invariably present during normal respiratory excursions are not present. Because a small tidal volume is used, there is less movement of the larynx, trachea, and lungs. This greatly facilitates the precise operation of the laser beam.

Although the reported incidence of pulmonary barotrauma in HFJV is low, it can lead to serious complications. Pulmonary barotrauma can result from high driving gas pressures and air trapping. Ventilators should initially be set at the lowest possible driving pressures and increased incrementally while carefully observing chest movements. There is a potential risk of barotrauma if the air pressures are not monitored. In addition to an injector catheter, Unzueta and associates used a second identical catheter placed 7 cm distal to the injector site to measure airway pressure continually.[146] Continuous monitoring of end-expired CO_2 and O_2 by conventional methods is difficult to interpret because of fast respiratory rates and high gas flow rates. However, there is a well-defined relationship between arterial CO_2 concentrations and end-tidal CO_2 concentration when expiratory gas is obtained by sidestream sampling during jet ventilation.[179] Observation of chest wall movements and blood gas analysis are reliable methods for assessing the adequacy of ventilation. Klein and coworkers suggested the use of a double-lumen jet catheter for respiratory monitoring.[168]

Air trapping and stacking of breaths are inherent problems in high-frequency ventilation because of short expiratory times.[180] In airways distal to the obstruction, injurious excess pressure can easily build up. Obstruction to gas outflow can easily occur because of the tumor and because of the presence of surgical instruments, bleeding, and mucosal edema. Light anesthesia or inadequate muscle relaxation can cause laryngospasm, closing the glottis and further obstructing the airflow. To prevent barotrauma, it is essential to ensure that there is adequate outflow.

c. COMBINED FREQUENCY JET VENTILATION

Oxygenation and CO_2 elimination may be improved by using low-frequency and high-frequency ventilation in combination (Fig. 40-34). In this method using combined (superimposed) frequencies of ventilation, the location of the gas inflow in the airway seems to influence the efficiency of jet ventilation. Supraglottic, combined-frequency ventilation seem to be superior to subglottic, monofrequent jet ventilation in providing an unobstructed view and access to glottis.[181] With intratracheal jet ventilation, aspiration and air entrapment are virtually absent. There is no clear advantage of one ventilation technique over the other.[182] In a study of 37 adult patients, supraglottic, combined-frequency ventilation was more efficient than subglottic, low-frequency or subglottic, combined-frequency ventilation.[181] However, in a bench model of laryngotracheal stenosis, supraglottic HFJV was

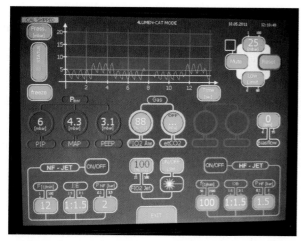

Figure 40-34 The combined-frequency jet ventilation monitor (Carl Reiner, Vienna, Austria) allows observation of the inspired oxygen concentration, measurement of end-tidal CO_2, and scrutiny of three- and four-lumen catheters. It has a laser-safe mode.

TABLE 40-9

Complications Associated with Jet Ventilation of the Lungs

Ventilation Related (n)*	Ventilation Unrelated (n)*
Major	
Pneumothorax (9)	None
Hypoxemia during anesthesia (6)	
Mediastinal air (2)	
Tension pneumothorax (1)	
Minor	
Carbon dioxide retention during anesthesia (3)	Prolonged mask support (10)
Subcutaneous emphysema (2)	Prolonged endotracheal intubation (5)
Gastric dilation (2)	Laryngospasm (5)
Airway bleeding (2)	Prolonged sleep or paralysis (2)
Recall of procedure (1)	

*Data from 15,701 patients were analyzed.
Adapted from Cozine K, Stone JG, Shulman S, Flaster ER: Ventilatory complications of carbon dioxide laser laryngeal surgery. *J Clin Anesth* 3:20, 1991.

associated with significantly larger end-expiratory pressures and peak inspiratory pressures.[183] Two risks are built in because of the location of the jet cannula: aspiration at the supraglottic location and barotrauma at the subglottic location.

High-frequency ventilation should be reserved for patients with severe airway obstruction or severe pulmonary dysfunction. Most cases do well with a variety of simpler techniques that are well established. They include ventilation with a laser-resistant tube or microlaryngoscopy tube, supraglottic jet ventilation with a jet needle, and subglottic jet ventilation with a catheter.[184]

There is no perfect mode of ventilation that suits all clinical conditions. Complications have been associated with various ventilation techniques in laser resections (Table 40-9). Table 40-10 suggests a general approach that is used in the pediatric population.

VIII. ANESTHETIC MANAGEMENT FOR TRACHEOBRONCHIAL TREE LASER SURGERY

Laser resection is the preferred method for removal of obstructive lesions from the trachea and bronchus. It is a safe and effective means of relieving central airway obstruction. With more than 4000 published interventions, the safety and efficacy of laser bronchoscopy has been well established.[142] Providing safe anesthesia for laser excision of lesions that are in the tracheobronchial tree can be challenging. Maintaining unhampered views of the operative field, gaining free and safe access to the laser, and supplying adequate ventilation are essential in choosing a method of anesthetic management, and these are not easy measures to provide for patients with an obstructed airway. The challenge is to preserve adequate gas exchange while maintaining good visualization and surgical access to the lesion.

The primary advantage of using a laser for recurrent benign tumors is that multiple resections can be safely performed in outpatients. This approach avoids the increased morbidity of open thoracotomy procedures. In cancer patients, endoscopic palliation helps in evaluation and staging of malignant tumors. These treatments reduce morbidity during chemotherapy without increasing surgical complications.[185] In cases of severe obstruction by unresectable tumors, a patent airway can be cored

TABLE 40-10

Techniques for Pediatric Laser Bronchoscopy

Site	Scope	Laser	Ventilation Method
Supraglottic or immediately subglottic	Direct laryngoscope	Carbon dioxide	Venturi ventilation through safe ETTs
Trachea, main stem bronchus	Rigid bronchoscope	Flexible KTP or argon laser	Manual ventilation through side arm of bronchoscope $FiO_2 < 0.5$
Distal to main stem bronchus	Flexible bronchoscope through a standard ETT	Flexible KTP or argon laser	Manual ventilation through standard $FiO_2 < 0.5$

ETT, Endotracheal tube; *FiO₂*, fraction of inspired oxygen; *KTP*, potassium titanyl phosphate.

with a laser.[186,187] The combination of laser and rigid bronchoscopy is ideal for treating central airway obstruction.[188] Relief of acute ventilatory distress is a major benefit of bronchoscopic laser resections.[189] Therapeutic bronchoscopy should be considered even in individuals with cancer requiring intubation and mechanical ventilation. Often, mechanical ventilation is successfully discontinued and death from suffocation postponed.[190]

When anesthesiologists and surgeons simultaneously handle the airway, they must have a predetermined plan for intraoperative and postoperative management. Good communication and cooperation are important, and development of a team approach is necessary for successful results.[191] Devising such a plan is made easier if the current problems are conceptualized in two broad categories: mechanical and patient-related issues. Mechanical issues deal with attaining good surgical access while simultaneously providing adequate gas exchange and anesthesia. Distal lesions pose a greater challenge because they can cause complete airway obstruction and are difficult to reach with laser treatment. An ideal treatment modality for endoscopic ablation provides secure airway protection, excellent visualization of the lesion, and delivery of safe and effective method of treatment. Use of a contact Nd:YAG fiberoptic laser system through a rigid bronchoscope has performed well in meeting these criteria.[192] Patient-related topics such as age, size, pulmonary function, and general health status should be the basis for all final decisions. It is important first to decide on the type of laser therapy, type of scope, and technique of ventilation. An anesthesia management plan can then be formulated on the basis of patient-related factors, available equipment, and expertise.

A. Rigid Ventilating Bronchoscopy

Although the rigid bronchoscope is an old instrument, it continues to play a major role in newer therapies for access to the airway.[193] Rigid bronchoscopy is the standard technique for anesthesia management during laser resection of severely obstructing tracheal masses.[194] The main advantage of the rigid bronchoscope is complete control of the airway. The bronchoscope ultimately functions as a rigid ETT. The area and clarity of the view of the surgical field with rigid scopes are superior to those with flexible scopes. However, the view is limited to the trachea, carina, and the main bronchi. Subglottic lesions can be visualized through a rigid bronchoscope. Compared with flexible bronchoscopes, rigid bronchoscopes have large-diameter instrument side channels. A variety of baskets, forceps, and grabbers that are used for a wide range of therapeutic procedures can pass easily through these wide channels. In the event of significant bleeding or tenacious secretions, the telescope can be withdrawn and suction catheters passed directly down the bronchoscope while maintaining oxygenation and control of the airway.

The rigid bronchoscope has a side port that can be attached to any conventional anesthesia delivery system. It substitutes for the ETT during the procedure. A removable eyepiece allows surgical interventions when open

and control of ventilation when in place. Usually, there is a variable leak around the scope, which can be compensated for by increasing the fresh gas flow.

The rigid bronchoscope provides an excellent view of the larynx, similar to the view provided by the direct laryngoscope. Ventilation can be provided through the rigid bronchoscope. Eliminating the ETT improves the access to the surgical field and reduces the risk of airway fire. With experience, rigid bronchoscopy is simple to use, is low cost, and is relatively safe when the proper precautions are observed.

Rigid bronchoscopy can be invaluable and life-saving in cases of severe obstruction because the bronchoscope can be pushed past the obstruction.[141,195] It is unsurpassed in evaluation, control, and therapeutic manipulation of the tracheobronchial tree.[196] A retrospective review of 300 patients over a 12-year period concluded that the use of rigid bronchoscopy offers certain advantages in ventilation during general anesthesia. Rigid therapeutic bronchoscopic intervention is increasingly accepted to treat patients with central airway obstruction. Laser resection is applicable when the obstruction is caused by malignant exophytic tracheobronchial lesions, benign granulation tissue, or tracheobronchial stenosis with scar tissue formation.[190] In one study, rigid bronchoscopy was preferred for proximal lesions and FOB used for distal lesions. Often, the rigid and flexible bronchoscopes were used together to maximum advantage.[197]

Drawbacks of rigid bronchoscopy include increased secretions and finite access to the distal airways and upper lobes. Conditions such as ankylosis of the jaw or rigid cervical spine, which make direct visualization of the larynx difficult, may preclude the use of a rigid bronchoscope. General anesthesia is often necessary for rigid bronchoscopy, whereas flexible bronchoscopy can be performed with sedation and topical anesthesia. Patients do not tolerate pressure on the soft tissues, and significant neck extensions are painful.[198]

B. Flexible Bronchoscopy

Flexible bronchoscopy is used to reach lesions in distal airways. Flexible fiberoptic scopes are more suited for procedures under sedation and local anesthesia.[161] Flexible bronchoscopes are built with bundles of optical fibers or a camera at the distal end. The fibers deliver light to the tip and transmit pixels. An image is constituted when all the pixels are reassembled. However, the image formed is not as good as the view from direct laryngoscopy. It is possible to visualize the entire airway because the tip of the bronchoscope can be flexed through an arc of 220 degrees. There is usually a working channel, which can be used for suction and for passing instruments. In adults, 5.5- to 6.0-mm flexible bronchoscopes are used, and in children, 3.6- and 2.2-mm scopes are popular. The disadvantage of the smaller scopes is that there is no instrument channel or, if present, it is too narrow. As technologic improvements occur in the design of smaller instruments and improved forceps, the therapeutic and diagnostic role of flexible bronchoscopes will become more prevalent in clinical practice.[199]

IX. CONCLUSIONS

Airway surgery is unique in that it involves an operation in which the anesthesiologist and surgeon are working in the same anatomical field. The addition of a laser beam (i.e., ignition source) into the airway may cause a catastrophic airway fire. An understanding of the fire triad and the steps that can be taken to avoid a fire is an essential requirement before undertaking laser airway surgery. General laser hazards include eye and skin injury, drape fires, and laser plumes. Airway fires occur when a laser strikes the unprotected surface of a tracheal tube or any other material within the airway that acts as a fuel source. Any high-energy source, such as diathermy, can act as an ignition source and can result in an explosive blowtorch fire.

Attempts to prevent fires from occurring have involved wrapping the tube in some form of protective covering. Metal foil tape wrapped around a standard tracheal tube is of historical interest but is not recommended. Specially manufactured laser tubes are most commonly used and vary in their protective coatings, number of cuffs, size, flexibility, and resistance to compression. All commercially available laser tubes can be involved in a laser fire if they are used outside their recommended protective range. Anesthetic gases and the flammability limits of potent inhaled anesthetics affect tube flammability.

The introduction of laser fibers through an FOB passed through an LMA was an important step, as was the use of LMAs during laser pharyngoplasty. Preoperative assessment aims to identify the size, mobility, and site of a lesion. Very mobile lesions may cause partial airway obstruction after induction of anesthesia, but total airway obstruction is extremely uncommon. Airway obstruction is worse in a spontaneously breathing patient after induction of anesthesia because of the loss of supporting tone in the oropharynx and hypopharynx. Supraglottic lesions, if mobile, can obstruct the airway or make visualization of the laryngeal inlet difficult. Subglottic lesions may allow a good view of the laryngeal inlet but cause difficulty during the passage of an ETT. The traditional teaching of inhalational induction and maintenance of spontaneous ventilation in obstructed airways has been questioned.

During anesthesia, a closed system with a laser tube may be used, or an open system may be employed using a spontaneous ventilation technique, intermittent apnea, or jet ventilation technique. With an open airway, it is not possible to produce a sustained fire, regardless of the laser power and oxygen concentration, because no fuel source is present in the airway. A tube, catheter, stent, or any foreign material introduced into the airway may act as a fuel source and complete the fire triad, which may result in a catastrophic airway fire if precautions are not taken.

X. CLINICAL PEARLS

- Good communication, cooperation, and the development of a team approach are essential requirements for successful laser airway surgery. The surgeon and anesthesiologist should be familiar with the principles of a laser, the types of laser available, hazards of laser use, the management of an airway fire, and the advantages and disadvantages of the various anesthetic techniques available.

- For an airway fire, three components of the fire triad are needed: fuel source, oxidant sources, and ignition source. Removal of one of these components prevents or reduces the risk of an airway fire, which in practice means removing or protecting the fuel sources, minimizing the oxidant sources, and not using an ignition source.

- Oxygen and nitrous oxide support combustion very well, and dilution of oxygen by nitrous oxide makes no difference to the flammability risk. In clinical practice, air and oxygen are most frequently used during laser airway surgery, with the oxygen concentration kept as low as clinically feasible while the laser is near the tube.

- All manufactured laser tubes have laser-resistant properties, providing some degree of protection against a laser strike, and these limits are provided by the manufacturer in the product literature, which describes the types of laser the tube has protection from and the limits of power settings for different lasers. Laser tubes vary in the material used, protective coating, relative size, and the number of cuffs. All laser tubes can result in an airway fire or blowtorch fire if used outside of their limits.

- The preoperative evaluation attempts to identify factors that may cause difficulty during the perioperative course. It involves a thorough medical evaluation of all patients before surgery. At the end of the preoperative assessment, the anesthesiologist should have some idea of the size, mobility, and location of the lesion. Recognition of a compromised or anatomically distorted upper airway is paramount in the preoperative assessment of these patients.

- Premedication to reduce secretions and anxiety may be useful in patients with minor airway lesions, but it should be avoided in patients with severe airway compromise. Thick secretions may block narrowed airways further, may be difficult to cough out by the patient, and may in extreme circumstances totally obstruct critically narrowed airways.

- Jet ventilation techniques are suitable for ventilation during laser surgery of most adult vocal cord lesions. The main limitation for their use is the experience of the anesthesiologist and the absence of suitable equipment. Life-threatening barotrauma is the most serious complication, and it occurs when room air is not entrained. This results in the delivery of very high driving pressures, leading to pneumomediastinum, pneumothorax, and surgical emphysema.

Acknowledgments

I would like to acknowledge Mitchel B. Sosis, MD, Lorraine J. Foley, MD, and Roy D. Cane, MD, for the parts of this chapter that are sourced from their work in previous editions.

SELECTED REFERENCES

All references can be found online at expertconsult.com.

1. Caplan RA, Barker SJ, Connis RT, et al: Practice advisory for the prevention and management of operating room fires. A report by the American Society of Anesthesiologists task force on operating room fires. *Anesthesiology* 108:786, 2008.

43. Puttick N: Anesthesia for laser airway surgery. In Oswal V, Remacle M, editors: *Principles and practice of lasers in otolaryngology and head and neck surgery*, The Hague, 2002, Krugrer, pp 63–76.

101. Rampil IJ: Anesthesia for laser surgery. In Miller RD, editor: *Miller's anesthesia*, ed 7, Philadelphia, 2010, Churchill Livingstone, pp 2405–2418.

109. Hunsaker DH: Anesthesia for microlaryngeal surgery: The case for subglottic jet ventilation. *Laryngoscope* 104(Suppl 65):1, 1994.

110. Ossoff RH: Laser safety in otolaryngology–head and neck surgery: Anesthetic and educational considerations for laryngeal surgery. *Laryngoscope* 99(Suppl 48):1, 1989.

134. Chee WK, Benumof JL: Airway fire during tracheostomy: Extubation may be contraindicated. *Anesthesiology* 89:1576, 1998.

135. Van Der Spek AF, Spargo PM, Norton ML: The physics of lasers and implications for their use during airway surgery. *Br J Anaesth* 60:709, 1988.

140. Sher M, Brimacombe J, Laing D: Anaesthesia for laser pharyngoplasty—A comparison of the tracheal tube with the reinforced laryngeal mask airway. *Anaesth Intensive Care* 23:149, 1995.

153. Calder I, Yentis SM: Could "safe practice" be compromising safe practice? Should anaesthetists have to demonstrate that face mask ventilation is possible before giving a neuromuscular blocker? *Anaesthesia* 63:113, 2008.

161. Conacher ID: Anaesthesia and tracheobronchial stenting for central airway obstruction in adults. *Br J Anaesth* 90:367, 2003.

Chapter 41

The Traumatized Airway

CALVIN A. BROWN III | ALI S. RAJA

I. DEFINING THE PROBLEM

A. The Clinical Challenge

Airway management in the trauma patient can be particularly challenging because of the presence of a difficult airway with the need for rapid action. The traumatized airway is often anatomically disrupted, obstructing direct laryngoscopy, and the presence of blood in the upper airway confounds attempts at fiberoptic intubation. Manual in-line stabilization of the cervical spine (C-spine) is required in most patients with blunt trauma, compounding the airway difficulties. Although trauma patients are often intubated outside the operating room (OR), usually in the emergency department (ED) resuscitation area, they can also present to the OR requiring intubation for emergency surgery. In the ED, trauma patients are intubated primarily by emergency physicians, but patients with direct trauma to the airway may be managed using a team approach, with emergency physicians, anesthesiologists, and surgeons working in concert to achieve the best possible results. In the OR or other units within the hospital, trauma airway management is typically the responsibility of the anesthesiologist, although surgeons may be called on to assist when the airway is disrupted.

Trauma patients needing airway intervention require a rapid evaluation for potentially difficult airway attributes, development of an airway management plan (including rescue techniques in the event of failure), and a willingness to act quickly with incomplete information. In most cases, the need to intervene is apparent, but certain situations can mislead the evaluating physician into thinking that an airway is not at risk. Many trauma patients initially appear to be stable; they maintain a patent airway and breathe spontaneously until some process causes them to deteriorate rapidly. Soft tissue swelling, hematomas, or subcutaneous air can cause dramatic and potentially lethal airway distortion, even though external findings remain unremarkable, until the patient suddenly decompensates. Any patient with a traumatized airway requires early assessment and decisive action. Delay or observation, although initially seeming prudent, can lead to catastrophic airway compromise and make airway intervention much more difficult than if it had been undertaken earlier.

1. Emergency Department or Trauma Resuscitation Room

Patients who have been subjected to acute blunt or penetrating trauma can present with a spectrum of injuries, ranging from minor and localized insults to catastrophic and multisystem trauma. In the trauma resuscitation room, intubation may be indicated by direct trauma to the head, face, neck, or airway; respiratory compromise due to thoracic injury; or overall management strategy, as in the critically injured patient with hypovolemic shock.

In most cases, the usual paradigms of airway management used in elective anesthesia are not applicable. Care of the acute, severely injured trauma patient is best done using a team approach with a clearly designated team captain, who controls the decision making, sequence, and flow of the entire resuscitation.

Airway management decisions are not driven only by the need for operative intervention; the decision about when and how to control a patient's airway is based on a complex series of considerations related to the patient's specific injuries and overall condition, the risk of deterioration, and the need for transport to locations in the hospital where resuscitation is not easily undertaken (e.g., angiography suite). This type of decision making about the airway is often more complicated than that involved in elective surgery, and a unique approach to airway intervention is needed. In smaller hospitals, where a trauma team approach cannot be used due to staffing limitations, decisions regarding resource allocation and prioritization of interventions are even more challenging.

2. Early Hospital Care of the Traumatized Patient

Trauma and burn patients frequently undergo surgery that is not related to their acute resuscitation but is required during the first few days of their hospital stay. Burn débridement and grafting, fracture fixation, complex wound revision and repair, and other procedures are often required hours or days after the patient has been stabilized and more acute, life-threatening problems have been controlled. Decision making in this setting is easier with respect to airway management because the decision to intubate is driven by the need for surgery and anesthetic management; however, careful preoperative assessment remains essential. In addition to the usual comorbidities that can make airway management difficult, trauma patients often have other complicating factors, such as direct airway injury, pulmonary injury with rapid oxyhemoglobin desaturation, persistently tenuous hemodynamic status, or cerebral injury with elevated intracranial pressure (ICP). Patients with significant total body surface area burns, crush injuries, or spinal cord injuries develop acetylcholine receptor upregulation, with its attendant risk of hyperkalemia if succinylcholine is administered.[1] Although classic teaching posits that this vulnerability to succinylcholine-induced hyperkalemia begins on postinjury day 7, some effect is seen as early as day 3.[2] This combination of considerations—specifically unresolved or unrecognized traumatic injuries, the potential for hyperkalemia, and the patient's preexisting comorbidities—can make airway management in this intermediate-term window anything but routine. A careful approach, including detailed consideration of possible difficult airway management protocols and relevant comorbidities, is essential.

3. Delayed Surgery

Traumatized patients frequently require multiple operative repairs or revisions before and during the rehabilitation phase. Delayed operations often are performed between 1 and 6 months after injury, and they may involve many of the considerations outlined previously, particularly those related to succinylcholine-induced hyperkalemia. However, because these patients usually are stable and most have already undergone procedures that require endotracheal intubation, most airway difficulties have been identified. Although the management of these patients raises important issues, this chapter focuses on the acutely traumatized patient and issues related to airway management in that setting.

B. The Decision to Intubate

The decision to intubate is the most important resuscitative decision, but it is often the one with which the provider struggles the most. Trauma patients present anxiety-provoking situations because their airway difficulty is often exaggerated by C-spine immobility, direct airway trauma, overall physiologic compromise, and the propensity for clinical deterioration. Early definitive airway management must be performed in a logical and safe fashion to continue evaluation and resuscitative efforts for these patients. Decision making must be based on a consistent, reproducible series of principles that accounts for the patient's current condition, likelihood of deterioration, planned diagnostic and therapeutic interventions (including transport), preinjury comorbidity, and the resources and expertise available in the resuscitation area.

Answers to three fundamental questions inform the decision to undertake emergency intubation:

1. Is there a failure to maintain or protect the airway?
2. Is there a failure of oxygenation or ventilation?
3. Is there a need for intubation based on the anticipated clinical course?

Questions 1 and 2 are relatively straightforward in the setting of the trauma patient. Failure to maintain the airway is clinically obvious. Loss of airway protection usually occurs in the setting of depressed mental status caused by head trauma, hypovolemic shock, or ingestion of drugs or alcohol and is a condition with which the ED physician and anesthesiologist are familiar. Airway protection is best tested by evaluation of the patient's ability to phonate (if possible). Phonation requires an unobstructed upper airway and the ability to execute complex, coordinated maneuvers. After phonation, the patient's ability to swallow and handle secretions is assessed. The ability to sense the pooling of secretions in the posterior pharynx and to perform the coordinated series of neurologic and muscular maneuvers to swallow requires a high degree of function and connotes airway protection. The gag reflex, long advocated as the test by which the need for intubation can be judged, should never be performed in a critically injured, supine, immobilized trauma patient. The wisdom of inserting a tongue blade or other device to stimulate the patient's posterior oral pharynx in this state is questionable, because vomiting is easily provoked and difficult to deal with.

The gag reflex is much less reliable than phonation and swallowing, and it is absent in up to 25% of the normal adult population.[3] The presence of a gag reflex does not equate to airway protection, nor does its absence indicate a need to intubate. The presence or absence of the gag reflex is better thought of as a neurologic evaluation (i.e., cranial nerves IX and X) rather than as part of an airway evaluation. The Glasgow Coma Scale is a better tool for predicting intubation.[4]

The ability of a patient to maintain appropriate oxygenation and ventilation can be assessed clinically and supported by pulse oximetry and capnography. Although arterial blood gas values are useful in evaluating the trauma patient with respect to identification of occult acidosis that may represent more severe shock than is clinically apparent, these determinations have little or no role in the decision to intubate. Evaluation of the patient's respiratory effort and the overall sense of the patient's injuries in the context of pulse oximetry readings are more important to the intubation decision than arterial blood gas values. Patients with compromised ventilation or oxygenation should receive high-flow face mask oxygen (O_2) with a reservoir, and all reversible issues should be addressed. Hemothorax, pneumothorax, flail chest, and opioid overdose are examples of reversible conditions that compromise oxygenation and ventilation. Most cases of hypoxemia or hypoventilation in multi-trauma patients are multifactorial and do not respond to simple interventions. In these cases, early intubation usually is indicated.

Most trauma patients can maintain and protect their airways and exhibit adequate or correctable oxygenation and ventilation. For them, it is the anticipated clinical course that guides the decision to intubate. This is the most sophisticated and most important of the decisions facing the airway manager or trauma captain. A patient may appear stable at the time of evaluation, but deterioration can be predicted as a natural course of the injuries. For example, the patient with burns from a closed-space fire with significant inhalation of superheated air (see Chapter 44) may present with a somewhat hoarse voice or a simple cough but has an otherwise patent airway. Failing to recognize the likelihood of progressive obstruction of the airway, which has been subjected to toxic and thermal insults, and to intervene in a timely fashion can lead to disaster. Although the patient may not meet the criteria for emergency intubation related to airway maintenance and protection, oxygenation, or ventilation, the likelihood of deterioration is alone sufficient to warrant airway intervention.[5] It is the predictability of the deterioration that determines the decision to intubate. Alternatively, the upper airway can be examined by fiberoptic laryngoscopy, informing the airway manager of the stability or fragility of airway patency. Similarly, the patient with a crushed pelvis, open femur fracture, and hypotension is inevitably intubated, even though there is no immediate threat to airway patency or oxygenation. The need for advanced imaging, aggressive pain control, and operative repair of obvious injuries dictates that the patient be intubated early and in a more controlled fashion than trying to manage a chaotic intubation from behind the computed tomography (CT) scanner.

Consideration of the patient as a whole, of the individual injuries and how they interact, of the effects of these injuries on the patient and on the patient's comorbidities, and of the need for interventions (including transport) frequently guides a prudent and rational decision to intubate, even when the patient does not have an immediate airway problem and when oxygenation and ventilation are adequate.

Preventing morbidity or mortality as it relates to trauma airway management refers to delaying intubation rather than to a mishap occurring during intubation. It is better to err on the side of intubating early and securing a potentially threatened airway than observing the patient with a false sense of security born from adequate oxygenation and ventilation at that moment. The purpose of observation is to see whether obstruction or airway failure ensues, but if either occurs, the results may be disastrous.

II. ANATOMY OF THE AIRWAY: TRAUMA CONSIDERATIONS

Although airway anatomy is discussed in Chapter 1, the following is a brief description of elements to consider in the trauma setting. The airway begins at the nares or lips and ends with the terminal bronchioles and alveoli of the lungs. The upper airway consists of the oral and nasal cavities and the pharynx, which provide a conduit for the movement of gases to the larynx, through the glottis, and into the trachea. The nasopharynx, oropharynx, and hypopharynx (Fig. 41-1) form a continuous space that conducts air from the outside world to the glottic aperture. The nasopharynx is protected anteriorly and laterally by the maxillary bones, the nasal bones, and nasal cartilage. Direct injury to the face, particularly from an impact with an object of high mass, high velocity, and low surface area (e.g., baseball bat), can collapse the maxillary structures into the nasopharynx and cause extensive hemorrhage, threatening the airway and complicating attempts to manage it. Similarly, the oropharynx is protected by the maxillary bones, alveolar ridges, and

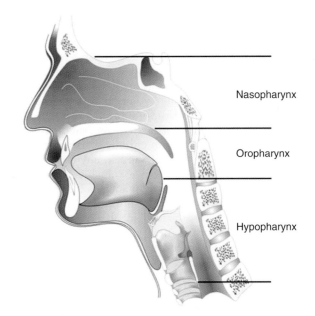

Figure 41-1 Airway anatomy. (From Redden RJ: Anatomic considerations in anesthesia. In Hagberg CA, editor: *Handbook of difficult airway management,* Philadelphia, 2000, Churchill Livingstone, p 11.)

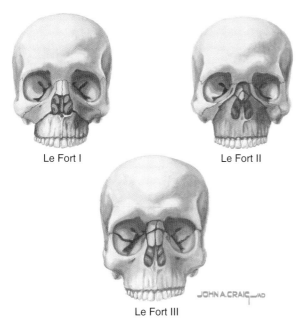

Le Fort I Le Fort II

Le Fort III

JOHN A. CRAIG _AD

Figure 41-2 Le Fort classification. (From the Netter Collection of Medical Illustrations; Website. Available at http://www.netterimages. com (accessed February 2012). Copyright Elsevier Inc.; all rights reserved.)

mandible but is subject to the same sort of intrusive injuries. Blows to the face producing Le Fort I, II, or III fractures (Fig. 41-2) can simultaneously threaten the airway and complicate airway management.

The larynx and trachea are essentially subcutaneous structures in the anterior neck. The larynx is separated from the skin only by subcutaneous fat and the anterior cervical fascia. The thyroid notch, cricothyroid membrane, and cricoid cartilage can be easily palpated to provide the critical landmarks for surgical access to the airway (see Chapter 31). The airway is mobile in the neck but is fairly firmly anchored by the strap muscles and cervical fascia. Tracheal deviation as a result of pneumothorax or hemothorax may occur in patients who are severely compromised.[6] Tracheal deviation is not helpful as a sign of pneumothorax because it usually occurs only when the pneumothorax is at an advanced state and easily identifiable by auscultation. Tracheal deviation can result from disruption of the neck anatomy caused by hemorrhage or extensive subcutaneous emphysema. It is also seen with chronic scarring, such as that related to previous radiotherapy. In any case, palpation of the trachea and larynx is a valuable exercise in the event that surgical airway management becomes necessary. It also can establish the position of the airway in the neck, even if orotracheal intubation is contemplated. Orotracheal intubation can be extraordinarily difficult or impossible when the trachea or larynx is displaced laterally.

Vascular structures in the neck, such as the carotid artery and jugular vein, do not have a direct bearing on the airway. Nonetheless, they can be the cause of significant airway compromise when vascular injury from blunt or penetrating trauma creates hemorrhage that displaces or otherwise changes the configuration of the airway. The

nerves supplying sensation to the supraglottic larynx and the remainder of the airway are rarely injured by trauma.

Knowledge of the anatomy of the upper airway is no more or less important in the management of the multitrauma patient than in any other setting in which emergency airway management is required. When specific trauma to the maxillofacial area or neck threatens and disrupts the airway, however, anatomic knowledge and the ability to improvise an approach may be key determinants of success.

III. SPECIFIC CLINICAL CONSIDERATIONS IN TRAUMA

A. Direct Airway Trauma

Direct trauma to the airway can be broadly classified as blunt or penetrating trauma. Each of these categories can be considered in the context of direct injury to the airway itself versus compromise or threat to the airway caused by the proximity of an injury in the neck. Injury to the airway can occur at one or more levels. Maxillofacial trauma can compromise the upper airway; direct injury to the neck can compromise the airway from the hypopharynx to the trachea; and injuries to the thorax can disrupt the lower trachea, main stem bronchi, or other smaller bronchi. The approach to airway management is dictated by the clinical presentation of the patient and the best judgment of the operator.

1. Penetrating Neck Trauma

Penetrating neck injuries range in scope from stab or other puncture wounds to major lacerations due to both low-velocity (e.g., BBs, pellets) and high-velocity (e.g., crossbows, firearms) projectile injury. The consequences of these various mechanisms can vary drastically. The overall mortality rate due to penetrating neck injuries is 2% to 6%, with a significantly lower mortality rate for low-velocity injuries.[7-9] The patient with a stab wound to the neck usually has identifiable anatomy and can undergo a planned airway evaluation and early intubation under controlled circumstances. Patients with high-velocity injuries often have significant vascular and hollow-structure injuries, and anatomic distortion can make airway management challenging.[10] These injuries mandate urgent airway management, but the approach is confounded by the myriad injuries caused by the missile.[11]

For the purposes of classification of penetrating injury, the neck is divided into three zones (Fig. 41-3). Zone 1 extends from the clavicles inferiorly to the level of the cricoid cartilage. Zone 2 extends from the cricoid cartilage to a line drawn through the angles of the mandible, and zone 3 is the area above the angles of the mandible. This classification is most useful for low-velocity penetration, such as from a stab or long-distance birdshot, but it has also been applied to high-velocity injuries, such as rifle wounds.[10] These zones were designated because of their unique anatomic characteristics.[12] Zone 1 is dominated by the major vascular structures at the root of the neck, specifically the carotid arteries, internal jugular veins, subclavian arteries and veins, and innominate arteries and veins. The airway at this level is relatively

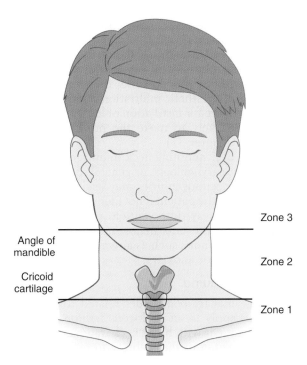

Angle of
mandible

Cricoid
cartilage

Zone 3

Zone 2

Zone 1

Figure 41-3 Zones of the neck.

inaccessible except by tracheotomy. Zone 1 injuries are relatively uncommon (<10% of penetrating neck injuries) but are often associated with major vascular injuries or injuries to the dome of the lung.[13] Patients with zone 1 injuries often require emergency airway management because of direct airway compromise by hemorrhage or the anticipated clinical course predicted by the profound shock that typically develops. There is little literature to guide the selection of airway management techniques for zone 1 penetrating injuries. Most information is limited to small case series of subsets of larger series that are dominated by zone 2 injuries. The approach to airway management is dictated more by the nature of the threat to the airway than by the location of the inciting wound. The overall approach to airway management in penetrating neck injuries is outlined subsequently.

Zone 2 is the most common location for penetrating neck injuries, accounting for most reported cases.[14] Zone 2 injuries require emergency airway intervention in approximately one third of the cases, with a large proportion of the remainder undergoing subsequent intubation related to evaluation or surgical repair. The area of concern in zone 2 extends from the anterior margins of the paravertebral muscles bilaterally. In this area, major vascular structures (e.g., common carotid arteries, internal jugular veins) and their associated sympathetic ganglia and the hypopharynx, esophagus, larynx, and trachea are all at risk. The most common cause of airway compromise in zone 2 injuries is external distortion by hemorrhage related to vascular injuries or direct injuries to the airway.[15]

Zone 3 injuries are uncommon (<10% of all penetrating neck injuries) because of the very small area involved and the protection provided by the mastoid processes posteriorly, the mandible anteriorly, and the base of the skull superiorly. The area, however, is rich with major

vascular structures (i.e., carotid arteries and internal jugular veins) and provides easy access to the pharynx. Surgical repair of injuries in this area is difficult, and most of these patients undergo extensive evaluation by angiography, with stenting of vascular injuries often the intervention of choice. Because zone 3 injuries involve the pharynx, direct airway compromise is uncommon except by hemorrhage into the airway from a through-and-through injury to the carotid artery. In these rare circumstances, immediate airway intervention is required and may be difficult because of the torrential hemorrhage. Orotracheal intubation is usually successful in these cases, however, particularly if the patient is positioned head down to prevent the blood from entering the operator's view. After the airway is secure, the mouth can be packed tightly with gauze to control the internal hemorrhage while direct external pressure is simultaneously applied as the patient is transported to the OR.

The approach to the airway in the patient with penetrating neck trauma is guided by the same principles that were outlined earlier in this chapter. Compromised airway patency or protection because of hemorrhage, for example, is an indication for active airway management. Similarly, severe shock with overall obtundation of the patient and an inability to protect the airway or ventilate and oxygenate adequately makes the intubation decision fairly straightforward. The difficulty lies in the patient who has evidence of injury to the neck, but who does not have an obviously compromised airway at the initial evaluation. It is in these cases that judgment is most important and that most tactical errors are made.

The best approach is to consider two specific issues. The first is whether there is evidence of a direct injury to an air-containing structure in the neck. Subcutaneous air indicates injury to an air-filled structure in the neck,[16] such as the airway (including the hypopharynx or pharynx) or the esophagus. In severe cases, particularly patients with injury to both vascular and air-filled structures, airway obstruction can occur rapidly, requiring emergency cricothyrotomy.[17] In less threatening cases, it is virtually impossible to tell whether the esophagus or airway is involved, and early direct or fiberoptic examination of the airway is indicated. Sedation and topical anesthesia allows the operator to determine the severity and location of any airway injury. Preparation with a small to moderate-size endotracheal tube (ETT) (e.g., 6.0- to 7.0-mm inside diameter) mounted on the scope before initiating endoscopy facilitates prompt intubation if the injury is found to be significant. If the scope has been placed successfully distal to the injury, the patient can be gently intubated over the flexible fiberoptic bronchoscope (FFB), because it is best to secure the airway distal to the injury. This at least ensures that the patient is safe until he or she can be transported to the OR for further evaluation by an otolaryngologist or general surgeon. Although tracheostomy is often necessary, in these cases, temporary oral endotracheal intubation over an FFB ensures airway control and minimizes the subsequent leakage of air into the tissues, facilitating later repair.[16] If no airway injury is identified and there is no evidence of increase in the subcutaneous emphysema in the neck during spontaneous or assisted ventilation, the injury can be presumed to be esophageal.[18] If, however, circumstances change and subcutaneous emphysema begins to increase, even slightly, intubation is recommended since development of large amounts of subcutaneous emphysema can distort airway anatomy such that subsequent intubation or surgical airway management becomes difficult or impossible. As with all penetrating neck injuries, early intubation, even in patients who do not appear to immediately require it, is the most prudent course.

The second issue is whether there is evidence of significant vascular injury to the neck. All penetrating neck wounds have some external bleeding, although it can be surprisingly modest. The issue with respect to airway management is whether injury has occurred to any of the major vascular structures in the neck (e.g., carotid arteries, jugular veins). A hematoma of any size, external hemorrhage, or any evidence of displacement of the airway structures can serve as evidence of direct vascular injury. As soon as it has been established that direct vascular injury has occurred, active airway management should be undertaken.[19,20] Most of these patients present early in the course of their injuries, when anatomy is preserved and orotracheal intubation is likely to be relatively easy to achieve. Waiting to determine whether the hematoma is expanding is perilous, because most of the hemorrhage into the neck occurs into the deep tissue planes, distorting and displacing the airway without external evidence until a crisis occurs. The time-honored dictum that hematomas of the neck should be observed to see whether they are expanding is not rational, and any evidence of direct vascular injury to the neck is sufficient justification for intubation. Early intubation can proceed using a rapid-sequence intubation (RSI) technique if a careful examination for difficult airway attributes fails to identify problems and there is a sound rescue strategy planned in the event of intubation failure.[21] Early intervention allows the operator to intubate in a controlled fashion rather than scrambling to secure an emergency airway later in the patient's course, when airway obstruction is imminent or has already occurred.

If there is doubt regarding oral access, three approaches can be considered. The first option is to perform oral RSI under a double setup with preparations and personnel in place to perform immediate surgical cricothyrotomy if orotracheal intubation is not successful. This approach should only be undertaken only if the preintubation airway assessment indicates that orotracheal intubation, although potentially difficult, is still likely to be successful. Similarly, there must be confidence that bag-mask ventilation (BMV) will be successful in maintaining the patient's oxygenation, if required. If visualization is suboptimal during conventional direct laryngoscopy, the use of a bougie or video laryngoscope can be considered.

The second option is to perform fiberoptic intubation under sedation and topical anesthesia, as described earlier. This allows the operator to use the FFB to identify and enter the airway, even if the anatomy has become distorted. If this is undertaken early in the patient's course, there is typically sufficient time and control to yield a high success rate. However, a distorted and bloodied airway makes fiberoptic intubation technically challenging, and the most experienced operator should perform the procedure.

The third option is to proceed directly with a planned surgical cricothyrotomy. This requires that the airway be identifiable with clear landmarks to permit a surgical approach. Local anesthetic infiltration and direct transcricothyroid puncture for instillation of local anesthesia into the airway are likely to make the procedure easier to perform (see Chapter 31).

In all cases of penetrating neck trauma, early consultation with an otolaryngologist or general surgeon is essential. Initially innocuous injuries may lead to catastrophic consequences for the patient if not identified and managed early.[22] Early airway intervention permits controlled resuscitation and prevents major morbidities related to penetrating neck injury, such as airway compromise with resultant hypoxia or anoxia.

2. Blunt Neck Trauma

Many of the management issues related to penetrating neck trauma apply in an analogous fashion to management of the patient with blunt neck trauma. The primary difference is related to the inability to precisely localize the injury (i.e., no obvious skin penetration to identify the point of injury) and the fact that blunt injury is usually more diffuse. Initial evaluation of the patient with a blunt neck trauma should include identification of bruising or ecchymosis related to the external injury. The oropharynx should be inspected to ensure that there is no injury to the tongue or dentition. The external neck should then be palpated carefully from the mandible to the clavicle. Palpation is focused on three findings:

1. Identification of swelling, hemorrhage, or subcutaneous emphysema
2. Evaluation for tenderness (if possible) of the neck, particularly the airway structures
3. Evaluation of the anatomy of the upper airway for direct airway injury and for the anatomic landmarks that are important if a surgical airway must be placed (see Chapter 31).

Because subcutaneous emphysema may be occult, it requires careful palpation. Extensive ecchymosis suggests blunt vascular injury with free hemorrhage (which is usually venous) or formation of a pseudoaneurysm. Extensive ecchymosis or extensive swelling strongly suggests impending airway compromise, and urgent airway intervention is advisable.[23] Infrequently, direct blunt neck trauma can cause laryngeal fracture or tracheal transection. The latter is often rapidly fatal, but patients may arrive in the trauma resuscitation area alive because of incomplete transsection.[24] In these cases, there is usually subcutaneous air, often accompanied by swelling, and pain elicited by palpation of the anterior airway. Although a trial of BMV may be tempting, it is likely to exacerbate the subcutaneous emphysema and accelerate the patient's deterioration. When such an injury is identified, the best approach is prompt transfer to the OR for surgical exploration of the anterior neck and establishment of the airway by tracheostomy distal to the transsection. Often, however, airway management must be undertaken before the surgery, and careful awake fiberoptic intubation over a small FFB after inhalational induction may be the least of all evils. If the airway must be secured in the ED, for example, before transportation to a level I trauma center, the same approach is used, substituting intravenous sedation and topical anesthesia for inhalational anesthesia because the latter is not available in the ED.

As with penetrating neck injuries, the key error in the management of the patient with blunt neck trauma is observing an already distorted airway to determine if the condition worsens. If the patient exhibits evidence of significant neck injury, it can be assumed that the airway is threatened. When this threat advances to actual airway compromise, it threatens the patient's life and thwarts subsequent attempts at airway management. As with penetrating trauma, early airway management is indicated when there is evidence of significant blunt injury to the neck.

Airway management is complicated by the fact that patients with blunt anterior neck trauma must be presumed to have a C-spine injury. Up to 50% of patients with blunt airway injury have a C-spine injury,[25] which is discussed here in the context of airway management.

In clothesline injuries, in which the neck is struck, usually transversely, by a fence wire or similar object, the central neck area may be significantly but deceptively disrupted from the impact.[17] Although these injuries can be dramatic and often require immediate airway management, the airway itself is often intact, signified by identification of intact structures and the absence of air bubbling or gurgling during negative-pressure or positive-pressure ventilation. Early intubation from above, preferably over an FFB, is best in these cases. If the airway has been breached, and gurgling or subcutaneous air is evident in the tissues of the neck, positive-pressure BMV is not likely to be successful in oxygenating the patient, and attempts at BMV may result in insufflation of large amounts of air into the soft tissues of the neck, further compromising the airway and the attempts at securing it. The best approach in these cases is to attempt to secure the airway over an FFB using sedation and topical anesthesia, with a plan to progress directly to a cricothyrotomy or emergency tracheostomy, if fiberoptic intubation is unsuccessful.

3. Maxillofacial Trauma

Mandibular fractures are usually isolated injuries, but they can occur in the setting of multitrauma, particularly in unrestrained occupants in motor vehicle collisions and victims of severe assault. They rarely threaten the airway unless the anterior mandible is fractured, which allows the tongue to fall back and obstruct the airway. Usually, this obstruction is easily relieved by pulling the anterior segment of the mandible forward. This maneuver also remedies any interference with endotracheal intubation by the posteriorly displaced tongue. Patients with fractures of the angle of the mandible or the mandibular condyles often have limited mouth opening due to pain and to anatomic restriction. Because the deformity is bony, it is often not abolished by neuromuscular blockade (NMB). Although it is always important to establish the extent of mouth opening and whether it is adequate to permit intubation before administering NMB agents, this is especially true in patients with mandibular fractures.

Maxillary fractures usually occur in one of the classically described Le Fort patterns. Although the precise location of the Le Fort fracture pattern is sometimes difficult to remember, the Le Fort I, II, and III fractures can be thought of as follows (see Fig. 41-2). The Le Fort I fracture represents separation of the roof of the mouth from the face, with the fracture extending through the alveolar ridge to the base of the nose and separating the alveolar ridge and hard palate from the rest of the face. The Le Fort II fracture is separation of the central face from the rest of the face and cranium. The fractures extend from the base of the nasal bones through the medial orbits down through the maxilla to the posterior molars, effectively creating a free-floating central face fragment. The Le Fort III fracture is separation of the face from the skull. This fracture extends from the base of the nasal bones through the orbits to the lateral orbital rims and then through the zygomatic arch and down through the pterygoid plate.

Le Fort I fractures rarely cause airway compromise. If the fracture fragment has displaced posteriorly, it can easily be pulled forward by gripping the upper incisors or alveolar ridge. Le Fort II fractures similarly do not compromise the airway unless extensive hemorrhage is present. The fracture fragment, although free floating, rarely displaces posteriorly enough to compromise the airway. In the absence of hemorrhage, the mouth and oral pharynx are usually patent and functional. However, Le Fort III fractures can significantly compromise the airway due to posterior displacement of the entire central face, compromising the oral and nasal pharynx. Similarly, extensive swelling or hemorrhage related to the fractures may threaten the airway. In all cases, careful oral inspection and suctioning to determine the patency and adequacy of the oral cavity, followed by early intubation for airway protection and overall management of the patient, are advisable.

An uncommon but disastrous presentation of maxillofacial injury occurs when an attempted suicide fails because the gun (usually a shotgun) is oriented in such a way as to have the mass of the shot pass upward through the face rather than on a posterior trajectory through the brainstem. This often happens when the patient places a rifle or shotgun under the chin and then tries to reach downward for the trigger. This movement naturally leads to extension of the neck, and the trajectory of the missile is altered, causing it to pass upward through the face (Fig. 41-4). Although such injuries occur with massive facial distortion, airway management can range from easy to virtually impossible. Destruction of the mandible, tongue, palate, and nasopharynx often makes orotracheal intubation impossible, and hemorrhage is usually extensive. Primary surgical airway management is usually the method of choice. However, the injury can be predominantly anterior, sparing the airway, and the mandible and tongue can be displaced forward, permitting adequate oral access for orotracheal intubation. Nonetheless, efficient suctioning is usually required because the hemorrhage can be significant.

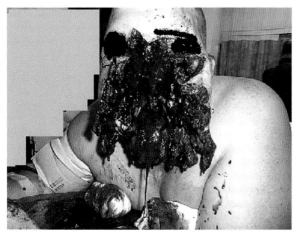

Figure 41-4 Facial trauma.

B. Cervical Spine Injury

Unstable injury to the C-spine presents a particular hazard with respect to airway management because of the potential to cause or exacerbate spinal cord injury. C-spine injury usually occurs when there is high-energy transfer, such as in a motor vehicle collision, but it can occur with relatively minor trauma in patients with significant degenerative disease of the C-spine, such as rheumatoid arthritis or osteopenia. Motor vehicle collisions are the greatest cause of spinal injury, accounting for about 50% of these injuries, followed by falls, athletic injury, and interpersonal violence.[26]

In the trauma resuscitation room, all patients who have been subjected to significant blunt trauma should be assumed to have a C-spine injury until it has been excluded. Penetrating trauma can also cause spinal injury, but creation of an unstable spinal injury without concomitant spinal cord injury is exceedingly rare. With penetrating injury, it is usually apparent whether spinal injury has occurred because the patient sustained a neurologic disability. Barring this finding, C-spine immobilization in a patient with isolated penetrating trauma is typically unnecessary and may even be harmful.[27-29]

One of the significant challenges related to airway management in patients with blunt trauma is the inability to determine definitively whether the patient has a C-spine injury before intubation is required. Fortunately, most patients with a C-spine injury do not require intubation during the acute phase of resuscitation. However, those who have the most severe trauma are likely to require intubation, and this is the same population who is at highest risk for spinal injury.[30] It has been estimated that 2% to 14% of all patients with serious blunt trauma have a significant C-spine injury.[31,32]

The decision about whether to obtain portable C-spine imaging before intubation must take into account two radiographic principles. First, a single, portable, lateral, cross-table radiograph is highly insensitive for significant C-spine injury. At least 25% of lateral C-spine radiographs fail to visualize the cervical-thoracic junction (C7-T1).[33] Even if the lateral radiograph is adequate, it should be considered no more than 80% sensitive for C-spine injury.[34] A complete three-view C-spine series fails to

identify about 15% of significant C-spine injuries, and it is difficult to obtain adequately for patients in cervical collars.[35] In consideration of this information, no plain radiograph should be interpreted as indicating that the C-spine is free of injury and that movement can be undertaken with impunity during intubation.

Second, the severe limitations of portable C-spine radiographs question their value before intubation. Current guidelines recommend the use of CT for C-spine evaluation of patients with trauma.[36] Given the limitations of portable cross-table plain radiographs of the spine and the danger of remote imaging before airway management, it is prudent to presume a C-spine injury and intubate with in-line C-spine stabilization without imaging.

Only patients who will not be obtaining CT imaging before emergency surgical management should have a lateral C-spine radiograph in the trauma bay. In other words, C-spine injuries should be presumed for all patients with blunt trauma needing airway management (and precautions should be taken accordingly), with CT imaging obtained for those thought to be stable enough for the scanner. However, in patients proceeding directly to the OR after intubation, a lateral C-spine x-ray (along with portable chest and pelvis radiographs) can be obtained to screen for the presence of catastrophic C-spine injury. In these cases, however, only a positive C-spine radiograph can be considered to provide additional information. The incidence of a false-negative radiograph despite significant injury is high enough that no reassurance should be taken from a negative study result.

Airway management in the patient with C-spine injury must be undertaken with strict attention to C-spine immobilization. This is best performed by a second operator whose sole function is to maintain the alignment of the head, neck, and torso. The best immobilization technique is one that allows the person performing the immobilization to have direct contact with the head and the torso.

Two common methods of immobilization are described. In one method, the assistant approaches the head from the thorax, resting his or her forearms on the upper chest and clavicles and passing the wrists and hands up alongside the neck bilaterally, so that the hands (with fingers spread) can grip and immobilize the occipital-parietal area of the head. This allows the assistant to prevent and detect any change in the angle of the head on the neck or the neck on the body during laryngoscopy and intubation. The assistant must provide direct feedback to the intubator of any motion.

In another method, the assistant crouches below the operating table, usually to the intubator's left side. The assistant then reaches up over the head of the table and immobilizes the base of the occiput with the heels of both hands. The fingers extend down alongside the neck to the top of the patient's shoulders, permitting the assistant to immobilize the head and neck and allowing detection of movement.

Intubation should be performed with the anterior portion of the cervical collar open because it may limit laryngoscopy. Leaving the collar intact has not been shown to reduce significant C-spine movement during intubation, and is not a substitute for manual in-line stabilization.[37-39] Although cricothyrotomy can be performed through the openings in most cervical collars, it is often technically challenging, and it is preferable to remove the anterior one half of the collar before undertaking surgical airway management. The debate regarding nasotracheal intubation versus various awake intubation techniques versus RSI in the trauma patient is discussed in "Principles of Airway Management in the Trauma Patient."

C. Intracranial Injury

Intracranial injury commonly occurs with blunt and penetrating forms of trauma. In penetrating trauma, injuries are obvious because the penetration must occur proximate to the cranial vault. With blunt trauma, however, the presence of intracranial injury can be much more difficult to establish. Although the Glasgow Coma Scale (GCS) score is widely used in trauma, it is at best a crude instrument. However, in the absence of a reversible cause (e.g., opioid overdose), a GCS score of 8 or less indicates coma and mandates intubation on the basis of airway protection and anticipated deterioration. Any patient with a GCS score of 12 or less should be considered to have significant head injury until cranial CT scanning can prove otherwise. These patients may have elevated ICPs, and all patients with a GCS score of 8 or less should be presumed to have elevated ICPs with loss of cerebral autoregulation. This approach has some impact on the agents selected for intubation and, to a lesser degree, the methods used.

Airway management in the patient with intracranial injury is dictated by an often-conflicting series of choices between limiting the adverse responses in the brain related to intubation and maintaining overall management of the patient's hemodynamic status and resuscitation. In patients with an elevated ICP, stimulation of the upper airway structures by a laryngoscope or other device results in an increase in the ICP.[40] The ICP appears to increase by two mechanisms: First, a release of sympathetic adrenergic transmitters results in elevation in heart rate and blood pressure, which translates to an elevation in ICP in the nonautoregulated brain.[41] Second, a direct reflexive increase in ICP is caused by laryngeal stimulation, although the mechanism is not precisely defined.[42]

Succinylcholine, which is the drug of choice for RSI of the multitrauma patient, is believed to cause an elevation in ICP, although this has been disputed.[43-45] The mitigation of these potential elevations in ICP is an important theme in the airway management of the trauma patient with presumed intracranial injury. Avoidance of hypoxia and hypercarbia and maintenance of adequate perfusion are vital for producing the best possible patient outcome.

Lidocaine has been studied in the context of prevention of the ICP response that is sympathetically mediated and the ICP response that is considered reflexive. Its use during RSI in the context of head injury continues to be controversial. Best-evidence reviews of patient outcomes and lidocaine use during airway management in head injured patients showed that no good evidence exists evaluating this specific issue.[46-48] Several small, randomized trials have found conflicting results with respect to the ability of lidocaine to attenuate spikes in ICP during laryngoscopy and intubation.[41,49-54] Overall, there is insufficient evidence to strongly recommend the use of lidocaine for the purpose of suppression of sympathetic discharge during intubation. However, lidocaine given intravenously at a dose of 1.5 mg/kg has been shown to blunt the direct ICP response to tracheal suctioning and laryngeal stimulation in hypocarbic patients with elevated ICP.[51,53] Lidocaine's wide therapeutic margin, familiarity, safety profile, and ready availability make it a reasonable choice when administered at 1.5 mg/kg intravenously for 3 minutes before the induction agent when undertaking RSI of a patient with known or presumed elevated ICP. Used in this manner, lidocaine may have a beneficial effect on the direct ICP response to laryngoscopy and intubation.

The sympathetic response to intubation has been extensively studied, and synthetic opioids and beta-blockers have been shown to attenuate the reflex sympathetic response to laryngoscopy. Administration of a beta-blocker to a trauma patient may worsen hemodynamic instability and is rarely desirable, except in certain cases of isolated head trauma. Similarly, administration of full sympathetic-blocking doses of the synthetic opioids, such as fentanyl, can have adverse effects, particularly in patients with hypovolemia, who depend on sympathetic drive. Fentanyl, in a dose of 2 to 3 μg/kg as a pretreatment agent, has been shown to attenuate the reflex sympathetic response to laryngoscopy and should have minimal adverse cardiovascular effects.[55] Care must be used, however, to ensure that the fentanyl does not cause respiratory depression with resulting hypercarbia and that the patient has sufficient hemodynamic stability to tolerate even this small dose.

Competitive NMB agents, such as rocuronium, achieve intubating conditions almost as rapidly as succinylcholine, but without the attendant rise in ICP.[56,57] However, the duration of paralysis when 1.0 mg/kg of rocuronium is used for intubation is about 45 minutes.[58] For this reason, succinylcholine, with its ultrarapid onset and shorter duration of action, remains the drug of choice for emergency intubation of trauma patients, including those with elevated ICP. The exacerbation of the ICP elevation by succinylcholine, however, is clearly not desirable. Evidence is poor supporting the administration of a defasciculating dose of a nondepolarizing NMB before succinylcholine to attenuate an increased ICP and is not recommended.

In summary, when RSI is planned, and there is no contraindication, 1.5 mg/kg of intravenous lidocaine and 3 μg/kg of intravenous fentanyl should be considered before the administration of succinylcholine. Defasciculating doses of non-depolarizing NMB drugs should not be used until further study clarifies their role. Laryngoscopy and intubation should be as gentle and atraumatic as possible. There is evidence that minimizing laryngeal stimulation helps to reduce the hemodynamic and ICP responses to laryngoscopy and intubation. Several devices have been evaluated to see whether they are less traumatic than direct laryngoscopy. Intubations through a laryngeal mask airway (LMA) and with the use of the Trachlight stylet appear to be less stimulating than intubation by direct laryngoscopy.[59,60] Studies comparing intubation over a lighted stylet with direct laryngoscopy indicate that the placement of the ETT into the trachea is more stimulating than the laryngoscopy itself.[61]

D. Intraocular Injury

Most patients with open globe injuries can be intubated in the OR under controlled conditions. Penetrating globe injuries usually are isolated and are caused primarily by implements (e.g., sticks, children's toys) or by low-velocity missiles (e.g., BBs, pellets). Occasionally, open globe injury occurs in the context of multitrauma and requires intubation in the trauma bay. Decisions related to overall management of the patient's multiple injuries should take precedence over management of the eye injury. Whether the intubation occurs in the trauma resuscitation bay or in the OR, the concern related to managing open globe injuries is whether succinylcholine, which causes a transient rise in intraocular pressure, may cause extrusion of intraocular contents.[62] There has never been a single case report of vitreous extrusion after the use of succinylcholine in a patient with an open globe injury.[63] The paramount consideration therefore appears to be prevention of straining, coughing, or bucking during the intubation, arguing for RSI. It has been recommended that a defasciculating dose of a competitive NMB agent be given 3 minutes before administration of succinylcholine in patients with open globe injuries to mitigate the elevation of intraocular pressure, but this approach has never been subjected to study. It appears that defasciculation is appropriate for patients with open globe injuries receiving succinylcholine unless there is a contraindication, such as severe respiratory compromise.

E. Thoracic Injury

Blunt and penetrating injuries can cause sufficient compromise of respiration or oxygenation to mandate intubation. The extent of injuries associated with penetrating trauma depends on the implement or missile used and the location and path of the object involved. High-velocity gunshot wounds to the chest are often fatal, causing disruption of the major vasculature, main stem bronchi, or the heart.[64] Lower-velocity gunshot wounds, especially those more peripherally placed, often cause much less blast injury to the chest, resulting in minor pulmonary contusions and a surprisingly low incidence of hemothorax or pneumothorax.[65] Pneumothorax is common in penetrating injury, whether caused by missile or implement, and cardiac injury with pericardial tamponade can occur. Blunt chest trauma tends to be more diffuse and is more often associated with pulmonary contusion, disruption of the chest wall with concomitant rib fractures, costochondral separation, hemothorax or pneumothorax, and if severe, disruption of a main stem bronchus or of the aorta.

In addition to a thorough physical examination and a determination of vital signs (including O_2 saturation), early, portable, anterior-posterior chest radiography is invaluable in assessing patients who are victims of thoracic trauma. However, obvious life-threatening conditions, such as tension pneumothorax, should be treated before radiographic confirmation. A patient presenting with external evidence of chest trauma (e.g., motor vehicle crash victim with multiple rib fractures and subcutaneous air) who has signs compatible with tension pneumothorax (e.g., hypotension, tachycardia, tachypnea, O_2 desaturation) should have immediate decompressive thoracostomy before radiographic studies. The finding of tracheal deviation occurs only in the final stages of tension pneumothorax when the patient is in extremis, and the presence of a midline trachea should never be used to exclude tension pneumothorax. If there are not sufficient personnel to manage all of the necessary tasks simultaneously, a needle thoracostomy can be done, pending insertion of the chest tube. Needle thoracostomy, however, is strictly a short-term temporizing measure, and tube thoracostomy with a 34-Fr or larger chest tube should be performed at the earliest opportunity. The objective is to release sufficient air such that diminished venous return and cardiac contractility are temporarily relieved. Release of tension pneumothorax also facilitates choice of the induction agent for intubation as hemodynamics typically improve significantly after needle or tube thoracostomy. Mitigation of the intrathoracic pressure helps to avoid the hypotension that may occur when positive-pressure ventilation is instituted after intubation.

Thoracic injuries have three effects on airway management. First, the intrathoracic injuries may be the primary reason for intubation. Pulmonary contusion, bilateral hemothorax, flail chest with respiratory compromise, pulmonary hemorrhage, and major life-threatening intrathoracic injury are all indications for early intubation.

Second, the thoracic injuries may compromise preoxygenation before intubation and promote rapid oxyhemoglobin desaturation after paralysis. Preoxygenation is essential when performing RSI, and patients with severe pulmonary injury may not preoxygenate well. It may be difficult to obtain O_2 saturations greater than 90%, even with high-flow O_2. Rapid oxyhemoglobin desaturation can be anticipated, and these patients may require BMV throughout the intubation sequence to maintain adequate oxygenation. This approach is particularly important in the patient with concomitant head injury.

Third, hypotension related to thoracic injuries may limit agent selection. Some induction agents, such as sodium thiopental and propofol, are potent venodilators and negative inotropes. When they are given to patients with hemodynamic compromise related to thoracic or multisystem injuries, the hypotension can be severe and prolonged. This effect often precludes the use of such agents or necessitates a significant reduction in dosage.

The intubation technique for patients with thoracic trauma is dictated by their overall status. Rarely does the thoracic trauma alone determine the technique. RSI usually is preferred, but care must be taken to preoxygenate the patient adequately and to maintain adequate oxygenation throughout the procedure. After the patient is intubated, positive-pressure ventilation may further compromise venous return and mean arterial blood pressure, and the mechanical ventilation should be adjusted to maintain adequate oxygenation with the least effective tidal volume until the patient-specific hemodynamic effects of the positive-pressure ventilation can be determined. Patients with pulmonary injury, such as pulmonary contusion, usually do better with modest amounts of positive end-expiratory pressure (5 to 10 mm Hg), but this has the potential to further compromise venous return and must be instituted with caution.

F. Hemorrhagic Shock

The patient in profound hemorrhagic shock has significant metabolic debt, experiences rapid muscle fatigue, is susceptible to respiratory compromise and failure, and usually requires intubation with positive-pressure ventilation unless the underlying process can be reversed. In addition to contributing to the need for intubation, hemorrhagic shock greatly limits the choice of agents for intubation. Induction agents such as sodium thiopental and propofol have significant adverse hemodynamic consequences.[65] These agents should be used in greatly reduced doses or avoided altogether in patients with hemorrhagic shock. Ketamine releases catecholamines and is the most stable of the induction agents. Ketamine can be used in a reduced dose of 1 mg/kg, even in patients with significant hemodynamic compromise. In frank shock, however, ketamine, like every other induction agent, depresses myocardial contractility and must be used with extreme caution.[66,67] It has been implicated in transient elevations of ICP, but the evidence in this regard is highly conflicted.[68] In the context of head injury with significant hypovolemia, ketamine's superior hemodynamic characteristics outweigh its potential to cause small, transient rises in ICP. Although caution is advised in administering ketamine to patients with head injury and to those in shock, it may be the least of all evils if given in a reduced dose in these patients.

Etomidate, an imidazole derivative, has remarkable hemodynamic stability.[69] In the induction dose of 0.3 mg/kg, it causes virtually no change in mean arterial blood pressure in normal and hypovolemic patients. In very large doses (two or three times the induction dose), etomidate consistently causes hypotension.[70] In morbidly obese trauma patients, dosing should be based on their lean body weight, not total body weight. For patients with frank shock, the dose should be reduced to between 0.15 and 0.2 mg/kg. Etomidate appears to have some cerebral protective effect and can significantly lower ICP without adverse effects on perfusion pressure.[71] It is therefore a rational agent for use in patients with multisystem trauma and hypovolemic shock.

Midazolam is infrequently used as an induction agent in multitrauma patients. It exhibits many of the same adverse hemodynamic effects as propofol and Pentothal. If it is used, the dose should be greatly reduced to 0.1 mg/kg in patients in frank shock. However, compared with other readily available agents, midazolam has a slower onset and longer clinical half-life, and at greatly reduced doses, it may not provide adequate amnesia for the patient.[72]

In addition to influencing the decision to intubate and the choice of agents, hemorrhagic shock greatly complicates overall management. Drug circulation times can be longer, and the physician may have to allow more time between the administration of succinylcholine and the first attempt at intubation. Succinylcholine itself is remarkably stable, although an increased or repeated dose may be required because of poor drug distribution in patients who have hemorrhagic shock. Pretreatment agents usually are avoided in hemorrhagic shock, with the exception of lidocaine for elevated ICP.

Isotonic fluid resuscitation must occur in parallel with preparation for intubation. The use of a high-flow blood-infusing unit can provide warmed packed red blood cells at a rate as high as 500 mL/min.[73] Care must be taken not to overshoot the resuscitation, particularly in the presence of penetrating injuries and those thought to be associated with ongoing bleeding. The goal is maintenance of an adequate perfusion pressure to support the brain and vital organs until surgical repair can be undertaken. There is no evidence that restoration of the blood pressure to a normal range is beneficial, and evidence suggests that permissive hypotension may instead be preferable.[74-76] Crystalloid can be infused as the first 2 L of fluid during resuscitation, but it should be rapidly replaced with blood if shock is ongoing. A urinary catheter may be helpful to monitor urine output, and lactic acid or base deficit values can help to monitor the overall treatment of shock.[77] If the patient is not going to be transported promptly to the OR, placement of an arterial line is highly advisable.

IV. PRINCIPLES OF AIRWAY MANAGEMENT IN THE TRAUMA PATIENT

A. Control of the Combative Patient

Trauma patients, particularly those who are intoxicated or who have sustained head injury, are frequently agitated or combative on arrival to the ED. In some cases, this agitation is a result of an overwhelming combination of confusing sensory inputs to the patient. Intoxication, head injury, disorientation, and severe pain can contribute to combative behavior. The patient's mental status may be an extension of a medical condition that precipitated the injury. Hypoglycemia, stroke, syncope, and seizure should be considered when the patient's mental status is significantly altered or when prehospital reports suggest a minor mechanism or minimal vehicular damage.

Initially, attempts should be made to reassure the patient and to help him or her orient to the chaotic environment of the resuscitation room. An agitated and confused patient may be helped by the physician placing his or her face relatively close to the patient's and speaking in a clear, firm, reassuring voice. Although this may have some initial calming effect, physical and chemical restraints are often necessary to facilitate an orderly, efficient, and safe trauma assessment. These patients are often restrained on a long spine board with a cervical collar, tape, and sandbags, but these constraints are temporary, and the patient's ability to move and to exert significant forces on the potentially injured spine often warrants further action.

The decision about whether to sedate a patient or to intubate for behavioral control should be made on the basis of the patient's overall injuries. If intubation is inevitable, even without combative behavior, based on the patient's injuries and expected clinical course, early intubation is the best approach. RSI allows protection of the C-spine, complete control of the patient, and treatment of multiple injuries without further disruption or pain. If the patient's overall injuries are deemed to be relatively modest and intubation would not be indicated in the absence of the combative behavior, chemical restraint without intubation is the best approach. Repeated, titrated doses of a butyrophenone, such as haloperidol, can rapidly achieve control of the patient without compromising respiration or significantly altering the neurologic examination. In the hemodynamically stable patient, 5 mg of haloperidol can be given intravenously in repeated doses every 5 minutes, with observation for effect.[78] Most patients calm rapidly under the influence of the haloperidol, and management can then proceed in a more orderly fashion. Haloperidol has been rumored to lower the seizure threshold and therefore be contraindicated in patients with head trauma, but this is close to a medical fairy tale. There are no well-controlled studies proving this association, and the remainder of the literature is a heterogenous mixture of rat studies and case reports.[79] There is no human evidence to support this often-cited contraindication. Droperidol was equally effective and commonly used for this purpose before the U.S. Food and Drug Administration (FDA) issued a highly controversial black box warning about QT interval prolongation, which greatly curtailed its use.[80]

Benzodiazepines are often used but have the potential for significantly more respiratory depression than haloperidol. Benzodiazepines must be used with great caution, particularly in patients with concomitant alcohol intoxication. The practice of using haloperidol in combination with benzodiazepines complicates matters by giving two drugs when one drug would do. Haloperidol has stood the test of time in trauma patients, who remain hemodynamically stable, and it can be given in large doses when necessary. Haloperidol does not alter the need to investigate the cause of the patient's combative behavior with CT, neurologic examination, and metabolic testing, but it does rapidly help to achieve control of the patient and permit ongoing evaluation.

B. Prevention of Aspiration

All trauma patients are considered to be at high risk for aspiration. Compromised airway protection from head injury or from intoxication, prone position, and a non-fasted state make aspiration a paramount concern. Reasonable precautions should be taken to prevent aspiration, particularly of gastric contents, during overall trauma management and particularly during airway management. The initial intubation method depends on the constellation of patient injuries, hemodynamic status, and the

equipment and expertise available. Most patients, however, will undergo RSI. Induction and the use of NMB drugs that occurs during RSI place the patient at risk for passive regurgitation. Early and generous suction, particularly when hemorrhage exists, reduces the aspiration of blood.

Routine application of posterior cricoid pressure (i.e., Sellick's maneuver) held throughout laryngoscopy was widely accepted dogma because it was thought to prevent aspiration through compression of the upper esophagus against the anterior cervical vertebral bodies. Although it seemed logical, it was never supported by firm evidence.[81,82] Misapplication of cricoid pressure is common among a variety of operators, and it can result in more difficult mask ventilation, direct laryngoscopy, and tracheal tube passage.[83-86] Moreover, regurgitation is often seen despite Sellick's maneuver being applied.[87-90] Advanced imaging suggests the cervical esophagus is positioned lateral to the cricoid ring in many patients, a relationship that is exaggerated by posterior pressure rarely resulting in esophageal obstruction.[91] C-spine motion may occur during cricoid pressure and introduce unnecessary risk for patients with known or suspected unstable C-spine injuries. If applied correctly however, Sellick's maneuver may reduce gastric insufflation during BMV.[92-94] On balance, the best approach is to consider posterior cricoid pressure optional during laryngoscopy and intubation and to remove it immediately if the laryngeal view is poor or tube passage is difficult. It should be routinely performed during prolonged rescue BMV.

If the patient vomits while on the spine board, the patient and the board should be rolled together into the right lateral decubitus position to permit suctioning and evacuation of the vomitus from the mouth. Vomiting is an indication for early intubation in patients who require immobilization on a spine board and who may be relatively helpless to manage the vomitus after it is in the mouth. When applying awake intubation techniques, adequate sedation and topical anesthesia should be used to prevent gagging and emesis. If the patient vomits during awake intubation, there is increased risk of aspiration because of the topical anesthesia of the supraglottic area and the vocal cords. Prompt suctioning and repositioning of the patient, if necessary, should help reduce this risk. There is no evidence that one particular device or technique is more likely to prevent aspiration than any other. RSI, developed as the cornerstone of emergency airway management because of its ability to reduce aspiration, has recently been challenged in this regard.[95]

C. Choice of Technique

The issues related to approach to the airway are discussed in detail in the individual sections earlier in this chapter. Overall, the choice of technique must balance the physiologic status of the patient, the nature of the injuries, predicted airway difficulty, the urgency of the airway intervention, and the availability of various devices and surgical backup. Historically, the Advanced Trauma Life Support (ATLS) course developed by members of the American College of Surgeons advocated blind nasotracheal intubation for patients with suspected C-spine injuries because it was believed to be less likely to cause C-spine movement. This belief was unfounded, and blind nasotracheal intubation has fallen out of favor as a method of airway management in the trauma patient because of slower intubation times, higher complication rates, and greater O_2 desaturation.[96-98] RSI is the preferred method for most intubations. There was early objection, however, due to suspicion of dangerous degrees of C-spine motion during unrestricted direct laryngoscopy and that residual muscle tone in nonparalyzed patients provided valuable splinting support. As a result of these two fundamentally incorrect beliefs, trauma intubations through the 1970s and 1980s were largely performed by awake intubation. Cadaver studies and those done in living patients have failed to support this contention. There is no evidence that careful laryngoscopy performed with in-line stabilization subjects the C-spine to any risk, although intubation should not be forceful or prolonged. There is good evidence that manual in-line stabilization combined with a careful oral laryngoscopy and RSI does not pose any risk to the cervical spinal cord.[99-101]

Unrelaxed patients present the potential for significantly more C-spine motion as a result of coughing, bucking, gagging, or other movement during an awake intubation attempt. RSI has been successful and frequently used during trauma intubations. In a published report of almost 9000 ED intubations from phase II of the National Emergency Airway Registry showed that 82% of trauma patients underwent RSI and 11% were intubated with no medications; they were mostly patients in full arrest or near-full arrest who were completely unresponsive on presentation and underwent immediate direct laryngoscopy with intubation and manual in-line stabilization. Less than 1% of patients underwent unassisted nasotracheal intubation.[102]

D. The Difficult Airway

Trauma patients represent a group with high-risk, exceptionally difficult airways. Acquired characteristics, such as airway trauma, C-spine immobility, hemodynamic compromise, and other potentially life-threatening injuries, can exacerbate inherently difficult airway markers, necessitating clarity of thought and error-free decision making during intubation. An efficient but detailed difficult airway assessment is necessary before NMB in the multitrauma patient. Conventional assessments that occur during a preoperative visit may not be possible in the trauma bay. It is rarely possible to obtain a prior surgical anesthetic history from the patient. Creators of the national *Emergency and the Difficult Airway Course: Anesthesia* have developed a four-pronged rapid assessment tool that can be quickly applied to virtually any patient.[103] Portions of this tool have been externally validated in emergency populations, and it is currently subject to further validation in the third phase of the National Emergency Airway Registry multicenter registry.[104] The LEMON mnemonic is used as shown in Box 41-1 to identify one or more attributes of a difficult airway in a patient.

The tool is overly sensitive at the cost of specificity, but that is more desirable than the converse. If a difficult

---

BOX 41-1 LEMON Mnemonic

L Look externally
E Evaluate the 3-3-2 rule
M Mallampati
O Obstruction
N Neck mobility

From Murphy MF, Walls RM: Identification of the difficult and failed airway. In Walls RM, Murphy MF, Luten RC, editors: *Manual of emergency airway management*, ed 3, Philadelphia, 2008, Lippincott Williams & Wilkins, pp 81–93.

---

intubation is anticipated, physicians use an algorithmic approach that is dictated by how stable the patient is and how urgently he or she needs to be intubated (Fig. 41-5). The easiest surrogate is the best attainable O_2 saturation measurement, because it defines the time available to consider alternative approaches. If the patient is well oxygenated and is reasonably stable (i.e., does not need to be intubated in the next 2 to 3 minutes), a methodic stepwise plan can be made. If the patient is critically desaturated and highly unstable, it is probably necessary to proceed directly with some form of airway intervention promptly without the luxury of a planned approach to the difficult airway. In this scenario, a double-setup RSI, in which the anterior neck is prepared for a surgical airway as RSI drugs are administered, is most appropriate. RSI gives the operator the best chance of intubation success, and if a *cannot intubate, cannot ventilate* (CICV)

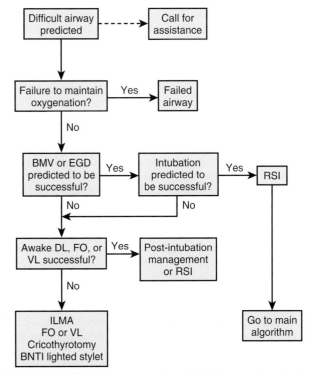

Figure 41-5 Difficult airway algorithm. *BMV,* Bag-mask ventilation; *BNTI,* blind nasotracheal intubation; *DL,* difficult laryngoscopy; *EGD,* extraglottic device; *FO,* fiberoptic; *ILMA,* intubating laryngeal mask airway; *RSI,* rapid-sequence intubation; *VL,* video laryngoscopy. (From Walls RM: *Manual of emergency airway management,* ed 3, Philadelphia, 2008, Lippincott Williams & Wilkins.)

BOX 41-2   MOANS Mnemonic

M   Mask seal
O   Obstruction or obesity
A   Age > 55 years
N   No teeth
S   Stiff lungs

From Murphy MF, Walls RM: Identification of the difficult and failed airway. In Walls RM, Murphy MF, Luten RC, editors: *Manual of emergency airway management*, ed 3, Philadelphia, 2008, Lippincott Williams & Wilkins, pp 81–93.

scenario develops, a cricothyrotomy should be immediately performed. Primary cricothyrotomy may be the primary method used, usually when orotracheal and nasotracheal intubation is predicted to be difficult or impossible. Rarely, other devices such as the FFB or intubating LMA (ILMA) are useful.

When there is sufficient time ($SaO_2 > 90\%$) to plan the intubation approach carefully, the patient should be evaluated for the likelihood of success with BMV and laryngoscopy. Predicted success with BMV is a necessary precursor to consideration of paralysis. The MOANS mnemonic (Box 41-2) contains a well-validated collection of patient attributes that contribute to difficult mask ventilation.[105] If it is the intubator's judgment that the patient cannot be BMV successfully, a technique using NMB is out of the question unless it is part of a double setup with an immediate ability to move to a surgical airway if the first attempt at laryngoscopy is unsuccessful. Next, the operator must decide whether laryngoscopy and intubation are likely to be successful. If it is thought that the patient is likely to be successfully intubated by direct laryngoscopy despite the difficult airway attributes, taking into consideration that the patient should successfully undergo BMV, RSI can be planned with a surgical backup, as necessary. For example, the assault patient requiring strict C-spine precautions because of a dislocated jaw and active upper airway bleeding would be challenging or impossible to manage with direct laryngoscopy because of a severely reduced mouth opening, neutral head position, and airway bleeding. However, a normal-sized patient who was stabbed in the abdomen and was placed in a C-spine collar by emergency medical services but who has little likelihood of a neck injury would routinely warrant a laryngoscopic attempt. Both patients meet criteria for a difficult airway, but successful direct laryngoscopy is reasonable in the second patient but not in the first patient. With the advent of the video laryngoscope, traditional difficult laryngoscopy predictors may not apply, and what constitutes a difficult video laryngoscopic attempt has not been defined. As our knowledge and experience with video laryngoscopy develops, our threshold for NMB in these patients may change.

In most circumstances, difficult airway attributes are identified in trauma patients, but the operator can still be confident that BMV and direct laryngoscopy will be successful, thereby permitting RSI. If, however, in the opinion of the operator, BMV or direct laryngoscopy is unlikely to be possible, it is better to proceed with an awake technique. This involves administration of sedation and use of topical anesthesia to permit awake evaluation of the airway by a direct, video-assisted, or fiberoptic technique (see Chapter 11). Awake laryngoscopy is a common approach that has three possible outcomes: the cords are well visualized, and the patient is intubated; the cords are well visualized, and the decision is made that RSI is possible (in this case, awake laryngoscopy is terminated, and the patient undergoes RSI); or awake laryngoscopy determines that orotracheal intubation will likely be difficult or impossible, and an alternative approach is necessary.

If, after awake direct laryngoscopy, it is determined that the patient cannot be intubated orally, there are several alternative techniques, which are described elsewhere in this textbook. In the trauma patient, the most useful of these is video laryngoscopy. Although it is susceptible to soiling from airway secretions and bleeding, the mechanical limitations inherent in direct laryngoscopy virtually vanish with video laryngoscopy, and glottic visualization nearly always improves.[106,107] Surgical cricothyrotomy, flexible fiberoptic intubation, video laryngoscopy, a lighted stylet technique, and an ILMA may be useful in selected cases. Supralaryngeal or retroglottic airways, such as the LMA, King LT, and others, can be used as a rescue device in the setting of a failed airway, but they are rarely preferred as a primary management tool in trauma patients because of the uncertainty about their ability to protect against aspiration. The goal in managing the trauma patient, even with an identified difficult airway, is to achieve endotracheal intubation with an inflated cuff to protect against aspiration. Placement of a device that does not achieve this is normally considered only in circumstances in which there has been a failed airway or the patient has precipitously arrested and definitive airway management is not possible (see "The Failed Airway").

E. Pharmacologic Considerations

Injured patients are most often managed with RSI and several factors commonly observed for trauma victims should be considered when finalizing the pharmacologic menu. Rapidly selecting the appropriate induction agent, NMB agent, and pretreatment agents to secure the airway with the least likelihood of adverse effect is paramount.

Trauma patients are frequently hypovolemic, even if their initial mean arterial blood pressure is normal. Drug selection must go hand in hand with volume resuscitation and other appropriate interventions, such as tube thoracostomy, control of external hemorrhage, and pelvic stabilization. The individual decisions related to choice of pretreatment and induction agents are discussed throughout this chapter, but a few points should be emphasized.

Induction agents should be chosen to provide the best possible intubating conditions (used in conjunction with succinylcholine) with the least likelihood for adverse hemodynamic consequences. Etomidate, in a dose of 0.3 mg/kg, is remarkably hemodynamically stable, appears to provide some degree of cerebral protection, and has an onset-duration profile similar to that of succinylcholine. Although etomidate has been associated with adrenal cortical suppression, this is not clinically significant when a single dose is used for induction for intubation.[108] Its safety during RSI in trauma patients has been challenged, although these studies have fatally flawed methodology and low patient numbers, making the results hard to interpret and impossible to apply to clinical practice.[109,110] Etomidate can cause myoclonic jerks during its onset, but use of a rapidly acting NMB agent, such as succinylcholine, mitigates this effect substantially. Ketamine is an appropriate induction agent for hypotensive trauma patients. Ketamine's role in head injury has been questioned because of its tendency to cause elevated ICP, but it is likely that the preservation of cerebral perfusion by maintenance of mean arterial blood pressure in hemodynamically unstable patients is more important than any theoretical risk to the brain caused by ketamine's tendency to increase cerebral activity and ICP.[64,111] Other induction agents, such as propofol and pentothal, have much more tendency to cause hypotension and should be used in reduced doses and with caution in compromised or elderly trauma patients. Patients in shock with an immediate need for intubation should be given reduced (one-third to one-half) doses, regardless of the induction agent. Choice of a paralytic is not altered by the presence or absence of trauma. Succinylcholine and rocuronium are both appropriate and result in near-equivalent intubating conditions and first-pass success, depending on the dose used.[112,113]

The choice of agents for sedation and awake intubation is influenced by the patient's general status. It is advisable to use the agent with which the operator is most familiar for sedation. For example, if the operator typically sedates patients for painful procedures using propofol, it may be the best choice to sedate the trauma patient for awake laryngoscopy. In the absence of operator preference, ketamine may be ideally suited, especially when combined with an antisialagogue because of its ability to preserve respirations and hemodynamic status.[114] Overall, familiarity with the drugs and the ability to titrate them carefully are probably more important than the drug's pharmacodynamic characteristics.

F. The Failed Airway

In managing the severely traumatized patient, it is important to have a clear definition of airway failure and a prepared action plan. The most widely accepted definition of a failed airway and the one used in the *Emergency and the Difficult Airway Course: Anesthesia* states that a failed airway exists when "(1) there have been three failed attempts by the most experienced operator, or (2) there has been one failed attempt by an experienced intubator combined with an inability to maintain adequate oxygen saturation despite airway adjuncts, maximal supplemental oxygen, and a bag and mask."[115]

In either case, it is necessary to recognize that, with the current method and device being used, orotracheal intubation is not going to succeed, and the operator must move on to a rescue technique. If three attempts have failed, but oxygenation can be maintained with BMV, the operator should quickly evaluate why

intubation was unsuccessful. Despite solid direct laryngoscopic technique, inadequate glottic exposure is often the culprit and results from the additive effect of poor C-spine mobility, reduced mouth opening, and oral secretions and blood. The modern difficult airway manager should have within his or her immediate reach a device designed to overcome these limitations and see around corners. Many options exist, although video laryngoscopy has shown the most promise, resulting in improved laryngeal views in almost every conceivable scenario in OR studies and ED populations.[106,107,116,117] In the CICV scenario, the most appropriate rescue device is surgical cricothyrotomy. One parallel attempt at oxygenation may occur by rapid, blind insertion of a rescue supralaryngeal airway, such as a King LT or LMA, but only in concert with preparation for a surgical approach. If the patient's oxygenation improves, other options can be explored. There should, however, be no hesitation for performing a cricothyrotomy if the slightest hint of supralaryngeal airway failure exists. An algorithm for managing a failed airway was developed for the *Emergency and the Difficult Airway Course: Anesthesia* and is shown in Figure 41-6.[115] The theme of the algorithm is that decisions are driven by whether there is sufficient

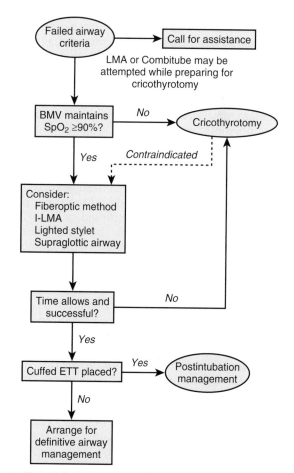

Figure 41-6 Failed airway algorithm. *BMV,* Bag-mask ventilation; *ETT,* endotracheal tube; *I-LMA,* intubating laryngeal mask airway; *LMA,* laryngeal mask airway; *SpO₂,* oxygen saturation measured by pulse oximetry. (From Walls RM: *Manual of emergency airway management,* ed 3, Philadelphia, 2008, Lippincott Williams & Wilkins.)

time to consider alternatives. If a CICV scenario arises at any time, the pathway leads to cricothyrotomy.

G. Rescue Techniques

The ultimate rescue technique for a failed airway in the trauma patient is surgical cricothyrotomy (see Chapter 31). When intubation has failed but ventilation is possible (i.e., *cannot intubate but can ventilate* scenario), several devices warrant consideration. They appear in the central box of the algorithm in Figure 41-6.

If direct laryngoscopy alone has been used, the operator should consider video laryngoscopy. The Glidescope video laryngoscope (GVL) and Macintosh video laryngoscope have been shown to improve laryngeal view compared with direct laryngoscopy in heterogeneous patient populations. Use of the GVL is associated with high levels of intubation success after failed direct laryngoscopy, although it may not be as effective in patients with significantly altered upper airway anatomy.[118] Video laryngoscopy should be considered early as a backup or principal intubating device for significantly difficult trauma airways. Optically enhanced devices, such as the Airtraq, are understudied in trauma populations, although, early data suggest the Airtraq may be effective for patients requiring C-spine precautions.[119]

If these tools are not available, many supralaryngeal airways can be tried. The Combitube has been evaluated as a primary airway management device and as a rescue device. Numerous studies have shown that emergency medical technicians can successfully insert Combitubes with a high likelihood of success.[120,121] When studied in a cadaver unstable C-spine model, the Combitube produced more posterior C-spine displacement than the LMA or fiberoptic methods. This suggests that in-line stabilization is equally important during Combitube insertion as during direct laryngoscopy.[122] Insertion with a cervical collar in place, however, has yielded mixed results. One study showed a high insertion success rate, and another reported successful blind insertion in only one third of patients with a semirigid collar on.[123,124] Ventilation with the Combitube, however, usually is highly successful.[124] The primary use of the Combitube is as a rescue device in the cannot intubate but can ventilate scenario in which other airway devices are thought unlikely to be successful. The Combitube is a less desirable choice because it does not place a cuffed ETT in the trachea when located in the esophageal position, but it usually suffices for ventilation and oxygenation. Another role for the Combitube is as a temporizing measure during preparations for cricothyrotomy. In this circumstance, only a single, expeditious attempt at placement is warranted.

Patients may arrive in the trauma bay with the Combitube inserted, inflated, and functioning. Because the Combitube does not provide a definitive airway (defined as a cuffed ETT in the trachea), it is advisable in most circumstances to intubate the patient and remove the Combitube. Details of insertion and use of the Combitube are discussed in Chapter 27, but there is a specific technique that must be used to intubate when the

Combitube is in place. The Combitube has two cuffs, which are inflated through two separate channels. The proximal (pharyngeal) cuff is the larger of the two and is indicated by the blue filling valve. After ensuring that the patient is stabilized and adequately preoxygenated, this proximal cuff should be deflated. The Combitube should then be moved to the left corner of the patient's mouth to permit access from the right side for laryngoscopy. Because the Combitube is almost always placed in the esophagus, it can remain in place while laryngoscopy proceeds. If difficulty arises, video laryngoscopy may be performed.[125] After the patient is intubated with the ETT cuff inflated and tube position confirmed by end-tidal CO_2 detection, the distal cuff on the Combitube can be deflated, and the Combitube can be removed. In the few cases in which the Combitube is inserted in the trachea, it can serve as a definitive airway, and tracheal placement is identified because successful ventilation and CO_2 detection are occurring through its second port. It has been recommended that a nasogastric tube be passed and the stomach decompressed before removal of the Combitube. It is possible for regurgitation to occur after removal of the Combitube, particularly if BMV occurred before placement of the Combitube in the prehospital setting.

In the ED and trauma resuscitation room, the ILMA is preferable to the Classic LMA. The ILMA is equally or more easily inserted and allows a conduit for subsequent intubation, with a significantly higher success rate than for the Classic LMA.[126,127] The ILMA has also been used to facilitate fiberoptic intubation and lighted stylet intubation.[128] The standard LMA and the LMA ProSeal have reasonable insertion success rates in the context of C-spine immobilization, but this situation has not been evaluated for the ILMA.[129] The ILMA has two main uses in the trauma patient. It can be used as the primary intubation method in a patient with an identified difficult airway. In the trauma patient, however, particularly one with an immobilized C-spine, the ILMA typically is not the first device selected. More commonly, the ILMA is used as a rescue device in a cannot intubate but can ventilate scenario. Placement of the ILMA allows ongoing ventilation with a very high success rate and facilitates endotracheal intubation. Like the Combitube, the ILMA can be placed as a temporizing measure during preparation for a cricothyrotomy in a CICV situation, as long as the placement and attempted ventilation through the ILMA do not delay initiation of surgical cricothyrotomy. Although less studied, the King LT shows promise as an effective rescue device and offers advantages of speed and success over the Combitube when used by prehospital providers.[130]

The lighted stylet has not been studied specifically in trauma as a primary intubating device or as a rescue device. In controlled settings and experienced hands, the lighted stylet can have a high intubation success rate. However, the possible need for reduced lighting during a trauma resuscitation, the lack of supporting evidence in managing trauma, and the availability of more effective video devices make this tool an option best left on the shelf.

V. CONCLUSIONS

The trauma airway is a subset of the difficult airway. In addition to the standard markers, specific issues such as anatomic disruption, brisk bleeding, and polytrauma must be managed along with global trauma resuscitation, making trauma airways particularly challenging. The fundamental principles that are applied to all patients with difficult airways must be applied to trauma patients. The foundation for success is an orderly approach, including prioritization of resuscitation steps, evaluation of the specific characteristics of the difficult airway, careful selection of pharmacologic agents, early use of video or optically enhanced airway tools, and coordination with other members of the resuscitation team.

VI. CLINICAL PEARLS

- Many trauma patients may initially appear to be maintaining their airways well, but because of progressive airway obstruction or multisystem traumatic comorbidities, they can deteriorate rapidly.

- Intubating a trauma patient should be part of an overall team-based approach to resuscitation. Although intubation may not be necessary to maintain airway patency, the patient's expected clinical course or need for emergent surgical intervention may prompt intubation.

- The gag reflex should not be used to gauge airway protection in any patient, especially those with trauma, who are typically secured on a backboard in a cervical collar and prone to aspiration. If these patients do vomit, they should be rolled with the board into a lateral decubitus position.

- Current evidence supports a strategy of not immobilizing the C-spine in patients with isolated penetrating trauma who do not have signs of neurologic compromise.

- CT images, not radiographs, should be obtained for all patients with suspected C-spine injury who are stable enough for travel to a CT scanner.

- Advent of the video laryngoscope has changed the management of difficult airways. Improved glottic visualization and high success rates for intubation support its use as an early rescue tool and principal intubating device.

- Sellick's maneuver does not prevent aspiration and may make intubation more difficult. It should be routine during bag-mask ventilation (BMV) but optional (at best) during intubation.

- Proceed with caution using induction agents, such as propofol or full-dose benzodiazepines, in patients with significant hemorrhage or shock.

- Predictors of a difficult airway, such as those contained in the LEMON mnemonic, should be applied to all trauma patients.

- A variety of effective rescue airway devices are available for use in trauma patients. Airway specialists should become familiar with and practice several of them to maximize the options available in case of a failed airway.

SELECTED REFERENCES

All references can be found online at expertconsult.com.

40. Adachi YU, Satomoto M, Higuchi H, et al: Fentanyl attenuates the hemodynamic response to intubation more than the response to laryngoscopy. *Anesth Analg* 95:233–237, 2002.
56. Perry J, Lee J, Wells G: Rocuronium versus succinylcholine for rapid sequence induction intubation. *Cochrane Database Syst Rev* (1):CD002788, 2003.
60. Maharaj CH, Buckley E, Harte BH, et al: Endotracheal intubation in patients with cervical spine immobilization. *Anesthesiology* 107:53–59, 2007.
82. Ellis DY, Harris T, Zideman D: Cricoid pressure in emergency department rapid sequence tracheal intubations: A risk-benefit analysis. *Ann Emerg Med* 50:653–665, 2007.
91. Smith KJ, Dobranowski J, Yip G, et al: Cricoid pressure displaces the esophagus: An observational study using magnetic resonance imaging. *Anesthesiology* 99:60–64, 2003.
95. Neilipovitz DT, Crosby ET: No evidence for decreased incidence of aspiration after rapid sequence induction. *Can J Anesth* 54:748–764, 2007.
102. Walls RM, Brown CA III, Bair AE, et al: Emergency airway management: A multi-center report of 8937 emergency department intubations. *J Emerg Med* 41:347–354, 2011.
103. Murphy MF, Walls RM: Identification of the difficult and failed airway. In Walls RM, Murphy MF, Luten RC, editors: *Manual of emergency airway management*, ed 3, Philadelphia, 2008, Lippincott Williams & Wilkins, pp 81–93.
105. Langeron O, Masso E, Hurax C, et al: Prediction of difficult mask ventilation. *Anesthesiology* 92:1229–1236, 2000.
106. Brown CA III, Bair AE, Pallin DJ, et al: Improved glottic exposure in adult emergency department tracheal intubations. *Ann Emerg Med* 56:83–88, 2010.

Chapter 42

The Difficult Airway in Neurosurgery

IRENE P. OSBORN | LARA FERRARIO

I. INTRODUCTION

Airway management in the neurosurgical patient is sometimes a challenging endeavor. In achieving and maintaining a patent airway, it is important to consider its impact on the central nervous system and the well-being of the patient. This chapter reflects the authors' experiences anesthetizing neurosurgical patients in several institutions. The 1990s were declared "the decade of the brain," and since then the variety of neurosurgical procedures, anesthetic techniques, and airway devices has increased dramatically. The evolution of neurosurgical practice and the growth of complex spine surgery provide a myriad of clinical challenges.

This chapter reviews the range of airway considerations faced daily by the neuroanesthesia practitioner. The goal is to address issues specific to the dedicated neuroanesthesiologist, as well as those related to the neurosurgical patient that might be encountered by the generalist anesthesiologist. This discussion reflects the ever-changing considerations in airway management of the neurosurgical patient and offers solutions to common clinical problems that occur in this patient population.

II. THE NEUROSURGICAL PATIENT

The American Academy of Neurological Surgeons (AANS) estimates that almost 1 million neurosurgical procedures are performed annually in the United States. Spine procedures are performed at three times the rate of cranial surgeries.[1] When considering the range of potential neurosurgical procedures, the variety of patient pathophysiology is substantial. A patient presenting for neurosurgery may appear to be completely normal or can present with clinical symptoms of intracranial hypertension. The airway might be assessed as "normal" but the patient's head is fixed in a frame. Also, the patient may present with acromegaly for pituitary surgery or may have a previous history of difficult intubation. Additionally, the unanticipated difficult airway becomes an even greater challenge in patients at risk for cerebral aneurysm rupture. Other challenges include the spine surgery patient in the prone position and considerations for extubation after prolonged surgery. Patients with central nervous system (CNS) disease can be sensitive to the effects of hypnotic agents, rendering them susceptible to apnea when premedication is given.

Neurosurgical procedures comprise only 7% of cases in the American Society of Anesthesiologists (ASA) closed-claims database but are associated with settlements that are 1.6 to 4 times more than general surgical procedures.[2] Understanding the patient's physiologic requirements, in addition to the surgeon's plan, is extremely important in these patients. It is wise to have a number of techniques for achieving, maintaining, and rescuing the neurosurgical airway.

A. Intracranial Dynamics and the Airway

Intracranial pressure (ICP) is the pressure within the rigid skull. Airway management in the face of intracranial hypertension is a frequent challenge for the neuroanesthesiologist, as well as the emergency physician. The patient who does not require immediate airway control may benefit from the simple maneuver of elevating the head. The head-up position may have beneficial effects on ICP through changes in mean arterial pressure (MAP), airway pressure, central venous pressure, and cerebrospinal fluid displacement.[3] Cerebral perfusion pressure (CPP) is the effective perfusion pressure driving blood through the brain, defined as the difference between mean arterial and intracranial pressures (CPP = MAP – ICP). A frequent consideration in the neurosurgical patient is the need to balance and maintain intracranial dynamics, avoiding increases in ICP, yet maintaining cerebral perfusion. Although head elevation may reduce ICP, raising the head above 30 degrees may place the patient at risk for venous air entrainment and should be done with caution.

Ventilation is intimately related to cerebral blood flow (CBF) and is an integral part of neuroanesthesia management. The avoidance of hypercarbia is essential in management of patients with intracranial hypertension. Carbon dioxide dilates the cerebral blood vessels, increasing the volume of blood in the intracranial vault and therefore increasing ICP. Periarteriolar hydrogen ion concentration, [H$^+$], powerfully influences cerebral arteriolar tone, and as the arterial carbon dioxide tension (PaCO_2) rises, [H$^+$] increases, causing arteriolar dilatation. This leads to a concomitant decrease in cerebrovascular resistance, causing an increase in CBF, and an increase in cerebral blood volume (CBV).[4] Difficult mask ventilation may quickly lead to hypercarbia, hypoxemia, and increased CBF. Hypoxia also remains one of the more potent arteriolar cerebrovascular dilators. Changes in the arterial oxygen tension (PaO_2) are associated with late increases in CBF. Hypoxia or ischemia leads to marked vasodilation, increased arterial vascular volume, and intracranial hypertension.[5]

Laryngoscopy and intubation, if performed with difficulty or improperly, can severely compromise intracranial dynamics and increase morbidity. Both the sympathetic and the parasympathetic nervous system mediate cardiovascular responses to endotracheal intubation.[6] Acute increases in ICP and MAP during laryngoscopy and endotracheal intubation have been well documented.[7] In 1975, Burney and Winn[8] measured ICP in 12 patients undergoing craniotomy and two patients for carotid arteriography. ICP did not change in response to the injection of contrast medium but increased significantly and dramatically in response to laryngoscopy and intubation. The increase appeared related to the initial ICP of these patients, possibly representing exhaustion of compensatory mechanisms. Special attention must be given to this factor during manipulation of the larynx in neurosurgical patients with initially increased ICP or space-occupying intracranial lesions.

Techniques to blunt this sympathetic response have included (1) an additional dose of thiopental or propofol, (2) use of beta-blockers or other antihypertensive agents, and (3) use of intravenous (IV) lidocaine. Esmolol or lidocaine as an IV bolus of 1.5 mg/kg before laryngoscopy and intubation did not completely prevent the increase in MAP and ICP.[9,10] Etomidate has been shown to cause an early "burst" suppression pattern on the electroencephalogram (EEG), minimal changes in CPP, and a marked reduction in ICP. This decrease in ICP was maintained during the first 30 seconds and the following 60 seconds after intubation, as MAP and heart rate remained unchanged.[11] Although not practical, this approach demonstrates the extent of efforts often made to obtund this response. Numerous methods have been advocated to prevent undesirable cardiovascular disturbances at intubation.[12] Whereas the cardiovascular response can be dramatic and substantial, the ICP response may lag behind and persist longer. Once the patient is intubated, ventilation parameters may be adjusted to the clinical situation.

III. CLINICAL STRATEGIES FOR THE NEUROSURGICAL PATIENT

Airway assessment of the neurosurgical patient requires similar considerations as described in other chapters of this textbook. The patient who has undergone previous surgery and has a history of difficult intubation warrants particular attention. A review of the anesthetic record should reveal which techniques produced success or failure. Difficult mask ventilation is of particular concern because of the potential for causing hypercarbia and the detrimental changes previously described.

A. Patient for Craniotomy

Patients who are neurologically intact may demonstrate no evidence of intracranial pathology or alteration. In addition to the history and physical examination, preoperative computed tomography (CT) or magnetic resonance imaging (MRI) scans of the head may give valuable information, because lesions associated with greater than 10 mm in midline shift or cerebral edema usually indicate intracranial hypertension.[13] These patients should be appropriately managed to avoid undue increases in ICP and CBF. Such measures include proper head positioning, preoxygenation, and appropriate dosing of induction agents and relaxants to achieve a smooth intubation. The primary challenge in anesthetizing a patient with a supratentorial mass lesion is to avoid further increases in ICP when one has limited intracranial compliance. There is no "ideal anesthetic" for this group of patients, and the perioperative management should be individualized. However, the practitioner should be aware of the effects of anesthetic agents on intracranial dynamics.

The preoperative use of midazolam for anxiety in these patients should not cause harm if they are carefully observed. A 1-mg to 2-mg dose of IV midazolam in adult patients may facilitate the induction of anesthesia without altering intracranial dynamics.[14] Opioids, on the other hand, should be restricted to very small amounts and given preoperatively under constant supervision because of possible hypercarbia and resultant effects. The efficacy of depth of anesthesia was recognized early on as a technique for avoiding intracranial hypertension.[15] Deep inhalation anesthesia was replaced by a combination of intravenous induction agents, notably thiopental, in combination with fentanyl. Thiopental produces a dose-dependent reduction in CBF and cerebral metabolic rate of oxygen consumption ($CMRO_2$). Other barbiturates, such as pentobarbital and methohexital, essentially have similar effects. ICP is reduced by barbiturates, likely because of the reduction in CBF and CBV. *Propofol* has largely replaced thiopental as the induction agent of choice for neuroanesthesia. Despite initial concerns about decreasing MAP and CPP, propofol provides a smooth transition to unconsciousness without an increase in heart rate, as observed with thiopental. This often produces less hypertension with laryngoscopy and intubation.[16]

Clinical doses of most opioids have minimal to modest depressive effects on CBF and $CMRO_2$. Early studies demonstrate that ICP is either not elevated or slightly decreased with fentanyl alone or in combination with droperidol. Reported ICP increases in patients with space-occupying lesions have been attributed to hypercapnia. The variability in response to opioids appears to be caused by the background anesthetic. When vasodilating drugs are used as part of the anesthetic management, the effect of the opioid is consistently that of a vasoconstrictor. *Sufentanil* was thought to produce an increase in ICP in patients with intracranial mass effect, but this was later attributed to a decrease in MAP.[17] *Alfentanil* produces little changes or slight decreases in CBF.[18] The beneficial effect of synthetic opioids is their ability to blunt the hemodynamic response to laryngoscopy and intubation without affecting intracranial dynamics. *Remifentanil* produces the most profound and consistent response, with lack of hypertension, tachycardia, or increase in ICP.[19] A continuous infusion throughout induction may provide the most effective hemodynamic control, while adequate ventilation is maintained.

The volatile agents, including nitrous oxide, can be considered dose-dependent cerebral vasodilators.[20] As a component of neuroanesthesia, volatile agents are typically used in moderate doses, in combination with opioids and hypnotic agents. The effects on cerebral circulation and metabolism of sevoflurane and desflurane are largely comparable to isoflurane. Both induce a direct vasodilation of the cerebral vessels, resulting in a less pronounced increase in CBF, compared to the decrease in cerebral metabolism.

Induction may be followed by hyperventilation with a volatile agent to deepen the anesthetic, decrease $CMRO_2$ (and CBF), and provide bronchodilation in patients with asthma or chronic obstructive pulmonary disease. Sevoflurane is useful in both pediatric and adult patients by allowing inhalation induction without the adverse effects of coughing or breath-holding.[21] A frequently employed technique in the cooperative patient is the use of active hyperventilation before induction, to initiate hypocapnia and decrease CBF as the patient loses consciousness. The use of topical anesthesia applied to the larynx and trachea can also prevent further response to laryngoscopy and intubation.[22] The large number of techniques recommended to suppress cardiovascular responses indicates that no single method has gained widespread acceptance (Table 42-1).

The obtunded patient with symptoms of intracranial hypertension requires additional attention to detail, avoiding premedication and maneuvers that increase coughing. If a rapid-sequence induction is not indicated

TABLE 42-1

Anesthetic Techniques to Avoid Increased Intracranial Pressure

Technique	Precaution(s)
Avoid hypercapnia.	Be vigilant of patient's respiratory status.
	Avoid undue sedation.
Avoid hypoxia.	Supplemental oxygen use mandatory.
	Be vigilant of patient's respiratory status.
	Take precautions to avoid aspiration.
	Preoxygenation before induction of anesthesia or tracheal intubation.
Avoid marked hypertension.	Be vigilant to changes in degree of painful stimulation.
	Ensure adequate depth of anesthesia before intubation attempts or surgical/procedural attempts.
Avoid severe neck rotation.	Attempt to maintain neck in neutral position.
	Be vigilant to head positioning of patient during surgery.
Avoid compression of jugular veins.	Consider avoiding internal jugular neck lines when possible.
Elevate head.	If backup position not possible, use reverse Trendelenburg (avoid hypotension).
Decrease blood viscosity and intracerebral vascular volume.	Avoid rapid infusion of mannitol, which may paradoxically increase intracranial pressure.
Avoid sustained increases in intrathoracic pressure.	Use maneuvers or pharmacologic agents to avoid bucking, movement, and vomiting.
	Avoid high ventilatory pressures when possible.
	Avoid PEEP when possible.
Avoid cerebral venodilators.	Consider beta-blocker use to treat hypertension.
	Consider calcium channel blockers.
	Avoid nitroglycerine and nitroprusside, if possible.

PEEP, Positive end-expiratory pressure.

and the patient's airway anatomy is adequate for laryngoscopy, anesthetic induction may proceed with voluntary hyperventilation with 100% oxygen by mask, if possible. After loss of consciousness, manual hyperventilation should occur both before and after administration of muscle relaxant. Opioid administration may begin at this time to prevent the sympathetic response to laryngoscopy. IV lidocaine (1 mg/kg) may be administered to blunt the hemodynamic and ICP response to laryngoscopy. Alternatively, a beta-blocker or an additional dose of propofol may be given. Esmolol or lidocaine, 1.5 mg/kg as an IV bolus before laryngoscopy and intubation, does not completely prevent the increase in MAP and ICP. Complete neuromuscular blockade should be verified before laryngoscopy to prevent cough and associated increases in ICP. Proper airway management is essential to avoid the twin insults of hypoxia and hypercarbia. An obstructed airway may also lead to a rise in intrathoracic pressure. This may produce an elevated venous pressure, increase in intracranial blood volume, and elevated ICP. If the patient can be mask-ventilated but intubation is difficult, one may choose to proceed with an alternative device to facilitate intubation.

Alternative devices, such as the lightwand, can be useful in failed intubation, particularly in patients with a small chin or limited mouth opening. Because a lightwand is inserted without use of a laryngoscope, there is potential for less hypertension and tachycardia. This finding was demonstrated by Nishikawa and associates[23] in 60 patients undergoing awake intubation for emergency surgery. Its successful use in the difficult airway requires experience and practice. Brimacombe and Kihara[24] compared the hemodynamic responses of the lightwand and intubating laryngeal mask airway (ILMA) to direct laryngoscopy in hypertensive and normotensive patients. In their series, both the ILMA and the lightwand attenuated the hemodynamic stress response to tracheal intubation compared with direct laryngoscopy in hypertensive, but not in normotensive, anesthetized paralyzed patients. Optical stylets, such as the Shikani Optical Stylet scope or the Clarus Video System, have similar characteristics and insertion technique with the added benefit of laryngoscopic viewing (Fig. 42-1) The ILMA is particularly useful in the failed intubation sequence, and the ability to ventilate is extremely important in neurosurgical patients. The success of the ILMA as a ventilatory device has been impressive, as demonstrated in several of the early evaluation studies.[25,26] It is also extremely useful in the setting of a failed fiberoptic intubation.[27]

The patient for aneurysm surgery who presents with a difficult airway is particularly problematic. If the airway is anticipated or known to be difficult, fiberoptic intubation is often the method of choice. This is assuming that one is skillful using the fiberoptic scope and is prepared to perform this technique in the awake, cooperative patient (see Chapter 11). IV fentanyl and midazolam may be carefully administered if the patient does not exhibit signs of intracranial hypertension. An arterial line is generally placed before induction. Additional techniques include remifentanil infusion (0.05 µg/kg/min) and dexmedetomidine infusion.[28,29] Both techniques require careful patient monitoring and may be useful. Once the glottis is viewed, a dose of lidocaine may be given via the fiberoptic scope to prevent coughing and "bucking" with intubation.

Alternative techniques for failed sedation or topicalization include awake placement of the ILMA or other techniques that do not produce excessive hemodynamic responses. The concomitant administration of beta-blockers or vasodilators may be necessary for blood pressure control. Essentially, the ASA Difficult Airway Management Algorithm should be followed with close monitoring of blood pressure and heart rate at all times until the airway is secured.

B. Head-Injured Patient

Traumatic brain injury (TBI) remains a prevalent disease in the United States and the world. The incidence of TBI is 175 to 300 per 100,000 population and accounts for 56,000 deaths per year in the United States.[30] With the increased use of seatbelts, motor vehicle crashes are now secondary to gunshot wounds as the leading causes of TBI. Early intubation of the head-injured patient is critical and is often established in the field if providers are so trained. It is essential for optimal management of the patient, providing for efficient ventilation and oxygenation, helping to prevent aspiration of gastric contents, and allowing for suction of the lungs and pulmonary toilet. However, patients who are unconscious and breathing adequately may be transported with oxygen by mask throughout their initial assessment. This is intuitive in the apneic and unresponsive patient with a Glasgow Coma Scale (GCS) score of 8 or less.

The anesthesiologist caring for the patient with TBI must understand that although primary mechanisms of injury *(primary insults)* are a large determinant of patient outcome, attention to *secondary insults*, such as hypoxia, hypotension, intracranial hypertension, and decreased CPP, can impact dramatically on morbidity, mortality, and quality of life of the TBI patient.[31] Evidence supports this, with mortality from TBI nationally decreasing over the decades.[32] *Hypoxia* in TBI patients is a frequent occurrence, particularly in the prehospital setting. Interestingly, hypoxia was identified in 44% of patients with TBI on

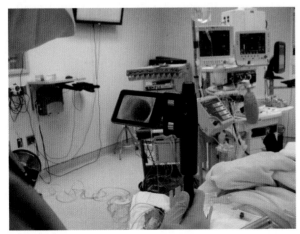

Figure 42-1 Intubation using the Clarus video system (Clarus Medical, Minneapolis, MN).

arrival in the emergency department.[33] Similarly, Jeremitsky and colleagues[34] report that hypoxia is one of three predictors of mortality in adult brain-injured patients (with hypothermia and hypoperfusion). Hypoxia dramatically impacts morbidity and mortality in TBI, and hypercapnia further increases mortality.

Hypotension is the secondary insult that has been most frequently cited as contributing to poor outcome after TBI. Hypertension is independently related to mortality in multivariate analysis.[34] Information from the Traumatic Coma Data Bank shows that a systolic blood pressure less than 80 mm Hg was one of five factors that worsened patient outcome at 6 months.[35] Hypotension during any phase in the brain trauma patient's hospital course is associated with a greater likelihood of severe disability and vegetative state.[36] However, early in the course of brain trauma, especially when combined with hypoxia, hypotension is devastating. When hypotension and hypoxia occur together, mortality is 75%.[35]

Techniques minimizing head movement should be used in TBI patients and by the most skilled clinicians. However, concern about a cervical fracture should never take precedence over relieving hypoxemia. It is of critical importance to ensure that appropriate monitoring is present throughout airway maneuvers. Nasal intubation should be avoided in head injury, particularly in patients with known or suspected basilar skull fractures and sinus injuries. Alternative airway devices, such as video laryngoscopes, any of the indirect rigid laryngoscopes, ILMA, or fiberoptic stylets, may be useful when the head must remain immobilized.[37] Most emergency patients are assumed to have a "full stomach," so it is important to weigh the risk of aspiration, which is a potential problem during laryngoscopy and intubation. If the situation warrants, surgeons should be prepared to perform a rapid cricothyrotomy if intubation attempts fail and ventilation becomes impossible.

C. Patient with Cervical Spine Disease

1. Management of Acute Injury and the Unstable Spine

Spinal injuries occur in approximately 13% to 30% of polytrauma patients, and cervical spine injury (CSI) represents about 0.9% to 3% of all polytrauma patients.[38,39] The relative risk of CSI is increased in the presence of severe head injury by a factor greater than 8.[40] In the United States, cervical trauma has an incidence of approximately 5 per 10,000 population annually, making up 4% of all blunt trauma. In trauma victims with a GCS score of 13 to 15, the incidence of CSI is 1.4%, but this rises dramatically to 10.2% if the GCS score is less than 8. It is of vital importance to capture all injuries in the unconscious polytrauma patient within an emergent time frame. If a CSI is missed or its detection delayed, the incidence of secondary neurologic deficit increases from 1.4% to 10.5%. For this reason, the Advanced Trauma Life Support (ATLS) protocol was created, constantly updated, and broadly followed in most trauma centers.[41] When a diagnosis of CSI is delayed, almost one third of patients may develop permanent neurologic deficit.[42] One of the areas of controversy is how best to "clear" the cervical spine in the trauma patient. Detection of CSI requires a variety of modalities that vary in sensitivity, including clinical evaluation, plain radiography, CT, MRI, and dynamic fluoroscopy.

Clinical Evaluation. To clear the cervical spine clinically, the following criteria must be met:

1. GCS score of 15, with the patient alert and oriented
2. Absence of injuries that may draw attention away from a CSI
3. Absence of drugs or intoxicants that may interfere with the patient's sensorium
4. Absence of signs or symptoms on examining the neck, specifically:
   a. No midline pain or tenderness
   b. Full range of active movement
   c. No neurologic deficit attributable to the cervical spine

Clearly, there will only be a small number of trauma patients who fulfill these criteria.

Plain Radiography. The cross-table lateral view alone, even if technically adequate and interpreted by an expert, will still miss 15% of cervical injuries. Of cross-table lateral films taken in emergency rooms, approximately a quarter of the films are anatomically inadequate, necessitating further imaging modalities for evaluation, usually of the cervicothoracic junction. A three-view cervical series includes the cross-table lateral view, open-mouth odontoid view, and anteroposterior (AP) view (Figs. 42-2 to 42-4). Using these views, the sensitivity increases to detect 90% of those with an actual injury. Again, anywhere from 25% to 50% of these series may be inadequate anatomically. In low-risk patients, plain radiography is an efficient diagnostic examination with specificity of 100%. In high-risk patients, plain radiography is a good adjunctive screening test in conjunction with a CT scan, with sensitivity of 93.3% and specificity of 95%.

Computed Tomography. CT scanning, either of the entire cervical spine or directed at areas missed by plain radiographs, provides a complementary approach when used in addition to the three-view cervical series, reducing the risk of missing a CSI to less than 1%. In the evaluation of the cervical spine, a helical CT scan has higher sensitivity and specificity than plain radiographs in the moderate-risk and high-risk trauma population, but it is more costly. In fact, a helical CT scan is the preferred initial screening test for detection of cervical spine fractures among moderate- to high-risk patients seen in urban trauma centers, reducing the incidence of paralysis resulting from false-negative imaging studies and institutional costs, when settlement costs are taken into account.[42]

a. INTUBATION

The anesthesiologist or emergency physician may be confronted with a patient with CSI who requires intubation. In one series, 26% of patients admitted to a large trauma center required intubation over the first day of admission. Furthermore, a growing body of literature indicates that

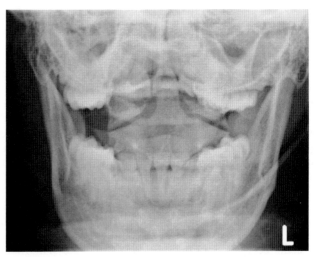

Figure 42-4 Normal odontoid cervical spine x-ray view. (Courtesy of Prasanna Vibhute, MD, Department of Radiology, Mount Sinai Medical Center.)

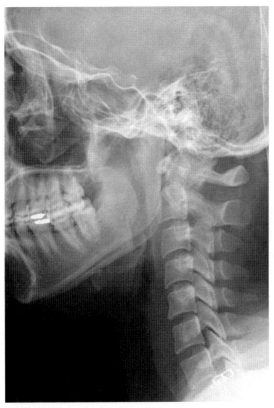

Figure 42-2 Normal lateral cervical x-ray view. (Courtesy of Prasanna Vibhute, MD, Department of Radiology, Mount Sinai Medical Center.)

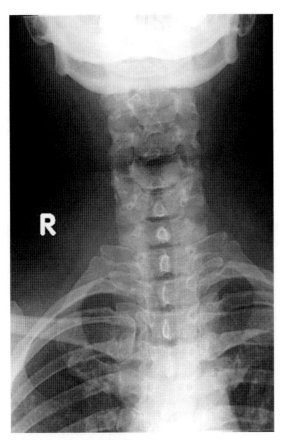

Figure 42-3 Normal anteroposterior cervical spine x-ray view. (Courtesy of Prasanna Vibhute, MD, Department of Radiology, Mount Sinai Medical Center.)

any patient with a CSI above C5 should be intubated electively, early in the course of presentation.[43] The following survey reviews airway devices and assigns utility based on clinical presentation of cervical injury.

i. **DIRECT LARYNGOSCOPY.** If performed appropriately, direct laryngoscopy is safe in the patient with CSI.[44-46] No neurologic sequelae were noted in a review of 73 patients with known cervical spine fractures intubated after rapid-sequence induction with the application of cricoid pressure and manual in-line stabilization (MILS) of the head and neck and direct laryngoscopy.[47] When intubating the patient with direct laryngoscopy, the anterior portion of the hard cervical collar can be removed to facilitate opening of the mouth at intubation.

The major concern during the initial management of patients with potential CSI is the further deterioration of the neurologic function caused by pathologic motion of the injured vertebrae. Therefore, to protect the spinal cord, it is crucial to maintain spinal alignment and preserve spinal stability by establishing early immobilization of the spine. Techniques to provide cervical spine immobilization include sandbag-tape immobilization and cervical collars of various consistency.[48] The same rationale is applied when management of the airway is required in the patient with suspicious CSI. The goal is to achieve endotracheal intubation as quickly as possible with the least amount of cervical motion. Although thorough evaluation for respiratory failure is necessary, current consensus is that early intubation is mandatory in patients with complete CSI, and evidence of respiratory failure should prompt immediate airway intervention.[49] As currently recommended by ATLS protocol, direct laryngoscopy with MILS is most often performed and has been extensively investigated.[50]

The effects of direct laryngoscopy have been studied in a range of patients, including those with normal neck anatomy under anesthesia, as well as in cadavers, including those with cervical lesions caused to simulate fractures at a variety of levels. In the anesthetized patient with normal cervical anatomy, using neuromuscular blockade and a no. 3 Macintosh blade, a variety of movements occur. On elevation of the blade to obtain a view of the larynx, there is superior rotation of the occiput and C1 in the sagittal plane, C2 remains near-neutral, and there is mild inferior rotation of C3 to C5.[51] The most significant movement is produced at the atlanto-occipital and atlantoaxial joints.[45] In cadaveric models of unstable cervical segments (C1-C2), the movements associated with maneuvers such as chin lift and jaw thrust are greater than those produced by the intubation itself. The application of cricoid pressure produced no significant movement at the site of injury in these patients.[6]

ii. **IMMOBILIZATION.** In view of the risk of secondary neurologic injury to the acutely injured, unstable cervical spine, it is widely viewed as standard of care to immobilize the cervical spine when this is suspected. The most common measures include manual in-line immobilization, immobilization of the head between two sandbags, and placement of a rigid cervical collar and a spinal board. This management is itself associated with significant morbidity and mortality. It may increase the difficulty of intubation or increase the likelihood of airway compromise and risk of aspiration. Nonetheless, the use of manual in-line immobilization (not traction) is the best means to minimize movement of the cervical spine during airway manipulations and should always be practiced. It should be recognized, however, that the presence of a cervical collar does not necessarily protect against movement at the occipitocervical and cervicothoracic junctions.[52]

In all these studies, a certain degree of movement of the cervical spine was detected during direct laryngoscopy with MILS. The magnitude of the reported displacement was within the physiologic ranges. In addition, no difference was detected in the movements recorded by using three different blades (Macintosh, Miller, McCoy). Santoni and colleagues[53] recently reported a direct correlation between the worsening of the glottic view caused by MILS and the increase in maximum applied pressure by the laryngoscope blade. They concluded that this increase in the force applied through the laryngoscope could worsen cervical instability. In the presence of cervical instability, impaired glottic visualization and secondary increases in pressure application with MILS have the potential to increase pathologic craniocervical motion.

The laryngoscopic pressure, which reflects a degree of difficulty in glottic visualization, can be significantly diminished by using video laryngoscopes, such as the Airtraq and the Pentax AirwayScope[54,55] (Fig. 42-5). These channeled video laryngoscopes allow for indirect laryngoscopy and provide optimal view of the glottis without alignment of the oropharyngeal and orotracheal axes. For these reasons, they have been successful in allowing tracheal intubation in the presence of cervical collars. The GlideScope is a widely used video laryngoscope with a record of success in cervical spine immobilization.[56,57] Using cinefluoroscopy, Robaitaille and colleagues[58] found that the GlideScope did not produce less cervical spine movement than the Macintosh blade but did provide an improved laryngoscopic view and successful intubation (Fig. 42-6).

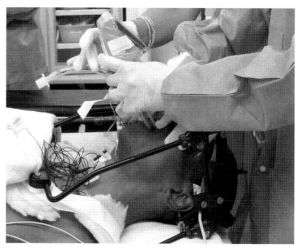

Figure 42-5 Intubation using the Pentax AWS videolaryngoscope (Pentax Ricoh Imaging, Tokyo).

iii. **AWAKE INTUBATION.** In a cooperative patient, awake fiberoptic intubation can be performed. One of the benefits of this technique is that it allows for the patient to be intubated without movement of the cervical spine. It may be performed with a hard collar in place. The patient's airway may be topicalized, but this may, in theory, increase the potential for aspiration in patients at risk for regurgitation and aspiration. Ovassapian and others,[59] however, found no evidence of aspiration in 105 patients at risk. Awake fiberoptic intubation may prove to be time-consuming and requires expert topicalization and operator skills for success. Because of the lack of assurance of expedient intubation and the risk of aspiration, we advocate that the fiberoptic scope be used in the cooperative patient in the urgent situation and in the nonurgent patient who is not at risk of aspiration. This recommendation is a general guideline, and expertise with any given airway device must be considered when using an airway technique in a specific clinical situation.

iv. **LARYNGEAL MASK AIRWAY.** Another alternative to direct laryngoscopy is the intubating LMA. Waltl and

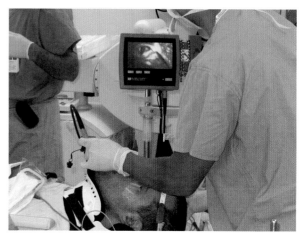

Figure 42-6 Intubation using the GlideScope in a cervical collar (Verathon, Bothell, Wash).

associates[60] reported that the ILMA produced less extension of the upper cervical spine than direct laryngoscopy.[61] Ferson and colleagues,[62] in 254 difficult-to-manage airways, reported that 70 patients with acutely unstable necks were all successfully intubated with the ILMA, 92.6% on the first attempt and 7.4% on the second attempt.[62] There was no report of worsening neurologic outcome or aspiration as a result of this intervention. The authors were skilled users of the device and practicing anesthetists who had vast clinical experience with the ILMA. Other studies were not as successful. Bilgin and Bozkurt[63] reported that optimum conditions for ventilation through the ILMA could be achieved at the first attempt only in 59% of the patients wearing a semirigid neck collar, and that two to four attempts were necessary in 42% of the patients. Successful blind intubation could be performed in all patients, but only 53% at the first attempt. On the contrary, first-attempt and overall success rates were reported to be higher than with blind techniques using a flexible fiberoptic scope or lightwand-guided tracheal intubation under vision through the ILMA. The clear disadvantage of this approach was the prolonged intubation time.[63]

This information must be viewed, however, in light of cadaveric experiments in which the intubating LMA has been demonstrated to create posterior pressure on the midportion of the cervical spine.[64] This may be particularly relevant in cervical flexion injuries. If the ILMA is to be used in a patient in a hard cervical collar with cricoid pressure, one should be aware of difficulties described in this scenario. Wong and associates[65] presented two cases where the ILMA was used in awake topicalized patients with unstable cervical spine without difficulty. In light of these studies indicating that the ILMA may produce cervical motion and excessive pressure on the cervical spine, and that it is difficult to place with application of cricoid pressure and the presence of a hard cervical collar, the ILMA cannot be recommended as a primary device in the patient with acute cervical injury. It should be viewed as a rescue device if direct or fiberoptic intubation fails.

v. **CRICOTHYROTOMY.** Although suggested as an alternative to direct laryngoscopy in patients with cervical neck trauma,[66] cricothyrotomy may produce a small but significant movement of the cervical spine.[67] Although often suggested as a primary mode of intubation of the unstable patient with CSI, the procedure is associated with a high complication rate.[68] In one study of long-term complications in emergency departments in the United Kingdom, only 41.5% survived to hospital discharge. A mere 25.9% of these patients who survived experienced no long-term complications (10.9% of all patients receiving emergency cricothyrotomy).[69] This high incidence of complications may be related to the decreasing number of cricothyrotomies performed and the unfamiliarity of many physicians with the procedure. The incidence of emergency surgical airway in the setting of trauma has decreased over the past several decades. Therefore, emergency cricothyrotomy should be reserved as a rescue procedure in the management of the airway in patients with acute cervical spine injuries.

Box 42-1	**Airway Techniques for Patients with Unstable Cervical Spine**

Awake fiberoptic intubation
Nasal intubation
Indirect rigid laryngoscopy
Bullard, Wu, and Upsher laryngoscopes
    Video laryngoscope and DCI systems
    Airtraq and Pentax AWS laryngoscopes
Direct laryngoscopy with in-line stabilization
Fiberoptic intubation using LMA as conduit
    LMA Classic
    LMA-Fastrach
Lightwand or fiberoptic lighted stylets
    Trachlight
    Shikani Optical Stylet, and Bonfils Retromolar Intubation
      Fiberscope
    Clarus video system
Retrograde intubation
Surgical airway
    Cricothyrotomy
    Tracheostomy

DCI, Direct coupled interface; *LMA,* laryngeal mask airway.

vi. **ALTERNATIVE STRATEGIES.** Optimal airway management strategies in patients with an unstable CSI remain controversial. Additional alternative devices to the laryngoscopes are a lightwand or an intubating fiberoptic stylets, such as the Shikani Optical Stylet and the Bonfils Retromolar Intubation Fiberscope. These tools are designed to allow blind tracheal intubation, avoiding hyperextension of the neck. However, few objective data guide the selection of appropriate devices. Different study series report that intubation with the Trachlight was successful at first attempt in 90% of patients. Inoue and colleagues[70] conducted a prospective randomized study of 148 patients receiving general anesthesia for procedures related to clinical and radiographic evidence of cervical abnormality. Trachlight or ILMA was used for tracheal intubation, with the head and neck held in a neutral position. In the Trachlight group, intubation was successful at the first attempt in 67 of 74 patients (90.5%) and at the second attempt in five (6.8%). In contrast, in the ILMA group, 54 of 74 patients (73.0%) were intubated within the protocol. The mean time for successful tracheal intubation at the first attempt was significantly shorter in the Trachlight group than in the ILMA group. The Trachlight may be more advantageous for orotracheal intubation in patients with CSI than the Fastrach with respect to reliability, rapidity, and safety. Skill and experience with the device are essential to achieving this success (Box 42-1).

b. **SUMMARY**

As can be appreciated from the previous discussion, the problem with airway management in patients with CSI is that the techniques normally employed to secure the airway have the potential to cause movement and thereby risk causing secondary neurologic injury. Although a strategy for "clearing" the cervical spine is previously outlined, the emergent nature of management of these often–multiply injured patients may mean that time does not permit this to be performed. Therefore, a group of patients remain whose cervical spinal integrity is uncertain and who must be managed as if their cervical spine is, in fact, injured. It is essential to proceed in the most expedient manner with the techniques that have been carefully practiced.

2. Chronic Spine Disease with Myelopathy

In the same manner as patients with ischemic heart disease present for noncardiac surgery, patients with cervical spine disease present for surgery for non-neurosurgical procedures. As such, their airway management is of interest to all, not solely those providing anesthesia for complex spinal surgery. One of the problems in relation to this patient group is predicting difficulty with intubation, both by direct laryngoscopy and fiberoptic intubation.[71]

Regarding fiberoptic intubation (FOI), the traditional bedside tests used to predict difficult direct laryngoscopy may not necessarily be predictive of difficulty in FOI. Difficulty with visualizing the vocal cords in FOI has been extensively documented and is most often caused by secretions and blood in the airway, distortion of the upper airway, and of particular relevance, resistance to passage of the endotracheal tube (ETT) in a high proportion of cases. This ETT problem has been linked to the size of the fiberoptic scope in relation to the ETT and indeed, the design of the ETT itself. Patients with rheumatoid arthritis may pose additional difficulty because of alteration in the plane of their vocal cords. Efforts at establishing which patient features influence difficulty in the passage of the ETT, or impingement, have been directed at examining radiologically common features. Neither the Mallampati grade nor the thyromental distance correlated with the degree of impingement on passage of the tube. There was, however, a positive correlation with the size of the epiglottis and the size of the tongue. In particular, the thickness was more important than the length of the tongue, an issue of particular relevance in patients with acromegaly.

Difficult intubation (DI) is well recognized as more common in patients with cervical spine disease. In particular, ankylosing spondylitis, rheumatoid arthritis, and Klippel-Feil abnormality present additional difficulty.[72] One of the problems with predicting DI is its incidence and the sensitivity and specificity of the tests used to detect it.[73] DI in the undifferentiated anesthesia community has an incidence of approximately 1%. The positive predictive value (PPV; proportion of difficult cases predicted to be difficult) of the common tests such as Mallampati or Wilson Risk Sum is about 8%, and the PPV of the tests used in combination is approximately 30%.[74] Tests predicting DI with sensitivity of 95% and specificity of 99% will have a 51% false-positive rate. However, if the prevalence of DI is theoretically 10%, the problem of false-positive cases would decrease to 8.7% (with sensitivity of 95% and specificity of 99%). One might therefore expect prediction of DI to be more rewarding in a patient subgroup with a high incidence of DI, such as those with cervical spine disease.

A number of important correlates have emerged from this examination. As previously discussed, when performing direct laryngoscopy, the most significant movement is produced at the atlanto-occipital and atlantoaxial joints.[45] Not surprisingly, therefore, patients with reduced mobility at this level present increased difficulty of intubation.[75] However, a highly significant association exists between disease of the occipito-atlanto-axial complex and impaired mandibular protrusion. This is mainly, but not uniquely, caused by rheumatoid disease. Also, extension at the craniocervical junction is needed to open the mouth fully, another limiting factor with direct laryngoscopy.

a. RHEUMATOID ARTHRITIS

Three especially relevant areas in which rheumatoid arthritis (RA) affects the airway and cervical spine are cricoarytenoid arthritis, temporomandibular arthritis, and atlantoaxial instability.[76] Laryngeal involvement in RA has a prevalence of 45% to 88%. Depending on the investigation, 59% of patients with RA show laryngeal involvement on physical examination, 14% show extrathoracic airway obstruction on spirometry, and 69% show one or more signs of laryngeal involvement. Of the latter, 75% have symptoms of breathing difficulty. For these RA patients, the greatest risk is after extubation. Intubation, even if of brief duration, can lead to sufficient mucosal edema to cause postextubation stridor and airway obstruction. Interestingly, the incidence of postextubation stridor is much lower after FOI (1%) than after direct laryngoscopy (14%).[77]

Up to two thirds of patients with long-standing RA may have limited temporomandibular joint (TMJ) mobility with consequent limited mouth opening. Of those with severe TMJ destruction, up to 70% may undergo episodes of airway obstruction similar to that seen in patients with micrognathia or obstructive sleep apnea syndrome.[78]

Atlantoaxial instability is present in about 25% of all patients with RA and is more likely in those with severe peripheral rheumatoid involvement. Symptoms correlate poorly with radiologic findings, and a serious concern is that some series have found atlantoaxial instability in approximately 5% of RA patients presenting for elective orthopedic surgery. The direction of the instability is variable, and a significant percentage will exhibit vertical subluxation, or cranial "settling." This can also result in impingement of the odontoid peg on the brainstem.[79]

b. SUMMARY

The patient who presents for elective surgery, with symptoms of cervical myelopathy, deserves careful airway management to avoid further injury. Intubation techniques described for the CSI patient are appropriate and best performed by experienced practitioners. When possible, awake intubation, followed by demonstration of extremity movement, is ideal and recommended. When this is not possible, a technique that produces minimal head movement and airway maintenance is acceptable. A thoughtful approach is based on patient anatomy, risk of intubation difficulty, and a rescue plan for intubation or ventilation failure.

IV. FAILED INTUBATION OR ANTICIPATED DIFFICULT AIRWAY

A. Patient in a Halo Frame or Stereotactic Headframe

Early halo immobilization is a common practice in patients with potentially unstable cervical injuries and may facilitate the diagnostic work-up and treatment of trauma patients with multiple injuries.[80] The halo device provides the most rigid form of external cervical immobilization. Although the halo frame is an effective form of cervical immobilization, complications can occur. This cumbersome device prevents easy access to the patient's airway and also prevents extension of the head.

Patients treated with halo fixation present unique challenges in terms of airway control. The halo frame prevents proper positioning for laryngoscopy by restricting atlanto-occipital extension. Oral intubation is often possible, but it is a function of other variables, such as mouth opening, tongue size, upper dentition, and ability to prognath the lower jaw forward. In the nonemergent setting, fiberoptic bronchoscopy can overcome the difficulties in intubating these patients,[81] but in an emergency setting, these intubations can be extremely difficult. Sims and Berger[82] reported a retrospective survey of 105 patients managed with halo fixation at a level 1 trauma center. In this series, 14 of the patients (13%) required emergent or semiemergent airway control with almost half the patients dying in the attempts or shortly after. Based on their findings, the authors suggest that early tracheostomy be considered in hospitalized trauma patients requiring halo fixation who present with a high Injury Severity Score (ISS), history of cardiac disease, or a condition requiring intubation on arrival. Patients who are intubated on arrival may be more likely to require emergent reintubation during their hospital stay. Older patients and those with a history of cardiac disease are more at risk for arrest-related death (Box 42-2).

Respiratory failure or airway obstruction in the patient wearing a halo frame becomes a serious emergency. If the airway needs to be secured and tracheal intubation has failed, use of adjuncts may be life-saving. The halo frame immobilizes the head and neck and prevents use of the "sniffing position" for laryngoscopy or assisted ventilation. Case reports have described a variety of techniques for airway rescue in the patient wearing halo fixation. The Bullard laryngoscope has been used after failed laryngoscopy in a patient who additionally had a difficult airway.[83]

The ILMA was successfully used in an awake patient when a fiberoptic scope was unavailable.[84] This device was also used by one of the authors after a failed intubation attempt following a respiratory arrest. A Combitube was used in a 78-year-old patient with respiratory deterioration after extubation when LMA insertion proved impossible.[85] In recent reports, 15 patients in halo-vest fixation were electively intubated for surgery under general anesthesia using the GlideScope, and a 14-year-old patient unable to tolerate awake FOI was successfully intubated with the Pentax AWS[86,87] (Fig. 42-7).

Patients who present for elective surgery in halo fixation should be approached carefully with a plan for intubation. The techniques described earlier for the anticipated difficult airway should be employed. It is imperative that (1) clinicians involved have skills and equipment for alternative intubation techniques, (2) a neurosurgeon or professional can safely remove the halo if necessary, and (3) a rescue plan is prepared in case of failed ventilation in these challenging patients.

Stereotactic Headframes. Stereotactic localization is widely used in neurosurgery and has revolutionized practice over the past 30 years. The term *stereotactic* originated from the Greek words *stereo* meaning "three-dimensional" and *tactos* meaning "touched." Lars Leksell is best known as the neurosurgeon who brought stereotaxis into clinical use, although it was originally described by Horsley and Clarke in 1908.[88] In 1949, Leksell designed the first instrument to be based on the arc-center principle, a system that provided precise mechanical three-dimensional control in intracranial space. It served to identify the target and to calculate the angles and distances to be used with the frame. The stereotactic system has undergone many refinements over the years. The early stereotactic frames produced by Leksell provided head fixation but significantly interfered with airway access. The later frames have a cross-bar that may be directed cephalad for easier access to the nose and mouth. The cross-bar can be removed by unscrewing two screws with an Allen wrench (which should always be available). Newer designs feature a movable front piece (Fig. 42-8).

Box 42-2	Recommendations for Early Tracheostomy in Trauma Patients with Halo Fixation

High cervical injury score
History of cardiac disease
Age >60 years
Intubated on arrival
Previous history of difficult intubation
Anticipated length of intubation greater than 1 week
Capability of surgical airway not available

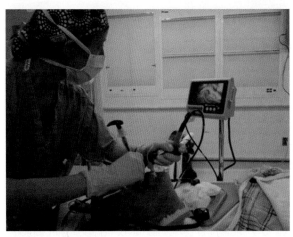

Figure 42-7 Patient in a halo fixation vest intubated using the GlideScope (Verathon).

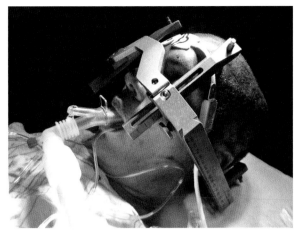

Figure 42-8 Leksell frame allows placement of a laryngeal mask airway (LMA Supreme; LMA North America, San Diego).

Despite moderate access to the airway, head positioning and fixation to the table can make proper positioning for airway management extremely challenging.

Applications of stereotaxis are increasing and are presently used for biopsy, craniotomy, and procedures for movement disorders. Neuronavigational techniques require the acquisition of radiologic studies, such as CT or MRI, while the patient is wearing the stereotactic frame. Stereotactic neurosurgery may require general anesthesia or conscious sedation. Cooperative patients who are neurologically intact may easily tolerate frame placement under sedation with local anesthetic applied at the pin sites. Conscious sedation is desirable when patients must be transported for diagnostic radiologic procedures in the headframe (Fig. 42-9). This is the anesthetic technique appropriate for intracranial biopsies and the surgical treatment of movement disorders and Parkinson's disease. The use of intravenous sedation must be carefully monitored, and the agents chosen should provide analgesia, sedation, and cardiovascular stability.[89] Oxygen should be administered by nasal cannula, and monitoring of capnography is extremely useful. It is essential to monitor head positioning during frame

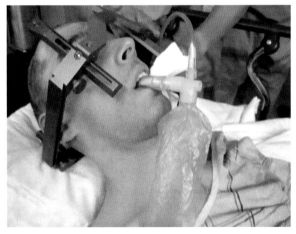

Figure 42-9 Patient in Leksell frame for transport with supraglottic airway and (Patil) intubation guide, "whistle" for management during transport (Elekta, Stockholm).

fixation to the operating table. Excessive head flexion may lead to airway obstruction when sedative agents are given.[90]

Potential complications of the surgical procedure include bleeding and the potential for air entrainment. Air entrainment may occur from the surgical site if near the venous sinuses or from the pins sites if placed near diploic veins.[91] This is usually noted by the development of coughing, dyspnea, and decreased oxygen saturation. It is important to make the diagnosis and inform the surgeon, who should immediately flood the operative field to prevent further air entry. Another and more serious risk is internal bleeding. Postoperatively, patients usually undergo a CT scan to check for signs of hemorrhage or hematoma formation.

Patient cooperation is an important factor in these procedures; pediatric patients, obtunded patients, and those at risk for seizures present increased management challenges. The obese patient or the patient prone to airway obstruction requires careful consideration for the stereotactic headframe technique, perhaps performed under general anesthesia. When this decision is made, the patient is anesthetized and intubated before frame placement and must be ventilated, sedated, and monitored for transport to and from a diagnostic radiologic area. Alternatively, a cooperative patient may tolerate placement of the headframe and diagnostic radiology, although the lesion is in the occipital region, requiring prone positioning. This problem may be solved by awake intubation in the headframe, followed by positioning after anesthesia is induced. If awake intubation fails, an alternative technique may be used. The LMA is extremely useful in this scenario and may be used as the sole airway in smaller patients having the procedure in the supine position. It is important to be familiar with a number of airway techniques and to have a plan for alternative methods of airway management should these challenges occur[92] (Box 42-3).

B. Patient for Awake Craniotomy or Embolization Procedures

Craniotomy in the awake state has been performed since ancient times. Current indications include resection of a lesion in the eloquent or speech center of the brain. Surgical procedures for the treatment of epilepsy, tumors, or arteriovenous malformation are sometimes performed in the awake patient. With refinement of neurophysiologic monitoring techniques, awake craniotomies are necessary in only a small percentage of patients. However, surgery for movement disorders has again increased the use of this technique. Intraoperative complications of awake craniotomy include restlessness and agitation.[93] This may occur when the patient is oversedated but experiences discomfort. More serious complications are hypoventilation, nausea, and seizures.[94] Changing the level of sedation will often resolve these problems. It is important to maintain the good rapport with the patient established preoperatively. Comfortable positioning of the patient to avoid discomfort, allowing surgical access and avoiding a claustrophobic atmosphere, is essential and requires cooperation of the entire operating room (OR) staff.

The evolution of anesthetic technique has progressed from fentanyl/droperidol to the current use of propofol infusion with alfentanil or remifentanil or dexmedetomidine.[95,96] Intraoperative nausea is rare with the use of propofol infusions. A newer agent is *dexmedetomidine* (Precedex), a selective α_2-adrenergic agonist used for continuous IV sedation. Dexmedetomidine has been shown to produce sedation and analgesia without respiratory depression. The onset is slower than with propofol, and dexmedetomidine must be administered by infusion. This may be beneficial for the older patient, pediatric patient, or potentially debilitated patient and has been used throughout intraoperative testing. Seizure control is sometimes necessary; methohexital (1 mg/kg) or a benzodiazepine (midazolam) is effective. Terminating the seizure requires careful titration of sedatives to avoid apnea.

If necessary, general anesthesia may be required for the uncooperative or the very young patient.[97] The "asleep-awake-asleep" technique has been used by some centers in an effort to minimize patient discomfort and provide better operating conditions for the surgeon. The patient undergoes a "light general anesthetic" with additional local anesthesia and is awakened intraoperatively for testing at the appropriate time.

Airway management can be challenging, and several maneuvers have been reported. Huncke and colleagues[98] used awake fiberoptic intubation, which was accomplished in 10 patients. This effective but arduous technique required significant skill and a special catheter to deliver local airway anesthetic. Some clinicians have also used nasal airways and blind nasal intubation, assuming that bleeding or significant discomfort is avoided. The most useful technique in recent years has been the laryngeal mask airway for control of the airway.[99] The LMA has been described in several reports and can be achieved (with skill) without having to remove drapes or change patient position.[100] In our experience, using the LMA Classic and the LMA-ProSeal, patients could be induced and re-anesthetized for the resection after intraoperative testing. This allows the surgeon a "quiet field," because many patients become hypercarbic while awake and sedated. The LMA-ProSeal is particularly advantageous for the ability to provide positive-pressure ventilation and deliberate entry into the gastric tract.[101]

Embolization Procedures. The endovascular treatment of intracranial aneurysm and arteriovenous malformation (AVM) is now an option for many patients. This new therapy offers significantly reduced morbidity, mortality, and hospital stay compared with craniotomy.[1] In patients with acute subarachnoid hemorrhage (SAH),

considerations must be made for the likelihood of increased ICP, changes in transmural pressure, and cerebral ischemia. During endovascular treatment, the two most serious potential complications are cerebral infarction and hemorrhage. Endovascular coiling may be safely applied within hours of the aneurysm rupture with low probability of aneurysm perforation. General anesthesia is preferred for patients with acute SAH. Despite concern for neurologic evaluation, most neuroradiologists now prefer general anesthesia for optimal imaging of studies and techniques. Airway control through an ETT or LMA allows for improved oxygenation, anesthetic administration, and a motionless patient. Radiologic imaging methods include high-resolution fluoroscopy and high-speed digital subtraction angiography (DSA) with a "roadmapping" function.[2] The computer superimposes images onto live fluoroscopy so that the progress of the radiopaque catheter tip can be seen. Any motion during this stage of the procedure profoundly degrades the image. The anesthesiologist is typically off to the side of the patient and must negotiate around the myriad of monitors and equipment, which are part of this terrain. One benefit of this environment is the ability to obtain fluoroscopic confirmation of ETT positioning, confirm proper central line location, if placed, or make the diagnosis of atelectasis.

Although the radiology suite may be in a remote location, the patient with an anticipated difficult airway should be approached in the same manner as in the OR. A potential limiting factor is the flat table, which does not allow the patient's head to be raised. Supporting blankets should be used to produce the optimal position for laryngoscopy or awake intubation, if necessary. The techniques described earlier apply in this setting, and we have used the fiberoptic bronchoscope, ILMA, lightwand, and GlideScope in the radiology suite. Emergence from anesthesia should be smooth, avoiding excessive coughing and "bucking." Hypertension should be controlled to prevent potential cerebral edema and bleeding at the femoral cannulation site. There is minimal pain, but patients are required to remain supine for a time.

C. Patient with Acromegaly

Acromegaly is a rare condition afflicting 3 to 4 per 1 million people.[102] After Marie's 1882 description of the disease,[103] Chappel[104] reported the death of an acromegalic patient secondary to airway obstruction in 1886. Airway obstruction is one of several mechanisms associated with DI in these patients. The association between difficult airway management and acromegaly has long been recognized in the anesthesiology community. Compared with the nonacromegalic population, acromegalic patients have a higher incidence of DI, unpredictable difficult airway, and problematic mask ventilation.

The occurrence of the difficult airway in acromegaly is well described, and the incidence of difficult laryngoscopy in these patients ranges from 9% to 33%.[105] The hypersecretion of growth hormone characterizing acromegaly results in a number of alterations in airway anatomy. Patients develop hypertrophy of the facial bones with coarsening of the features. The hypertrophy of the mandibular bone leads to prognathism. In addition to significant macroglossia, hypertrophy of laryngeal and pharyngeal soft tissues and structures (e.g., vocal cords, arytenoepiglottic and ventricular folds) is well documented. Schmitt and associates[106] found a 26% incidence of Cormack and Lehane grade III views on direct laryngoscopy in acromegalic patients.

Past case reports described the inability to ventilate and intubate the acromegalic patient, but heightened awareness and preparation have led to increased success with these patients.[107] Preinduction airway assessment may not correlate with difficulty of intubation. Although Mallampati classification may be helpful, the thyromental distance is an insensitive indicator of DI. The lack of large prospective studies on acromegaly precludes an absolute statement regarding predictive value of preoperative assessment to difficulty of intubation at this time. Sharma and colleagues[108] recently compared the modified Mallampati classification with the upper lip bite test as predictor for difficult laryngoscopy in acromegalic patients, concluding that "sensitivity and accuracy of both tests were less in the acromegalic population than the non-acromegalic controls."

Airway management in the agromegalic patient remains problematic. Some advocate the use of awake fiberoptic intubation in patients with acromegaly to avoid the creation of a surgical airway.[109,110] This approach is gradually changing. While awake FOI remains the present standard of care for difficult airways, acromegalic patients have considerable redundant tissue and large tongues. Hakala and colleagues[111] reported that FOI may prove difficult or fail in patients with acromegaly. When considering awake FOI, the increased incidence of coronary artery disease in patients with acromegaly should also be considered.[112] An anesthetic plan must be formulated to balance the risks of losing the airway and precipitating myocardial ischemia. The plan should include (1) a second anesthesiologist if a difficult airway is anticipated, (2) a difficult airway cart, and (3) a surgeon skilled in performing a surgical airway.

In addition to difficulty with intubation of acromegalic patients, ventilation may also be challenging. Various explanations have been described as the reason for difficulty in ventilating these patients. The prognathic jaw may impede proper mask placement; the large tongue or redundancy of soft tissue may lead to airway obstruction with recumbency and use of muscle relaxants; and the decreased range of neck motion secondary to cervical osteophyte formation may impede the attainment of proper sniffing position. There is a 16% to 30% incidence of upper airway obstruction diagnosed by spirometry in patients with acromegaly.[113] Additionally, the incidence of sleep apnea is increased in these patients.[114] A history of obstructive sleep apnea, hoarseness, or stridor should alert the anesthesiologist to possible glottic and infraglottic involvement and the potential for difficulty with intubation and ventilation. This propensity toward airway obstruction must also be considered in the immediate postoperative period, especially in the patient with bilateral nasal packing.[115,116] Postoperative negative-pressure pulmonary edema has been described in acromegalic patients from partial obstruction after extubation (Box 42-4).

Box 42-4 Airway Considerations in Patients with Acromegaly

Prognathic jaw
Macroglossia
Osteophyte formation of cervical spine; decreased range of motion of neck
Thickening of pharyngeal and laryngeal soft tissue
Thickening of vocal cords
Recurrent laryngeal nerve paralysis
Decrease in width of cricoid arch
Hypertrophy of arytenoepiglottic folds
Hypertrophy of ventricular folds
Central sleep apnea

The ILMA has been advocated as an adjunct for intubating patients with acromegaly, but the failure rate may be too high for its use as a primary tool. Law-Koune and others[117] reported a 47.4% first-attempt failure rate with the ILMA in acromegalic patients induced with propofol, concluding that the "rate of failed blind intubation through the ILMA precludes its use as a first choice for elective airway management." Further research is required to address if the use of the ILMA as a conduit for light-wand- or fiberoptic-assisted intubation will improve the success rate. As a rescue strategy in failed laryngoscopic or fiberoptic intubation, the ILMA may be an option, if awakening the patient is not a realistic alternative. Also, we used FOI with the LMA Classic (sizes 5 and 6) in two patients with acromegaly when the ILMA did not allow successful intubation.

Use of video laryngoscopy is likely to be beneficial in acromegalic patients. Prospective studies are lacking, but we continue to have excellent results at our institutions using the GlideScope and the McGrath video laryngoscopes as primary or secondary instruments for intubating patients with acromegaly (Fig. 42-10). The construction of most blade-type video laryngoscopes allows easy navigation around the large tongue and usually provides excellent visualization of the glottic opening.[118] Experience with video laryngoscopy is recommended in normal airways before attempting use in a potentially difficult airway.

D. Role of Laryngeal Mask Airway in Neurosurgery

Although use of both the LMA and the intubating LMA for neurosurgical procedures has been previously described, this section addresses additional issues and further details their use in the neurosurgical patient population. Although the LMA cannot substitute for the ETT, it can be used in a number of situations where an ETT would be difficult or impossible to insert. In addition, the beneficial effects on cardiovascular and intracranial reflexes make the LMA a wise choice in certain neurosurgical procedures. This assumes that the clinician is skilled in LMA placement and manages the anesthetic appropriately. Several case reports describe LMA use in craniotomy, but these were scenarios of failed intubation and the necessity for an airway in fasted patients.[119,120] Although the intubating LMA has been discussed

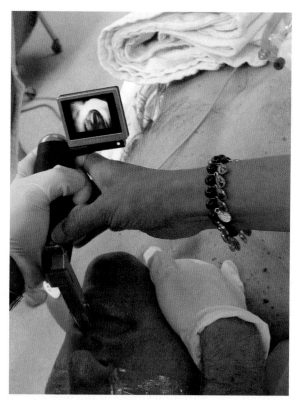

Figure 42-10 Intubation of acromegalic patient with McGrath Series 5 video laryngoscope (LMA North America).

extensively as a device for airway management in patients with limited neck movement, Combes and colleagues[121] demonstrated its role in the failed-intubation scenario. In their prospective study of unanticipated difficult intubation, they concluded that the ILMA and the gum elastic bougie effectively solve most problems occurring during unexpected difficult airway management.[121] This is particularly important for the neurosurgical patient, who may not easily tolerate repeated laryngoscopy attempts, inadequate ventilation, and excessive hypertension and tachycardia.

The LMA can also be used as a conduit for FOI and as a rescue airway technique that is preferred by some clinicians rather than the ILMA.[122] The LMA, as well as the ILMA, can be inserted in a variety of patient positions. This becomes useful in the dreaded situation of extubation in the prone position, as well as loss of the airway in a sedated patient fixed in a headframe.[120] Assuming the mouth opening is adequate, the device can be easily placed by facing the patient and using the thumb to insert along the hard palate. A case report describes anesthetic induction and management in the prone position for a penetrating spine injury at C1-C2 using a LMA.[123] Elective use in the prone position, although considered controversial by some, can be safely performed in appropriate patients with proper positioning. There is a growing body of experience and literature on the utility of this technique with the LMA Supreme. Studies have shown the ease of insertion with the patient positioned prone for surgery. This obviates the need for turning an anesthetized patient and allows for efficient use of OR time.[124,125]

Hypertension, coughing, and bucking preferably are avoided in the neurosurgical patient. When these are a particular consideration or the patient has severe asthma or chronic obstructive pulmonary disease (COPD), extubation may be facilitated by exchanging the ETT for the LMA (using LMA as "bridge to extubation").[126] This is performed while the patient is still deeply anesthetized, without airway reflexes. The exchange technique is also useful when an elaborate head draping is required and excessive neck movement will likely provoke coughing and bucking. The technique is also known as the "Bailey maneuver," used at the Royal Throat, Nose and Ear Hospital in London.[127] The laryngeal mask provides a number of airway options for the neurosurgical patient and should always be readily available.

V. POSTOPERATIVE CONSIDERATIONS

A. Airway Injury and Function after Neurosurgery

A range of airway problems is possible in the patient who has undergone neurosurgery. Potential risks include an intraoperative seizure, hypoxia, and hypoperfusion of an ischemic penumbral area, which may produce an obtunded postoperative state. These factors, along with the residual effects of anesthetic drugs, may render the patient unable to maintain the airway safely. Patients undergo neurosurgery in a variety of positions other than supine, and the effects of gravity, venous pressure, and fluid administration may alter the integrity of the airway structures. Thus, although the airway itself may not be considered a difficult airway, there are reasons why airway function may not automatically return immediately after neurosurgery. In addition to this global effect on the ability to maintain the airway, there are specific risks of alteration in airway function after neurosurgery.

1. After Supratentorial Craniotomy

In addition to general issues regarding impaired level of consciousness, as previously mentioned, patients may present with airway problems who have previously undergone temporoparietal or pterional craniotomy. When these patients subsequently present for surgery, either further neurosurgery or other non-neurosurgical procedures, they may now have a difficult airway because of limited mouth opening not evident at the original craniotomy. This is as a consequence of scar formation in the region of the temporalis muscle.[128] This is much more likely to occur in those who have had a period of sedation and ventilation in the intensive care unit following their original craniotomy, because they do not resume normal eating and talking activities. Even patients extubated immediately after craniotomy and who do resume normal eating and talking are at risk of developing restricted mouth opening if, for reasons of excessive pain, they themselves limit jaw movement and subsequently develop restrictive scarring. Kawaguchi and associates[129] were able to characterize postcraniotomy changes in mouth opening that occurred in 92 patients after surgery. The postoperative reduction in maximal mouth opening was greater in the group who underwent frontotemporal craniotomy (vs. parietal or occipital regions). Limited mouth opening resolved after 3 months in most patients. Supratentorial craniotomies separated by short intervals can increase the risk of limited mouth opening, which may result in a difficult intubation.

There is a risk that anesthesiologists may be lulled into a false sense of security in this setting, if they limit their assessment of the airway to reviewing the previous anesthesia chart. This will only describe the grade of laryngoscopy at that time, and if they do not perform a new, postcraniotomy assessment of the airway, with particular reference to mouth opening, they may find a critical reduction in ease of laryngoscopy.

2. After Cervical Spine Surgery

The intraoperative management of the patient scheduled for cervical spinal surgery is considered in detail earlier. A significant number of the problems, however, present themselves only on completion of the surgery. Although the surgical goals included alleviating spinal cord compression, reduction of dislocation, or fixation of instability, almost invariably these procedures result in a reduced range of cervical movement. Consequently, on emergence, it may be difficult to maintain the airway in the presence of residual anesthesia because airway maneuvers possible after induction of anesthesia are no longer viable.

Anterior cervical spinal surgery may result in recurrent laryngeal nerve injury or hematoma, causing airway obstruction after extubation. The most common cause of vocal cord paralysis is compression of the recurrent laryngeal nerve within the endolarynx. Monitoring of ETT cuff pressure and release after retractor placement may prevent injury to the recurrent laryngeal nerve.[130] Edema may also develop in the tissues of the neck because the esophagus and trachea are retracted during these procedures to obtain access to the cervical spine. In contrast to problems associated with recurrent laryngeal nerve injury, such as angioedema or hematoma, which tend to occur early, this edema may not develop for 2 to 3 days postoperatively. Common features in these patients require reintubation with an increasing number of levels manipulated; the higher the operated levels, the longer the surgery, and the greater the intraoperative blood loss, the greater is the risk for reintubation. If these patients require reintubation, it is often difficult to perform, with significant rates of mortality and hypoxic sequelae. Consequently, attempts have been made to identify the risks previously described and the strategies to predict at-risk groups and plan alternative management, as discussed next.

Sagi and colleagues[131] demonstrated that 19 patients (6.1%) had an airway complication, six patients (1.9%) required reintubation, and one patient died. Symptoms developed on average 36 hours postoperatively. All complications except for two were attributable to pharyngeal edema. Variables found to be statistically associated with an airway complication were exposing more than three vertebral bodies; intraoperative blood loss greater than 300 mL; exposures involving C2, C3, or C4; and surgery longer than 5 hours. A history of myelopathy, spinal cord injury, pulmonary problems, smoking, anesthetic risk

factors, and the absence of a drain did not correlate with an airway complication. Thus, patients with prolonged procedures (5 hours), exposing more than three vertebral levels that include C2, C3, or C4 and with more than 300-mL blood loss, should remain intubated or should be extubated over an airway exchange catheter and watched carefully for respiratory insufficiency.

Swallowing difficulties and dysphonia may occur in patients undergoing anterior cervical discectomy and fusion. The etiology and incidence of these abnormalities are not well defined. Once again, there is a tendency for patients undergoing multilevel surgery to demonstrate increased incidence of swallowing abnormalities on postoperative radiographic studies.[132] Patients undergoing multilevel procedures are at an increased risk for these complications, in part because of soft tissue swelling in the neck. Although more rare, the risk of migration of the bone, synthetic graft, or plate into the airway or compressing the airway with resultant obstruction may also occur. In addition to necessitating reintubation, this has the added hazards of intubation being required in a patient with a potentially unstable cervical spine and the need for further surgery.[133,134]

The issues surrounding airway complications of *posterior* cervical spinal surgery, which are additional to those of *anterior* cervical spinal surgery, relate mainly to anesthesia conducted with the patient in the prone position, as discussed next.

3. After Posterior Fossa Surgery

Because of the position of the lower cranial nerves in relation to the posterior fossa, the patient's ability to maintain the airway may be compromised postoperatively. Performance of a careful history preoperatively may unmask subtle impairment of gag reflex with increased episodes of choking on food, and family members may have noticed changes in character of speech. Duration of surgery, proximity of the surgical site to the lower cranial nerves, and the presence of either edema or hematoma in relation to these nerves may result in both loss of gag reflex and loss of the ability to maintain and protect the airway after posterior fossa surgery. Because of the proximity of the brainstem, further hazards are presented postoperatively because central control of respiration may be jeopardized, and these factors will dictate the safety of timing of extubation.[135,136]

Potential postoperative airway problems divide essentially into those of the prone and sitting position, and those related to surgery on the structures in the posterior fossa. Basically, patients are at risk even before the end of these surgeries because securing the ETT in this setting is problematic because secretions and skin preparation solutions are ongoing threats to its security. Even if securely fastened to the skin, facial edema may result in the ETT migrating out of the trachea, especially in children in whom the distance between endobronchial intubation and extubation is small. Facial edema itself is not necessarily hazardous to the airway, but macroglossia and oropharyngeal edema clearly are problematic.[134]

A variety of mechanisms have been proposed to account for the macroglossia seen after posterior cervical spinal and posterior fossa surgery.[137] Clearly, if the tongue becomes inadvertently trapped between the teeth, lingual edema will result. The venous drainage of the tongue may be obstructed by the presence of an oropharyngeal airway, and if an esophageal stethoscope is there along with an oral ETT, these further risk impairing the venous and lymphatic drainage of the tongue in the prone position. Other factors that may contribute to the formation of edema are lateral rotation of the head and neck and flexion of the neck, because these two maneuvers may impair venous drainage of the head and neck.[138] The duration of surgery, as well as blood loss and fluid replacement, should also be taken into account as to the likelihood of developing macroglossia.[139]

In all these settings, although macroglossia may be immediately apparent and may preclude extubation, the oropharyngeal airway and the ETT may be the only elements maintaining the airway, and only on their removal does the edema become apparent, risking airway compromise. A rarer neurologic complication impacting on airway function after surgery in this position is quadriplegia. This may be caused by a combination of prolonged hyperflexion, overstretching of the cord, and compromised blood supply to the cord.[140] The devastating complication of quadriplegia has been reported as another risk of surgery in the seated position. Clearly, extubation of the neurosurgical patient after prolonged surgery requires careful consideration, a review of the patient's intraoperative course, and assessment of airway and neurologic responses. Patients who appear to have obvious facial or airway swelling with minimal response to the ETT are best left intubated until they are fully recovered and meet all criteria for extubation.

VI. CONCLUSIONS

The scope of airway considerations in the neurosurgical patient is vast. General and specific concerns in patient management include airway assessment and emergency airway algorithms. These patients often present with a number of disease processes, which must be considered in relation to the anesthetic as well as to airway management. This task becomes more challenging as patients become older, live longer, and present with multiple medical problems. Additionally, neurosurgical procedures, both in and outside the operating room, are becoming more complex with time. Some procedures will be done with the neurosurgical patient in prone, lateral, or sitting position. Others will require the patient to be awake temporarily and then anesthetized. The approach to airway control is a decision made by the anesthesiologist, often in collaboration with the surgeon. It is important for the practitioner to explore new airway devices and techniques and to gain skill in those that will benefit the neurosurgical patient population. Many problems may occur in the patient after neurosurgery, and thus vigilance both intraoperatively and postoperatively is essential. Anesthesiologists' role as perioperative physician requires that they provide close observation of the patient throughout the perioperative period and render the safest care possible.

VII. CLINICAL PEARLS

- In addition to airway assessment, a neurologic examination or communication with the surgeon is invaluable before induction of anesthesia for neurosurgical procedures.

- Patients with an unstable cervical spine may be unable to cooperate with an awake fiberoptic intubation because of intoxication, hypoxia, or head injury. The need for a CSI patient's airway to be secured is often urgent because of the cervical spine injury or associated head or facial injury.

- A rigid cervical collar may make airway management difficult, impeding mouth opening and application of cricoid pressure. Therefore, with manual in-line immobilization in place, the front part of the collar should be removed or opened before attempted intubation.

- Patients with acromegaly frequently have obstructive sleep apnea and should be induced and ventilated with caution. Direct laryngoscopy and video laryngoscopy are the most effective intubation techniques.

- Elective patients who demonstrate neurologic symptoms of the extremities with neck flexion or extension should have awake, topicalized endotracheal intubation.

- Become familiar with alternative airway devices and practice in normal airways before treating patients with difficult airways.

- Be attentive and inspect the degree of neck flexion in patients positioned prone, lateral, or in any head fixation device.

- A cuff leak test may be helpful before extubation after prolonged surgery in the prone position; always have reintubation strategies and plans.

SELECTED REFERENCES

All references can be found online at www.expertconsult.com.

30. Bedell E, Pough DS: Anesthetic management of traumatic brain injury. *Anesthesiol Clin North Am* 20:417–439, 2002.
56. Bathory I, Frascarlo P, Kern C, et al: Evaluation of the GlideScope for tracheal intubation in patients with cervical spine immobilization by a semi-rigid collar. *Anaesthesia* 64:1337–1341, 2009.
60. Waltl B, Melischek M, Schuschnig C: Tracheal intubation and cervical spine excursion: direct laryngoscopy vs. intubating laryngeal mask. *Anaesthesia* 56:221–226, 2001.
79. Paus AC, Steen H, Røislien J: High mortality rate in rheumatoid arthritis with subluxation of the cervical spine: a cohort study of operated and nonoperated patients. *Spine (Phila Pa 1976)* 33:2278, 2008.
82. Sims CA, Berger DL: Airway risk in hospitalized trauma patients with cervical injuries requiring halo fixation. *Ann Surg* 225:280–284, 2002.
105. Nemergut EC, Zuo Z: Airway management in patients with pituitary disease: a review of 746 patients. *J Neurosurg Anesthesiol* 18:73–77, 2006.
115. Spiekermann BF, Stone DJ, Bogdonoff DL: Airway management in neuroanaesthesia. *Can J Anaesth* 43:820–834, 1996.
131. Sagi HC, Beutler W, Carroll E, Connolly PJ: Airway complications associated with surgery on the anterior spine. *Spine* 27:949–953, 2002.
134. Bruder N, Ravussin P: Recovery from anesthesia and postoperative extubation of neurosurgical patients: a review. *J Neurosurg Anesth* 11:282–293, 1999.

Chapter 43

Obesity, Sleep Apnea, the Airway, and Anesthesia

BABATUNDE OGUNNAIKE | GIRISH P. JOSHI

I. INTRODUCTION

Up to 80% of people with obstructive sleep apnea (OSA) are obese, and with obesity at epidemic proportions worldwide,[1] OSA remains a major contributing factor to airway management difficulties. Numerous studies have reported major respiratory complications, including brain damage and death, in surgical patients with OSA.[2,3] These disastrous outcomes result from failure to secure the airway during the induction of anesthesia, airway obstruction immediately after tracheal extubation, and respiratory arrest after the administration of opioids or sedation in the postoperative period.

The prevalence of OSA is about 20% in the U.S. population. It occurs as a result of partial or complete airway obstruction during sleep,[4] and it is associated with episodic hypoxemia and hypercarbia.[5-7] However, with the U.S. population aging and becoming obese, the prevalence of OSA is expected to increase significantly. Among the surgical population, patients with morbid obesity and OSA tend to be overrepresented due to the higher rates of obesity and OSA-related complications requiring

surgical therapy.[3,8] More than 75% of patients with OSA are undiagnosed or untreated.

II. DEFINITIONS OF OBESITY AND OBSTRUCTIVE SLEEP APNEA

Obesity is a degree of excess weight associated with adverse health consequences.[9] It is defined as a body mass index (BMI, or weight in kg divided by height in m²) greater than 29, and overweight is defined as a BMI of 25 to 29.9.[9] A BMI of 40 or greater is classified as morbid obesity, and a BMI of 50 or greater designates super-obesity. Morbid obesity is associated with an increased risk of comorbidities,[10] which may influence perioperative morbidity and mortality.[11]

OSA is a disorder characterized by repetitive upper airway collapse during sleep. Airflow ceases for more than 10 seconds, five or more times per hour, despite continuing ventilatory effort. It usually is associated with a decrease in arterial oxygen saturation (SaO_2) of more than 4%.[12] Obstructive sleep hypopnea is a greater than 50% decrease in airflow for more than 10 seconds occurring

15 times or more per hour of sleep. It is usually associated with a decrease of 4% or more in SaO₂.

III. PATHOPHYSIOLOGY OF OBSTRUCTIVE SLEEP APNEA

A. Pharyngeal Muscle Activity and Airway Patency

Three pharyngeal segments—nasopharynx (i.e., retropalatal pharynx), oropharynx (i.e., retroglossal pharynx), and laryngopharynx (i.e., retroepiglottic pharynx)—form the upper airway, which is a long, soft-walled tube that lacks bony support on the anterior and lateral walls, which makes it collapsible (Fig. 43-1).[6] The transmural pressures across the pharyngeal walls (i.e., difference between extraluminal and intraluminal pressure) determine the patency of the upper airway. Activation of pharyngeal dilator muscles—the tensor veli palatini, the genioglossus, and the muscles of the hyoid bones (geniohyoid, sternohyoid, and thyrohyoid)—during inspiration counteracts the narrowing effects of reduced intraluminal pressure associated with inspiration. In addition to this inspiration-associated activation, tonic activity of these muscles during wakefulness helps to stabilize the pharyngeal walls.

Upper airway collapse is caused by a reduction in pharyngeal dilator muscle activation, which likely results from the loss of stimulatory effect of wakefulness (i.e., induction of sleep), reduction in respiratory drive, depression of negative pressure reflexes, and the loss of lung volume, which decreases longitudinal traction on the pharyngeal walls.

B. Sleep Pattern, Airway Obstruction, and Arousal

Normal sleep consists of four to six cycles of non–rapid-eye-movement (NREM) sleep followed by rapid-eye-movement (REM) sleep. The four stages of NREM sleep and one stage of REM sleep represent progressive slowing of the electroencephalographic waves. Rhythmic activity of the upper airway muscles decreases during deeper stages of sleep, which is accompanied by significant increase in upper airway resistance and consequent upper airway collapse.[13]

Contraction of the diaphragm during inspiration creates a subatmospheric pressure within the airway that may lead to narrowing of the collapsible segments of the pharynx.[14] As pharyngeal pressure becomes more

Figure 43-1 Airway obstruction during sleep apnea. *Top,* The schematic drawing shows the important upper airway anatomy. The nasopharynx ends at the tip of the uvula; the oropharynx extends from the tip of the uvula to the epiglottis; and the laryngopharynx extends from the tip of the epiglottis to the posterior cricoid cartilage. *Middle,* The drawing shows the action of the most important dilator muscles of the upper airway. The tensor palatine, genioglossus, and hyoid muscles enlarge the nasopharynx, oropharynx, and laryngopharynx, respectively. *Bottom,* The drawing shows collapse of the nasopharynx at the palatal level, the oropharynx at the glottic level, and the laryngopharynx at the epiglottic level. (From Benumof JL: Obstructive sleep apnea in the adult obese patient: implications for airway management. *J Clin Anesth* 13:144–156, 2001.)

UPPER AIRWAY ANATOMY

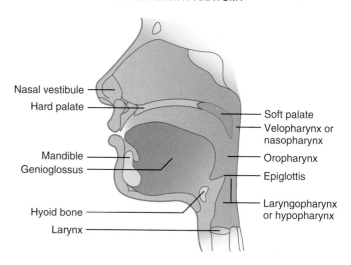

ACTION OF THE UPPER AIRWAY DILATOR MUSCLES

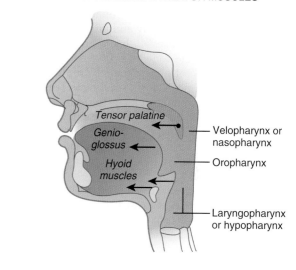

SITES OF OBSTRUCTION DURING SLEEP APNEA

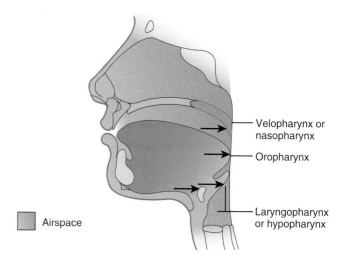

PATHOPHYSIOLOGY OF OBSTRUCTIVE SLEEP APNEA

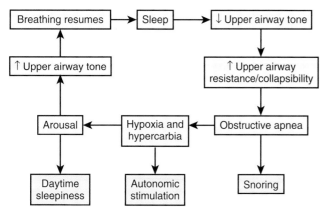

Figure 43-2 Pathophysiology of obstructive sleep apnea.

negative, pharyngeal collapse progressively increases. The lateral pharyngeal walls, a major site of pharyngeal adipose tissue deposition, are the most compliant and therefore the most common site of pharyngeal collapse.[15] In obese patients, deposition of fat around the pharyngeal walls narrows the upper airway and increases the extraluminal pressure and collapse.[16,17] For a given degree of loss of pharyngeal muscle tone and pharyngeal muscle collapse, a greater degree of pharyngeal obstruction is observed in patients with a posteriorly set tongue (caused by micrognathia and retrognathia or a receding mandible), large tongue, large tonsils, and nasal obstruction. Other factors that contribute to upper airway narrowing and subsequent collapse during sleep include: large neck circumference, anatomic or craniofacial abnormalities affecting the airway, and age.[18,19]

Airway collapse leads to obstructive apnea and consequently causes a decrease in arterial oxygen tension (PaO_2) and increase in arterial carbon dioxide tension ($PaCO_2$), which increases neural traffic in the reticular activating system, progressively increasing ventilatory efforts[20,21] and causing arousal from sleep. Arousal, expressed as extremity twitching, gasping or snorting, vocalization, and increased electroencephalographic activity, reactivates the pharyngeal muscles and opens the upper airway. As the upper airway opens, ventilation resumes, which corrects hypoxia and hypercarbia.[22] Hyperventilation after arousal reverses the blood gas disturbance to correspondingly decrease the central drive. The cycle repeats itself when the patient again falls asleep (Fig. 43-2).

Frequent arousals result in sleep disruption and excessive daytime somnolence, and oxygen desaturation, sympathetic hyperactivity, and a systemic inflammatory response may contribute to cardiovascular comorbidities such as systemic hypertension, cardiac arrhythmias, myocardial ischemia, pulmonary hypertension, and heart failure.[23]

IV. DIAGNOSIS OF OBSTRUCTIVE SLEEP APNEA

Because OSA is undiagnosed in an estimated 60% to 70% of patients and failure to recognize OSA preoperatively is one of the major causes of perioperative

---

BOX 43-1 **STOP-BANG Scoring System**

S = Snoring. Do you snore loudly (louder than talking or loud enough to be heard through closed doors)?
T = Tiredness. Do you often feel tired, fatigued, or sleepy during daytime?
O = Observed apnea. Has anyone observed you stop breathing during your sleep?
P = Pressure. Do you have or are you being treated for high blood pressure?
B = Body mass index >35 kg/m^2
A = Age >50 yr
N = Neck circumference >40 cm
G = Male gender

Risk of Obstructive Sleep Apnea

High risk: ≥3 questions answered yes
Low risk: <3 questions answered yes

From Chung F, Yegneswaran B, Liao P, et al: STOP questionnaire: A tool to screen patients for obstructive sleep apnea. *Anesthesiology* 108:812–821, 2008.

complications,[5-7] all patients must be screened for OSA. Obtaining a thorough history and physical examination helps to determine a presumptive diagnosis of OSA, and polysomnography can confirm the diagnosis and severity of OSA and can determine the need for and level of continuous positive airway pressure (CPAP).

A. Clinical Diagnosis

A presumptive clinical diagnosis of OSA may be made from an observation of components that make up the classic triad of sleep disordered breathing (i.e., history or observation of apnea or snoring with hypopnea during sleep), arousal from sleep (i.e., extremity movement, turning, vocalization, or snoring), and daytime sleepiness (i.e., easily falling asleep during quiet times of the day) or fatigue. Because arousals may not be readily apparent, diagnosis of OSA is commonly based on two of the three components, sleep disordered breathing and daytime somnolence.

A systematic review and meta-analysis of clinical screening tests for OSA reported that the STOP-BANG screening tool was easy to use and a good predictor of severe OSA (i.e., apnea-hypopnea index [AHI] >30) (Box 43-1).[24,25] The STOP-BANG questionnaire has a sensitivity of 93% and specificity of 43% at an AHI greater than 15 and a sensitivity of 100% and specificity of 37% at an AHI greater than 30.[25] Other questionnaires, including the Berlin questionnaire and the American Society of Anesthesiologists (ASA) checklist, are also in clinical use and have a similar predictive accuracy for OSA.[26-28]

When the cricomental space, defined as the perpendicular distance from a line between the cricoid cartilage and the inner mentum to the skin of the neck, is more than 1.5 cm, the diagnosis of OSA can be excluded with a negative predictive value of 100%.[29] A decision rule developed to diagnose OSA using three predictors (i.e., cricomental space ≤1.5 cm, pharyngeal grade greater than II, and presence of an overbite) has a positive predictive value of 95% and may provide an alternative to polysomnography.[29]

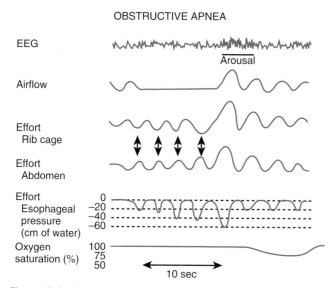

Figure 43-3 Upper airway closure with obstructive apnea. Increasing ventilatory effort is seen in the rib cage, the abdomen, and the level of esophageal pressure (measured with an esophageal balloon), despite lack of oronasal airflow. Arousal recorded on the electroencephalogram *(EEG)* is associated with increasing ventilatory effort, as indicated by the esophageal pressure. Oxyhemoglobin desaturation follows the termination of apnea. During apnea, the movements of the rib cage and the abdomen *(effort)* are in opposite directions *(arrows)* as a result of attempts to breathe against a closed airway. After the airway opens in response to arousal, rib cage and abdominal movements become synchronous. (From Strollo PJ, Rogers RM: Obstructive sleep apnea. *N Engl J Med* 334:99–104, 1996.)

B. Polysomnography

Polysomnography remains the gold standard in the diagnosis of OSA. Polysomnography consists of monitoring the electroencephalogram (EEG), electrooculogram (EOG), and submental electromyogram (EMG) for staging sleep. Oral and nasal airflow, respiratory efforts (i.e., inductance or impedance pneumography to monitor thoracoabdominal motion or the diaphragmatic EMG), oximetry, and capnography are also monitored. Body position, sound, arterial blood pressure, and the electrocardiogram are monitored (Fig. 43-3).[30]

The results of a sleep study are reported as events and indices. Events include apnea (no airflow ≥10 seconds), hypopnea (tidal volume [V_T] ≤50% of the control awake value ≥10 seconds), desaturation (>4% decrease in SaO_2), and arousal, which may be detected clinically (i.e., vocalization, turning, or extremity movement) or by an electroencephalographic burst.[12] Indices are measured as events per hour, which include the AHI (i.e., number of times a patient was apneic or hypopneic per hour), oxygen desaturation index (i.e., number of times a patient had a more than 4% decrease in SaO_2 per hour), and arousal index (i.e., number of times a patient was aroused per hour). If the patient has OSA, the entire sleep study is repeated with CPAP titration to determine the level of CPAP that causes a significant decrease in the AHI.

Because polysomnography may not always be available, other screening devices with single or multiple channels have been explored and may represent alternative methods to diagnose OSA. One study suggested that

an O_2 saturation value of more than 94% on room air in the absence of other causes should lend consideration to the diagnosis of long-standing OSA.[31] The American Academy of Sleep Medicine recommended that the portable monitoring used as an alternative to a polysomnogram must record airflow, respiratory effort, and blood oxygenation. The device also must allow display of raw data with a capability for manual scoring or editing of automated scoring.[32]

It is unclear whether a routine preoperative sleep study (i.e., polysomnogram or home sleep study) could improve perioperative outcomes, because the optimal duration of preoperative CPAP therapy before proceeding with elective surgical procedures is unknown, and compliance with CPAP varies. For those suspected of having OSA based on clinical criteria, anesthesiologists may elect to proceed with a presumptive diagnosis of OSA, unless the patients have significant comorbidities.[5,7]

The severity of OSA is best expressed in terms of the AHI; an AHI of 6 to 20 is considered mild, an AHI of 21 to 40 is moderate, and an AHI greater than 40 is severe OSA. Different sleep laboratories use different criteria for defining the severity of OSA. Because determination of OSA severity based on clinical criteria may be difficult, it may be prudent to treat these patients as if they have moderate or severe OSA.

V. OBESITY, OBSTRUCTIVE SLEEP APNEA, AND THE AIRWAY

Obesity (determined by the BMI) is considered a predictor of difficult mask ventilation (DMV) and difficult intubation (DI).[33] Morbidly obese patients have deposits of excess adipose tissue in the neck, breast, thoracic wall, and abdomen that may impede patency of and access to the upper airway. Magnetic resonance imaging studies of obese patients found greater amounts of fat in areas surrounding the collapsible segments of the pharynx in those with OSA,[34,35] which may explain the difficulty in airway management in obese patients with OSA but not in all obese patients. The distribution pattern of body fat may be a more relevant factor contributing to difficult airway management than the BMI itself.[34] Clinical studies have found that BMI alone is not a good predictor of a difficult airway.[36-40]

Patients with severe OSA (AHI ≥40) have been shown to be at a significantly higher risk for DMV and DI, leading to speculation that they may have different anatomic characteristics compared with patients who have less severe OSA.[41] Obese patients with OSA have larger neck circumferences than equally obese patients (i.e., similar BMI) without OSA.[16,42] This neck "mass loading" (up to 28% increase in neck soft tissue) may be responsible for a more collapsible airway, leading to DMV and DI.[16] Men have a higher percentage of soft tissue and fat in the neck compared with women,[43,44] which may explain greater airway difficulties in male OSA patients compared with female OSA patients. A logistic regression model identified neck circumference at the level of the thyroid cartilage as the single most predictor of problematic intubation.[45] Probability of a DI increases significantly with a neck circumference of 40 cm or more.[45,46]

Neck circumference corrected for height (i.e., neck circumference/height) is sensitive and specific for detecting OSA compared with neck circumference alone.[47] Racial differences in craniofacial anatomy may contribute to the severity of OSA and to a DI.[48,49] Other factors that may contribute to difficult airway management include diabetes mellitus and abnormal facial morphology.[50,51]

Ultrasonography has been used to quantify neck soft tissue at the level of the vocal cords and suprasternal notch to determine potential predictors of difficult laryngoscopy in morbidly obese patients.[52] The amount of pretracheal soft tissue was found to be a strong measure distinguishing an easy laryngoscopy from a difficult one.[52] Lateral head and neck radiography can easily identify caudal soft tissue displacement, which shifts the hyoid bone caudally to increase the distance between the mandible and the hyoid bone. When this distance is more than 20 mm, the presence of OSA and a possible difficult airway should be suspected.[53] Radiographic evaluation has affirmed strong relationships among DI and higher Mallampati scores, OSA, greater mandibular depth, and smaller mandibular and cervical angles.[54]

VI. EFFECTS OF ANESTHESIA AND SURGERY ON POSTOPERATIVE SLEEP

Sedatives/hypnotics, opioids, and muscle relaxants impair neural input to the upper airway muscles and therefore may worsen or even induce OSA. These drugs also decrease the ventilatory response to hypoxemia and hypercarbia, further exaggerating OSA. In contrast to natural sleep, in which OSA patients are aroused in response to asphyxia, drug-induced airway obstruction and apnea lack the ability to arouse and respond adequately to asphyxia. This situation may have life-threatening consequences.

Other factors that influence sleep patterns and can exacerbate sleep disorders include the stress response to surgical insult and postoperative anxiety, pain, and opioids.[55] These factors reduce REM sleep in the immediate postoperative period, which is followed by a rebound REM sleep that can last for several days after surgery.[56] The rebound REM sleep makes patients with OSA even more vulnerable to airway obstruction. Postoperative sleep disturbances appear to be related to the location and invasiveness of the surgical procedure.[57] For example, fewer sleep disturbances occur after mild or moderately invasive surgery than after major surgical procedures.

VII. PERIOPERATIVE RISKS OF OBESITY AND OBSTRUCTIVE SLEEP APNEA

Factors that determine the perioperative risks in obese and OSA patients include the degree of obesity (i.e., BMI) and the severity of OSA, invasiveness of anesthesia and surgery, and postoperative opioid requirements.[27] The ASA practice guidelines propose a scoring system that may be used to estimate whether an OSA patient is at increased risk for perioperative complications[27] and to determine perioperative management (Box 43-2).

Patients who are at significantly increased risk for perioperative complications (score ≥ 5) are not considered to

---

BOX 43-2 **American Society of Anesthesiologists Scoring System for Estimating Perioperative Complications**

A. Severity of sleep apnea is based on sleep study (i.e., AHI) results or clinical indicators if a sleep study is not available:
   None = 0
   Mild OSA = 1
   Moderate OSA = 2
   Severe OSA = 3
   Subtract a point for patients using CPAP or BiPAP preoperatively and postoperatively.
   Add a point for a patient with a $PaCO_2$ greater than 50 mm Hg.
B. Invasiveness of surgery and anesthesia:
   Superficial surgery under local or peripheral nerve block anesthesia without sedation = 0
   Superficial surgery with moderate sedation or general anesthesia or peripheral surgery under spinal or epidural anesthesia (with no more than moderate sedation) = 1
   Peripheral surgery with general anesthesia or airway surgery with moderate sedation = 2
   Major surgery or airway surgery under general anesthesia = 3
C. Requirement for postoperative opioid:
   None = 0
   Low-dose oral opioids = 1
   High-dose oral opioids or parenteral or neuraxial opioids = 3
D. Estimation of perioperative risk:
   Overall score = score of A plus larger score of B or C.
   Patients with an overall score of 4 may be at increased perioperative risk from OSA.
   Patients with an overall score of 5 or greater may be at significantly increased perioperative risk from OSA.

AHI, Apnea-hypopnea index; *BiPAP,* bi-level positive airway pressure; *CPAP,* continuous positive airway pressure; *OSA,* obstructive sleep apnea; *PaCO_2,* arterial partial pressure of carbon dioxide.
Adapted from Gross JB, Bachenberg KL, Benumof JL, et al: Practice guidelines for the perioperative management of patients with obstructive sleep apnea: A report by the Task Force on Perioperative Management of patients with obstructive sleep apnea. *Anesthesiology* 104:1081–1093, 2006.

---

be good candidates for ambulatory surgery. Patients with mild OSA who are undergoing superficial or minor surgical procedures under local, regional, or general anesthesia and who are expected to have a minimal postoperative opioid requirement may undergo ambulatory surgery. Ambulatory surgery is not recommended for patients undergoing airway surgery or upper abdominal laparoscopic surgery. Because the ASA scoring system needs validation, it should serve only as a guide.

VIII. INTRAOPERATIVE CONSIDERATIONS

The major concerns during induction of anesthesia or sedation/analgesia technique in obese and in OSA patients include DMV, DI, and increased risk of regurgitation of gastric contents and potential pulmonary aspiration.[58] General anesthesia with a secure airway is

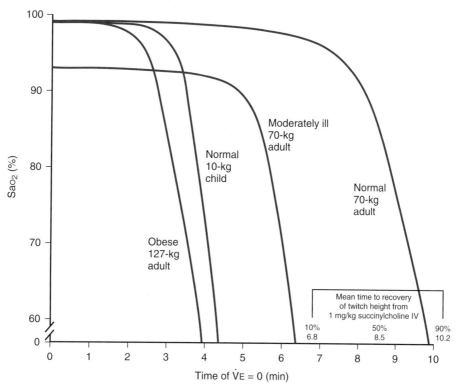

Figure 43-4 Arterial oxygen saturation *(Sao₂)* versus time of apnea for various types of patients. Mean times to recovery from 1 mg/kg of intravenous succinylcholine *(lower right corner)*. Critical hemoglobin desaturation occurs before return to an unparalyzed state after 1 mg/kg of intravenous succinylcholine. (From Benumof JL, Dagg R, Benumof R: Critical hemoglobin desaturation will occur before return to unparalyzed state following 1 mg/kg intravenous succinylcholine. *Anesthesiology* 87:979–982, 1997.)

considered preferable to deep sedation without an airway,[27] which is increasingly used in modern anesthesia practice.[59]

A. Preinduction Considerations

Alterations in pulmonary function (e.g., reduced functional residual capacity [FRC] and O₂ reserves) in obese patients may result in severe hypoxemia even after short periods of apnea (Fig. 43-4).[60,61] Positioning of the patient in the head-elevated laryngoscopy position (HELP), which can be achieved by stacking blankets or a specially designed foam pillow (Troop Elevation Pillow, CR Enterprises, Frisco, TX)[62] or the inflatable Rapid Airway Management Positioner (RAMP, Airpal Inc., Center Valley, PA),[63] can compensate for the exaggerated flexed position from posterior cervical fat. The objective of this maneuver is to elevate the head, upper body, and shoulders above the chest so that an imaginary horizontal line connects the sternal notch with the external auditory meatus to create a better alignment among the oral, pharyngeal, and laryngeal axes (see Fig. 9-1 in Chapter 9). This position structurally improves maintenance of the passive pharyngeal airway, facilitates bag-mask ventilation, and improves the success of endotracheal intubation.

Other techniques used to avoid postinduction hypoxemia include preoxygenation with 100% O₂ until the end-tidal oxygen value is at least 90% and use of 10 cm H₂O of CPAP or bi-level positive airway pressure (BiPAP)

ventilation (i.e., intermittent positive-pressure ventilation [PPV] with positive end-expiratory pressure [PEEP]) with the patient in a 25-degree head-up position.[60,64-66] Preinduction techniques followed by 10 cm H₂O of PEEP during bag-mask ventilation and after intubation can reduce post-intubation atelectasis and improve arterial oxygenation.[67] A poorly sealed preoxygenation system results in difficulty with achieving adequate preoxygenation within a reasonable period of time (Fig. 43-5).[6]

B. Awake Endotracheal Intubation

One of the critical decisions regarding induction of general anesthesia in the obese patient with OSA is to determine whether awake intubation should be performed. Awake intubation should be considered when any component of the triple maneuver (i.e., mandible advancement, neck extension, and mouth opening) is unattainable.[68] Obese OSA patients typically are more difficult to intubate than their non-OSA counterparts,[51] but obesity by itself has not been largely associated with difficult laryngoscopy or DI.[36,37,41,68] A retrospective analysis performed to identify patient characteristics that influence the choice of awake fiberoptic intubation or intubation after general anesthesia in obese patients revealed that awake intubation patients were more likely to be male, have a BMI of 60 kg/m² or greater, and be assigned to a Mallampati class of III or IV.[69] Because no single factor predicts DMV or DI, it may be prudent to combine multiple predictors, such as Mallampati class III

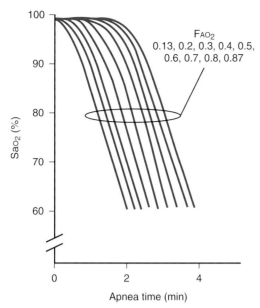

Figure 43-5 Arterial oxygen saturation (SaO₂) versus time of apnea for a patient with a body mass index of 40 kg/m² for various initial preapnea concentrations of the fraction of alveolar oxygen (FAO₂). An FAO₂ of 0.87 (*right-most curve*) corresponds to a fraction of inspired oxygen (FIO₂) of 1.0, and an FAO₂ of 0.13 (*left-most curve*) corresponds to an FIO₂ of 0.21. (From Benumof JL: Obstructive sleep apnea in the adult obese patient: Implications for airway management. *J Clin Anesth* 13:144-156, 2001.)

or IV,[70] neck circumference of 40 cm or larger, limited mandibular protrusion,[38] and severe OSA (AHI ≥40), to determine the need for awake intubation.

During awake intubation, sedatives and opioids, although desirable, should be minimized or totally avoided if possible, because airway obstruction can occur while the airway is being secured.[6] Dexmedetomidine is a highly selective α₂-adrenergic agonist with sedative, amnestic, analgesic, and sympatholytic properties that does not cause respiratory depression.[71] It reduces salivary secretions through sympatholytic and vagomimetic effects, which should improve visualization during fiberoptic intubation and facilitate awake intubation. The addition of ketamine with dexmedetomidine may further improve a patient's tolerance to awake intubation without impairing respiration.[72]

Topical anesthesia applied to facilitate awake intubation may compromise the airway patency.[73,74] In the upper airway, topical anesthesia may impair neural compensatory mechanoreceptors necessary for the arousal response and cause narrowing of the pharyngeal cross-sectional area, which may induce and prolong apneic episodes.[73,74] The spray-as-you-go technique for topicalization of the local anesthetic during awake intubation is often performed to minimize the time of obtundation of laryngeal reflexes.

C. Endotracheal Intubation After Induction of Anesthesia

If endotracheal intubation is planned after induction of anesthesia, adequate preparation must be made for a difficult airway based on the ASA difficult airway management guidelines.[75] Emergency airway equipment (e.g., video laryngoscopes, supralaryngeal airways, flexible fiberoptic bronchoscopes) and additional help must be immediately available. Video laryngoscopes offer superior viewing of the glottis and reduce the duration of performing endotracheal intubation, thereby preventing significant desaturation in morbidly obese patients.[76-78] The laryngeal mask airway is an effective rescue device for the difficult airway or failed airway, even in obese patients.[79,80] However, the increased intra-abdominal pressures associated with obesity may increase the risk of gastric aspiration with the use of the laryngeal mask airway, because it does not completely seal the airway. Restrictive pulmonary disease in obese patients can increase the peak inspiratory pressures and cause leaks around the laryngeal mask airway cuff, leading to hypoventilation and gastric insufflation.[81,82]

Because of concerns about aspiration and a difficult airway, rapid-sequence induction of general anesthesia with propofol and succinylcholine or rocuronium and cricoid pressure constitute the standard of care for morbidly obese patients. However, it is important to ensure sufficient depth of anesthesia, because inadequate anesthesia predisposes to regurgitation of gastric contents and pulmonary aspiration.

A short-acting muscle relaxant (e.g., succinylcholine) is recommended because it allows a rapid recovery, which may allow rapid return of spontaneous breathing. However, even with low-dose succinylcholine, recovery of breathing and pharyngeal patency may not occur before development of severe hypoxemia because morbidly obese patients can desaturate rapidly.[61] A higher dose of succinylcholine has been recommended for optimal intubating conditions in morbidly obese patients.[83,84]

Use of high-dose rocuronium may allow rapid intubating conditions, but its longer duration of action may be detrimental during a DI or DMV. Sugammadex (not available in the United States) can rapidly reverse rocuronium-induced muscle relaxation in case of impossible bag-mask ventilation or endotracheal intubation to avoid disastrous consequences.[85] However, it does not reverse unconsciousness induced by the intravenous anesthetic agent, and airway patency therefore may not be restored.

The need for rapid-sequence induction in the obese patient with no other risk factors (e.g., diabetes, history of significant reflux) is being questioned.[5,86] Controlled induction of general anesthesia allows appropriate titration of intravenous anesthetic, prevents hemodynamic instability that can occur from a predetermined dose, allows adequate ventilation, and avoids hypoxia between induction and endotracheal intubation. However, these benefits should be weighed against the risks of DMV and DI with rapid development of severe O₂ desaturation when faced with minimal risk of aspiration.

D. Mechanical Ventilation

The aim of mechanical ventilation in obese patients is to prevent progressive atelectasis that is commonly seen in this patient population.[87] Proposed ventilatory strategies for obese patients include the use of lower inspired oxygen concentrations (FIO_2) to maintain physiologic oxygenation,[88] low V_T (6 to 8 mL/kg ideal body weight),[89] application of PEEP (5 to 10 cm H_2O), and inclusion of recruitment maneuvers (i.e., large manual or automatic lung inflations).[90-93] Recruitment maneuvers to adequately open up the collapsed alveoli may require airway pressures of up to 55 cm H_2O, which may have deleterious effects on hemodynamics and therefore should be performed only after hemodynamic stabilization and be maintained for only a short period.[94] Use of pressure-controlled ventilation may allow improved distribution of gases and lower peak airway pressure.[95,96] Hyperventilation should be avoided because hypocapnia may cause metabolic alkalosis and postoperative hypoventilation.[87]

IX. POSTOPERATIVE CONSIDERATIONS

There is a high risk of post-extubation airway obstruction in obese patients with OSA, which is further increased after airway surgery with subsequent nasal packing. The ASA Closed Claims Project database analysis of lawsuits involving loss of airway after tracheal extubation found that those cases resulted in higher incidences of brain death and death than loss of airway during induction of anesthesia.[97] In 67% of the lawsuits, the patients were obese, and 28% had a history of OSA.[97]

The effects of obesity on respiratory mechanics, including a reduction in FRC, a decrease in lung compliance, expiratory flow limitation, and development of intrinsic PEEP, act together to elevate the work of breathing at rest and increase the risk of perioperative pulmonary complications.[98,99] This situation may be compounded by the negative respiratory effects induced by sedative/hypnotics and muscle relaxants that can persist for several hours after anesthesia.[100,101]

Factors to consider when determining whether to leave the patient intubated after surgery include BMI, severity of OSA, associated cardiopulmonary disease, ease of bag-mask ventilation and intubation at induction of anesthesia, type and duration of surgical procedure, and the intraoperative course. Patients with OSA should be extubated in a semirecumbent position after they are fully awake (i.e., rational, oriented, and responding to commands in a quick and unambiguous manner) and after verification of complete reversal of neuromuscular blockade. A nasopharyngeal or oropharyngeal airway may prevent post-extubation airway obstruction.[102]

A. Postoperative Noninvasive Positive-Pressure Ventilation

CPAP is the most commonly used form of noninvasive PPV in OSA patients. It works by acting as a pneumatic splint to prevent airway collapse during sleep, thereby reducing the work of breathing by counteracting auto-PEEP to reduce respiratory muscle load, improving lung function (particularly FRC), and improving gas exchange.[103,104] Auto-CPAP, delivered by a self-titrating device, uses algorithms to detect variations in the degree of obstruction and adjusts to the pressure level to restore normal breathing, thereby compensating for factors

modifying upper airway collapsibility, including stage of sleep, posture during sleep, and the use of drugs that affect upper airway muscle tone.[105] However, it has not been confirmed that auto-CPAP is more effective than fixed CPAP.[106,107]

CPAP or BiPAP should be applied as soon as possible after surgery to patients who are receiving it preoperatively. It should be instituted when nausea, vomiting, post-extubation suctioning, level of consciousness, communication, facial edema, and drug depression issues are minimal or nonexistent.[27] The use of CPAP immediately after tracheal extubation may improve postoperative pulmonary function.[108]

B. Postoperative Disposition

Requirements for postoperative monitoring depend on patient-specific factors (e.g., high BMI, severe OSA, associated cardiopulmonary disease), invasiveness of the anesthetic technique, the type and duration of surgery, and the intraoperative course.[31] Patients with severe OSA undergoing an extensive surgical procedure that requires significant opioid analgesia may require close monitoring in a monitored environment (e.g., intensive care unit, step-down unit). Creation of intermediate care (observational) units with higher nursing ratios has been suggested as the most rational solution for postoperative care of morbidly obese patients with OSA who have moderate disease and whose conditions are not severe enough to qualify for an intensive care unit.

The scientific literature regarding the safety of ambulatory surgery in OSA patients is sparse and of limited quality,[5] and the suitability of these procedures remains controversial. The ASA practice guidelines propose a scoring system that may be used to determine the suitability for ambulatory surgery (see Box 43-2).[27] Patients who are at significantly increased risk for perioperative complications (score ≥ 5) are not good candidates for ambulatory surgery.[27] OSA patients should be monitored for a median of 3 hours longer than their non-OSA counterparts before discharge from the facility.[27] Monitoring should continue for a median of 7 hours after the last episode of airway obstruction or hypoxemia while breathing room air in an unstimulated environment. Unfortunately, the recommendation for longer postoperative stays is not based on any scientific evidence and may be the major limitation on performing surgical procedures in an ambulatory setting.

X. CONCLUSIONS

Airway management and general anesthesia for patients with obesity and OSA remains a challenge to anesthesiologists and other health care professionals. Understanding the pathophysiology of the disease with respect to how OSA complicates the status of various body systems and presents difficulties to the anesthesiologist is important in providing optimal care and improving perioperative outcomes. Because life-threatening situations may be encountered in this patient population, adequate preparation cannot be overemphasized.

The possible presence of OSA must be confirmed by a proper diagnosis obtained clinically or through a comprehensive sleep study. This is a primary step in ensuring that adequate surgical preparation is made. Preoperative diagnosis may improve the perioperative outcome because perioperative management can be modified appropriately, including delay of surgery to confirm and quantitate the diagnosis with a sleep study and use of appropriate anesthesia technique. It is necessary to develop protocols that allow much earlier identification and evaluation of OSA and preparation of an appropriate perioperative management plan. Postoperatively, the OSA patient must be watched closely because the risk of pharyngeal collapse and life-threatening airway obstruction lingers for several days after surgery, especially when opioids are used.

XI. CLINICAL PEARLS

- Clinical diagnosis of obstructive sleep apnea (OSA) may be made by observing the components of the classic triad of sleep-disordered breathing (i.e., history or observation of apnea or snoring with hypopnea during sleep), arousal from sleep (i.e., extremity movement, turning, vocalization, or snoring), and daytime sleepiness (i.e., easily falling asleep during quiet times of the day) or fatigue.

- A high body mass index (BMI) is a weak but statistically significant predictor of difficult intubation (DI) or failed endotracheal intubation and of difficult mask ventilation (DMV). The distribution pattern of body fat, rather than the BMI value, may be a more relevant factor in a difficult laryngoscopy. Measuring the neck circumference at the level of the thyroid cartilage is a useful addition to the normal daily practice of measuring weight or BMI during preoperative airway evaluation.

- A lateral head and neck radiograph demonstrating caudal soft tissue displacement that shifts the hyoid bone caudally to increase the distance between the mandible and the hyoid bone to more than 20 mm suggests the presence of obstructive sleep apnea (OSA) and possible difficult airway.

- General anesthesia with a secure airway is preferable to deep sedation without an airway for superficial procedures and for OSA patients undergoing procedures involving the upper airway.

- Intubation under general anesthesia should be carried out with the patient fully preoxygenated to prevent hypoxia because the relatively low functional residual capacity (FRC) found in obese patients causes them to desaturate more rapidly.

- The head-elevated laryngoscopy position (HELP) significantly elevates the head, upper body, and shoulders above the chest so that an imaginary horizontal line connects the sternal notch with the external auditory meatus to create a better alignment among the three axes.

- Intravenous anesthetic agents, except for ketamine, significantly decrease inspiratory negative airway pressure by depressing the chemical drive. Ketamine has a less depressant effect on pharyngeal dilating muscle activity, but it increases pharyngeal secretions, thereby offsetting the beneficial effect.

- A short-acting muscle relaxant, such as succinylcholine, does not ensure recovery of muscle function or pharyngeal patency before development of severe hypoxemia in morbidly obese patients with significantly decreased FRC.

- Rapid-sequence intubation is often recommended in obese patients because of the high prevalence of lower esophageal sphincter hypotonia, which increases the prevalence of gastroesophageal reflux disease, but the benefits should be weighed against the risks of DMV or DI.

- The aim of mechanical ventilation in obese patients is to keep the lungs open during the entire respiratory cycle to counteract the negative effects of respiratory modifications induced by general anesthesia and paralysis, which can persist for a few days postoperatively.

- The endotracheal tube should be left in place, or extubation should be carried out over an airway exchange catheter if any doubt exists about the ability of the patient to breathe spontaneously or the ability of the practitioner to reintubate in an emergency.

- Tracheal extubation should occur in the semi-upright or head-up position only after the obese OSA patient regains full consciousness after general anesthesia and after confirming airway patency and verification of complete reversal of neuromuscular blockade. Continuous positive airway pressure (CPAP) should be applied as soon as possible after surgery in patients who are receiving it preoperatively, but it should be instituted when nausea, vomiting, post-extubation suctioning, level of consciousness, communication, facial edema, and drug depression issues are minimal or nonexistent.

- Obese OSA patients should be cared for in a monitored environment because of an increased risk of opioid-induced postoperative upper airway obstruction.

SELECTED REFERENCES

All references can be found online at expertconsult.com.

5. Joshi GP: The adult obese patient with sleep apnea for ambulatory surgery. ASA refresher courses in anesthesiology. *Anesthesiology* 35:97–106, 2007.
6. Benumof JL: Obesity, sleep apnea, the airway and anesthesia. *Curr Opin Anaesthesiol* 17:21–30, 2004.
7. Adesanya AO, Lee W, Greilich NB, et al: Perioperative management of obstructive sleep apnea. *Chest* 138:1489–1498, 2010.
8. Chung SA, Yuan H, Chung F: A systemic review of obstructive sleep apnea and its implications for anesthesiologists. *Anesth Analg* 107:1543–1563, 2008.
18. Tsuiki S, Isono S, Ishikawa T, et al: Anatomical balance of the upper airway and obstructive sleep apnea. *Anesthesiology* 108:1009–1015, 2008.
24. Ramachandran SK, Josephs LA: A meta-analysis of clinical screening tests for obstructive sleep apnea. *Anesthesiology* 110:928–939, 2009.

25. Chung F, Yegneswaran B, Liao P, et al: STOP Questionnaire: A tool to screen patients for obstructive sleep apnea. *Anesthesiology* 108:812–821, 2008.
27. From Gross JB, Bachenberg KL, Benumof JL, et al: Practice guidelines for the perioperative management of patients with obstructive sleep apnea: A report by the Task Force on Perioperative Management of patients with obstructive sleep apnea. *Anesthesiology* 104:1081–1093, 2006.

68. Isono S. Obstructive sleep apnea of obese adults: Pathophysiology and perioperative airway management. *Anesthesiology* 110:908–921, 2009.
87. Gertler R, Joshi GP: Modern understanding of intraoperative mechanical ventilation in normal and diseased lungs. *Adv Anesth* 26:15–33, 2010.

Chapter 44

Airway Management in Burn Patients

BETTINA U. SCHMITZ | JOHN A. GRISWOLD

I. INTRODUCTION

The airway of the burn patient presents ongoing challenges and special considerations during the period of initial burn injury and throughout the patient's hospital course. As a consequence of their injuries, some burn patients have airway difficulties throughout the remainder of their lives.

The National Burn Repository reports 181,000 hospital admissions for burn injury for 1998 through 2007 in 73 U.S. burn centers. The overall mortality rate during this period was 4.9%.[1] A 2006 report of the National Burn Repository indicated an incidence of inhalational trauma of 5.7% during the previous 10 years.[2] Inhalational burn trauma was associated with a 27.3% mortality rate, compared with a rate of 4.5% for burned patients without inhalational injury.[2] A review of 850 children admitted with inhalational injury during a 10-year period at the four Shriner's Pediatric Burn Centers in the United States found a mortality rate of 16.4%.[3] Consequently, inhalational burns contribute significantly to mortality among the burn population. Although the outcomes for survival after burns and the quality of life of burn victims have improved, respiratory complications are an ongoing source of burn morbidity and mortality.

II. AIRWAY MANAGEMENT IN THE ACUTELY BURNED PATIENT

A. Evaluation of the Patient after Acute Burn Injury and Indication for Airway Management

1. Assessment at the Scene

First responders have a crucial role in the early management of burn patients. In addition to the usual trauma assessments, emergency medical service (EMS) staff must determine whether the patient's condition warrants immediate intubation in the field or the patient can be observed. Indications for intubation at the trauma scene include the following[4,5]:

- Unconsciousness and altered mental status (with incumbent aspiration risk)
- Respiratory distress (e.g., desaturation with supplemental oxygen [O_2], tachypnea)
- Thermal airway injury
- Hoarseness, stridor, dysphagia, or drooling
- Burn injury to the neck and face after fire or smoke exposure in a closed space or carbonated sputum

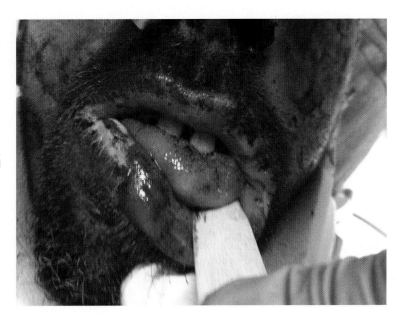

Figure 44-1 Carbonaceous sputum, singed nasal hairs, and facial burns indicate possible upper airway thermal injury.

- Prolonged transport to the hospital of the patient with possible airway injury
- Extensive burn injury
- Additional traumatic injuries

Patients with a flame injury from a barbecue or fire in an open space may have burns to the neck and face but no airway involvement and therefore do not require early intubation.

In addition to initial medical management of the patient, EMS staff gathers information about the type of injury and the patient's medical history. The information should be recorded for transport with the patient to a specialized burn center.

The practice of prehospital intubation of the burned patient has been questioned. Eastman and colleagues[6] reviewed the charts of 1272 patients admitted after field intubation over a period of 23 years and found that 69% of them survived. However, 30% of the survivors were extubated on admission or on the second day after the burn. None required reintubation. Klein and associates[7] reviewed the charts of patients admitted to the Washington Burn Center after a transport of more than 90 miles for the period of 2000 through 2003. They examined parameters such as duration of transport, error in burn severity estimation, fluid management, appropriateness of intubation, and transport complications. Of 1877 patients, 424 were transported more than 90 miles to the burn center. No patient died during transport, and 111 patients arrived intubated, with only 61% having inhalational burns. More than 50% of patients were extubated within the first 24 hours after admission.

Failure to secure an airway was one of the most common complications occurring during patient transport. The fact that airway obstruction can develop very quickly in burn patients and that the experience and equipment of EMS are often limited supports intubation in the field before transport in the patient with a potential for respiratory compromise.

2. Assessment in the Hospital

Roughly 10% of burn patients also present with other traumatic injuries. All burn patients are considered trauma patients and consequently undergo a primary trauma survey (i.e., the ABCDE algorithm: airway, breathing, circulation, disability, and exposure).[8] The extent and surface area of the burn are noted, other traumatic injuries identified and treated, and the airway secured if indicated. The incidence of inhalational trauma, length of hospital stay, and mortality rate are increased for patients presenting with burns and other traumatic nonburn injuries.[9]

On arrival of the patient at the burn center, the tube position is confirmed with carbon dioxide (CO_2) monitoring and auscultation of the lung fields. Uncertainty about endotracheal tube (ETT) placement should be remedied by direct laryngoscopy or fiberoptic bronchoscopy. The mouth, pharynx, and larynx are examined by laryngoscopy to assess edema and identify any burned mucosa and the presence of soot (Fig. 44-1). A radiograph is obtained to verify the ETT position and identify other potential injuries, such as a pneumothorax. Lung parenchymal injuries usually are not immediately detectable by radiography immediately after injury. Patients presenting with a supralaryngeal airway (SLA) on arrival at the hospital require endotracheal intubation or a surgical airway.

In the unintubated patient, the presence of soot in the sputum, dyspnea, tachypnea, hoarseness, and stridor are signs of impending airway obstruction. Fiberoptic endoscopy is the gold standard for the diagnosis of inhalational trauma.[10-17] In the awake patient, a nasal fiberoptic examination under local anesthesia can be performed to evaluate the larynx and confirm the presence or absence of edema and soot. Patients with altered mental status, dyspnea, hoarseness, or stridor require immediate intubation.

A relevant history for airway management after burn injury includes the following information:

- Location and type of injury (e.g., flame, steam, chemical, electrical, vehicular)
- Mental and physical condition at the scene of injury and changes during transport
- History of a difficult airway
- Circumstances of the burn (e.g., open space, closed space)
- Other traumatic injuries
- Other medical history[10,12,18,19]

Rarely, inhalation of hot steam and hot fluids can lead to a rapidly progressive upper airway edema. Chemical fires can have more complex sequelae because the chemicals themselves can injure tissues after extinction of the fire. The circumstances of the burn injury and its duration can help to discern the likelihood of carbon monoxide (CO), cyanide (CN), and other toxicities.

3. Altered Mental Status

An isolated burn injury usually does not produce a mental status change early in the disease course. A disoriented, stuporous, or unconscious burn patient should be closely examined for additional trauma. Burn-related reasons for altered mental status include inhalation-induced hypoxemia, CO poisoning, CN toxicity, and electrical injury. Other sources of altered mental status include head trauma, alcohol or drug ingestion, metabolic disorders, seizures, and psychosis. Patients with altered mental status should be intubated and ventilated with 100% O_2 until CO poisoning and CN toxicity can be ruled out. Intubation should be performed using maneuvers to stabilize the cervical spine (C-spine) if neck injury has not been ruled out.[10,12,17,20,21]

4. Cardiovascular Abnormalities

Cardiovascular instability, dysrhythmia, and cardiac arrest can be consequences of CO intoxication. Cardiac disturbances can also result from innate cardiac disease combined with the response to traumatic injury. Hypotension is often caused by fluid loss associated with burns. Hemorrhagic and neurogenic shock can also lead to hypotension in these patients as a consequence of nonburn injuries. The airway should be secured in hemodynamically unstable patients.[10,17,22]

5. Neck and Face Burns

Extensive burns of the face and neck produce facial edema, making direct laryngoscopy difficult or impossible. These patients may have pharyngeal and laryngeal edema, further complicating intubation (Fig. 44-2). Delay in securing the airway can lead to a "cannot intubate, cannot ventilate" situation. Surgical airways must be performed in this instance.[10,17,21,23]

6. Extensive Burns

Patients with large body surface area burns frequently have airway burns as well (Fig. 44-3). Edema after resuscitative efforts can make intubation impossible. After massive burns, patients develop a hypermetabolic state leading to increased CO_2 production requiring ventilator support. Some physicians suggest prophylactic

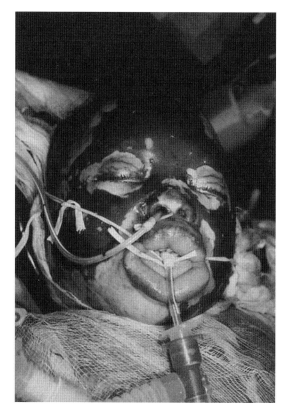

Figure 44-2 Severe airway edema continues to progress for several days after initial injury and intubation.

intubation for total body surface area burns greater than 30%.[10,12,17,22]

7. Additional Injuries

Burn injuries can occur in explosions. In this setting, blast injuries, including pneumothorax and eardrum perforation, must be addressed. To escape a fire, victims often jump from windows, sustaining fractures. Burns caused by vehicular trauma can be associated with other traumatic injuries. Electrical high-voltage contact can be accompanied by brain edema, cardiac dysrhythmias, myonecrosis, and rhabdomyolysis with renal injury. C-spine injury should be ruled out as expeditiously as possible in the course of patient management, depending on the nature of the primary injury.

B. Inhalational Injury

Approximately 20% to 30% of patients admitted to regional burn centers have some degree of inhalational injury and are at risk from toxic gases.[19,24] Edelman and colleagues[25] reviewed 829 patients admitted to a burn center between 2000 and 2004 and found that 28% had an inhalational injury. Although the mortality rate for patients with solely a thermal injury was 3% and was 12% for those with an isolated inhalational injury, patients with combined thermal and inhalational injuries had a mortality rate of 14.6%.[25] Box 44-1 summarizes smoke inhalational injuries.

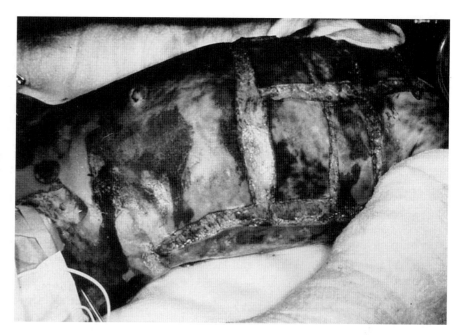

Figure 44-3 Extensive burns to the chest and neck can require immediate escharotomy to facilitate ventilation.

1. Injury to the Respiratory Tract

a. UPPER AND LOWER AIRWAY INHALATION SMOKE INJURY

Inhalational injury of the airway can be caused by steam, carbenoids, chemicals, and the toxic products of combustion. In most patients, the entire airway is involved, and several toxic agents are inhaled. Inhalational injury results from thermal injury (heat) to the upper airway, toxic chemicals in the respiratory tract, and CO and CN toxicities.

Thermal injury and inhaled chemical toxins cause burn injuries by different mechanisms. In an enclosed environment, temperatures can exceed 800° C, with an O_2 concentration of just 10% and CO concentrations greater than 0.5%.[26,27] Injuries are often described by the area of the tracheobronchial tree affected. The upper airway lies above the vocal cords, whereas the lower airway consists of the tracheobronchial tree, including terminal bronchi and alveoli.

The upper airway consists of the nasal and oral cavities, the pharynx, and laryngeal structures such as the epiglottis, false vocal cords, and true vocal cords. Direct injury

of the upper airway with steam, superheated air, or hot liquid is rare. The heat-conducting capacity of air is low, reducing the potential for injury. Reflex closure of the glottis usually protects the structures below the vocal cords from steam injury. Signs of upper airway injury by heated air and steam include erythema, edema, ischemia, and pharyngeal ulcerations. Although the initial presentation of injury may be unimpressive, these lesions can quickly lead to airway edema and obstruction.

The lower airway includes the tracheobronchial system and the lung parenchyma. Most injuries of the upper and lower airway result from the chemical toxins produced by combustion. Burned rubber and plastics release ammonia, chloride, sulfur, and nitrogen dioxides. Cotton and wool fires produce toxic aldehydes, including formaldehyde. Laminated structures produce cyanide.[16,21,22,28-30]

b. PATHOPHYSIOLOGY OF SMOKE INHALATIONAL INJURY

Different mechanisms contribute to the pulmonary changes after smoke inhalation. An increase in bronchial perfusion contributes to the development of pulmonary edema, as does the increased permeability of the pulmonary vasculature caused by an increase in nitric oxide (NO).

NO formed from arginine by nitrous oxide synthetase (NOS) has an important role in pulmonary changes after smoke injury. Smoke inhalation stimulates vasomotor and sensory nerve endings in the tracheobronchial tract, releasing neuropeptides with bronchoconstricting properties. Neutrophil activation produces reactive oxygen species (ROS), increasing the activity of NOS.[31]

Increased NO in the lung reduces hypoxic pulmonary vasoconstriction, leading to ventilation-perfusion ($\dot{V}/\dot{Q}$)) mismatch and edema formation. O_2 and NO react to form peroxynitrite. Peroxynitrite causes cellular injury and damage to cell membranes that results in increased pulmonary vascular permeability and pulmonary edema.

BOX 44-1   Smoke Inhalational Injuries

- Inhalation injury occurs in 20% to 30% of burn patients.
- Inhalation injury increases burn mortality.
- The leading cause of immediate death from burns is inhalational injury, not the burn itself.
- Heat injury is confined above the vocal cords.
- Inhalation damage is caused by toxic chemicals and thermal injury.
- Sequelae of inhalational burns include pulmonary edema, $\dot{V}/\dot{Q}$ mismatch, atelectasis, airway obstruction, and pneumonia.
- Carbon monoxide (CO) and cyanide (CN) systemic toxicities should be suspected with burns in confined areas.

Peroxynitrite, other reactive O_2 species, and reactive nitrogen (N_2) species damage DNA. In an effort to repair damaged DNA, poly(ADP-ribose) polymerase (PARP) is activated. PARP uses ATP energy reserves to repair damaged DNA. Depletion of ATP by PARP activity results in cell death.[32-35]

The coagulation cascade is activated, leading to fibrin deposition in the airway. Airway casts are formed, often obstructing the airway and impairing gas exchange in the lungs. Inhibition of surfactant leads to alveolar collapse, atelectasis, and $\dot{V}/\dot{Q}$ mismatch.[11,16,21,28,34,36]

c. SYMPTOMS

Ninety percent of patients with burns to the face and neck have an airway injury. Indicators for airway injury after burn include the following:

- Facial burn with singed nasal and facial hair
- Soot in the oropharynx
- Soot in the sputum
- Dysphonia
- Stridor
- Rhonchi
- Bronchospasm
- Respiratory distress
- Hypoxia
- Loss of consciousness

Absence of facial burns does not rule out an airway injury. However, carbonated sputum does not necessarily indicate injury below the vocal cords, because it can be drained from the nasal cavity.[10,12,13,16,17,21,23]

d. DIAGNOSIS

The gold standard for the diagnosis of an inhalational injury is direct or fiberoptic inspection of the larynx and tracheobronchial tree. Initial evaluation should document the presence and extent of injury to establish a baseline of the airway injury. Recurrent examinations are needed to evaluate the course of injury and to remove necrotic tissue to prevent airway obstruction and atelectasis.[10-17]

Flow-volume curves are difficult to obtain and depend on the patient's effort, making them less useful for discerning airway obstruction and compromise in the acute burn patient.[10,16] The arterial blood gas determination may not demonstrate any abnormalities during the early stage of airway injury,[10,16] and the radiograph obtained at presentation may not reveal any pathologic changes caused by the burn. Previous changes and nonburn injuries, however, are evident. Radioisotope evaluation of the lungs can demonstrate injury to the lung parenchyma and small airways. After intravenous injection of xenon 133 or inhalation of technetium 99, the healthy lung can rapidly clear the isotopes, but injured parenchyma clears isotopes in a delayed and uneven manner. This type of testing is not practical in the acutely injured patient.[16,17,21]

2. Systemic Toxicity from Inhalational Injury

a. CARBON MONOXIDE POISONING

CO is a product of combustion. It is a colorless, odorless, tasteless gas. Burn victims injured in a confined space should always be evaluated for possible CO poisoning. CO has great avidity for the iron of hemoglobin and cytochrome oxidase. CO's affinity for hemoglobin is 200 times greater than that of O_2. Moreover, carboxyhemoglobin shifts the O_2 dissociation curve to the left, impeding the delivery of O_2 to the tissues. CO binds to cytochrome oxidase in the mitochondria, impairing O_2 use on a cellular level and producing tissue hypoxia and acidosis.[6,10,13,21,28]

CO poisoning is the leading cause of poisoning death in the United States.[37] It is often missed because the signs and symptoms are nonspecific, including fatigue, headache, weakness, dizziness, confusion, and loss of consciousness.[10,38] A history, examination, and laboratory studies are required to make the diagnosis of CO poisoning and to plan treatment.[39-43]

The history should elicit the circumstances of burn (e.g., closed-space fire), time of exposure, and source (e.g., internal combustion engines in closed space, smoke inhalation, stoves, furnaces). The examination should take into account the pathophysiology of burn injuries, including an affinity of CO for hemoglobin that is 240 times more than that of O_2, reduced hemoglobin O_2 carrying capacity, tissue hypoxia, and the leftward shift of the hemoglobin dissociation curve.

Laboratory tests include pulse oximetry and O_2 saturation, but O_2 partial pressure does not reflect CO poisoning.[10,13,17] Carboxyhemoglobin is measured and normally is less than 2% in nonsmokers. The carboxyhemoglobin level is slightly higher in pregnant patients due to fetal CO. The concentration of carboxyhemoglobin is chronically 3% to 8% in smokers and more than 10% to 15% after smoking.

Symptoms of CO poisoning include headache, nausea, fatigue, and dizziness with carboxyhemoglobin levels between 10% and 20%. Few symptoms occur with levels lower than 10%. Disorientation may occur with carboxyhemoglobin levels between 20% and 40%; stupor or coma with levels between 40% and 60%; and death with levels greater than 60%. Pets exposed to CO can likewise be affected.

Treatment includes 100% O_2 administered to all burn victims. This level of O_2 accelerates the dissociation of CO from hemoglobin by 50% every 30 minutes. Patients with CO-hemoglobin levels between 20% and 25% should be intubated. Hyperbaric O_2 therapy increases the elimination of CO and can be considered for unconscious patients.[11,13,22,28] No data suggest that hyperbaric O_2 therapy mitigates any long-term sequelae of CO poisoning. Limited availability of these chambers and difficulties accessing the patient while in the chamber impede the use of hyperbaric therapy for acute care of burned patients.

Sequelae include delayed neurologic symptoms such as ataxia, mental degradation, and incontinence, which are seen in 12.5% of patients with high initial CO-hemoglobin levels. Computed tomography (CT) can demonstrate decreased density of the globus pallidus.[10,11,13,16,17,21]

b. CYANIDE POISONING

CN is the product of burning plastics containing high amounts of nitrogen, such as polyurethane, polyacrylonitrile, and acrocyanate. CN causes asphyxia at the cellular level by inhibiting cytochrome oxidase and preventing mitochondrial respiration. O_2 consumption is reduced through interruption of the tricarboxylic acid cycle, and anaerobic metabolism occurs with the development of a lactic acidosis.[10,11,13,16,44]

A history, examination, and diagnostic studies are required to determine CN poisoning and its treatment. Inhalational injury in a confined space makes CN poisoning more likely, as does an increased CO-hemoglobin concentration. Measurement of blood CN concentration can be made but may not be immediately available. Levels between 0.5 and 1 mg/L are considered toxic, and levels above 1 mg/L are thought to be lethal.[13,44,45]

The symptoms, including headache and confusion, are similar to those of CO poisoning. Electrocardiographic changes may be seen, and seizures may occur. Loss of consciousness is often transitory in CO poisoning but is sustained in CN poisoning. Bradypnea occurs in CN poisoning but is not found in CO poisoning. Pupillary dilatation may occur in CN poisoning but is not frequently found in CO poisoning.

Therapy includes amyl nitrite and sodium nitrite to induce methemoglobinemia, which binds with CN. Thiosulfate is a substrate in the metabolism of CN into less toxic thiocyanate by hepatic rhodanese. Hydroxycobalamin also binds with CN, forming nontoxic cyanocobalamin. Hydroxycobalamin has minimal side effects, whereas methemoglobinemia reduces tissue O_2 delivery to patients with impaired use of O_2 at the cellular level.[44,46-51]

C. Airway Management Approaches

1. Airway Management in the Field

Intubation when indicated should be performed at the scene according to locally established management protocols. Video-assisted intubation can be performed if the equipment is available. Depending on the nature of the injury, C-spine precautions should be employed. All patients should have a rapid-sequence induction.

If intubation is difficult in the upper airway patent, an SLA (e.g., laryngeal mask airway [LMA], King LT, Easytube, Combitube) can be employed as needed. Unfortunately, none of these devices protects the airway from aspiration. Moreover, with time, airway and laryngeal edema make ventilation with an SLA progressively difficult, and when necessary, a surgical airway should be employed.[30]

2. Airway Management in the Hospital

Airway assessment is performed as previously described using fiberoptic bronchoscopy. Signs of airway injury include the following:

- Airway soot
- Erythema, edema, or ulceration
- Mucosal fragility
- Increased secretions
- Loss of cough reflex (indicates greater depth of mucosal injury)
- Mucosal necrosis

Evaluation of the lower airway requires airway topicalization and sedation. Evaluation of the upper airway can determine the need for intubation. After intubation, fiberoptic evaluation of the tracheobronchial tree can proceed. Patients with significant soot, hyperemia, and edema are intubated immediately. Patients without such symptoms can be observed and undergo serial airway examinations. Anesthetic agents to facilitate intubation must be selected on an individual basis. Combined propofol and ketamine may be useful to facilitate intubation with minimal perturbations of the patient's hemodynamics.

Rapid-sequence intubation techniques should be employed because the patients are unlikely to have been fasted before their burn. Succinylcholine is considered safe to administer in the first 24 hours after a burn. After this 24-hour window, succinylcholine use is contraindicated due to the development of immature nicotinic receptors over the muscle membrane, which can lead to hyperkalemia after succinylcholine administration.[52] These receptors occur at the neuromuscular junction and over the entire muscle membrane. Moreover, the prolonged channel opening time of these receptors contributes to the release of potassium from the myocyte. Over time, the number of receptors returns to baseline as the burn heals; however, the patient may be at risk for hyperkalemia for up to 2 years.[53,54]

In patients with severe neck burns, laryngoscopy can be impossible, necessitating a surgical airway. The precise airway tools to employ depend on the individual practitioner's preference. Fiberoptic intubation limits movement of the head and neck but may be impossible in the sooty, bloody airway of the burn patient with a smoke inhalation injury. Various video laryngoscopes can be used to provide airway visualization, especially when in-line stabilization is employed for patients at risk for C-spine injury. Surgical airway approaches should always be considered and employed when needed.

In patients presenting with a LMA in place, fiberoptic intubation through the LMA can be performed. The Aintree intubation catheter can be placed with fiberoptic endoscopy into the trachea, the LMA removed, and an ETT passed into the trachea. Chapter 50 further explains this technique.

In patients arriving with an Easytube, Combitube, or VBM Laryngeal Tube in place, an Airtraq intubation device can be inserted between the tongue and the laryngeal tube, and after partial deflation of the laryngeal tube cuff, the Airtraq can be advanced until the cords are visualized. Other devices, such as any of the video laryngoscopes, flexible fiberoptic laryngoscopes, or fiberoptic stylets can be used in the same fashion. Leaving the SLA in place permits O_2 delivery while intubation is attempted. Direct laryngoscopy with in-line stabilization when indicated can also be employed. Surgical airways should be performed when intubation appears doubtful and is needed. Surgical airways should not be delayed for multiple attempts at direct or video laryngoscopy. The same considerations that complicate intubation also complicate the performance of a surgical airway in the burn patient. An SLA often can be employed to provide ventilation while a definitive surgical airway is obtained. A cart for the management of a difficult airway should be available with a variety of devices, catheters, video laryngoscopes, and a surgical airway tray when inhalation burn patients are treated.

3. Airway Management in Burned Children

Because of their small airway diameters, even a modest degree of airway edema in pediatric patients can lead to airway collapse. Because the resistance to flow is inversely proportional to the fourth power of the radius of the tube, decreasing the radius by one half increases resistance 16-fold.

Loss of airway and aspiration is the fourth most common cause of death cited in a study of pediatric burn patients.[55,56] Intubation may be indicated when the amount of resuscitative fluid is predicted to be more than 180 mL/kg.[57] Intubation with a Miller blade is often successful in children because the high position of the larynx requires lifting of the epiglottis. Cuffed ETTs are preferred because they allow the delivery of higher ventilator pressures and eliminate the need for repeated laryngoscopy and exchanges of the endotracheal tube if the leak is too great.[56,58]

4. Tracheotomy

Tracheotomy is performed in burn patients when laryngoscopy and intubation attempts fail. Elective tracheotomy for burn patients who need prolonged periods of positive-pressure ventilator support has been associated with airway strictures and stenosis after recovery.[10,13,37,59] However, most studies do not identify an increased risk of tracheotomies in burn patients compared with other populations.[60-63] In a retrospective study, Namdar and colleagues[64] demonstrated that tracheotomy permitted the use of lung-protective ventilation strategies in burn patients. However, Saffle and assocates[65] found no benefit for early tracheotomy as far as duration of ventilator support, length of stay, infection complications, or survival. In the pediatric population, tracheotomy caused no increased risk of complications.[38,66,67] The potential loss of the airway is less in children with a tracheotomy than those with an ETT in place. Some studies have found that percutaneous tracheotomy has reduced mechanical ventilation, hospital stay, and cost compared with traditional surgical tracheotomy.[61,68-71]

5. Securing the Artificial Airway

Securing the ETT of the burned patient can be challenging. Ideally, the ETT should be fixed without producing additional facial injuries and adjust to facial swelling. Taping usually is ineffective in securing the ETT. Suturing the tube to the gums, wiring it to a tooth, wiring it to brackets anchored to the enamel of the incisors, and circumferential fixation devices have all been employed.[72] Tying the tube with sling ribbon (umbilical tape) or even use of a disposable surgical free mask can secure it to the head. Care must be taken so that the items tied about the head do not lacerate the corners of the mouth or the ears. The tape stops must be checked routinely because facial edema can expand and pull the tube out of the

trachea. If a leak develops, fiberoptic laryngoscopy can be used to guide the ETT back into the trachea. The ETT's position and taping should be checked frequently, especially during changes in patient position and after patient transport.

6. Extubation of the Burn Patient

a. EXTUBATION OF THE BURNED PATIENT AFTER 12 HOURS OF INTUBATION

After a burn injury, patients are at risk for strictures, granulomas, and airway stenosis. Patients can be symptomatic immediately after ETT removal, or strictures can develop over time, leading to progressive airway stenosis.

Before extubation, the upper airway should be assessed for patency. Fiberoptic inspection of the larynx and airway is useful to identify potential sources of immediate extubation airway loss. The patient's other critical illnesses also should be corrected before considering extubation. Any gastric feedings should be discontinued at least 4 hours before extubation, and the patient should be free of ileus and gastrointestinal bleeding. All burn patients should pass a CPAP trial, fulfill routine extubation criteria, and have a leak around the deflated ETT cuff.[73]

Extubation should be delayed if the patient requires an increased fraction of inspired oxygen (FIO_2) of more than 40%, pressure support of more than 10 cm H_2O, high minute ventilation, or a positive end-expiratory pressure (PEEP) greater than 5 cm H_2O to maintain an arterial oxygen saturation (SaO_2) of 94%. Routine intensive care unit ventilatory management parameters must always be considered.

In patients at high risk for airway compromise after extubation, the anesthesiologist and surgeon can be at the bedside to reintubate or provide a surgical airway if the extubation effort fails. A Cook catheter can be placed in the airway and left in position after extubation to serve as a reintubation guide.

After extubation, speech and swallowing consultants can help to restore the voice and assist in preventing aspiration. Because airway stenosis can occur, prolonged extubation follow-up and fiberoptic evaluation is indicated.[14,16,20,28,60,69,74-76] Video stroboscopic vocal cord evaluation can be used as a screening tool to decide whether further airway evaluation by an ear, nose, and throat specialist is required.

Extubation failure occurs with a higher incidence in the burn population than among other critically ill patients (30% versus 23%).[77] Usually, the cause of failure is poor pulmonary toilet. Extubation failure is associated with burn size, inhalational trauma, and age of the patient.

b. EXTUBATION AFTER BURN SURGERY

Patients without airway injuries can be managed according to usual anesthesia practices. If significant edema exists in the face or airway, extubation after surgery is delayed until it subsides. If other airway difficulties occur, extubation in a controlled manner is undertaken as described earlier.[13,16,78]

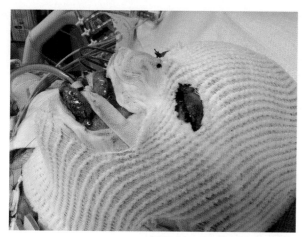

Figure 44-4 Dressings on the face can make bag-mask ventilation difficult or impossible. A supraglottic device can be used to ventilate the patient until the muscle relaxant takes effect and the trachea can be intubated.

III. AIRWAY MANAGEMENT DURING THE LATER STAGES OF BURN MANAGEMENT

Burn patients require multiple procedures after their initial intensive care course. Close airway evaluation is required in this population. SLAs and regional anesthetics can be employed when indicated.[79-81] As always, the patient's airway history is reviewed and an examination completed. Even weeks after extubation following a prolonged intubation, a patient can develop strictures and granulomas, which can complicate airway management.[71] Availability of adjuvant airway management devices should be considered when the recovering burn patient is brought to surgery during a long-term convalescence (Fig. 44-4).

IV. CONCLUSIONS

Burn patients present challenges in management in the field, in the hospital, in the intensive care unit, and during recovery. All burn patients are considered to have difficult airways, and management protocols are adjusted accordingly.

V. CLINICAL PEARLS

• Additional traumatic injuries should be ruled out in every burn patient.

• Intubation in the acutely burned patient with a traumatic C-spine injury should be performed using C-spine precautions.

• A variety of devices, including video laryngoscopes and fiberoptic endoscopes, should be available for intubation of the acutely burned patient and the previously burned patients; the ASA difficult airway algorithm should be applied in treating a patient with a difficult airway.

• Direct thermal injury to the upper airway can result in a fast-developing massive edema, compromising the airway and impeding intubation.

• Inhalation smoke injury causes direct injury to the upper and lower airways and can cause systemic toxicity through toxic smoke components, such as carbon monoxide and cyanide.

• Fiberoptic endoscopy is the gold standard for the diagnosis of inhalation smoke injury.

• Airway obstruction through edema formation can rapidly develop in children because of their smaller-diameter airways.

• Meticulous endotracheal tube (ETT) fixation and adjustment is crucial in the presence of facial edema formation. Loss of airway at the peak of edema formation can easily result in a "cannot ventilate, cannot intubate" situation.

• Before extubation, pathologic changes such as scars, stenosis, and webs should be excluded in patients after direct thermal or inhalation smoke injury to the upper airway.

• Airway management in the later stages after a burn injury can be complicated by pathologic changes such as scars and webs in the airway and by scars and contractures of the face and the neck.

SELECTED REFERENCES

All references can be found online at expertconsult.com.

3. Palmieri TL, Warner P, Mlcak RP, et al: Inhalation injury in children: A 10 year experience at Shriners Hospital for Children. *J Burn Care Res* 30:206–208, 2009.

6. Eastman AL, Arnoldo BA, Hunt JL, et al: Pre-burn center management of the burned airway: Do we know enough? *J Burn Care Res* 31:701–705, 2010.

9. Santaniello JM, Luchette FA, Esposito TJ, et al: The year experience of burn, trauma and combined burn/trauma injuries comparing outcomes. *J Trauma* 57:696–701, 2004.

32. Maybauer MO, Rehberg S, Traber DL, et al: Pathophysiology of acute lung injury in severe burn and smoke inhalation injury. *Anaesthesist* 58:805–812, 2009.

50. Barillo DJ: Effects/treatment of toxic gases: diagnosis and treatment of cyanide toxicity. *J Burn Care Res* 30:148–152, 2009.

51. Borron SW, Baud FJ, Barriot P, et al: Prospective study of hydroxycobalamin for acute cyanide poisoning in smoke inhalation. *Ann Emerg Med* 49:794–801, 2007.

53. Martyn JA, Fukushima Y, Chon J-Y, et al: Muscle relaxants in burns, trauma, and critical illness. *Int Anesthesiol Clin* 44:123–142, 2006.

55. Gore DC, Hawkins HK, Chinkes DL, et al: Assessment of adverse events in the demise of pediatric burn patients. *J Trauma* 63:814–818, 2007.

56. Fidkowski CW, Fuzaylov G, Sherdan RL, Coté CJ: Inhalation burn injury in children. *Paediatr Anaesth* 19:147–154, 2009.

58. Silver GM, Freiburg C, Halerz M, et al: A survey of airway and ventilator management strategies in North American pediatric burn units. *J Burn Care Rehabil* 25:435–440, 2004.

Chapter 45

Regional Anesthesia and the Difficult Airway

JACQUES E. CHELLY | JESSEN MUKALEL

I. INTRODUCTION

Regional anesthesia is recognized as an effective alternative to general anesthesia and is included in the American Society of Anesthesiologists (ASA) difficult airway algorithm as an alternative to failed intubation (Fig. 45-1).[1] The anesthesiologist should carefully balance the risks and benefits of using regional anesthesia compared with those of securing the airway before the administration of anesthesia in a patient with an established difficult airway. The anesthesiologist has a responsibility to provide safe anesthetic care, including maintaining appropriate conditions to manage the airway effectively during the perioperative period. Morbidity and mortality as a consequence of mismanagement or lack of proper management of the airway represent major concerns for anesthesiologists worldwide.

Many factors must be considered by the anesthesiologist managing a patient with a difficult airway. Although management of the airway is most often easily performed before surgery, serious consideration should be given to the increased difficulty associated with the need to control the airway during the course of surgery, especially in a patient with an established difficult airway. Intraoperative block failure because of a change in the surgical plan or excess duration of surgery is a concern that must be taken into consideration when considering the use of regional anesthesia on the difficult airway patient. The anesthesiologist must determine on an individual basis what is most appropriate, whether it is preoperative management of a difficult airway or the use of regional anesthesia, and must assess the risks associated with management of the airway during the course of surgery.

II. PRACTICE GUIDELINES FOR MANAGEMENT OF THE DIFFICULT AIRWAY

Irrespective of the final decision, an appropriate assessment of the patient's airway represents the first step. Although the ability to predict accurately a difficult airway preoperatively would be of great value, it is evident from the literature that no single airway assessment can reliably predict a difficult airway.[2] Nevertheless, a preoperative airway history and physical examination should be performed in order to facilitate the choice and management of the difficult airway, as well as reduce the likelihood of adverse outcomes (see Chapter 9).[3]

Langeron and colleagues have established five factors that are frequently associated with difficult airway management.[4] They separated difficult airway into difficult mask ventilation and difficult intubation; the former is the more deleterious of the two. It is well established that airway management may be more difficult in trauma cases and in patients with comorbidities, such as severe rheumatoid arthritis, morbid obesity, metabolic diseases, deformities, or pregnancy. Rocke and colleagues demonstrated that the incidence of difficult airway is 10 times higher during pregnancy than in the general population. They documented the potential risk factors for difficult airway in the obstetric patient.[5] The risk factors included short neck, missing protruding incisors, receding mandible, facial edema, and high Mallampati scores. The relative risk of experiencing a difficult intubation compared with an uncomplicated class I airway assessment has been established as follows: class II, 3.23; class III, 7.58; class IV, 11.3; short neck, 5.01; receding mandible, 9.71; and protruding maxillary incisors, 8.0. Using the probability

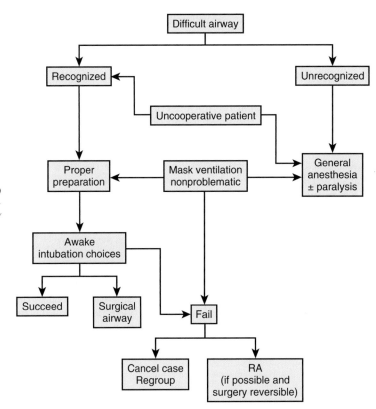

Figure 45-1   In the airway algorithm, regional anesthesia *(RA)* represents an acknowledged alternative to a failed intubation. (From Hagberg CA, editor: *Handbook of difficult airway management*, Philadelphia, 2000, Churchill Livingstone.)

index or a combination of risk factors, or both, showed that for a combination of class III or IV plus protruding incisors, short neck, or receding mandible, the probability of difficult laryngoscopy was more than 90%.

The concept of a difficult airway has different meanings for different physicians. Although most anesthesiologists agree that a patient with very limited mouth opening, Mallampati IV classification, and a very short neck has a difficult airway, there is more controversy about the relative difficulty of managing the airway in a patient with cervical trauma or obesity. This in part reflects the increased expertise in airway management of anesthesiologists and the increased number of airway devices designed to facilitate airway management. For example, Hagberg and colleagues demonstrated that Cormack-Lehane grade 3 airways assessed by laryngoscopy were reduced to grade 2 and even grade 1 when using the video laryngoscope.[6,7] The experience of the anesthesiologist with difficult airway management and access to certain airway management devices represent important factors in establishing the relative difficulty of managing the airway of a given patient.

Kheterpal and colleagues followed Langeron's work by determining the incidence and predictors of difficult mask ventilation and impossible bag-mask ventilation in relation to a difficult intubation.[8] Kheterpal later observed in more than 50,000 patients[9] that 25% of impossible bag-mask ventilations (*n* = 19) also had difficult intubations and that 10% (*n* = 2) required surgical airways. The incidence of impossible bag-mask ventilations was 0.15%. Radiation-induced changes in the neck, male sex, obstructive sleep apnea, Mallampati class III or IV, and presence of a beard were identified as independent predictors. Despite the low incidence, the anesthesiologist must anticipate and recognize differences for difficult mask ventilation and difficult intubation while also exercising sound judgment in conducting regional anesthesia in this patient population.

III. USE OF REGIONAL ANESTHESIA VERSUS PREOPERATIVE MANAGEMENT OF THE AIRWAY

In the past few years, interest has increased in using regional anesthesia as the primary anesthesia technique, especially in patients undergoing gynecologic or obstetric; plastic; ear, nose, and throat; trauma; and orthopedic surgery. The literature supports using various techniques for performing regional anesthesia as the primary anesthetic on patients with difficult airways.[10-12] We do not recommend performing these cases unless the anesthesiologist has a level of certainty about performing the block. Because of the more expanded use of regional anesthesia, anesthesiologists have become better accomplished at these techniques (e.g., higher success rate, lower frequency of complications). However, no regional technique provides a 100% success rate or is completely free of complications. Regional anesthesia complications include hematoma, nerve injury, and local anesthetic–associated complications, such as cardiac arrest, seizures, and death. When deciding whether to perform a regional technique in lieu of securing the airway preoperatively, these complications should be considered because they may trigger the need for immediate and urgent control of the airway because of a sudden loss of respiratory function (total spinal) or the development of local anesthesia–related complications (e.g., cardiac arrest, seizures).

Occurrence of these complications may be delayed, even if in most cases they occur within minutes after performance of a block. Anesthesiologists must be prepared to control the airway during the entire perioperative period. Although any regional technique intrinsically carries the risk of complications, the relative risk is different for each regional technique. For example, the use of an ulnar block at the wrist for an open reduction and internal fixation of the fifth finger performed using 5 to 6 mL of 0.5% ropivacaine is associated with a much lower risk of local anesthetic toxicity than the use of a transarterial axillary block performed with 40 mL of 0.5% bupivacaine. The specific type of approach, technique (e.g., transarterial, neurostimulator, paresthesia), volume of local anesthetic, and relative proximity of the injection site to a vessel or the central nervous system are some of the factors associated with the risks of toxicity associated with the use of regional anesthesia. Several considerations are important in making the decision to use regional anesthesia in a patient with an established difficult airway (Box 45-1). Knapik and colleagues demonstrated the ability to perform regional anesthesia for valvular heart surgery using a thoracic epidural on a patient with severe pulmonary disease, precluding the use of general endotracheal anesthesia.[13] However, during cardiopulmonary bypass, the patient required ventilatory support with a mask technique, a feat that would have been ill advised if difficult mask ventilation was anticipated.

A. Selection of Patients

Not all patients are good candidates for regional anesthesia, especially anyone with an established difficult airway. The use of regional anesthesia as the plan of anesthetic management rather than securing the airway may be considered in adult patients who are calm, possess good communication skills, and understand and accept the risks and benefits of a regional technique over general anesthesia. Consent for regional anesthesia should include consent for the perioperative management of the airway in the case of a failed block or other uncertainty arising during surgery. It is therefore important to consider the patient's psychological status and not perform regional anesthesia in a patient who consents to regional anesthesia to avoid an awake fiberoptic intubation (e.g., negative previous experience); has a history of claustrophobia, a condition that may be exacerbated by the need to place a surgical sheet over the face of the patient; is unable to remain still, especially in the context of minimal sedation use, because of preexisting medical or surgical conditions (e.g., severe rheumatoid arthritis, back pain, prostate hypertrophy, hyperactive bladder, poor peripheral circulation); or has a psychiatric condition, such as severe depression, hysteria, psychosis, or Alzheimer's disease. It is also important to evaluate the patient's sensitivity to sedation. For example, it is unlikely that opioid-tolerant patients with a history of chronic or cancer pain would be sensitive to sedation. The increased requirement for the sedative or anesthetic may represent a contraindication for the use of regional anesthesia.

BOX 45-1 Regional Anesthesia Versus Control of the Airway in Patients with Established Difficult Airways

Patient

Informed consent
Cooperative and calm
Hemodynamically stable
Ability to tolerate sedation, if required
Ability to communicate with anesthesiologist throughout procedure
No history of claustrophobia
Adequate intravenous access

Anesthesiologist

Expertise in both RA and DA management
Enough preoperative time to perform RA technique
Appropriate RA technique for surgical procedure
Prepared for alternative plans for DA

Surgeon

Dependable and reliable
Willing and able to supplement RA with local anesthetics, if necessary
Cooperative with primary and alternative plans for DA management

Types of Surgery

Nonemergent (except cesarean section)
Short duration
Patient's position allows good airway access
Can be interrupted for DA management
Limited or moderate blood loss

Support

Availability of appropriate equipment for RA and DA management
Staff (anesthesiologists, operating room nurses)

DA, Difficult airway; *RA,* regional anesthesia.

B. Anesthetic Environment

1. Anesthesiologist's Expertise

The use of regional anesthesia as an alternative to the preoperative management of the airway in a patient with a known difficult airway can be considered only if the anesthesiologist has appropriate expertise with regional techniques and difficult airway management. Peripheral nerve blocks can be classified according to the degree of difficulty (Box 45-2).

a. REGIONAL ANESTHESIA

Before considering the use of regional anesthesia in patients with an established difficult airway, it is necessary to verify that regional anesthesia is not contraindicated. General contraindications for the use of regional anesthesia include coagulopathy and infection. Specific contraindications must also be considered, such as chronic obstructive pulmonary disease (COPD) for an interscalene block. Although the use of regional anesthesia is associated with intrinsic risks, evidence also supports the concept that appropriate expertise in regional anesthesia represents an important determinant for the success of the procedure and for reducing the risk of complications.

Expertise includes proper experience in the chosen technique; appropriate knowledge of the relevant anatomy, especially innervation; knowledge of the equipment; and knowledge of the pharmacology of local anesthetics and any medications added to a local anesthetic mixture or given for sedation.

The use of neurostimulator and ultrasound techniques is preferred to the use of paresthesia or transarterial techniques, or both, in the performance of regional anesthesia to increase the likelihood of success and minimize the required dose of local anesthetics, thereby minimizing the risk of seizures related to an intravascular injection. The smallest needle possible should be used to avoid intrathecal placement of the needle when performing an interscalene or a lumbar plexus block. Table 45-1 shows the needle sizes related to the practice of the most common peripheral nerve blocks.

TABLE 45-1	
Needle Length for Most Common Peripheral Nerve Blocks	
Type of Block	**Length (cm)**
Interscalene and supraclavicular blocks at the elbow and the wrist	2.5
Axillary, high humeral, posterior popliteal Infraclavicular (coracoid) and femoral blocks	5.0
Lumbar plexus, lateral sciatic, gluteal, and infragluteal	10.0
Posterior sciatic, anterior sciatic, and high lateral sciatic blocks	15.0

Although the literature provides information about the relative success rate of each technique for a given surgical procedure, the anesthesiologist's personal experience is more important in deciding which regional anesthesia technique is most appropriate. To optimize the success rate and minimize the risk of complications associated with the use of regional anesthesia in a patient with an established difficult airway, the anesthesiologist should favor the techniques that he or she is most comfortable with for a given surgical procedure rather than base the choice on the literature. For example, it is established that most shoulder or knee operations can be performed using an interscalene or a combined sciatic and femoral nerve block, respectively. However, if the anesthesiologist responsible for the care of the patient does not routinely use peripheral nerve blocks for these operations, preoperative management of the airway is preferable.

REGIONAL ANESTHESIA COMPLICATIONS. In the case of a patient with an established difficult airway, the likely complications are those that would lead to the immediate need to secure the airway because of total spinal block, cardiac arrest, or seizure. Among regional techniques, neuraxial blocks have a higher rate of complications.[14-19] Closed claim studies have demonstrated that young, healthy patients undergoing surgery during spinal anesthesia can experience sudden cardiac arrest.[20] In obstetrics, 70% of the regional anesthesia–related deaths occurred among women who had epidural anesthesia, and the remaining 30% were associated with spinal anesthesia. These deaths resulted when the block became too high for adequate ventilation, and the airway could not be secured, leading to hypoxia or aspiration, or both.[21,22]

The ASA study of closed claims in obstetrics also showed that about 25% of the anesthesia-related maternal deaths were associated with regional anesthesia. Ananthanarayan and associates presented a case of difficult intubation with brainstem anesthesia after retrobulbar block.[23] After failed endotracheal intubation, the airway was secured using a laryngeal mask airway.[23] Among the peripheral nerve blocks, lumbar plexus block,[24-26] interscalene and axillary brachial plexus block,[27-34] intercostal block, and retrobulbar block are those most often associated with complications requiring immediate control of the airway.[23] This possibility also exists with the performance of any peripheral nerve block, especially when relatively large volumes of local anesthetic are injected rapidly or when there is a vein or artery located near the nerve.

LOCAL ANESTHETICS. The choice of the local anesthetic mixture, its volume and concentration, and the mode of administration deserve serious consideration. Although the choices are dictated by the technique (e.g., major conduction blockade versus peripheral nerve blocks), selection of the local anesthetic mixture should be based even more on the safety of patients with a difficult airway, with special focus on possible complications requiring immediate airway intervention. Local anesthetics that have the highest safety profile and provide adequate anesthesia covering the entire surgical period are most

TABLE 45-2
Maximum Dose of Commonly Used Local Anesthetics

Anesthetic	Maximum Dose (mg)	pH
Lidocaine	300	6.5
Mepivacaine	500	4.5
Bupivacaine	150	4.5-6
Ropivacaine	225-300	4.6

suitable. The maximum dose of local anesthetics should be determined to decrease the risk of toxicity. Table 45-2 shows various local anesthetics and their maximum accepted doses.

b. EXPERTISE IN MANAGEMENT OF THE DIFFICULT AIRWAY

Because perioperative management of the airway may be required during the course of the procedure in a patient undergoing surgery under regional anesthesia, the anesthesiologist should be appropriately trained and experienced in difficult airway management. Use of regional anesthesia in a patient with an established difficult airway cannot be considered an appropriate alternative for the inexperienced or unprepared anesthesiologist.

2. Proper Anesthetic Setting

In addition to proper expertise in regional anesthesia and difficult airway management, the proper equipment for difficult airway management should be in good order and readily accessible during the entire perioperative period. Support should be available because calling for help is one of the first steps according to the revised version of the airway algorithm.[3] The time commitment to manage the airway appropriately should be weighed against the relative availability of the anesthesiologist during the entire perioperative period, because management of the airway may be required intraoperatively. This is especially important when the anesthesiologist supervises more than one location. An anesthesiologist who is supervising residents or certified registered nurse anesthetists or who is on call is not as available as when he or she supervises one location.

C. Surgical Environment

1. Type of Surgery

Use of a regional anesthesia technique is not appropriate for all types of operations. For a patient with an established difficult airway, a successful block does not obviate intraoperative management because the patient becomes uncomfortable or there are major hemodynamic changes or bleeding. Regional anesthesia should be considered for shorter procedures with minimal expected blood loss. For example, a short abdominal procedure may benefit from a spinal, epidural, or in some cases, bilateral paravertebral blocks. Diaphragmatic function is not blocked by a spinal or epidural anesthetic, which explains why most anesthesiologists favor the use of neuraxial blocks for low abdominal procedures. In orthopedics, it is important to consider all surgical requirements, especially those related to the use of a tourniquet. Although in surgical procedures of less than 30 minutes' duration, tourniquet pain

TABLE 45-3
Regional Anesthesia Versus Preoperative Management for Difficult Airways

Approach	Surgical Application
Surgeries That Might Be Performed Using Regional Anesthesia	
Peripheral nerve blocks	Minor orthopedic trauma of the upper and lower extremity
	Open reduction with internal fixation of the small finger, elbow, and ankle and wrist fracture
	Minor arthroscopy surgery (e.g., shoulder, knee, ankle)
Neuraxial blocks	Gynecologic surgery
	Cesarean section
Surgeries More Suitable for Preoperative Management	
Airway management for long operations associated with major blood loss	Major or multiple trauma
	Major abdominal surgery
	Revised total hip surgery
	Major orthopedic oncology surgery
Airway management for long operations performed in the prone position	Spinal surgery
	Achilles' tendon surgery
Airway management for blocks unlikely to provide adequate anesthesia	Interscalene block for high humeral fracture
	Lumbar plexus block for hip surgery

is usually not an issue, the mechanism of tourniquet pain should be well understood and managed, because it usually requires sedation or analgesics, or both, that are often contraindicated in patients with unsecured difficult airways (Table 45-3).

2. Cooperation Between Surgeon and Anesthesiologist

Especially in the case of a patient with an established difficult airway, the anesthesiologist and the surgeon must agree that the operation can be performed using regional anesthesia alone or with supplementation of the block by local anesthesia during the procedure. The anesthesiologist should be familiar with the surgeon, the surgical procedure, and the surgical environment, including the availability of surgical equipment and support staff. For example, for joint replacement procedures, many hospitals and surgery centers depend on the presence of a prosthesis representative. Availability of these representatives may involve significant time delays, imposing significant limitations on the use of regional anesthesia. In a patient with an established difficult airway, the use of regional anesthesia requires the surgical procedure to be well defined, because prolonged surgical time, hemodynamic instability, or blood loss can lead to significant problems. If regional anesthesia is preferred, the surgeon should proceed only after careful determination that the patient is properly anesthetized and that inflation of a tourniquet, if used, is well tolerated. Because of the relationship between cuff inflation pressure and tourniquet pain, it is important to minimize the pressure level at which the tourniquet is inflated. Although it is well established that pain associated with a tourniquet can occur immediately at the time of the inflation or be delayed, it is critically important to verify that the tourniquet is tolerated at the time of inflation. In short procedures, delayed tourniquet pain represents a lesser concern.

3. Positioning of the Patient

The patient's position during surgery is a critical element in the choice between preoperative management of the airway and the use of regional anesthesia. Prone and lateral positions are more likely to make management of the airway during surgery more difficult. The sitting position is also unfavorable for the use of regional anesthesia unless it is possible to convert quickly to the supine position (e.g., patient undergoing shoulder surgery in a beach chair position under an interscalene block). Although it is always possible to change to the supine position urgently, it is far from optimal medical management. Of all the positions, the supine position allows the best access to the airway. When considering the patient's positioning for a surgical procedure, it is important to consider the relationship between the surgical preparation and the patient's positioning, even when supine. For example, during an open reduction and fixation of an elbow fracture, the elbow is often elevated and flexed over the patient and then draped. Pediatric or claustrophobic patients may react to this positioning with significant stress and anxiety, a situation favoring preoperative management of the airway rather than regional anesthesia.

The anesthesiologist can proceed with the performance of regional anesthesia if it is found to be an appropriate alternative to preoperative management of the airway. The chosen technique can be physically performed outside or inside the operating room, depending on the specific block and the facility's preference. Enough time should be available for performance of the block and evaluation of its effects. Because complications do occur, it is necessary to be prepared for cardiovascular and central nervous system resuscitation. Certain positions, such as sitting for epidural or paravertebral blocks, have risks of serious complications, such as vasovagal syncope, that may require ventilatory support.

IV. CONCLUSIONS

The use of regional anesthesia in patients with an established difficult airway remains the exception rather than the rule in current practice. Regional anesthesia represents an acceptable alternative to preoperative management of the airway if certain conditions are met: establishment of proper indications for the use of regional anesthesia, appropriate consent obtained from the patient, an anesthesiologist who is experienced in regional anesthesia and difficult airway management and who is available during the entire perioperative period, and equipment

and support that are readily available during the full perioperative period.

V. CLINICAL PEARLS

- The decision to perform regional anesthesia should include the surgeon's opinion.

- Choosing regional anesthesia is easier when intraoperative management of the airway can be easily accomplished during surgery (e.g., lower extremity surgery with the patient in the supine position).

- Performing a regional technique before surgery may help to assess the patient's level of anxiety and agitation and to confirm whether the choice is the right one.

- The reliability of the surgeon and the type of surgery should weigh heavily in determining whether a regional anesthesia approach is appropriate.

- If regional anesthesia is chosen, it is important to wait for the surgical block to be confirmed.

- The block should be performed as close as possible to the start of surgery.

- The duration of a block is shorter in young patients than in elderly patients.

SELECTED REFERENCES

All references can be found online at expertconsult.com.

10. Delgado Tapia JA, Garcia Sánchez MJ, Priéto Cuellar M, et al: Infraclavicular brachial plexus block using a multiple injection technique and an approach in the cranial direction in a patient with anticipated difficulties in tracheal intubation. *Rev Esp Anestesiol Reanim* 49:105–107, 2002.
14. Auroy Y, Narchi P, Messiah A, et al: Serious complications related to regional anesthesia: Results of a prospective survey in France. *Anesthesiology* 87:479–486, 1997.
15. Caplan RA, Ward RJ, Posner K, et al: Unexpected cardiac arrest during spinal anesthesia: A closed claims analysis of predisposing factors. *Anesthesiology* 68:5–11, 1988.
19. Liguori GA, Sharrock NE: Asystole and severe bradycardia during epidural anesthesia in orthopedic patients. *Anesthesiology* 86:250–257, 1997.
23. Ananthanarayan C, Cole AF, Kazdan M: Difficult intubation and brain-stem anaesthesia. *Can J Anaesth* 44:658–661, 1997.
26. Pousman RM, Mansoor Z, Sciard D: Total spinal anesthetic after continuous posterior lumbar plexus block. *Anesthesiology* 98:1281–1282, 2003.
27. Baraka A, Hanna M, Hammoud R: Unconsciousness and apnea complicating parascalene brachial plexus block: Possible subarachnoid block. *Anesthesiology* 77:1046–1047, 1992.
28. Cook LB: Unsuspected extradural catheterization in an interscalene block. *Br J Anaesth* 67:473–475, 1991.
29. Durrani Z, Winnie AP: Brainstem toxicity with reversible lock-in syndrome after intrascalene brachial plexus block. *Anesth Analg* 72:249–252, 1991.
30. Dutton RP, Eckhardt WF III, Sunder N: Total spinal anesthesia after interscalene blockade of the brachial plexus. *Anesthesiology* 80:939–941, 1994.
33. McGlade DP: Extensive central neural blockade following interscalene brachial plexus blockade. *Anaesth Intensive Care* 20:514–516, 1992.
34. Ross S, Scarsborough CD: Total spinal anesthesia following brachial-plexus block. *Anesthesiology* 39:458, 1972.

Chapter 46

Airway Management in Intensive Care Medicine

KURT RUETZLER | PETER KRAFFT | MICHAEL FRASS

I. INTRODUCTION

A major responsibility of the anesthesiologist or critical care physician is the maintenance of adequate ventilation and pulmonary gas exchange in critically ill patients. In the operating room (OR) the incidence of airway catastrophes resulting in emergency tracheostomy, brain damage, or death ranges from 0.01 to 2 cases per 10,000 procedures. Emergency airway management is often even more challenging in the intensive care unit (ICU) setting. The increasing demand for critical care medicine makes it necessary to focus on specific airway problems encountered in ICU patients.

Major differences exist between airway management in a controlled setting such as the OR and airway management in the ICU. Difficult laryngoscopy and endotracheal intubation is often successful after multiple attempts in the OR because of adequate patient preparation and positioning. To the contrary, endotracheal intubation of the "crashing" critically ill patient with poor cardiopulmonary reserve in a relatively uncontrolled environment requires a different approach to prevent serious problems.

This chapter briefly describes noninvasive and "invasive" airway management with special respect on the recommendations of the American Society of Anesthesiologists Task Force on Management of the Difficult Airway (ASA algorithm) first presented in 1991.[1] The basic principles of the ASA algorithm are meticulous patient evaluation before sedation or anesthesia induction, awake intubation if problems are suspected, and preparation of an alternative approach in case of failure.

Those recommendations are at least in part valuable for the management of ICU patients as well. Unfortunately, the ASA algorithm has a number of characteristics that prevent direct application to the ICU situation. Airway management in ICU patients is usually urgent or emergent, often depriving the physician of the time necessary to evaluate the patients and plan the life-saving intervention. The patient is presumed to have a full stomach and must therefore undergo awake airway management or rapid-sequence induction. The option of reemergence from anesthesia to resume spontaneous ventilation if difficulty is encountered is mostly unfeasible. However, at least part of the algorithm is of major importance for ICU airway management and is therefore presented in detail.

Intensive care unit airway management is complex; this chapter focuses on the most important topics to provide the reader with the information required for daily ICU practice. The chapter begins with a brief overview over noninvasive airway management (including continuous positive airway pressure via mask or helmet) and proceeds with prelaryngoscopic airway assessment. This special aspect is extensively addressed because many airway catastrophes can be prevented only by adequate evaluation and preparation of the patient before the administration of sedatives. The gold standard techniques for the performance of direct laryngoscopy and oral or nasal endotracheal intubation are then presented. Alternative methods to direct laryngoscopy (especially awake endotracheal intubation!) are discussed and the control of patients' airways in emergency situations is presented: One of four emergency techniques must be chosen immediately—laryngeal mask airway, esophageal-tracheal Combitube, transtracheal jet ventilation, or surgical airway—to prevent cerebral hypoxia. For planned as well as emergency ICU airway management, the alternative methods or techniques must be readily available before sedation and must be practiced in routine cases.

Long-term translaryngeal intubation might result in serious laryngeal damage, including ulcer formation or tracheal stenosis. Therefore, indication, timing, and recent techniques of tracheostomy are discussed, with advantages and drawbacks. Airway management in ICU patients is a matter of ongoing research and discussion. For example, the percentage of patients undergoing tracheostomy and the timing of tracheostomy underwent dramatic changes after the introduction of percutaneous dilatational tracheostomy (PDT) in the 1980s. Regardless of the technique used, PDT can quickly be performed at bedside, has a relatively low incidence of complications in trained hands, and is cost-effective, with excellent cosmetic results. After presenting routine airway care maneuvers (e.g., tracheal suctioning), this chapter closes with an often-overlooked problem in ICU airway management, difficult extubation, often encountered in patients after ear-nose-throat (ENT) procedures or other causes of pharyngeal-laryngeal swelling or distortion. Close interaction is needed with the attending ENT specialist, with coping strategies to prevent catastrophes during extubation. Special topics of ICU airway management are also detailed in other chapters (see Contents and Index).

II. NONINVASIVE AIRWAY MANAGEMENT

Invasive ventilation using an endotracheal tube (ETT) was once the gold standard for ventilatory support of critically ill patients. However, longer duration of invasive ventilation increases the risk of complications such as ventilator-associated pneumonia (VAP).[2] Noninvasive ventilation (NIV) preserves the patient's ability to speak and cough and has been shown to reduce complications related to intubation, especially VAP.[3-5] For this reason, use of NIV has become widely accepted, especially in patients with chronic obstructive pulmonary disease (COPD) and patients with cardiac failure, since weaning from respirator and ETT may become extremely difficult. In selected patients with respiratory failure, noninvasive positive pressure ventilation helps to reduce an increased respiratory rate, augments tidal volumes and reduces work of breathing.[6,7] Therefore, NIV is a promising approach to ventilatory support of ICU patients and might become even more important as a "weaning as well as a therapeutic procedure" in the near future.

A. Indications and Contraindications of Noninvasive Ventilation

Basically, NIV is applied in three different areas: in acute respiratory failure, as a weaning strategy, and in the management of the difficult airway.

1. Acute Respiratory Failure

Over the past decade, *noninvasive positive-pressure ventilation* (NPPV) has increased in popularity in the patient with acute exacerbations of COPD. In these patients, based on evidence derived from multiple randomized trials, NIV should be considered as first-line therapy.[8-12]

In a systematic review, Keenan and colleagues[13] assessed the effect of NPPV on rate of endotracheal intubation, length of hospital stay, and in-hospital mortality in patients with an acute exacerbation of COPD. The addition of NPPV to standard care in patients with COPD exacerbation decreased the rate of endotracheal intubation (risk reduction [RR], 28%; 95% confidence interval [CI], 15%-40%), length of hospital stay (absolute reduction, 4.57 days; CI, 2.30-6.83 days), and in-hospital mortality rate (RR, 10%; CI, 5%-15%). However, subgroup analysis showed that these beneficial effects occurred only in patients with severe exacerbations, not in those with milder exacerbations of COPD.

A similar approach was used by the Cochrane Database group, presenting a systematic review on the effectiveness of NPPV in management of acute COPD exacerbations.[14] Only randomized controlled trials (RCTs) were selected by two independent reviewers. NPPV not only decreased mortality (RR 0.41; 95% CI 0.26, 0.64), but also decreased the need for intubation (RR 0.42; CI 0.31, 0.59) and treatment failures (RR 0.51; CI 0.39, 0.67). In addition, complications associated with treatment (RR 0.32; CI 0.18, 0.56) and length of hospital stay (−3.24 days; CI −4.42, −2.06) were also reduced in the NPPV group. The reviewers concluded that NPPV should be used as the first-line intervention in all patients with respiratory failure secondary to an acute exacerbation of COPD. NPPV should be considered early in the course of respiratory failure, to avoid endotracheal intubation, reduce mortality, and avoid treatment failure.

Carlucci and associates[15] evaluated the changes in the practice of NIV for the treatment of COPD patients between 1992 and 1999. In this special patients' collective, the failure rate of NPPV was constant over the years (17%). Although the severity of acute respiratory failure (ARF) episodes increased (defined by pH and APACHE II at admission), the risk of failure for a patient with pH less than 7.25 was threefold lower in the period 1997-99 compared with 1992-96. Furthermore, a significantly higher percentage of patients (pH >7.28) were treated at the normal ward and not in the ICU, which allowed a significant cost reduction.

Based on strong evidence (level 1), recent clinical studies support the use of NIV to treat ARF related to COPD exacerbations, treat cardiogenic pulmonary edema, and facilitate weaning and extubation in patients with COPD and immunosuppressed patients.[8,16] The future will show whether this trend away from "invasive" toward noninvasive ventilatory support in routine patient care will be sustained.

2. Weaning Strategy

Weaning from the ventilator is difficult in up to 20% of all patients. Already the consequent use of standardized weaning strategies (regardless of their content) has increased the success rates after extubation. In this context, Udwadia and coauthors[17] described the use of NIV as a weaning strategy first in 1992. In 2003, Burns and coworkers[18] performed the first meta-analysis of NIV as a weaning strategy, including five clinical trials and 171 patients. NIV showed significant benefit for duration of in-hospital-stay, total duration of ventilation, reduced mortality, and lower VAP rate compared with conventional weaning using endotracheal intubation. In a 2010 systematic review that included 12 randomized and quasi-randomized studies, Burns and others[19] compared NIV and invasive weaning strategy in 530 COPD patients.[19] This meta-analysis showed that NIV weaning in COPD patients is associated with decreased mortality, decreased incidence of VAP, reduced length of stay in ICU and hospital, and decreased total duration of ventilation and duration of endotracheal intubation.

Current studies on NIV weaning, predominantly focused on COPD patients, propose a potential reduction in mortality and VAP.[20] In fact, further clinical research is necessary to clarify potential benefits of NIV as weaning strategy versus conventional weaning via ETTs or cannulas.

3. Difficult Airway Management

Critically ill patients are characterized by limited physiologic reserves, possibly resulting in catastrophic complications during airway management, including cardiac arrest. After a systematic review of airway management

in critically ill patients in 2007, Walz and colleagues[21] proposed adaptations to the ASA Difficult Airway Algorithm. In this algorithm, NIV serves as a valuable adjunct to conventional invasive airway management.

4. Contraindications

Absolute contraindications to NIV include respiratory arrest and the inability to tightly fit the face mask. The physician must consider potential clinical benefits as well as potential drawbacks for the following relative contraindications:

- Hemodynamic instability or uncontrollable dysrhythmias
- Any type of coma
- Mentally confused, agitated, or uncooperative patient
- Swallowing impairment or excessive secretions
- Increased risk of pulmonary aspiration
- Injuries or upper airway surgery

B. Different Types of Noninvasive Devices

Various types of face masks and helmets are widely used for administering NIV (Fig. 46-1).

1. Noninvasive Positive-Pressure Ventilation via Face Mask

Noninvasive PPV can be administered by face masks covering the mouth and nose (and eyes) or by nasal masks covering only the nose. Either technique includes a mask that is pressed against the patient's face using an elastic band (e.g., Classen band). The patient may now be supported by either continuous positive airway pressure (CPAP), pressure support ventilation (PSV), or volume-cycled or pressure-cycled systems, such as bi-level positive airway pressure (BiPAP). However, dyspneic ARF patients tend to breathe through their mouth, causing air leaking and reducing the efficacy of nasal NPPV. Face masks are preferable in these patients, and application seems to be easy. However, the pressure of the face mask against the face, especially the root of the nose, causes significant discomfort and skin lesions, and several patients refused prolonged application.[22,23] Further disadvantages are potential gastric inflation followed by vomiting (risk of aspiration), claustrophobia, and difficult speaking.[16]

2. Noninvasive Positive-Pressure Ventilation via Helmet

The helmet consists of a cylindrical transparent part that is drawn over the patient's head (e.g., CaStar, Starmed, Italy). While the helmet is closed, the lower part contains an elastic ring to ensure a tight seal at the patient's neck (Fig. 46-2). Two openings with sideways fittings to ventilatory tubing allow supportive ventilation such as continuous flow or pressure support. The helmet is a noninvasive means of ventilation; the patient has a free view through the transparent helmet and can even wear glasses, with no fogging from the circulating air. A new model of the Castar helmet includes an additional round opening with a diameter of about 10 cm for nursing the patient's face. This helmet was used as first-line intervention to treat patients with hypoxemic ARF, compared with NPPV via standard face mask.[24] Thirty-three

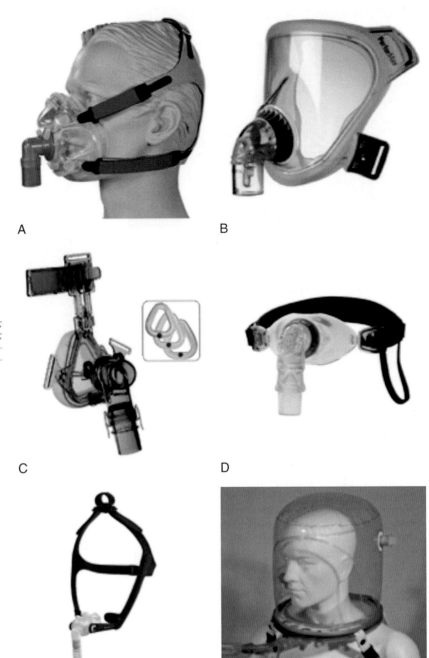

Figure 46-1   A, Full face mask; **B,** total face mask; **C,** nasal mask; **D,** mouthpiece; **E,** nasal pillows; **F,** helmet. (From Nava S, Hill N: Noninvasive ventilation in acute respiratory failure. *Lancet* 374:250–259, 2009.)

A   B

C   D

E   F

consecutive patients without COPD and with hypoxemic ARF (defined as severe dyspnea at rest, respiratory rate >30 breaths/min, PaO_2/FiO_2 <200, and active contraction of the accessory muscles of respiration) were enrolled. The 33 patients and the 66 controls had similar characteristics at baseline. Eight patients (24%) in the helmet group and 21 patients (32%) in the facial mask group ($P = .3$) failed NPPV and were intubated. No patients failed NPPV because of intolerance of the technique in the helmet group, versus eight patients (38%) in the mask group ($P = .047$). Complications related to the technique (skin necrosis, gastric distention, eye irritation) were fewer in the helmet group compared with the mask group (no patients vs. 14 patients (21%), $P = .002$). The

helmet allowed continuous application of NPPV for a longer period ($P = .05$). NPPV by helmet successfully treated hypoxemic ARF, with better tolerance and fewer complications than face mask NPPV.

In another prospective clinical investigation in a general ICU, the feasibility and safety of fiberoptic bronchoscopy (FOB) with bronchoalveolar lavage (BAL) was tested during NPPV delivered by helmet in patients with ARF and suspected pneumonia.[25] Four adult patients with ARF underwent NPPV via the helmet and required fiberoptic BAL for suspected pneumonia. NPPV was delivered through the helmet in the pressure support ventilation mode. The specific seal connector placed in the plastic ring of the helmet allowed the passage of the

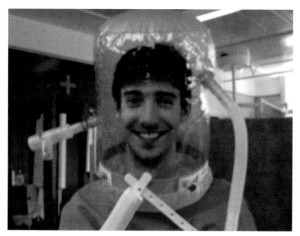

Figure 46-2 Application of Castar helmet in healthy volunteer.

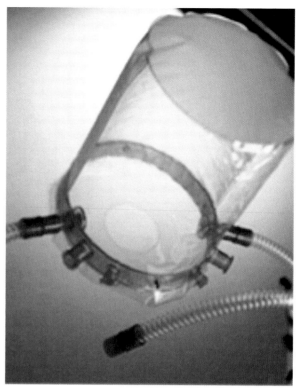

Figure 46-3 Rüsch 4Vent helmet. (Courtesy of Rüsch, Vienna, Austria.)

bronchoscope, maintaining assisted ventilation. Arterial blood gas levels, pH, oxygen saturation, respiratory rate, heart rate, and mean arterial blood pressure (BP) were monitored during the study. Helmet NPPV avoided gas exchange deterioration during FOB and BAL, with good tolerance. During the procedure, heart rate increased by 5% and mean arterial BP by 7% over baseline; these levels returned to prebronchoscopy values immediately after the withdrawal of the bronchoscope. Endotracheal intubation was never required during the 24 hours after the procedure. BAL yielded diagnostic information in three of four patients. NPPV through the helmet allows a safe diagnostic FOB with BAL in patients with hypoxemic ARF, avoiding gas exchange deterioration, and endotracheal intubation.

Several special aspects of the helmet, such as the effects of direct exposure of external and middle ear to positive airway pressure, remain to be determined. Cavaliere and others[26] recommended earplugs in select NPPV patients treated with the helmet, especially during long-term support at high airway pressures. NPPV has become an integral part of daily ICU care for many patients with acute and chronic respiratory failure. However, the potential effectiveness of NPPV varies among different patient populations. The greatest benefit is seen in patients with pure *hypercapnic* respiratory failure, as seen in COPD patients. The more severe hypoxemia becomes, the less beneficial the effects observed. Clearly, further studies are necessary to identify patients with hypoxemic ARF who might benefit from NPPV.[27]

The Rüsch 4Vent (Kernen, Germany) allows unrestricted field of view and minimum level of noise. Tubing and accessories are connected to the rigid ring of the 4Vent. Diffusers prevent the stream of gas from blowing directly into the patient's face. Filters reduce the noise inside the helmet. Similar to the Castar helmet, the patient is able to speak and take liquid food and drinks. The supple material allows the helmet also to be worn lying down (Fig. 46-3).

Advantages of NPPV include few air leaks, minimal cooperation required, and absence of nasal or facial skin damage. Disadvantages include rebreathing, gastric inflation followed by vomiting, dry eyes, noise, and asynchrony with pressure support ventilation, as well as shoulder discomfort induced by the straps.[16]

III. ENDOTRACHEAL INTUBATION IN INTENSIVE CARE

A. Prelaryngoscopy Airway Assessment

Any factor in the patient's history suggesting a difficult airway must be known before anesthesia induction, especially all diseases resulting in pharyngeal or laryngeal deformities (congenital abnormalities, surgical or traumatic deformities, laryngeal trauma, edema or tumors, goiter). As a first and rapid orientation, the simple "rule of threes" can be applied: if three fingers can be placed between the teeth, between the mandible and the hyoid bone, and between the thyroid cartilage and the sternal notch in neutral position, direct laryngoscopy should be straightforward.[28] Furthermore, more or less complex tests and scoring systems have been suggested to predict a difficult airway before anesthesia induction. The most frequently used tests are the Mallampati classification, thyromental distance, mobility of the cervical spine, and combined scoring systems (e.g., Wilson test) or multivariate risk indices[29-31] (Table 46-1).

Mallampati classification is the most common diagnostic test and is based on the evaluation of the relationship of tongue size relative to pharynx size, as follows[31]:

Class I: uvula, faucial pillars, and soft palate visible
Class II: faucial pillars and soft palate visible
Class III: only soft palate visible

TABLE 46-1
Airway Assessment

Assessment	0 Points	1 Point	2 Points
1. Interincisor gap	>4 cm	<4 cm	Cannot open mouth
2. Mallampati classification	Class I	Class II	Class III
	A Class I	B Class II	C Class III
3. Head/neck movement	>90 degrees	90 degrees	<90 degrees
4. Buck teeth	Can be prognathic or edentulous	Can approximate teeth only	Cannot approximate teeth
5. Thyromental distance	>6.5 cm	6.0-6.5 cm	<6.0 cm
6. Body weight	<90 kg	90-110 kg	>110 kg
7. History of difficult intubation	None	Questionable	Definite
Airway score (AS) range: 0-14	0	7	14

The operator should be aware that the risk of difficult airway is increased in class II and especially class III patients. In the original publication, Mallampati and colleagues[31] reported excellent statistical results on the performance of the classification system. However, later investigations could not replicate these findings and report a high incidence of false-positive results.[32,33]

Thyromental distance (according to Patil) is defined as distance between thyroid cartilage (Adam's apple) and the mandible with the patient's head and neck maximally extended. The authors measured thyromental distance before anesthesia induction in 75 patients and reported a minimum distance of 6.5 cm being necessary for a successful laryngoscopic approach. At a thyromental distance less than 6.0 cm, direct laryngoscopy is impossible; between 6.0 and 6.5 cm, the operator should be prepared for a difficult airway. Sensitivity of this test varies according to definition of the "danger zone" (i.e., thyromental distance <7.0 or <6.5 cm) and is reported in the range of 30% to 90%. In most studies, specificity ranges between 80% and 97%.[32,34] Thyromental distance is a useful diagnostic test with a relatively low intra- and inter-observer variation. However, the lacking stratification for patient height and weight makes data interpretation difficult.

Direct laryngoscopy without *extension of the atlanto-occipital joint* is impossible. Decreased mobility of the upper cervical spine (e.g., in patients with rheumatoid arthritis) is a major factor responsible for failed attempts of endotracheal intubation.[35] Nichol and Zuck[30] clearly demonstrated that a reduced atlanto-occipital distance is a major factor for a limited extension of head and neck. Assessment of cervical spine mobility is performed with the patient looking straight ahead and maximum mouth opening. The patient is now urged to flex and extend the head and neck. The angle between the extreme positions should be at least 90 degrees; otherwise, a difficult laryn-goscopy must be assumed, with high specificity in the 90% range.

The range and freedom of mandibular movement and the architecture of the teeth have pivotal roles in facilitating laryngoscopic intubation, so Khan and colleagues[36] proposed the *upper lip bite test*. Patients were grouped according to the following findings: lower incisors can bite the upper lip above the vermilion line (class I); lower incisors can bite the upper lip below the vermilion line (class II); and lower incisors cannot bite the upper lip (class III). In 300 elective patients, the authors evaluated the new test with the Mallampati classification. Negative predictive value for both test groups was similar (98%), but the positive predictive value of the lip bite test was better (29% vs. 13%). To improve positive and negative predictive values of those screening tests, several authors proposed the combination of various risk scores. In 1988, Wilson and associates[29] published a screening test system, including patient weight, mobility of the cervical spine, and anatomic-physiologic parameters of the stomato-gnathic system (Table 46-2). According to the authors, difficult airways must be suspected with 2 or more cumulative points. This scoring system requires more extensive evaluation but results in improved statistical performance. In patients with a cumulative result of 2 points, sensitivity of 75% was observed.[29] Oates and coauthors[32] reported specificity of 92%.

El-Ganzouri and associates[37] proposed a *multivariate risk index*, similar to the Wilson test. The authors recommend the following approach:

- Airway score (AS) of 0: proceed with routine management, no difficulties are expected.
- AS of 1 to 2 points: proceed with routine management, check fiberoptic availability, and prepare a special plan B.

TABLE 46-2
Wilson's Test

Risk Factor	Criterion	Points
Body weight	<90 kg	0
	90-110 kg	1
	>110 kg	2
Head and neck movement	>90 degrees	0
	90 degrees (±10)	1
	<90 degrees	2
Jaw movement	MMO >5 cm or LJ in front of UJ	0
	MMO <5 cm and LJ = UJ	1
	MMO <5 cm and LJ behind UJ	2
Receding mandible	Normal	0
	Moderate	1
	Severe	2
Buck teeth	Normal	0
	Moderate	1
	Severe	2

MMO, Maximum mouth opening; *LJ,* lower jaw; *UJ,* upper jaw.
From Wilson ME et al: Predicting difficult intubation. *Br J Anaesth* 61:211-216, 1988.

- AS of 3 to 4 points: have the fiberoptic scope on standby at bedside, and call for help; prepare for asleep or awake fiberoptic intubation.
- AS greater than 5 points: perform awake intubation (most practitioners prefer awake fiberoptic intubation).

Statistical results demonstrate a relatively weak performance in clinical routine. Even combinations of tests or scoring systems combining several risk factors are prone to misjudgment for the individual patient.[34] The upper airway is a complex structure and consists of many anatomically relevant variables. Also, statistical performance of these tests is still unsatisfying; the operator might be warned of trouble. Closely evaluating the patient before anesthesia induction might prevent catastrophic "cannot intubate, cannot ventilate" situations.

B. Oral vs. Nasal Endotracheal Intubation

Oral intubation and especially nasal intubation are characterized by special advantages and complications, with orotracheal intubation being currently favored by most anesthesiologists. Box 46-1 lists the contraindications for nasal intubation in critically ill patients.

The most common complication of *nasotracheal intubation* is nasal bleeding, occurring in about 45% of

Box 46-1 **Contraindications to Nasal Intubation**

Severe coagulopathy
High-dose systemic anticoagulation
Known nasal or paranasal pathologies
Infection of paranasal sinuses
Basilar skull fractures
Traumatic brain injury with leakage

patients.[38] The incidence of bleeding can be reduced with adequate preparation (vasoconstrictors). In most cases, bleeding is self-limited, and no further intervention is needed. Other complications are necrosis of the tip or wing of the nose (up to 4% of patients) and complications induced by the impaired drainage of paranasal sinus secretions.[39] Nasotracheal intubation impairs the drainage of the maxillary sinus, resulting in congestion of secretions, followed within a few days by bacterial overgrowth and sinusitis. This typical complication of intensive care occurs within 8 days in 25% to 100% of transnasally intubated patients.[40,41] The incidence is closely related to the duration of endotracheal intubation, from 37% after 3 days to 100% after 1 week, with the majority resolving within 1 week after extubation.[42] Therefore, in all ICU patients presenting with fever of unknown origin, a high index of suspicion for sinusitis must be maintained. Radiologic or ultrasound studies, including computed tomography (CT) scans, may be necessary to demonstrate the presence of fluid or inflammation. Bacterial sinus infection may ultimately lead to bacteremia and systemic inflammatory response. These infections tend to be polymicrobial, but often display a predominance of gram-negative bacilli (particularly *Pseudomonas aeruginosa*), *Staphylococcus aureus*, or fungi. Treatment includes removal of all nasal tubes and institution of appropriate antibiotic therapy, along with decongestant therapy. In some cases, surgical drainage may be necessary. Serious, but rare complications after nasotracheal intubation are accidental turbinectomy, intracranial placement, and retropharyngeal dissection.[43-45]

Oral intubation, on the other hand, interferes greatly with oral and pharyngeal hygiene, and even small lesions of oral soft tissues may result in extensive bacterial or viral soft tissue infections (e.g., herpetic lesions).[46] Most authors agree that all complications typically seen with nasal intubation may also occur during orotracheal intubation, although at a significantly lower incidence. Therefore, *oral endotracheal intubation* is the preferred route of tube passage, and nasal intubation is reserved for special indications, mainly short-term ventilatory support in oral surgery. For patients requiring intubation for more than 7 days, the nasotracheal route should always be avoided.[47]

C. Choosing the Correct ETT Size

According to literature, there is a clear association between endotracheal tube diameter and the incidence of laryngeal complications. Injury is located mainly in the posterior part of the glottis, where pressures up to 200 or 400 mm Hg are exerted by poorly deformable ETTs.[48] This pressure is reduced by the use of softer ETTs with a smaller diameter. In routine anesthesia patients, use of a smaller ETT reduces the incidence of postoperative sore throat, presumably because of the decreased pressure at the ETT-mucosal interface. Stout and associates[49] studied 101 patients randomized to larger (9 mm for male, 8.5 female) or smaller (7 mm for male, 6.5 mm for female) endotracheal tubes, and the incidence of postoperative sore throat was 48% (large ETT) versus 22% (small ETT). No ventilatory difficulties were observed in either group.

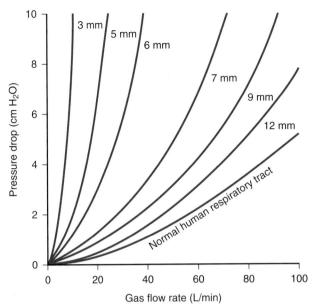

Figure 46-4 Driving pressure required to produce a flow rate of air versus internal diameter (ID) of endotracheal tubes. (From Nunn JF: *Applied respiratory physiology,* ed 3, Boston, 1987, Butterworths.)

The limiting factor for minimizing ETT diameter is the increased flow resistance and work of breathing. The pressure gradient required to generate gas flow can be calculated according to the Hagen-Poiseuille relationship, in which the rapidity of gas flow is directly proportional to the square of the ETT diameter (D) and the pressure (P) and indirectly to the ETT length and gas viscosity (valid only in laminar flow conditions). In other words, the pressure gradient through the airways proportionally rises with flow, viscosity, and ETT length but increases exponentially when ETT radius decreases. Viscosity of the gas administered has clinical consequences; with lower viscosity, a lower pressure gradient necessarily results in a lower airflow resistance. For example, gas mixtures with a high percentage of helium are often used to overcome upper airway obstruction (e.g., from tracheal compression or stenosis) and to treat the most severe status asthmaticus.[50,51]

In all patients, endotracheal intubation artificially increases airway resistance, because ETT inner diameter (ID) is smaller than tracheal diameter. Usually, ETT length exceeds length of the natural airways. Resistance is further increased by the curved design of the tubes necessary to resemble the patient's airway. Resistance measured using curved tubes is about 3% higher compared with straight tubes.[52] Therefore, the pressure gradient to generate gas flow is minimized by using an ETT with a larger diameter, short length, and straight design. Flow resistance can be translated in work of breathing, which is inversely proportional to ETT diameter (Fig. 46-4). The non-elastic work of breathing is increased twofold by using 7.0 mm–ID ETT and onefold by using an 8.0 mm–ID ETT versus a 9.0 mm–ID ETT.[53] With respect to gas flow, it is warranted to use as large an ETT as is practical for patients presenting with respiratory dysfunction; a short tracheal cannula with ID of 9.0 to 10 mm is best.

Clinical Implications. Using a smaller ETT seems to reduce laryngeal damage. The use of an ETT with an ID of 6.0 mm or less does not present a problem in anesthetized patients without spontaneous ventilation, because relatively low gas flow velocities are necessary to maintain adequate ventilation. However, gas flow resistance drastically increases, especially in spontaneously breathing patients in respiratory distress, who benefit from larger ETTs. Therefore, ETTs with ID of 7.0 to 8.0 mm seem appropriate for women and 8.0 to 9.0 mm for men.

An interesting aspect of ETT selection is airway management for professional singers. Powner[54] sent a written survey to all physician members of the Voice Foundation on airway management in professional singers. A strong consensus (76%) favored a smaller ETT for singers (6- to 7-mm ID for males and 6.0-mm ID for females) via the oral (46%) versus nasal (36%) route. Intubation/extubation by the most expert/experienced personnel was emphasized to minimize laryngeal trauma. Preferences for an early tracheostomy (6 days) versus their usual time (10 days) were approximately equal (44% vs. 50%, respectively).

The tracheal cuff has also been implicated as a cause of tracheal damage following long-term ventilatory support. Red-rubber ETTs equipped with low–residual volume, high-pressure cuffs exert high pressures to the tracheal mucosa and are thought to be damaging.[55] Using an experimental study design in rabbits, Nordin and coauthors[56] investigated tracheal mucosal perfusion and cuff-to-tracheal wall pressures exerted by low–residual volume, high-pressure cuffs and compared the results to those obtained with high-volume, low-pressure cuffs. Blood flow to the tracheal mucosa adjacent to the high-pressure cuff ceased beyond 30 mm Hg. Using high-volume cuffs, mucosal blood flow did not cease up to intracuff pressures of 80 to 120 mm Hg. However, cautious recommendations were made, and cuff pressure should be maintained below 30 cm H_2O.[55]

Conditions in ICU patients differ from routine anesthesia patients. ICU patients are mainly breathing spontaneously or on partial ventilatory support. Spontaneous breathing results in cuff pressure changes; cuff pressure decreases during inspiration and increases during expiration. Active changes in pleural pressure by forced inspiratory efforts combined with direct modulation of tracheal musculature result in marked increases of tracheal diameter and a fall in cuff pressure, even toward 0 cm H_2O.

Prolonged airway support using ETT or tracheal cannula might result in severe damage to the tracheal mucosa and increased incidence of late complications. Tracheal stenosis might be induced by direct trauma or by the pressure exerted by the ETT cuff. The presence of an ETT sutured to canine tracheal mucosa induced erythematous laryngeal mucosa in less than 1 day, proceeding to mucosal ulceration and loss of airway architecture in less than 1 week.[57] Damage was generally severe after 1 week, but no further tendency to aggravation after 1 week was observed.

The tracheal vascular supply to the tracheal submucosa is oriented in a circumferential direction anteriorly and longitudinally in the posterior part of the trachea. Seegobin and van Hessalt[58] investigated tracheal mucosal blood flow in 40 routine surgery patients using an endoscopic photographic technique while varying cuff inflation pressure. They suggested that tracheal blood flow is almost normal at 25 cm H_2O. Increasing cuff pressure results in a pale appearance of the tracheal mucosa at 40, blanched at 50, and flow is completely absent at 60 cm H_2O. Thus, it was recommended that cuff inflation pressure should not exceed 30 cm H_2O (22 mm Hg).

Joh and colleagues[59] observed similar results, measuring tracheal mucosal blood flow in an experimental model using the hydrogen clearance method. No significant depression in mucosal blood flow was observed with the cuff inflated to a maximum of 20 mm Hg. Increasing cuff pressures to 30 or even 45 mm Hg resulted in significant reduction in mucosal blood flow, and the authors concluded that cuff pressures should be kept at or below 20 mm Hg. Incorrect cuff pressure settings may result in tracheomalacia and subglottic stenosis (too high pressures) or late-onset nosocomial pneumonia (insufficient pressures). Several authors suggested that microaspirations might thereby be facilitated and recommended the use of automatic cuff-pressure regulators.[60] In a randomized study in 130 patients, Pothmann and associates[61] reported a significant reduction in late-onset pneumonias by a microprocessor-controlled automatic cuff-pressure regulator. However, the few studies covering small numbers of patients means that the devices described cannot currently be recommended for routine patient care.[60,62]

D. Drugs Used for Sedation and Analgesia

In general, less is more in conscious sedation for airway management. Drugs must be administered in dosages not interfering with protective reflexes and patient cooperation. Therefore, short-acting drugs with a potential antidote should be used.

The presumption of a "full stomach" in emergency intubations dictates the use of a rapid-sequence induction (RSI) technique. Cricoid pressure and laryngoscopy at the earliest possible moment place increased demands on the physician preparing to intubate the patient.[63] The ICU patient presents with even more risk factors than the routine OR patient. With facial distortion, swelling, secretions, and mandibular or cervical spine injury, ICU patients present the most challenging airway management problems.

Stimulation of the airway with a laryngoscope and ETT presents an extremely noxious stimulus.[64] This stimulation causes "pressor response" and results in hypertension and tachycardia. In critically ill patients with limited reserves for adequate tissue oxygenation, this pressor response may induce myocardial and cerebrovascular injury.[65] This physiologic stress after airway management may unmask relative hypovolemia or vasodilatation and may result in post-intubation hypotension.[66] Endotracheal intubation also can provoke bronchospasm and coughing, possibly aggravating underlying conditions such as asthma, intraocular hypertension, and intracranial hypertension. Patients at risk for adverse events from airway manipulation benefit from pre-induction drugs.[67]

We prefer the combination of low-dose midazolam (0.1 µg/kg) and an opioid such as fentanyl (2 µg/kg). *Fentanyl* is the most frequently used opioid because of its rapid onset and short duration of action. Fentanyl and its derivatives, sufentanil and alfentanil, can cause rigidity of chest wall, but this rigidity seems to be associated with higher doses and rapid opioid injection. Fentanyl can be antagonized rapidly using naloxone,[68] whereas midazolam can be antagonized using flumazenil.

Remifentanil is a novel µ-receptor agonist that has been used in surgical and obstetric analgesia for more than a decade. Its pharmacokinetics suggests that remifentanil may be an ideal opioid. Notably, its unique features include rapid onset of action (~1 minute), rapid degradation by tissue and plasma esterases, and half-life of approximately 3 minutes.[69,70] Infusion of 0.05 to 0.1 µg/kg/min produces blood concentrations of 1 to 3 ng/mL. Rapid onset and elimination of remifentanil facilitate its effective and safe use during airway management in the ICU. Several studies focused on remifentanil as a sole sedative and analgesic agent in the ICU setting. Puchner and coworkers[71] prospectively studied remifentanil (0.1-0.5 µg/kg/min) alone versus fentanyl plus midazolam for fiberoptic intubation. Fiberoptic nasal intubation was possible in all patients, with a better-suppressed hemodynamic response and tolerance of ETT advance in the remifentanil group. Recall was significantly more common in the remifentanil group. A combination of remifentanil and midazolam or propofol is a valuable approach.[72]

Lallo and coworkers[73] recently studied 60 patients requiring fiberoptic nasotracheal intubation, randomized to target-controlled infusions of propofol or remifentanil. Both agents can be rapidly titrated to achieve good intubating conditions and patient comfort. In addition, remifentanil preserves patient cooperation, making it safer when spontaneous ventilation is paramount. Yeganeh and associates[74] enrolled 22 patients who had cervical trauma and semi-elective maxillofacial surgery and administered remifentanil with target-controlled or manually controlled infusion techniques. They recommended remifentanil infusion to provide good conscious sedation, but target-controlled remifentanil infusion seems to provide better conditions compared with manually controlled remifentanil infusion and is easier to use.

Alternative drugs suitable for ICU airway management and even awake fiberoptic intubation are (S+)-ketamine and propofol.[75] *Propofol* is a rapid-acting, lipid-soluble induction drug that induces hypnosis in a single arm-brain circulation time. In patients with cardiac comorbidities and limited physiologic reserve, the use of propofol can be associated with significant hypotension. Causes of hypotension are reduced systemic vascular resistance and possibly depressed inotropy.[76] In an analysis of 4096 patients undergoing general anesthesia, Reich and associates[77] reported that the use of propofol was a statistically significant predictor of hypotension. Furthermore, in 2406 patients with retrievable outcome data, prolonged in-hospital stay and death were more common in those who experienced hypotension.[77] Therefore, use of propofol may have special risks in high-risk patients with known cardiac dysfunction.[78]

Ketamine is a rapid-acting, dissociative anesthetic agent (similar to phencyclidine) with potent amnestic, analgesic, and sympathomimetic effects.[67] Ketamine can cause realistic hallucinations and extreme emotional distress. This may be prevented with the obligatory combination of a benzodiazepine. The sympathomimetic effects of ketamine may produce cardiac ischemia by increasing cardiac output. Consequently, use of ketamine should be avoided in patients with cardiac dysfunction. Leykin and others[79] found that the administration of ketamine resulted in excellent intubation conditions in patients undergoing elective surgery compared with sodium pentothal. In a prospective, randomized clinical trial, Ledowski and Wulf[80] reported that the combination of ketamine with rocuronium and etomidate resulted in superior intubation conditions. This combination may be useful in treating hemodynamically unstable patients in the ICU setting, when succinylcholine is contraindicated.[21] The use of ketamine in patients with increased intracranial pressure is only recommended in mechanically ventilated patients.[81] Ketamine is associated with realistic and truthful nightmares. In this context, the combination with midazolam seems to be an obligatory recommendation. Currently, an S(+) enantiomer of ketamine is available. This enantiomer seems to be free of these clinically relevant side effects although use of these S(+) enantiomers is still recommended in combination with midazolam.

Etomidate provides good intubation conditions with only moderate hemodynamic depression in patients undergoing RSI.[82] Etomidate inhibits adrenosteroid production through the inhibition of mitochondrial hydroxylase, after continuous or even single administration.[83-85] Cuthbergson and colleagues[86] recruited 500 patients to a multicenter, randomized, double-blind, placebo-controlled trial. The use of bolus etomidate was associated with an increased incidence of inadequate response to corticotrophin and is likely associated with an increase in mortality. Therefore, the authors recommend extreme caution in the use of etomidate in critically ill patients with septic shock.[86] Roberts and Redman[87] and Bloomfield and Noble[88,89] also questioned any use of etomidate in critically ill patients.

Dexmedetomidine is increasingly used as a sedative for monitored anesthesia. Advantages include its analgesic properties, "cooperative sedation," and lack of respiratory depression. Dexmedetomidine is also increasingly used in RSI and awake intubation, with promising studies showing a beneficial effect.[90,91] However, long-term observational studies are still lacking, and the current scientific level is too weak to recommend routine use of dexmedetomidine.

Muscle relaxants are also used in emergency airway management in the ICU. If endotracheal intubation fails, the merits of preserving spontaneous ventilation versus optimized intubating conditions using non-depolarizing muscle relaxants should be considered.

Succinylcholine is a very-rapid-acting, polarizing muscle relaxant enabling excellent intubation conditions in less than 1 minute.[92] Unfortunately, it has serious side effects, including the possibility of triggering malignant hyperthermia. The use of succinylcholine is contraindicated in patients with acute major burns, upper or lower neuronal lesions, prolonged immobility, massive crush injuries, and various myopathies.[21] Benumof and associates[93] clearly demonstrated that even the short duration of action of succinylcholine is too long, and critical hemoglobin desaturation will occur before return to an unparalyzed state, even after a 1-mg/kg dose.[93]

Rocuronium is the most widely used non-depolarizing neuromuscular blocking agent. The recommended dosage of "normal" intubation is 0.6 mg/kg. For RSI, higher dosages up to 1.2 mg/kg are necessary and provide excellent intubation conditions within 1 minute.[94] A meta-analysis by the Cochrane Collaborative Group concluded that succinylcholine created superior intubation conditions compared with rocuronium.[95] The only absolute contraindication against the use of rocuronium is allergy to aminosteroid neuromuscular drugs. A major advantage of rocuronium is the possibility of rapid and complete reversal of even deep neuromuscular block by the administration of sugammadex.[96] Based on a systemic review by Chambers and others,[97] the use of sugammadex in combination with high-dose rocuronium is efficacious.

E. Awake Endotracheal Intubation

Successful awake intubation depends on proper patient preparation. Extensive psychological support and clear explanation about reason for and management of awake intubation are necessary and helpful in the ICU setting.

The airway is topically anesthetized with 5% to 10% lignocaine, which is sprayed with a flexible nozzle into the posterior pharynx to reduce coughing and buckling during intubation. If a fiberscope is used, the larynx is then sprayed with 2 mL of lignocaine 2% administered through the working channel of the fiberscope, after which the scope is advanced into the trachea. Thereafter, a second spray is applied into the trachea before the ETT is advanced. Alternative approaches include blockade of superior laryngeal nerve or lingual nerve and transtracheal anesthesia.

Once the patient is properly prepared, any of the intubation techniques listed in Box 46-2 can be chosen according to the operator's preference.[98-102]

In case the first attempt of awake intubation fails because of equipment/operator failure or poor patient cooperation, the following options should be considered: a modified method for awake intubation (e.g., change from blind nasal to fiberoptic approach), induction of general anesthesia, and transition to a fiberoptic-guided

---

Box 46-2   Nonsurgical Techniques for Awake Intubation

Fiberoptic intubation (oral, nasal)
Intubation using rigid fiberoptic scopes (e.g., Bullard, Wu)[98,99]
Blind intubation through LMA Fastrach[100]
Direct rigid laryngoscopy
Retrograde techniques (with or without fiberoptic scope)
Trachlight or other lighted stylets (lightwands)[101]
Blind nasal intubation[102]

intubation method. We believe that the first choice for awake airway management is fiberoptic oral or nasal intubation. If oral intubation is performed, a conduit (i.e., Ovassapian fiberoptic intubating airway) may be used to facilitate fiberscope and ETT insertion. Additionally, a 4 × 4 gauze pad may be used to pull the tongue forward.

A valuable alternative approach is the insertion of the intubating laryngeal mask airway (ILMA) under local anesthesia and light sedation. Intubation is then performed blindly or using a fiberscope inserted through the LMA. Langeron and coworkers[103] prospectively compared ILMA intubation with fiberoptic intubation in patients with difficult airway and reported similar success rates (>90%) and durations for both techniques. Another interesting approach is the combination of Fastrach and lighted stylet. Dimitriou and associates[104] studied 44 of 11,621 patients in whom three attempts of direct laryngoscopy failed. In all these patients, an ILMA was inserted and sufficient ventilation was possible in all patients after a maximum of two attempts. Thereafter, a well-lubricated silicon ETT loaded with a flexible lightwand was introduced. Lightwand intubation was successful at the first attempt in 38 of 44 patients, at the second attempt in three patients, and at the third to fifth attempt in two. Intubation failed in only one patient. Finally, if all those alternatives fail, the establishment of a surgical airway should be considered.

F. Assessment of Correct ETT Placement

Esophageal intubation is a major complication of airway management and can result in severe brain damage or even death. Evaluating the U.S./American closed-claims database (5480 claims), Cheney and colleagues[105] reported the changing trends in anesthesia-related death and permanent brain damage. In the 1980s, 11% of claims associated with death or brain damage involved esophageal intubation, fortunately decreasing to 3% in the 1990s. This reduction was attributed to the introduction of end-tidal carbon dioxide partial pressure (P_{ETCO_2}) monitoring in the 1990s (Fig. 46-5).

Esophageal intubation is an issue even in sufficiently equipped ICUs. Schwarz and colleagues[106] studied almost 300 emergency intubations in an ICU setting and reported esophageal intubation in 8% of cases (ETT misplacement was corrected in all patients before the onset of hypoxemia).

Techniques for clinical evaluation of ETT position include the following:

- Direct visualization of the ETT between the vocal cords[107,108]
- Ventilation-bag compliance[109]
- Auscultation of breath sounds over lungs and epigastrium[110]
- Observation of symmetrical chest excursions
- ETT condensation[111]
- Lighted stylet (lightwand)[112]
- Esophageal detector device and self-inflating bulb[113-115]
- Acoustic reflectometry[116,117]
- Fiberoptic bronchoscopy
- Chest radiograph

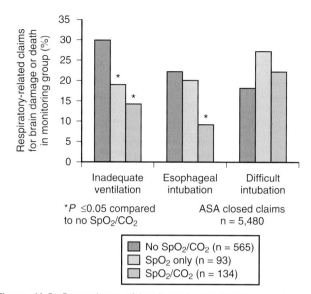

Figure 46-5 Percentage of inadequate ventilation, esophageal intubation, and difficult intubation events associated with death or brain damage in anesthesia-related insurance claims. (From Cheney FW. Changing trends in anesthesia-related death and permanent brain damage. *ASA Newslett* 66.6–8, 2002.)

- Colorimetric end-tidal CO_2 detector and P_{ETCO_2} measurement[115,118]

Radiographic investigation is of limited value because of the delay in diagnosis. Fiberoptic evaluation needs special equipment and preparation and is time-consuming. Acoustic reflectometry is a promising new approach with excellent results, at least in experienced hands. Rafael and coworkers[117] studied acoustic reflectometry in 200 adult intubated patients and reported a 99% correct tracheal and a 100% correct esophageal identification rate. Currently, CO_2 monitoring comes closest to the ideal monitor of correct ETT positioning. CO_2 monitoring can be performed either colorimetrically by relatively inexpensive single-use CO_2 detectors (e.g., Easy Cap, Tyco Healthcare; or Colibri, ICOR AB, Bromma, Sweden) or by capnography using infrared absorption.[118,119] Ventilation is assessed as P_{ETCO_2} approximates arterial CO_2 partial pressure (Pa_{CO_2}) within 2 to 6 mm Hg in normal lungs. Unfortunately, in many disease states, this discrepancy increases significantly. The concentration of CO_2 expired is determined by CO_2 production (e.g., body temperature, muscle tone), CO_2 transport (e.g., circulation, pulmonary perfusion), and CO_2 elimination (pulmonary and airway integrity). Therefore, absence of P_{ETCO_2} indicates esophageal intubation, circuit disconnection, cardiac arrest, or airway obstruction. A false-positive result may be obtained after gastric inflation with CO_2 containing gas or digestion of carbohydrate-enriched beverages. ETT-misplacement can be excluded by observing a normal P_{ETCO_2} waveform for three to six consecutive breaths.

Knapp and associates[120] investigated four different methods—auscultation, capnographic P_{ETCO_2} determination, self-inflating bulb, and transillumination using Trachlight—for the verification of correct ETT positioning in 152 examinations in an ICU setting. Only P_{ETCO_2}

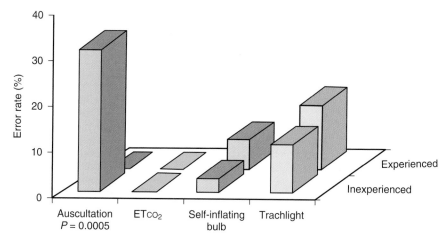

Figure 46-6 Error rates of experienced and inexperienced examiners obtained by evaluating endotracheal tube placement using one of four methods: auscultation, end-tidal carbon dioxide pressure *(ETCO₂)*, self-inflating bulb, and Trachlight. (From Knapp S, Kofler J, Stoiser B, et al: The assessment of four different methods to verify tracheal tube placement in the critical care setting. *Anesth Analg* 88:766–770, 1999.)

monitoring was reliable for the verification of tracheal ETT placement (Fig 46-6). A poorer performance was only reported for prehospital and in-hospital cardiac arrest patients. However, end-tidal CO_2 concentrations are closely correlated with resuscitation outcome in this special setting.[121]

In conclusion, correct tracheal ETT placement can therefore only unequivocally be assured by a physiologic $P_{ET}CO_2$ signal for several consecutive breaths (eventually combined with an esophageal detector device in the prehospital setting), by direct visualization of the ETT between the vocal cords, or by fiberoptic visualization of tracheal cartilaginous rings and carina. All other techniques may provide useful additional information but are prone to errors and misinterpretation.

IV. DIFFICULT AIRWAY MANAGEMENT IN INTENSIVE CARE

Critically ill patients with preexisting hypoxia and poor cardiopulmonary reserve have a higher risk of adverse events during airway management.[122] Consequently, emergency endotracheal intubation in critically ill patients is associated with a significant incidence of major complications. Airway management in intensive care patients differs significantly from endotracheal intubation done for routine surgical procedures in the OR. Airway management in the ICU is often carried out in deteriorating patients in respiratory failure, shock, or cardiopulmonary arrest, and little time may be available for patient evaluation, examination, and preparation. Therefore, the ICU physician should approach the patient with the following four questions in mind[123]:

• Will mask ventilation likely to be successful, when general anesthesia is induced before securing the airway?
• Will endotracheal intubation likely to be successful, when general anesthesia is induced before securing the airway?
• Are there any obstacles making awake fiberoptic intubation difficult?
• In case troubles are encountered, what is plan B?

In a prospective investigation of 297 endotracheal intubations in an emergency ICU setting, Schwartz and coauthors[106] reported major complications in a significant number of patients. Among the problems encountered were difficult intubations (8%), esophageal intubations (8%), pulmonary aspiration (4%), and an associated mortality of 3%. The authors also reported that 3% of hospitalized critically ill patients die within 30 minutes of emergency intubation.

In another observational multicenter study performed in French ICUs, at least one severe complication occurred in 28%: severe hypoxemia (26%), hemodynamic collapse (25%), and cardiac arrest (2%).[124] The other complications were difficult intubation (12%), cardiac dysrhythmia (10%), esophageal intubation (5%), and aspiration (2%).

The initial step in difficult airway management might be the most important: assessing the patient's airway. Afterward, the determination of need for invasive or noninvasive ventilatory support must be done. If invasive airway management is needed, the physician performing airway management must be prepared for two serious complications.

Difficult Mask Ventilation. Difficult ventilation has been defined as the inability of a trained anesthetist to maintain the oxygen saturation greater than 90% using a face mask for ventilation and 100% inspired oxygen, provided that the preventilation oxygen saturation level was within the normal range.[125] Langeron and coauthors[126] prospectively studied 1502 patients and observed difficult mask ventilation (DMV) in 75 patients (5%). DMV was anticipated by the anesthesiologist in only 13 patients (17% of DMV cases). Using a multivariate analysis, five criteria were recognized as independent factors for a DMV (age >55, BMI >26 kg/m², beard, lack of teeth, history of snoring), with the presence of two indicating high likelihood of DMV (sensitivity, 0.72; specificity, 0.73). The implication for clinical practice is to avoid the administration of intravenous induction agents in patients with a high risk of DMV and secure the airway awake (Table 46-3). The risk factors for DMV include age over 55 years, body mass index (BMI) greater than 26 kg/m², lack of teeth, male gender, Mallampati class IV airway, presence of beard, and a history of snoring.[21,126,127]

TABLE 46-3

Anatomic Factors Associated with Difficult Ventilation

Site	Airway Issue	Intervention
Face	Facial wasting, beard, edentulous, snoring history	Patient positioning: sniffing position, and/or jaw thrust; ensure proper fit of mask to face; variety of different mask sizes; oropharyngeal and nasopharyngeal airways; team ventilation, with one person "bagging" while other ensures proper seal; leave in dentures while ventilating patient.
Upper airway	Abscess, hematoma, neoplasm, epiglottitis	Assist ventilation and avoid neuromuscular paralysis; awake intubation, possible fiberoptic with preparation for emergency cricothyrotomy; call for help if upper airway obstruction is suspected.
Lower airway	Reactive airways	Preinduction administration of bronchodilators, nitrates, and diuretics
	Airspace disease: pneumonia, ARDS, pulmonary edema, hemo/pneumothorax	PEEP valve for oxygenation in pulmonary edema, ARDS, and pneumonia; decompress pneumothorax if you are going to apply positive-pressure ventilation.
Thorax-abdomen	Ascites, obesity, hemoperitoneum, abdominal compartment syndrome	Use of bag-valve-mask with PEEP valve may help oxygenation and ventilation.

ARDS, Adult respiratory distress syndrome; *PEEP,* positive end-expiratory pressure.
From Reynolds SF, Heffner J: Airway management of the critically ill patient: rapid-sequence intubation. *Chest* 127:1397–1412, 2005.

Difficult or Impossible Intubation. Difficult intubation (DI) has been defined by the need for more than three intubation attempts or attempts at intubation that last more than 10 minutes. Difficult laryngoscopy and intubation are common phenomena even during routine patient care in the OR. Several investigations clearly demonstrated that minor problems necessitating a second intubation attempt are encountered in up to 8% of patients.[128-130] Grade 3 laryngoscopy, requiring multiple attempts at intubation, occurs in 1% to 4% among all patients.[131-133] Inability to intubate due to grade 3 or 4 laryngoscopic views is present in 0.05% to 0.35% of routine anesthesia cases.[131,134,135] Fortunately, the "cannot ventilate, cannot intubate" situation is rare in the OR and occurs in approximately 2 in 10,000 cases.[125,136,137] Christie and others[138] recapitulated several clinical indicators (Table 46-4).

In addition, Reed and colleagues[139] demonstrated that patients with large incisors, a reduced mouth opening and a reduced thyroid-to-floor-of-mouth distance are more likely to have a poor glottic view during laryngoscopy.

Management of the difficult airway in the emergency department (ED) and in the ICU has not been studied as well as in the OR. Sakles and associates[140] performed a 1-year study on 610 patients requiring airway control in the ED. Rapid-sequence induction was used in 84%, and a total of 98.9% were successfully intubated. In 33 patients (5.4%), inadvertent esophageal intubation occurred. Seven (1.2%) patients could not be intubated and underwent cricothyrotomy. Three patients experienced sustained cardiac arrest after intubation. In a prospective observational study on failed intubation attempts in the ED, Bair and colleagues[102] identified 7712 patients undergoing emergency intubation. In seven patients, a definitive airway could never be established. A total of 207 patients (2.7%) with failed endotracheal intubation were then included in the study. The majority of failed intubations occurred when RSI was not used as first choice (i.e., oral intubation under sedation, oral

TABLE 46-4

Clinical Indicators for Difficult Intubation

Airway Exam Component	Non-Reassuring Findings
Length of upper incisors	Relatively long
Relation of maxillary and mandibular incisors during normal jaw closure	Prominent "overbite" (maxillary incisors anterior to mandibular incisors)
Relation of maxillary and mandibular incisors during voluntary protrusion	Patient cannot bring mandibular incisors anterior to (in front of) maxillary incisors
Interincisor distance	<3 cm
Visibility of uvula	Not visible when tongue is protruded with patient in sitting position (e.g., Mallampati class >II)
Shape of palate	Highly arched or very narrow
Compliance of mandibular space	Stiff, indurated, occupied by mass, or nonresilient
Thyromental distance	Less than three ordinary finger breadths
Length of neck	Short
Thickness of neck	Thick
Range of motion of head and neck	Patient cannot touch tip of chin to chest or cannot extend neck.

From Christie JM et al: Unplanned endotracheal extubation in the intensive care unit. *J Clin Anesth* 8:289–293, 1996.

intubation without sedation, or blind nasotracheal intubation). The most common rescue technique was RSI (49%), followed by a surgical airway (21%). The authors concluded that invasive airway techniques are still important, and rescue airway techniques should be emphasized in ongoing medical education.

Schwartz and others[106] investigated the complications of 297 consecutive endotracheal intubations in 238 adult critically ill patients in the ICU, studied prospectively over 10 months; 89% of intubations were accomplished at the first attempt, and 8% of patients met criteria for DI. Four percent of intubations were only possible after four or more attempts. Esophageal intubation was observed in 8% of intubations but all were recognized before any adverse sequelae resulted. New and/or unexplained pulmonary infiltrates were regarded as indicative

for pulmonary aspiration of gastric contents and occurred in 4% of patients. Seven patients (3%) died during or within 30 minutes of the procedure.

The ASA Difficult Airway Algorithm helps reduce the incidence of severe or catastrophic events during airway management, especially for anesthesia patients.[1] The basic principles of this approach are meticulous patient evaluation before anesthesia induction, awake intubation if problems are suspected, and preparation of an alternative approach in case of failure (Fig. 46-7). Those recommendations are also valuable for the management of critically ill patients. As mentioned, the ASA algorithm has characteristics that prevent direct application to the practice of ICU airway management. Airway management in the ICU is usually urgent or emergent, often depriving the physician of the time necessary to evaluate

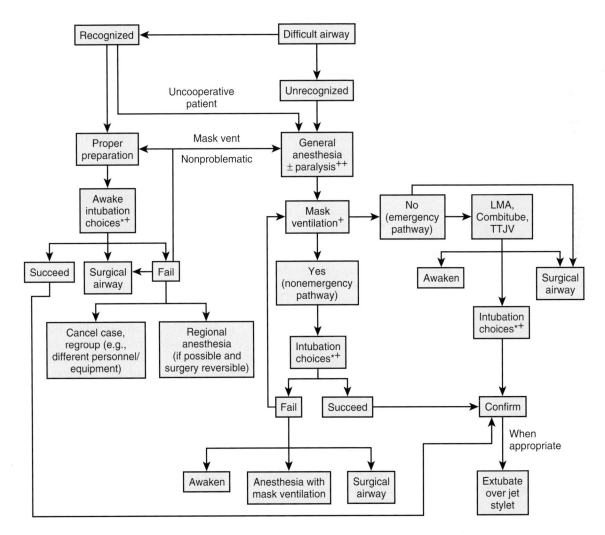

+Always consider calling for help (e.g., technical, medical, surgical etc.) when difficulty with mask ventilation and/or tracheal intubation is encountered

++Consider the need to preserve spontaneous ventilation

*Nonsurgical tracheal intubation choices consist of laryngoscopy with a rigid laryngoscope blade (many types), blind orotracheal or nasotracheal technique, fiberoptic/stylet technique, retrograde technique, illuminating stylet, rigid bronchoscope, percutaneous dilational tracheal entry.

Figure 46-7 American Society of Anesthesiologists Difficult Airway (DA) Algorithm. *LMA,* Laryngeal mask airway; *TTJV,* transtracheal jet ventilation. (From Benumof JL: Laryngeal mask airway and the ASA Difficult Airway Algorithm. *Anesthesiology* 84:686–699, 1996.)

the patient and plan the life-saving intervention. The patient is presumed to have a full stomach and therefore must undergo awake airway management or RSI. The option of reemergence from anesthesia to resume spontaneous ventilation if difficulty is encountered is often impossible. Therefore, modified algorithms with more specific considerations of the special circumstances encountered in ICU and emergency patients have been suggested ("crash airway" or "failed airway" algorithm).[141] Although lacking prospective evaluation, these guidelines might represent a more appropriate application of principles and constraints to airway management in the ED setting.[63]

The best means for coping with the problem of *failed airway* is to prevent its occurrence. This requires the optimization of the initial attempt of laryngoscopy, to prevent multiple attempts causing bleeding and swelling. The net result might be a vicious circle, with each attempt leading to greater likelihood of failed intubation and ventilation, with potentially disastrous consequences. Optimizing laryngoscopy requires appropriate positioning of the patient, use of a laryngoscope blade best fitting the situation, optimal external laryngeal pressure (BURP maneuver: backward, upward, rightward pressure on cricoid cartilage), and eventually effective muscle relaxation.[63] When all these factors are taken into account, the first attempt of laryngoscopy is likely to be the best attempt.

According to the ASA Difficult Airway Algorithm and most other recommendations, there are only four appropriate options for the management of "cannot mask-ventilate, cannot intubate" situations[142] (Fig. 46-7): immediate insertion of laryngeal mask airway or esophageal-tracheal Combitube, manual transtracheal jet ventilation, or surgical access to the patient's airway (tracheostomy or cricothyrotomy).[1] A rational and well-considered approach in difficult airway management is elementary. Strict adherence to airway management guidelines (e.g., ASA algorithm) is essential and reduces failed airway attempts.

A. Esophageal-Tracheal Combitube

The esophageal-tracheal Combitube (ETC) is a double-lumen airway ("pharyngeal" and "distal" lumen) invented by Frass and coworkers,[143] equipped with a pharyngeal balloon and a distal cuff (Covidien, Mansfield, Mass). The ETC is designed for blind insertion into the patient's esophagus or trachea. In more than 95% of all *blind* insertions, the ETC enters the esophagus. After insertion, the pharyngeal balloon is inflated (maximum, 85/100 mL air) and seals against the oral cavity, while the distal cuff (5-12/15 mL air) prevents gastric inflation. Test ventilation is started via the pharyngeal lumen (i.e., supraglottic ventilation). Absence of breath sounds and gastric inflation indicate the rare case where the ETC has blindly entered the trachea. Ventilation is attempted via the distal lumen, the distal cuff blocked with the minimum amount of air providing adequate seal, and the ETC used as a conventional ETT. Two different ETC sizes are available: a small-adult model (37 French, Combitube SA) for

women and men ranging in height from 120 to 200 cm and a 41-F model for taller patients.[144,145]

The ETC has been used extensively in emergency situations, as well as during routine surgery.[144,146,147] The authors recommend sufficient training during elective surgery before using the airway in emergency situations.[145,148,149] In routine cases, the ETC might be inserted using a standard laryngoscope to reduce the risk of tissue injury.[150,151] Contraindications for the use of the ETC are esophageal pathologies, ingestion of caustic substances, and central airway pathologies. Disadvantages are the lack of access to the patient's airways (suctioning of tracheal secretions impossible), lack of a pediatric ETC, and risk of venous stasis and soft tissue (tongue) swelling after prolonged use. The former limitations will be eliminated by the introduction of a redesigned ETC enabling fiberoptic access to the patient's airways and a pediatric version of the ETC.[152,153]

Advantages of the Combitube include protection against aspiration of gastric contents and the applicability of high airway pressures.[154] The ETC might stay in place for up to 8 hours, providing time for further decision making.[155] Changing the ETC for a definitive airway (regular ETT or tracheal cannula) might be done by an attempt of direct laryngoscopy, fiberoptically, or surgically (elective tracheostomy or cricothyrotomy).[152,156]

Recently, the EasyTube has been released (Teleflexmedical Ruesch). It is similar to the Combitube but offers certain advantages: The "pharyngeal" lumen of the Easy-Tube ends just below the oropharyngeal balloon. Therefore, the "tracheo-esophageal" lumen is thinner than that of the Combitube, which carries the two lumens down to the end. Since the distal single lumen of the EasyTube is significantly thinner, the potential danger of mucosal damage is minimized. Furthermore, the oropharyngeal balloon is latex free. The EasyTube comes in two sizes. The 28-F EasyTube ("pediatric size") is available for patients ranging in height from 90 to 130 cm; the 41-F EasyTube is designed for patients taller than 130 cm. A fiberscope can be passed through the so-called pharyngeal lumen because it is open at the distal end. This feature allows inspection of the trachea and possible replacement of the EasyTube using a guidewire, in addition to a larger suction catheter via both lumens (14-F suction catheter in 41-F EasyTube). The EasyTube has been used in a few cases of difficult intubation at the ICU (see Chapter 27).

B. Laryngeal Mask Airway

The laryngeal mask airway (LMA North America, San Diego) was presented in 1983, gained widespread popularity, and is currently used extensively during general anesthesia.[142,157,158] The LMA may be placed for three different reasons: as a routine airway and ventilatory device, as an emergency airway in cannot-intubate, cannot-ventilate situations or as a conduit for endotracheal intubation. Advantages of LMA use as a routine airway have been demonstrated clearly over conventional face mask ventilation. Tidal volumes administered were higher and problems associated with airway management (difficulties in maintaining airway or $SpO_2 \geq 95\%$) less frequently encountered during LMA use compared with regular face mask.[159] LMA works well under these circumstances, because exact positioning is not crucial for a clinically acceptable patent airway.

Furthermore, the potential use of this recent airway in respiratory emergency situations has been recognized early.[160] Leach and associates[161] described use of the LMA as the immediate airway in cardiopulmonary resuscitation, and their findings were confirmed by a larger investigation.[162] A multicenter study was undertaken to assess the potential value of the LMA when inserted by ward nurses during resuscitation as a method of airway management, prior to the arrival of the advanced life support team with endotracheal intubation capability; 130 nurses were trained and 164 cases of cardiac arrest studied. The LMA was inserted at the first attempt in 71% and at the second attempt in 26% of patients. Satisfactory chest expansion occurred in 86%. The mean interval between cardiac arrest and LMA insertion was 2.4 minutes. Regurgitation of gastric contents occurred before airway insertion in 20 patients (12%) and during insertion in three (2%).[162]

Therefore, the LMA has been incorporated into the ASA algorithm and might be inserted as a conduit for fiberoptic endotracheal intubation in the awake or anesthetized patient who cannot be conventionally intubated (mask ventilation may or may not be possible) and as a non-emergency or emergency airway in the anesthetized patient[142] (Fig. 46-8).

Especially for those patients with supraglottic pathologies and unfavorable anatomy for face mask ventilation or endotracheal intubation, an early LMA insertion should be considered. Drawbacks of the LMA include the lack of access to the patient's central airways, risk of aspiration, limited positive airway pressures due to the often inadequate seal, and the need for training. Moreover, the LMA is a supraglottic airway device and thereby unable to establish adequate gas exchange in patients with central airway obstruction.

In the meantime, several modifications of the LMA have been proposed and have been or will be introduced into clinical routine. The ILMA differs from conventional LMAs by having a wider, shorter stainless steel tube; a handle to steady the device; and an epiglottic elevating bar (movable flap fixed to upper rim of mask). The ILMA is accepting cuffed ETTs up to ID of 8.5 mm, enabling blind or fiberoptic intubation using the correctly placed ILMA as a conduit. Success rates for blind ILMA intubation in the 75% to 90% or greater range have been reported.[103,163,164]

The ILMA has therefore been recommended as a rescue device for emergency airway management. Ferson

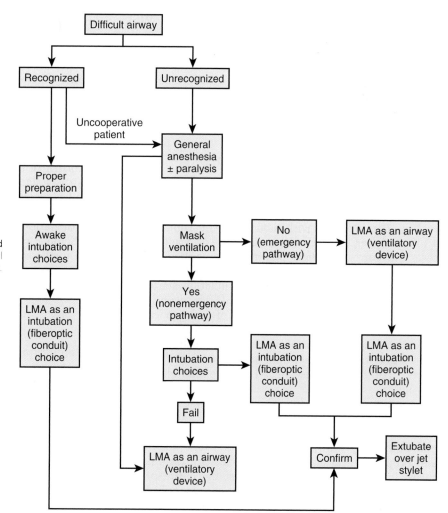

Figure 46-8 Laryngeal mask airway *(LMA)* and ASA DA algorithm. *(From Benumof JL: Laryngeal mask airway and ASA Difficult Airway Algorithm. Anesthesiology 84:686–699, 1996.)*

and colleagues[163] used the ILMA in 254 patients with different types of difficult airway. Insertion of the ILMA was accomplished in three attempts or fewer in all patients. The overall success rates for blind and fiberoptically guided intubations through the ILMA were 96.5% and 100.0%, respectively. Repeated "blind" intubation attempts with the ILMA resulted in esophageal perforation in one elderly patient.[165] Therefore, for blind ILMA intubation, the specially designed silicon tube with rounded bevel should be preferred, because success rates exceed those encountered with standard reinforced tubes.[166] Muscle relaxation is not needed for blind ILMA intubation but increases success rates.[166]

Laryngeal Mask Airway vs. Combitube. Sealing capacities and protection against regurgitation of gastric contents of the intubating LMA seem to be inferior to those of the Combitube (ETC), with average leak fractions of the LMA of 20% to 25% during positive-pressure ventilation and airway pressures of 20 to 30 cm H_2O.[167] Use of the ETC offers higher peak airway pressures and permits positive end-expiratory pressure (PEEP) ventilation, thereby enabling higher tidal ventilation and maintenance of adequate gas exchange, even in those patients with severe underlying pulmonary pathology (e.g., aspiration of gastric contents).[168] In contrast to the ETC, blind or fiberoptic intubation is possible through the LMA lumen (using conventional ETTs up to ID of 6.5 mm) and especially through the ILMA (up to 8.5 mm). With the currently available ETC model, no blind or fiberoptic access to the patient's airway is necessary. Krafft and others[152] modified the standard ETC model and created a larger ventilation hole, which can be used for fiberoptic intubation or tracheal cleansing. However, the redesigned model is currently not available, and it is uncertain whether it will be produced in the near future.

C. Transtracheal Jet Ventilation

In brief, transtracheal jet ventilation (TTJV) is performed using a 16- or 14-gauge catheter, and a 1.5- to 3.5-bar oxygen source (equipped with pressure regulator) in combination with noncompliant tubing. The TTJV catheter is inserted through a cricothyroid puncture, and correct tracheal placement is verified by the aspiration of 20 mL of free air. Noncompliant tubing is then connected and manual oxygen inflation started at an inspiratory rate less than 1 second (~0.5 second) and an inspiratory/expiratory time ratio of 1:3 (to ensure enough time for passive exhalation). Alveolar ventilation is achieved by bulk flow of oxygen through the cannula, as well as translaryngeal entrainment of room air (Venturi effect). For example, use of a 16-gauge cannula and a driving pressure of 3.5 bar results in a gas flow of approximately 500 mL/sec.[169] Therefore, facilitation of passive exhalation by maintaining patency of natural airways is of major importance to avoid overinflation and pulmonary barotrauma. Therefore, nasopharyngeal and oropharyngeal airways are inserted, maximum jaw thrust is well maintained throughout the entire procedure, and expiratory chest movements are observed continuously.

Performed in elective as well as emergency situations, the major indications for TTJV are lack of equipment for conventional airway management, the "cannot ventilate, cannot intubate" situation, ventilatory support during upper airway surgery, or support during endotracheal intubation by other techniques (e.g., ventilation during prolonged fiberoptic intubation). Complications of TTJV during *elective* application are rare but occur frequently during *emergency* TTJV (mainly limited to tissue emphysema). Monnier and colleagues[170] used high-frequency TTJV for ventilatory support during elective laser surgery for laryngeal and subglottic lesions and observed only one complication in 65 patients (mediastinal emphysema). Smith and coworkers,[171] however, reported a 29% complication rate in 28 emergency TTJV patients (exhalation difficulty in 14%, subcutaneous emphysema in 7%, mediastinal emphysema in 4%, arterial perforation in 4%). Other complications of TTJV (e.g., esophageal puncture, bleeding, hematoma formation) have been reported but rarely occur.

D. Emergency Surgical Airway

Rapid-sequence induction is the standard for emergency airway management in ICUs and EDs. Reported success rates of RSI are 97% to 99%, and an emergency surgical airway is only necessary in 0.5% to 2% of patients.[140,172] Sakles and associates[140] evaluated 610 patients requiring emergency airway management in the ED during a 1-year period; RSI was used in 515 (84%). A total of 603 patients (98.9%) were successfully intubated, and only seven patients could not be intubated and underwent cricothyrotomy. Therefore, anesthesiologists and intensive care physicians have only limited experience with surgical airway management. The ASA algorithm has proved to be an invaluable tool, but only briefly addresses the circumstances when a patient must be intubated immediately regardless of the difficulties presented. Since performance of a surgical airway is the final pathway of all airway algorithms, cricothyrotomy must be mastered by all clinicians involved in emergency airway management. Surgical airway management comprises percutaneous dilatational cricothyrotomy or tracheostomy using the Seldinger technique, surgical cricothyrotomy, or surgical tracheostomy. In emergency situations and in cases of unexpected intubation failure in the ICU, surgical or percutaneous cricothyrotomy using the Seldinger technique is preferred over tracheostomy and enables rapid and easy airway access and restoration of adequate gas exchange and ventilation.

1. Percutaneous Cricothyrotomy

Several commercial kits are available for emergency cricothyrotomy, implying easy insertion and high success rates (e.g., Melker or Arndt set, Cook Critical Care, Bloomington, Ind). *Seldinger technique* cricothyrotomy is achieved by performing cricothyroid puncture with a medium-sized needle, passing a wire through the needle, and then passing a dilator and airway over the wire (analogous to insertion of central venous line). Advertisement and promotion claim that percutaneous cricothyrotomy is a quick and easy procedure; in fact, after identification of the cricothyroid membrane, the Seldinger approach is no faster than open cricothyrotomy.[173] Furthermore, none of the percutaneous techniques provides a cuffed tube within the trachea.

Eisenburger and colleagues[174] compared Seldinger technique emergency cricothyrotomy with conventional surgical approach in human cadavers. Tracheal placement of the tube was achieved in 60% ($n = 12$) in the Seldinger group versus 70% ($n = 14$) in the open group ($P = ns$). Furthermore, five attempts in the Seldinger group had to be aborted because of kinking of the guidewire. No differences in the time necessary to perform the procedures were registered. Chan and coworkers[173] performed a similar study in cadavers but observed higher success rates. Airway placement was accurate in 13 of 15 cases for the standard technique (87%) and in 14 of 15 cases for the wire-guided technique (93%). Comparing wire-guided versus standard techniques, no differences were seen in complication rates or performance times. However, one must remember that all these results are obtained in an unstressed elective situation in the morgue; one assumes that results in true emergency situations might be even poorer.

A newer cricothyrotomy device, the Portex Cricothyrotomy Kit (PCK), is based on the concept of mechanical detection of the posterior wall of the larynx (see Chapter 30, Fig. 30-15). In a comparison of two emergency cricothyrotomy kits in 40 human cadavers, the use of PCK was responsible for more lesions and more failures than the standard set, in which cricothyrotomy was based on the Seldinger technique.[175]

2. Surgical Cricothyrotomy

The vasculature is rich overlying the cervical trachea but is strikingly absent over the cricothyroid membrane (CTM). Surgical cricothyrotomy can be performed only after correct identification of the CTM between thyroid and cricoid cartilage; the vertical length of the membrane is about 0.7 to 1.0 mm. The set of instruments used should be simple: scalpel with no. 11 blade, tracheal hook, Trousseau dilator, and cuffed tracheostomy tube. The most common technique is the "no drop" technique, where the larynx and trachea are immobilized by the operator's hand throughout the procedure. Other techniques have been proposed (e.g., four-step technique), but the no-drop technique has proved its value with the following six steps (Fig. 46-9)[176]:

Step 1: Identify the CTM. Key landmark is the laryngeal prominence (Adam's apple), which is easier to palpate in men than in women. It can be identified in the midline at the junction of upper and middle third of the anterior neck. Thumb and long finger stabilize the larynx, while the index finger is run down the anterior surface of the thyroid cartilage until the concavity of the CTM is reached.

Step 2: Immobilize the larynx by holding the superior horns of the thyroid between thumb and long finger, and incise the skin *vertically* (vertical incision 2-3 cm in length provides maximum flexibility and minimum trauma). Vertical skin incision should be made through skin and subcutaneous tissues and not into the airway. Thereafter, the CTM is again identified using the index finger. Several authors prefer to leave the index finger in the wound even during the dissection of the membrane (enables the membrane incision directly caudal to the index finger).

Step 3: Incise the CTM transversely in its distal third whenever possible (avoidance of superior thyroid artery). The incision should be wide enough to permit easy insertion of the cannula (1.5-2 cm).

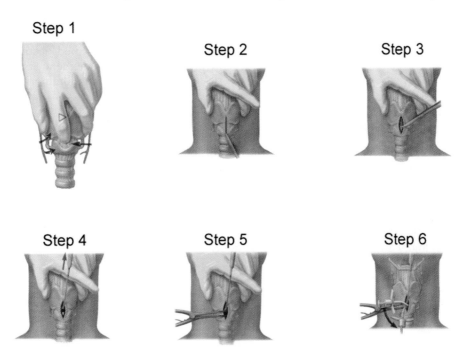

Figure 46-9 Six steps in performing surgical cricothyrotomy. (From Walls RM, Gibbs MA: Surgical airway. *Semin Anesth Periop Med Pain* 20:183-192, 2001.)

Step 4: Insert the tracheal hook transversely into the incised membrane, then rotate it 90 degrees to the midline (some authors waive use of tracheal hook in open cricothyrotomy). The hook strictly immobilizes the larynx and brings the opening within the membrane closer into the field of view.

Step 5: Insert the Trousseau dilator into the airway for several millimeters, then open it to dilate the airway. Some prefer opening the branches in a rostrocaudal direction because most resistance to cannulation is encountered between thyroid and cricoid. However, transverse dilation is also possible.

Step 6: Insert the respective tracheal cannula with the right hand between the prongs opened with the operator's left hand. Slight twisting of the cannula, with a 90-degree rotation of the Trousseau dilator, may be necessary to advance the tracheal cannula safely.

As mentioned, Seldinger as well as open cricothyrotomy are characterized by several pitfalls; both techniques require training in the manikin or better, in human cadavers, and the individual operator must choose the preferred technique. Several authors prefer the open approach because a cuffed cannula can be used, and endotracheal suctioning or bronchoscopy is possible.

In conclusion, the ASA Difficult Airway Algorithm was approved by the ASA House of Delegates in October 1992 and became effective July 1993.[1] Every patient needs to be screened for difficult airways before anesthesia induction, and when difficulties are expected, airways need to be secured with the patient still awake (using fiberoptic scope in most cases). If difficulties are encountered with the patient already anesthetized, refrain from repeated and forceful attempts at direct laryngoscopy, and instead consider alternative methods. If a "cannot ventilate, cannot intubate" situation is encountered, either LMA or Combitube must be inserted immediately. Further alternatives are institution of TTJV or immediate surgical access to the patient's airway. The most important point is to be alert and have a plan B and C prepared in case difficulties arise.

V. COMPLICATIONS OF TRANSLARYNGEAL INTUBATION

In a recent report on 3423 emergent non-OR endotracheal intubations, Martin and associates[177] found that the total incidence of difficult intubations was 10.3%. Complications occurred in 4.2%, including aspiration (2.8%), esophageal intubation (1.3%), dental injury (0.2%), and pneumothorax (0.1%). This report confirms that airway management in the hospital environment is also associated with increased risk of airway complications.

Hoarseness is a common complication after translaryngeal intubation and is reported to occur in 20% to 42% of patients.[55,178] Jones and colleagues[179] prospectively studied the incidence of hoarseness in 167 patients undergoing anesthesia, endotracheal intubation, and surgery. Fifty-four patients (32%) complained about postoperative hoarseness, with all except five returning to normal within 7 days. Vocal cord granuloma was observed in two patients. The site of granuloma is typically at the tip of the vocal processes of the arytenoid cartilages because of their incessant movement.[180]

In a prospective study of 226 endotracheal intubations in 143 adult patients, Stauffer and associates[46] reported that 62% of all patients developed at least one complication of long-term translaryngeal intubation. The main complications, in anatomic order, are nasal and paranasal as well as laryngeal and tracheal injuries. Laryngeal injury is a common complication even after short-term translaryngeal intubation. Kambic and Radsel[181] examined 1000 patients at the end of anesthesia. Severe intubation lesions were registered in 6.2% of patients, with most injuries resolving within a few days. However, 1% of patients sustained vocal cord dysfunction even after short-term translaryngeal intubation (Table 46-5).

In about 4% to 10% of patients, severe damage to the vocal apparatus is encountered (e.g., vocal cord paralysis, granuloma, subluxation of arytenoid cartilage).[182] Most severe complications are observed within the trachea itself (e.g., ulcerations, hematomas up to necrosis, tracheomalacia).[39,46] These complications occur infrequently but may require extensive surgical interventions (i.e., resection of trachea)[183] (Figs. 46-10 and 46-11).

Laryngeal or tracheal trauma is even more common during acute airway management in emergency situations. Maxeiner[184] performed postmortem examinations involving 294 cases of emergency intubation. Acute macroscopic sequelae (mucosal hemorrhage or injury, deeper tissue hemorrhage in false vocal cords) were observed in 18% of those resuscitated outside the hospital and in 16.9% of in-hospital patients. Soft tissue hematomas were observed at the laryngeal opening (31%), vocal cords (37%), laryngeal opening and vocal cords (17%), in the subglottic region (17%), and in the hypopharynx (29%). Lesions at the laryngeal aperture were mainly located at the right part of the larynx.

TABLE 46-5

Outcome of Laryngeal Injury 3 Months after Short-Term Intubation

	Total	Cured	Cicatrix	Synechia
Vocal cord hematoma	45	38	7	—
Hematoma of supraglottic region	7	7	—	—
Laceration of vocal cord mucosa	8	7	—	1
Laceration of vocal muscle	1	—	1	—
Subluxation of arytenoid	1	1	—	—
TOTAL	**62**	**53**	**8**	**1**

From Kambic V, Radsel Z: Intubation lesion of the larynx. *Br J Anaesth* 50:587–590, 1978.

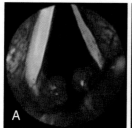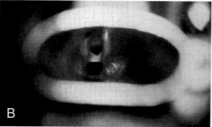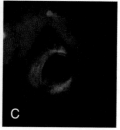

Figure 46-10 Laryngeal damage induced by long-term translaryngeal (ETT) intubation. **A,** Papilloma; **B,** synechia; **C,** subglottic stenosis. (From Denk DM et al: Glottic bridge synechia following intubation, *Otolaryngol Nova* 3:41–44, 1993.)

Other serious complications of translaryngeal intubation have also been reported. Lim and coworkers[185] reported three cases of recurrent laryngeal nerve palsy in three patients after short-term intubation for surgery unrelated to the neck. Pressure neuropraxia resulted from an overinflated ETT cuff compressing the peripheral anterior branches of the right recurrent laryngeal nerve. Frink and Pattison[186] and Castella and coworkers[187] reported posterior arytenoid dislocation after uneventful endotracheal intubation and anesthesia. Furthermore, both pharyngeal and esophageal perforation have been reported after repeated attempts at intubation, especially using a rigid stylet.[188] The tip of the rigid stylet therefore should never protrude from the distal tip of the ETT.

In addition, endotracheal intubation may result in reduced clearance and retention of mucous secretions, bacterial colonization, and ventilator-associated pneumonia.[189] In a survey of 9080 ventilated patients, VAP developed in 842 patients (9.3%).[190] The mean interval between ICU admission and diagnosis of VAP was 4.5 ±7.5 days, and independent risk factors for the development of VAP were male gender and trauma admission. However, VAP seems to be a complication more of endotracheal intubation and not of ventilatory support, because recent studies show a reduced incidence in patients undergoing noninvasive mechanical ventilation.[191] A prospective, randomized study evaluated whether a closed suctioning (CS) system (TrachCare) influences crossover contamination between bronchial system and gastric juices, as well as frequency of VAP, compared with an open suctioning (OS) system. Five cross-contaminations were observed in the OS group on day 3 versus day 1; the 5 strains shared common genotypes as determined by random amplification of polymorphic DNA. No cross-contaminations were seen in the CS group (P = 0.037). VAP occurred in five patients of the OS group but in none of the CS group patients (P = 0.037). Arterial oxygen saturation (SpaO2) decreased significantly in the OS group compared with presuctioning values, the opposite of the CS group. Whereas presuctioning values were comparable between groups, postsuctioning SpaO2 was significantly higher in the CS group. CS significantly reduced cross-contamination between bronchial system and gastric juices and reduced the incidence of VAP when compared with OS. Hypoxic phases can be reduced by the help of CS.[192]

VI. AIRWAY MANAGEMENT FOR PROLONGED MECHANICAL VENTILATION (TRACHEOSTOMY)

Tracheostomy is one of the oldest surgical procedures performed in history. Transcutaneous insertion of a cannula into the patient's trachea was first described in Egyptian and Hinduistic literature between 2000 and 1000 BC.[193] The first description of "modern" tracheostomy was by the Italian surgeon Fabricius of Aquapendente in the 17th century using a tracheal cannula.[194] Development of tracheostomy continued, with many case reports on alternative techniques reported in the next three centuries.[195,196]

The currently used technique for "conventional" surgical tracheostomy was first described by Jackson[197] in 1909. Until several years ago, "open" surgical tracheostomy was the one and only method and therefore the gold standard for the long-term airway management in intensive care medicine. However, the conventional approach has several disadvantages, such as need to transfer the patient to the OR and early and late complications (e.g., bleeding, stoma infection). Therefore, Shelden and colleagues[198] reported a percutaneous access to the trachea. However, this procedure was relatively complicated and was followed by deadly complications.[199] Not until 1985 did Ciaglia and associates[200] propose a percutaneous approach using the Seldinger technique and increasingly larger-sized dilators for progressive tracheal dilation, as supposed by Sanctorius[201] in the 17th century.

Note the following definitions:

Tracheostomy: Surgical incision of the upper third of the anterior tracheal wall to insert a cannula.

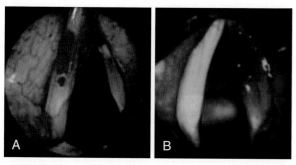

Figure 46-11 A, Acute laryngeal damage during airway management; **B,** hematoma of the true vocal cords after traumatic intubation attempts.

TABLE 46-6

Major Complications of Prolonged Translaryngeal Intubation

Complication	Rate (%)	Reference
Supraglottic Laryngeal Injury (Ulceration, Scarring, Stenosis)		
Laryngitis	3	323
Mucosal ulceration/edema of epiglottis	7-12	46
Mucosal ulceration/edema of larynx	29-51	46
Submucosal hemorrhage of epiglottis/larynx	5-12	46
Supraglottic laryngeal stenosis	12*	260
Glottic Injury		
Glottic ulceration	51	46
Glottic scarring and stenosis	12-18*	260
Bilateral vocal cord paralysis (rare)	Few reported cases	323
Posterior commissure syndrome	6	260
Subglottic Injury		
Subglottic stenosis/scarring	12*	260
Tracheal injury		
Tracheal stenosis (<50% stenosis)	19	46
Tracheal dilation/tracheomalacia	N/A	N/A
Tracheoesophageal fistula†	0.5-5*	324

*After 10 days of endotracheal intubation.
†From 0.5% to 5% of all tracheoesophageal fistulas are caused by endotracheal intubation.
NA, Not available.
From Shirawi N, Arabi Y: Bench-to-bedside review: early tracheostomy in critically ill trauma patients. *Crit Care* 10:201, 2006.

Tracheostoma: Artificial opening into the trachea through the neck to the outside created by tracheostomy or tracheotomy.
Tracheotomy: Surgical technique to create a permanent epithelialized tracheostoma.
Cricothyrotomy: Surgical incision of the cricothyroid membrane for the insertion of a cannula.
Coniotomy: Percutaneous emergency cricothyrotomy using special single-use sets.

A. Reasons for Performing Tracheostomy

Tracheostomy (or tracheotomy) is one of the most frequently performed elective surgical procedures in ICU patients, done in almost 10% of intubated patients. Tracheostomy is generally done for the following four reasons[202]:

- To relieve upper-airway obstruction caused by tumor, surgery, trauma, foreign body, or infection
- To prevent laryngeal and upper airway damage caused by prolonged translaryngeal intubation
- To allow easy or frequent access to the lower airway for suctioning and secretion removal
- To provide a stable airway in a patient who requires prolonged mechanical ventilation or oxygenation support[203] (Table 46-6)

The issue of long-term translaryngeal intubation versus tracheostomy now favors secondary tracheostomy, although the adequate time point is still under discussion. In 2010, Durbin[202] listed benefits of changing from a translaryngeal ETT to a tracheostomy tube in patients who require prolonged intubation. However, the evidence level for most topics discussed is "poor" and comes mainly from uncontrolled trials (Table 46-7).

B. Timing of Tracheostomy

In 1989, at the Consensus Conference on Artificial Airways in patients receiving mechanical ventilation, the indications for nasal or oral ETTs and tracheostomy tubes were forged; "if the need for an artificial airway is

TABLE 46-7

Benefits of Changing from Translaryngeal Endotracheal Tube to Tracheostomy Tube in Patient Requiring Prolonged Intubation

Benefit	Type/Quality of Evidence Showing Benefit
Improved patient comfort	Uncontrolled reports, clinical opinion
Less need for sedation	Several RCTs
Lower work of breathing	Theoretical analysis, one small study
Improved patient safety	Clinical belief but minimal data, some contradictory
Improved oral hygiene	Clinical observation
Oral intake more likely	Opinion only
Earlier ability to speak	Uncontrolled reports
Better long-term laryngeal function	Large uncontrolled reports
Faster weaning from mechanical ventilation	One RCT
Lower risk of ventilator-associated pneumonia	Controversial, data support for both sides
Lower mortality	One RCT supports, many do not, but large RCT supports no increased mortality with tracheostomy
Shorter intensive care unit and hospital stay	Several meta-analyses

RCT, Randomized controlled trial.
From Durbin CG Jr: Tracheostomy: why, when, and how? *Respir Care* 55:1056–1068, 2010.

TABLE 46-8

Early vs. Delayed Percutaneous Dilatational Tracheostomy

Outcome Measurement	Early Tracheotomy (n = 60)	Prolonged Translaryngeal Intubation (n = 60)
Died (%)	19 (31.7)	37 (61.7)*
Pneumonia (5)	3 (5)	15 (25)*
Days in intensive care unit (±SD)	4.8 (±1.4)	16.2 (±3.8)†
Days mechanically ventilated (±SD)	7.6 (±4.0)	17.4 (±5.3)†
Days sedated (±SD)	3.2 (±0.4)	14.1 (±2.9)†
Days on high-dose pressors	3.5 (±4)	3.0 (±4.5)
Organism(s) causing pneumonia: Methicillin-resistant *Staphylococcus aureus, Pseudomonas aeruginosa* mixture	1	5

*P <.005.
†P <.001.
There was a significant difference between the early tracheotomy groups and the prolonged translaryngeal intubation group in outcome measures. Some patients were sent to a step-down while still on mechanical ventilation.
From Rumbak MJ et al: A prospective, randomized study comparing early percutaneous dilational tracheotomy to prolonged translaryngeal intubation (delayed tracheotomy) in critically ill medical patients. *Crit Care Med* 32:1689-1694, 2004.

anticipated to be greater than 21 days, a tracheostomy should be preferred."[204] With the introduction of percutaneous methods, the issue of translaryngeal intubation versus tracheostomy shifted to the best time point to perform tracheostomy.

In a prospective multicenter randomized trial, Rumbak and coworkers[205] assigned 120 patients to *early* (within 48 hours after arrival at ICU) and *delayed* (14-16 days after arrival) percutaneous dilatational tracheostomy. Early tracheostomy was associated with significantly less mortality, nosocomial pneumonia, unplanned extubation, oral and laryngeal trauma, and a shorter duration of mechanical ventilation and ICU admission (Tables 46-8 and 46-9). Prospective studies by Arabi,[206] Bouderka,[207] and Rodriguez[208] and their associates approved the shorter duration of mechanical ventilation in patients with earlier tracheostomy. In a systemic review and meta-analysis of five randomized trials, Griffith and colleagues[209]

TABLE 46-9

Cause of Death in Critically Ill Medical Patients Receiving Early Tracheotomy or Delayed Translaryngeal Intubation*

Cause of Death	Early Tracheotomy (n = 19)	Delayed Translaryngeal Intubation (n = 37)
Ventilator-associated pneumonia	2	9
Gastrointestinal bleed	1	3
Acute myocardial infarction	2	4
Pulmonary embolus	1	1
Intractable septic shock	4	8
Withdrawal of life support	2	1
Respiratory failure	7	11

*More patients died of ventilator-associated pneumonia in the prolonged translaryngeal group than the early tracheotomy group.
From Rumbak MJ et al: A prospective, randomized study comparing early percutaneous dilational tracheotomy to prolonged translaryngeal intubation (delayed tracheotomy) in critically ill medical patients. *Crit Care Med* 32:1689-1694, 2004.

found that early tracheostomy is associated with 8.5 fewer days of mechanical ventilation and 15 fewer days in the ICU. However, there were no significant differences in mortality or nosocomial pneumonia rates.

In contrast, most studies could not demonstrate definitive advantages of early (days 3-5) versus later (days 10-14) tracheostomy.[210,211] In a systematic review, Maziak and colleagues[212] identified 48 possibly relevant articles of 8153 citations; five of the 48 articles met the inclusion criteria. After data review, the authors found no significant advantages of early (days 2-7) versus late (>days 4-14) tracheostomy, concluding insufficient evidence exists to support that the timing of tracheostomy alters the duration of mechanical ventilation or extent of airway injury. In a 2006 meta-analysis comparing early and late tracheostomy in ICU trauma patients, Dunham and Ransom[213] found no differences in mortality, nosocomial pneumonia, duration of mechanical ventilation, laryngotracheal pathology rates, or length of stay in hospital.

In a questionnaire answered by 48 Swiss ICUs (1995-1996; 90,412 patients and 243,921 ventilator-days), 10% of all patients who were ventilated longer than 24 hours underwent tracheostomy.[214] The majority of tracheotomies (35%) were performed in the second week of critical illness. However, 68% of all interviewed physicians would also perform an early (<day 7) tracheostomy if indicated (expected longer ICU course). The authors concluded that tracheostomy in Swiss ICUs is far from being standardized with regard to indication, timing, and choice of technique.

A randomized prospective study is required to examine the need for and the timing of tracheostomy in patients requiring prolonged mechanical ventilation. The findings of such a study would have significant impact on the clinical practice and hospital costs.[212] Until then, the following recommendations of the Consensus Conference of 1989 are still valid[204]:

- Patients with an estimated duration of intubation longer than 7 to 10 days are managed by translaryngeal intubation.
- Reevaluation of the patient at day 7: extubation possible within the next 7 days? If yes, continue

translaryngeal intubation (cumulative duration of translaryngeal intubation <14 days).

- All patients with slow recovery or deterioration with an estimated duration of intubation longer than 14 days should undergo tracheostomy.
- Early elective tracheostomy (days 3-5) in patients with an estimated duration of intubation longer than 21 days
- Patients in whom estimation of ventilator days is difficult should undergo daily evaluation of the pros and cons of tracheostomy and continued translaryngeal intubation.[215]

C. Tracheostomy Techniques

Basically, two approaches are available for performing tracheostomy: conventional *surgical tracheostomy* (ST) and *percutaneous dilatational tracheostomy* (PDT). During the past 15 years, standard tracheostomy using an open surgical approach and the percutaneous techniques were used in parallel. Meanwhile, the use of PDT is still expanding, and several experts suggest PDT as the new gold standard for securing definitive airways in prolonged-ventilated adult patients. This might be true, but exceptions include neuroscience patients requiring prolonged cannula care. Furthermore, anesthesiologists must keep in mind that any procedure in airway management is influenced by individual experience and preference.

1. Conventional Surgical Tracheostomy

Tracheal dissection to provide relief from airway obstruction resurfaced in the diphtheria epidemic in the 19th century. The current technique for "conventional" ST was first described by Jackson[197] in 1909. Many variations exist in technique, but ST is preferably performed in the OR.[216] In critically ill patients for whom transport seems too risky, tracheostomy can also be performed in the ICU bed, although mainly under inferior surgical conditions. Positioning the patient with head and neck extended and a small pillow under the shoulders is a major part of successful technique. Overextension of the head should be avoided; the airway might be narrowed further, and the tracheostomy site might be erroneously too low (near innominate artery). The operating field should be prepared according to aseptic conditions. Patients who do not tolerate this position may assume a sitting or semirecumbent position.

After proper preparation, palpate the landmarks (e.g., thyroid and sternal notch, cricoid cartilage), and make a 3-cm vertical skin incision extending inferior to the cricoid cartilage. Some advocate a horizontal incision because of the better cosmetic results. Subcutaneous fat can be resected using electrocautery, and the inferior limit of the surgical field should be screened for the proximity of the innominate artery. Dissect platysma until the midline raphae between the strap muscles are identified. Strictly adhere to the midline to avoid bleeding and paratracheal structures. After retracting the strap muscles laterally, the pretracheal fascia and the thyroid isthmus are exposed. The thyroid may be retracted out of field, but a resection is recommended due to the reduced incidence of postoperative bleeding

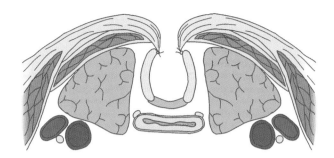

Figure 46-12 Permanent epithelialized tracheostoma. (From Hartung, Osswald, Petroianu, editors: *Die Atemwege*. Wissenschaftliche Verlagsgesellschaft, Stuttgart, 2001, p 159.)

complications. Securing the cricoid cartilage with a hook and superior traction improves control of the tracheal entry. Tracheal incision should be performed between the second and third or the third and fourth tracheal rings. The first tracheal ring should always be left intact to protect the cricoid cartilage.

Several options for a semipermanent tracheostomy exist; a T-, U-, or H-shaped tracheal opening can be made, with the tracheal flaps sutured to the neck skin. Creation of a U-shaped flap ("Björk flap") is not recommended because of the increased risk of flap necrosis. No tracheal cartilage should be resected, to reduce the risk of tracheal stenosis.

A permanent tracheostoma is necessary for patients who indefinitely require secure transluminal access (e.g., head injury). For the creation of a permanent stoma, a small portion of the anterior tracheal wall is resected, and skin flaps are sutured to the rectangular tracheal opening (Fig. 46-12).

2. Percutaneous Dilatational Tracheostomy Techniques

During the 1990s, a dramatic change in airway management for long-term ventilatory support occurred with the introduction of percutaneous approaches to the trachea. Percutaneous tracheostomy was first described by Shelden and colleagues[198] in 1955, but the approach never became popular because of severe complications.[199] With the introduction of the Seldinger technique by Ciaglia and others,[200] a triumphant advance of percutaneous tracheostomy began because of presumed advantages (Box 46-3).

Simpson and associates[217] showed that the number of critically ill patients at their facility undergoing tracheostomy had increased from 8.5% to 16.8% of all critically ill patients since the introduction of PDT. This represents a doubling of the proportion of ICU patients undergoing tracheostomy. Tracheostomy was

Box 46-3	Major Advantages of Percutaneous Approach to Tracheostomy

1. Bedside procedure
2. Easy to learn
3. Reduced personnel
4. Reduced incidence of wound infection

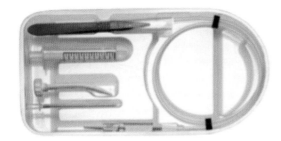

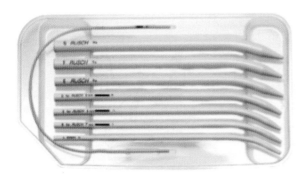

Figure 46-13 PercuQuick set for percutaneous tracheostomy. (Courtesy of Rüsch, Essilengen, Germany.)

also performed significantly earlier, at a median of 4 days versus 8 days of mechanical ventilation. Of approximately 31,000 tracheostomies performed in Germany (~80 million population), more than 50% were PDTs.

The question of which technique, ST or PDT, is better for tracheostomy remains to be answered definitively.

a. PERCUTANEOUS DILATATIONAL TRACHEOSTOMY ACCORDING TO CIAGLIA

Pasquale Ciaglia introduced PDT in 1985 as an alternative approach to conventional ST.[200] Using the original Ciaglia technique, the correct puncture site in the midline between first or third tracheal ring is identified, the trachea punctured (free aspiration of 20 mL air possible), and a guidewire inserted. Over this guidewire, special dilators are introduced, and the anterior wall of the trachea is dilated until an opening with a diameter of approximately 36 French is achieved (Fig. 46-13). Advantages of this method are short duration of the procedure

and bedside performance. However, contraindications must be considered (Box 46-4).

To enhance patient safety, Marelli and colleagues[218] proposed that the entire procedure be monitored fiberoptically. The use of a FOB prevents endotracheal insertion out of the anterior midline or injury to the posterior tracheal wall, particularly during dilatation. A drawback of FOB control is that its insertion into the airway results in a partial obstruction of the ventilatory path thereby compromising ventilation.[219]

For performing PDT, the anesthetized patient is positioned with the head and neck extended. The anterior part of the neck is cleaned and draped in accordance with thyroid surgery guidelines. The FOB is then introduced through the tracheal tube in place, and the correct puncture site is identified. For this purpose, the ETT must be drawn back toward the glottic opening, and the FOB must be inside the ETT to prevent erroneous puncture of the scope (after the procedure, the scope must undergo a complete evaluation to prevent water intrusion).[220]

After puncturing the trachea in the midline between the first and third tracheal ring, a guidewire is inserted under fiberoptic vision (Fig. 46-14A). Puncturing must be done in the midline, in the middle between the tracheal cartilages. Puncture near a tracheal ring must be prevented because cartilage damage or fractures are associated with late complications such as tracheal stenosis (Fig. 46-14B). Thereafter, a guidance cannula is slid over the guidewire and a 1.5-cm skin incision made. The puncture site is then dilated with seven (hydrophilic) plastic dilators up to a diameter of 36 F (12 mm) (Fig. 46-14C). Lastly, the tracheal cannula (maximum ID of 9 mm) is inserted as guided by a medium-sized dilator (Fig. 46-14D). A slight resistance is often encountered during cannula insertion, which is overcome by using sufficient

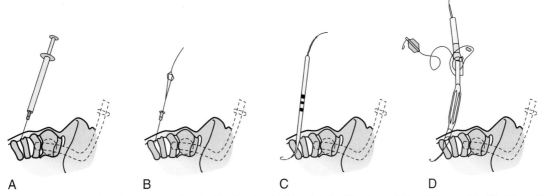

A   B   C   D

Figure 46-14 Percutaneous tracheostomy according to Ciaglia. See text for details. (Courtesy of Rüsch, Vienna. Modified from Ciaglia P et al: Elective percutaneous dilatational tracheostomy: a new simple bedside procedure—preliminary report. *Chest* 87:715–719, 1985.)[201]

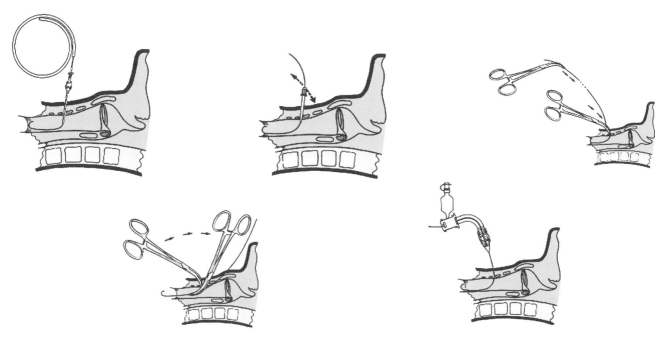

Figure 46-15 Percutaneous tracheostomy according to Griggs. (Courtesy of Rüsch, Vienna. Modified from Griggs WM et al: A simple percutaneous tracheostomy technique. *Surg Gynecol Obstet* 170:543–545, 1990.)

lubricating fluid and rotating movements during insertion. After cannula insertion, the FOB is removed from the ETT and inserted into the tracheal cannula, to verify correct placement, optimize cannula insertion depth, and remove bloody secretions from trachea and bronchi.

b. PERCUTANEOUS DILATATIONAL TRACHEOSTOMY ACCORDING TO GRIGGS

In 1989, Schachner and associates[221] presented a single-dilatation tracheostomy forceps over a guidewire (Rapitrach; Fresenius, Runcom, Cheshire, UK), which carried a relatively high incidence of injury of the posterior tracheal wall. In 1990, Griggs and coauthors[222] developed another guidewire dilating forceps (Portex, Kent, England) with a smooth rounded tip (modified Howard-Kelly forceps with blunt edge). The procedure is characterized by a similar approach as the Ciaglia technique with transillumination (diaphanoscopy), puncturing of the trachea (18-gauge needle), guidewire insertion, and skin incision (Fig. 46-15). All neck structures are slightly dilated by one small dilator. Next, the specially designed forceps is inserted through the guidewire until the trachea is reached, and the skin and pretracheal tissues are dilated by opening the blades. The forceps is carefully advanced into the trachea under fiberoptic control, with the tip of the forceps pointing toward the carina. By pulling both branches of the forceps apart, the trachea is also dilated. According to the Ciaglia technique, the tracheal cannula chosen is then inserted by means of an adequate dilator over the guidewire.

c. TRANSLARYNGEAL TRACHEOSTOMY ACCORDING TO FANTONI

The translaryngeal approach for tracheostomy (TLT) was introduced in 1996 by Fantoni sind coworkers.[223,224] In contrast to all other percutaneous techniques, the initial

puncture of the trachea is directed cranially (Fig. 46-16). After tracheal puncture, a guidewire is passed through the needle and passed toward the oropharynx alongside or inside the tracheal tube. The patient is then reintubated with the kit's 5-mm-ID tube, and the wire is connected with the tracheal cannula. The cannula is then advanced through the pharynx into the trachea by constantly pulling on the guidewire. The pointed head is then pulled out the anterior tracheal wall and soft tissues of the neck. Next, the pointed head is cut off, and the cannula is to be rotated 180 degrees downward using a plastic obturator. Thereafter, the fiberoptic scope is inserted through the cannula to check correct positioning in the trachea.

The major advantage of this approach is that minimal or no skin incision is necessary, minimizing the bleeding risk. Typical problems encountered with TLT are: difficulties with the intratracheal rotation of the cannula, the need for changing the ETT, and potential contamination of the tube during oropharyngeal passage.

Byhahn and coworkers[225] investigated practicability and early complications of Fantoni's TLT technique in 47 ICU patients. No severe complications (aspiration or bleeding) were observed; only oxygenation deteriorated in about one fourth of the patients. The authors concluded that TLT is a valuable alternative technique to Ciaglia's approach, but should be performed only in patients requiring a fraction of inspired oxygen concentration (F_{IO_2}) of less than 0.8. Westphal and associates[226] compared TLT with the Ciaglia approach in a prospective study of 90 patients. Although success and complication rates were similar between the groups, problems during the procedure were far more common with the TLT technique, especially in positioning the guidewire correctly. Cantais and others[227] prospectively compared forceps-dilational and translaryngeal technique in 100 adult critically ill patients. Fantoni's translaryngeal

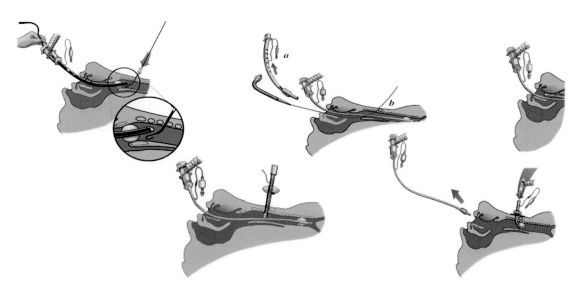

Figure 46-16   Percutaneous tracheostomy according to Fantoni. (Courtesy of Rüsch, Vienna.) (Modified from Fantoni A, Ripamonti D: A nonderivative, non-surgical tracheostomy: the translaryngeal method. *Intensive Care Med* 23:386–392, 1997.)

technique took nearly twice as long as forceps-dilation (13 vs. 7 minutes, respectively). Although minor bleeding episodes were less in the Fantoni group, major complications were more common, and unsolvable technical problems were encountered in 23% of patients. Nevertheless, the authors concluded that both techniques are safe, and physicians should be able to choose their preferred technique.

d. ROTATING DILATATIONAL TRACHEOSTOMY (PERCUTWIST)

The PercuTwist technique (Teleflexmedical Ruesch, Kernen, Germany) offers an alternative real single-step percutaneous tracheostomy approach (Figs. 46-17 and 46-18). Preparation, puncturing of the trachea, and guidewire insertion are performed according to the Ciaglia and Griggs techniques (Fig. 46-17, 1 and 2). After needle removal, an 8-mm to 10-mm skin incision is made (Fig. 46-17, 3), and a special hydrophilic dilation screw (suited for either 8 or 9 mm ID tracheal cannulas) is slid over the guidewire until the skin incision is reached (Fig. 46-17, 4). Using slight pressure, the dilator is turned clockwise until the first threads are advanced into the pretracheal soft tissues (Fig. 46-17, 5). The PercuTwist is then carefully advanced without pushing until the tip of the screw is fiberoptically visualized inside the trachea (Fig. 46-19). The screw is then advanced into the trachea twist by twist under gentle elevation of the anterior tracheal wall. The dilator is removed by counterclockwise rotation, and the tracheal cannula is inserted using an insertion dilator guided by the in situ guidewire (Fig. 46-17, 6 and 7).

Frova and Quintel[228] reported the use of the PercuTwist system in 50 consecutive ICU patients and found a 100% success rate without serious complications. Tracheal ring fractures were observed in 4 of 50 patients (8%), but no posterior tracheal wall injury. Westphal and coworkers[229] studied 10 consecutive patients and reported no early complications besides minor bleeding (<20 mL) in two patients. In a prospective randomized study in 70

consecutive patients, Byhahn and associates[230] compared safety and efficacy of PercuTwist and Blue Rhino tracheostomy. In the PercuTwist group, complications occurred in 12 patients, including posterior wall tears, tracheoesophageal fistula, false cannula passage, and four failures to insert the cannula, compared with seven complications in the Blue Rhino group. However, no statistically significant differences in minor and overall complications were observed between the two techniques. This major complication rate of 33% in the PercuTwist group was in vast contrast with the results of Sengupta and coauthors,[231] who observed about 90 patients over 20 months of routine use of PercuTwist. All procedures performed were graded as having absent or minimal bleeding, although six patients had abnormal clotting profiles. Grundling and colleagues[232] also reported no severe complications in 54 patients of a prospective observational clinical study. A rare complication of tracheostomy is tracheal ring fracture, which was also described with the PercuTwist technique.[233]

Yurtseven and others[234] reported on 130 patients undergoing tracheostomy using three different techniques. The main finding was that PercuTwist ($n = 45$) was associated with minimal complications (two patients with longitudinal tracheal abrasion) and appears to be an easy to perform and practical alternative to standard PDT ($n = 44$, four longitudinal abrasions, one posterior tracheal wall injury, and one tracheal ring rupture) and the guidewire dilating forceps (GWDF) group ($n = 41$; two cases of longitudinal tracheal abrasions, one posterior tracheal wall injury). Furthermore, operating times using PercuTwist were significantly shorter than in the other groups (9.9 ± 1.1, 6.2 ± 1.4, and 5.4 ± 1.2 minutes in PDT, GWDF, and PercuTwist groups, respectively).

Imperiale and associates[235] reported on intracranial pressure changes during tracheostomy using PercuTwist. Use of PercuTwist did not cause secondary intracranial hypertension insult and therefore could also be considered safe in a select population of brain-injured patients.

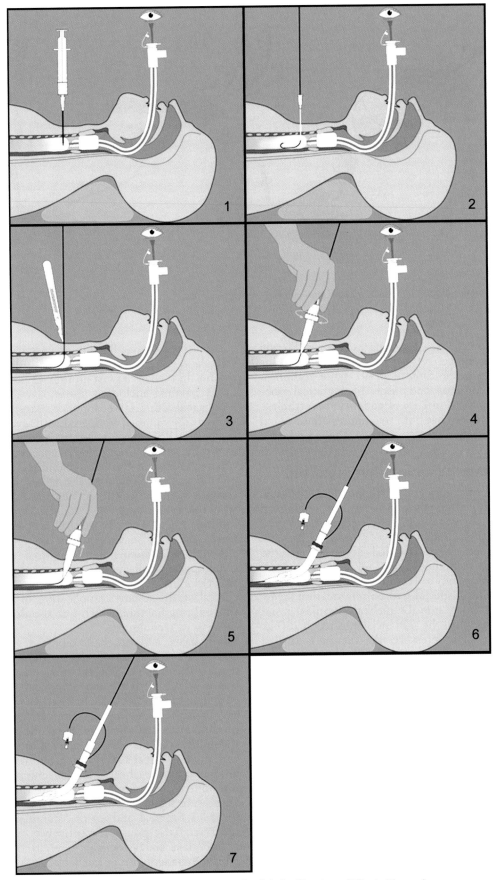

Figure 46-17 PercuTwist. See text for details. (Courtesy of Rüsch, Vienna.)

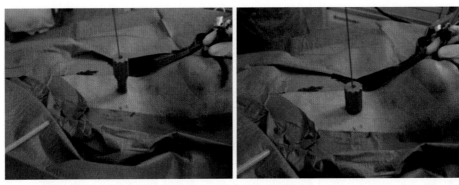

Figure 46-18 Performance of PercuTwist tracheostomy. (Courtesy of Rüsch, Vienna.)

A distinct advantage of the PercuTwist technique over all other percutaneous approaches is that the stoma remains open after removal of the screw, and immediate emergency intubation of the stoma with a small tracheal tube is possible. With all other devices, dilated stoma closes by the tissue pressure immediately after removal of the dilators.

e. CIAGLIA BLUE RHINO

The technique of PDT has constantly been evolving. In 1998 a modification was introduced called Ciaglia Blue Rhino (Percutaneous Tracheostomy Introducer Kit, Cook Critical Care). The standard multiple dilators were replaced by a single, sharply tapered dilator shaped similar to the horn of a rhino (Fig. 46-20). The dilation process can be performed in a single step, without the need to change dilators (Fig. 46-21). Therefore, the risk of injury to the posterior tracheal wall, bleeding episodes, and impaired oxygenation by repeated airway obstruction during the dilation process may be reduced.[236]

The Percutaneous Tracheostomy Introducer Set consists of a puncture needle, guidewire, small dilator and special Blue Rhino dilator, and three curved stylets for placement of the tracheostomy tube. Instructions are as follows[237]:

1. Withdraw the ETT under fiberoptic control to a level above the assumed puncture site.
2. Make a horizontal skin incision and puncture the trachea in the midline between the second and third tracheal cartilage rings.
3. Introduce the guidewire using the Seldinger technique.
4. Withdraw the needle, and introduce the guiding catheter.

5. Predilate the puncture canal with the small dilator.
6. To increase the dilator's external smoothness, moisten the Blue Rhino dilator with a few milliliters of saline solution or distilled water.
7. Advance the wet dilator over the guidewire and guiding catheter through the soft tissues and into the trachea up to its marking of 38-F external diameter. The dilation should require a minimum of force because of the dilator's smoothness (Fig. 46-21A and B).
8. Ensure the Blue Rhino PDT set contains three hard-rubber stylets of different sizes with cone-shaped tips. The tracheostomy tube should be armed with its corresponding stylet.
9. Advance this perfectly fitting unit into the trachea (Fig. 46-21C).
10. Afterward, withdraw the stylet and confirm the correct position of the tracheostomy tube using fiberoptic bronchoscopy.
11. Connect the tube with the respirator, and remove the ETT.

In a small, prospective, randomized study in 2000, Byhahn and others[237] compared the classic PDT with the Blue Rhino in 50 critically ill patients and reported a relatively high incidence of cartilage damage (9 of 25 cases), but no life-threatening complications with either

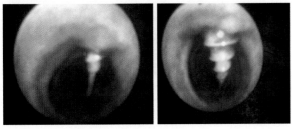

Figure 46-19 Fiberoptic control of the PercuTwist technique. (Courtesy of Teleflexmedical Ruesch, Vienna.)

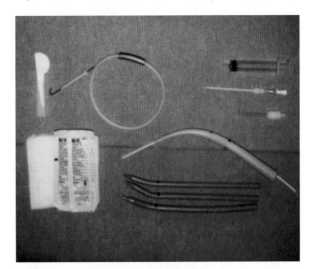

Figure 46-20 Ciaglia Blue Rhino dilator set for percutaneous tracheostomy. (Courtesy of Rüsch, Vienna.)

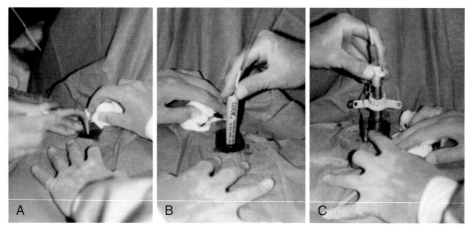

Figure 46-21 Single-step Ciaglia Blue Rhino: a modified technique for percutaneous dilatational tracheostomy. See text for details. (Modified from Byhahn C et al: [Ciaglia Blue Rhino: a modified technique for percutaneous dilatation tracheostomy—technique and early clinical results]. *Anaesthesist* 49:202–206, 2000.)

method. In 2002, Fikkers and associates[238] assessed perioperative, early, and late complications in 100 consecutive Blue Rhino tracheostomies. Success rate was 98%, with minor and major complications observed in 30% and 12%, respectively. Tracheal stenosis was observed in one patient (over 6-12 months). In 2003, Dongelmans and others[239] showed that the use of Blue Rhino in an ICU environment is associated with a very low rate of major and minor complications.[240] In a retrospective study of 318 tracheostomies, Bhatti and associates[240] reported a low complication rate similar to open surgical tracheostomy, concluding that the complication rate of PDT can be reduced further with experience and use of strict protocols, making it even safer than an open ST.

In 2005, Kost and colleagues[241] evaluated 500 adults; 309 underwent PDT using Ciaglia Blue Rhino (single dilator), and 191 used the Ciaglia Percutaneous Tracheostomy Introducer Kit (multiple dilator). Total complication rate was 9.2% (6.5% in Blue Rhino and 13.6% in multidilator group). The most frequent intraoperative complications were brief oxygen desaturation (14 patients) and bleeding (12 patients). This study also identified ASA class IV patients as having a significantly increased risk of complications. Johnson[242] and Ambesh[243] and coworkers showed that the single-dilator technique decreased operative time compared with the serial-dilator technique. In both studies, complication rates were not increased by single-step dilation. In 2007, De Leyn and colleagues[244] performed a systematic review and recommended the modified Blue Rhino as the technique of choice, based on its simplicity and short procedure time (level 2c). In 2010, Dempsey and colleagues[245] reported a prospective evaluation of the single-tapered-dilator technique, with tracheostomies performed in 589 patients (2003-2009). PDT was attempted in 576 patients and successfully completed in 572. Four attempts were stopped due to bleeding. In 149 patients (26%) intraoperative technical difficulties were encountered. Early complications occurred in 16 patients (3%). Significant late complications occurred in four patients; in two patients, a trachea-innominate fistula was found and led to the death of both patients. The mortality directly attributable to PDT was 0.35%.

Based on clinical studies and personal experience, the single-step PDT currently is the most widely used technique.[245-248]

f. CIAGLIA BLUE DOLPHIN

In 2009, Gromann and associates[249,250] studied a modified PDT called Blue Dolphin, a balloon dilation technique that exerts mainly radial force to widen the tracheostoma. This force may reduce complications such as fracture of tracheal cartilage rings or injuries to the posterior tracheal wall (Fig. 46-22).

Surgical Procedure

1. Ensure optimal placement of patient with full extension of head and neck.
2. Perform surgical disinfection and sterile covering of the operative area.
3. Manually examine the cricoid cartilage.
4. Make a 1-cm to 2-cm, horizontal surgical incision.
5. Puncture the trachea at the level between the second and third tracheal cartilages.

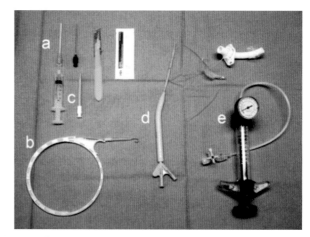

Figure 46-22 Ciaglia Blue Dolphin set balloon percutaneous tracheostomy introducer: *a,* introducer needle; *b,* wire guide; *c,* 14-F dilators; *d,* balloon-tipped catheter loading dilator assembly; *e,* Cook inflation device. (From Gromann TW et al: Balloon dilatational tracheostomy: initial experience with the Ciaglia Blue Dolphin method. *Anesth Analg* 108:1862–1866, 2009.)

6. Ensure puncture of the trachea using bronchoscopy.
7. Place the guidewire using the Seldinger technique.
8. Enlarge the puncture canal with the blue, short introducing dilators.
9. Attach the prepared inflation device to the balloon port on the balloon-catheter assembly.
10. Remove the introducing dilators; the guidewire remains in situ.
11. Introduce the prepared tracheostomy tube.
    a. Fill up the balloon with normal saline using the inflation pump (max pressure, 11 atm).
    b. Hold this pressure for at least 15 seconds.
    c. Deflate the balloon.
    d. Simultaneously insert the balloon-catheter assembly, loading dilator, tracheostomy tube, and guidewire.
    e. When tracheostomy tube is in place, remove the rest of the assembly.
    f. Inflate the tracheal tube–balloon cuff.
    g. Verify by bronchoscopy.

In the primary study by Gromann,[250] 20 patients underwent this procedure at the ICU bedside, and surgery averaged 3.3 ±1.9 minutes. There were no injuries of the posterior tracheal wall, no bleeding requiring treatment, or wound infections. One patient had a fracture of a tracheal ring, and another patient had subcutaneous emphysema.

In 2010, Cianchi and others[251] compared this new Blue Dolphin system with the Ciaglia Blue Rhino system in 70 ICU patients. Surgical procedure time in the Blue Rhino group was significantly shorter than in the Blue Dolphin group (1.5 vs. 4 minutes). Limited intratracheal bleeding requiring no intervention was more frequent in the Dolphin group. Although Blue Rhino was associated with fewer tracheal injuries and time for procedure was shorter, the authors concluded that PDT using the Ciaglia Blue Dolphin technique is a feasible and viable option in ICU patients.

D. Airway Management During Tracheostomy

During puncture of the trachea, the endotracheal tube must be withdrawn just below the vocal cords to protect the bronchoscope and tube cuff. Therefore, alternative approaches such as ventilatory support using a laryngeal mask airway or a Fastrach have been suggested.[252-254] In an RCT, Dosemeci and colleagues[255] studied LMA as an alternative airway for management during PDT in 60 patients, concluding that LMA is an effective and successful ventilatory device. It improves visualization of the trachea and larynx during fiberoptic-assisted PDT and prevents the difficulties associated with use of the ETT, such as cuff puncture, tube transection by the needle, and accidental extubation. However, Ambesh and associates[256] clearly demonstrated that changing ETT to LMA might result in potentially life-threatening complications, including loss of the airway during PDT. In a prospective randomized study, they compared the safety and efficacy of ETT versus LMA ventilation during PDT in 60 critically ill patients. Although the complication rate

Box 46-5	Complications of Percutaneous Dilatational Tracheostomy

Early
Bleeding
Wound infection
Pneumothorax, pneumomediastinum
Tracheoesophageal fistula
Malpositioning of cannula
Damage to tracheal cartilages

Late
Infection
Pneumonia
Aspiration
Granulation tissue
Tracheal stenosis
Persisting fistula after decannulation
Tracheoesophageal fistula
Tracheomalacia

was low in the ETT group (7% ETT impalement, 7% cuff puncture, and 3% accidental extubation), a high rate of complications was observed in the LMA group (33% incidence of airway loss, inadequate ventilation, and gastric distention). A change of the ETT for an LMA during the performance of tracheostomy therefore cannot be recommended and may only be an alternative method for patients not intubated before the procedure.

E. Perioperative and Early Complications of Tracheostomy

A number of potential complications may occur during or immediately after PDT (Box 46-5). Bleeding is the most common perioperative complication, with incidence up to 4%.[257] After controversial statements, routine chest radiography for identifying complications at an early stage is not longer recommended after tracheostomy placement, unless there are signs of unexpected compromise of air exchange.[258,259] Ambesh and associates[243] compared two percutaneous single-dilator techniques (Blue Rhino, Griggs dilating forceps) in 60 consecutive patients. Percutaneous access to the trachea was possible in all patients, with significantly more difficult cannulations in the Griggs group (30% vs. 7%). Overdilatation of the stoma occurred more frequently in the Griggs group (23% vs. 0%), whereas Blue Rhino was often associated with tracheal ring fractures (30% vs. 0%). Some variation in complications is seen with different techniques for PDT. The single-dilator technique (Blue Rhino) appears to be fast and incurs no more risk than the multiple-dilator technique of Ciaglia.[238,242]

F. Late Complications of Tracheostomy

Many mechanisms may cause late complications after tracheostomy.[46] The most important factors may be placement of the tube, especially prolonged intubations; leaving the tube in place for prolonged periods, possibly related to inflated cuff; and abnormal healing at the site of injured tracheal mucosa. Clinically relevant late

TABLE 46-10

Long-Term Complications of Surgical Tracheostomy (ST) vs. Percutaneous Dilatational Tracheostomy (PDT) in Critically Ill Patients

| Study | PROPORTION AVAILABLE FOR LONG-TERM FOLLOW-UP (%) | | Duration of Follow-Up | REPORTED COMPLICATIONS | | |
	ST	PDT		Complication	ST (%)	PDT (%)
Hazard et al.[325]	8/24 (33)	11/22 (50)	1.5-3 mo	Delayed closure	3 (38)	0 (0)
				Tracheal stenosis	5 (63)	2 (18)
				Cosmetic deformity	2 (25)	1 (9)
Gysin et al.[326]	20/35 (57)	10/35 (29)	3 mo	Delayed closure	2 (10)	1 (10)
				Tracheal cartilage lesion	1 (5)	0 (0)
				Unesthetic scar	8 (40)	2 (20)
Raine et al.[327]	26/50 (52)	24/50 (48)	4 mo	Tracheal stenosis	11 (46)	7 (27)
				Scar requiring surgical revision	5 (21)	2 (8)
Heikkinen et al.[328]	11/56 (20)	11/56 (20)	18 mo	Delayed closure	1	0
				Airway symptoms*	2	2
				Dysphagia	1	0
Wu et al.[329]	12/42 (29)	15/41 (37)	2-4 yr	Tracheal malacia	1 (8)	0 (0)
Melloni et al.[330]	13/25 (52)	15/25 (60)	6 mo	Tracheomalacia	0 (0)	1 (7)
				Tracheal stenosis	0 (0)	1 (7)
Antonelli et al.[331]	13/72 (18)	18/67 (27)	12 mo	Delayed closure	7 (54)	7 (39)
				Airway symptoms*	6 (46)	5 (28)
				Tracheal stenosis	2 (11)	1 (6)
				Need for stomaplasty	3 (16)	1 (6)
Silvester et al.[332]	42/100 (42)	29/100 (29)	20 mo	Airway symptoms*	10 (24)	12 (41)
				Stridor	2 (5)	0 (0)
				Vocal cord paralysis	1 (2)	0 (0)
				Unesthetic scar	2 (5)	0 (0)

*Airway symptoms included hoarseness, feeling of a lump in the throat, cough, dyspnea, and subjective phonetic or respiratory problems.
From Delaney A et al: Percutaneous dilatational tracheostomy versus surgical tracheostomy in critically ill patients: a systematic review and meta-analysis. *Crit Care* 10:R55, 2006.

complications after tracheostomy occur in up to 65% of patients.[260-263] The most common and important complication is development of granulation tissue. *Granulation tissue* occurs subclinically or presents as failure to wean patients from ventilator, failure to decannulate, or as upper airway obstruction with respiratory failure after decannulation.[264] Further late complications include tracheal stenosis, aspiration pneumonia, tracheomalacia, and tracheoesophageal fistula[265] (Table 46-10).

After its introduction by Ciaglia in 1985,[200] many investigators have reported their experience with the technique and have concluded that PDT is safe and cost-effective. Vigliaroli and others[266] reported their clinical experience with Ciaglia's dilational tracheostomy over 6 years in 304 patients, 41 of whom were evaluated for late complications. No perioperative death occurred, and early complication rate was 5%. No late complications (e.g., tracheal stenosis) were observed in any of the fiberoptically investigated patients during follow-up to 180 days.

Escarment and associates[267] evaluated the safety and complication rates of the Griggs technique in a consecutive series of 162 ICU patients. Early intraoperative complications occurred in 17%, being minor technical difficulties without morbidity (e.g., inadvertent extubation, difficult cannulation, hemorrhage). Average cannulation duration was 25 days, and stoma closure was effective in all patients after about 3 to 4 days. Follow-up was available in 81 patients, and endoscopic evaluation of the airways 3 months after decannulation was

performed in 73 patients; 62 (85%) were normal, seven (10%) had granulation tissue at the stoma site, and four (5%) had tracheal stenosis, with dyspnea in two patients (3%).

Norwood and colleagues[268] determined the incidence of tracheal stenosis and other late complications after PDT in 422 patients undergoing tracheostomy between 1992 and 1999 (Ciaglia approach). Of the 340 survivors, 100 were interviewed and further evaluated by fiberoptic laryngotracheoscopy and tracheal computed tomography. CT scans identified mild stenosis (11%-25%) in 21% of patients (all asymptomatic), moderate stenosis (26%-50%) in 8%, and severe stenosis (>50%) in 2% of patients (Fig. 46-23; see also Fig. 46-11A).

Hotchkiss and coworkers[269] performed a cadaver study to evaluate the stoma and surrounding insertion site for laryngotracheal injury in six fixed cadaver specimens. Puncture and dilation were performed using the Blue Rhino technique, and no fiberoptic control of the procedure was used. Puncture level was accurately predicted in only 50% of cadavers. Anterior tracheal internal wall mucosal injury was observed in all specimens. Cartilaginous injury was severe in five of six specimens that sustained multiple comminuted injuries to two or more adjacent tracheal rings. The authors concluded that the injuries observed may significantly contribute to the development of tracheal stenosis. However, no data are presented on the potential impact of bronchoscopic guidance on the incidence of these complications.

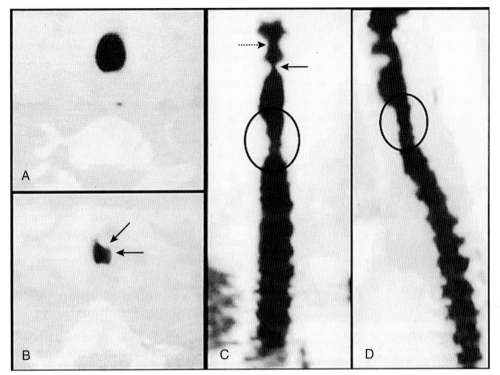

Figure 46-23 Patient with 45% tracheal stenosis. **A,** Axial view of normal trachea just above stoma level. **B,** Axial view of stoma level; arrows denote areas of anterior and lateral stenosis. **C,** Coronal view with circled area of stenosis; dotted arrow denotes false vocal cords; solid arrow indicates true vocal cords. **D,** Sagittal view with circled area of stenosis. (From Norwood S et al: Incidence of tracheal stenosis and other late complications after percutaneous tracheostomy. *Ann Surg* 232:233–241, 2000.)

Leonard and others[270] assessed the late outcome following forceps tracheostomy in a prospective observational study of 49 patients. Tracheal stenosis was observed in one patient (2%), whereas other, minor complications (e.g., change in voice, 49%) were observed frequently. However, whether this was caused by the preceding translaryngeal intubation or the technique of tracheostomy could not be determined.

The main problem of PDT leading to tracheal stenosis is that tracheal rings are forced into a position that creates the opening for the cannula. This maneuver is capable of deforming the tracheal cartilage so that it protrudes into the airway (Fig. 46-24).

Koitschev and associates[271] reported on three patients with severe tracheal stenosis/obliteration after PDT (Figs. 46-25 and 46-26). In all patients, tracheal narrowing occurred above the level of the stoma. The authors speculated the cause was a procedure-related mechanism (tracheal ring invagination and consecutive development of granulation tissue) rather than a mechanism based on the duration of cannulation (normally producing stenosis below the stoma).

In conclusion, PDT seems to be a safe, relatively simple, and quick procedure that can performed at bedside. Early complications and infection rate (~2%) might be even lower and cosmetic results better than with surgical tracheostomy. However, PDT must be performed by an experienced operator at the correct puncture site, straight in the midline between two tracheal rings, and may never be performed without fiberoptic guidance.[272] All special techniques proposed are characterized by special drawbacks or complications. The Blue

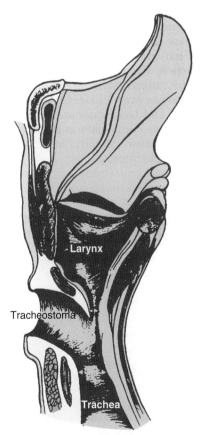

Figure 46-24 Suprastomal stenosis. Anterior tracheal wall is invaginated into the lumen. (From Koitschev A, et al: Tracheal stenosis and obliteration above the tracheostoma after percutaneous dilational tracheostomy. *Crit Care Med* 31:1574–1576, 2003.)

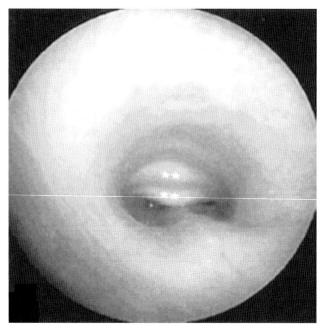

Figure 46-25 Endotracheal view revealing invagination of the cartilage rings. (From Koitschev A, et al: Tracheal stenosis and obliteration above the tracheostoma after percutaneous dilational tracheostomy. *Crit Care Med* 31:1574-1576, 2003.)

Rhino technique is associated with a relatively high incidence of tracheal ring fractures (~30%), whereas the PercuTwist approach has a higher risk of posterior tracheal wall injury. It is therefore difficult to compare "percutaneous dilatational tracheostomy" to the conventional surgical approach, since these are completely different techniques with different success and complication rates. Much larger studies over a longer time studying clearly defined patients and techniques are necessary to clarify the incidence of late complications after PDT. Currently, it is too early to draw definitive conclusions on PDT versus surgical tracheostomy.

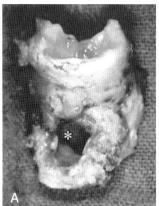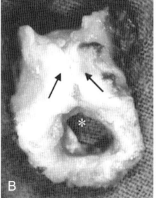

Figure 46-26 Anatomic specimen of resected trachea: front **(A)** and back **(B)** views. Arrows indicate scar tissue above the stoma. (From Koitschev A, et al: Tracheal stenosis and obliteration above the tracheostoma after percutaneous dilational tracheostomy. *Crit Care Med* 31:1574-1576, 2003.)

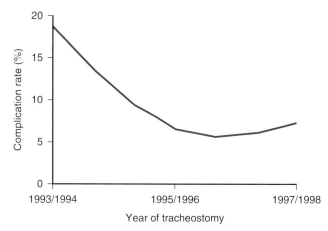

Figure 46-27 Learning curve for perioperative complications during percutaneous dilatational tracheostomy. (From Petros S: Percutaneous tracheostomy. *Crit Care* 3:R5-R10, 1999.)

G. Conventional (Surgical) vs. Percutaneous Tracheostomy

Comparing PDT with historical data of complications of ST is erroneous and may give a biased picture. Moreover, varying definitions and different techniques used by the authors make interpretation of data difficult. Complication rates for ST vary widely, between 6% and 66%, with mortality of 2%.[273] To reduce this incidence of complications and to perform a bedside procedure, the different percutaneous techniques have been proposed.

Special reference to early complications shows that serious bleeding can occur with either ST or PDT, but appears to be less frequent with PDT.[274] Considerable danger arises in the significant rate of posterior tracheal wall perforation with development of tension pneumothoraces when using PDT.[275] To avoid posterior tracheal wall injury, guidewire and guiding catheter should be firmly stabilized during PDT, and fiberoptic visualization of the entire process is obligatory. In common, pneumothorax is infrequent when using PDT but occurs in 1% to 3% when using ST.[276]

Numerous studies suggest minimal difference in acute serious complications between ST and PDT,[277] while others propose a learning curve and a significantly lower complications rate thereafter. Petros[257] clearly showed a learning curve in performing tracheostomy after prospectively evaluating 234 PDTs (Fig. 46-27).

Massick and colleagues[278] performed a prospective analysis of complication incidence for the first 100 PDTs (Ciaglia) performed in a local community hospital. The authors clearly demonstrated a learning curve, with the first 20 patients exhibiting a significantly higher incidence of perioperative as well as late complications. Furthermore, patients with suboptimal anatomy were found to have significantly increased complication rates independent of operator and institutional experience. PDT has a steep learning curve, with most perioperative, postoperative, and late complications occurring in the first 20 patients.

Beiderlinden and others[279] assessed the incidence of early complications of fiberoptically guided PDT beyond the learning curve (all investigators performed >100

PDTs). With 133 consecutive patients undergoing PDT (114 conventional Ciaglia technique and 22 Blue Rhino), tubes were fixed at the skin, and no routine tube exchanges were performed. Insertion of the tracheal tube was easy or modestly difficult in 87%, and no procedure-related deaths occurred. The incidence of tube-related complications (e.g., tracheal wall lesion, bleeding, cannula misplacement) was low, 0.7%. Fracture of tracheal rings was observed in 24%. Despite this finding, the authors concluded that with experience in performing PDT, fixation of the tracheal cannula, and omission of routine tube changes, the complication rate is low.

Several studies compared ST and PDT technique, in addition to multiple reviews and four meta-analyses.[265,280-282] At present, no consensus exists as the optimal approach in terms of minimizing complications.

Dulguerov and associates[280] performed a meta-analysis comparing surgical and percutaneous access to the trachea. Study patients were grouped as having surgical tracheostomy from 1960 to 1984 (17 investigations in 4185 patients), surgical tracheostomy from 1985 to 1996 (21 studies in 3512 patients), or PDT (27 studies in 1817 patients). The highest perioperative and postoperative complication rates were observed in the "older" surgical studies (9% and 33%, respectively). Although perioperative complication rates were higher in the percutaneous studies (10% vs. 3%), postoperative complications were lower compared with the surgical approach (7% vs. 10%). However, this meta-analysis was criticized because studies on percutaneous tracheostomy without fiberoptic control were also included. Furthermore, it is difficult to perform a meta-analysis on this topic because not only percutaneous versus surgical approaches were compared. The percutaneous group is a mix of several different procedures and techniques used (i.e., with or without fiberoptic control, Ciaglia or Griggs technique).

Subsequently, Delaney and coauthors[265] performed a systematic review and meta-analysis, including 17 RCTs involving 1212 patients. Pooled analysis showed no statistical difference in mortality or major complications. The rate of wound and stoma infections was low, 6.6%, but infections were significantly less common in the PDT group. Unfortunately, studies rarely include long-term follow-up, and significant late complications may be missed.

In a meta-analysis, Freeman and associates[281] examined five studies (236 patients) and found that PDT was associated with a lower overall postoperative complication rate, less perioperative bleeding, and lower incidence of stomal bleeding and stomal infection. In addition, PDT was quicker than ST by 9.84 minutes. The meta-analysis of Higgins and Punthakee[282] included 973 patients from 15 RCTs (490 PDTs and 483 STs). The author found significantly fewer complications in PDT with respect to wound infection and unfavorable scarring. Consequently, overall complications trended toward favoring the percutaneous technique. PDT appeared to be more cost-effective by freeing up OR resources, including time and personnel; providing greater feasibility in terms of bedside capability; and allowing nonsurgeons to perform the procedure

safely[282,283] (Tables 46-11 and 46-12). Most authors reported lower complication rates with the individual percutaneous technique used[272,284] (Table 46-11). Tracheostomy is increasingly performed outside the OR and by PDT rather than ST technique.[285]

Bowen and colleagues[286] performed a retrospective medical chart review. Over 23 months, 213 patients received ST ($n = 74$) or PDT ($n = 139$). Perioperative complications occurred in five of 74 patients (6.76%) during PDT (whereas three patients, 4.1%, required emergent operative exploration of the neck) versus three of 139 patients (2.2%) during ST. Surgical time for PDT in the ICU was significantly shorter and cost less than ST performed in the OR.

In conclusion, all studies clearly show that adequate training and teaching is the major factor reducing complications with PDT. Until those issues are cleared, PDT can be recommended with some exceptions. Especially in patients presenting with a short thick neck, goiter, or difficult airway, PDT should be performed only by an experienced physician, with a physician prepared for ST present.[287] The most important part is fiberoptic control of the entire procedure, since erroneous punctures or direct trauma of the esophagus or tracheal wall are prevented or recognized early.[288]

VII. ROUTINE AIRWAY CARE IN MECHANICALLY VENTILATED PATIENTS

Tracheal suctioning is an intervention to remove accumulated mucus from endotracheal tube, trachea, and lower airways in patients requiring intubation for mechanical ventilation. Intubation, ventilation, and especially sedation impair the transport of mucus in the airways. Accumulated mucus in the subglottic space is a well-proven cause of ventilator-associated pneumonia. Prevention of VAP includes aspiration of secretion by suctioning.[289-291] Furthermore, coughing is impaired from ETT interference with glottic closure.

Tracheal suctioning, an essential aspect of airway management, is a potentially life-threatening procedure that can lead to hypoxia, cardiac dysrhythmias, trauma, and atelectasis.[292] Traditionally, tracheal suctioning is performed by disconnecting the patient from the respirator, applying manual hyperinflation ("bagging"), inserting a suctioning catheter into the patient's airways, and applying negative pressure to remove secretions.[293] Saline may be instilled to dilute secretions and facilitate suctioning. Tracheal suctioning is intended as a beneficial procedure, but few studies have been performed on this topic. To the contrary, several investigations reported adverse effects.[294,295] Stone and colleagues[294] reported cardiac dysrhythmias in post–cardiac surgery patients. Aldkofer and Powaser[295] reported a decrease in oxygen tension of 20 mm Hg.

Therefore, tracheal suctioning should be performed "on demand," and the need for suctioning and the effectiveness of the procedure must be determined by chest auscultation.[1] Suctioning on a routine schedule (e.g., every 4-6 hours) should be abandoned. Prior to the procedure, the patient must be properly informed, because tracheal suctioning is a frightening and unpleasant

TABLE 46-11

Comparison of Overall Complications for Open vs. Percutaneous Tracheostomy, Including Adjusted Values for Minor Hemorrhage

Review: New review
Comparison: 02 overall complications
Outcome: 02 adjusted overall complications (minor bleeding)

Study or sub-category	Percutaneous n/N	Open n/N	OR (fixed) 95% CI	Weight %	OR (fixed) 95% CI
Antonelli	33/67	45/72		20.76	0.58 [0.30, 1.14]
Crofts	2/25	5/28		4.09	0.40 [0.07, 2.28]
Freeman	10/40	4/40		2.83	3.00 [0.85, 10.54]
Friedman	8/26	21/27		13.45	0.13 [0.04, 0.44]
Gysin	22/35	17/35		5.95	1.79 [0.69, 4.65]
Hazard	6/22	24/24		15.88	0.01 [0.00, 0.15]
Heikkinen	3/30	2/26		1.82	1.33 [0.21, 8.67]
Holdgaard	6/30	0/30		0.37	16.18 [0.87, 301.62]
Massick	12/50	2/50		1.43	7.58 [1.60, 35.93]
Melloni	3/25	11/25		9.13	0.17 [0.04, 0.73]
Porter	7/12	3/12		1.18	4.20 [0.74, 23.91]
Raine	20/50	29/50		16.41	0.48 [0.22, 1.07]
Sustic	0/8	2/8		2.23	0.15 [0.01, 3.77]
Tabaee	6/29	1/14		1.01	3.39 [0.37, 31.34]
Wu	3/41	4/42		3.45	0.75 [0.16, 3.58]
Total (95% CI)	490	483		100.00	0.75 [0.56, 1.00]

Total events: 141 (Percutaneous), 170 (Open)
Test for heterogeneity: Chi^2 = 50.73, df = 14 (P < 0.00001), I^2 = 72.4%
Test for overall effect: Z = 1.97 (P = 0.05)

0.1 0.2 0.5 1 2 5 10

Favors percutaneous   Favors open

OR, Odds ratio; CI, confidence interval.
From Higgins KM, Punthakee X: Meta-analysis comparison of open versus percutaneous tracheostomy. *Laryngoscope* 117:447-454, 2007.

experience; for many patients, it is the only remembrance on their ICU stay.

To prevent hypoxemia and resulting complications, preoxygenation at an FiO$_2$ of 1.0 should be started 1 minute before suctioning. Suctioning is an invasive procedure, and sterile gloves should be worn during the process. Catheter selection is also important; the external diameter of the suction catheter should not exceed one-half the ETT internal diameter.[296] Larger catheters are traumatic, whereas smaller catheters are often insufficient at removing viscous secretions.

Much confusion surrounds normal saline instillation (NSI) to facilitate tracheal suctioning. NSI is reportedly beneficial in removing thick, tenacious secretions in patients receiving mechanical ventilation. Currently, no data confirm beneficial effects of saline irrigation. To the contrary, increasing literature focuses on harmful effects of routine tracheal NSI.[297,298] Despite the use of NSI for 25 years, many questions remain, such as the volume of saline to instill. Volumes instilled in adult patients vary between 2 and 5 mL, 5 and 10 mL, and up to 40 mL.[298] Volume of saline used has never been evaluated in controlled research studies. Investigating unretrieved saline, Hanley and others[299] instilled saline tagged with technetium 99m in two subjects. Only 20% of saline instilled was retrieved by suctioning, and the authors concluded that NSI at the proximal end of the ETT only sprinkles

the trachea. Part of the remaining saline may be "blown out" during brisk coughing, and instillation at the distal end of the ETT might minimize this risk.

Furthermore, NSI has a major impact on physiologic parameters: Gray and coauthors[300] assessed minute volume and forced vital capacity in 15 patients suctioned with or without NSI. No statistically significant differences were found between the groups. However, Kinloch[297] could show that oxygenation status (i.e., mixed venous oxygen saturation) of patients suctioned using 5 mL of normal saline was poorer than in patients suctioned without saline instillation. In a systematic review, Blackwood[298] concluded that after 25 years of inconsistent practice in trying to remove tenacious secretions, it is time to focus on techniques to prevent thick and tenacious secretions.

Suctioning should be performed with continuous negative pressure at 80 to 150 mm Hg applied only during catheter withdrawal.[292,301] Higher pressures can cause hypoxemia, atelectasis, or catheter adherence to the tracheal mucosa. Duration of a single suctioning pass should not exceed 10 to 15 seconds, and the number of suctioning passes should not exceed three during one suctioning episode.[302] To minimize the risk of postsuctioning desaturation, the patient should be reconnected to the oxygen supply immediately (maximum, 10 seconds) after suctioning. To evaluate effectiveness of suctioning, a

TABLE 46-12

Mortality and Complication Rates for Surgical Tracheostomy (Open) and Percutaneous Dilatational Tracheostomy (PDT)

Study	Tracheostomy Type	No.	Operative Mortality	Stenosis Rate*	Overall Complications
Dayal and el Masri	Open	50	0% (0/50)	0% (0/6)	38% (19/50)
Stauffer et al.	Open	51	2% (1/51)	11% (2/18)[†]	63% (32/51)
Miller and Kapp	Open	84	1.2% (1/84)	8% (4/51)	45% (40/84)
Skaggs and Cogbill	Open	147	5% (7/147)	0% (0/57)	48% (71/147)
Schusterman et al.	Open	214	0.5% (1/214)	(>4% (9/?))	26% (56/214)
Mulder and Rubush	Open	428	5.1% (22/428)	8% (20/261)	45% (193/428)
Average complication rates for open tracheostomy			3.2% (31/974)	6.6% (26/393)	42% (411/974)
Hazard et al.	PDT	55	0% (0/55)	0% (0/14)	10.9% (6/55)
Marelli et al.	PDT	61	1.6% (1/61)[‡]	0% (0/13)	11.5% (7/61)
Winkler et al.	PDT	71	0% (0/71)	0% (0/12)	5.5% (4/72)
Friedman and Mayer	PDT	100	1.0% (1/100)[§]	3% (1/37)	19% (19/100)
McFarlane et al.	PDT	121	0% (0/121)	5% (4/77)	19% (19/100)
Ciaglia and Graniero	PDT	170	0% (0/170)	0% (0/30)	11% (19/170)
Present study	PDT	356	0.3% (1/356)	3.7% (8/214)	19% (69/356)
Average complication rates for PDT			0.3% (3/934)	3.3% (13/397)	15% (124/814)

*Percentage represents clinically symptomatic tracheal stenosis or radiographic evidence of >50% stenosis without clinical symptoms (total number of patients with stenosis/total number of patient with cannulas removed).

[†]Death caused by cardiac arrhythmia in one patient.

[‡]One patient died because of tracheoinnominate artery fistula 6 days after PDT.

[§]Nine of 18 patients who had cannulas removed in this series had tracheal stenosis of >11% as determined by follow-up tomography studies (i.e., 65% overall stenosis rate). One patient had obstructive symptoms caused by a 60% stenosis and died. One patient had >50% stenosis without symptoms.

Modified from Hill BB et al: Percutaneous dilational tracheostomy: report of 356 cases. *J Trauma* 41:238–244, 1996.

comprehensive respiratory assessment is recommended after suctioning.[301]

Minimally invasive endotracheal suctioning has been recommended as an alternative approach. "Minimally invasive" means that the suction catheter never reaches the trachea, no saline is installed, no bagging is performed, and suctioning is only performed when clinically indicated. In an RCT of 383 ICU patients, van de Leur and associates[293] compared routine suctioning (n = 197) with the proposed minimally invasive approach (n = 186). No differences were found in duration of intubation, ICU stay, pulmonary infection, or mortality. However, suctioning-related adverse effects (e.g., desaturation, BP elevation, blood in mucus) were significantly less in the minimally invasive group. In another study, the same group evaluated patients' recollection of the suctioning procedure; 208 patients were interviewed within 3 days after ICU discharge, and the level of discomfort was quantified using a visual analogue scale.[303] A significantly lower prevalence of recollection of airway suctioning was found in the minimally invasive treated patients. Further studies are needed to prove those findings, but reconsidering the individual suctioning techniques seems to be valuable.

Furthermore, closed suctioning (CS) systems have been recommended. A reduced incidence of VAP was reported.[304] "Classic" open suctioning (OS) is routinely performed by disconnecting the patient from the ventilator and introducing a regular suctioning catheter through the ETT into the upper airways.[305] Alternatively, suctioning can be accomplished with a CS system attached between ETT and ventilatory tubing, allowing introduction of the suctioning catheter into the airways without disconnecting the patient from the ventilator.[306,307] CS

has some advantages compared to the conventional OS technique. CS can be helpful in limiting environmental, personnel, and patient contamination and in preventing the loss of lung volume and the alveolar derecruitment associated with standard suctioning in the severely hypoxemic patient. However, the impact of CS on the incidence of ventilator-associated pneumonia, as well as its cost-effectiveness, remains to be determined.[305]

An interesting approach using a visualized ETT has been suggested by Frass and colleagues.[308] The so-called visualized endotracheal tube (VETT system; Pulmonx, Palo Alto, Calif) corresponds to a standard ETT with incorporated fiberoptic fibers, continuously displaying a view of patient's trachea and carina. The device worked effectively until extubation (mean duration, 137 hours), although the lens had to be rinsed approximately four times daily. Online monitoring of ETT position and amount of retained secretions is possible. Furthermore, targeted suctioning of right or left lung can be performed under visual control. The authors assumed that the frequency of suctioning maneuvers can be reduced by using this new technique.[308] However, the VETT system is not commercially available.

In recent years, *continuous aspiration of subglottic secretions* (CASS) has become increasingly popular, although few randomized prospective studies have compared CASS and conventional suctioning.[309-312] The results have been inhomogeneous and the conclusions on VAP prevention contradictory, with most studies based on a limited number of patients. Bouza and associates[291] performed a randomized comparison of conventional aspiration and CASS during a 2-year period; 359 patients underwent CASS, and 331 patients underwent conventional suctioning. The results of this important study are

TABLE 46-13

Continuous Aspiration of Subglottic Secretions (CASS): Clinical Outcome in All Randomized Patients (per Protocol Analysis)

Variables	CASS (*n* = 331)	Conventional Suction (*n* = 359)	*p* Value
VAP (%)	12 (3.6)	19 (5.3)	0.2
Episodes of VAP/1000 days of MV (no.)	17.9	27.6	0.18
Duration of mechanical ventilation (days)	1.0 (1.0-1.0)	1.0 (1.0-1.0)	0.4
Length of ICU stay, (days)	3 (2-5)	3 (2-5)	0.3
Length of hospital stay (days)	8 (7-12)	9 (8-13)	0.9
Mortality	23 (6.9)	26 (7.2)	0.5
Hospital antibiotic use in daily defined doses	1213.5 (1145.7-1283.2)	1932.5 (1846.8-2020.1)	<0.001
Episodes of *Clostridium difficile*–associated diarrhea	3 (0.9)	5 (1.4)	0.4

VAP, Ventilation-associated pneumonia; *MV*, mechanical ventilation.
From Bouza E et al: Continuous aspiration of subglottic secretions in the prevention of ventilator-associated pneumonia in the postoperative period of major heart surgery. *Chest* 134:938–946, 2008.

presented in Table 46-13. No agreement has been reached in this area, however, and more research is needed to clarify the potentially beneficial effects of CASS. Furthermore, prospective research is needed to clarify the role of continuous cuff pressure monitoring, removal of biofilm formation in the ETTs, and routine saline instillation before tracheal suctioning.[313]

VIII. DIFFICULT EXTUBATION IN CRITICALLY ILL PATIENTS

Extubation of the trachea of ICU patients represents a special challenge to the attending physician. Every routine extubation (difficult airway absent) can be associated with severe complications, including hemodynamic decompensation and cardiac failure, breath-holding, laryngospasm, aspiration, or increased intracranial pressure. Factors that result in a relatively high incidence of difficult extubation in intensive care include special surgical procedures (head and neck surgery), swelling of laryngeal or pharyngeal tissues, limited airway access (maxillomandibular fixation, cervical immobilization, tracheal resection), and long-term ventilatory support with muscle fatigue.

In patients with preexisting difficult airway, one should be aware that emergent reintubation is an entirely different situation. Extubation of these patients might result in airway catastrophes. However, few studies have focused on this integral part of difficult airway management, and evidence is insufficient to permit critical evaluation of extubation strategies. The ASA Task Force on Management of the Difficult Airway recommended that each anesthesiologist and critical care physician have a preformulated strategy for extubation of patients with a difficult airway.[314] The preformulated strategy should include the following:

- Evaluation for general clinical factors that may produce an adverse impact on post-extubation ventilation
- Formulation of an airway management plan that can be implemented if the patient is not able to maintain adequate ventilation after extubation
- Consideration of short-term use of a guide that can serve as guidance for reintubation

By decreasing upper airway tract diameter, laryngeal edema increases airway resistance and manifests as stridor and respiratory distress. Reintubation may be required if the patient is unable to sustain the increased respiratory work. To discern patients with and without significant laryngeal edema, de Bast and associates[315] described the "cuff leak test." Leak was evaluated immediately before extubation in 76 patients, expressed as the difference between expired tidal volume (assisted control mode) measured with the ETT cuff inflated and deflated. The authors concluded that a cuff leak greater than 15.5% can be used as a screening test to limit the risk of reintubation in laryngeal edema.

Reintubation under emergency conditions in the ICU-bed is entirely different from the controlled circumstances in the OR. In ICU patients, use of "tracheal tube exchangers" (e.g., Cook Critical Care) may be indicated. This type of device is lubricated and then inserted through the lumen of the ETT into the trachea before the tube is removed. Oxygen may be delivered continuously through the hollow lumen of a tracheal tube exchanger using the by-packed adapter. If severe respiratory insufficiency occurs, another ETT is slid over this guiding bar into the trachea, blindly or under direct laryngoscopy. Alternatively, extubation may also be performed using a fiberoptic bronchoscope left inside of the trachea, in addition to a bite block. This procedure enables directed suctioning of tracheal secretions, especially during the sensible post-extubation phase. Fiberoptically controlled reintubation is possible at any time point; this approach may be advantageous in ENT and maxillofacial patients.

Not only the extubation procedure, but the entire post-extubation period, approximately 48 hours, is of utmost importance for patient outcome. It is well known that the receptors associated with swallowing are altered by the presence of an ETT.[316] The reason for swallowing dysfunction after extubation of the trachea seems to be a combination of "muscle freezing" from non-use and loss of proprioception from superficial mucosal lesions. Leder and others[317] investigated the incidence of aspiration after extubation in 20 consecutive trauma patients. All subjects underwent bedside transnasal fiberoptic endoscopic evaluation of swallowing 24 ±2 hours after extubation to determine objectively aspiration status. Aspiration was identified in 9 of 20 subjects (45%) and 4 of these 9 (44%) were silent aspirators. The authors concluded that trauma patients have an increased risk of aspiration after orotracheal intubation and prolonged mechanical ventilation. Moreover, silent aspiration was suggested as an occult cause of post-extubation pneumonia. This high incidence of aspiration could not be verified by a consecutive prospective study by the same group. Barquist and coworkers[318] found an aspiration rate of only 10% and delayed enteral nutrition in those patients. However, no beneficial effect of fiberoptic post-extubation monitoring was observed in this small prospective study of 70 patients.

Another important factor is the impact of accidental extubation (with or without reintubation) on pneumonia risk and patient outcome. *Unplanned extubation* (UEX) accounts for about 10% of extubations and requires reintubation in 60% of cases.[138,319] In a prospective multicenter trial on predisposing factors and complications of UEX in more than 400 patients, Boulain[319] reported an incidence of 10.8%, which means 1.6 UEXs per 100 ventilated days. Multivariate analysis determined four factors contributing to UEX: chronic respiratory failure, ETT fixation with only thin adhesive tape, orotracheal intubation, and lack of intravenous sedation. The rates of mortality, laryngeal complications, and length of mechanical ventilation were similar in UEX and non-UEX patients. Patients were more often reintubated after UEX, every second versus every tenth non-UEX patient. The authors hypothesized that simple measures such as strong fixation of ETT, adequate sedation, and particular attention to orally intubated patients should minimize UEX.

Reintubation has been identified as a major risk factor for nosocomial pneumonia.[320] In a case-control study, Epstein and associates[321] found that either form of UEX (successfully tolerated or failed during weaning or ventilatory support) was associated with longer ICU stay but did not increase mortality. Recently, de Lassence and colleagues[322] prospectively evaluated a 2-year database, including 750 mechanically ventilated patients from six ICUs. *Accidental extubation*, but not self-extubation or reintubation after weaning, increased the risk of nosocomial pneumonia. It is essential to recognize that the difficult airway has not been successfully managed until the trachea is safely extubated and reintubation is prevented for at least 48 hours.

IX. CONCLUSIONS

Critical care physicians manage the airway with great efficacy for the vast majority of patients. However, in up to 10% of patients, difficulties in laryngoscopy occur, caused by unfavorable anatomy of face, airway, or cervical spine. Failed intubation can result in life-threatening hypoxia and must be prevented by strict adherence to recent recommendations (ASA algorithm). The main factors for successful emergency airway management are being prepared and having a plan B ready and securing the airway awake when trouble is suspected. Awake airway management using the fiberoptic scope is the most secure technique, leaving the patient's protective reflexes intact and exerting only minor effects on the cardiocirculatory system.

Recognizing the difficult airway situation only after anesthesia induction may result in "cannot intubate, can ventilate" or catastrophic "cannot intubate, cannot ventilate" situations. The latter situation requires immediate intervention (LMA, Combitube, TTJV) or performing a surgical airway (mainly emergency cricothyrotomy). All those techniques must be practiced in routine cases in order to be performed successfully in emergency situations.

Concerning airway management for long-term ventilatory support, tracheostomy is currently popular because of the introduction of percutaneous dilatational tracheostomy into clinical routine. Long-term translaryngeal intubation might cause severe damage to the laryngeal apparatus and trachea (granuloma formation, stenosis). In patients requiring long-term ventilatory support, we recommend tracheostomy between the first and second week on the ventilator, to reduce the incidence of long-term damage to the laryngeal structures. The technique of tracheostomy used depends on physician preference and experience. However, one should be aware that both conventional surgical tracheostomy as well as PDT require training and knowledge and are characterized by distinct learning curves. PDT should only be performed by experienced operators and under continuous fiberoptic control (best using a TV monitor to observe the entire procedure). Complications of long-term airway management are common and have a discernible morbidity.

Therefore, from the decision to intubate until extubation of the patient, we should always keep in mind that *first, do no harm.*

X. CLINICAL PEARLS

- Noninvasive ventilation techniques in the ICU are increasingly used.

- Adequate and proper positioning of patients for airway management is essential.

- A thorough airway assessment should be performed on all patients before any airway intervention.

- Never act before adequate preoxygenation.

- Each intubation could be a difficult intubation; stay attentive.

- Endotracheal intubation remains the gold standard in invasive airway management, but alternate devices (e.g., supraglottic) are potentially live-saving alternatives.

- Medications are often needed, but be prepared for any potential side effects.

- Awake tracheal intubation is an established approach, but skill and experience are required.

- Timing for tracheostomy remains controversial.

- From intubation until extubation of the patient, do no harm.

SELECTED REFERENCES

All references can be found online at expertconsult.com.

20. Burns KE, Adhikari NK, Keenan SP, et al: Use of noninvasive ventilation to wean critically ill adults off invasive ventilation: meta-analysis and systematic review. *BMJ* 338B:1574, 2009.

86. Cuthbertson BH, Sprung CL, Annane D, et al: The effects of etomidate on adrenal responsiveness and mortality in patients with septic shock. *Intensive Care Med* 35:1868–1876, 2009.

124. Jaber S, Amraoui J, Lefrant JY, et al: Clinical practice and risk factors for immediate complications of endotracheal intubation in the intensive care unit: a prospective, multiple-center study. *Crit Care Med* 34:2355–2361, 2006.

168. Frass M, Staudinger T, Losert H, et al: Airway management during cardiopulmonary resuscitation: a comparative study of bag-valve-mask, laryngeal mask airway and Combitube in a bench model. *Resuscitation* 43:80–81, 1999.

174. Eisenburger P, Laczika K, List M, et al: Comparison of conventional surgical versus Seldinger technique emergency cricothyrotomy performed by inexperienced clinicians. *Anesthesiology* 92:687–690, 2000.

177. Martin LD, Mhyre JM, Shanks AM, et al: 3,423 emergency tracheal intubations at a university hospital: airway outcomes and complications. *Anesthesiology* 114:42–48, 2011.

202. Durbin CG, Jr: Tracheostomy: why, when, and how? *Respir Care* 55:1056–1068, 2010.

209. Griffiths J, Barber VS, Morgan L, et al: Systematic review and meta-analysis of studies of the timing of tracheostomy in adult patients undergoing artificial ventilation. *BMJ* 330:1243, 2005.

285. Engels PT, Bagshaw SM, Meier M, et al: Tracheostomy: from insertion to decannulation. *Can J Surg* 52:427–433, 2009.

313. Lorente L, Blot S, Rello J: New issues and controversies in the prevention of ventilator-associated pneumonia. *Am J Respir Crit Care Med* 182:870–876, 2010.

PART 6

Postintubation Procedures

Chapter 47

Endotracheal Tube and Respiratory Care

THOMAS C. MORT | JEFFREY P. KECK JR. | LEAH MEISTERLING

I. INTRODUCTION

The earliest recorded use of airway manipulation with an artificial device dates back to early Roman civilization when Asclepiades performed a tracheostomy for laryngeal edema. Today it is clear that the role of the endotracheal tube (ETT) in medicine is as invaluable as that of any other medical device created to date. The establishment of a definitive airway via the ETT in both elective and emergency situations has allowed for the delivery of immediate life-sustaining therapies during resuscitation, the maintenance of oxygenation and ventilation in prolonged illness, and the (temporary) delivery of inhaled anesthesia.[1] This chapter begins with a brief history of the development of the ETT. It describes the various ETTs available along with their indications for use and respective limitations. It reviews basic airway anatomy with regard to ETT placement, proper positioning and stabilization of the ETT, and complications attributed to its use. Finally, it addresses respiratory care of the intubated and mechanically ventilated patient.

II. PROPERTIES OF THE ENDOTRACHEAL TUBE

A. Anatomy of the Endotracheal Tube

Between the time of Asclepiades and the present, ETTs have been constructed of a variety of materials, including reed, brass, and steel. Eventually, in 1917, Magill and Rowbotham manufactured them from rubber for the purpose of administering anesthesia.[2] In 1928, when Guedel and Waters added a protective cuff to prevent aspiration, the modern ETT was born. Rubber, however, had limitations in this application, such as increased stiffness with rising temperature and limited adhesive properties with different polymers, which required the cuffs to be manufactured from the same polymer as the tube.[3] These shortcomings led to the search for alternative materials. In 1967, polyvinyl chloride (PVC) was popularized by Dr. S.A. Leader, and it has since been the material most commonly used. One property that makes PVC attractive is that it provides stiffness to an ETT at room temperature to assist with intubation yet becomes more malleable with the increased temperature in situ. Other properties include the ability to embed radiopaque lines in the material to assist with positioning and recognition on a radiograph. Because it accepts many materials, the addition of an exteriorized inflation line to connect the pilot balloon to the cuff can allow for varied cuff materials. Finally, it simply is much lower in cost than other available materials.[3]

The 15-mm adapter allows for universality between ventilating devices such as a bag-mask ventilation system, anesthesia circuit, or ventilator circuit. The adapter fits ETTs as large as 12 mm internal diameter and as small as 3 mm, thereby providing further commonality among multiple ETTs and ventilating devices. Having one standard size also allows for interchange between devices made for tracheostomies or ETTs. The adapter is removable to allow for passage of intraluminal devices (e.g., bronchoscope, suction catheter) or to allow passage of the ETT via a supraglottic airway device such as a laryngeal mask airway (LMA, LMA North America, San Diego, CA). Adapter removal may facilitate the extraction of extensive biofilm accumulation or mucus plugs. Additionally, some clinicians choose to resize (shorten) the ETT.[4]

The Murphy eye, so named for Peter Murphy, an English anesthetist, is designed to provide an extra (secondary) portal for ventilation should the most distal lumen become opacified by bodily fluids, foreign bodies, or soft tissue prolapse. The most typical manifestation of this phenomenon occurs when the distal lumen abuts soft tissue of the tracheal tree, thereby occluding distal flow, or when secretion build-up occludes the distal opening. However, both native and foreign materials are also capable of creating such a dilemma, including mucus, blood, and foreign bodies. Management of such an obstruction is discussed later in this chapter.

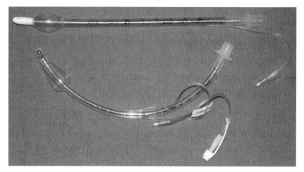

Figure 47-1 Structural comparison of the intubating laryngeal mask airway (ILMA) high-pressure, low-volume (HPLV) cuff *(top)* and a high-volume, low-pressure (HVLP) cuff *(bottom)*. (Courtesy of LMA North America, San Diego, CA.)

The cuffs on the early ETTs were, like the tubes themselves, composed of rubber. The rubber ETT cuffs had limitations such as the need for elevated inflation pressures (high pressure, low volume [HPLV]) to fill the cuff and occlude the airway surrounding the ETT. These high inflation pressures result in the transmission of high lateral pressures to the tracheal wall, albeit in a very minimal contact area, to maintain a seal. The trachea is not circular but rather D–shaped. HPLV cuffs inflate in a circular manner, thereby altering the structure of the trachea; the high pressure exerted on the tracheal wall impairs capillary pressure and possibly results in greater mucosal ischemia.[5] The most commonly used HPLV cuffs in today's practice are the reusable silicone ETTs found with intubating LMAs (ILMAs) (Fig. 47-1). Caution should be exercised when using these ETTs for prolonged periods, given their inherent risk of tracheal mucosal damage. The introduction of PVC-based cuffs reduced this problem because the cuff wall was more supple and thinner, allowing the cuff to accommodate high volume and low pressure (HVLP) and thus providing an adequate seal with lower lateral wall pressures.[3,5,6] The main value of the HVLP cuff is its ability to conform to the irregular borders of the trachea.[7-9] Polyurethane is even thinner and more pliable, with increased tensile strength, allowing for higher volumes, larger contact areas, and minimal mucosal pressures.[10] Foam-based cuffs exist and provide maximal conformation to the tracheal walls, but they do little for the prevention of microaspiration.[9]

Remodeling of the cuff has been particularly driven by the desire to improve prevention of ventilator-associated pneumonia (VAP), and the shape of the cuff has also been altered. The Mallinckrodt TaperGuard Evac ETT (Covidien, Boulder, CO) is a new option that has been demonstrated in randomized, controlled trials to reduce microaspiration by as much as 83%, compared with traditional HVLP barrel shaped cuffs (Fig. 47-2).[8] It is postulated that a barrel-shaped tube tends to wrinkle and fold in an attempt to conform to the tracheal wall, allowing small channels for potential microaspiration, whereas the bulbous, conical shape of the TaperGuard ETT may reduce wrinkling and thus decrease the incidence of microaspiration. Continued work in this area may lead to improved tracheal wall sealing capabilities at safe levels

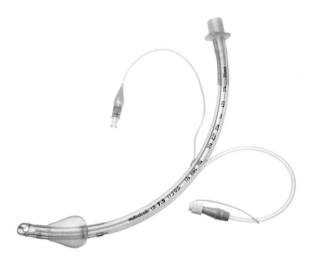

Figure 47-2 Taperguard endotracheal tube cuff. (Courtesy Covidien, Boulder, CO.)

of pressure while minimizing potential pathways for the translocation of oronasal and gastric secretions, which is thought to be the prime etiologic pathway for VAP.[11]

The pilot balloon of an ETT functions as an indirect volume gauge for the ETT cuff, relative to the amount of air located in the cuff (inflated or deflated). The pilot balloon does not provide information about the absolute volume insufflated or the pressure exerted on the tracheal mucosa. When a pilot balloon fails or is an impediment to an intubation, options are generally limited to a tracheal tube exchange.[12-14] Pilot balloon failures have multiple causes. Shearing along the ETT connection (usually due to contact with dentition), cracked inflation valves (from syringe manipulation or trauma), material aging, and pilot tubing laceration due to biting all cause the ETT cuff to lose air over time.[15-18] Simple techniques have been described to replace a pilot balloon in a variety of clinical situations using equipment readily available in the operating room. Needles or intravenous catheters with stopcocks or claves, epidural clamp connectors, and commercially available repair kits (Fig. 47-3) provide reliable

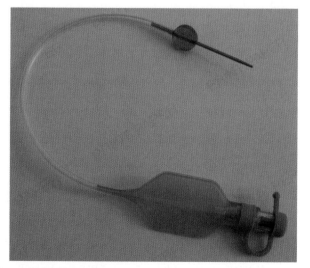

Figure 47-3 Pilot balloon repair device. (Courtesy Instrumentation Industries, Bethel Park, PA.)

substitutions for incompetent pilot balloons when they are connected to the pilot-cuff inflation line.[19,20] The procedure for replacing an incompetent valve is as follows: cut the inflation tube distal to the pilot balloon; insert a needle or intravenous catheter into the cut end (or affix the hub of an epidural catheter to the cut end); and use a stopcock or clave (an item capable of stemming the entrance of air) on the needle or catheter after insufflation, paying careful attention not to overinflate.

B. Development and Properties of the Endotracheal Tube

The purpose of the ETT has always been the same, and it has always had the same inherent problems. Technology continues to advance the standard ETT for improved function and decreased physiologic insult. Rather than compensate for the resistance produced by a rubber or PVC ETT, a newly designed ETT has been produced of ultrathin polyurethane that is reinforced with wire to resist collapsing and kinking. This wire is unique in that it has an elastic shape memory to prevent deformation. The internal diameter is increased without compromising the rigid shape of the ETT. The result is a tube with a resistance similar to that of the upper airway that is lighter, offers less airflow resistance, and, when compressed, forms an egg shape rather than an oval.[21] Experimentally, this new design has been shown to decrease inspiratory and expiratory resistance by 60% each and the inspiratory, expiratory, and total work of breathing (WOB) by 70%, 47%, and 45%, respectively.[22,23]

The use of the ETT continues to expand. No longer is it expected to be simply a conduit for ventilation. As the technology has advanced, the original ETT has steadily been outfitted with a host of successful innovations to improve patient care, whether for convenience or necessity. For example, modifications to the cuff to improve occlusion of the trachea in an effort to prevent microaspiration, coupled with an extra subglottic suctioning port (and other patient care maneuvers), have served to vastly reduce the incidence of VAP.[7-9] Another example is the modification of the surfaces of the ETT to minimize bacterial adhesion and thereby minimize biofilm accumulation.[24] As for bells and whistles, there are ETTs with fiberoptic cameras distally, allowing for ease of placement and the possibility of continued intratracheal surveillance. Another example is the addition of multiple sensors, for so-called bioimpedance cardiography, that are capable of monitoring stroke volume variation, cardiac output, systemic vascular resistance, and arterial pressures (due to the close proximity of the ETT and the aorta) and thereby, at least theoretically, preventing the need for further invasive technologies. Continued study of these modifications may provide justification to adapt these technologies to patient care.

C. Physiologic Effects of Endotracheal Tube Placement

The placement of an ETT, whether oral, nasal, or translaryngeal, is unnatural. Certain physiologic changes occur that must be addressed, including those created by the

ETT itself and those modified by its presence. The properties inherent to the ETT are relatively obvious: it causes a partial obstruction, resulting in a decrease in the normal airway circumference and the possibility of turbulent air flow patterns. Additionally, the narrowed conduit leads to higher pressure relationships with lower flows, possibly leading to damaged mucosa distally. The presence of the ETT is a nidus for the inflammatory cascade. Despite its relatively hypoallergenic profile, it is still a recognizable foreign body and as such triggers well-defined host responses. Placement of the device, regardless of the care used in placing it, still results in mechanical trauma to all of the periglottic mucosalized regions and therefore decreases the ability of the respiratory mucosa to protect itself. Finally, the ETT may cause airway alteration secondary to pressure injury.

The body's response to the ETT is also multifaceted, affecting mechanics, structure, and physiologic function. Loss of humidity and heat is the most obvious effect of replacing the regular mucosa with a foreign conduit. The gas that is delivered is already dry and cool, but bypassing the patient's natural ability to heat and humidify leads to problems more distally, including reduced ciliary function, inspissated secretions, and increased mucus plugging. The normally motile respiratory cilia are essentially paralyzed, leading to impaired secretion management. The body lacks its normal ability to move debris in a proximal direction, and collection sites develop within the tracheobronchial tree, leading to multiple potential areas for infection. Additionally, these partially or completely occluded areas may result in lobar collapse and, consequently, a ventilation-perfusion mismatch. This obstruction can also create an inability to completely exhale, leading to breath stacking and auto-PEEP (positive end-expiratory pressure) and possibly resultant barotrauma.

D. Complications of Endotracheal Tube Placement

Complications associated with ETT placement should be grouped into three major subcategories: those that occur at intubation, those that occur with the ETT in situ, and postextubation sequelae.[25] The problems associated with placement are numerous and can be worsened in emergencies, with multiple attempts, use of a variety of devices, or inexperience of the operator.[26] Problems at placement include dental and oral problems, maxillofacial damage, displacement of the arytenoid cartilages, vocal cord ulceration or dysfunction, airway perforation, autonomic hyperactivity, and, of course, failed intubation. Structural damage is unlikely to be repaired until the patient no longer requires intubation, unless the damage interferes with ventilation and oxygenation. Problems that occur as a result of an in situ ETT include those related to the ETT, such as aspiration, vocal cord paralysis, or transient nerve palsy; ulceration and granuloma formation in the trachea and on the cords; tracheal synechiae; subglottic stenosis; laryngeal webbing; tracheomalacia; tracheoesophageal, tracheoinnominate, or tracheocarotid fistula; and recurrent and superior laryngeal nerve damage.[27] Other complications are related to

mechanical ventilation facilitated by the ETT and include aspiration, barotrauma (pneumothorax, pneumomediastinum), VAP, and dislodgement.[28] Finally, postextubation complications can lead to long-term morbidity or the urgent need for reintubation. Many of the postextubation culprits have already been encountered as complications of ETT placement or presence, particularly subglottic stenosis, vocal cord injury, and hoarseness.[28,29]

III. ENDOTRACHEAL TUBES AND OTHER AIRWAY ADJUNCTS

A. Choice of Endotracheal Tube Size

In selecting an ETT, consideration must be given to the functional reason for placement as well as patient-specific factors such as body height, gender, airway integrity, airway pathology, and previous airway manipulation or instrumentation. Theoretically, short-term placement for anesthesia should be different than placement for prolonged support with mechanical ventilation or for fiberoptic bronchoscopy to aid therapy. Generally, the trachea of an adult female accepts a tube of 7.5 to 8.0 mm and that of a male accepts one of 8.5 to 9.0 mm, but typically a 7.0-mm ETT is used for females and an 8.0-mm tube for males, at least in the United States. It is also generally accepted that an ETT of at least 8.0 mm is needed for competent use of an adult-based bronchoscopic investigation.[30]

1. Small Tubes and Airway Resistance

The physics of laminar gas flow through a conduit are described by the Hagen-Poiseuille equation, which reflects the relationship of resistance varying inversely with the fourth power of tube radius. Despite the fact that gas flow through ETTs is often turbulent rather than laminar, the effect on resistance to gas flow represented by each millimeter decrease in tube size is considerable, ranging from 25% to 100%.[31] Airway resistance is affected by more than tube diameter: the presence of secretion within the tube, ETT kinking, and positioning of the head and neck can also increase the tendency for turbulent flow.[32,33] The fundamental principle of which to be mindful is that airway resistance induced by an ETT is inversely proportional to the tube size—hence, the mantra that the largest tube is usually the best size.[34]

Airway resistance increases with decreasing ETT diameter, whether due to internal occlusion, smaller size, or external compression. As airway resistance increases, WOB also increases.[31] The increase in WOB associated with a 1-mm reduction in ETT diameter varies in accordance with tidal volume and respiratory rate at a given minute ventilation and can range from 34% to 154%.[31] When ventilation is controlled, the increase in WOB related to ETT resistance is seldom of any consequence, because it is overcome by ventilator adjustments. However, small-diameter tubes create greater difficulty for patients in weaning from ventilatory support due to the higher levels of resistance encountered when attempting to breathe spontaneously.[35,36] It has been suggested that an inability to spontaneously ventilate due to the increased WOB imposed by a 7-mm ETT might indicate that extubation will fail regardless of tube size.[37,38]

Increased airway resistance associated with a smaller-diameter ETT may also be associated with inadvertent PEEP. Patients with high oxygen consumption, increased carbon dioxide production, or ventilation-perfusion relationships that produce high dead space ventilation often require higher minute ventilations to achieve appropriate ventilation and oxygenation. The gas flows necessary to maintain such a minute ventilation are also quite high, and the resistance imposed by a smaller-diameter ETT further prohibits the completion of expiratory flow before initiation of the subsequent inspiration. This breath stacking results in air trapping and unwanted PEEP, magnifying the risk of mechanical ventilation because barotrauma and subsequent intrathoracic over-pressure could result in circulatory compromise.[39]

The restriction to gas flow through any ETT increases dramatically when devices such as a suction catheter or bronchoscope are placed in the lumen. The cross-sectional area of the tube is effectively reduced by an amount equal to the cross-sectional area of the device inserted into the tube. The limitation of gas flow has consequences for both the inspiratory and expiratory phases: inspiratory flow may be inadequate to maintain oxygenation and ventilation during the procedure, and retarded expiratory flow may lead to overdistention resulting in barotrauma or circulatory compromise.[40]

2. Large Tubes and Trauma

Whereas smaller-diameter ETTs have disadvantages related to gas flow and airway resistance, larger tubes are more frequently associated with traumatic placements and damage to both the laryngeal structures and the tracheal mucosa.[37,38,41] Larger ETTs are associated with a higher incidence of sore throat after general anesthesia, compared with smaller-diameter tubes, but this difference is relatively negligible with long-term intubation.[42] With prolonged intubation, laryngeal trauma is more likely. Women, because of the inherently smaller size of their airway, are more susceptible to injury than men.[43,44]

Laryngeal structures at particular risk for trauma are the arytenoid cartilages and the cricoid cartilage. Trauma results not only from the shape discrepancy between the round ETT and the angular, wedge-shaped glottic opening but also from direct contact and pressure on these structures and from repetitive tube movement, which leads to ulceration or erosion of the protective mucosa.[44-46] Tracheal mucosal injury can also occur because of the irregular surfaces created by wrinkling and folding of the ETT cuff or the externalized pilot tube used to fill the ETT cuff. If the tracheal lumen is "overcrowded," airway injury is more likely to occur when large tubes are used and little cuff volume is required to seal the airway.[47]

B. Potentially Beneficial Alternatives to the Standard Endotracheal Tube

1. Preformed and Reinforced Tubes

Modifications to the ETT that are made in the operating room setting to accomplish specific surgeries are often developed in response to interference and access issues. The ability to work without disturbing the ETT has led to several variations of the ETT that can be placed safely

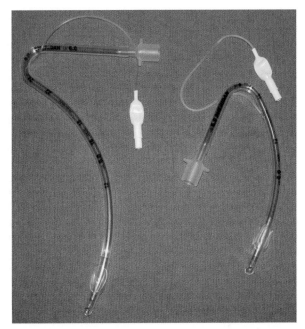

Figure 47-4 Nasal *(left)* and oral *(right)* Ring-Adair-Elwyn (RAE) preformed endotracheal tubes. *(Courtesy Covidien, Mansfield, MA.)*

and remove the risk of inadvertent advancement, dislodgement, kinking, or obstruction. ETTs used in remote locations also have airway access issues associated with tube kinking and partial occlusion, which typically are related to positioning problems and associated comorbidities. In part because of less stringent vigilance, unintended consequences of ETT use outside the operating room may result in more drastic outcomes. In response to these dilemmas, a variety of tubes have been developed to maintain their shape and patency in locations where distortion might cause kinking and occlusion.

Rigid, preformed tubes such as those developed for long-term use in tracheostomy were known to maintain their patency despite the need for angulation. Preformed tubes have been developed for specific application in anesthesia practice as well. The Ring-Adair-Elwyn (RAE) tubes (Mallinckrodt Inc., Pleasanton, CA), both oral and nasal (Fig. 47-4), maintain a fixed contour similar to the average facial profile, allowing for head and neck surgery while minimizing surgical field interference. Their contour also reduces the risk of pressure injury to the posterior pharynx when repositioning is desired. The intra-airway length is tied to the size of the ETT, with a relatively appropriate depth based on the average size of a patient for whom the tube might be selected.[48,49]

An anode or armored tube with an embedded wire coil is designed to minimize kinking even with quite severe position-induced angulation. Armored tubes are popular for use in head and neck surgery where remote airway access and the potential for kinking of the ETT are concerns. Placement of an armored tube through a tracheostomy for procedures such as laryngectomy is a common practice; it allows placement during surgical procedures such that the tube can be mobilized or the circuit draped away from the field without a high risk of tube kinking. The other common use of a wire-reinforced tube is with the ILMA. These tubes are designed to facilitate placement through the device and to be used for short periods of time. The HPLV cuff and the theoretical possibility of kinking and resultant airway obstruction make the long-term use of ILMAs risky.

The embedded wire concept of the armored ETT has also been developed for long-term tracheostomy use. Although the armored tracheostomy tube is not free of risks, one advantage is that its flexibility allows its length and intratracheal depth to be adjusted, which may be beneficial if tracheomalacia at the level of the cuff develops.[50] These tracheostomy tubes are also popular for use in morbidly obese patients, in whom, because of the depth of tissue, preformed tracheostomy tubes may not have the shape required to fit an individual patient. One major consequence of this type of reinforced ETT may occur when external pressure is applied to the wire-reinforced component (i.e., by patient biting). Once a compression threshold is reached, the luminal support provided by the wire may be compromised, and a permanent, irreparable dent remains that can significantly endanger ventilation and suctioning capabilities.

2. Laser Tubes

Progress in laser technology has advanced surgical capabilities, particularly for airway surgery. To protect patients and health care providers from laser-induced injury to eyes and airways, special precautions are required. Fire is the most serious danger associated with the use of lasers in the operating room, especially when a laser is used in airway surgery.[30,51-53] A major complication related to the use of lasers for laryngeal surgery is ignition of the ETT.[54] The laser beam may ignite the tube by direct penetration or indirectly if burning tissue is inhaled into the tube.[30,51,52,55] The ease of ignition is related to the ETT material, the concentration of oxygen in use, and any other adjunctive materials or gases that could support combustion.[30,52,55] Most ETTs are constructed of PVC, which is highly flammable. Ideally, PVC tubes should not be used for airways when a laser is employed.[51,55,56]

ETTs can be laser-proofed or protected from the laser beam by wrapping them with either reflective metal tape or muslin. Ideally, they should be constructed from noncombustible materials. In particular, the ETT cuff is vulnerable to puncture by the laser beam and should be filled with saline or water, which allows more energy to be absorbed before disruption.[30,52,55] One trick to enhance appreciation of a penetrated, defective cuff, is to place a dye indicator, such as methylene blue, into the solution that is instilled into the cuff. Any leakage will clearly mark the airway and alert the provider to the potential dangers.[57] Protecting the tube from the laser beam by wrapping it with a foil tape has proved effective (commercial devices are available) (Fig. 47-5).[58] Tubes made of materials such as metal and silicone and those with special double cuffs also reduce the risk of airway fires and injury during laser airway surgery.[51,58]

3. Subglottic Suctioning Evac Endotracheal Tubes

Hospitalized patients who require mechanical ventilation are susceptible to the development of aspiration pneumonia. VAP is known to increase hospital length of stay, health care costs, and mortality.[59] Organisms that grow in pooled subglottic secretions above the inflated cuff of

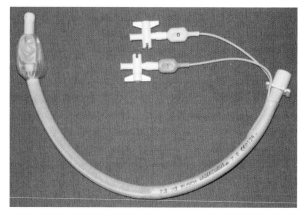

Figure 47-5 Rusch Lasertubus laser-safe endotracheal tube. (Courtesy Teleflex Medical, Durham, NC.)

the ETT, but beneath the glottis, have previously been unmeasurable with any reliability and are now demonstrated to be a major impetus for VAP. Several nursing care measures may be taken to reduce the incidence of VAP caused by this route, including improved oral care, patient positioning by elevating the head of the bed past 30 degrees, frequent suctioning, and ensuring postpyloric tube feedings, but none of these measures completely stops the production.[60]

The presence of these pooled collections has led to the development of specific ETTs that possess a dedicated suction system capable of emptying this area of debris. Drainage of subglottic secretions has been shown to prevent VAP.[61-64] The currently available subglottic drainage ETTs have a suction lumen that opens on the external (posterolateral) surface of the ETT immediately above the cuff (Fig. 47-6). The lumen is attached to constant or intermittent suction for active drainage of the space. Although these ETTs are beneficial, their efficacy is not 100%, and therefore all of the aforementioned nursing care actions remain vital to good hygiene and prevention of VAP. The subglottic drainage tubes have been further developed to include variations in cuff construction (materials, shapes, volumes, locations) that help to prevent aspiration of the subglottic debris.

Subglottic secretions are not the only recognized cause for VAP. Biofilm is an accumulation of debris adhered to the internal circumference of the ETT that is composed of tissue, secretions, mucus, and undetermined bacteria load. Biofilm can be aspirated, leading to a nidus for infection or causing an area of obstruction to airflow. Biofilm removal and reduction by hygiene care are currently

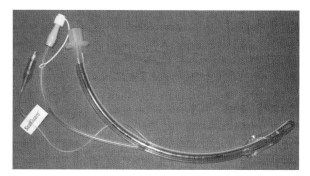

Figure 47-6 Mallinckrodt Sealguard Evac Endotracheal Tube. (Courtesy Covidien, Mansfield, MA.)

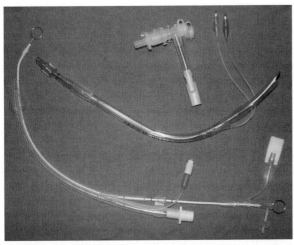

Figure 47-7 Endobronchial blocking devices for lung isolation. Mallinckrodt Endobronchial Tube *(top)*. (Covidien, Mansfield, MA); Fuji TCB Univent Tube *(bottom)*. (Phycon Products, Tokyo, Japan).

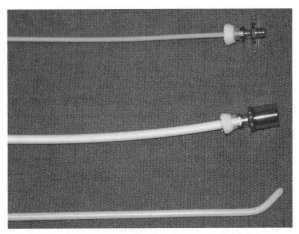

Figure 47-8 A selection of airway exchange catheters. Double-lumen airway exchange catheter *(top)*, Aintree Intubation Catheter *(center)* and Portex Single-Use Bougie *(bottom)*. (Aintree Courtesy Cook Medical, Bloomington, IN; Portex Courtesy Smiths Medical, Carlsbad, CA.)

better researched than prevention. However, there is a growing interest in the reduction of biofilm through construction of ETTs impregnated with antimicrobial agents.[65-67] The ability of such developments to affect the incidence of VAP has not yet been proved.

4. Double-Lumen Endotracheal Tubes

The uses of a double-lumen endotracheal tube (DLT) (Fig. 47-7) can be separated into relative and absolute indications. The absolute indications are isolation, to avoid soilage or contamination of the contralateral lung tissue when dealing with infections or frank hemoptysis from a unilateral location, bronchoalveolar lavage, and one-lung ventilation (OLV). The most common reason for placement is OLV for surgical exposure, but OLV can also be important in cases of bronchopleural or broncho-cutaneous fistula, unilateral pulmonary hemorrhage, giant unilateral bulla or cyst, and severe unilateral ventilation-perfusion mismatch. The relative indications all deal with surgical exposure. Complementing the DLT as another option for lung isolation, particularly if a DLT cannot be placed, are bronchial blocking devices. However, the DLT has an advantage because of the ability to pass suctioning catheters or fiberoptic devices into the area on collapse without drastically jeopardizing OLV or contaminating the contralateral side.

Relative contraindications to the placement of a DLT are fairly minimal. They include patient refusal (likely due to risk of trauma secondary to the large size), a known difficult airway, and the speed with which an isolated airway must be established. In patients with difficult airways, specially designed airway exchange catheters (Cook Medical, Bloomington, IN) (Fig. 47-8) can be used after placement of a conventional ETT to facilitate DLT placement. Additionally, some makers of video laryngoscopic technologies have developed specific DLT devices. The time required for placement is usually the biggest detractor to their use. Situations such as frank hemoptysis may be better served by a rapid-sequence induction and placement of a contralateral, main stem, single-lumen ETT for stabilization.

This technique is not ideal for long-term management. The long-term use of the DLT in the intensive care unit

(ICU) setting (>24 to 48 hours) must be approached with caution, because the two smaller-diameter lumens are at significantly increased risk for partial or complete occlusion. Consideration should be given to close monitoring of luminal patency with fiberoptic evaluation on a regular basis and optimization of luminal hygiene to reduce mucus or biofilm accumulation.

5. Supraglottic Airways

Supraglottic devices are continually coming onto the market. Largely designed for shorter surgical procedures to deliver general anesthesia, their use seems to be growing past their original intent. Supraglottic airways (Fig. 47-9) such as the LMA, the esophageal-tracheal Combitube (ETC, Tyco Healthcare, Mansfield, MA), the King LT (King Systems, Noblesville, IN), and other variants have provided valuable means of establishing an (unsecured) airway in an emergency. Equally important is their ability to function as a conduit for endotracheal intubation. For example, the ILMA is a blind passage

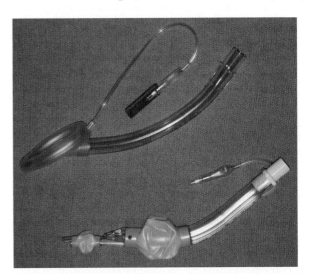

Figure 47-9 Supraglottic devices. LMA Unique *(top)*, (Courtesy USA) King LT Supraglottic Device *(bottom)*. (LMA Unique courtesy LMA North America Inc., San Diego, CA; King LT courtesy King Systems, Noblesville, IN.)

device that is designed to place an ETT through the LMA. Recently, use of the LMA as a conduit for fiberoptic bronchoscopy and subsequent ETT placement has also been demonstrated in emergency situations.[68] Although these devices do not provide classically definitive airways, their utility is unsurpassed in helping to manage the difficult airway.

IV. PROPER SAFEGUARDING OF THE AIRWAY

A. Airway Evaluation: Predicting the Difficult Airway

The decision to intubate, whether for airway protection, ventilatory failure, inadequate oxygenation, or medication delivery, is often difficult, but equally difficult can be the decision of how to intubate. Each patient and airway is unique, as is the clinical setting and the judgment, skill, and equipment of the airway team that responds. Outside the operating room, time often does not allow a comprehensive evaluation and establishment of a plan complete with contingencies before the decision to intubate must be made. Performance of a proper airway evaluation before intubation is attempted can dramatically improve outcomes.

However, a difficult airway should be assumed when one approaches the patient outside the controlled setting of the operating room. An airway physical examination is paramount to predicting a successful attempt. Criteria such as dental status, mouth opening, thyromental distance, cervical range of motion, Mallampati score, and neck circumference are all standard examination points. However, the emergent intubation presents a host of new, potentially detrimental issues not seen in operating room intubations. For example, hemodynamics may not allow for the controlled process typically seen in the operating room. Trauma patients may have actively unstable facial fractures or cervical vertebral injuries that merit inline stabilization and modified techniques for tube placement. Neurosurgical patients may have external fixators to stabilize injuries or intracranial monitoring devices that make it difficult to position the head. The type of bed a patient is in can also create access issues with intubation. A bariatric bed with an inflatable mattress can be very difficult to properly ramp, thereby making positioning suboptimal. Last, but not least, is the patient with failed extubation who must be reintubated. Issues with anxiety, hypoxemia, decreased functional residual and closing capacities, copious secretions, residual airway edema, and subglottic stenosis all make a repeat attempt more difficult than the first pass.[28]

B. Identifying Proper Position of the Endotracheal Tube

1. Detection of Esophageal Intubation

Once the clinician has deemed intubation necessary and has performed the intervention, confirmation of proper ET placement must be provided expeditiously. An incorrectly positioned ETT can produce adverse effects, especially in an already apneic patient. Unrecognized

esophageal intubation can have disastrous consequences with a reported incidence as high as 8% in critical patients.[69] Therefore, a brief discussion of verification of ETT placement is warranted.

Once intubation has been accomplished, confirmation of proper placement of the ETT in the trachea needs to be achieved, ideally by the detection of end-tidal carbon dioxide ($EtCO_2$) in expired gases using capnography or other capnometric (colorimetric) methods.[70] The detection of $EtCO_2$ is not fail-safe and does not guarantee that the ETT is positioned within the tracheal lumen (e.g., the tip may lie above the vocal cords). After three to five breaths, the absence of $EtCO_2$ suggests a nontracheal placement. Blockage or soilage of the $EtCO_2$ detection device can hamper efforts. $EtCO_2$ detection should be complemented with indirect maneuvers such as auscultation, ETT misting or fogging, bag compliance, chest wall excursions, lack of phonation, and improved oxygen saturation. The dependence of any $EtCO_2$ detection device on adequate cardiac output has spurred utilization of an esophageal detector device (Fig. 47-10). It is essentially an air-filled bulb placed on the end of an in situ ETT. After a vacuum has been created by squeezing the bulb, immediate re-expansion should occur when the bulb is placed on an ETT in the trachea (any column of air). If the ETT is esophageal, the suction created by the bulb will draw the pliable esophageal tissue into the distal lumen of the ETT, preventing full expansion of the bulb on top of the ETT (column of soft tissue).[71-73]

If intubation is to occur in a patient with cardiac arrest, capnometry may be fallible given the amount of down time and the lack of any life-sustaining cardiac output. If cardiopulmonary resuscitation (CPR) is adequate, this technicality is likely to be moot. However, esophageal bulb detectors can be helpful in this situation, although false-positives and false-negatives do occur and confound ETT verification. Still other methods that are independent of carbon dioxide and cardiac output exist, such as a tracheal whistle to verify correct placement (Box 47-1), but not one is without limitations.[72-77] Ideally, two methods are to be considered fail-safe: direct or indirect visualization of the ETT traversing the vocal cords and fiberoptic verification via the ETT lumen. The limitation of direct laryngoscopy is the operator's line of sight to the glottic opening. The key is to identify the ETT

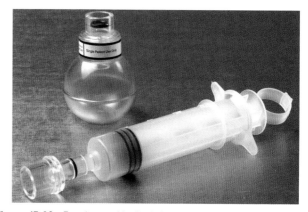

Figure 47-10 Esophageal bulb detector and a homemade syringe device. (Courtesy Wolfe-Tory Medical, Inc.)

Box 47-1	Methods Used to Verify Endotracheal Tube Placement

Sustainable, exhaled CO_2 by capnography or colorimetric methods

Fiberoptic visualization of carina

Videolaryngoscopic visualization of translaryngeal endotracheal tube position

Direct laryngoscopic visualization of translaryngeal position

Positive response with esophageal bulb detector device or syringe method

Auscultation of breath sounds in bilateral lung fields and absence of same in epigastric area

Visualization of chest wall movement with spontaneous patient efforts

Reservoir bag synchrony with spontaneous patient efforts

Palpable ballottement of cuff in suprasternal notch

Acoustic reflectometry

Transtracheal illumination

Chest roentgenogram

Condensation in endotracheal tube

Lack of phonation in the nonparalyzed, semiconscious patient

Bougie passage to distinguish between tracheobronchial tree and esophagus

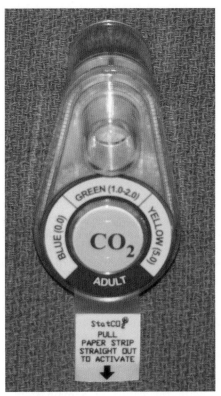

Figure 47-11 Example of a colorimetric capnometric device. (Courtesy Mercury Medical, Clearwater, FL.)

positioned in the glottis, not simply to see it go in. An indirect method such as video laryngoscopy does improve the validity of ETT passage. Fiberoptic verification is hampered by equipment availability at the bedside, any airway or ETT soilage, time constraints, and operator skill. Chest rise and condensation from expired gas found in the ETT have also been used, but these signs may occur in esophageal intubations as well.[77] Therefore, the gold standard used today is the presence of $EtCO_2$ in expired gases as demonstrated by capnography or other colorimetric techniques.[70]

Capnography yields quantifiable measurements of inspired and expired gases in addition to a waveform generated with each tidal volume. Although not without limitations (e.g., lack of portability, need for a power source), capnography reliably identifies initial proper placement of the ETT (nonesophageal) and provides a continuous verification of ETT security. If esophageal intubation has occurred, a gradual reduction in height of the capnograph waveforms is observed with successive breaths. False-positive results during esophageal intubations may occur in situations of ingested CO_2-containing or -liberating substances (e.g., carbonated beverages) before intubation, bag-mask ventilation with inflation of expired air into the stomach, or intubation of the supralaryngeal hypopharynx.[78] Inappropriate extubations may occur due to misinterpretation of a false-negative situation because an $EtCO_2$ waveform is lacking despite proper placement. This error may occur with unrecognized circuit disconnections, an obstructed or kinked ETT, a disconnected or contaminated gas sampling line (water, secretions, entrainment of room air), equipment failure, severe bronchospasm, or inadequate cardiac output. Unquestionably, capnography is dependent on pulmonary blood flow. In the absence of perfusion (e.g., cardiac arrest), the utility of capnography can be limited; however, even in very low-flow states (e.g., CPR, separation from

cardiopulmonary bypass), it has been shown to provide effective detection. Ornato and colleagues used an animal model to evaluate the relationship between cardiac output (CO) and $EtCO_2$. Through manipulation of CO, with inotropes or controlled hemorrhage, a logarithmic relationship between CO and $EtCO_2$ was demonstrated.[50] This finding shows that capnography is useful in cardiac resuscitation to assist with evaluation of low-flow states and adequacy of perfusion.

To alleviate the logistic concerns with capnography in emergency situations—mainly the lack of portability and the need for a power source—a portable and reliable means of detecting $EtCO_2$ was developed. Colorimetric $EtCO_2$ uses a detector impregnated with metacresol purple (Fig. 47-11). This indicator is pH sensitive and changes color, from purple to yellow, in the presence of CO_2. The devices are disposable, attach between the ETT and the circuit or bag, and provide a rapid and reliable indication of CO_2 concentration on a graded scale: A (purple) corresponds to an $EtCO_2$ level of 0.5%, B (tan) to a level of 0.5% to 2%, and C (yellow) to a level greater than 2%.[70,77] Limitations of this method are that it is ineffective with exposure to humidified gases, vomitus, or secretions and in cases of prolonged cardiac arrest or low-perfusion states. False-positive results can occur as well, just as in capnography. Delays in recognition of esophageal intubation with colorimetric capnometry have been reported far more often than with capnography, particularly in patients with prolonged bag-mask ventilation or ingestion of $EtCO_2$-containing substances before intubation. Therefore, capnography simply is the best method for detection of esophageal intubation.[79]

As mentioned previously, the esophageal bulb detector capitalizes on the physical characteristics of the esophagus, which, unlike the trachea, collapses when negative pressure is applied. Commercial devices exist, but a homemade version can be improvised using a syringe that attaches to the end of the ETT. When the plunger is withdrawn, resistance is appreciated if an esophageal intubation has occurred, because the walls of the esophagus collapse around the ETT. Unencumbered aspiration of the plunger occurs with proper tracheal placement.[71] Bulb detector devices are reported to be reliable and effective, with one study demonstrating a sensitivity of 100% and a specificity of 99%.[72] However, other studies have reported limitations and false-negative results in patients with copious or aspirated secretions, gastric distention, vomitus in the airway, morbid obesity, or reduced functional residual capacity.[71,80-83]

A little used but highly effective method of detecting proper ETT location is the passage of a catheter (e.g., bougie) via the ETT to decipher a straight smooth muscle pathway (esophagus without pathology) or a more rigid, angulated tube with reduction in the luminal diameter (tracheobronchial tree). A bougie can be used in this fashion, particularly at the time it is being used as an adjunct to intubation, or later if necessary. Gentle advancement to 28 to 34 cm (in adults) typically results in contact with the carina or a main stem bronchus. Further advancement down a main stem bronchus should be limited by the secondary lobar carina. Gentle unopposed advancement of the bougie beyond 35 cm suggests esophageal placement (assuming no esophageal pathology).

2. Confirmation of Appropriate Depth of Insertion

After correct tracheal placement of the ETT has been verified, it is imperative to identify the correct depth of the ETT to ensure adequate ventilation of each lung.[49] Before addressing the various methods that assist in confirmation of appropriate ETT depth, a brief discussion of what is considered to be the correct depth is warranted. Malpositioning of ETTs occurs frequently, with unrecognized right main stem intubation occurring in approximately 4% of chest radiographs.[49,69,84] The generally accepted depth of insertion of the ETT is between 2 and 7 cm above the carina, optimally between 4 and 7 cm above the carina with the head and neck in a neutral position.[49,77,85-87] It is important to realize this, because flexion-extension movements of the neck can displace the ETT upward or downward with resultant extubation or main stem intubation, respectively. Typically the right main stem bronchus is entered, given its straighter trajectory in relation to the trachea. If endobronchial intubation remains undetected, an inadvertent hyperinflation of the ipsilateral lung can occur with subsequent pneumothorax and concomitant atelectasis of the hypoventilated contralateral lung. Indeed, it has been reported that up to 15% of chest radiographs reveal malpositioned ETTs in intubated patients.[84,88,89] This is more frequently seen after difficult airway management.

In the operating room, chest radiographs are not used to confirm proper position; rather, indirect clinical assessment methods are used (i.e., auscultation of bilateral breath sounds, visualization of equal chest expansion, and direct visualization of the ETT tip placed just below the vocal cords). The ETT is also manufactured with distance measurements to aid with the depth of insertion. In orally intubated patients, a depth of 23 cm at the teeth or corner of the mouth has been advocated for men and 21 to 22 cm for women.[90,91] In nasotracheal intubations, a depth of 26 cm at the nares in women and 28 cm in men should be sufficient for proper tracheal position.[92] Other methods used include direct visualization of the ETT tip in reference to the carina with a fiberoptic scope or catheter,[69] transtracheal illumination, and ballottement of the ETT cuff in the suprasternal notch.[93-96]

3. Cuff Pressure Monitoring

Probably the most often overlooked parameter in daily airway care is cuff pressure.[97,98] Almost universally, this measurement is neglected in operating room intubations. However, it is well documented that excessive forces applied to the tracheal mucosa can cause necrosis and ulceration.[9,99,100] Cuff pressures of 30 cm H_2O for 4 hours have been shown to damage ciliary motility for at least 3 days.[100-102] In addition, animal studies have revealed diminished circulation in the tracheal mucosa with a pressure of just 20 cm H_2O, exaggerated greatly in the presence of hypotension.[103]

Normal occlusive pressures should be between 20 and 30 cm H_2O to avoid complications while maintaining an adequate seal in the tracheal lumen circumferentially around the cuff to prevent microaspiration and ultimately VAP.[100] Depending on the type of cuff used, the same pressure range seems to be effective at accomplishing this task both in vitro and during in vivo animal studies. For example, standardized HVLP cuffs have been demonstrated to be ineffective at preventing microaspiration with pressures as high as 60 cm H_2O,[7] whereas polyurethane tubes seem to be effective down to 15 cm H_2O.[7,10,104]

As was previously discussed, ETTs are not without risks. However, it appears that most of the morbidity is related to either inappropriate inflation of an ETT cuff or a defective ETT cuff.[98-100] An often dreaded scenario that leads to increased morbidity is frequent ETT exchanges for suspected cuff leaks. Trended values for cuff pressure could help to alleviate some of these unnecessary procedures. Most importantly, it has been demonstrated that manual palpation of the cuff or instillation of a standard volume of air often underestimates the actual occlusive pressure delivered, leading to unrecognized complications.[97,98,100] Therefore, it is recommended that frequent examination of the cuff pressure be documented and trended using manometry.

Reusable aneroid manometers can be onerous to calibrate and are often difficult to locate; in addition, they pose a recurring risk of cross-contamination for each patient. The manometers currently in use in most ICUs provide only a single data point at the time of collection. A commercially available disposable, precalibrated device that constantly measures airway cuff pressures is available. The PressureEasy device (Smiths Medical, St. Paul, MN), among others, attaches to the pilot balloon and exhibits a mark in a fixed window when the measured

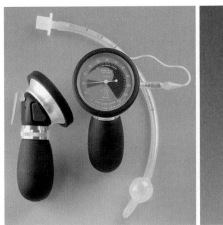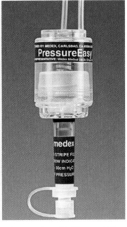

Figure 47-12 Posey Cufflator aneroid manometer *(left)* and the PressureEasy Pressure Controller Device *(right)* for monitoring endotracheal tube cuff pressure. (Cufflator courtesy Posey Company, Arcadia, CA; PressureEasy courtesy Smiths Medical, Dublin, OH.)

cuff pressure is in the optimal range of 20 and 30 cm H_2O (Fig. 47-12).[97-100]

4. Evaluation of an Audible Cuff Leak

Although ETT cuff leaks pertain most often to the ICU or postanesthesia care unit (PACU) setting and longer-duration intubations, short-term tracheal intubation in the operating room may also fall prey to an apparent leak. The most relevant question is, When is a cuff leak really a cuff leak? The audible leak implies that air is escaping from the presumably closed ETT system. The leak may be caused by a defective ETT cuff that has failed, ripped, or is microperforated (in which case the pilot balloon deflates spontaneously). Equally possible is a defective pilot balloon–line assembly. The valve on the pilot balloon may be faulty and incompetent, the balloon may have a perforation, the line may be cracked or broken or may become disjointed at the tube end or the valve end. Moreover, the intermittent or continuous audible leak may represent an ETT cuff that fails to seal the airway due to malpositioning, deranged shape, or laxity and deformation of the tracheal wall (e.g., tracheomalacia,

tracheitis, tracheal erosion). The ETT cuff (intact pilot balloon) may be subglottic, between the vocal cords, or supraglottic, having been displaced during patient movement, transport, repositioning, "tonguing" (dislodging the ETT by moving it with the tongue) of the ETT, excessive coughing, excessive tension on the ETT by the ventilator circuit, or, commonly, positioning for radiography. Once the ETT is partially displaced upward, an audible leak may prompt further ETT cuff insufflation, leading to further displacement. Head and neck movement by the patient may be all that is required to further displace the ETT into the hypopharyngeal region. This must be diagnosed before disaster strikes.

The various sources of a suspected cuff leak require investigation because each necessitates a different solution. Any one solution, incorrectly applied, may lead to morbidity or mortality. For example, a cuff leak resulting from a herniated cuff above the vocal cords may prompt the team to order a chest radiograph. Further displacement may take place during lifting and repositioning of the patient for the examination. Conversely, if an ETT is malpositioned in the hypopharynx (intact pilot balloon) but is assumed to be a properly positioned ETT with a cuff perforation, an exchange catheter passed via the ETT (presumably into the trachea) may exit the supraglottic ETT and enter the esophagus, leading to airway compromise. Table 47-1 highlights the possible causes and potential solutions, with relevant risk assessments for an apparent cuff leak evaluation.

5. Documentation of Placement

Clinicians who care for patients who are intubated for long periods in the ICU may find it onerous to obtain pertinent airway management details. This can be especially detrimental to future care providers who are faced with a patient with a known or suspected difficult airway. This situation could result for a number of reasons: lack of relevance (routine intubation before the patient's surgery), lack of continuity (the intubator is no longer involved in the patient's care), or an incomplete or total lack of documentation.

As an ICU course progresses, the details surrounding the original ETT placement may prove less relevant

TABLE 47-1

Causes and Solutions for Apparent ETT Cuff Leaks

Problem	Solution	Risk Level
Cuff perforation (pilot balloon deflation)	Exchange ETT (only feasible choice)	High
Incompetent pilot valve	Exchange ETT	High
	Clamp line (Kelly, hemostat)—short term solution	Low
	Place stopcock or cap on valve	Low
	Replace pilot balloon–line assembly	Low
Broken pilot line	Exchange ETT	High
	Clamp line (Kelly, hemostat)—short-term solution	Low
	Replace pilot balloon line assembly (homemade vs. commercial)	Low
Displaced ETT (intact pilot balloon)	Perform fiberoptic evaluation—diagnostic	Low-moderate
	Blindly advance ETT	Very high
	Videolaryngoscopy evaluation	Low-moderate
	Blindly pass airway exchange catheter	High
	Perform direct laryngoscopy (suboptimal line of sight)	Low-moderate

ETT, Endotracheal tube.

because the patient's clinical status and airway are dynamic, not static. A previously easy airway may remain so, but difficulty often increases as edema, trauma, secretion management, and patient status decline to confound an airway intervention. Anatomic abnormalities may be hidden or exaggerated by excessive fluid administration or a capillary leakage phenomenon in the critically ill patient, and examination of the airway may become impossible. Appreciation of the airway adjuncts that have been attempted is imperative for the incoming airway team. Immediate availability of pertinent historical airway management details may prove helpful in delivering better care. Documentation of airway interventions and procedures on a specific sheet (Fig. 47-13) may provide the incoming airway team perspective on what to expect in a single concise location.

C. Stabilization of the Endotracheal Tube

After verification and confirmation of proper tracheal placement and position have been achieved, care should be focused on securing the ETT in its proper position, and frequent assessments should be made to recognize malpositioning.[105,106]

At the most basic level, recording and confirming the depth of the ETT at the patient's teeth or lips in centimeters should be routine. This measurement should be documented on the respiratory care flow sheet. In patients requiring prolonged mechanical ventilation, the depth should be assessed and documented frequently (e.g., every shift, every 4 hours), along with clinical assessments of ETT patency and hygiene, appropriate chest expansion, and auscultation findings.

Securing and surveillance of the ETT are important not only to ensure proper depth and positioning but also to reduce the incidence of inadvertent extubation.[105] Unplanned extubation is primarily a problem in the ICU. It has a reported incidence of approximately 2% to 16%, with 80% of those extubated requiring reintubation, and contributes to a higher rate of airway-related complications, hemodynamic alterations, patient morbidity, and mortality.[48,107-109] The most frequently identified cause is inadequate sedation of a mechanically ventilated patient, and only a few studies have specifically addressed techniques used to secure ETTs. In a study comparing four such techniques, Levy and Griego concluded that the use of simple adhesive tape split at both ends and secured to both the ETT and patient's face was more effective than proprietary methods and allowed more effective nursing care, improved oral hygiene, and greater comfort for the patient.[106] However, Barnason and colleagues found no statistical difference between two methods studied in preventing unplanned extubation, allowing oral hygiene, or maintaining facial skin integrity.[110]

Attention to proper ETT stabilization primarily focuses on the reduction of unplanned extubation, improved comfort for the patient with prolonged ventilatory requirements, minimization of iatrogenic complications related to the method of fixture, and ease of nursing and respiratory care. One study addressed massive air leaks and contributing factors. The authors defined a massive air leak as one that requires extubation. Over a

2-year period, 18 ETTs were removed for massive air leaks, of which 61% were found to be free of mechanical defects (intact cuff). Fourteen of the 18 patients required reintubation; 2 of them aspirated gastric contents on replacement, and 1 suffered severe epistaxis from a blind nasal reintubation, resulting in a 21% complication rate.[111] The authors concluded that malpositioning was the most plausible explanation for the apparent air leaks. This study reinforces the importance of securing the ETT and daily vigilance to ensure that proper depth and positioning are confirmed and maintained.

Despite these studies, no consensus exists concerning the best method of securing the ETT.

1. Taping

The classically described methods are a "barber's pole" technique for operating room intubations, a simple split tape technique (Fig. 47-14), and a more secure "four-point" technique for intubations anticipated to last for 24 hours or longer. In each of these methods, tape is used to anchor the ETT to the face. Moisture, in the form of sweat, secretions, or vomitus, can jeopardize the integrity of the bond between adhesive and skin, putting the security of the ETT at risk.[105] Additionally, patient comfort is an issue when tape is used for this purpose. Skin breakdown due to allergic reactions, pressure necrosis, or repetitive trauma has been documented as a potential problem from the use of this method. The four-point method is more secure than the barber's pole technique because the tape encircles the patient's head and is not as susceptible to moisture because it is anchored to itself as well as to the patient's skin.

2. Commercially Available Devices

Although several options are available, a proprietary device has been developed to help secure the ETT and provide increased patient comfort while facilitating airway care. This device, the AnchorFast (Hollister Inc., Libertyville, IL) (Fig. 47-15), incorporates an ergonomically designed frame to minimize well-known pressure points, a latex-free adhesive on a pad, and a padded Velcro-style retaining strap that encircles the head. Preliminary studies comparing this device against classic adhesive tapes showed reduced skin breakdown, fewer lip ulcers, and improved patient comfort.[106,112]

Another commercial device used to secure the ETT has been postulated; it mimics the nasal bridling technique used for nasogastric tubes. This product is still in development.

3. Stapling for Facial Burns

The overall incidence of burn patients in most practices is very small, and this creates an unfamiliarity with their care, particularly as it relates to airway management. The focus of this section is to discuss the unique situation presented by the facial burn. Aside from the obvious difficulties of tube placement initially, replacement of an ETT after a burn resuscitation is far more challenging due to a multitude of unique injuries. The two major problems with securing an ETT for the patient with a facial burn are the increased (and increasing) edema due to ongoing inflammatory processes and continued

Department of Anesthesiology Airway Management Note

Airway Management Procedure:

[ ] Elective   [ ] Urgent   [ ] Emergent

[ ] Cardiac or Respiratory Arrest

[ ] Intubation   [ ] ETT Exchange   [ ] Extubation   [ ] Other: _____

Date: _____ **Call Time:** _____ **Arrival Time:** _____

Location: _____ **Staff:** _____

Height: _____ **Weight:** _____ **NPO Status:** _____

BP: _____ **HR:** _____ **Oxy Sat:** _____ on… _____ %

[ ] Room Air   [ ] Nasal   [ ] Facemask   [ ] NRB   [ ] NIPPV

Isolation Precautions: [ ] Contact   [ ] Droplet   [ ] Airborne

                                     [ ] Vector   [ ] Common Vehicle

Condition Upon Arrival (check all that apply):

[ ] Awake   [ ] Hypoxemic   [ ] Dyspnea   [ ] Secretions

[ ] Sedated…   [ ] Hypercarbic   [ ] Tachypnea   [ ] Vomitus

[ ] Agitated   [ ] Stridorous   [ ] Bradypnea   [ ] Blood

[ ] Unconscious   [ ] Wheezing   [ ] Apnea   [ ] Foreign Matter…

[ ] Other/Comments: _____

Underlying Pathologies/Co-Morbidities (if known, mark all that apply):

Neurologic: [ ] CVA   [ ] Increased ICP   [ ] ICH/SDH   [ ] Seizure

                       [ ] SCI   [ ] Δ Mental Status   [ ] Drug Overdose

Pulmonary: [ ] Asthma   [ ] COPD   [ ] ARDS   [ ] OSA   [ ] PE

                       [ ] PNA…   [ ] CAP   [ ] VAP   [ ] Pulm. Contusion

                       [ ] Pneumo/Hemothorax   [ ] Upper Airway Issue…

                       [ ] Post-operative Respiratory Failure   [ ] NPPE

Cardiac: [ ] AMI   [ ] CHF   [ ] Dysrhythmia…   [ ] Tamponade

Metabolic: [ ] Acidosis…   [ ] Electrolyte…   [ ] Alcohol Withdrawal

                     [ ] UGIB or LGIB   [ ] SBO   [ ] Mesenteric Ischemia

Infectious: [ ] Immune compromised   [ ] Sepsis   [ ] PTA

                    [ ] Tonsil/Epiglottitis   [ ] Tracheitis/Bronchitis

Trauma: [ ] Cranial/Spinal…   [ ] Thoracic…   [ ] Abdominal…

                [ ] Orthopedic…

Other/Comments: _____

_____

_____

Airway Management Procedural Documentation:

Preoxygenation: [ ] Room Air   [ ] Facemask/NRB   [ ] 100%, Bag-Mask

Ventilation: [ ] Assisted   [ ] Controlled   [ ] Easy   [ ] Difficult

                   [ ] Oral Airway   [ ] Nasal Airway   [ ] Two-person

Positioning: [ ] Supine   [ ] Ramped   [ ] Elevated HOB

                 [ ] Sitting   [ ] Other: _____

Induction: [ ] Awake   [ ] Sedated   [ ] General Anesthesia   [ ] None

               [ ] Topical Anesthesia   [ ] Airway Block…   [ ] Paralysis…

               [ ] Rapid Sequence Induction   [ ] Cricoid Pressure

               [ ] Other: _____

Medications: [ ] Etomidate _____ mg   [ ] Propofol _____ mg

                 [ ] Ketamine _____ mg   [ ] Other: _____ mg

                 [ ] Succinylcholine _____ mg   [ ] Rocuronium _____ mg

1st Attempt: [ ] DL: MAC _____ MILLER _____ [ ] Glidescope/VL   [ ] FOB

               Other: _____

               C-L View: [ ] 1   [ ] 2a   [ ] 2b   [ ] 3a   [ ] 3b   [ ] 4

                                     [ ] Secretions   [ ] Blood   [ ] Edema

               AirwayAdjuncts: [ ] Bougie   [ ] ILMA   [ ] LMA

               Other/Comments: _____

Figure 47-13 Example of a detailed airway record for emergency intubations.

Continued

2nd Attempt: [ ] DL: MAC_____ MILLER_____   [ ] Glidescope/VL   [ ] FOB

Other:_____

C-L View: [ ] 1   [ ] 2a   [ ] 2b   [ ] 3a   [ ] 3b   [ ] 4
              [ ] Secretions   [ ] Blood   [ ] Edema

AirwayAdjuncts: [ ] Bougie   [ ] ILMA   [ ] LMA

Other/Comments: _____

_____

_____

3rd Attempt: [ ] DL: MAC_____ MILLER_____   [ ] Glidescope/VL   [ ] FOB

Other:_____

C-L View: [ ] 1   [ ] 2a   [ ] 2b   [ ] 3a   [ ] 3b   [ ] 4
              [ ] Secretions   [ ] Blood   [ ] Edema

AirwayAdjuncts: [ ] Bougie   [ ] ILMA   [ ] LMA

Other/Comments: _____

_____

_____

Airway Device Ultimately Placed: [ ] ETT...   [ ] LMA...   [ ] Combitube

Size:_____ Type: [ ] Standard   [ ] ORAE   [ ] NRAE
                             [ ] Subglottic EVAC   [ ] ECOM

Placement Location: _____ cm @ lip

Confirmation: [ ] Esophageal bulb device   [ ] ETCO$_2$ [ ] Direct Visual
                      [ ] Bilateral BS   [ ] Bronchoscopy   [ ] Chest X-ray

Post-Procedure Vital Signs:

BP: _____ HR: _____ Oxy Sat:_____ on..._____ %

Other/Comments: _____

_____

_____

_____

_____

_____

_____

_____

_____

_____

Signature:_____ Date/Time: _____

Figure 47-13, cont'd

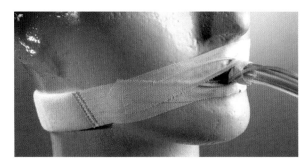

Figure 47-14 The split-tape method of taping the endotracheal tube.

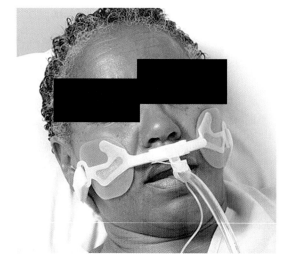

Figure 47-15 The AnchorFast system for endotracheal tube stabilization. (Courtesy of Hollister Inc., Libertyville, IL.)

resuscitation, which makes the face ever expanding, and the actual burned skin, which is constantly weeping and often débrided or sloughing. It should be obvious that adhesive devices, both simple tape and proprietary devices, are ineffective in this situation. A well-documented and accepted method in these patients is to secure the ETT with tape and anchor it to the skin by stapling the tape to the burned areas. This is surprisingly well tolerated, but more importantly it is very reliable to maintain the airway and is easy to care for.

One important airway management caveat should be understood regarding proper ETT position at the gum line or lips in all intubated patients: the ETT marking at these locations only assures the location of the proximal end; it does not guarantee the depth and location of the distal ETT tip. Although this problem pertains most often to the ventilated PACU or ICU patient, an ETT located at 25 cm at the gum line and seemingly secured by tape or a commercial device does not guarantee tracheal intubation (with or without a cuff leak). Typically, a continuous or intermittent apparent cuff leak leads to further insufflation of the pilot balloon to fix the leak. An intact (inflated) pilot balloon, in this clinical situation, should arouse suspicion that the distal tip is abnormally located outside the glottis. The potential for an airway catastrophe is extreme, especially in the patient with a difficult airway, compounded by significant mechanical ventilatory requirements. Proper assessment of the ETT position, preferably with flexible bronchoscopy for diagnostic and therapeutic maneuvers, is indicated.

D. Rapid Response Cart for Airway Emergencies

Areas in which care for intubated patients is provided need to have a dedicated set of supplies to establish emergency airways in the event of primary respiratory failure or cardiac arrest to reestablish lost, previously secured airways. The responding airway team must be knowledgeable and competent in advanced management techniques and provided with immediate access to such equipment. Infrequent or casual airway managers should ask for assistance early in the management process or even immediately, before starting. The American Society of Anesthesiologists difficult airway algorithm (Fig. 47-16) should be close at hand to guide less experienced individuals who encounter problems.[113] Supplies on the cart may differ based on personal preference and facility purchase, but there are some items that must be present to help save a life.

Laryngoscopy, ETT exchange, pulmonary toilet, and a "cannot intubate, cannot ventilate" (CICV) scenario must all be covered in the equipment selection. Laryngoscopy includes both conventional (direct) and video laryngoscopy; it is used to assist the team with replacing the ETT after an inadvertent extubation, augmenting the exchange of a damaged ETT over an airway exchange catheter, improving the ability to assess ETT location within the airway, and interrogating the physiologic integrity of an airway slated for extubation.[114]

An airway exchange catheter, coupled with video laryngoscopy, greatly reduces the complication rates for necessary airway exchanges in ICU patients, thereby earning its place in an airway response cart within the ICU.[114] A fiberoptic bronchoscope should be available for confirmation purposes, for awake intubation procedures, and for deeper pulmonary toilet needs to improve ventilation and oxygenation.[115] Supraglottic airway devices should be available for situations in which mask ventilation is difficult or as a conduit to facilitate the placement of an endotracheal airway.[116] Lastly, equipment for the placement of a surgical airway must be provided. Despite all of the options available, a scalpel may be the only device capable of establishing the airway. In cases of a known or suspected difficult airway, it is helpful to immediately contact someone with the ability to place a surgical airway should other conventional or advanced noninvasive means fail.

Box 47-2 delineates the contents of a proposed difficult airway cart, which should be readily available in case of any airway catastrophe.

V. MAINTENANCE OF THE ENDOTRACHEAL TUBE

There is currently no alternative to the placement of an oral, nasal, or transtracheal ETT, whether to maintain airway patency, perform ventilation, improve oxygenation, remove secretions, or deliver necessary therapies. However, the ETT is only as good as its most pristine state. Despite the unavoidable decision, some still look on the placement of an ETT as a necessary evil. The conundrum arises in preserving or remastering the physiologic function of the host tissues while combating their inherent defenses aimed at reacting to the new artificial airway and protecting the new foreign device to maintain its optimized function as in its original condition.

The presence of the ETT bypasses the host defenses of the upper airway, eliminates the humidification of inspired gases, increases the WOB, limits the administration of medications, and prevents prophylactic oral hygiene. All of these changes promote bacterial colonization, inflammation, and sputum production. Inability to actively clear secretions because of a poor cough or increased difficulty of passive removal by health care personnel can lead to plugging of proximal and distal airways as well as the ETT. These retained secretions may result in the formation of atelectasis, ventilation-perfusion mismatching in the form of a shunt or dead space, hypoxemia, and increased respiratory load, thereby prolonging the duration of mechanical ventilation.[117,118] Therefore, aggressive respiratory care must be provided for the intubated patient to avoid these complications and further morbidity.

A. Heat and Humidity of Inspired Gas

During normal breathing, the air is delivered to the carina at a temperature of 32° C and an absolute humidity of 30.4 mg H_2O/L.[119] The insertion of an ETT via the nose, mouth, or trachea bypasses the upper airway and causes the natural ability to heat and humidify inspired gas to be lost. The American Association for Respiratory Care states that devices should provide a minimum of 30 mg

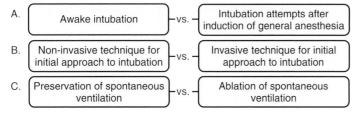

DIFFICULT AIRWAY ALGORITHM

1. Assess the likelihood and clinical impact of basic management problems:
   A. Difficult ventilation
   B. Difficult intubation
   C. Difficult with patient cooperation or consent
   D. Difficult tracheostomy

2. Actively pursue opportunities to deliver supplemental oxygen throughout the process of difficult airway management

3. Consider the relative merits and feasibility of basic management choices:

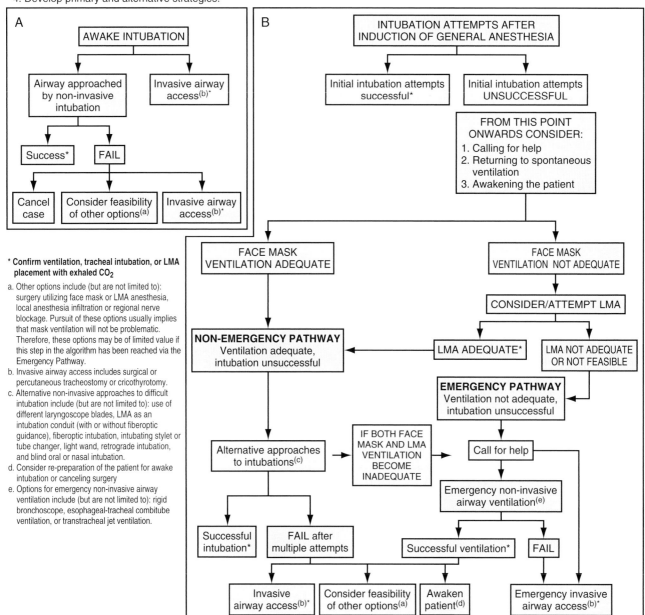

Figure 47-16 American Society of Anesthesiologists difficult airway algorithm. *LMA,* Laryngeal mask airway. (Courtesy of American Society of Anesthesiologists, Park Ridge, IL.)

Fiberoptic bronchoscope and video monitoring system (optional), adult and pediatric sizes
Magill and Krause forceps
Solution atomizer
Ovassapian and Williams airways
Video laryngoscopy (various products available) blades, sizes for neonate to large adult
Direct laryngoscopy Miller and Macintosh blades, sizes 1-4
Intubating laryngeal mask airways, sizes 3-5 (or equivalent)
Standard laryngeal mask airways, sizes 3-5 (or equivalent)
Esophageal-tracheal Combitube (or King LT or EasyTube by Rüsch)
Gum elastic bougies (various manufacturers)
Airway exchange catheters, multiple sizes
Endotracheal tubes, sizes 6-9, standard and Evac types (pediatric sizes if appropriate)
Capnometric devices
Cricothyroidotomy kit (purchased or hospital standardized)
Retrograde intubation kit (Cook Critical Care)
Percutaneous tracheostomy kit
Medications kit (etomidate, propofol, ketamine, succinylcholine, rocuronium, intravenous and viscous lidocaine, atropine)

of H_2O/L of delivered gas at 30° C.[120] If inspired air is not warmed and humidified, the result is a dry, cool gas that is damaging to the respiratory tract and impedes mucociliary function. Secretions may become dry and inspissated, possibly leading to partial or complete occlusion of the ETT lumen. If left unrecognized, this occlusion may lead to barotrauma and death.[93] The most common method to protect against this situation is the use of an active heated humidifier or a passive heat and moisture exchanger (HME) (Fig. 47-17).[121]

HMEs are typically cylindrical devices that are fitted to the ventilator circuit, usually just proximal to the ETT connector and the Y-piece, with limited changes on airway mechanics.[122,123] This is the most effective HME placement for maximizing humidity and temperature retention in the patient circuit.[121,124] The materials provide heat, humidification, and filtering properties, earning the device the nickname, "artificial nose."[125] They are lightweight and inexpensive, require no power source, and reduce circuit condensation, making them attractive alternatives to the more expensive heated humidifiers.

Use of heated humidifiers is associated with the production of almost 100% humidity in the inspiratory gas and is thus more effective than use of HMEs. These units require an external power source and additional circuitry, increasing cost. Accidental overheating can occur and may create additional damage to the airway if temperatures are not frequently monitored. There is no consensus about the proper duration of use of these implements. Multiple studies have failed to show a correlation of increased incidence of pneumonia with heated humidifiers versus HMEs or with frequent changes of HMEs or heated humidifiers. Therefore, frequent changes (i.e., more often than every 7 days) of ventilator circuits, unless they are visually soiled, is neither cost-effective nor medically efficacious.[73,126-129]

B. Suctioning

Perhaps the simplest and most logical means of assisting with secretion clearance is direct suctioning. This modality is safe, but when it is performed carelessly, complications may occur, including soft tissue or airway trauma, aspiration, laryngospasm, increased intracranial pressure, bronchospasm, hypoxemia, and cardiac dysrhythmias.[130] Hypoxemia can be minimized with preoxygenation using a fraction of inspired oxygen (Fi_{O_2}) of 100%. In patients with intracranial hypertension, mild hyperventilation or blunting of the cough reflex with instilled intravenous lidocaine just before suctioning may reduce the risks of additional increases in intracranial pressure. The evacuation procedure should be brief and intermittent. The vacuum should be applied only after the suction catheter has been advanced to its distal position. After each pass of the catheter, lung re-expansion with a few gentle manual breaths should be administered. Suctioning can be applied by a single-use open system in which the catheter is unprotected and open to the environment or by a closed system (Fig. 47-18) that sheathes the catheter in a sterile protective covering.

Closed systems are usually incorporated into the ventilator breathing circuit at the junction of the Y-piece and

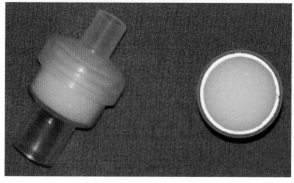

Figure 47-17   A heat and moisture exchanger.

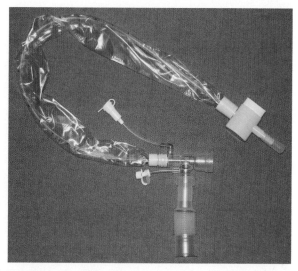

Figure 47-18   The Ballard closed endotracheal tube suctioning system.

the ETT or tracheostomy tube, allowing continued ventilation during suctioning with no need to disconnect the circuit. The advantage of not having to disconnect is important for patients who require aggressive ventilator management (e.g., high PEEP therapy), making them less susceptible to alveolar derecruitment compared with open suctioning. The retractable catheter does not add any additional restriction to airflow (when not deployed). There are concerns that colonization of these devices with aspiration of bacterial particles and cross-contamination may predispose to VAP.[131] Such concerns have led to differing opinions on the appropriate timing of any system changes. Kollef and coworkers randomly assigned patients to scheduled changes every 24 hours or to no change except when there was a malfunction or visible soiling.[132] In both groups, 15% of patients developed VAP. The only difference was in total cost: $11,016 USD in the group with scheduled changes and $837 USD in the group with no scheduled changes.[132,133]

C. Subglottic Care

Secretion management has, by necessity, moved beyond the ETT lumen. Suctioning of secretions that are pooled above the ETT cuff, in the subglottic space, is an important step in good tracheal care and is paramount in the prevention of VAP.[111,132-137] Subglottic suctioning has been shown to decrease the incidence of VAP in the ICU from 16% to 4%.[135] Specialized ETTs with dedicated subglottic suctioning ports are more expensive ($15 compared with $1 for a standard ETT).[138] An interesting cost analysis done in 2003 demonstrated that despite this increased cost, the estimated cost benefit of an ETT with a subglottic suction port was $4,992 per case of VAP saved.[138] The U.S. Centers for Disease Control and Prevention (CDC) universally recommends the use of subglottic suctioning tubes in the ICU to help reduce the rate of VAP.[139]

Subglottic suctioning can be done with small suction catheters that are advanced down the trachea until resistance is met from the ETT cuff. Another option is using ETTs with a subglottic port positioned just above the cuff. These specialized ETTs are certainly not infallible and do not replace vigilant airway care. It has been demonstrated that dysfunction of the suction lumen can occur almost 50% of the time.[140] In 43% of cases, the cause of the suction loss was determined to be prolapse of the tracheal mucosa into the subglottic suction port.[140]

D. Bronchoscopy

The use of fiberoptic bronchoscopy for routine secretion management is not advocated. It is expensive, requires proficient training, and may produce complications such as barotrauma secondary to a marked reduction or cessation in expiratory airflow (depending on the relative airway caliber) in intubated patients.[4] It should be reserved for assisting with lobar collapse caused by mucus plugging or inspissated secretions not amenable to conventional mucolysis, to perform so-called pulmonary toilet bronchoscopy that may be needed after an inhalation injury to evaluate for tracheobronchial injury, to aid in the diagnosis of significant hemoptysis, or to assist with specimen procurement when clinical suspicion merits sampling.

E. Biofilm Management

Biofilm and adherence of secretions (Fig. 47-19) within the ETT have been implicated in the development of VAP, increased WOB, delays in extubation, and other complications.[141-144] Biofilm can easily be identified by bronchoscopy on insertion of the scope into the ETT. Newer technologies using acoustic reflectometry have also been developed to help with monitoring the accumulation of biofilm and evaluating the integrity of the intubated airway. The SonarMed airway monitoring device (SonarMed, Indianapolis, IN) employs this technology to assess ETT positioning and movement as well as ETT patency hampered by either internal or external agents.

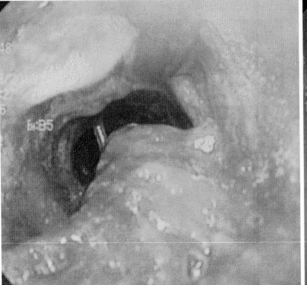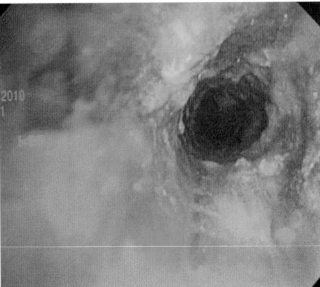

Figure 47-19 Examples of biofilm accumulation inside the lumen of an endotracheal tube.

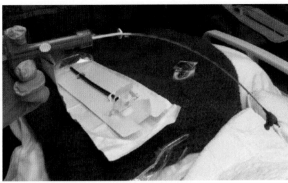

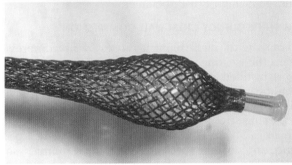

Figure 47-20 The Omneotech Complete Airway Management (CAM) Rescue Cath catheter. (Courtesy of Omneotech, Tavernier, FL.)

Traditional methods used to manage biofilm include catheter suctioning, bronchoscopic lavage, and ETT exchange. Catheter suctioning is often ineffective for biofilm removal, because its presence frequently evades detection as the suction catheter navigates the patent channel formed by the biofilm concretions, thereby leaving the impression that the lumen is patent. Bronchoscopic lavage and ETT exchange are hampered by significant costs and hazards for both practitioners and patients. Another option is a device that essentially scrapes the biofilm from the luminal surface of the ETT. The Complete Airway Management (CAM) Rescue Cath by Omneotech (Tavernier, FL) (Fig. 47-20) resembles a Fogarty catheter used to remove a thrombus. This product has an inflatable balloon at the distal end of a catheter that is encased in a latticed netting to provide "traction" and atraumatic "abrasion" of the lumen. It is introduced into the ETT and advanced to the distal end (based on ETT and CAM depth markings); the balloon is then inflated, and the catheter is fully withdrawn back out through the proximal end of the catheter, along with any luminal biofilm. This device and procedure may prove to be a useful option in already hypoxic or PEEP-dependent patients in whom time-consuming bronchoscopies could be hazardous. The CAM Rescue Cath is also a good option for patients with a potentially difficult airway, in whom ETT exchange can pose a considerable risk.[145]

Information on the prevention of biofilm formation is rife with conflicting data. One study showed no difference in rate of *Pseudomonas aeruginosa* and *Staphylococcus epidermidis* biofilm formation among different ETT materials including PVC, silicone, stainless steel, and sterling silver.[146] More recently, however, ETTs coated in silver and chlorhexidine showed significantly reduced rates of biofilm colonization in a nonclinical setting.[23,147] The preventive management of biofilm may not be far in the future, but chlorhexidine-coated ETTs are currently not available. For now, the best strategy to manage biofilm is increased vigilance, fastidious respiratory care, and new technologies aimed at minimization and safe clearance.

VI. RESPIRATORY THERAPIES FOR THE INTUBATED PATIENT

A. Secretion Clearance and Control Therapies

1. Mucolytic Agents

Agents used to decrease the viscosity of tracheobronchial secretions and assist with their reduction and clearance have been used for decades. The primary agent in use is *N*-acetylcysteine (NAC, Mucomyst). NAC is a sulfhydryl-containing compound; therefore, it is classified as a thiol. It has extensive first-pass metabolism in the gastrointestinal tract and liver when administered orally and is almost completely absorbed; only minimal amounts are excreted in the feces. The plasma half-life is approximately 2 hours, with virtually no detectable NAC at approximately 12 hours.[148]

Most of NAC's biochemical effects appear to be related to its sulfhydryl group, which reduces the production hydroxyl radicals.[148,149] This effect has provided many uses for NAC beyond that of a mucolytic agent, including hepatic protection in acetaminophen overdose and renal protection against contrast-induced nephropathy.[52,150] NAC's effects on mucus viscosity result from its ability to disrupt the disulfide bridges and render them more liquid.[133,148] NAC is usually delivered by nebulizer in combination with a β_2-adrenergic agonist because it can induce bronchospasm.[151] Clinically, its effects have been variable in patients with chronic bronchitis, for whom oral NAC is used to assist with exacerbations and symptomatic relief.[152-154] Direct instillation of NAC during bronchoscopy may assist in secretion removal.

Another important factor in mucus viscosity is DNA content. DNA contributes to secretion viscosity because it accumulates from the degradation of bacteria and neutrophils. An agent that is considered mostly a mucokinetic agent, recombinant deoxyribonuclease (DNase, Pulmozyme), has been used in nebulized form in patients with bronchiectasis caused by cystic fibrosis with good results; however, it is expensive, and its use beyond this population of patients is not indicated.[117,155,156]

One interesting therapy used in the population of burn patients who have an associated inhalation injury is nebulized heparin. Heparin assists with decreasing and removing bronchial casts that form with inhalation injury. Heparin's anticoagulant effects assist with removal of casts, and it may act as a free radical scavenger with anti-inflammatory effects. Although studies have not consistently shown a significant change in pulmonary function, cast formation and removal are favorably altered.[157,158]

2. Chest Physiotherapy

Chest physiotherapy encompasses a variety of techniques that include position changes, percussion and vibration of the chest wall, and stimulation of a cough response. These are relatively dogmatic approaches that have historically provided poor results. They also tend to be burdensome to both the respiratory therapist and the patient. Newer, alternative techniques show promising results.

a. PERCUSSION AND POSTURAL DRAINAGE

Used extensively in patients with cystic fibrosis, the technique of percussion with postural drainage utilizes external percussion of the chest wall overlying the affected lung region. Percussion can be applied manually with a cupped hand or by an automated, usually pneumatic, device. The application of percussion or vibration, or both, to the chest wall functions to loosen the secretions in the bronchi and facilitate their mobilization.[94,159] A steep Trendelenburg position of 25 degrees or more is employed—less if the patient cannot tolerate that angle—to facilitate the gravitational effects on mucus clearance.[77,160]

Relative contraindications to the postural component of this therapy are the presence of increased intracranial pressure; the possibility of an unprotected airway and the potential for aspiration; recent esophageal, ophthalmic, or intracranial surgery; congestive heart failure; and uncontrolled hypertension.[120] As for the application of percussion or vibration, placement of the technique over recent surgical sites (e.g., split-thickness skin grafts, rib fractures or chest trauma, pulmonary contusions, burns, unstable spine fractures) or in the presence of coagulopathies, subcutaneous emphysema, or bronchospasm are all relative contraindications.[160] Hazards include hypoxemia and accidental extubation.

Clinically and experimentally, the use of percussion with postural drainage in cystic fibrosis patients is well supported.[161-163] However, patients' compliance remains a concern, because the technique is burdensome for patients and caregivers.

b. POSITIVE END-EXPIRATORY PRESSURE THERAPY

PEEP therapy, as a secretion clearance technique, creates a restriction to expiratory flow by means of a face mask or mouthpiece. The resistance is adjusted to 10 to 20 cm H_2O of back pressure during expiration, which allows airflow to move into distal airways and associated lung units, forcing past secretions and causing them to move toward the larger airways, where suctioning is more feasible. The maneuver is used with gentle and forceful coughs lasting up to 20 minutes and aerosolized medications that can be administered concurrently. Patients with an increased WOB or severe dyspnea may have difficulty performing this technique due to temporary lapses in ventilation. PEEP therapy is at least as effective for secretion clearance as percussion with postural drainage, if not more effective, and patient satisfaction is markedly more favorable.[125,164,165]

c. INTRAPULMONARY PERCUSSIVE VENTILATION

Intrapulmonary percussive ventilation (IPV) can be delivered through a mouthpiece or to the end of the ETT.

Its high-frequency percussive oscillations function to loosen retained secretions, expand airways and lungs, and reduce atelectasis. Conceptualized and designed by Dr. Forrest Bird, IPV uses a "phasetron"—a sliding venturi device capable of providing 5 to 35 cm H_2O pressure during oscillations of 2 to 5 Hz.[166] Aerosolized medications may also be delivered during IPV treatments. Favorable results have been reported for secretion clearance and lung expansion in patients with cystic fibrosis, as well as in other disorders with an increased incidence of thickened secretions.[167,168] IPV offers an advantage to patients who lack the ability to perform percussion with postural drainage or high PEEP therapies.

d. HIGH-FREQUENCY CHEST WALL COMPRESSION

Therapy with high-frequency chest wall compression entails the wearing of an inflatable vest around the chest. Air is instilled into the vest bladder and then rapidly withdrawn in a cyclic manner, essentially creating an artificial cough. The high-frequency oscillations that are produced range from 5 to 25 Hz and can generate pressures as high as 50 cm H_2O. These oscillations create a gentle "squeezing" of the patient's chest that mimics small coughs. The frequency of the oscillations can be adjusted, and sensors in the vest can reduce the pressure delivered when the patient's chest expands (as with a sigh breath or a deep cough).[141] Secretion clearance and improvement in mucus rheology have also been reported.[169,170] Perhaps the biggest drawback of this method is its cost, estimated at $15,900 USD for each unit.

B. Overcoming Work of Breathing Imposed by Endotracheal Tubes, Tracheostomy Tubes, and Ventilator Circuits

With any translaryngeal intubation, the upper airway is bypassed and the resistance it imparts is thereby removed; however, there is still a substantial amount of work performed by the patient in an effort to ventilate. WOB is minimal during normal, quiet breathing, accounting for about 5% of the total oxygen consumption at rest. With increases in WOB, oxygen consumption can be markedly increased to as much as 30% or more.[155] This newly acquired increased demand may not be well tolerated by the critically ill patient. The additional WOB (WOB$_{add}$) imposed by the artificial airway and ventilator apparatus not only hinders weaning and liberation from mechanical ventilation but also impairs tissue oxygenation and alters critical blood flow, which may lead to worsened organ dysfunction.[86] To initiate a "breath" from the ventilator, a pressure differential across the ETT and circuit must be produced. The patient must overcome this resistance to initiate the demand flow needed for ventilation to occur. It has been shown experimentally that the ETT, the ventilator circuit, and the ventilator itself all add varying degrees of additional work for the patient to overcome, on top of the problems that initially necessitated intubation and mechanical ventilation.[32,171]

1. Pressure Support

Various modalities have been designed to overcome WOB$_{add}$ imposed by the artificial airway and ventilator.[155]

One is pressure support (PS), which is used as either an adjunct or as a mode of ventilation to help the spontaneously breathing patient overcome the WOB$_{add}$ imposed by an artificial airway.[21,168,172] A preset, flow-triggered inspiratory pressure chosen by the clinician is added to the airway opening pressure when inspiration is triggered by the patient. Because it is flow cycled, the patient can control the duration and depth of inspiration, and the PS ceases when some preset gas flow has diminished, usually about 25% of the maximal peak flow achieved.[173] PS has been shown to decrease WOB$_{add}$ even with normal lungs.[173,174] However, in patients with obstructive pulmonary disease and expiratory flow limitation, breath stacking, or auto-PEEP, flow may not decelerate quickly enough, and active exhalation may be necessary to terminate the PS, thereby creating additional WOB.[175] The amount of inspiratory pressure added is usually 4 to 15 cm H$_2$O. Currently, it is recommended that PS be applied for all spontaneously breathing, intubated patients to assist with overcoming the resistance of the ETT or tracheostomy tube.[176] Additional PS may be necessary if tidal volumes or respiratory rates, or both, are inadequate to support oxygenation. Most patients tolerate PS well, but decreased tolerance in patients susceptible to expiratory flow limitation must be appreciated and accounted for in any management strategy.

2. Continuous Positive Airway Pressure

Continuous positive airway pressure (CPAP) is applied at end-exhalation in spontaneously breathing patients. Much like PEEP, CPAP is designed to offset the degree of atelectasis that occurs inherently in the intubated, supine patient. CPAP ranging from 4 to 10 cm H$_2$O should be provided for all spontaneously breathing patients in an effort to compensate for the loss of expiratory lung volumes and further promote oxygenation. So-called physiologic PEEP, an amount thought to rectify the aforementioned atelectasis, is theoretical but is estimated to be equivalent to 4 cm H$_2$O in the normal lung. The reduction in WOB seen with CPAP has been appreciated primarily in the setting of expiratory airflow reductions; in such cases, CPAP offsets the auto-PEEP, thereby reducing the work required to generate the next inspiratory effort.[177] The type of flow-triggered mechanism and the location at which the flow differential is measured (typically at the tracheal end of the ETT) have been shown experimentally to decrease the inspiratory WOB as well.[178] CPAP is usually applied in combination with added PS.

3. Automatic Tube Compensation

As stated previously, the ETT imposes a substantial degree of resistance to inspiration. The modalities described thus far assist with decreasing some of the work needed to overcome this burden. Added PS and PS ventilation help compensate for the resistance primarily encountered during inhalation but not during exhalation, and they are not consistently provided because of the varying flow across the ETT during normal breathing.[179] Much resistance to exhalation is also produced by the presence of an ETT. Indeed, the internal diameter of the ETT greatly affects this phenomenon, as do other factors

such as gas flow rates, gas density and viscosity, and luminal secretions adherent to the ETT wall. Automatic tube compensation (ATC) is a feature on some newer ventilators. It is designed to assist with the resistance imposed by the ETT or tracheostomy tube during both the inspiratory and expiratory phases of the respiratory cycle. By altering the PS delivered—raising it during inspiration and lowering it during expiration according to the pressure-flow characteristics of the ETT—ATC adjusts for the resistance and the pressure drop across the ETT during spontaneous breathing. A computer assists by calculating the pressure difference across the ETT (ΔP^{ETT}) based on ETT size, measuring gas flow and airway pressure, and selecting the resistive properties of the ETT.[179] Unlike PS, ATC cannot be used as a ventilatory mode; it is merely an adjunct component to mechanical ventilation.

One drawback to ATC is the inability to correct for the reductions in airway diameter that can occur with secretions or kinking. This limitation results in an inaccurate measurement of ΔP^{ETT} such that ATC undercompensates for the pressure difference across the airway. A high index of suspicion is necessary to monitor for this possibility. Clinically, ATC has been shown to decrease the WOB$_{add}$ encountered with ETTs and tracheostomy tubes.[28] When these modalities were used to assist with weaning and extubation of patients in a T-piece trial, there was no difference in the workload encountered with ATC and T-piece alone, whereas adding PS to the T-piece trial at 7 cm H$_2$O unloaded this additional work.[180]

C. Pharmacologic Treatments

1. Inhalation Drug Delivery

The presence of an ETT does not limit drug delivery to the lungs and may actually enhance it. Many clinicians take advantage of this route of administration. The two predominant methods used to deliver agents are metered-dose inhalers (MDIs) and nebulizers. The drugs delivered by these devices are most commonly bronchodilators, mucolytics, corticosteroids, and antibiotics. For pulmonary ailments, inhaled drugs achieve efficacy comparable to or exceeding that of systemically delivered drugs with a smaller dose.[181-183] Tracheal administration of some traditionally systemic drugs often requires much higher doses to ensure absorption.

Inhalation drug delivery has other advantages over systemic administration. Systemic side effects can be reduced, because systemic absorption is markedly decreased. Variable reports regarding penetration and distribution of an aerosol to the lower respiratory tract range from 0% to 42% with nebulizers and 0.3% to 98% with MDIs. However, when the delivery method was standardized, the amount delivered in either method was similar, about 15%.[184-186]

Particle size also plays an important role in delivery. The larger the particle, the less likely it is to be delivered distally to the alveoli. Aerosol particles ranging between 1 and 5 μm are optimal for proper deposition.[181,182,185,187] The density of the gas carrying the aerosol also influences the delivery in an inverse relationship. Improvement in delivery has been reported when a mixture of helium and oxygen was used in the ventilator circuits of both MDIs and nebulizers.[183,188]

a. NEBULIZERS

The performance of a nebulizer depends on multiple factors including the model, operating pressure, flow rate, and volume of diluent utilized. Nebulizers are capable of generating aerosols with particle sizes of 1 to 3 µm, and the size produced is inversely influenced by the flow rate or pressure used: the greater the flow rate, the smaller the particle.[181,182] Nebulizers may be used continuously or intermittently. Intermittent use appears to be more efficient than continuous delivery, with less waste of aerosol demonstrated.[189] Placing a nebulizer upstream from the Y-piece and ETT also increases drug delivery.[187,189,190] Interestingly, the use of continuous drug nebulization may impair the ability of the patient to initiate a negative-pressure inspiratory effort in the PS mode of ventilation, thereby leading to hypoventilation.[168,191]

b. METERED-DOSE INHALERS

An MDI delivers medication in combination with a mixture of pressurized propellants, preservatives, flavoring agents, and surfactants. The final concentration of active drug constitutes about 1% of the total volume in the canister.[181] When the stem on the MDI canister is depressed, a finite amount of drug is released at a certain velocity, and a spray cloud develops. Various adapters are available that fit in line with the ventilator circuit or on the end of the ETT as so-called elbow adapters to aid in the administration of inhalational therapies. Chambers or spacers appear to provide better delivery of aerosol compared with the more commonly used elbow adapters.[192] MDIs typically cause more aerosol deposition on the ETT than nebulizers do, decreasing the amount of drug delivered. These particles, in turn, adhere to the ETT. This problem can be reduced by using a spacer and performing the administration with meticulous attention to timing of the ventilatory cycle: it is most effective during inspiration and when synchronized with the patient's spontaneous effort. Dhand and Tobin reported excellent results with their technique of MDI delivery.[189]

When comparing the overall efficacy of nebulizers versus that of MDIs, several factors favor the use of MDIs in mechanically ventilated patients. Nebulizers may become colonized with bacteria and help to deliver an aerosolized inoculum. Bowton and colleagues reported a potential saving of $300,000 USD annually with the use of MDIs compared with nebulizers.[193]

2. Inhaled Bronchodilators

Airway reactivity is a ubiquitous consequence of airway manipulation that hinders respiratory function and prolongs the duration of mechanical ventilation. Additional pathophysiologic processes attributed to persistent bronchospastic disease that serve to prolong mechanical ventilation include mucosal inflammation that persists and promotes further mucus production, airway hyperemia and resultant edema, and the consequent narrowing of small airways leading to an increase in closing

volume. These processes adversely affect oxygenation as functional residual capacity is decreased and CO_2 elimination, as expiratory flow, is limited. At extremes of expiratory flow limitation, generous amounts of intrinsic PEEP (auto-PEEP) are generated; this can impede cardiac filling by reducing preload, and hypotension and cardiac arrest may result. The physical effects of auto-PEEP are not limited to the cardiovascular system. The obvious effects of alveolar overdistention include an increased physiologic dead space and the potential for barotrauma, especially when controlled positive-pressure mechanical ventilation is instituted. Pneumothorax, pneumomediastinum, and pneumoperitoneum may all occur as a result, as may patient-ventilator dysynchrony.

Many maneuvers are available to reduce the effects of bronchospasm (and higher airway pressures), including decreasing the respiratory rate, prolonging the expiratory time, decreasing the tidal volume, and increasing the inspiratory flow rate. Pharmacologically, the use of β-adrenergic agonists, specifically β2-agonists such as albuterol, is the mainstay therapy. β2-receptors on bronchial smooth muscle promote relaxation and dilation of the airway diameter when stimulated. Systemic methylxanthines such as theophylline do not add much benefit in the acute stage of treating bronchospasm or reactive airways. Their narrow therapeutic window and vast side effect profile increase potential toxicity.

β2-agonists also have a beneficial effect on respiratory cilia in that they cause an increase in ciliary beat frequency.[194] This phenomenon is mediated by β-adrenergic receptors and can be attenuated with nonselective beta-blocking agents. An increase in the frequency of ciliary beating promotes mucus clearance over the respiratory epithelium. Other effects include increased water secretion onto the airway surface, which facilitates mucus clearance.[195] Indeed, the beneficial effects of β-agonists on bronchial reactivity and mucociliary clearance are evident. However, there are data suggesting a more robust effect in healthier airways than in chronically diseased airways such as those seen in patients with chronic bronchitis, possibly due to downregulation and chronic attenuation.[196] Newer formulations of inhaled β-agonists such as levalbuterol may have reduced side effect profiles and possibly improved outcomes.

3. Anticholinergics

Although inhaled β-agonists are pivotal in the reduction of airway reactivity, the use of inhaled anticholinergics such as ipratropium bromide or the newer tiotropium bromide needs to be emphasized, given their obvious synergistic effect with β-agonists. It is well appreciated that many of the mechanisms of airway reactivity and inflammation associated with bronchospastic disease are cholinergically mediated. In patients with chronic obstructive pulmonary disease, the use of these agents alone or in combination with β-agonists is the foundation for rescue therapy and a mainstay in chronic management.[183]

4. Corticosteroids

Inhaled glucocorticoid therapy has become a mainstay of treatment in various obstructive respiratory ailments, including chronic obstructive pulmonary disease and asthma. This class of medicines unquestionably has disease-specific effects at the target organ. Equally interesting is the fact that administration in an aerosol preparation magnifies their effects while markedly reducing their side effect profile, leading to a lower risk-benefit value. Targeted efficacy with minimal adverse effects helps to quantify an appropriate risk-benefit value.[197,198] High lung deposition or targeting, high receptor binding, longer pulmonary retention, and high lipid conjugation are among the pharmacokinetic parameters that lead to improved efficacy of these compounds and should be considered. A low or negligible oral bioavailability, smaller particle size leading to a relatively inactive drug at the oropharynx, higher plasma protein binding, increased metabolism rates, higher clearances, and lower systemic concentrations are associated with lower risks for adverse effects.[197-199]

For individuals who require long-term care with inhaled glucocorticoids during ventilator dependency, therapy should be continued to minimize the underlying disease process and thereby decrease the number of new variables, including adrenal insufficiency, in the treatment equation with inhaled or intravenous formulations.[200] Despite all of these perceived benefits, inhaled glucocorticoids do not seem to reduce mortality.[201] Acute exacerbations tend to be treated with intravenous or oral preparations due to the higher doses required.

5. Inhaled Antibiotics

Inhaled antibiotics have been used for decades, falling in and out of favor over the years. They are used primarily for treatment and suppression of chronic airway bacterial colonization. Their theoretical advantages are improved drug delivery and higher concentrations at the site of infection, leading to improved efficacy and better bacterial eradication compared with systemic administration.[90,202-204] The primary concern with this therapy is development of bacterial resistance.

Results differ on efficacy. Inhaled antibiotics, mainly aminoglycosides, have been used extensively in cystic fibrosis patients with good results.[90,202-205] Palmer and colleagues reported a marked reduction in the volume of airway secretions and a decrease in the laboratory markers of inflammation in a prospective study of mechanically ventilated patients with chronic respiratory failure.[90,205] However, their study lacked power and was not randomized.

Other studies have failed to show similar benefits but rather have demonstrated poor, unpredictable drug delivery.[206] Unequal ventilation, atelectasis, lobar collapse, and consolidation impair even drug distribution. Bronchospasm with chest tightness has also been reported.[134] Use of inhaled antibiotics should be limited to selected patients, such as those with cystic fibrosis. Routine use to assist with secretion reduction and clearance in the mechanically ventilated patient is not recommended.

D. Positioning of the Patient

The appropriate position in which to maintain the patient requiring mechanical ventilation has been debated.

Current recommendations from the CDC state that elevating the head 30 to 40 degrees reduces the risk of VAP. A study examining head elevation and the rate of VAP concluded early after interim analysis showed an incidence of microbiologically confirmed pneumonia of 5% in semirecumbent patients versus 23% in supine patients.[207] The semirecumbent position has also been supported with regard to facilitating nursing care and decreasing gastric reflux and resultant aspiration. It has not been shown to have an effect on the hemodynamic status of the patient, although this remains a common theoretical concern.[208]

Special beds that provide continuous lateral rotation have been used for patients who cannot be repositioned easily, such as those with severe head or traumatic brain injury, bariatric patients, and those who are pharmacologically paralyzed (e.g., patients with acute respiratory distress syndrome [ARDS]). These beds are advertised to enhance skin care, reduce thrombotic events, and improve pulmonary function. Their use is proposed to reduce atelectasis and, hence, pneumonia formation; however, studies' results have remained conflicting.[209,210]

Occasionally, in severe cases of ARDS, alternative positioning (prone) may be necessary to facilitate ventilation and oxygenation. This method attempts to combat the physiologic shunt that is responsible for the observed hypoxemia. The prone position improves oxygenation by increasing lung volume, recruiting posterior lung fields, and redistributing perfusion.[211] No statistical difference was shown in a meta-analysis of the data for prone positioning of patients, although a small subset of patients with severe ARDS has been shown to benefit.[212,213] However, prone positioning is not without risks, particularly an increased risk for bed sores and ETT complications such as dislodgement.[212] Recently, a bed has become commercially available that possesses the ability to fully prone the patient, making use of this potentially beneficial intervention more dependent on necessity than caregiver feasibility. (Rotoprone, KCI Therapeutic Support Systems, San Antonio, TX.)

VII. CONCLUSIONS

The establishment and maintenance of a secure and dependable airway is paramount in the care of the critically ill patient. From the very onset of admission to the ICU, care of the airway should begin with surveillance and a determination of which airways will be difficult to secure or difficult to maintain. The proper choice of an artificial airway not only facilitates ventilatory requirements for improved oxygenation but protects the patient from untoward iatrogenic problems encountered with instrumentation. Regardless of the intervention, an unfettered vigilance is the key to improved outcomes. Proper ETT care, early performance of a tracheostomy (when indicated), frequent pulmonary hygiene, and the use of established protocols and proven preventive measures should help to ensure safe and successful outcomes in critically ill patients.

VIII. CLINICAL PEARLS

- Polyurethane endotracheal tube (ETT) cuffs that have high-volume, low-pressure (HVLP) cuffs are capable of conforming to the irregular borders of the tracheal lumen and therefore are more effective at preventing microaspiration.

- ETT placement has mechanical and physiologic consequences. Vigilant surveillance of skin hygiene, airway patency, cuff integrity, and ventilatory support must be realized to minimize injury and maximize support.

- Confirmation of ETT placement is necessary to aid in proper resuscitation efforts. Verification by the presence of end-tidal carbon dioxide, whether by capnography or capnometry or by direct or indirect visualization, is mandatory to ensure appropriate placement.

- Cuff leak evaluation is a multifaceted endeavor requiring vigilance, diligence, and skill. An appropriate analysis of the potential cause, scrutinized against the risks and benefits of ETT exchange, must occur with limited interference to homeostasis.

- ETT exchange, whether for biofilm accumulation and luminal obstruction, ETT cuff damage (cuff leak), or other ETT mechanical failure (e.g., kinking) is a high-risk ordeal. The decision to exchange an ETT should be assessed against newer, currently available technologies, such as biofilm extraction, that are designed to salvage damaged ETTs. Should the decision to perform an exchange arise, airway adjuncts such as an airway exchange catheter and video laryngoscopy have proved invaluable for achieving higher success rates.

- Once an ETT is in place, efforts must be aggressive and perpetual to decrease the risk of ventilator-associated pneumonia (VAP); these efforts range from acid-suppression therapies to use of specially designed ETTs to advanced nursing care regimens. VAP appears to be more multifaceted than previously believed. Subglottic suctioning and biofilm management are just the beginning steps.

- Any area of a facility that deals with intubated patients should have a readily accessible difficult airway cart. The cart should be well outfitted but tailored to the types of airways managed and familiar as well as specific for the providers who respond to such emergencies.

- As with pulmonary artery catheters, it is not the difficult airway cart that manages the airway but the personnel who utilize it.

- It is better to investigate any perceived ETT problem electively than to deal with its consequences after it becomes an acute emergency.

- The landscape of ETT design, construction, and maintenance has changed and will continue to change over the next decade. Not all variations will prove effective, but improved patient care will take place.

SELECTED REFERENCES

All references can be found online at expertconsult.com.

9. Spiegel JE: *Endotracheal tube cuffs: Design and function. Anesthesiology News Guide to Airway Management*, New York, 2010, McMahon Publishing, pp 51–58.

21. Kuhlen R, Max M, Dembinski R, et al: Breathing pattern and workload during automatic tube compensation, pressure support and T-piece trials in weaning patients. *Eur J Anaesthesiol* 20:10–16, 2003.

25. Divatia JV, Bhowmick K: Complications of endotracheal intubation and other airway management procedures. *Indian J Anaesth* 49:308–318, 2005.

26. Mort TC: Emergency tracheal intubation: Complications associated with repeated laryngoscopic attempts. *Anesth Analg* 99:607–613, 2004.

61. Berra L, De Marchi L, Panigada M, et al: Evaluation of continuous aspiration of subglottic secretion in an in vivo study. *Crit Care Med* 32:2071–2078, 2004.

62. Dezfulian C, Shojania K, Collard HR, et al: Subglottic secretion drainage for preventing ventilator-associated pneumonia: A meta-analysis. *Am J Med* 118:11–18, 2005.

91. Salem MR: Verification of endotracheal tube position. *Anesthesiol Clin North Am* 19:813–839, 2001.

100. Sengupta P, Sessier DI, Maglinger P, et al: Endotracheal tube cuff pressure in three hospitals and the volume required to produce appropriate cuff pressure. *BMCAnesthesiol* 4(1):8, 2004.

104. Lorente L, Lecuona M, Jiménez A, et al: Influence of an endotracheal tube with polyurethane cuff and subglottic secretion drainage on pneumonia. *Am J Respir Crit Care Med* 176:1079–1183, 2007.

113. American Society of Anesthesiologists Task Force on Difficult Airway Management: Practice guideline for management of the difficult airway. *Anesthesiology* 98:1269–1277, 2003.

135. Smulders K, van der Hoeven H, Weers-Pothoff I, et al: A randomized clinical trial of intermittent subglottic secretion drainage in patients receiving mechanical ventilation. *Chest* 121:858–862, 2002.

137. Coffin SE, Klompas M, Classen D, et al: Strategies to prevent ventilator associated pneumonia in acute care hospitals. Supplement Article SHEA/ISDA Practice Recommendation. *Infect Control Hosp Epidemiol* 29(Suppl 1):S31–S40, 2008.

139. Tablan OC, Anderson LJ, Besser R, et al: Guidelines for preventing health-care associated pneumonia, 2003. Recommendations of CDC and the Healthcare Infection Control Practices Advisory Committee. *MMWR Recomm Rep* 53(RR-3):1–36, 2004.

140. Dragoumanis CK, Vretzakis GI, Papaloannou VE, et al: Investigating the failure to aspirate subglottic secretions with the Evac endotracheal tube. *Anesth Analg* 105:1083–1085, 2007.

141. Kapadia FN: Factors associated with blocked tracheal tubes. *Intensive Care Med* 27:1679–1681, 2001.

145. Mort T, Aldo F, Kopp GW: Managing the unusual airway—Case studies in complexity: Clearing luminal occlusions. *Anesthesiology News* 36(8):64–65, 2010.

146. Jarrett WA, Ribes J, Manaligod JM: Biofilm formation on tracheostomy tubes. *Ear Nose Throat J* 81:659–661, 2002.

164. Shah C, Kollef MH: Endotracheal tube intraluminal volume loss among mechanically ventilated patients. *Crit Care Med* 32:120–125, 2004.

212. Kopterides P, Siempos II, Armaganidis A: Prone positioning in hypoxemic respiratory failure: Meta-analysis of randomized controlled trials. *J Crit Care* 24:89–100, 2009.

Chapter 48

Mechanical Ventilation

MARK A. WARNER | BELA PATEL

I. INTRODUCTION

Mechanical ventilation is frequently used to provide respiratory support in times of critical illness or in patients undergoing general anesthesia. The main goals of mechanical ventilation are oxygenation and carbon dioxide elimination, which are ensured by maintaining adequate tidal volumes and respiratory rates. Since the foot-pump ventilation apparatus was designed by Fell O'Dwyer in 1888, significant advances have been made in positive-pressure ventilation. Because the mechanical ventilator can injure the lung, safe application to limit ventilator-induced lung injury (VILI) and negative interactions with other organ systems is fundamental in managing patients. This chapter reviews different modes of mechanical ventilation and describes their characteristics, attributes, and shortcomings.

When describing mechanical ventilation, we refer only to positive-pressure ventilation, which is used in contemporary settings. Negative-pressure ventilation was employed with the advent of mechanical ventilation to treat patients affected by poliomyelitis, but it is no longer used and not discussed in this chapter.

Esteban and colleagues reviewed the use of mechanical ventilation in intensive care units (ICUs) in North America, South America, Spain, and Portugal. Among the indications for mechanical ventilation, acute respiratory failure was the most common (66% of patients), followed by coma (15%), exacerbation of chronic obstructive pulmonary disease (COPD, 13%), and neuromuscular weakness (5%). The principal causes of acute respiratory failure across all centers were pneumonia (16%), sepsis (16%), postoperative infection (15%), heart failure (12%), acute respiratory distress syndrome (ARDS, 12%), trauma (12%), unspecified causes (13%), and aspiration (3%). Endotracheal tubes were used three times more often than tracheostomies to provide artificial airways. There was some variability in the modes of ventilation used in the different countries participating in the study. Assist-control ventilation (ACV) was the most common worldwide, followed by synchronized intermittent mandatory ventilation (SIMV) with pressure support and by pressure-support ventilation (PSV) alone. However, in North American ICUs, ACV and SIMV were used equally.[1]

To initiate mechanical ventilation, the patient must have in place an artificial airway with which to interface with the ventilator. Various types of airway devices are discussed in other chapters of this textbook. Patients are connected to a mechanical ventilator with an orotracheal tube (i.e., endotracheal tube), nasotracheal tube, or tracheostomy.

Common reasons for insertion of an artificial airway are to maintain airway patency, to prevent aspiration, to facilitate clearance of secretions, and to allow mechanical ventilatory support.[2] There are several indications for mechanical ventilation:

- Hypoxemic respiratory failure
- Hypercapnic respiratory failure
- Mixed respiratory failure
- Altered mentation with inability by the patient to protect the airway
- Hemodynamic instability
- Maintenance of adequate oxygenation and ventilation during deep sedation, anesthesia, or neuromuscular blockade

II. INITIATION OF MECHANICAL VENTILATION

Mechanical ventilation can be delivered to the patient by invasive or noninvasive methods. Noninvasive positive-pressure ventilation (NIPPV) is delivered by an external nasal or a naso-oral interface such as a face mask. The decision to use invasive or noninvasive mechanical ventilation depends on the severity and rapid anticipated reversibility of the underlying condition and the mental status of the patient. NIPPV is useful in cases of hypercapnic respiratory failure, especially associated with COPD; obstructive sleep apnea; cardiogenic pulmonary edema; and hypercapnic respiratory insufficiency in persons with adequate mental status to remain communicative.[3-5] Application of NIPPV requires frequent assessments to ensure that the desired goal of oxygenation or ventilation is being achieved.

After the deciding to initiate invasive positive-pressure mechanical ventilation, several variables must be considered for effective implementation. They include tidal volume, respiratory rate, positive end-expiratory pressure (PEEP), fraction of inspired oxygen (F_{IO_2}), peak flow, plateau pressure, trigger sensitivity, flow rate, and flow pattern.

A. Tidal Volume

Tidal volume is the volume of air delivered to the lungs with each breath by the mechanical ventilator. Historically, initial tidal volumes were set at 10 to 15 mL/kg of actual body weight for patients with neuromuscular diseases. Over the past 2 decades, VILI has been associated with excessive tidal volume leading to alveolar distention.[6,7] The mechanism of lung injury includes regional overinflation,[8] stress of repeated opening and closing of lung units,[9,10] and sheer stress between adjacent structures with differing mechanical properties.[11]

The low-tidal-volume strategy, which uses 6 mL/kg of predicted body weight, has become the standard of care for patients with ARDS, following the Acute Respiratory Distress Syndrome Network (ARDS Network) publication in 2000.[12] The ARDS Network prospectively studied intubated patients with acute lung injury (ALI) or ARDS to determine whether a low-tidal-volume strategy, compared with a traditional-tidal-volume strategy, could improve mortality and decrease the total number of ventilator days. The final analysis showed a 23% reduction in all-cause mortality and a 9% absolute decrease in

mortality with the use of a tidal volume of 6 mL/kg of predicted body weight and plateau pressures of 30 cm H_2O or less, compared with the usual practice of 12 mL/kg of predicted body weight and plateau pressures of 50 cm H_2O or less. Low tidal volume or so-called lung protective ventilation is recommended for all patients with ARDS. In patients without ARDS, a retrospective review demonstrated the relationship between ALI and the use of tidal volumes greater than 10 mL/kg of predicted body weight.[13] Considering the current evidence, tidal volumes greater than 10 mL/kg of predicted body weight should not be routinely used in the care of the mechanically ventilated patient.[12,13]

B. Respiratory Rate

The respiratory rate setting depends on the desired minute ventilation. Minute ventilation is a product of the respiratory rate and the tidal volume, and it is expressed in liters per minute. After a patient is intubated and placed on the mechanical ventilator, it is important to ensure adequate minute ventilation since the underlying pathophysiology or pharmacologic interventions can suppress the patient's ability to compensate for metabolic demands. In most scenarios, the rate is determined by observing the patient's native respiratory rate before intubation. The normal rate of minute ventilation is 5 to 7 L/min. In patients with sepsis or diabetic ketoacidosis, the native minute ventilation may be as high as 12 to 15 L/min, requiring a high respiratory rate. To adequately compensate for the acid-base derangements and ensure adequate minute ventilation, it is necessary to titrate the set respiratory rate until the desired pH and Pa_{CO_2} goals are met. Permissive hypercapnia (i.e., allowing the Pa_{CO_2} to increase intentionally to achieve other goals) may be appropriate in certain clinical conditions. Auto-PEEP (i.e. intrinsic PEEP) must be evaluated to ensure it remains at less than 5 cm H_2O. After the goal is achieved, it is a safe practice to set the rate at 4 breaths/min below the spontaneous breathing rate in the event that intrinsic or extrinsic factors suppress respiration. In patients on SIMV, the rate is initially set to meet up to 80% of the minute ventilation demands. Initial respiratory rates are usually 12 to 16 breaths/min, but rates of breaths per minute in the high 20s to low 30s may be required in patients with ARDS. In those with obstructive lung disease (e.g., asthma), a lower respiratory rate is desired, with significant risk of developing auto-PEEP. Assessment and management of auto-PEEP are discussed separately.

C. Positive End-Expiratory Pressure

PEEP is the alveolar pressure above the atmospheric pressure at end-expiration. Applied PEEP (i.e., extrinsic PEEP) through mechanical ventilation allows delivery of positive pressure at the end of expiration to keep the unstable lung units from collapse.[14] PEEP increases the peak inspiratory pressure, which directly overcomes the opening pressure of the unstable lung units. Low levels of PEEP (3 to 5 cm H_2O) are routinely used in patients on mechanical ventilation. It can decrease alveolar collapse at end-expiration and may reduce the incidence of

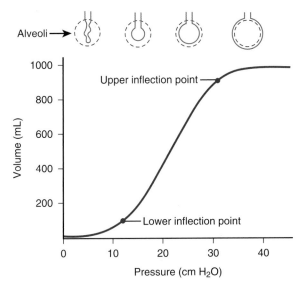

Figure 48-1 Calculation of optimal positive end-expiratory pressure (PEEP). Mechanical ventilation delivers low levels of PEEP to keep unstable alveoli from collapse at end expiration. The volume-pressure curve can be used to assess changes in lung compliance and to determine a ventilation strategy by identifying the lower inflection point, which is the critical opening pressure of collapsed alveoli, and the upper inflection point, which indicates a state of lung overinflation. (From Haitsma JJ: Physiology of mechanical ventilation. *Crit Care Clin* 23:117–134, 2007.)

ventilator-associated pneumonia.[15] Higher levels of PEEP are employed to improve oxygenation in patients with hypoxic respiratory failure. Goals in managing ARDS are to optimize alveolar recruitment and decrease cycles of recruitment and derecruitment of alveolar lung units. Several strategies are used to determine optimal PEEP, but there are limited data to support their routine use. Determining the lower inflection point of the pressure-volume curve (P_{flex}), which reflects the transition from low to higher compliance, and applying PEEP of 2 cm H_2O greater than this point may be used to estimate the appropriate level of applied PEEP (Fig. 48-1).[16]

Because it is often impractical to routinely obtain pressure-volume curves, algorithms have been developed

(e.g., in ARDS Network trials), with PaO_2/FIO_2 ratios to set the recommended PEEP (Table 48-1).[12] Measuring esophageal pressures to estimate transpulmonary pressures has been studied as a method to determine the appropriate applied PEEP in patients with ARDS, and this approach has demonstrated improvement in oxygenation and compliance.[17] Trials of increasing or decreasing PEEP can also be used.[18,19] Higher levels of PEEP in postoperative patients have had no benefit.[20]

Lung injury in patients with hypoxic respiratory failure is heterogeneous. Since the collapse and repeated opening and closing of unstable lung units leads to further injury, its prevention would be the optimal ventilator strategy. High PEEP has been used mitigate alveolar collapse and cyclic alveolar stress. Several trials demonstrated that high PEEP increased oxygenation but did not improve mortality rates.[21,22] However, a meta-analysis of high PEEP trials indicated a mortality benefit for patients with a PaO_2/FIO_2 ratio of less than 200.[23] The optimal method of applying adequate PEEP has not been established.[14] Trials in ARDS patients demonstrate PEEP requirements are usually between 12 and 20 cm H_2O.

D. Fraction of Inspired Oxygen

On initiation of mechanical ventilation, the FIO_2 usually is set at 1.0. The goal is to rapidly reduce the FIO_2 to the target PaO_2 and SpO_2 to limit the consequences of supplemental oxygen. In most patients, a target PaO_2 of 60 mm Hg and SpO_2 of 90% meets oxygenation requirements. However, some patients may have higher PaO_2 targets based on their underlying cardiopulmonary status (e.g., myocardial ischemia, pulmonary hypertension). In patients with ARDS, targeting a PaO_2 as low as 50 mm Hg may be appropriate to limit alveolar injury.[24] A prolonged high level of FIO_2 has been associated with airway and parenchymal injury, atelectasis from nitrogen washout, and increased risk of diffuse alveolar damage, which is even higher in patients receiving bleomycin therapy.[25,26] If the need for supplemental FIO_2 remains greater than 0.6, FIO_2 should be reduced with strategies such as applied PEEP and alternative ventilator modes.

TABLE 48-1														
Combinations of PEEP and FIO₂ Used in the ARDS Network Trials														
Component	**Allowable Combinations of PEEP and FIO₂***													
Lower-PEEP Group														
FIO₂	0.3	0.4	0.4	0.5	0.5	0.6	0.7	0.7	0.7	0.8	0.9	0.9	0.9	1.0
PEEP	5	5	8	8	10	10	10	12	14	14	14	16	18	18-24
Higher-PEEP Group†														
FIO₂	0.3	0.3	0.3	0.3	0.3	0.4	0.4	0.5	0.5	0.5-0.8	0.8	0.9	1.0	
PEEP	5	8	10	12	14	14	16	16	18	20	22	22	22-24	
Higher-PEEP Group‡														
FIO₂	0.3	0.3	0.4	0.4	0.5	0.5	0.5-0.8	0.8	0.9	1.0				
PEEP	12	14	14	16	16	18	20	22	22	22-24				

*Combinations of positive end-expiratory pressure (PEEP in cm H_2O) and fraction of inspired oxygen (FIO_2) used in the Acute Respiratory Distress Syndrome (ARDS) network trials.
†Before the protocol changed to use higher levels of PEEP.
‡After the protocol changed to use higher levels of PEEP.
Adapted from National Heart, Lung and Blood Institute ARDS Clinical Trials Network. Higher versus lower positive end-expiratory pressures in patients with the acute respiratory distress syndrome. *N Engl J Med* 351:327–336, 2004.

E. Peak Pressure

Peak airway pressure is a measurement of the maximum pressure felt by the airways on inspiration. In the passive patient, peak airway pressure, or peak pressure, depends on the respiratory rate, tidal volume, and inspiratory flow rate in volume-targeted modes of mechanical ventilation. When awake and active, the patient's effort contributes to the peak pressure. In pressure-targeted ventilator modes, the peak pressure is directly related to the inspiratory pressure that is set and the inspiratory flow rate.[27] Studies have not consistently shown barotrauma to be an adverse consequence of increased peak pressures.[28,29] The peak airway pressure typically is higher than the plateau pressure, and the difference indicates airway resistance.

F. Plateau Pressure

Plateau pressure is the pressure that is applied by the mechanical ventilator to the small airways and alveoli. The plateau pressure is measured at end-inspiration with an inspiratory hold maneuver on the mechanical ventilator that is 0.5 to 1 second. Meta-analysis demonstrated a significant correlation between plateau pressures greater than 35 cm H_2O and the risk of barotrauma.[30] In the ARDS Network trial, lower tidal volume ventilation with plateau pressures less than 30 mm Hg was associated with a lower mortality rate than that found for conventional tidal volume using plateau pressures less than 50 mm Hg.[12]

Common reasons for increased plateau pressures are the use of high PEEP, inspiratory flow, and tidal volume. Adverse consequences of high plateau pressures are barotrauma, resulting in ventilator-associated lung injury, pneumothorax, pneumomediastinum, and subcutaneous emphysema. If barotrauma develops, it may be beneficial to reduce the plateau pressures further by decreasing the tidal volume, PEEP, or flow or by increasing the patient's sedation.

G. Trigger Sensitivity

Sensors on the ventilator detect the patient's effort in terms of negative inspiratory pressure applied to the circuit by the patient or inspiratory flow of air from the patient. This is referred to as "triggering the ventilator" or "triggering a breath." Pressure trigger sensitivity typically is set between −1 and −3 cm H_2O, and a breath is triggered when a negative inspiratory effort is greater than the set sensitivity. A flow-triggered breath is delivered when the return flow is less than the delivered flow. When the patient does not provide adequate negative inspiratory pressure or flow rate to trigger breaths, the ventilator provides mandatory breaths to the patient at the set parameters. The breaths are initiated by the ventilator at the set time, as determined by the set respiratory rate, and it delivers the breath at the prescribed flow rate until the desired tidal volume has been achieved, after which the ventilator cycles off for passive exhalation.

H. Flow Rate

Flow rate, or peak inspiratory flow rate, is the maximum flow at which a set tidal volume breath is delivered by the ventilator. Most modern ventilators can deliver flow rates between 60 and 120 L/min. Flow rates should be titrated to meet the patient's inspiratory demands.[31] If the peak flow rate is too low for the patient, dyspnea, patient-ventilator asynchrony, and increased work of breathing may result. High peak flow rates increase peak airway pressures and lower mean airway pressures, which may decrease oxygenation.[27]

In most patients, peak flow rates of 60 L/min are adequate. Higher flow rates are required in patients with higher ventilator demands.[31] Higher peak flow rates may also be necessary in patients with obstructive lung disease to decrease inspiratory time, thereby increasing the expiratory time and reducing the risk of developing auto-PEEP.[32,33]

I. Flow Pattern

Modern mechanical ventilators can deliver various inspiratory flow patterns. The constant or square waveform is a description of the inspiratory flow that is delivered by the mechanical ventilator. It correlates with volume-cycled breaths, in which the inspiratory flow remains constant until the desired tidal volume is delivered and then remains at that level until expiration. In this pattern of inspiratory flow, the airway pressure varies and depends on the patient's effort and compliance of the lung. The sinusoidal wave flow gradually increases and decreases throughout the respiratory cycle. In the decelerating ramp wave (i.e., saw-tooth wave), the flow rate begins maximally and decreases until the end of inspiration. It parallels normal inspiratory pattern most closely. The ramp wave yields the most homogenous distribution of ventilation in most conditions, decreases peak airway pressures, and improves carbon dioxide (CO_2) elimination.[34] For patients who are triggering the ventilator, this strategy of ventilation is recommended (Fig. 48-2).

III. COMMON MODES OF MECHANICAL VENTILATION

The three most commonly used modes of mechanical ventilation are ACV, SIMV, and PSV. Each mode describes whether breaths are volume constant or pressure constant; which are mandatory or spontaneous, or both; and which variables determine a change in function. All three modes have uses throughout the spectrum of stabilization of ventilation, maintenance of ventilation, and weaning from mechanical support.

Choice of the type of mechanical ventilation is most often determined by whether resting of respiratory muscles is indicated. Patients who are hemodynamically compromised, patients with severe oxygenation or ventilation derangements, and those undergoing general endotracheal anesthesia qualify for a rest of respiratory muscles. In these cases, it is prudent to choose a mode of ventilation that accomplishes ventilation without the need for

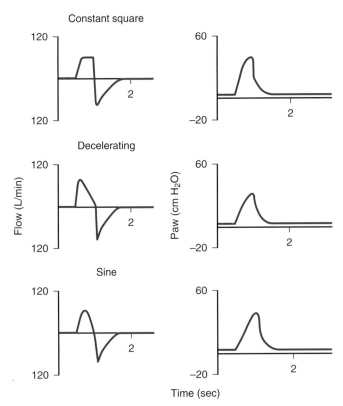

Figure 48-2 The three most common inspiratory flow patterns in humans *(left)* are compared with their corresponding pressure versus time curves *(right)*. (From Yang SC, Yang SP: Effects of inspiratory flow waveforms on lung mechanics, gas exchange and respiratory metabolism in COPD patients during mechanical ventilation. *Chest* 122:2096–2104, 2002.)

spontaneous respirations; ACV is most often used. However, if use of muscles of respiration is desired, SIMV or PSV should be considered. Patients in whom the use of respiratory muscles is desired are usually those being weaned from mechanical ventilation or undergoing assessment of muscle strength and adequacy of spontaneous work of breathing. PSV is the only mode of the three that entirely relies on the patient spontaneously breathing. Table 48-2 shows the set and variable parameters in each common mode of ventilation. Control mode of ventilation (CMV) is the original mode of ventilation. In CMV, the patient receives a positive-pressure breath at a set rate without the ability to influence how it is delivered.

A. Assist-Control Ventilation

Volume assist-control ventilation (VACV) is the most frequently used initial mode of ventilation, and it has

several advantages in stabilization and maintenance of adequate ventilation. Using VACV allows adequate oxygenation and ventilation, and it decreases the work of breathing while treating a pathologic process. It is commonly used in patients expected to be passive, as in routine use in the operating room for general anesthesia and in comatose patients.

VACV is a combination mode of ventilation in which the preset tidal volume is delivered in response to the inspiratory effort or if no patient effort occurs within a set period of time. The period is determined by the backup respiratory rate set on the ventilator. A patient-triggered breath is sensed by a change in airway flow or pressure. When the change reaches the trigger threshold, the ventilator delivers the predetermined tidal volume. In ACV, the limit variable that increases to the set threshold before inspiration ends is volume or flow, or both. The cycle variable that ends inspiration is volume or time. Peak inspiratory airway pressure and plateau pressure are variable in this setting. In patients with deep sedation or neuromuscular blockade, the ACV mode functions like CMV. The advantage of ACV is that it substantially decreases the work of breath and decreases myocardial oxygen demand. The disadvantages of ACV in the active patient are that it is less comfortable than spontaneous breathing and that it can induce respiratory alkalosis and breath-stacking (Table 48-3).

When ACV is used in a volume-targeted mode, airway pressures vary. When patients with severe hypoxemia (e.g., ARDS) require high PEEP and FIO_2 settings to maintain adequate oxygenation, the airway pressures that are generated to deliver the desired tidal volume increase. This increasing pressure can be measured as the peak inspiratory pressure, the mean airway pressure, or the plateau pressure, all of which attempt to describe the pressures that are transmitted through the airways at different levels and at different points in the respiratory cycle. As the plateau pressures increase, reflecting increasing alveolar pressure, it may be prudent to use a pressure-control variant of the ACV mode.

Similar to volume-targeted ACV, the pressure-targeted ACV mode requires the user to input the frequency (i.e., desired respiratory rate), PEEP, and FIO_2, but instead of a desired tidal volume, the user sets the upper limit of the inspiratory pressure that is allowable. As the ventilator delivers a breath, the inspiratory flow continues until the maximum pressure or allotted time is reached, and the flow then ceases. In pressure-targeted ACV, the tidal volume varies, and consistency is sacrificed to prevent barotrauma by high pressures (Table 48-4).[35] Figure 48-3 depicts the differences in VACV and pressure

TABLE 48-2

Set and Variable Parameters for Common Modes of Mechanical Ventilation

Ventilation Mode	Respiratory Rate	Tidal Volume	Peak Inspiratory Pressure	PEEP	FIO₂
ACV	Set	Set	Set/variable	Set	Set
SIMV	Set	Set	Variable	Set	Set
PSV	Variable	Variable	Variable	Set	Set

ACV, Assist-control ventilation; *FIO₂,* fraction of inspired oxygen; *PEEP,* positive end-expiratory pressure; *PSV,* pressure-support ventilation; *SIMV,* synchronized intermittent mandatory ventilation.

TABLE 48-3

Advantages and Disadvantages of Conventional Modes

Ventilation Mode	Advantages	Disadvantages
ACV	Predictable tidal volumes	Uncomfortable for the awake patient
	Mandatory respiratory rate	Respiratory alkalosis possible
	Useful for reliable ventilation	Breath-stacking, auto-PEEP
	Good for stabilization of hypoxemia	Not a weaning mode
	Decreases work of breathing	Usually requires sedation
SIMV	More comfortable	Spontaneous breaths vary
	Allows respiratory muscle work	Increases weaning time
PSV	More comfortable	No guaranteed respiratory rate
	Allows for evaluation of spontaneous work of breathing	No guaranteed tidal volume
	Weaning mode	Apnea can be disastrous

ACV, Assist-control ventilation; *PEEP,* positive end-expiratory pressure; *PSV,* pressure-support ventilation; *SIMV,* synchronized intermittent mandatory ventilation.

TABLE 48-4

Comparison of Volume-Targeted and Pressure-Targeted Assist-Control Ventilation

Parameter	Volume-Targeted Ventilation	Pressure-Targeted Ventilation
Frequency (rate)	Set	Set
Tidal volume	Set	Variable
Inspiratory flow	Set	Set
Peak inspiratory pressure	Variable	Set
PEEP	Set	Set
FiO_2	Set	Set

PEEP, Positive end-expiratory pressure; *FiO₂,* fraction of inspired oxygen.

assist-control ventilation (PACV) in graphs of pressure versus time and airflow versus time.

ARDS is commonly seen in medical and surgical patients and presents dilemmas in treatment.[36] According to the 1994 American-European Consensus Conference definition, ARDS is recognized as a spectrum, which includes ALI, as defined by a ratio of the partial pressure of arterial oxygen to the fraction of inspired oxygen (PaO_2/FiO_2) of 300 or less, and ARDS, which is defined as a PaO_2/FiO_2 ratio of 200 or less. Other characteristics of ARDS are the acute onset of bilateral pulmonary infiltrates and a pulmonary capillary wedge pressure of less than 18 mm Hg (or no evidence of elevated left atrial pressure). ARDS is synonymous with noncardiogenic pulmonary edema.[37] ALI has many direct and indirect causes. Examples of direct injury are pneumonia, orogastric fluid aspiration, and inhalation injury; indirect causes of injury include severe sepsis, shock, pancreatitis, blood product transfusion, and narcotic overdose.[38]

Ventilatory strategies for the management of ARDS rest on the results of the ARDS Network studies, which demonstrated that patients given tidal volumes of 6 mL/kg of predicted body weight had improved mortality rates compared with patients with tidal volumes of 12 mL/kg of predicted body weight. Another finding was that plateau pressures less than 30 cm H_2O protect the lung (Fig. 48-4 and Table 48-5).[12] In 1998, Amato and colleagues demonstrated the mortality benefit of lower tidal volumes and a lower rate of barotraumas (Fig. 48-5).[16] Two meta-analyses demonstrated decreased mortality rates with the use of low tidal volume ventilation (i.e., lung-protective ventilation).[39,40] In ARDS management, plateau pressures should be less than or equal to 30 cm H_2O or the lowest possible level. A high-PEEP strategy decreased the mortality rate in a meta-analysis of 2299 ARDS patients.[23] Randomized trials of ventilation in ARDS patients are summarized in Table 48-6.

B. Synchronized Intermittent Mandatory Ventilation

SIMV is a frequently used mode of ventilation in hospital medical and surgical units. SIMV has some features that incorporate characteristics of ACV and PSV. SIMV uses

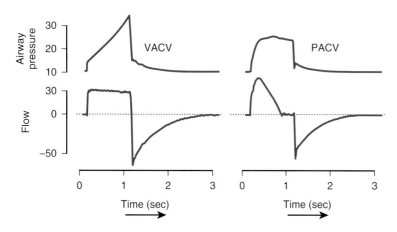

Figure 48-3 Graphs of airway pressure versus time and airflow versus time compare volume assist-control ventilation *(VACV)* and pressure assist-control ventilation *(PACV).* (From Marini JJ: Point: Is pressure assist-control preferred over volume assist-control mode for lung protective ventilation in patients with ARDS? Yes. *Chest* 140:286–290, 2011.)

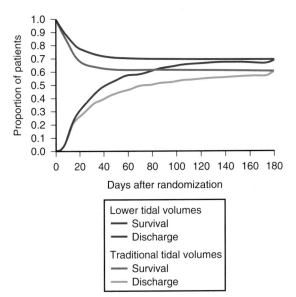

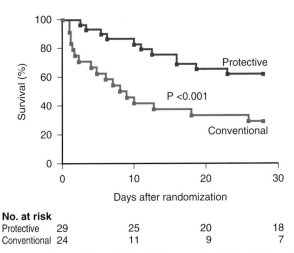

Figure 48-4 The Kaplan-Meier curve from the ARDS Network study compares survival to 180 days and discharge to home without breathing assistance in the lower tidal volume group and the traditional tidal volume group. (From Acute Respiratory Distress Syndrome Network: Ventilation with lower tidal volumes as compared with traditional tidal volumes for acute lung injury and the acute respiratory distress syndrome. *N Engl J Med* 342:1301–1308, 2000.)

Figure 48-5 Comparison of the 28-day survival of patients with acute respiratory distress syndrome (ARDS) assigned to protective or conventional mechanical ventilation. (From Al-Saady N, Bennett ED: Decelerating inspiratory flow waveform improves lung mechanics and gas exchange in patients on intermittent positive-pressure ventilation. *Intensive Care Med* 11:68–75, 1985.)

the same settings as ACV: frequency, tidal volume, PEEP, and FiO_2, but it also has a setting for a prescribed pressure support for a spontaneous breath. The purpose of the two types of breaths (i.e., mandatory and spontaneous) is to allow increased diaphragmatic activity and increased work of breathing by the patient when triggering spontaneous breaths. SIMV is sometimes used as a weaning mode, but it can prolong mechanical ventilation and is therefore not routinely recommended for weaning.[41]

When a patient is deeply sedated or paralyzed, SIMV functions the same as ACV. The patient receives the set number of mandatory breaths as determined by the set frequency at the prescribed tidal volume with the set PEEP and FiO_2. However, in patients who are more awake, SIMV can assist the patient when he or she triggers a mandatory breath and can support the patient with the prescribed pressure support and PEEP in spontaneous breaths that are above the number of mandatory breaths set. The advantage of this mode is that it allows the patient to get the set number of mandatory breaths by controlling the breaths (if the patient is not initiating inspiration) or assisting breaths (if the patient is triggering the start of inspiration), and the patient is allowed to make an effort at spontaneous breaths. The use of SIMV also may reduce sedation requirements (see Table 48-3).[42]

TABLE 48-5

Main Outcome Variables in the Acute Respiratory Distress Syndrome (ARDS) Network Trial of Low Tidal Volumes versus Traditional Tidal Volumes in Patients with ARDS

Outcome Variable	Group Receiving Lower Tidal Volumes	Group Receiving Traditional Tidal Volumes	P Value
Death before discharge home and breathing without assistance (%)	31.0	39.8	0.007
Breathing without assistance by day 28 (%)	65.7	55.0	<0.001
No. of ventilator-free days, days 1 to 28 (%)[†]	12 ± 11*	10 ± 11*	0.007
Barotrauma, days 1 to 28 (%)[‡]	10	11	0.43
No. of days without failure of nonpulmonary organs or systems, days 1 to 28[§]	15 ± 11*	12 ± 11*	0.006

*Mean ± SD.
[†]The number of ventilator-free days is the mean number of days from day 1 to day 28 during which the patient had been breathing without assistance for at least 48 consecutive hours.
[‡]Barotrauma was defined as any new pneumothorax, pneumomediastinum, or subcutaneous emphysema or a pneumatocele that was more than 2 cm in diameter.
[§]Circulatory failure was defined as a systolic blood pressure of 90 mm Hg or less or the need for treatment with any vasopressor; coagulation failure as a platelet count of 80,000/mm³ or less; hepatic failure as a serum bilirubin concentration of at least 2 mg/dL (34 µmol/L); and renal failure as a serum creatinine concentration of at least 2 mg/dL (177 µmol/L).
From The Acute Respiratory Distress Syndrome Network: Ventilation with lower tidal volumes as compared with traditional tidal volumes for acute lung injury and the acute respiratory distress syndrome. *N Engl J Med* 342:1301–1308, 2000.

TABLE 48-6

Summary of Randomized, Controlled Trials of Ventilatory Strategies Used for Adult Patients Who Have or Are at Risk for Acute Respiratory Distress Syndrome to Prevent Ventilator-Associated Lung Injury

Study Component	Amato et al.[16] (N = 53)	Brochard et al.[111] (N = 108)	Brower et al.[112] (N = 52)	Stewart et al.[113] (N = 120)	NIH* (N = 861)
Population					
Entry criteria	LIS > 2.5 PAWP < 16 mm Hg MV < 7 d	LIS > 2.5 MV < 3 d	PaO_2/FIO_2 < 200 MV < 1 d	PaO_2/FIO_2 < 250 MV < 1 d	PaO_2/FIO_2 < 300 MV < 36 hr
Exclusion criteria	Coronary insufficiency, prior lung disease, barotrauma, uncontrolled acidosis intracranial hypertension, terminal disease	Left heart failure, acute or chronic organ failure, chest wall abnormality, intracranial hypertension, head injury, terminal disease	Age <18, left heart failure, acute neurologic disease, chronic lung disease, thoracic surgery	Age <18, left heart failure, myocardial ischemia, acute or chronic neurologic disease, PIP > 30 for 2 hr, terminal disease	Age <18, left heart failure, acute neurologic disease, life expectancy <6 mo, hepatic failure
Characteristics at Inclusion					
APACHE II	28 vs 27	18 vs 17	90 vs 85 (APACHE III)	22 vs 21	
PaO_2/FIO_2	112 vs 134	144 vs 155	129 vs 150	123 vs 145	
LIS	3.4 vs 3.2	3.0 vs 3.0	2.7 vs 2.8		
Targeted Settings					
Intervention	V_T < 6 mL/kg PIP < 40 cm H_2O $P_{driving}$ < 20 cm H_2O CPAP recruiting	$P_{plateau}$ ≤ 25–30 cm H_2O V_T = 6–10 mL/kg	$P_{plateau}$ ≤ 30 cm H_2O V_T ≤ 8 mL/kg IBW	PIP < 30 cm H_2O V_T ≤ 8 mL/kg IBW	V_T ≤ 6 mL/kg IBW Reduce V_T if $P_{plateau}$ > 30 cm H_2O
Control	V_T = 12 mL/kg $PaCO_2$, 35–38 mm Hg PIP unlimited	V_T = 10–15 mL/kg, PIP < 60 cm H_2O	$P_{plateau}$ ≤ 45–55 cm H_2O V_T = 10–12 mL/kg IBW	PIP ≤ 50 cm H_2O V_T = 10–15 mL/kg IBW	V_T = 12 mL/kg IBW Reduce V_T if $P_{plateau}$ > 50 cm H_2O
PEEP (cm H_2O)					
Intervention	2 above P_{flex}	0–15, titrated to best P/F ratio	5–20 titrated to best P/F ratio	5–20 titrated to best P/F ratio	Titrated to gas exchange
Control	Titrated to P/F ratio	Titrated to P/F ratio	Titrated to P/F ratio	Titrated to P/F ratio	Titrated to gas exchange
Resulting Settings†					
$P_{plateau}$ (cm H_2O)	30 vs 37	26 vs 32	25 vs 32	22 vs 28	25 vs 32–34
PEEP (cm H_2O)	16 vs 7	11 vs 11	10 vs 9	9 vs 7	8–9, both groups
V_T (mL or mL/kg)	350 vs 770 mL	7 vs 10 mL/kg	7 vs 10 mL/kg	7 vs 11 mL/kg	6.2 vs 11.8 mL/kg
PaO_2 (mm Hg)	55 vs 32	60 vs 41	50 vs 40	54 vs 46	
Outcomes					
Mortality	13/29 (45%) vs 17/24 (71%)	47% vs 38%	13/26 (50%) vs 12/26 (46%)	30/60 (50%) vs 28/60 (47%)	31 vs 39%
Barotauma‡	2 (7%) vs 10 (42%)	8 (14%) vs 7 (12%)	1 (4%) vs 2 (8%)	6 (10%) vs 4 (7%)	No difference

APACHE II, Acute Physiology and Chronic Health Evaluation II; *CPAP*, continuous positive airway pressure; *FIO_2*, fraction of inspired oxygen; *IBW*, ideal body weight (formulas used for calculation were not uniform across studies; Brochard and coworkers used "dry weight" to determine tidal volume); *LIS*, lung injury score; *MV*, mechanical ventilation; *PaO_2*, partial pressure of arterial oxygen; *$P_{driving}$*, driving pressure; *PEEP*, positive end-expiratory pressure; *P/F*, *PaO_2/FIO_2*, fraction of inspired oxygen; *P_{flex}*, pressure at the lower inflection point of the pressure-volume curve; *PIP*, peak inspiratory pressure; *PAWP*, pulmonary artery wedge pressure; *$P_{plateau}$*, plateau pressure; *V_T*, tidal volume.

*National Institutes of Health (NIH) Acute Respiratory Distress Syndrome (ARDS) Network Trials, as reported on the NIH Web site (www.nih.gov).

†Precise comparison of resulting settings across the studies is difficult, because there is variation in the schedule of reporting; we attempted to compare mean values on days 1 through 3.

‡Barotrauma was defined by Amato and coworkers as clinical barotrauma; by Brower and colleagues as pneumothorax; by Stewart and coworkers as pneumothorax, pneumomediastinum, subcutaneous emphysema, and lung cysts on a chest radiograph; and by Brochard and colleagues as pneumothorax requiring a chest tube.

Adapted from American Thoracic Society, European Society of Intensive Care Medicine, and Societé de Réanimation de Langue Française: International Consensus Conference in intensive care medicine: Ventilator-associated lung injury in ARDS. *Am J Respir Crit Care Med* 160:2118–2124, 1999.

C. Pressure-Support Ventilation

PSV is used for patients who are awake enough to accomplish spontaneous breathing. PSV was initially developed to reduce work of breathing in SIMV but evolved into a stand-alone mode of ventilation. PSV augments the patient's spontaneous inspiratory efforts with the selected level of positive airway pressure. The inspiratory pressure is delivered until the flow decreases to a predetermined level (usually 25% of peak flow). PSV allows the user to control the desired pressure support, PEEP, and F_{IO_2}. This mode relies entirely on spontaneous breaths by the patient, who must have an intact ventilatory drive. The work of breathing of PSV is inversely proportional to the level of pressure support and the flow rate.[43] Because no tidal volume is guaranteed by this mode of ventilation, pressure support must be titrated to help the patient achieve an adequate tidal volume. However, any change in lung compliance or airway impedance results in a change in tidal volume. A certain level of pressure support is needed to overcome the resistance of the ventilator circuit and endotracheal tube. This typically is less than 10 cm H_2O, but it can be higher with narrower endotracheal tubes.[44] Pressure support above that needed to overcome resistance supplements the achieved tidal volumes. Typical pressure support settings are 5 to 25 mm H_2O. When full ventilator support is needed for the patient, PSV may not be the ideal mode because it requires a higher work of breathing and minute ventilation is not guaranteed (see Table 48-3).

D. Pressure-Regulated Volume Control

Pressure-regulated volume control (PRVC) can be employed with ACV or SIMV. With PRVC, the ventilator monitors the patient's effort and varies the peak inspiratory pressure that is allowed with the inspiratory flow to achieve the set tidal volume. The ventilator provides a breath at a low pressure and then calculates the peak pressure necessary to deliver the set tidal volume. That pressure level is delivered during the next breath. If the target is not attained, the peak pressure is adjusted by 1 to 3 cm H_2O for the next breath. This allows breath-to-breath correction and enables increased airway pressure control. Because the inspiratory time and flow are auto-regulated, it results in a smaller increase in plateau airway pressures with a given tidal volume. Because the ventilator responds to the patient's effort in PRVC, as the patient's ventilator demand increases, the inspiratory pressure decreases, thereby increasing the patient's work of breathing.[45]

IV. UNCOMMON MODES OF VENTILATION

A. Inverse-Ratio Ventilation

Inverse-ratio ventilation (IRV) is positive-pressure ventilation with an inspiratory-expiratory (I:E) ratio of greater than 1. It has been used in the management of severe ARDS to improve oxygenation when PEEP has been optimized.[46] I:E ratios usually range from 1:2 to 1:5,

whereas in IRV, they may be 1:1, 2:1, or higher. Increasing the inspiratory time increases mean airway pressure without increasing the inspiratory plateau pressure, which may improve oxygenation.[47,48] This application is most commonly used with time-cycled pressure-control ventilation (PCV), but it can also be used with volume-cycled ventilation. The improvements in oxygenation are modest, and carbon dioxide elimination is preserved or enhanced[48,49]; however, not all studies have shown benefit.[50] Development of auto-PEEP is common in IRV, and it may be responsible for some of the improvements in oxygenation, but it also increases the risk of barotrauma. Because the benefits of IRV are controversial, it should be limited to use in patients with severe ARDS with refractory hypoxemia.[51]

B. Airway Pressure–Release Ventilation

Airway pressure–release ventilation (APRV) is similar to a blend of inverse-ratio PCV and SIMV. APRV offers two levels of continuous positive airway pressure (CPAP) ventilation, in which it uses high and low pressures to aid in recruitment of atelectatic lung units and allows spontaneous breathing.[52,53] The continuous high positive pressure (P_{high}) is delivered by the ventilator for a prolonged duration (T_{high}) and then drops to the lower pressure (P_{low}) for a short duration (T_{low}). Spontaneous breathing can occur during high and low pressures. Overall, the lower pressure is set to manage hypoxemia and the upper level to promote CO_2 elimination. When the patient cannot initiate breaths, the mode is identical to inverse-ratio PCV.[54] One study of 24 patients with ARDS showed that when APRV was compared with PSV, APRV improved oxygenation and cardiac parameters, along with improvements in ventilation-perfusion matching in the lung.[55]

APRV can decrease peak airway pressures, improve oxygenation, improve alveolar recruitment, and improve cardiac output, but the findings have been inconsistent, and there has been no evidence of mortality benefit.[56-59] During periods of transition between low and high pressures, patient ventilator dyssynchrony can occur. APRV is not recommended for patients with obstructive lung disease or high levels of minute ventilation (Figs. 48-6 and 48-7).

Bi-level ventilation is similar to APRV but has additional features.[60] The transitions from low and high pressures are coordinated with the patient's effort to reduce dyssynchrony. T_{low} usually is longer in bi-level ventilation, which allows for more spontaneous breaths to occur at this pressure level. As in APRV, bi-level ventilation has been used primarily in patients with ALI or ARDS, and it should be avoided in patients with obstructive lung disease because of the risk of auto-PEEP due to shortened expiratory times.

C. High-Frequency Ventilation

There are many types of high-frequency mechanical ventilation. High-frequency ventilation is positive-pressure ventilation with tidal volumes near the anatomic dead space and flow rates greater than 60 breaths/min. The

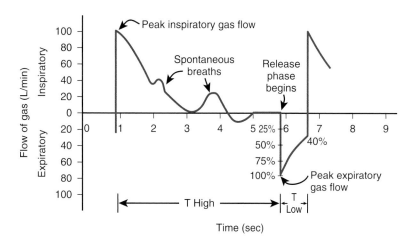

Figure 48-6 Inspiratory and expiratory flow of gas in airway pressure release ventilation. *T High*, Number of seconds spent at the higher pressure; *T Low*, number of seconds spent at the lower pressure. (From Frawley PM, Habashi NM: Airway pressure release ventilation: Theory and practice. *AACN Clinical Issues* 12:234-246, 2001.)

theoretical advantages over conventional ventilation are that the tidal volumes of 1 to 3 mL/kg and the higher levels of PEEP reduce the risk of cyclical alveolar injury and collapse and limit alveolar overdistention. The ability to maintain high mean airway pressures and lower plateau pressures can improve oxygenation.

High-frequency oscillatory ventilation (HFOV), sometimes called the *oscillator,* is a means of improving oxygenation by providing an oxygen-rich and CO_2-poor gas at high respiratory rates that rapidly mixes with sinusoidal flow at stroke volumes that approximate anatomic dead space. HFOV is the most commonly used high-frequency ventilator in adults. HFOV uses a pump to generate a respiratory frequency of 3 to 6 Hz or 180 to 360 breaths/min. In a 1984 publication, Chang described five mechanisms of oxygen delivery by high-frequency oscillation: direct alveolar ventilation of proximal airways; bulk convective gas mixing in conductive airways by recirculation of air among neighboring airways in different cycles of opening and closing of the alveolus; convective transport of gases; longitudinal dispersion by airway turbulence; and molecular diffusion.[61] Additional work is needed to delineate the exact mechanisms involved in gas exchange in high-frequency ventilation.

Selection guidelines for HFOV do not exist, but patients with ARDS who develop refractory hypoxemia on conventional ventilation are sometimes considered.[62-64] In patients with ALI that progresses to ARDS, high PEEP and FiO_2 values may be required to sustain oxygenation. HFOV uses high airway pressures during very short time intervals to help recruit and oxygenate atelectatic lung.

The mean airway pressure is set by manipulation of the inspiratory flow rate and an expiratory back-pressure valve. A multicenter trial of 148 patients with ARDS compared conventional ventilation with high-frequency oscillatory ventilation. Patients were randomized to receive conventional mechanical ventilation or high-frequency oscillatory ventilation and were followed to compare 30-day ventilator-free survival. Results demonstrated improved 30-day mortality rates in the HFOV group, but it did not rise to statistical significance, nor did various secondary end points, including rates for 6-month mortality and duration of mechanical ventilation.[63] HFOV in patients with obstructive lung disease (e.g., COPD, asthma) may lead to significant auto-PEEP.

The oscillator requires vigilance on the part of the physician and respiratory therapist because patients are usually hypoxemic at the initiation of HFOV. Because the oscillator is uncomfortable for patients, they usually require increased sedation and often need pharmacologic paralysis. Careful titration of inspiratory pressure and frequency are needed to obtain optimal settings. During HFOV, ventilation is a passive process, and the patient must have the endotracheal tube cuff deflated to allow for passive exhalation of CO_2. Overall, HFOV appears to be equivalent to conventional ventilation in ARDS patients and useful in the management of refractory hypoxemia and severe air leaks (Fig. 48-8).[65]

In high-frequency jet ventilation (HFJV), a pressurized gas is introduced by inserting a cannula from the HFJV device into the endotracheal tube. An initial pressure of 35 pounds per square inch is set with a rate of

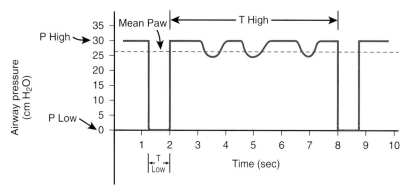

Figure 48-7 Pressure-time curve for airway pressure release ventilation. *Paw,* Airway pressure; *P High,* higher pressure used for respiration on bilevel (e.g., 30 cm H_2O); *P Low,* lower pressure used on bilevel (e.g., 0 cm H_2O); *T High,* number of seconds in the respiratory cycle spent at the higher pressure; *T Low,* number of seconds spent at the lower pressure. (From Frawley PM, Habashi NM: Airway pressure release ventilation: Theory and practice. *AACN Clinical Issues* 12:234-246, 2001.)

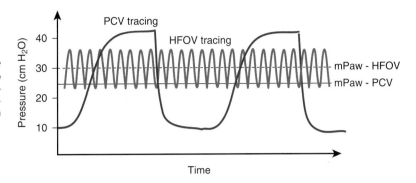

Figure 48-8 The pressure-time curve for high-frequency oscillatory ventilation *(HFOV)* is superimposed on the tracing for pressure-control ventilation *(PCV)* for comparison. (From Chang KP, Stewart TE, Mehta S: High-frequency oscillatory ventilation for adult patients with ARDS. *Chest* 131:1907–1916, 2007.)

100 to 150 breaths/min and an inspiratory fraction of 30%.[66] HFJV is more commonly employed in pediatric patients, but it has some use in laryngeal surgery. The drawback of conventional jet ventilators is there is not an adequate measure of intrapulmonary pressure in the circuit, and the patient may be at risk for volutrauma from overdistention of distal airways.

High-frequency pressure ventilation (HFPV) is a time-cycled, pressure-limited mode of ventilation that delivers subphysiologic tidal volumes at rates as high as 500 breaths/min.[67] HFPV has been used in burn units, specifically for patients with inhalation lung injury, and for salvage therapy in patients with severe ARDS.[68] The basic tenets are the same as for HFOV, but it oscillates at two different pressure levels. A Phasitron valve at the end of the endotracheal tube delivers small tidal volumes at frequencies of 200 to 900 breaths/min superimposed on PCV. Whereas the HFOV uses rapid oscillations of small volumes at high frequencies that transiently reach high airway pressures, the HFPV prolongs the application of high airway pressure at high frequencies to assist in clearance of mucus and in sloughing airway secretions. A single-center, prospective, randomized trial comparing HFPV with low tidal volume ventilation in burn patients with ALI demonstrated no difference in mortality rates or ventilator-free days.[69]

V. NONINVASIVE VENTILATION

NIPPV provides ventilatory support through an external interface such as a nasal or oronasal mask that is firmly secured to the face. The physiologic effect of NIPPV rests in its ability to provide positive pressure into the nasopharynx or oropharynx that splints open the airway and is then transmitted downstream to the lungs, where it increases lung volume. Several cardiovascular effects are seen with NIPPV in this setting. Decreased venous return occurs, and the increased intrathoracic pressure can decrease afterload and thereby increase cardiac output. Figure 48-9 details the interaction of the effects of NIPPV on the cardiopulmonary system.

Patient selection is paramount in the decision to initiate NIPPV. NIPPV is not recommended for patients with upper airway obstruction, cardiac arrest, hemodynamic instability, respiratory arrest, injury of the face, massive gastrointestinal bleeding, a high risk of aspiration, significantly depressed mentation, or an inability to clear secretions (Table 48-7).[70-72]

NIPPV has been useful in many situations, including exacerbations of COPD with hypercapnia,[73-75] cardiogenic pulmonary edema,[76-79] hypercapnic respiratory failure (i.e., Glasgow Coma Scale score greater than 10), and hypoxic respiratory failure.

NIPPV can be delivered by a standard ventilator through a face mask, nasal mask, or nasal plugs. Heated humidification increases the patient's comfort.[80] Common modes of ventilation used to deliver NIPPV are CPAP, bi-level positive airway pressure (BPAP), PSV, proportional-assist ventilation (PAV), and ACV. Modes of NIPPV may be selected on the basis of patient characteristics. For example, patients who require greater support in reducing the work of breathing should be placed on ACV mode, or the patient's comfort may be increased with PSV.[81] There was no difference in mortality rates between these modalities for various disease states.[82-85] The patient should be monitored very closely after initiation of NIPPV. If prompt improvement is not evident within 1 or 2 hours, the physician should proceed to intubation.[86] In a prospective, multicenter, cohort study, NIPPV failed in 30% of patients. The highest intubation rates occurred in patients with ARDS (51%) or community-acquired pneumonia (50%), and the lowest rates were for those with pulmonary contusion (18%) or cardiogenic pulmonary edema (10%) (Fig 48-10).[87]

NIPPV improves mortality rates and length of stay for patients with severe COPD exacerbations.[4] A meta-analysis

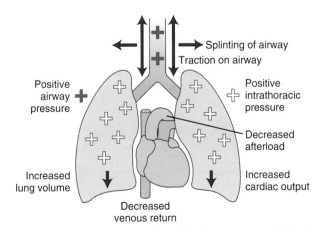

Figure 48-9 Physiologic effects of positive airway pressure. (Adapted from Antonescu-Turcu A, Parthasarathy S: CPAP and Bi-level PAP therapy: New and established roles. *Respir Care* 55:1216–1228, 2010.)

TABLE 48-7

Factors for Success or Failure of Noninvasive Positive-Pressure Ventilation

Success	Failure
• High PaCO$_2$ with low A-a gradient • Improvement in pH, PaCO$_2$, and decreased respiratory rate after 1 hour of NIPPV • Good level of consciousness	• High APACHE score • Pneumonia on chest radiograph • Copious secretions • Edentulous • Poor nutrition status • Confusion or delirium

A-a, Alveolar to arterial; *APACHE,* Acute Physiology and Chronic Health Evaluation; *PaCO$_2$,* arterial partial pressure of carbon dioxide; *NIPPV,* noninvasive positive-pressure ventilation.

of patients with severe COPD exacerbations and mild COPD exacerbations demonstrated no mortality benefit for the patients with milder COPD exacerbations.[74] In cases of cardiogenic pulmonary edema, NIPPV decreases the rate of intubation, but the mortality benefit is uncertain because of conflicting study results.[3,88] Patients with hypoxic respiratory failure and asthma exacerbations may benefit from NIPPV. NIPPV use in post-extubation failure has been studied.[89,90] If NIPPV is used immediately on extubation in patients with hypercapnia during the spontaneous breathing trial, it may prevent reintubation and is associated with a reduction in mortality rates.[91] NIPPV use in patients after the development of post-extubation failure did not reduce reintubation rates and increased mortality rates, with a longer median time from failure to reintubation in the NIPPV group.[92]

In patients with severe COPD exacerbations and cardiogenic pulmonary edema, NIPPV should be attempted if no contraindications exist. In other causes of respiratory failure, such as hypoxic respiratory failure, NIPPV can be considered if the patient does not meet the criteria for intubation. However, if the patient does not stabilize in the first 2 hours, management should rapidly progress to intubation and invasive mechanical ventilation.

VI. WEANING FROM MECHANICAL VENTILATION

The process of weaning from mechanical ventilation is a continuum from decreasing support provided by the

ventilator to assessment of readiness using multiple variables, and discontinuation from the mechanical ventilator.

In 2001, a collective task force from the American College of Chest Physicians, the American Association of Respiratory Care, and the American College of Critical Care Medicine examined the issue of discontinuation of mechanical ventilation and defined patients who required prolonged mechanical ventilation and strategies to liberate them from the mechanical ventilator. They found that patients who are mechanically ventilated spend approximately 42% of their ventilator time undergoing the weaning process. The task force offered 12 recommendations to standardize practice for discontinuing mechanical ventilation, including searching for causes of respiratory failure; early discontinuation of sedation of postoperative patients; ensuring daily spontaneous breathing trials for patients who meet the criteria for hemodynamic, pulmonary, and mental stability; outlining criteria for evaluation of patients on a spontaneous breathing trial; and strategies for prolonged weaning and daily spontaneous breathing trials assisted by nonphysician practitioners within the health care organization.[93] The clinical criteria outlined by the task force includes clinically improving cause of respiratory failure, adequate oxygenation (defined as PaO$_2$/FiO$_2$ greater than 150 mm Hg or oxyhemoglobin saturation greater than 90%, while receiving FiO$_2$ less than or equal to 0.4 and a PEEP less than or equal to 5 cm H$_2$O); hemodynamic stability (absent or low-dose vasopressors and no signs of myocardial ischemia); arterial pH greater than 7.25; and a patient that is able to initiate a spontaneous inspiratory effort.[93]

A study of 300 patients published in 1996 demonstrated the value of daily screening of patients by trials of spontaneous breathing. In the study, patients were assessed daily by the nurse and respiratory therapist, and if preset guidelines were met, patients underwent a 2-hour spontaneous breathing trial. If the patient passed the trial, the physician was notified, and the patient was extubated. The study demonstrated a decrease in ventilator days; a decrease in the number of complications, including reintubation; and lower hospital cost.[94] Another study showed a decrease in the number of ventilator days and ICU days with daily weaning of sedation.[95]

In 2007, a second task force produced the Statement of the Sixth International Consensus Conference on

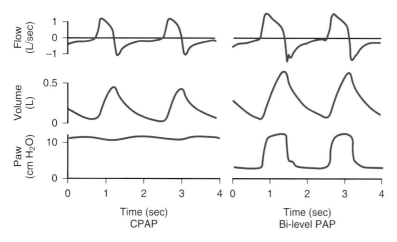

Figure 48-10 Airflow, volume, and airway pressure *(Paw)* versus time tracings for continuous positive airway pressure *(CPAP)* and bi-level positive airway pressure *(Bi-level PAP)*. (From Antonescu-Turcu A, Parthasarathy S: CPAP and Bi-level PAP therapy: New and established roles. *Respir Care* 55:1216–1228, 2010.)

TABLE 48-8

Time from Initiation of Weaning to Successful
Extubation with Various Ventilation Modes

Weaning Technique	Median (days)	First Quartile (days)	Third Quartile (days)
Intermittent mandatory ventilation	5	3	11
Pressure-support ventilation	4	2	12
Intermittent trials of spontaneous breathing	3	2	6
Once-daily trial of spontaneous breathing	3	1	6

From Esteban A, Frutos F, Tobin MJ, et al: A comparison of four methods of weaning patients from mechanical ventilation. Spanish Lung Failure Collaborative Group. *N Engl J Med* 332:345–350, 1995.

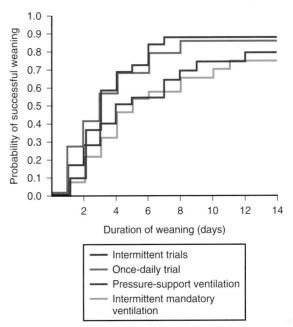

Figure 48-11   The Kaplan-Meier curve shows the probability of successful weaning from mechanical ventilation for pressure-support ventilation versus intermittent mandatory ventilation and for intermittent trials of spontaneous breathing versus once-daily trials of spontaneous breathing. (From Esteban A, Frutos F, Tobin MJ, et al: A comparison of four methods of weaning patients from mechanical ventilation. Spanish Lung Failure Collaborative Group. *N Engl J Med* 332:345–350, 1995.)

Intensive Care Medicine, which answered five important questions about ventilator weaning: What is known about the epidemiology of weaning problems? What is the pathophysiology of weaning failure? What is the usual process of initial weaning from the ventilator? Is there a role for different ventilator modes in more difficult weaning? How should patients with prolonged weaning failure be managed? Based on the answers to these questions, important recommendations were made to help identify the characteristics that predicted favorable and unfavorable weaning outcomes and determine which modes of ventilation should be used when a patient fails the spontaneous breathing trial.

The task force also addressed the use of noninvasive ventilation and prolonged ventilator dependence. Successful weaning was defined as 48 hours free of the ventilator; weaning as early as possible, using spontaneous breathing trials; avoidance of SIMV as a weaning mode; and use of PSV or AC after a failed weaning attempt. NIPPV should not routinely be used after failed extubation; it should be used only in patients with hypercapnia, although CPAP may be useful in preventing hypoxemia in postoperative patients (Table 48-8).[96]

In 1995, the Spanish Lung Failure Collaborative Group prospectively compared the use of intermittent mandatory ventilation (IMV), PSV, intermittent trials of spontaneous breathing, and once-daily spontaneous breathing trials. The study showed that spontaneous breathing trials in either form were superior to IMV or PSV in terms of time from initiation of weaning to successful extubation and probability of successful weaning (Fig 48-11).[41]

To illustrate the interaction of spontaneous breathing trials with daily interruption of sedation, the Awakening and Breathing Trial in 2008 showed that after randomizing 336 patients to the standard protocol or to daily discontinuation of sedation and daily spontaneous breathing trials, the intervention group had 3 fewer days on the mechanical ventilator, fewer ICU days, shorter hospital days, and improved survival rates compared with the standard protocol (Figs. 48-12 and 48-13).[97] Numerous weaning parameters have been studied to hasten liberation from mechanical ventilation, but none have been shown to be superior to using clinical criteria combined with an algorithmic approach to discontinuation of sedation and ventilation.

VII. COMPLICATIONS OF MECHANICAL VENTILATION

A. Mechanical Complications

Mechanical ventilation may produce complications from use of an orotracheal or nasotracheal tube and complications of using positive-pressure ventilation. Common complications of artificial airways are laryngeal edema and irritation, tracheal stenosis, sinusitis, vocal cord damage, and paralysis. Complications of positive-pressure ventilation include barotrauma, which may lead to alveolar rupture and a continuum of pneumothorax, pneumomediastinum, and subcutaneous emphysema. The lungs are susceptible to alveolar distention due to high tidal volumes delivered by the ventilator to alveoli as a result of preset volumes. Due to the heterogenous nature of the lung, even lower volumes may be disproportionally delivered to open alveoli. Atelectotrauma, or cyclic atelectasis, is sheer-force trauma resulting from repeated opening and collapsing of the alveolus in response to positive-pressure ventilation (Fig. 48-14).

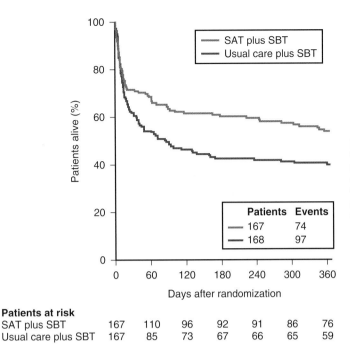

Figure 48-12 Survival at 1 year after randomization to usual care with trials of spontaneous breathing *(SBT)* or to trials of spontaneous awakening *(SAT)* with SBT. (From Girard TD, Kress JP, Fuchs BD, et al: Efficacy and safety of a paired sedation and ventilator weaning protocol for mechanically ventilated patients in intensive care (Awakening and Breathing Controlled trial): A randomised controlled trial. *Lancet* 371:126–134, 2008.)

Volutrauma and atelectotrauma are within the spectrum of ill-defined entities of ventilator-associated lung injury (VALI), which appears to be more common in lungs of patients with ARDS or ALI. Although causation has not been determined, VALI has been observed in patients who have undergone mechanical ventilation. VILI is an entity well described in animal models. It is a syndrome of diffuse alveolar damage that is morphologically identical to ARDS and that is caused by mechanical ventilation.[98] Alveolar injury results in increased permeability, loss of functional surfactant, release of cytokines, and alveolar collapse (Fig. 48-15). Other factors that may be associated with an increased risk for VALI include immunosuppression,[99] high ventilator rates,[100] supine body position, and hyperthermia.[101]

1. Auto-PEEP

Intrinsic PEEP or auto-PEEP results from incomplete alveolar emptying before the initiation of the next breath.[102] The alveolar pressures remain positive relative to atmospheric pressures at end-expiration. High minute ventilation from high tidal volumes or respiratory rates is a common cause. When high respiratory rates exist, expiratory time may be decreased to a point at which the full tidal volume is not exhaled before the next breath. High tidal volumes are less likely to be exhaled entirely before the next breath. Patients with obstructive lung diseases such as COPD and asthma often have auto-PEEP while on mechanical ventilation due to disease-related limited expiratory flow.[103] Expiratory resistance from any obstruction of the endotracheal tube (e.g., kinks, secretions) or patient-ventilator asynchrony can lead to auto-PEEP. Auto-PEEP can result from high tidal volumes, a high respiratory rate, or a decreased expiratory time relative to inhalation time in any disease state (Table 48-9).

2. Consequences of Auto-PEEP

Auto-PEEP can decrease venous return, reduce ventricular compliance, and induce hypotension.[104] Hypovolemic patients are at increased risk for PEEP-related hypotension. Alveolar distention from auto-PEEP can lead to barotrauma, worsening oxygenation from ventilation-perfusion ($\dot{V}/\dot{Q}$) mismatch, and VALI. Auto-PEEP increases the work of breathing by raising the pressure the patient must generate to trigger a ventilator breath. If the breath is triggered at -2 cm H_2O and the auto-PEEP is 6 cm H_2O, the patient needs to overcome both (-8 cm H_2O of negative pressure) to initiate a breath. Auto-PEEP increases peak and plateau pressures in volume-controlled modes and decreases tidal volume in pressure-cycled ventilation.[24] Auto-PEEP also increases peak and plateau pressures, which can lead to an overestimation of thoracic compliance. Increased plateau pressures can be transmitted to the intrathoracic vessels and can lead to an overestimation of the central venous pressures and the pulmonary artery occlusion pressure (Table 48-10).

Auto-PEEP can be monitored in several ways but sometimes can be difficult to detect. The graphs of flow versus time demonstrate initiation of a new breath before the expiration reaches zero flow. End expiratory alveolar pressure, measured by introducing an end-expiratory breath-hold and subtracting applied PEEP, can quantitate auto-PEEP. The breath-hold allows the pressure in the proximal airways to equilibrate with alveolar pressure. Auscultation for airflow at the end of expiration is also useful.[105]

Management of auto-PEEP is targeted at promoting alveolar emptying and increasing expiratory time. Reducing minute ventilation by targeting tidal volume or the respiratory rate, or both, and by increasing inspiratory flow can be effective measures in reducing auto-PEEP.

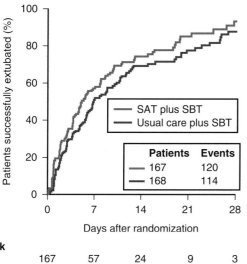

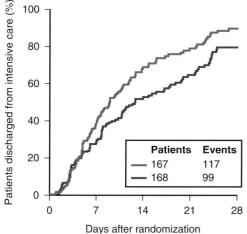

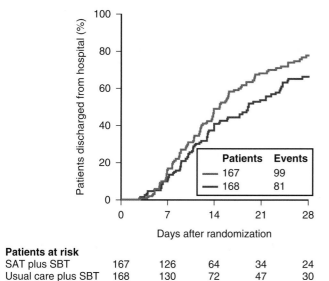

Patients at risk

SAT plus SBT	167	57	24	9	3
A Usual care plus SBT	168	68	30	18	8

Patients at risk

SAT plus SBT	167	89	35	20	10
B Usual care plus SBT	165	102	52	33	18

Patients at risk

SAT plus SBT	167	126	64	34	24
C Usual care plus SBT	168	130	72	47	30

Figure 48-13 Probability of successful extubation **(A),** discharge from intensive care **(B),** or discharge from hospital **(C)** within the first 28 days after randomization. *SAT,* Spontaneous awakening trials; *SBT,* spontaneous breathing trials. (From Girard TD, Kress JP, Fuchs BD, et al: Efficacy and safety of a paired sedation and ventilator weaning protocol for mechanically ventilated patients in intensive care (Awakening and Breathing Controlled trial): A randomised controlled trial. *Lancet* 371:126–134, 2008.)

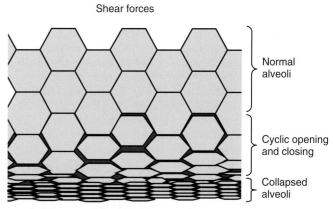

Figure 48-14 Atelectotrauma (i.e., cyclic atelectasis) results from the sheer forces generated by repeated opening and collapsing of the alveoli in response to positive-pressure ventilation. (From Papadokos PJ, Lachmann B: The open lung concept of mechanical ventilation: The role of recruitment and stabilization. *Crit Care Clin* 23:241–250, 2007.)

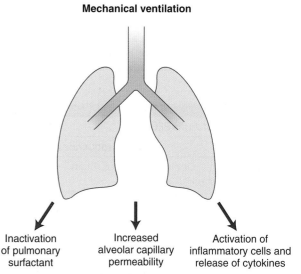

Figure 48-15 Downstream effects of lung injury from mechanical ventilation. (From Papadokos PJ, Lachmann B: The open lung concept of mechanical ventilation: The role of recruitment and stabilization. *Crit Care Clin* 23:241–250, 2007.)

TABLE 48-9
Auto-PEEP Factors

Causes of Auto-PEEP	Factors
High minute ventilation	High tidal volume
	High respiratory rate
Expiratory flow limitation	Airway narrowing from bronchospasm, collapse, inflammation, or remodeling
Expiratory resistance	Patient-ventilator asynchrony
	Narrow or obstructed endotracheal tube
	Secretions

PEEP, Positive end-expiratory pressure.

Management of the underlying condition is important, especially for patients with obstructive lung diseases treated with bronchodilators, steroids, and antimicrobial therapies. In patients with COPD or asthma, the limited expiratory flow can be counterbalanced by application of extrinsic PEEP.[106] Small amounts of extrinsic PEEP can decrease intrinsic PEEP by keeping the small airways open at end-expiration. However, the applied PEEP should be less than intrinsic PEEP to prevent an increase in alveolar pressures.[107]

B. Infectious Complications

Ventilator-associated pneumonia (VAP), a type of hospital-acquired pneumonia (HAP), is defined as a diagnosis of pneumonia 48 to 72 hours after endotracheal intubation. Studies of management with noninvasive ventilation show a decreased incidence of pneumonia when endotracheal intubation is avoided.[91] The earlier pneumonia is diagnosed after onset of mechanical ventilation, the better the prognosis. Pneumonia diagnosed later in the course of mechanical ventilation is more likely to be caused by a drug-resistant organism and carries a worse prognosis. Several practices can help to minimize the occurrence of pneumonia on the ventilator, including elevating the head of the bed to the semirecumbent position of 30 to 45 degrees, aggressive weaning of sedation, use of orotracheal and orogastric tubes to decrease the potential for sinusitis, daily assessments to liberate from mechanical ventilation, avoiding gastric

TABLE 48-10
Consequences of Auto-PEEP

Affected System	Consequences
Cardiac	Decreases venous return
	Hypotension
	Overestimation of CVP and PCWP
Pulmonary	Alveolar overdistension
	Barotrauma or pneumothorax
	Increases peak and plateau in pressure ventilation
	Increases work of breathing
	Underestimation of thoracic compliance

CVP, Central venous pressure; *PCWP,* pulmonary capillary wedge pressure; *PEEP,* positive end-expiratory pressure.

overdistention, avoiding unplanned extubations, oral care with antiseptic solution, and limiting contamination of ventilator tubing.[108,109] Once a VAP occurs, there is no difference in mechanical ventilation–free days, the length of ICU days, the number of organ failure–free days and mortality rates on day 60 between the groups receiving between 8 days and 15 days of treatment with appropriate antibiotics.[110]

VIII. CONCLUSIONS

Various modes of mechanical ventilation can be used to provide respiratory support in critical illness or in patients undergoing general anesthesia. Safe application to limit VALI and negative interactions with other organ systems is fundamental in managing patients receiving mechanical ventilation. NIPPV can be safely and effectively applied to patients with acute respiratory failure from COPD, pulmonary edema, or other diseases. Mechanical ventilation selection using common or uncommon modes is determined by several factors, including hemodynamical instability, severe oxygenation or ventilation derangements, general anesthesia, and patient comfort. A lung-protective strategy incorporating tidal volumes of 6 mL/kg of predicted body weight and plateau pressures of 30 cm H_2O or improves outcomes in ARDS. Tidal volumes greater than 10 mL/kg of predicted body weight should not be routinely used in managing other lung states. PEEP can be applied to improve oxygenation and to limit collapse and repeated opening and closing of unstable units, which can lead to lung injury. Plateau pressures greater than 35 cm H_2O have been associated with increased risk of barotrauma and VALI. Auto-PEEP should be monitored to avoid related complications. Measures to reduce the risk of VAP should be instituted on initiation of mechanical ventilation.

Daily trials of spontaneous breathing expedite weaning and liberation from mechanical ventilation. Ventilator weaning algorithms that allow for non-physician providers to assess the readiness of patients for extubation when they meet certain preset criteria are often useful. Daily interruption of sedation facilitates liberation from the mechanical ventilation.

IX. CLINICAL PEARLS

- The indications for mechanical ventilation include hypoxemic and hypercapnic respiratory failure, altered mentation with patient inability to protect the airway, hemodynamic instability, and to maintain adequate oxygenation and ventilation during deep sedation, anesthesia, or neuromuscular blockade.

- Positive end-expiratory pressure (PEEP) improves oxygenation in patients with hypoxic respiratory failure, optimizes alveolar recruitment and decreases cycles of recruitment and derecruitment of alveolar lung units.

- Assist-control ventilation (ACV) can be volume targeted, upon initiation of mechanical ventilation, or pressure targeted when increased oxygenation is required, but there is concern about increasing airway pressures.

- A lung-protective strategy should be employed in all patients with acute lung injury (ALI) or acute respiratory distress syndrome (ARDS). Using low tidal volumes of 6 mL/kg of predicted body weight with plateau pressures of 30 cm H2O or less has become the standard of care for patients with ARDS.

- Synchronized intermittent mandatory ventilation (SIMV) incorporates some characteristics of ACV and pressure-support ventilation (PSV). The purpose of the two types of breaths (mandatory and spontaneous) is to allow increased diaphragmatic activity and increased work of breathing when triggering spontaneous breaths.

- Airway pressure–release ventilation (APRV) uses high and low pressures to aid in recruitment of atelectatic lung units and allows spontaneous breathing. It can decrease airway pressures and improve oxygenation, alveolar recruitment, and cardiac output.

- High-frequency ventilation, sometimes called the *oscillator*, improves oxygenation by providing oxygen-rich and CO_2-poor gas that rapidly mixes with sinusoidal flow at stroke volumes that approximate anatomic dead space. Each type of high-frequency ventilation—high-frequency jet ventilation, high-frequency oscillatory ventilation, and high-frequency percussive ventilation—has its subtleties and specific indications.

- Noninvasive positive-pressure ventilation (NIPPV) is useful in many situations, including exacerbations of COPD, cardiogenic pulmonary edema, and hypercapnic respiratory failure in patients with a Glasgow Coma Scale score of more than 10.

- During weaning from mechanical ventilation, daily interruption of sedation (unless contraindicated by severe hypoxemia or the need for neuromuscular blockade) and daily trials of spontaneous breathing should be employed for all patients.

SELECTED REFERENCES

All references can be found online at expertconsult.com.

12. Acute Respiratory Distress Syndrome Network: Ventilation with lower tidal volumes as compared with traditional tidal volumes for acute lung injury and the acute respiratory distress syndrome. *N Engl J Med* 342:1301–1308, 2000.

13. Gajic O, Dara SI, Mendez JL, et al: Ventilator associated lung injury in patients without acute lung injury at the onset of mechanical ventilation. *Crit Care Med* 32:1817–1824, 2004.

16. Amato MB, Barbas CS, Medeiros DM, et al: Effect of protective-ventilation strategy on mortality in the acute respiratory distress syndrome. *N Engl J Med* 338:347–354, 1998.

21. Brower RG, Lanken PN, MacIntyre N, et al: National heart, lung, and blood institute ARDS clinical trials network. Higher versus lower positive end-expiratory pressures in patients with the acute respiratory distress syndrome. *N Engl J Med* 351:327–336, 2004.

23. Briel M, Meade M, Mercat A, et al: Higher vs lower positive end-expiratory pressure in patients with acute lung injury and acute respiratory distress syndrome: Systematic review and meta-analysis. *JAMA* 303:865–873, 2010.

41. Esteban A, Frutos F, Tobin MJ, et al: A comparison of four methods of weaning patients from mechanical ventilation. Spanish Lung Failure Collaborative Group. *N Engl J Med* 332:345–350, 1995.

63. Derdak S, Mehta S, Stewart TE, et al: Multicenter oscillatory ventilation for acute respiratory distress syndrome trial (MOAT) study investigators. *Am J Respir Crit Care Med* 166:801–808, 2002.

87. Antonelli M, Conti G, Moro ML, et al: Predictors of failure of noninvasive positive pressure ventilation in patients with acute hypoxemic respiratory failure: A multi-center study. *Intensive Care Med* 27:1718–1728, 2001.

97. Girard TD, Kress JP, Fuchs BD, et al: Efficacy and safety of a paired sedation and ventilator weaning protocol for mechanically ventilated patients in intensive care (Awakening and Breathing Controlled trial): A randomised controlled trial. *Lancet* 371:126–134, 2008.

108. American Thoracic Society/Infectious Disease Society of America: Guidelines for the management of adults with hospital-acquired, ventilator-associated, and healthcare-associated pneumonia. *Am J Respir Crit Care Med* 171:388–416, 2005.

Chapter 49

Monitoring the Airway and Pulmonary Function

NEAL H. COHEN | DAVID E. SCHWARTZ

I. INTRODUCTION

The patient with a potentially compromised airway or altered respiratory function presents many clinical challenges, such as identifying the cause of the derangement and choosing the most appropriate therapeutic and supportive interventions. Although a comprehensive physical assessment remains one of the most valuable methods for assessing the patient and determining whether the patient is responding appropriately to clinical interventions, several monitoring techniques can be valuable adjuncts to the clinical assessment.

During the past 20 years, the number and variety of monitors have increased, providing clinically relevant and useful information about gas exchange, pulmonary function, and the ventilator-patient interface. Some monitors, such as the pulse oximeter, have become routine equipment in the operating room (OR), intensive care unit (ICU), and other clinical settings. Others are used more selectively to monitor specific clinical situation or physiologic changes. To select the right device and use it to its full potential, the physician should understand the mechanism, benefits, and limitations of each monitor. The clinician should know how to interpret the information provided, correlate the data with the clinical situation, and in some cases, reconcile differences in information

about the patient that is provided by different monitors to make appropriate clinical decisions.

Although most monitoring devices provide useful information, some are easier to use than others. Some data suggest that the devices that are easiest to use and for which the data are easiest to interpret are the most clinically useful devices.[1] In many situations, the information provided by monitors that is thought to be straightforward requires a comprehensive understanding of its physiologic basis. For example, although the pulse oximeter provides a straightforward measurement of oxygen (O_2) saturation, which can be easily interpreted in most cases, the information in many clinical situations does not accurately reflect the O_2 saturation (in the presence of carbon monoxide) or O_2 tension (when the patient is severely acidotic or alkalotic).[2,3] Interpretation requires an understanding of the patient's physiology and the method by which the monitor reports the data. The same caveats are true for almost every monitor that is used clinically to guide diagnosis, management, and response to therapy. The clinician must know what monitors are available and when the information provided by the monitor is clinically useful and must know how to interpret the data and understand the limitations of each device.

This chapter describes techniques for monitoring and evaluating the airway, gas exchange, and pulmonary function. It provides an overview of the monitors used to assess the patient and describes specific monitors that are useful in assessing the appropriateness of mechanical ventilatory support. Because the modes of ventilation have changed considerably and the options for providing mandatory and spontaneously initiated modes of ventilation have become available, monitoring pulmonary function and the patient-ventilator interface has become increasingly important.[4] The benefits and limitations of each monitoring technique are discussed.

II. MONITORING THE AIRWAY

A. Non-intubated Patient

Monitoring the airway is a critical component of clinical assessment for any patient requiring sedation, analgesia, or ventilatory support. As a result of underlying anatomic abnormalities, physiologic alterations in the level of consciousness, edema of the airway, or administration of respiratory depressants, a patient can develop upper airway dysfunction with life-threatening consequences. Assessment of the airway should include the clinical evaluation that is routinely performed by the anesthesiologist before initiating anesthesia or by the critical care practitioner before performing endotracheal intubation. In many cases, the assessment must be performed rapidly under challenging circumstances, but if possible, the evaluation should include a brief and focused history and physical examination. The patient should be asked about snoring or episodes of airway obstruction during sleep; previous experiences with endotracheal intubation, including difficult intubation, hoarseness after airway manipulation, and hoarseness with exercise; previous lengthy endotracheal intubation; and a history of tracheostomy or tracheal abnormalities, including stenosis or tracheomalacia. Patients with rheumatoid arthritis should be questioned about upper airway problems, particularly those related to potential arthritic changes in the cricoarytenoid joints. Patients who have had previous neck or mediastinal surgery should be carefully evaluated for evidence of unilateral or bilateral vocal cord dysfunction. For patients unable to provide a history, discussion with family members or the nurse caring for the patient, a review of the medical record, or direct observation of the airway and ventilatory pattern while preparing equipment for intubation or other interventions can provide useful information to guide management decisions. In selected patients, a lateral neck radiograph can provide useful information about the upper airway and presence of masses in the airway or epiglottic edema, although in most cases, upper airway compromise necessitates emergent intubation without the benefit of a radiologic evaluation.[5]

Examination of the airway for any patient presenting with respiratory insufficiency mandates a thorough assessment of the upper airway, including evaluation of mobility of the jaw, chin, and neck, and estimation of the potential ease or difficulty of endotracheal intubation based on the size of the mandible and visualization of the airway (i.e., Mallampati classification). The clinical assessment usually can be performed while providing supplemental O_2 or positive airway pressure by mask while preparing for the intubation. For patients with challenging abnormalities of the upper airway that may make routine laryngoscopy difficult, alternative methods to secure the airway should be considered, and the appropriate equipment should be readily available to allow rapid control using a standard laryngoscope, laryngeal mask airway (LMA), fiberoptic technique, lightwand, video laryngoscope, or in emergent situations, cricothyroidotomy or tracheostomy.

B. During Endotracheal Intubation

Although there are several situations in which the airway can be monitored and noninvasive ventilatory support provided, many patients require placement of an artificial airway for airway protection or to facilitate ventilatory support. A variety of airway devices are available, including different types of LMAs, endotracheal tubes (ETTs), and tracheotomy tubes. In some cases, the LMA can provide initial airway support to facilitate subsequent endotracheal intubation. In other cases, such as for selected surgical procedures, the LMA is sufficient to provide partial protection of the airway while allowing spontaneous ventilation. When an LMA is placed, positioning of the airway must be verified. Direct visualization of LMA placement is usually not required, and positioning can be confirmed on the basis of clinical signs. If the patient is breathing comfortably without evidence of obstruction, the LMA is usually in a good position. For the spontaneously breathing patient, this clinical assessment is sufficient. When positive-pressure ventilation may be required, better confirmation of the correct position is desirable because of the potential risks. Positive-pressure ventilation may cause a leak around the LMA, compromising the ability to provide an adequate tidal volume (V_T). Ventilation through the LMA does not prevent entrainment of gas into the stomach, and the risk of regurgitation and aspiration must be considered. In this situation, the correct position of the LMA must be confirmed, and if there is any question about the appropriate placement, its position must be verified by direct visualization, or the LMA must be replaced with an ETT by placing the ETT through the LMA or removing the LMA and intubating the trachea directly.

Although a variety of masks and other devices are available to facilitate ventilatory support without tracheal instrumentation, the patient requiring airway protection or positive-pressure ventilation usually undergoes endotracheal intubation through transoral or transnasal routes or through a surgical airway (see Chapter 17). When endotracheal intubation is required, confirmation of correct placement is essential. The most reliable method to assess the location of an artificial airway within the trachea is direct visualization of the tube passing through the vocal cords at the time of intubation. Physical examination is also important to ensure that both lungs are being ventilated after placement of the airway. Auscultation over the lung fields (particularly the apices of the lungs) and stomach should routinely be performed to assess ETT placement. When the ETT is within the trachea, equal breath sounds should be heard over both lung fields while listening over the apices. Auscultation over the upper lung fields minimizes the likelihood of hearing sounds transmitted from the stomach. For most adult patients, if the ETT is located within the trachea, no breath sounds should be heard over the stomach. Unfortunately, auscultation can be misleading. Occasionally, particularly in children, breath sounds are transmitted to the stomach even when the ETT is properly positioned. For patients with extensive parenchymal lung disease, effusions, or endobronchial lesions, breath sounds may not be heard equally over both lung fields even when the ETT is properly positioned within the trachea.

Other clinical signs can be useful in determining whether the ETT is within the trachea. They include identifying mist within the lumen of the ETT during exhalation, palpation of the cuff of the ETT in the suprasternal notch, and the normal "feel" of a reservoir bag during manual ventilation. Despite the clinical usefulness of these methods, none is infallible, and false-positive and false-negative evaluations have been reported.[6]

A more reliable monitor for confirming that the artificial airway is within the trachea is identification of carbon dioxide (CO_2) in exhaled gas. If the airway is within the trachea and the patient is ventilating spontaneously or receiving positive-pressure ventilation, CO_2 should be eliminated by the lungs. The presence of CO_2 or measurement of CO_2 concentration can be used to determine the location of the ETT. Several devices are available to monitor CO_2 in expired gases. In the OR, CO_2 can be measured using an infrared device,[7] Raman effect scattering, or mass spectrometry. In the ICU, emergency department (ED), or other settings, including out-of-hospital locations, colorimetric techniques can successfully estimate the CO_2 concentration, or infrared devices can accurately measure the CO_2 concentration in expired gases.[8,9] As a result of the ease of use and widespread availability of these devices, the documentation of CO_2 in exhaled gas after placement of an artificial airway (i.e., capnography) has become the standard of care in anesthesia practice and is routinely used during emergency airway management in many hospitals and emergency settings. A detailed description of capnography is provided on page 1011. Unfortunately, even these devices can provide misleading information, and the information they provide is not foolproof.[10,11]

Capnography is a useful monitor to confirm correct placement of the ETT, but it is not uniformly reliable and can be misleading.[12] For example, when the patient has been ventilated by mask before intubation, CO_2-containing gas may remain in the stomach. A capnograph may indicate the presence of CO_2 in the expired gas, but it does not reflect CO_2 from the airway. This problem is even more common when capnography is used to monitor the patient who has recently received bicarbonate-containing solutions or has been drinking CO_2-containing beverages before placement of the artificial airway. In these situations, CO_2 is eliminated from the stomach during the first few breaths provided through the ETT. The presence of CO_2 from exhaled gas therefore should be monitored for at least a few breaths.

If CO_2 continues to be eliminated through the ETT after four or five breaths, endotracheal placement of the tube can be ensured.[11] Another problem with capnography when used to confirm ETT placement is that CO_2 elimination occurs only if the patient has sufficient cardiac output to deliver CO_2 to the lungs. If the patient has suffered a cardiac arrest and cardiac output is very low or absent, no CO_2 is delivered to the lung. The capnogram reveals neither a digital display of CO_2 from exhaled gas nor, if the CO_2 waveform is being monitored, a capnographic display, even when the ETT is within the trachea.[13-16] During cardiopulmonary resuscitation, the presence of CO_2 in exhaled gas provides confirmation that the cardiac output has improved and CO_2 is being eliminated from the lungs. Sometimes, even when cardiac output is inadequate, chest compressions are effective at eliminating enough CO_2 from the lungs to confirm ETT placement.

Another technique to confirm placement of the ETT in the trachea at the time of intubation is use of a self-inflating bulb. This technique was advocated as an easy way to confirm the proper position of the ETT in out-of-hospital intubations. The technique uses a bulb that is applied to the ETT. Self-inflation of the bulb within 4 seconds determines that the ETT is in proper position. Although the technique has some proponents, most studies are unable to confirm that this is a reliable method to verify ETT placement.[17]

When the position of the ETT within the trachea has been confirmed, it is important to assess the exact location of the tube within the trachea to avoid placement too proximal (increasing the risk of accidental extubation) or too distal (endobronchial). Incorrect positioning of the ETT has been associated with several complications, including pneumothorax and death.[18] The location of the ETT should be confirmed at the time of placement and be regularly assessed while the artificial airway remains in place, because the position can change even after the ETT is secured. Flexion of the neck moves the ETT toward the carina, and extension moves the tube up toward the vocal cords. In adult patients, flexion and extension of the head changes the position of the ETT tip by as much as 2 cm.[18] As the ETT softens or the patient manipulates the ETT with the tongue, the tube position changes. As a result of changes in ETT position, patients are at risk for self-extubation, even when the tube is secured at the mouth and the extremities are restrained.

Several techniques can be used to assess the correct position of the ETT within the trachea. For example, placement of the ETT to a predetermined distance has been advocated as a way to minimize the likelihood of endobronchial intubation. Owen and Cheney suggested that the tube be placed to a depth of 21 cm in women and 23 cm in men when referenced to the anterior alveolar ridge or the front teeth. In their study using this approach, endobronchial intubation was avoided.[19] Subsequent studies have not confirmed that this technique prevents endobronchial intubation in critically ill adults or that it is predictive of the relationship between the position of the ETT at the teeth and the tube's position relative to the carina.[20-22]

Fiberoptic bronchoscopy has been used to determine proper positioning of the ETT.[23] When a flexible fiberoptic bronchoscope is readily available, it can be used to confirm the location of the tip of the ETT within the trachea.[24] Because many ORs and ICUs have "difficult airway carts" readily available, the use of the flexible fiberoptic bronchoscope to assist with intubation and confirm the tubes's location has become more common. The technique is useful, although it is not without some risk. Insertion of the flexible fiberoptic bronchoscope reduces the effective cross-sectional area of the ETT, potentially compromising ventilation and oxygenation.[25] Peak inspiratory pressure increases. Partial obstruction of the ETT results in an increase in airway resistance, which may lead to the development of occult end-expiratory pressure and increase the risk of pneumothorax or cause hemodynamic compromise.[26] Despite these limitations, in experienced hands, the assessment can be completed rapidly and without complications. It is a particularly useful way of documenting the location of the ETT within the trachea in the patient for whom the specific location of the tube is critically important, such as one with abnormal tracheal anatomy, the patient at risk for obstruction of the right upper lobe bronchus, or one with specific needs related to the planned surgical procedure.

Capnography can be used to identify endobronchial migration of an ETT.[27] With distal migration of the tube, the EtCO$_2$ falls. The change is usually associated with an increase in peak inspiratory pressure. These changes, although not always reliable, can provide early evidence of ETT migration because the CO$_2$ changes precede a change in arterial blood gases (ABGs) or other signs of displacement.

Probably the most commonly used method to assess the location of the ETT within the trachea is the routine post-intubation chest radiograph. The distance of the ETT from the carina can be measured from a portable anteroposterior radiograph obtained at the bedside. Although many clinicians have questioned whether the cost of chest radiography warrants its routine use for documentation of ETT placement, it remains the most useful and reliable method to determine the appropriate depth of the ETT within the trachea.[20-22]

One special clinical situation warrants additional monitoring of the artificial airway. Some patients require placement of a double-lumen tube to facilitate a unilateral surgical procedure of the lung, to provide differential lung ventilation, or to protect one lung from contamination with blood or infected secretions from the other lung. In these cases, proper placement of the double-lumen tube must be ensured. Physical examination alone and other monitoring techniques are usually insufficient to confirm proper positioning. Fiberoptic evaluation is most often required to confirm the ETT position after initial placement and to reevaluate placement after the patient is repositioned for a surgical procedure or while requiring differential lung ventilation in the ICU.[28] Direct visualization of the tip of the double-lumen tube and the relationship between the tracheal and bronchial lumens ensures that the tube is in the proper position and that the two lungs are isolated. Other techniques can be used to diagnose malpositioning of double-lumen tubes, although there are few studies that confirm their value. Capnography, which has been useful in identifying endobronchial migration of a single-lumen ETT,[27] may provide information about the location of a double-lumen tube, particularly if only one lung is being ventilated at the time of evaluation. Spirometry, which can be obtained from in-line monitoring devices added to the anesthesia circuit or monitoring techniques provided by critical care ventilators, can also provide early detection of double-lumen tube malpositioning.[29] As the ETT migrates, expiratory flow obstruction, as can occur with malpositioning of the tube, can be detected as a change in the shape of the expiratory limb of the flow-volume loop. Inspiratory obstruction is best diagnosed by a change in the pressure-volume loop.

C. During Weaning

Careful evaluation and monitoring of the patient's airway are required before and immediately after tracheal extubation. After the patient is weaned from ventilatory support and is being prepared for extubation, the patient's ability to protect and maintain the airway after tracheal extubation must be assessed, although it can be difficult to do so with the ETT in place. Various clinical criteria have been used to determine whether the intubated patient can protect the airway. The most common criteria are a normal gag response and a strong cough. If the patient gags when the back of the throat is stimulated and coughs during suctioning, most clinicians feel confident that the patient will be able to prevent aspiration after extubation. These criteria, however, have never been subjected to scientific evaluation. Some patients who have a poor gag or cough with the ETT in place are able to handle secretions and to cough effectively after endotracheal extubation. Others, who seem to have a satisfactory cough or gag before extubation, are still unable to protect the airway when extubated. The problem with airway protection may become clinically apparent only when the patient begins to eat, because pharyngeal function may remain abnormal for several hours to days after endotracheal intubation.[30] Nonetheless, these criteria continue to be the most commonly used to determine whether the patient can be extubated safely.

After a decision is made that the patient can protect the airway, the airway size and vocal cord function must be assessed before ETT removal. Most commonly for patients intubated for a straightforward surgical procedure, routine clinical evaluation is sufficient; no formal assessment of airway size is required before extubation. However, if the patient develops significant edema of the head and neck during surgery or has a surgical procedure of the head or neck that may compromise the airway, a more thorough assessment is required. A common technique used to assess airway size is to determine whether the patient can breathe around the ETT when its cuff is deflated and the tube occluded. When the patient is able to breathe around the ETT, the patient can be successfully extubated; however, this approach may not provide sufficient justification for keeping the patient intubated.

Many patients cannot breathe around the occluded ETT because of the increased resistance with the tube in place. As a result, alternative methods have been suggested. The leak test assesses the airway pressure required for a leak to develop around the cuff when positive-pressure ventilation is applied through the ETT with the cuff deflated.[31] Although the specific pressure at which the leak develops has not been well correlated with successful extubation, some clinicians require that a leak occur when the airway pressure is low, usually less than 15 cm H_2O, before extubation. Unfortunately, some studies, including a systematic review of the literature that included more than 2300 patients, have been unable to confirm the value of the leak test at all nor a specific leak pressure or volume above which extubation is contraindicated.[32] If the airway pressure required to identify a leak during positive-pressure inspiration is high, probably 20 to 25 cm H_2O, the patient may have sufficient upper airway edema to warrant leaving the ETT in place until the edema resolves.

D. After Tracheal Decannulation

After the ETT is removed, the airway must be closely monitored. For most surgical patients, the risk of airway compromise after extubation of the trachea is small. Occasionally, airway edema can become a problem. Less commonly, vocal cord dysfunction or cricoarytenoid dislocation can cause hoarseness or airway obstruction. Patients at risk for upper airway edema include those who have required large amounts of fluid or blood products for resuscitation in the OR or ICU and patients who were cared for in the prone position.

Most of these patients do not have the ETT removed until the edema resolves. However, even after external signs of edema resolve, assessment of the airway lumen and competency can be challenging. With the ETT in place, the airway is stented open; after removal, the airway may no longer be patent or of sufficient size to allow normal spontaneous ventilation. Sometimes, the narrowing of the airway becomes apparent only when the patient's inspiratory flow increases, resulting in stridor and increased airway resistance. If stridor develops and edema of the airway is suspected, aerosolized vasoconstrictors can be used to reduce airway swelling. Nebulized racemic epinephrine has been used successfully. The vasoconstrictive effects of the epinephrine reduce the edema and improve the cross-sectional area of the airway. When epinephrine is required, it must be administered with caution. After discontinuation of the epinephrine, rebound hyperemia can occur. If repeated epinephrine treatments are required, the epinephrine dose and frequency of treatment should be tapered (in frequency or dose) rather than abruptly withdrawn. Systemic steroids can be used to reduce upper airway edema, but their onset of action is slow. If upper airway edema is suspected and steroids are to be administered, they should be administered 6 to 8 hours before the anticipated extubation. When edema does not respond to therapy or the patient has evidence of other abnormalities, including tracheomalacia, emergent intubation may be required. For patients for whom the clinical assessment is not

entirely clear but the risks of extubation are outweighed by the benefits, special equipment, including fiberoptic intubation equipment and cricothyroidotomy kits, should be readily available to facilitate emergent intubation.

Vocal cord function can be impaired after surgery. Postoperative vocal cord dysfunction can be caused by direct trauma at the time of endotracheal intubation or edema. Recurrent laryngeal nerve dysfunction can also occur, most commonly caused by nerve retraction or transection during surgery or direct trauma from high intratracheal pressure transmitted from the ETT cuff.[33] Unfortunately, it is difficult to assess vocal cord function with the ETT in place. The evaluation usually requires that the ETT be removed (see Chapter 50). After extubation, evaluation of laryngeal and vocal cord function can be assessed fiberoptically. In some patients, evaluation of the airway can be performed by inserting the fiberoptic device through the ETT and then removing the tube over the fiberoptic shaft to allow visualization of the airway. Assessment requires that the patient breathe spontaneously, so that the movement of the vocal cords can be visualized. Although the assessment can be performed in the ICU, the more common approach is to perform the evaluation under more controlled conditions in the OR, where all of the emergency airway and surgical equipment is available to secure the airway. Evaluation and extubation can be performed after the patient is anesthetized with a volatile anesthetic agent and is breathing spontaneously. If severe stridor or airway obstruction develops with removal of the ETT, the patient can be reintubated or have a tracheostomy performed for long-term airway maintenance (see also Chapter 31). In most cases, even when there is injury to a recurrent laryngeal nerve or one vocal cord, the patient is able to breathe normally without stridor, unless the patient's inspiratory flows are excessive. The greater risk exists for the patient who suffers bilateral vocal cord palsies. While still sedated, the patient may not have stridor or evidence of airway obstruction. However, as the patient awakens and inspiratory flows increase, the stridor becomes obvious and usually requires emergent endotracheal intubation or, more commonly, tracheostomy.

Stridor can occur as a result of dislocation of the cricoarytenoid joint. The risk of cricoarytenoid dislocation is greatest in patients with rheumatoid arthritis, in whom the joint may be affected. However, dislocation should be suspected in any difficult intubation patient who requires multiple attempts and extensive manipulation of the airway.

III. MONITORING RESPIRATORY FUNCTION

A. Clinical Assessment

The clinical examination remains one of the most important and valuable methods to monitor a patient's respiratory status. Too often, attention is placed on technologically sophisticated monitoring devices, and the physical examination is cursory, or the clinical findings are undervalued. Nonetheless, much information about actual or potential airway problems and abnormalities in pulmonary mechanical function or gas exchange can be obtained from a carefully performed and thorough examination. Many of the early signs of respiratory failure are apparent on physical assessment (see Chapter 9) before the abnormalities are apparent by other means. For example, the respiratory rate provides important information about respiratory reserve, dead space, and respiratory drive, particularly when interpreted in conjunction with arterial carbon dioxide tension ($PaCO_2$). Tachypnea is frequently the earliest sign of impending respiratory failure. The patient's pattern of breathing should be evaluated. Subtle changes in the respiratory rate, V_T, and pattern of breathing may provide an early indication of increased work of breathing (as may occur with reduced lung compliance, increased airway resistance, or phrenic nerve dysfunction) or altered ventilatory drive. Although inspiratory flow and minute ventilation ($\dot{V}_E$) are difficult to quantify by clinical examination alone, respiratory distress often manifests as the patient attempts to increase alveolar ventilation by taking larger, more rapid inspirations.

Upper airway obstruction, as may occur after manipulation of the airway, in association with epiglottitis or a mass in or around the airway can be assessed by careful clinical evaluation. Nasal flaring, stridor, and chest wall movement in the absence of airflow suggest upper airway obstruction. If the patient is making respiratory efforts and has abdominal expansion during inspiration without chest excursions, he or she has upper airway obstruction and may require manipulation of the upper airway, including a jaw thrust, initiation of positive-pressure ventilation support with continuous positive airway pressure (CPAP) or bi-level positive airway pressure (BiPAP), and endotracheal intubation. When the patient presents with stridor, the physical evaluation is also useful in identifying the location of airway compromise. When the stridor occurs primarily during inspiration, it is caused by extrathoracic obstruction; when it occurs during exhalation, it reflects an intrathoracic obstruction. If the stridor occurs during both inspiration and exhalation, the obstruction is fixed, such as may occur with tracheal stenosis. The fixed obstruction is rarely amenable to conservative treatment, and endotracheal intubation is most likely to be required until a more definitive therapy can be provided. In selected patients, helium therapy can be used as a temporizing intervention until a more definitive treatment can be provided.[34]

Respiratory dyssynchrony is an early and critical indicator of respiratory muscle fatigue and impending respiratory failure.[35,36] Respiratory dyssynchrony (when the patient has no evidence of upper airway obstruction) is identified by assessing chest wall and abdominal movement during normal tidal breathing. A paradoxical respiratory pattern suggests that the patient may have inadequate muscle strength to sustain spontaneous respiration and that positive-pressure ventilation support may be required. Tobin and colleagues found that respiratory muscle dyssynchrony could occur before the development of fatigue,[37,38] although fatigue of the respiratory muscles did not always result in the development of dyssynchrony.[39]

Clinical observation of the patient should include careful assessment of the respiratory muscles as a way of assessing the patient's respiratory reserve. Use of accessory muscles, including the sternocleidomastoid and scalene muscles, is commonly seen in patients with long-standing respiratory failure associated with chronic obstructive pulmonary disease (COPD).[40] The position of the diaphragm and diaphragmatic motion are also affected in patients with severe COPD. The patient who relies on accessory muscles and has minimal diaphragmatic excursion does not have any respiratory reserve. The patient is at risk for recurrent respiratory failure and presents a significant challenge during weaning when mechanical ventilatory support is required.

The routine physical examination of the lungs should be performed as part of the assessment for every patient. The examination can provide evidence of parenchymal lung abnormalities and cardiopulmonary pathology. Palpation of the chest and auscultation of the lungs can provide useful information about the presence of pleural effusions, pneumothorax, or other extrapulmonary air, and it can assess the location of the diaphragms. The examination can provide information about potential physiologic abnormalities and guide the selection of other monitoring techniques, including ABGs and chest radiography.

Although the physical examination is useful and should be performed routinely, some of the physical signs and symptoms of respiratory failure are not diagnostic, but instead reflect the physiologic manifestations of the underlying problem. The greatest value of the physical examination is that it provides an initial baseline assessment of the patient, and subsequent examinations can clarify the response to clinical interventions. The physical examination combined with other monitoring modalities remains an important monitor of respiratory status.

B. Radiologic Evaluation

The chest radiograph is another important monitor of the pulmonary status, although it represents a static picture of the clinical situation. The chest radiograph can confirm proper placement of central venous and other catheters, the ETT,[22] and pacemakers. Routine portable chest radiography usually provides evidence of pulmonary infiltrates and pulmonary edema. Radiographic findings that suggest pulmonary edema include bronchial cuffing, perihilar pulmonary infiltrates, and Kerley B lines. Although these findings are helpful, in many critically ill patients, differentiation of diffuse, bilateral infiltrates caused by infection from pulmonary edema can be difficult. When underlying pulmonary diseases such as COPD coexist with acute pulmonary edema, the classic bilateral, fluffy pulmonary infiltrates may not be present. In these circumstances, the x-ray findings must be correlated with other clinical data to explain the radiographic findings.

The chest radiograph can occasionally identify possible abnormalities in the larger airways, including tracheal stenosis and dilatation (as may occur when the ETT cuff is overinflated), although confirmation of the suspected findings usually requires computed tomography (CT) or magnetic resonance imaging (MRI). The presence of tracheomalacia is more difficult, because the airway may look normal on a routine chest radiograph. The tracheal abnormality is more evident on clinical examination (i.e., stridor with forced exhalation) or on a dynamic radiographic study, such as a cine-CT scan.

The routine chest radiograph has limitations when used as a monitor of respiratory status. Radiographic findings do not always correlate with other clinical and physiologic monitors because the radiologic changes can be delayed in onset and resolution. The radiologic technique also influences the value of the chest radiograph as a monitor. Most commonly, a portable anteroposterior radiograph is obtained with the patient in the supine position. When it is performed in this manner, interpretation of heart size, differentiation of atelectasis and pleural effusions, and detection of pneumothoraces may be difficult. When trying to identify any of these abnormalities, other views, including upright or lateral decubitus x-ray films, should be requested, depending on the suspected pathology. Occasionally, an ultrasound or CT scan of the chest may be required to confirm the presence of pleural effusions, pulmonary abscesses, or other abnormalities.

Other radiologic evaluations can be useful to assess abnormalities observed on the chest radiograph or physical examination. Ventilation-perfusion ($\dot{V}/\dot{Q}$) scans have been used to detect pulmonary emboli, although the $\dot{V}/\dot{Q}$ scans are often inadequate or impossible when assessing a mechanically ventilated, critically ill patient for possible pulmonary emboli. For the ICU patient with suspected pulmonary emboli, pulmonary arteriograms or, more commonly, spiral CT scans are performed because they can be completed quickly and provide better diagnostic information than the $\dot{V}/\dot{Q}$ scan alone.

CT and MRI can assess the airways and pulmonary parenchyma. They can identify the location, extent, and character of upper airway abnormalities, including mass lesions, pulmonary intraparenchymal lesions, pleural effusions, and other pulmonary and extrapulmonary abnormalities.

C. Assessment of Gas Exchange

One of the most important goals in monitoring pulmonary function is to determine whether the lung is able to sustain satisfactory oxygenation and ventilation. Invasive and noninvasive monitors of gas exchange are used routinely. Although noninvasive devices are useful and provide important information about oxygenation and ventilation, the ABG determination remains the most frequently used monitor of oxygenation, ventilation, and acid-base abnormalities.[41]

1. Blood Gas Monitoring

ABG measurement remains an essential component of respiratory monitoring. It provides direct measurement of arterial oxygen tension (PaO_2), $PaCO_2$, and pH. From these measured parameters, bicarbonate concentration (HCO_3^-), oxygen saturation (SaO_2), and base excess or base deficit are calculated. The measured and calculated parameters define adequacy of gas exchange, acid-base balance, and overall cardiorespiratory status.

ABGs, including PaO_2, $PaCO_2$, and pH, are used routinely in the OR, ICU, and ED and occasionally in other clinical settings to evaluate gas exchange and respiratory

reserve. Direct measurement of PaO_2 from a sample of arterial blood obtained from a direct arterial puncture or from an indwelling arterial catheter has been the traditional method for assessing oxygenation. To interpret PaO_2 accurately requires an understanding of normal pulmonary physiology and the influences of alterations in ventilation and perfusion on the predicted value of arterial oxygen tension. Normal PaO_2 declines with age. The normal PaO_2 can vary over time by as much as ±10%, and the PaO_2 measured by a blood gas machine can vary by ±10%. Hypoxemia can result from several factors, including inadequate inspired O_2 (i.e., low PaO_2), $\dot{V}/\dot{Q}$ mismatch, shunt, or inadequate cardiac output (i.e., low mixed venous oxygen tension [$P\bar{v}O_2$]). Documentation of an acceptable PaO_2 is reassuring, although it is important to put the PaO_2 value into context. It alone does not ensure that a patient's O_2 delivery is sufficient. To assess the adequacy of O_2 delivery, additional studies are necessary, including evaluation of acid-base status, measurement of serum lactate and mixed venous O_2 content, and cardiac output measurement.

The $PaCO_2$ is used to assess adequacy of ventilation, differentiating whether ventilation is normal or abnormal (too high or too low). The normal $PaCO_2$ is 40 mm Hg. If the $PaCO_2$ is less than 40 mm Hg, the patient is hyperventilating; if the $PaCO_2$ is more than 40 mm Hg, the patient is hypoventilating. However, the $PaCO_2$ alone is only one measure of the adequacy of ventilation. It must be interpreted in relation to the pH. In response to changes in pH, ventilatory drive changes. When a patient develops a metabolic alkalosis, as might occur after a bicarbonate infusion or the administration of large quantities of citrated bank blood, the ventilatory drive is decreased. The $PaCO_2$ rises, but the decrease in $\dot{V}E$ is appropriate and is not an indication of respiratory failure. Similarly, the patient who has a significant metabolic acidosis should increase $\dot{V}_E$ to normalize the pH. In interpreting whether the patient is ventilating appropriately and has a normal ventilatory drive, the $PaCO_2$ and pH must be evaluated simultaneously. For example, if a patient has a normal $PaCO_2$ of 40 mm Hg, but the pH is below normal (e.g., 7.25), the ventilatory effort is inadequate, suggesting inadequate respiratory compensation due to drugs that are suppressing ventilatory drive or underlying respiratory failure.

When arterial blood cannot be obtained, venous blood sampling (peripheral or central) has been used to estimate arterial $PaCO_2$, although it is not a useful way to evaluate oxygenation. In some clinical situations, the difference between $PaCO_2$ and $P\bar{v}CO_2$ is small, and $P\bar{v}CO_2$ can be used as an estimate of $PaCO_2$. However, the exact relationship between arterial and venous $PaCO_2$ is not consistent from patient to patient or within a single patient as the clinical conditions change. $P\bar{v}CO_2$ cannot be used as a substitute for $PaCO_2$.

Although monitoring gas exchange using ABG measurements is important, the technique has some limitations. Blood gas monitoring is invasive, and samples must be drawn from an indwelling arterial catheter or an arterial puncture. Frequent blood gas sampling can result in significant blood loss, which may be a clinical problem for any unstable patient, particularly the pediatric patient or anemic adult. Placement and maintenance of an arterial catheter have associated risks, including hemorrhage, hand ischemia, arterial thrombosis and embolism, infection,[42,43] and development of a radial artery aneurysm.[44]

Blood gas monitoring usually is obtained by intermittent sampling from an arterial puncture or indwelling arterial catheter. When a patient's respiratory status is unstable or is rapidly evolving or when frequent adjustments in ventilatory support are required, intermittent monitoring may be insufficient. In these clinical situations, continuous monitoring is preferable. Continuous intra-atrial blood gas monitors can provide useful real-time data regarding gas exchange and acid-base status,[45,46] although the clinical utility of these monitors has not been validated, and the technology is not widely available.[47,48] These monitors use fluorescence-based probes placed through an arterial catheter to provide a continuous assessment of PaO_2, $PaCO_2$, and pH. The information obtained from these instruments should provide more immediate information about changes in gas exchange or acid-base balance. However, the probes and monitors are more expensive than intermittent blood gas analysis and have not become routine monitors.

2. Noninvasive Monitoring

Assessment of gas exchange using noninvasive techniques has revolutionized clinical care, particularly for anesthesiologists and intensive care providers. Because clinical evaluation of gas exchange is unreliable and often a late sign of deterioration,[49] noninvasive devices that continuously monitor oxygenation and ventilation are valuable tools. Several noninvasive methods are available for evaluating oxygenation and ventilation. The most commonly used devices include the pulse oximeter for monitoring oxygenation and the capnograph for evaluating ventilation.

a. PULSE OXIMETRY

Pulse oximetry provides a rapid, continuous, and noninvasive estimation of the O_2 saturation of hemoglobin in arterial blood, and it is used routinely to monitor clinical care involving airway management in the OR, ED, and ICU.[50-53] It has become the standard monitor of oxygenation during administration of sedation for procedures and during general medical care.[54-57] With routine use of this monitor, a high prevalence of clinically undetected hypoxemia in adults and children has been demonstrated.[50,57-59] These episodes of desaturation may affect morbidity and mortality.[60,61] With severe and sustained hypoxemia (i.e., oxygen saturation from pulse oximetry [SpO_2] is less than 85% for more than 5 minutes), patients with known cardiac disease were twice as likely to have perioperative ischemia after noncardiac surgery.[61] Among medical patients, those who experienced episodes of hypoxemia within the first 24 hours of hospitalization were three times more likely to die 4 to 7 months after discharge.[60]

It is logical to assume that the routine use of pulse oximetry has made caring for patients safer by increasing the detection of hypoxemia, better understanding its causes, and allowing more rapid and effective interventions to correct the pathophysiologic causes. Some clinicians have suggested that the early detection of arterial oxygen desaturation with the use of pulse oximetry may improve outcomes.[61-64] Although clinical studies do not confirm this belief, they do not negate the presumed benefit of this monitoring tool.[65-68] A systematic review of the Cochrane database found no evidence of an outcome benefit of the use of pulse oximetry in anesthesia practice.[69] Despite the lack of good outcome data to document that value of pulse oximetry, its use is considered standard of care for critically ill patients and patients receiving moderate or deep sedation or anesthesia.

To measure the O_2 saturation of hemoglobin in arterial blood, pulse oximetry uses two fundamental principles: the differential light absorption of oxyhemoglobin (O_2Hb) and reduced hemoglobin (Hb) and the increase in light absorption produced by pulsatile blood flow compared with that of a background of connective tissue, skin, bone, and venous blood.[56,70] The spectrophotometric principle that forms the basis for oximetry is the Lambert-Beer law (Equation 1), which allows determination of the concentration of an unknown solute in a solvent by light absorption.

$$I_1/I_0 = e^{-alc} \tag{1}$$

where

I_1 = intensity of the light out of the sample
I_0 = intensity of the incident light
a = absorption coefficient of the substance
l = distance the light travels through the material (i.e., path length)
c = concentration of the absorbing species
e = base of the natural logarithm

Use of the Lambert-Beer law allows the determination of the concentration of a solute in a solvent as long as the extinction coefficient is known. It also follows that for a solution with multiple solutes, a separate wavelength of light is needed for differentiation of the solutes. For a solution with four solutes, four wavelengths of light are required.

The commercially available pulse oximeters use light-emitting diodes (LEDs) that transmit light at specific wavelengths: 660 nm (red) and 940 nm (infrared). These wavelengths were selected because the absorption characteristics of O_2Hb and reduced Hb are sufficiently different at these wavelengths to allow differentiation of O_2Hb and Hb (Fig. 49-1).

The pulse oximeter determines arterial saturation by timing the measurement to pulsations in the arterial system. During pulsatile flow, the vascular bed expands and contracts, creating a change in the light path length.[51] These pulsations alter the quantity of light transmitted to the sensor and provide a plethysmographic waveform.[71] This timing of the signal allows the pulse oximeter to differentiate arterial oxygen saturation from venous saturation on the basis of the ratio of pulsatile and baseline absorption of red and infrared light (Fig. 49-2).

The pulse oximeter displays the O_2 saturation based on a ratio (R) of pulsatile and baseline absorption at the two wavelengths transmitted (i.e., 660 and 940 nm) in the tissue bed. The relationship is shown in Equation 2:

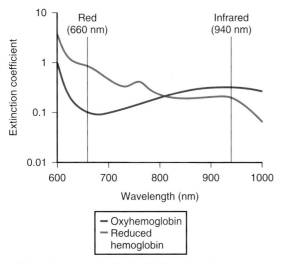

Figure 49-1 Absorption (extinction) characteristics of oxyhemoglobin and reduced hemoglobin are shown. There are marked differences between the two at light wavelengths of 660 nm (red) and 940 nm (infrared). (From Tobin MJ: Respiratory monitoring. *JAMA* 264:244–251, 1990.)

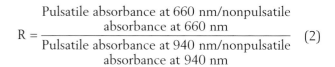

$$R = \frac{\text{Pulsatile absorbance at 660 nm/nonpulsatile absorbance at 660 nm}}{\text{Pulsatile absorbance at 940 nm/nonpulsatile absorbance at 940 nm}} \quad (2)$$

The O_2 saturation displayed by the pulse oximeter is empirically related to this calculated value on the basis of calibration curves derived for healthy, nonsmoking adult men breathing O_2 at various concentrations. Most commercially available pulse oximeters are calibrated over the range of 70% to 100%. The accuracy of pulse oximetry in determining the SaO_2 of Hb has been excellent over this range,[51] with an error of ±3% to 4%.[57]

Although pulse oximetry has become a ubiquitous monitoring device, particularly to confirm adequacy of oxygenation during airway management, it has limitations. First, the measurement of O_2 saturation does not provide a direct assessment of oxygen tension. Because of the shape of the oxygen-hemoglobin dissociation curve, at higher levels of oxygenation measurements of SpO_2 are insensitive in detecting significant changes in PaO_2 (Fig. 49-3). Second, the pulse oximeter is not accurate when oxygen saturation is less than 70%. The inaccuracy results from the limited range of O_2 saturations

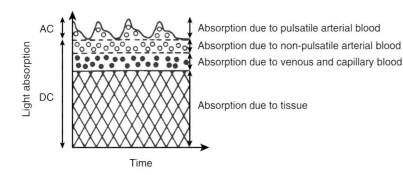

Figure 49-2 Schematic representation of light absorption through living tissue. Notice that the alternating current *(AC)* signal results from the pulsatile component of arterial blood and that the direct current *(DC)* signal comprises all the nonpulsatile absorbers of light in the tissue, including nonpulsatile blood in the veins and capillaries and nonpulsatile blood in all other tissues. (From Tremper KK, Barker SJ: Pulse oximetry. *Anesthesiology* 70:98–108, 1989.)

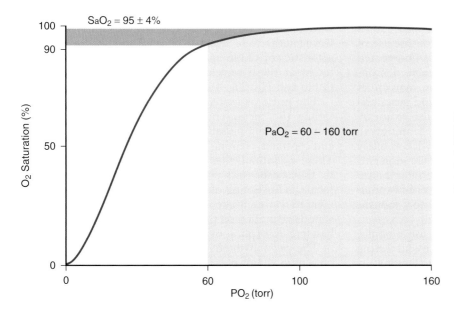

Figure 49-3 Oxygen dissociation curve. Because pulse oximeters have 95% confidence limits for SaO_2 of ±3% to 4%, an oximeter reading of 95% can represent a PaO_2 of 60 mm Hg (saturation of 91%) or 160 mm Hg (saturation of 99%). (From Tobin MJ: Respiratory monitoring in the intensive care unit. *Am Rev Respir Dis* 138:1625–1642, 1988.)

used in the calibration process and the difficulty in obtaining reliable human data at these low oxygen saturations.[71,72]

The accuracy of pulse oximeters during hypoxemia has been extensively studied and reviewed.[37,73-76] Most of these studies have been performed on healthy volunteers who had desaturation induced by breathing hypoxic gas mixtures for short periods. Pulse oximeters from different manufacturers varied in their accuracy during hypoxemia; the direction of error differs among these devices, with some overestimating and some underestimating true arterial O_2 saturation. Some study results documented problems with the calibration curves and caused revision of the algorithms by the manufacturers.[72-77] These modifications to the algorithms have improved performance of the oximeters.[57]

Other factors affect the performance of pulse oximeters. The response characteristics of pulse oximeters are clinically important, particularly in situations in which the saturation may be changing rapidly, as can occur during management of the difficult airway. Investigators have studied the response characteristics of pulse oximetry in clinical practice.[72-77] West and colleagues studied five obese, nonsmoking men with sleep apnea syndrome.[78] During spontaneous desaturation, the pulse oximeter underestimated the minimum SaO_2, and during spontaneous resaturation, there was an overshoot of the maximum SpO_2. The location of the probe also influences the response time for the pulse oximeter. Probes placed on the ear respond more quickly to sudden decrease in SaO_2 than probes placed on a digit.[75] The response time to changes in O_2 saturation of the pulse oximeter also depends on heart rate. For fingertip sensors, as heart rate increases, the response to an acute change in saturation is faster; for ear or nasal probes, the relationship is reversed, and as heart rate increases, the response to changes in SaO_2 is slower.[78]

Accuracy of the pulse oximeter is altered in several situations (Box 49-1). Excessive light, such as fluorescent or xenon arc surgical lights, bilirubin lights, and heating lamps, can cause falsely low or high SpO_2 values.[57,72,79] Covering the probe with an opaque material helps to eliminate this problem. Electrocautery devices can produce significant electrical interference, which results in improper functioning of the pulse oximeter.[56] The infrared pulse waves used by neurosurgical image guidance systems interfere with the signal quality and O_2

saturation detection by pulse oximetry.[80] The use of aluminum foil as a shield was effective in restoring the accuracy of six brands of pulse oximeters when exposed to the infrared signal generated by a neuronavigation device.[81] Misalignment of disposable pulse oximeter probes may cause falsely low O_2 saturation to be displayed by pulse oximeters, even though the plethysmographic tracing is of excellent quality, and this can change anesthetic management.[82] In 100 patients entering the postanesthesia care unit (PACU) at Massachusetts General Hospital, only 6 had perfect placement of the probes, and for the remaining 94, the average misalignment distance was 5.4 mm (range, 0 to 23 mm).[82] In a single case report, a Massimo Signal Extraction Technology (Massimo SET; Irvine, CA) pulse oximeter using SatShare technology with a Datex-Ohmeda AS/3 monitor displayed an uninterrupted waveform and normal O_2 saturation during asystole in a patient undergoing abdominal surgery.[83]

Motion of the probe, such as when a patient or caregiver moves the digit on which the oximeter probe is placed, can cause artifactual readings from the pulse oximeter. Vibration of the sensor delays the detection time for hypoxemia and causes spurious decreases in SpO_2.[84] Movement can result in errors of as much as 20%.[85] In a large, prospective study, patients' motion was the major reason for abandoning the use of a pulse oximeter in the PACU.[86] In pediatric patients, 71% of all alarms were false.[87] Attempts have been made to minimize the effect of motion by timing the measurement of SpO_2 to the electrocardiogram (ECG). Pulse oximeters that possess ECG linkage and time the measurement of arterial saturation to the ECG have performed better during vibration than those without this feature.[84] Although this ECG interface is helpful, it has not completely eliminated motion as a problem, particularly in very active or agitated patients. Another approach to decreasing the effect of patients' motion on the accuracy of oximetric data has been to reject motion artifact retrospectively using changes in the plethysmographic waveform that immediately preceded the questionable event.[85] This results in fewer detected episodes of false O_2 desaturation, although at the price of missing true events.[88]

Several manufacturers have added technology designed to minimize motion artifact and to extract a more accurate (true) signal. The Masimo SET uses unique sensor designs and software algorithms to reduce the incidence of false alarms. When the performance of oximeters using this technology was compared in volunteers with that of the Nellcor N-3000 Symphony with improved low-signal performance (Oxismart) and the older Nellcor N-200, the oximeters using Masimo SET were superior in error and signal dropout rate.[89] Baker and colleagues compared the functioning and accuracy of 20 pulse oximeter models in volunteers with hypoxemia during motion and found that the Masimo SET had the best overall performance.[90] When used in the neonatal ICU, Masimo SET resulted in dramatically fewer false alarms and captured more true events than the Nellcor N-200.[91] Oximeters using Masimo SET were more reliable in detecting bradycardia and hypoxemic episodes in patients in the neonatal

---

BOX 49-1	Conditions Affecting the Accuracy of Pulse Oximetry

External light sources
Electrocautery
Motion of the probe
Dyshemoglobinemias: carboxyhemoglobin, methemoglobin
Dyes and pigments: indocyanine green, methylene blue, indigo carmine
Nail polish
Severe anemia
Low perfusion, low perfusion index
Excessive venous pulsations

ICU than the N-3000.[92] This is evidence that more reliable data from oximetry can improve the process of care in a cost-effective manner. In adults after cardiac surgery, the use of more reliable oximeters (those with Masimo SET) compared with conventional oximeters resulted in a more rapid reduction in fraction of inspired oxygen (FIO_2) and the need for fewer ABG determinations during mechanical ventilation.[93] Petterson and colleagues have reviewed the various technologies used to prevent the effects of motion artifacts on the accuracy of pulse oximeters.[94]

Another problem with the pulse oximeter is its inability to differentiate oxyhemoglobin from other hemoglobins, such as methemoglobin and carboxyhemoglobin. An oximeter is able to differentiate only as many substances as the number of wavelengths of light it emits.[56,77] Commercially available oximeters can detect only two types of hemoglobin, reduced and oxygenated (Hb and O_2Hb). Pulse oximeters derive a functional saturation of hemoglobin, which is defined in Equation 3:

$$\text{Functional saturation} = \frac{O_2Hb \times 100\%}{O_2Hb + Hb} \qquad (3)$$

This functional saturation does not account for other hemoglobins, such as methemoglobin (MetHb) or carboxyhemoglobin (COHb). To assess the presence of these other hemoglobin species, two additional wavelengths of light must be incorporated into the measuring device. Spectrophotometric heme oximeters (CO-oximeters) that use four or more wavelengths of light are able to measure other hemoglobin species and calculate the fractional saturation using Equation 4:

$$\text{Fractional saturation} = \frac{O_2Hb \times 100\%}{O_2Hb + Hb + MetHb + COHb} \qquad (4)$$

When COHb or MetHb is present, the pulse oximeter does not provide a true measurement of oxygen saturation.[95,96] The presence of COHb causes a false elevation in the SpO_2 measurement.[95] As shown in Figure 49-4, COHb has minimal light absorption at 940 nm, and at 660 nm, its absorption coefficient is almost identical to that of O_2Hb. The pulse oximeter cannot differentiate COHb from O_2Hb; it overestimates the O_2Hb.[95] The SpO_2 displayed by the pulse oximeter approximates the sums of COHb and O_2Hb. This problem with pulse oximeters is important to consider when assessing oxygenation in patients who have sustained smoke inhalation or patients who have smoked just before proposed airway management. COHb can also be present in long-term ICU patients because carbon monoxide (CO) is a metabolic product of heme metabolism.[97,98] The influence of this potential endogenous source of CO on the accuracy of SpO_2 in the critically ill patient requires further evaluation. In any case, when high CO levels are suspected, O_2 saturation should be measured using a CO-oximeter rather than a pulse oximeter.

MetHb also interferes with pulse oximeter measurements.[96,99] As MetHb levels exceed 30% to 35%, SpO_2 becomes independent of the MetHb level, approaching

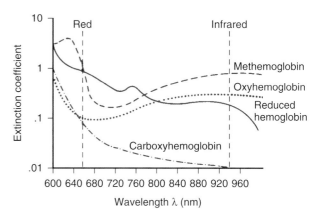

HEMOGLOBIN EXTINCTION CURVES

Figure 49-4 Transmitted light absorbance spectra of four hemoglobin species: oxyhemoglobin, reduced hemoglobin, carboxyhemoglobin, and methemoglobin. (From Tremper KK, Barker SJ: Pulse oximetry. *Anesthesiology* 70:98–108, 1989)

85%. This inaccuracy occurs because the MetHb absorption coefficient at 660 nm is almost identical to that of reduced hemoglobin, whereas at 940 nm, it is greater than that of other hemoglobins (see Fig. 49-4). The pulse oximeter therefore overestimates or underestimates the true SaO_2, depending on the level of MetHb.[77] Some causes of high MetHb levels include administration of nitrates, local anesthetics (e.g., lidocaine, benzocaine), metoclopramide, sulfa-containing drugs, ethylenediaminetetraacetic acid (EDTA), and diaminodiphenylsulfone (Dapsone) and primaquine phosphate used to treat patients with acquired immunodeficiency syndrome (AIDS). Some patients can also have congenitally high MetHb levels.

The continuous and noninvasive detection of oxygenated and deoxygenated hemoglobin, as well as COHb, MetHb, and total hemoglobin, has become possible with the development of oximetric technology. The devices used to monitor these parameters are referred to as pulse CO-oximeters. These newer devices use 8 to 12 wavelengths of light. Devices developed by Massimo Corporation, the Rainbow Set Radical 7 pulse CO-oximeter and the Rad 57 pulse CO-oximeter, can detect and accurately measure the concentrations of COHb and MetHb.[100] An advantage of these devices is the ability to continuously monitor the level of dyshemoglobinemia and monitor the response to treatment.[101-105] The clinical value of this technology has been documented in numerous case reports of detection of carboxyhemoglobinemia and methemoglobinemia. However, the specific algorithms used to detect the dyshemoglobins impacts the accuracy of these devices. For example, the accuracy of the Massimo Radical 7 Pulse CO-oximeter in measuring MetHb during coincident hypoxemia ($SaO_2 < 95\%$) was poor in 14 healthy adults with overestimation of MetHb levels by 10% to 40%.[106] After the company made modifications of the software and separated the optical sensors for MetHb and COHb, the accuracy for measuring MetHb concentrations improved considerably.[107]

Pulse CO-oximetry can also be used to continuously determine the hemoglobin concentration in arterial blood

(SpHb).[108] Macknet and colleagues used a Masimo Radical 7 with a spectrophotometric adhesive sensor using 12 wavelengths of light to measure SpHb in 20 healthy volunteers undergoing hemodilution (with removal of 500 mL of whole blood) compared with the standard total hemoglobin (tHb) measurement using a laboratory CO-oximeter.[109] The investigators found that the average difference between SpHb and tHb to be –0.15 g/dL, with a standard deviation of 0.92 g/dL, and they concluded that SpHb is accurate within 1.0 g/dL. In 20 patients undergoing spinal surgery, Miller and colleagues compared SpHb with tHb and with hemoglobin measured with a point-of-care device, the HemoCue.[110] There was an overall tendency for the SpHb to overestimate the corresponding tHb, especially when the perfusion index (PI) was higher than 1.4, the manufacturer's threshold value for accuracy of SpHb. This study also calls into question the utility of using SpHb in making clinical decisions, because 22% of the pulse CO-oximeter tests determined hemoglobin values were more than 2.0 g/dL different from the tHb values.[110] However, other investigators have found the monitor to be a useful guide to clinical decision making. In a preliminary study of 350 patients undergoing orthopedic surgery, the use of noninvasive, continuous hemoglobin monitoring reduced the frequency of blood transfusions and decreased the number of units of blood transfused compared with standard hemoglobin measurement.[111] Although these studies have documented the value of SpHb monitoring in some clinical situations, the clinical value for guiding transfusion decisions for the patient with rapid, acute blood loss, large fluid shifts, or poor PI will require further investigation.

Fetal Hb does not affect the accuracy of the pulse oximeter.[56,57,79] The effect of other dyshemoglobinemias, such as sulfhemoglobin, on the accuracy of pulse oximetry has not been investigated.[79] Other pigments that interfere with the accuracy of pulse oximeter measurements include indocyanine green, methylene blue, and indigo carmine.[79] These dyes cause transient artifactual falls in saturation; the extent of the problem depends on the absorption characteristics of the dye. Skin pigmentation has minimal effect on pulse oximeter readings, although very dark pigmentation can result in a slight decrease in accuracy.[112,113] Jaundice has caused artificially low and artificially high pulse oximeter readings.[94] In most studies, however, even very high bilirubin levels have had no effect on the accuracy of the SpO_2.[103,114]

Certain shades of nail polish can alter significantly the accuracy of pulse oximetry when the sensor is placed directly over the nail bed. The extent to which accuracy is affected depends on the absorption characteristics of the nail polish at 660 and 940 nm. Black, blue, and green polishes can falsely lower the measured SpO_2 by up to 6%; red nail polish has little effect on pulse oximeter measurements.[79,115,116] If a patient has a darkly pigmented polish, it should be removed from the nail bed that is going to receive the probe, or the probe should be placed over the sides of the digit, thereby avoiding transmission of the signal through the nail bed.[79,116] Darker skin pigments can produce falsely high readings of arterial O_2 saturation by many pulse oximeters during hypoxemia.

The positive bias in patients with dark skin may be as much as 8% when arterial O_2 saturation is less than 80%, and it is less pronounced in patients with intermediate pigmentation and smallest in those with the lightest skin.[117] This may be explained by the use of light-skinned individuals for the testing and calibration of pulse oximeters. However, not all oximeters produce this result. The Masimo Radical oximeter with an adhesive, disposable probe was found to underestimate oxygen saturation in hypoxic subjects.[118]

Severe anemia can affect the accuracy of the pulse oximeter. Lee and coworkers demonstrated that the pulse oximeter was inaccurate when the hematocrit was less than 10%.[119] Vegfors and colleagues also found that the pulse oximeter is not accurate when the hematocrit is very low,[120] but they suggested that the problem was caused by poor perfusion rather than the hematocrit level alone. Of more importance in the management of the severely anemic patient is the assessment of O_2 delivery, rather than O_2 saturation, even when the pulse oximeter is accurate. SpO_2 reflects only O_2 saturation and does not provide a guide to adequacy of the oxygen-carrying capacity of the blood or O_2 delivery. In patients with sickle cell anemia, pulse oximetry correlates well with SaO_2 measured by CO-oximeter, although with a clinically insignificant bias toward underestimation.[121]

When patients become hypotensive, hypovolemic, or markedly vasoconstricted, the peripheral pulse diminishes. This results in an additional problem with the performance of the pulse oximeter because the monitor works only when the patient has adequate arterial pulsations. When the patient's peripheral perfusion is poor, the pulse oximeter may be unable to measure SpO_2. In one study of patients with poor perfusion after cardiopulmonary bypass, only 2 of 20 brands of pulse oximeters were able to give SpO_2 values within 4% of that obtained using a CO-oximeter.[122] Attempts to improve the accuracy of pulse oximeters in hypoperfused conditions have not adequately solved the problem. Alternative probe locations, such as the nose or ear, and reflectance, rather than transmittance, techniques have been tried with various degrees of success.[123,124] Investigators have evaluated pulse oximetry using probes placed in the esophagus.[125-127] When placed esophageally or in other internal tissue sites, the measurement of SpO_2 depends on reflectance and not on detection of the transmitted signal on the side opposite the emitter, as in standard transmission pulse oximetry.[128,129] Esophageal location of the pulse oximeter probe in critically ill surgical patients results in more consistent SaO_2 readings than with standard surface probes, and the function of probes was not affected by changes in perfusion or temperature.[127] Esophageal pulse oximetry has also been used successfully in neonatal and older pediatric patients.[130] Fetal pulse oximetry uses reflectance technology.[131] Unfortunately, the expected reduction in the rate of cesarean delivery with the use of fetal oximetry has not occurred.[132] In patients with peripheral vascular disease undergoing vascular surgery, the use of a forehead reflectance probe was shown to be an acceptable alternative to the standard transmission probe placed on the earlobe.[128]

The accuracy of SpO_2 measurements in hypothermic patients has not been rigorously evaluated, but it seems to depend primarily on the presence or absence of an adequate pulse signal rather than temperature itself.[133] In one study, active warming of patients improved the ability of pulse oximeters to detect a signal and decreased the incidence of false alarms.[134]

Pulsations other than arterial pulsations interfere with the performance of the pulse oximeter. When venous pulsations are pronounced, for example, the pulse oximeter may underestimate the true arterial oxygen saturation of hemoglobin.[135] In a group of patients with severe tricuspid insufficiency, pulse oximetry underestimated the O_2 saturation by up to 11%. Other clinical situations in which venous pulsations may be important include patients with severe congestive heart failure and patients who require very high venous pressure, such as after a Fontan procedure performed as treatment for tricuspid atresia.

Severe burns and injury to the digits of both hands and feet have been reported from the application of pulse oximeter probes.[136-138] Frequently rotating the site of application and increasing vigilance can minimize these events. Burns of the skin have occurred with the application of pulse oximeters to patients after photodynamic therapy with the porfimer sodium (Photofrin).[139] During intraoperative photochemotherapy with verteporfin, frequent rotation of the site of the pulse oximeter at intervals of 7 to 15 minutes during the 6-hour procedure prevented cutaneous injury.[140]

The plethysmographic waveforms produced by many pulse oximeters have been evaluated as a noninvasive method to determine blood pressure, intravascular volume, and perfusion.[115,141-147] Respiratory-induced changes in photoplethysmography, as a predictor for volume responsiveness in mechanically ventilated patients, is similar to that seen in the arterial pressure waveform, and these dynamic measurements are superior to the static measurements obtained from intravascular catheters.[148-150] Some patient conditions may limit the use of these dynamic indicators of volume responsiveness, including dysrhythmias, a requirement for positive-pressure ventilation with a V_T greater than 8 mL/kg, and low levels of positive end-expiratory pressure (PEEP).[151] Plethysmographic variations induced by the use of positive-pressure ventilation were more reliable in predicting fluid responsiveness than central venous pressure or pulmonary artery occlusion pressure in mechanically ventilated cardiac surgery patients postoperatively.[152] Photoplethysmographic pulse variation of more than 9% produced by mechanical ventilation identified patients who were likely to respond to fluid administration with an increase in cardiac output.[148] In this study, there was no relationship between arterial pressure measured directly and the amplitude of the photoplethysmogram. Respiratory changes in the amplitude of the plethysmographic pulse were found to be as accurate as changes in pulse pressure from an arterial catheter produced by mechanical ventilation in septic patients for the prediction of fluid responsiveness.[153] The use of respiratory variations in photoplethysmography has been as reliable and as accurate an indicator of mild hypovolemia (up to a 20% decrease in estimated circulating blood volume) as the use of arterial waveform analysis in hemodynamically stable, mechanically ventilated patients undergoing autologous hemodilution.[154] On the contrary, Landsverk and colleagues found that there are larger intraindividual and interindividual variability in critically ill patients in indices derived from pulse oximeter technology than from those using arterial waveforms and that this may limit the reliability of predicting volume responsiveness using the pulse oximeter.[155]

The use of the respiratory-induced waveform variation (RIWV) in photoplethysmography may be useful in detecting hypovolemia in spontaneously breathing humans.[156,157] In a study of trauma patients in the prehospital setting, Chen and colleagues found that photoplethysmography RIWV was independently correlated with major hemorrhage and that it may enhance detection of hypovolemia beyond the use of standard vital signs.[156] In a study of volunteers, McGrath and colleagues progressively reduced central blood volume using lower body negative pressure up to −100 mm Hg and investigated the pulse shape features of the photoplethysmographic patter obtained from sensors placed on the finger, forehead, and ear to determine which might serve as indicator of hypovolemia.[157] The investigators found that reductions in pulse amplitude, width, and area under the curve of the pulse oximeter waveform from the ear and forehead were strongly correlated with reductions in stroke volume with the forehead sensor having the best performance. These changes in waveform were seen before reductions in arterial blood pressure. The increased sympathetic activity that accompanies hypovolemia and the concomitant peripheral vasoconstriction were thought by the investigators to reduce the ability of the photoplethysmogram obtained from the finger probe to function as well as the probes in other locations in detecting hypovolemia.

The Massimo Corporation developed a proprietary algorithm, the Pleth Variability Index (PVI), which allows continuous and automated calculation of respiratory-induced variations of the photoplethysmographic waveform. PVI is a dynamic measure of the changes in the perfusion index (PI) that occur over a complete respiratory cycle. The PI is the ratio of pulsatile absorption of the pulse oximeter signal (AC) to that obtained during the baseline nonpulsatile signal (DC), and it reflects the amplitude of the plethysmographic waveform.[115] To calculate PI, the pulsatile signal is indexed to the nonpulsatile blood flow and expressed as a percentage: $PI = (AC/DC) \times 100$. The PVI calculation uses the maximal (PI_{max}) and minimal (PI_{min}) PI values over the respiratory cycle: $PVI = [(PI_{max} - PI_{min})/PI_{max}] \times 100$, expressed as a percentage.[158]

Studies have investigated the usefulness of the PVI to predict fluid responsiveness in patients and guide patient management.[159-161] In patients after cardiac surgery, PVI was able to predict the reduction in cardiac output produced by the application of PEEP of 10 cm H_2O when patients were mechanically ventilated with a V_T greater than 8 mL/kg.[158] When patients were ventilated with a V_T of 6 mL/kg, the PVI and the change in respiratory variation in arterial pulse pressure (ΔPP) were unable to accurately assess the hemodynamic effects of PEEP. In a study of goal-directed fluid management, PVI was used to assess volume responsiveness in 82 patients undergoing abdominal surgery. The use of PVI resulted in a decrease in the volume of fluid administered in the OR and reduced lactate levels in the intraoperative and post-operative periods.[160] Zimmermann and colleagues found that PVI is comparable to stroke volume variation as an indicator of volume responsiveness.[162] PVI also can predict fluid responsiveness (i.e., increase in cardiac output of ≥15%) in mechanically ventilated critically ill patients with circulatory insufficiency after a 500-mL colloid bolus.[161] In this study, a higher PVI at baseline was associated with a larger change in cardiac output after fluid administration.

The PI that is provided in some pulse oximetric monitoring systems correlates with peripheral perfusion. Lima and colleagues found that the PI correlated with changes in the core-to-toe temperature difference in critically ill patients and suggested that it might be clinically helpful to monitor changes in PI in this population of patients.[144]

In the postoperative period, continuous pulse oximetry can be a useful surveillance monitor, and it can reduce respiratory complications. One commercially available system uses a paging system to alert the nursing staff when preset physiologic alarm limits are breached. In one study that evaluated the clinical benefits of the Patient SafetyNet System (Massimo Corp.), careful selection of the alarm limits reduced the number of false alarms but provided notification to the nurse of changes in physiologic parameters, including O_2 saturation. The investigators demonstrated a decrease in ICU transfers and reduced need for rescue events (i.e., activation of rapid response team, cardiac arrest team, or stat airway team) compared with before implementation of the system.[163] Further investigation of the clinical value of these systems is needed to justify widespread implementation.

b. CAPNOGRAPHY

Capnography provides a noninvasive method to assess ventilation and ventilation-perfusion relationships.[164-166] A capnograph provides a continuous display of the CO_2 concentration of gases from the airways. The CO_2 concentration at the end of normal exhalation ($EtCO_2$, $PETCO_2$) is a reflection of gas from the distal alveoli; it therefore represents an estimate of the alveolar CO_2 concentration ($PACO_2$). When ventilation and perfusion are well matched, the $PACO_2$ closely approximates the $PaCO_2$, and $PACO_2 \cong PaCO_2 \cong PETCO_2$. The normal gradient between $PaCO_2$ and $PETCO_2$ ($P[a - ET]CO_2$) is more than 6 mm Hg. The gradient between $PaCO_2$ and $PETCO_2$ increases when pulmonary perfusion is reduced or ventilation is maldistributed.

The capnogram is a waveform that graphically represents the CO_2 concentration over time. The capnogram provides information about adequacy of ventilation, potential airflow obstruction, and in conjunction with other monitors, $\dot{V}/\dot{Q}$ relationships. A normal capnogram has four components, the ascending limb, alveolar plateau, descending limb, and baseline (Fig. 49-5). The ascending limb represents the CO_2 concentration of the gas in rapidly emptying alveoli. The alveolar plateau occurs

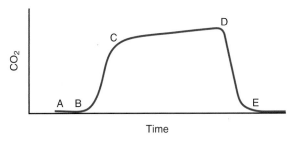

Figure 49-5 Normal capnogram. Exhalation begins at point A and continues to point D. Segment *C-D* is the alveolar plateau. Point *D* represents the end-tidal carbon dioxide. Inspiration is represented by rapid, descending limb of segment *D-E*, which reaches the zero baseline.

because the CO_2 concentration from uniformly ventilated alveoli is relatively constant. The $PETCO_2$ is the point at which the CO_2 concentration is highest, representing the CO_2 concentration approximating true alveolar gas. The rapid, descending limb of the capnogram signals inspiration. The baseline represents the CO_2 concentration of inspired gas.

Various methods of gas analysis are commercially available, including mass spectrometry, Raman scattering, and infrared absorption spectrometry. The most commonly used method is infrared spectrophotometry. It is based on the principle that CO_2 absorbs infrared light. As the infrared light is passed through a sample of gas, the amount of infrared light absorbed is proportional to the concentration of CO_2 in the sample.

Two different sampling techniques are used for capnography: mainstream and sidestream devices. The mainstream (in-line) capnograph has a transducer that is connected to the patient's ETT. The transducer contains the infrared light source and a photodetector. The mainstream capnograph has a faster response time because no gas is withdrawn from the patient's airway. Secretions usually do not prevent accurate measurement because they are easily removed from the sensor site. The mainstream device does have some limitations, including the weight of the connectors, the increased equipment dead space (as much as 20 mL), and the inability to use mainstream devices in extubated patients.

The sidestream (diverting) capnograph aspirates gas from the patient's airway to the capnograph through a sampling tube. Analysis of the CO_2 concentration is performed in the monitor rather than at the airway adapter. Because the analysis is not done at the airway, the airway connector is smaller and adds no significant dead space or weight to the Y connection between the ETT and ventilator circuit. The sidestream device can also be used with a modified nasal cannula to monitor CO_2 concentrations in the airway of nonintubated patients. The response time of the sidestream capnograph is slower because it aspirates gas from the airway. The sampling can be compromised by significant water condensation in the catheter and pulmonary secretions.

Capnography has important applications during airway management and mechanical ventilatory support. It is a useful monitor during endotracheal intubation and to confirm placement of the ETT within the trachea. It can document adequacy of ventilation during mechanical

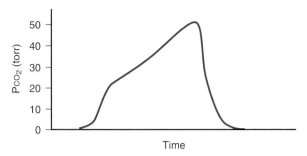

Figure 49-6 Capnograph waveform in a patient with airflow obstruction demonstrates lack of an alveolar plateau.

ventilatory support, spontaneous ventilation in intubated and nonintubated patients, and adequacy of cardiopulmonary resuscitation. Capnography can also be used to monitor the nonintubated patient using a nasal cannula that aspirates the exhaled gas and analyzes the CO_2 concentration. This technique is useful when evaluating the patient with a tenuous airway or gas exchange who may require urgent or emergent endotracheal intubation and mechanical ventilatory support.

The capnographic waveform provides a graphic display of the CO_2 concentration over time. The waveform can be used to identify significant inspiratory or expiratory airway obstruction, including intrinsic airway obstruction or a kinked ETT (Fig. 49-6). With expiratory obstruction, the waveform does not have a normal alveolar plateau. By continuously monitoring the capnographic waveform, the response to bronchodilator therapy can be visually confirmed. The capnographic waveform can also be used to diagnose rebreathing of CO_2; with rebreathing, as can occur when fresh gas flow is inadequate, the baseline (inspired) CO_2 concentration increases.

Despite its clinical utility, capnography has significant limitations as a monitor of ventilation for patients with impaired pulmonary function or hemodynamic instability. The biggest problem is that the correlation between $PaCO_2$ and $PETCO_2$ varies and is sometimes poor in patients with low cardiac output or altered $\dot{V}/\dot{Q}$ relationships. The correlation varies as the patient's clinical condition changes, making interpretations of ventilation from $PETCO_2$ measurements alone unreliable. This has been documented in patients suffering severe traumatic injury, particularly those with traumatic brain injury for whom hypocapnia and hypercapnia should be avoided.[167,168] In a study of 180 trauma patients presenting to an ED, the correlation between $PETCO_2$ and $PaCO_2$ was poor (R^2 = 0.277).[169] Following common recommendations for ventilation in these patients to maintain $PETCO_2$ values between 35 and 39 mm Hg resulted in significant hypoventilation. The $PaCO_2$ was more than 40 mm Hg in 80% of cases and more than 50 mm Hg in 30% of cases. The correlation between $PETCO_2$ and $PaCO_2$ was best for patients with only traumatic brain injury and poor for those with chest injuries or decreased perfusion. An increased difference between $PaCO_2$ and $PETCO_2$ in patients with traumatic brain injury was observed for those with coexistent severe chest trauma, hypotension, and metabolic acidosis. For patients without significant extracranial trauma, the $PaCO_2$ and $PETCO_2$ were 100%

concordant.[170] Capnography may be used to guide ventilatory therapy in patients with traumatic brain injury, but only if there is limited injury to other organ systems. It can provide useful noninvasive information in patients undergoing apnea testing to confirm brain death,[171] although most clinicians perform confirmatory ABG analysis to document the $PaCO_2$ before declaring brain death.

IV. MONITORING RESPIRATORY FUNCTION DURING MECHANICAL VENTILATORY SUPPORT

Assessment of pulmonary mechanical function can be performed using a variety of monitoring techniques for the patient who is breathing spontaneously and for the mechanically ventilated patient.[172-175] The techniques are useful for optimizing ventilatory support in the critically ill patient, determining the extent to which the patient can initiate spontaneous ventilation, guiding the use of supportive modes of ventilation (e.g., pressure support ventilation), and determining when and how to initiate weaning from mechanical ventilatory support. With several new modes of ventilation and supportive techniques to augment patient-initiated breaths, these monitoring techniques have become an essential component of respiratory management.

A. Assessment of Pulmonary Mechanical Function

Assessment of dead space ventilation ($\dot{V}_D$) is critical to understanding the nature of a patient's respiratory dysfunction and defining the ventilatory needs of the patient. The $\dot{V}_D$ represents wasted ventilation in that it increases the work of breathing without contributing to gas exchange.

Most clinicians measure $PaCO_2$ to determine whether the patient has adequate ventilation, defined as effective removal of CO_2 by the lungs. $PaCO_2$ is an essential measure of respiratory function and cardiorespiratory relationships, although interpretation of $PaCO_2$ requires an understanding of respiratory function, acid-base status, and compensatory mechanisms by which the patient may adjust to decreased alveolar ventilation ($\dot{V}_A$). Evaluating the adequacy of ventilation requires an understanding of $\dot{V}_A$ and $\dot{V}_D$. The determinants of $PaCO_2$ are represented in Equation 5:

$$PaCO_2 = k\dot{V}CO_2/\dot{V}_A \qquad (5)$$

where
k = 0.863
$\dot{V}CO_2$ = carbon dioxide production (mL/min)
$\dot{V}_A$ = alveolar ventilation (L/min)

The equation assumes that inspired CO_2 is zero. CO_2 elimination through the lung depends solely on the $\dot{V}_A$, the area within the lung where gas exchange occurs.[175] The remainder of the lung and large airways represent dead space, the volume of gas that does not participate in gas exchange; $\dot{V}_D$ has no effect on CO_2 elimination.

The required $\dot{V}_E$ to maintain CO_2 homeostasis depends on the relationship between $\dot{V}_A$ and $\dot{V}_D$. As the dead space increases, the work of breathing (respiratory rate or V_T) must increase to compensate for the wasted ventilation and maintain a normal $PaCO_2$. For the clinician caring for the patient with respiratory failure, having knowledge of a patient's dead space provides important information about the $\dot{V}_E$ that is required to maintain a normal $PaCO_2$ and therefore whether the patient is a candidate for weaning from mechanical ventilatory support. $\dot{V}_E$ is the sum of $\dot{V}_A$ and $\dot{V}_D$, as shown in Equation 6:

$$\dot{V}_E = \dot{V}_A + \dot{V}_D \qquad (6)$$

Dead space is composed of anatomic dead space, alveolar dead space, and dead space imposed by equipment used to maintain the airway and ensure ventilation. The anatomic dead space is the volume of gas within the conducting airways; in a normal, 70-kg man, it averages about 156 mL (about 1 mL/lb).[176] The volume of the anatomic dead space increases with increases in lung volume and decreases in the supine position.[177-180] Intubation of the airway with an ETT decreases the anatomic dead space by about 50% because of the elimination of the extrathoracic airway (the nose and mouth, which do not contribute to gas exchange).[179,181] Depending on the intraluminal volume of the ETT and any additional apparatus dead space, the actual reduction of the anatomic dead space that occurs after endotracheal intubation may be inconsequential. Alveolar dead space is defined as the amount of gas that penetrates to the alveolar level but does not participate in gas exchange. In healthy individuals, this volume is minimal; however, alveolar dead space is increased in patients with $\dot{V}/\dot{Q}$ inequalities, such as those with pulmonary emboli or severe lung injury. The physiologic dead space is the sum of the anatomic and alveolar dead spaces and is represented by the total volume of gas in each breath that does not participate in gas exchange.

The portion of each breath that is dead space can be determined by calculating the ratio of dead space volume to tidal volume (V_D/V_T). The V_D/V_T is a useful clinical monitor of the overall work of breathing. It can be estimated using the Bohr equation:

$$V_D/V_T = PaCO_2 - PeCO_2/PaCO_2 - PiCO_2 \qquad (7)$$

where
$PaCO_2$ = alveolar carbon dioxide tension
$PeCO_2$ = carbon dioxide tension in mixed expired gas
$PiCO_2$ = inspired carbon dioxide tension

The V_D/V_T can be estimated more easily by assuming that $PiCO_2$ is zero and estimating alveolar CO_2 as arterial CO_2. This simplified formula represents the Enghoff modification of the Bohr equation[70,72,181]:

$$V_D/V_T = PaCO_2 - PeCO_2/PaCO_2 \qquad (8)$$

The normal V_D/V_T is 0.3 at rest; it decreases during exercise, primarily as a result of an increase in V_T, a more efficient way to increase alveolar ventilation with increasing O_2 consumption and CO_2 production.[179,181] Patients with severe respiratory failure may have a V_D/V_T value as high as 0.75, even with an ETT in place. In this situation, the patient's work of breathing is so high that discontinuation of some level of ventilatory support is not possible,[182] although modes of ventilation that increase V_T without an accompanying increase in work of breathing, such as pressure support ventilation, may facilitate spontaneous ventilatory work.

From a measurement of $PeCO_2$ and $PaCO_2$, the V_D/V_T can be calculated. $PeCO_2$ can be measured by collecting expired gas in a large-volume reservoir (e.g., Douglas bag, meteorologic balloon) for 3 to 5 minutes (depending on the $\dot{V}_E$) and measuring the CO_2 tension of a sample of this gas.[181,183] $PaCO_2$ is measured from blood gas obtained simultaneously during the collection of the expired gas.

Some technical factors must be taken into account when measuring V_D/V_T in mechanically ventilated patients. A correction must be made for gas compression within the ventilator, connecting tubing, and any additional dead space from the apparatus.[184] If the compression volume is ignored, the true physiologic dead space is underestimated by as much as 16%. Newer ventilators adjust the V_T to take into account the compression volume of the ventilator circuit. Several ventilator parameters can influence the accuracy of the measurement of V_D. For example, physiologic dead space was found to increase markedly when the duration of inspiration during mechanical ventilation was decreased from 1 to 0.5 second in paralyzed patients.[185] A nomogram of the relationship between $\dot{V}_E$, V_D/V_T, and $PaCO_2$ in mechanically ventilated patients was developed to aid in the titration of ventilatory support, assess the response to medical therapy, and increase the precision of the therapeutic management of critically ill patients.[186]

A simpler method for estimating V_D/V_T has been described. Measurement of the carbon dioxide pressure (PCO_2) in the condensate of expired gas in the collection bottle from the expiratory limb of the mechanical ventilator is equivalent to the cumbersome technique of collecting the mixed expired gas.[183] This PCO_2 value can be substituted for $PeCO_2$, greatly simplifying the measurement of physiologic dead space in mechanically ventilated patients.

Another approach to the noninvasive assessment of the physiologic V_D/V_T ratio substitutes $PetCO_2$ for $PaCO_2$. For normal subjects, the relationship between $PetCO_2$ and $PaCO_2$ is well established.[187,188] At rest, $PetCO_2$ underestimates $PaCO_2$ by 2 to 3 mm Hg. However, with exercise, $PetCO_2$ can overestimate $PaCO_2$. The difference between $PetCO_2$ and $PaCO_2$ varies directly with V_T and cardiac output and inversely with respiratory rate.

For patients undergoing general anesthesia or with respiratory failure, the gradient between arterial and end-tidal CO_2 ($P[a - et]CO_2$) increases.[179,189] This increase reflects more ventilation to lung units with high $\dot{V}/\dot{Q}$ relationships. For patients with normal pulmonary function who are mechanically ventilated during general anesthesia, the $P[a - et]CO_2$ averages 5 mm Hg; the $P[a - et]CO_2$ can be as high as 15 mm Hg in the supine position. The average P[a – ET]CO$_2$ increases to 8 mm Hg when these patients are placed in the lateral decubitus position.[190] In patients with respiratory failure, the P[a – ET]CO$_2$ can be even greater. In patients with respiratory failure, there is a close correlation between P[a – ET]CO$_2$ and V$_D$/V$_T$.[189] The P[a – ET]CO$_2$ can therefore be used as an indicator of the efficiency of ventilation.

In patients with acute lung injury, an increase in V$_D$/V$_T$ correlates with increased mortality and with a decrease in ventilator free days. As a result, the V$_D$/V$_T$ can be used as a marker of severity of disease.[191,192] Frankenfield and colleagues[193] developed and validated an equation that uses clinically available data to estimate V/V$_T$: V$_D$/V$_T$ = 0.32 + 0.0106 (PaCO$_2$ – EtCO$_2$) + 0.003 (respiratory rate) + 0.0015 (age in years). The equation was constructed from data obtained from 135 patients and validated on an additional 50 patients (R^2 = 0.67). Volumetric capnography, also called the single-breath test for CO$_2$, can be used to estimate physiologic dead space.[189] Volumetric capnography enlists a plot of the expired CO$_2$ against the exhaled volume of a single breath. Volumetric capnography in combination with D-dimer testing has been used in the ED to help evaluate patients with suspected pulmonary emboli and to select the optimal level of PEEP in anesthetized, morbidly obese patients.[194,195]

1. Airway Resistance and Lung-Thorax Compliance

In the intubated, ventilated patient, airway resistance and lung-thorax compliance can be differentiated by evaluating peak and plateau pressures and by the difference between them (Fig. 49-7). The peak airway pressure generated by the ventilator reflects the pressure necessary to overcome airway resistance and compliance of the lung and chest wall. The peak pressure is elevated when airway resistance is increased, as may occur with increased pulmonary secretions or a kinked ETT or when lung-thorax compliance is reduced.[196] The peak pressure is influenced by other factors, including ventilator parameters, such as inspiratory flow rate and pattern, V$_T$, and the ETT size. The ratio of the V$_T$ delivered divided by the pressure change, the difference between the peak inspiratory pressure and PEEP, is the dynamic compliance. Dynamic

compliance is reduced when airway resistance is increased or lung-thorax compliance is reduced.

To differentiate the cause for reduced dynamic compliance and increased peak airway pressure, the static compliance must be calculated. Static compliance can be assessed by determining the plateau pressure, the pressure achieved in the airways when the lung is inflated to a specific V$_T$ under conditions of zero gas flow. Static compliance is measured when inspiration is complete and the lung remains inflated with no further gas flow. Most mechanical ventilators have the capability to provide an inspiratory pause (hold) that allows measurement of the plateau pressure. The pressure generated in the lung during the inspiratory pause is the pressure required to overcome lung and chest wall compliance. Because there is no gas flow at the time of measurement, airway resistance does not contribute to the measured pressure. The static compliance can be estimated by dividing the V$_T$ by the difference between the plateau pressure and PEEP. The normal static compliance measured using this method is 60 to 100 mL/cm H$_2$O. The static compliance is reduced in patients with an extensive pulmonary infiltrate, pulmonary edema, atelectasis, endobronchial intubation, pneumothorax, or any decrease in chest wall compliance, as may occur with chest wall edema or subcutaneous emphysema.

2. Intrinsic Positive End-Expiratory Pressure

Hyperinflation (overdistention) of the lung occurs in some mechanically ventilated patients because of air trapping. Gas can be trapped within the lung during the expiratory phase because of dynamic airflow limitation (e.g., associated with asthma) or inadequate expiratory time, as may occur when the inspiratory flow is so low that it causes a high inspiratory-to-expiratory (I:E) ratio. The hyperinflation that results has been called auto-PEEP, intrinsic PEEP (PEEPi), or occult PEEP.[26,197] The presence of auto-PEEP increases the risk of barotrauma, compromises hemodynamics by reducing venous return, increases the patient's work of breathing, and can result in unilateral lung hyperinflation.[26,184,197]

Identification of PEEPi is difficult. PEEPi is not reflected in the pressure measured on the manometer of the ventilator at the end of exhalation, because at end expiration, the exhalation valve is open to atmospheric pressure (PEEP = 0 cm H$_2$O) or reflects the level of PEEP provided by the ventilator (Fig. 49-8). PEEPi can be quantitated by occluding the expiratory port of the ventilator circuit at the end of exhalation immediately before the next breath is delivered. The pressure in the lungs and ventilator circuit equilibrates. The level of PEEPi is then displayed on the manometer. Although this approach provides an estimate of the magnitude of gas trapping, it is technically difficult and hard to reproduce. Another method to determine whether PEEPi is present, but not to quantitate it, uses evaluation of the expiratory flow waveform. If expiratory flow does not fall to zero before the next inspiration, gas is trapped within the lung, creating PEEPi (Fig. 49-9). When PEEPi is identified using this method, the flow waveform can be monitored while adjusting ventilator parameters to minimize PEEPi.

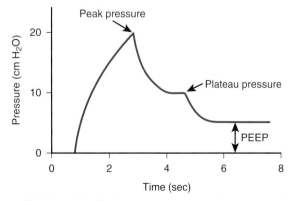

Figure 49-7 Graphic display of airway pressure in a mechanically ventilated patient. Peak inspiratory pressure is achieved during gas flow into lung. Plateau pressure is achieved by temporary occlusion of expiratory tubing. From these pressures, dynamic and static compliance can be calculated. *PEEP,* Positive end-expiratory pressure.

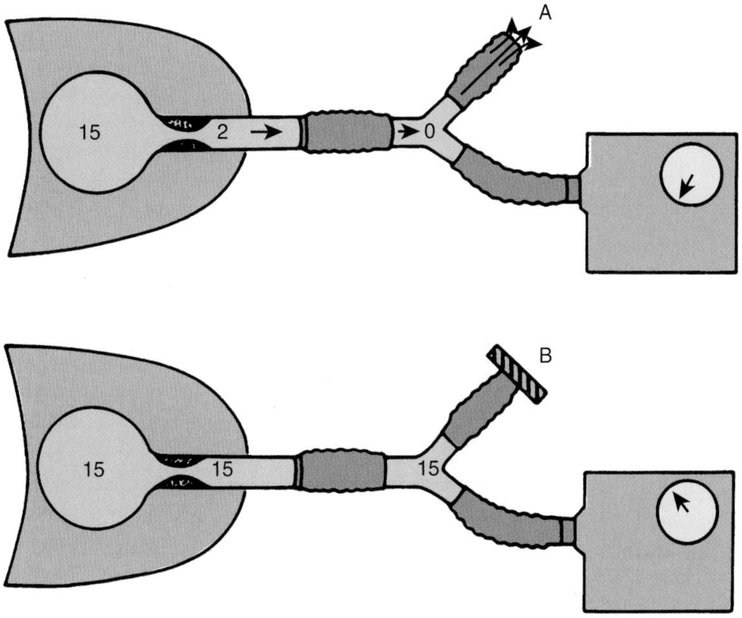

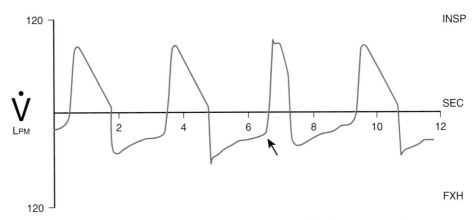

Figure 49-8 *A,* Auto–positive end-expiratory pressure (PEEP) is detected by occlusion of the end-expiratory port just before initiation of the next ventilator inflation cycle. *B, The* ventilator's manometer measures alveolar pressure (auto-PEEP) only when pressures are allowed to equilibrate by occlusion of the expiratory port and end exhalation. (From Pepe PE, Marini JJ: Occult positive end-expiratory pressure in mechanically ventilated patients with airflow obstruction: The auto-PEEP effect. *Am Rev Respir Dis* 126:166–170, 1982.)

3. Ventilatory Waveform Analysis

Ventilatory waveform analysis is a useful method to assess airway patency, pulmonary function, and the patient-ventilator interface. Most critical care ventilators have a variety of waveform monitoring capabilities; for applications in which the ventilators do not have integrated waveform monitoring capability, separate monitors are available to assess waveform, work of breathing, capnography, and other useful monitoring parameters, such as O_2 consumption, CO_2 production, and calculated energy expenditure. Although all of these measures help in the care of critically ill patients, the waveforms are particularly useful in assessing the patient's air movement, identifying the presence of gas trapping, and for many patients, providing critically important information about the adequacy of the ventilatory parameters used to optimize gas exchange. Evaluating the flow-time and pressure-time curves can provide information about whether the patient is able to trigger the ventilator to initiate spontaneously supported breaths (e.g., pressure

support) and to determine whether the peak inspiratory flow and flow pattern are adequate to meet the patient's needs.[198-200] When the patient appears agitated or dyssynchronous with the ventilator, the waveforms can be useful in giving direct feedback about whether the problem is related to inappropriately low inspiratory flow or other ventilator-dependent parameters or inadequate analgesia or sedation.[201-203]

In many cases, modifications to the ventilator can improve the clinical situation and minimize the need for excessive sedation. In addition to displaying inspiratory and expiratory flow patterns, the ventilator displays pressure-volume and flow-volume loops, both of which can be useful in assessing whether the peak inspiratory flow is too high or too low or the V_T is too high, putting the patient at risk for pulmonary volutrauma.[204] For patients with adult respiratory distress syndrome, in whom we recognize the deleterious effects of high V_T and high airway pressures, analysis of the waveforms can help in adjusting ventilator parameters to optimize gas exchange without increasing the risk of lung

Figure 49-9 Flow-time curve demonstrates expiratory flow continuing until initiation of inspiration *(arrow).* In a normal patient, expiratory flow falls to zero, indicating complete emptying to functional residual capacity. Continued expiratory flow indicates gas trapping.

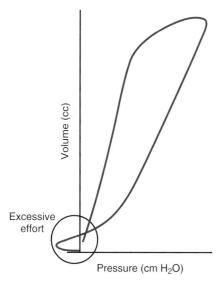

Figure 49-10 Pressure-volume curve identifies excessive effort by the patient to initiate a patient-triggered breath. Excessive effort is required to initiate a breath for assist-control ventilation or pressure-support ventilation. (From Novametrix Medical Systems: *Bedside respiratory mechanics monitoring*, Wallingford, CT, 1998, Novametrix Medical Systems.)

disruption.[205] Figure 49-10 illustrates waveforms that identify excessive work of breathing during patient-initiated breaths. While monitoring the waveforms, adjustments can be made in ventilator parameters to optimize flow patterns and minimize airway pressures, PEEPi, and work of breathing.

4. Work of Breathing

The work of breathing is another important monitor of a patient's respiratory status, respiratory reserve, and likelihood of being successfully weaned from mechanical ventilatory support. The patient's work of breathing (WOBp) can be assessed by clinical evaluation at the bedside or calculated using data obtained from an esophageal balloon and flow transducer at the airway.[177,206] The clinical evaluation of WOBp, although useful, can be misleading. Some patients who appear to have excessive WOBp indicate that they are comfortable. Others with a low $\dot{V}_E$ and slow respiratory rate are already working maximally, and although they appear comfortable at the current level of ventilatory support, they cannot tolerate any further increase in their WOBp.

To better assess the WOBp and monitor the patient's efforts more closely while adjusting the level of ventilatory support, the WOBp can be measured directly using bedside monitors. The monitors require placement of an esophageal balloon to measure esophageal pressure as an estimate of intrapleural pressure. The WOBp is calculated by integrating the area under the pressure-volume loop. With an understanding of each of the components of WOBp, flow-resistive, elastic, and apparatus-induced modifications can be made in ventilator parameters to minimize the patient's WOBp. This monitoring technique has been recommended as a way to adjust pressure support ventilation to optimize gas exchange while minimizing WOBp. Although the additional information about the patient-ventilator interface has resulted in

modifications of methods of ventilating critically ill patients, no studies have documented which parameters are most useful to monitor and which modifications to ventilator management result in the best outcomes.

B. Assessment of Pulmonary Function During Weaning

Several measures of pulmonary mechanical function are used to evaluate the likelihood of weaning success in the mechanically ventilated ICU patient.[182] Vital capacity (VC) and maximum inspiratory pressure (MIP or Pimax) are commonly employed to evaluate pulmonary mechanical function. A VC of 10 mL/kg and Pimax more negative than −20 cm H_2O have been useful predictors of weaning success for some patients. Other measures of mechanical function that have been used to predict weaning success include maximum voluntary ventilation (MVV) greater than two times the resting level and $\dot{V}_E$ less than 10 L/min. A V_D/V_T greater than 0.6 has predicted weaning failure consistently. Unfortunately, although each of these parameters can be used to assess pulmonary mechanical function, several studies have demonstrated that none predicts weaning success.

Other monitoring techniques have been employed to predict weaning success, including continuous measurement of O_2 consumption.[207] Although many studies have attempted to define key factors in predicting weaning success, changes in mechanical ventilatory capabilities and our understanding of the risks and benefits of mechanical ventilatory support have had a major impact on methods for assessment and monitoring of patients. The use of pressure support ventilation and noninvasive modes of ventilatory support have made interpretation of the studies and recommendations difficult. One of the key components in the decision-making process about weaning and discontinuation of mechanical ventilatory support is related to the patient's ability to protect the airway and the need for intensive respiratory care rather than specific respiratory mechanical parameters. Many patients previously thought to be unweanable can be weaned from mandatory ventilatory support and provided with ventilatory assistance using pressure-support ventilation through an ETT or using noninvasive ventilation, BiPAP by mask, or mask CPAP. The traditional methods for assessing weaning may no longer apply. Nonetheless, an understanding of the various methods that have been used to assess weaning potential is critical to defining the most effective way to have a patient make the transition from positive-pressure ventilation to spontaneous ventilation.

1. Weaning Indices

Several indices have been developed to predict when a patient can be successfully weaned from mechanical ventilatory support. These indices combine multiple individual parameters to predict weaning success; some incorporate indices of gas exchange. One study evaluated multiparameter indices, including the rapid shallow breathing (RSB) index, the ratio of respiratory frequency divided by V_T in liters, and the CROP index (i.e., thoracic *c*ompliance, *r*espiratory rate, arterial *o*xygenation, Pimax), which incorporates measures of dynamic lung compliance, respiratory rate, gas exchange, and inspiratory pressure.[208] An RSB index of less than 105 was shown to have a high predictive value for weaning success, whereas the CROP index and more traditional indices had poor predictive values. A study could not confirm these findings and demonstrated that an RSB index of less than 105 did not predict failed weaning.[209]

2. Breathing Pattern Analysis

Respiratory impedance plethysmography (RIP) can be used to assess the breathing pattern by measuring V_T, respiratory frequency, inspiratory time, and the contribution of the rib cage and abdomen to lung volume changes.[37,38] Using RIP, the relationship between rib cage and abdominal contributions to V_T (i.e., respiratory muscle dyssynchrony) has been quantitated. RIP is useful for evaluating changes in functional residual capacity and level of PEEPi as ventilator parameters are adjusted. As a method for predicting weaning success, the technique has had variable success.

3. Airway Occlusion Pressure

The airway occlusion pressure has been used as an index of respiratory drive, although it is rarely used as a routine monitor of ventilatory drive. Airway occlusion pressure is the pressure generated 0.1 second ($P_{0.1}$) after initiating an inspiratory effort against an occluded airway. The $P_{0.1}$ in normal subjects usually is less than 2 cm H_2O. Some studies suggest that a $P_{0.1}$ value greater than 6 cm H_2O is incompatible with successful weaning for patients with COPD.[210] Few studies have confirmed the value of airway occlusion pressure as a predictor of successful weaning success,[211,212] and its clinical utility remains unclear.

V. CONCLUSIONS

Several methods are available to monitor the airway and pulmonary function in the patient who requires endotracheal intubation and mechanical ventilatory support. Monitoring techniques include clinical assessment, monitors of gas exchange, and a variety of methods to evaluate pulmonary mechanical function. Selection of the most appropriate monitors for each patient depends on an understanding of the clinical situation, the available monitoring techniques, the information each monitor provides, and the limitations of the monitors. The challenge for the physician is to identify and appropriately use techniques that optimize clinical management and reduce morbidity and mortality, rather than using any monitor simply because it is available.

VI. CLINICAL PEARLS

- The most reliable method for determining the intratracheal location of an artificial airway is direct visualization of the device passing through the vocal cords; fiberoptic assessment can define the specific location of the endotracheal tube in the airways.

- When using CO_2 detection in exhaled gas from an artificial airway to document whether the endotracheal tube is within the trachea, CO_2 should be present for four or five breaths.

- Respiratory dyssynchrony (i.e., abdominal expansion during inspiration without chest excursions) in a patient without upper airway obstruction is an early and critical indicator of respiratory muscle fatigue and impending respiratory failure.

- The accuracy of pulse oximetry is altered by several factors, including external light sources, motion, poor perfusion, and dyshemoglobinemias.

- Analysis of the plethysmographic waveform from a pulse oximeter has clinical utility in the hemodynamic assessment of patients and evaluation of intravascular volume status.

- In patients with traumatic brain injury, adjustment of ventilatory parameters based on end-tidal CO_2 values may be unreliable.

- V_D/V_T can be used as a marker of disease severity in patients with acute lung injury.

SELECTED REFERENCES

All references can be found online at expertconsult.com.
1. Tobin MJ: Respiratory monitoring. *JAMA* 264:244–251, 1990.
4. deWit M: Monitoring of patient-ventilator interaction at the bedside. *Respir Care* 56:61–72, 2011.
24. Salem MR: Verification of endotracheal tube position. *Anesthesiol Clin North Am* 19:813–839, 2001.
56. Schnapp LM, Cohen NH: Pulse oximetry: Uses and abuses. *Chest* 98:1244–1250, 1990.
166. Szaflarski NL, Cohen NH: Use of capnography in critically ill adults. *Heart Lung* 20:363–372, 1991.
181. Nunn JF: *Nunn's applied respiratory physiology*, Oxford, UK, 1993, Butterworth-Heinemann.
193. Frankenfield DC, Alam S, Bekteshi E, et al: Predicting dead space ventilation in critically ill patients using clinically available data. *Crit Care Med* 38:288–291, 2010.
199. Hess DR: Ventilator waveforms and the physiology of pressure support ventilation. *Respir Care* 50:166–186, 2005.
200. Fernandez-Perez ER, Hubmayr RD: Interpretation of airway pressure waveforms. *Intensive Care Med* 32:658–659, 2006.
203. Nilsestuen O, Hargett KD: Using ventilator graphics to identify patient-ventilator asynchrony. *Respir Care* 50:202–234, 2005.

Chapter 50

Extubation and Reintubation of the Difficult Airway

RICHARD M. COOPER | SOFIA KHAN

I. INTRODUCTION

Tracheal extubation has received relatively limited critical scrutiny compared with that accorded to intubation. Textbooks, reviews, and conferences focusing on the airway frequently ignore this aspect of management, despite the observation that airway complications are significantly more likely to be associated with extubation than intubation.[1] These complications range from the relatively minor, such as coughing and transient breath holding that have little impact on outcome, to those that are life-threatening. The American Society of Anesthesiologists (ASA) Closed Claims Project analyzed adverse respiratory events and found that 17% of brain injuries and deaths occurred after extubation in the operating room or postanesthesia care unit (PACU).[2] Complications associated with extubation in critical care areas are likely to occur more frequently and have more serious consequences.[3,4]

The ASA Task Force on Management of the Difficult Airway and the Canadian Airway Focus Group recommended a preformulated strategy for extubation of the difficult airway and an airway management plan for dealing with post-extubation hypoventilation.[5,6] This chapter classifies the complications associated with routine and more complex tracheal extubation or reintubation, proposes a risk stratification for extubation and reintubation in various clinical settings, and suggests strategies that may prove helpful in reducing serious complications or death.

Low-risk or routine extubations have been reviewed elsewhere and are not the focus of this chapter. Although they are dealt with only briefly, concerns include the adequacy of recovery from neuromuscular blockade, depressant effects of narcotics and residual volatile or intravenous sedatives, level of consciousness, hemodynamic stability, adequate ventilation and oxygenation, normothermia, freedom from noxious stimulation, and airway patency.[7-10] The controversy about deep versus awake extubation has been addressed elsewhere,[10-12] and most of the present discussion concentrates on extubation of more challenging airways and strategies that may increase the probability of success.

II. EXTUBATION FAILURES AND CHALLENGES

Extubation fails when an attempt to remove a tracheal tube is unsuccessful. Reintubation failure occurs when extubation is followed by an immediate or delayed but unsuccessful attempt to reintubate the trachea. There is no agreement about how to define failure, and because there is no consensus about the time frame, reported incidences may vary. It is reasonable to consider the failed extubation in two separate clinical settings: the intensive care unit (ICU), where such failures are relatively common, and the operating room or PACU, where they are far less common.

In the ICU, the ability to predict readiness for extubation is imprecise despite a host of predictive criteria.[13-16] To minimize the risks, discomfort, and expense of prolonged intubation, a trial of extubation is occasionally attempted, but it may be followed sometime thereafter by a need to reintubate. The incidence of required reintubation ranges from 6% to 20%, and it depends on the clinical mix of patients,[15,17,18] their critical acuity, critical care resources, and the threshold levels for extubation. Even if reintubation is successful, patients who failed their initial extubation had increased rates of ICU mortality and cost of care, prolonged ICU stay, and hospital length of stay.[19] Compared with routine postoperative patients, intensive care patients are more likely to fail extubation because neurologic obtundation may leave them unable to protect their airways. Debilitation and impaired mucociliary clearance may interfere with pulmonary toilet, and diminished strength, altered pulmonary mechanics, increased dead space, and venous admixture may result in hypercapnic or hypoxemic respiratory failure.

Although the complications associated with extubation of postoperative patients may be more common than those associated with intubation, they rarely require reintubation. Studies involving a wide case mix of postoperative patients show a high degree of concordance regarding the incidence of required reintubation. Combining the results of four large studies enrolling more than 150,000 patients, the incidence ranged from 0.09% to 0.19%.[20-23] The reintubation rate appears to be significantly higher (1% to 3%) after selected surgical procedures such as panendoscopy[20] and a variety of head and neck procedures.[24-28]

Postoperative reintubation, although uncommon, may offer some unexpected challenges, including anatomic distortion, physiologic instability, incomplete information concerning the patient, lack of essential equipment and time, and inexperienced personnel. These problems may convert a previously easily managed airway into a life-threatening disaster. A difficult airway adequately managed during a controlled intubation is completely different from the difficult airway in an agitated, hypoxemic, and hypotensive patient.

III. EXTUBATION RISK STRATIFICATION

Risks related to extubation fall into two broad categories: the risk of extubation failing and the risk of reintubation failing. Within each category, there is a continuum from low to high risk. Like the prediction of a difficult intubation, this is an inexact science; it is probably safest to err on the cautious side. Most extubations are expected and turn out to be uneventful, but even these routine extubations may be associated with complications (Box 50-1).

The causes of a failed extubation can be classified as a failure of oxygenation, failure of ventilation, inadequate clearance of pulmonary secretions, or loss of airway patency. We cannot always predict which patients will require reintubation, and if reintubation is likely to be difficult, it is prudent to employ strategies expected to maximize the likelihood of success. In this discussion, if reintubation is expected to be difficult, we regard such extubations as intermediate- or high-risk extubations, although such designations are based on probability and clinical judgment.

BOX 50-1 **Complications of Routine Extubations**

- Unintended extubation
- Fixation of endotracheal tube
- Hypertension, tachycardia
- Coughing, breath-holding
- Laryngeal injury
- Laryngospasm or vocal cord paralysis
- Stridor, airway obstruction
- Negative pressure pulmonary edema
- Laryngeal incompetence
- Aspiration

A. Routine Extubations

A retrospective database review from The University of Michigan analyzed 107,317 general anesthetics administered between 1994 and 1999.[23] It identified 191 required reintubations in the operating room or PACU, 112 (58.6%) of which were for respiratory reasons. The most common respiratory causes were hypercapnic or hypoxemic respiratory insufficiency (60%), respiratory obstruction (20.5%), and laryngospasm or bronchospasm (19.5%). Failed extubations from a respiratory cause occurred at a rate of 112/107,301 or 0.1%. Unintended extubation accounted for 25 of 191 reintubations, all of which occurred in the operating room. Surgical complications, including neck hematoma, pneumothorax, laryngeal nerve paralysis, and bleeding, accounted for 16 of 191 reintubations. Contrary to their expectations, the investigators found that excessive narcotics (9 cases) and prolonged neuromuscular blockade with pancuronium (2 cases) were responsible for only 11 of 191 reintubations. This self-reported information was retrospective, and sometimes required interpretation of the causes from the therapies applied (e.g., narcotic antagonists, additional doses of anticholinergics).

A prospective study from Thailand found a rate of reintubation occurring within 24 hours of 27 per 10,000 patients.[29] This was twice the rate observed in the University of Michigan study.[23] The precipitating factor in the Thai study was thought to be residual neuromuscular weakness in almost three quarters of cases requiring reintubation in the operating room or PACU. In a Taiwanese database that surveyed almost 138,000 patients undergoing general anesthesia between 2005 and 2007, 83 reintubations were performed after intended extubation.[30] Overall, this represented a rate of 6 reintubations per 10,000 patients. Comparing these patients with a matched cohort not requiring reintubation, the investigators identified the following factors as most predictive of a need for reintubation: chronic obstructive pulmonary disease (odds ratio [OR] = 7.17; 95% confidence interval [CI], 1.98 to 26.00), pneumonia (OR = 7.94; 95% CI, 1.03 to 32.78), ascites (OR = 13.86; 95% CI, 1.08 to 174.74), and systemic inflammatory response syndrome (OR = 11.90; 95% CI, 2.63 to 53.86).

1. Hypoventilation Syndromes

The ASA Closed Claims Project found that 4% of 1175 closed claims resulted from critical respiratory events in the PACU. The highest proportion was attributed to inadequate ventilation, and many of these patients died or suffered brain damage.[31]

Many clinical conditions may give rise to postoperative ventilatory failure. A multicenter, prospective survey in France that looked at almost 200,000 general anesthetics administered between 1978 and 1982 found that postoperative respiratory depression accounted for 27 of 85 respiratory complications that were life-threatening or had serious sequelae. These complications were responsible for seven deaths and five cases of hypoxic encephalopathy.[32] A respiratory rate of less than 8 breaths/min was observed by PACU nurses among 0.2% of 24,000 patients after general anesthesia.[22]

Hypoventilation may be mediated centrally at the level of the upper motor neuron, anterior horn cell, lower motor neuron, neuromuscular junction, or respiratory muscles. Clinical correlates include central sleep apnea, carotid endarterectomy,[33] medullary injuries, demyelinating disorders, direct injury to peripheral nerves, poliomyelitis, Guillain-Barré syndrome, motor neuron disease, myasthenia gravis, and botulism. Hypoventilation may result from the loss of lung or pleural elasticity, diaphragmatic splinting caused by abdominal pain or distention, thoracic deformities such as kyphoscoliosis, or multifactorial entities such as morbid obesity and severe chronic obstructive pulmonary disease. Rarely, hypercapnia results from excess carbon dioxide production or a marked increase in physiologic dead space.

The residual effects of anesthetic drugs contribute to inadequate postoperative ventilation.[34-36] It may be aggravated by incomplete reversal of neuromuscular blockers,[37] hypocalcemia or hypermagnesemia, or the administration of other drugs, including antibiotics, local anesthetics, diuretics, and calcium channel blockers, which may potentiate neuromuscular blockade.

2. Hypoxemic Respiratory Failure

A review of the many causes of postoperative hypoxemia is beyond the scope of this chapter, but it can occur because of hypoventilation, a low inspired oxygen concentration, ventilation-perfusion mismatch, right-to-left shunting, increased oxygen consumption, diminished oxygen transport, or rarely, an impairment of oxygen diffusion. These events are more likely in some clinical situations because of preexisting medical conditions or anesthetic and surgical interventions. If sufficiently severe, there may be a requirement for continuous positive airway pressure (CPAP) or reintubation and mechanical ventilation.

3. Inability to Protect the Airway

ICU or postoperative patients may be unable to protect the airway because of preexisting obtundation, neurologic injury, or the effects of residual anesthesia. In the latter case, it may be possible to temporize by turning patients on their sides, altering their positions (head up or head down) or by reversing residual medications with antagonists. These measures may not restore airway competency, and lack of resolution may necessitate reintubation.

4. Failure of Pulmonary Toilet

Inadequate clearance of pulmonary secretions may result from a depressed level of consciousness with impaired airway reflexes, overproduction of secretions, alteration of sputum consistency leading to inspissation and plugging, impaired mucociliary clearance, or inadequate neuromuscular reserve. These problems may result in atelectasis or pneumonia with attendant hypoxemic respiratory failure. Alterations in pulmonary mechanics may also lead to hypercapnia, necessitating reintubation.

5. Inadvertent Extubations

Inadvertent extubations may result from movement of or by the patient with an inadequately secured tracheal tube. Intraoperatively, this may occur in the prone position, when the airway is shared with the surgeon, when the head and neck are extended, when draping obscures the view, or when drapes adhere to the endotracheal tube (ETT) or circuit and are carelessly removed. In the ICU, extubation may occur when the patient is repositioned for a radiograph or routine nursing care. Patients insufficiently sedated are at greater risk for deliberate self-extubation,[38] but those more heavily sedated are more likely to require reintubation.[39] Fastidious attention to securing and supporting the ETT and breathing circuit is essential. Self-extubation may occur during emergence from anesthesia, when the patient is confused, agitated, and distressed, which promotes premature extubation. In the ICU, it may not be possible to know whether a self-extubation is accidental or deliberate, but many of these patients require reintubation,[40] are more likely to exhibit post-extubation stridor, and may need multiple intubation attempts, increasing the likelihood of esophageal intubation and death.[41-43]

6. Entrapment

The tracheal tube may become entrapped due to an inability to deflate the cuff,[44,45] or there may be difficulties with the pilot tube.[46,47] Difficulties include a crimped pilot tube, a defective pilot valve, and fixation of the tracheal tube by Kirschner wires,[48] screws,[49] ligatures,[50] or entanglement with other devices.[51,52] Entrapment can also occur during a percutaneous tracheostomy.[53] Mechanical obstruction of an entrapped tube is a life-threatening complication. Partial transection of the tracheal tube by an osteotome during a maxillary osteotomy has resulted in the partially cut tube forming a barb that caught on the posterior aspect of the hard palate.[54] One report of tube entrapment with fatal consequences involved a Carlens tube that was inadvertently sutured to the pulmonary artery.[55] Lang and colleagues recommended routine intraoperative testing for tracheal tube movement when fixation devices are used in proximity to the airway.[49] Uncertainty about tube movement should prompt fiberoptic examination before emergence from general anesthesia.

7. Hypertension and Tachycardia

Transient hemodynamic disturbances accompany extubation in most adults. These responses may be prevented by deep extubation,[56] insertion of a laryngeal mask airway (LMA) before emergence, or attenuated by concurrent medication.[57-59] Most healthy patients not on antihypertensive agents or other cardioactive drugs exhibit increases in heart rate and systolic blood pressure of more than 20% in association with extubation.[60] After coronary artery bypass surgery, these changes tend to be transient, lasting 5 to 10 minutes, and they usually are not associated with electrocardiographic evidence of myocardial ischemia.[61] Coronary sinus lactate extraction measurements, however, indicate that among patients with poor cardiac function, extubation may be associated with myocardial ischemia.[62] Patients with inadequately controlled hypertension, carcinoid, pheochromocytoma, hypertension associated with pregnancy, or hyperthyroidism may be expected to display even greater increases in blood pressure in response to tracheal extubation. The specific strategies needed to attenuate these usually transient changes are dictated by the clinical context. The strategies, which are not universally effective, include the use of intracuff,[63-65] intratracheal,[66] or intravenous lidocaine[61,67,68]; beta-blockers[60,69-71]; dexmedetomidine[72,73]; and nitrates.

8. Intracranial Hypertension

Tracheal intubation and suctioning are associated with a rise in intracranial pressure. Extubation probably is associated with comparable or even greater increases in intracranial pressure. There is evidence, albeit contradictory, that intravenous and endotracheal lidocaine attenuate this effect.[74,75]

9. Intraocular Pressure

Madan and colleagues compared the intraocular pressure changes of tracheal intubation and extubation in children with and without glaucoma.[76] They observed significantly greater increases 30 seconds and 2 minutes after deep extubation compared with the corresponding times after uncomplicated intubations. These differences were seen in both groups of children. It is likely that significant increases in intraocular pressure observed after deep extubation would have been even higher had extubation occurred after recovery of consciousness. Lamb and coworkers observed similar effects of extubation on intraocular pressure in adults and commented that this increase could be prevented by using an LMA rather than a tracheal tube.[77]

10. Coughing

Coughing on emergence from general anesthesia is virtually ubiquitous, particularly when an ETT is used.[78] No difference between smokers and nonsmokers is observed. Although coughing is a protective reflex, it can be particularly troublesome in the setting of ophthalmologic, neurologic, oropharyngeal, and neck surgery.

Several strategies have been proposed to minimize coughing, including deep endotracheal extubation, primary use of or conversion to an LMA,[57,79,80] use of the sedative dexmedetomidine,[73] intravenous or topical application of a local anesthetic to the vocal folds, and use of intracuff lidocaine.[63,65,67,81] However, coughing on emergence is common and relatively benign for most patients.

The emergence of severe acute respiratory syndrome (SARS) and the high prevalence of drug-resistant droplet or airborne diseases in some locales make coughing potentially hazardous to the airway manager. In 2003, Toronto was the North American epicenter for SARS, and coughing assumed life-threatening proportions for medical personnel.[82-87] Patients with cough, fever, and pulmonary infiltrates were dangerous, and coughing on emergence was not protective, but rather posed a threat by dispersing infectious respiratory droplets on those in the patient's vicinity. The strategies adopted at that time have been largely relaxed, although they may again become necessary when new risks threaten patients and care providers.

11. Laryngeal Edema

Several of the complications of endotracheal intubation do not become apparent until after extubation occurs.[88] Glottic or tracheal injury may occur despite a good laryngeal view or during awake fiberoptic intubation.[89-91] Anatomic or functional laryngeal problems are more likely to develop as a consequence of a difficult or prolonged intubation attempts.[22] Possible airway injuries include laryngeal edema, laceration, hematoma, granuloma formation, vocal fold immobility, and dislocation of the arytenoid cartilages.[92]

Glottic edema has been classified as supraglottic, retroarytenoidal, and subglottic.[93] Supraglottic edema may result in posterior displacement of the epiglottis, reducing the laryngeal inlet and causing inspiratory obstruction. Retroarytenoidal edema restricts movement of the arytenoid cartilages, limiting vocal cord abduction on inspiration. Subglottic edema, a particular problem in neonates and infants, results in swelling of the loose submucosal connective tissue that is confined by the non-expandable cricoid cartilage. In neonates and small children, this is the narrowest part of the upper airway, and small reductions in diameter result in a significant increase in airway resistance. In children, laryngeal edema is promoted by a tight-fitting ETT, traumatic intubation, intubation longer than 1 hour, coughing on the tracheal tube, and intraoperative alterations of head position.[94] Koka and coworkers found an incidence of 1% among children younger than 17 years. Laryngeal edema should be suspected when inspiratory stridor develops within 6 hours of extubation. Management of laryngeal edema depends on its severity. Treatment options include head-up positioning, supplemental humidified oxygen, racemic epinephrine, helium-oxygen administration, reintubation, and tracheostomy.

Clinical studies of children and adults that evaluated the role of prophylactic corticosteroids in the prevention of post-extubation stridor have yielded contradictory findings.[95-98] In the setting of adult ICUs, a large, multi-center, prospective, randomized, double-blind trial of methylprednisolone (20 mg administered 12 hours before and every 4 hours until extubation) versus placebo found that steroids significantly reduced post-extubation laryngeal edema (11 of 355 versus 76 of 343, $P < 0.0001$) and required reintubation due to laryngeal edema (8% versus 54%, $P = 0.005$). Laryngeal edema was defined by any two of stridor, inspiratory prolongation, and use of

accessory muscles. It was classified as severe if reintubation was required within 36 hours. Laryngoscopy was not performed unless reintubation was required. Factors associated with a greater risk of laryngeal edema included female sex, shorter height, larger-diameter ETT, admission for trauma, and shorter duration of intubation. The absence of pretreatment with methylprednisolone was associated with a hazard ratio of more than 8.[99] It is possible that the benefits of steroids are restricted to high-risk populations and require administration of multiple doses.[100, 101] Contradictory findings may relate to risk factors in the study populations and variability of dosage regimens.

An alternative classification has been proposed for laryngotracheal injury after prolonged intubation.[102-104] Immediate post-extubation airway obstruction results from glottic and subglottic granulation tissue, which may swell on removal of the ETT. Posterior glottic and subglottic stenosis due to contracting scar tissue results in increasing obstruction weeks or months after extubation. Benjamin found that fiberoptic evaluation or laryngoscopy with the tube in situ was of limited value.[102] An ETT obscures the view of the posterior glottis and subglottis. These lesions were best identified using rigid telescopes with image magnification during general anesthesia. This approach permitted anticipation of problems and development of a management strategy.

12. Laryngospasm

Laryngospasm is believed to be a common cause of post-extubation airway obstruction, particularly in children.[105] Even in adults, Rose and colleagues found that it accounted for 23.3% of critical postoperative respiratory events, although the diagnosis was presumptive.[106] Olsson and Hallen observed an increased incidence among patients presenting for emergency surgery, those requiring nasogastric tubes, and patients undergoing tonsillectomy, cervical dilation, hypospadias correction, oral endoscopy, or excision of skin lesions.[105] A variety of triggers are recognized, including vagal, trigeminal, auditory, phrenic, sciatic, and splanchnic nerve stimulation; cervical flexion or extension with an indwelling ETT; or vocal cord irritation from blood, vomitus, or oral secretions.[107] A risk assessment questionnaire was used in a study to prospectively evaluate almost 10,000 children undergoing general anesthesia. A positive history of nocturnal dry cough, exertional wheezing, or more than three wheezing episodes in the prior 12 months was associated with a fourfold increase in the risk of laryngospasm in the PACU and a 2.7-fold increased risk of airway obstruction during surgery or in the PACU.[108] Twice as many children were managed with an LMA than an ETT, and an equal number had their devices removed awake and asleep. The depth of anesthesia at the time of device removal did not influence the incidence of laryngospasm.

Laryngospasm involves bilateral adduction of the true vocal folds, vestibular folds, and aryepiglottic folds that outlasts the duration of the stimulus. This is protective to the extent that it prevents aspiration of solids and liquids. It becomes maladaptive when it restricts ventilation and oxygenation. The intrinsic laryngeal muscles are the main mediators of laryngospasm, and they include the cricothyroids, lateral cricoarytenoids, and thyroarytenoid muscles. The cricothyroid muscles are the vocal cord tensors, an action mediated by the SLN. Management of laryngospasm consists of prevention by either extubating at a sufficiently deep plane of anesthesia or awaiting recovery of consciousness.[56] Potential airway irritants should be removed and painful stimulation should be discontinued. If laryngospasm occurs, oxygen by sustained positive pressure may be helpful, although this may push the aryepiglottic folds more tightly together.[109] Larson described a technique of applying firm digital pressure anteriorly directed to the "laryngospasm notch" between the ascending mandibular ramus and the mastoid process and observed that this technique is rapid and highly effective.[110] Very small doses of a short-acting neuromuscular blocker with or without reintubation may be necessary.[111,112]

13. Macroglossia

Massive tongue swelling may complicate prolonged posterior fossa surgery performed with the patient in the sitting, prone, or park bench position.[113-116] It is also seen with very steep or prolonged Trendelenburg positioning, hypothyroidism, acromegaly, lymphangioma, idiopathic hyperplasia, metabolic disorders, amyloidosis, cystic hygroma, neurofibromatosis, rhabdomyosarcoma, sublingual or submandibular infections, and chromosomal abnormalities such as the Beckwith-Wiedemann syndrome.[117]

The most common and dramatic presentation of macroglossia results from angioedema.[118] It can be congenital or acquired. Hereditary angioedema results from a deficiency of C1 esterase inhibitor; acquired C1 esterase deficiency is associated with histamine release, a physical stimulus, or most commonly, a reaction to angiotensin-converting enzyme inhibitors or angiotensin receptor blockers.[118,119] Although involvement of the tongue is the most obvious manifestation, the uvula, soft tissues, and larynx may also be involved.

In the ICU setting, macroglossia may be seen as a complication of extreme volume overloading or tongue trauma, particularly when it is further complicated by a coagulopathic state. If this occurs or progresses after extubation, it can lead to partial or complete airway obstruction, making reintubation necessary but difficult or impossible.[114] Lam and Vavilala postulate that positioning in most cases results in venous compression leading to arterial insufficiency and subsequent reperfusion injury.[115] Alternatively, local compression may cause venous or lymphatic obstruction with resultant immediate and typically milder tongue swelling. The latter form is less severe but more apparent, and extubation is likely to be postponed.

14. Laryngeal or Tracheal Injury

Airway injuries, such as lacerations, edema, arytenoid dislocation, and vocal fold paralysis, may occur from the lips to the distal trachea. The lip or tongue may become entrapped between the laryngoscope blade and the mandibular teeth, resulting in swelling or bleeding, although this is unlikely to be severe enough to complicate extubation. The glottis may be injured as a result of insertion of a round tube through a triangular opening. The trachea can be lacerated or penetrated by the ETT or its introducer or by ischemic compression by the cuff on the tracheal mucosa. Palatopharyngeal injuries have been described as a consequence of blind insertion of an ETT during video laryngoscopy.[120-127] Although these injuries are not often apparent at the time of laryngoscopy, they have been managed conservatively and should not complicate extubation. The epiglottis can be downfolded during intubation, but the consequences of downfolding, even if prolonged, are unknown.[128]

Laryngeal injuries accounted for 33% of all airway injury claims and 6% of all claims in the ASA Closed Claims Project database.[129] They range from transient hoarseness to vocal fold paralysis. Even when direct laryngoscopy provides a satisfactory glottic view or intubation is facilitated by fiberoptic instrumentation,[89,91] airway injury can occur and go unsuspected until after the ETT is removed. Airway injuries are presumed to be less likely if intubation is easy, but analysis of the ASA Closed Claims Project revealed that 58% of airway trauma and 80% of laryngeal injuries were associated with intubations that were not difficult.[129,130] Judging from the findings of the Closed Claims Project, difficult intubations were more likely to result in pharyngeal and esophageal than tracheal injuries.

Vocal fold immobility may result from injury to the recurrent laryngeal nerve or the arytenoid cartilages.[92,131-139] Arytenoid immobility has resulted from seemingly uneventful Macintosh and McCoy direct laryngoscopy,[137,140] double-lumen tube insertion, and lightwand intubation.[134] The mechanism of this injury is uncertain. It may be a consequence of a subluxation or a hemarthrosis with subsequent resolution or fixation. Prolonged or stressful contact between the ETT and the posteromedial aspects of the vocal cords, arytenoids, or posterior commissure may result in ulceration of the perichondrium, which heals with fibrous adhesions that produce an immobile glottis. This complication may be more common than the literature indicates.[92,141] Persistent post-extubation hoarseness, a breathy voice, and an ineffective cough should prompt assessment by an otolaryngologist. The diagnosis is confirmed by endoscopic visualization of an immobile vocal cord associated with a rotated arytenoid cartilage.[88] If the diagnosis is made early, before the onset of ankylosis, it may be possible to manipulate the arytenoid back into position.

Vocal fold paralysis results from injury to the vagus or one of its branches (i.e., recurrent laryngeal nerve [RLN] or external division of the superior laryngeal nerve [ex-SLN]) and may resemble arytenoid dislocation or ankylosis. Differentiation may require palpation of the cricoarytenoid joints under anesthesia or laryngeal electromyography.[88] When vocal fold paralysis occurs as a surgical complication, it is usually associated with neck, thyroid, or thoracic surgery. The left RLN can also be compressed by thoracic tumors, aortic aneurysmal dilatation, left atrial enlargement, or during closure of a patent ductus arteriosus. Occasionally, a surgical cause cannot be implicated. Cavo and coworkers postulated that an over-inflated ETT cuff might result in injury to the anterior divisions of the RLN.[142]

The RLN supplies all of the intrinsic laryngeal muscles except the cricothyroid, the true vocal cord tensor, which is innervated by the ex-SLNs. Unilateral ex-SLN injury results in a shortened, adducted vocal fold with a shift of the epiglottis and the anterior larynx toward the affected side. This produces a breathy voice but no obstruction and usually resolves within days to months. Bilateral ex-SLN injury causes the epiglottis to overhang, making the vocal folds difficult to visualize. If seen, they are bowed. This produces hoarseness with reduction in volume and range but no obstruction. Unilateral RLN injury causes the vocal fold to assume a fixed paramedian position and produces a hoarse voice. There may be a marginal airway with a weak cough. Bilateral RLN injury results in both vocal folds being fixed in the paramedian position and inspiratory stridor, often necessitating a surgical airway.[143]

Pharyngeal, nasopharyngeal, and esophageal injuries include perforation, lacerations, contusions, and infections. These injuries may be associated with difficult laryngoscopy or intubation, but they may also result from the blind passage of a gum elastic bougie,[144] nasogastric tube,[145] nasotracheal tube,[146] suction catheter, esophageal stethoscope transesophageal echo probe, or temperature probe.[147] Penetrating injuries can communicate with the esophagus, resulting in a tracheoesophageal fistula, or with the mediastinum, which may go unrecognized and result in mediastinitis, retropharyngeal abscess, and death.[131] After a brief intubation, soft tissue injuries resulting in airway obstruction are more likely to result from edema or hematoma than infection. Most of the described injuries do not significantly complicate extubation. Laryngeal and tracheal stenoses are serious complications, but they are rarely evident at the time of extubation.

15. Airway Injury

Burn patients can have intrinsic and extrinsic airway injuries. Circumferential neck involvement is an example of an extrinsic injury. Smoke inhalation or thermal injuries are examples of intrinsic injuries. Burn patients are at particular risk of requiring reintubation. They can have bronchorrhea, impaired mucociliary clearance and local defenses, laryngeal and supraglottic edema, increased carbon dioxide production, and progressive acute respiratory distress syndrome. Carbon monoxide may also diminish their level of consciousness and the ability to protect their airway. It may be difficult to secure the tracheal tube because of involvement of the adjacent skin, and burn victims may be agitated or uncooperative, increasing the risk of unintended extubation.[148] Kemper and coworkers reported their management of 13 burn patients younger than 15 years, 7 of whom exhibited post-extubation stridor. Patients treated with helium-oxygen mixtures had lower stridor scores than patients treated with an air-oxygen mixture.[149] They found that 11 of 30 extubated burn victims required treatment for stridor after extubation, consisting of racemic epinephrine, helium-oxygen, reintubation (n = 5), or tracheostomy (n = 1). The absence of a cuff leak was considered to be the best predictor of failure, with a sensitivity of 100% and a positive predictive value of 79%.[149]

A variety of conditions may lead to airway edema severe enough to result in post-extubation stridor. It occurred in 2% to 37% of ICU patients after "prolonged intubation."[150] A test was sought to predict patients with sufficient airway swelling to compromise safe extubation. The cuff-leak test was initially proposed for children with croup.[151] The concept is that marked airway swelling is likely if air does not escape around the deflated ETT cuff when the ETT is occluded as the patient exhales. The cuff-leak test was the best predictor of successful extubation in a pediatric burn and trauma unit, and although sensitive, it was not specific for predicting stridor, necessitating reintubation in 62 adults.[152,153]

The test has been refined by evaluating cuff-leak volume as the difference between inspiratory and expiratory tidal volumes during assist-control ventilation after cuff deflation.[41,154] Two studies found the cuff-leak volume could predict post-extubation stridor. In one study, 8 of 45 patients exhibited stridor, 4 of whom required reintubation.[154] In the other study involving 88 adult medical ICU patients, 6 patients exhibited stridor, 3 of whom required reintubation.[41] They observed a significantly smaller cuff leak in patients who subsequently developed stridor, concluding that this measurement was the best predictor of the presence or absence of stridor. However, a study of 561 consecutive cardiothoracic patients who were extubated within 24 hours (median, 12 hours) defined a the cuff leak as the difference between the inspired and expired tidal volumes during assist-controlled ventilation. None of the (20) patients with leaks <110 mL developed stridor whereas one patient with a leak of 350 mL did and required reintubation. This led the investigators to conclude that the quantitative cuff-leak test was not reliable in this patient population.[155]

In another study involving 110 trauma victims, cuff leaks of less than 10% had a 96% specificity for predicting post-extubation stridor or the need for reintubation.[156] De Bast and colleagues studied 76 adults in a combined medical-surgical ICU.[157] An equal number of patients had been intubated for more or less than 48 hours. Assist-control ventilation was reinstituted after cuff deflation, and the percentage of cuff leak was determined. Receiver operating characteristic (ROC) curves yielded a cutoff value of 15.5% cuff leak to equalize the false positives and false negatives for reintubation due to laryngeal edema, but this study was relatively small. Among patients intubated for more than 48 hours, only 2 of 22 with large-volume leaks and 6 of 16 with small-volume leaks required reintubation for laryngeal edema.

Kriner and colleagues evaluated the cuff-leak test for its ability to predict post-extubation stridor among 462 adult patients intubated for longer than 24 hours.[150] They evaluated the two thresholds previously described; a positive test was defined as a cuff-leak volume of 110 mL or less or of 15.5% or less of the exhaled tidal volume. Ten of 82 patients with leak volumes of 110 mL or less developed post-extubation stridor, and 10 of 380 with larger leaks developed post-extubation stridor, giving a positive predictive value for stridor of 0.12 and negative predictive value of 0.97. The sensitivity and specificity of the test under these conditions were 0.50 and 0.84, respectively.[150] With leak volumes of 15.5% or less, 7 of 48 patients developed post-extubation stridor, and 13 of 414 patients with volumes greater than 15.5% developed stridor, yielding positive and negative predictive values of 0.15 and 0.97, respectively. The sensitivity and specificity of this test for post-extubation stridor were 0.35 and 0.91, respectively. The prevalence of post-extubation stridor was 20 of 462. Seven of these patients required reintubation; 15 were managed with racemic epinephrine or helium-oxygen mixtures, or both, and 2 of the 15 failed, requiring intubation. The investigators concluded that neither threshold adequately predicted post-extubation stridor or could justify delaying extubation.

The reported variability of post-extubation stridor (2% to 37%) results in part from inconsistent diagnostic criteria,[150] but undoubtedly there are many other factors at play. Factors increasing the risk of post-extubation stridor include longer duration of intubation,[150] trauma and burns,[14,148,154,158] pediatric age group,[158] female gender,[95,97,150] traumatic or emergent intubations, periods of hypotension, agitation, persistent attempts at phonation, inadequate ETT fixation, aggressive tracheal suctioning, highly positive fluid balance, low plasma oncotic pressure, gastroesophageal reflux, increased ETT diameter, and the presence of a nasogastric tube.[95,97,150]

In summary, it appears that despite the intuitive appeal of the cuff-leak test, neither the qualitative nor quantitative test adequately predicts adult patients who will develop stridor after extubation.[150,155,159] It did not predict where patients were likely to require reintubation. Deem argued that absence of a cuff leak might result in an unnecessary delay of extubation, whereas a large cuff leak might produce false reassurance that there will be no difficulties.[159] At least in adults, the value of this test is uncertain.

16. Postobstructive Pulmonary Edema

Severe airway obstruction from any cause may complicate extubation and lead to postobstructive pulmonary edema, also called negative-pressure pulmonary edema.[160] This edema occurs when a forceful inspiratory effort is made against an obstructed airway (i.e., Mueller maneuver), often a closed glottis, generating large negative intrapleural pressures that promote venous return. The increase in venous pressure is aggravated by a lowered alveolar pressure, resulting in transudation of fluids into the pulmonary interstitium and alveoli. It may also result in a rightward shift of the interatrial and interventricular septa, raising left atrial and ventricular pressures. Some instances may be complicated by a permeability defect with exudative fluid and inflammatory cells.[161-166]

Postobstructive pulmonary edema usually occurs in adult patients with upper airway tumors, severe laryngospasm, or rarely, bilateral vocal cord palsy,[167] whereas in children, it occurs most commonly as a complication of croup or epiglottitis.[168] The onset may be within minutes of the development of airway obstruction. It typically resolves with relief of the obstruction and supportive treatment for pulmonary edema.[166]

B. Higher-Risk Extubations

Although the previously described complications may follow a routine extubation, two additional groups of patients may be affected: those with a higher risk for reintubation and those in whom accomplishing reintubation can be challenging or impossible. Patients at higher risk for reintubation have preexisting medical conditions that reduce their physiologic reserve, ranging from moderate disability to an extremely marginal state. The possibility of higher-risk extubations also exists for a continuum of patients, from those in whom mask ventilation and reintubation should be easily achieved to those in whom both would pose a significant challenge. They may have their jaws wired shut or have a neck that is very poorly suited for emergent surgical access.[169,170]

Chronic pulmonary or cardiac disease may compromise spontaneous ventilation and necessitate intubation. The patient with an ineffective cough or increased secretions may have a need for pulmonary toilet. An obtunded patient may be unable to protect his airway. A list of higher-risk extubations is provided in Table 50-1.

Any reintubation is fundamentally different from the original intubation, because it is likely to occur in an urgent or emergent setting with limited information, personnel, and equipment. The patient is more likely to be hypoxic, acidotic, agitated, and hemodynamically unstable, and the procedure may be done in haste by the available personnel. A preemptive strategy is appropriate to manage these patients.

IV. CLINICAL SETTINGS OF COMPLICATIONS

A. Operative Conditions

1. Laryngoscopic Surgery

Mathew and colleagues looked at 13,593 consecutive PACU admissions from 1986 through 1989.[21] Twenty-six (0.19%) of these patients required reintubation while in the PACU; seven of them had undergone ear, nose, and throat procedures. Of the seven patients, three had laryngeal edema, one was obstructed from a large thyroid, two bled at the operative site, and one developed postobstructive pulmonary edema after a tonsillectomy.

Patients undergoing laryngoscopy and panendoscopy (i.e., laryngoscopy, bronchoscopy, and esophagoscopy) are at an increased postoperative risk for airway obstruction and are approximately 20 times as likely to require reintubation as patients undergoing a wide variety of other surgical procedures.[20] Reviewing the records of 324 diagnostic laryngoscopies and 302 panendoscopies, Hill and colleagues found that patients who had undergone laryngeal biopsy were at the greatest postoperative airway risk. Thirteen (5%) of 252 patients required reintubation, most within 1 hour of extubation. Twelve of 13 had undergone laryngeal biopsy. Most of these patients had chronic obstructive pulmonary disease, and their need for reintubation was attributed largely to this.

Robinson prospectively studied 183 patients who had 204 endoscopic laryngeal procedures.[171] Seven patients had tracheostomies before or after their surgery because of high-risk airways. Two of the remaining patients developed postoperative stridor; one required reintubation, and the other required a delayed tracheostomy. Indirect

TABLE 50-1

Complications of Higher-Risk Extubations

Complication	Surgical and Medical Settings
Inability to Tolerate Extubation and Required Reintubation	
Airway obstruction	Laryngeal injury or hypopharyngeal swelling after laryngoscopy
	Paradoxical vocal cord motion
	After thyroidectomy, anterior cervical surgery, or carotid artery surgery
	Wound swelling, hematoma
	Vocal cord injury (e.g., recurrent laryngeal nerve)
	Hypoglossal nerve injury
	After palatoplasty
	Maxillofacial swelling
	Macroglossia
	Obstructive sleep apnea
	Rheumatoid arthritis
	Parkinson's disease
	Prolonged intubation
Inadequate ventilation	Central sleep apnea
	Severe chronic obstructive pulmonary disease
	Residual sedation or neuromuscular blockade
	Preexisting neuromuscular disorder
	Diaphragmatic splinting
	Relative hypoventilation (e.g., increased CO_2 production)
Inadequate oxygenation	Inadequate inspired oxygen concentration
	Ventilation-perfusion mismatch
	Right-left shunt
	Increased O_2 consumption
	Decreased O_2 delivery
	Impaired pulmonary diffusion
Failure of pulmonary toilet	Obtundation
	Pulmonary secretions
	Quantity
	Quality (inspissated)
	Impaired mucociliary clearance
	Neuromuscular impairment
Inability to protect airway	Obtundation
	Neuromuscular disorder
Difficulty Reestablishing the Airway	
Airway injury	Thermal injury, smoke inhalation
	Blood or trauma obscuring the view
	Blood or trauma obstructing the airway
Previous airway difficulties	Known prior difficulties (e.g., multiple attempts, devices, or operators)
	Cormack-Lehane class ≥ 3 for laryngeal view
Limited airway access	Maxillomandibular fixation
	Cervical immobilization, unstable cervical spine, or halo fixation
	Tracheal resection (e.g., guardian suture)
	Major head and neck surgery
Emergent setting	Lack of knowledge regarding prior or potential difficulties
	Lack of expertise
	Insufficient time to prepare personnel, equipment, and medications

laryngoscopy carried out 4 to 6 hours after surgery revealed mucosal hemorrhage or laryngopharyngeal swelling in 32% of cases. Because the patients undergoing tracheostomy were not described, it is possible that the low incidence of reintubation resulted from an aggressive approach to preemptive tracheostomy.

2. Thyroid Surgery

A variety of airway-related injuries can be associated with thyroidectomies, including SLN and RLN injuries, wound hematoma, and tracheomalacia. Lacoste and colleagues retrospectively reviewed the records of 3008 patients who underwent thyroidectomies between 1968 and 1988.[27] The RLN had been identified intraoperatively in 2427 of these patients. Indirect laryngoscopy was performed on the third or fifth postoperative day. The RLN was damaged in 0.5% of patients with benign goiters and 10.6% of patients with thyroid cancer. RLN injury produces hoarseness, persistent coughing with phonation, and risk of aspiration. Unilateral RLN palsy was observed in 1.1% of patients. Three patients had bilateral RLN palsy and required tracheostomy. Six of a total of 16 deaths during the first 30 postoperative days were attributed to respiratory complications. One death occurred after failed intubation due to a deviated, constricted trachea. A second death was attributed to difficulties performing a tracheostomy. Two deaths resulted from aspiration or pneumonia, possibly related to RLN dysfunction.

SLN injury is more challenging to diagnose. It produces dysphonia and vocal fatigue, particularly in the higher registers. In a 5-year, multicenter study involving 42 centers and almost 15,000 thyroid operations, the diagnosis was suspected in 3.7% and confirmed in 0.4% of patients.[172]

Local hemorrhage or hematoma occurs postoperatively in 0.1% to 1.6% of patients undergoing thyroid surgery and in 0.36% of the patients cared for by Lacoste and colleagues.[27,172-174] These complications occurred 5 minutes to 3 days postoperatively. Re-exploration within the first day was required only twice. Airway obstruction may result from significant laryngeal and pharyngeal edema, and wound evacuation may be of limited value in the relief of airway obstruction.[173,175,176] It may result from or be aggravated by ligature slippage, coughing, vomiting,[174] coagulopathies, and reoperation.[173] The prophylactic placement of surgical drains likely reduces the incidence of this complication. Wound evacuation may result in significant improvement; however this is not always the case. If time permits or intubation fails, wound evacuation should be considered.[176] Laryngeal edema may persist after the wound has been evacuated, necessitating postoperative intubation.

Tracheomalacia is rarely diagnosed after thyroidectomies, even in patients with significant retrosternal tracheal compression, although it may exist subclinically.[177-181] Although symptoms, computed tomography (CT), and pulmonary function test results make it easy to recognize airway compression preoperatively, tracheomalacia may be difficult to predict or even detect from the surgical field, and it does not become apparent until after the ETT is removed and spontaneous ventilation has resumed.[182]

3. Carotid Artery Surgery

Neck swelling or hematoma formation after carotid endarterectomy may be relatively common. The New York Carotid Artery Surgery (NYCAS) study analyzed 9308 procedures performed between 1998 and 1999 at 167 hospitals.[183] A hematoma was identified in 5% of patients, substantially increasing the risk of death (OR = 4.30; 95% CI, 2.72 to 5.00) and stroke (OR = 3.89; 95% CI, 2.82 to 5.38). Hematoma occurrence reported in the literature ranges from 1.2% to 12%, depending on the definition used.[183] The overall rate of wound hematomas in the North American Symptomatic Carotid Endarterectomy Trial (NASCET), involving 1415 patients was 7.1%, 3.9% of which cases were considered to be mild (i.e., no delay in discharge), 3.0% were moderate (i.e., delay in discharge), and 0.3% were severe (i.e., permanent functional disability or death). The moderate and severe cases required re-exploration or wound evacuation (3.3%). Hematoma contributed to the death of four patients.[184] When wound hematomas are identified by a comparison of preoperative and postoperative CT scans, it occurs far more frequently (26%).[185] The postoperative reintubation or exploration rate is 1% to 3.3%.[184,186]

Kunkel and colleagues described 15 patients who developed wound hematomas after carotid endarterectomy.[187] Eight of these were evacuated under local anesthesia. In six of seven cases in which general anesthesia was induced before opening the wound, difficulties arose with airway management, resulting in two deaths and one patient with severe neurologic impairment. O'Sullivan and coworkers reported a similar experience for six patients with airway obstruction after carotid endarterectomy.[188] Stridor was not relieved by wound evacuation. Administration of muscle relaxants made manual mask ventilation and tracheal intubation virtually impossible due to marked glottic or supraglottic edema. Cyanosis and extreme bradydysrhythmias or asystole occurred in four patients. The providers endorsed Kunkle's recommendation for wound evacuation but thought that much of the airway compromise was caused by edema from venous or lymphatic congestion. They emphasized that the outward appearance may lead to an underestimation of the situation's gravity. Voice changes are early signs of danger and may be relatively subtle. Rapid clinical deterioration can occur after stridor develops.[189]

Studies by Carmichael and colleagues provided additional evidence for the role of swelling and bleeding in a small but elegant study. They compared the CT scans of 19 patients before and after carotid endarterectomy surgery.[185] Clinically, 1 patient had severe swelling, 4 had moderate swelling, and 3 had mild swelling, but 10 were deemed normal. However, postoperative CT scans demonstrated significant swelling of the retropharyngeal space and a reduction of the anteroposterior and transverse airway diameter, particularly at the level of the hyoid. Compared with preoperative CT scans, the calculated volume reduction averaged 32% ± 7% for extubated patients. The scans revealed a wound hematoma estimated to be greater than 10 mL (range, 44 to 94 mL) in 5 of 19 patients. Patients who remained intubated postoperatively showed a significantly greater volume reduction of 62% ± 9% ($P < 0.025$). Those remaining intubated as a result of swelling had contralateral extension of the swelling. These observations may help to explain why opening the wound frequently fails to provide benefit in many patients. Nonetheless, it may be difficult to clinically differentiate bleeding from swelling. After radiologic demonstration of swelling, the same group evaluated the benefits of prophylactic dexamethasone but failed to demonstrate any clinical benefit.[190]

A 10-year, retrospective review of 3224 carotid endarterectomies performed at The Mayo Clinic revealed that 44 (1.4%) patients required wound exploration within 72 hours of surgery, despite the nonreversal of heparin.[191] In two patients, re-exploration occurred before the initial extubation. The decision to re-explore was made in the PACU for 7 patients; the remaining 35 were identified in the ICU or ward. Only one patient required a surgical airway when direct laryngoscopy failed in the ICU. Several techniques were initially employed: awake bronchoscopic intubation (15 of 20 of which were successful), direct laryngoscopy after induction (13 of 15 were successful), and awake direct laryngoscopy (5 of 7 were successful). When awake bronchoscopy failed, direct laryngoscopy was successful whether the patient was awake (3 of 3) or asleep (2 of 2). When direct laryngoscopy initially failed after induction in two patients, it succeeded after opening the incision. When awake direct laryngoscopy failed, one patient required a surgical airway; in the other, direct laryngoscopy succeeded after opening the incision. Despite the size of this series, it is not possible to draw conclusions about which techniques are most successful. Success likely depends on the skill and judgment of the airway manager. It is also possible that this study differed from the other studies in that the decision to re-explore was made earlier and patients had less airway distortion.

Several nerve injuries can result from carotid artery surgery or the anesthetic technique. The range reported in the literature is 3% to 23%, although most of these cases resolve within 4 months of surgery.[192] In the NYCAS study, cranial nerve palsies occurred in 514 (5.5%) of 9308 patients and involved, in descending order, the hypoglossal nerve (170), producing tongue deviation to the operative side; a branch of the facial nerve (126), resulting in lip or facial droop; the glossopharyngeal nerve (41); a branch of the vagus, which may involve the RLN and produce vocal cord paresis (31); the trigeminal nerve (19); a branch of the cervical plexus (10); or more than one nerve group (117).[183]

Bilateral vocal cord and bilateral hypoglossal nerve palsies have been described after staged, bilateral carotid endarterectomies.[24,25] In the latter case, the first procedure, performed under regional anesthesia, had been complicated by a wound hematoma, resulting in numbness over the anterior neck and diminished sensation in the C2 and C3 distribution. The subsequent endarterectomy, done 4 weeks later under deep cervical plexus block with subcutaneous infiltration, caused intraoperative airway obstruction and asystole. The airway was secured, but repeated attempts at extubation resulted in persistent obstruction due to bilateral hypoglossal nerve palsy. In another case, performed under cervical plexus block, the patient developed bilateral vocal cord paralysis that required intubation and subsequent tracheotomy. It is suspected that she had a previously unrecognized contralateral vocal cord palsy from a prior thyroidectomy.[193] In this case, the vocal cord dysfunction was co-incident with retraction of the carotid sheath—although it can also be induced by a cervical plexus block—but it raises the importance of the preoperative assessment of patients who have had prior head and neck surgery.

4. Cervical Surgery

Cervical spine procedures may be followed by airway-related complications, including vocal cord paralysis and airway obstruction. Vocal cord dysfunction was seen in 5% of 411 patients undergoing anterior cervical discectomy and fusion.[194] Stridor was observed in one patient with bilateral vocal cord paralysis who required a tracheostomy. Fifteen of 17 patients had recovered by 12 months. One additional patient had recovered by 15 months, and the remaining patient was lost to follow-up.

Emery and colleagues studied the records of 133 patients who underwent cervical corpectomies with arthrodesis between 1974 and 1989.[26] The patients had undergone an anterior approach to achieve a three-level vertebral body and disc resection with bone grafting. This surgical approach requires tracheal and esophageal retraction toward the opposite side to permit exposure. Drains were placed, and all patients were immobilized by a halo vest or a rigid head-cervical-thoracic orthosis. They identified seven patients (5.3%) who required postoperative reintubation, and although they did not compare these patients with those not requiring reintubation, they attempted to identify common features that increased the risk of postoperative airway compromise. Three patients were immediately reintubated in the operating room, and four were reintubated 12 to 91 hours postoperatively. Severe hypopharyngeal swelling was observed at reintubation in four of seven patients and possibly in a fifth. Five of the seven reintubations had no serious sequelae; these patients were extubated within 2 to 8 days. One patient required a cricothyroidotomy, but delay resulted in hypoxic encephalopathy and death. Another patient was reintubated but developed and succumbed to severe adult respiratory distress syndrome. The investigators think that preexisting pulmonary disease, moderate or severe preoperative myelopathy, extensive multilevel decompression with prolonged surgery, and tissue retraction were risk factors for postoperative airway obstruction, but there were no controls.[26] They recommended 1 to 3 days of elective intubation postoperatively, a cuff-leak test, and direct laryngoscopy at extubation.

Venna and Rowbottom reviewed the records of 180 patients who had undergone a variety of cervical surgical procedures.[28] Based on the Emery study, they had made the decision to keep high-risk patients intubated until they met specified criteria, including a demonstrable cuff leak and the absence of significant airway edema on laryngoscopy. The average time to extubation was 33.5 hours. Despite the delay and the aforementioned criteria, 12 patients (6.6%) demonstrated post-extubation stridor

and breathing difficulties, and 5 (2.7%) required reintubation. Two patients required tracheostomy, and two deaths were attributed to airway obstruction and unsuccessful reintubation.

Sagi and coworkers conducted a retrospective chart review of 311 anterior cervical procedures in an effort to identify the factors associated with airway complications.[195] In this series, 19 (6.1%) of patients had airway complications, but only 6 (1.9%) required reintubation. Most of these complications were attributed to pharyngeal edema. Risk factors included increased intraoperative bleeding, prolonged surgery (>5 hours), and exposure of more than three vertebral bodies, particularly when they included C2, C3, or C4. Reviewing the literature, these investigators identified an airway complication rate of 2.4% (from 1615 cases), 35 of whom required reintubation or tracheostomy. On average, those requiring reintubation did so at 24 hours.

Epstein and coworkers developed a collaborative protocol involving the neurosurgeon and anesthesiologist. Their objective was avoidance of reintubations.[196] Although their study enrolled only 58 patients, they required high-risk, lengthy procedures involving several cervical levels and significant blood loss. All patients remained electively intubated overnight and underwent fiberoptic airway examination before considering extubation. Most patients were extubated the day after surgery, but three remained intubated until day 7. Only one patient required reintubation. This reintubation rate was essentially the same as that observed by Emery and colleagues,[26] but Epstein's cohort appeared to undergo higher-risk surgery.

In an effort to better understand the mechanism of postoperative airway obstruction, Andrew and Sidhu compared the soft tissue changes on the preoperative and postoperative cervical spine radiographs of 32 consecutive patients after a one- or two-level anterior cervical discectomy and fusion.[197] They found that the swelling was maximal at the C3-C4 level, corresponding to the area where Emery observed pharyngeal edema. None of their patients experienced dyspnea despite mean differences of 9.4 mm (95% CI, 7.41 to 11.09 mm) to 10.7 mm (95% CI, 7.8.82 to 12.58 mm) between the preoperative and postoperative radiographs at C3 and C4, respectively. It appears that this area is most vulnerable, regardless of the level operated on. Compared with Sagi's study, these patients underwent much shorter and more limited procedures.

Extubation criteria after anterior cervical spine surgery were discussed at length in the Society for Airway Management online Forum in 2011. The groups who perform this surgery frequently tend to extubate most of their patients at the conclusion of surgery, except when the blood loss is high (e.g., >500 mL), the surgery is prolonged (e.g., >5 hours), the operation involves more than three levels, the airway was difficult or expected to be difficult, or comorbidities exist, such as severe cervical myelopathy, obesity, and obstructive sleep apnea (OSA). Patients with multiple risk factors are cared for in an ICU and are extubated over an airway exchange catheter (AEC) (personal communication from C.A. Hagberg, SAM Forum, February 2011).

Patients undergoing posterior cervical surgery may face the risk of macroglossia and significant retropharyngeal and hypopharyngeal swelling, which may be aggravated by fixation of the cervical spine and make intubation more difficult.[198] There is a low probability (1.1% to 1.7%) that reintubation will be required,[196,198] but accomplishing this may be very difficult.

5. Maxillofacial Surgery and Trauma

Maxillary and mandibular surgery produces conspicuous and often worrisome swelling. Anxiety regarding postoperative care may be heightened by limited airway access, fear that airway intervention may disrupt the surgical repair, and anecdotal reports of near misses or actual fatalities. Because many of these patients are young and otherwise healthy and are undergoing elective surgery for functional or cosmetic improvement, there may be concerns about litigation. It is speculative about whether this results in more or less aggressive care.

Although these concerns demand special attention, deaths rarely occur. In a review of 461 perioperative deaths reported to the Ontario, Canada, coroner between 1986 and 1995, the investigators found only one death associated with orthognathic surgery, although they were unable to determine how many such cases had been performed (see "In Vivo Studies").[199] They were unable to identify nonlethal complications. Meisami and others performed magnetic resonance imaging (MRI) approximately 24 hours after maxillary or mandibular surgery in 40 patients.[200] Despite the significant facial swelling seen in almost all the patients, none exhibited soft tissue swelling from the base of the tongue to the glottis.

Complete airway obstruction after elective orthognathic surgery has been reported. Dark and colleagues described a case involving a young woman who underwent seemingly uneventful mandibular and maxillary osteotomies with submental liposuction.[201] Immediately after extubation, she developed airway obstruction requiring reintubation. Repeated fiberoptic examination and CT showed severe and extensive edema from the tongue to the trachea, which was maximal at the level of the hyoid. By the fourth postoperative day, a cuff leak was detected, and the patient was successfully extubated over a tube exchanger. Hogan and Argalious described a patient in whom maxillomandibular advancement was performed for OSA.[202] The procedure lasted 9 hours, during which he received 7200 mL of crystalloid and 500 mL hetastarch. He remained intubated overnight, and after demonstrating adequate spontaneous ventilation and a cuff leak, he was extubated (over a 19-F AEC). Extubation was immediately followed by clinical evidence of airway obstruction, and he was reintubated. The obstruction was attributed to fractured hardware and a hematoma in the piriform fossa that caused extrinsic compression. This could easily have resulted from periglottic edema. The investigators concluded that patients undergoing this type of surgery face a high risk of airway complications and recommended nasopharyngolaryngoscopy before extubation.

Clinical assessment of airway edema is unreliable,[200] and studies indicate that the cuff-leak test is neither sufficiently sensitive nor specific to determine when to extubate these patients. Endoscopic assessment may help to identify patients who harbor occult clots (i.e., "coroner's clot") behind the soft palate or adjacent to the glottis, but it may miss or itself give rise to troublesome bleeding.

Maxillofacial injuries often result from unrestrained occupants of motor vehicles encountering an unyielding dashboard, windshield, or steering wheel. Gunshot wounds or physical altercations also cause maxillofacial injury. Airway obstruction is a primary cause of morbidity and mortality in these patients, and many die before they reach the hospital.[203] Those with less life-threatening injuries are likely to present with a full stomach, and many have associated head and neck injuries, lacerations, loose or avulsed teeth, intraoral fractures, and fractures extending into the paranasal sinuses, into the orbit, or through the cribriform plate. They may also have an unstable cervical spine or damage to the neural axis. Injuries to the lower face raise the possibility of a laryngeal fracture. Intermaxillary fixation may be part of the surgical plan, necessitating a nasal intubation or a surgical airway. Timing of tracheal extubation is complex and must take into consideration factors such as the patient's level of consciousness, ability to maintain satisfactory gas exchange, coagulation status, and integrity of protective airway reflexes. Attention must be paid to the difficulties originally encountered in securing the airway and an evaluation of whether reintubation would be easier or more difficult after surgery and resuscitation. Most of the trauma literature about airway management addresses intubation and offers little help with extubation, making cooperation between the anesthesiologist,[204,205] surgeon, and critical care physician essential. Intermaxillary fixation requires wire cutters to be immediately available and personnel to know which wires to cut. A flexible bronchoscope, provisions for an emergency surgical airway, and the required expertise should be immediately available at the time of extubation. Alternatives include prophylactic tracheotomy, submental intubation,[206-208] nasal intubation, and bronchoscopic airway evaluation performed before extubation,[209] although assessment may be limited to supraglottic structures and exclusion of tube entrapment. Ideally, extubation should be accomplished in a reversible manner, permitting supplemental oxygenation, ventilation, and reintubation if needed (see "Extubation Strategies").

6. Deep Neck Infections

Infections involving the submandibular, sublingual, submental, prevertebral, parapharyngeal, and retropharyngeal spaces are significant airway management challenges, whether intubation is achieved for surgical drainage or for protection during medical management. In expert hands, bronchoscopy-assisted intubation can often be achieved.[210] When this is unsuccessful or constitutes a significant risk of rupturing the abscess, a surgical airway before incision and drainage may be called for.[211] Potter and colleagues retrospectively compared the outcomes of 34 patients in whom a tracheotomy was performed with 51 patients who remained intubated after surgical drainage.[212] All patients had undergone surgical drainage for impending airway compromise and required airway support postoperatively. It was not always evident to the investigators why a particular strategy was chosen, and these groups were not likely identical. Airway loss occurred more commonly in the intubated patients, but this characteristic was not statistically significant. Two deaths occurred, one resulting from an unintended extubation and the other from post-extubation laryngeal edema and an inability to reestablish the airway. The latter patient had a cuff leak before extubation, and signs of obstruction developed 30 minutes after the ETT was removed. Surgical drainage rarely results in immediate airway improvement, and reintubation or emergent placement of a surgical airway, if required, may be complicated by edema, tissue distortion, and urgency.

7. Posterior Fossa Surgery

Posterior fossa surgery can cause injury to cranial nerves, bilateral vocal cord paralysis, brainstem or respiratory control center injury, and macroglossia.[114,115,167,213-216] Because the nerve roots may be very close to the operative site, the resultant injuries may be bilateral, extensive, and transient or permanent. Gorski and coworkers suggested that tolerance of the ETT and the absence of a gag reflex on oral suctioning should arouse suspicion of such an injury.[214] Howard and colleagues described a patient with a recurrent choroid plexus papilloma involving the fourth ventricle.[215] Preoperatively, the patient displayed bulbar dysfunction. His extubation on the first postoperative day was complicated by complete airway obstruction, hypoxia, and a seizure. Laryngoscopy performed after neuromuscular blockade revealed mildly edematous vocal cords. After reintubation and elective tracheostomy, fiberoptic examination showed the vocal folds in a neutral position. Nocturnal ventilation and tracheostomy were still required at 1 and 3 months, respectively. This patient demonstrated central apnea and bulbar dysfunction with hypoglossal paralysis and unopposed vocal fold adduction.

Artru and colleagues described a patient with a cerebellar mass, severe papilledema, and bulbar signs.[213] Despite recovery of consciousness and strength, the patient remained apneic and required ventilatory support for 7 days. The investigators cautioned that the dorsal pons and medulla are the sites of the cardiovascular and respiratory centers that control hemodynamics and ventilation. The area is also host to several cranial nerve nuclei. Damage to these areas can result from edema, disruption, ischemia, or compression and may cause a loss of respiratory drive or airway obstruction.

Dohi and coworkers described a patient who developed bulbar signs, including bilateral vocal cord paralysis after excision of a recurrent cerebellopontine angle tumor.[167] Negative-pressure pulmonary edema developed as a consequence of a bilateral, presumably central RLN injury, and a tracheostomy was required until recovery 3 months later. During the initial intubation, the glottis could not be seen by direct laryngoscopy, and blind intubation was performed. The details of three subsequent unsuccessful extubations and reintubations were not described. Trials of extubation in a patient known to be a difficult (direct) laryngoscopy case are life-threatening and cannot be justified. A tracheostomy

was performed, and vocal cord function recovered after 3 months.

Early vocal cord evaluation after extubation has been advocated along with the involvement of a neurosurgeon, otolaryngologist, speech therapist, and intensivist to manage patients who have developed laryngeal dysfunction.[216] A tracheostomy and an enteral feeding tube may be needed. A more preemptive approach (described later in more detail) involves flexible laryngoscopic assessment through a supraglottic airway (SGA) after removal of the ETT.

8. Stereotactic Surgery and Cervical Immobilization

Stereotactic neurosurgical and neuroradiologic procedures are finding increasing applications. When head frames are used, they may impede access for SGA placement or laryngoscopy. Similarly, patients in cervical immobilization devices for spinal cord protection may undergo high-risk surgical procedures.[116] Careful planning for their extubation is critical because reintubation may be difficult, and rapid surgical access may be virtually impossible. Full recovery of strength and consciousness, persistence of respiratory drive, the presence of a cuff leak, preservation of protective reflexes, and absence of significant tongue swelling are the essential prerequisites for extubation. Postoperative seizures, vomiting, elevated intracranial pressure, and neurologic obtundation may make extubation particularly hazardous. Several of the strategies described subsequently should be given serious consideration in managing these patients.

9. Tracheal Resections

Patients with moderate or severe tracheal stenosis may come for surgical tracheal resection. These patients usually have tracheal stenosis or tracheomalacia, often caused by prolonged intubation or occasionally caused by a retrosternal mass. Some patients may have compromised preoperative respiratory function. After an end-to-end anastomosis, the surgeon may elect to place a "guardian suture" from the chin to the chest, maintaining the head and neck in flexion and thereby minimizing traction on the suture lines (Fig. 50-1).[217,218] The preference is for early extubation to avoid positive pressure, coughing, and presence of a foreign body in the airway.[217-221] A cough-free extubation is highly desirable, as is avoidance of a need for reintubation, which if required could prove very challenging.

10. Palatoplasty

A variety of surgical procedures have been employed to treat OSA, including uvulopalatopharyngoplasty, midline glossectomy, mandibular advancement, limited mandibular osteotomies with genioglossal advancement, and hyoid bone suspension.[222] Pepin and colleagues published a critical analysis of the literature on the risks and benefits of surgical treatment of snoring and OSA.[223] They identified "at least five deaths" after uvulopalatopharyngoplasty and found that few studies had adequate numbers to allow conclusions to be drawn regarding their outcomes. Less than one half of the studies commented on the frequency of complications. A retrospective review of 101 uvulopalatopharyngoplasties identified an early postoperative respiratory complication rate of 10%.[224] Ten of

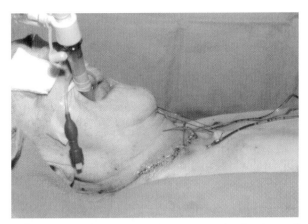

Figure 50-1 This patient has undergone a cricotracheal resection. Cervical extension is restricted by a chin-to-chest guardian suture. The patient has been extubated, and a laryngeal mask airway has been introduced before reversal of neuromuscular blockade or awakening. This reduces coughing on emergence, allowing gradual recovery and assessment of spontaneous respiratory function while minimizing the potential distraction of the surgical anastomosis. It also provides the optimal means of performing flexible laryngobronchial examination under controlled conditions. (Courtesy of Patrick Gullane, MD, University Health Network, Toronto, Ont.)

11 patients required reintubation, and 1 death resulted from airway obstruction.

Uvulopalatopharyngoplasty was introduced to deal with retropalatine collapse. However, in approximately one half of the adult patients with OSA, obstruction occurs at the retrolingual pharynx. Tongue suspension is one of several approaches introduced to manage the latter group of patients.[225] The procedure involves placement of an anchoring screw in the genial tubercle and attachment of a suture through the base of the tongue. Szokol described a morbidly obese patient with OSA in whom this procedure was performed.[222] Laryngoscopy and bag-mask ventilation had been difficult. At the conclusion of the procedure, the patient was fully awake, was able to sustain a head lift for 5 seconds, demonstrated a negative inspiratory pressure of 40 cm H_2O, and was extubated. Stridor was observed immediately, and bag-mask and laryngeal mask ventilation were ineffective. Attempts to reintubate the patient were unsuccessful, necessitating a cricothyroidotomy. Subsequent direct laryngoscopy showed a markedly swollen epiglottis and grossly edematous laryngeal and hypopharyngeal tissues. The patient developed negative-pressure pulmonary edema, and a tracheostomy was performed 2 days later because of persistent swelling. Tracheal decannulation occurred uneventfully 2 weeks later. The physicians speculated that airway manipulation during the surgery was the cause of this patient's swelling. They did not consider that the swelling might have resulted from or at least been aggravated by repeated attempts at laryngoscopy.

Palatoplasty, alone or in combination with other procedures, may be performed on patients with cleft palates or other congenital abnormalities. In one study, 14 (5.7%) of 247 patients undergoing palatoplasty had postoperative airway problems, 12 of whom required reintubation. One half of the patients experiencing complications had Pierre Robin sequence; three of the patients required reintubation 24 to 48 hours postoperatively.[226]

B. Preexisting Medical Conditions

1. Paradoxical Vocal Cord Motion

Paradoxical vocal cord motion (PVCM) is the quintessential example of a situation wherein reintubation will be required. Intubation is not more difficult; extubation is the challenge. This uncommon and poorly understood condition is frequently mistaken for refractory asthma or recurrent laryngospasm.[227-229] The diagnosis is both overlooked and overused, leading to confusion.[230] It also is called vocal cord dysfunction, Munchausen stridor, psychogenic stridor, factitious asthma, pseudoasthma, and irritable larynx syndrome.[230,231] Normal vocal cord motion involves inspiratory abduction and 10% to 40% adduction on expiration. With PVCM, adduction of the true vocal cords occurs on inspiration or expiration, or both. The false vocal cords and the posterior laryngeal wall may further contribute to the airway obstruction.[231-234] This condition may be associated with psychosocial disorders, stress, exercise, gastroesophageal reflux, irritant exposure, or airway manipulation. Pulmonary function tests show normal expiratory but flattened inspiratory flow loops. It is important to differentiate this condition from asthma, laryngospasm, anaphylaxis, angioedema, gastroesophageal reflux, and vocal cord paralysis. The incidence of PVCM is unknown.

Harbison and coworkers described two patients who had post-extubation stridor after thyroidectomies.[235] This is a particularly challenging situation with a complex differential diagnosis, especially because one of the patients had unilateral vocal cord paralysis preoperatively. In that patient, post-extubation stridor developed 24 hours postoperatively and could be observed while awake and asleep. Fiberoptic examination under sedation showed paradoxical motion of the mobile cord. She was managed successfully with speech therapy. They speculated that these cases might have resulted from surgical manipulation of the RLN during the thyroidectomies.

Hammer and colleagues described a 32-year-old woman with recurrent episodes of stridor,[236] sometimes associated with cyanosis, despite normal flow-volume loops and pulmonary function tests. The diagnosis of PVCM was made endoscopically and managed with relaxation techniques. After preoperative sedation, topical lidocaine, and bilateral SLN blocks, she underwent an awake fiberoptic intubation. At the conclusion of surgery, extubation was performed after she was fully awake, but sustained inspiratory stridor ensued, resulting in reintubation. A subsequent attempt the next day confirmed inspiratory vocal fold adduction, and a tracheostomy was required for 58 days. In the absence of features predicting a challenging intubation, there seems little justification for awake intubation, and it may contribute unnecessarily to an anxiety disorder.

PVCM imposes no special requirements for intubation. The abnormality is functional rather than anatomic. Appropriate management depends on having the correct diagnosis, which requires clinical suspicion and endoscopic confirmation of inspiratory adduction of the vocal cords. Adequate oxygenation, consideration of CPAP or helium-oxygen administration, positioning, reassurance, and support may suffice, although sedation may be required after the diagnosis is confirmed. Speech therapy, psychotherapy, hypnosis, and reassurance may be helpful in the long-term management,[237] but such is not always the case.[227] Some reports have recommended electromyographically guided botulinum toxin injection into the thyroarytenoid muscle for recalcitrant cases. The optimal anesthetic management of these patients is unknown. Regional anesthesia avoids airway intervention, but it does not ensure that a condition that may be stress related will not occur. Familiarity with this condition, calm reassurance when there is prior suspicion, and perhaps deep extubation seem prudent.

2. Parkinson's Disease

Susceptibility to aspiration is common among patients with Parkinson's disease and is the most common cause of death. Dysphonia, most frequently hypophonia, occurs in approximately 70% to 90% of patients with Parkinson's disease.[238,239] Video stroboscopic findings include laryngeal tremor, vocal fold bowing, and abnormal glottic opening and closing.[239] Several neurodegenerative diseases, including multiple system atrophy, have some features in common with Parkinson's disease, including dysphonia, and these patients may exhibit bilateral abductor vocal fold paresis. Typically, symptoms in patients with Parkinson's disease progress insidiously, are not recognized by the patient, and may be associated with nocturnal stridor. These features resemble those of OSA identified by polysomnography. Many of these patients may benefit from nocturnal CPAP or bi-level positive airway pressure (BiPAP).[238]

Blumin and Berke described seven patients, only one of whom presented for surgery. This patient underwent a transurethral prostate resection under general anesthesia, and 2 weeks after surgery, he returned with biphasic stridor that necessitated an emergent tracheostomy. It is unclear whether there was a relationship between the surgery or anesthesia and subsequent airway obstruction.

Patients with multiple system atrophy have daytime hypoxemia associated with abnormal laryngopharyngeal movements, including obstruction at the arytenoids, epiglottis, base of the tongue, and soft palate. The significance of these problems is unclear, but they may contribute to complications after extubation.[240]

Vincken and colleagues studied 27 patients with extrapyramidal disorders.[241] Twenty-four had flow-volume loops, many of which demonstrated saw-toothed oscillations, even in the absence of respiratory symptoms. They observed oscillations with rhythmic (4 to 8 Hz) or irregular movements of the glottis and supraglottic structures. Ten patients exhibited intermittent upper airway obstruction. Four patients had stridor or dyspnea. The investigators believed that the upper airway was the primary site of involvement. In a subsequent report, they observed symptomatic improvement with levodopa despite persistence of the oscillatory pattern on flow-volume loops.[242] Inspiratory and expiratory flows after levodopa increased from 1.40 to 3.50 L/sec and 0.95 to 5.05 L/sec, respectively. Bronchodilators provided no additional benefit. This case may have important implications for the perioperative management of patients with Parkinson's disease.

Easdown and colleagues described a patient with Parkinson's disease who had a respiratory arrest 60 hours after surgery.[243] Before that event, the patient had episodic desaturation, labored breathing, and progressive hypercapnia in the absence of tremor or rigidity. Treatment with bronchodilators produced no benefit, and his condition improved immediately after intubation. With the ETT, compliance and resistance appeared normal. This patient's levodopa or carbidopa had not been resumed postoperatively, and the investigators speculated that this caused or contributed to upper airway obstruction. Because most patients with Parkinson's disease are elderly and may have comorbidities that can make the diagnosis uncertain, it is important to consider involvement of the upper airway and the dramatic effect withdrawal and reinstatement of medications can have on their clinical course. This concern is reinforced by a case report describing a patient who developed airway obstruction and acute respiratory acidosis requiring intubation preoperatively because five doses of his antiparkinsonian medications were withheld while he was being fasted.[244] Easdown and colleagues emphasized the importance of continuing these medications, and avoidance of dopamine antagonists throughout the perioperative period.[243]

Backus and colleagues described a patient with long-standing Parkinson's disease who became aphonic, developed stridor, and suffered respiratory arrest shortly after taking cough medication.[245] Complete upper airway obstruction recurred with vocal fold apposition immediately after extubation. Four days later, the patient extubated herself with no further complications. The investigators interpreted this spontaneous laryngospasm as a manifestation of Parkinson's disease. Others have observed upper airway dysfunction, airflow limitation, and bilateral abductor vocal cord paralysis in association with Parkinson's disease. The first episode might not have been spontaneous but instead a consequence of aspiration of the cough medicine. Nonetheless, there remains a possibility that these patients are more prone to laryngospasm, whether spontaneous or induced by glottic stimulation.

Liu and coworkers described airway obstruction during induction of anesthesia.[246] Despite being unable to visualize the larynx, they attributed the obstruction to laryngospasm. The obstruction resolved with awake, blind nasal intubation but recurred 24 hours later on extubation. At that point, fiberoptic examination showed inspiratory vocal fold adduction, necessitating reintubation. It is unclear whether they were observing manifestations of Parkinson's disease or PVCM, but extubation was uneventful 24 hours later after increasing the dosage of levodopa or carbidopa.

Parkinson's disease is a common disorder, but only 13 cases of stridor have been attributed to it.[239] The pathogenesis of upper airway obstruction is unknown. It may be mediated by the basal ganglia and nucleus ambiguus. A similar phenomenon involving esophageal spasm has been associated with Parkinson's disease. One theory invokes laryngeal hypertonicity, which may be triggered by copious secretions.

3. Rheumatoid Arthritis

In patients with rheumatoid arthritis, the airway manager needs to be concerned about three joint areas: the cervical spine, the temporomandibular joint (TMJ), and the cricoarytenoid joint.[247] Autopsy studies suggest that 30% to 50% of patients with rheumatoid arthritis have significant cervical spine involvement. Cervical subluxation has been identified clinically in 43% to 86% of these patients and may represent a serious neurologic risk during intubation with flexion or extension.[145,247-249] The spectrum of cervical involvement ranges from ligamentous destruction with subluxation and impaction to extreme limitations in the range of motion because of fibrosis and ankylosis. These patients may have a narrowed glottic aperture, limited mouth opening due to involvement of the TMJs, micrognathism, laryngeal deviation, and cricoarytenoid and cricothyroid involvement.[250,251] Kohjitani and colleagues retrospectively described four patients undergoing bilateral TMJ replacement; three had glottic erythema and swelling on endoscopy, three had OSA, and three experienced laryngospasm at intubation and after extubation.[251] TMJ involvement may result in loss of ramal height and micrognathia with or without ankylosis and associated OSA.

Cricoarytenoid arthritis and its consequences have long been recognized in the anesthesia and general medical literature.[252-256] Although rheumatoid arthritis is the most common cause of this condition, it also may be associated with bacterial infections, mumps, diphtheria, syphilis, tuberculosis, Reiter's syndrome, ankylosing spondylitis, systemic lupus erythematosus, gout, progressive systemic sclerosis, and other conditions.[257] The cricoarytenoid joint has a synovial lining and bursa. Its mobility is vital for speech, respiration, and protection from aspiration. Inflammatory changes may include effusion, pannus formation, joint erosion, and ankylosis, any of which may compromise the joint's functions. Its involvement may be unsuspected or mistaken for asthma until intubation or after extubation and may necessitate a surgical airway.[258,259] Dysphonia, dyspnea, or stridor should raise suspicion of this possibility. Complete airway obstruction is a well-described but uncommon complication, despite involvement of the cricoarytenoids in 26% to 86% of patients with rheumatoid arthritis.[251,259] Laryngoscopy may reveal a rough and thick mucosa with narrowing of the vocal chink. Although airway obstruction occurs most commonly in patients with long-standing rheumatoid arthritis with polyarticular and systemic involvement, laryngeal stridor has been described as the sole manifestation of this disease.[260]

Keenan and coworkers described tracheal scoliosis, which consisted of tracheal deviation, laryngeal rotation, anterior angulation, and vocal fold adduction seen fiberoptically and on CT scans.[255] It was presumed to result from the loss of vertical height and asymmetrical bony erosions.

Wattenmaker and colleagues studied patients with rheumatoid arthritis undergoing posterior cervical spine procedures.[250] Their primary objective was to compare the perioperative airway complications seen in rheumatoid arthritis patients when intubation was performed by direct laryngoscopic or flexible bronchoscopy. Retrospectively reviewing 128 consecutive posterior cervical procedures, upper airway obstruction characterized by stridor occurred in 9 of 128 patients, 1 of 70 patients intubated with bronchoscopic guidance, and 8 of 58 patients intubated otherwise (i.e., direct laryngoscopy or blind nasotracheal technique). Five patients (all in the nonbronchoscopic group) required emergency reintubation that proved to be very difficult, with two near fatalities and one death. Although the two groups were similar with regard to age, gender, American Rheumatology Association classification, ASA physical status, duration of surgery and anesthesia, fluid balance, and postoperative immobilization, there were significant differences in time to extubation. Seven of the patients could not be intubated by flexible bronchoscopy and were therefore intubated by a nonfiberoptic technique. The patients were not randomized to different methods; criteria for the method of intubation and techniques were not described; all patients were intubated awake; and the study was carried out over an 11-year period.[261] Although it is not possible to draw firm conclusions from this study, there was a high incidence (7%) of post-extubation stridor and difficult or failed reintubations, regardless of the intubation technique.

Patients with rheumatoid arthritis qualify as higher-risk extubation cases because they may have a fixed or unstable cervical spine, TMJ ankylosis, difficult intubations by direct or flexible laryngoscopy, and increased risk of post-extubation airway obstruction. Several investigators have recommended postponing extubation until the patient is wide awake. Unfortunately, this provides increased protection against nothing other than laryngospasm and aspiration. The prevailing wisdom is that patients with limited mouth opening and a potentially unstable cervical spine should be intubated with a flexible bronchoscope.[250] This method involves blind passage of the ETT through the cords, which may be traumatic,[91,261] particularly in the face of preexisting cricoarytenoid arthritis. Regional anesthesia should be considered as an alternative to general anesthesia when appropriate. When intubation cannot be avoided, proposed extubation strategies include a preemptive tracheostomy or a method that increases the reversibility of extubation. Neither strategy has been prospectively evaluated in this population.

4. Tracheomalacia

Tracheomalacia is a dynamic airway obstruction resulting from loss of the cartilaginous tracheal support. This results in the posterior membranous wall bulging anteriorly when the intratracheal pressure is reduced or the intrathoracic pressure is increased.[141] Although rare, it should be considered when the patient has dyspnea on exertion with difficulty clearing secretions and a seal-like, incessant cough.[141,262]

Patients frequently are misdiagnosed with asthma and fail to respond to escalating therapy. Pulmonary function tests (i.e., forced expiratory volume at 1 second, forced vital capacity, and peak expiratory flow) show severely diminished expiratory flow with relative preservation of the inspiratory flow. The diagnosis may be confirmed fiberoptically during spontaneous breathing. Tracheomalacia may be congenital[263] or result from vascular compression,[264] an intrathoracic goiter,[265] chronic obstructive pulmonary disease, or prolonged intubation. The latter may be caused by ETT cuff-induced erosion of the tracheal cartilage with or without extension to the membranous trachea.

The severity of the dynamic obstruction is proportional to the expiratory force. It may be unapparent during quiet breathing but disabling in a distressed patient. Positive pressure or bypassing the lesion with a tracheal tube provides temporary relief while further management options are considered. They may include medical management, surgical resection, or placement of a stent.[262] Additional suggestions for the extubation of a patient with suspected tracheomalacia are described later.

Relapsing polychondritis is an example of extensive tracheobronchomalacia. It is a rare, multisystem disease characterized by episodic inflammation of cartilaginous structures resulting in tissue destruction.[262,266] Laryngeal and tracheal tract involvement occurs in approximately one half of patients. It usually occurs early in the course of the disease and may manifest as hoarseness, nonproductive cough, shortness of breath, and stridor. Upper airway obstruction is usually diffuse and may progress to involve the glottis, subglottic area, trachea, and bronchial cartilages. Histologically, there is evidence of perichondral inflammation and replacement of cartilage by fibrous tissue that manifests as inflammatory swelling and progressive destruction of cartilage. The clinical manifestations range from bronchorrhea and recurrent pneumonia to airway collapse. Medical management consists of steroids, nonsteroidal anti-inflammatory drugs, and immunosuppressant agents, but their benefit varies. Surgical management consists of external airway splinting or self-expanding metallic stents. These patients may present for bronchoscopy, tracheostomy, tracheal or nasal reconstruction, aortic valve replacement, or stent placement.[264,267-271] Airway collapse after extubation should be anticipated and may be temporarily dealt with by CPAP.[272,273]

5. Obstructive Sleep Apnea Syndrome

In the ASA Closed Claims Project analysis of adverse respiratory events, 65 of the 156 perioperative events involved obese patients; for the claims specifically related to extubation, 12 of the 18 were obese, and 5 of these patients had been diagnosed with OSA.[2] OSA correlates positively with age and obesity, both of which are becoming increasingly prevalent. The pathophysiology and perioperative airway management of OSA in obese patients has been comprehensively reviewed.[274-276] Many surgical patients have undiagnosed or untreated OSA. OSA syndrome is associated with an increased risk of gastroesophageal reflux, difficult mask ventilation[276-278] and laryngoscopic intubation,[279-282] and accelerated arterial oxygen desaturation.[276,283] The risk of airway obstruction after surgery is increased for patients with OSA; life-threatening post-extubation obstruction occurred in 7 (5%) of 135 patients.[279,284] Rapid desaturation, difficult mask ventilation, and difficult direct laryngoscopy make this a particularly high-risk setting.[285] The ASA practice guidelines

for the management of patients with OSA provided limited guidance beyond a strong recommendation that they be fully awake and that the airway manager verify that neuromuscular blockade is completely reversed before extubation. If possible, extubation and recovery should be carried out in the lateral or semi-upright position,[286] nasal CPAP should be available or routinely implemented, and consideration should be given to extubation over a tube exchanger.[274,276,280,284,287] These strategies have been associated with better outcomes, and anecdotal comparisons are compelling, but they have not been subjected to controlled, randomized trials, and they were not addressed by the ASA Task Force.

6. Laryngeal Incompetence

Laryngeal function may be disturbed for at least 4 hours after tracheal extubation.[288] Immediately after extubation, 8 (33%) of 24 patients aspirated swallowed radiopaque dye; 5 showed radiologic evidence of massive aspiration. Four hours after extubation, 4 (20%) of 20 patients aspirated dye; 3 had massive aspirations. At 24 hours, the rate was reduced to 5%. In this study, patients had been intubated for 8 to 28 hours during and after cardiac surgery. Although the investigators did not observe a relationship between duration of intubation (8 to 28 hours) and aspiration, it is unclear whether the presumed laryngeal incompetence occurs after brief intubation or is more common and severe with prolonged intubation. The mechanism of laryngeal incompetence was postulated to be primarily sensory because patients who aspirated dye did not cough.

Residual neuromuscular paralysis is a common problem in postoperative patients and may result in hypoventilation, hypoxemia, pharyngeal and laryngeal dysfunction, or increased pulmonary aspiration.[264,289] Pharyngeal function was impaired in conscious volunteers receiving a continuous infusion of vecuronium and resulted in laryngeal penetration of contrast medium proportional to the degree of blockade.[290] Relaxation of the upper esophageal sphincter was also observed. None of the volunteers coughed or had respiratory symptoms. Berg and colleagues found a higher incidence of postoperative pulmonary complications (i.e., pulmonary infiltrate or atelectasis associated with cough, sputum, or shortness of breath) among patients randomly assigned to receive a long-acting or intermediate-acting neuromuscular blocker.[291] It is intriguing to speculate on how residual neuromuscular blockade may contribute to laryngeal incompetence.

7. Pulmonary Aspiration of Gastric Contents

Although more patients are being diagnosed with gastroesophageal reflux, the diagnosis of perioperative pulmonary aspiration has not increased.[292,293] Aspiration is estimated to complicate 1 of 2000 to 3000 general anesthetics and was responsible for only 3 of 156 perioperative events in the ASA Closed Claims Project review.[2,293,294] Nonetheless, it is the leading cause of pneumonia in the ICU and a common cause of acute respiratory distress syndrome.[295] Many of these cases are ventilator-associated pneumonia and occur with the ETT in situ. Factors predisposing a surgical patient to aspiration include emergency surgery, pain, obesity, narcotics, nausea, ileus, bowel obstruction, pregnancy, some surgical positions, depressed level of consciousness, inadequate depth of anesthesia, postoperative drowsiness, and residual neuromuscular blockade. Despite the ubiquity of these conditions, perioperative aspiration is not commonly identified. Before intubation, difficult bag-mask ventilation may result in gastric distention, which may be further complicated if laryngoscopy proves difficult because it may delay securing the airway. Repeated laryngoscopic attempts may cause edema, thereby increasing glottic resistance. Aspiration may also result from obtundation or conditions that impair vocal cord apposition (e.g., vocal cord paralysis, laryngeal incompetence, residual neuromuscular blockade, granulomas). Aspiration can cause serious morbidity and death.[292-295]

Although most incidents of aspiration seem to occur at induction, many occur during maintenance and recovery from anesthesia.[296] Numerous strategies have been described to reduce the risk at induction, but relatively little information is available on how best to prevent this later. Premature extubation, postoperative nausea, delayed gastric emptying, residual neuromuscular blockade, relaxation of the esophageal sphincters, decreased level of consciousness, gagging on an ETT, supine recovery, and impaired laryngeal competence may make emergence from anesthesia and tracheal extubation as problematic as induction. A kinked or clamped nasogastric tube may promote regurgitation and aspiration. Evidence-based recommendations on an extubation strategy to reduce aspiration are not available. It would seem logical to minimize the contributing factors: postoperative nausea and vomiting, residual neuromuscular blockade, decreased level of consciousness and associated diminished protective airway reflexes, and gastric evacuation. We do not know whether gastric decompression reduces aspiration; a well-seated i-gel SGA[297] or ProSeal LMA may or may not offer some protection from aspiration.[298-300] With the current information, it is not appropriate to recommend the elective use of these devices in a patient at increased risk for aspiration.

V. FACTORS AFFECTING INTUBATION AND EXTUBATION

A. Previously Encountered Airway Difficulties

Multiple attempts at laryngoscopy by experienced personnel, a need for alternative airway management techniques due to failure of direct laryngoscopy, and prior difficulty prompting the primary use of alternative techniques are settings in which reintubation may be problematic. In urgent or emergent circumstances, methods that had previously been successful may not be available or appropriate. The required equipment, necessary skills, or time required to perform alternative techniques may not be available. Uncertainty regarding the ease of ventilation or intubation may correctly lead to disinclination to administer paralytic and sedating drugs. Although they may facilitate ventilation and intubation, failure will result in an apneic patient who can neither be ventilated nor intubated. Knowledge of prior difficulties may result in intubation conditions that are less favorable to success. Repeated attempts at laryngoscopy are associated with a significant increase in the risk of hypoxemia, esophageal intubation, regurgitation, aspiration, bradycardia, and cardiac arrest.[2,301] To avoid this risk, flexible bronchoscopic intubation may be considered, but in an agitated, hypoxic patient with secretions or blood in the airway, it may be difficult to achieve adequate topical anesthesia, and the procedure may be difficult or impossible.

B. Limited Access

Limited access to the airway is exemplified by intermaxillary fixation, severe cervical restriction, instability, or immobilization, and the chin-to-chest guardian suture (see Fig. 50-1) to prevent traction tracheal resection. More commonly, this situation may arise in the confining space of a PACU, ICU, or patient room where access is limited. In each case, there may be additional risks related to oxygenation, ventilation, airway obstruction, or pulmonary toilet. For example, after cervical fixation or orthognathic surgery, the patient may have macroglossia or supraglottic edema. A patient requiring tracheal resection may be unable to clear blood or secretions from the airway.

C. High-Risk Cases

A higher-risk extubation exists when there is an increased likelihood that reintubation will be necessary or an increased risk that reestablishing the airway will be difficult. The increased need to reintubate may result from failure of oxygenation, ventilation, pulmonary toilet, or loss of airway patency. These risks cannot always be anticipated, but there are often identifiable patients with less reserve. The clinical conditions previously discussed, including OSA; rheumatoid arthritis; cervical, tracheal, thyroid, or carotid surgery; and intermaxillary fixation, are higher-risk settings because reintubation may be challenging.

The clinical playing field may not be level at all hours of the day. The immediate availability of highly trained primary and support personnel, equipment, and the necessary clinical information may be problematic at night or during periods of intense activity. The ASA Task Force on Management of the Difficult Airway and the Canadian Airway Focus Group recommended a preformulated strategy for extubation of the difficult airway.[5,6] The ASA Closed Claims Project supported the need for such a strategy.[2] Patients at risk for hypoventilation, hypoxemia, and loss of airway patency have been discussed. The remainder of this chapter addresses specific extubation strategies.

VI. EXTUBATION STRATEGIES

If any of the higher-risk extubation conditions exists or is anticipated, the clinician should consider a strategy that does not cut off access to the airway. Ideally, the strategy should permit continued administration of oxygen or ventilation of a failing patient even while the airway is being reestablished. These objectives are consistent with the ASA Task Force and Canadian Airway Focus Group recommendations.[5,6]

Extubation risk stratification is largely based on intuition, anecdotal reports, and limited clinical series. The proposed classification and strategies are becoming broader and deeper with time. Because most patients—even those at high risk—can be successfully extubated, any proposed strategy must entail less risk than removing the tracheal tube and hoping for the best. It should also involve minimal discomfort, have an acceptable cost, and facilitate oxygenation, ventilation, and reintubation.

A. Deep versus Awake Extubation

Extubations may be performed before or after recovery of consciousness. Deep extubation ordinarily occurs after full recovery of neuromuscular function and the resumption of spontaneous ventilation. Its purported advantage is avoidance of the adverse reflexes associated with extubation, such as hypertension, dysrhythmias, coughing, laryngospasm, and increased intraocular or intracranial pressures. The fundamental disadvantage of deep extubation is the patient's inability to protect his airway against obstruction and aspiration. When deep extubation is improperly executed, laryngospasm and its attendant complications are more likely to occur. Although not having to wait for the recovery of consciousness may accelerate operating room turnover, this approach is more difficult to justify when anesthetic agents having a faster elimination time are available. Delays in recovery usually are brief. Unscavenged volatile anesthetic agents may also represent an occupational health hazard. A significant proportion of American anesthesiologists practice the technique, at least some of the time, but there are few data for adults that compare the safety of deep extubation with that of awake extubation.[12] Koga and colleagues compared three small groups of adult patients who underwent deep extubation, awake extubation, or deep extubation after the insertion of an LMA.[80] Straining occurred in a high (but comparable) proportion of patients whether the ETT was removed before or after recovery of consciousness.

Current strategies include extubation on low-dose propofol or remifentanil and intracuff or intravenous lidocaine, which may reduce coughing and straining on extubation. Deep extubation followed by LMA insertion (with 2% to 3% isoflurane) is discussed later. Deep extubation is contraindicated when mask ventilation was or is likely to be difficult, the risk of aspiration is increased, endotracheal intubation was difficult, or airway edema is likely.

B. Extubation with a Laryngeal Mask or Other Supraglottic Airway

On emergence from general anesthesia, most patients tolerate an LMA with less coughing and changes in intraocular, intracranial, and arterial pressures (see Fig. 50-1).[57,77,80,302,303] Silva and Brimacombe substituted an LMA for the ETT in a small series of patients while still asleep and paralyzed after completion of neurosurgical procedures.[304] Muscle relaxation was then reversed, and the anesthetic was discontinued. The LMAs were removed when the patients resumed spontaneous ventilation and obeyed commands. None of the 10 patients coughed, and changes in the rate-pressure product (indicating cardiac oxygen requirements) were minimal. The investigators concluded that the technique might prove useful in patients undergoing other types of surgical procedures. They stressed that this substitution should be performed only by those skilled in LMA insertion. Patients must be at a sufficient depth of anesthesia or coughing, breath-holding, laryngospasm, and the very pressor responses this substitution is intended to avoid may occur. Bailey and others recommended that the LMA be inserted before removal of the ETT to prevent losing the airway after tracheal extubation.[80,305] Compared with deep tracheal extubation followed by Guedel airway insertion, there was a lower incidence of coughing and requirement for airway manipulation.[305] Koga and coworkers compared this technique with deep and awake tracheal extubation.[80] They observed no difference in recovery conditions between patients in whom the ETT was removed by deep or awake methods; however, they noticed a significant improvement in recovery conditions when the LMA substitution was performed. This technique is useful but can jeopardize a secure airway if not properly executed. It should be practiced on routine airways before use in higher-risk extubations.[306] Brimacombe suggested (personal communication, December 2010) that a ProSeal LMA or LMA Supreme with a gum elastic bougie inserted through the drainage tube could produce a more secure substitution for an ETT.[307]

Sometimes, it is desirable to perform the exchange of an ETT for an SGA in reverse. Several types of tube exchanges have been described. Asai wanted to replace a damaged ETT in a patient who had been a difficult intubation.[308] He inserted an LMA Classic behind the existing ETT. A fiberoptic bronchoscope (FOB) with a replacement 7-mm ETT was introduced through the LMA; the FOB was advanced through the vocal cords, and the original ETT was removed. The new ETT was then advanced over the FOB, which was removed. To extend the length of the ETT to enable its removal from the LMA, another ETT was inserted into the proximal end of the replacement ETT.[308] This technique was complicated and could easily have failed.

Matioc and Arndt wished to substitute an ETT for a ProSeal LMA.[309] Using an Arndt Airway Exchange Catheter Set (Cook Critical Care, Bloomington, IN) (see Fig. 50-6), they introduced an FOB through the ProSeal LMA into the trachea. The set comes with a 144-cm extrastiff Amplatz guidewire, which was passed through the FOB, and the latter was removed. An 11-F, 70-cm, Cook airway exchange catheter (CAEC) was introduced over the guidewire and the ProSeal LMA was removed. The replacement ETT was then advanced over the exchange catheter.

A simpler approach involving the Aintree intubation catheter (Cook Critical Care) has been described with a variety of SGAs, including the cuffed oropharyngeal airway (COPA),[310] the LMA Classic,[311-313] the LMA

ProSeal,[314,315] and the LMA Supreme.[316] The Aintree intubation catheter is 56 cm long and has an internal diameter (ID) of 4.7 mm; its outer diameter (OD) is 6.3 mm (19 F). A bronchoscope (<4 mm) can be inserted through the device, leaving 3 or 4 cm protruding beyond its tip. A 7-mm or larger ETT can be advanced over it. Only the distal 3 to 4 cm of the protruding bronchoscope is flexible, but it is usually sufficient to allow successful maneuvering into the trachea, after which the SGA is removed and a replacement ETT is advanced over the Aintree catheter. A Rapi-Fit adapter is provided to enable positive-pressure ventilation while the substitution is performed. The Aintree intubation catheter and FOB are inserted together through the SGA. There are several advantages of this technique.[315,317] It can be used to facilitate conversion from an unmodified LMA to an oral ETT of adequate size. Sufficient length allows the LMA to be removed with minimal risk of losing the airway. The Aintree intubation catheter fits tightly to the insertion cord of the FOB and to the ETT, thereby reducing the size discrepancy that often results in difficult glottic passage. The catheter can be used as a conduit for manual or jet ventilation during an exchange. An LMA Classic, inserted as a rescue device (for "cannot intubate, cannot ventilate" cases) can facilitate safe tube exchange without the need for an intubating LMA.

C. Extubation or Reintubation over a Fiberoptic Bronchoscope or Laryngoscope

When tube entrapment is a possibility, extubation over an FOB can avert a disastrous outcome. For a spontaneously breathing patient, extubation over an FOB provides the opportunity of visually assessing the trachea and laryngeal anatomy and function. This can help in the patient suspected of having tracheomalacia, vocal cord paresis, or PVCM. It also permits assessment of supraglottic structures.[318] These opportunities can be maximized by reassuring the patient and by providing judicious sedation, an antisialogue, and the use of a Yankauer sucker for oral secretions. The oropharynx is suctioned, taking care to avoid inducing a gag reflex. The FOB is placed above the carina, and the cuff is slowly deflated to minimize coughing. The ETT is slowly withdrawn into the oropharynx, followed by very gradual withdrawal of the FOB to the supraglottic region. After the patient is comfortable, the FOB is further withdrawn to a position just above the vocal cords. Even with this deliberate technique, the exercise is frequently frustrated by excessive secretions, coughing, swallowing, or poor tolerance with insufficient opportunity of visualizing the structures of interest.

If the technique is successful, it may identify problems and anticipate complications. When significant abnormalities are identified, a decision must be made about whether to immediately reinsert the ETT or withdraw the FOB and manage the patient with agents such as corticosteroids, racemic epinephrine, and helium-oxygen.[149,152] This technique is not practical for performing a trial of extubation, in part because such a trial lasts only seconds or minutes.

Watson endorsed the use of an FOB to exchange ETTs, citing the advantages of minimal sedation, risk of aspiration, hemodynamic embarrassment, and uncertainty about tube placement.[319] His technique involved passing the loaded FOB alongside the existing ETT. He had used this technique successfully in 13 of 15 attempts. Dellinger suggested that use of an FOB to perform tube exchanges offered the greatest likelihood of reintubation success and recommended techniques for conversion from nasal to oral, oral to nasal, and oral to oral ETT exchange in addition to extubation.[318] We have found this method of extubation to be unreliable and one that demands immediate and often incorrect clinical judgment.

D. Extubation with a Supraglottic Airway with or Without a Bronchoscope

Extubation of a difficult airway over an FOB or SGA has the limitations previously described, but the combination of these devices offers significant advantages. Replacement of an ETT with an SGA provides an excellent means of performing a fiberoptic assessment of glottic and subglottic anatomy and function. After the substitution is performed and the patient is under anesthesia or a suitable degree of sedation, muscle relaxation can be reversed and spontaneous ventilation allowed to resume. An FOB is then passed through the SGA, and vocal fold movement and appearance can be assessed while the concentrations of oxygen and volatile agents (if necessary) can be controlled. The view is protected from oral secretions, and inadequate ventilation can be supplemented. PVCM or tracheomalacia can be visually and functionally evaluated, although both may be minimal if the patient is deeply anesthetized.

This technique is useful in patients with recurrent post-extubation stridor or those at risk for static or dynamic tracheal stenosis. We frequently employ this technique in patients undergoing thyroidectomy when tracheomalacia or vocal fold paralysis is suspected.[181]

E. Use of a Gum Elastic Bougie or Mizus Endotracheal Tube Replacement Obturator

Finucane and Kupshik described an awake, blind nasal intubation in a patient with cervical instability, but the cuff became damaged, requiring a tube exchange.[320] They used the 63-cm-long, 4-mm-OD plastic sleeve from a brachial central venous catheter as a tube exchanger. Others have used a gum elastic bougie to achieve similar objectives.[321-324]

Cook Critical Care designed the Mizus Endotracheal Tube Replacement Obturator (METTRO) for the replacement of endotracheal and tracheostomy tubes (Fig. 50-2). It is available in two sizes: 70 cm long (7.0 F, 2.3 mm) for replacement of ETTs as small as 3 mm and 80 cm long (19 F, 6.3 mm) for passing through tubes 7 mm or larger. The METTRO is a single-use, flexible, radiopaque, solid device with a tapered tip and distance markings. The package insert instructs the user to advance this device until resistance is encountered, but this recommendation can result in coughing, discomfort,

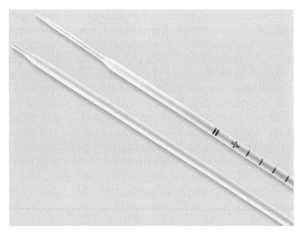

Figure 50-2 The Mizus Endotracheal Tube Replacement Obturator (METTRO) is a solid device that is tapered at the end. It is available in two diameters (7 and 19 mm) and two lengths (70 and 80 cm). The figure shows the proximal (bottom) and distal (top) ends of one of these. (Courtesy of Cook Critical Care, Bloomington, IN.)

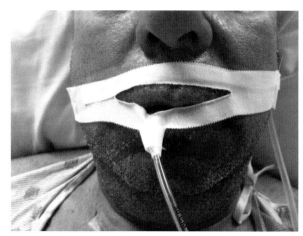

Figure 50-3 An Endotracheal Ventilation Catheter (ETVC) properly secured tube exchanger.

hypertension, and tachycardia. Tracheal perforation has been reported using different devices but following similar recommendations.[325,326]

The smaller airway obturator has been used to maintain airway access during tracheostomies in 22 patients and for "tentative extubations" in 7 patients.[327] The smaller-caliber device was preferred by Audenaert and colleagues because patient discomfort was minimal during tube exchanges and the device was unobtrusive during surgical tracheostomies. The obturator was removed when it was apparent that the patient was unlikely to require reintubation. The 19-F obturator was not conducive to spontaneous breathing. Chipley and coworkers used a METTRO in an obese patient with a fractured occipital condyle recovering from respiratory failure.[328] They left this in place for 48 hours, removing it when extubation appeared to be successful. They also described the use of the obturator to stimulate coughing, although this might have been ill advised given the possibility of tracheal perforation. The METTRO obturator is being phased out and will soon be unavailable.

In a modification of the Eschmann gum elastic bougie (Intubation Guide, Smiths Medical, Keene, NH), both ends of the bougie were amputated, exposing a hollow core. A cannula, syringe, and ETT connector enabled this assembly to be connected to an oxygen source.[329]

F. Use of Jet Stylets

The ubiquitous nasogastric tube has been used as an exchange catheter,[330] but these devices are specifically formulated to become softer as they are warmed. This thermolability is not a desirable characteristic for a tube exchanger.

Bedger and Chang coined the term *jet stylet* to refer to a self-fashioned, 65-cm-long, plastic catheter with a removable 15-mm adapter at the proximal end. It could be connected to an anesthesia machine or jet injector.[331] They created three side ports cut into the distal 5 cm to minimize catheter whip during jet ventilation. They used the stylet for extubation or reintubation of 59 patients.

It also functioned adequately in patients when it was used for jet ventilation and oxygen insufflation. Although no complications were described in this series, in an earlier report, Bedger and Chang described tension pneumothoraces in 3 of 600 patients ventilated through a 3.5-mm-OD pediatric chest tube at 15 psi.[332] This stylet had been used to provide airway access and ventilation during direct laryngoscopy. They speculated that the pneumothoraces might have resulted from endobronchial migration of the catheter. They did not consider the possibility that barotrauma occurred as a result of jet ventilation against apposed vocal cords as the patients were recovering from neuromuscular blockade.

G. Use of Commercial Tube Exchangers

Several commercial products incorporate many of the features described by Bedger and Chang.[331] They are long, hollow catheters that may include connectors for jet or manual ventilation. Most have distance and radiopaque markers. They also have end and distal side holes. They can be introduced through an existing ETT, permitting its withdrawal. Oxygen insufflation or jet ventilation can be provided through the tube exchanger. Respiratory monitoring can be achieved by connection to a capnograph. Spontaneous breathing may take place around the device. In most reports, these catheters have been tolerated well enough that they can be left in situ until it is unlikely that reintubation will be required. They must be properly secured to ensure that they do not come out prematurely (Fig. 50-3). Even with the catheter in place, most patients will be able to talk or cough.

If reintubation or a tube exchange is required, it can be facilitated with gentle laryngoscopy, not necessarily to reveal the glottis but to retract the tongue. Reintubation using a tube exchanger is similar to intubation over an FOB, and the difference of diameters between the tube exchanger and the advancing ETT may predict the relative ease of tube advancement. It is wise to delegate someone to secure the exchange catheter during reintubation. If resistance is encountered, ETT rotation may successfully release the tube from the piriform fossa, "vocal cord," or arytenoid cartilage, but it is best to minimize the size discrepancy by choosing a larger-diameter tube exchanger or a smaller-diameter ETT.

These devices are consistent with practice guidelines from the ASA Task Force and Canadian Airway Focus Group recommendations regarding the extubation of the difficult airway.[5,6] They increase the probability that reintubation will succeed; if difficulty is encountered, the device can provide a conduit for oxygen insufflation. Jet ventilation, if necessary, can be accomplished while alternative techniques are explored. This may be thought of as a reversible or staged extubation. With the device in place, other options can be pursued, including evaluation of the benefits of helium-oxygen mixtures or inhalation of racemic epinephrine. Knowing that the patient is satisfactorily oxygenated and ventilated, the airway manager can recruit additional information, equipment, and expertise.

The differences between these commercial products are far less important than the concept of a reversible extubation. In our opinion, reintubation of the high-risk patient may be unlikely, but it must have a high probability of success.

1. Tracheal Tube Exchangers

The most basic commercial tube exchangers are the Sheridan T.T.X. (Hudson Respiratory Care Inc. [RCI], Temecula, CA) (Fig. 50-4) and the JEM Endotracheal Tube Changer (Instrumentation Industries Inc., Bethel Park, PA). The T.T.X. devices are available in four ODs (2.0-, 3.3-, 4.8-, and 5.8-mm) and two lengths (56 and 81 cm). The smallest can be inserted into tracheal tubes with IDs as small as 2.5 mm. A longer, 100-cm endobronchial exchanger (Sheridan E.T.X.) is available for exchanging double-lumen tubes. They are firm—Shore hardness of 85, the same durometer measurement as the CAEC and Cardiomed International's Endotracheal Ventilation Catheter (ETVC)—although thermolabile and therefore subject to softening with heat. They are frosted to minimize drag and have a radiopaque stripe and distance

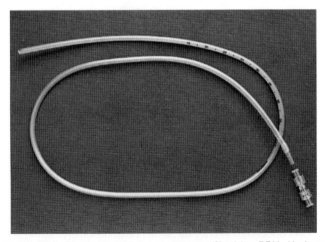

Figure 50-4 The tracheal tube exchanger (Sheridan T.T.X., Hudson RCI) is a simple catheter with no proximal or distal modifications. These devices are available in four diameters and two lengths. If the device is to be used for ventilation, it must be adapted by the user. There are no distal side ports, which makes jet injection potentially hazardous. (*From Cooper RM: The difficult airway-II. Anesthesiol Clin North Am 13:683-707, 1995.*)

markings. They have no side holes or connectors. An alternative product, the Sheridan JETTX Exchanger, is a longer device (100 cm), but it is available in only a single OD that is suitable for ETTs greater than 6.5-mm ID. It incorporates a proximal slip-fit connector that can be connected by a Luer-Lok to a jet ventilator. As with the T.T.X., there is only a single, distal end hole.

The JEM devices are available in nine sizes and are compatible with ETTs from 2.5- to 7.5-mm ID (JEM 325 to 400). These are single-use, high-density, polyethylene devices without proximal connectors or distal side holes.

2. Cook Airway Exchange Catheters

Cook Critical Care has developed a family of hollow stylets known as CAECs (Fig. 50-5A). They are available in 8.0-, 11-, 14-, and 19-F sizes, corresponding to 2.7-, 3.7-, 4.7-, and 6.3-mm ODs, respectively. They can be used to exchange ETTs with IDs of 3, 4, 5, and 7 mm, respectively. The 8-F CAEC is 45 cm long, and the others are 83 cm long. The devices are radiopaque, have distance markings between 15 and 30 cm from the distal end, and have two distal side holes and an end hole. Proximally, two types of connectors are secured and released by a patented Rapi-Fit adapter (see Fig. 50-5B). They provide a 15-mm connection or a Luer-Lok jet ventilation attachment and were designed for rapid removal and reattachment while the tracheal tube is being off-loaded and replaced. The length and IDs (1.6 to 3.4 mm) make manual ventilation with a resuscitation bag possible but useful only for short periods because resistance is very high. The Luer-Lok jet Rapi-Fit connector allows jet ventilation, but the paucity of distal side holes potentially increases catheter whip and the risk of barotrauma.[333]

Atlas and Mort examined the relationship between the diameter of the two larger CAECs and tolerance, as well as the ability to phonate and cough.[334] It is unclear whether their patients were randomly assigned to specific sizes of catheters. Phonation and discomfort were similar in both groups, with only 3 of 101 patients experiencing significant discomfort. Cough effort tended to be reduced with the larger CAEC, but this did not achieve significance. Atlas and colleagues also looked at a larger tube exchanger (JEM 400 Endotracheal Tube Changer, Instrumentation Industries Inc.), which they reasoned would have a higher degree of success as a tube exchanger. This device has an OD of 6.35 mm and is said to be stiffer. They adapted the JEM 400 using the Rapi-Fit connector from the CAEC 19-83 to enable jet ventilation.[335] This device, like the Sheridan JETTX, has only a single end-hole and is not recommended for jet ventilation.

Mort evaluated the concept of reversible extubation in patients with difficult airways.[336] From an institutional database, he identified patients who were extubated in the operating room, PACU, or ICU with a CAEC. The tube exchanger was left in place until the need for reintubation was considered unlikely. Over a 9-year period, 354 patients qualified. Two groups emerged: those who required reintubation while the AEC was still in place and another group who required reintubation within 7 days but after the AEC had been removed. Airway-related complications were compared for the two groups. The AEC dwell time was a mean of 3.9 hours (range, 5

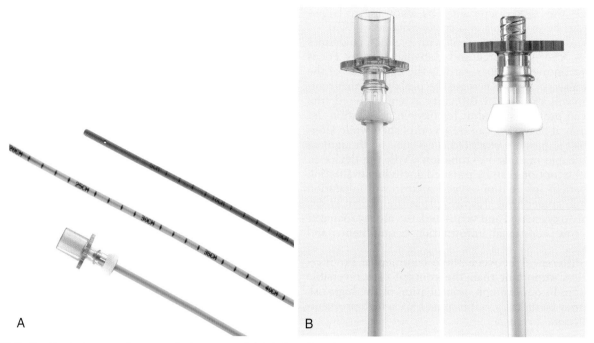

Figure 50-5 The Cook airway exchange catheters are available in four diameters and two lengths. They are radiopaque and have distance markings at each centimeter throughout the working length. **A,** The proximal Rapi-Fit adapter, the middle section, and the distal end of a flexible-tip exchange catheter (available only on the double-lumen exchange catheter). Notice that there are two distal side holes and one end hole. **B,** Two Rapi-Fit adapters: a Luer-Lok jet adapter *(right)* and a 15-mm connector *(left)*. (Courtesy of Cook Critical Care, Bloomington, IN.)

minutes to 72 hours). Of 354 patients, 288 were extubated in the ICU and had previously required three or more laryngoscopic attempts or alternative devices to achieve intubation. Comparing the overall success rate in the two groups, 47 of 51 patients in the AEC group were successfully reintubated, 87% on the first attempt. The four failures in this group resulted from inadvertent removal of the AEC in three; one patient was rescued with an intubating LMA and flexible bronchoscope. Mild (SpO$_2$ < 90%) and severe hypoxia (<70%) were experienced by three and four patients, respectively. Of the 37 patients requiring reintubation without an AEC, the first pass success rate was only 14%, with mild and severe hypoxia in 50% and 19%, respectively; three or more laryngoscopy attempts in 28 of 36 patients; and the need for a rescue device in 32 of 36 patients.[336] In all cases, reintubation was attempted by a member of an anesthesia airway team: an attending anesthesiologist or a resident under direct supervision. Although reintubation over an AEC does not guarantee first-pass success, this strategy was strikingly more effective (87% versus 14% first-pass success) and had far fewer life-threatening complications.

3. Arndt Airway Exchange Catheter

The Arndt Airway Exchange Catheter (Cook Critical Care), a radiopaque exchange catheter, consists of an extrastiff Amplatz guidewire with positioning marks, a Rapi-Fit adapter, a bronchoscopic port, and a distally tapered 14-F (4.7-mm-OD), 70-cm-long AEC. It was designed for the exchange of LMAs, endobronchial tubes, and ETTs (Fig. 50-6). Bronchoscopy is performed through the existing airway device. The flexible end of the Amplatz

guidewire is introduced through the working channel of the bronchoscope and under visual control and is advanced to the level of the carina. The bronchoscope is removed over the wire, taking care that it is neither advanced nor withdrawn. The Arndt AEC is advanced over the guidewire to the appropriate depth, determined by aligning the distance markings on the airway device with that of the AEC. The original airway is carefully

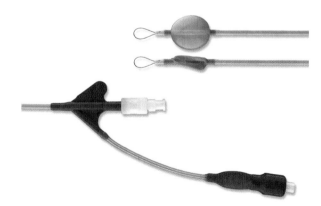

Figure 50-6 The Arndt Airway Exchange Catheter Set (Cook Critical Care, Bloomington, IN) consists of a bronchoscopic adapter, a stiff Amplatz guidewire, a tapered airway exchange catheter, and two Rapi-Fit adapters. The adapter permits continuation of positive pressure ventilation while a bronchoscope is introduced through the original endotracheal tube (ETT). The guidewire is inserted through the bronchoscope's working channel, and the original ETT and bronchoscope are withdrawn. A tapered exchange catheter is advanced over the guidewire, and it may be connected with a 15-mm or jet Rapi-Fit adapter to provide ventilation. The replacement ETT is then advanced over the exchange catheter.

removed, and its replacement is advanced over the AEC.[309]

4. Endotracheal Ventilation Catheter

Cardiomed's Endotracheal Ventilation Catheter (Lindsay, Ontario, Canada) is made of a hybrid plastic (Fig. 50-7). It is 85 cm long and has a 4-mm OD (12 F) and 3-mm ID. It has a radiopaque stripe along its entire length and distance markings at 4-cm intervals. Proximally, it has a male hose barb with a threaded adapter welded into the catheter. These attachments have been constructed to prevent restriction of the catheter's ID. The threaded adapter connects to an easily removed Luer-Lok adapter. Distally, it is blunt ended with one end hole and eight helically arranged side holes to minimize catheter whip and jet ventilation pressures. Unpublished studies by the manufacturer found no significant softening over time at body temperature. This is desirable for a product that may remain in situ and be required to serve as a stylet. A metal guidewire is available to provide additional stiffness, but we have not found this to be necessary.

The ETVC was designed to facilitate reversible extubation.[337] We have used it in at least 600 patients, the

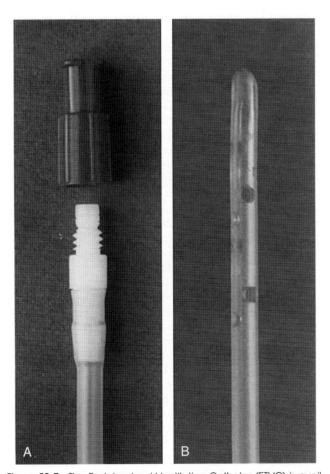

Figure 50-7 The Endotracheal Ventilation Catheter (ETVC) is available in one length (85 cm) with an outside diameter of 4 mm. It is nonthermolabile and has a radiopaque stripe along its length. There are distance markings every 4 cm. **A,** Proximally, there is a welded, barbed, plastic connector with a threaded Luer-Lok adapter for jet ventilation. **B,** Distally, there is a blunt end hole with eight helically arranged side holes, which minimize catheter whip and reduce the jet injection pressure.

first 202 of whom has been reported.[338] Although the ETVC had been used to facilitate reintubation, this was not required in most cases. In the original series, reintubation or tube exchange was performed in 32 (16%) of 202 cases, a rate that was very similar to that reported by others.[339] In both series, the ETVC[338] and the CAEC[339] were used primarily to maintain airway access. In the original publication, the ETVC was used for oxygen insufflation (31 patients), jet ventilation (45 patients), and post-extubation capnography (54 patients).[338]

Reintubation was successful in 20 (91%) of 22 attempts. One failure occurred with a softer prototype. The second failure resulted when an inexperienced and unsupervised operator attempted a tube exchange. Difficulty was occasionally encountered advancing the ETT through the glottis, similar to that experienced when using an FOB to intubate.[340] Tongue retraction with a laryngoscope blade should always be attempted when possible. ETT rotation or the use of an ETT such as the Parker Flex-Tip (Parker Medical, Boulder, CO) may prove useful. Because the ETVC has a relatively small OD, use of a smaller-diameter ETT is recommended.

Oxygen insufflation was achieved by connecting the male component of the ETVC to an oxygen flowmeter with 1 to 2 L/min flow rate, which was titrated to the arterial saturation. Jet ventilation is discussed later.

Complications included barotrauma, intolerance, unintended dislodgment, and tracheal perforation. Intolerance occurred in 2 of 202 patients (typically because of carinal irritation) and in 1 patient recently recovered from status asthmaticus. Intolerance should prompt reassessment of the depth of insertion. If the depth is clinically or radiographically appropriate, and the ETVC (or other AEC) continues to be required, tolerance usually can be achieved by instilling lidocaine through the device. Most patients, including those with reactive airways, have tolerated the ETVC without difficulty. Dislodgement occurred when the ETVC was inadequately secured or the patient "tongued" the catheter out. Proper fixation is essential (see Fig. 50-3). Tracheal or bronchial perforation with different instrumentation has been described.[325,326] In our case, it occurred in a patient with obstructing, proliferative tracheal papillomatosis and a chronic tracheostomy. A rigid prototype catheter was inserted alongside the tracheostomy, penetrating the posterior tracheal wall. Jet ventilation resulted in fatal barotrauma. Aspiration and laryngospasm have not been observed.

H. Exchange of Double-Lumen Tubes

Double-lumen tubes are selected for procedures requiring lung isolation. Although the resistance through a larger double-lumen tube does not preclude postoperative ventilation or weaning, it may be desirable to replace it with a single-lumen tube, particularly if care is to be transferred to an area where familiarity is lacking or ventilatory support may be prolonged. The double-lumen tube may have to be changed because of damage to a cuff or because the initial tube was an inappropriate size. Substitution can often be achieved by direct or indirect (e.g., video) laryngoscopy. While the larynx is in view, the double-lumen tube is withdrawn and immediately replaced with a single-lumen tube or replacement double-lumen tube. Occasionally, this cannot be accomplished.[341] Whether the substitution is a single- to double-, double- to single-, or double- to double-lumen tube, the requirements are similar, and the previously described tube exchangers may not be sufficiently long or firm.[342,343]

The Sheridan E.T.X. Exchanger is 100 cm long and was designed for use with the Sheri-Bronch double-lumen tube (35 to 41 F). It has one distal end hole. There are distance markings and tracheal and bronchial markings to indicate when the distal tip of the E.T.X. is at the opening of the distal lumen. This device lacks a connector for manual ventilation, and the manufacturer recommends against the use of jet ventilation.

Extra Firm with Soft Tip tube exchangers (Cook Critical Care) are available in 11- and 14-F sizes. They are 100 cm long and were designed specifically for the exchange of double-lumen tracheal tubes (designations C-CAE-11.0-100-DLT-EF ST and CAE-14.0-100-DLT-EF ST). These devices have ODs of 3.7 mm and 6.3 mm, respectively. The *soft tip* refers to the distal 7-cm segment of the catheter.

1. Visually Assisted Tube Exchange

It is difficult to imagine a safer or more secure confirmation of a tube exchange than seeing one tube replace another. This is not always possible, but it sometimes may be achieved by combining techniques, such as indirect laryngoscopy (video laryngoscopy) with a tube exchanger, thereby providing security, visual verification, and a means of correcting difficulties with tube advancement.

The recently discontinued WuScope (Achi Corp., Fremont, CA, and Asahi Optical, Tokyo, Japan) has been used to exchange double-lumen tubes and conventional ETTs in patients with difficult airways.[344-346] The WuScope provided a good glottic view in a morbidly obese patient with adult respiratory distress syndrome and permitted insertion of a suction catheter anterior to the existing nasotracheal tube. The nasotracheal tube was withdrawn, and the replacement oral ETT was easily advanced over the suction catheter with minimal interruption of mechanical ventilation. We think that a visually direct tube exchange with a WuScope, Bullard Scope (Circon, Santa Barbara, CA), Upsher UltraScope (Mercury Medical, Clearwater, FL), or video laryngoscope is preferable to blind passage of an ETT over a flexible bronchoscope or tube exchanger. A hollow tube exchanger, however, would have permitted oxygen insufflation or jet ventilation had desaturation or difficulties with tube advancement occurred. A supraglottic view (in contrast to the infraglottic view provided by a flexible bronchoscope) of the exchange enables identification and correction of an ETT impingement or the outward migration of the exchange catheter.[347]

The concept of visually direct tube exchange was assessed retrospectively in a population in whom no view of the larynx could be obtained by direct laryngoscopy.[348] Using one of three indirect laryngoscopes—the Glidescope (Verathon Medical, Bothell WA), Airtraq (Prodol Meditec, Vizcaya, Spain), or McGrath Series 5 (Aircraft Medical, Edinburgh, Scotland)—in conjunction with an AEC, 51 exchanges were performed. Four of the cases involved a double-lumen tube converted to a conventional ETT or a nasal to oral conversion. Thirty-seven patients had previously difficult intubations requiring multiple attempts or a rescue technique. Most of the patients were obese or morbidly obese and had a positive fluid balance of more than 10 L over the previous 4 days. The intention of the study was not to compare the specific devices but rather to evaluate the advantages of visually directing the tube exchange. Mort reported that this was achieved on the first attempt in 47 of 49 patients.[348] In the two failures, use of the Glidescope video laryngoscope afforded an excellent view of the AEC migrating cephalad, allowing rapid reintubation with a styletted ETT. He pointed out that had the tube exchange been performed blindly, the replacement would have failed, with potentially serious consequences. Others have made similar observations.[349,350] These findings and our personal experiences are consistent with Mort's recommendations.

2. Conversion from Nasal to Oral Intubation

Blind or bronchoscopically assisted nasal intubation is sometimes performed when oral approaches are difficult or unsuccessful. The nasal tube may have to be converted to an oral one because of complications or the intended surgery. Whenever possible, this should be done under visual control, assisted by a flexible bronchoscope,[351] rigid fiberoptic device, or video or optical laryngoscope.[344,348] The more anatomically or physiologically challenging the patient, the more compelling the case for including a tube exchanger.

Gabriel and Azocar described a patient in halo fixation in whom the connector was detached and the nasotracheal tube was advanced deeper into the trachea.[352] The tube was then grasped close to the uvula with forceps and digitally extracted through the mouth. Novella used a Sheridan T.T.X. to convert a nasal to an oral tube in a patient with Klippel-Feil syndrome who first underwent orthognathic surgery and subsequent septorhinoplasty.[353] After completion of orthognathic surgery, the T.T.X. was inserted into the nasal tracheal tube, and the latter was withdrawn. The T.T.X. was then grasped with two Magill forceps; the caudal one was used to stabilize the catheter, and the cephalad one was used to withdraw the proximal end out of the mouth. An oral tube was then railroaded over the T.T.X. Cooper described a similar maneuver in a patient in whom oral fiberoptic intubation could not be accomplished, but fiberoptic nasal intubation was achieved.[354] He passed an ETVC through the existing nasal tube and removed the latter. The ETVC was then stabilized with caudal Magill forceps and withdrawn through the mouth with the cephalad forceps. Oxygen insufflation was provided through the ETVC, which was then used to thread an oral tube into the trachea. In this case, oxygen desaturation was avoided, although the procedure was easily and quickly accomplished.

3. Conversion from Oral to Nasal Intubation

During efforts to convert from an oral to a nasal tracheal tube, Sumiyoshi and coworkers used negative-pressure ventilation during the tube exchange.[355] Their patient was in a halo and chest cast due to a cervical injury, and laryngoscopy had been unsuccessful. An attempt to introduce a 4.8-mm FOB adjacent to the existing tube (with a tube exchanger through it) was unsuccessful. A subsequent effort involved a 3.5-mm FOB and a 7-F METTRO using negative pressure to achieve ventilation. A smaller, hollow tube exchanger might have been successful and could have avoided the risk of negative-pressure pulmonary edema resulting from an ETT and FOB occupying a small glottic opening.[356] Smith and Fenner performed an oral to nasal conversion using a 4.0-mm-OD, flexible bronchoscope, which they inserted through the glottis and anterior to an oral tube.[357] The oral tube was withdrawn, and a nasal tube was advanced over the FOB. Many of the difficulties in performing a tube exchange can be avoided with the use of indirect (fiberoptic or video) laryngoscopes, ideally in combination with AECs.

4. Conversion from Supraglottic Airways to Endotracheal Tubes

A discussion of the conversion of various SGAs to ETTs is beyond the scope of this chapter, but the process is addressed elsewhere. Whenever possible, this conversion should be facilitated by visual guidance, using direct laryngoscopy or an indirect technique. These techniques include the use of a flexible bronchoscope and Aintree catheter or a video laryngoscope.[358,359]

5. Changing Tracheostomy Tubes

A tracheostomy tube may need to be replaced because of tube damage, such as cuff rupture, occlusion with secretions, or conversion to another type or size of tracheostomy tube. If the tracheostomy was recently performed, the tissue is friable. In patients in whom a false passage has been created during the original procedure, in those with poor tissue integrity, or those highly dependent on supplemental oxygen, exchanging the tracheostomy tube can be difficult and fraught with complications. The Weinmann Tracheostomy Exchange Set (Cook Critical Care) (Fig. 50-8), consists of a Ciaglia Blue Rhino tracheostomy dilator, a CAEC, Rapi-Fit adapter, and two loading dilators (26 and 28 F). The 45-cm-long exchange catheter is passed through the tracheostomy tube to be replaced; its cuff is deflated, and the tube is removed over the exchange catheter. The replacement tracheostomy

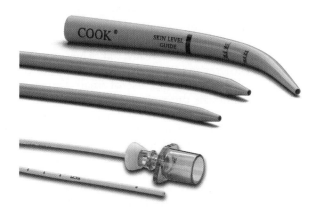

Figure 50-8 Weinmann Tracheostomy Exchange Set. (Courtesy of Cook Critical Care, Bloomington, IN.)

tube and its loading dilator are placed over the AEC, which is connected to the Rapi-Fit adapter, permitting ventilation as required. The loading catheter and tracheostomy catheter are advanced using the AEC as a guide. If stomal dilatation is required, the set is equipped with Ciglia Blue Rhino dilators (32 to 38 F).[360] The only description of this device advocates jet ventilation and high-flow oxygen insufflation. AEC insertion must be atraumatic, confirmed with a carbon dioxide (CO_2) tracing, and the depth verified to ensure it is not beyond the carina. Only the amount of oxygen (O_2) required to prevent significant oxygen desaturation should be supplied.

VII. JET VENTILATION THROUGH STYLETS

The preceding sections stressed the importance of being able to supplement oxygenation during a tube exchange. In most circumstances, a patient's oxygen content can be adequately sustained with insufflation, obviating the need for high-pressure jet ventilation. If oxygen requirements are high before a tube exchange, the equipment should be immediately available to provide jet ventilation. This equipment consists of a manually cycled, Venturi-type jet ventilator with a Luer-Lok adapter and an in-line pressure-reducing valve (see Fig. 50-8).[361] The objective of jet ventilation is to correct life-threatening hypoxemia—not to normalize arterial blood gases. Although the achievement of normal $PaCO_2$ may be attainable, the risks quite likely exceed the benefits.[343] Barotrauma has occurred through such misguided objectives, and it has been fatal in some cases.

As an example of the risks, the Chief Coroner of Ontario, Canada, investigated the death of a man who had intermaxillary fixation after orthognathic surgery. He was awake and comfortable at the conclusion of surgery. He was extubated over an AEC, through which oxygen was insufflated at 5 L/min. On arrival in the PACU, he was distressed and complained of back pain and difficulty breathing. Shortly thereafter, he had a cardiac arrest. Needle thoracentesis revealed a tension pneumothorax, and although the initial resuscitation restored a pulse, he developed hypoxic encephalopathy and died. It is unclear whether the insertion was traumatic (although the autopsy did not reveal a laceration or perforation at the distal tip location), whether the flows were at some point much higher, or whether jet ventilation had been employed at any time. The specific device, its size, and details regarding its insertion and fixation are unknown, but it is advisable to obtain a capnographic tracing before applying oxygen insufflation or jet ventilation. The lowest possible flows and driving pressures should be used.

A. In Vitro Studies

Transtracheal jet ventilation by means of an intravenous catheter or intratracheal ventilation using a stylet or tube exchanger has been advocated in the management of the "cannot intubate, cannot ventilate" patient.[5,362] The inspiratory volume depends on the driving pressure, injection time, respiratory compliance and resistance, and resistance of the tube exchanger. The latter is determined by the catheter's ID and length. The expiratory volume depends on exhalation time, elastic recoil of the lungs, and airways resistance.[361,363] Mismatch between inspiratory and expiratory volumes can have serious consequences.

In vitro studies using jet stylets have been conducted to determine flow, pressure, and entrainment characteristics. Using an in vitro model, with three sizes of Sheridan T.T.X. catheters, Dworkin and colleagues measured the inspiratory and expiratory flows resulting from a 50-psi injection as the simulated upper airway resistance, lung compliance, gas flow rate, and injection times were varied.[363] The upper airway resistance was determined by the effective tracheal diameter, which they defined as a computed difference between the OD of the T.T.X. and the tracheal diameter. They simulated upper airway obstruction by using various sizes of ETT adapters (11- to 3.5-mm ID) in the proximal airway. The gas flows through the large, medium, and small tube exchangers, when connected to a pressure source of 50 psi, were 63, 33, and 12 L/min, respectively. In their model, if the difference between the tracheal and T.T.X. diameters resulted in an effective tracheal diameter that was greater than 4 to 4.5 mm, air trapping did not occur. Because increased upper airway resistance and reduced effective tracheal diameter resulted in larger tidal volumes, they concluded that jet ventilation through a long catheter that was positioned close to the carina caused little Venturi effect or air entrainment. Placement of the catheter close to the carina may ensure a higher oxygen concentration by reducing room air entrainment, but it also increases the risk of distal catheter migration and barotrauma.

In another in vitro model, calculations based on oxygen dilution and direct measurement using a pneumotachograph revealed that air entrainment accounted for 0% to 31% of the inspired volume.[364] The largest T.T.X. and lung compliance resulted in the greatest entrainment. Gaughan and colleagues used a high driving pressure (50 psi), long inspiratory time (1 second), and brief expiratory time (1 second).[364] Even within a low-compliance system, the large T.T.X. was associated with excessive tidal volumes.

Prolonging expiratory time reduces the minute ventilation by reducing the respiratory rate. This technique still exposes the lungs to potentially injurious tidal volumes. An alternative approach is to reduce the driving pressure. Gaughan and coworkers assessed the tidal volumes and air entrainment in a model lung with a range of compliance sets ventilated by high- and low-flow regulators through 14- and 16-gauge intravenous catheters.[365] Their high-flow regulator at steady state produced flow rates of 320 L/min at 100 psi, whereas the low-flow regulator produced flows up to 15 L/min at 9 to 5 psi. Intravenous catheters, because of their short length, offer considerably less resistance to flow. Their proximity to the upper airway also results in greater air entrainment (15% to 74%). Both high- and low-flow regulators allowed adequate minute ventilation in the setting of normal tracheal and bronchial diameters and normal compliance. The investigators recommended that during transtracheal jet ventilation, when low-flow regulators were used, an inspiratory-to-expiratory (I:E) ratio of 1:1 should be used because it yields the greatest minute ventilation. Although this observation is undoubtedly true, it remains to be determined whether such high minute volumes are clinically necessary or safe.[343,361]

B. In Vivo Studies

Chang and colleagues provided intraoperative jet ventilation using a 3.5-mm chest tube as a jet catheter.[332] They ventilated with 15 psi at 10 to 16 breaths/min and continued until spontaneous ventilation was deemed adequate. The patient recovered but had a left pneumothorax that was attributed to catheter migration and unilateral ventilation. The investigators mentioned that they had encountered three cases of pneumothoraces and one pneumoperitoneum in approximately 600 similar procedures. They drew attention to the importance of catheter placement and advised that even brief airway obstruction can result in barotrauma. However, they failed to mention that vocal fold apposition occurring during recovery might promote this complication. In a subsequent paper, the same investigators stated that the jet stylet had been used for the ventilation of six patients, resulting in normocarbia and adequate ventilation.[331] Baraka described a patient with a poor laryngeal view in whom an ETT exchange was facilitated using a CAEC.[366] This was advanced until resistance was encountered. Jet ventilation at 50 psi was commenced before withdrawal of the ETT or deflation of its cuff. The result was right-chest expansion but incomplete deflation, but within three breaths, asystole was observed. A needle thoracotomy confirmed the diagnosis of tension pneumothorax, and sinus rhythm was restored.[366]

Egol and colleagues described pneumothoraces and a pneumoperitoneum in three patients using a variety of delivery devices and driving pressures.[333] They included an 18-F suction catheter at 50 psi, a nasogastric sump tube at 20 psi (inspiratory time at 30%), and a fiberoptic laryngoscope at 40 psi. They attributed the barotrauma observed to incorrect catheter placement, ventilation during phonation, and possible direct mucosal penetration from jet injection. They examined the relationship between the number of distal side holes in the tube exchanger and the pressure at the catheter tip. At any given driving pressure, the more side holes, the lower the pressure at the catheter tip. They recommended vigilance regarding the location of the catheter tip, including avoidance of direct mucosal contact and insertion into orifices where exhalation might be restricted. They advocated securing the catheter to minimize migration, use of catheters with multiple side holes, use of small-diameter jet catheters to minimize the resistance to exhalation, and use of the minimal effective driving pressure. They encouraged the development and use of an effective pressure sensor and pressure-cutoff device.

The ETVC has an end hole and eight distal side holes (see Fig. 50-7). Its use to provide jet ventilation during general anesthesia with muscle relaxation on 45 occasions was described.[338] Its attachment to a handheld jet ventilator with a pressure-reducing valve is shown in Figure 50-9. Between 1991 and 1993, Irish and coworkers

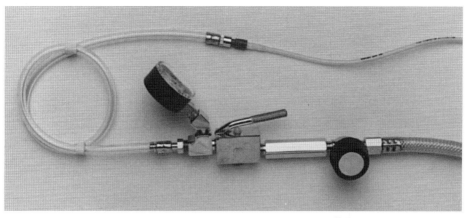

Figure 50-9   An Endotracheal Ventilation Catheter (ETVC) is connected to a handheld jet injector. The Rapi-Fit adapter or the Sheridan JETTX exchanger can be similarly attached. A pressure-reducing valve enables the operator to select a driving pressure that yields adequate chest expansion while minimizing the risk of barotrauma.

used this device with a driving pressure of 50 psi in 25 anesthetized and paralyzed patients undergoing percutaneous dilatational tracheostomies.[367] They observed barotrauma in one patient. Arterial blood gases in 12 consecutive, critically ill patients revealed a pH of 7.37 ± 0.09, $Paco_2$ of 45.5 ± 10.8, and Pao_2 of 256 ± 126 (mean ± SD). In a subsequent report, a patient ventilated for 90 minutes at only 20 psi developed a pneumothorax.[343] Chan and Manninen also described use of the ETVC to provide jet ventilation.[368] After performing a fiberoptic intubation in a patient with an unstable cervical spine, they discovered that the cuff of the ETT had been damaged. They inserted a flexible bronchoscope through the other nostril and advanced it through the vocal cords anterior to the original ETT. They then passed an ETVC through the original ETT and provided three breaths of jet ventilation at 50 psi. The patient developed a pneumothorax. Unfortunately, they used a high driving pressure through an exchange catheter that might have been too deeply inserted in the setting of near-complete glottic occlusion (i.e., partial cuff deflation, 6-mm ETT, and an FOB passing through the vocal cords).

These cases reinforce the general principles previously stated.[343,369] The need for jet ventilation should always be weighed against its possible risks. It should be immediately available and used when there is evidence of deteriorating oxygenation. If a 15-mm connector is available, capnography should be used to confirm intratracheal placement. An in-line pressure-reducing valve should be used, and ventilation should begin with the lowest pressure capable of producing adequate chest expansion. The duration of inspiration should be minimized while the duration of exhalation is determined by observing the return of the thoracic diameter to its position before inspiratory. The depth of catheter insertion should be far enough from the carina that distal migration does not occur but not so proximal that jet ventilation results in the catheter's ejection from the glottis. Multiple distal side holes can reduce catheter whip and the distal catheter pressure during jet ventilation. Every effort must be taken to minimize expiratory resistance.

VIII. CONCLUSIONS

Successful airway management does not end with tracheal intubation, any more than a safe flight is only concerned only with the take-off. Although respiratory complications are more common at extubation than during intubation, most are relatively minor and do not require reintubation. However, the need for reintubation cannot always be predicted. Reintubation may prove to be difficult and dangerous in a variety of circumstances. The ASA Task Force and the Canadian Airway Focus Group have recommended that each anesthesiologist have a preformulated strategy for extubation of the difficult airway. A risk stratification scheme can be used to identify patients for whom special extubation precautions seem to be warranted. Although many strategies are available, their benefits have not been subjected to rigorous evaluation. A reversible extubation can be performed with a tube exchanger. Use of a stylet does not guarantee that reintubation will succeed. The probability of a successful tube exchange may be enhanced if it can be performed under visual control using direct or indirect laryngoscopy. Carefully used, however, it should enhance patient safety by providing oxygen insufflation and jet ventilation while other avenues are explored.

IX. CLINICAL PEARLS

- Careful planning of tracheal extubation or tube exchange is as vital as the planning required for intubation. Airway complications are as common after tube removal as during insertion.

- Extubation carries the risk of reintubation and the risk of failed reintubation.

- Reintubation may be required because of an airway obstruction or because of failure of oxygenation, ventilation, clearance of secretions, or airway protection.

- Anticipating a successful extubation is an inexact science. Any emergent reintubation is likely to be more complex due to urgent conditions and physiologic instability.

- Reintubation may fail because of inadequate access to the airway (e.g., halo fixation, maxillomandibular fixation), preexisting anatomic features (e.g., retrognathism, prominent incisors), inadequate preparation, lack of expertise or insufficient information (e.g., emergencies), a rapidly deteriorating clinical state, or blood, secretions, or swelling obscuring the visual field.

- Many threatening circumstances can be anticipated and managed preemptively with an extubation strategy.

- Extubation strategies include deep extubation, bronchoscopic examination under anesthesia through a supraglottic airway (SGA), substitution of an endotracheal tube with an SGA, and extubation over a tube exchanger.

- The safest extubation strategy may be a surgical airway.

- A supraglottic device or tube exchanger should be left in place until it is likely that reintubation will not be required. Premature withdrawal is a common mistake.

- A reintubation strategy may include the judicious administration of oxygen by insufflation or jet ventilation; advancement of an endotracheal tube over the tube exchanger, preferably with tongue retraction; or indirect laryngoscopy.

SELECTED REFERENCES

All references can be found online at expertconsult.com.

8. Miller KA, Harkin CP, Bailey PL: Postoperative tracheal extubation. *Anesth Analg* 80:149–172, 1995.
23. Lee PJ, MacLennan A, Naughton NN, O'Reilly M: An analysis of reintubations from a quality assurance database of 152,000 cases. *J Clin Anesth* 15:575–581, 2003.
99. Francois B, Bellissant E, Gissot V, et al: 12-h pretreatment with methylprednisolone versus placebo for prevention of postextubation laryngeal oedema: A randomised double-blind trial. *Lancet* 369:1083–1089, 2007.
103. Benjamin B, Cummings CW, Fredrickson JM, et al: Laryngeal trauma from Intubation: Endoscopic evaluation and classification. In Otolaryngology: Head and neck surgery, vol 3, St. Louis, 1998, Mosby–Year Book, pp 2018–2033.
150. Kriner EJ, Shafazand S, Colice GL: The endotracheal tube cuff-leak test as a predictor for postextubation stridor. *Respir Care* 50:1632–1638, 2005.
172. Rosato L, Avenia N, Bernante P, et al: Complications of thyroid surgery: Analysis of a multicentric study on 14,934 patients operated on in Italy over 5 years. *World J Surg* 28:271–276, 2004.
270. Biro P, Rohling R, Schmid S, et al: Anesthesia in a patient with acute respiratory insufficiency due to relapsing polychondritis. *J Clin Anesth* 6:59–62, 1994.
330. Steinberg MJ, Chmiel RA: Use of a nasogastric tube as a guide for endotracheal reintubation. *J Oral Maxillofac Surg* 47:1232–1233, 1989.
342. Hannallah M: Evaluation of tracheal tube exchangers for replacement of double-lumen endobronchial tubes. *Anesthesiology* 77:609–610, 1992.
363. Dworkin R, Benumof JL, Benumof R, Karagianes TG: The effective tracheal diameter that causes air trapping during jet ventilation. *J Cardiothorac Anesth* 4:731–736, 1990.

Chapter 51

Complications of Managing the Airway

JAN-HENRIK SCHIFF | ANDREAS WALTHER | CLAUDE KRIER | CARIN A. HAGBERG

I. COMPLICATIONS IN MANAGING PATIENTS WITH DIFFICULT AIRWAYS

Difficulty in managing the airway is the most important cause of anesthesia-related morbidity and mortality. In the American Society of Anesthesiologists (ASA) Closed Claims Project, 6% of all claims concerned airway injury.[1] Difficult intubation was a factor in only 39% of airway injury claims. Eighty-seven percent of the airway injuries were temporary, and 8% resulted in death. In 21%, the standard of care was inappropriate (Table 51-1). Female patients, elective surgery, and outpatient procedures had higher rates of injury. There was no difference in ASA physical status classification and obesity among those with airway injuries during general anesthesia.

TABLE 51-1

Severity of Injury and Standard of Care

Site of Injury (N)	SEVERITY OF INJURY		STANDARD OF CARE	
	Nonfatal n (%)	Fatal n (%)	Standard n (%)	Substandard n (%)
Larynx (87)	86 (99)	1 (1)	74 (96)	3 (4)
Pharynx (51)	46 (90)	5 (10)	29 (71)	12 (29)
Esophagus (48)	39 (81)	9 (19)	25 (60)	17 (40)
Trachea (39)	33 (85)	6 (15)	20 (63)	12 (38)
TMJ (27)	27 (100)	0	21 (100)	0
Nose (13)	13 (100)	0	11 (85)	2 (15)

TMJ, Temporomandibular joint.
Modified from Domino KB, Posner KL, Caplan RA, Cheney FW: Airway injury during anesthesia: A closed claims analysis. *Anesthesiology* 91:1703, 1999.

International studies exploring the incidence of complications during general anesthesia have been published in the United Kingdom,[2,3] Australia,[4] and France.[5] The procedural problems and airway complications found in these studies are summarized in Table 51-2.

The inability to secure the airway and subsequent failure of oxygenation constitute a life-threatening complication. In absence of major oxygen (O_2) reserves, failure of oxygenation leads to hypoxia, followed by brain damage, cardiovascular breakdown, and death. As soon as oxygenation is no longer achievable, tissue damage is initiated, and irreversible injury occurs in a few minutes. The ultimate goal of airway management is oxygenation of the patient, not placement of an endotracheal tube (ETT).

Some complications are dramatic and immediately life-threatening (e.g., unrecognized esophageal intubation, tracheal rupture); some are severe and long-lasting (e.g., nerve injuries), and some are painful for the patient (e.g., sore throat). Good clinical practice aims to avoid all of these complications.

A. History of the Patient and Examination

Serious complications of airway management may result from not recognizing the level of airway difficulties. For example, it is impossible to clear an airway problem at the level of the vocal cords or the upper trachea when using a supralaryngeal airway device (SAD). These cases should be managed with endotracheal intubation or with a transglottic or transtracheal airway. Similarly,

fiberoptically guided intubation may not prove beneficial in cases of bleeding and vomiting.

To minimize injury to the patient, the anesthesiologist should examine the airway carefully, identify potential problems, devise a plan that involves the least risk for injury, and have a backup plan that can be instituted immediately if needed. Common sense should prevail at all times. Lessons learned from difficult cases should be used to modify daily practice and minimize future problems associated with airway management.

The first step in managing patients with difficult airways is to establish a specific algorithm for the anesthesia department by accepting the existing ASA algorithm or adapting it to the requirements of the specific patient population of the department. The first step in this algorithm is identification of patients with difficult airways during the preoperative examination. Most patients have the typical physical signs or history of a difficult airway and are easily identified. Although a few patients have none of these signs, they remain at risk for a difficult airway, and we should focus on them. Unfortunately, a reliable test for detecting all patients at risk does not exist. The sensitivity and specificity of all existing tests are rather low. The anesthesiologist must be alert to all possibilities, because airway difficulties may occur at any time.

All tests should be performed in a standardized manner for every patient to prevent errors in the results. Practitioners should understand the functions and limits of each test. Combinations of simple tests or the application of more complex tests may increase the predictive value

TABLE 51-2

Procedural Problems and Airway Complications Encountered During General Anesthesia

Respiration	Equipment	Drugs	Management
Difficult intubation	Substandard monitoring	Missing drugs	Insufficient training
Difficult ventilation	Defective apparatus	Mixup of drugs	No specialist on call
Failed intubation	Equipment not available	Drug overdosage	Inadequate assistance
Aspiration		Drug hangover	Insufficient diagnostic
Laryngospasm			Nonfasted patient
Bronchospasm			
Pneumothorax			
Airway trauma			
Airway obstruction			
Respiratory depression			

Data from references 2-5.

of the preanesthesia examination findings.[6,7] In uncertain cases, the preoperative evaluation of the airway can use fiberoptic devices under local anesthesia. Test and physical examination results must be documented, especially when the examiner is not the person administering anesthesia during the procedure.

B. Omission, Commission, and Communication

In anesthesia practice, errors of omission are more common than errors of commission. Errors of omission include failure to recognize the magnitude of a problem, make appropriate observations, or act in a timely manner. Errors of commission include trauma to the lips, nose, or laryngotracheal mucosa; forcing sharp instruments into areas in which they do not belong; and introducing air or secretions into regions of the body in which further complications will ensue. The primary goal of anesthesiologists is to ensure the safety and well-being of their patients, and they are usually careful in performing the technical aspects of their jobs. The most frequent cause of fatal errors in medical practice, especially in the field of airway management, is to ignore inadequate experience and skills and not call for help.

C. Planning and Scheduling

Many complications of airway management result from insufficient communication between the members of the medical team and improper coordination of patients in the operating room schedule. A patient with known difficult airway problems should be scheduled at a time when the most experienced anesthesiologists and surgeons are available. Communication among the entire staff is paramount to create optimal conditions for the patient's safety.

Delayed recognition of complications leads to delayed therapy. Inadequate monitoring, nonfunctional equipment, and untrained staff have been linked to airway catastrophes. For optimal airway management, a difficult airway cart must be available, as recommended in the ASA guidelines. The cart should include additional devices and specialized equipment for managing all airway problems.

II. COMPLICATIONS WITH SUPRALARYNGEAL AIRWAY DEVICES

A. Mask Ventilation

The difficult mask ventilation is an underestimated aspect of managing a difficult airway. Ventilation using a bag-mask breathing system is an essential task of the trained anesthesiologist, and it may be life-saving for the patient. The "cannot intubate, cannot ventilate" (CICV) scenario represents the most extreme type of airway problem.[8] Mask ventilation is used at the beginning of most cases of general anesthesia. Although the mask and the technique may seem benign, each can cause problems.

1. The Sterilization Process

Many of the devices used to ventilate the patient and secure the airway are disposable, but some equipment is reusable. All devices should be checked before use, and reusable items should be free of residual cleaning agents. Masks may have pinhole defects in their air-filled bladders, allowing air leaks or extravasation of cleaning fluid. In one case report, the fluid caused severe burning and irritation to the patient's eyes,[9] and another patient contracted chemical conjunctivitis from residual glutaraldehyde on an anesthesia mask.[10] If ethylene oxide, a common cleaning solution, adheres to reusable surfaces, it can cause serious mucosal injury. Water added to ethylene oxide forms ethylene glycol, a known irritant. Residual glutaraldehyde on an improperly rinsed laryngoscope blade caused massive tongue swelling and life-threatening allergic glossitis.[11] Care must be taken to thoroughly rinse the suction channel of a fiberoptic bronchoscope (FOB) after cleaning. Residual agents may drip out of the FOB port into the larynx or trachea, causing severe chemical burns.

2. Mechanical Difficulties

A mask is typically applied to a patient's face *before* induction of general anesthesia. Preoxygenation of the patient is the first step in securing the airway. The mask should be applied during spontaneous breathing, before drugs are given. During placement, direct contact of the rigid parts of the mask with the bridge of the nose or mandible should be avoided because they are at particular risk for compromised blood flow.[11] Bruising and soft tissue damage may occur in these regions with excessive pressure, and pressure damage to the mental nerves as they exit from the foramina has been implicated in lower lip numbness in two patients.[12] Care must be taken to avoid contact with the eyes to prevent corneal abrasions, retinal artery occlusions, and blindness. As induction proceeds, firmer mask pressure and stronger lifting pressure on the angle of the mandible become necessary to maintain a tight mask fit and secure the airway. Pressure on the soft tissue of the submandibular region may obstruct the airway, especially in small children, or it can damage the mandibular branch of the facial nerve, resulting in transient facial nerve paralysis.[13]

Occasionally, the base of the tongue may fall back into the oral pharynx during induction and obstruct the airway. Oropharyngeal airways must be gently inserted into the mouth to avoid injury, such as broken teeth or mucosal tears. Improper placement may worsen airway obstruction by forcing the tongue backward. Equal care should be given to the placement of nasopharyngeal airways to avoid bleeding and epistaxis.

Before insertion of an oropharyngeal or nasopharyngeal airway, the oropharyngeal space should be enlarged. During conventional mask ventilation, the mandible is pressed against the maxilla, blocking condylar motion and hindering sufficient mouth opening and maximal extension of the base of the tongue. The mouth is opened and the mandible gently drawn forward and upward to displace the base of the tongue to a ventral position and increase the oropharyngeal space.

The lifting pressure applied to the angle of the mandible is sometimes sufficient to subluxate the temporomandibular joint (TMJ). Patients may experience persistent pain or bruising at these points and may have chronic dislocation of the jaw, which can cause severe discomfort.

Positive airway pressure can force air into the stomach instead of the trachea, producing gastric distention, difficult ventilation, and increased likelihood of regurgitation. Cricoid pressure can help to reduce the amount of air being forced into the stomach. The ability to achieve adequate mask ventilation should be assessed preoperatively. Independent risk factors for difficult mask ventilation are the presence of a beard, increased body mass index, lack of teeth, age older than 55 years, history of snoring or sleep apnea, limited mandibular protrusion test, male gender, Mallampati class III or IV (used to predict ease of intubation), and airway masses or tumors.[14]

Other factors may make mask ventilation difficult or impossible, such as large tongues, facial burns or deformities, stridor, or nasal polyposis. In these cases, it may be best to avoid mask ventilation and perform awake fiberoptic intubation. Patients with trauma to the pharyngeal mucosa may be at risk for subcutaneous emphysema.

Laryngoceles may manifest as or cause upper airway obstruction during induction of anesthesia. Congenital factors contribute to development of laryngoceles, and persons who play wind instruments also may be at risk because high intrapharyngeal pressures can weaken soft tissue and cause laryngoceles in the lateral pharynx.[15,16]

3. Prolonged Mask Ventilation

Because mask ventilation offers no protection against silent regurgitation, the anesthesiologist should be vigilant for questionable airway noise, coughing, or bucking. Transparent masks allow visualization of the mouth and early identification of vomitus. Extra care should be taken to avoid undue pressure on vulnerable parts of the face. When continuous positive airway pressure (CPAP) is applied to patients with basilar skull fractures, pneumocephalus may occur.[17,18] At least one case report identified positive airway pressure as the cause of bilateral otorrhagia.[19]

Mask ventilation is relatively contraindicated in nonfasting patients, intestinal obstruction, head-low position, extreme obesity, tracheoesophageal fistula, and massive naso-oropharyngeal bleeding, although it may be lifesaving when other airway devices fail. Especially in pediatric cases, it may be necessary to avoid hypoxia.[20]

Adequate monitoring during mask ventilation includes observation of chest movement, pulse oximetry, measurement of end-tidal carbon dioxide (ETCO2), and breathing pressure control. In infants, a precordial placed stethoscope is recommended.

B. Laryngeal Mask Airway

The laryngeal mask airway (LMA), a device designed for upper airway management, is a cross between a face mask and an ETT. The LMA has been used in millions of patients and has been accepted as a safe technique in many types of surgical procedures. With use of the LMA,

muscle relaxation is unnecessary, laryngoscopy is avoided, and hemodynamic changes are minimized during insertion. The LMA has a clear advantage when laryngeal trauma must be minimized (e.g., in operatic singers), when a standard mask fit is impossible, and when light planes of anesthesia are desired.[21] It has proved valuable in situations in which mask ventilation is unexpectedly difficult and direct laryngoscopy impossible, and it may be used as a conduit for a fiberoptic intubation with a standard ETT.[22] Use of the device is an integral part of the ASA difficult airway algorithm.[23]

Placing the LMA correctly can be difficult in some patients. The mask may fold on itself, and pressure on the epiglottis can push the device down into the glottic opening, or the epiglottis may become entrapped in the laryngeal inlet of the mask. The tip of the epiglottis may fold into the vocal cords, increasing the work of breathing and producing coughing, laryngospasm, or complete airway obstruction. Excess lubricant can leak into the trachea, promoting coughing or laryngospasm.[24] Regardless of the problems encountered in placing the LMA, airway patency is usually maintained. An inadequate mouth opening (<1.5 cm), inadequate anesthesia depth, insertion with a not fully deflated cuff, inadequate size of LMA, inadequate force during insertion, and inadequate volumes for cuff inflation can cause malpositioning of the LMA.

Numerous complications are associated with the LMA. Perhaps the greatest limitation is the inability of the LMA to protect against pulmonary aspiration and regurgitation of gastric contents. Because the LMA does not isolate the trachea from the esophagus, its use is risky when the patient has a full stomach or when high airway pressures are necessary for positive-pressure ventilation. The overall risk of aspiration and regurgitation using the LMA seems to be in the same low range as endotracheal intubation when the indications and contraindications for the LMA are respected.[25] The risk of aspiration, which is a consequence of the device's design, should be weighed against the advantages of the LMA in cases of difficult intubation and ventilation. Other complications have been reported with the use of the LMA. Their incidence and severity depend on the user's skills and experience, depth of anesthesia, and anatomic or pathologic factors.[26]

Failure to insert the LMA results from inadequate anesthesia depth, suboptimal head and neck position, incorrect mask deflation, failure to follow the palatopharyngeal curve during insertion, inadequate depth of insertion, cricoid pressure, and oral variations such as large tonsils. Laryngeal spasm and coughing result from inadequate anesthesia depth, tip impaction against the glottis, and aspiration. Mask leaks or the inability to ventilate the lungs results from inadequate anesthesia depth, malpositioned mask, inadequate size of the mask, and high airway pressure. A displacement of the LMA after insertion is caused by inadequate anesthesia depth, a pulled or twisted tube, and inadequate mask size. Problems during recovery are removal of the LMA at an inappropriate anesthesia depth, laryngospasm and coughing when oral secretions enter the larynx after cuff deflation, tube occlusion caused by biting, and regurgitation. Effects on pharyngolaryngeal reflexes such as laryngeal spasm, coughing, gagging, bronchospasm, breath-holding, and retching may be associated with LMA use.

The incidence of sore throat with this device is between 17% and 26%.[27] The incidence of failed placement is 1% to 5%, although this rate tends to decrease with increasing operator experience.[28] The LMA cuff is permeable to nitrous oxide and carbon dioxide, which results in substantial increases in cuff pressure and volume during prolonged procedures.[29,30]

Several case reports mention edema of the epiglottis, uvula, posterior pharyngeal wall, and vocal cords; in the worst cases, these conditions have led to airway obstruction.[31-33] Nerve paralysis (i.e., lingual, recurrent, hypoglossal, and glossopharyngeal), postobstructive pulmonary edema, tongue cyanosis, and transient dysarthria have been reported. Cuff-pressure control can reduce at least some of these complications.[27,34-37] Other problems with the LMA include dislodgment, kinking, and foreign bodies in the tube, leading to airway obstruction.[38]

Newer designs of the LMA were developed to increase comfort, handling, or safety in various situations. To minimize the risk of aspiration and regurgitation, the ProSeal laryngeal mask airway (PLMA), which has an esophageal vent, was released in 2000.[39] It isolates the glottis from the upper esophagus when correctly positioned, which further protects the airway.[40,41] Some cases with gastric insufflation with a malpositioned PLMA were reported.[42,43]

The intubating laryngeal mask airway (ILMA) was designed to overcome unexpected difficult laryngoscopic intubation. Use of the ILMA has been successful in patients with difficult airways.[44,45] Tracheal intubation through the ILMA using special ETTs is easier than with the standard LMA, and the success rate for blind insertion of a tube through the ILMA is more than 90%.[46,47] Branthwaite reported a case of larynx perforation leading to mediastinitis and the patient's death.[48] Fiberoptically guided insertion of an ETT through an LMA has had the highest success rate for intubation and the lowest rate for damage of laryngeal structures.

Modifications of extraglottic airways combine features of various LMAs. For example, the LMA Supreme combines the Fastrach intubating laryngeal mask airway (ILMA-Fastrach) shape with the PLMA gastric port, resulting in a higher rate of success on first attempt at insertion and lower leak pressures, and the LMA I-Gel supraglottic airway is a single-use device without an inflatable cuff.[49,50] Other devices, such as the LMA C-Trach, use integrated fiberoptic channels to visualize the glottic region.[51] Overall rates of complications are similar to those described earlier.

Classic contraindications to using an LMA include nonfasted patients, extreme obesity, necessity of high breathing pressures (20 to 25 cm H_2O) in the presence of low pulmonary compliance or chronic obstructive pulmonary disease (COPD), acute abdomen, hiatal hernia, Zenker's diverticulum, trauma, intoxication, airway problems at the glottic or infraglottic level, and thoracic trauma. Nevertheless, the LMA's successors, particularly those with a channel for the insertion of a gastric tube, have led to more liberal use of LMA devices.[52-54]

C. Esophageal-Tracheal Combitube

The esophageal-tracheal Combitube is an esophagotracheal, double-lumen airway designed for emergency use when standard airway management measures have failed.[55,56] Use in elective surgery has been reported.[57-60]

The device is inserted blindly into the mouth and advanced to preset markings. The distal tube is usually positioned within the esophagus at this point. A distal cuff is inflated within the esophagus, and a large-volume proximal cuff is inflated inside the pharynx. Ventilation is then attempted through the esophageal tube because esophageal intubation occurs in approximately 96% of insertions. If ventilation through this lumen fails, ventilation is attempted through the tracheal lumen. The device is designed for single use, but a study of multiple uses of the Combitube found no problems with the reprocessing.[61] Another study warned against reuse because insufficient cleaning may lead to transmission of iatrogenic infections.[62]

The 37-F (small adult) Combitube is not recommended for patients shorter than 120 cm, and the 41-F Combitube is not recommended for patients shorter than 150 cm. Disregarding those recommendations may induce serious esophageal injury. Further contraindications to using a Combitube are intact gag reflexes, ingestion of caustic substances, known esophageal disease, airway problems at the glottic or infraglottic level, and latex allergy.[56]

The Combitube has major disadvantages because of its design. It can be used for a maximum of 8 hours (tracheobronchial care is difficult through the Combitube), suctioning of the trachea is not possible with the device in the esophageal position (may become problematic with copious tracheal secretions), it may injure pharyngeal and esophageal soft tissues, and no pediatric sizes are available.

Complications have been reported with use of the Combitube. In two patients, the device was inserted too far, causing the large pharyngeal cuff to lie directly over the glottis and obstruct the upper airway.[63] This was easily resolved by partially withdrawing the Combitube until breath sounds were auscultated. Tongue discoloration has been reported while the pharyngeal cuff was inflated, but it usually resolves immediately without further adverse sequelae after the cuff is deflated. The Combitube has been linked to glossopharyngeal and hypoglossal nerve dysfunction, esophageal rupture, subcutaneous emphysema, pneumomediastinum, pneumoperitoneum, and tracheal and esophageal injury and bleeding.[64-66] Esophageal lacerations were most likely caused by incorrect use; in both cases, the distal cuff was overblocked, and the larger Combitube (41 F) was used in a small patient. Despite their disadvantages, the Combitube and the EasyTube are widely accepted as devices for managing the difficult airway.

D. Other Supraglottic Airway Devices

Many devices are available for managing the airway at the supraglottic level: cuffed oropharyngeal airway (COPA), laryngeal tube (LT), LaryVent, glottic aperture seal airway (GO2 airway), Cobra perilaryngeal airway (CobraPLA), and King Laryngeal Tube Suction (LTS).[67-69] Overall, they seem to cause complications and physiologic alterations similar to those found with the LMA.[70,71] The devices were designed for separating the airway from the esophagus but do not efficiently protect the airway from regurgitation and aspiration. They share several advantages and disadvantages. Contraindications include nonfasted patients, gastroesophageal reflux, hiatal hernia, pregnancy, obesity, reduced pulmonary compliance, glottic and infraglottic stenosis, and a mechanical obstruction of the oropharynx. Most complications arise from dislodgment, overblocking the cuff, and insufficient depth of anesthesia. Most of the devices were developed in the past few years, and acceptance in routine practice has varied.

Another concern is the wide range of supraglottic devices. In addition to the limited storage space provided on the airway management cart, it seems impossible to maintain regular and sufficient training with all devices for all practitioners. Many complications in airway management are caused by operator inexperience and by inadequate or nonfunctional equipment. The recommendation for all anesthesiologists is to select a few devices that are used routinely or for which practitioners are well trained.

III. COMPLICATIONS WITH INTUBATION

A. Endotracheal Intubation

1. Anatomic Requirements

Successful oral intubation requires four anatomic traits: adequate mouth opening, sufficient pharyngeal space (determined by visualization of the hypopharynx), compliant submandibular tissue (determined by measuring the thyromental distance), and adequate atlanto-occipital extension.[72] If the patient's anatomy is compromised in any of these factors, intubation will be difficult. For optimal conditions, a free view to the vocal cords is necessary, and introduction of the ETT should be easily performed.

The opening to the airway may prove inadequate because of facial scars, TMJ disease, macroglossia, or dental disease. Nasal intubation techniques, such as blind or fiberoptic approaches, may overcome this problem. A fiberoptic technique is preferred because blind techniques are associated with a high incidence of complications.

The pharyngeal space may be limited by tumors, abscesses, edema, and surgical or traumatic disruption. If the anatomy is distorted, the anesthesiologist must optimize the view of the vocal cords. Awake intubation may be necessary, and it should be considered whenever the pharyngeal space is limited. If direct laryngoscopy is performed, the patient should be placed in the sniffing position, and a styletted ETT should be considered. Every effort—backward-upward-rightward pressure (BURP) or optimal external laryngeal manipulation (OELM)—should be made to optimize visualization and identification of the laryngeal and pharyngeal structures.[73,74]

Compliance of the submandibular space is essential to ensure that the tongue can be placed out of the way to view the glottis. Compliance may be decreased by scarring, changes caused by radiation, or localized infections. Extension of the atlanto-occipital region is necessary to lift the epiglottis off the posterior pharyngeal wall during direct laryngoscopy. A fused, fixed, or unstable spine may be rigid enough to impede visualization of the glottic structures. Awake intubation or fiberoptic techniques should be considered in these instances.

2. Laryngoscope Modifications and Rigid Optical Instruments

Laryngoscopes are designed for visualization of the vocal cords and for placement of the ETT into the trachea under direct vision. The two main types are the curved Macintosh blade and the straight blade (i.e., Miller with a curved tip and Wisconsin or Foregger with a straight tip). All blades are available in different sizes for every age of patients. The main injury caused by using laryngoscopes is damage to the teeth. In cases of inadequate visualization of the vocal cords, a change of the patient's head position may lead to success. In some cases, a blade of inadequate size is responsible for intubation failure. An external laryngeal manipulation (e.g., BURP, OELM) may move the vocal cords into the line of vision and facilitate intubation.

Obtaining a view of the vocal cords with a conventional laryngoscope requires optimal positioning of the patient. With a flexible fiberscope, positioning is not an issue, and damage to the teeth is less likely. Similarly, with innovations such as the Glidescope video laryngoscope, Airtraq laryngoscope, McGrath video laryngoscope, Pentax Airway Scope (Pentax AWS), and Truview video laryngoscope, a video image of the oropharynx and the laryngeal inlet is transmitted from the camera in the tip of the blade and allows laryngoscopy and intubation in positions other than the sniffing position. The advantages of these instruments help to reduce the number of difficult or failed intubations and the incidence of dental damage. In studies on mannequins or patients with normal airways, these devices have been evaluated as better than or equal to the Macintosh laryngoscope, and data demonstrate successful intubation of patients with known or suspected difficult airways.[75,76] Although visualization of the vocal cords has become easier, insertion of the intubation tube can be tricky. The monitor view reveals only the laryngeal inlet, and advancing the tube into the larynx may requires an introducer or a built-in guiding channel, which can make the instrument bulky and the technique more complicated than with a conventional laryngoscope. Several cases of pharyngeal injuries have been reported with the rigid stylet of the Glidescope.[77] Increased awareness of potential complications, better training and supervision, and appropriate equipment and patient selection can reduce the incidence of complications.

Laryngoscopy requires deep anesthesia because it causes strong stimulation of physiologic reflexes, and respiratory, cardiovascular, and neurologic adverse effects are possible.[78] Hypertensive patients, pregnant patients with hypertension, and patients with ischemic heart disease are particularly at risk. Deep anesthesia, application of topical anesthetics, prevention of the sympathoadrenal response with drugs such as atropine or intravenous lidocaine, and minimizing mechanical stimulation can attenuate the adverse effects.

Laryngoscopes have been modified to optimize visualization of the vocal cords. The Corazelli-London and McCoy-Mirakuhr flexible-tip blades may achieve a better view of the glottis by drawing the epiglottis up.[79]

Rigid optical instruments such as the Bonfils retromolar intubation fiberscope and its modifications,[80] the Bullard laryngoscope, and the intubation tracheoscope[81] are not commonly used in anesthesiology. They require skilled handling, and experience should be gained in routine cases to apply to difficult airway situations. The rigid intubation tracheoscope, a familiar device in ear, nose, and throat surgery, has special indications and may be useful in the hands of anesthesiologists. Available in two sizes (child and adult), it consists of a battery-filled handle and a straight, rigid tube with a connection to a breathing bag or circuit. The rigid tracheoscope is useful for tumors, scars, and abscesses in the oropharynx, base of the tongue, and larynx and for aspirated foreign bodies.

The disadvantages of these instruments are a relatively closed view through the tube, a high risk of damage to the teeth and laryngeal structures, possible perforation of the hypopharynx, and risk of aspiration. High-flow oxygen insufflation through a port induced subcutaneous cervical and facial emphysema in one patient.[82]

3. Difficult Intubation

Despite optimal positioning of the head and neck, the glottis is sometimes impossible to visualize, even in patients without obvious predisposing features.[83-85] Risk factors for difficult tracheal intubation include male sex, age between 40 and 59 years, and obesity.[72] Anesthesiologists should be aware of the potential for a difficult intubation in the following circumstances:

- Posterior depth of the mandible greater than 2.7 cm (which limits submandibular displacement of the soft tissues)
- Anterior depth of the mandible greater than 4.8 cm
- Correlation between effective length of the mandible and a posterior depth less than 3.6
- Distance between the occiput and spinous process of C1 of about 2.6 mm
- Distance between the spinous processes of C1 and C2 of about 2.6 mm (which narrows the limits of head extension)
- Longer maxilla with protruding teeth
- Caudally positioned hyoid bone (increasing the mandible-hyoid distance)
- More rostrally positioned angle of the mandible (a phenotypical receding mandible)[83,86-89]

A chin-to-thyroid cartilage distance of less than three finger breadths (about 7 cm) hampers visualization of the glottis.[90] A combination of tests may increase the predictive value of the preanesthesia examination results.[6,7] Causes for difficulty in securing the airway are shown in Box 51-1.[25,91] Computerized analysis of facial structure provides an accurate approach to predicting difficult

Box 51-1	Miscellaneous Causes of Difficult Securing of the Airway

Symptoms

Dumpling voice
Hoarseness
Pathologic respiratory sound
Foreign body feeling
Odynophagia

Constitutional Factors

Mouth opening <3 cm
Microstomia
Dental abnormalities
Macroglossia
Receding mandible
Obesity
Buffalo neck
Moon face
Beard

Diseases

Limited temporomandibular joint mobility
Limited atlanto-occipital and atlantoaxial joint mobility
Unstable cervical spine
Limited laryngeal mobility
Postoperative or post-traumatic rigidity of the soft tissue of mouth and neck
Congenital, postoperative, post-traumatic anomalies of face and neck
Abscesses and tumors in face and neck
Paradontosis
Phlegmon of the floor of the mouth and of the neck
Epiglottitis
Mediastinitis
Stenosis of the upper airway
Enlarged goiter

Modified from Krier C, Georgi R: Airway management: Is there more than one "gold standard"? *Anasthesiol Intensivmed Notfallmed Schmerzther* 36:193–194, 2001.

intubation.[92] Patients who proved difficult to intubate should be told about it and given written documentation so that they can notify future anesthesiologists. Patients should be registered with the MedicAlert Foundation.

4. Nasotracheal Passage

a. CRANIAL INTUBATION

Nasotracheal intubations are potentially hazardous. In patients with basilar skull fractures or certain facial fractures (e.g., LeFort II or III fractures), the ETT may be inadvertently introduced into the cranial vault (Fig. 51-1).[93] Fractures of the frontal part of the skull base with cerebrospinal rhinorrhea, intranasal abscesses or abscesses with intranasal expansion, choanal atresia, hyperplastic tonsils, tendency to uncontrollable nasal bleeding, and coagulopathies are considered contraindications to nasotracheal intubation. In a case of nasotracheal intubation, asystole occurred after the tube was introduced into the orbit.[94] However, if care is taken, the complication rates of oral and nasal intubation are not different.[95] Nasal intubation in a patient with a known or suspected skull

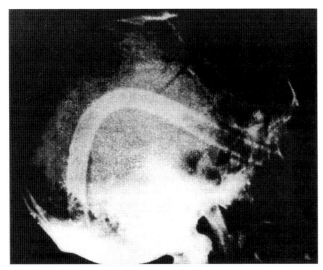

Figure 51-1 Intracranial nasotracheal tube (computer enhanced). (From Horellou MF, Mathe D, Feiss P: A hazard of naso-tracheal intubation. *Anaesthesia* 33:73, 1978.)

fracture should be performed only by using fiberoptic bronchoscopy and with extreme caution in the inferior nasal meatus. For midfacial fractures with intact dura mater, it is possible to open the dura by manipulation during nasotracheal intubation.

b. NASAL INJURY

Nasotracheal intubation may be problematic in the presence of hypertrophic turbinates, extreme deviation of the nasal septum, prominences on the nasal septum, chronic infections in the nasal cavity, and nasal polyposis. Minor bruising occurs in 54% of nasal intubations and most commonly involves the mucosa overlying the inferior turbinate and the adjacent septum.[96] If epistaxis occurs, the ETT cuff should be inflated and remain in the nostril to tamponade the bleeding.

The nasal mucosa must be vasoconstricted before instrumentation.[97] Some agents used for this purpose are 0.5% phenylephrine in 4% lidocaine or 0.1% xylometazoline. A 4% solution of cocaine may be associated with severe adverse effects and is no longer recommended for vasoconstriction. The risk of nasal injury can be minimized with the use of a small, well-lubricated ETT with a flexible tip that has been soaked in warm water.[98]

Possible complications of nasotracheal intubation are dislodgment of nasal polyps,[88] dislodgment of nasal turbinates,[99,100] adenoidectomy, injury of the nasal septum, perforation of the piriform sinus, and the epiglottic vallecula. In case of injury to the piriform sinus, the internal branch of the superior laryngeal nerve, soft tissue of the pharynx, the larynx, and the superior laryngeal vessels may be damaged. Tears in the pharyngeal mucosa can mature into retropharyngeal abscesses.[101] Nasotracheal tubes may dissect and run behind the posterior pharyngeal wall. Patients with an obstructed nasal passage due to convoluted turbinates are at increased risk for this complication. One case of external compression of the nasotracheal tube due to the displaced bony fragments of multiple Le Fort fractures was reported.[102]

Delayed complications of nasotracheal intubation include pharyngitis, rhinitis, and synechia between the nasal septum and inferior turbinate bone. After the tube is secured in the trachea, ensure that it is also secured properly at the level of the nostril. Distortion of the nares can lead to ischemia, skin necrosis, or nasal adhesions.

Even without gross trauma, mechanical damage to the superficial epithelial layers caused by nasal intubation results in mucociliary slowing in 65% of patients and bacteremia in another 5.5%.[103,104] The most common organisms introduced into the blood are nasopharyngeal commensal organisms (e.g., *Streptococcus viridans*), which can cause endocarditis and systemic infection. Even short-term intubation has caused nasal septal and retropharyngeal abscesses. Acute otitis media has occurred in 13% of nasally intubated neonates.[105] Paranasal sinusitis has been reported, most commonly occurring with nasal intubation for more than 5 days.[106,107] Infection may be related to sustained edema and occlusion of the sinus drainage pathways. Prompt diagnosis is critical, and paranasal sinusitis should be suspected in any patient with facial tenderness, pain, or purulent nasal discharge or in any nasally intubated patient who develops sepsis with no other obvious source. A careful examination of the patient is necessary, but the success of a previous cosmetic operation should not be endangered. The nasal structures must be checked again postoperatively.

c. FOREIGN BODIES

The nostrils are common sites for entry of foreign bodies. Small children, known for placing small objects into their orifices, find the nostrils one of the most accessible sites. More than 80% of patients who aspirated a foreign body are children, and most were between 1 and 3 years old.[108-110] Foreign body aspiration is the cause of death of 7% of children younger than 4 years.

Smith and colleagues reported a rhinolith that was dislodged during nasotracheal intubation.[111] The mass had formed around the rubber tire of a toy car that the patient had placed in his nose 30 years earlier. Nasotracheal intubation can dislodge similar foreign bodies that may obstruct the ETT, pharynx, or trachea. If a nasal foreign body is known or suspected, it should be gently dislodged, advanced into the oral pharynx, and retrieved before intubation. Mask ventilation may also dislodge foreign bodies to the lower parts of the airway.

5. Traumatic Intubation

Difficult intubations often are traumatic intubations. In a case of difficult intubation, the practitioner tends to increase the lifting forces of the laryngoscope blade, which may damage the intraoral tissues and osseous structures. When the operator continues to intubate the patient many times without changing his approach or technique, difficult intubation is changing to traumatic intubation. Use of increasing forces causes swelling, bleeding, or perforation, and the intubation becomes more and more difficult. It may end in a CICV situation. We recommend a maximum of three attempts to achieve intubation using a laryngoscope. If intubation fails after three attempts, another airway-securing technique should be used following the airway management algorithm.

a. LIP TRAUMA

Lip injuries, which are typically found on the right upper lip, include lacerations, hematomas, edema, and teeth marks. They are usually caused by inattentive laryngoscopy performed by inexperienced practitioners, the laryngoscope blade, and the teeth. Although these lesions are annoying to the patient, they are usually self-limited.

b. DENTAL TRAUMA

The incidence of dental injuries associated with anesthesia is greater than 1 case in 4500 procedures.[112] Maxillary central incisors are most at risk; 50% of these injuries happen during laryngoscopy, 23% after extubation, 8% during extubation, and 5% in the context of regional anesthesia. Dental injuries are also associated with the use of LMAs and oropharyngeal airways. With insufficient anesthesia, depth biting against the tube is possible. Dental injuries are most common in small children, patients with periodontal disease (in which structural support is poor) or fixed dental work (e.g., bridges, capped teeth), protrusion of the upper incisors (i.e., overbite), carious teeth, and cases of difficult intubation. Preexisting dental pathology should be explored, and all loose, diseased, chipped, or capped teeth must be documented in the chart before anesthesia induction and intubation.[113] The patient must be advised of the risk of dental damage. Tooth guards may be used, but they can be awkward and obstruct vision,[114] although the time for intubation is not significantly longer.[115]

Fragments of chipped or partially broken teeth and completely avulsed teeth should be located and retrieved. Care should be taken to ensure that no foreign bodies slip into the pharynx to later become lodged in the esophagus or the larynx. Avulsed teeth should be saved in a moist gauze or in normal saline without cleaning them. Tooth aspiration may cause serious complications requiring rigid or flexible bronchoscopy for removal. With a rapid response from an oral surgeon or a dentist, an intact tooth often can be reimplanted and saved. The optimal time is within the first hour; thereafter, reimplantation success diminishes with increasing time.[116]

c. TONGUE INJURY

Massive tongue swelling, or macroglossia, has been reported in adult and pediatric patients.[117,118] Some cases occurred while a bite block was in place, some happened with an oral airway and soft tissue compression of the chin, and some occurred with no protective device. The common denominator was that they all occurred when there was substantial neck flexion during endotracheal intubation and surgery was prolonged. Macroglossia results from obstructed venous and lymphatic drainage of the tongue, and it has been associated with angiotensin-converting enzyme inhibitors.[119] In each case, the ETT might have severely compromised the circulation on the affected side of the tongue. One report described the sudden onset of tongue swelling after prolonged surgery to repair a cleft palate,[120] during which the tongue was retracted extensively. Obstruction of the submandibular duct by an ETT may lead to massive tongue swelling.[121] Reduced sense of taste, cyanosis, or loss of tongue sensation is possible after compression of the lingual nerve or by lingual artery compression during forced intubation or associated with an oversized, malpositioned, or overinflated LMA.

d. DAMAGE TO THE UVULA

Uvula trauma is usually associated with the use of ETTs, oropharyngeal and nasopharyngeal airways, LMAs,[122] or Combitubes and with overzealous blind use of a suction catheter.[123] The results of damaging the uvula are edema and necrosis.[124] Sore throat, odynophagia, painful swallowing, coughing, foreign body sensation, and serious life-threatening airway obstruction are reported.[125]

e. PHARYNGEAL MUCOSAL DAMAGE

A postoperative sore throat (POST) likely represents a broad constellation of signs and symptoms. The incidence of POST after intubation is higher than POST after LMA use and after face mask ventilation.[126,127] The incidence of sore throat associated with the use of the Combitube was 48%.[128] Aggressive suctioning is probably a mitigating factor. The incidence is substantially higher in women and in patients undergoing thyroid surgery. No correlation was seen with factors such as age, use of muscle relaxants, type of narcotic used, number of intubation attempts, or duration of intubation. Small tube and cuff size and topical treatment and inhalation of steroids have a positive impact on POST.[129] However, pain on swallowing usually lasts no more than 24 to 48 hours and can be relieved in part by having the patient breathe humidified air.

f. LARYNGEAL TRAUMA AND DAMAGE TO THE VOCAL CORDS

Trauma to the larynx may occur after endotracheal intubation. It depends on the intubator's skill and the degree of difficulty. In one large study, 6.2% of patients sustained severe lesions, 4.5% had hematoma of the vocal cords, 1% had hematoma of the supraglottic region, and 1% sustained lacerations and scars of the vocal cord mucosa.[130] Recovery typically is prompt with conservative therapy.[131] Hoarseness may appear 2 weeks postoperatively.[132]

Granulations usually occur as a complication of long-term intubation. However, a small but significant number of patients sustain laryngeal injuries during short-term intubation.[133] Intubation can cause various degrees of laryngeal trauma, including thickening, edema, erythema, hematoma, and granuloma of the vocal folds.[134,135] Injuries of the laryngeal muscles and suspensory ligaments are possible. The larynx should be inspected for injury before insertion of the ETT to document and treat preexistent lesions. Anesthesiologists should be vigilant in all cases of hoarseness, and patients should be examined by an otorhinolaryngologist preoperatively.

Arytenoid dislocation and subluxation have been reported as a rare complication of intubation.[136] Mitigating factors include traumatic and difficult intubations, repeated attempts at intubation, and attempted intubation using blind techniques such as light-guided intubation,[137] retrograde intubation, and use of the McCoy laryngoscope.[138] Early diagnosis and conservative or operative treatment are necessary,[139] because fibrosis with subsequent malpositioning and ankylosis may occur after 48 hours.

The vocal process of the arytenoid is the most common site of injury by the ETT because it is positioned between the vocal cords. Granuloma formation most commonly occurs at this site. The degree of injury worsens with increasing tube size and duration of intubation.[140]

Many investigators have reported unilateral or bilateral vocal cord paralysis after intubation, which is usually temporary.[141-144] One report associated vocal cord paralysis with use of ethylene oxide to sterilize ETTs.[145] Hoarseness occurs with unilateral paralysis, whereas respiratory obstruction occurs with bilateral problems. The most likely source of injury is an ETT cuff malpositioned in the subglottic larynx with pressure on the recurrent laryngeal nerve.[142,143] Permanent voice change after intubation because of external laryngeal nerve trauma has been reported in up to 3% of patients undergoing surgery at sites other than the head or neck. The incidence may be decreased by avoiding overinflation of the ETT cuff and by placing the ETT at least 15 mm below the vocal cords.[142] Eroded vocal cords may adhere to one another, eventually forming synechiae. This is a potential problem when airflow between the vocal cords has been compromised as a result of tracheostomy.[146] Surgical correction is usually necessary.

g. TRACHEOBRONCHIAL TRAUMA

Tracheal trauma has many causes.[147] Injury may result from an overinflated ETT cuff, inadequate tube size, or malpositioned tube tip, laryngoscope, stylet, tube exchanger, or related equipment. Predisposing factors include anatomic difficulties; blind or hurried intubation; inadequate positioning; poor visualization; and most commonly, inexperience of the intubator. The presence of an ETT may lead to edema, desquamation, inflammation, and ulceration of the airway.[148] The severity of the injury may be related to the duration of intubation, although this relationship is not well established.[149] Any irritating stimulus, such as pressure from an oversized ETT, dry inhaled gases, allergic reactions to inhaled sprays, or chemical irritation from residual cleaning solutions, can initiate an inflammatory response and cause mucosal edema in the larynx or trachea. Edema after extubation limits the lumen diameter and increases airway resistance. Small children are most susceptible to this problem, in which a sudden increase in airway resistance results from laryngotracheobronchitis or croup. Almost 4% of children 1 to 3 years old develop croup after tracheal intubation.[150,151] Mechanical trauma may result from sharp objects within the trachea, such as a stylet tip that extends beyond the length of the ETT. Tracheal ruptures, especially after emergency intubation, were reported.[152] One case of a bronchial rupture caused by an ETT exchanger was reported.[153]

ETT cuffs inflated to a pressure greater than that of the capillary perfusion may devitalize the tracheal mucosa, leading to ulceration, necrosis, and loss of structural integrity.[154] Ulceration can occur at even lower pressures in hypotensive patients. The need for increasing cuff volumes to maintain a seal is an ominous sign that heralds tracheomalacia.[155] Massive gastric distention in an intubated patient may signal the presence of a tracheoesophageal fistula as the cuff progressively erodes into the

esophagus.[156] Any patient with more than 10 mL of blood in the ETT without a known cause should be assessed for a tracheocarotid fistula.[157] The various nerves in this region of the neck are also at risk. Erosion of the ETT into the paratracheal nerves may result in dysphonia, hoarseness, and laryngeal incompetence. Tracheomalacia results from erosion confined to the tracheal cartilages. The anesthesiologist must inflate the ETT cuff only as much as necessary to ensure an adequate airway seal. When nitrous oxide is used during a lengthy surgical procedure, the pressure in the cuff should be checked by a cuff pressure control device. In the presence of 70% nitrous oxide, intracuff pressures take an average of 12 minutes to increase to levels that are potentially high enough to cause tracheal ischemia.[154] The cuff pressure should not exceed 25 cm H_2O. Increasing cuff pressure caused by surgical manipulations can be observed and prevented by using a cuff pressure control device.

Tracheal intubation may erode the tracheal mucosa, leading to scar tissue, which ultimately retracts and leads to stenoses of the trachea, larynx, or nares. The reported incidence of granulomas is 1 case in every 800 to 20,000 intubations.[158,159] They are more common in women than in men and occur rarely in children. The most common site of erosion is along the posterior laryngeal wall, where granulation tissue easily overgrows. Side effects of granulomas include cough, hoarseness, and throat pain. The growths may be prevented by minimizing the trauma associated with laryngoscopy and intubation. When granulomas occur, surgical excision is usually required.

Membranes and webs may eventually replace tracheal and laryngeal ulcers. These growths are commonly thick and gray. Care should be taken while intubating patients with these lesions because inadvertent detachment may result in respiratory obstruction or bleeding into the airway. With time, the inflammatory process associated with laryngeal ulcers may extend to the laryngeal cartilage. If this occurs, the cartilage may become inflamed (i.e., chondritis) or softened (i.e., chondromalacia).

Several months after prolonged tracheal intubation, tracheal stenosis and fibrosis may occur. This usually represents the end stage of a progression from tracheal wall erosion to cartilaginous weakening to healing with fibrosis.[147] Stenoses typically occur at the site of an inflated cuff, although they may occur at the ETT tip. Symptoms include a nonproductive cough, dyspnea, and signs of respiratory obstruction. Dilation of the stenosis is curative in its early stages. However, surgical correction may be necessary after the tracheal lumen has been reduced to 4 to 5 mm.[160,161]

Supraglottic complications induced by long-term intubation may be prevented by early tracheostomy. There is no evidence supporting an ideal time for tracheostomy in long-term ventilated patients.

h. BAROTRAUMA

Barotrauma results from high-pressure distention of intrapulmonary structures. High-flow insufflation techniques in which small catheters are used distal to the larynx are most often associated with barotrauma. These problems are common in microlaryngeal surgery when jet ventilation is used.[162-166] Direct impingement of the catheter tip on the tracheal mucosa may also cause barotrauma.[164] Edema or hematoma may occur if the jet of air strikes the mucosa of the larynx or the vocal cords, leading to laryngospasm. When air leaks into the peribronchial tissues, it can traverse into the subcutaneous space, the lung interstitium, or the pleural and pericardial cavities. Pneumomediastinum or tension pneumothorax and possibly tamponade are the results, and chest tubes may be necessary. Progressive accumulation of air may cause loss of pulmonary compliance, loss of ventilatory volume, or if the accumulation is large enough, overdistension of lung tissue with cardiopulmonary compromise and, finally, impossible ventilation. Safety mechanisms should be in place to prevent high-pressure airflow in the event that intrapulmonary pressures become excessive. For diseased pulmonary tissue, the least possible airway pressure should be used to prevent parenchymal blowout. This advice also applies to patients with blunt thoracic trauma who have subcutaneous emphysema. They should be presumed to have a bronchial leak unless proved otherwise. Barotrauma may also result from upper airway obstruction during jet ventilation.[167]

i. NERVE INJURIES

Laryngoscopy and cuffed supraglottic airway devices may cause periodic or permanent nerve injury. Lingual, recurrent, hypoglossal, and glossopharyngeal nerve paralysis have been described for LMA devices, and neuropraxia with weakness, numbness, or paralysis of the tongue can occur after laryngoscopy.[34] After damage to the internal branch of the superior laryngeal nerve during a difficult intubation, two patients had signs of aspiration.[168]

Malposition of the cuff or tube may be one reason for this rare damage. Ahmad and Yentis postulated that lingual nerve injury may occur where the nerve distal to its gingival branch is compressed by the LMA tubing against the side of the tongue.[169] In addition to the cases previously described, we observed one case of permanent anosmia after nasotracheal intubation with no pathologic findings.

j. SPINAL CORD AND VERTEBRAL COLUMN INJURY

Airway managing techniques such as chin lift, jaw thrust, and direct laryngoscopy transmit movement to the cervical spine. When a patient's neck is fused, adequate neck extension may be impossible to obtain. Attempting to hyperextend the necks of these patients may result in cervical fractures and quadriplegia.[170] A head that is fixated in a cervical collar or halo does not allow neck extension and limits the successful use of direct laryngoscopy. Using a fiberoptic device to assist intubation should be considered in these cases. If immediate intubation is necessary, patients with an acute fracture of the back and neck may be supported by in-line cervical stabilization during careful intubation while protecting the head against excessive movement and fixing it in a safe position by a second person.[171] C1 and C2 fractures seem to be particularly vulnerable because any degree of extension may compromise spinal cord function. Between 10% and 25% of spinal cord injuries occur because of improper immobilization of the vertebral column after trauma, and neurologic deterioration was

associated with direct laryngoscopy in a patient with a cervical spine injury.[172-175]

Several conditions, such as Down syndrome and rheumatoid arthritis, are associated with atlantoaxial instability.[176,177] Excessive neck extension in a patient with an undiagnosed Arnold-Chiari malformation may cause worsening of cerebellar tonsil herniation.[178] Patients with underlying diseases such as connective tissue disorders, lytic bone tumors, and osteoporosis should be intubated carefully, and extreme neck extension should be avoided in every patient because of loss of muscle tone by curarizing drugs. A range-of-motion test and an assessment of neck extension should be performed before inducing anesthesia. A case of quadriplegia after bag-ventilation, direct laryngoscopy, and cricothyrotomy in a patient with an unrecognized cervical spine injury was reported.[175] Hastings found in a review of records of 150 patients with unstable cervical spine injury a 1.3% incidence of neurologic deterioration after elective surgery with tracheal intubation. Inadequate airway management may result in disaster of permanent spinal cord injury. Awake fiberoptic intubation should be considered when neck extension cannot be achieved without the risk of damage and time is not crucial. It is considered the safest method for airway management in patients with cervical spine injury, followed by LMA and the Combitube.[171]

k. EYE INJURIES

The ASA Closed Claims Project reported that the eye injuries were responsible for 3% of all claims; of these, 35% were related to corneal injuries, with corneal abrasions being the most common eye complication.[179] They are primarily caused by a face mask being placed on an open eye or by the eyelids not being completely closed during anesthesia.[180,181] Jewelry, identification cards, and loose-fitting watch bands have been implicated in scratching the eyeball.[182] A stethoscope hanging from the neck of a clinician can fall forward and strike the patient's eyes or forehead. Prevention consists of vigilance on the part of the anesthesiologist and application of adhesive tape over the closed eyelids. Especially during head and neck surgery, the eyelids should be taped closed, and the eyes should be covered carefully with soft eyepads.[183] Some clinicians routinely apply lubricating ointment to the inside of the eyelids, although this has not been proved to increase efficacy.

Although these injuries typically heal within 24 hours, they are usually painful and can lead to corneal ulceration. An immediate ophthalmologic consultation is recommended. Local anesthetics should not be applied because they can delay regeneration of the epithelium and may promote keratitis. Treatment consists of allowing the injured eye to rest by use of an eye patch and applying an antibiotic ointment.

l. TEMPOROMANDIBULAR JOINT INJURIES

TMJ anatomy is special in that one side cannot be moved without the other side. Both joints represent a functional unit, and injuries to one TMJ affect the other side. Opening the mouth is a combination of rotary and translational movement in the joint. The rotary movement allows only a mouth opening of about 25 mm; the

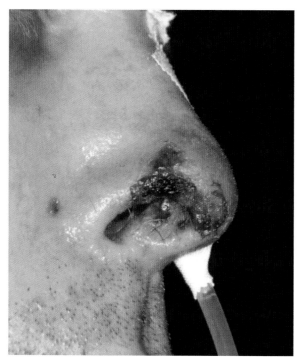

Figure 51-2 Necrosis of right nasal wing after 3 days of intubation with an anatomic, preformed tube.

maximal opening is achieved by the translational movement. Pathologic changes such as bone cysts, rheumatid arthritis, and atrophy of the mandible due to age can reduce the joint mobility and may lead to fractures. Rupture of the lateral ligament is possible. TMJ injuries are caused by increasing forces during laryngoscopy to optimize the view of the vocal cords. Limited mouth opening, pain in the joint, lateral deviation of the mandible (e.g., unilateral luxation), protrusion of the mandible (e.g., bilateral luxation), and lockjaw (e.g., fixation after joint luxation) may occur. Most reported cases of TMJ injury were not associated with difficult airway.[184]

m. DAMAGE TO THE NOSE

Some injuries to the nose and endonasal structures were described previously. Using anatomically preformed tubes for head and neck surgery or compression of the nasal wing may lead to necrosis in the worse cases (Fig. 51-2). Wrapping the tube with foam material at the nasal wing level and careful nursing in cases of long-term intubation may reduce or avoid this complication.

6. Esophageal Intubation

a. ENDOTRACHEAL TUBE PLACEMENT

When visualization of the glottis is difficult, the ETT may inadvertently be introduced into the esophagus. Esophageal intubation is more common among inexperienced practitioners, but it may also occur in the hands of experienced stuff members. Intubating the esophagus is not disastrous, but failing to detect and correct the condition is. Recognition of this error must be rapid to avoid the adverse effects of prolonged hypoxia. A closed claims analysis of adverse anesthesia events reported that 18%

of respiratory-related claims involved esophageal intubation.[185] Preoxygenation can help alleviate this problem by allowing a longer apneic period for tracheal intubation and by delaying the onset of hypoxemia. End-tidal CO_2 capnography is essential in confirming endotracheal placement of the tube. Capnography should be available wherever intubation is performed. In out-of-hospital practice and emergency medicine, where capnography may not be available, calorimetric single-use CO_2 detectors or an esophageal detector device can help to identify failed intubation in 94.6%.[186] Esophageal intubation can briefly produce an end-tidal CO_2 capnogram (e.g., in presence of CO_2-containing drinks in the stomach), but the waveform diminishes rapidly after three to five breaths.[187,188] Fiberoptic control is another safe way to confirm the correct position of the tube. Other signs, such as equal bilateral breath sounds, symmetrical bilateral chest wall movement, epigastric auscultation and observation, and tube condensation, are potentially misleading.[189] A misplaced tube should remain in place while the trachea is correctly intubated. This helps to identify the correct orifice for intubation and protects the trachea from invasion by regurgitated stomach contents. Once proper endotracheal intubation is achieved after an esophageal intubation, the stomach should be suctioned to minimize vomiting, gastric perforation, or compromise of ventilation.

b. ESOPHAGEAL PERFORATION AND RETROPHARYNGEAL ABSCESS

Perforation of the esophagus has been reported on several occasions.[190-198] It seems most likely to occur when inexperienced clinicians handle emergency situations, when intubation is difficult, or in presence of esophageal pathology. Perforation occurs most commonly over the cricopharyngeus muscle on the posterior esophageal wall, where the esophagus is narrow and thin. Subcutaneous emphysema, pneumothorax, fever, cellulitis, cyanosis, throat pain, mediastinitis, empyema, pericarditis, and death can occur. Early detection and treatment of the condition are critical because the mortality rate of mediastinitis is more than 50%. An esophageal perforation should be suspected in any patient with a fever, sore throat, and subcutaneous emphysema after a difficult intubation.

A case report identified a traumatic tracheal perforation through the esophagus in a patient with a difficult intubation.[199] Cases of esophageal perforation have been associated with the use of an esophageal-tracheal Combitube.[65,66]

7. Bronchial Intubation

a. USE OF AN ENDOTRACHEAL TUBE

Bronchial intubation is common and sometimes difficult to identify. Asymmetrical chest expansion, unilateral absence of breath sounds (especially on the left side), and eventual arterial blood gas abnormalities are diagnostic features. Bronchial intubation (preferentially right-sided) is more common in newborns and children, because of the small distance between the carina and the glottis. The position of the tip of the tube should be carefully

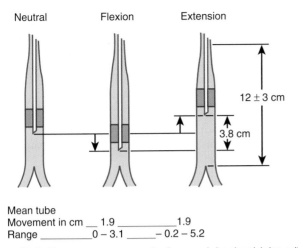

Neutral   Flexion   Extension

12 ± 3 cm

3.8 cm

Mean tube
Movement in cm __ 1.9 _____ 1.9
Range _____ 0 – 3.1 _____ – 0.2 – 5.2

Figure 51-3 The mean movement of an endotracheal tube with flexion and extension of the neck from a neutral position. The mean tube movement between flexion and extension is one third to one fourth of the length of a normal adult trachea (12 ± 3 cm). (From Conrardy PA, Goodman LR, Lainge F, et al: Alteration of endotracheal tube position: Flexion and extension of the neck. *Crit Care Med* 4:8, 1976.)

monitored in children. If bronchial intubation goes undetected, it may lead to atelectasis, hypoxia, and pulmonary edema.[200] Transillumination of the neck with a lightwand can assist in tube location,[201] although not in cases of obesity and large goiter. Fiberoptic control is the best tool to detect proper position of the tube. The ETT may be deliberately advanced into a main stem bronchus and withdrawn until bilateral breath sounds are auscultated.

The tip of the ETT may move between 3.8 and 6.4 cm during flexion or extension of the patient's head as the patient is positioned for surgery (Fig. 51-3).[202] It is easy to remember that the tip of the ETT moves in the same direction as the patient's nose. If the patient's neck is flexed, the nose is pointed downward, and the ETT advances farther into the trachea. The tube moves away from the carina an average of 0.7 cm during lateral rotation of the head. Care should be taken in case of cleft palate surgery or tonsillectomy. Special blades used by the surgeon to achieve a direct view may move the ETT forward during positioning the blade. A stethoscope placed on the left chest helps to identify an endobronchial tube that is being displaced.

When inadvertent bronchial intubation is discovered, the tube should be withdrawn several centimeters and the lungs inflated sufficiently to expand any atelectatic areas. In cases of chronic atelectasis, bronchoscopy may be required to remove mucous plugs. This problem can be avoided by measuring the length of the ETT alongside the patient before intubation. The tip of the tube should ideally be at least 2 cm above the carina, which may be approximated at the sternal angle (of Louis) adjacent to the junction of the sternum with the second rib. Appropriate orotracheal tube depths are 21 cm from the teeth in adult women and 23 cm in adult men, and nasotracheal tube depths are 25 cm in women and 27 cm in men from the nares.[203]

b. USE OF A DOUBLE-LUMEN TUBE

Safe limits for the placement of double-lumen tubes have been outlined by Benumof and colleagues.[204] Modern FOBs have removed the guesswork surrounding endotracheal-bronchial tube tip location. The double-lumen tube may be inserted blindly into the appropriate bronchus, followed by bronchoscopic confirmation of its position, or the bronchoscope may be inserted initially and used as a stylet over which the double-lumen tube is advanced. Fiberoptic bronchoscopy significantly reduces malposition of the double-lumen tube, and its routine use is recommended after intubation, changing patient's position, increasing ventilation pressure, and irregular auscultation sounds. However, even in the best of hands, tracheobronchial injuries occur.[205] Bronchial rupture is a serious complication that requires immediate attention. Using double-lumen tubes that are too large may be the cause of bronchial trauma.[206] The 37- to 39-F double-lumen tubes are recommended for women, and the 39- to 41-F tubes are recommended for men.

B. Maintenance of the Endotracheal Tube

1. Airway Obstruction

A patent airway is an absolute requirement for safe anesthesia. Airway obstruction can occur at any time during administration of general anesthesia, particularly in prolonged operations or in patients with predisposing anatomic abnormalities. Airway obstruction should be considered when an intubated patient has diminished breath sounds associated with increasing peak inspiratory pressures. Obstruction can result from diverse factors,[207] including a sharp bend or kink in the ETT, a tube that has been bitten closed, or a tube that is obstructed with mucus, blood, foreign bodies, or lubricant.[208,209] The ETT may become warm with continued use during prolonged procedures; under these circumstances, the tube may kink and become obstructed. Many clinicians mistakenly treat the patient for bronchospasm when the turbulent air movement comes from the ETT, not from the patient. At least two cases have been reported in which the plastic coating on a stylet sheared off and occluded the lumen of an ETT.[210,211] In another case, a tube was obstructed by the prominent knuckle of an aortic arch.[212] Nitrous oxide can cause expansion of gas bubbles trapped in the walls of an ETT, leading to airway obstruction.[213]

The cuff of an ETT can cause airway obstruction. An overinflated cuff may compress the bevel of the ETT against the tracheal wall, occluding its tip.[214] The cuff may also herniate over the tip of the tube and cause an obstruction.[215] When faced with any of these problems, the best solution is to pass a suction catheter or an FOB down the lumen of the ETT and attempt to clear it. If the tube is totally obstructed, passage of a stylet may be tried. Total obstruction that cannot be remedied quickly requires removal of the tube, and the patient should be reintubated as rapidly as possible. The ETT and connecting hoses should be supported and, if necessary, taped to prevent kinking caused by their own weight. Inspiratory gases should be humidified during long anesthesia to prevent tube obstruction from dried secretions.

Unusual causes of airway obstruction have been reported. In two patients, complete airway obstruction occurred secondary to achalasia and esophageal dilation.[216,217] Two cases of tension hydrothorax that caused airway obstruction during laparoscopic surgery have been reported. The first patient had malignant ascites that, when combined with a pneumoperitoneum, led to a rapid accumulation of pleural fluid with respiratory and cardiovascular compromise.[218] The second case occurred during operative hysteroscopy when a large volume of glycine was absorbed through opened myometrial vessels under high intraabdominal pressure.[219] In each case, more than 1.5 L of clear fluid was drained once chest tubes were placed.

2. Disconnection and Dislodgment

A common and serious complication of tracheal intubation is disconnection of the ETT from the remainder of the anesthesia circuit. This was identified as the most common critical incident in a study of anesthesia-related human errors and equipment failures.[220] A trained anesthesiologist usually identifies this problem immediately. The low-pressure alarm sounds first, and the patient's breath sounds become absent. However, if the ventilator continues to function normally, the physician may be unaware of the nature of the problem. Disconnections are most likely to occur if the connections are made of dissimilar materials, if the patient's head is turned away from the anesthesiologist, or if the airway connections are hidden beneath the surgical drapes. Alarms to signal airway disconnection are included on all modern anesthesia machines, and their signals should be taken seriously.

Connections between the ETT and the breathing circuit should be checked and reinforced at the outset, before the anesthesiologist loses visual control of the airway. There should be no tension on the connections from the weight of the corrugated tubing or the drapes on the tubing. Members of the surgical team should be discouraged from inadvertently leaning on any portion of the breathing circuit. The exact site of disconnection should be ascertained rapidly by checking each connection, beginning at the patient's airway and moving proximally back to the machine.[221] Nonetheless, the anesthesiologist must have a prearranged plan in mind in the event that an airway is inadvertently disconnected or dislodged during surgery.

3. Circuit Leaks

Leaks in an air delivery circuit can cause hypoventilation and dilution of the inspired gases by entry of room air into the system. With an ascending bellows system, such as that found in newer models of anesthesia machines, the bellows do not rise completely during exhalation if there is a leak. This situation indicates that the circuit leak exceeds the inflow of fresh gas. Older machines with a descending bellows system do not provide such a visual clue and appear to function normally. The anesthesiologist should be vigilant at all times for signs of a circuit leak. The inspired oxygen concentration measured at the gas sampling port is reduced because of dilution with room air, and the partial pressure of end-tidal CO_2

increases. Cyanosis, decreased oxygen saturation (SpO_2), or hypertension and tachycardia associated with hypercapnia may be the presenting signs, although each of these is typically a late finding.

Mnemonics such as COVER ABCD–A SWIFT CHECK may help to diagnose and treat the conditions[222]:

C   Circulation, capnograph, and color (saturation)
O   Oxygen supply and oxygen analyzer
V   Ventilation of intubated patient and vaporizers (include analyzers)
E   Endotracheal tube (position, orientation, and patency) and eliminate machine problems
R   Review monitors and equipment
A   Airway (with face or laryngeal mask)
B   Breathing (with spontaneous ventilation)
C   Circulation (in detail)
D   Drugs (consider all given or not given)
A   Awareness of air and allergy
SWIFT CHECK of patient, surgeon, process, and responses

4. Laser Fires

Lasers are frequently used in the operating room to ablate benign and neoplastic tissues in the airway. The use of special laser-guarded or metal tubes is recommended, and all inflammatory materials such as prosthetic teeth and nasogastric tubes should be removed. One of the most catastrophic events associated with their use is an airway fire, which occurs when the laser ignites the ETT.[223-225] The risk that a laser beam will contact the wall of an ETT is $1:2$.[226] Perforation of the tube may occur and produce a blowtorch-like flame. Oxygen-rich inspired gas concentrations fuel brisk ignition of the plastic in the ETT and can fuel a fire in both directions. The ETT acts as a blowtorch; the fire is fed by the combustible walls of the tube and is intensified by the high rate of oxygen flow. The heat and fumes of the burning plastic may cause severe damage to the airway. Treatment consists of immediately disconnecting the circuit from the ETT and removing the burning tube from the airway. If the tube is not burning or if complete loss of the airway may occur with removal of the tube, leaving the tube in situ should be considered. The fire should be extinguished with saline, and the patient should be supported by face mask ventilation. The airway should be evaluated for damage with bronchoscopy, and the appropriate supportive respiratory care should be given.

Many precautions can reduce the risk for an airway fire. If possible, placement of an ETT may be avoided altogether if air can be delivered through a ventilating laryngoscope, a jet ventilation system, or by intermittent apneic ventilation.[227] If a tracheostomy tube is in place, ventilation may occur distal to the site of laser surgery. The choice of laser tubes should be consistent with the type of laser used. Blocking cuffs are particularly vulnerable to the laser beam. Covering the tube with saline-soaked gauze or noncombustible tape, using a positive end-expiratory pressure (PEEP) of 5 to 10 cm H_2O to prevent aspiration of material in case of cuff puncture, and filling the cuff with saline to act as extinguisher in the event of puncture are measures that can protect the patient's airway.[228,229] Placing a dye, such as methylene blue, in the saline can further alert the anesthesiologist, because in the event of a fire, a stream that is the color of the dye will be emitted.

Nitrous oxide should be avoided because it supports combustion. Oxygen concentrations should never exceed 40% for the same reason.[230,231]

C. Special Techniques

1. Fiberoptic Intubation

Fiberoptic intubation is the method of choice in all cases of anticipated difficult airway. It combines direct vision with flexibility to view the pharynx when direct laryngoscopy is considered difficult or impossible. Use of the FOB is not a quick technique, and it probably should not be considered when speed is required. Although the device can be used in many different situations involving airway management and preoperative evaluation of critical patients, it also has several limitations and potential complications.

Intubation with an FOB should not be attempted when the pharynx is filled with blood or saliva, when inadequate space exists within the oral cavity to identify pharyngeal structures, or when time is critical and creating a surgical airway is the priority. Relative contraindications include marked tissue edema, distortion of the oropharyngeal anatomy, narrowed nasal passages, soft tissue traction, and a severe cervical flexion deformity. Operator experience with the technique and proper preparation are essential. Connecting the device to a video system can help with guidance by a more experienced bystander particularly in training situations.[232]

Potential complications associated with the FOB include bleeding, epistaxis (especially if a nasal airway is attempted), laryngotracheal trauma, laryngospasm, bronchospasm, and aspiration of blood, saliva, or gastric contents. Another possible hazard is associated with the practice of insufflating oxygen through the suction channel. Although this technique can help to keep the tip of the bronchoscope clean and provide for a high volume of forced inspiratory oxygen, it can also cause high-pressure submucosal injection of oxygen if the tip cuts into the pharyngeal mucosa. If this sequence occurs, the result may be pronounced subcutaneous emphysema of the pharynx, face, and periorbital regions.[233]

2. Lighted Stylets

The lighted stylet may be used to facilitate intubation under local and general anesthesia. A light at the tip of a flexible stylet is used to transilluminate the soft tissues of the pharynx. The device can be used blindly or as an aid when direct laryngoscopy is difficult. It may also confirm that the tip of an ETT is still within the cervical trachea and establish that the tube has not been advanced too far.[234]

Because use of the lighted stylet is a blind technique, the pharyngeal pathologic condition cannot be visualized or avoided. This method should not be used in patients with suspected abnormalities of the upper airway, such as tumors, polyps, infections (e.g., epiglottitis, retropharyngeal abscess), trauma, or foreign bodies. The lighted stylet should be used with caution in patients in whom transillumination of the anterior neck is limited, such those with dark skin pigmentation, morbid obesity, limited neck mobility, a large tongue, and a long epiglottis. If placement of the stylet is difficult, the anesthesiologist should consider abandoning the technique for fear of worsening a pathologic process.

Several real and potential complications have been reported with the use of this device. Sore throat, hoarseness, mucosal damage, and arytenoid subluxation are possible. Several cases have been reported in which the light fell off of the end of the stylet. In another instance, the protective tubing was not removed from the stylet and had the potential to become dislodged within the trachea. Heat damage to the tracheal mucosa in prolonged intubation is a potential risk with inappropriate handling. To avoid heat damage, the Trachlight's bulb flashes on and off after 30 seconds.[235]

Recommendation for use in emergency cases cannot be given because the risk of regurgitation is high, cricoid pressure may affect the ease of intubation, and in some cases, more than one attempt is necessary. The transillumination technique is not suitable for verification of the ETT's position because of misinterpretations.

3. Submandibular and Submental Approach for Tracheal Intubation

The oral route for tracheal intubation can interfere with some maxillofacial surgical procedures, and the nasal route can be contraindicated or impossible. Nasotracheal intubation is contraindicated in patients with fractures in the cribriform plate of the ethmoid, which frequently accompany Le Fort II and III maxillary fractures, because of the potential complications of infection and the possibility of cranial intubation. Tracheostomy is the usual solution in these circumstances, but it also carries complications. An alternative method is to introduce the tracheal tube through a submental or a submandibular incision, bypassing the surgical area and avoiding the complications of tracheostomy. Damage to adjacent structures with bleeding, tube displacement, aspiration, and hypoxia when passing the tube through a submental excision and infections have been reported.[236,237]

IV. COMPLICATIONS WITH INFRAGLOTTIC PROCEDURES

Infraglottic airway access is the last step in the ASA airway management algorithm. When tracheal intubation is impossible, a patient's airway is compromised, and the patient's condition deteriorates into a CICV situation threatening brain damage or death, life-saving steps must be undertaken immediately. There are no contraindications for infraglottic procedures in these critical situations. The most severe complication is failure to establish an airway before damage or death occurs. Complications arise because the decision to progress to a surgical airway is not made soon enough or because the procedure is performed too slowly. In all cases of difficult airway, the practitioner should evaluate the possibility of an infraglottic airway access. Difficult anatomic situations, marked scars, abscesses, and morbid obesity may limit infraglottic access techniques.

Infraglottic airway techniques are suitable for emergency situations, and they are indicated for oxygenation and ventilation of anesthetized patients. Surgical procedures of the upper airway, laryngeal surgery, and diagnostic procedures have been successfully managed with this technique.

A. Translaryngeal Airway

1. Retrograde Wire Intubation

Retrograde wire intubation is an excellent technique for securing a difficult airway. It can be used when anatomic limitations obscure the glottic opening. Because the technique is blind, it is important to exercise caution and not worsen any preexisting conditions. The technique has variations, such as using the FOB by passing the wire through the suction channel or through a tube exchanger.[238]

Although simple in concept, the basic technique has numerous problems and potential complications. The procedure takes some time to perform and should not be considered under emergency circumstances unless the practitioner is very experienced. The tip of the ETT has been known to get caught on the glottic structures. The problem may be alleviated somewhat by using a tapered dilator inside the ETT or by using an epidural catheter as the wire to assist with passing the ETT through the glottis. Bleeding may occur at the site of the tracheal puncture in quantities sufficient to cause a tracheal clot or airway obstruction. Cases of severe hemoptysis with resultant hypoxia, cardiopulmonary arrest, arrhythmias, and death after retrograde wire intubation have been reported.[239-242] Subcutaneous emphysema localized to the area of the transtracheal needle puncture is common but usually self-limited. In severe cases, the air may track back through the fascial planes of the neck, leading to tracheal compression with resultant airway compromise, pneumomediastinum, and pneumothorax.[243,244] Laryngospasm may result from irritation by the retrograde wire unless the vocal cords are anesthetized or relaxed. Other, less common complications include esophageal perforations, tracheal hematoma, laryngeal edema, infections, tracheitis, tracheal fistulas, trigeminal nerve injury, and vocal cord damage.[245,246] The complications reported with retrograde wire intubation were most often associated with multiple attempts, large-gauge needles, and untrained staff members in emergency settings.[247]

2. Cricothyrotomy

Two methods are described: the surgical cricothyrotomy (using a scalpel) and the needle cricothyrotomy (using a needle set). In both procedures, the cricothyroid membrane must be perforated. Acute complications include bleeding (especially during surgical cricothyrotomy), misplacement of the tube (especially after needle cricothyrotomy), failure of airway access, wound infection, displaced cartilage fractures, and laryngotracheal separation.[248] Other complications include breaking and bending of the needle, subcutaneous emphysema, pneumothorax, pneumomediastinum, and pneumopericardium.

When cricothyrotomy is performed in the case of total upper airway obstruction, barotrauma may occur because of expiratory blockade.

Granulation tissue around the tracheostomy site, subglottic stenosis, massive laryngeal mucosa trauma, endolaryngeal hematoma and laceration, vocal cord paralysis, hoarseness, and thyroid cartilage fracture with dysphasia are direct long-term complications. Indirect long-term complications include brain damage or mental impairment due to hypoxia when the cricothyrotomy takes more than 2 to 3 minutes.

Every emergency translaryngeal airway should be changed to a formal tracheostomy as soon as possible. Subglottic stenosis is a delayed complication, especially in children.

B. Transtracheal Airway

1. Transtracheal Jet Ventilation

One emergency method is transtracheal jet ventilation (TTJV), which is accomplished by introducing a small, percutaneous catheter into the trachea and insufflating the respiratory tract with high-pressure oxygen over a jet ventilator or a hand jet device (e.g., VBM Manujet). Although this technique may be helpful in critical situations, life-threatening problems are associated with it.

To accomplish TTJV, a long, large-bore catheter is advanced through the cricothyroid membrane into the trachea. If this catheter is displaced from the trachea, subcutaneous emphysema, hypoventilation, pneumomediastinum, pneumothorax, severe abdominal distention, or death may result.[164] On the basis of normal skin compliance, a 4-inch catheter may be pulled into the subcutaneous space by applying traction to its proximal end. The hub of the TTJV catheter must be continuously pressed firmly against the skin.

Barotrauma is a potential complication of TTJV.[249,250] Oxygen delivered through a transtracheal catheter must be able to escape the lungs freely, or overdistention and pulmonary rupture may occur.[251,252] Any changes in breath sounds, chest wall expansion, or hemodynamics should be considered to result from pneumothorax. In cases of total airway obstruction, the risk for pneumothorax is greatly increased because gas cannot escape from the lungs in a normal manner. Strong consideration should be given to placing a second transtracheal egress catheter in these circumstances. Laryngospasm can impede the outward flow of oxygen from the trachea. It should be prevented by providing adequate local anesthesia to the neighboring structures or by relaxing the patient.[250] If the larynx is obstructed by a foreign body, only low-flow oxygen should be delivered until safe egress of gas is established. Inadvertent placement of a gas delivery line into the gastrointestinal tract may result in complications and may cause gastric rupture, esophageal perforation, bleeding, hematoma, and hemoptysis.[253,254]

Damage to the tracheal mucosa may occur in patients who are managed with long-term TTJV, especially if the gas is not humidified.[255] The possibility of tracheal mucosal ulceration should be considered in any patient if nonhumidified TTJV is attempted through single-orifice catheters for a prolonged period.

2. Percutaneous Dilatational Tracheostomy

Percutaneous dilatational tracheostomy is not primarily recommended for emergency use. With further development, these insertion techniques became faster and appeared to be suitable for emergency situations in skilled hands.[256-260] Different sets are available.

Bleeding, subcutaneous and mediastinal emphysema, pneumothorax, airway obstruction, aspiration, infection, and death are early complications. Accidental extubation is a serious complication, because replacement of the cannula may be impossible. In this situation, orotracheal intubation or a translaryngeal oxygenation is required.[261] Bacteremia also has been reported.[262]

Delayed complications include tracheal stenosis, scars, hoarseness, and tracheoesophageal and tracheocutaneous fistulas. The incidence of injury for percutaneous dilatational tracheostomy is 2%, which is lower than for formal tracheostomy.

3. Formal Tracheostomy

A formal tracheostomy is rarely recommended in emergency situations. Various types of instruments, assistance, and sterile conditions are required, and the tracheostomy should be performed only by a trained surgeon.

Bleeding is a complication of all surgical procedures, including airway access procedures. Minitracheostomy occasionally results in excessive bleeding into the airway, necessitating progression to full surgical tracheostomy.[263] The inflated cuff used in formal tracheostomy prevents pulmonary aspiration of blood. In rare cases, the innominate artery can rupture into the trachea because of excessive pressure from the tracheostomy tube, with resultant massive hemorrhage into the airway. Air embolism during operative procedure is possible.

If an air leak occurs and the cervical skin has healed around the tracheostomy tube, air can escape into the subcutaneous spaces of the neck, resulting in subcutaneous emphysema. If the condition goes unrecognized and the patient is maintained on high-pressure mechanical ventilation, the air may track to other locations. Air escaping into the paratracheal spaces can result in a pneumomediastinum. Air released into the pleural cavity can result in a tension pneumothorax.

Tracheal stenosis is a complication of long-term tracheostomy. A tracheostomy tube can cause tracheal erosion, particularly into the esophagus (i.e., tracheoesophageal fistula) or the brachiocephalic artery. These tubes typically sit low in the trachea and are designed with a fixed curve. Tube pressure can damage the skin at the insertion site.

Accidental extubation and dislodgment of the cannula occurs occasionally, most often in the early postoperative period. If the cannula is inadvertently removed from a fresh tracheostomy, it should be replaced as quickly as possible. Infection, mediastinal sepsis, tracheal stenosis, and tracheomalacia are rare late complications.

V. PHYSIOLOGIC RESPONSES

The larynx has the greatest afferent nerve supply of the airway. Airway reflexes are important in protection of the airway. They must be suppressed for stress-free airway management, especially for endotracheal intubation. Intensive autonomic response may occur during placement, maintenance, and removal of all airway management devices.

A. Hemodynamic Changes

Direct laryngoscopy and tracheal intubation are potent stimuli that may instigate an intense autonomic response.[264,265] Tachycardia, hypertension, arrhythmias, bronchospasm, and bronchorrhea are common; hypotension and bradycardia occur less often. Patients with preexisting hypertension are even more at risk when they are under stress.

Oczenski and colleagues showed that the insertion of a Combitube was associated with a significantly higher and longer-lasting increase in systolic, diastolic, and mean arterial pressure; heart rate; and plasma catecholamine concentration compared with insertion of a LMA and laryngoscopic endotracheal intubation (Fig. 51-4).[266] Hemodynamic and catecholamine responses to insertion of an LMA are minimal.[267,268] The apparently sympathetically mediated responses to mechanical stimulation of larynx, trachea-carina, and bronchi may be completely or partially blocked by topical or intravenous lidocaine.[269] The magnitude of stimuli to the upper airway depends on the number of attempts and the duration of intubation. In cases of difficult airway situations a higher increase of hemodynamic responses is anticipated. The hemodynamic response may also be blunted by giving opioids or short-acting selective β_1-blockers before laryngoscopy and intubation.[270] Because many patients have coexisting cardiovascular disease and cannot meet increased myocardial oxygen demands, large hemodynamic responses must be prevented. More than 11% of patients with myocardial disease develop some degree of myocardial ischemia during intubation.[271] The key is to provide an adequate depth of anesthesia with intravenous or inhalational agents before instrumentation of the airway.

Fiberoptic intubation performed under sufficient local anesthesia and conscious sedation is an appropriate technique to prevent major hemodynamic changes during intubation. Minor hemodynamic changes and minor increases of plasma catecholamine concentration are nevertheless apparent in this technique. Fiberoptic intubation using a special mask adapter shows fewer hemodynamic changes than those caused by laryngoscopy after induction of anesthesia. The lowest cardiovascular responses were documented in patients after insertion of an LMA.[272]

B. Laryngospasm

Laryngospasm is a protective reflex mediated by the vagus nerve. This reflex is an attempt to prevent aspiration of foreign bodies into the trachea. It may be provoked by movement of the cervical spine, pain, vocal cord irritation by secretions, or sudden stimulation while the patient is still in a light plane of anesthesia.[273]

In some cases of laryngospasm, the patient makes respiratory efforts but cannot move air in or out of the

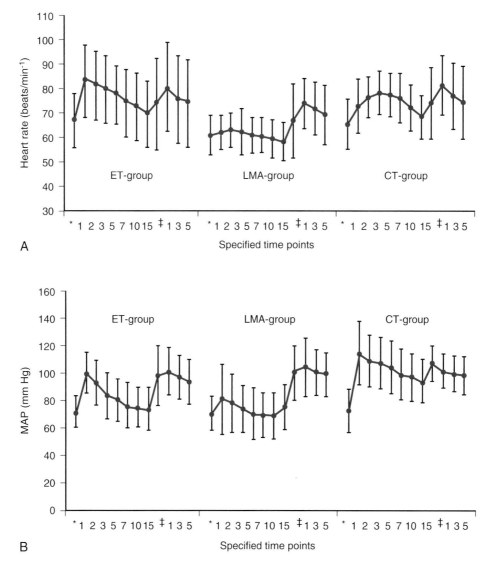

*(Baseline): immediately before intubation/insertion of the airway
‡Immediately before extubation/removal of the airway

Figure 51-4 **A** and **B,** Heart rate and mean arterial blood pressure *(MAP)* at specified times (mean ± SD, *n* = 73) during insertion of the endotracheal tube *(ET),* laryngeal mask airway *(LMA),* and Combitube *(CT).* (From Oczenski W, Krenn H, Dahaba AA, et al: Hemodynamic and catecholamine stress responses to insertion of the Combitube, laryngeal mask airway or tracheal intubation. *Anesth Analg* 88:1389, 1999.)

lungs. If direct laryngoscopy was performed, the vocal cords would be completely adducted. However, laryngospasm involves more than spastic closure of the vocal cords. An infolding of the arytenoids and the aryepiglottic folds occurs; these structures are subsequently covered by the epiglottis.[274] Malpositioning, incorrect insertion of an LMA, secretions or blood in the airway, and inadequate depth of anesthesia during intubation or extubation of the LMA or tracheal tube may induce laryngospasm. It may also occur during fiberoptic intubation performed in unanesthetized or subanesthetized laryngeal structures. A firm jaw thrust can sometimes break the spasm—the hyoid is elevated, thereby stretching the epiglottis and aryepiglottic folds to open the forced closure.

The stimulus should be removed, a change of airway should be considered, and secretions should be suctioned away. Positive mask pressure with 100% oxygen may help by distending the pharynx or vocal cords, but this technique is not always adequate. Gentle chest compression in children may also help.[275] Deepening the anesthesia with small doses of propofol (0.25 to 0.8 mg/kg given intravenously can treat laryngospasm in 76.9%) or treatment with a short-acting muscle relaxant (0.1 to 3 mg/kg of succinylcholine) are the most promising ways to break the spasm.[276]

C. Bronchospasm

Tracheal irritation from the ETT can cause bronchospasm that is sufficiently severe to prevent air movement throughout the lungs.[277] Approximately 80% of the measurable resistance to airflow occurs in the large central airways; the remaining 20% occurs in the smaller peripheral bronchioles.[278] The incidence of intraoperative bronchospasm is almost 9% with endotracheal intubation, 0,13% with an LMA, but almost 0% with mask ventilation.[279,280] Poor correlation is seen with age, sex, duration or severity of reactive airway disease, duration of anesthesia, or the forced expiratory volume in 1 second.[279] Other factors that may contribute to bronchospasm include inhaled stimulants, release of allergic mediators, viral infections, exercise, or pharmacologic factors (including beta-blockers, prostaglandin inhibitors, and anticholinesterases). Bronchospasm may occur during fiberoptic intubation if parts of subglottic airway are insufficiently anesthetized. The spasm can be treated with inhalation of epinephrine or isoproterenol or a β_2-agonist (e.g., albuterol, metaproterenol, or terbutaline) or by deepening the level of a volatile anesthetic.

D. Coughing and Bucking

Two additional adverse responses to intubation are coughing and bucking on the ETT.[281] These responses are potentially hazardous in cases of increased intracranial pressure,[282] intracranial vascular anomalies, open-globe injuries, or ophthalmologic surgery or in cases in which increased intra-abdominal pressure may rupture an abdominal incision.[283] Intubating a patient only when an adequate depth of anesthesia has been achieved helps to prevent this reflex.

Coughing and bucking occur less frequently with the LMA. However, in the case of lubricant globules on the anterior surface of the cuff, light anesthesia, and malpositioning, they may be observed.

E. Vomiting, Regurgitation, and Aspiration

The overall incidence of aspiration during general anesthesia has been reported as 1 in 2131 procedures (in Sweden) to 1 in 14,150 procedures (in France). The incidence in the United States was 1 in 3216 procedures. The associated mortality rate was 1 in 71,829 cases in the United States.[284] A meta-analysis of 547 publications concerning use of the LMA suggested that the overall incidence of pulmonary aspiration was about 2 in 10,000 cases.[285]

The ETT and Combitube are most effective in preventing pulmonary aspiration. To reduce the risk of pulmonary aspiration, some airway management devices, such as the ProSeal-LMA and the Laryngeal Tube S, were redesigned.

In any patient considered to have a full stomach, the likelihood of vomiting in response to irritation of the airway is increased, and aspiration of stomach contents is a constant concern. Aspiration leads to coughing, laryngospasm, and bronchospasm, assuming that protective reflexes are intact. Hypertonia, bradycardia, asystole, and hypoxia may occur. The magnitude of pulmonary reactions depends on the type and quantity of the aspirated material.[286]

The Sellick maneuver, or cricoid pressure (CP), is controversial. Although some strongly endorse the technique and trust its effectiveness, others think that CP should be abandoned because it adds to patients' risks with no evidence of gained benefit. Other practitioners apply CP because they think it is a low-risk technique that may work in some patients. The future of CP use lies in the answer to the question of whether it is effective in preventing regurgitation or an unnecessary hazard. Because aspiration is a rare event, a study to confirm the preventive effect of CP may not be feasible.

It is possible to completely obstruct the airway with CP. CP has resulted in airway obstruction in patients with lingual tonsils, lingual thyroid glands,[287] and undiagnosed laryngeal trauma.[288] If any doubt exists about the success of an oral intubation, awake techniques should be considered under these circumstances.[289]

F. Intraocular Pressure Changes

Intraocular pressure increases during direct laryngoscopy and extubation, but not during LMA insertion.[290,291] Decreased intraocular pressure was observed under tracheal intubation during general anesthesia with propofol and with sevoflurane, both combined with remifentanil.[292]

Sufentanil is effective in preventing intraocular pressure increases caused by rapid-sequence induction with succinylcholine; alternatively rocuronium can be used.[293] Increased intraocular pressure should be strictly avoided in patients with penetrating eye injuries.

G. Intracranial Pressure Changes

Intracranial pressure markedly and transiently rises during laryngoscopy and endotracheal intubation. Patients with head injury are at risk from this increase because it reduces cerebral perfusion and may increase the likelihood of secondary brain damage.[294] Fiberoptic bronchoscopy produces a substantial but transient increase of intracranial pressure.[295] Deep anesthesia during induction can prevent these adverse effects.

H. Apnea

Apnea may be a reflex response to tracheal irritation from the ETT or other airway techniques. Extraneous reasons for the apnea—for example, if the patient is a premature or term neonate,[296] has had induction drugs or excessive narcotics, or has a reflux response to light levels of anesthesia—should be ruled out initially. If no clear reason exists for the patient's lack of respiratory effort, mechanical ventilation can be initiated, and spontaneous ventilation can be attempted later.

I. Latex Allergy

Of anaphylaxis episodes occurring during surgical procedures, 16.6% are related to latex allergies.[297] To prevent anaphylaxis during anesthesia and surgery, the patient's history should be evaluated preoperatively. There is no therapy for latex allergy, and avoidance of latex-containing products is mandatory for predisposed individuals.[298] Latex allergy affects 8% of the U.S. general population and has a prevalence of 30% among health care workers.[299,300] There has been an increase in the incidence of type I and IV latex sensitivity in the general population, from 1% in 1980 to 8% in 1996.[301] The prevalence

Box 51-2 Pathophysiologic Effects of Tracheal Extubation

Primary Local Effects

Airway
  Obstruction
  Coughing
  Breath-holding
  Damage to the vocal cords
  Arytenoid dislocation/luxation

Primary Systemic Effects

Cardiovascular System
  Tachycardia
  Increased systemic arterial pressure
  Increased pulmonary arterial pressure

Secondary Effects

Central Nervous System
  Increased intracranial pressure
Eyes
  Increased intraocular pressure

Modified from Hartley M: Difficulties in tracheal extubation. In Latto IP, Vaughan RS, editors: *Difficulties in tracheal intubation*, London, 1997, Saunders.

of latex sensitivity among anesthesiologists is about 12.5%, and the prevalence of allergy is 2.4%.[302]

Patients with spina bifida, rubber industry workers, atopic patients, and patients with a history of many operations are most at risk.[303] Patients with certain exotic food allergies may also have a coexisting latex allergy[304]; in one study, the rate was 86%.[305]

Patients with type I hypersensitivity are at risk for anaphylaxis with hypotension, rash, and bronchospasm. Type I hypersensitivity symptoms are localized contact urticaria with pruritus and edema. Generalized reactions are rash or hives, tearing, rhinitis, hoarseness, dyspnea, nausea, vomiting, bronchospasm, abdominal cramping, and diarrhea.

Contamination with latex during anesthesia is possible through direct contact by face mask, endotracheal and gastric tubes, gloves, syringes, and electrodes; through inhalation from contaminated circuits and room air; and through the parenteral path with latex-containing intravenous administration sets.

Most airway management devices are available as latex-free products. The oropharyngeal cuff of the Combitube contains latex; therefore, it is contraindicated in patients with known latex allergy. All anesthesiology departments should have a special latex-safe cart with all medical supplies and devices.

VI. COMPLICATIONS WITH EXTUBATION

Primary and secondary responses to extubation are possible. The primary effects are local and systemic responses (Box 51-2). The same responses after intubation may be observed at extubation. During intubation, the patient is more protected by anesthesia induction than during extubation, and the cardiovascular responses may be even more exaggerated. The most serious complication after extubation is acute airway obstruction. Decreased consciousness with central respiratory depression, decreased muscle tone, and tongue retraction to the postpharyngeal wall may lead to inspiratory or expiratory stridor, dyspnea, cyanosis, tachycardia, hypertension, agitation, and sweating. Laryngospasm is also possible, and urgent treatment is necessary to prevent hypoxia, brain damage, and death. Other complications after extubation are not caused by the removal of the tube itself; they are consequences of the previous intubation and the duration of tube placement, such as laryngitis, edema, ulcerations, granuloma, or synechia of the vocal cords. The quality of tracheal intubation contributes to laryngeal morbidity, and excellent conditions are less frequently associated with postoperative hoarseness and vocal cord sequelae.

A. Hemodynamic Changes

Hemodynamic changes, including a 20% increase in heart rate and blood pressure, occur in most patients at the time of extubation,[306,307] and symptoms that are associated with sympathoadrenal activity should be expected. These changes are usually transient and rarely require treatment. Although most patients tolerate these hemodynamic responses well, patients with cardiac disease,[271] pregnancy-induced hypertension,[308] and increased intracranial pressure may be at particular risk for life-threatening ischemic myocardial episodes.[309] Patients with cardiac disease have had decreased ejection fractions at the time of extubation.[310] Management consists of extubation under deep anesthesia or pharmacologic therapy. Deep extubation is inappropriate for patients with a difficult airway, those at high risk for aspiration, and those with compromised airway access. Pharmacologic strategies emphasize the importance of decreasing the heart rate, such as with short-acting beta-blockers.[311] Cerebral hemorrhage is possible. Using an LMA may significantly reduce local and cardiovascular responses at removal if the cuff pressure is minimized to avoid overstimulation of the patient.[26]

B. Laryngospasm

In a computer-aided study of 136,929 patients, the incidence of laryngospasm was 50 cases per 1000 children with bronchial asthma or airway infection and 25 cases per 1000 in children 1 to 3 months old after tracheal intubation had been performed.[312]

The optimal course for treating laryngospasm is to avoid it in the first place. Treatment was described earlier. When laryngospasm is anticipated, the patient may undergo a deep extubation. A patient undergoing deep extubation should be placed in the lateral position with the head down to keep the vocal cords clear of secretions during emergence. It is best to extubate patients during a positive-pressure breath to remove residual secretions. Extubation during positive-pressure breath is the procedure of choice in children. A study showed that children could be safely extubated in deep anesthesia from a 1.5 minimum effective alveolar anesthetic concentration of sevoflurane or desflurane.[313] The study of Koga and colleagues showed that the rate of airway obstruction in patients extubated during deep anesthesia (17 of 20) was not higher than in patients extubated after regained consciousness (18 of 20).[314]

C. Laryngeal Edema

Laryngeal edema is an important cause of post-extubation obstruction, especially in neonates and infants. This condition has various causes and is classified as supraglottic, retroarytenoidal, or subglottic.[315] Supraglottic edema most commonly results from surgical manipulation, positioning, hematoma formation, overaggressive fluid management, impaired venous drainage, or coexisting conditions (e.g., preeclampsia, angioneurotic edema). Retroarytenoidal edema typically results from local trauma or irritation. Subglottic edema occurs most often in children, particularly neonates and infants. Factors associated with development of subglottic edema include traumatic intubation, intubation lasting longer than 1 hour, bucking on the ETT, changes in head position, or tight-fitting tubes. Laryngeal edema usually manifests as stridor within 30 to 60 minutes after extubation, although it may start as late as 6 hours after extubation. Regardless of the cause of laryngeal edema, management depends on the severity of the condition. Therapy consists of humidified oxygen, nebulized epinephrine, head-up positioning, and occasionally reintubation with a smaller ETT. The practice of administering parenteral steroids with the goal of preventing or reducing edema after long-term (>36 hours) ventilation may prove beneficial for adult patients, but routine administration for anesthesia is controversial.[316]

D. Laryngotracheal Trauma

Unlike trauma during intubation, airway trauma at the time of extubation is not well described. Arytenoid cartilage dislocation has been reported after difficult and routine intubations.[122,317] Symptoms become apparent soon after extubation and may be mild (e.g., difficulty swallowing, voice changes) or major (e.g., complete airway obstruction). Management depends on the severity of the condition. Options include reintubation, arytenoid reduction, and tracheostomy. If laryngotracheal trauma is suspected, an otolaryngology consultation is warranted.

E. Bronchospasm

In patients at risk for bronchospasm, the timing of extubation is important. These patients may be extubated during deep anesthesia (if this approach can be used safely) or when they are fully awake and their own airway reflexes are present. Although the degree of spasm in this condition may be severe, it is usually self-limited and short-lived.

F. Negative-Pressure Pulmonary Edema

When airway obstruction occurs after extubation in the case of laryngospasm, negative-pressure pulmonary edema may occur in a spontaneously breathing patient. As a result of inspiratory effort against the closed glottis, these patients generate negative intrapleural pressure of more than 100 cm H_2O. Rib retraction with poor air movement, laryngospasm, and stridor may lead to the rare diagnosis. Increased left ventricular preload and afterload, altered pulmonary vascular resistance, increased adrenergic state, right ventricle dilation, intraventricular septum shift to the left, left ventricular diastolic dysfunction, increased left heart loading conditions, enhanced microvascular intramural hydrostatic pressure, negative pleural pressure, and transmission to the lung interstitium may result in a marked increase in transmural pressure, fluid filtration into the lung, and development of pulmonary edema.[318]

Negative-pressure pulmonary edema is seen within minutes after extubation. Hemoptysis and alveolar hemorrhage are rare symptoms. Management involves removing the obstruction, supporting the patient with oxygen, monitoring the patient closely, and reducing the afterload. CPAP therapy is useful, and reintubation is rarely necessary. Most cases resolve spontaneously without further complications.

G. Aspiration

Pulmonary aspiration of gastric contents is a constant threat for any patient who has a full stomach or is at risk for postoperative vomiting. Laryngeal function is altered for at least 4 hours after tracheal extubation.[319] Coughing is a physiologic response to protect the airway from aspiration. Depression of reflexes, along with the presence of residual anesthetic agents, places most recently extubated patients at risk. Aspiration is probably more prevalent than is currently thought. Most cases are so minor that they do not affect the patient's postoperative course. Reducing gastric contents by suctioning through a gastric tube and extubation with the patient placed in the lateral position with a head-down tilt is the safest protection against aspiration. Perioperative problems, if they do occur, are usually attributed to factors such as atelectasis. Management consists of supportive measures. Depending on the extent of aspiration, measures include supportive care, ranging from administration of oxygen through a nasal cannula to reintubation with mechanical ventilation, and PEEP.

H. Airway Compression

External compression of the airway after extubation may lead to obstruction. An excessively tight postoperative neck dressing is a cause of external compression that is easily resolved. A more ominous situation is a rapidly expanding hematoma close to the airway. This may occur after certain operations, such as carotid endarterectomy, and must be quickly diagnosed and treated before total airway obstruction occurs.[320] Immediate surgical re-exploration is indicated, although the airway concerns for these patients should be approached with extreme caution. To minimize airway distortion, general anesthesia should be avoided until the wound is evacuated under local anesthesia. However, even after surgical drainage, airway obstruction may occur as the result of venous or lymphatic congestion. Any use of muscle relaxants during anesthesia induction in these patients may result in catastrophe, regardless of whether the wound was previously drained. Conservative options for managing the airway in this situation include awake fiberoptic intubation, surgical airways, or inhalation induction. Muscle relaxants should be avoided until the airway is secured.

External compression of the neck, such as chronic compression of a goiter, may also result from tracheomalacia.[321] This condition is usually seen after the goiter has been removed, although cases were reported in which the airway collapsed with induction or after extubation.[322,323] Airway obstruction in these patients becomes apparent soon after extubation. Management includes reintubation, surgical tracheal support (i.e., stenting), or tracheostomy below the level of obstruction.

I. Difficult Extubation

Occasionally, ETTs are difficult to remove. Possible causes are failure to deflate the cuff, use of an oversized tube,[324] adhesion of the tube to the tracheal wall,[325] or transfixation of the tube by an inadvertent suture to a nearby organ, a wire, a screw placed in an oromaxillofacial operation, or a broken drill.[326-329,340] Possible sequelae of these complications include airway leak, aspiration, tube obstruction, and trauma from attempts at forceful extubation. One case was reported in which a nasogastric tube made a loop around the ETT.[330] In most cases, the problem arises from an inability to deflate the cuff, commonly as a result of failure in the cuff-deflating mechanism. If this problem occurs, the cuff should be punctured with a transtracheal needle. If tube fixation is suspected, the passage of the tube should be checked with a suction catheter or a fiberscope. Forceful removal of an ETT with the cuff inflated may result in damage to the vocal cords and arytenoid dislocation.

J. Accidental Extubation

Accidental extubation during anesthesia has been reported with disposable tonsillectomy instruments,[331] change of the patient's head position, and in neurosurgery with the patient in the knee-elbow position.[332] Most accidental extubations were reported from intensive care unit patients, for whom self-extubation was the most common incident (77% to 85%).[333-335] The rate of reintubation was 37% to 57%.[333-335] The requirement for reintubation is higher for patients with full ventilatory support than those during the weaning phase.

Patients at risk for accidental extubation are characterized by the absence of physical restraints, a high nurse-to-patient ratio, trips out of the intensive care unit (59%), light sedation (43%), use of bedside portable radiography, accidental removal of the nasogastric tube or tugging on the ETT, oral intubation, and insufficient sedation.[336] Complications after accidental extubation may be hypoxia, hypercarbic respiratory failure, aspiration, retention of pulmonary secretion, arrhythmia, and tachycardia. To avoid unplanned extubation, tubes can be secured

with special tube holders,[337] with waterproof tape, and with fixation using a knot or a bow.[338,339]

Reintubation may be very difficult, especially after a difficult intubation. The use of a Combitube or an LMA is required in some cases of inadequate access to the patient's head in the intensive care setting.[340]

VII. CONCLUSIONS

Anesthesiologists face many challenges and complications when managing airways. Errors may be technical or judgmental. By learning from the mistakes of the past, we can avoid or minimize them by anticipating problems, devising safe primary and backup plans for every patient, maintaining vigilance throughout all operative procedures, and using common sense at all times.

VIII. CLINICAL PEARLS

- The final goal of airway management is oxygenation of the patient, not placement of an endotracheal tube (ETT).

- Serious complications of airway management result from not recognizing the level of airway difficulties.

- To minimize injury to the patient, the anesthesiologist should examine the patient's airway carefully, identify potential problems, devise a plan that involves the least risk for injury, and have a backup plan immediately available. Common sense should prevail at all times.

- In daily anesthesia practice, errors of omission are more common than errors of commission. Errors of omission include failure to recognize the magnitude of a problem, failure to make appropriate observations, and failure to act in a timely manner. Errors of commission include actions such as trauma to the lips, nose, or laryngotracheal mucosa; forcing sharp instruments into areas in which they do not belong; or introducing air or secretions into regions of the body in which further complications will ensue.

- Many complications in airway management result from insufficient communication between the members of the medical team and improper coordination of the patients in the daily operating room schedule. A patient with known difficult airway problems should be scheduled at a time when the most experienced anesthesiologists and surgeons are available.

- Delayed recognition of complications leads to delayed therapy. Inadequate monitoring, nonfunctional equipment, and an untrained staff can contribute to airway catastrophes.

- The overall risk of aspiration and regurgitation using the laryngeal mask airway (LMA) is about that for endotracheal intubation when the indications and contraindications for the LMA are respected. The risk of aspiration, which is a consequence of the airway device's design, should be weighed against the advantages of the LMA in cases of difficult intubation and ventilation.

- Because of the increased risk associated with multiple attempts of any airway technique, a maximum of three attempts is recommended to minimize trauma to the airway.

- Any airway device technique may cause movement and subsequent injury to the patient with an injured cervical spine.

- A patent airway is an absolute requirement for safe anesthesia. Airway obstruction can occur at any time during administration of general anesthesia, particularly in prolonged operations or in patients with predisposing anatomic abnormalities. The most serious complication after extubation is the occurrence of acute airway obstruction.

SELECTED REFERENCES

All references can be found online at expertconsult.com.

14. El-Orbany M, Woehlck HJ: Difficult mask ventilation. *Anesth Analg* 109:1870, 2009.
27. Seet E, Yousaf F, Gupta S, et al: Use of manometry for laryngeal mask airway reduces postoperative pharyngolaryngeal adverse events: A prospective, randomized trial. *Anesthesiology* 112:652, 2010.
34. Brimacombe J, Clarke G, Keller C: Lingual nerve injury associated with the ProSeal laryngeal mask airway: A case report and review of the literature. *Br J Anaesth* 95:420, 2005.
46. Benumof JL: Laryngeal mask airway and the ASA difficult airway algorithm. *Anesthesiology* 84:686, 1996.
54. López AM, Valero R, Brimacombe J: Insertion and use of the LMA Supreme in the prone position. *Anaesthesia* 65:154, 2010.
74. Benumof JL, Cooper SD: Quantitative improvement in laryngoscopic view by optimal external laryngeal manipulation. *J Clin Anesth* 8:136, 1996.
76. Mihai R, Blair E, Kay H, Cook TM: A quantitative review and meta-analysis of performance of non-standard laryngoscopes and rigid fibreoptic intubation aids. *Anaesthesia* 63:745, 2008.
171. Ghafoor AU, Martin TW, Gopalakrishnan S, Viswamitra S: Caring for the patients with cervical spine injuries: What have we learned? *J Clin Anesth* 17:640, 2005.
183. Martin DP, Weingarten TN, Gunn PW, et al: Performance improvement system and postoperative corneal injuries: Incidence and risk factors. *Anesthesiology* 111:320, 2009.
275. Al-Metwalli RR, Mowafi HA, Ismail SA: Gentle chest compression relieves extubation laryngospasm in children. *J Anesth* 24:854, 2010.
276. Al-alami AA, Zestos MM, Baraka AS: Pediatric laryngospasm: Prevention and treatment. *Curr Opin Anaesthesiol* 22:388, 2009.
289. El-Orbany M, Connolly LA: Rapid sequence induction and intubation: current controversy. *Anesth Analg* 110:1318, 2010.
335. Tanios MA, Epstein SK, Livelo J, Teres D: Can we identify patients at high risk for unplanned extubation? A large-scale multidisciplinary survey. *Respir Care* 55:561, 2010.

PART 7

Societal Considerations

Chapter 52

Teaching Airway Management Outside the Operating Room

SEBASTIAN G. RUSSO | STEPHEN F. DIERDORF

I. BACKGROUND

Management of the airway is the most important and potentially the most life-saving (or life-threatening) task that an anesthesiologist, emergency department (ED) physician, or intensivist performs. Missteps in airway management can result in mortality or significant morbidity. In 1985, the American Society of Anesthesiologists (ASA) Committee on Professional Liability began to analyze closed-claim malpractice cases to objectively assess adverse outcomes from anesthesia. The initial analysis of the data, published in 1990, revealed that respiratory events accounted for 34% of the claims (522/1541 cases) and that 85% of the respiratory events resulted in permanent neurologic injury or death.[1] Three mechanisms of adverse outcome from respiratory events accounted for 73% of the events: inadequate ventilation (38%), esophageal intubation (18%), and difficult endotracheal intubation (DI; 17%).

The reviewers concluded that 90% of the cases of inadequate ventilation and esophageal intubation could have been prevented if monitoring with capnography and pulse oximetry had been employed. It was also concluded that only 36% of the cases of DI were easily preventable. In response to this finding, the Task Force on Management of the Difficult Airway (DA) was formed by the ASA. After an exhaustive search and evaluation of the medical literature concerning airway management published between 1973 and 1991, the task force published *Practice Guidelines for Management of the Difficult Airway*

in March, 1993.[2] These guidelines included recommendations for evaluation of the airway, basic preparation for DA management, strategy for intubation of the DA, and postoperative care. The Task Force also developed an algorithm for management of the DA. Updated guidelines, based on information accrued since 1993, were published in 2003.[3] It can be anticipated that future updates based on experience with new airway devices will occur.[4] Other organizations with interest in airway management have also published airway management guidelines.[5]

A. Is There Evidence That the Difficult Airway Guidelines Have Been Effective in Reducing Adverse Airway Events?

A review of the closed claims database in 1999 revealed a decline in claims for adverse respiratory events, primarily related to a reduction in claims for inadequate ventilation and esophageal intubation.[6] Claims for adverse events secondary to DI remained relatively constant, and claims for trauma to the upper airway increased. The claims for pharyngeal and esophageal trauma were frequently associated with DI. Another study, published in 2005, compared claims for DA management during two time periods: 1985–1992 (before DA guidelines) and 1993–1999 (after DA guidelines). Claims for adverse respiratory outcomes (death or brain death) during induction of anesthesia decreased by 67% during the latter period compared with the former. However, claims for similar adverse respiratory outcomes occurring during the maintenance phase of anesthesia, at extubation, or during recovery did not change.[7]

Although respiratory events are more likely to result in an adverse outcome, the incidence of patients with a DA in clinical anesthesia practice is actually quite low. The incidence of *failure to intubate the trachea* in a large series of surgical patients was only 0.3%.[8] Although the most comprehensive published data have concerned perioperative airway management, airway management in the prehospital setting, in the ED, and in the intensive care unit (ICU) is no less important and must be included in any airway education program.[9] Airway management is not an easy skill to learn, and educators must give careful consideration to the complexity of airway management and the ability of different types of health care providers to manage ventilation and endotracheal intubation.

Objectives for education in airway management include the theoretical and practical aspects of airway devices and techniques and a time-based environment that mimics actual clinical situations. The student must also gain an appreciation of the relationship between the practitioner and the patient and the effects that clinical decisions may have on outcome.[10] The teaching program must allow the learner in a nonclinical environment to make choices that may result in an adverse outcome.

II. MILLER'S LEARNING PYRAMID

An airway teaching program must teach simple maneuvers (e.g., performing a jaw thrust) as well as complex skills such as awake fiberoptic intubation (FOI). The design of a successful education program begins with the development of clear objectives. What has to be taught, to whom, and how? The program must also address different knowledge and skill levels. Miller's learning pyramid for assessment of clinical skills has four stages of ability: *Knows, Knows How, Shows How,* and *Does* (Fig. 52-1).[11]

An example of this pyramid can be applied to use of the laryngeal mask airway (LMA). The first level, *Knows,* is the knowledge that there is a need for airway management and that the LMA can be used for that purpose. *Knows How* is the knowledge of how to prepare and insert the LMA. At the next competence level, the learner *Shows* that he or she is capable of inserting the LMA. The highest competence level, *Does,* reflects transfer of the new skill (LMA use) to the clinical situation. The first three levels of the learning pyramid can be achieved with didactic lectures, video observation, computer programs, and skill-training with mannequins, animal models, or cadavers.

Because skills and scientific information gained during simulator training may not be easy to transfer directly to clinical practice, the clinical environment is the best environment for developing airway management skills.[12] Practicing techniques such as airway assessment, bagmask ventilation (BMV), supralaryngeal airway (SLA) insertion, direct laryngoscopy, and FOI in actual patients would be ideal. The highest competence level (*Does*) in airway management ultimately requires practice in the

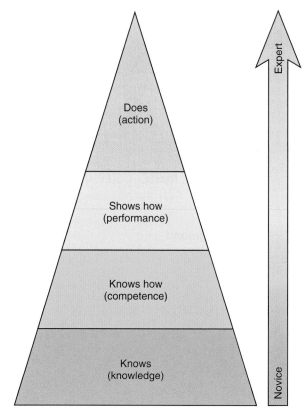

Figure 52-1 Level of competence based on clinical assessment. The highest level of competence, *Does,* is ultimately achieved with clinical performance. (Adapted from Miller GE: The assessment of clinical skills/competence/performance. *Academic Medicine* 65, S63–S67, 1990.)

clinical environment. There are, however, a number of barriers to training exclusively in the clinical arena (Box 52-1). Training outside the operating room (OR) or ICU is done to minimize the risk to patients and promote efficient clinical learning.

III. COMPUTER-BASED LEARNING

The pace of development of interactive computer-assisted instructional programs has surpassed simulation development over the past 10 years. Computer-assisted

---

BOX 52-1 Barriers to Teaching Difficult Airway Management in the Clinical Environment

Infrequent opportunities for certain skills
- Retrograde intubation
- Transtracheal jet ventilation
- Percutaneous tracheostomy

Time pressure in the clinical setting

Difficulty in matching knowledgeable teachers and the right patient with the trainee

Perceived risks of practicing on patients when the technique is not indicated

Ethical considerations
- High risk and high cost of management failure by an inexperienced trainee
- Use of new methods before adequate experience with the method is obtained

instruction can facilitate the organization and linkage of information directly applicable to clinical situations.[13] A major advantage of computer-based instruction is the low cost after development and the lack of need for a human instructor. The learner can use the program at his or her own pace and as many times as necessary to achieve mastery of the subject. The increased power of laptop computers has reduced the need for computer centers and provides the learner with exceptional mobility. Computer-assisted instruction can also provide alternative learning methods for students who do not learn well with traditional teaching methods.

A clinical department can develop its own instructional programs or access existing programs via the Internet. The number of Web sites relevant to anesthesia continues to grow, and the Internet provides rapid access for users in remote locations.[14] However, Internet programs are not peer-reviewed, and quality can be variable.[15] The transition from Web 1.0 to Web 2.0 has encouraged more interactivity and improved the quality of Web-based education.[16] The disadvantages of Web-based education, such as insufficient feedback and instructional ambiguity, can be overcome by providing local faculty input to supplement the Web-based program.

Technical assistance may be required for the clinical faculty to facilitate in-house program development. The potentially daunting task of program assembly and maintenance must not be an obstacle to the faculty.

There are several objectives of an interactive airway management program (Box 52-2). One is to familiarize the learner with the anatomy and physiology of the upper airway. The complexity of the upper airway is often overlooked, and understanding of upper airway function can provide an early warning of impending respiratory difficulty. The structure and function of various airway devices can be displayed with diagrams, photographs, and videotapes. Computer-based multimedia programs can demonstrate device function and technique with a much

more effective presentation than a traditional lecture format.

After the basic principles of airway management have been presented, interactive programs can be directed to elucidate the intricacies of the DA algorithm so that the learner understands the critical decision points during the course of airway management. A library of actual airway abnormalities can be loaded onto the computer as an additional teaching tool. Most modern video laryngoscopes (VLs) and flexible fiberoptic bronchoscopes (FFBs) can record airway examinations and airway device insertion. The combination of text material and narration with imported diagrams, photographs, and videotapes can be used to explain concepts and airway management techniques in considerable detail. More advanced interactive programs can simulate the clinical environment and present actual clinical scenarios in a real-time environment that permits the student to halt the program and access information that may affect the decision process. Such scenario-based learning is becoming increasingly important in medical education.

IV. EFFICACY OF SIMULATION IN EDUCATION

Simulation has been used for decades to address training problems in high-risk disciplines such as military science and aviation. Medical simulation began in the mid-1990s and has grown rapidly.[17] Simulator training programs incorporate psychomotor and decision-making skills that address the highest level of competence in Miller's pyramid: *Does*. When the programs are appropriately designed, simulation can close the gap between acquisition of skills and meaningful use of the acquired skills (Fig. 52-2). This may be especially true for rare situations. Because the incidence of the DA is low in clinical practice, two questions must be addressed: How can an anesthesiologist in clinical practice learn new airway skills? and How can the ramifications of critical decision points in airway management be learned?

The inherent nature of airway management includes uncertainty, complexity, time pressure, and high costs for failure. Simulation provides the ideal method for closely replicating the clinical situation and may help to scientifically evaluate strategies, decision points, and algorithm adherence.[18,19] The efficacy of education with medical simulation is well established, but its effect on reducing the incidence of adverse patient outcomes is more controversial.[18,20-24] It is easy to prove the effect of a theoretical lecture or workshop with a pretest and post-test. It is not easy to prove the effect of simulation on patient outcome in rare but life-threatening situations such as the DA. Nevertheless, there is evidence in the literature that simulator- and scenario-based training improves patient care.

BOX 52-2   Instructional Components of an Airway Management Educational Program

Upper airway anatomy and physiology
Principles of the airway examination
- Recognition of the abnormal airway
Structure and function of airway devices
- Bag-mask ventilation (BMV)
- Pharyngeal airways
- Supralaryngeal airways (SLAs)
- Conventional direct laryngoscopes
- Video laryngoscopes (VLs)
- Flexible fiberoptic bronchoscopes (FFBs)
- Emergent invasive techniques
Static simulation practice (e.g., mannequin)
Examples of upper airway pathology
Critical decision points in the difficult airway algorithm
- Indications for awake intubation
- Cannot intubate, can ventilate
- Cannot intubate, cannot ventilate
Real-time clinical simulation

V. TYPES OF SIMULATORS

Simulators can be classified as low-fidelity (static) or high-fidelity (dynamic).

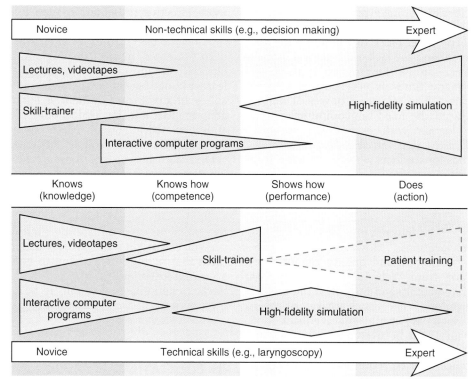

Figure 52-2 Indications for use of different training tools in the acquisition of technical and nontechnical skills based on Miller's learning pyramid. The width of the pyramid should reflect the benefit of the distinct training tool on the indicated level of competency.

A. Low-Fidelity Simulators

Skill-trainers or mannequins are available for most airway devices, such as conventional laryngoscopes, SLAs, and FFBs. Skill-trainers are designed to teach specific motor skills, such as direct laryngoscopy, the fundamentals of FFB guidance, or SLA insertion.

Mannequins do not always accurately replicate human anatomy and cannot be altered to represent abnormal anatomy. Such low-fidelity simulators provide neither physiologic data nor clinical feedback for the learner. Despite these shortcomings, however, effective skill transference to clinical use may be facilitated.[25]

B. High-Fidelity Simulators

High-fidelity simulators, more commonly referred to as human patient simulators, offer many advantages over low-fidelity simulators. Physiologic parameters such as blood pressure, heart rate, pulse oximetry, capnography, breath sounds, peripheral pulses, and temperature can be programmed into the simulator. High-fidelity simulators cannot accommodate the variations in human anatomy.[26] This is especially true for DI scenarios in which insertion of an SLA may be clinically effective. The reason is that the DI scenario in the simulator is created by supraglottic obstruction rather than laryngeal displacement.

Current simulators have pre-programmed clinical scenarios that require no program assembly and minimal technical expertise on the part of the instructor. The teaching programs present time-based physiologic changes in the simulator that accurately reflect actual clinical events. The programs allow the learner many different management choices, and the instructor can vary the simulator's physiologic responses based on the learner's selection of techniques. Human performance deteriorates during periods of stress, and there is a tendency to revert to old behavior patterns. Translated to airway management, this may result in repetitive attempts to use airway techniques that have previously failed (e.g., rigid direct laryngoscopy) while the patient's condition continues to worsen. Simulation can be used to teach new management techniques, and permits the learner to apply those techniques in a simulated environment in which the adverse effects of a poor choice will be evident. Repetitive simulated encounters can then be employed until the new technique becomes part of the learner's management armamentarium. High-fidelity medical simulation can create a learning environment that supports experiential and reflective learning. For this purpose, a realistic scenario based on a real-life situation is introduced into an authentic environment, followed by a structured debriefing about strategies the learner chose. Appropriate simulation teaching programs help the student develop integrated emotional, cognitive, and psychomotor abilities that effect a change in behavior and performance in the clinical setting. These advantages offset the initial capital investment, need for training space, and operational costs.

Many medical institutions and health care consortiums have invested in multipurpose simulation centers to provide training for different types of health care providers. These centers replicate ORs, ICU beds, ward beds, examination rooms, and ambulance bays to provide a realistic setting for trainees (Fig. 52-3). Simulation centers

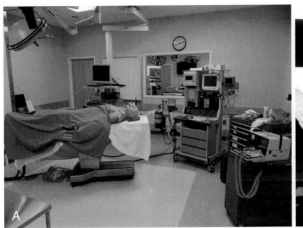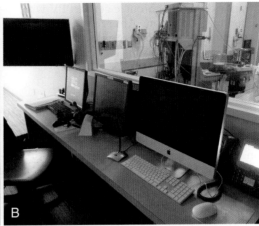

Figure 52-3   A, A simulated operating room (OR) equipped with a high-fidelity human patient simulator. **B,** The control room of the simulated OR. The trainer can orchestrate the simulator session from the control room while observing the trainee's performance through the one-way mirror.

can employ full-time technicians to manage the technical aspects of simulation. This allows the teaching faculty to concentrate their efforts on curriculum development and the direction of simulation sessions.

Trainees from many disciplines need experience with simulation education. Licensure and board accreditation examination systems are rapidly incorporating an evaluation of performance with high-fidelity simulation.[27-29]

VI. AIRWAY MANAGEMENT SKILLS

There are several skills that the experienced airway provider must acquire in order to provide comprehensive airway management. Airway management skills are not easy to learn, the time to apply those skills to the apneic patient is short, and the risks of failure include death or permanent neurologic injury.[30] Traditional educational programs depend on the accumulation of clinical experience, which may take years. Structured simulation-based teaching should provide a broader experience in a shorter period of time, thereby improving the airway management skills of a greater number of providers.

The instructor must determine what level of skill a particular provider must possess to meet his or her expected need. A gastroenterologist administering or supervising the administration of medications for conscious sedation does not require the same level of airway management expertise as the ED physician or the anesthesiologist. There is considerable variation in the airway skills of first responders, and the rescue airway techniques that are to be applied by first responders must be determined in the early planning phase of the teaching program. The instructor must design an educational program that meets the objectives for each type of student. The program will consist of the didactic material that explains the theory of the skill and describes how the technique is employed. After the theory is understood, the student can learn and demonstrate proficiency with static simulators (mannequins). For some skills, proficiency with a static mannequin is all that is required; other skills may require additional simulation experience before clinical application.

One of the challenges in designing a course for airway instruction is the myriad of devices and techniques that are commercially available. It is not possible for an institution to have all devices available, nor is it possible for an individual to be proficient with every device. Practitioners need to be selective in choice of airway devices based on the patient population served and the resources available from the institution. Proficiency with one type of device from each category is satisfactory for most situations.

A. Bag-Mask Ventilation

BMV is an important airway management technique that does not receive as much attention as it deserves. A major determinant of successful resuscitation of an apneic patient is the rapidity with which the first responder can establish effective ventilation. The student should know the effect of the unconscious state (whether drug or disease induced) on the upper airway and how this produces airway obstruction. Relaxation of the pharyngeal muscles and tongue obstructs the hypopharynx and allows the epiglottis to obstruct the glottic inlet. Elevation of the mandible lifts the tongue off the posterior pharyngeal wall and moves the epiglottis away from the glottic inlet, thereby opening the airway. Compression of the face mask against the face to produce an airtight seal permits positive-pressure ventilation (PPV) via the unobstructed airway. After the student understands these basic principles, instruction with a static mannequin demonstrates the actual technique of BMV. When the learner can demonstrate proficiency with the mannequin, he or she is ready to apply the skill to patients.

Since the LMA entered clinical practice, there has been concern about loss of BMV skills. Practice of this technique can occur in the OR while neuromuscular blockade takes effect. Also, very short procedures could continue to be performed with mask ventilation rather than light ventilation.

An additional exercise that is highly instructive is teaching the students to use BMV on each other. Augmented ventilation of the conscious patient allows the student to learn how to synchronize gentle PPV with the subject's inherent inspiration. After a short period of supplemental hyperventilation, the learner can completely control the conscious subject's ventilation.

B. Pharyngeal Airways

Pharyngeal airways, including oropharyngeal and nasopharyngeal airways, are designed to provide a patent passage through the mouth and hypopharynx by elevating the tongue and epiglottis. Pharyngeal airways are simple in design but extremely effective for alleviating upper airway obstruction. Insertion of a pharyngeal airway and two-person ventilation can provide effective ventilation in some of the most challenging DA cases. The use of pharyngeal airways can be easily integrated into the instructional program for BMV. Any medical provider who may encounter upper airway obstruction should be proficient with the use of pharyngeal airways.

C. Supralaryngeal Airways

Effective use of SLAs requires a higher level of expertise than the use of pharyngeal airways. There are many manufacturers that supply SLAs, and insertion techniques vary. All SLAs are purported to provide a secure airway with a seal adequate for PPV. However, many SLAs have not undergone rigorous investigation before market release. Such devices may not survive the rigors of clinical practice and may be withdrawn from the market subsequently. Course design should focus on the concepts that are central to all SLA devices. Didactic material presented to the learner should explain the rationale for the device's design and provide complete description of the insertion technique and correct positioning of the SLA in the upper airway. The learner must also understand the procedures for confirmation of correct placement and potential complications before clinical application of the technique. Users with an incomplete knowledge of potential difficulties are likely to encounter some complications. Despite the risk of complications, SLAs have a high success rate for establishing effective ventilation during resuscitation.

The LMA has been shown to be an effective device for emergency ventilation when used by relatively inexperienced providers. First responders should be trained in use of the LMA as an early intervention. The medical literature concerning effectiveness of the LMA during resuscitation is extensive. Whether such effectiveness can be achieved with other SLA devices has not yet been proven, but the supposition seems likely.

Information that the learner should acquire during the initial phase of the training program includes the structural function of the device and correct insertion and positioning. Common to all SLA devices is their insertion over the tongue, into the hypopharynx, and above the glottic inlet. Although the type of SLA employed varies from institution to institution, it is beneficial to provide training with different SLA devices. There are several mannequins available for SLA insertion training, but performance varies, and the instructor must select one that is suitable for the particular device used.[31]

The depth and intensity of SLA training depends on the level of performance that is desired, and the goals for each type of medical provider must be clearly delineated. Anesthesiologists, who require the highest level of performance, must invest considerable time in mastering the use of the LMA. There are two learning curves: an initial learning phase consisting of 50 to 75 insertions, and a slower learning phase encompassing hundreds of insertions.[32-34]

D. Conventional Direct Laryngoscopy

Conventional direct laryngoscopy has been a mainstay for airway management for decades and is considered by many to be the gold standard for emergency airway management. Skill development for direct laryngoscopy is difficult and requires more experience than previously thought.[35] Numerous studies have demonstrated that alternative airway techniques, such as placement of an SLA, actually result in more rapid and effective ventilation than endotracheal intubation with conventional direct laryngoscopy. Such observations have caused many airway educators to change how they teach emergency airway management.[36]

The rigid, direct laryngoscope is designed to align the three axes—oral cavity, hypopharynx, and larynx—so as to establish a line of sight for passage of an endotracheal tube. Line of sight is achieved by depressing the tongue and sublingual tissue with the rigid laryngoscope blade into the submandibular space. Anatomic variations such as abnormal or carious dentition, a small mandible, lingual tonsillar hyperplasia, reduced cervical mobility, and obesity may reduce the effectiveness of the rigid laryngoscope in developing a line of sight. The application of excessive force to the upper airway can cause significant injury. Insertion of the laryngoscope blade and points of force application require subtle skills that are not easily appreciated by the novice with mere observation. A methodical instruction program that includes guided clinical experience is necessary. It is no longer acceptable for learners to begin direct laryngoscopy by intubating patients.

A training course for providers who have little or no experience with conventional direct laryngoscopy should begin with lecture material that includes upper airway anatomy and physiology, the mechanics of direct laryngoscopy, and sequential instruction on the intubation process. Models have been developed that can be adjusted to reflect anatomic variants so that the student can see the effects of these variants on intubation technique.[37] Mannequin practice with a VL has been shown to improve the success rate for intubation of patients.[38] A clinical instructor should expect all novices to have extensive simulated experience before patient exposure. Selection of appropriate patients (such as lean, edentulous patients followed by patients with normal dentition) enhances the experience while reducing the likelihood of patient injury. Endotracheal intubation of patients who are likely to have rapid arterial oxygen desaturation, such as obese patients or children, should be done only after the learner has accumulated significant experience.

E. Video Laryngoscopy

Advances in imaging technology have spawned a new class of intubation devices, the VLs.[39] VLs continue to be refined and may in the future become the instrument of choice for all endotracheal intubations. The Bullard laryngoscope was introduced many years ago and was perhaps the first VL to have significant clinical application. The refinement of other imaging techniques has generated an increase in the number of different VLs now available. The basic components of all VLs are a rigid, anatomic blade and an imaging device that provides a view of the larynx without requiring line of sight. The important advantage of such a design is that it permits a reduction in the force that must be exerted by the laryngoscope blade on the patient's upper airway in order to see the glottic inlet.

Although the blade of the VL resembles the blade of a conventional direct laryngoscope, the insertion techniques for the two devices are different. A conventional direct laryngoscope blade is inserted in the right side of the mouth with the tip of the blade directed toward the right tonsil bed. The blade is then redirected toward the midline and advanced until the epiglottis is seen. Once the epiglottis is visualized, the blade can be advanced into the vallecula or underneath the epiglottis to expose the glottis. The VL, on the other hand, should be passed over the tongue in the midline and advanced until the epiglottis appears. The blade is then advanced into the vallecula and rotated slightly anterior, which elevates the epiglottis and permits a good view of the glottis.

Even experienced laryngoscopists do not appreciate the differences in technique when they first use a VL. Comparative studies of various laryngoscopes provide information about performance in different scenarios, and students should be exposed to several VLs so they can determine which one is best for them.[40,41] Once the technique of video laryngoscopy has been mastered, many prefer it to conventional direct laryngoscopy for even routine endotracheal intubations.

F. Fiberoptic-Assisted Endotracheal Intubation

Fiberoptic-assisted endotracheal intubation (FOI) has revolutionized management of the DA. FFBs for airway management began to be used in anesthesia practice in the 1970s but initially did not gain widespread acceptance. The problem was a lack of effective training of anesthesiologists. In most cases, the FFB was used only when a DA was anticipated and the plan was for an awake intubation. The clinical situation, consequently, was an inexperienced endoscopist, an abnormal airway, and an awake, uncomfortable patient. The outcome was not likely to be pleasant or successful. It was not until creative airway management teachers developed effective teaching programs that FOI became a routine part of resident education.[42,43] Although much progress has been made with resident education, there is still inconsistency among residency programs with respect to FOI.[44]

Performance of FOI is a skill that every advanced airway management provider should master. Although the process by which providers are taught this skill has not been standardized, there is sufficient evidence in the medical literature to provide guidance for instructional development. A department's or institution's ultimate training system may be influenced by financial and manpower resources. There are low-tech and high-tech models and simulators that can be used. Do skills learned with models and simulators transfer to clinical performance? Resolution of this question is central to the efficacy of medical simulation education and remains controversial.[45] The preponderance of evidence concerning FOI affirms the theory that there is significant skill retention and transference.[46-48]

The course for FOI should begin with didactic material that describes upper airway anatomy, FFB construction and operation, and the fundamentals of FFB manipulation. This material may be presented in a traditional lecture format or via a computer program. The next phase of the program must permit the learner to practice FOI. This can be accomplished with static mannequins of the head and neck or with simple, nonanatomic models that require the learner to recognize objects or numbers after FFB manipulation. These models can be constructed with boxes or tubes that require the learner to visualize the images through the FFB during the process of FOI (Fig. 52-4). More realistic static mannequins are also available (Fig. 52-5). The video bronchoscope is a very useful device because the instructor can observe the intubation process on the monitor and offer suggestions to the learner as the intubation progresses (Fig. 52-6). Modern video bronchoscopes produce a high-resolution, wide-angle image of the airway. Teaching with a video bronchoscope improves the rapidity and success of endotracheal intubation by anesthesiology residents.[49]

There are high-fidelity simulators specifically designed for FFB training. These simulators accurately reproduce the responses to the user's manipulations, including mucosal bleeding, coughing, and laryngeal motion with respiration. Goldman and associates demonstrated that virtual reality–trained novices quickly learned FFB manipulation, and after a short training period, they performed as well as experienced attending anesthesiologists.[50] A high-fidelity simulator can replace the need for practice with animal and cadaver models. High-fidelity

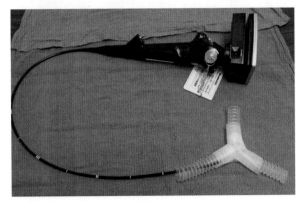

Figure 52-4 An inexpensive and easily constructed model of a tracheobronchial tree made from anesthesia circuit tubing.

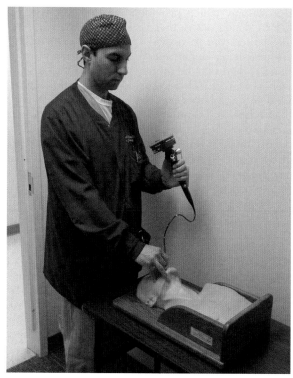

Figure 52-5 An anesthesiology resident practicing fiberoptic intubation with a static mannequin.

simulators are expensive and may not offer significant advantages over less expensive models. Virtual reality computer programs may provide the same benefits as high-tech bronchoscopic simulators.[51]

After the student has mastered the extraoperative phases of the training program, he or she is ready to begin clinical training with oral FOI of lean patients with normal airways receiving general anesthesia.[52,53] This part of the training emphasizes FFB navigation, management of secretions in the airway, and passage of an endotracheal

tube over the FFB. This teaching program works just as well for pediatric patients.[54] The time required to become competent with FOI varies from resident to resident. Some may be very capable after 10 to 15 successful intubations, whereas others may require 25 to 50 intubations.[55] After a resident is competent with FOI of normal patients, he or she can progress to patients that can be easily ventilated after induction of anesthesia but in whom laryngoscopy is difficult.

After proficiency with FOI of anesthetized patients can be demonstrated, the learner is ready to progress to awake intubation. The entire educational process can be completed in 4 to 6 weeks by most anesthesiology residents—a relatively short time to acquire such a valuable skill (Box 52-3). The challenge for residents from other specialties is having enough clinical opportunities after completing simulator training. Collaborative efforts among anesthesiologists; intensivists; ED physicians; ear, nose, and throat surgeons; and pulmonologists are required to meet the educational needs of all the appropriate disciplines.

Education of practicing clinicians who did not have formal training in FOI remains a significant challenge, because the pressures of clinical practice may not allow time for graded patient experience. Many attendees of educational fiberoptic workshops report an extremely low rate of clinical application after the workshop. The ultimate solution for this group of clinicians may be high-fidelity simulation training at a simulation center followed by experience with more recently trained clinicians as they join the practice group.

G. Invasive Airway Techniques

Invasive airway techniques are difficult to practice because of limited clinical opportunities. Although mannequins do not accurately replicate the clinical scenario for most invasive airway techniques, mannequin practice does allow the learner to practice the sequence of steps for emergency invasive airway management. Some institutions employ fresh cadavers, isolated animal tracheas,

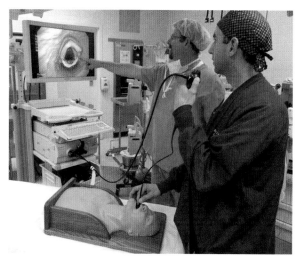

Figure 52-6 A resident practicing guidance with a flexible fiberoptic video bronchoscope on a mannequin under faculty supervision.

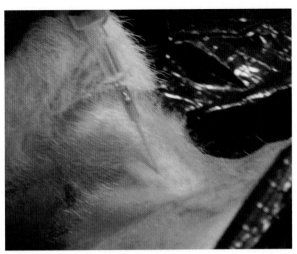

Figure 52-7   Percutaneous identification of the trachea with needle aspiration through the cricothyroid membrane of a human cadaver. This is the initial step in emergency cricothyrotomy.

or anesthetized animals as models for invasive airway insertion (Fig. 52-7).[56,57]

The necessity for emergency invasive airway procedures has undoubtedly been diminished by the development of SLAs and VLs.[58] This is fortunate in that providers with minimal invasive experience do not have a high success rate with invasive airway techniques and can encounter significant complications when performing them.[59] However, there are still situations in which all noninvasive methods have failed and an emergent, invasive airway technique is required.

H. Comprehensive Airway Management

The final step for educating individual medical providers who need broad airway skills, such as anesthesiologists, ED physicians, and critical care physicians, is a clinical rotation focused on airway management problems. The traditional approach to clinical airway training was based on the concept that each resident would acquire sufficient exposure to airway cases during residency (apprenticeship model). This teaching model promotes inconsistency among programs and individual inconsistencies within programs. Professional anesthesiology organizations have failed to provide specific guidelines for training in airway management. More progressive educators have instituted airway rotations in their residency programs to expose all residents to a wide variety of airway devices and techniques.[60] As more clinicians who have had comprehensive airway training enter clinical practice, their training should provide a springboard for further professional development.[61]

Simulation can be employed to evaluate team performance and institutional protocols.[62,63] This methodology will assume increasing importance as health care institutions merge into larger organizations and become more process oriented. For many processes it is yet unknown whether patient outcome is significantly improved, therefore a validation of their merit is required. Multidisciplinary simulated exercises may expose deficiencies in institutional procedures for management of high-risk patient events.

VII. CONCLUSIONS

Clinical teaching of airway management on actual patients is irreplaceable. However, the risk of complications is increased when novices are being taught airway management methods. Learning the fundamentals of airway management outside the OR, ED, or ICU better prepares the learner for clinical experience. The educator will find that outside instruction renders the clinical teaching experience more efficient with reduced patient risk. The development of powerful personal computers and high-fidelity simulators permits the construction of interactive programs with realistic clinical scenarios that mimic actual patient experiences. These tools allow the learner to participate in simulated airway events and to practice repeatedly until the management concepts and airway techniques are mastered.

It is imperative that instructional courses be tailored to the skill level of the learner and that clear objectives be elucidated during the process of course design. Extraoperative instruction can occur with an integration of traditional teaching methods, computer programs, lowfidelity and high-fidelity simulators, and animal models. The development of virtual reality computer programs and simulators is progressing at a rapid pace. Some airway management skills are difficult to learn, and robust instructional programs must become an integral part of residency training. Coordination of nonclinical and clinical instructional programs will ensure effective acquisition of airway management skills with minimal risk to patients.

Training programs should develop simulation-based education curricula.[64] Instruction in airway management is well suited for simulation. An alternative to developing an in-house simulation center is to use established simulation centers. The ASA has developed a process for simulation center endorsement, and the network of endorsed simulation centers continues to expand. There is little doubt that medical simulation at all levels of complexity has become an integral part of medical education.

VIII. CLINICAL PEARLS

- The first step in developing a simulation program is construction of a curriculum with clear educational objectives.

- The technology of the simulator should not interfere with teaching objectives.

- The type of simulator (low-fidelity or high-fidelity) should be matched to the educational plan.

- Simulation should replicate the clinical environment as closely as possible.

- Licensure and accreditation may in the future require measurement of performance on simulators.

SELECTED REFERENCES

All references can be found online at expertconsult.com.

9. Martin LD, Mhyre JM, Shanks AM, et al: 3,423 Emergency tracheal intubations at a university hospital. *Anesthesiology* 114:42–48, 2011.

10. McGaghie WC, Issenberg SB, Petrussa ER, et al: A critical review of simulation-based medical education research. *Med Educ* 44:50–63, 2010.

12. Rai MR, Popat MT: Evaluation of airway equipment: Man or manikin? *Anaesthesia* 66:1–3, 2011.

18. Borges BC, Boets S, Siu LW, et al: Incomplete adherence to the ASA difficult airway algorithm is unchanged after a high-fidelity simulation session. *Can J Anaesth* 57:644–649, 2010.

19. Eich C, Timmerman A, Russo SG, et al: A controlled rapid-sequence induction for infants may reduce unsafe actions and stress. *Acta Anaesthesiol Scand* 53:1167–1172, 2009.

20. Bruppacher HR, Alam SK, LeBlanc VR, et al: Simulation-based training improves physicians' performance in patient care in high-stakes clinical setting of cardiac surgery. *Anesthesiology* 112:985–992, 2010.

22. Russo SG, Eich C, Barwig J, et al: Self-reported changes in attitude and behavior after attending a simulation-aided airway management course. *J Clin Anesth* 19:517–522, 2007.

27. DeMaria S, Levine AI, Bryson EO: The use of multi-modality simulation in the retraining of the physician for medical licensure. *J Clin Anesth* 22:294–299, 2010.

35. Mulcaster JT, Mills J, Hung OR, et al: Laryngoscopic intubation: Learning and performance. *Anesthesiology* 98:23–27, 2003.

42. Roberts JT: Preparing to use the flexible fiber-optic laryngoscope. *J Clin Anesth* 3:64–75, 1991.

60. Crosby E, Lane A: Innovations in anesthesia education: The development and implementation of a resident rotation for advanced airway management. *Can J Anaesth* 56:939–959, 2009.

Chapter 53

Airway Management Instruction in the Operating Room

ROBERT WONG | ROBERT T. NARUSE | ELIZABETH C. BEHRINGER

I. INTRODUCTION

Airway management of either the routine or the difficult airway remains a critical aspect of both anesthesiology training and lifelong anesthetic practice. Anesthesiologists remain the most recognized "airway management specialists" and are routinely involved in elective and emergency procedures involving securing the airway throughout the hospital. Anesthesiologists may be asked to provide a secure airway as an application of advanced cardiac life support during cardiorespiratory arrest, as part of an elective or emergency surgical or radiologic procedure, or in the intensive care unit (ICU).

The American Society of Anesthesiologists (ASA) closed-claims analyses are a series of publications that review closed malpractice claims against anesthesiologists gleaned from the databases of 35 medical liability insurance carriers. The initial 1990 report reviewed adverse respiratory events associated with anesthesia care during the 1970s and 1980s.[1] In the 1970s, 55% of all claims of death or brain damage were caused by anesthetic-associated adverse respiratory events. Respiratory events during anesthetic care leading to adverse outcomes were the largest group of injuries resulting in malpractice litigation. This landmark study highlighted the three mechanisms associated with adverse outcomes: inadequate ventilation, unrecognized esophageal intubation, and difficult endotracheal intubation. Other events noted in a subsequent study included airway trauma, pneumothorax, aspiration of orogastric contents, and bronchospasm. These less common adverse respiratory events can be associated with anesthetic care as well.[2]

In 1998, a follow-up study noted a significant change in airway-related closed claims during the 1990s.[3] During this decade, a 10% decrease in the incidence of anesthetic-related adverse respiratory events was noted. This dramatic decline can be attributed to the routine use of pulse oximetry, use of capnography, and the advent and widespread use of the ASA Difficult Airway Algorithm in continuing education.[4,5] Additional factors that play vital roles include residency training specifically focused on airway management, continuing education in airway management, and scientific literature on management of the difficult airway.[6]

II. IMPORTANCE OF LIFELONG LEARNING IN AIRWAY MANAGEMENT

The importance of clinical education in airway management during residency training and in the postgraduate setting can be underscored by a brief review of airway management in the ICU. Anesthesiologists are often consulted for airway management in the ICU during both residency training and postgraduate practice.[7] Nayyar and Lisbon[8] surveyed anesthesiology residency training programs with regard to emergency airway management practices outside the operating room (OR). In the vast majority of programs surveyed, anesthesiologists performed most of the intubations on the hospital ward, including the ICU. This study supports the importance of tailoring airway practice to the patient environment, as supported by the scientific literature.

Mort[9] reviewed the incidence of hemodynamic and airway complications associated with tracheal reintubation after unplanned extubation in the ICU. The 57 patients reintubated after self-extubation were examined over a 27-month period; 93% of reintubations occurred within 2 hours of self-extubation. Of these patients, 72% had hemodynamic compromise or airway-related complications such as hypotension (35%), tachycardia (30%), hypertension (14%), multiple laryngoscopic attempts (22%), difficult laryngoscopy (16%), difficult intubation (14%), hypoxemia (14%), and esophageal intubation (14%). One patient required a surgical airway. One case of "cannot ventilate, cannot intubate" leading to cardiac arrest and death occurred. Less than one third of the patients studied had a "mishap-free" reintubation in the ICU.[9] Thus, it was recommended that individual ICUs develop strategies to decrease the rate of self-extubation based on patient safety and the impact of emergency airway management.

Mort[10,11] reported two additional studies of airway management in remote settings pertinent to clinical practice. The first study used an emergency intubation database from 1990 to 2002 in support of the ASA guidelines for difficult airway management, concluding that when conventional intubation techniques fail after three attempts, advanced airway devices should be used and immediately available.[10] The database was divided into two periods. Period A (1990-1995) included 340 intubations in which accessory airway devices, such as the laryngeal mask airway (LMA), bougie, Combitube, or fiberoptic bronchoscope, were not routinely available. Period B (1995-2002) included 437 patients for whom these devices were readily available. The relationship between the use of any accessory airway devices and airway and hemodynamic complications, including number of intubation attempts, hypoxemia, regurgitation, aspiration, bradycardia, and dysrhythmia, was determined. Intubations were performed in the surgical ICU, medical ICU, hospital ward, neurosurgical or trauma ICU, coronary care ICU, emergency department, and postanesthetic care unit. The study found a 33% reduction in hypoxemic episodes (oxygen saturation [SpO_2] <90%) and a 50% reduction in severe hypoxemic episodes (SpO_2 <70%) in group B patients, for whom accessory airway devices were readily available. Regurgitation was reduced from 4% to 1.7%, aspiration from 2.1% to 0.2%, bradycardia from 5% to 2%, dysrhythmia from 9.1% to 3.7%, and multiple intubation attempts from 30% to 15% in group A and B patients, respectively. The use of accessory airway devices increased from 5% in Group A patients to 42% in Group B patients. Notably, LMA use increased 21-fold. The aggressive approach of incorporating the ASA difficult airway management guidelines by early intervention with accessory airway devices led to a remarkable reduction in multiple attempts at laryngoscopy and a decreased incidence of airway and hemodynamic complications. This study confirms the importance of application of the ASA algorithm outside the OR setting and also justifies the immediate availability of a well-stocked difficult airway cart in all hospital locations where emergency airway management is performed, especially the ICU

setting. It also illustrates the importance of familiarity with and experience in the use of accessory airway devices as a mandatory part of the standard of care in routine anesthetic practice.

In the second study, Mort[11] reviewed the utility of exchanging an endotracheal tube (ETT) in the ICU by two methods: direct laryngoscopy (DL) or airway exchange catheters (AECs). ETT exchanges from an 8-year quality improvement database were reviewed. Patients with an uncompromised glottic view (Cormack-Lehane views 1 and 2) were divided by method of exchange: DL ($n = 99$) versus AEC, Cook 14 or 19 French ($n = 34$). Hypoxemia, intubation attempts, esophageal intubation, bradycardia, cardiac arrest, and the need for a surgical airway were compared. Successful ETT exchange on the first attempt was higher with use of an AEC (95% AEC vs. 62% DL). The need for multiple attempts at laryngoscopy was higher in the DL group (26% DL vs. 2.9% AEC). In addition, rescue airway techniques were used more frequently in the DL group (16 of 99 cases; a surgical airway was necessary in 5 of the 16 DL-rescued airways). No rescue maneuvers were necessary in the AEC group. Hypoxemia and severe hypoxemia, esophageal intubation, bradyarrhythmias, and cardiac arrest during DL for ETT exchange were also more frequent in the DL group. It was determined that use of an AEC during ETT exchange in the ICU lowered the risk of complications considerably, even in the presence of a previously uncompromised view of the glottic inlet. This study also highlights the importance of familiarity with alternative techniques to DL as part of safe airway management and anesthetic practice.

Mort[12] also studied the hazards of repeated attempts at laryngoscopy in critically ill patients, with 2833 critically ill patients entered in an emergency intubation quality improvement database. Patients had cardiovascular, pulmonary, metabolic, neurologic, or traumatic injuries. In this retrospective review, the practice analysis documented in the database was evaluated for both airway and hemodynamic complications. These variables were correlated with the number of laryngoscopic attempts required for successful intubation. All the patients required emergency intubation outside the OR setting. A statistically significant increase was seen in airway-related complications when the number of laryngoscopic attempts increased to two or more intubation attempts. The incidences of hypoxemia, regurgitation of gastric contents, aspiration of gastric contents, bradycardia, and cardiac arrest were significantly higher when the number of attempts at conventional laryngoscopy increased. This study supports the recommendation of the ASA Task Force on Management of the Difficult Airway guidelines to limit the number of laryngoscopy attempts and to be facile and familiar with alternative techniques of difficult airway management.[12]

These studies highlight the importance of committed, lifelong learning in the variety of techniques in advanced airway management available to the anesthesiologist. This chapter focuses on the means available to accomplish this goal by review of pertinent supporting literature.

III. TEACHING AIRWAY MANAGEMENT—THE COMPONENTS

The topic of teaching airway management skills can be divided into several components, including anatomy, evaluation of the airway, and teaching materials, such as airway simulators (see Chapter 52). In addition, the scientific literature supports teaching techniques in mask airway management, direct laryngoscopy, fiberoptic intubation, supraglottic airway ventilation or assisted intubation, video laryngoscopy, and surgical airway management. The scientific literature also highlights the utility of instruction in airway management during anesthesiology residency training and postgraduate courses.

Several authors advocate review of basic anatomy as essential groundwork for mastery of difficult airway management. Gaiser[6] published a review of teaching airway management skills, advocating use of an anatomy textbook as a valuable teaching tool. Review of basic airway anatomy can be achieved in lecture format or self-study.[6,13,14] Katz and colleagues[15] used videotapes to review basic airway anatomy as a part of their learning module in fiberoptic intubation (FOI). Haponik and associates[16] used a computer software program to teach tracheobronchial anatomy as a preparation for a virtual training course on FOI. Evaluation of the airway for potential difficulty is an integral part of difficult airway management. The second iteration of the ASA practice guidelines stresses the importance of a thorough history and physical examination of each patient for anticipated difficulty.[5] This evidence-based guideline incorporates 11 physical examination points related to the airway that provide a succinct set of predictors of potential airway difficulty (see Chapter 10). The current guidelines for management of the difficult airway may also be found at the ASA website, www.asahq.org.

Although practicing anesthesiologists and anesthesiology residents have unlimited access to techniques for evaluation of potential difficulty in airway management, other physicians do not. The American College of Obstetricians and Gynecologists (ACOG) emphasizes the importance of identifying parturients at risk for possible difficult intubation (DI) during emergency delivery: "The obstetric care team should be alert to the presence of risk factors that place the parturient at risk for complications from general anesthesia."[17] At the Hospital of the University of Pennsylvania, Gaiser and associates[18] studied the ability of obstetricians to recognize parturients at risk for DI in light of the ACOG policy statement. The 160 parturients had an airway examination conducted by four separate physicians, an attending and resident obstetrician, as well as an attending and resident anesthesiologist. The physicians were asked to complete a questionnaire about DI, use of antepartum consultation, and the choice of labor analgesia after each patient's examination. During the first 80 airway examinations, the obstetricians did not receive any guidance or education on recognition of the difficult airway and complications associated with it. For the following 80 airway examinations, the obstetricians received a 30-minute tutorial on methods to examine the airway for potential difficulty, as well as the complications of DI. The anesthesiologists' responses were used as the standard. The sensitivity, specificity, and positive and negative predictive values were calculated for the responses of the other physicians. Unfortunately, brief, 30-minute tutorials did not affect the results of the obstetricians' ability to assess the airway. Instruction did not affect the number of consultations requested by either resident or attending obstetricians for possible DI. However, attending obstetricians were significantly more likely to utilize epidural analgesia for 2 cm of cervical dilation in women with a possible difficult airway.[18] This study highlights the importance of discussing airway management and its potential complications with surgical colleagues because it can affect clinical judgment, in this case, a change in the choice and timing of labor analgesia in parturients with a suspected difficult airway.

IV. INSTRUCTION IN SPECIFIC TECHNIQUES OR DEVICES

The scientific literature is replete with studies pertaining to mastery of specific devices and techniques of airway management, and a brief review of supraglottic airways, fiberoptic intubation, and the surgical airway is warranted.

A. Laryngeal Mask Airway

The past 30 years has seen a proliferation of supraglottic airway devices. Starting with the laryngeal mask airway described in 1983 by Brain,[19] 14 different supraglottic devices were listed by Cook[20] in 2003. Recommended training for the use of these devices varies according to idiosyncrasies of the individual device. The LMA remains the prototypical supraglottic airway.

Brimacombe[21] provides an excellent review of educational considerations with the LMA, summarizing the myriad sources detailing skills acquisition using the various versions of the LMA. Gurman and coauthors[22] compared retention of airway management skills in 47 medical students instructed in the use of direct laryngoscopy, LMA, and Combitube placement during a 2-week rotation in anesthesiology. Mannequins were used for teaching and testing. The authors noted no diminution in skill with any device over a 6-month period following training.

Dickinson and Curry[23] studied the efficacy of mannequin training for proper LMA insertion in paramedics attending an Advanced Cardiac Life Support (ACLS) training course.[23] A high success rate in the use of the LMA led to the conclusion that this was a suitable alternative to live training in patients. Ferson and coworkers[24] studied 20 anesthesiologists over 2 months, examining the efficacy of instruction in the use of the LMA by comparing manual or videotape training with hands-on training by an experienced anesthesiologist using a mannequin. More than 90% of participants in the hands-on training group achieved passing scores for LMA insertion technique after 17 insertions. Less than 30% of the group using manual videotape training achieved this score.

Brimacombe[21] suggests that four phases of education are required to incorporate the LMA into clinical practice (Box 53-1). Phases 2 to 4 are enhanced when a mentor

Box 53-1 **Phases of Education for Incorporation of Laryngeal Mask Airway (LMA) into Clinical Practice**

Phase 1: Reading and viewing instructional material to gain an understanding of basic concepts on LMA use.
Phase 2: Mannequin or cadaver training to develop basic motor skills for LMA use.
Phase 3: Use of LMA clinically in simple, elective cases to acquire basic clinical skills.
Phase 4: Use of LMA in more complex cases to acquire advanced clinical skills.

(e.g., experienced LMA user) is available to the novice for individualized training. Coulson and coauthors[25] showed that digital insertion of the ProSeal LMA (pLMA) using inexperienced personnel after mannequin-only training was as successful as in anesthetized adults. Success rates of approximately 90% after 2 minutes were found in each group.

The I-gel (Intersurgical, Workingham, UK) is another supraglottic airway device (SAD) with demonstrated promise. Wharton and associates[26] demonstrated an 82.5% success rate in mannequins and 80% success rate in anesthetized patients on the first attempt by novice users (medical students, non-anesthesia physicians, allied health professionals). Roberts[27] concluded that mannequin-only training in the emergency technique for LMA insertion is as effective as live patient training. However, Rai and Popat[28] note the limitations of mannequin-only studies and training, emphasizing that even advanced, high-fidelity simulation mannequins are unable to recreate the "feel" and finer aspects of human airway anatomy.

B. Fiberoptic Intubation

In an early study of clinical competence in the performance of fiberoptic laryngoscopy and endotracheal intubation, Johnson and Roberts[29] hypothesized that an acceptable level of technical expertise in fiberoptic intubation could be acquired within 10 intubations while maintaining patient safety. The learning objectives included an intubation time of 2 minutes or less and greater than 90% success on the first intubation attempt. Ninety-one ASA class I or II patients with normal laryngeal anatomy undergoing general anesthesia were intubated orally with an Olympus LF-1 fiberoptic scope after induction of general anesthesia. The mean time for intubation was 1.92 (±1.45) minutes. Four anesthesiology residents without prior fiberoptic experience intubated at least 15 patients each. A learning curve was generated using logarithmic analysis of the mean (±SD) time for intubation of patients 1 to 15 for all residents combined. The learning curve noted that the mean intubation time decreased from 4.00 (±2.91) minutes to 1.52 (±0.76) minutes within the first 10 intubations. After the tenth asleep FOI, the mean intubation time was 1.53 minutes, with greater than 95% success rate for the first attempt. No clinically significant changes in oxygen saturation (So_2), mean arterial pressure, or heart rate were noted

during asleep FOI in this study. An acceptable level of technical expertise in FOI can be achieved safely by performing at least 10 elective asleep FOIs by novice anesthesiologists.[29]

Erb[30] evaluated teaching orotracheal FOI in 100 anesthetized, spontaneously breathing patients. Five anesthesia residents without prior experience in FOI participated in this study. Each resident randomly intubated 10 spontaneously breathing patients (group A) and 10 paralyzed patients (group B) tracheally. An overall success rate of 96% was defined as successful endotracheal intubation in two attempts or less. No difference was found between the two groups. During FOI, So_2 remained over 95% in group A, whereas 2 of 10 patients in group B had So_2 fall below 95% during fiberoptic attempts. The authors noted that FOI under conditions of spontaneous respiration is a well-established, standard-of-care technique of difficult airway management. This study demonstrated a feasible and safe method to train novices in the skill of FOI under conditions of general anesthesia and spontaneous ventilation.[30]

At the Children's Memorial Hospital at Northwestern University, Wheeler and colleagues[31] performed a study teaching residents pediatric FOI. Twenty clinical anesthesia second-year (CA-2) residents were randomly assigned to the traditional teaching group (FOI with standard eyepiece) or the video-assisted group (FOI using integrated camera and video screen). All residents were novices in pediatric FOI. One of two attending anesthesiologists supervised each resident during the elective FOI of 15 healthy children ages 1 to 6 years. Variables included time from mask removal to confirmation of successful endotracheal intubation by end-tidal carbon dioxide detection and FOI attempts up to 3 minutes or three attempts. The primary outcome of time to success or failure was compared between the two groups. Failure rates, as well as the number of attempts, were also compared. Of 300 intubations attempted; eight failed. On average, the group using video-assisted FOI as a training tool was faster and three times more likely to achieve successful FOI. The video-assisted group also had significantly fewer attempts at intubation than the residents in the traditional group. The authors concluded that a video-assisted system, where the attending anesthesiologist is able to provide real-time feedback during FOI of pediatric patients, was superior as a teaching method to the traditional teaching model.[31] The newer generations of video FOI equipment are especially useful in such teaching situations. This type of equipment allows for viewing by multiple persons, as well as capture of still images and videos for later review (Olympus MAF-Type GM, TM, LF-V).

Ovassapian[32] provides a succinct review of learning fiberoptic intubation techniques, emphasizing the following points to encourage more frequent use of the fiberscope in anesthesia and critical care practice[8] (Boxes 53-2 and 53-3:

1. The techniques of FOI are not difficult to learn. Mastery of the art of fiberoptic airway management readily develops with time and experience.
2. The technique of FOI is different from rigid laryngoscopy. Without formal training, the anesthesiologist

---

Box 53-2 Guidelines for Successful Fiberoptic Intubation

1. Organize a functional fiberoptic cart.
2. Maintain a functional fiberscope.
3. Follow a checklist prior to each use.
4. Skillfully manipulate the fiberscope.
5. Follow approaches and steps of fiberoptic intubation.

---

should not expect immediate and successful use of the fiberscope for endotracheal intubation.

3. No anesthesiologist should perform a new technical task without studying and developing the required base of knowledge involved in its performance.
4. The fiberscope is a simple but sophisticated airway management tool. It should be utilized to its full diagnostic and therapeutic potential in airway management. The greater the experience of the anesthesiologist in using the fiberscope under a variety of clinical circumstances, the greater is the degree of skill that develops with time.
5. The essential steps for successful use of the fiberscope include organizing and maintaining a functional fiberoptic cart, setting up an instrument and intubation checklist, and practicing on models to develop the skills necessary for fiberoptic maneuvering.

Naik and coauthors[33] attempted to determine if FOI skills learned outside the OR on a simple model could be transferred to the clinical setting. Twenty-four first-year anesthesiology and second-year internal medicine residents were recruited for this study. Residents were randomly allocated to a didactic teaching group ($n = 12$) or a model-training group ($n = 12$). The didactic teaching group received a detailed lecture from an expert in FOI. The model-training group was expertly guided through the tasks performed on a simple model designed to refine fiberoptic manipulation skills. After the training session, residents performed a fiberoptic orotracheal intubation on healthy, consenting, anesthetized, paralyzed female patients who were undergoing elective surgery. Patients were predicted to be easy laryngoscopic intubations. Two "blinded" anesthesiologists evaluated each patient. The authors found that the model-training group outperformed the didactic group in the OR when evaluated with a global rating scale, as well as a

---

Box 53-3 Knowledge Base for Performing Fiberoptic Intubation (FOI)

- How the fiberscope functions
- How to avoid damaging the fiberscope
- Indications for FOI
- Limitations of FOI
- How to recognize abnormal airway anatomy
- Appropriate preparation of the patient
- How to provide safe conscious sedation
- How to provide good topical anesthesia of the airway
- How to monitor the patient adequately
- Causes of failure of FOI
- Complications of fiberoptic airway endoscopy

---

preparatory checklist. The model-trained residents completed fiberoptic orotracheal intubation significantly faster and more often than didactic-trained residents. The authors concluded that training fiberoptic orotracheal intubation skills using a simple model is more effective than conventional didactic instruction, when incorporating skills in the clinical setting. They suggested that incorporation of model-based training in FOI may greatly reduce the time accompanying subsequent training in the OR.[33]

In a study of an educational resource specific to the acquisition and maintenance of endoscopic skills, Marsland and colleagues[34] describe the use of DEXTER. This nonanatomic, endoscopic dexterity–training system is designed to encourage practice in fiberoptic endoscopy as well as establish and maintain a state of procedural readiness. Educational training systems such as DEXTER help to maintain these skills even if the anesthesiologist's clinical exposure to difficult airway management is sporadic.

The pulmonary literature also addresses the issue of training in fiberoptic bronchoscopy. In a study of "virtual reality" bronchoscopic training, Colt and colleagues[13] hypothesized that novice trainees in the procedure of flexible fiberoptic bronchoscopy could rapidly acquire basic skills using a virtual-reality skill center. Furthermore, these trainees would compare favorably with senior colleagues who had been conventionally trained on live patients. Five novice bronchoscopists entering a pulmonary–critical care training program were studied prospectively. Flexible fiberoptic bronchoscopic inspection of the tracheobronchial tree was taught using a virtual-reality bronchoscopic skill center, including a proxy flexible bronchoscope, robotic interface device, and personal computer with monitor and simulation software (PreOp Endoscopy Simulator; Immersion Medical, Gaithersburg, Md). The proxy bronchoscope, modeled after a conventional fiberoptic bronchoscope, provides realistic images to the users as they navigate through virtual tracheobronchial anatomy.[13] The authors measured dexterity, speed, and accuracy using the skill center as well as an inanimate airway model before and after 4 hours of group instruction and 4 hours of individual unsupervised practice. The results of this group were compared with those of a control group of four skilled physicians. Each of these pulmonologists had performed at least 200 bronchoscopies during 2 years of training. They found that novice bronchoscopists significantly improved dexterity and accuracy using either the virtual or inanimate airway model. After training, fewer bronchial segments were missed, and fewer contacts with the tracheobronchial wall occurred. Speed and total time spent with unvisualized bronchial anatomy did not change. After training, novice performance equaled or surpassed that of skilled physicians. Novices tended to perform more thorough examinations of the tracheobronchial tree. They missed significantly fewer bronchial segments in both the inanimate and virtual simulation models. The authors concluded that a short, focused course of instruction and unsupervised practice using a virtual bronchoscopy simulator enabled novices to achieve a level of technical skill similar to that of colleagues with several years of experience.[13] These skills were reproduced in an inanimate airway training model that mimics direct care of patients.

Conversely, Crabtree and associates[35] showed that simulator performance may not be a good indicator of FOI performance in the clinical setting. Chandra and colleagues[36] concluded that there was no added benefit from training on costly virtual-reality models compared with low-fidelity, nonanatomic models designed to refine FOI skills with respect to transfer of skills to actual patient care.

C. Surgical Airway

Lack of experience is the main source of procedural failure with cricothyrotomy, although hands-on training is also lacking. A study evaluating difficult airway instruction found that although 80% of American anesthesiology residency training programs taught cricothyrotomy, 60% of these courses consisted of only lectures.[37] As a result, many physicians lack the necessary skills to perform a cricothyrotomy correctly or expeditiously.

Correct and safe performance of cricothyrotomy is life-saving in patients who cannot be ventilated or intubated successfully. Eisenburger and coworkers[38] compared conventional surgical technique (group 1) versus Seldinger technique (group 2) emergency cricothyrotomy performed by inexperienced clinicians in adult human cadavers. The ease of use and times to locate the cricothyroid membrane, to tracheal puncture, and to first lung ventilation were compared. Participants were allowed a single attempt at the procedure. A pathologist dissected the neck of each cadaver to assess the correct position of the tube and any injury to the airway. Subjective assessment of the technique on a visual analog scale (1 = easiest to 5 = most difficult) was conducted. The age, height, and weight of the cadavers used in this study were uniform. Subjective assessment of each method as well as anatomy of the cadavers was not statistically different between the two groups. Correct tracheal placement of the tube was achieved in 70% of surgical cricothyrotomies ($n = 14$) and 60% of Seldinger cricothyrotomy ($n = 12$). Five attempts in group 2 (Seldinger) were aborted because of kinking of the guidewire. Time intervals between start of the procedure and location of the cricothyroid membrane, tracheal puncture, and first ventilation were not statistically different. Thus, in this limited study, each method showed equally poor performance and suggested that further study be undertaken to define the learning curve of this life-saving procedure.[38]

McCarthy and colleagues[39] attempted to define the accuracy of cricothyrotomy performed in canine versus human cadaver models during surgical skills training. Thirty-three advanced trauma life support (ATLS) physician students performed cricothyrotomy in canine models. Ten flight nurses performed a bimonthly surgical skills practicum on similarly prepared animals. Neck specimens of the euthanized animals were excised, fixed, and mapped by the authors. Subsequent courses in ATLS used human cadavers and similarly prepared trainees. In these models, cricothyrotomy sites were mapped in situ.

In canine models, 47 neck specimens of 52 attempted cricothyrotomies were inspected and mapped. Four specimens were excluded from the final analysis because of multiple attempts at cricothyrotomy. Thirteen of the 43 analyzed canine models had a misplaced cricothyrotomy (30.2%). Cricothyrotomy attempts were correct 27 of 28 times in the human cadaver model (96.4%). The authors concluded that placement accuracy in the canine model was low, and that human cadaver models were superior for realistic training.[39]

Wong and associates[40] attempted to determine the minimum training experience required to perform surgical cricothyroidotomy in 40 seconds or less in mannequins. The 102 anesthesiologists participating in this study were shown a video demonstrating the Seldinger technique of cricothyrotomy. They then performed 10 consecutive cricothyrotomy procedures on a mannequin using a preassembled percutaneous dilatational cricothyrotomy set (Melker Emergency Percutaneous Dilatational Set; Cook Critical Care, Bloomington, Ind). Each attempted procedure was timed from initial palpation of the skin to successful lung insufflation. Cricothyrotomy was considered successful if performed in 40 seconds or less. Cricothyrotomy time was considered to have reached a plateau when there was no significant reduction in time in three consecutive attempts. A significant reduction in time for successful cricothyrotomy was found over the 10 attempts. The cricothyrotomy time reached a plateau by the fourth attempt. Success rate reached a plateau by the fifth attempt. The authors concluded that mannequin practice for percutaneous dilational cricothyrotomy led to a reduction in cricothyrotomy time and improved success rates of this procedure. By the fifth attempt, 96% of participants were able to perform a cricothyrotomy successfully in 40 seconds or less. The authors recommended that clinicians providing emergency airway management should be trained on mannequins for at least five attempts or until performance times of 40 seconds or less are achieved. Clinical correlation and optimal retraining intervals for this procedure have yet to be determined.[40]

Friedman and colleagues[37] compared cricothyrotomy skills acquired in a simple inexpensive model to those learned on a high-fidelity simulator using valid evaluation instruments and testing on cadavers. First-year and second-year anesthesia residents were recruited. All performed a pretest videotaped cricothyrotomy on cadavers. Subjects were then randomized into two groups. The high-fidelity group ($n = 11$) performed two cricothyrotomies on a full-scale simulator with anatomically accurate larynx. The low-fidelity group ($n = 11$) performed two cricothyrotomies on a low-fidelity model constructed from corrugated tubing. Within 2 weeks, all subjects performed a post-test. Two blinded examiners graded and timed the performances using a checklist and global rating scale. The results showed no significant difference between the two groups. The authors concluded that skills acquired using the simple model were not significantly different from those acquired using the expensive simulator.[37] Skills acquired from both models transferred effectively to cadaver performance.

V. RESIDENT TRAINING IN ADVANCED AIRWAY MANAGEMENT

Anesthesiologists are physicians specialized in advanced airway management, including ventilation and endotracheal intubation. Despite extensive exposure to advanced airway management, challenges to intubation and ventilation may be encountered in daily practice. It is vital to provide trainees experience in the recognition and management of the difficult airway. Formal, organized rotations in advanced airway management better prepare future physicians in management of a difficult airway. Training programs with a comprehensive difficult airway rotation are associated with decreased respiratory morbidity and less need for emergency surgical airways.[41]

Since the introduction of the ASA Practice Guidelines for Management of the Difficult Airway in 1993, surveys have assessed if training programs are incorporating a difficult airway module in their core curriculum. A recent survey, conducted by a Society of Airway Management (SAM) task force, showed that 43 of 88 ACGME- and ACUDA-approved residency programs offered a formal airway rotation, a significant increase from 33% of residency training programs in 2003.[42,43]

Despite an improved emphasis on teaching trainees the recognition and management of the difficult airway, there remains a lack of uniformity with regard to minimum requirements for competencies with a variety of airway devices or techniques. As a result, a trainee's experience in advanced airway management may vary dramatically from one training program to another. The following reviews discuss factors that are important considerations in the development of a useful and successful difficult airway management curriculum.

In 1995, a survey on formal training in advanced airway management techniques was sent to the program directors of 169 anesthesiology residency training programs in the United States; 143 directors responded.[44] Formal rotations in advanced airway management were brief and often limited to didactic lectures. Only 27% of responding programs had a formal advanced airway management course in their curriculum, and 60% of these courses were less than 2 weeks in duration.

Subsequently, a number of academic anesthesiology departments published their specific rotations in advanced airway management. Cooper and Benumof[45] described the University of California–San Diego Department of Anesthesiology's advanced airway rotation. The goal of this rotation was to create nonurgent, nonstressful learning situations where a number of airway management techniques can be mastered in patients. The rotation includes the administrative responsibilities of starting an airway rotation. Administrative aspects include (1) approval of the residency program director, the departmental education committee, or both; (2) selecting experienced faculty to serve as instructors; (3) careful scheduling; (4) formulating the didactic program; and (5) having the appropriate equipment available (e.g., a dedicated difficult airway cart). Residents receive a syllabus containing classic and current articles on both airway management devices and techniques before the rotation. The syllabus is the foundation for both formal

didactic teaching and informal teaching in the OR.[45] Before use in any patient, any new or unfamiliar airway device or technique is discussed thoroughly with regard to theory, description, insertion technique, and current clinical practice. Subsequently, the individual device is used in models, mannequins, or both. When invasive techniques are introduced (e.g., retrograde intubation, transtracheal jet ventilation, or percutaneous cricothyrotomy), a special workshop is held at the anatomy laboratory of the medical school. Human cadavers serve as models for instruction in the necessary technical skills involved in the procedure.

Patient selection is critical during this rotation. According to the authors, straightforward patients are ideal, including ASA class I or II patients undergoing elective general anesthesia without the need for extensive monitoring or setup. These patients undergo surgery in the supine position, with ready access to the airway throughout the procedure. Patients with head or neck injury, in whom there is competition for the airway, are generally avoided unless the patient requires an awake intubation technique. Patients with a known or suspected difficult airway are prioritized to the resident on the airway management rotation. A goal of this rotation is to perform advanced airway management techniques for 40 to 50 patients during the 1-month rotation.[45] Didactic teaching includes performance of a thorough evaluation of the airway based on the current ASA recommendations on difficult airway management.[5] The findings of every airway examination are discussed with the supervising faculty. Residents are instructed in proper preparation of the patient for awake intubation techniques. In addition, they garner experience in devices such as the LMA, Combitube, lighted stylets, and advanced rigid fiberoptic laryngoscopes. The adjunct use of the fiberoptic bronchoscope (FOB) is encouraged. Once a patent airway is established, the resident is encouraged to identify all pertinent tracheobronchial anatomy by inserting an FOB through a bronchoscope adapter.[45]

Dunn and colleagues[46] at Baystate Medical Center in Springfield, Massachusetts, described their resident training in advanced airway management. They developed a formal advanced airway management program consisting of two separate 1-month rotations. Each rotation has a separate focus. One month occurs during the later half of the CA-1 year. The second month occurs during the CA-2 year. Residents are given a set of objectives, a required reading list, and a required number of procedures unique to advanced airway management. These procedures must be performed during the course of the rotation. This rotation consists of a core faculty group with expertise in airway management. According to the authors, five issues must be addressed in order to implement an airway rotation: (1) equipment, (2) core faculty, (3) curriculum, (4) time commitment, and (5) faculty development.[46]

The Baystate Medical Center rotation uses seven difficult airway (DA) carts distributed in five anesthetizing locations. The carts are uniformly set up and stocked. The authors believe that uniformity of *equipment* enhances physician performance of emergent airway management. Each cart and its contents cost approximately $30,000.[46]

Contents of the DA carts include a variety of face masks, different sizes of the LMA, Combitube, and transtracheal puncture equipment. Each DA cart is equipped with the three modalities of difficult airway management thought to be the most helpful: flexible FOB, intubating LMA (Fastrach; LMA North America, San Diego), and a variety of rigid fiberoptic laryngoscopes. Each cart incorporates a video system, which improves teaching and is an integral part of the program.

Core faculty members are proficient in all modalities of airway management. The size of the core faculty group is sufficient to ensure coverage during vacations, other clinical commitments, and so forth. At least one faculty member is available each day of the rotation. Contact with a core group of faculty ensures that residents master each technique in an adequately supervised fashion.[46]

The *curriculum* for this rotation includes a required reading list. Each of these publications requires discussion with a core faculty member to demonstrate adequate knowledge of the contents. The first month's rotation for CA-1 residents focuses on the ASA airway management algorithm, as well as techniques of FOB. The second month's rotation for CA-2 residents has a separate reading list and focuses on alternative techniques of advanced airway management as well as complications.[46] Requirements for successful completion of the first month of the rotation include no fewer than 10 fiberoptic intubations, 10 Bullard Scope intubations, and six LMA Fastrach intubations. In the second month of the airway rotation, the resident is required to perform at least 10 additional fiberoptic intubations (at least two pediatric fiberoptic intubations), 10 Bullard intubations, and six LMA Fastrach intubations. Residents in both months of the rotation are encouraged to seek out "known difficult airway" cases on the elective schedule, as well as participate in the preoperative consultation of these patients. A worksheet detailing each difficult airway case is kept by the resident and "signed off" by the core faculty. The authors detail the importance of departmental commitment to advanced airway management training, as well as the development of faculty interested in advanced airway management.[46]

Hagberg and colleagues[43] at the University of Texas Medical School at Houston reviewed the instruction of airway management skills during anesthesiology residency training. This study, a follow-up to Koppel and Reed's study,[44] was conducted 3 years after the mandate of the Accreditation Council for Graduate Medical Education (ACGME) requiring that residents have significant experience in specialized techniques of airway management, such as fiberoptic intubation, double-lumen tube placement, and LMA use.[43] A survey of all directors of anesthesiology residency programs listed in the Graduate Medical Education Directory for the years 1998 and 1999 was conducted. The survey was sent by both e-mail and fax to each program director. A second copy was sent to non-responders 4 weeks after the initial mailing. Of the 132 program directors surveyed, 79 (60%) replied. Of the 79 respondents, 26 reported programs (33%) that had a difficult airway rotation. Interestingly, this number had increased only slightly since prior publications and the ACGME mandate.[43] An advanced airway

management rotation was offered throughout the clinical base years of training in 13 (49%) programs of respondents. The rotation was 1 week in duration in 16 (61%) of the cases offering a program. Formal instruction was given before the start of the rotation in 18 (69%) programs. Instruction usually occurred using surgical patients (in 22 or 85% of programs), using ASA I or II patients (in 20 or 77% of programs), and was conducted by select faculty (in 20 or 78% of programs).

The most frequently taught airway management modalities included the flexible FOB and the LMA. Invasive techniques such as percutaneous cricothyrotomy or tracheostomy were taught infrequently. There was a time limitation of 2 to 5 minutes or a maximum number of attempts in device-specific airway management in five programs (19%). A required case number for each device was found in five of the programs surveyed (19%). In this survey, instruction in advanced techniques of airway management occurred most often in the form of video, written instruction, and practice on actual patients undergoing surgical procedures. Nontraditional methods of instruction, such as computer-assisted instruction or patient simulators, were used infrequently. Residents received both skills and written evaluation in 63% of the programs with a specific rotation in advanced airway management.[43]

This study raised several questions about the instruction of advanced airway management, suggesting further study on the efficacy of different training techniques. The authors are proponents of a future clinical certification process for training in advanced airway management for all anesthesiologists. They suggest that the residency review committees for anesthesiology and the ACGME should establish number requirements for specific airway-related procedures to ensure standardization of resident training. Follow-up studies are warranted when such mandates are established, because standardization of training in these techniques may further decrease airway-related morbidity and mortality.[43]

Allen and Murray[47] addressed the issue of *patient consent* when teaching airway management skills, suggesting that any procedure that deviates significantly from the standard of care should invoke patient consent. In the authors' practice, substitution of laryngoscope blades or use of the LMA or lightwand does not require specific patient consent. However, use of the Combitube, FOI, any retrograde technique, or elective repeated instrumentation with several different devices requires patient consent. Most important, the authors stress that constant supervision of residents by experienced faculty is of paramount importance to minimize patient risk. Initial experience in advanced airway management in a simulated environment may further reduce patient risk.[47]

Benumof and Cooper's reply[48] to Allen and Murray[47] stated that special consent was not necessary for well-established and accepted airway management techniques, especially in the presence of experienced faculty. Constant supervision by experienced faculty ensures against undue force or rough handling of the airway and offers the ability to abort or change an initial airway management technique as needed. In Benumof and Cooper's published experience of approximately 1000 faculty–airway rotation resident cases, only three adverse outcomes occurred. In two cases, intubation through the self-sealing FOB adapter on an intubating anesthesia mask resulted in a piece of the blue diaphragm being inadvertently carried into the trachea; thus, these adapters were no longer used. In each case, the complication was recognized immediately by the supervising faculty. Bronchoscopy forceps were used in both cases through the FOB's working channel to retrieve the piece of plastic, without incident. The third event occurred when an improperly sterilized LMA was used. The LMA was inadvertently cleaned in Cidex, and perilaryngeal edema ensued in the patient. The patient was tracheally intubated and experienced no long-term morbidity. The cleaning impropriety was corrected. The authors stress that careful use of accepted methods under strict and expert supervision does not mandate patient consent.[48]

Learning in the OR or emergency room environment is not ideal, because it imposes stressors on both the patient and the student. Possible dental trauma, aspiration, and bruised or lacerated soft tissue can occur, even under close patient supervision. Factors that may hinder the learning process for the resident include concerns of harming the patient and increased performance pressure with watchful OR staff (nurses, surgeons). In addition, time constraints, such as impending oxygen desaturation, delay of the start of surgical case, and increased pressure to maintain the OR schedule, can interfere with the airway management learning process and limits opportunity for instruction and criticism.[49] Furthermore, students are rarely given a second chance if they fail the first time, especially if the patient is a difficult intubation. This further hinders the learning process for the student. Conversely, other procedures are simply not reasonable to practice on healthy patients, such as cricothyrotomy. Despite these limitations, the performance of various airway management skills in the elective patient or simulated setting are vitally important to the success in more urgent or unanticipated settings.

In a 2007 *Chest* article, Kory and associates[50] evaluated the teaching of airway management in medicine residents, challenging the traditional belief of "learning by doing" for resident training. The authors hypothesized that the "see one, do one, teach one" method is not appropriate in high-risk, low-frequency events such as respiratory arrest and difficult intubation patients. Although most programs offer simulation technology, it is not yet a standard component of residency training programs. Studying scenario-based training (SBT) and computerized patient simulator (CPS) versus traditionally trained (TT), the authors found that SBT-trained and CPS-trained internal medicine residents performed better than TT internal medicine residents in airway management skills.[50] This study focused on internal medicine residents, but its basic principles can theoretically be extrapolated to the training of any medical specialty in difficult airway management.

Training using simulators can be helpful for more advanced airway skills such as FOI and the intubating laryngeal mask airway (ILMA). Simulation facilitates the learning process in airway management and also offers other advantages, such as no risk of patient injury.

Simulation allows for the performance of multiple attempts and types of interventions, allowing for errors because patient harm is avoided. Interventions can be stopped for feedback from trainers, uncommon scenarios can be created for serial practice, and interventions can be repeated after feedback for reinforced teaching. Simulator training decreases the amount of time performing the actual task on patients. This is useful for new trainees, whose skills are generally limited, and reduces the potential for patient injury. Naik and associates[33] show that acquired skills from a simple training model are transferable to the clinical environment. Compared with basic didactic training, those who trained with a basic model for FOI demonstrated a faster intubation time, improved intubation success rate, and better technique. Further discussion of the role of simulation in advanced airway management is discussed in Chapter 52.

Model trainings can also be beneficial for tasks that are infrequently encountered on actual patients. Kory and others[50] studied the progression of two groups: medical students trained by the traditional method of experience as clinical opportunities arose vs. students trained through patient simulator and SBT. The simulator group outperformed the TT group.

Another option for practice in infrequently performed airway management techniques involves the use of recently deceased individuals. Advantages include the ability to practice invasive procedures such as cricothyrotomy in a realistic setting. Consent from family members is obtained for this practice. Olsen and colleagues[51] found that obtaining consent from family to perform postmortem procedures is a valid option. The most common reason for refusal is personal and religious beliefs. After consent in this study, a cricothyrotomy was performed by emergency medicine resident physicians, supervised by an attending physician.

To develop successful skills in airway management, anesthesia residents should use mannequins and simulators suitable for the intricacy of the training objective. Simple models are sufficient in gaining basic skills and knowledge. Once a trainee becomes more comfortable with the device or technique, more detailed models and simulators may be helpful in conveying more complex goals and objectives. At Penn State's training program, anesthesia residents use mannequins for practice in cricothyrotomy. However, mannequin training alone is not sufficient for developing intubation skills or management of a difficult airway with most devices. One study showed that only 53 of 103 intubations by emergency medical technicians (EMTs), solely using mannequin practice, were successful, with many requiring more than one attempt.[52]

Laryngoscopy and intubation are fundamental skills of all anesthesiologists. However, it is necessary to be proficient with other adjunctive airway management skills to have a variety of methods to secure a difficult airway successfully. Connelly and associates[53] conducted a retrospective study of unanticipated difficult airways and found higher success rates with LMA and FOI, when compared to repeated direct laryngoscopy. National surveys of anesthesia programs find that more than one skill set is needed to be effective in managing a difficult airway. This is partly the result of the variation in accessibility of certain equipment from place to place.[43] In addition to basic laryngoscopy and mask ventilation, proficiency with FOI and ILMA use are both deemed essential in training.[49]

Skill in providing ventilation through basic face mask skills is often overlooked during residency training. Effective mask airway can salvage a difficult intubation in emergency settings, but it is also used for adequate preoxygenation and to control ventilation as part of initial resuscitation. Areas of focus include proper mask selection, proper mask placement to provide a good seal, and proper neck extension and jaw thrust, to facilitate mask ventilation and prevent associated complications, such as gastric distention or aspiration, soft tissue injury, and corneal abrasions.[54] Equally important is the recognition of patient characteristics associated with difficult mask ventilation and use of an oral/nasal airway, when needed.

Laryngoscopy is a basic skill all anesthesia residents must acquire during their residency. A study of first-year anesthesia residents by Konrad and colleagues[55] found that successful intubation increased rapidly during the first 20 attempts, and the learning curve reached 90% success rate after a mean of 57 attempts. However, even after 80 intubations, 18% of residents still required assistance. Mulcaster and associates[56] investigated skill with direct laryngoscopy by nonanesthesia individuals and found similar results, with an average of 47 intubation attempts needed to reach a 90% success rate. Mannequin training alone was not sufficient to adequately prepare nonanesthesia individuals for successful direct laryngoscopy. A majority of the individuals studied had difficulties with direct laryngoscopy performed on patients despite 20 successful intubations on mannequins. Hirsch-Allen and coworkers[57] found that the year of training and type of residency were associated with multiple tracheal intubation attempts. Anesthesia residents had the lowest reintubation rate, regardless of their year of training. This important study emphasizes that a higher number of intubations is needed to obtain a 90% successful rate for nonanesthesia physicians who desire to master the technique of direct laryngoscopy and endotracheal intubation.

In a study of LMAs placed by EMTs, insertion was 100% successful in mannequins but only 64% successful in the field.[58] This emphasizes the performance of LMA insertion on live patients and deemphasizes the importance of mannequin training as a sole teaching tool.

Video-enabled technology is another tool in the airway management armamentarium[59] and another vital skill that residents should acquire during residency training. Video-enabled airway technology includes the integration of existing intubation equipment (laryngoscope, fiberscope) with a video system, allowing the image to be projected onto a monitor. Recording the resident's attempt at intubation enables supervising faculty to provide insight on the performance, allows for review and correction of technical inadequacies by guiding the resident's hand during the attempt, and allows for feedback afterward. Instructors are able to visualize what the trainee sees during laryngoscopy or FOI. By doing so, the video system allows both mentor and student to share the same view of anatomy and to follow the progress of the airway management technique employed.[60]

Video-enabled systems may be superior in the successful intubation of some difficult airway patients compared with conventional direct laryngoscopy.[59] Jungbauer and colleagues[61] prospectively studied tracheal intubation of 200 patients with Mallampati scores of 3 or 4 using the Berci-Kaplan video laryngoscopy (Storz) system, versus direct laryngoscopy. The video system provided a superior view of the cords, had a higher success rate, had faster time to intubation, and required fewer optimizing maneuvers than direct laryngoscopy.[61] Marrel and associates[62] studied video laryngoscopy and direct laryngoscopy in 80 morbidly obese patients. They found that the view achieved with the video system was significantly better in 28 patients and duration of intubation shorter.

Numerous studies support the routine use of alternatives to direct laryngoscopy in the setting of failed and known difficult intubation. Studies support the use of salvage interventions in the setting of an unanticipated difficult intubation with a practiced alternative, because these are likely to be associated with better outcomes compared with persistent direct laryngoscopy. Video laryngoscopy is emerging as a vital tool in both anticipated and unanticipated difficult intubation.[59] Residents should be familiar and trained to use one or more of the commercially available video laryngoscopes during their training. Video laryngoscopes are necessary tools for difficult airway management when direct laryngoscopy fails and also serve as invaluable tools in teaching advanced airway management.

VI. CONCLUSIONS

Anesthesiologists are recognized as airway management specialists in most aspects of modern medical practice. With this recognition comes responsibility. Anesthesiologists should make a career-long commitment to foster expertise in the recognition and management of the difficult airway through proficient examination of the patient, communication and documentation of airway management concerns with physician colleagues, and appropriate application of specialized techniques of advanced airway management, when applicable. Fortunately, a variety of different methods are available for training and experience in advanced airway management. The key to learning and skill acquisition remains the interest and commitment of the individual.

VII. CLINICAL PEARLS

- Hands-on training with laryngeal mask airway insertion is associated with higher success rates than manual or videotape training. However, even the most advanced mannequins are unable to recreate human airway anatomy.

- Novice anesthesiologists can safely achieve an acceptable level of technical expertise in fiberoptic intubation by performing at least 10 elective, asleep fiberoptic intubations.

- The main cause of failure with cricothyrotomy is lack of experience and hands-on training. Ten attempts on a manikin decreases time and improves success in percutaneous dilatational cricothyrotomy.

- Establishment of an airway rotation requires proper equipment, core faculty, curriculum, time commitment, and faculty development.

- Constant faculty supervision provides patient safety and the ability to abort or change airway management.

- Learning in the OR is not ideal. Training using simulators can be helpful with more advanced airway skills, such as fiberoptic intubation and intubating LMA. Skills achieved with simple training models are transferable to the clinical environment.

- Laryngoscopy is a basic skill all anesthesia residents should master during training.

- Video-enabled technology can be beneficial in the training of residents in difficult airway management.

- Residents should be familiar with various intubating devices during training. Salvage interventions for unanticipated difficult intubation are associated with better outcomes than persistent direct laryngoscopy.

- Use of airway exchange catheters during endotracheal tube exchange in the ICU lowers the risk of complications, even with a previously uncompromised view of the glottic inlet.

SELECTED REFERENCES

All references can be found online at expertconsult.com.

11. Mort TC: Exchanging an ETT in the presence of an uncompromised view: direct laryngoscopy vs. the airway exchange catheter. *Crit Care Med* 30: Research citation K, 2003.

24. Ferson DZ, Bui TP, Arens JF: Evaluation of the effectiveness of two methods of training for the insertion of the laryngeal mask airway. *Anesthesiology* 93:A558, 2000.

29. Johnson C, Roberts JT: Clinical competence in the performance of fiberoptic laryngoscopy and endotracheal intubation: a study of resident instruction. *J Clin Anesth* 1:344, 1989.

31. Wheeler M, Roth AG, Dsida RM, et al: Teaching residents pediatric fiberoptic intubation of the trachea: traditional fiberscope with an eyepiece versus video-assisted technique using a fiberscope with an integrated camera. *Anesthesiology* 101:842, 2004.

33. Naik VN, Matsumoto ED, Houston PL, et al: Fiberoptic orotracheal intubation on anesthetized patients: do manipulation skills learned on a simple model transfer into the operating room? *Anesthesiology* 95:343, 2001.

37. Friedman Z, You-Ten KE, Bould MD, et al: Teaching lifesaving procedures: the impact of model fidelity on acquisition and transfer of cricothyrotomy skills to performance on cadavers. *Anesth Analg* 107:1663–1669, 2008.

38. Eisenburger P, Laczika K, List M, et al: Comparison of conventional surgical versus Seldinger technique emergency cricothyrotomy performed by inexperienced clinicians. *Anesthesiology* 92:687, 2000.

40. Wong DT, Prabhu AF, Coloma M, et al: What is the minimum training required for successful cricothyroidotomy? A study in mannequins. *Anesthesiology* 98:349, 2003.

46. Dunn S, Connelly NR, Robbins L: Resident training in advanced airway management. *J Clin Anesth* 16:472, 2004.

48. Benumof JL, Cooper SD: Reply. *Anesthesiology* 85:438, 1996.

49. Crosby E, Lane A: Innovations in anesthesia education: the development and implementation of a resident rotation for advanced airway management. *Can J Anaesth* 56:939–959, 2009.

55. Konrad C, Schupfer G, Wietlisbach M, et al: Learning manual skills in anesthesiology: is there a recommended number of cases for anesthetic procedures? *Anesth Analg* 86:635–639, 1998.

56. Mulcaster JT, Mills J, Hung OR, et al: Laryngoscopic intubation: learning and performance. *Anesthesiology* 98:23–27, 2003.

57. Hirsch-Allen AJ, Ayas N, Mountain S, et al: Influence of residency training on multiple attempts at endotracheal intubation. *Can J Anaesth* 57:823–829, 2010.

59. Behringer EC, Kristensen MS: Evidence of novelty versus benefit of new intubation equipment. *Anaesthesia* 66(Suppl):57–64, 2011.

60. Kaplan MB, Ward DS, Berci G: A new video laryngoscope: an aid to intubation and teaching. *J Clin Anesth* 14:620–626, 2002.

Effective Dissemination of Critical Airway Information: The MedicAlert Foundation* National Difficult Airway/Intubation Registry

LYNETTE J. MARK, MD | LORRAINE J. FOLEY, MD

I. OVERVIEW

Dissemination of critical airway information traditionally has been accomplished by documentation in the medical record, by verbal communication to patients and physicians, by letter, or by a combination of these. Significant shortcomings of these types of communication include questionable understanding by the patient or future care provider of the significance of the airway difficulty, non-uniformity of documentation, and an inability to access the information at a later date, particularly during an emergency. Even the emergence of the electronic health record (EHR) has not yet provided an answer to the need for universal access to emergency medical information. However, a solution that is already in place is the non-profit MedicAlert Foundation, the oldest and foremost national and international emergency medical information and identification service. Founded in 1956, MedicAlert Foundation International, headquartered in Turlock, California, relays critical, life-saving medical

---

information through a live 24/7 service for its 4 million members.

In 1992, the MedicAlert Foundation National Difficult Airway/Intubation Registry was begun to facilitate uniform documentation and effective dissemination of standardized critical information related to complex airway management. The Registry was created by the Anesthesia Advisory Council of the MedicAlert Foundation, a volunteer multidisciplinary team of anesthesiologists, otolaryngologists, and experts in quality assurance and risk management. According to Andrew Wigglesworth, President and CEO of MedicAlert Foundation International, Registry contained almost 11,700 patients with identified difficult airway or difficult intubation in 2010 (personal communication, May 14, 2010).

This chapter focuses on how critical airway information can be effectively disseminated to future care providers through the MedicAlert Foundation and the National Difficult Airway/Intubation Registry. The components and benefits of the MedicAlert Foundation and this Registry are compared with those of in-house anesthesia documentation, letters to the patient, airway registries, commercially available for-profit medical alert information systems, and the yet-to-be realized universal EHR. Information on how patients can join the MedicAlert Foundation and enroll in the National Difficult Airway/Intubation Registry can be found in Appendix A.

II. DIFFICULT AIRWAY/INTUBATION: A MULTIFACETED PROBLEM

Complex airway management is a multifaceted problem involving practitioners in a variety of clinical settings. The consequences of failed airway management can be devastating to the patient, the practitioner, and the health care system. Critical issues include (1) identification of patients with difficult airway/intubation, (2) use of practice guidelines and a difficult airway/intubation algorithm for airway management, (3) use of a difficult airway/intubation team, and (4) the consequences of difficult airway/intubation.

A. Identification of Patients

Controversies regarding predictors and definitions of "difficult" cases exist both within and among medical specialties that deal with difficult airway/intubation. This is a consequence of the complex interactions among patient variables, the clinical setting, and the skills of the practitioner.[21] Historically, the anesthesiology literature has cited an incidence of 1% to 3% unanticipated difficult airway/intubation in patients undergoing general endotracheal anesthesia in the operating room.[2-5] More recently, incidences up to 18% have been reported.[6,7] In non–operating room emergent intubations, the reported incidence of difficult intubation has ranged from 6% to 10%.[8,9]

At a local level, if a 1% to 3% incidence is applied, then an institution in which 25,000 general endotracheal anesthetic procedures are performed annually could have 250 to 750 unanticipated difficult airway/intubations per year. On a national level, based on an American Society of Anesthesiologists (ASA) membership of 44,000 and assuming that a full-time practicing anesthesiologist is likely to encounter at least one unanticipated difficult intubation per year,[10] there could be 44,000 unanticipated difficult airway/intubations annually in the United States. These numbers do not take into account intubations that occur in clinical settings other than the operating room or are performed by anesthesia care providers who are not members of the ASA. Consideration of the possible number of unanticipated difficult airway/intubations on an international level further shows that the scope of this problem and its impact on patients and the health care system warrants vigorous efforts to identify solutions.

B. Multidisciplinary Practice Guidelines and Difficult Airway/Intubation Algorithms

The ASA first developed and published practice guidelines for management of the difficult airway in 1993.[2] These guidelines heightened practitioners' awareness of the scope and magnitude of problems related to complex airway management and encouraged familiarity with a standardized clinical airway algorithm. At that same time, the Johns Hopkins Department of Anesthesiology and Critical Medicine initiated a collaborative effort with the Department of Otolaryngology—Head and Neck Surgery to develop and modify airway management techniques and clinical algorithms.[11]

More recently, other organizations and countries have proposed and tested their own strategies and algorithms for managing difficult airway/intubation cases.[12-15] Some algorithms incorporate the use of new airway devices,[16] whereas others are designed for use in settings other than the operating room.[8,17] A text on emergency department airway management has recommended a universal algorithm in addition to algorithms for specific circumstances.[18,19] Guidelines developed for anesthesiologists in the operating room cannot reasonably be applied to emergent intubation in the field, and the most successful algorithms have been developed at a local level by a multidisciplinary team.[20]

The creation of these various algorithms is still in harmony with the purpose of the ASA practice guidelines: (1) the practice guidelines are not intended as standards or absolute requirements; (2) they are subject to revision as warranted by the evolution of medical knowledge, technology, and practice; and (3) their recommendations may be adopted, modified, or rejected according to clinical needs and constraints.[1] Considering all of these variables tends to move airway management farther away from one standardized difficult airway/intubation algorithm. This leads to the inevitable conclusion, as noted in an ASA editorial, that optimal or preferred tracheal intubation techniques and devices will be different for each individual patient and depend on the skill and experience of the practitioner in that particular clinical setting.[21]

C. A Difficult Airway/Intubation Team

Strategies for improving the response to difficult airway/intubation during an emergency code situation can include the use of a difficult airway response team (DART) and a DART equipment cart such as the one developed in 2008 at the Johns Hopkins Medical Institutions. This multidepartmental educational and operational program involved anesthesiology, otolaryngology, trauma surgery, and the emergency department; clarified unclear roles of the various providers; and initiated facility-wide quality improvement of problems such as difficulty accessing specific equipment.[22] A retrospective review at this institution of cases from 1992 through 2006 demonstrated an annual frequency of approximately 6.5 emergency surgical airways (cricothyrotomy or tracheostomy). Two years after initiation of a comprehensive DART program, the annual frequency was approximately 2.2, despite an increase in the number of patients reported to have difficult airway/intubation.[23] Implementation of the DART program also reduced the number of airway sentinel events from several in the preceding 2 years to none in the first 2 years of the DART program. In addition, no claims related to airway events were paid during this time.[24]

D. Consequences of Difficult Airway Management

The consequences of a difficult airway or difficult intubation can include minor or major adverse medical events or death, professional liability to the practitioner, and direct and indirect costs to the patient and the health care system. In 1988, the ASA Committee on Professional Liability closed claims study found that respiratory events were the most common cause of brain damage and death during anesthesia, with difficult intubation being the likeliest category for risk reduction. The median payment for respiratory claims was $200,000.[25] In a 1992 loss analysis study conducted by the Physicians Insurers Association of America, files from 43 physician-owned malpractice insurance companies (representing approximately 2000 anesthesiologists nationally) ranked "intubation problems" as the third most prevalent misadventure. The average paid indemnity for 175 of 339 files was $196,958.[26] In an analysis of approximately 5000 claims filed in Maryland over a 15-year period that named an anesthesiologist as a defendant, insertion of an endotracheal tube was the sixth most common medical procedure leading to a liability claim. One malpractice claim was filed for every 7.5 patient injuries that occurred from difficult airway events and adverse outcomes, and a single claim in 1994 resulted in a jury award of $5 million (Laura Morlick, Johns Hopkins Medical Institutions, Baltimore, MD, personal communication, July 17, 1994). A study of the ASA closed claims database from 1985 to 1999 revealed that 67% of claims of difficult airway liability were associated with intubation.[27]

During airway management, repeated intubation attempts cause swelling and bleeding, with each attempt creating a greater likelihood of failed intubation and ventilation leading to potentially disastrous consequences, even brain damage or death.[18,27,28] Prolongation of the airway management process has been shown to increase the rate complications up to 70% with multiple tracheal intubation attempts.[8,29]

Most complaints initiated against physicians are unrelated to the physician's technical skill but arise because of inadequate records or poor communication. More complete documentation and communication may be the practitioner's best defense.[30] A 1994 survey of patients who were enrolled by Johns Hopkins in the MedicAlert National Difficult Airway/Intubation Registry found that, despite experiencing adverse outcomes (cancellation of surgery, dental trauma, soft tissue trauma, desaturation, cardiovascular compromise, and cricothyrotomy or tracheostomy), 100% felt that the enrollment gave them a sense of comfort in that future care providers would understand the significance of their difficult airway/intubation. Enrollment in the Registry and documentation of enrollment in the patient's medical record is a positive reflection of the provider's concern for the patient's future safety.[31] In a fall 2010 survey conducted by the MedicAlert Foundation of more than 700 members already enrolled in the National Difficult Airway/Intubation Registry, 69.6% of respondents said that a physician had recommended that they enroll, and 92.7% said that what they expected to gain from enrolling was peace of mind knowing that their difficult airway/intubation information would be available in an emergency (A. Wigglesworth, personal communication, September 23, 2010).

III. DIFFICULT AIRWAY/ INTUBATION: DOCUMENTATION OF CRITICAL INFORMATION

The communication of successful and unsuccessful airway management techniques consists of two parts: (1) documentation at the time of the event (preanesthesia, anesthesia, postanesthesia) for concurrent care providers during that episode of care, and (2) dissemination of that information to future care providers during subsequent episodes of care. This section deals with documentation to concurrent care providers during an episode of care.

A. Documentation in Medical Records

In the past, no standardized, uniform, readily available document existed to precisely record airway events. Traditionally, difficult airway/intubation information was recorded in the paper anesthesia record as a nonstandardized, handwritten, free text entry. This information was not included in the operative report or on the face sheet of the medical record; it was hidden and seldom accessed by physicians and nurses caring for the patient in the intensive care unit or nursing unit. In addition, this information was department specific in that it was not shared with other departments (emergency; ear, nose, and throat) within the institution that also encountered patients with difficult airway or difficult intubation.

In 1987, Martin L. Norton and colleagues at the University of Michigan pioneered efforts to more fully evaluate patients with complex airway problems by establishing the University of Michigan Airway Clinic.

This is believed to be the first formally established clinic specifically for patients with difficult airway/intubation. Clinical documentation consisted of a handwritten airway clinic record sheet and photodocumentation.[32] Since that time, the standard of care for documentation of difficult airway/intubation information has been steadily evolving. In 1992, Lynette Mark and colleagues in the Johns Hopkins Anesthesiology and Critical Care Medicine Department developed the Anesthesiology Consultant Report. This two-page report fully described the preoperative evaluation of a difficult airway/intubation, including intraoperative airway techniques and management and a narrative description of the events. The Anesthesiology Consultant Report raised the standard of documentation during a patient's initial episode of care in that its detailed airway management documentation was a more accessible part of the patient's medical record. Care providers were also alerted by a highly visible wristband.[11]

In 1993 and 2003, the ASA practice guidelines recommended that anesthesiologists document more fully in the medical record and include a description of the nature of the airway difficulties, the various airway management techniques that were employed, and the extent to which each of these techniques was beneficial or detrimental in managing the difficult airway.[1,2]

B. Documentation in In-House Electronic Medical Records

At the Johns Hopkins Medical Institutions, the 1992 Anesthesia Consultant Report evolved into an Anesthesia Consult form that contained a template and free-text entry as part of the in-house Johns Hopkins computerized medical record. In 1995, at Beth Israel Deaconess Medical Center in Boston, patients' difficult airway/intubation information was entered into the nurse's assessment section, and a "difficult airway/intubation" notice was placed in the computerized patient record.[33]

At present, the electronic medical record (EMR) is, by definition, limited to a single health system. The University of Michigan Department of Anesthesiology and many other facilities use a perioperative clinical information software system such as Centricity (General Electric Healthcare, Waukesha, WI) to collect difficult airway/intubation information in an airway management record that contains required fields, a drop-down menu, and a comment section for free text. This information is available at bedside workstations throughout the facility, including the floor and intensive care units, as part of the EMR.[9] Other institutions have developed their own EMR systems for in-house use, with multiple terminals that allow access throughout the hospital.

Recording in the EMR that the patient has a difficult airway or difficult intubation triggers the use of a difficult airway/intubation wristband and an alert on the facesheet similar to that for allergies. A commercially developed or in-house EMR system can ensure that a patient with difficult airway/intubation is recognized as such during the remainder of the hospital stay and subsequent hospital stays.

IV. DIFFICULT AIRWAY/ INTUBATION: DISSEMINATION OF CRITICAL INFORMATION

The communication of successful and unsuccessful airway management techniques consists of documentation at the time of the event and dissemination of that information to future care providers. This section deals with dissemination of that critical information.

A. ASA Recommendations for Dissemination of Information

Before the creation of the ASA practice guidelines, there was little or no literature discussing the benefits of patient notification of difficult airway management.[7] The 1993 ASA practice guidelines recommended that the anesthesiologist inform the patient (or responsible person) of the airway difficulty that was encountered and that notification systems, such as a written report or letter to the patient or communication with the patient's surgeon or primary caregiver, could be considered.[2] The 2003 ASA practice guidelines added a recommendation for a bracelet or equivalent identification device that could be kept with the patient at all times.[1]

B. Dissemination of Information via Paper Medical Records

Traditionally, difficult airway/intubation information was housed in the patient's paper medical record. Even when this written documentation was adequate, it usually could not be disseminated to care providers during subsequent episodes of care because it was difficult or impossible to retrieve paper-based records from storage, particularly in the event of an emergency.

C. Verbal Dissemination of Information

Most anesthesiologists inform the patient of a difficult airway/intubation in the postanesthesia care unit. However, this verbal communication of difficult airway information to the patient is unreliable. Communication can be hindered by the patient's intubation or by postoperative pain or sedation. Family members present are usually more concerned about the patient's surgical findings and recovery from anesthesia and surgery.[7] One study found that 50% of patients informed verbally did not recall or were unsure about ever having had a postoperative conversation with their anesthesiologist.[34]

Difficult airway/intubation information relayed verbally can be miscommunicated because of patients' lack of understanding of medical words or because anxiety related to their medical condition prevents them from assimilating this information. In addition, providers may underrepresent the severity of the difficult airway/intubation to allay patients' anxiety or because of fear of liability exposure. When these patients reenter the health care system, the previous verbal communication about difficult airway/intubation may not be remembered, and they may deny any difficult airway history or relate a vague history. In an emergency situation, patients who are unconscious cannot relate any difficult airway/intubation information they may have been told.

D. Dissemination of Information via Letters

Beginning in 1992, the Johns Hopkins Anesthesia Consultant Report (described previously) was distributed by letter to the patient's surgeon and referring physician.[11] In 2000, the Department of Anesthesiology at Mayo Clinic Scottsdale began providing written notification to patients about their difficult airway in the form of letters mailed 1 week postoperatively. However, in a follow-up survey 2 years later, 20% of patients could not recall receiving the letter. To improve communication, the Clinic followed up with a telephone call to confirm receipt of the letter and to emphasize the importance of the difficult airway/intubation. A MedicAlert Foundation brochure was also included in the letter. The survey found that of those patients who remembered receiving a difficult airway/intubation letter, 41% had informed their primary care physician of their difficult airway, and 95% who subsequently had surgery had informed their surgeons or anesthesiologist or both. The survey concluded that the patients were able to inform subsequent care providers that they had a difficult airway even though most of them did not understand how "difficult airway" affected their subsequent anesthesia and airway management.[34]

More recently, various publications have reiterated the need for some type of standard written notification or airway alert form to be distributed to the patient, the primary care provider, and the surgeon.[7,35]

E. Dissemination of Information via Difficult Airway/Intubation Registries

In some facilities, after a patient has been identified as having a difficult airway or difficult intubation and the airway management information has been entered in a hospital-wide information system, the patient's name is entered into an in-house difficult airway/intubation registry.

In 1987, the Norton and colleagues at the University of Michigan established a permanent in-house Airway Clinic (described previously) linked to an Airway Registry and an information response center for dissemination of critical airway information. As the Registry grew in size, it became increasingly apparent that the response center could not accommodate 24-hour emergency requests for difficult airway/intubation information, so Registry patients were enrolled in the MedicAlert Foundation registry.[36] In 1992, Mark and colleagues at the Johns Hopkins Medical Institutions established a permanent in-house Difficult Airway/Intubation Registry.[11] This registry still exists, and all patients who are identified as having difficult airway/intubation are entered into this in-house database; a note or flag is placed in their electronic record, and they receive a follow-up letter that includes a brochure and recommendation that they enroll in the MedicAlert Foundation. In 1995, in response to the ASA Difficult Airway Task Force practice guidelines

and the Anesthesia Advisory Counsel of the MedicAlert Foundation, an in-house computerized Difficult Airway Registry was initiated at Beth Israel Deaconess Medical Center.[36]

The purpose of an in-house registry is to disseminate critical airway information during subsequent episodes of care at that facility. A review of 119 patients in the Beth Israel Deaconess Medical Center difficult airway registry from 1995 to 1997 found that 31 (26%) had returned for surgery one or more times and that the registry provided valuable information for subsequent airway management.[37] However, in-house difficult airway/intubation registries are not common, even at tertiary-level institutions, and the information they contain is available only within that institution.

F. Dissemination of Information via Electronic Medical Records and Electronic Health Records Systems

In 1991, the Institute of Medicine set a goal of 10 years for widespread use of computerized patient records. In 1994, the Computer-Based Patient Record Institute announced that it would seek major funding to finalize the development of standards for health care informatics. Since then, the EMR has been implemented in some places; however, its scope is limited to a single health system.

More recently, there has been a push to implement an EHR system in American health care, with an increase in motivation provided by funding from the American Recovery and Reinvestment Act of 2009 (ARRA) directed at supporting such implementation. In an EHR system, the patient's complete health record would be captured across all health care institutions. This is the focus of the ARRA funding, as reinforced by Meaningful Use requirements (explicit criteria for receiving Medicare payments for provision of medical care). In 2011, Beth Israel Deaconess Medical Center became the first hospital to have its in-house–developed EHR system certified as meeting Meaningful Use requirements.[38] Part of the certification involved having the capacity to provide patients with an electronic copy of their health information within 3 business days (if they request it). The goal is to provide patients access to information that is important to them, when they need it, and to allow patients to be treated holistically through coordination with other providers.[39] However, an electronic copy of the record provided 3 business days after discharge may not provide access to critical information when patients need it and does not automatically ensure coordination of care with other providers.

A survey found that only 1 in 7 consumers could access their medical records electronically; even when access was possible, 40% were unable to see certain documents (e.g., laboratory reports, prescription history, immunization records).[40] In 2009, the Health Information Technology for Economic and Clinical Health (HITECH) Act was passed in an effort to improve the health of Americans and the performance of the health care system. Some of its programs included support for state initiatives for health information exchange and creation of a common platform for health information exchange across the country: the National Health Information Network (NHIN).[41]

One state program is the Chesapeake Regional Information System for Our Patients (CRISP) in Maryland. Its goal is to deliver the right health information to the right place at the right time. However, not all Maryland hospitals are included in the CRISP program, and the program does not access medical information on a national level, does not provide emergency information to Maryland residents who travel outside of the state or internationally, and does not cover new residents who have moved into the state and whose medical information is housed elsewhere.[42] Over time, it is hoped that this and other state programs can be expanded to form the envisioned (NHIN). The emergence and encouraged development of an EHR system in the United States cannot, at present, provide an answer to the need for immediate national or international access to emergency medical information. However, a solution that is already in place and fully operational can be found with the MedicAlert Foundation.

V. THE MEDICALERT FOUNDATION

The MedicAlert Foundation pioneered and maintains the foremost national and international emergency medical information and identification services system that provides immediate access to critical medical information.

A. History of the MedicAlert Foundation

The MedicAlert Foundation is a 501(c)3 nonprofit organization that was founded in 1956 by Dr. Marion C. Collins, a physician, and his family because of his daughter's life-threatening allergy. The MedicAlert Foundation has been endorsed by more than 50 organizations, including the ASA in 1979, the World Federation of Societies of Anaesthesiologists (WFSA) in 1992, and the American Academy of Otolaryngology–Head and Neck Surgery Foundation (AAO-HNS) in 1993. Many of the founding members of the Society for Airway Management (SAM) in 1995 were already members of the MedicAlert Foundation's Anesthesia Advisory Council. In 1996, on the occasion of the MedicAlert Foundation's 40th anniversary, the wife of its founding physician, Chrissie Collins, was awarded the American Medical Association's highest honor, the Citation for Distinguished Service.

The MedicAlert Foundation has nine international affiliates providing services in 25 countries and in 140 different languages. The MedicAlert Foundation, headquartered in the United States, has been in operation since 1956 and is still the only nonprofit agency providing emergency medical information and identification services. Its mission is to protect and save lives by disseminating critical patient information immediately and accurately, when needed, for its 4 million members (2.3 million in the United States and 1.7 million worldwide).

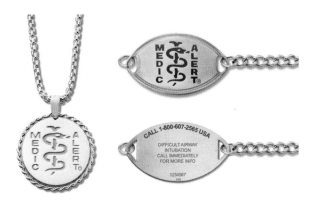

Figure 54-1 MedicAlert medical IDs. The MedicAlert medical ID as a necklace and a bracelet. The reverse side of the medical ID shows the MedicAlert Foundation's telephone numbers (toll-free nationally and internationally without charge to the caller), the Difficult Airway/Intubation designation, and the patient's unique MedicAlert Foundation identification number. (Courtesy of the MedicAlert Foundation, Turlock, CA.)

B. Services Provided by the MedicAlert Foundation

The MedicAlert Foundation's core services comprise a four-part system: a personalized and custom-made MedicAlert medical ID worn as a bracelet or necklace (Fig. 54-1), a personalized MedicAlert wallet card (Fig. 54-2), an Emergency Medical Information Record (EMIR), and the MedicAlert live 24/7 Emergency Response Service Center. The MedicAlert medical ID and MedicAlert wallet card immediately alert a care provider that the patient has a specific medical condition, such as an allergy, autism, asthma, diabetes, or difficult airway/intubation. Engraved on the medical ID and printed on the wallet card is the toll-free emergency phone number, 1-800-607-2565. For members who travel internationally, MedicAlert recommends that they also have engraved on the medical ID and printed on the wallet card the International Call Collect number, 209-634-4917. The Emergency Response Center accepts all international collect calls and is staffed by a team of medically trained personnel who respond to calls 24 hours a day, 7 days a week, in more than 140 languages.

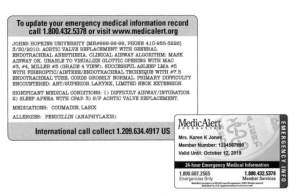

Figure 54-2 The MedicAlert Wallet Card. This card contains a narrative of the patient's medical diagnoses and specific successful and unsuccessful airway techniques that have been used. (Courtesy of the MedicAlert Foundation, Turlock, CA.)

In 1990, the MedicAlert Foundation expanded member information to include Advance Directives and information about medical devices. The Foundation has partnered with the Alzheimer's Association since 2007 and with the Autism Society of America since 2009 to provide life-saving services to high-risk patients.

The MedicAlert Foundation has always been on the cutting edge of information-providing services. In the 1970s, it computerized all of its members' records and was the first registry to use a scan form system to reduce the costs of data entry.[43] Since 1990, the MedicAlert Foundation has offered members their own personal EMIR). Looking to the future, the EHR system envisions seamless, immediate, and simultaneous access by more than one health care provider to all parts of a patient's record regardless of where those parts were created or stored. Far from competing with the envisioned EHR system, the MedicAlert Foundation has anticipated it and embraced the goal of enabling the dissemination of information to any EHR system. This could be as simple as an HL7 text message or as complicated as a set of discrete data detailing specific medical information. By serving as a central repository in a web of interconnected EHR systems, the MedicAlert Foundation could play a key role in providing critical life-saving information to the clinical systems directly involved in a patient's care. Finally, as patients continue to become more engaged in managing their own health care through the use of personal health records (PHRs)—as provided by Microsoft, Google, and other vendors—the MedicAlert Foundation will be able to keep patients' PHRs updated with the latest medical information.

The MedicAlert Foundation maintains the privacy and confidentiality of member's information. All electronic data are securely encrypted and backed up in earthquake-, fire-, and flood-proof locations. Overall security is reviewed by a third party. Financial information is used only for MedicAlert billing and is never shared with any other person or organization for other purposes.

At the time of member enrollment, the MedicAlert Foundation obtains prior approval for storage and transfer of members' information to emergency responders. Personal and medical information remains secure and confidential and is used solely for its authorized and intended purpose. The MedicAlert Foundation may release de-identified member information for valid medical research. The release of identifiable member information for medical research or clinical trials requires the member's informed consent in accordance with applicable laws and regulations for human subject trials. For more than 50 years, there have been no claims against the MedicAlert Foundation for breach of confidentiality or dissemination of incorrect medical information. Although the MedicAlert Foundation is not defined as a "covered entity" under the Health Insurance Portability and Accountability Act (HIPAA) of 1996, the organization's information privacy and security standards complement the HIPAA provisions and are fully compliant with the requirements of the Federal Trade Commission and those of the European Union SafeHarbor framework.

C. Membership in the MedicAlert Foundation

MedicAlert Foundation membership is $35/year for adults. This allows members to manage their own personal EMIR, with no limit on the number of updates per year. Members can update their information 24 hours a day by logging on to their own personal secure online account. An annual membership for children is $20/year. A MedicAlert Gold membership is available for $9.95/ month; members with this status can consolidate all of their paper records (e.g., laboratory reports, immunization records, radiology reports, electrocardiography results) in an electronic format. Members each have a unique Document Center that can receive faxed medical records from their physicians. The faxed documents are then converted into a PDF file and are available 24 hours a day from any Internet-connected computer. Information on how patients can enroll in the MedicAlert Foundation is presented in Appendix A.

VI. THE MEDICALERT FOUNDATION NATIONAL DIFFICULT AIRWAY/ INTUBATION REGISTRY

For years, anesthesiologists have recognized the value of the MedicAlert Foundation's emergency response system for patients with malignant hyperthermia (Index Zero hotline). They have also encouraged patients to enroll in the MedicAlert Foundation under a general designation of "difficult airway."

A. History of the Registry

In 1992, the ASA and others recommended the creation of a national difficult airway registry for the United States.[1] At that time, the Anesthesia Advisory Council, a volunteer, multidisciplinary team of anesthesiologists, otolaryngologists, and experts in quality assurance and risk management (see Appendix B), joined together to address the following questions: (1) When an airway event happens, is there consistency in documentation? and (2) Is there a central, accessible database for dissemination of critical airway information? The Council identified only two existing airway databases, those at the University of Michigan Airway Clinic and the MedicAlert Foundation. The Anesthesia Advisory Council recommended the creation of the National Difficult Airway/ Intubation Registry within the MedicAlert Foundation to facilitate uniform documentation and effective dissemination of standardized critical information related to complex airway management. The Council selected the category "difficult airway/intubation" as a standard nomenclature to be engraved on the MedicAlert medical ID.

In 1995, the SAM was founded, and the Anesthesia Advisory Council passed the torch to the SAM to take the MedicAlert National Difficult Airway/Intubation Registry into the next millennium.[44] Today, it is the only difficult airway/intubation registry that exists at a national level in the United States.

On an international level, Austria established the Austrian Difficult Airway/Intubation Registry (ADAIR) in 1999,[45] and Denmark established the Danish Difficult Airway Registry in 2005.[46] These registries are not international in scope. Only the MedicAlert Foundation National Difficult Airway/Intubation Registry is truly international, because it is able to disseminate critical information to care providers anywhere in the world 24 hours a day, 7 days a week, in 140 different languages.

B. Objectives of the Registry

The major objectives of the Anesthesia Advisory Council for the National Difficult Airway/Intubation Registry were (1) to develop and implement mechanisms for uniform documentation and dissemination of critical information, (2) to establish a central database of airway management information for research purposes, (3) to conduct long-term tracking of patients to assess implications of adverse outcomes for future management, and (4) to determine whether rapid and economical dissemination of critical airway information could have a positive impact on the future care of patients and overall costs to the health care system.

C. Components of the Registry

The components of the National Difficult Airway/Intubation Registry include information for health care providers and patients, a specialized enrollment form, a secure database, the supporting services of the MedicAlert Foundation (i.e., medical ID, wallet card, EMIR, and 24/7 Emergency Response Service Center), and a follow-up letter sent to the primary care physician or specialist (as indicated by the patient on the enrollment form). In 2003, the ASA practice guidelines recommended that a notification bracelet or equivalent identification device be included as part of a notification system for difficult airway/intubation patients.[1] This has always been a part of the MedicAlert system since its beginning in 1956.

The National Difficult Airway/Intubation Registry specialized enrollment form is in a PDF format. The anesthesiologist downloads the form from the website (www.medicalert.org [accessed April 2012]) and prints it out, or the MedicAlert Foundation can send it to the anesthesiologist as a PDF attachment to an e-mail. The anesthesiologist completes and signs the airway database section (Fig. 54-3) of the enrollment form. This section includes the hospital name, patient's medical record number, surgical procedure, date of procedure, clinical anesthesia profile, nature of difficulty encountered, reasons for difficulty, successful and unsuccessful techniques, best visualization of airway anatomy, clinically applied algorithm, and clinical outcome. With the exception of specific airway requirements (related to tracheal surgery, stenosis, or other conditions requiring specific sizes of endotracheal tubes), recommendations for future airway management are not included, so as to avoid conflict with future practitioners' choices of airway management techniques. The form is then given to the patient to complete (including the name of the primary care

physician), sign, and mail in (or fax to) the MedicAlert Foundation along with a check or credit card information for the enrollment fee. The amount of the enrollment fee depends on which type of membership the patient selects. For patients who are unable to pay for membership, the MedicAlert Foundation will enroll them for free if the completed enrollment form is accompanied by a statement of financial need that is written on official letterhead paper and signed by the anesthesiologist or other provider.

D. Characteristics of Registry Patients

Between 1992 and 1994, more than 250 adult and pediatric patients throughout the United States were enrolled in the MedicAlert Foundation National Difficult Airway/Intubation Registry. Their characteristics were as follows: ASA classes I and II, 54%; ASA classes III and IV, 46%; ASA class V, 0%. For airway management in these patients, conventional laryngoscopy was successful only about 20% of the time. These patients had 39 reported adverse outcomes: cancellations, 9 (23%); dental trauma, 3 (8%); desaturation, 7 (18%); soft tissue trauma, 11 (28%); cardiovascular compromise, 2 (5%); and other, 7 (18%). Patients were enrolled from private and academic institutions, from outpatient surgical centers, and by self-referral.[47] By 2003, there were approximately 7020 patients enrolled in the MedicAlert National Difficult Airway/Intubation Registry.[34]

As of 2010, there were almost 11,700 patients enrolled in the MedicAlert National Difficult Airway/Intubation Registry (A. Wigglesworth, personal communication, May 14, 2011). The MedicAlert Foundation, the Anesthesia Advisory Council, and SAM are in the process of analyzing this registry, and efforts are underway to expand the enrollment form in the future to an international query.

E. Benefits of the Registry

Benefits of the National Difficult Airway/Intubation Registry include patient safety, practitioner security, and cost savings. With enrollment, the patient's primary care physician and specialists are notified of the patient's difficult airway/intubation status to facilitate local continuity of care. The patient is also protected during subsequent episodes of care. A 2010 survey of more than 700 members in the MedicAlert Foundation National Difficult Airway/Intubation Registry found that 11.2% had had another episode of care in which difficult airway/intubation was a factor (A. Wigglesworth, personal communication, October 2010).

The Registry provides a chronology of the patient's airway events over time, reflecting changes in pathophysiology and airway management. This chronology assists future care providers in their decision-making process and allays any concerns about mistakenly labeling a patient as having a difficult airway or difficult intubation. The patient's MedicAlert medical ID or wallet card provides a visible or easily accessible reminder of the difficult airway/intubation status, and the MedicAlert Foundation's toll-free phone number provides access to the

5. TO BE FILLED OUT BY PRACTITIONER (Patient should proceed to question 6): Not placed on Medic Alert computer record until validated by physician.

1. _____

HOSPITAL NAME   MEDICAL RECORD # (Very important)

2. Clinical profile: ❏ Anesthesiologist ❏ CRNA ❏ Otolaryngologist ❏ ED
    Other _____
    ASA classification   ❏ I   ❏ II   ❏ III   ❏ IV   ❏ V   ❏ E
    HT _____ Wt/kg _____
    Site: ❏ OR ❏ Non-OR ❏ Ward ❏ ED   Other _____
    Monitors utilized: ❏ Capnography ❏ Oximetry Other _____

3. The difficult airway was: ❏ Anticipated ❏ Unanticipated

4. If anticipated, how was the difficulty discovered?
❏ Airway history by patient/family interview ❏ Physical exam
❏ Documentation in medical record   ❏ Diagnostic tests/consultations
    Specify _____

5. What type of difficult airway was encountered?
❏ Mask/ventilation ❏ Intubation ❏ Extubation   Other _____

6. The difficulty encountered was primarily:
❏ Small mouth ❏ Tongue ❏ Dentition ❏ Ant/superior larynx
❏ Limited jaw opening/mobility ❏ Limited neck extention ❏ C-spine stability
❏ Distorted anatomy ❏ Infection ❏ Pregnancy   Other _____

7. Visualization (check all that apply)
❏ Complete glottic opening   ❏ Partial glottic opening   ❏ Arytenoids
❏ Tip of epiglottis

_____ ___/___/_____
PROCEDURE   Mo Day Year

8. What equipment/techniques were successful in airway management?
(Circle all that apply)
Awake • Asleep • Nasal • Oral • Blind nasal • Laryngeal mask • MAC #1 2 3 4 •
MILLER #1 2 3 4 • Fiberoptic • Intubation guide • Retrograde • Lightwand •
Jet ventilation • Cricothyrotomy • Existing trach/surgical airway •
Percutaneous crico/trach • Bougie • Combitube • Tracheotomy •
Specialized laryngoscope, blade and size (specify) _____
Endotracheal tube and size (specify) _____
Other and size (specify) _____

9. What equipment/techniques were unsuccessful in airway management?
(Circle all that apply)
Awake • Asleep • Nasal • Oral • Blind nasal • Laryngeal mask • MAC #1 2 3 4 •
MILLER #1 2 3 4 • Fiberoptic • Intubation guide • Retrograde • Lightwand •
Jet ventilation • Cricothyrotomy • Existing trach/surgical airway •
Percutaneous crico/trach • Bougie • Combitube • Tracheotomy •
Specialized laryngoscope, blade and size (specify) _____
Endotracheal tube and size (specify) _____
Other and size (specify) _____

10. What was the outcome? ❏ No adverse outcomes ❏ Cancel procedure
    ❏ Dental trauma ❏ Soft tissue/nasal trauma ❏ Laryngeal trauma ❏ Desaturation
    ❏ Vocal chord trauma ❏ Tracheal trauma ❏ Cardiovascular compromise ❏ Aspiration
    Other: _____

Specify clinically applied algorithm, number of attempts and pertinent findings. _____

Recommendations for colleagues: _____

Physician or anesthetist's signature _____   Print name/phone # _____
                                                        Include on wallet card? ❏ Yes ❏ No

6. **SELECT YOUR EMBLEM:** Indicate style and metal type desired.

STYLE	METAL	FEE**:
❏ Small bracelet	❏ Stainless steel	$35
❏ Standard bracelet	❏ Sterling silver	$50
❏ Necklace	❏ Gold filled	$75
	❏ Designer silver	$115

(Fees and terms subject to change without notice)

7. **BRACELET SIZE:** ❏ 6" ❏ 6 ½" ❏ 7" ❏ 7 ½" ❏ 8" ❏ 8 ½" ❏ 9"

8. **PAYMENT CALCULATION**
** REGISTRATION FEE: $ _____
(Tax deductible medical expense.)
Includes issuance of ID number, wallet card
and one custom engraved emblem with chain.
ANNUAL MEMBERSHIP FEE: $15 $ _Ø_
(First year free.) Includes 24-hour, year-round
emergency hot line service and free updating
of your computer record.
CONTRIBUTION: (Tax deductible) $ _____
*MedicAlert, a nonprofit foundation, is partially
supported by contibutions for professional and
public education programs.*
TOTAL AMOUNT ENCLOSED: $ _____

9. **METHOD OF PAYMENT**
❏ Check ❏ Mastercard ❏ Visa ❏ Discover ❏ Money order *(No other cards accepted.)*
No CODs. Payment must accompany order.
Send to: **Medic Alert, 2323 Colorado Ave., Turlock, CA 95382**

Card number: _____

Expiration date: _____
Note: Your signature and payment or card information must be indicated to enroll by mail.

10. SIGNATURE OF MEMBER

_____

I understand and accept the legal statement printed on the back of this form.

1844

Figure 54-3 The MedicAlert Foundation National Difficult Airway/Intubation Registry Enrollment Form, showing the airway database section from the original (1994) Registry enrollment form. In 2011, the Society for Airway Management (SAM) began revising this section, and the updated version will be available in the near future on the MedicAlert Foundation's Web site and possibly on the SAM Web site. (Courtesy of Lynette J. Mark, MD.)

details of the patient's airway management information 24/7, no matter where the patient travels in the world.

The Registry increases practitioner protection from liability by improving provider-patient communication. Enrollment gives providers an opportunity to inform patients of their airway difficulties and adverse events while offering a way to protect them during subsequent events, and this is perceived as a positive reflection of the provider's concern. As described previously, a 1994 survey of Johns Hopkins patients found that, despite experiencing adverse outcomes, 100% of patients felt that enrollment in the Registry gave them a sense of comfort that future care providers would understand their condition.[31] In the operating room, this difficult airway/intubation knowledge may help avoid adverse outcomes and malpractice suits.

The cost of initial enrollment in the Registry may be justified by future cost savings realized by the patient and the provider or institution. Knowing that a patient was previously identified as having a difficult airway or difficult intubation and what techniques were used could promote the cost-effective use of equipment and operating room time and decrease the incidence of cancellations. A 10-month study of 690 patients undergoing coronary artery bypass surgery at the Johns Hopkins Medical Institutions as the first procedure of the day looked at charges for anesthesia preparation time (i.e., anesthesiologist's professional fee, anesthesia resident's charge, drug and supply charges, and operating room time charges). Of these patients, 684 had no airway difficulty (control group) and 6 had difficult airway/intubation and were subsequently enrolled in the National Difficult Airway/Intubation Registry. There was a mean charge of $990.71 for the control group patients and a mean charge of $1578.24 for the difficult airway/intubation patients, representing a 59% increase over the control group.[48]

VII. OTHER EMERGENCY MEDICAL RESPONSE SYSTEMS

There are currently more than 600 commercial, for-profit emergency response systems that are available to consumers. Of these, some offer a visible medical ID in the form of a necklace or bracelet or a separate wallet card, but none offers that final link of a live 24/7, toll-free national and international hotline to disseminate critical medical information in an emergency situation. The MedicAlert Foundation is the only nonprofit organization that offers this comprehensive program of services and the only organization that has an ongoing Difficult Airway/Intubation Registry (A. Wigglesworth, personal communication, May 14, 2011).

VIII. CONCLUSIONS

Information is the lifeblood of modern medicine, and health information technology is its circulatory system.[49] Quality improvements in the process of managing difficult airway/intubation situations (methods to identify patients, algorithms, equipment, airway teams) should be vigorous and ongoing but should be accompanied by improvements in how airway information is documented and disseminated. Once a patient with a difficult airway/intubation is identified, documentation of the airway management is critical and should include the specifics of successful and unsuccessful techniques, the skill level of the practitioner, and the clinical setting where the event occurred. The patient's in-house EMR, which can be accessed by multiple care providers and is linked to a difficult airway/intubation patient wristband and an alert on the facesheet, ensures that the patient is recognized as such throughout the initial episode of care.

After a difficult airway/intubation event has occurred, a critical issue is how this patient-specific information can be disseminated to future care providers in a timely manner during a subsequent episode of care. This is important because the availability of documentation of successful and unsuccessful airway management techniques can decrease the number of intubation attempts that are associated with complications (including death and brain damage), thereby improving patient safety and decreasing practitioner liability. ASA recommendations for dissemination of this information include informing the patient (or responsible person) of the presence of a difficult airway and the reasons for difficulty with (1) a written report or letter to the patient, (2) a report in the medical record, (3) a chart flag, (4) communication with the patient's surgeon or primary caregiver, and (5) a notification bracelet or equivalent identification device.

Informing the patient via verbal communication of difficult airway/intubation information should always be done, but this should not be regarded as a reliable way to disseminate critical information. Even when patients relay the fact of difficult airway/intubation to the next anesthesiologist, the details of successful and unsuccessful airway management techniques may not be included. Written communication of difficult airway information in the form of a letter to the patient is an effective strategy, but some patients will not remember receiving the letter, and others will lose or misplace the letter over time. In the event of an emergency, it is highly unlikely that patients would have those letters in their possession or that their primary care providers could access those letters in a timely way in their medical records. In-house difficult airway/intubation registries can successfully provide critical airway management information but only for a select group of patients who return to the same facility. It is evident that even with implementation of each of the first four ASA recommendations and other strategies, the patient's critical airway information may not be readily available outside the immediate scope of the hospital or primary caregiver.

Although an EHR system is under development and much progress has been made, the complexity and scope of issues to be addressed makes the time frame for accomplishing this goal uncertain. At present, difficult airway/intubation information in a patient's EMR record may be available at some hospitals or through a small network of related facilities but not comprehensively throughout a region or state and not nationally or internationally. At present, none of these methods of dissemination of information can fulfill the need for immediate access to emergency medical information whenever and wherever it is needed.

It is only by implementing the fifth ASA recommendation for a notification bracelet or equivalent identification device—a visible medical ID that speaks for itself—that the presence of the patient's difficult airway/intubation can be made known to any future care provider in any setting. And to be most effective, this medical ID must be linked to a database that provides patient-specific difficult airway/intubation information on demand at any time, anywhere in the world.

Fortunately, this solution is already in place and fully operational in the MedicAlert Foundation. Only the MedicAlert Foundation fulfills the need for immediate access to and dissemination of emergency medical information, nationally or internationally. The visible

MedicAlert difficult airway/intubation medical ID speaks for itself and is recognized by care providers around the world. The medical ID is linked to an Emergency Response Center that is staffed by a team of medically trained personnel who respond to calls from care providers 24 hours a day, 7 days a week, in more than 140 languages, and the MedicAlert Foundation National Difficult Airway/Intubation Registry provides the critical details of a patient's prior airway management to future care providers anywhere and at any time they are needed.

IX. CLINICAL PEARLS

- The MedicAlert Foundation, founded in 1965 and endorsed by the American Society of Anesthesiologists (ASA) in 1979, is the only 501(c)(3) nonprofit organization that provides a comprehensive medical service to members, in the form of visible medical ID, a separate wallet card, a Web-accessible personal health record, and a 24/7 live emergency response service.

- In 1992, the MedicAlert Foundation National Difficult Airway/Intubation Registry was created to facilitate uniform documentation and effective dissemination of standardized critical information related to complex airway management.

- The ASA Practice Guidelines for the Difficult Airway recommend the following components for dissemination of critical airway information: (1) a written report or letter to the patient, (2) a report in the medical record, (3) a chart flag, (4) communication with the patient's surgeon or primary caregiver, and (5) a notification bracelet or equivalent identification device. MedicAlert is currently the only organization that can readily provide this service.

- The consequences of a difficult airway/intubation may include minor or major adverse medical events or death, professional liability to the practitioner, and direct and indirect costs to the patient and health care system. Difficult airway/intubation still accounts for the highest percentage of closed claims in anesthesia.

- By 2010, the MedicAlert National Difficult Airway/Intubation Registry included more than 11,000 active members with the condition of "difficult airway."

- Individuals can become members of the MedicAlert Foundation by calling 1-800-ID-ALERT or by visiting the Web site (www.medicalert.org [accessed April 2012]). There is an annual enrollment fee, but if a person cannot afford the fee, a health care provider may contact MedicAlert and request that the fee be waived.

- The Foundation plans to have an updated National Difficult Airway/Intubation Registry form available on both their Web site and that of the Society for Airway Management (www.samhq.com [accessed April 2012]) by the summer of 2012.

SELECTED REFERENCES

All references can be found online at expertconsult.com.

1. American Society of Anesthesiologists Task Force on Management of the Difficult Airway: An updated report by the American Society of Anesthesiologists Task Force on Management of the Difficult Airway. *Anesthesiology* 98:1269–1277, 2003.
7. Koenig HM: No more difficult airway, again! Time for consistent standardized written patient notification of a difficult airway. *Anesthesia Patient Safety Foundation Newsletter* Summer:1–6, 2010.
11. Mark LJ, Beattie C, Ferrell CL, et al: The difficult airway: Mechanisms of effective dissemination of critical information. *J Clin Anesth* 4:247–251, 1992.
31. Cherian M, Mark L, Schauble J, et al: *The national MedicAlert(r) difficult airway/intubation registry: Patient safety and patient satisfaction [abstract].* Presented at the Annual Meeting of the American Society of Anesthesiologists, San Francisco, CA, October 1994.
34. Trentman TL, Frasco PE, Milde LN: Utility of letters sent to patients after difficult airway management. *J Clin Anesth* 16:247–261, 2004.
37. Foley LJ, Sands D, Feinstein D, et al: Effect of difficult airway (DA) registry on subsequent airway management experience in the first 2 years of a DA registry. *Anesthesiology* 89:A1220, 1996.
41. The Office of the National Coordinator for Health Information Technology: HITECH program. Available at http://www.healthit.hhs.gov (accessed April 2012).
44. Roman P, Dahab Y, Herzer K, et al: *MedicAlert(r) national registry for difficult airway/intubation: A 1992–2010 perspective [abstract].* Presented at the Annual Meeting of the Society for Airway Management, Chicago, IL, September 16, 2010.
48. Mark LJ, Schauble J, Turley SM, et al: *The MedicAlert(r) national difficult airway/intubation registry: Technology that pays for itself [abstract].* Presented at the Annual Meeting of the Society for Technology in Anesthesia, Phoenix, AZ, January 1995.

Persons can become members of the MedicAlert® Foundation by:
1. Calling the MedicAlert® Foundation at 1-800-ID-ALERT™ (1-800-432-5378)
2. Visiting the MedicAlert® Foundation Web site at www.medicalert.org
3. E-mailing the MedicAlert® Foundation at customer_service@medicalert.org

Completed National Difficult Airway/Intubation Registry enrollment forms can be:
1. Mailed to the MedicAlert® Foundation, 2323 Colorado Ave., Turlock, CA 95382
2. Faxed to the MedicAlert® Foundation, fax: 1-800-863-3429

Additional National Difficult Airway/Intubation Registry enrollment forms can be obtained by:
1. Visiting the MedicAlert® Foundation Web site at www.medicalert.org

2. E-mailing the MedicAlert® Foundation at customer_service@medicalert.org
3. Calling the MedicAlert® Foundation at 1-800-ID-ALERT™ (1-800-432-5378)

For additional information regarding the National Difficult Airway/Intubation Registry:
1. Visit the MedicAlert® Foundation website at www.medicalert.org
2. Call MedicAlert® Foundation, 1-800-ID-ALERT™ (1-800-432-5378)
3. Contact Lynette J. Mark, MD, Associate Professor, Department of Anesthesiology and Critical Care Medicine, The Johns Hopkins University School of Medicine, 600 North Wolfe St., Tower 711, Baltimore, MD 21287-8711

Telephone: 410-955-0631
Fax: 410-955-0994
E-mail: lmark@jhmi.edu

Anesthesia Advisory Council of the MedicAlert® Foundation

Founding Members, 1992

Lynette Mark, MD

Charles Beattie, PhD, MD

Charles W. Cummings, MD

Paul W. Flint, MD

Robert Forbes, MD

Gordon Gibby, MD

Paul Goldiner, MD

J. S. Gravenstein, Sr., MD

Martin L. Norton, MD, JD

Andranik Ovassapian, MD, FAC

A. Thomas Pedroni, Jr., Esq

Ellison C. Pierce, Jr., MD

J. G. Reves, MD

James Roberts, MD

Mark C. Rogers, MD

Henry Rosenberg, MD

James F. Schauble, MD

Alan Jay Schwartz, MD, MS Ed

Richard S. Wilbur, MD, JD

John F. Williams, Jr., MD

Chapter 55

Medical-Legal Considerations: The ASA Closed Claims Project

KAREN L. POSNER | ROBERT A. CAPLAN

I. HISTORICAL PERSPECTIVE

Anesthesiologists have a long-standing appreciation for risks associated with airway management. During the past 60 years, a variety of studies have demonstrated that events involving the respiratory system are a prominent cause of adverse outcomes in anesthesia practice.[1-8] A few examples help illustrate this point. The Anesthesia Study Commission, which investigated anesthesia-related fatalities in metropolitan Philadelphia during the period 1935–1944, identified respiratory factors such as airway obstruction, hypoxia, and aspiration as the probable cause of death in approximately 19% of cases.[7] A large, multicenter study by Beecher and Todd, conducted about a decade later when curare and other muscle relaxants were first entering clinical practice, led to the recognition of excess mortality associated with perioperative respiratory depression.[1] In the 1970s, Utting and colleagues analyzed a 7-year series of anesthesia accidents reported to the Medical Defence Union of the United Kingdom (UK).[8] Of 227 cases resulting in death or brain damage, 36% involved adverse respiratory events such as esophageal intubation, ventilator misuse, and aspiration.

Critical-incident studies have offered a similar picture. A landmark study in the late 1970s by Cooper and colleagues revealed that 29% of reported incidents were related to respiratory events such as airway mismanagement or failure and misuse of ventilators and breathing circuits.[2] A decade later, the Australian Incident Monitoring Study provided a detailed analysis of the first 2000

cases voluntarily submitted since the late 1980s.[6] In their collection of critical incidents, problems with ventilation accounted for 16% of reports from anesthesiologists in Australia and New Zealand.

II. THE CLOSED CLAIMS PERSPECTIVE

Closed medical malpractice claims represent an important resource for the study of professional liability associated with airway management. To better appreciate this resource, it is helpful to describe some basic features of claims data.

A medical malpractice claim is a demand for financial compensation by an individual who has sustained injury in connection with medical care. Resolution of a claim usually occurs by an out-of-court process or by litigation. Once a claim is resolved, its file is closed. A closed claim file typically contains a broad assortment of documents related to the adverse outcome. These documents may include medical records, narrative statements by the involved health care personnel, expert and peer reviews, deposition summaries, outcome and follow-up reports, and the cost of settlement or jury award.

Claims represent only a small fraction of all adverse outcomes arising from medical care. The Harvard Medical Practice Study of patients in New York State in 1984 reported that approximately 4% of patients sustained an iatrogenic injury during hospitalization,[9] but only 1 of every 8 injured patients filed a malpractice claim. Similar

TABLE 55-1

Most Common Damaging Events in U.S. Closed Anesthesia Claims*

	Total (n = 8157)	1970s (n = 655)	1980s (n = 2871)	1990s (n = 3393)	2000s (n = 1146)
Respiratory events	24%	35%	28%	18%	23%
Block-related events	13%	9%	10%	15%	14%
Cardiovascular events	13%	11%	11%	14%	16%
Equipment problems	11%	9%	10%	10%	15%
Wrong drug or dose	5%	4%	5%	6%	5%

*Total anesthesia claims = 8954. Claims for chronic pain management are excluded. Claims with unknown year of event and miscellaneous events are not shown.
Data from ASA Closed Claims Database, 2008.

findings were described 10 years earlier by the Medical Insurance Feasibility Study in California.[10] These small fractions make it unlikely that claims can be regarded as representing a cross section of all adverse outcomes.

Although claims may not serve as a representative sample of the entire population of adverse outcomes, these cases have a direct and important implication for the study of professional liability: the cost of claims plays an important role in determining the cost of medical malpractice premiums. By studying a large collection of claims, it may be possible to identify types of adverse events that consistently make a large contribution to insurance costs. This information helps focus research and risk management strategies on areas of clinical practice associated with the greatest losses. Successfully reducing losses may lead to lower premiums, with accompanying savings for physicians, patients, and associated third-party participants. Because many types of adverse outcomes are relatively rare, claims files also represent an enriched environment for collecting information about infrequent but catastrophic events. Examination of a large set of rare or unusual adverse outcomes with a common theme provides an opportunity to generate hypotheses of causation and remedy that may not be evident to anesthesiologists who experience such cases as isolated events.

Since 1985, the Committee on Professional Liability of the American Society of Anesthesiologists (ASA) has engaged in a structured analysis of closed anesthesia claims in the United States, known as the ASA Closed Claims Project. Cases involving adverse anesthetic outcomes are retrieved from the closed claims files of U.S. medical-liability insurance carriers who voluntarily participate in the project. Claims for dental injury are not included in the ASA Closed Claims Project, and the data reported in this chapter also exclude claims associated with chronic pain management. In aggregate, the participating carriers provide coverage for approximately 36% of U.S. anesthesiologists. Because several years often elapse between the occurrence of an adverse event and the closure of its associated claim, the majority of cases span an interval from the 1980s to the early 2000s. The database now contains more than 8000 cases.

A detailed description of data collection procedures for the Closed Claims Project has been reported previously.[11,12] In brief, each claim file is reviewed by a practicing anesthesiologist, and a standardized form is used to record detailed information on characteristics of patients, surgical procedures, anesthetic agents and techniques, involved personnel, sequence of events, standard of care,

critical incidents, clinical manifestations, responsibility, and outcome. Standard of care is rated on the basis of reasonable and prudent practices at the time of the event. Practice patterns that may have evolved at a later date are not retrospectively applied when the standard of care is rated. An adverse outcome is deemed preventable with better monitoring if the reviewer finds that the use—or better use—of any monitor would probably have prevented the outcome, whether or not such a monitor was available at the time of the event. An acceptable level of interrater reliability has been established for reviewer judgments on the standard of care and preventability of adverse outcomes with better monitoring.[13]

A. Principal Features of Adverse Respiratory Outcomes and High-Frequency Adverse Respiratory Events

1. Basic Features

Adverse respiratory events constitute the single largest source of injury in the Closed Claims Project (Table 55-1). A detailed analysis of these events was initiated when the database reached a total of 1541 claims.[14] The contrast between adverse respiratory events and other claims was particularly unfavorable. Respiratory event–related claims were (and still are) characterized by a high frequency of devastating outcomes and costly payments (Table 55-2).

Just three mechanisms of injury accounted for almost two thirds of all claims for adverse respiratory events (Table 55-3). These mechanisms were inadequate ventilation (24% of cases), esophageal intubation (12%), and difficult intubation (DI; 24%). In the 1990s, after the adoption of pulse oximetry and end-tidal CO_2 ($EtCO_2$) as monitoring standards, DI (28%) and inadequate ventilation (18%) remained the most common adverse respiratory events, but esophageal intubation (5%) had decreased greatly compared with earlier decades (see Table 55-3). Evaluation of claims from the early 2000s suggests that this profile of adverse respiratory events is staying the same.

Aspiration was the third most common adverse respiratory event in the 1990s and 2000s. The remaining adverse respiratory events were produced by a variety of low-frequency mechanisms including airway obstruction, bronchospasm, premature and unintentional extubation, endobronchial intubation, inadequate inspired oxygen delivery, and equipment failure. Special features of low-frequency events are discussed later in this chapter.

TABLE 55-2

Comparison of Respiratory and Nonrespiratory Events*

	TOTAL		1970S		1980S		1990S		2000S	
	Respiratory (n = 1928)	All Others (n = 6229)	Respiratory (n = 232)	All Others (n = 423)	Respiratory (n = 811)	All Others (n = 2060)	Respiratory (n = 597)	All Others (n = 2796)	Respiratory (n = 267)	All Others (n = 879)
Incidence	24%	76%	35%	65%	28%	72%	18%	82%	23%	77%
Death or brain damage[†]	75%	31%	88%	38%	79%	31%	66%	29%	69%	34%
Preventable[†]	43%	9%	71%	20%	59%	12%	19%	6%	24%	9%
Substandard care[†]	60%	28%	73%	34%	67%	30%	51%	24%	51%	34%
Payment frequency[†]	67%	48%	79%	58%	71%	52%	60%	43%	64%	52%
Median payment[†] (2008 dollars)	474,000	174,950	690,525	222,750	532,000	142,500	378,075	177,530	380,750	244,000

*Total anesthesia claims = 8954. Claims for chronic pain management are excluded. Claims with unknown year of event are not shown.
[†]$P < 0.05$ for respiratory compared with nonrespiratory events in all time periods and overall (chi square for proportions and Kolmogorov-Smirnov test for payments).
Data from ASA Closed Claims Database, 2008.

A detailed display of outcome and payment data for the three most common types of adverse respiratory events since 1990 (inadequate ventilation, DI, and aspiration) is shown in Table 55-4. Death and permanent brain damage were more frequent in claims for respiratory events compared with nonrespiratory events ($P < 0.05$). Claims for inadequate ventilation exhibited the highest proportion of death and brain damage (89%, see Table 55-4). Overall, payment for respiratory-related claims ranged from $1260 to $11 million (in 2008$). Most claims (61%) resulted in payment. Claims for adverse respiratory events typically involved healthy adults undergoing nonemergency surgery with general anesthesia (GA) (Table 55-5).

The reviewers judged that better monitoring would have prevented the adverse outcome in 20% of the 867 claims for adverse respiratory events since 1990. In contrast, only 7% of nonrespiratory claims were judged preventable with better monitoring ($P < 0.01$). Half (54%) of all claims for inadequate ventilation were considered preventable with better monitoring, as opposed to 5% of claims for DI and only 1% of claims for aspiration.

For the claims considered preventable with better monitoring, the reviewers pointed to pulse oximetry, capnometry, or both in most cases. Data on the role of better monitoring in the prevention of adverse outcomes must be interpreted with particular care, because the reviewers were not asked to consider confounding factors such as equipment malfunction, diversion of attention, or the impact of false-positive and false-negative results. Therefore, the reviewers' judgments should be regarded as a near-maximum (and probably unattainable) estimate of the efficacy of better monitoring. It should also be noted that this analysis is based on claims for events that occurred after the adoption of pulse oximetry and $EtCO_2$ as ASA standards.

2. Inadequate Ventilation

The largest class of adverse respiratory events was inadequate ventilation. The distinguishing feature in this group of claims was the reviewer's inability to identify a specific mechanism of injury. In part, the inability to assign a mechanism of injury may reflect uncertainty on the part of the original health care providers. Because

TABLE 55-3

Most Common Adverse Respiratory Events as Proportion of All Respiratory Events in Decade*

Respiratory Event	Total (n = 1928)	1970s (n = 232)	1980s (n = 811)	1990s (n = 597)	2000s (n = 267)
Inadequate ventilation and/or oxygenation	24%	37%	24%	18%	25%
Difficult intubation	24%	15%	24%	28%	22%
Esophageal intubation	12%	15%	18%	5%	6%
Aspiration	11%	7%	7%	15%	19%
Airway obstruction	8%	6%	9%	9%	7%
Premature extubation	8%	4%	6%	12%	8%
Bronchospasm	4%	7%	5%	3%	1%

*Other adverse respiratory events (inadvertent extubation, inadequate fraction of inspired oxygen, endobronchial intubation) exhibited an overall incidence of <5% of all respiratory events. Total anesthesia claims = 8954. Claims for chronic pain management are excluded. Claims with unknown year of event are not shown.
Data from ASA Closed Claims Database, 2008.

TABLE 55-4

Outcome, Payment, and Frequency for the Most Common Adverse Respiratory Events Occurring in 1990 or Later*

	Difficult Intubation (*n* = 232)	Inadequate Ventilation (*n* = 174)	Aspiration (*n* = 140)	All Respiratory Events[†] (*n* = 867)	All Nonrespiratory Events (*n* = 3681)
Outcome					
Death	46%	63%	56%	53%	22%
Permanent brain damage	9%	26%	8%	14%	8%
Payment (2008 dollars)					
Range	$1370-$11,060,000	$21,875-$8,040,000	$3600-$5,490,000	$1260-$11,060,000	$124-$32,168,000
Median	$306,000	$548,700	$297,000	$378,075	$197,750
Payment frequency	63%	64%	55%	61%	45%

*Total anesthesia claims = 8954. Claims for chronic pain management and all claims for events prior to 1990 are excluded.
[†]*P* < 0.05 compared with nonrespiratory events in all outcome and payment categories.
Data from ASA Closed Claims Database, 2008.

most adverse events occurred before the widespread use of pulse oximetry and capnometry, the uncertainty may be due to the limitations of traditional clinical signs, such as chest excursion, reservoir bag motion, and breath sounds. With increasing use of quantitative measures of ventilation, fewer cases have been assigned to the category of inadequate ventilation. These events have declined in occurrence from 37% of all respiratory events in the 1970s to 25% in the 2000s (see Table 55-3). It is also possible that a delayed rather than contemporaneous approach to the investigation of adverse outcomes is not powerful enough to provide an understanding of many events.

3. Esophageal Intubation

Prompt detection of esophageal intubation is a key concern in anesthesia practice. At present, anesthesiologists

TABLE 55-5

Basic Clinical Features of Cases Involving Adverse Respiratory Events Occurring in 1990 or Later*

Feature	Respiratory Events (*n* = 867)	All Others (*n* = 3681)
Age in years (mean ± SD)	47.2 ± 19.8	45.5 ± 18.7
Pediatric	8%	5%
ASAPS 1-2	42%	53%
Emergency	26%	18%
Gender		
Female	51%	59%
Male	49%	41%
Primary anesthetic		
General	81%	62%
Regional	4%	27%
Monitored anesthesia care (MAC)	8%	6%
Other[†]	7%	6%

P < 0.05 for respiratory compared with nonrespiratory events in all categories (chi square test for proportions, *t*-test for age). Total anesthesia claims = 8954. Claims for chronic pain management and all claims prior to 1990 are excluded.
[†]Includes combined regional and general anesthesia, standby, and unknown.
ASAPS, American Society of Anesthesiologists Physical Status; *SD,* standard deviation.
Data from ASA Closed Claims Database, 2008.

rely primarily on capnometry to confirm endotracheal intubation. The ASA Closed Claims Project database provides an important lesson about the pitfalls of less quantitative methods.

In 1990, we performed an in-depth analysis of 94 closed claims for esophageal intubation.[14] Almost all (92%) of these claims occurred during the period 1975–1985, before routine use of intraoperative capnometry. The single most striking finding was that detection of esophageal intubation required at least 5 minutes in most cases (97%). Our immediate reaction was simply, "What took so long?" We wondered whether such delays in detection were caused by incompetence or negligence (e.g., intubation performed by a legally blind physician, minimal attention to the patient during the procedure), but we found only eight claims (9%) that could be explained in such a way.

A closer look at the esophageal intubation claims suggested that reliance on indirect tests of ventilation may have been an important factor contributing to delay. For example, auscultation is a test that is traditionally used during the first few minutes after intubation. In our set of claims, auscultation of breath sounds was documented in 62 of the 94 claims for esophageal intubation (63%). In 3 (5%) of these cases, breath sound auscultation led to a correct diagnosis of esophageal intubation. In 30 cases (48%), auscultation led to the erroneous conclusion that the endotracheal tube (ETT) was located in the trachea when it was actually in the esophagus. This result was termed a misdiagnosis of endotracheal intubation.

The diagnostic error in such cases was recognized in a variety of ways, including later reexamination with direct laryngoscopy, absence of any object in the trachea at the time of an emergency tracheostomy (despite ongoing "ventilation" through an ETT), resolution of cyanosis after reintubation (often by a second participant), and discovery of esophageal intubation at autopsy. In 29 (47%) of the 62 claims in which auscultation was documented, the records did not contain sufficient information to determine how the auscultatory findings were interpreted. In another 32 cases (34%), there was no information about the use of auscultation.

Using this information, we constructed a best-case scenario by assuming that auscultation led to a correct diagnosis in the 3 cases in which it actually did so, as well as in the 61 cases in which there was no information about its role or the information was unclear. Using this approach of constructing a hypothetical situation to demonstrate the greatest possible benefit, auscultation is still associated with a misdiagnosis rate of 32% (30 of 94 cases). Although the limitations of auscultation are well known,[15] we think these claims emphasize the importance of confirming intubation with the quantitative and ongoing information provided by capnometry.

Another indirect test of ventilation is cyanosis. Almost all of the esophageal intubation claims that we studied took place before pulse oximetry became part of the ASA Standards for Basic Anesthetic Monitoring. The human eye is relatively insensitive to the changes in skin color that occur during arterial desaturation,[16,17] so it is not surprising that cyanosis preceded the recognition of esophageal intubation in only 34% of cases. One might also expect cardiovascular clues to accompany hypoxemia or hypercarbia and that these clues might alert the anesthesiologist to the possibility of esophageal intubation. Indeed, at least one major hemodynamic derangement was recorded in 79 (84%) of the 94 claims for esophageal intubation, and this knowledge preceded the recognition of esophageal intubation in 60 claims (65%). In order of frequency, the abnormalities included bradycardia, asystole, hypotension, unspecified dysrhythmia, tachycardia, and ventricular fibrillation (Table 55-6). Such changes certainly have the potential to serve as cues, but when they are extremely severe (e.g., ventricular fibrillation, asystole) they draw attention away from the underlying problem and leave very little time for effective remedies. These features point to the importance of confirmatory tests that provide early, direct, and ongoing confirmation of ventilation through the ETT.

Is injury from undetected esophageal intubation no longer a concern? As shown in Table 55-3, claims for esophageal intubation decreased considerably in the 1990s and later compared with the prior two decades. A few claims for esophageal intubation still enter the database, but they usually involve cases in which capnometry was unavailable or not used or the procedure took place in a remote location.[18]

4. Difficult Intubation

Claims for DI in the ASA Closed Claims Project were distinguished by a relatively small percentage of cases in

TABLE 55-6
Major Hemodynamic Derangements Accompanying Esophageal Intubation Claims*

Hemodynamic Derangement	Percent of Claims ($n = 94$)
Bradycardia	57
Asystole	55
Hypotension	49
Unspecified dysrhythmia	10
Tachycardia	5
Ventricular fibrillation	1

*Percentages sum to more than 100 because of multiple derangements. Total anesthesia claims = 1541.
Data from ASA Closed Claims Database, 1990. Table adapted from Caplan RA, Posner KL, Cheney FW, et al: Adverse respiratory events in anesthesia: A closed claims analysis. *Anesthesiology* 72:828, 1990.

which care was considered less than appropriate (46%, compared with more than 80% for inadequate ventilation and esophageal intubation) and by a similarly small percentage of cases in which better monitoring would have prevented the complication (19%, again compared with more than 80% for inadequate ventilation and esophageal intubation). Although these findings seem outwardly favorable, the comparisons are not so attractive from the perspective of risk reduction. If most cases of DI cannot be linked to obvious inadequacies in care or deficiencies in monitoring, it is unlikely that claims analysis alone can point to effective or broad-based remedies. Simulators, algorithms, and drill routines have generated considerable interest in recent years. These newer educational tools and management strategies may provide an important opportunity for clinicians to gain concentrated exposure to relatively infrequent events.

An evidence-based guideline for management of the difficult airway (DA) has been developed by the ASA.[19] Key features of this guideline are discussed in Chapter 10. The impact of this set of guidelines on claims involving DA management was studied in the ASA Closed Claims Project.[20] DA problems were encountered during all phases of anesthesia management, including preinduction, induction, maintenance, emergence, postanesthesia care unit (PACU) care, and intensive care unit settings. Death and brain damage were more common in DA claims arising from procedures performed outside the operating room (OR) or the PACU and in the settings of difficult mask ventilation (DMV); "cannot intubate, cannot ventilate" (CICV) emergencies; or persistent intubation attempts.[20]

5. Aspiration

An in-depth analysis of claims for pulmonary aspiration was conducted in 1991, when such claims accounted for 3% of the database (56 cases).[21] Almost all cases (95%) occurred in patients who received GA. The aspirated material was gastric contents in 88% of these cases; other cases involved aspiration of blood, pus, or teeth. Approximately one third (34%) of aspirations took place during anesthetic induction just before endotracheal intubation. In 6 of these cases, aspiration occurred during a rapid-sequence induction; in another 6, the aspiration occurred under circumstances in which the reviewer believed that rapid-sequence induction was indicated but in which it was not used. Another one third of aspiration cases (36%) took place during the maintenance phase of mask GA. Only 2 cases (4%) occurred during the maintenance phase of endotracheal GA. Aspiration occurred in one of these cases when the ETT was removed to facilitate the passage of a nasogastric tube. In the other instance, aspiration occurred while an ETT with a leaking cuff was being replaced with a new tube. The remaining cases (18%) took place during emergence from anesthesia.

Two clinical factors—pregnancy and emergency surgical status—were particularly prevalent in claims for aspiration. Obstetric patients accounted for 12% of the overall database but represented 29% of all aspiration claims ($P < 0.05$) in the 1991 study.[21] This trend changed dramatically in subsequent years, with aspiration occurring in fewer than 1% of obstetric claims from 1990 or

TABLE 55-7

Low-Frequency Adverse Respiratory Events

Type of Claim	n (% of Total)	Death (%)	Brain Damage (%)	Payment Frequency (%)	Payment Median ($)
Airway trauma	97 (4.7)	12	0	60	22,000
Pneumothorax	67 (3.3)	24	10	63	19,000
Airway obstruction	56 (2.7)	64	23	63	300,000
Aspiration	56 (2.7)	45	5	66	60,000
Bronchospasm	40 (1.9)	70	18	53	218,000
All infrequent respiratory events*	300 (14.6)	37[†‡]	10[†]	60[†‡]	60,000[†]
Other respiratory events	462 (22.6)	70	23	75	233,000
All nonrespiratory events	1284 (63.7)	22	9	59	40,000

*Because >1 adverse respiratory event occurred in 16 claims, the total number of claims for 316 events is 300. Total no. of claims = 2046.
[†]$P < 0.01$ compared with other respiratory claims.
[‡]$P < 0.01$ compared with nonrespiratory claims.
Data from ASA Closed Claims Database, 1991. Table adapted from Cheney FW, Posner KL, Caplan RA, et al: Adverse respiratory events infrequently leading to malpractice suits: A closed claims analysis. *Anesthesiology* 75:932, 1991.

later.[22] Emergency surgery patients accounted for 19% of the database in 1991 but represented 45% of all aspiration claims ($P < 0.01$). It is also noteworthy that 23% of aspiration claims involved a problem with airway management, such as DI (9 cases) or esophageal intubation (4 cases). This relationship was previously reported by Olsson and colleagues.[23]

Overall, aspiration accounted for only 3% of claims in the database. This is consistent with the observation by Warner and colleagues that the incidence of aspiration in more than 200,000 patients who underwent elective or emergency surgery during 1985–1991 was very low (1 in 3216).[24] These observations suggest that current strategies used to prevent aspiration in the United States are generally successful, particularly in obstetric patients.

B. Low-Frequency Adverse Respiratory Events

1. Basic Features

The foregoing discussion focused on the most common mechanisms of respiratory injury in the closed claims database. A formal study of low-frequency adverse respiratory events was conducted in 1991, when the ASA Closed Claims Project database had reached 2046 cases.[21] Although these events were much less common (each

category representing no more than 5% of the overall database), sufficient claims were collected to permit the identification of recurrent themes that might contribute to liability. Five categories of events have been studied in depth, each category containing at least 40 claims and together encompassing 300 claims, or about 15% of the overall database. These categories are airway trauma, pneumothorax, airway obstruction, aspiration, and bronchospasm. Death or brain damage occurred in almost half (47%) of these cases, and the median payment was $60,000 (Table 55-7). Airway trauma was reanalyzed in detail in 1999.[25] Aspiration now represents one of the most common adverse respiratory events.

2. Airway Trauma

Airway trauma was the most common type of low-frequency airway event, accounting for 266 of 4460 claims, or 6% of the overall database, in the 1999 study.[25] DI was associated with 103 (39%) of these claims. The most frequent sites of injury were the larynx, pharynx, and esophagus (Table 55-8), which together accounted for 70% of injuries associated with airway trauma claims. Esophageal and tracheal injuries were more likely than other airway trauma claims to be associated with DI. In contrast, laryngeal and temporomandibular joint (TMJ) injuries were rarely associated with DI. Pharyngeal and

TABLE 55-8

Distribution of Airway Trauma Sites and Presence of Concomitant Difficult Intubation

	Location of Injury (% of Total)	Difficult Intubation (% of Site)
Larynx	87 (33%)	17 (20%)*
Pharynx	51 (19%)	26 (51%)
Esophagus	48 (18%)	30 (62%)*
Trachea	39 (15%)	25 (64%)*
Temporomandibular joint	27 (10%)	0 (0%)*
Nasopharynx, nose	13 (5%)	4 (31%)

*$P < 0.05$ compared with other sites combined. Total anesthesia claims = 4460.
Data from ASA Closed Claims Database, 1999. Table adapted from Domino KB, Posner KL, Caplan RA, et al: Airway injury during anesthesia: A closed claims analysis. *Anesthesiology* 91:1703, 1999.

esophageal injuries most commonly consisted of lacerations or perforations leading to mediastinitis or mediastinal abscess. The most common laryngeal injuries were vocal cord paralysis (30 cases), granuloma (15 cases), and arytenoid dislocation (7 cases). None of the 27 TMJ injuries was associated with DI.

These claims provide several useful insights. Circumstances surrounding DI clearly put the tissues of the pharynx and esophagus at risk. The clinical implication is that patients in whom endotracheal intubation has been difficult should be observed for, or told to watch for, the development of signs and symptoms of pharyngeal abscess or mediastinitis. Because soft tissue infections may develop slowly over a period of days, an apparent lack of complications in the first few hours after surgery should not be regarded as a definitive outcome in patients who have experienced DI. This is especially important to remember in the ambulatory surgery setting.

Although it is easy to understand how DI may lead to trauma of the larynx, it is less apparent why laryngeal injuries appeared to be so infrequently associated with DI. The reasons for vocal cord paralysis, granuloma, and arytenoid dislocation with routine intubation were not apparent from the data available in the claim file. Similarly, it is curious that TMJ injury was present only with routine intubation. One might expect that TMJ injury would be more commonly associated with DI, in which forces applied to the jaw during airway manipulation and laryngoscopy might be more intense or prolonged than those encountered during routine intubation. These observations suggest that many injuries to the larynx and TMJ may be related to predisposing factors or underlying characteristics of patients that we do not yet understand. A similar phenomenon was observed in the review of closed claims for peripheral nerve injuries.[26,27]

3. Pneumothorax

Pneumothorax was the second most common type of low-frequency airway event.[21] Clinical activities that were not directly or clearly related to airway management were associated with 43 (64%) of the 67 claims for pneumothorax (Table 55-9). In particular, five types of nerve blocks (supraclavicular, intercostal, stellate ganglion, interscalene, and suprascapular) were responsible for 40% of pneumothorax claims. Airway instrumentation was associated with pneumothorax in 19% of cases. The actual mechanism of pneumothorax was not anatomically proved in most cases but was usually attributed to laryngoscopy, ETT placement, or bronchoscopy on the basis of clinical events and reviewer judgments. Barotrauma was the cause of pneumothorax in 11 claims (16%), mostly arising from obstruction of the expiratory limb of a mechanical ventilator or the use of excessive tidal volumes (7 cases).

A notable feature of pneumothorax claims was the marked disparity in outcome between events associated with airway instrumentation and events arising from nerve blocks or central-line placement. In the subset of 24 claims involving airway instrumentation, the outcome in 16 cases (67%) was death or permanent brain damage. In contrast, there were no instances of death or brain damage in the 16 cases of pneumothorax that arose after nerve blocks or central-line placement. We speculate that this difference may be due at least in part to the more rapid compromise of respiratory and circulatory function that occurs under conditions of mechanical ventilation and positive-pressure gas delivery. Not surprisingly, the median payment for pneumothorax associated with nerve block or central-line placement was only $6000, whereas that for cases associated with airway instrumentation was $75,000.

4. Airway Obstruction

Airway obstruction accounted for 56 claims, or approximately 3% of the database.[21] Most cases (89%) occurred during GA. Obstruction was attributed to an upper airway site in 39 claims (70%), although an exact cause or site was identifiable in only half of these claims. Laryngospasm was the most common cause of upper airway obstruction, accounting for 11 (28%) of 39 cases. Other causes of upper airway obstruction included foreign body (4 cases), laryngeal polyps (2 cases), laryngeal edema (1 case), and pharyngeal hematoma (1 case). In 10 cases of upper airway obstruction, emergency tracheostomy was performed.

Causes of lower airway obstruction (21% of claims) included blood clots or mucus plugs in the tracheal lumen and external compression related to mediastinal tumor masses or blood. ETT obstruction accounted for 9% of cases and was attributed to blood clots in the lumen of the ETT or to kinking of the tube itself. Other factors associated with claims for airway obstruction included concurrent DI (17 cases, 30%), operation on the airway (13 cases, 23%), and pediatric age group (10 cases, 18%). The outcome in almost all claims for airway obstruction (87%) was death or brain damage.

5. Bronchospasm

Adverse outcomes arising from bronchospasm accounted for 40 claims, or almost 2% of the database.[21] Most of these claims (80%) occurred during the administration of GA as the primary anesthetic technique. Almost half (48%) of the patients had a medical history that included asthma, chronic obstructive pulmonary disease, smoking, or some combination of these. In cases involving the

TABLE 55-9		
Clinical Factors Associated with Pneumothorax Claims*		
Clinical Factor	**Claims**	**Total (%)**
Airway Related		
Airway instrumentation	13	19
Barotrauma	11	16
Non-airway Related		
Regional block	27	40
Central line	5	7
Spontaneous or unknown	5	7
Other	6	9
Total	67	100

*Total anesthesia claims = 2046.
Data from ASA Closed Claims Database, 1991. Table adapted from Cheney FW, Posner KL, Caplan RA, et al: Adverse respiratory events infrequently leading to malpractice suit: A closed claims analysis. *Anesthesiology* 75:932, 1991.

administration of GA, the first occurrence of bronchospasm was more often at the time of intubation (69%) than during maintenance (25%) or emergence (6%).

Twenty percent of claims for bronchospasm were associated with the conduct of regional anesthesia. In most of these cases, bronchospasm occurred during cesarean section when endotracheal intubation was required for management of a failed block or a high block in a patient with a history of asthma. These cases illustrate the concept that regional anesthesia does not, in itself, obviate the risk associated with intraoperative management of reactive airway disease. In particular, the risk of bronchospasm may be especially pronounced in this setting, because relatively modest doses of intravenous agents are often used in an effort to minimize anesthetic effects on the fetus.

Bronchospasm claims were also notable in cases that involved a difficult differential diagnosis. The claims files in the 1991 study indicated that clinicians had difficulty distinguishing between bronchospasm and the presence of esophageal intubation (6 cases) or pneumothorax (4 cases). $EtCO_2$ monitoring was not used in any of the 6 cases in which the failure to make a correct and timely differential diagnosis between esophageal intubation and bronchospasm led to an adverse outcome. $EtCO_2$ is now an ASA standard for verification and monitoring of ETT placement, and bronchospasm appears to be on a steadily declining trend (see Table 55-3). However, it is important to recognize that failure to differentiate between bronchospasm and esophageal intubation may still occur in cases in which bronchospasm is so severe that ventilation is impossible and CO_2 cannot reach the detector in clinically useful amounts. In this circumstance, fiberoptic bronchoscopy can be helpful.

C. Emerging Trends from the ASA Closed Claims Project

The database of the Closed Claims Project is now sufficiently large that it can be studied for evidence of changing trends in the overall distribution of adverse events and outcomes. In doing so, two key limitations must be emphasized. First, these data cannot be used to generate any general estimates of risk. This limitation arises from a lack of denominator data, a probable bias toward severe outcomes, and partial reliance on the observations of direct participants. Second, the resolution of a claim is a lengthy process. Typically, this leads to a delay of approximately 5 years between the occurrence of a claim and its entry into the database. Therefore, the most recent trends (which are usually of greatest interest) must be viewed as especially tentative because they may change considerably as additional claims are resolved and processed.

In 1999, an examination of trends was conducted.[11] At that point, the database consisted of more than 4000 claims drawn from 35 U.S. insurance organizations. Two major trends were evident. First, there was a general decrease in the severity of injury that was specifically characterized by a declining incidence of claims for death and brain damage. For example, 56% of claims between 1970 and 1979 involved death or brain damage, compared with only 31% of those between 1990 and 1994.

Second, the contribution of adverse respiratory events to death and brain damage declined. During the earliest interval, 1970–1979, 56% of claims for death and brain damage arose from respiratory system events. This percentage decreased to 49% in 1980–1989 and to 38% from 1990 onward.

Some tentative associations can be postulated. In the 1990s, there were several changes in monitoring and clinical practice that may have had an impact on adverse respiratory events. Pulse oximetry and end-tidal capnometry have been widely available since the mid-1980s. Moreover, the ASA Standards for Basic Intraoperative Monitoring specified the use of pulse oximetry for basic intraoperative monitoring beginning in 1990 and $EtCO_2$ for verification of endotracheal intubation beginning in 1991.

Is the presence of these monitors reflected in the pattern of liability for closed claims? This question was explored in 2006, when the overall database contained 6894 cases.[28] Claims for death and brain damage between 1975 and 2000 were analyzed. Respiratory events declined from approximately 50% of death and brain damage claims before 1986 to 28% by 1992. A downward trend in claims for death and brain damage and a similar downward trend in the proportion of respiratory events leading to these claims preceded the introduction of pulse oximetry and $EtCO_2$ monitoring into anesthetic practice. These decreases seemed to be unrelated to the increase in the proportion of claims in which these monitors were used.[28]

New trends in adverse respiratory events are now emerging outside the traditional arena of GA in the OR. An analysis of closed claims from 1990 or later that were associated with monitored anesthesia care (MAC) revealed that respiratory depression after an absolute or relative overdose of sedative or opioid drugs was the most common specific mechanism leading to claims (21%).[29] Most of these claims involved death or brain damage. Improved respiratory monitoring (capnography, improved vigilance, audible alarms) might have prevented almost half of these claims. One quarter of these claims arose from procedures performed in the endoscopy suite.

Analysis of claims from 1990 or later associated with procedures outside the OR found that adverse respiratory events were more common in remote locations and were often judged as preventable by better respiratory monitoring.[18] A 2009 ASA Statement on Respiratory Monitoring During Endoscopic Procedures provided guidance on CO_2 monitoring and airway management during endoscopic procedures.[30] Since July 2011, the ASA Standards for Basic Anesthetic Monitoring have provided additional specificity about the use of CO_2 monitoring: "During moderate or deep sedation the adequacy of ventilation shall be evaluated by continual observation of qualitative clinical signs and monitoring for the presence of exhaled CO_2 unless precluded or invalidated by the nature of the patient, procedure, or equipment.[31]

As mentioned previously, evidence-based guidelines for management of the DA have been developed by the ASA.[19] Clinicians often worry that the proliferation of practice guidelines will lead to a general increase in liability. It is important to remember that modern, evidence-based guidelines have a relatively flexible place in medical practice that differs from that of standards. Standards are typically used for straightforward aspects of care that command high levels of agreement and acceptance. Noncompliance implies an action that is outside a clearly recognized norm; in some instances, such actions may be accompanied by sanctions. Guidelines are employed for more complex aspects of care that cannot be precisely codified and accepted in a near-uniform fashion. Guidelines are intended as recommendations that can assist the anesthesiologist and the patient in making decisions about health care. Guidelines may be accepted, modified, or even rejected according to specific clinical needs and constraints. This means that not following a guideline, under some clinical conditions, can still be a decision that is consistent with reasonable and prudent practice. In DA malpractice claims, the ASA guideline for management of the DA has rarely been an issue in litigation. In the few claims in which the guideline was a factor, it was used for the defense more often than for the plaintiff.[20]

III. CONCLUSIONS

The database of the ASA Closed Claims Project indicates that adverse events involving the respiratory system continue to constitute an important source of liability in anesthetic practice. These events represent a particularly urgent target for research and preventive strategies because they are characterized by a high frequency of severe outcomes and costly payments.

Inadequate ventilation and DI account for almost one half of all adverse respiratory events. The occurrence of injuries related to inadequate ventilation has been decreasing, but DI remains a recurring problem. The use of capnography to confirm ETT placement seems to have reduced the severity of outcomes associated with delayed recognition of esophageal intubation. Aspiration is emerging as the third most common adverse respiratory event leading to malpractice claims.

The in-depth analysis of low-frequency respiratory events also provides valuable lessons. Complications associated with airway trauma may not manifest in the immediate postoperative period. This suggests that explicit follow-up plans and communication are particularly important for outpatients who have experienced airway management difficulties.

Overall, reviewers have found that a large proportion of claims involving adverse respiratory events might have been prevented by the use of pulse oximetry and capnography (either alone or in combination). Even after the widespread adoption of these two modalities, however, 19% to 24% of adverse respiratory events were considered preventable by better monitoring. It is difficult to know whether this perception is accurate in its own right or whether it reflects wishful hindsight and unrealistic expectations. However, recent studies of claims arising during MAC and in locations outside of the OR underscore the preventive potential of respiratory system monitoring.

IV. CLINICAL PEARLS

- Anesthesiologists have a long-standing appreciation for risks associated with airway management.
- Adverse respiratory events constitute the single largest source of injury in the ASA Closed Claims Project database.
- Claims for adverse respiratory events are characterized by devastating patient injuries and high liability payments.
- The most common adverse respiratory events in claims since 1990 are difficult intubation (DI), inadequate ventilation, and aspiration
- The occurrence of injuries related to inadequate ventilation has been decreasing, but DI remains a recurring problem.
- Adverse respiratory events are emerging as a source of patient injury during monitored anesthesia care (MAC), especially in remote locations outside the operating room (OR).

Acknowledgments

The ASA Closed Claims Project is supported by funds from the American Society of Anesthesiologists. The Project committee gratefully acknowledges the contributions of insurance companies who have granted access to closed claims files and of those members of the American Society of Anesthesiologists who have served as reviewers of closed claims and as participants in studies of peer review.

The opinions expressed herein are those of the authors and do not represent the policy of the American Society of Anesthesiologists.

SELECTED REFERENCES

All references can be found online at expertconsult.com.

11. Cheney FW: The American Society of Anesthesiologists Closed Claims Project: What have we learned, how has it affected practice, and how will it affect practice in the future? *Anesthesiology* 91:552–556, 1999.
14. Caplan RA, Posner KL, Ward RJ, et al: Adverse respiratory events in anesthesia: A closed claims analysis. *Anesthesiology* 72:828–833, 1990.
18. Metzner J, Posner KL, Domino KB: The risk and safety of anesthesia at remote locations: The US closed claims analysis. *Curr Opin Anaesthesiol* 22:502–508, 2009.
19. Practice guidelines for management of the difficult airway: An updated report by the American Society of Anesthesiologists Task Force on Management of the Difficult Airway. *Anesthesiology* 98:1269–1277, 2003.
20. Peterson GN, Domino KB, Caplan RA, et al: Management of the difficult airway: A closed claims analysis. *Anesthesiology* 103:33–39, 2005.
21. Cheney FW, Posner KL, Caplan RA: Adverse respiratory events infrequently leading to malpractice suits: A closed claims analysis. *Anesthesiology* 75:932–939, 1991.
25. Domino KB, Posner KL, Caplan RA, et al: Airway injury during anesthesia: A closed claims analysis. *Anesthesiology* 91:1703–1711, 1999.
28. Cheney FW, Posner KL, Lee LA, et al: Trends in anesthesia-related death and permanent brain damage: A closed claims analysis. *Anesthesiology* 105:1081–1086, 2006.
29. Bhananker SM, Posner KL, Cheney FW, et al: Injury and liability associated with monitored anesthesia care: A closed claims analysis. *Anesthesiology* 104:228–234, 2006.

Index